AAOS
AMERICAN ACADEMY OF ORTHOPAEDIC SURGEONS

THIRTEENTH EDITION

Emergency

Care and Transportation of the Sick and Injured

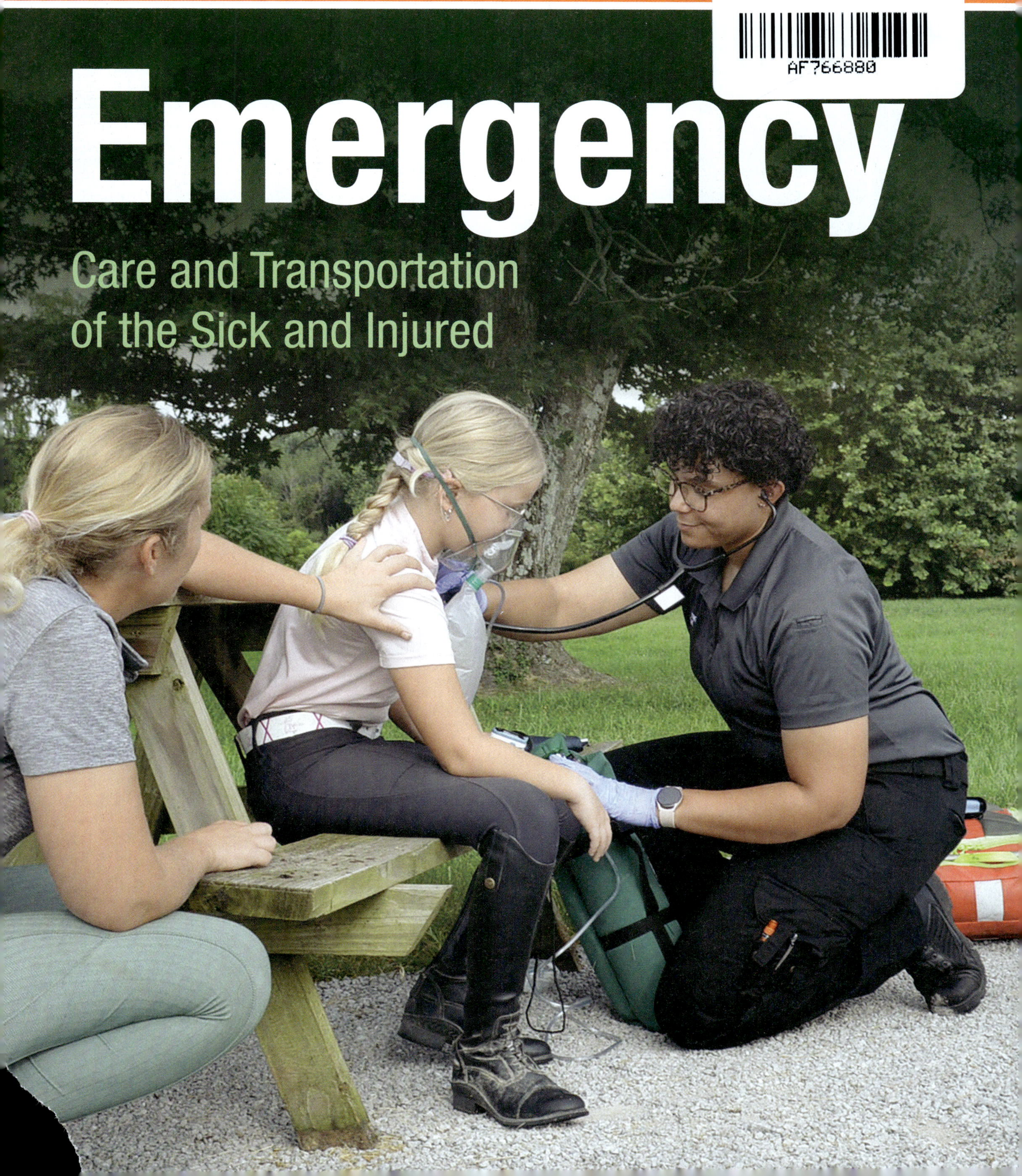

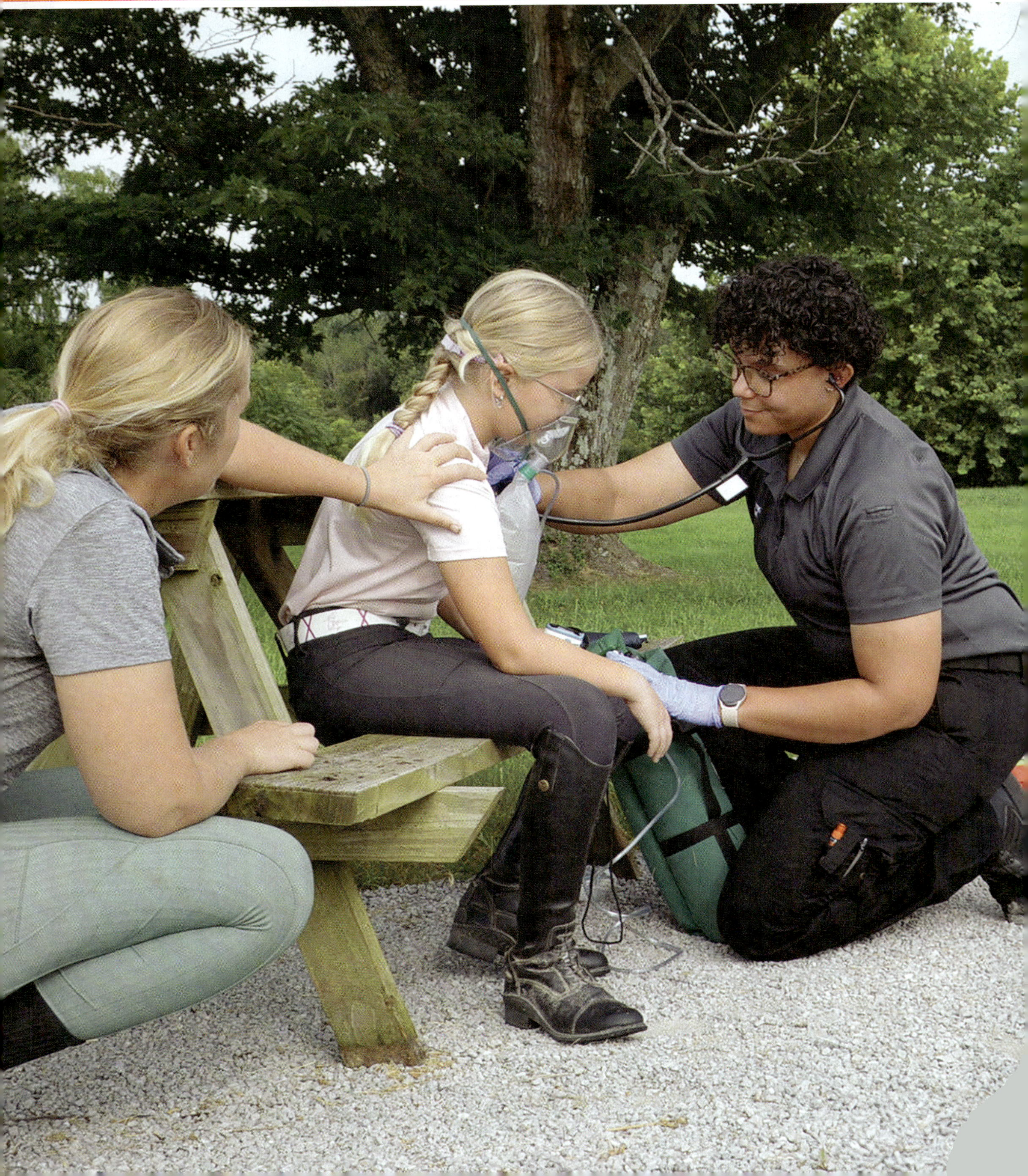

THIRTEENTH EDITION

Emergency

Care and Transportation of the Sick and Injured

AAOS
American Academy of Orthopaedic Surgeons

Series Editor:
Alfonso Mejia, MD, MPH, FAAOS

Lead Editors:
Dennis Edgerly, MEd, EMT-P
Kim D. McKenna, PhD, MEd, RN, NRP

JONES & BARTLETT LEARNING

World Headquarters
Jones & Bartlett Learning
25 Mall Road
Burlington, MA 01803
978-443-5000
info@jblearning.com
www.jblearning.com
www.psglearning.com

Editorial Credits
Chief Commercial Officer: Anna Salt Troise, MBA
Director, Publishing: Hans J. Koelsch, PhD
Senior Manager, Editorial: Lisa Claxton Moore

30119-9

Production Credits
Vice President, Innovative Learning and Assessment Solutions: Ada Woo
Senior Director, Content Production and Delivery: Christine Emerton
Director, Product: Cathy Esperti
Product Manager, EMS: Jameel Sylvia
Manager, Content Development: Tiffany Sliter
Content Manager: Carly Mahoney
Developmental Editor: Mike Boblitt
Manager, Intellectual Properties and Content Production: Kristen Rogers
Content Production Manager: Dan Stone
Content Production Manager: Michael Lepera
Senior Intellectual Property Specialist (eBook): Angela Dooley
Director, Marketing: Andrea DeFronzo
Director, Sales, Public Safety Group: Brian Hendrickson
Senior Product Marketing Manager: Elaine Riordan
Director, Product Fulfillment: Aaron McKinzie
Purchasing Manager: Wendy Kilborn
Composition: S4Carlisle Publishing Services
Cover Design: MPS Limited
Media Developer: Faith Brosnan
Intellectual Property Specialist: Robin Silverman
Cover Image (Title Page, Part Opener, Chapter Opener): © Jones & Bartlett Learning
Printing and Binding: Lakeside Book Company

Library of Congress Cataloging-in-Publication Data
Library of Congress Cataloging-in-Publication Data unavailable at time of printing.

LCCN: 2026000406

6048

Printed in the United States of America
30 29 28 27 26   10 9 8 7 6 5 4 3 2 1

Celebrating Over 50 Years of EMS Education and Innovation

In 1971, the American Academy of Orthopaedic Surgeons (AAOS) published the first edition of ***Emergency Care and Transportation of the Sick and Injured*** with its now-familiar orange cover, and laid the foundation of EMS training. Their commitment and dedication to excellence has transformed how EMS education is delivered throughout the world and helped develop and train countless world-class EMS clinicians.

In 1997, the AAOS partnered with Jones & Bartlett Publishers (now Jones & Bartlett Learning) to release ***Emergency Care and Transportation of the Sick and Injured, Sixth Edition***. Since the publication of that edition, the AAOS and the Jones & Bartlett Learning Public Safety Group have worked together to transform all levels of EMS training, from emergency medical responder to paramedic. This partnership has resulted in market-leading resources that go beyond initial training into assessment, continuing education, and professional resources to support EMS clinicians through every step of their education and career.

Today, the AAOS suite of EMS educational resources is the gold standard in training programs, with exceptional content and instructional resources that meet the diverse needs of today's educators and students.

The Jones & Bartlett Learning Public Safety Group is proud and honored to partner with the American Academy of Orthopaedic Surgeons on the "Orange Book," published for the first time over 55 years ago.

To explore other AAOS publications, programs, and products on orthopaedic trauma and other practice areas, please visit **www.aaos.org/Education**.

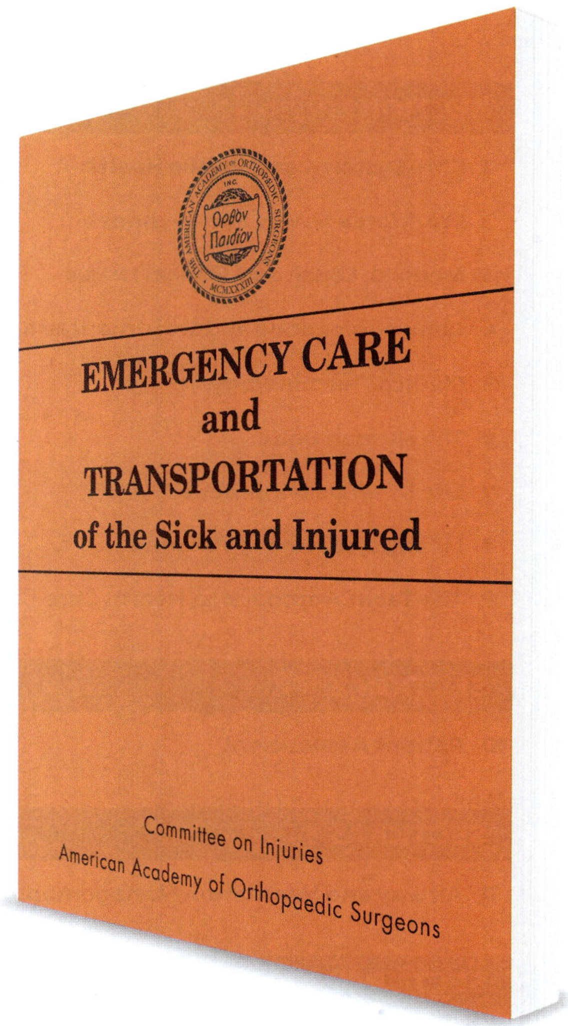

AAOS
American Academy of Orthopaedic Surgeons

PUBLIC SAFETY GROUP
A Jones & Bartlett Learning Brand

Brief Contents

SECTION 1 Preparatory 1

1 **EMS Systems and Public Health** 2

2 **Workforce Safety and Wellness** 26

3 **Medical, Legal, and Ethical Issues** 61

4 **Communications and Documentation** 96

5 **Medical Terminology** 147

6 **The Human Body** 173

7 **Life Span Development** 233

8 **Lifting and Moving Patients** 256

9 **The Team Approach to Health Care** 299

SECTION 2 Patient Assessment 319

10 **Patient Assessment** 320

SECTION 3 Airway 399

11 **Airway and Ventilation Management** 400

SECTION 4 Pharmacology 487

12 **Principles of Pharmacology and Medication Administration** 488

SECTION 5 Shock and Resuscitation 531

13 **Shock** 532

14 **BLS Resuscitation** 560

SECTION 6 Medical 611

15 **Medical Overview** 612

16 **Respiratory Emergencies** 639

17 **Cardiovascular Emergencies** 688

18 **Neurologic Emergencies** 729

19 **Gastrointestinal and Urologic Emergencies** 763

20 **Endocrine and Hematologic Emergencies** 789

21 **Allergy and Anaphylaxis** 816

22 **Toxicology** 835

23 **Behavioral Health Emergencies** 869

SECTION 7 Trauma 895

24 **Trauma Overview** 896

25 **Bleeding** 928

26 **Soft-Tissue Injuries** 955

27 **Face and Neck Injuries** 999

28 **Head and Spine Injuries** 1032

29 **Chest Injuries** 1086

30 **Abdominal and Genitourinary Injuries** 1111

31 **Orthopaedic Injuries** 1138

32 **Environmental Emergencies** 1193

SECTION 8 Special Patient Populations 1241

33 **Gynecologic Emergencies** 1242

34 **Obstetrics and Neonatal Care** 1256

35 **Patients With Special Challenges** 1298

SECTION 9 EMS Operations 1339

36 **Transport Operations** 1340

37 **Vehicle Extrication and Special Rescue** 1380

38 **Incident Management** 1402

39 **Terrorism Response and Disaster Management** 1446

Glossary 1481

Index 1526

Contents

SECTION 1 Preparatory 1

1 EMS Systems and Public Health 2

Introduction 3
Purpose and History of EMS 3
Freedom House Ambulance 4
Standardization of EMS Practice and Education 5
National Levels of EMS Training 6
Becoming an EMT 8
Education and Training 8
Certification 9
Licensure 10
Credentialing 10
Roles and Responsibilities of the EMT 11
Professional Attributes 11
Overview of the EMS System 13
EMS System Components 14
Legislation and Regulation 14
Public Access 15
Public BLS and Immediate Aid 15
Responding Agencies and Workforce 15
Medical Oversight 16
Quality Management 16
EMS Research 18
EMS and Public Health 18
Social Drivers of Health and Health Equity 18
Mobile Integrated Health 19
Public Health Surveillance 19
Prevention and Education 19

2 Workforce Safety and Wellness 26

Introduction 27
General Wellness Principles 27
Nutrition 28
Exercise and Relaxation 29
Sleep 30
Stress Management 31
Disease Prevention and Health Promotion 32
EMT Mental Health 33
Balancing Work, Family, and Health 33
Burnout and Compassion Fatigue 34
Potentially Psychologically Traumatizing Events and Posttraumatic Stress 34
Resilience and Posttraumatic Growth 35
Understanding and Addressing Risk for Suicide 36
Prevention of Physical Work-Related Injury and Illness 37
Safe Lifting Practices 38
Infectious and Communicable Disease Precautions 38
Additional Response Safety Considerations 51
Violence Against EMS Clinicians 53
Inclusive Workplace Considerations 53
Combatting Incivility in the Workplace 53
Sexual Harassment 54
Cultural Diversity on the Job 54

3 Medical, Legal, and Ethical Issues 61

Introduction 62
Consent 62
Expressed Consent 64
Implied Consent 64
Involuntary Consent 65
Minors and Consent 65
Forcible Restraint 66
The Right to Refuse Treatment 67
Confidentiality 69
Health Insurance Portability and Accountability Act 69
Social Media 70
Advance Directives 71
Physical Signs of Death 73
Presumptive Signs of Death 73
Definitive Signs of Death 74
Medical Examiner Cases 74
Special Situations 75
Organ Donors 75
Medical Identification Insignia 76
Scope of Practice 76
Standards of Care 76
Standards Imposed by Local Custom 77
Standards Imposed by Law 77
Professional or Institutional Standards 77
Standards Imposed by Textbooks 78
Standards Imposed by States 79
Duty to Act 79
Negligence 79
Abandonment 80
Assault and Battery and Kidnapping 80
Defamation 81
Good Samaritan Laws and Immunity 81
Records and Reports 82
Special Mandatory Reporting Requirements 83
Abuse of Children, Older People, and Others 83
Injury During the Commission of a Felony 83
Drug-Related Injuries 83
Childbirth 83
Other Reporting Requirements 83
Scene of a Crime 84
The EMT in Court 84
Ethical Responsibilities 86

4 Communications and Documentation 96

Introduction 97
Therapeutic Communication 98
Health Literacy 99
Medical Fear 99
211 Call Line 99
Age, Culture, and Personal Experience 99
Nonverbal Communication 100
Verbal Communication 102
Interpersonal Skills 106
Mission-Critical Communications 112
Communicating With Critically Ill and Injured Patients 114
Death and Dying 115
Written Communications and Documentation 118
Patient Care Report 118
Types of Forms 120
Standardized Narrative Formats 121
Reporting Errors 125
Documenting Refusal of Care 126
Special Reporting Situations 129
Communications Systems and Equipment 129
Base Station Radios 130
Mobile and Portable Radios 130
Repeater-Based Systems 131
Digital Equipment 131
Cellular/Satellite Telephones 132
Other Communications Equipment 132
Radio Communications 133
Responding to the Scene 134
Communicating With Medical Direction and Hospitals 137
Maintenance of Radio Equipment 139

5 Medical Terminology 147

Introduction 148
Anatomy of a Medical Term 148
Word Roots 148
Prefixes 148
Suffixes 148
Combining Vowels 148
Word Building Rules 149
Plural Endings 149
Special Word Parts 149
Numbers 149
Colors 150
Positions and Directions 150
Common Direction, Movement, and Position Terms 151
Directional Terms 151
Movement Terms 153
Other Directional Terms 153
Anatomic Positions 154
Breaking Terms Apart 155
Abbreviations and Symbols 155
Abbreviations 155
Symbols 157
Master Tables 157

6 The Human Body 173

Introduction 174
Topographic Anatomy 174
The Planes of the Body 174
From Cells to Systems 175
The Skeletal System: Anatomy 175
Bones 175
Joints 176
The Axial Skeleton 177
The Appendicular Skeleton 179
The Pelvis 179
The Lower Extremities 180
The Skeletal System: Physiology 181
The Musculoskeletal System: Anatomy 181
Skeletal Muscle 182
The Musculoskeletal System: Physiology 182
The Respiratory System: Anatomy 184
The Upper Airway 184
The Lower Airway 185
Mechanics of Breathing 186
The Respiratory System: Physiology 188
Respiration 188
Ventilation 190
Characteristics of Normal Breathing 191
The Circulatory System: Anatomy 191
The Heart 191
Arteries 194
Capillaries 194
Veins 195
Blood Composition 196
The Spleen 196
The Circulatory System: Physiology 196
Normal Circulation in Adults 197
Inadequate Circulation in Adults 198
The Function of Blood 199
Nervous System Control of the Cardiovascular System 200
The Nervous System: Anatomy and Physiology 201
The Central Nervous System 201
The Peripheral Nervous System 204
The Integumentary System (Skin): Anatomy 205
The Integumentary System (Skin): Physiology 206
The Digestive System: Anatomy 206
The Abdomen 206
Mouth 208
Oropharynx 208
Esophagus 209
Stomach 209
Pancreas 209
Liver 209
Small Intestine 210
Large Intestine 210
Appendix 210
Rectum 210
The Digestive System: Physiology 210
The Lymphatic System: Anatomy and Physiology 211
The Endocrine System: Anatomy and Physiology 211
The Urinary System: Anatomy and Physiology 213
The Genital System: Anatomy and Physiology 214
The Male Reproductive System and Organs 214
The Female Reproductive System and Organs 215
Life Support Chain 215
Pathophysiology 217
Respiratory Compromise 217
Shock 218
Alteration of Cellular Metabolism 220

7 Life Span Development 233

Introduction 234
Vital Signs 234
Newborns (Birth to 1 Month) and Infants (1 Month to 1 Year) 235
Physical Changes 235
Psychosocial Changes 237
Assessment Considerations for Newborns and Infants 238
Toddlers (1 to 3 Years) and Preschoolers (3 to 6 Years) 239
Physical Changes 239
Psychosocial Changes 240
Assessment Considerations for Toddlers 241
Assessment Considerations for Preschoolers 242
School-Age Children (6 to 12 Years) 242
Physical Changes 242
Psychosocial Changes 243
Assessment Considerations for School-Age Children 243
Adolescents (12 to 18 Years) 243
Physical Changes 244
Psychosocial Changes 244
Assessment Considerations for Adolescents 245
Early Adults (18 to 40 Years) 246
Physical Changes 246
Psychosocial Changes 246
Middle Adults (40 to 65 Years) 246
Physical Changes 246
Psychosocial Changes 247
Older Adults (65 Years and Older) 247
Generational Considerations 247
Physical Changes 248
Psychosocial Changes 251

8 Lifting and Moving Patients 256

Introduction 257
Principles of Moving and Positioning the Patient 258
Anatomy and Body Mechanics 258
Directions and Commands 265
Patient Positioning 266
Personnel Considerations 267
Emergency Moves 267
Urgent Moves 270
Nonurgent Moves 275
Equipment for Lifting and Moving Patients 276
The Wheeled Ambulance Stretcher 276
Backboards 284
Scoop Stretchers 284
Vacuum Mattresses 284
Stair Chairs 288
Neonatal Isolettes 290
Binder Lifts 291
Slipp Patient Movers 291
Portable/Folding Stretchers 291
Flexible Stretchers 292
Basket Stretchers 293
Short Backboards 293
Decontamination 294

9 The Team Approach to Health Care 299

Introduction 300
The Culture of Safety in EMS 300
Just Culture 300
Interdisciplinary Collaboration 301
An Era of Team Health Care 301
Community Paramedicine and Mobile Integrated Healthcare Teams 302
Differences Among Teams 302
Types of Teams 302
Regular Teams 302
Temporary Teams 302
Special Teams 302
Principles of Effective Team Performance 303
A Shared Goal 303
Clear Roles and Responsibilities 303
Diverse and Competent Skill Sets 303
Effective Collaboration and Communication 304
Supportive and Coordinated Leadership 305
Effective Team Membership 305
Crew Resource Management 306
Transfer of Patient Care 308
General Guidelines 308
BLS and ALS Clinicians Working Together 309
ALS Assist 309
Where BLS Care Ends and ALS Care Begins 310
Critical Thinking and Clinical Decision Making in EMS 310
Stages of the Decision-Making Process 311
Decision Traps 312
Troubleshooting Team Conflicts 312
The Team Approach to Behavioral and Mental Health Calls 313

SECTION 2 Patient Assessment 319

10 Patient Assessment 320

Introduction 324
Scene Size-up 325
Ensure Scene Safety 326
Determine Mechanism of Injury/Nature of Illness 327
Take Standard Precautions 329
Determine Number of Patients 330
Consider Additional/Specialized Resources 330
Geriatric Patients: Considerations During Scene Size-up 331
Primary Assessment 332
Identify and Treat Life Threats 332
Form a General Impression 333
Scan for Signs of Uncontrolled External Bleeding 334
Assess Level of Consciousness 334
Assess the Airway 336
Assess Breathing 336
Assess Circulation 338
Assess and Control External Bleeding 342
Pediatric Patients: Considerations During Primary Assessment 343
Geriatric Patients: Considerations During Primary Assessment 346
Determine Priority of Patient Care and Transport 346
History Taking 348
Investigate the Chief Complaint or Chief Concern (History of Present Illness) 349
Identify Pertinent Negatives 352

Secondary Assessment 355
General Systematic (Head-to-Toe) Assessment 356
Focused Systematic Assessment 362
Reassessment 388
Repeat the Primary Assessment 388
Reassess Vital Signs 388
Reassess the Chief Complaint or Chief Concern 389
Recheck Interventions 389
Identify and Treat Changes in the Patient's Condition 389
Reassess Patient 389
Pediatric Patients: Considerations During the Reassessment 389
Special Challenges in Completing a Patient Assessment 389
Silence 389
Overly Talkative 389
Multiple Symptoms 390
Intoxication 390
Crying 390
Confusing Behavior or History 390
Limited Cognitive Abilities 390
Cultural Challenges 391
Language Barriers 391

SECTION 3 Airway 399

11 Airway and Ventilation Management 400

Introduction 402
Anatomy of the Respiratory System 402
Anatomy of the Upper Airway 402
Anatomy of the Lower Airway 404
Physiology of Breathing 407
Ventilation 408
Oxygenation 411
Respiration 411
Pathophysiology of Respiration 413
Factors in the Nervous System 413
Ventilation/Perfusion Ratio and Mismatch 413
Factors Affecting Pulmonary Ventilation 414
Factors Affecting Respiration 415
Circulatory Compromise 416
Patient Assessment 416
Recognizing Adequate Breathing 416
Recognizing Abnormal Breathing 416
Assessment of Respiration 419
Opening the Airway 424
Head Tilt–Chin Lift Maneuver 426
Jaw-Thrust Maneuver 427
Opening the Mouth 428
Suctioning 428
Suctioning Equipment 428
Techniques of Suctioning 429
Basic Airway Adjuncts 431
Oropharyngeal Airways 431
Nasopharyngeal Airways 434
Maintaining the Airway 436
Supplemental Oxygen 437
Supplemental Oxygen Equipment 437
Procedures for Operating and Administering Oxygen 440
Hazards of Supplemental Oxygen 442
Oxygen-Delivery Equipment 443
Nonrebreathing Masks 443
Nasal Cannulas 444
Partial Rebreathing Masks 444
Venturi Masks 444
Tracheostomy Masks 445
Humidification 445
Assisted and Artificial Ventilation 445
Assisting Ventilation in Respiratory Distress/Failure 446
Artificial Ventilation 446
Continuous Positive Airway Pressure 454
Mechanism 455
Indications 456
Contraindications 456
Application 456
Complications 459
Stomas and Tracheostomy Tubes 459
Foreign Body Airway Obstruction 461
Recognition 462
Emergency Medical Care for Foreign Body Airway Obstruction 463
Dental Appliances 464
Facial Bleeding 464
Pediatric Airway Management 464
Airway Adjuncts 465
Oxygen Delivery Devices 467
Assisting With ALS Airway Procedures 469
Assisting With Intubation 469
Assisting With Supraglottic Airway Placement 474

SECTION 4 Pharmacology 487

12 Principles of Pharmacology and Medication Administration 488

Introduction 489
How Medications Work 490
Medication Names 492
Routes of Administration 492
Medication Forms 495
Tablets and Capsules 495
Solutions and Suspensions 497
Metered-Dose Inhalers 497
Topical Medications 497
Transdermal Medications 497
Gels 498
Gases for Inhalation 498
General Steps in Administering Medication 498
Medication Administration Cross-Check Procedure 500
Medication Administration and the EMT 501
Medications Used by EMTs 501
Oral Medications 506
Sublingual Medications 507
Intramuscular Medications 509
Intranasal Medications 515
Inhalation Medications 516
Patient Medications 520
Implications for EMS Clinicians 520
Medication Errors 524

SECTION 5 Shock and Resuscitation 531

13 Shock 532

Introduction 533
Pathophysiology 533
 Perfusion 533
Causes of Shock 536
Types of Shock 536
 Cardiogenic Shock 536
 Obstructive Shock 537
 Distributive Shock 540
 Hypovolemic Shock 542
The Progression of Shock 543
Patient Assessment for Shock 544
 Scene Size-up 544
 Primary Assessment 544
 History Taking 545
 Secondary Assessment 545
 Reassessment 546
Emergency Medical Care for Shock 546
 Treating Cardiogenic Shock 547
 Treating Obstructive Shock 549
 Treating Distributive Shock 550
 Treating Hypovolemic Shock 550
Treating Shock in Infants and Children 551
 Circulation Emergencies and Management 551
 Dehydration Emergencies and Management 553
Treating Shock in Older Patients 554

14 BLS Resuscitation 560

Introduction 562
Principles of BLS 562
 The Goal of CPR 562
 Recognizing the Need for CPR 563
 The Chain of Survival 564
Performing CPR 566
 Positioning the Patient 566
 Checking for Adequate Breathing and a Pulse 566
 Performing External Chest Compressions 566
 Opening the Airway in Adults 569
 Providing Artificial Ventilations 571
One-Rescuer Adult CPR 572
Two-Rescuer Adult CPR 572
 Switching Positions 575
Automated External Defibrillation 576
 Overview of AEDs 576
 AED Use 577
 Patient Care Following AED Use 581
 AED Maintenance 583
 Medical Direction and Incident Review Relating to AED Use 583
Additional Devices and Techniques to Assist Circulation 583
 Mechanical Piston Device 585
 Load-Distributing Band CPR or Vest CPR 585
Infant and Child CPR 586
 Determining Responsiveness 588
 Checking for Breathing and Pulse 588
 Opening the Airway in Children 591
 Providing Rescue Breathing to Children 593
 Using an AED in Infants and Children 594
Interrupting CPR 594
Determining Not to Start CPR 594
Stopping CPR 595
Foreign Body Airway Obstruction in Adults 596
 Recognizing Foreign Body Airway Obstruction 596
 Removing a Foreign Body Airway Obstruction in an Adult 597
Foreign Body Airway Obstruction in Infants and Children 599
 Removing a Foreign Body Airway Obstruction in Children 600
 Removing a Foreign Body Airway Obstruction in Infants 601
Special Resuscitation Circumstances 603
 Opioid Overdose 603
 Cardiac Arrest in Pregnancy 603
 Lazarus Syndrome 603
Grief Support for Family Members and Loved Ones 604
Education and Training for the EMT 605
Education and Training for the Public 605

SECTION 6 Medical 611

15 Medical Overview 612

Introduction 613
Types of Medical Emergencies 613
Patient Assessment 614
 Scene Size-up 615
 Primary Assessment 615
 History Taking 617
 Secondary Assessment 618
 Reassessment 620
Management, Transport, and Destination 620
 Scene Time 621
 Type of Transport 621
 Destination Selection 622
Infectious Diseases 623
 General Assessment Principles 623
 General Management Principles 624
 Epidemic and Pandemic Considerations 624
Common or Serious Communicable Diseases 624
 Influenza 624
 Herpes Simplex 625
 HIV Infection 625
 Hepatitis 626
 Meningitis 628
 Tuberculosis 629
 Pertussis 630
 Methicillin-Resistant *Staphylococcus aureus* 631
 Global Health Issues 631
 Travel Medicine 631
Conclusion 632

16 Respiratory Emergencies 639

Introduction 640
Anatomy of the Respiratory System 641
 The Pediatric Respiratory System 641
 The Geriatric Respiratory System 643
Physiology of Respiration 643
Pathophysiology 644
 Carbon Dioxide Retention and Hypoxic Drive 645
 Causes of Dyspnea 647
 Upper or Lower Airway Infection 648

Patient Assessment 649
Scene Size-up 649
Primary Assessment 649
History Taking 654
Secondary Assessment 655
Reassessment 657
General Care for Respiratory Emergencies 657
Administering Oxygen 658
Using Metered-Dose Inhalers and Small-Volume Nebulizers 658
Recognition and Management of Specific Conditions 664
Respiratory Infections 664
Acute Pulmonary Edema 668
Chronic Obstructive Pulmonary Disease 670
Asthma and Anaphylaxis 671
Spontaneous Pneumothorax 675
Pleural Effusion 676
Obstruction of the Airway 676
Pulmonary Embolism 677
Hyperventilation 678
Environmental/Industrial Exposure 679
Carbon Monoxide Poisoning 679
Cystic Fibrosis 679

17 Cardiovascular Emergencies 688

Introduction 689
Anatomy and Physiology 689
Circulation 691
The Geriatric Circulatory System 697
The Pediatric Circulatory System 697
Pathophysiology 698
Atherosclerosis 698
Acute Coronary Syndrome 699
Cardiogenic Shock 702
Heart Failure 702
Hypertensive Emergencies 705
Patient Assessment 706
Scene Size-up 706
Primary Assessment 706
History Taking 708
Secondary Assessment 709
Reassessment 711
Emergency Medical Care for Chest Pain or Discomfort 711
Administering Nitroglycerin 712
Cardiac Monitoring 714
Placing the Electrodes 714
Performing Cardiac Monitoring 715
Reviewing the ECG Tracing 718
Heart Surgeries and Cardiac Assistive Devices 718
Automatic Implantable Cardiac Defibrillators 719
External Defibrillator Vest 720
Ventricular Assist Devices 720
Cardiac Arrest 722

18 Neurologic Emergencies 729

Introduction 730
Anatomy and Physiology 730
Pathophysiology 731
Headache 732
Stroke 734
Types of Stroke 734
Signs and Symptoms of Stroke 737
Conditions That May Mimic Stroke 738
Seizures 738
Causes of Seizures 740
The Importance of Recognizing Seizures 741
The Postictal State 742
Syncope 742
Altered Mental Status 743
Causes of Altered Mental Status 743
Patient Assessment 745
Scene Size-up 745
Primary Assessment 746
History Taking 748
Secondary Assessment 749
Stroke Assessment 749
Reassessment 752
Emergency Medical Care 755
Headache 755
Stroke 756
Seizure 757
Altered Mental Status 757

19 Gastrointestinal and Urologic Emergencies 763

Introduction 764
Anatomy and Physiology 764
The GI System 764
Additional Abdominal Organs 765
The Genital System 765
The Urinary System 765
Pathophysiology 766
Abdominal Pain 767
Causes of Acute Abdomen 768
Urinary System Dysfunction 773
Problems Relating to the Female Reproductive Organs 774
Age-Related Considerations 774
Patient Assessment 776
Scene Size-up 776
Primary Assessment 776
History Taking 777
Secondary Assessment 778
Reassessment 779
Emergency Medical Care 780
Dialysis Emergencies 781

20 Endocrine and Hematologic Emergencies 789

Introduction 790
Endocrine Emergencies 790
Anatomy and Physiology 790
Pathophysiology 792
Patient Assessment of Diabetes 799
Scene Size-up 799
Primary Assessment 799
History Taking 800
Secondary Assessment 800
Reassessment 801
Emergency Medical Care for Diabetic Emergencies 803
Administering Glucose 803
Transporting the Patient 804
Reassessing the Patient After Administering Glucose 804
The Presentation of Hypoglycemia 805
Seizures 805

Altered Mental Status 805
Misdiagnosis of Neurologic Dysfunction 806
Relationship to Airway Management 806
Hematologic Emergencies 806
Anatomy and Physiology 806
Pathophysiology 807
Patient Assessment of Hematologic Disorders 809
Scene Size-up 809
Primary Assessment 810
History Taking 810
Secondary Assessment 810
Reassessment 811
Emergency Medical Care for Hematologic Disorders 811

21 Allergy and Anaphylaxis 816

Introduction 817
Anatomy and Physiology 817
Pathophysiology 817
Common Allergens 819
Patient Assessment of an Immunologic Emergency 820
Scene Size-up 820
Primary Assessment 820
History Taking 822
Secondary Assessment 823
Reassessment 824
Emergency Medical Care of Immunologic Emergencies 825
Epinephrine 825

22 Toxicology 835

Introduction 836
Identifying the Patient and the Poison 836
How Poisons Enter the Body 838
Inhaled Poisons 839
Absorbed and Surface Contact Poisons 841
Ingested Poisons 842
Injected Poisons 843
Patient Assessment 844
Scene Size-up 844
Primary Assessment 845
History Taking 846
Secondary Assessment 847
Reassessment 847
Emergency Medical Care 847
Specific Poisons 848
Alcohol 849
Opioids 850
Sedative-Hypnotic Drugs 853
Inhalants 854
Hydrogen Sulfide 854
Sympathomimetics 855
Synthetic Cathinones (Bath Salts) 856
Cannabis 856
Synthetic Marijuana 857
Hallucinogens 857
Anticholinergic Agents 857
Cholinergic Agents 858
Miscellaneous Drugs 858
Food Poisoning 859
Plant Poisoning 860
Special Populations 862
Considerations for Geriatric Patients 862
Considerations for Pediatric Patients 862

23 Behavioral Health Emergencies 869

Introduction 870
Mental Illness Versus Behavioral Health Emergency 870
Defining Mental Illness 870
Defining a Behavioral Health Emergency 870
Mental Health Crisis Care Systems 870
Conditions That Resemble Behavioral Health Emergencies 871
Common Behavioral Health Emergencies 871
Depression 871
Bipolar Disorders 872
Schizophrenia 873
Suicide 873
Posttraumatic Stress Disorder 875
Dementia 876
Delirium 876
Substance Use Disorders 877
Acute Psychosis 877
Scene Safety Considerations 878
Patient Assessment 880
Scene Size-up 880
Primary Assessment 880
History Taking 881
Secondary Assessment 882
Reassessment 883
De-escalation and Restraint 884
The Process of Restraining a Patient 886
The Potentially Violent Patient 888
Medicolegal Considerations 890

SECTION 7 Trauma 895

24 Trauma Overview 896

Introduction 897
Energy and Trauma 897
Newton's Laws of Motion 899
Newton's First Law 899
Newton's Second Law 899
Newton's Third Law 899
MOI Profiles 900
Blunt Trauma 900
Vehicular Crashes 901
Car Versus Pedestrian 907
Car Versus Bicycle 907
Motorcycle Crash 907
Falls 908
Penetrating Trauma 909
Blast Injuries 911
Types of Primary Blast Injury 913
Multisystem Trauma 914
Patient Assessment 914
Injuries to the Head 915
Injuries to the Neck and Throat 915
Injuries to the Chest 915
Injuries to the Abdomen 916
Management: Transport and Destination 916
Scene Time 916
Destination Selection 916
Type of Transport 918
Trauma Scoring Systems 918
Revised Trauma Score 920

25 Bleeding 928
Introduction 929
Anatomy and Physiology of the Cardiovascular System 929
The Heart 929
Blood Vessels and Blood 929
Pathophysiology and Perfusion 931
External Bleeding 932
The Significance of External Bleeding 932
Characteristics of External Bleeding 933
Internal Bleeding 935
Mechanism of Injury for Internal Bleeding 935
Nature of Illness for Internal Bleeding 935
Signs and Symptoms of Internal Bleeding 935
Patient Assessment for External and Internal Bleeding 936
Scene Size-Up 936
Primary Assessment 937
History Taking 938
Secondary Assessment 938
Reassessment 939
Emergency Medical Care for External Bleeding 940
Wound Packing and Hemostatic Dressings 941
Tourniquets 944
Junctional Tourniquets 946
Pelvic Binder 947
Bleeding From the Nose, Ears, and Mouth 947
Emergency Medical Care for Internal Bleeding 948

26 Soft-Tissue Injuries 955
Introduction 956
Anatomy and Physiology of the Skin 956
Anatomy 957
Physiology 958
Pathophysiology of Closed and Open Injuries 958
Closed Injuries 959
Open Injuries 961
Patient Assessment of Closed and Open Injuries 965
Scene Size-Up 966
Primary Assessment 966
History Taking 969
Secondary Assessment 970
Reassessment 970
Emergency Medical Care for Closed Injuries 972
Emergency Medical Care for Open Injuries 972
Abdominal Wounds 973
Impaled Objects 974
Neck Injuries 975
Bites 975
Burns 977
Pathophysiology of Burns 977
Complications of Burns 977
Burn Assessment 978
Patient Assessment of Burns 981
Scene Size-up 981
Primary Assessment 981
History Taking 983
Secondary Assessment 984
Reassessment 985
Emergency Medical Care for Burns 985
Management of Specific Burns 987
Dressing and Bandaging 992
Sterile Dressings 992
Bandages 993

27 Face and Neck Injuries 999
Introduction 1000
Anatomy and Physiology 1000
The Eye 1002
Injuries of the Face and Neck 1003
Soft-Tissue Injuries 1004
Patient Assessment 1004
Scene Size-Up 1004
Primary Assessment 1005
History Taking 1006
Secondary Assessment 1006
Reassessment 1007
Emergency Medical Care 1008
Emergency Medical Care for Specific Injuries 1010
Injuries of the Eyes 1010
Epistaxis and Injuries of the Nose 1020
Injuries of the Ear 1021
Facial Fractures 1023
Dental Injuries 1024
Injuries of the Cheek 1024
Injuries of the Neck 1025

28 Head and Spine Injuries 1032
Introduction 1033
Anatomy and Physiology 1033
Nervous System 1033
How the Nervous System Works 1036
Skeletal System 1037
Head Injuries 1038
Scalp Lacerations 1039
Skull Fracture 1039
Traumatic Brain Injuries 1041
Intracranial Pressure and Herniation 1042
Intracranial Hemorrhage 1042
Concussion 1044
Brain Contusion 1045
Other Brain Injuries 1045
Spine Injuries 1045
Patient Assessment 1046
Scene Size-Up 1046
Primary Assessment 1047
History Taking 1050
Secondary Assessment 1050
Reassessment 1054
Emergency Medical Care of Head Injuries 1055
Managing the Airway 1056
Managing Circulation 1056
Emergency Medical Care of Spinal Injuries 1057
Managing the Airway 1058
Performing SMR 1058
Preparation for Transport 1062
Supine Patients 1062
Sitting Patients 1070
Standing Patients 1072
SMR in Children 1072
Helmet Removal 1074

29 Chest Injuries 1086
Introduction 1087
Anatomy and Physiology 1087
Mechanics of Ventilation 1089
Injuries of the Chest 1089
Signs and Symptoms of Chest Injury 1091

Patient Assessment 1092
Scene Size-Up 1092
Primary Assessment 1092
History Taking 1094
Secondary Assessment 1094
Reassessment 1096
Complications and Management of Chest Injuries 1097
Pneumothorax 1097
Hemothorax 1100
Cardiac Tamponade 1100
Rib Fractures 1102
Flail Chest 1102
Other Chest Injuries 1103
Pulmonary Contusion 1103
Other Fractures 1103
Traumatic Asphyxia 1104
Blunt Myocardial Injury 1104
Commotio Cordis 1105
Laceration of the Great Vessels 1105

30 Abdominal and Genitourinary Injuries 1111

Introduction 1112
Anatomy and Physiology of the Abdomen 1112
Abdominal Quadrants 1112
Hollow and Solid Organs 1113
Abdominal Injuries 1115
Closed Abdominal Injuries 1115
Open Abdominal Injuries 1116
Hollow Organ Injuries 1117
Solid Organ Injuries 1118
Patient Assessment of Abdominal Injuries 1119
Scene Size-Up 1119
Primary Assessment 1119
History Taking 1121
Secondary Assessment 1122
Reassessment 1124
Emergency Medical Care of Abdominal Injuries 1124
Closed Abdominal Injuries 1124
Open Abdominal Injuries 1125
Anatomy of the Genitourinary System 1126
Injuries of the Genitourinary System 1127
Injuries of the Kidneys 1127
Injuries to the Urinary Bladder 1128
Injuries of the External Male Genitalia 1129
Injuries of the Female Genitalia 1129
Patient Assessment of the Genitourinary System 1129
Scene Size-Up 1130
Primary Assessment 1130
History Taking 1131
Secondary Assessment 1131
Reassessment 1132
Emergency Medical Care of Genitourinary Injuries 1132
Kidneys 1132
Urinary Bladder 1132
External Male Genitalia 1132
Female Genitalia 1133
Rectal Bleeding 1133
Sexual Assault and Rape 1133

31 Orthopaedic Injuries 1138

Introduction 1139
Anatomy and Physiology of the Musculoskeletal System 1139
Muscles 1139
The Skeleton 1140
Pathophysiology of the Musculoskeletal System 1143
Children 1143
Older Adults 1144
Musculoskeletal Injuries 1145
Mechanism of Injury 1145
Fractures 1146
Dislocations 1149
Sprains 1150
Strains 1151
Amputations 1151
Patient Assessment 1151
Scene Size-up 1152
Primary Assessment 1152
History Taking 1153
Secondary Assessment 1154
Reassessment 1155
Emergency Medical Care 1156
Handling Injured Extremities 1157
Splinting 1157
Transport 1162
Specific Musculoskeletal Injuries 1163
Injuries of the Clavicle and Scapula 1163
Dislocation of the Shoulder 1165
Fracture of the Humerus 1166
Elbow Injuries 1167
Fractures of the Forearm 1169
Injuries of the Wrist and Hand 1170
Fractures of the Pelvis 1172
Dislocation of the Hip 1173
Fractures of the Proximal Femur 1174
Femoral Shaft Fractures 1175
Injuries of Knee Ligaments 1181
Dislocation of the Knee 1181
Fractures Involving the Knee 1182
Dislocation of the Patella 1183
Injuries of the Tibia and Fibula 1183
Ankle Injuries 1183
Foot Injuries 1184
Sprains and Strains 1185
Amputations 1185
Compartment Syndrome 1186

32 Environmental Emergencies 1193

Introduction 1194
Factors Affecting Exposure 1194
Cold Exposure 1196
Hypothermia 1197
Local Cold Injuries 1199
Assessment of Cold Injuries 1201
Scene Size-up 1201
Primary Assessment 1201
History Taking 1202
Secondary Assessment 1202
Reassessment 1202
Management of Cold Emergencies 1203
Emergency Care of Local Cold Injuries 1204
Cold Exposure and the EMS Clinician 1205
Heat Exposure 1205
Heat Cramps 1206
Heat Exhaustion 1206
Heatstroke 1207
Assessment of Heat Emergencies 1208
Scene Size-up 1208
Primary Assessment 1208

History Taking	1209
Secondary Assessment	1209
Reassessment	1209
Management of Heat Emergencies	1210
Heat Cramps	1210
Heat Exhaustion	1210
Heatstroke	1212
Drowning	1212
Spinal Injuries in Submersion Incidents	1213
Hypothermia in the Context of Submersion	1215
Scuba Diving Emergencies	1217
Descent Emergencies	1217
Emergencies at the Bottom	1217
Ascent Emergencies	1217
Assessment of Drowning and Scuba Diving Emergencies	1218
Scene Size-up	1218
Primary Assessment	1219
History Taking	1219
Secondary Assessment	1220
Reassessment	1220
Emergency Care for Drowning or Scuba Diving Emergencies	1221
Drowning Emergencies	1221
Scuba Diving Emergencies	1221
Prevention	1222
High Altitude	1223
Lightning	1224
Emergency Medical Care	1225
Bites and Envenomation	1225
Spider Bites	1225
Hymenoptera Stings	1227
Snake Bites	1228
Scorpion Stings	1232
Tick Bites	1233
Injuries From Marine Animals	1234

SECTION 8 Special Patient Populations 1241

33 Gynecologic Emergencies 1242

Introduction	1243
Anatomy and Physiology	1243
Pathophysiology	1245
Pelvic Inflammatory Disease	1245
Sexually Transmitted Infections	1246
Vaginal Bleeding	1247
Patient Assessment	1247
Scene Size-up	1247
Primary Assessment	1248
History Taking	1248
Secondary Assessment	1249
Reassessment	1251
Emergency Medical Care	1251

34 Obstetrics and Neonatal Care 1256

Introduction	1257
Anatomy and Physiology of the Female Reproductive System	1258
Normal Changes in Pregnancy	1260
Complications of Pregnancy	1261
Diabetes	1261
Hypertension in Pregnancy	1261
Bleeding	1262
Abortion	1264
Substance Use Disorder	1264
Maternal Cardiac Arrest	1265
Trauma and Pregnancy	1265
Cultural Value Considerations	1267
Teenage Pregnancy	1267
Patient Assessment	1267
Scene Size-up	1268
Primary Assessment	1268
History Taking	1268
Secondary Assessment	1269
Reassessment	1270
Stages of Labor	1270
Normal Delivery Management	1271
Preparing for Delivery	1271
The Delivery	1275
Postdelivery Care	1280
Neonatal Assessment and Resuscitation	1282
Additional Resuscitation Efforts	1283
The Apgar Score	1283
Complicated Delivery Emergencies	1287
Shoulder Dystocia	1287
Breech Delivery	1287
Presentation Complications	1288
Spina Bifida	1289
Multiple Gestation	1289
Preterm Birth	1290
Postterm Pregnancy	1290
Fetal Death	1291
Postpartum Complications	1291

35 Patients With Special Challenges 1298

Introduction	1299
Developmental Disability	1300
Autism Spectrum Disorder	1301
Down Syndrome	1301
Brain Injury	1302
Interacting With Patients Who Have a Developmental Disability	1302
Sensory Disabilities	1303
Visual Impairment	1303
Hearing Impairment	1304
Physical Disabilities	1306
Cerebral Palsy	1306
Spina Bifida	1307
Paralysis	1308
Orthotic and Prosthetic Devices	1308
Bariatric Patients	1308
Interacting With Patients Who Have Obesity	1309
Transporting a Patient With Obesity	1309
Patients With Medical Technology Assistance	1309
Tracheostomy Tubes	1310
Home Oxygen	1310
Mechanical Ventilators	1310
Apnea Monitors	1312
Internal Cardiac Pacemakers and Defibrillators	1313
Ventricular Assist Devices	1313
External Defibrillator Vest	1314
Central Venous Catheter	1314
Gastrostomy Tubes	1315
Shunts	1315
Vagus Nerve Stimulators	1316
Colostomies, Ileostomies, and Urostomies	1316

Emergencies Involving Infants 1316
Sudden Unexpected Infant Death 1316
Brief Resolved Unexplained Event 1317
Patients Who Have Experienced Abuse or Neglect 1318
Child Abuse and Neglect 1318
Human Trafficking 1320
Elder Abuse and Neglect 1321
Sexual Assault and Rape 1323
Care for Patients in Special Settings 1326
Nursing and Skilled Care Facilities 1326
Home Care 1328
Hospice Care and Terminally Ill Patients 1328
Poverty and Homelessness 1329
The Expanding Role of EMS in Addressing Special Populations 1330

SECTION 9 EMS Operations 1339

36 Transport Operations 1340

Introduction 1341
Emergency Vehicle Design 1342
Phases of an Ambulance Call 1344
The Preparation Phase 1344
The Dispatch Phase 1352
En Route to the Scene 1353
Arrival at the Scene 1354
The Transfer Phase 1357
The Transport Phase 1357
The Delivery Phase 1358
En Route to the Station 1358
The Postrun Phase 1359
Safe Emergency Vehicle Operation 1360
Mental and Emotional Fitness 1360
Safety Restraints 1361
Vehicle Handling 1363
Siren Risk–Benefit Analysis 1364
Driver Anticipation 1364
The Cushion of Safety 1365
The Problem of Excessive Speed 1366
Recognition of Siren Syndrome 1366
Weather and Road Conditions 1367
Laws and Regulations 1368
Specific Driving Situations 1369
Distractions 1370
Driving Alone 1370
Air Medical Services 1370
Calling for Air Medical Services 1371
Establishing a Landing Zone 1372
Ensuring Safety During Landing and Patient Transfer 1373
Avoiding Communication Issues 1375
Special Considerations 1375

37 Vehicle Extrication and Special Rescue 1380

Introduction 1381
Safety 1381
Vehicle Safety Systems 1381
Fundamentals of Extrication 1382
Preparation 1383
En Route to the Scene 1384
Arrival and Scene Size-up 1384
Hazard Control 1386
Support Operations 1388
Gaining Access 1388
Emergency Care 1391
Removal of the Patient 1391
Transfer of the Patient 1392
Termination 1392
Specialized Rescue Situations 1393
Technical Rescue Situations 1393
Search and Rescue 1394
Trench Rescue 1395
Tactical Emergency Medical Support 1395
Structure Fires 1397

38 Incident Management 1402

Introduction 1403
National Incident Management System 1404
Incident Command System 1404
ICS Roles and Responsibilities 1405
Communications and Information Management 1408
Mobilization and Deployment 1408
EMS Response Within the ICS 1409
Preparedness 1409
Scene Size-up 1409
Establishing Command 1411
Communications 1411
The Medical Branch of Incident Command 1411
Triage Supervisor 1411
Treatment Supervisor 1411
Transportation Supervisor 1412
Staging Supervisor 1412
Physicians on Scene 1413
Rehabilitation Supervisor 1413
Extrication and Special Rescue 1413
Morgue Supervisor 1413
Mass-Casualty Incidents 1414
Triage 1415
Triage Categories 1415
Triage Tags 1416
Triage Systems 1417
Triage Special Considerations 1419
Destination Decisions 1420
Disaster Management 1420
Introduction to Hazardous Materials 1421
Recognizing a Hazardous Material 1422
Occupancy and Location 1423
Senses 1423
Containers 1423
The Department of Transportation Marking System 1426
Other Considerations 1427
Identification 1430
Hazmat Scene Operations 1432
Classification of Hazardous Materials 1434
Personal Protective Equipment Level 1435
Caring for Patients at a Hazmat Incident 1435

39 Terrorism Response and Disaster Management 1446

Introduction 1447
What Is Terrorism? 1447
Active Shooter Events 1448
Weapons of Mass Destruction 1450
Chemical Terrorism/Warfare 1451
Biologic Terrorism/Warfare 1451
Nuclear/Radiologic Terrorism 1451

EMT Response to Terrorism 1451
Recognizing a Terrorist Event (Indicators) 1451
Response Actions 1452
Chemical Agents 1454
Vesicants (Blister Agents) 1455
Pulmonary Agents (Choking Agents) 1456
Nerve Agents 1457
Metabolic Agents (Cyanides) 1460
Biologic Agents 1463
Viruses 1463
Bacteria 1464
Neurotoxins 1466
Other EMT Roles During a Biologic Event 1469
Radiologic/Nuclear Devices 1469
What Is Radiation? 1469
Sources of Radiologic Material 1470
Radiologic Dispersal Devices 1471
Nuclear Energy 1471
Nuclear Weapons 1471
Symptomatology 1471
Protective Measures 1472
Medical Management 1472
Incendiary and Explosive Devices 1473

Glossary 1481

Index 1526

Skill Drills

Skill Drill 2-1	Proper Glove Removal Technique	44
Skill Drill 2-2	Managing a Potential Exposure	47
Skill Drill 8-1	Performing the Power Lift	261
Skill Drill 8-2	Performing the Rapid Extrication Technique	272
Skill Drill 8-3	Performing the Extremity Lift	276
Skill Drill 8-4	Log Rolling a Patient on the Ground	280
Skill Drill 8-5	Loading a Stretcher Into an Ambulance	283
Skill Drill 8-6	Using a Scoop Stretcher	285
Skill Drill 8-7	Performing the Diamond Carry	286
Skill Drill 8-8	Performing the One-Handed Carry	287
Skill Drill 8-9	Carrying a Patient on Stairs Using a Backboard or Similar Transport Device	289
Skill Drill 8-10	Using a Stair Chair	290
Skill Drill 10-1	Performing the Secondary Assessment	357
Skill Drill 10-2	Obtaining Blood Pressure by Auscultation	371
Skill Drill 10-3	Obtaining Blood Pressure by Palpation	373
Skill Drill 10-4	Assessing Neurovascular Status	377
Skill Drill 10-5	Assessing Blood Glucose Level	385
Skill Drill 11-1	Applying the Pulse Oximeter	421
Skill Drill 11-2	Positioning the Unconscious Patient	425
Skill Drill 11-3	Suctioning a Patient's Airway	430
Skill Drill 11-4	Inserting an Oropharyngeal Airway With a 90° Rotation	433
Skill Drill 11-5	Inserting an Oropharyngeal Airway With a 180° Rotation	434
Skill Drill 11-6	Inserting a Nasopharyngeal Airway	435
Skill Drill 11-7	Placing an Oxygen Cylinder Into Service	441
Skill Drill 11-8	Performing One-Rescuer Bag-Mask Ventilations	451
Skill Drill 11-9	Using CPAP	457
Skill Drill 11-10	Inserting an Oropharyngeal Airway in a Pediatric Patient	466
Skill Drill 12-1	Drawing Medication From a Vial	511
Skill Drill 12-2	Administering Medication via the Intramuscular Route	513
Skill Drill 14-1	Performing Adult Chest Compressions	567
Skill Drill 14-2	Performing One-Rescuer Adult CPR	573
Skill Drill 14-3	Performing Two-Rescuer Adult CPR	574
Skill Drill 14-4	Using an AED	578
Skill Drill 14-5	Performing Infant Chest Compressions	589
Skill Drill 14-6	Performing CPR on a Child	590
Skill Drill 14-7	Removing a Foreign Body Airway Obstruction in an Unresponsive Child	602
Skill Drill 16-1	Assisting a Patient With a Metered-Dose Inhaler	662
Skill Drill 16-2	Assisting a Patient With a Small-Volume Nebulizer	663
Skill Drill 17-1	Administering Nitroglycerin	713
Skill Drill 17-2	Performing Cardiac Monitoring	716
Skill Drill 21-1	Using an EpiPen Auto-injector	827
Skill Drill 21-2	Using a Neffy Intranasal Device	829
Skill Drill 23-1	Restraining a Patient	888
Skill Drill 25-1	Controlling External Bleeding	942
Skill Drill 25-2	Packing a Wound	943

Skill Drill 25-3 Applying a Commercial Tourniquet 946
Skill Drill 25-4 Controlling Epistaxis 949
Skill Drill 25-5 Controlling Internal Bleeding 950
Skill Drill 26-1 Stabilizing an Impaled Object 974
Skill Drill 26-2 Caring for Burns 986
Skill Drill 27-1 Removing a Foreign Object From Under the Upper Eyelid 1011
Skill Drill 27-2 Stabilizing a Foreign Object Impaled in the Eye 1013
Skill Drill 27-3 Controlling Bleeding From a Neck Injury 1026
Skill Drill 28-1 Performing Manual In-Line Stabilization 1059
Skill Drill 28-2 Applying a Cervical Collar 1060
Skill Drill 28-3 Securing a Patient to a Long Backboard 1063
Skill Drill 28-4 Placing a Patient on a Full-Body Vacuum Mattress 1066
Skill Drill 28-5 Securing a Patient Found in a Sitting Position 1070
Skill Drill 28-6 Performing SMR for a Pediatric Patient 1073
Skill Drill 28-7 Performing SMR for a Patient in a Car Seat 1075
Skill Drill 28-8 Removing a Helmet 1078
Skill Drill 31-1 Applying a Rigid Splint 1160
Skill Drill 31-2 Applying a Vacuum Splint 1162
Skill Drill 31-3 Splinting the Hand and Wrist 1171
Skill Drill 31-4 Applying a Hare Traction Splint 1177
Skill Drill 31-5 Applying a Slishman Traction Splint 1179
Skill Drill 32-1 Treating for Heat Exhaustion 1211
Skill Drill 32-2 Stabilizing a Suspected Spinal Injury in the Water 1216
Skill Drill 34-1 Putting on Sterile Gloves 1274
Skill Drill 34-2 Delivering the Newborn 1276

Acknowledgments

AMERICAN ACADEMY OF ORTHOPAEDIC SURGEONS

The American Academy of Orthopaedic Surgeons and the Public Safety Group would like to thank the editors, authors, and reviewers of previous editions of *Emergency Care and Transportation of the Sick and Injured*, as well as acknowledge those involved in the thirteenth edition.

Series Editor

Alfonso Mejia, MD, MPH, FAAOS
Program Director, Orthopedic Surgery Residency Program
Vice Head, Department of Orthopedic Surgery
University of Illinois at Chicago College of Medicine
Medical Director
Tactical Emergency Medical Support Physician
South Suburban Emergency Response Team
Chicago, Illinois

Lead Editors

Dennis Edgerly, MEd, EMT-P
Director, EMS Academy
Arapahoe Community College
Littleton, Colorado

Kim D. McKenna, PhD, MEd, RN, NRP
Consultant Paramedic
St. Louis, Missouri

Contributors

Andrew Bartkus, JD, MSN, RN, NRP, CEN, CCRN, CFRN, Esq
Lovelace Westside Hospital
Albuquerque, New Mexico

Chris Coughlin, PhD, NRP, NEMSEC
Contra Costa College
California

Remle Crowe, PhD, NREMT
ESO
Austin, Texas

David L. Dalton, BS, Paramedic
St. Charles County Ambulance District
St. Peters, Missouri

Rommie L. Duckworth, MPA, LP, EFO, FO
Ridgefield Fire Department
Ridgefield, Connecticut

Dennis Edgerly, MEd, EMT-P
Arapahoe Community College
Littleton, Colorado

Jason Ferguson, EdD, NRP
Central Virginia Community College
Lynchburg, Virginia

Rhonda J. Hunt, MEd, NRP
Albany State University, Darton College of Health Professions
Albany, Georgia

Michael Kaduce, MPS, NRP
The Falck Health Institute
Orange County, California

Mike McEvoy, PhD, NRP, RN, CCRN
Albany Medical Center
Albany, New York

Kim D. McKenna, PhD, MEd, RN, NRP
Consultant Paramedic
St. Louis, Missouri

Katie O'Connor, MPP, NRP
Santa Rosa Junior College
Santa Rosa, California

Stephen J. Rahm, NRP, FcEHS
Centre for Health Sciences
Bulverde, Texas

Michael Tarantino, MAS, BA
Bergen County EMS Training Center
Paramus, New Jersey

Bryan Ware, BS, EMT-P
Beulah Fire Protection and Ambulance District
Beulah, Colorado

Brittany Williams, DHSc, RRT-ACCS, NPS, AE-C, REMT-P
Santa Fe College
Gainesville, Florida

Reviewers

Aref Abdellatif, MS, BS, Firefighter/Paramedic, LI
Oakton College
Skokie, Illinois

Robert Aguilar, BT, NRP, CCP-C
Oklahoma State University–Oklahoma City
Oklahoma City, Oklahoma

Joseph Baldwin, NYS EMT, NREMT, NYS CIC
FDNY EMS Academy
Fort Totten, New York

Shelly Beck, MS, AEMT
University of Utah
Salt Lake City, Utah

Jon Blank, BS, NRP
Roanoke County Fire and Rescue Department
Roanoke, Virginia

James Blivin, AS, NRP
Emergency Health Services Federation
New Cumberland, Pennsylvania

Robert W. Bowen, MS, NRP
Arlington County Fire Department
Arlington, Virginia

Jason Brooks, EdD, NRP
University of South Alabama Department of Emergency Medical Services
Mobile, Alabama

Brian W. Buzzella, AS
Broward College
Davie, Florida

Anthony Caliguire, AS, CIC
Hudson Valley Community College Paramedic Program
Troy, New York

Sharon F. Chiumento, BSN, EMT-P
Monroe Community College
Rochester, New York

Heidi P. Cordi, MD, MPH, MS, EMT-P, FACEP, FAADM
Albany Med Health System
Albany Medical Center
Albany, New York

Kent Courtney, NRP
Essential Safety Training and Consulting
Rimrock, Arizona

Sean Davis, MEd, CICNRP, F&E Instructor II
Auburn Career Center
Concord, Ohio

John A. Dorn, Jr., AAS, NRP, EMT-P, EMT-Instructor
RWJ Barnabas Health, Mobile Health
Somerville, New Jersey

Glenn Faught, MS, NRP
Arkansas State University Mid-South
West Memphis, Arkansas

Timothy N. Fonger, NRP, EMT-P, EMS I/C, USCG (Ret.)
Dorsey College
Grand Rapids, Michigan

Adam C. Fritsch, NRP, CCP
Advanced Professional Healthcare Education
Delafield, Wisconsin

Braiden Green, MPA, CCP, NCEE
College of Southern Nevada
Las Vegas, Nevada

Kevin M. Gurney, MS, CCEMT-P, I/C
Delta Ambulance
Waterville, Maine

Kirk Hallett, RN, NRP, FNP
Vital Knowledge Group
Richmond, Virginia

Jennifer Hannigan, MEd, NRP, CIC, NEMCEC
Suffolk County EMS
Yaphank, New York

Anthony S. Harbour, MEd, BSN, RN, NRP
Virginia Commonwealth University School of Medicine
Center for Trauma and Critical Care Education
Richmond, Virginia

Keith B. Hermiz, NRAEMT
Grafton Rescue Squad
Grafton, Vermont

Connie Holder, MS, AEMT
University of Utah
Salt Lake City, Utah

Evan Holtz, MBA, BSN, RN, EMT(I), NCEE
NJ Association of EMS Educators
Jersey City, New Jersey

Matt Hunt, BSEd, EMT-P
Albany State University
Albany, Georgia

Joseph Hurlburt, BS, NREMT-P
Northwest Wexford Emergency Authority
Mesick/Buckley, Michigan

Scott Jaeggi
Rio Hondo Fire Academy
Santa Fe Springs, California

Erik D. Jesse, MPA, MPsy, NRP, FP-C, CCEMTP
Volunteer State Community College
Gallatin, Tennessee

Joe Kalilikani, Jr., BAS, EMT
Pasadena City College
Pasadena, California

Timothy M. Kimble, BA, AAS, NRP, CEM
Camp Rock Enon Scout Reservation (BSA)
Gore, Virginia

Mark A. King, MS, MEMS (Ret.)
Kennebec Valley Community College
Fairfield, Maine

Blake E. Klingle, MS, RN, CEN, CCEMT-P
Waukesha County Technical College
Pewaukee, Wisconsin

Karen (Keri) Wydner Krause, RN, EMT-P, CCRN
Lakeshore Technical College
Cleveland, Wisconsin

Kevin Kurzweil, BS, MICP, EMT-I, CHSE
New Jersey Association of EMS Educators
Flemington, New Jersey

Lance Lopez, NRP
Rocky Mountain Resuscitation
Fredericksburg, Virginia

Michael McDonald, BSN, RN, NRP
Loudoun County Combined Fire Rescue System
Leesburg, Virginia

Steve McGraw, MHSA, NRP
City of Fairfax Fire Department
Fairfax, Virginia

Lucian Mirra, EdD(c), MEd, NRP
Albemarle County Fire Rescue
Charlottesville, Virginia

Joseph J. Ogershok, Jr., BS, NRAEMT
Hollidaysburg American Legion Ambulance Service
Hollidaysburg, Pennsylvania

Alan Ottarson, MSc, NRP
Gloucester Fire and Rescue
Gloucester, Virginia

Laura Pieslewicz, BS Emergency Management, BS Fire Science
Pima Community College
Emergency Medical Technology
Tucson, Arizona

Ian Pleet, NREMT
Virginia Department of Fire Programs
Manassas, Virginia

Victor T. Podbielski, MBA, NRP, IPMA-CP
Fredericksburg Fire Department
Fredericksburg, Virginia

Robert Policht, MA, LT, EMT
City of Passaic Fire Department
Passaic, New Jersey

Steven T. Powell, AAS, NRP
Rockingham County Fire and Rescue
Harrisonburg, Virginia

Michael A. Pruitt, MPA, BS, NRP
Carilion Clinic Patient Transportation
Roanoke, Virginia

Douglas Randell, BS, NRP
Hendricks Regional Health EMS
Danville, Indiana

Dustin E. Ridings, BA, FF/EMT-P, NRP
Green Bay Metro Fire Department
Green Bay, Wisconsin

Jamie Rossborough, NRP, CCP-C, FP-C,
South Davis Community Hospital/Western Peaks Specialty Hospital
Bountiful, Utah

Dennis Russell, MEd, ATC, NRP, I/C
United Ambulance Service/ United Training Center
Lewiston, Maine

Richard M. Saalsaa, EMT
Philomath Fire and Rescue
Philomath, Oregon

Michael R. Schulz, MA EdL, LP
Truckee Meadows Community College, Department of Public Safety Programs
Reno, Nevada

Jeb Sheidler, DMSc, PA-C, ATC, NRP, TP-C, WP-C, CP-C
Medical College of Georgia at Augusta University
Augusta, Georgia

Sara Sproule, NRP, CCEMT-P
Prince William County Department of Fire and Rescue
Prince William County, Virginia

Andrew W. Stern, MPA, MA, NRP, CCEMT-P
Hudson Valley Community College Paramedic Program
Troy, New York

Frank Strange, Jr., MEd, NRP
Oklahoma State University–Oklahoma City
Oklahoma City, Oklahoma

Russell D. Stuart, EMT-I
RWJ Barnabas Health
Somerville, New Jersey

Jameel Sylvia, MPA, NRP
David Geffen School of Medicine at UCLA
Los Angeles, California

Michael Tarantino, MAS, BA
Bergen County EMS Training Center
Paramus, New Jersey

Scott Tomek, EdS, MA, FP-C, CCP-C, C-NPT
University of Minnesota Medical School, Department of Emergency Medicine
Minneapolis, Minnesota

Brian Turner, RN, CCEMT-P
Princeton, Iowa

Rekeisha Watson-Love, MBA, NRP, IC
Milwaukee, Wisconsin

Thomas Worthington, MEd, EMT-P, EMSIC
Schoolcraft College, Department of Emergency Medical Technology
Livonia, Michigan

Photoshoot Acknowledgments

We would like to thank the following people and institutions for their collaboration on the photoshoots for this project. Their assistance is greatly appreciated.

Rhonda J. Hunt
Albany State University, Darton College of Health Professions
Albany, Georgia

John Luker
Baptist Health La Grange/ Oldham County EMS
La Grange, Kentucky

Kevin Mahoney
Aura Prep, Rescue Training International
Elmont, New York

Stephen J. Rahm
Centre for Health Sciences
Bulverde, Texas

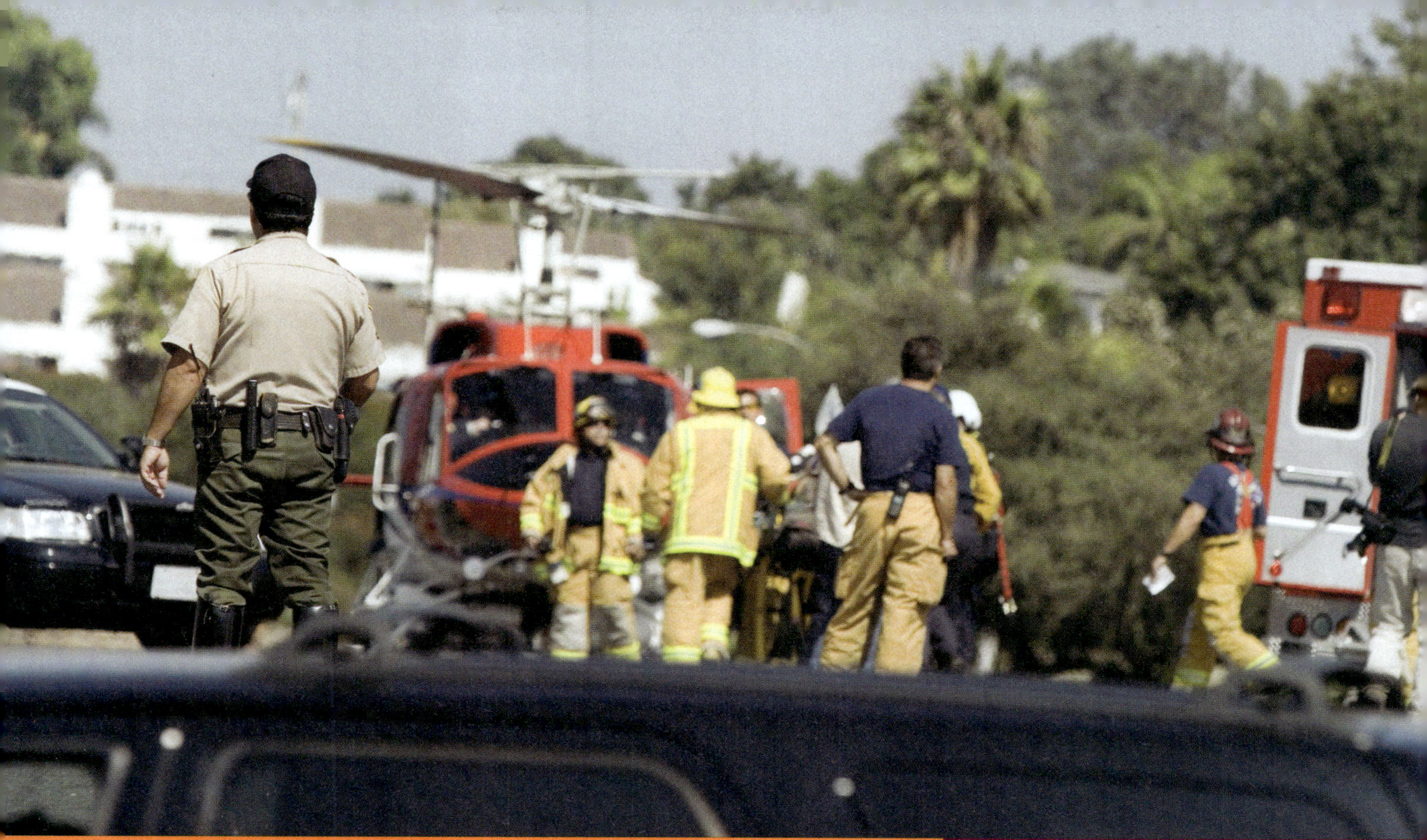

SECTION

1

Preparatory

1 EMS Systems and Public Health
2 Workforce Safety and Wellness
3 Medical, Legal, and Ethical Issues
4 Communications and Documentation
5 Medical Terminology
6 The Human Body
7 Life Span Development
8 Lifting and Moving Patients
9 The Team Approach to Health Care

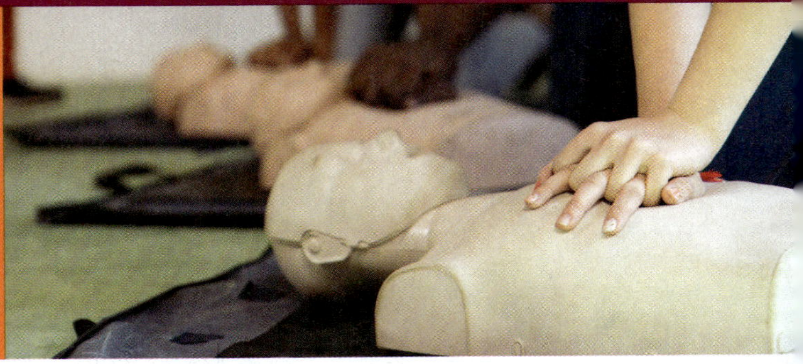

Chapter 1

EMS Systems and Public Health

NATIONAL EMS EDUCATION STANDARD COMPETENCIES

Preparatory

Applies knowledge of the emergency medical services (EMS) system, safety/well-being of the emergency medical technician (EMT), and medical/legal and ethical issues to the provision of emergency care.

EMS Systems

- EMS systems (pp 13–18)
- Roles, responsibilities, and professionalism of EMS personnel (pp 11–13)
- Quality improvement vs. quality assurance (pp 16–18)
- Role of medical oversight (p 16)
- Culture of safety/patient safety (Chapter 9, *The Team Approach to Health Care*)
- Continuum of care (Chapter 9, *The Team Approach to Health Care*)
- History of EMS (pp 3–5)
- Systems of care (eg, stroke, trauma, pediatrics) (Chapter 17, *Cardiovascular Emergencies*; Chapter 24, *Trauma Overview*)
- Mobile integrated healthcare/community paramedicine (MIH/CP) and other EMS-related specialty roles (pp 18–20)

Research

- Impact of research on EMT care (p 18)
- Data collection (pp 16–18)
- Evidence-based decision making (p 18)

Public Health

Applies knowledge of the principles of public health epidemiology including public health emergencies, public health monitoring, health promotion, and illness and injury prevention.

Public Health Overview

- EMS roles in public health (pp 18–20)
- Infection prevention and control (Chapter 2, *Workforce Safety and Wellness*)
- Human trafficking (Chapter 35, *Patients With Special Challenges*)
- EMS electronic health record (EHR) reporting and data collection (p 16)
- Governmental/nongovernmental roles and resources (pp 14–18)
- Public health mission and goals (p 18)
- Social, geographic, economic, and demographic determinants of health (pp 18–19)
- Patient and community education (pp 19–20)
- Injury prevention and wellness (Chapter 2, *Workforce Safety and Wellness*)
- Unique pediatric, geriatric, and special population public health concerns (Chapter 15, *Medical Overview*; Chapter 35, *Patients With Special Challenges*)
- Screenings and vaccinations/immunizations (Chapter 2, *Workforce Safety and Wellness*)

KNOWLEDGE OBJECTIVES

1. Define emergency medical services (EMS) systems. (p 3)
2. Discuss the historical background of the development of the EMS system. (pp 3–5)
3. Name the four national levels of EMS training and certification. (pp 6–7)
4. Describe the four national levels of EMS certification in terms of sets of knowledge, skills, and abilities needed for each. (pp 6–7)
5. Explain the differences between EMS training, certification, licensure, and credentialing. (pp 8–11)
6. Describe the roles and responsibilities of the EMT. (pp 11–12)
7. Describe the attributes an EMT is expected to possess. (pp 11–13)
8. Discuss the guiding principles of EMS Agenda 2050. (p 14)
9. Discuss the importance of documentation for research and quality improvement. (p 16–18)
10. Explain how quality assurance differs from quality improvement. (p 16)
11. Describe the role of medical oversight in an EMS system. (p 16)
12. Discuss social drivers of health and their influence on a person's health. (p 18–19)
13. Characterize the EMT's role in disease and injury prevention, public education, and health surveillance in the community. (pp 18–20)
14. Define mobile integrated health care. (p 19)

SKILLS OBJECTIVES

There are no skills objectives for this chapter.

Introduction

You are about to enter an exciting field. As an **emergency medical technician (EMT)**, you will be a critical part of the **emergency medical services (EMS)** system. Traditionally, EMS has been defined as a team of health care professionals who provide emergency care and transportation for the sick and injured; however, EMS is evolving into a versatile mobile community health resource that is an essential part of a larger system to prevent and treat not only acute illness and injury, but also chronic ailments.

While the chapters that follow in this text will prepare you with the knowledge to evaluate and treat patients who are experiencing a wide variety of medical and traumatic conditions, you already possess the most important characteristics to be successful in EMS: a natural liking for people and a natural inclination to tell the truth. Good EMS clinicians are good caregivers who respect people, what they worry about, what hurts them, and what scares them. Speaking of what scares them, fear is an important element of every emergency. Learning to address a patient's fear can greatly improve communication and ultimately the care you provide. Not every call for care will involve a life-threatening emergency. As the great EMS educator Thom Dick explains in his book *People Care*, it is important to understand that emergencies are defined by their owners and not their responders. It is critical that you remember to always serve as a caregiver, not a judge. The compassion, kindness, gentleness, professionalism, and skill you bring will have a tremendously positive effect on each patient you encounter.

Words of Wisdom

You are embarking on a special career in EMS. As educator Thom Dick wrote, "You're going to be there when a lot of people are born, and when a lot of people die. In most every culture, such moments are regarded as sacred and private, made special by a divine presence. No one on Earth would be welcomed, but you are personally invited. What an honor that is."[1]

Purpose and History of EMS

As an EMT, you will join a long tradition of people who provide emergency medical care to their fellow human beings. EMS as we know it today had its origins in 1966 with the publication of *Accidental Death and Disability: The Neglected Disease of Modern Society*.[2] This report, prepared jointly by the Committees on Trauma and Shock of the National Academy of Sciences/National Research Council, shed light on an alarmingly high number of preventable deaths, particularly on US roadways as a result of motor vehicle collisions. The report also revealed to the public and Congress the serious inadequacy of prehospital emergency care and transport, citing serious deficiencies in prehospital training, and recommended the development of national standard courses and texts. In short order, Congress passed a series of legislation that led to the creation of what is now the National Highway Traffic Safety Administration (NHTSA), under the US Department of Transportation (DOT). Primarily viewed by the government as an emergency transportation service, EMS was assigned to the DOT, where the federal Office of EMS resides today.

Because EMS operations affect so many aspects of government, in 2005 Congress established the Federal Interagency Committee on Emergency Medical Services (FICEMS). The goal of FICEMS is to promote coordination between EMS and the Department of Defense, Department of Health and Human Services, Department of Homeland Security, Federal Communications Commission, and Department of Transportation.[3] Two years later, the National EMS Advisory Council (NEMSAC) was formed as a means for representatives from citizens' groups and from the EMS community to advise the NHTSA and the FICEMS on policy issues.[4]

Special Populations

EMS INITIATIVES TO IMPROVE PEDIATRIC CARE IN EMS

In 1984, Congress established the Emergency Medical Services for Children (EMSC) program. The goal of the EMSC is to improve the care of children and to reduce pediatric death and disability related to illness or injury. States are funded to develop programs and initiatives to support the EMSC goals. The EMSC develops education programs, quality and process improvements, and policy recommendations; it also funds research related to the emergency care of children.[5]

Freedom House Ambulance

As recently as the 1960s and early 1970s, emergency ambulance services and prehospital care varied widely across the United States. In many areas, the only emergency care and ambulance service was provided by the local funeral home using a hearse that could be converted to carry a cot and serve as an ambulance. In other places, police would rush people to the hospital in the back of a van, or a fire department may have used a station wagon that carried a cot and a first aid kit. In most cases, these vehicles were staffed with a driver and an attendant with limited basic first aid training.

Freedom House Ambulance Service was a pioneering project that established the first paramedic program in the United States in 1967 (**FIGURE 1-1**). This agency began as an improbable experiment after Phil Hallen, president of the Maurice Falk Medical Fund, met with Peter Safar, the renowned anesthesiologist often referred to as the "Father of CPR." Their goal was to improve care for residents of the Hill District, a predominantly African American neighborhood in Pittsburgh. They would achieve this goal by doing what was unthinkable at the time; they would train Black men from the Hill community to do what only physicians had done inside of hospitals until that point. Freedom House Paramedic John Moon was the first nonphysician to perform an endotracheal intubation in the field. These crews paved the way for many other prehospital medical developments, including electrocardiogram transmission and intravenous naloxone administration for patients experiencing opioid overdoses.

Freedom House Ambulance would not only save countless lives in Pittsburgh's most underserved

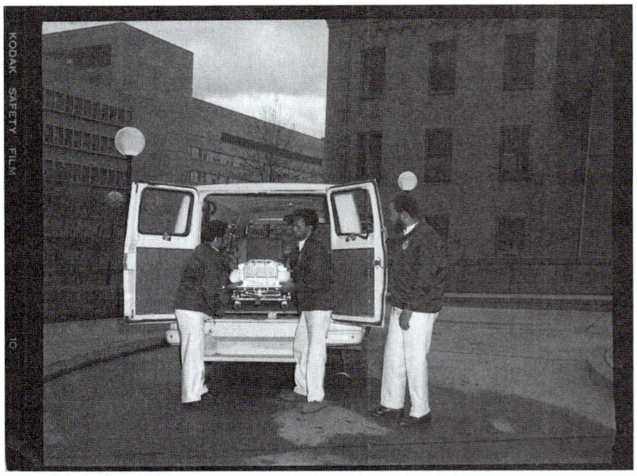

FIGURE 1-1 Freedom House EMTs in Pittsburgh, Pennsylvania, in 1970.

neighborhoods but would also serve as the blueprint for the nation's first paramedic textbook and the first set of national paramedic standards. Dr. Nancy Caroline, the first medical director of Freedom House Ambulance, developed the revolutionary first paramedic curriculum and authored the first paramedic textbook. In 1974, Freedom House Ambulance's training regimen was chosen by the DOT to serve as the national model for standardized paramedic training, fortifying a legacy for generations of EMS clinicians to come.

Standardization of EMS Practice and Education

In response to the wide variability in prehospital care and training, the National Registry of EMTs was established in 1970 to ensure uniform national practice standards and provide an independent certification examination process. In 1971, the DOT developed and published the first National Standard Curriculum (NSC) to serve as the guideline for EMT training. To support the EMT course, in 1971 the American Academy of Orthopaedic Surgeons published the first EMT textbook, *Emergency Care and Transportation of the Sick and Injured*, often called the Orange Book because of the cover's color. Through the 1970s, following the recommended training guidelines, each state developed the necessary legislation, and the EMS system expanded throughout the United States. During the same period, emergency medicine became a recognized medical specialty, and the fully staffed emergency departments (EDs) that we know today became the accepted standard of care.

In the late 1970s, the DOT developed the NSC for paramedic-level education and training. The NSC was prescriptive in terms of course planning and structure, objectives, detailed lesson plans, specific content material, and suggested hours of instruction. The NSC was expanded to additional EMS clinician levels and was revised several times over the years, until the 1996 EMS Agenda for the Future proposed a new vision for EMS education, based

Words of Wisdom

The National Highway Traffic Safety Administration (NHTSA) recognized the need for a symbol that would represent EMS as a critical public service and created the *Star of Life*. NHTSA holds priority rights to the use of this registered certification mark.

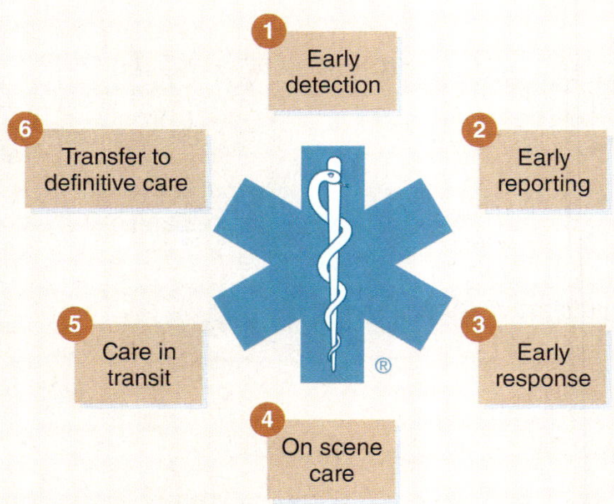

Adapted from the personal Medical Identification Symbol of the American Medical Association.

Adapted from the personal Medical Identification Symbol of the American Medical Association, each bar on the Star of Life represents one of six essential EMS functions:

1. Detection
2. Reporting
3. Response
4. On-scene care
5. Care in transit
6. Transfer to definitive care

The serpent and staff in the symbol portray the staff of Asclepius, an ancient Greek physician deified as the god of medicine. Overall, the staff represents medicine and healing, with the skin-shedding serpent indicating renewal.

The Star of Life has become synonymous with emergency medical care around the globe. This symbol serves as a means of identification on ambulances, emergency medical equipment, patches or apparel worn by EMS clinicians, and materials such as books, pamphlets, manuals, reports, and publications that either have a direct application to EMS or were generated by an EMS organization. It also appears on road maps and highway signs indicating the location of or access to qualified emergency medical care.

Adapted from US National Highway Traffic Safety Administration. http://www.ems.gov

on a systems approach and competency-based outcomes. This new vision led to the development of the National EMS Education Standards. The knowledge and skills you will learn in this course are part of this national movement toward a patient-centered EMS system that safely and efficiently meets the needs of an ever-changing health care industry.

National Levels of EMS Training

The EMT level of care is one of four nationally recognized out-of-hospital EMS clinician levels; the other three levels are **emergency medical responder (EMR)**, **advanced emergency medical technician (AEMT)**, and **paramedic**. The **National EMS Scope of Practice Model** describes the minimum expected entry-level practice expectations for each of the four EMS clinician levels.[6] **TABLE 1-1** shows some examples from this model. This model provides guidance for states in developing their legislation, rules, and regulations; however, each state maintains the authority to regulate EMS and determine the scope of practice of state-licensed EMS clinicians.

Aligned with the National EMS Scope of Practice Model, the **National EMS Education Standards** outline the knowledge and competencies that students should acquire to perform at entry level in each of these four EMS roles.[7]

TABLE 1-1 Examples From the Interpretive Guidelines: National EMS Scope of Practice Model

Note:
- An EMT can provide all of the skills listed in the EMR level.
- An AEMT can provide all of the skills listed in the EMR and EMT levels.
- A paramedic can provide all of the skills listed in the EMR, EMT, and AEMT levels.

EMR	EMT	AEMT	Paramedic
Examples of Airway/Ventilation/Oxygenation Skills			
Oral airway	Nasal airway	Supraglottic airway	Endotracheal intubation
Bag-mask device	CPAP	Tracheobronchial suctioning	Cricothyrotomy
Upper airway suctioning	Pulse oximetry	$ETCO_2$ monitoring	Airway obstruction removal by direct laryngoscopy
Nasal cannula	Oxygen humidifiers		High-flow nasal cannula
Examples of Cardiovascular/Circulation Skills			
Manual CPR	Mechanical CPR		Cardioversion, electrical
Automatic/semiautomatic defibrillation (AED use)	Acquisition and transmission of 12-lead ECG		Manual defibrillation Interpretation of 12-lead ECG
Examples of Medication Administration Routes			
Intramuscular auto-injector	Oral	Subcutaneous	Transdermal
Intranasal, premeasured	Sublingual	Intravenous	Rectal

Abbreviations: AED, automated external defibrillation; CPAP, continuous positive airway pressure; CPR, cardiopulmonary resuscitation; ECG, electrocardiogram; $ETCO_2$, end-tidal carbon dioxide

Note: The 2019 National EMS Scope of Practice Model serves as a foundation for states to build their own model. It is intended to illustrate the operation of each level of EMS clinician and the progression from one level to another. It is not inclusive of every skill a state may allow.

EMS courses are competency-based, meaning they are designed to help students reach a level at which they can apply their knowledge, skills, and abilities (KSAs) in meeting the minimum performance requirements of each certification level. The time to achieve this competence varies depending on factors such as prior student experience, program resources, and EMS educators' teaching methods. Thus, the total hours required to complete each level of the program vary and may be determined by state law.

Emergency Medical Responder

EMRs often arrive on scene before the EMTs and ambulance, bridging a critical gap between the onset of the emergency and the arrival of higher-level medical resources. EMR training provides the skills necessary to initiate immediate care, call for an ambulance if one has not already been called, and work with the EMTs and other EMS clinicians on their arrival. EMRs frequently have additional roles such as law enforcement officers, firefighters, park rangers, ski patrollers, or other organized rescuers (**FIGURE 1-2**).

Emergency Medical Technician

Although not always first to arrive, EMTs are expected to quickly assess the patient, provide immediate stabilizing measures, and request additional resources if needed. An EMT has additional depth and breadth of training in basic emergency care and transportation of sick and injured patients. EMT courses provide the essential knowledge and skills required to provide basic emergency care in the field. EMTs are often partnered with EMS clinicians trained at higher levels as part of an ambulance crew. However, depending on patient needs or system resources, EMTs are sometimes the highest level of out-of-hospital care a patient will encounter. EMTs may serve in a variety of roles beyond staffing an ambulance, including as members of a patient care team in a hospital or health care facility, or in a community setting providing home visits to help manage a patient's care and safety.

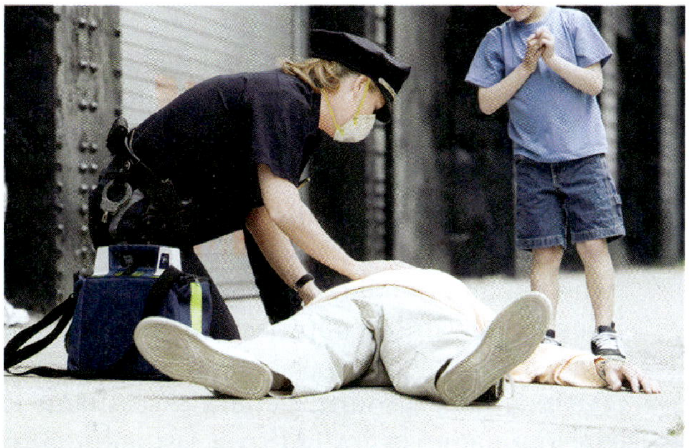

FIGURE 1-2 Emergency medical responders, such as law enforcement officers, are trained to provide immediate basic life support until emergency medical technicians arrive on the scene.

Advanced Emergency Medical Technician

An AEMT has additional preparation beyond the EMT level that includes training and education in specific aspects of **advanced life support (ALS)**, such as intravenous therapy, use of advanced airway adjuncts, and administration of certain emergency medications. The AEMT course is designed to add knowledge and skills in specific aspects of ALS to clinicians who have been trained and have experience in providing emergency care as EMTs. The purpose of this level of EMS clinician is to deliver an expanded range of skills beyond the EMT level. In some parts of the United States, the availability of paramedics is limited. AEMTs help to fill the gap by providing limited ALS care in regions where paramedics are not available.

Paramedic

The paramedic completes an extensive course of education and training that focuses on **basic life support (BLS)** and ALS assessments and treatments (**FIGURE 1-3**). This course is often divided between classroom and internship training. Increasingly, this training is offered within the context of an associate's degree or bachelor's degree college program. Paramedics obtain and interpret diagnostic findings to initiate advanced treatments to include invasive airway management, medication administration, and manual defibrillation. Paramedics may also work in roles outside of traditional emergency ambulance response, such as in community-based settings where they monitor the needs of disproportionately affected groups and work to prevent negative outcomes.

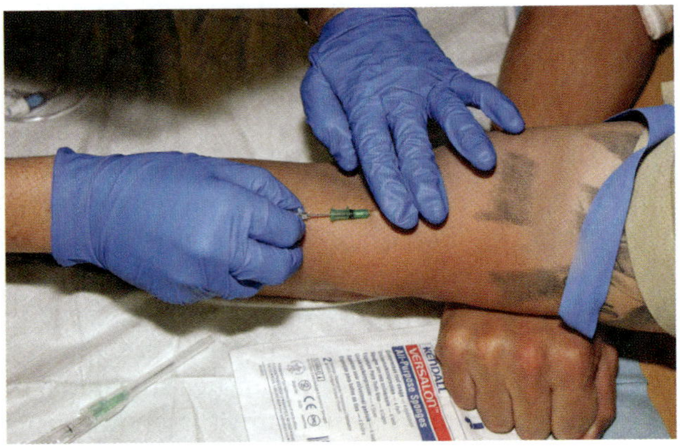

FIGURE 1-3 Paramedic education and training cover a wide range of advanced life support skills.

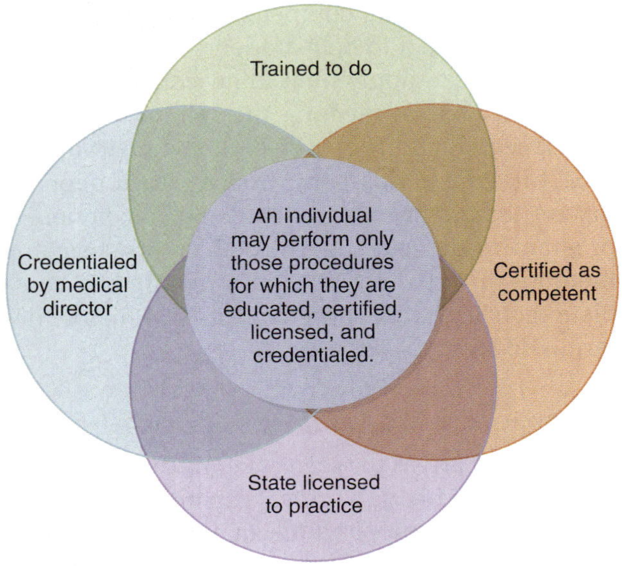

FIGURE 1-4 The relationship among emergency medical services education, certification, licensure, and credentialing.

Modified from The National EMS Scope of Practice Model. National Highway Traffic Safety Administration. 2007. https://one.nhtsa.gov/people/injury/ems/EMSScope.pdf.

Becoming an EMT

This course is the initial step in acquiring the critical KSAs to serve as an EMT. In addition to completing an EMT initial education program, a candidate must successfully complete certification, licensure, and credentialing processes to work as an EMT (**FIGURE 1-4**).

Education and Training

This text covers the practices and skills identified in the National EMS Education Standards. It also covers the information needed for EMTs to perform the skills outlined in the National EMS Scope of Practice Model. To supplement the required core content, this text includes additional information to help you understand and apply the knowledge and skills included in the EMT course. The goal is to apply the KSAs identified in this text to work in the field as an effective EMS clinician. To achieve this goal, it is essential that you complete the assigned reading. Simply attending class will not adequately prepare you to demonstrate the KSAs needed to complete each part of the course. Each class builds your ability to apply previous information. It is vital that you complete the readings and assignments to help you understand subsequent lessons and, ultimately, to be able to apply those lessons in real-world emergency situations. This approach is pivotal to your success in this course.

In class, your instructor will review the key parts of the reading assignment and clarify and expand on them. Further, your instructor will conduct activities to help you apply your new knowledge and deepen your understanding of it. Unless you carefully read the assignment and take notes before coming to class, you will not fully understand or benefit from the classroom presentations and discussions. Creating your own tools, such as flashcards, study questions, scenarios, and outlines, may help you retain important information (**TABLE 1-2**).

Some of the subjects discussed in this text include the following:

- **Scene size-up.** Scene size-up involves getting an overview of the situation at hand and an awareness of the presence and level of safety threats. During scene size-up, you must gain a big-picture perspective of the call, determine whether it is safe to proceed, determine whether additional resources are needed, and identify the initial approach to mitigate the emergency.
- **Patient assessment.** Patient assessment is the foundation of any EMS call. Using your understanding of anatomy, physiology, and the pathophysiology of diseases, you will perform effective assessment techniques to determine what might be wrong with your patient and identify life threats.

TABLE 1-2 Study Tips

- Determine the time of day when you can most effectively study.
- Make, and stick to, a study schedule that will allow you to master the information in small, digestible chunks.
- Find a place that is free from distractions and interruptions.
- Do not remain on call for work, family, or other obligations during study time.
- Turn off your devices so you are not taken out of the study zone by unnecessary alerts.
- Find a study group or partner. Work to help each other, and keep each other accountable.
- Before you begin, specify your study objectives. If necessary, write down specific questions you have about the material.
- Before reading an entire section, give it a quick overview to understand what you will be studying and how it will be presented.
- Study the most challenging information first, while you still have the most mental energy and drive.
- Group topics into manageable chunks to study.
- Think about each key learning point in terms of how you would explain it clearly to someone who was not in the class.
- Focus on learning and applying the information, not on examination grades.
- Consider making simple flowcharts or diagrams to better understand disease processes, assessment and care priorities, and decision making.
- Take advantage of additional learning tools, such as quizzes, simulations, or case studies, that allow you to test your knowledge and identify gaps in your learning.

- **Treatment.** As an EMT, you will identify the need for and prioritize patient care. In some cases, you may work to improve patient oxygenation and ventilation. In others, you may control bleeding or assist patients during childbirth. In addition to hands-on skills, you will learn how to treat patients who are in emotional crisis and how to calm patients to relieve some of their anxiety or fear.
- **Transport.** Most patients need to be transported to a facility. This could mean a hospital, clinic, or other medical care facility. Choosing the facility with the appropriate resources for a patient can have an important effect on their outcome. You will learn how to safely transport patients with a wide variety of illnesses and injuries.
- **EMS as a career.** Most of you are taking this course because you want to help people. To ensure all EMS clinicians have a long, healthy career, it is important for you to learn how to take care of yourself. You will learn about job stressors and successful ways to cope with them.

Certification

Following completion of an EMT education and training course, the next step is **certification**. This process verifies that a clinician meets the minimum required KSA competencies for safe and effective emergency operations and patient care. Certification examinations often use a variety of testing instruments, such as multiple-choice questions, multiple-select questions, drag-and-drop items, skills stations, and simulated emergency calls. These examinations are typically conducted or regulated by a state or military agency or by the National Registry of EMTs (often referred to as the NREMT or National Registry). The National Registry is a nongovernmental, not-for-profit organization whose mission is to support the EMS profession through partnerships, research, and lifelong assessment of clinical competence. Almost all states require National Registry certification for candidates to be eligible for a license to practice.

One of the functions of the National EMS Scope of Practice Model is to create stable foundations on which each level of EMS clinician is grounded. The net effect is to encourage a more consistent definition of "what is an EMT" so clinicians can move more freely about the country. National Registry certification often facilitates licensure in other states. The Interstate Commission for EMS Personnel Practice aims to increase the ability of EMS clinicians to practice in other states through the Recognition of EMS Personnel Licensure Interstate CompAct (REPLICA). REPLICA is not a form of EMS licensure reciprocity. It simply extends a privilege for EMS personnel from member states to practice on a short-term or intermittent basis under approved circumstances in other member states.

In 2020, the National Registry launched the National EMS-ID number system. An EMS-ID is a

12-digit identification number issued at no charge to all EMS professionals, from EMR to paramedic, and to students entering the profession. The number is automatically generated by the National Registry when a person creates an account. For EMS clinicians with an existing account, an EMS-ID is retroactively created. Unlike the certification number issued by the National Registry (Registry Number), EMS-IDs do not change as the person's certification level changes. Thus, the various certification numbers that individuals may obtain in their career are all tied back to the single EMS-ID.

Although not all states use the National Registry certification process, other EMS certification examinations may also be informed by the National Registry's EMS Practice Analysis. Approximately every 5 years, the National Registry surveys EMS clinicians of all levels from across the United States to understand the current real-world practice of out-of-hospital emergency care and to help create a blueprint for valid certification examinations. In effect, the Practice Analysis attempts to answer the question, "What is most important for EMS clinicians to know and be able to do to deliver safe and effective care?" In 2019, the Practice Analysis also used data from the **National EMS Information System (NEMSIS)** to understand the types of calls and interventions EMS personnel in the United States encounter in actual practice. From this information, the current Practice Analysis determines the certification test plan for each level of EMS clinician. The test plan lays out an approximate percentage of questions on each topic that students will encounter on National Registry certification examinations.

Licensure

After successfully completing the certification process, an EMS clinician is typically eligible for **licensure**, which is the legal authority to practice in their state. The standards for prehospital emergency care and the people who provide it are governed by the laws of each state. These laws are typically regulated by an office of EMS operating under the state's department of health. Although some states refer to this phase as certification, for the purposes of this text, the term *licensure* will be used. Obtaining licensure in a state does not grant an EMT an unrestricted right to practice.

To be licensed and function as an EMT, you must meet certain requirements. The specific requirements differ from state to state. Ask your instructor or your state EMS office about the requirements in your state. Generally, the criteria to be licensed and employed as an EMT include the following:

- High school diploma or equivalent
- Proof of immunization against certain communicable diseases
- Successful completion of a background check and drug screening
- Valid driver's license
- Successful completion of a recognized health care provider BLS/cardiopulmonary resuscitation (CPR) course
- Successful completion of a state-approved EMT course
- Successful completion of a state-recognized written certification examination (usually National Registry)
- Compliance with other state, local, and employer provisions

The **Americans With Disabilities Act (ADA)** of 1990 protects people who have a disability from being denied access to programs and services that are provided by state or local governments and prohibits employers from failing to provide full and equal employment to those with a disability. In addition, Title I of the ADA protects EMTs with disabilities seeking gainful employment under many circumstances. Employers with a certain number of employees are required to adjust processes so that a candidate with a disability can be considered for the position, and when possible, modify the work environment or how the job is normally performed. This allows EMTs who can perform the functional job skills with reasonable accommodations the opportunity to pursue a career in EMS.

One of the primary responsibilities of each state is to ensure the safety of its residents. As such, states have requirements prohibiting people with certain legal infractions from becoming EMS clinicians. The specific legal exclusions, either misdemeanors and/or felonies, are created on a state-by-state basis. Contact your state EMS office for more information.

Credentialing

The next phase toward working as an EMT is **credentialing**. Credentialing is the determination that authorizes a clinician to perform a skill or role. Credentialing may be a local or regional process, and it is typically directed and overseen by a physician medical director. In some cases, EMTs may be specifically credentialed to perform either fewer or additional techniques in their area or to work in certain types of care systems. Finally, the local medical director should provide regular oversight and support to EMS personnel. For example, the medications that will be carried on an ambulance or the locations where patients are transported are the day-to-day operational concerns on which the medical director, and often state, regional, or local EMS advisory boards, will have direct input.

Roles and Responsibilities of the EMT

As an EMT, you will often be the first health care professional to assess and treat the patient; as such, you have certain roles and responsibilities (**TABLE 1-3**) and are expected to possess certain attributes (**TABLE 1-4**). The guiding principle for EMS personnel is "everything you do needs to be done with the patient in mind." What is in the best interest of the patient? This approach is referred to as being a patient advocate.

Street Smarts

A patient may experience only once what you may witness hundreds of times. Understand and be empathetic to the patient's anxiety and fear. Although some calls may not appear to be an emergency to you, they are considered an emergency by your patients and their family members. Treat these individuals with respect. Your patients and their family members will always remember how you acted when you were with them.

Professional Attributes

As an EMT, whether you are paid or a volunteer, you are a health care professional. Part of your responsibility is to make sure patient care is given a high priority without endangering your own safety

TABLE 1-3 Roles and Responsibilities of the EMT

- Keep vehicles and equipment ready for an emergency.
- Ensure the safety of yourself, your partner, the patient, and bystanders.
- Operate the emergency vehicle in a safe manner.
- Be an on-scene leader.
- Evaluate the scene.
- Call for additional resources as needed.
- Gain patient access.
- Perform a thorough patient assessment.
- Provide emergency medical care to the patient.
- Give emotional support to the patient, the patient's family, and other responders.
- Engage in shared decision-making regarding the best destination or resource for the patient's next phase of care.
- Maintain continuity of care by working with other medical professionals.
- Resolve emergency incidents.
- Uphold medical and legal standards.
- Ensure and protect patient privacy.
- Give administrative support.
- Constantly continue your professional development.
- Cultivate and sustain community relations.
- Give back to the profession.
- Maintain continued competence.

YOU are the EMT

After successfully obtaining National EMT Certification and a state EMT license, you have just been hired as an EMT. As part of the credentialing process at your EMS agency, you are on duty with your Field Training Officer, who is a paramedic, and an AEMT partner. You are in the process of checking the ambulance when you are dispatched to a report of a 48-year-old woman with back pain. You and your crew proceed to the scene, approximately 6 miles away.

1. How does your training as an EMT compare to that of other EMS clinician certification/licensure levels?
2. How does your EMT certification differ from your state EMT license?

TABLE 1-4 Professional Attributes of EMTs

Attribute	Description
Integrity	Consistent adherence to a code of honest behavior
Empathy	Aware of and thoughtful toward the needs of others
Self-motivation	Ability to discover problems and solve them without direction
Appearance and hygiene	Ability to project a sense of trust, professionalism, knowledge, and compassion
Self-confidence	A state of being, in which you know what you know ***and*** know what you do not know; able to ask for help
Time management	Ability to perform or delegate multiple tasks, ensuring efficiency and safety
Communications	Ability to understand others and have them understand you
Teamwork and diplomacy	Ability to work with others and to know your place within a team; ability to communicate while giving respect to the listener
Respect	Regard for the importance of others; belief that others are more important than self
Patient advocacy	Ability to keep the patient's needs at the center of care
Careful delivery of care	Ability to attend to detail and ensure patient care is provided as safely as possible

or the safety of others. Professionalism extends beyond appearance and the activities you perform on a daily basis. As a professional, you have a responsibility to your partner, colleagues, patients, and profession to maintain a current level of knowledge. Your attitude and behavior must reflect that you are knowledgeable and sincerely dedicated to serving anyone who is injured or in an acute medical emergency.

A professional and compassionate manner helps to build confidence and ease the patient's anxiety (**FIGURE 1-5**). You are expected to perform under pressure with composure and self-confidence. Patients and families who are under stress need to be treated with understanding, respect, and compassion.

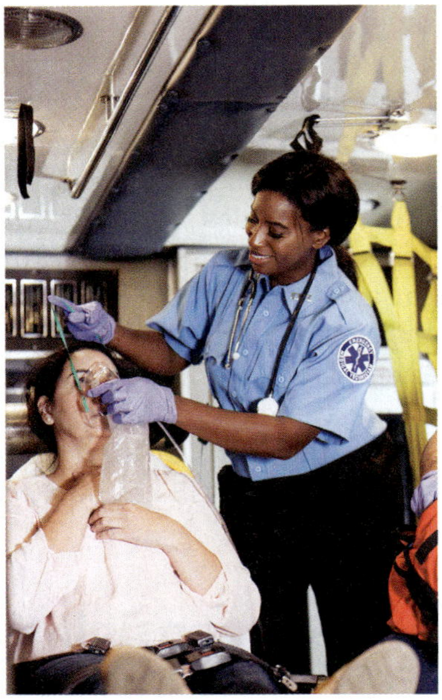

FIGURE 1-5 A professional and compassionate demeanor help build confidence and ease patient anxiety.

Most patients will treat you with respect and appreciation, but on the worst days of their lives, some will not. Some patients are uncooperative, demanding, unpleasant, ungrateful, and verbally abusive. You must be nonjudgmental and overcome your instincts to react poorly to such behavior. Remember, when people are hurt, ill, under stress, frightened, despondent, under the influence of alcohol or drugs, or feeling threatened, they will often react with inappropriate behavior, even toward those who are trying to help and care for them. All patients, regardless of their attitude, are entitled to compassion, respect, and the best care that you can provide.

Most people in this country can obtain proper routine medical care when they are ill and are supported by relatives and friends who will help to take care of them. However, when you are called to a home for a medical problem that is clearly not an emergency, remember that for some patients, calling an ambulance and being transported to the ED is the only way for them to obtain medical care.

In other cases, the reason a person says they called 9-1-1 is not the true reason. Consider a widow who just lost her husband of more than 50 years and is terrified to spend her first night alone, but calls 9-1-1 for chronic back pain. Performing a good assessment can help you understand the true reason you were called and help you do your best to address the patient's needs.

As a new EMT, you will be given a lot of advice and training from the more experienced EMTs with whom you serve. Some may voice a callous disregard for some types of patients. Do not be influenced by the unprofessional attitude of these clinicians, regardless of how experienced or skilled they appear.

As a health care professional and an extension of physician care, you are bound by patient confidentiality. You should not discuss your findings or any disclosures made by the patient with anyone but those who are treating the patient or in limited situations, as required by law, the police, or other social agencies. When discussing a call with others, you should be careful to avoid revealing any information that might disclose the name or identity of patients you have treated. Be careful not to gossip about calls and patients with others, even in your own home. Do not post on social media about calls and patients. Considerations relating to patient privacy, including requirements of the Health Insurance Portability and Accountability Act (HIPAA), are discussed further in Chapter 3, *Medical, Legal, and Ethical Issues.*

Overview of the EMS System

As an EMT, you will be joining a larger system. Operating at the intersection of health care, public health, emergency management, and public safety, EMS is uniquely integrated with other services to enhance community health and safety (**FIGURE 1-6**).

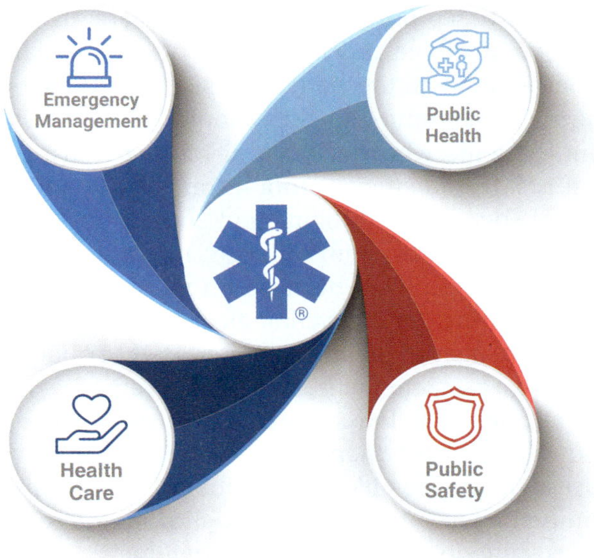

FIGURE 1-6 EMS is part of a larger system that includes health care, public health, emergency management, and public safety.

Courtesy of National Highway Traffic Safety Administration/U.S. Department of Transportation.

YOU are the EMT

You arrive at the scene, ensure it is safe to enter, and make contact with the patient, a 48-year-old woman. She is sitting on her couch, does not appear to be in obvious distress, and states her pain has been intermittent for about a month. She tells you and your crew that it is uncomfortable for her to walk. You assess the patient as your partner prepares to take her vital signs.

Recording Time: 0 Minutes	
Appearance	Seated on the couch; eyes open and follow EMS crewmembers
Level of consciousness	Conscious and alert
Airway	Open; clear of secretions or foreign bodies
Breathing	Adequate rate and depth
Circulation	Radial pulse, normal rate and rhythm; skin is baseline color, warm, and dry

3. In addition to potential medical emergencies, what else should you consider as you continue to assess this patient?

As the 1996 EMS Agenda for the Future set an aspiration for EMS systems to work toward, the 2019 release of EMS Agenda 2050 created a multidisciplinary national vision for EMS delivery.[8] The goal is to develop a more cohesive and consistent people-centered system across the country. The document features seven key aspects of a people-centered EMS system, as outlined in **TABLE 1-5**.

The vision of EMS Agenda 2050 is that of a people-centered EMS system, one in which people receive comprehensive, quality care in the most comfortable and convenient place. This care is based on sound research focused on producing the right outcomes. In this people-centered system, patients who need it will receive transport that is safe and efficient (not necessarily at a high rate of speed or with lights and siren[9]). Care in a people-centered system will focus not only on lifesaving interventions, but also on reducing physical, emotional, and psychological suffering. Such EMS systems will be an integrated part of a larger health care system focused on proactively preventing injuries and illnesses rather than reactively responding to treat them. EMS clinicians will have access to and be able to contribute to a patient's comprehensive medical record, allowing not only improvements of treatment for individual patients, but also updates in prevention, diagnosis, and treatments as our understanding and technology advance.

TABLE 1-5 EMS Agenda 2050 Components of a People-Centered EMS System

A People-Centered EMS System
1. Comprehensive, quality, convenient care
2. Evidence-based clinical care
3. Safe and efficient transport when needed
4. Holistic care that reduces physical, emotional, and psychological suffering
5. Integration with public health and preventive care
6. Comprehensive and easily accessible patient records
7. Comprehensive expert systems supporting prevention, diagnosis, and treatment

The EMS Agenda 2050 guiding principles include an EMS system design that is as follows[8]:

- Inherently safe and effective, so the entire system from start to finish is designed to minimize exposure to injury, infections, illness, or stress
- Integrated and seamless, where EMS is fully integrated with all other aspects of health care and is engaged with other emergency services and within the communities in which they operate
- Reliable and prepared, ensuring EMS care is delivered consistently and compassionately and is guided by sound research at all times, by all EMS clinicians, at all levels, or from all agencies
- Socially equitable, so that access to care and the quality of care are not determined by a patient's age, socioeconomic status, gender, ethnicity, or where they live
- Sustainable and efficient, meaning systems must be fiscally responsible, providing value to the community with a minimum of waste and a maximum of accountability
- Adaptable and innovative, evolving to meet the changing needs of the people whom they serve by continuously evaluating new tools and techniques, education programs, and system designs

EMS System Components

The structure of EMS systems, from response models to financing, varies across communities. Nevertheless, essential components of any EMS system include legislation and regulation, public access, public BLS and immediate aid, agencies and workforce, medical oversight, information systems and data, quality management, and research.

Legislation and Regulation

The state EMS office is responsible for authorizing, auditing, and regulating all EMS training institutions, courses, instructors, and clinicians within the state. In most states, the state EMS office obtains input from an advisory committee made up of representatives of the services, service medical directors, medical associations, hospitals, training programs, instructors' associations, EMS associations, and the public in that state.

Public Access

In time-sensitive emergencies, easy access to help is essential. In most of the country, an emergency communication center that dispatches fire, police, rescue, and EMS units can be reached by dialing 9-1-1. This communication center is sometimes called a **public safety access point (PSAP)**. At the communication center, trained call takers and dispatchers obtain the necessary information from the caller and, following dispatch protocols, dispatch the ambulance crew and other equipment and responders that may be needed. The EMS dispatch process is described further in Chapter 4, *Communications and Documentation.*

Public BLS and Immediate Aid

With the development of EMS and increased awareness of the need for immediate emergency care, millions of laypeople have been trained in BLS/CPR. In addition to CPR, many people take first aid courses and other task-specific courses such as Stop the Bleed that focus on bleeding control and other simple skills that may be required to provide immediate essential care. These courses are designed to train people so those in the workplace (teachers, coaches, child care providers, and others) can provide the necessary critical care in the minutes before EMTs or other responders arrive at the scene.

One of the most dramatic developments in prehospital emergency care is the increased availability of **automated external defibrillators (AEDs)** deployed in public places for use by untrained members of the general public. These devices, some no larger than a cell phone, detect treatable life-threatening cardiac dysrhythmias (ventricular fibrillation and ventricular tachycardia) and deliver the appropriate electrical shock to the patient without the need for a trained health care operator. Mobile apps are playing an evolving role by allowing laypeople trained in CPR to be alerted of a cardiac arrest in their area and connecting them with the location of the nearest public AED. For example, the PulsePoint AED app allows emergency call takers to locate any registered AED and relay its location to individuals on scene.

Responding Agencies and Workforce

The agencies and personnel who respond to emergencies are a key component of the EMS system. The types of agencies responding and how they respond vary across systems and types of calls. EMS systems depend on a highly trained, sufficiently staffed workforce to meet the community's needs.

YOU are the EMT

Your partner records the patient's vital signs on the patient care report as you ask the patient additional questions regarding her back pain. She tells you her lower back began hurting about a month ago; however, she has never been evaluated by a physician. She tells you that she currently does not have health insurance after losing her job. She tells you that she did not injure her back. She does not report any other symptoms or past medical history.

Recording Time:	4 Minutes
Respirations	16 breaths/min; regular and unlabored
Pulse	88 beats/min; strong and regular
Skin	Baseline color, warm, and dry
Blood pressure	126/66 mm Hg
Oxygen saturation (Spo_2)	99% (on room air)

Your assessment of the patient's back does not reveal any obvious deformities, swelling, or bruising, and her vital signs are stable. The patient requests you take her to the hospital.

4. How is patient care integrated across health systems when a patient is transported to the hospital?

Medical Oversight

Each EMS system has a physician **medical director** who authorizes the EMS clinicians in the service to provide medical care in the field. Although in some systems, the individual EMTs may not regularly encounter their medical director, in virtually all systems, the appropriate care for each injury, condition, or illness encountered in the field is determined by the medical director and is described in a set of written standing orders and protocols. Standing orders are part of protocols, and they designate what the EMT is allowed to do for a specific complaint or condition. Clinicians are not required to consult medical direction before implementing standing orders.

Medical oversight is provided either off-line (indirect) or online (direct), as authorized by the medical director.[8,10,11] Online medical oversight consists of guidance given over the phone or radio directly from the medical director or a designated physician, such as a base station physician at a receiving hospital. Medical oversight is sometimes used synonymously with the term medical direction, or medical direction may specifically refer to the person/agency delegated to perform the role. Off-line medical oversight consists of standing orders, training, and supervision authorized by the medical director. Each EMT must know and follow the protocols developed by the medical director.

Information Systems and Data

Before widespread computer use, patient care was documented by EMS clinicians on paper forms. Now, almost all EMS systems leverage the power of technology to enter patient care information into electronic patient care records (ePCRs). In nearly all states, this information is submitted to the National EMS Database hosted by NEMSIS. Funded by NHTSA, NEMSIS is responsible for developing and maintaining the national EMS data standard. The NEMSIS data standard consists of more than 150 core elements that all ePCR software providers must collect in a uniform manner. Having a core uniform dataset allows local, state, and national stakeholders to more easily and accurately assess EMS system needs and performance.

> **Words of Wisdom**
>
> What you document in your ePCR matters. This information will often be used for quality management and research. How you document also matters. Using the drop-down menus to record assessments and treatments makes it easy for your agency to evaluate system needs and performance, whereas the free-text narrative should be used to provide context that is not otherwise easily captured in the drop-down fields.

Quality Management

EMS systems continuously strive to become safer and more effective while delivering high-quality, evidence-based care. The widespread adoption of ePCRs and increasing availability of user-centered analytic tools have made it much easier to report on large quantities of data. However, more data does not directly translate into improvement. Focusing on measures that matter is a key aspect of improving quality. Formed in 2018, the National EMS Quality Alliance (NEMSQA) was formed to develop evidence-based quality measures for EMS and health care partners. NEMSQA has published a national suite of quality measures with clear definitions using the NEMSIS standard so that agencies can easily compare their performance over time as they work to improve care. These measures include treatment for clinical conditions such as asthma, hypoglycemia, and stroke as well as safety measures for EMS clinicians and the patients and communities they serve.

A robust quality management program is a key component of helping EMS systems continuously become safer and more effective. These programs may be implemented at the state, regional, or local levels. Quality management is an umbrella term that encompasses the distinct processes of **quality assurance (QA)** and **quality improvement (QI)**. The purpose of QA is to monitor compliance against a standard. Thus, QA is a reactive process that identifies problems after they have already occurred. Meanwhile, the goal of QI is to make meaningful improvements in desired outcomes. QI is a proactive approach that involves making changes to a system to improve performance.

There are many frameworks available for QI; however, one of the most popular models used in health care is the Model for Improvement. Published in 1996 and adopted by the Institute for Healthcare

Improvement, the Model for Improvement consists of three fundamental questions linked to Plan-Do-Study-Act cycles for testing changes (**FIGURE 1-7**). This framework involves a high level of collaboration, and your observations and experiences as a frontline clinician are valuable to this work.

A commitment to quality means that an EMS agency should not have a punitive culture where errors are treated by shame and blame. Instead, errors should be treated as learning opportunities. Many agencies have embraced **Just Culture** as an approach to quality management. This approach balances accountability and justice in a system that believes in learning from errors. At the same time, these agencies focus on identifying risks within their system and making design improvements to

Words of Wisdom

The terms *quality assurance* (QA) and *quality improvement* (QI) are often used interchangeably. However, these processes are distinct and have different goals. QA measures care against a predefined standard or benchmark and is inherently reactive, detecting problems after they have occurred. In contrast, QI is a proactive approach that involves making changes to the system to improve performance, preventing problems from happening.

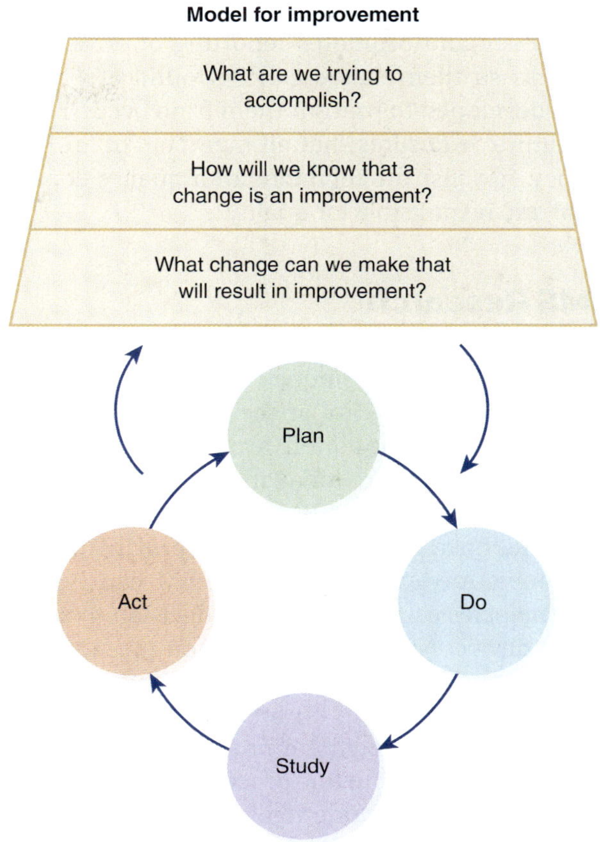

FIGURE 1-7 Model for Improvement

Reproduced with permission from "Model for improvement". Boston, Massachusetts: Institute for Healthcare Improvement; 2020. Available on https://www.ihi.org/resources/how-improve-model-improvement.

YOU are the EMT

The patient is placed onto the stretcher in a position of comfort, using pillows to support her back where she feels discomfort, and loaded into the ambulance. You and your Field Training Officer are in the back with the patient coaching her to relax as your AEMT partner drives to the hospital. You reassess the patient shortly after you begin transport to the hospital.

Recording Time: 12 Minutes	
Level of consciousness	Conscious and alert
Respirations	16 breaths/min; regular and unlabored
Pulse	90 beats/min; strong and regular
Skin	Baseline color, warm, and dry
Blood pressure	120/62 mm Hg
Oxygen saturation (Spo_2)	97% (on room air)

Within a few minutes, the patient tells you her back pain has begun to subside.

5. Why is it important that you document your assessments using the drop-down menus in the ePCR instead of in the free-text narrative?

ensure safety. A Just Culture encourages trust within the agency and promotes reporting of errors and mishaps so their causes can be found and measures developed to prevent them from occurring in the future. It ensures that all members of an EMS agency, not just the members of a quality department, are responsible for quality.

EMS Research

In the early days of EMS, expert opinion guided which tools and techniques EMS clinicians employed. While EMS care at the time was provided with the best information available, virtually all aspects of health care today incorporate **evidence-based medicine (EBM)**. EBM is focused on interventions that have proven useful in improving patient outcomes. An example of how EBM can benefit EMS agencies can be seen in the decision to adopt a new device. New devices are often promoted as important tools for EMS clinicians, and EMS has historically been quick to incorporate new products into practice. Before a product becomes part of the standard of care, the process for new product adoption should include rigorous impartial scientific evaluation of manufacturer claims. In this way, research can help agencies save money by not investing in interventions that may not provide benefit and protects patients from potential harm.

While not every aspect of EMS has enough research to be truly evidence-based, many EMS systems and states now consult the *National Model EMS Clinical Guidelines: Version 3.0* from the National Association of State EMS Officials.[12] These treatment guidelines are based on a review of current research and expert consensus. It is important to stay current on the latest advances in EMS care. The Prehospital Guidelines Consortium is a group of national organizations that have an interest in developing, implementing, and evaluating evidence-based guidelines. The Prehospital Guidelines Consortium is collaborating with the National Registry to identify peer-reviewed research to improve the knowledge of EMS clinicians regarding the most current science every 2 years. Its website provides the current EMS evidence-based guidelines and a reading list of EMS research.[13]

As an EMT, you will be involved in research through gathering data from every call you go on. Additionally, you may be involved in a specific research project. For example, you may be part of a study to determine how much oxygen should be given to patients with shortness of breath. Your job is to carefully follow the research protocol and record all of the pertinent information about these patients. The information gathered is analyzed by researchers to answer these questions and the results are shared with the rest of the EMS community to change patient care practices. Modern medical practice is based on such research.

Words of Wisdom

In the words of author, poet, and activist Maya Angelou, "Do the best you can until you know better. Then, when you know better, do better." The science of EMS is constantly evolving. As an EMT, you will need to continuously update your knowledge and stay up-to-date with the latest research. Remain ready to adapt your practice as the evidence base grows and evolves.

EMS and Public Health

Although television series and movies tend to portray EMS as constantly encountering patients in need of urgent medical attention, time-critical emergencies are actually a small proportion of what EMS does. Less than 10% of calls involve a potentially lifesaving intervention. While EMS plays an important role in these low-frequency, high-criticality encounters for patients with acute illnesses and injuries such as heart attacks, strokes, or major trauma, EMS can have an even larger influence on community health through its roles in public health. **Public health** examines the health needs of entire populations, with the goal of preventing health problems.

Social Drivers of Health and Health Equity

A person's overall health is influenced by many things beyond health care. Collectively, these non–health care factors are referred to as **social drivers of health**. These drivers are sometimes referred to as social "determinants" of health, though the term "drivers" is preferred over determinants, as determinants may imply predetermined or fixed conditions. These factors represent the nonmedical elements that influence health outcomes. The World Health Organization (WHO) defines social drivers of health as "the conditions into which people are born, live, grow, work, and age, and the wider set of forces and systems shaping the conditions of daily life."[14,15] Categories of social drivers of health include economic stability, education access and quality, health care access and quality, neighborhood, and community.

Words of Wisdom

Many people who live in lower income communities have limited access to healthy, fresh food. These areas are commonly referred to as food deserts. A lack of healthy food options negatively affects the overall health of a community.[16]

Closely related to social drivers of health is the concept of **health equity**, defined by the Centers for Disease Control and Prevention as "the state in which everyone has a fair and just opportunity to attain their highest level of health."[17] As out-of-hospital health care clinicians who encounter patients directly in the spaces where they live and work, EMS clinicians are uniquely positioned to understand and address the social factors that affect a patient's health and advance health equity.

Mobile Integrated Health

EMS clinicians have historically been responsible for care before and during transport to an ED. This is changing. **Mobile integrated health care (MIH)**, sometimes referred to as community paramedicine, is a method of delivering health care that uses the prehospital spectrum of care resources. In the MIH model, health care is provided within the community, rather than at a physician's office or hospital. An integrated team of health care professionals, including EMS clinicians, delivers health care services in the community and connects patients with other valuable resources such as social services. An advantage of this model is that it offers access to care for patients within communities who may have limited access to medical resources. In addition to the patient care services an EMS clinician would typically provide, services provided by MIH professionals may include performing health evaluations, completing home safety assessments, monitoring chronic illnesses or conditions, obtaining laboratory samples, administering immunizations, and serving as a patient advocate.

Words of Wisdom

To demonstrate how health inequities can affect medical care, consider the example of an asthmatic child whose parents have called 9-1-1 several times within 1 month. Although it may be tempting to think the parents are neglecting proper care for their child, social drivers of health could play a big role in this case. Both parents work but have no benefits. Because their combined annual income puts them just above the poverty guidelines, their family does not qualify for certain federal programs, including the Children's Medical Health Insurance Program (CHIP), which would ensure their children have a primary care physician.[18] In addition, the only housing they can afford is in an urban area with industrial pollution, which increases their child's risk for respiratory conditions such as infections, irritation, and lung damage. Empathetic care and possible referral to MIH resources may assist this family to manage their child's illness.

Public Health Surveillance

As an EMT, you may also be involved in the surveillance of illnesses and injuries. Information from the patient care reports generated by EMS clinicians can be used to determine if a serious, widespread condition exists. For example, EMS reports can provide statistical information to the local government about motor vehicle collisions. This type of injury surveillance data can be used to determine ways to improve a dangerous intersection, to prevent crashes from ever happening, or to limit the severity of injuries to drivers. EMS data are also often routinely used for surveillance of infectious diseases and opioid overdoses.

Prevention and Education

The primary focus of the public health arm of health care is prevention. Public health is proactive and works to prevent illness and injury. The concept of prevention applies to both the patient and the EMS clinician. Eating right, exercising, and using other stress management techniques can help prevent medical emergencies. It may seem strange, but the goal of education should be to create an environment where the need for EMS is decreased. Collaboration between EMS and public health is key to help reduce morbidity and mortality and promote population health, while preventing illness and injury.

EMS often works with public health agencies on both primary and secondary prevention strategies. **Primary prevention** focuses on strategies that will prevent the event from ever happening. Poliomyelitis (polio) was a devastating disease that caused death and disability for thousands of Americans in the early 1900s. A vaccine was developed to prevent the disease. In the span of one generation, the disease was virtually eliminated. Vaccinations are a good example of primary prevention within public health. In a **secondary prevention** strategy, the event has already happened. The question is, how can we decrease the negative effects of the event? Helmets and seat belts do not prevent the accident from happening, yet they do prevent serious injuries from occurring due to the accident. The next time you drive down a major roadway, take note of the construction of the guardrails. There have been significant changes in guardrail construction over the years as more information has become available on what happens during a vehicle collision.

There are several ways EMTs can contribute to public health prevention efforts. For example, you may engage in harm reduction initiatives by providing take-home naloxone kits or fentanyl testing strips for patients with opioid use disorder. As an EMT, you may be called on to assist with community education, a form of public health outreach. You can become involved in programs that educate the community about pool safety, proper car seat use, or fall prevention for older adults. Many EMS agencies engage communities in events to learn how to perform compression-only CPR, how to help a choking victim, how to identify a stroke, or how to stop serious bleeding (**FIGURE 1-8**). Public education increases public respect for EMS. When people understand what it means to work on an ambulance and provide care to the sick and injured, they are more likely to consider EMS a vital part of the public health care system. Remember, small actions can lead to big differences!

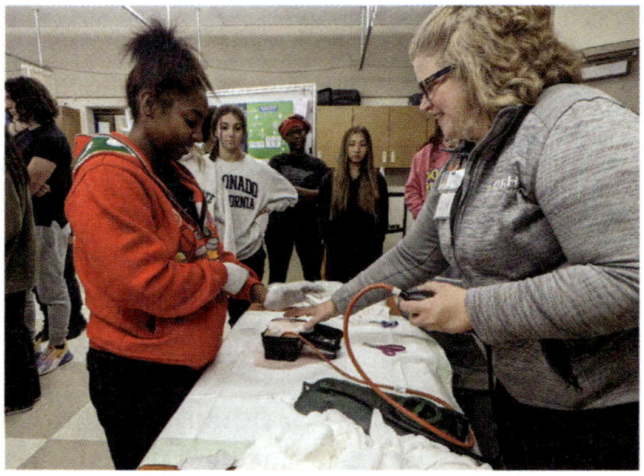

FIGURE 1-8 As an EMT, you can become involved in public health training in your community. For example, the Stop the Bleed campaign teaches bleeding-control techniques to laypersons, such as the high school students shown here.

YOU are the EMT

The patient's condition has remained stable throughout transport. After reassessing her, the paramedic asks you to call in your patient report to the receiving facility. Your estimated time of arrival is 8 minutes.

Recording Time: 19 Minutes	
Level of consciousness	Conscious and alert
Respirations	14 breaths/min; regular and unlabored
Pulse	70 beats/min; strong and regular
Skin	Baseline color, warm, and dry
Blood pressure	118/60 mm Hg
Oxygen saturation (Spo_2)	98% (on room air)

You deliver the patient to the ED in stable condition and give your verbal report to a staff nurse. The patient thanks you and your crew for taking such good care of her. You depart the hospital and return to service. On the way back to the station, the Field Training Officer reviews your documentation and your performance.

6. What is the purpose of reviewing an EMS call?

YOU are the EMT SUMMARY

1. How does your training as an EMT compare to that of other EMS clinician certification/licensure levels?

The National EMS Scope of Practice Model describes four levels of EMS practice, each with a different scope of practice and each requiring different types of education and training. The National EMS Education Standards outline the knowledge and competencies that should be taught to students in each of these four levels of EMS practice. The primary focus of EMR training is to provide immediate lifesaving care to patients while ensuring access to the EMS system. EMT training provides more depth than that of the EMR, including increased knowledge of anatomy, physiology, and pathophysiology; more comprehensive assessment skills; and additional treatment options to stabilize patients initially and provide fundamental care. AEMT training includes additional knowledge and skills, such as invasive techniques that include intravenous access and advanced airways, as well as additional medications that can be administered. Paramedic training includes even more in-depth knowledge, diagnostic skills, and advanced treatment (eg, intravenous drug administration).

2. How does your EMT certification differ from your state EMT license?

Certification is a process that verifies that an EMT meets the minimum entry-level competencies for providing safe and effective care. These examinations are typically conducted by the National Registry of EMTs or a state or military agency. This process does not directly translate to a right to practice as an EMT. Licensure refers to the legal authority to practice within a state. This process is typically regulated by the state's office of EMS. Licensure does not mean an unrestricted right to provide care and some regions or individual agencies have specific processes to credential EMS clinicians to provide care.

3. In addition to potential medical emergencies, what else should you consider as you continue to assess this patient?

Your role is to take care of patients, whether the situation is what you would personally consider an emergency or not. A patient may be experiencing distress beyond the main concern reported. Ask the patient about recent causes of stress. Also consider that not all patients have reliable access to primary care. For some, EMS may be the entry point to further health care. If the patient is transported to the hospital, an EMT will also need to consider which methods to most safely and comfortably move, carry, and transport the patient.

4. How is patient care integrated across health systems when a patient is transported to the hospital?

Delivering excellent and compassionate care and providing transportation to a higher level of care should be the norm. When a patient is transported to a hospital, the responsibility for the assessment and treatment of the patient started at the scene is transferred to a higher level of care. This integration of care can be enhanced by complete and detailed communication to the receiving staff of information from the scene and of history gathered by EMS personnel. This may start before arrival with prenotification when appropriate or by consultation with online medical direction about treatment options. Verbal reports to hospital staff on arrival at the hospital pass along essential details that may help staff to make preliminary decisions about laboratory tests, radiologic studies, or the need for immediate treatment. In addition, your report provides information about the treatment given before arrival and the results of that treatment. Your verbal report can then be followed by a more complete and detailed written report with additional details or explanations.

5. Why is it important that you document your assessments using the drop-down menus in the ePCR instead of in the free-text narrative?

Performance improvement and research initiatives rely on clear documentation by EMS clinicians. Drop-down fields ensure that data are collected in a consistent way following the NEMSIS standard. Furthermore, data entered in the drop-down menus of the ePCR can be easily queried in analytics platforms and summarized. This helps agency leaders evaluate and communicate the needs of patients and EMS systems with others, including local, state, and federal governments. Documentation using drop-down fields helps quality management personnel give credit for performance on key metrics and helps determine where to tailor future improvement work.

6. What is the purpose of reviewing an EMS call?

A review of an EMS call can provide feedback regarding how you cared for the patient and met the individual's physical and emotional needs. It should not be punitive or fault-finding; it is an educational tool to

YOU are the EMT SUMMARY continued

enhance your patient care skills. EMTs must be open to constructive criticism; this is how you learn and become a more skilled emergency care clinician. Informal reviews are ideal learning opportunities because information about the call is still fresh. Reviews may also be used in formal system QI initiatives to make changes to the system and drive meaningful change.

Prep Kit

Ready for Review

- EMS is an essential part of a larger system and sits at the intersection of emergency management, health care, public safety, and public health. EMS clinician roles are expanding to prevent and treat not only acute illness and injury, but also chronic ailments.
- The National EMS Scope of Practice Model provides overarching guidelines for the practices and minimum competencies for each of the four EMS clinician levels. Aligned with this model, the National EMS Education Standards outline the knowledge and competencies at each EMS clinician level.
- The standards for prehospital emergency care and the clinicians who deliver it are governed by the laws in each state and are typically regulated by a state office of EMS.
- Certification is a process to verify that an EMS clinician has met the minimum competencies for a given EMS clinician training level, whereas licensure refers to the legal authority to practice within a state, and credentialing authorizes clinicians to perform skills or roles.
- EMRs, such as law enforcement officers, firefighters, park rangers, ski patrollers, or other organized rescuers, often arrive at the scene before the ambulance and EMTs. This level of training is focused on providing immediate lifesaving care and ensuring access to the EMS system.
- EMTs have training in basic emergency care knowledge, skills, and attitudes; they focus on initial care and transport of patients that includes identification, assessment, and treatment of many emergency and nonemergency conditions.
- An AEMT has training in specific aspects of ALS care, such as intravenous therapy and the administration of certain emergency medications.
- A paramedic has extensive training in ALS, including endotracheal intubation, emergency pharmacology, cardiac monitoring, and other advanced assessment and treatment skills.
- After the EMTs size up the scene and assess the patient, they provide the emergency care and transport that is indicated based on their findings as outlined in the agency's standing orders and protocols or by the physician who is providing online medical direction.
- EMT attributes include compassion and motivation to reduce suffering, pain, and mortality in those who are injured or acutely ill; a desire to provide each patient with the best possible care; commitment to obtain the knowledge and skills that this position requires; and the drive to continually increase your knowledge, skills, and ability.
- Once you have completed the course, you must assume responsibility for directing your own study through continuing education provided by your service's training officer and medical director or through other opportunities available to you. Your commitment to

Prep Kit continued

continued learning is the key to being a good EMT.

- What you document in the ePCR matters and will be used for QI and research. Using the drop-down menus to record assessments and treatments ensures standardized documentation aligned with the NEMSIS standard and facilitates reporting and analysis.
- Quality management encompasses QA (monitoring compliance against a standard) and QI (making changes to systems to make measurable improvements). Robust quality programs avoid punitive cultures and see errors as learning opportunities.
- The evidence behind EMS practices is constantly evolving through research. EMTs should stay informed on the latest research and be ready to adapt their care to the latest evidence-based practices.
- A person's health is influenced by more than health care. These non–health care factors are known as social drivers of health and include the conditions in the environments in which people are born, live, learn, work, and age.
- The role of EMS in public health is important to help improve community health and safety and increase equity in care delivery and patient outcomes. Public health activities include prevention, public education, and surveillance.
- Mobile integrated health care is an example of how EMS roles are evolving to provide care within communities and connect patients with the right resources to meet their needs.

Vital Vocabulary

advanced emergency medical technician (AEMT) An individual who has training in specific aspects of advanced life support, such as intravenous therapy and the administration of certain emergency medications.

advanced life support (ALS) Advanced lifesaving procedures, such as advanced airway management, intravenous access, and medication administration.

Americans With Disabilities Act (ADA) Comprehensive legislation that is designed to protect people with disabilities against discrimination.

automated external defibrillators (AEDs) Devices that detect treatable life-threatening cardiac dysrhythmias (ventricular fibrillation and ventricular tachycardia) and deliver the appropriate electrical shock to the patient.

basic life support (BLS) Noninvasive emergency lifesaving care that is used to treat medical conditions, including airway obstruction, respiratory arrest, and cardiac arrest.

certification A process in which a person, an institution, or a program is evaluated and recognized as meeting certain predetermined standards to provide safe and ethical care.

credentialing An established process to determine the qualifications necessary to be allowed to perform a particular skill or role, or to function as an organization.

emergency medical responder (EMR) A professional, such as police officer, firefighter, lifeguard, or other rescuer, who may arrive first at the scene of an emergency to provide initial medical assistance and ensure access to EMS.

emergency medical services (EMS) A multidisciplinary system to provide out-of-hospital care to the sick and injured within communities.

emergency medical technician (EMT) An individual who has training in basic life support, including automated external defibrillation, use of a definitive airway adjunct, and assisting patients with certain medications.

evidence-based medicine (EBM) An approach to medicine where decisions are based on well-conducted research that is integrated with the expertise of the EMS clinician and the patient's wishes and needs.

Prep Kit continued

health equity As defined by the World Health Organization, "the absence of unfair and avoidable or remediable differences in health among population groups defined socially, economically, demographically, or geographically."

Just Culture An approach to quality management that strives to balance accountability and justice in a system that believes in learning from errors.

licensure The process whereby a competent authority, usually the state, allows people to perform a regulated act.

medical director The physician who authorizes or delegates to the EMT the authority to provide medical care in the field.

medical oversight Supervision of an EMS system or education program that includes instructions given directly by radio or cell phone (online/direct) to those on scene or indirectly by protocol/guidelines (off-line/indirect); also includes credentialing EMS clinicians and overseeing quality improvement activities as authorized by the medical director of the service or program.

mobile integrated health care (MIH) A method of delivering health care that involves providing health care within the community rather than at a physician's office or hospital.

National EMS Education Standards A set of professional standards published by the National Highway Traffic Safety Administration that define the knowledge and competencies that students should acquire to perform at entry level as an EMS clinician. Four levels are defined: emergency medical responder, emergency medical technician, advanced emergency medical technician, or paramedic.

National EMS Information System (NEMSIS) A system funded by the National Highway Traffic Safety Administration that is responsible for developing and maintaining the national EMS data standard.

National EMS Scope of Practice Model A document created by the National Highway Traffic Safety Administration (NHTSA) that outlines the minimum entry-level skills performed by EMS clinicians at each nationally recognized level.

paramedic An individual who has extensive training in advanced life support, including endotracheal intubation, emergency pharmacology, cardiac monitoring, and other advanced assessment and treatment skills.

primary prevention Efforts to prevent an injury or illness from ever occurring.

public health The branch of medicine that is focused on examining the health needs of entire populations with the goal of preventing health problems.

public safety access point (PSAP) A call center, staffed by trained personnel who are responsible for managing requests for police, fire, and ambulance services.

quality assurance (QA) A reactive process that involves monitoring compliance against a standard to identify problems that have already occurred.

quality improvement (QI) A proactive process that involves making changes to a system to improve performance.

secondary prevention Efforts to limit the effects of an injury or illness that has already occurred.

social drivers of health The conditions in which people live, including the forces and systems shaping their daily lives.

References

1. Dick T. *People Care: Perspectives and Practices for Professional Caregivers*. 3rd ed. HMP; 2018.
2. National Academy of Sciences and National Research Council. *Accidental Death and Disability: The Neglected Disease of Modern Society*. Washington, DC: National Academies Press; 1966.
3. Federal Interagency Committee on Emergency Medical Services (FICEMS). EMS.gov website. https://www.ems

Prep Kit continued

.gov/resources/federal-interagency-committee-on-ems-fic/. Updated November 14, 2023. Accessed October 4, 2024.

4. National EMS Advisory Council (NEMSAC). EMS.gov website. https://www.ems.gov/resources/national-ems-advisory-council-nemsac/. Updated March 26, 2024. Accessed October 4, 2024.
5. Emergency Medical Services for Children (EMSC). Health Resources and Services Administration website. https://mchb.hrsa.gov/programs-impact/emergency-medical-services-children-emsc. Published August 2023. Accessed October 4, 2024.
6. National Association of State EMS Officials. *National EMS Scope of Practice Model*. Washington, DC: National Highway Traffic Safety Administration; February 2019. Report No. DOT HS 812-666. https://www.ems.gov/assets/National_EMS_Scope_of_Practice_Model_2019.pdf. Accessed October 4, 2024.
7. National Highway Traffic Safety Administration. *National Emergency Medical Services Education Standards*. https://www.ems.gov/assets/EMS_Education-Standards_2021_FNL.pdf. EMS.gov website. Published January 2021. Accessed October 4, 2024.
8. National Highway Traffic Safety Administration. *EMS Agenda 2050: A People-Centered Vision for the Future of Emergency Medical Services*; 2019:58. Washington, DC: National Highway Traffic Safety Administration. ems.gov website. https://www.ems.gov/projects/ems-agenda-2050.html. Updated October 18, 2023. Accessed October 4, 2024.
9. Jarvis JL, Hamilton V, Taigman M, Brown LH. Using red lights and sirens for emergency ambulance response: how often are potentially life-saving interventions performed? *Prehosp Emerg Care*. 2021;25(4):549–555.
10. Physician oversight of emergency medical services. *Prehosp Emerg Care*. 2016;21(2): 281–282.
11. Levy M, Gallagher J. Medical oversight of EMS systems. In: Cone DC, Brice JH, Delbridge TR, Myers JB, eds. *Emergency Medical Services: Clinical Practice and Systems Oversight*. 3rd ed. Vol 2. Hoboken, NJ: Wiley-Blackwell; 2021:3–16.
12. National Association of State EMS Officials. *National Model EMS Clinical Guidelines: Version 3.0*. https://nasemso.org/wp-content/uploads/National-Model-EMS-Clinical-Guidelines_2022.pdf. Updated March 2022. Accessed October 4, 2024.
13. Prehospital Guidelines Consortium website [homepage]. https://prehospitalguidelines.org/ebg-resources/. Accessed October 4, 2024.
14. Social determinants of health. World Health Organization website. https://www.who.int/health-topics/social-determinants-of-health#tab=tab_1. Accessed October 4, 2024.
15. Michigan Center for Rural Health. Social drivers of health. Michigan State University website. https://mcrh.msu.edu/programs/Social-Drivers-of-Health. Accessed October 4, 2024.
16. Everything you need to know about food deserts. One New Humanity website. https://www.onenewhumanitycdc.org/blog/everything-you-need-to-know-about-food-deserts. Accessed October 4, 2024.
17. What is health equity? Centers for Disease Control and Prevention website. https://www.cdc.gov/health-equity/what-is/index.html. Published June 11, 2024. Accessed October 4, 2024.
18. Poverty guidelines. Assistant Secretary for Planning and Evaluation website. https://aspe.hhs.gov/topics/poverty-economic-mobility/poverty-guidelines. Accessed October 4, 2024.

Additional Resources

Caffrey SM, Barnes LC, Olvera DJ. Joint position statement on degree requirements for paramedics. *Prehosp Emerg Care.* 2019;23(3):434–437.

Choi BY, Blumberg C, Williams K. Mobile integrated health care and community paramedicine: an emerging emergency medical services concept. *Ann Emerg Med*. 2016;67(3):361–366.

Cone D, Brice JH, Delbridge TR, Myers JB. *Emergency Medical Services: Clinical Practice and Systems Oversight*. 3rd ed. Hoboken, NJ: John Wiley & Sons; 2021.

Faul M, Aikman SN, Sasser SM. Bystander intervention prior to the arrival of emergency medical services: comparing assistance across types of medical emergencies. *Prehosp Emerg Care.* 2016;20(3):317–323.

Goolsby C, Jacobs L, Hunt R, et al. Stop the Bleed Education Consortium: education program content and delivery recommendations. *J Trauma Acute Care Surg.* 2018;84(1):205–210.

PulsePoint overview: next generation AED management. PulsePoint website. https://www.pulsepoint.org/pulsepoint-aed. Accessed December 24, 2024.

Chapter 2

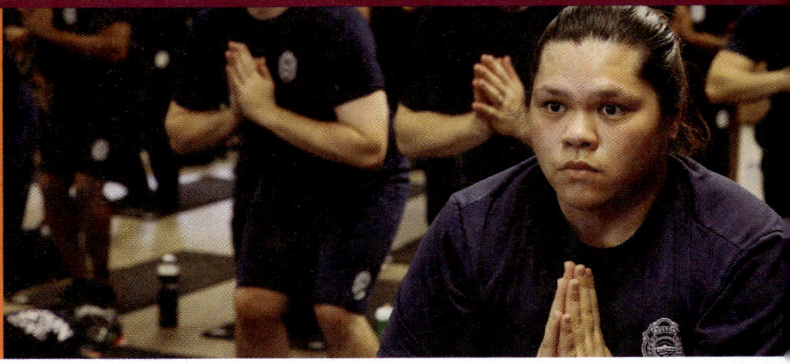

Workforce Safety and Wellness

NATIONAL EMS EDUCATION STANDARD COMPETENCIES

Preparatory

Applies knowledge of the emergency medical services (EMS) system, safety/well-being of the emergency medical technician (EMT), medical/legal, and ethical issues to the provision of emergency care.

Workforce Safety and Wellness

- Standard safety precautions (pp 40–46)
- Personal protective equipment (pp 40–46)
- Lifting and moving patients (Chapter 8, *Lifting and Moving Patients*)
- Crew resource management (Chapter 9, *The Team Approach to Health Care*)
- Stress management (pp 31–32, 34–37)
- Prevention of work-related injuries and illnesses (pp 37–53)
- Responder mental health, resilience, and suicide prevention (pp 33–37)
- Wellness principles (pp 27–33)
- Disease transmission (pp 38–51)

Public Health

Applies knowledge of the principles of public health epidemiology including public health emergencies, public health monitoring, health promotion, and illness and injury prevention.

Public Health Overview

- EMS roles in public health (Chapter 1, *EMS Systems and Public Health*)
- Infection prevention and control (pp 38–51)
- Human trafficking (Chapter 35, *Patients With Special Challenges*)
- EMS electronic health record (EHR) reporting and data collection (Chapter 1, *EMS Systems and Public Health*)
- Governmental/nongovernmental roles and resources (Chapter 1, *EMS Systems and Public Health*)
- Public health mission and goals (Chapter 1, *EMS Systems and Public Health*)
- Social, geographic, economic, and demographic determinants of health (Chapter 1, *EMS Systems and Public Health*)
- Patient and community education (Chapter 1, *EMS Systems and Public Health*)
- Injury prevention and wellness (pp 38–51)
- Unique pediatric, geriatric, and special population public health concerns (Chapter 10, *Patient Assessment*; Chapter 35, *Patients With Special Challenges*)
- Screenings and vaccinations/immunizations (pp 48–51)

KNOWLEDGE OBJECTIVES

1. Explain the components that contribute to wellness and resilience and their importance in managing stress. (pp 27–37)
2. Identify the risks and hazards of fatigue in EMS. (pp 30–31)

3. Recognize the physiologic, physical, and psychological responses to stress. (pp 31–32, 34–37)
4. Describe factors that contribute to burnout and compassion fatigue. (pp 34–35)
5. Explain potentially psychologically traumatizing events and strategies to mitigate their effects. (pp 34–35)
6. Explain posttraumatic stress disorder (PTSD) and steps that can be taken to decrease the likelihood that PTSD will develop. (pp 34–35)
7. Identify resources for positive mental health and suicide prevention. (pp 36–37)
8. State the routes of disease transmission. (pp 38–40)
9. Describe the specific routes of transmission and the steps to prevent and/or manage an exposure. (pp 38–51)
10. Apply the standard precautions used in treating patients to prevent infection. (pp 40–46)
11. Explain the steps to take for personal protection from airborne and bloodborne pathogens. (pp 40–46)
12. Differentiate infectious disease and communicable disease. (p 38)
13. Demonstrate proper handwashing techniques. (pp 40–42)
14. Explain the ways in which immunity to infectious diseases is acquired. (pp 48–50)
15. Summarize postexposure management of exposure to patient blood or body fluids, including completing a postexposure report. (pp 50–51)
16. Discuss the steps necessary to determine scene safety and to prevent work-related injuries at the scene. (pp 51–53)
17. Recognize the possibility of violent situations and the steps to take to deal with them. (p 53)
18. Discuss workplace issues such as incivility and sexual harassment. (pp 53–54)
19. Describe the benefits of a diverse and inclusive workplace. (pp 54–55)

SKILLS OBJECTIVES

1. Demonstrate how to properly remove gloves. (p 44, Skill Drill 2-1)
2. Demonstrate the steps necessary to manage a potential exposure situation. (p 47, Skill Drill 2-2)

Introduction

To be successful in a career that involves taking care of others requires that you first value and care for yourself. Developing habits to keep yourself safe and healthy are paramount. Although working as an emergency responder may involve increased risk compared to other professions, there are actions you can take to greatly reduce the probability of injury or illness. Likewise, burnout is not something that everyone in EMS needs to experience. Prioritizing your physical and mental well-being will enable you to spend a career taking great care of others.

You are not replaceable, and what you do for others really matters. As part of your EMT training, you will learn how to recognize risks to your health, safety, and well-being and that of your partners and your patients. You will also learn how, when possible, you can avoid such hazards, protect yourself and others from them, or minimize their effects.

Words of Wisdom

Good caregivers must first care for themselves. As educator Thom Dick wrote in his book *People Care*, "We're here to serve others, and they're important. But not more important than we are." Valuing ourselves and prioritizing our own health and safety ensure that we are able to provide the best care for others.

General Wellness Principles

Although many people might think of health simply as the absence of disease or physical injury, we now understand that health is a complex interaction among physical, mental, and emotional conditions. Because they are intertwined, chronic physical, mental, or emotional stresses can worsen or increase the likelihood that combinations of physical, mental, or emotional health conditions will develop. Fortunately, the opposite is also true.

Supporting good physical, mental, and emotional health can significantly lower the risk of chronic and acute health problems, permitting the EMS clinician to not only survive, but thrive.

Wellness is the active pursuit of a state of good health. It is crucial for EMS clinicians to understand that they must work to maintain their wellness in the same way that they must work to maintain their knowledge, skills, and attitudes to be effective emergency responders. Wellness is multifaceted. Maintaining good physical fitness is important, but by itself it is not enough to ensure wellness for an EMS clinician. Consistent wellness practices can help EMS clinicians prevent injury and illness not only in the moment, but throughout their careers and beyond.

Nutrition

As an EMT, your role requires peak physical and mental performance to provide the best care possible. Regular, well-balanced meals are essential to provide the nutrients that are necessary to keep your body fueled and help you maintain good health.

The scientific knowledge around nutrition is continuously evolving and many guiding resources exist. For example, the US Departments of Agriculture (USDA) and Health and Human Services collaborate to update and release the *Dietary Guidelines for Americans* every 5 years with the goal of promoting health and preventing disease. These guidelines provide a customizable healthy eating framework that can be adapted to meet personal and cultural needs.

Building a healthy eating routine includes consuming nutrient-dense forms of foods and beverages across food groups. The core elements that make up a healthy dietary pattern include the following:

- Vegetables of all types
- Whole fruits
- Grains, at least half of which are whole grains
- Protein, including lean meats, poultry, eggs, seafood, beans, peas, lentils, nuts, seeds, and soy products
- Dairy or dairy alternatives such as soy
- Oils, including vegetable oils and oils in food such as seafood or nuts

Key nutrition recommendations also include limiting foods and beverages that are higher in added sugars, saturated fats, and sodium, and alcoholic beverages. Added sugars should represent less than 10% of calories per day. Saturated fat should represent less than 10% of calories per day. Sodium should be less than 2,300 mg per day.[1]

A healthy eating routine involves more than our choices of food. It is important to focus on drink choices, too. When you are thirsty, reach for water first (**FIGURE 2-1**). Carrying a reusable water bottle to refill during your shift can help you stay hydrated. Avoid drinks with added sugars, including soda, energy drinks, sports drinks, sweetened waters, and sweetened coffee or tea drinks. Even low- and no-calorie sweeteners do not carry health benefits and may not help you meet your health goals. Eating whole fruits is recommended over drinking fruit juices, as the whole fruits contain fiber you need to stay healthy. If you drink juice, consider 100% fruit juice with no added sugars and limit servings to 4 ounces or less.

To help translate the scientific findings into actionable habits and create healthy eating

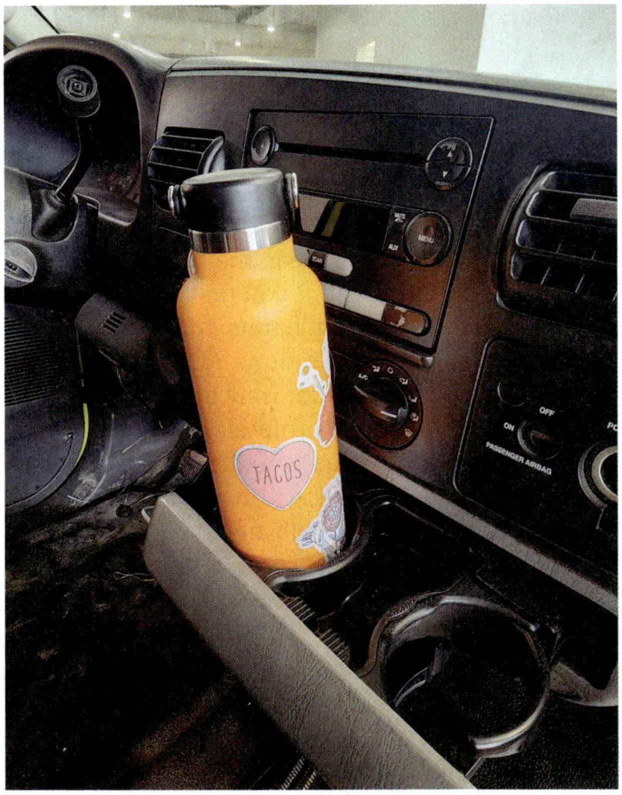

FIGURE 2-1 Maintain an adequate fluid intake by drinking plenty of water.

Courtesy of Remle Crowe.

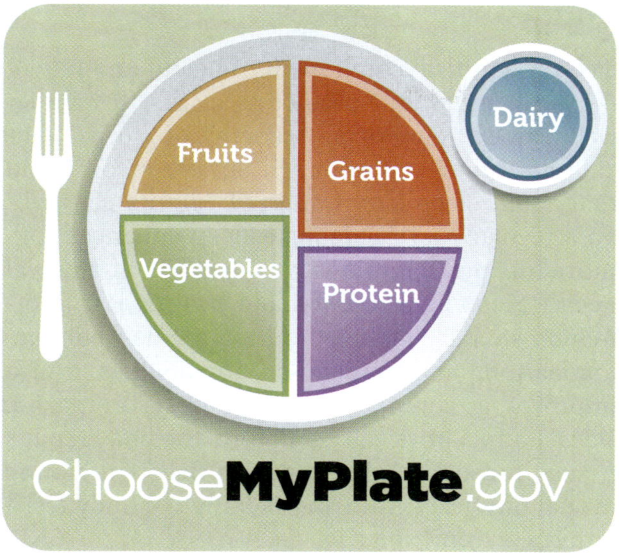

FIGURE 2-2 The USDA's MyPlate emphasizes healthy portions of vegetables, fruits, grains, proteins, and dairy and can be customized to fit individual dietary needs, preferences, cultural traditions, and budget. Access the personalized planning tool at MyPlate.gov.

Courtesy of the USDA Center for Nutrition Policy and Promotion.

routines, the USDA has developed MyPlate and a suite of associated tools (**FIGURE 2-2**). MyPlate replaces the 1992 Food Pyramid and provides a personalized approach to help individuals meet their health goals. Eating several small, healthy meals throughout the day can help keep your energy resources up, while overeating may reduce your physical and mental performance. Because EMS shift work can create challenges to maintaining a consistent meal schedule, consider carrying a supply of healthy snacks, such as whole fruits, vegetables, and nuts.

Ultimately, it is important to remember that nutrition is not an all-or-nothing proposition. Even small, healthy choices add up and contribute to overall health.

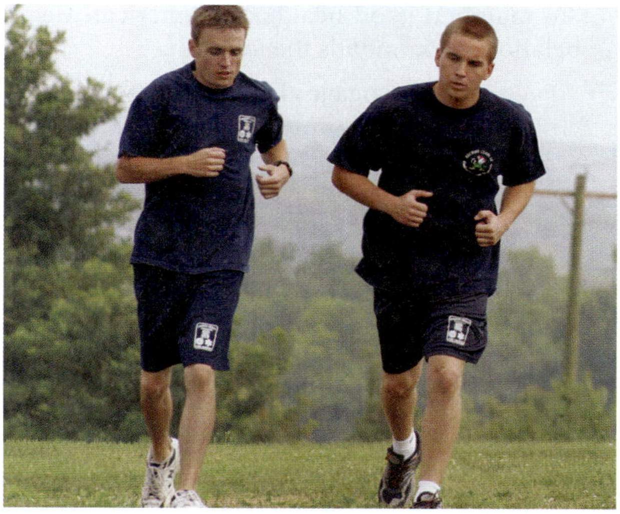

FIGURE 2-3 A regular program of exercise will increase strength and endurance.

© Jones & Bartlett Learning. Courtesy of MIEMSS.

Exercise and Relaxation

Regular exercise will enhance the benefits of maintaining good nutrition and adequate hydration, ensuring the body is able to handle the requirements that you will place on it by lifting patients, performing CPR, and moving heavy equipment. When you are in good physical condition, you can handle stress more easily and you are less likely to sustain injury. Regular exercise will increase your strength and endurance.

Your exercise routine should involve aspects of cardiovascular endurance, muscular strength building, mobility, and flexibility (**FIGURE 2-3**). Endurance will ensure your cardiovascular system is able to provide your muscles and brain with needed oxygen. Strength training, also known as resistance training, helps build muscles and protect joints. Mobility training and stretching improve your body's range of motion, flexibility, and functional movement, which can reduce joint deterioration and help you stay active and healthy.

YOU are the EMT

You have just finished orientation and field training as an EMT at your first EMS job. Tomorrow you will start working a 24-hour shift from 0600 to 0600 with your paramedic partner. You know that this system is very busy and you likely will not have a break during lunchtime to sit and eat.

1. How can you prepare yourself for this shift?

To maintain good health, the American Heart Association recommends the following[2]:

- Each week, engage in at least 150 minutes of moderate-intensity aerobic activity, 75 minutes of vigorous aerobic activity, or a combination of both, preferably spread across multiple days.
- At least 2 days per week, incorporate moderate- to high-intensity muscle-strengthening exercises.
- Limit the time you spend being sedentary. Even light-intensity exercise may improve your fitness level.
- Try to improve these minimum recommendations over time.

While achieving exercise goals may seem daunting, there are strategies you can use to set yourself up for success. Plan activities ahead of time and use strategies that make your exercise sessions convenient. When it comes to exercise, embrace the mindset of "all or something," not "all or nothing." It is okay to start small: Move a little every day; even a walk to the mailbox or 5 minutes of stretching may be an appropriate starting point for some people. Exercise should not be a punishment, so try to find activities you enjoy. For some, the key to maintaining a routine is working out with others. Doing so can increase your sense of accountability, increase your enjoyment of exercising, and build social relationships, which can also improve your emotional resilience.

Just as exercise is important for overall health, so is relaxation. Practices such as mindfulness and meditation can help the body and mind recover. Mindfulness activities have been shown to reduce stress and its associated symptoms in first responders.[3] An easy introduction to mindfulness practice can be found on the free UCLA Mindful app, which offers guided meditation activities that take as little as 3 minutes.[4] Additionally, practicing gratitude by routinely taking a moment to acknowledge and appreciate things that are meaningful or valuable to you can improve well-being. These practices may seem awkward at first, but they often turn into an enjoyable part of the day.

Street Smarts

It is critical that you are able to recognize when you are stressed and develop healthy coping skills to manage stress.

Sleep

Sleep is a critical component of health and one of the most important predictors of first responder wellness. The American Academy of Sleep Medicine and the Sleep Research Society recommend that adults sleep a minimum of 7 hours per night on a regular basis.[5] Adequate sleep enhances cognitive function, emotional well-being, and physical health. Sleep helps consolidate and process information we have gathered during the day, enhancing learning and problem-solving abilities. It also improves attention, focus, and decision-making skills. From a physical standpoint, the body repairs tissues, muscles, and cells during sleep, promoting overall physical health and helping the body resist or recover from injury.

Because of the nature of shift work, the intensity, and "around-the-clock" nature of emergency medical care, many EMS clinicians find themselves chronically fatigued and experiencing sleep deprivation. Research has found that one-half of EMS clinicians get less than 6 hours of sleep per 24 hours and report severe mental and physical fatigue. In the short term, fatigue can lead to medical errors, vehicle crashes, and other harm to patients, bystanders, and EMS clinicians. In the long term, sleep deprivation can lead to hypertension, sleep apnea, respiratory problems, diabetes, depression, and other medical conditions. Adequate sleep is as important as eating well and exercising in the maintenance of good health. Sleep should be regular and uninterrupted. Recommendations to improve sleep quality include the following[6,7]:

- Make sleep a priority by scheduling social activities and household tasks to allow you time for adequate rest. Inform others of your sleep schedule.
- Develop a sleep schedule and aim for 7 to 9 hours of sleep per 24 hours.
- Ensure your sleep environment is dark, quiet, and cool. If necessary, use blackout shades or an eye mask to block light, or earplugs or devices that produce white (or pink) noise to reduce disruptive noise.
- Establish a calming presleep routine. Find activities that help you wind down and feel relaxed and consistently engage in these activities before sleep. This routine could include taking a bath, reading a book, or practicing meditation or relaxation exercises.

- Avoid caffeine, alcohol, nicotine, and other chemicals that interfere with sleep for several hours before bedtime (some sources say up to 8 hours for caffeine and 3 hours for alcohol).
- Avoid heavy presleep meals. However, going to bed hungry can negatively affect sleep. Choose a lighter meal before sleep that will not cause indigestion or discomfort.
- Leave enough time after exercise to engage in your presleep routine before you try to fall asleep.
- Balance fluid intake. Stay hydrated, but avoid overhydration; you don't want your sleep to be interrupted by trips to the bathroom.
- Develop strategies for sleep problems. If you are unable to sleep after approximately 20 minutes, try additional calming presleep activities rather than "fighting" to get to sleep. If sleep problems occur more than three times in a row during 1 week, seek advice from a sleep professional.
- Use napping as a tool. Short naps (15 to 20 minutes) can boost alertness, while longer naps (90 minutes) can reduce sleep debt. Avoid longer naps in the 4 to 6 hours before your main sleep.
- Plan your transition to days off. When entering a block of days off, particularly after working night shifts, having a short sleep in the morning and going to sleep earlier than usual can help your body adjust. Where possible, expose yourself to natural light during your waking hours to maintain healthy sleep–wake cycles.

The Fatigue in EMS project was a 5-year project with the goal to understand and apply sleep science principles to the EMS workforce. This project, supported by the National Highway Traffic Safety Administration (NHTSA) through the National Association of State EMS Officials (NASEMSO), included partnerships with the University of Pittsburgh School of Medicine and the Institutes of Behavior Resources to develop evidence-based guidelines for fatigue management. The evidence-based recommendations for fatigue risk management in EMS include the following[8]:

- Fatigue/sleepiness survey instruments should be used to measure and monitor fatigue among EMS personnel.
- EMS personnel should work shifts shorter than 24 hours in duration.
- EMS personnel should have access to caffeine as a countermeasure to fatigue.
- EMS personnel should have the opportunity to nap while on duty to mitigate fatigue.
- EMS personnel should receive education and training to mitigate fatigue and fatigue-related risks.

Recommendations for individual clinicians to combat fatigue include the following[8]:

- Get an adequate duration (more than 7 hours) and quality of sleep.
- Where allowed, take 20- to 30-minute naps or rest breaks during shift work.
- Increase physical exercise such as stretching, walking, and jogging in place.
- Be careful about caffeine consumption. Caffeine can increase alertness but is not a replacement for sleep. In large quantities, caffeine can contribute to cardiac dysrhythmias, seizures, and increased stress and anxiety.
- Engage in mental exercise, such as having a conversation or playing a game.

Of course, the most effective way to combat fatigue is to ensure good sleep in the first place.

Stress Management

Managing stress is crucial for maintaining wellness among EMTs, who routinely face high-pressure situations. The Brabban and Turkington stress bucket analogy provides a helpful framework for understanding and managing stress.[9] In this analogy,

YOU are the EMT

You are now in the 18th hour of your 24-hour shift and have just been called to complete an interfacility transfer with a drive time of approximately 35 minutes. You realize that you are starting to feel tired.

2. What are some strategies you can use to combat fatigue and help you stay safe for the duration of this shift?

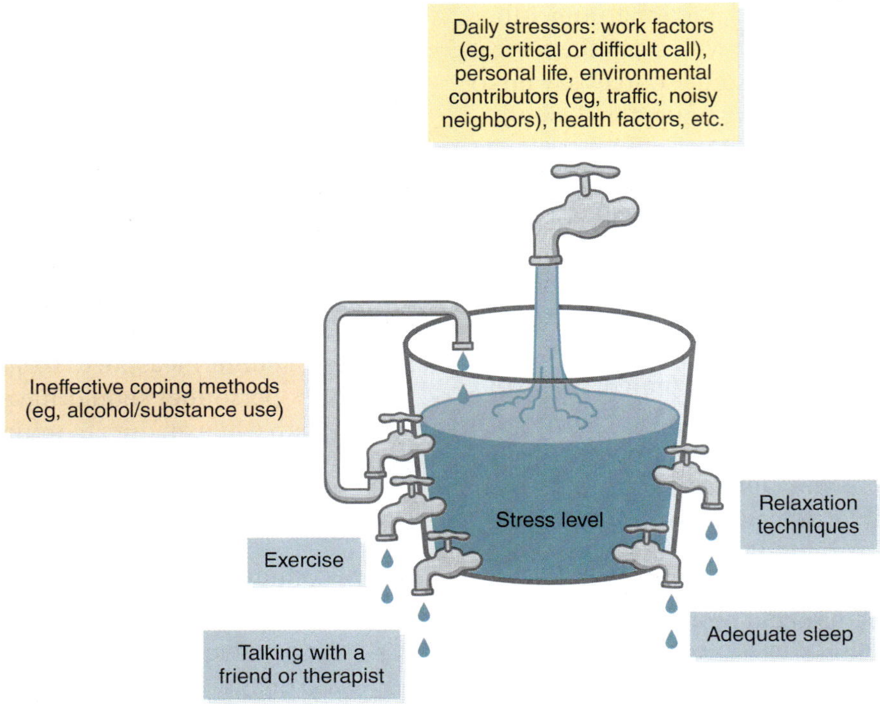

FIGURE 2-4 Stress bucket analogy.

each person has a "stress bucket" that collects water droplets (daily stressors). When the bucket overflows, it leads to overwhelming stress and negative health consequences. Effective stress management involves finding ways to empty the bucket, such as through relaxation techniques, exercise, talking to a trusted person or therapist, and ensuring adequate sleep (**FIGURE 2-4**). Recognizing personal stressors and implementing stress-relief activities can help keep the stress bucket from overflowing, thereby maintaining mental wellness.

Disease Prevention and Health Promotion

Another critical aspect of wellness involves disease prevention and health promotion. Strictly speaking, although both of these efforts involve personal practices and medical services, disease prevention focuses more on medical care to avoid or reduce the effect of disease on an individual. Meanwhile, health promotion is more focused on personal practices and social habits to improve one's health.

Examples of disease prevention include preventive and postexposure vaccinations, dental hygiene services, disease screening, and education and counseling relating to physical, mental, and emotional health risks. Examples of health promotion include education about and support for proper nutrition, physical exercise, tobacco and vaping cessation, and use of mental health and substance use disorder services.

Smoking, Vaping, or Chewing Nicotine

If you don't already use tobacco or vape, don't start. Use of tobacco products produces many of the most harmful cardiovascular and lung diseases that you will confront during your career. Smoking tobacco products is linked to many negative health consequences, including lung cancer, respiratory diseases (eg, chronic obstructive pulmonary disease), emphysema, chronic bronchitis, bladder cancer, and many others. Use of smokeless tobacco (dry or moist snuff) is also associated with health risks, including cancers of the throat, mouth, and pancreas. Vaping has been shown to produce significant negative effects on the cardiovascular and respiratory systems, contributing to elevated risk of heart disease and stroke. Severe cases of e-cigarette or vaping-associated lung injury resulting in death have been reported.

Alcohol Use

According to the **Centers for Disease Control and Prevention (CDC)**, excessive alcohol use caused nearly 180,000 deaths in the United States from 2020 to 2021, continuing an upward trend in the past 2 decades.[10] Definitions of excessive drinking are shown in **TABLE 2-1**. In all cases, drinking less is better for health than drinking more.

According to recommendations in the *Dietary Guidelines*, individuals who do not drink alcohol should not start for any reason. In the past, some studies touted the health benefits related to moderate consumption of alcohol, such as improved heart health from drinking red wine; however, more recently, influential studies note that "no level of alcohol consumption improves health."[11] The accumulation of much evidence suggests there is a relationship between alcohol use and the risk of heart disease, stroke, mental illness, and many other diseases.[12] Excessive alcohol use may also increase the risk of the development of various cancers, including those of the mouth, throat, breast, esophagus, and liver.

It is also important to note that some people, including those who are pregnant or might be pregnant, who have certain medical conditions or are taking certain medications that interact with alcohol, or who are recovering from alcohol use disorder, should not drink at all.

If you are of legal drinking age and choose to drink alcohol, drink in moderation. Moderate alcohol consumption is described as one drink or fewer per day for women and two drinks or fewer per day for men.

TABLE 2-1 Definitions of Excessive Alcohol Use[a]

	Binge Drinking	Heavy Drinking
Men	5 or more drinks during a single occasion	15 or more drinks per week
Women	4 or more drinks during a single occasion	8 or more drinks per week

[a]Any alcohol use by individuals younger than 21 years and pregnant individuals is considered excessive.

Data From: Division of Population Health, National Center for Chronic Disease Prevention and Health Promotion, Centers for Disease Control and Prevention (CDC). Alcohol use and your health. CDC website. https://www.cdc.gov/alcohol/data-stats.htm.

Cannabis Use

Cannabis, commonly known as marijuana, is a plant that contains a variety of chemical compounds called cannabinoids. Cannabinoids are active substances found in cannabis that interact with the body's endocannabinoid system, which regulates various physiologic processes including mood, memory, pain sensation, and appetite. The most well-known cannabinoids are THC (tetrahydrocannabinol), the primary psychoactive compound responsible for the "high" associated with cannabis use, and CBD (cannabidiol), which is nonpsychoactive and often used for its potential therapeutic effects. Despite the legalization in many states of cannabis and cannabinoid products for medicinal purposes or recreational use, cannabis use is not without risks. For example, cannabis hyperemesis syndrome, associated most commonly with long-term use, is a disorder characterized by bouts of nausea and vomiting.[13]

Cannabis use among EMTs poses important implications for workforce wellness. The cognitive and motor function effects can compromise the EMT's job performance, and research suggests that cannabis may have a prolonged effect on attention and cognitive function.[14] The question of whether EMS clinicians have the right to use cannabis off duty, where it is legal, without employment consequences remains unclear. Thus far, the law has favored employers who have disciplined or terminated employees for the use of cannabis, even when legal in the state. It is important that you know and understand your agency's policies related to cannabis use.

EMT Mental Health

Balancing Work, Family, and Health

As an EMT, you will often be called to assist patients who are sick and injured at any time of the day or night. Unfortunately, there is no way to predict the timing of illness, injury, or interfacility transfer. Volunteer EMTs may often be called away from family or friends during social activities. Shift workers may be required to be apart from loved ones for long periods of time. You should never let the job interfere excessively with your own needs. Find a balance between work and your personal life; you owe it to yourself and to your loved ones. It is important to make sure you have the time that you need to relax with family and friends. Taking time to rest, recharge, and connect with others can help prevent many mental health conditions sometimes associated with EMS work.

Burnout and Compassion Fatigue

The term **burnout** was first coined in the 1970s to describe extreme emotional and physical exhaustion attributed to one's work. Burnout often manifests as a combination of emotional exhaustion, cynicism, and reduced sense of personal accomplishment. According to the job demands–resources theory, burnout most often results when job demands exceed job resources for an extended period.[15] Examples of job demands include physical workload and time pressure. Examples of job resources include pay and benefits, performance feedback, and respect from supervisors and colleagues. In EMS, burnout has negative consequences for individuals and organizations. Among individuals, burnout has been linked to sleeplessness, depression, and hypertension.[16] At the organizational level, burnout has been linked to higher rates of absenteeism (sickness absence) and turnover.[17]

Burnout is not an inevitable consequence of working in EMS. Even if you do experience burnout, it does not have to be a permanent state. Burnout is a dynamic condition that can be managed and overcome by rebalancing resources and demands. One strategy to help maintain balance is to keep a scrapbook of positive memories throughout your career, like photos with colleagues or letters from patients. These memories can serve as a reminder of the meaningful effect your work has and help sustain your motivation and well-being.

Compassion fatigue, a term coined in 1992, is characterized by gradual lessening of compassion over time caused by prolonged exposure to traumatic events and the intense empathy required to care for those in **distress**.[18,19] Sometimes described as "the cost of caring," compassion fatigue is common among those who work in health care and disaster and emergency services.[19] This condition can manifest as a diminished ability to empathize with patients, increased irritability, and a sense of helplessness. Compassion fatigue is a reaction to caring for others who have experienced trauma. Regular self-care practices, seeking peer support, and professional counseling are strategies for mitigating the effects of compassion fatigue.

Potentially Psychologically Traumatizing Events and Posttraumatic Stress

EMS clinicians are exposed to trauma at much higher rates than the general population; however, it is important to recognize that these events do not always lead to mental health conditions. By reducing stigma and creating safe spaces for discussion around mental well-being, we can lessen the likelihood that job stress and exposure to trauma will result in negative mental health effects. This section will also discuss strategies to help maintain health and mitigate the effects of exposure to traumatic events.

Sometimes referred to as a critical incident, a **potentially psychologically traumatizing event** is any incident that deeply affects the mental and emotional well-being of an EMS clinician. While certain types of events may more often be associated with psychologically traumatizing events, such as incidents involving the death of a child or a person known to the responder, it is important to understand that *any* event can be a psychologically traumatizing event. These situations can cause moral injury, which refers to the psychological, behavioral, social, or spiritual distress that individuals may experience after being exposed to events that violate their own moral standards and expectations.[20,21]

It is the individual's response to the event, not the event itself, that determines whether it is a psychologically traumatizing event. How a person responds to a stressor can depend greatly on factors such as the person's overall mood, health, and other sources of stress that may be present at the same time. Because so many factors come into play, different people will react differently to the same stressors. Moreover, a person may react differently to the same stressor under different circumstances. Think back to the stress bucket analogy and consider how a person whose bucket is near overflowing may be able to cope with a traumatic event compared to a person whose bucket is at a lower level. You should not feel ashamed if you have a strong emotional reaction to an event, even if that event is not something that you think would typically be associated with psychological trauma.

Exposures to potentially psychologically traumatizing events have the potential to cause **posttraumatic stress disorder (PTSD)** and other trauma-related mental health conditions. PTSD is a mental health condition characterized by persistent and distressing symptoms that include intrusive memories, flashbacks, nightmares, severe anxiety, and uncontrollable thoughts about the event. Early recognition of PTSD and treatment are crucial for effective management and recovery. EMS clinicians should seek help from mental health professionals who specialize in trauma among first responders. Accessing help is nothing to be ashamed of, and many EMS organizations provide access to helpful resources, including counseling services and peer support programs.

A process called **critical incident stress management (CISM)** was developed to address potentially psychologically traumatizing situations and help reduce the likelihood that PTSD will develop after such an incident (**FIGURE 2-5**). The process theoretically is used to confront the responses to critical incidents and defuse them, directing the emergency services personnel toward physical and emotional equilibrium. CISM can occur formally, as a debriefing for those who were on scene. In such situations, trained CISM teams of peers and mental health professionals may facilitate the process. This debriefing process was believed to be the gold standard for assisting EMS clinicians following exposure to a psychologically traumatizing event.

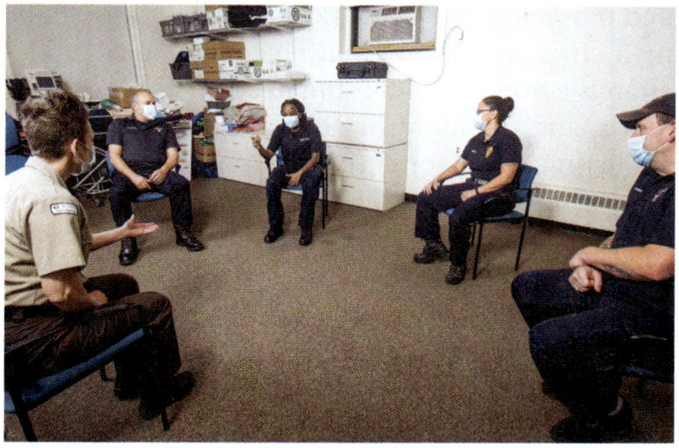

FIGURE 2-5 Critical incident stress management is sometimes used to help clinicians manage stress.

However, there is no one-size-fits-all approach, and the research continues to evolve on this topic as additional methods of supporting EMS clinicians have been developed. Mental health professionals should determine situations in which this type of intervention may be helpful versus those in which it has the potential to create harm.

Peer support involves trained members within an organization who seek out and talk with other peers about mental health concerns. Peer support may be formal or informal and can help lower stigma and build team cohesion. Professional counseling and therapy can also be helpful, especially when the professional has experience and expertise in treating traumatic stress in first responders.

Resilience and Posttraumatic Growth

When it comes to PTSD and other mental health conditions relating to psychologically traumatic experiences, prevention is the best medicine. Just as you focus on maintaining your physical health with proper nutrition and exercise to prevent injury, you can protect your mental health with proper attention and support. **Resilience** is the capacity of an individual to cope with and recover from distress. Although some people tend to be more resilient than others, a person's resilience may change. We have significant control over our ability to build resilience.[22] Strategies to build resilience include the following:

- Develop a support network by cultivating strong relationships with family, friends, and colleagues.
- Prioritize self-care through regular exercise, nutrition, sleep, and relaxation techniques. Sleep is especially key for processing memories and reducing the likelihood that a potentially psychologically traumatizing event results in harm by separating the emotion from the memory.
- Foster a positive mindset by practicing gratitude and focusing on the positive aspects of life, even in challenging times.
- Build emotional regulation by learning techniques such as deep breathing and mindfulness to stay calm and focused during times of stress.
- Stay connected to your purpose by engaging in activities that align with your values and give you a sense of meaning.

- Seek professional help when needed. Do not hesitate to seek support from mental health professionals.

At the core of resilience is the belief that within crisis lies an opportunity for growth. The term posttraumatic growth (PTG) was coined in the mid-1990s by psychologists Richard Tedeschi and Lawrence Calhoun.[23] PTG is the positive changes that arise from the struggle to cope with a traumatizing situation. Where resilience refers to bouncing back from trauma, PTG goes beyond to encompass growing from adversity.

Connection is critical for both resilience and PTG. Humans are hardwired for connection, with an innate need to belong. Social support requires meaningful connection to others and a feeling of safety. This is why coping mechanisms such as excessive alcohol use, substance use, and isolation can be so destructive. Avoidance and isolation fail to address, process, and resolve the psychologically traumatic experience.

Street Smarts

Box breathing or tactical breathing is a deep breathing technique that can help you manage stress and gain control of your emotions.[24] This process lowers your heart rate and allows you to focus during stressful situations. Visualize a box with a number on each side. Side 1 reminds you to breathe in for a count of 4; side 2, to hold your breath for a count of 4; side 3, to breathe out for a count of 4; and side 4, to again hold your breath for a count of 4. The process can then be repeated.

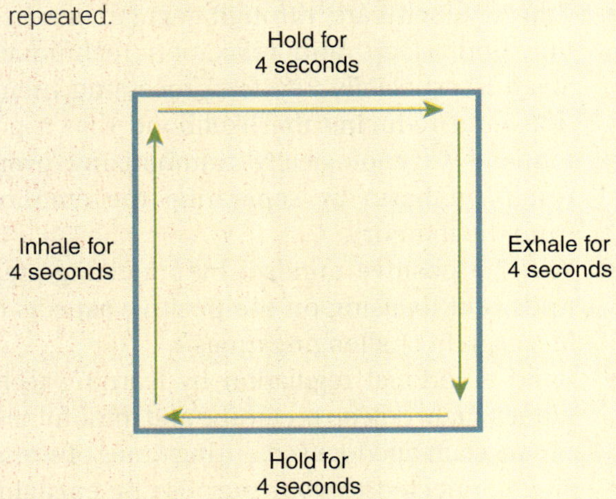

Understanding and Addressing Risk for Suicide

Suicide is increasingly recognized as a critical issue among EMS clinicians. Research suggests that EMS clinicians die by suicide at a higher rate than the general population.[25,26] Interpreting these statistics is challenging due to differences in demographics between EMS clinicians and the general population, underreporting, and misclassification of deaths.[27] Nonetheless, suicide is the 10th leading cause of death in the United States and ranks higher than line-of-duty deaths among EMS clinicians.[28]

High rates of suicide among EMS clinicians are often attributed to the nature of their work, including exposure to high levels of psychological stress. However, it is crucial to understand that correlation may not equal causation. The true causes of suicide are more complex, involving intersections among personal, organizational, and relationship issues. Attributing EMS suicide primarily to PTSD overlooks other significant factors and can lead EMS clinicians to feel that their stress is unworthy of attention, furthering feelings of alienation and isolation. In fact, factors most commonly associated with thoughts of suicide are marital/relationship issues, work-related issues, alcohol and substance use disorders, legal concerns, financial problems, and then PTSD.[29]

While signs such as expressing a desire to die, depression, increased alcohol or drug use, giving away possessions, or withdrawing from others are associated with death by suicide, an overemphasis on these warning signs can be problematic. Most people who experience thoughts of suicide do not die by suicide and those at highest risk often work hardest to hide their struggles and prevent detection. Suicidal ideation is common, with estimates that between one-fourth and one-third of people will have thoughts about suicide at some time.[19] Connection and belonging are fundamental human needs that can help individuals overcome thoughts of suicide by reducing feelings of isolation and fostering a sense of purpose and worth. Unfortunately, the culture within many EMS organizations has historically stigmatized mental health concerns, leading individuals to stay quiet and isolated, rather than seek help.

Changing this culture requires understanding factors that affect mental health and creating environments that encourage open discussion. As an

EMT, it is essential to speak out against exclusionary behaviors such as bullying in the workplace (discussed later in this chapter). Checking in on colleagues, creating safe spaces for open discussion, and encouraging help-seeking are key to preventing death by suicide. Many emergency response organizations offer their own access to stress management and mental health services along with peer support teams and employee assistance programs. In addition, numerous national services are available to first responders. The Code Green Campaign is a mental health and advocacy organization for first responders. Its website directs those in need of emotional support to many resources, including the following:

- CrewCare: www.crewcarelife.com/crisis-support/
- 988 Suicide and Crisis Lifeline: https://988lifeline.org
- Center for Firefighter Behavioral Health: www.cffbh.org
- Safe Call Now: www.safecallnowusa.org

By destigmatizing conversations around mental health and fostering a culture of understanding, support, and open communication, EMS organizations can reduce the risk of suicide among clinicians and ensure that those in need receive the help they deserve.

Words of Wisdom

Attitudes toward wellness are as important as knowledge and behaviors. An EMT can know about effective ways to deal with stress, but this knowledge will not help if the person's attitude is, "That doesn't apply to me. I'm fine." Experiencing stress or other mental health concerns is common and not a sign of weakness. Just as you rest, stay hydrated, and take medication to recover from a physical illness, you should practice self-care, seek support, and possibly engage in therapy to maintain and improve your mental health.

Safety Tips

Coworkers often notice a change in behavior or attitude before a supervisor does. This is especially true in EMS, where close relationships develop between people who work together and share rooms, meals, and social interactions. Being a friend means helping a friend. Talk to your partner about changes in behavior you have noticed and offer a safe space to listen. Likewise, if you are having trouble dealing with a crisis, remember, you are not alone. Reach out and talk with others.

Prevention of Physical Work-Related Injury and Illness

According to the Bureau of Labor Statistics, there are approximately 3.5 million serious injuries and 5,000 deaths each year in US workplaces.[30] EMS clinicians visit EDs for work-related injuries and exposures approximately 20,000 times each year.[31] As an EMT, you are most at risk for sprains and strains, exposures to blood and body fluids, and falls. In 2020, almost one-fourth of EMS-related injuries involved strains or sprains, and almost one-third of injuries resulted from overexertion.[32] Simple measures such as practicing safe lifting, using appropriate PPE, and wearing slip-resistant footwear can reduce the incidence of these visits.

Many EMS organizations have established injury and illness prevention programs to determine workplace hazards and implement a plan to mitigate those hazards. Each injury and illness prevention program should involve management and workers and include hazard identification, prevention, and control; education and training; and program evaluation.

YOU are the EMT

It is now 0400 and you receive a call to 14 Nightingale Street for an unconscious adult who is not breathing. You and your paramedic partner respond to the scene. This is your first call involving a critically ill patient.

3. How can you prepare yourself psychologically for this call?

Safe Lifting Practices

We have already discussed the importance of physical fitness for an EMT. Lifting 125 pounds (57 kg) can be difficult if you do not exercise regularly. Lifting is a job duty you will perform often, so safe lifting techniques are critical to your health and well-being. Back injuries are common in EMS work. For your health and well-being, remember these tips:

- Preplan the move.
- Bend your legs, not your waist.
- Keep the weight close to your body.
- Lift straight up, using your legs, not your back.

For a full discussion of this subject, see Chapter 8, *Lifting and Moving Patients*.

Infectious and Communicable Disease Precautions

As an EMT, you will be called on to treat and transport patients with a variety of infectious or communicable diseases. An **infectious disease** is a medical condition caused by the growth and spread of harmful organisms within the body. A **communicable disease** is a disease that can be spread from one person or species to another. Immunizations, simple handwashing, and other protective techniques can dramatically reduce the health care clinician's risk of **infection**.

Familiarize yourself with the following terminology related to infectious diseases. A **pathogen** is a microorganism that is capable of causing disease in a susceptible host. **Contamination** is the presence of pathogens or foreign bodies on or in objects such as dressings, water, food, needles, wounds, or a patient's body. **Exposure** is a situation in which a person has had contact with blood, body fluids, tissues, or airborne particles in a manner that may allow disease transmission to occur. **Personal protective equipment (PPE)** is protective equipment that an individual wears to prevent exposure to a pathogen or other hazardous condition.

Words of Wisdom

All communicable diseases are infectious, but not all infectious diseases are easily communicable. For example, *Salmonella* is an infectious bacterium that causes food poisoning, but the infection is not communicable to others. Hepatitis B is an infectious disease that is communicable to others through contact with body fluids. In contrast, airborne- or droplet-spread infectious diseases such as COVID-19 are easily spread to others.

Routes of Transmission

Whereas all infections result from an abnormal invasion of body spaces and tissues by germs, different germs use different means of attack, or mechanisms of transmission. **Transmission** is the way an infectious disease is spread. There are several ways infectious diseases can be transmitted: contact (direct or indirect), aerosolized (in droplets), foodborne, and vector-borne (transmitted through insects or parasitic worms).

Contact transmission is the movement of an organism from one person to another through physical touch. There are two types of contact transmission: direct and indirect. **Direct contact** occurs when an organism is moved from one person to another through touching, without any intermediary (**FIGURE 2-6**). As an example, suppose the driver of a vehicle involved in a motor vehicle collision has **hepatitis** C and is bleeding uncontrollably from an arm injury. The EMT caring for the patient will need to make contact with the blood to control the patient's bleeding. The EMT has a small unnoticed cut on their own arm, which comes into direct contact with the patient's bleeding arm. As the EMT touches

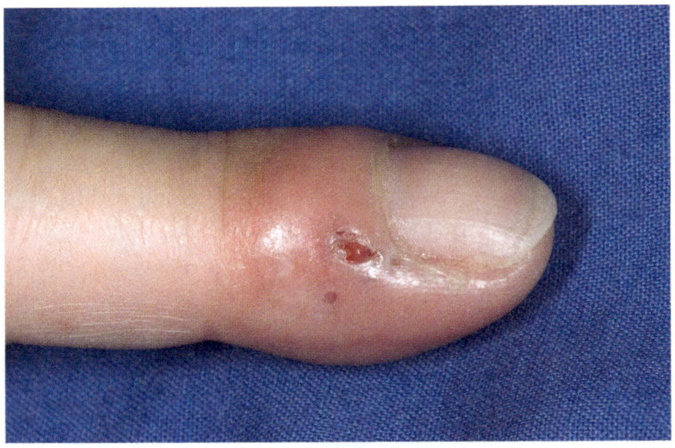

FIGURE 2-6 Finger infection resulting from not wearing gloves during contact with a patient.

the patient, the hepatitis C virus moves from the patient's blood into the EMT's body through the cut on their arm, thus infecting them. This is an example of direct contact, where blood is the vehicle. **Bloodborne pathogens** are microorganisms that are present in human blood and can cause disease in humans. Another example of transmission through direct contact is sexual transmission, in which the virus is transferred via body fluids such as semen and vaginal fluids. Some viruses, such as the **human immunodeficiency virus (HIV),** can be transmitted by multiple means, including both bloodborne and sexual transmission.

Indirect contact involves the spread of infection from the patient with an infection to another person through an inanimate object. The object that transmits the infection is called a *fomite*. Using the same patient from the previous example, as the EMT was caring for the patient, suppose some blood got onto the ambulance stretcher. If the stretcher is not properly cleaned afterward, the virus will remain on the stretcher and can be transmitted to someone else days later.

Words of Wisdom

Fungi are small, plantlike organisms such as yeast. Fungi cause many common conditions such as athlete's foot and jock itch. Protozoa are single-cell, animal-like microorganisms. Protozoa cause diseases such as malaria. Helminths are worms such as roundworms, pinworms, and hookworms. These worms are parasites that can infect people and cause serious health problems.

Needlesticks are another example of how infection spreads through indirect contact. In this case, the virus moves from the patient to the needle to the health care clinician. This route of transmission was more common many years ago, before the advent of safety equipment such as needleless intravenous systems.

Airborne transmission involves spreading an infectious agent through mechanisms such as droplets or dust. The common cold is caused by more than 200 different viruses, with the most common being rhinoviruses.[33] These viruses move from person to person by coughing and sneezing. Interestingly, when a person sneezes, the moisture from the airway moves forcefully and quickly through a narrow opening. If the moisture droplets are large, they travel short distances and can be involved in direct contact transmission. If the moisture droplets are tiny, they are turned into an airborne particle and can float in the air for long distances. Sneezing can actually transmit disease through direct contact *and* airborne routes (**FIGURE 2-7**). When the virus lands on a surface, it can survive for some time. If someone touches the surface and then touches their face or mouth, infection can occur via indirect contact.

Words of Wisdom

A type of coronavirus known as severe acute respiratory syndrome coronavirus 2 (SARS-CoV-2) was responsible for the coronavirus disease 2019 (COVID-19) pandemic. Its transmission occurs through airborne droplets, including those produced from coughing or sneezing.

Because of indirect contact transmission, it is unsanitary to use your hands to cover a cough or sneeze because the organisms travel onto your hands. If you then touch a cellphone, doorknob, or patient, the organisms will travel. Using a tissue to cover your mouth and nose when coughing or

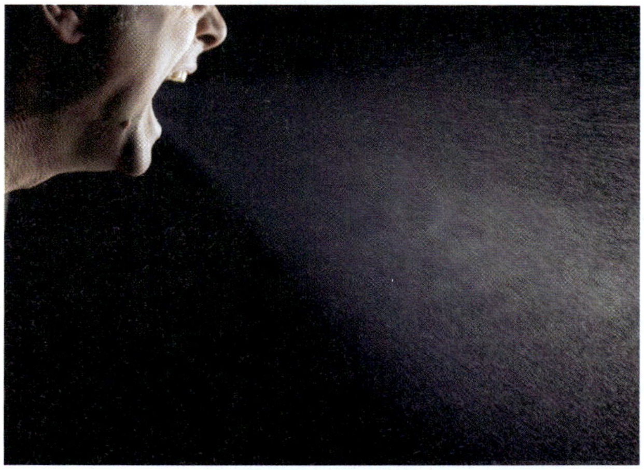

FIGURE 2-7 Coughing and sneezing create droplets and aerosols.

sneezing is better for controlling the spread of organisms.[34] You should then throw the tissue away and wash your hands with soap and water for at least 20 seconds or use an alcohol-based hand sanitizer. Remember, if you place the used tissue in your pocket, the tissue may repeatedly spread organisms to your hand, which your hand would then pass on to other surfaces. If you do not have a tissue, one of the best techniques to avoid contaminating your hands is to cough or sneeze into the crook of your elbow. Because you do not touch objects with your inner arms, the risk of moving organisms to an object or person is reduced (**FIGURE 2-8**).

Foodborne transmission involves the contamination of food or water with an organism that can cause disease. When food is prepared, it is important to ensure raw meats do not come into contact with other foods to prevent the spread of bacteria. It is also important that food is prepared and stored properly at all times to minimize the possibility of illness. Proper cleaning of food preparation surfaces before and after use also helps to decrease the likelihood of transmitting foodborne bacteria.

Vector-borne transmission involves the spread of infection by animals or insects that carry an organism from one person or place to another. An example of this method of transmission is the bubonic plague, which occurred in Europe and Asia in the Middle Ages. In the 14th century, this disease killed more than 25 million people in Europe alone.[35] This bacterial disease was caused by infected fleas that live on rats. As the rats moved, so did their fleas, carrying the bubonic plague. Other vector-borne diseases include avian influenza, rabies, and Lyme disease.

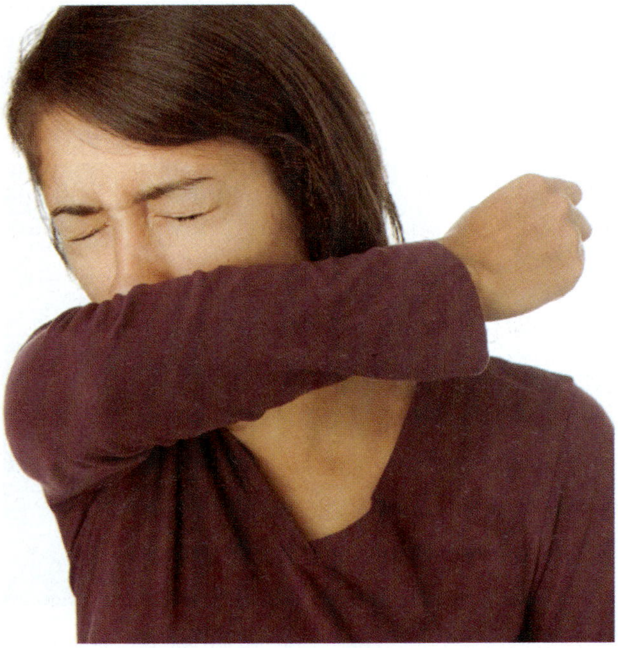

FIGURE 2-8 Coughing or sneezing into a tissue or your inner arm helps minimize the spread of germs.

Standard Precautions

The **Occupational Safety and Health Administration (OSHA)** develops and publishes guidelines concerning reducing hazards in the workplace. It is also responsible for enforcing these guidelines. OSHA requires all EMTs to be trained in handling bloodborne pathogens and in approaching a patient who may have an infectious or communicable disease. Training must be provided for issues including blood and body fluid precautions, airborne precautions, and contamination precautions.

Because health care workers are exposed to so many different types of infections, the CDC developed a set of **standard precautions** for health care workers to use in treating patients. Standard precautions are protective measures designed to prevent health care workers from coming into contact with objects, blood, body fluids, and other potential risks that could lead to exposure to germs. The CDC recommendation is to assume that every person is potentially infected or can spread an organism that could be transmitted in the health care setting[36]; therefore, you must apply **infection control** procedures to reduce infection in patients and other health care personnel. OSHA refers to the same concept using the term *universal precautions*. **TABLE 2-2** summarizes the CDC recommendations. You must also notify your **designated officer** if you are exposed.

Proper Hand Hygiene

Proper handwashing is the simplest yet most effective way to control disease transmission (**FIGURE 2-9**). You should always wash your hands before and after contact with a patient, even if you wear gloves. The longer the germs remain with you, the greater the chance they will get through your barriers. Any breaks in the skin such as tiny cuts and abrasions are potential access points for pathogens.

TABLE 2-2 Standard Precautions for the Care of All Patients, Including Those With Confirmed or Suspected COVID-19, in All Health Care Settings—Centers for Disease Control and Prevention

Component	Recommendations
Hand hygiene	• Perform after touching blood, body fluids, secretions, excretions, or contaminated items. • Perform immediately after removing gloves. • Perform between patient contacts. • For patients with highly communicable diseases, use an alcohol-based hand rub before putting on gloves.
Personal Protective Equipment (PPE)	
Gloves	• Wear if there is a possibility of touching blood, body fluids, secretions, excretions, or contaminated items. • Wear if touching mucous membranes and nonintact skin. • Wear for any patient contact involving a suspected communicable disease.
Gown	• Wear during procedures and patient care activities when contact of the EMT's clothing/exposed skin to blood, body fluids, secretions, excretions, or contaminated items is anticipated, particularly in the context of a communicable disease outbreak.
Mask, eye protection, face shield	• Wear during procedures and patient care activities likely to generate splashes or sprays of blood, body fluids, secretions, or excretions. Examples include suctioning or endotracheal intubation. • For patients with a communicable respiratory disease, N95 or higher masks, elastomeric half-piece respirators, or powered air-purifying respirators (PAPRs), are acceptable. A face shield or goggles are also required to avoid droplets getting into the eyes during high-risk activities.
Patient Care Environment	
Soiled patient care equipment	• Wear utility gloves when decontaminating equipment. • Handle equipment in a manner that prevents transfer of microorganisms to others and the environment. • Practice hand hygiene after removing gloves.
Environmental controls	• Have procedures for the routine care, cleaning, and disinfection of environmental surfaces. • Pay special attention to frequently touched surfaces within the ambulance (eg, handrails, seats, cabinets, doors).
Textiles and laundry	• Handle in a manner that prevents transfer of microorganisms to others and to the environment.
Needles and other sharp objects	• Do not recap, bend, break, or hand-manipulate used needles. • Use safety features when available (needleless intravenous systems). • Place sharps in puncture-resistant containers.
Special Circumstances	
Patient resuscitation	• Use a bag-mask device or other ventilation devices to prevent contact with mouth and oral secretions.
Respiratory hygiene/cough etiquette	• Instruct symptomatic patients to cover mouth/nose when sneezing or coughing. • If concern exists regarding the patient's ability to control spread of respiratory secretions, place a surgical mask on the patient. • If a mask cannot be used, maintain physical distance of at least 6 feet (1.8 m) if possible.

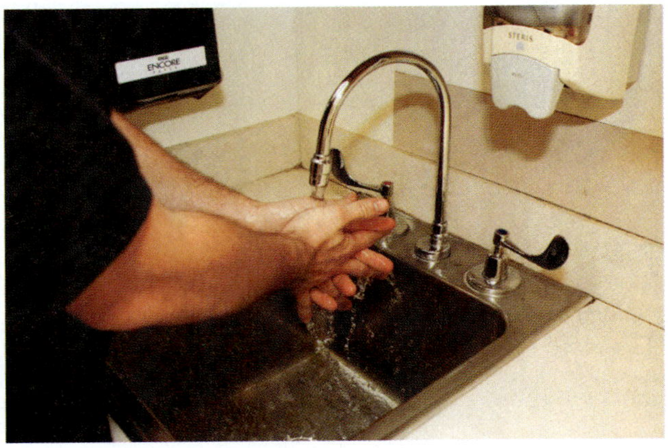

FIGURE 2-9 When washing your hands, rub your hands together for at least 20 seconds to work up a lather. Pay particular attention to your fingernails, the areas between fingers, and the back of the hands.

Words of Wisdom

In some cases when standard N95 masks are not available or long periods of care for a highly infectious patient are needed, a powered air-purifying respirator (PAPR) may be used. A PAPR provides positive airflow into a loose-fitting hood or tight-fitting facepiece through a filter or cartridge powered by a battery. Although these devices are often more comfortable to work in than the standard goggles and masks, they are expensive, take considerable room to store, and require special training. PAPRs may also limit the EMT's ability to have a full field of vision and to hear using a stethoscope. For these reasons, the PAPR is typically deployed only to special response teams in EMS systems rather than being readily available on every ambulance.

Although soap and water are not protective in all cases, in certain cases they provide excellent protection against further transmission from your skin to others.

Rinse your hands using warm water. If running water is not available, you may use waterless handwashing substitutes (**FIGURE 2-10**). These solutions can prevent many potential bacterial infections. If you use a waterless substitute in the field, make sure you wash your hands using soap and water as soon as possible. Finally, dry your hands with a paper towel, and use the paper towel to turn off the faucet.

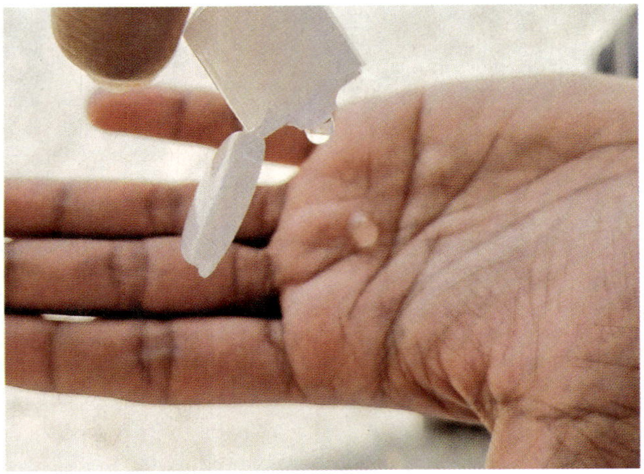

FIGURE 2-10 Use a waterless handwashing solution if running water is not available. Be sure to wash your hands with soap and water as soon as possible.

Safety Tips

Keep in mind that alcohol-based hand sanitizers do not kill some bacteria (eg, *Clostridioides difficile*), emphasizing the need to wear gloves and thoroughly wash the hands with soap and water as soon as possible.[37]

Gloves

Gloves and eye protection are the minimum standard for all patient care if there is any possibility of exposure to blood or body fluids. Vinyl, nitrile, and latex gloves provide adequate protection. Your department may prefer one type of glove over the other, or you may have the freedom to choose for yourself. You should evaluate each situation and choose the glove that works best. (Some patients and EMTs are allergic to latex. If you suspect you are allergic, consult your supervisor for options.) Vinyl gloves may be best for situations with minimal patient contact or nonsterile procedures, and nitrile or latex gloves may be best for invasive procedures where sterility is required. Change gloves if they have been exposed to motor oil, gasoline, or any petroleum-based product. Do not use petroleum jelly with latex gloves because it will degrade the latex's integrity. Wear double gloves if there is substantial bleeding. You may also wear double gloves if you will be exposed to large volumes of

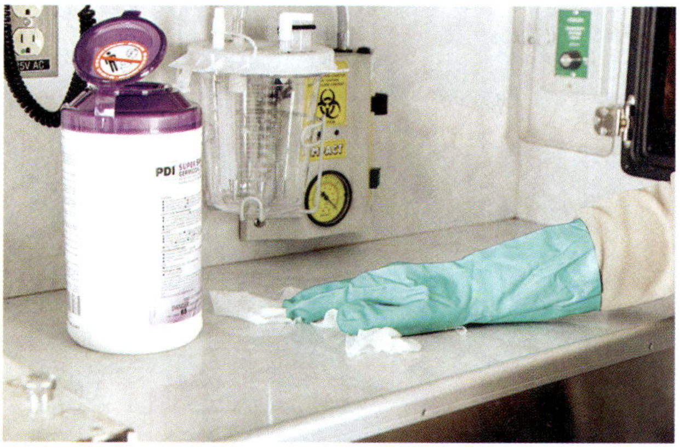

FIGURE 2-11 Use heavy-duty utility gloves to clean the unit. You should not use lightweight latex or vinyl gloves for cleaning.

other body fluids. Be sure to change gloves as you move from patient to patient. For cleaning and disinfecting the ambulance, you should use heavy-duty utility gloves (**FIGURE 2-11**). You should never use lightweight latex or vinyl gloves for cleaning.

Removing used latex or nitryl gloves requires following a methodical technique to avoid contaminating yourself with the materials on the outside of the gloves (**SKILL DRILL 2-1**).

1. Begin by removing one glove. With your other gloved hand, pinch the first glove at the wrist—being certain to touch only the outside of the first glove—and start to roll it back off your hand, inside out (**Step 1**).
2. Hold the removed glove in your gloved hand (**Step 2**).
3. To remove the second glove, slide two fingers of your bare hand inside the remaining glove at the wrist (**Step 3**).
4. Gently stretch the glove away from the hand and pull the glove off, keeping it inside out. The first glove remains inside the second glove (**Step 4**).
5. If possible, dispose of the gloves in a biohazard container or a sealed plastic bag. If one is not available, dispose in a trash can. Wash your hands with soap and running water. If they are not available, use an alcohol-based hand sanitizer.

Gloves are the most common type of PPE. In many EMS rescue operations, you must also protect your hands and wrists from injury. You may wear puncture-proof leather gloves, with latex gloves underneath. This combination will allow you free use of your hands with added protection from blood and body fluids. Remember that soiled latex or nitryl gloves are considered medical waste and must be disposed of properly. Leather gloves must be treated as contaminated material until they can be properly decontaminated.

Safety Tips

The daily physical and environmental conditions of your job can take a toll on your body. You can help safeguard your health by dressing appropriately and taking certain actions. Proper footwear is extremely important. Boots should be resistant to water penetration, punctures, and slip hazards. Because you will be on your feet all day, they should also be comfortable! Also consider your long-term health by wearing sunglasses and sunscreen to protect against exposure to ultraviolet light and wearing hearing protection (eg, foam earplugs) when working in noisy environments for extended periods.

Other protective clothing may be needed based on your job assignment. Examples include specialized cold weather gear, turnout gear (bunker gear) to protect against heat or fire, firefighting gloves to prevent hand injuries, and helmets with top and side protection and a chin strap in areas where falling objects may present a hazard.

Eye Protection and Face Shields

Eye protection is important in preventing blood or airborne droplets from entering your eyes (**FIGURE 2-12**). Blood splatters are a significant possibility in most trauma situations, and airborne droplets can cause disease transmission in many viral infections such as COVID-19. Wearing goggles or a full face shield is your best protection. Clinicians who wear prescription eyeglasses will also need additional protection for their eyes. Prescription eyeglasses offer insufficient side protection and are not considered appropriate for PPE. Contact lenses do not offer any added protection from splashing. Face shields will also provide good eye protection (**FIGURE 2-13**).

Gowns

Occasionally, you may need to wear a gown. A gown provides protection from extensive blood or other

Skill Drill 2-1 Proper Glove Removal Technique

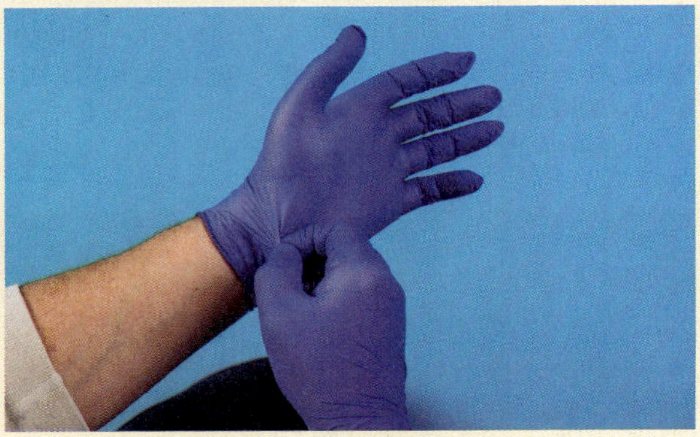

Step 1

Begin by removing one glove. Pinch one glove on the outside near the wrist.

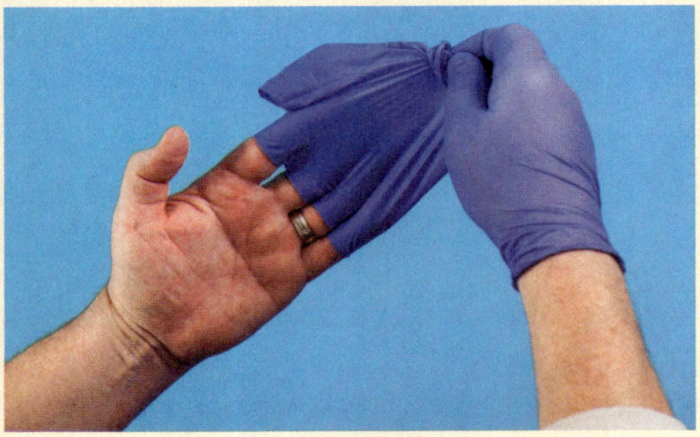

Step 2

Gently pull the glove off, turning it inside out as you pull with the hand that is still gloved. Hold the removed glove in your gloved hand.

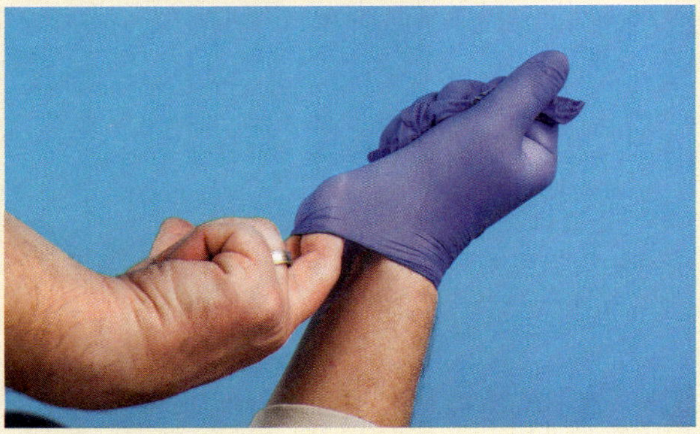

Step 3

To remove the second glove, slide two fingers of your bare hand inside the remaining glove at the wrist.

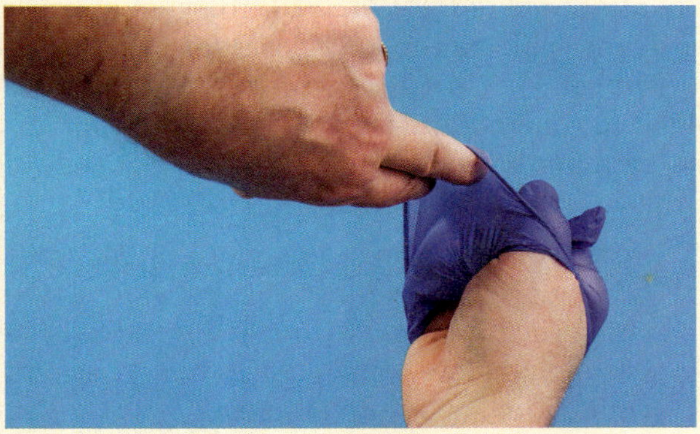

Step 4

Gently stretch the glove away from the hand and pull the glove off, keeping it inside out. The first glove remains inside the second glove.

body fluids splatter. Gowns may be worn in situations such as an **aerosol-generating procedure (AGP)** such as endotracheal intubation, field delivery of a baby, or major trauma. Your department will likely have a policy regarding gowns. Be sure you know your local policy. There are times when a change of uniform is preferred because trying to clean off contaminants is difficult and sometimes impossible without professional cleaning and disinfection; sometimes the uniform must be disposed of entirely.

Masks, Respirators, and Barrier Devices

Wearing masks is a complex issue. You should wear a standard surgical mask if blood or body fluid spatter is a possibility. If you suspect a patient has

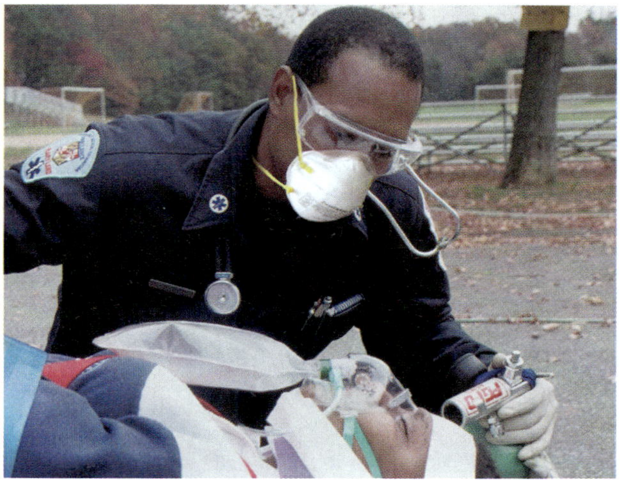

FIGURE 2-12 Wear eye protection with side shields to prevent blood splatter or airborne droplets from entering your eyes.

© Jones & Bartlett Learning. Courtesy of MIEMSS.

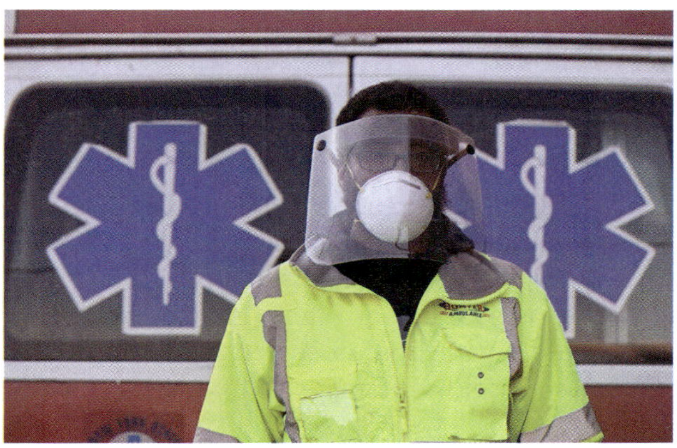

FIGURE 2-13 The surgical mask/face shield combination.

© Sipa USA/Alamy Stock Photo.

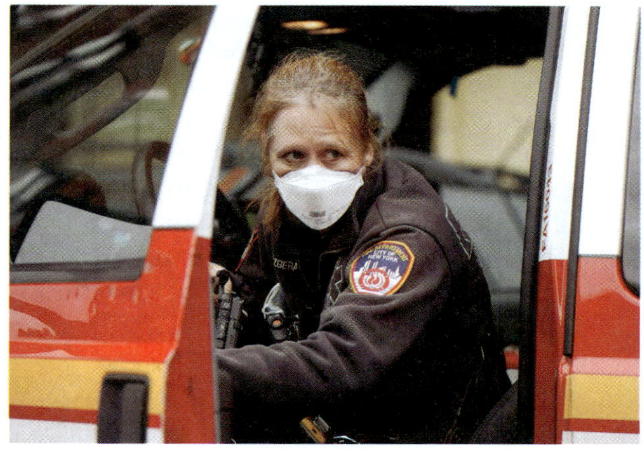

FIGURE 2-14 Wear a particulate respirator to protect yourself from airborne disease transmission.

© John Minchillo/AP Photo.

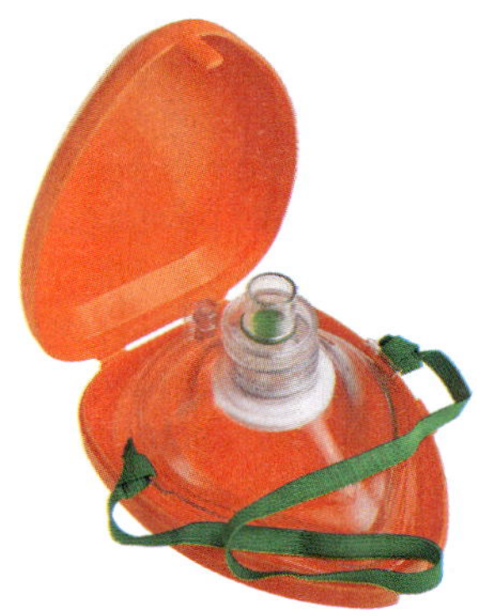

FIGURE 2-15 Barrier devices such as a pocket mask provide protection when providing mouth-to-mask ventilation. These devices should not be used, however, if there is active community spread of virus by airborne route.

© Bart J/ShutterStock.

an airborne- or droplet-spread disease such as tuberculosis or influenza, or in situations such as the COVID-19 pandemic, place a surgical mask on the patient and a particulate air respirator, such as an N95 mask, on yourself (**FIGURE 2-14**). Protective eyewear using safety glasses with side shields, goggles, or a full face shield is also needed. If the patient needs oxygen, place a nonrebreathing mask instead of a surgical mask on the patient and set the oxygen flow rate at 10 to 15 L/min. Do not place a particulate respirator on the patient; it is unnecessary and uncomfortable. A simple surgical mask will reduce the risk of transmission of germs from the patient into the air. Use of a particulate respirator should comply with OSHA standards, which state facial hair, such as long sideburns or a mustache, must be trimmed so it does not prevent a proper fit.[38] Particulate respirators must be fit-tested to ensure their efficacy.

Although there are no documented cases of disease transmission to rescuers as a result of performing unprotected mouth-to-mouth resuscitation on a patient with an infection, you should use a pocket mask if a bag-mask device is not readily available (**FIGURE 2-15**). Neither mouth-to-mouth nor mouth-to-mask resuscitation are recommended in a situation where there is an active community spread of a virus that can be transmitted by airborne route. Bag-mask ventilation is an AGP that requires use of a HEPA filter on the exhalation valve in epidemic scenarios such as COVID-19.

Remember, the outside surfaces of these devices are considered contaminated after they have been exposed to the patient. You must make sure gloves, masks, gowns, and all other PPE items that have been exposed to infectious processes or blood are properly disposed of according to local guidelines. If you are stuck by a needle, get blood or body fluids in your eye, or have significant body fluid contact with the patient, immediately report the incident to your supervisor.

Safety Tips

Putting on (donning) and taking off (doffing) the full complement of PPE in a consistent sequence is essential to reduce the risk of contamination. Although there are some variations, and additional PPE used in certain situations, the most common components of PPE are a mask, eyewear or full face shield, gloves, and gown. To ensure proper donning and doffing, the EMT should have a partner observe and assist with the process.

- **Donning PPE.** Always don the PPE in the same order based on your departmental policies.
  1. Apply the gown and secure the ties at the neck and waist.
  2. Put on the N95 mask and ensure there is a tight seal.
  3. Don appropriate wraparound eyewear, goggles, or full face shield.
  4. Don gloves last. Be sure to pull the cuffs up and over the sleeves of your gown.
- **Doffing PPE.** Regardless of the process used to doff PPE, the mask is the last item to be removed. Remove PPE carefully to ensure you do not contaminate yourself.
  1. Take off gloves as described previously and discard.
  2. Remove eye protection from the back, tilting it forward to remove. Decontaminate it later.
  3. Remove the gown by reaching around and untying it or breaking the ties. Then pull your arms out while pulling the gown inside out, being careful not to touch the contaminated side of the gown. Discard the gown and then clean your hands with an alcohol-based hand sanitizer.
  4. To remove the mask, reach around the back and pull the bottom strap over your head, then remove the top strap to pull the mask away from your face. Discard the mask and clean your hands again thoroughly.

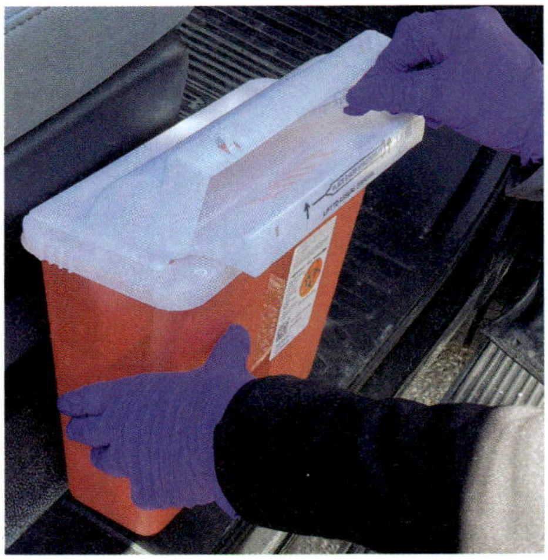

FIGURE 2-16 Properly dispose of sharps in a closed, rigid, marked container.

Proper Disposal of Sharps

Be careful when handling needles, scalpels, and other sharp items. The spread of HIV and hepatitis C in the health care setting can usually be traced back to careless handling of sharps.

- Do not recap, break, or bend needles. Even the most careful clinicians may expose themselves through an accidental needlestick.
- Dispose of all sharp items that have been in contact with human secretions in approved, closed, rigid containers (**FIGURE 2-16**).

Employer Responsibilities

While your employer cannot guarantee a 100% risk-free environment, you have a right to know about diseases that may pose a risk to you. OSHA regulations, especially for private and federal agencies, require that all employees be offered a workplace environment that reduces the risk for exposure. Note that in some states that have their own OSHA plans, state and municipal employees must also be covered.

In addition to OSHA guidelines, other national guidelines and standards, including those from the CDC and the National Fire Protection Agency, address reducing the risk of exposure to bloodborne pathogens and airborne diseases. These agencies set a standard of care for all fire and EMS personnel, and this standard applies whether you are a full-time paid employee or a volunteer. It is your responsibility to know your department's infection control plan and to use it. The plan may include the following components:

- Determination of exposure risk (describes people at risk and situations posing risk)
- Education and training (outlines how clinicians will receive safety instruction)
- PPE (lists availability and intended use of PPE items)
- Cleaning and disinfection practices (describes how to maintain vehicles and equipment)
- Immunization guidelines and testing policies (outlines frequency and methods of administering relevant immunizations and infection testing)
- Postexposure management (identifies whom to notify in case of exposure and proper response procedures)
- Compliance monitoring (describes how the department will ensure adherence to safety policies)
- Communication of hazards to employees (ensures employees receive initial and annual updates regarding exposure concerns and safety recommendations)
- Record keeping (lists documentation that must be retained, who is responsible for managing it, and who may access it)

Establishing an Infection Control Routine

Infection control should be an important part of your daily routine. Follow the steps in **SKILL DRILL 2-2** to manage potential exposure situations:

1. En route to the scene, make sure PPE is out and available (**Step 1**).
2. On arrival, identify and address safety hazards, then perform a rapid scan of the patient, noting whether any blood or body fluids are present.

Skill Drill 2-2 Managing a Potential Exposure

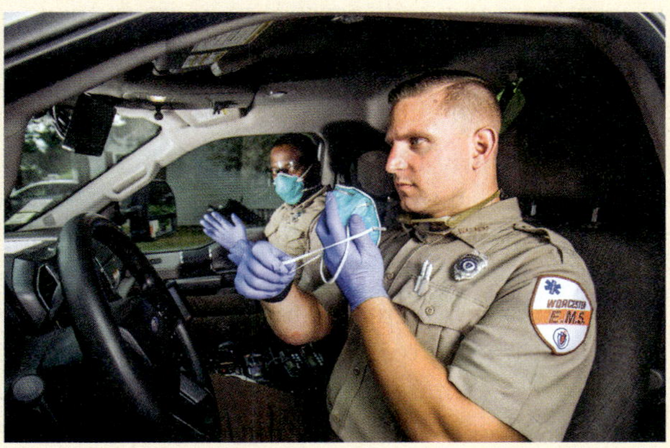

Step 1

En route to the scene, make sure that PPE is out and available to don when you arrive at the scene.

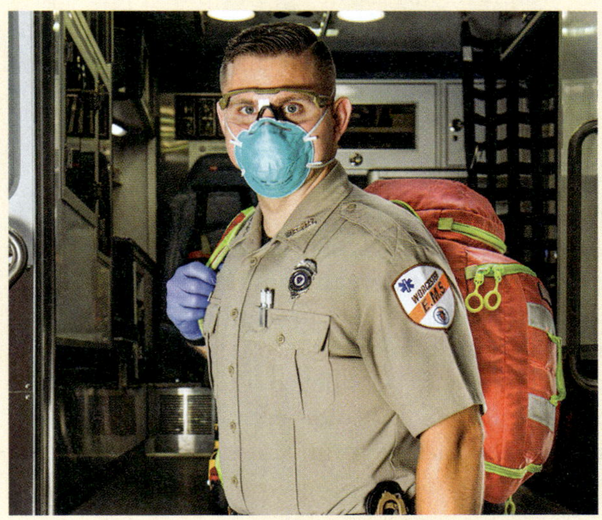

Step 2

On arrival, identify and address safety hazards, then perform a rapid scan of the patient, noting whether any blood or body fluids are present. Select the proper PPE according to the tasks you are likely to perform. Typically, gloves and protective eyewear will be used for all patient contacts.

3. Select the proper PPE according to the tasks you are likely to perform. Typically, gloves and protective eyewear will be used for all patient contacts (**Step 2**). A disposable gown and masks are often required during epidemic or pandemic situations, and the type of mask will depend on the transmission mode of the relevant pathogen.
4. Change gloves or remove the topmost layer of gloves if wearing multiple layers of gloves.
5. Wash hands or at the very least use hand sanitizer between patients; don PPE as quickly as possible to minimize time spent before initiating care. Remove gloves and other gear after contact with the patient, unless you are in the patient compartment. Remember that good hand hygiene is always necessary.
6. Limit the number of people who are involved in patient care if there are multiple injuries and a substantial amount of blood at the scene.
7. If you or your partner is exposed while providing care, try to relieve one another as soon as possible so that you can seek care, including basic first aid care such as cleaning and dressing a wound. Notify the designated officer and report the incident. This will also help to maintain confidentiality for both the patient and yourself.

Cleaning and Decontaminating the Ambulance and Equipment

Be sure to routinely clean the ambulance after each run and on a daily basis. Cleaning is an essential part of the prevention and control of communicable diseases, ensuring removal of surface organisms that may remain in the unit. You should clean your unit as quickly as possible so it can be returned to service. Address the high-contact areas, including surfaces that were in direct contact with the patient's blood or body fluids or surfaces that you touched while caring for the patient after having contact with the patient's blood or body fluids.

Any reusable medical equipment should be properly cleaned and sterilized per your department's standard operating procedures. Keep in mind that in hospitals, entire departments are devoted to sterilizing medical instruments. Proper sterilization requires the right tools and the right skills, so always carefully follow your department's procedures.

Learn the regulations defining medical waste in your area. The disposal of infectious waste, such as needles, sharps, and heavily soiled dressings, may vary from hospital to hospital and from state to state.

Maintaining Disease Immunity

Even if pathogens do reach you, you are not necessarily at risk for infection. For example, you may be **immune**, or resistant, to those particular germs. Immunity is a major factor in determining whether a **host** (the organism or the individual who is attacked by the infecting agent) will become ill from a particular germ (**TABLE 2-3**). One way to gain immunity from many diseases is to be immunized, or vaccinated, against them. Vaccinations have nearly eliminated some childhood diseases in the United States, such as measles and polio.

Another way in which the body becomes immune to a disease is when it recovers from an infection from that germ. Afterward, the body's immune system recognizes and repels that pathogen when it shows up again. After healthy people are exposed, lifelong immunity to many common pathogens will develop. For example, a person who contracts and becomes infected with the hepatitis A virus may be ill for several weeks, but because immunity will develop, the person will not get the illness again;

YOU are the EMT

The patient is an 86-year-old man who is apneic and pulseless. You note there is vomitus with blood near the patient's head. You and your partner are joined by another ALS crew. After performing resuscitative measures for more than 30 minutes, the team determines that termination of resuscitation is most appropriate. Resuscitation is stopped and a paramedic from the other crew calls medical control for the time of death. Your paramedic partner delivers the death notification to the patient's spouse and you start to clean up the scene.

4. What precautions should you take while cleaning up the scene?

TABLE 2-3 Immunity to Infectious Diseases

Type of Immunity	Characteristics	Examples	Comments
Lifelong	The illness will not recur.	Measles Mumps Polio Rubella Hepatitis A Hepatitis B	Infection or vaccination provides long-term immunity from getting a new infection. A live vaccine is required only for measles.
Partial	The person who has recovered from a first infection is unlikely to get a new infection from another person, but illness may develop from germs that lie dormant from the initial infection.	Chickenpox Tuberculosis	Infection or vaccination provides lifelong immunity to the patient from acquiring a new infection, but the original illness may reoccur, or it may reoccur in a different way. In the case of chickenpox, which is caused by the herpes zoster virus, an infection may reoccur years later in the form of shingles.
None	Exposure confers no protection from reinfection. The infection may wear down the patient's resistance.	Gonorrhea Syphilis Human immunodeficiency virus	No vaccine is available. Repeated infections are common. For example, there is effective immediate treatment for gonorrhea, and the germs may be eradicated; however, reinfection is likely if the high-risk practices continue (eg, unprotected sex). For syphilis, the lack of immunity allows the germs to continue to cause damage within the host.
Other/unknown	Some viruses change from year to year, making it difficult to develop vaccines or innate immunity.	Influenza virus strains	Although a vaccine is available for influenza and SARS-CoV-2 viruses, researchers must predict which strains will be prevalent 1 year or more in advance. This means that if a new strain occurs, the vaccine will not provide full protection in the community.
	In other cases, virus strains are new and little is known about them.	SARS-CoV-2 virus	In the case of a new virus, there will be many unknowns. Initially there will be no vaccine. Additionally, it takes time to know if having the disease or getting the vaccine confers temporary or lifelong immunity.

Abbreviation: SARS-CoV-2, severe acute respiratory syndrome coronavirus 2

however, sometimes the immunity is only partial. Although partial immunity protects against new infections, pathogens that remain in the body from the first illness still may be able to cause the same disease again when the body is stressed or has some impairment in its immune system. For example, tuberculosis can cause a mild, unnoticeable infection before the body builds up a partial immunity. If the infection is never treated, the infection may be reactivated when immunity is weakened; however, these people are protected against a new infection from another person. Humans seem unable to mount an effective immune response to some infections, such as HIV, which is an infection that can progress to acquired immunodeficiency syndrome (AIDS).

Remember, germs that cause no symptoms in one person may cause serious illness in another.

Immunizations and Testing

As an EMT, you are at risk for acquiring an infectious or communicable disease. Using basic protective measures can minimize the risk. You are responsible for protecting yourself, so take an active role in achieving that goal.

Prevention begins by maintaining your personal health. Annual health examinations should be required for all EMS personnel. A history of all your childhood infectious diseases should be recorded and kept on file. Childhood infectious diseases include chickenpox, mumps, measles, rubella, and whooping cough. You must be immunized against these diseases unless you already had the disease or have previously been vaccinated against it.

OSHA has developed requirements for protection from occupational exposure to bloodborne pathogens and needlesticks. Each employer whose employees may reasonably be expected to come in contact with blood or other potentially infectious materials must create an infection control plan designed to minimize occupational exposure. As part of these requirements, employers are required to offer the hepatitis B vaccine at no cost to employees with risk of occupational exposure. Employees who decline the vaccine must sign a waiver indicating their refusal to take the vaccine and may later decide to take the vaccine at the employer's expense. Furthermore, the CDC recommends the following immunizations for health care workers[39]:

- Hepatitis B (required by OSHA)
- Influenza (yearly)
- COVID-19 (yearly)
- Measles, mumps, and rubella (MMR) (typically a one-time vaccination)
- Varicella (chickenpox) vaccine or having had chickenpox
- Tetanus, diphtheria, pertussis (Tdap) (every 10 years)

Most of these vaccinations are given to infants and children as part of their routine series of immunizations. It is imperative that you keep all these vaccinations up to date to help protect you as well as your family and patients. Health care workers who are routinely exposed to meningitis (often those who work in an institutional setting) should receive one dose of meningococcal vaccine. Although hepatitis A immunization is not required by OSHA, you may consider vaccination as a preventive measure. Hepatitis A vaccination is not necessary if you have had hepatitis A in the past. All these vaccines are effective and rarely cause side effects.

You should also have a skin test for tuberculosis before you begin working as an EMT. The purpose of this test is to identify anyone who has been exposed to tuberculosis in the past. Testing should be repeated if there is an exposure to tuberculosis and at intervals recommended by your agency or state.[40]

General Postexposure Management

The likelihood that you will become infected during routine patient care is low. In the event that you are exposed to blood or other body substances despite all of your precautions, there are still measures that you can take to protect your health. If you are exposed to a patient's blood or body fluids, you should first turn over patient care to another EMS clinician. When it is safe to do so, clean the exposed area with soap and water. If your eyes were exposed, rinse them with water for at least 20 minutes as soon as possible.

Next, activate your department's infection control plan. This usually involves contacting a supervisor or your department's infection control officer to assist you. This person will help you to navigate the postexposure protocols.

You will need to be screened to determine whether there was a significant exposure to possible bloodborne pathogens. Just because you were exposed to a patient's blood or body fluids does not mean that there is a risk of infection. Typically, you will need a follow-up evaluation by a physician to determine whether a significant exposure occurred. If the exposure was significant, blood may be drawn from both you and the patient to determine whether any infectious agents were present.

You will have to complete an exposure report. Questions in the report may include: When did the event happen? What were you doing when you were exposed? What PPE were you wearing? What did you do after you were exposed? Completing this paperwork will help relay critical information to the right people, resulting in help for you and possibly new protocols to help prevent another incident in the future.

Time is important! If you are exposed, let your supervisor or infection control officer know immediately. Some diseases will act quickly, whereas others may lie dormant for a long time. The best way to reduce your risk of contracting a work-related disease is through early activation of your department's infection control plan.

In the case of diseases spread in the air or by droplets, you may not realize you have been exposed to the disease until the hospital notifies you. If you were wearing full PPE including gloves, gown, eye protection, and N95 mask, no further follow-up may be needed. In other cases, specific postexposure care or prophylaxis may be indicated. In the event that you have been exposed to COVID-19 without proper PPE, the CDC currently does not require work restrictions unless symptoms develop or you test positive for SARS-CoV-2.[41]

Postexposure Prophylaxis and Treatment for Significant Exposure

The last defense for an EMT who has had a significant exposure to an infectious disease is postexposure preventive measures or treatment. Unfortunately, these are not available for all diseases and are only offered if an investigation determines that you have had a significant exposure. Postexposure treatment for HIV includes treatment with a specific combination of antiretroviral medications. In the case of hepatitis B exposure, you will be tested to see if you already have antibodies if you have been vaccinated for the disease. If you have antibodies, no treatment is needed. If you do not have antibodies, you will receive an injection with hepatitis B immune globulin, which contains antibodies that will attack the virus in your body. However, this injection only confers temporary protection, so it is followed up with the series of three hepatitis B immunization shots. There is no treatment to prevent you from getting hepatitis C infection after an exposure. Follow-up blood testing will be conducted for 6 months to determine if you become infected.

Postexposure treatment for tuberculosis will not begin unless your tuberculin skin test is positive during the monitoring period. In those cases, a long period of treatment with oral antituberculin medicines will begin. A blood test to confirm the presence of tuberculosis will likely be performed prior to treatment.

There are very few infectious exposures for which you will receive antibiotics. Significant exposure to pertussis and some types of bacterial meningitis would be examples.

Street Smarts

You should be aware of the procedures you are required to follow if you are involved in an exposure during your clinical or field experience. If you do not know, ask your instructor immediately.

Additional Response Safety Considerations

The personal safety of all those involved in an emergency situation is important. In fact, it is so important that it is best that you internalize the steps necessary to preserve personal safety so these actions become automatic. You should begin protecting yourself as soon as you are dispatched. Before you leave the scene, begin preparing yourself mentally and physically. Make judicious use of lights and siren by weighing the risks and benefits like you would any clinical procedure. Wear seat belts, including both the lap belt and shoulder harness, en route to the scene whenever the vehicle is in motion, unless patient care makes doing so impossible (**FIGURE 2-17**). Many EMS units have mandatory

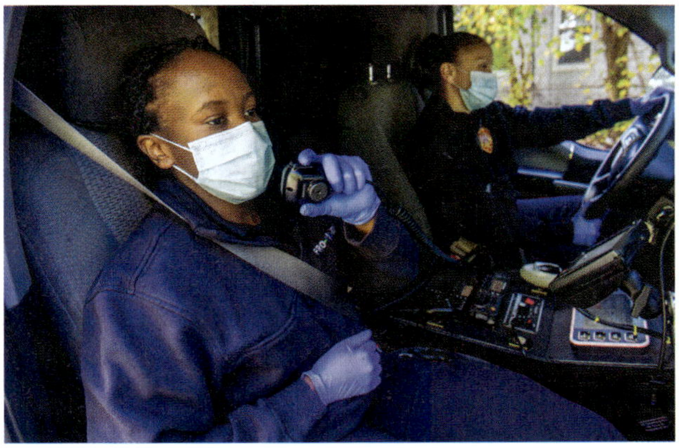

FIGURE 2-17 Wear seat belts whenever you are riding in the ambulance, including when you are responding on a call.

seat belt policies for the driver at all times, for all EMTs during transit to the scene, and for anyone who is riding with a patient. Don the appropriate PPE prior to departing the ambulance.

A scene that appears safe initially can develop into a hazardous situation at any moment. Be alert for any suspicious person or activity at the scene, because your first priority must be your own safety. A second accident at the scene or an injury to you or your partner creates more problems. Delays in emergency medical care for patients increase the burden on other EMTs and may result in unnecessary injury or death.

Safety Tips

An important safety measure is to always wear seat belts in the ambulance, including when you are en route to the scene and during transport.

The scene must be well marked (**FIGURE 2-18**). If law enforcement has not already done so, you should make sure the proper warning devices are placed at a sufficient distance from the scene to properly warn, slow, and divert oncoming traffic. This will alert motorists coming from both directions that a crash has occurred. When you must work in a traffic lane, park a heavy vehicle such as a fire engine (if available) in a position that blocks traffic in the lane where you are working. When working at night, you must have plenty of light. Poor lighting increases the risk of injury to both you and the patient. It also results in poor emergency medical care. Wearing a reflective vest or clothing will help to make you more visible at night and decrease your risk of injury (**FIGURE 2-19**). An ANSI-2 safety vest must be worn when working on a roadway, day or night.

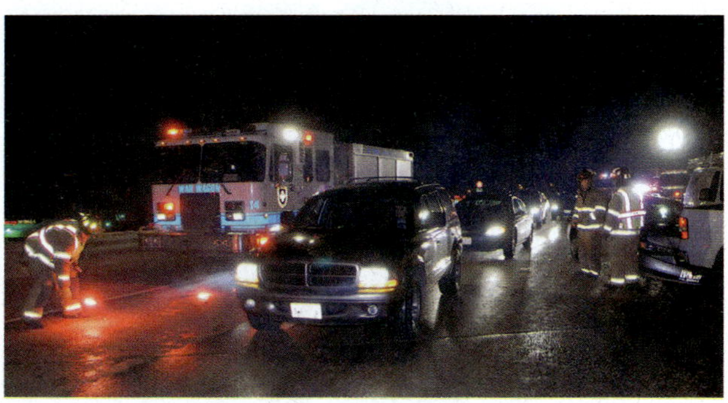

FIGURE 2-18 Make sure the crash scene is well marked to prevent a second crash that may damage emergency vehicles or result in injury to you, your partner, or the patient.

Certain types of emergency scenes may pose unique safety risks to responders. Guidance for working at these scenes is discussed in the following chapters:

- Chapter 36, *Transport Operations*, reviews safety precautions when driving to a scene or transporting a patient from a scene. It also outlines safe practices when helping with a helicopter landing or approaching a helicopter.
- Chapter 37, *Vehicle Extrication and Special Rescue*, discusses operations relating to particularly volatile scenes, such as those involving moving water, fire, or tactical response.
- Chapter 38, *Incident Management*, describes scenes involving disasters and hazardous materials, where the EMT may need to take special precautions and work within a larger system to remain safe and ensure the safety of others.
- Chapter 39, *Terrorism Response and Disaster Management*, discusses scenes with high

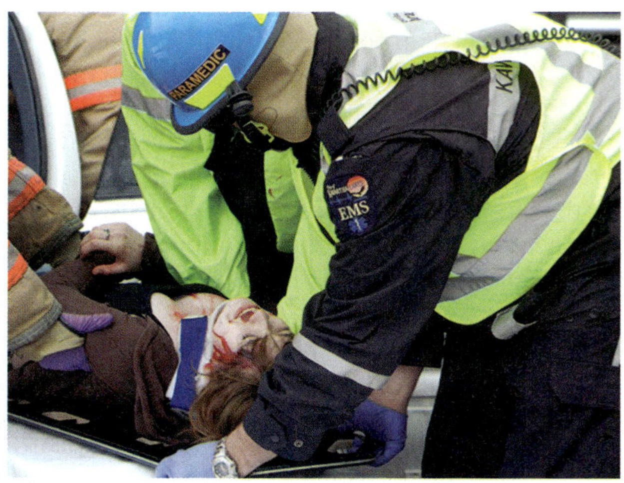

FIGURE 2-19 The American National Standards Institute (and International Safety Equipment Association) requires EMS personnel to wear reflective vests or clothing that meets class 2 or 3 standards on roadways. You can also wear emblems or clothing to help make you more visible at night and improve your safety in the dark.

potential for violence, including active shooters, weapons of mass destruction, and incidents involving biologic, nuclear, incendiary, chemical, and explosive threats.

Violence Against EMS Clinicians

In some cases, emergency responders might be the direct target of violence. The rate of violence-related injuries with work loss for emergency responders is 22 times higher than the overall rate for other employees in the United States.[42] Ensuring health and wellness in the face of violence against EMS clinicians demands strategies of prevention and strategies of protection.

Recommendations for the prevention of violence include the following:

- Training and practice in identifying scenes of potential violence
- Training and practice in deescalation strategies and techniques
- Training and practice to improve interpersonal communications
- Practice in ongoing scene assessment
- Dispatch identification and alerting of past or potential threats of violence

Recommendations for protection against violence include the following:

- Training and practice in self-defense and escape techniques
- Training and practice in physical restraint and sedation techniques
- Fitting and use of body armor
- Training and practice in operations with law enforcement personnel

EMTs who experience physical or verbal violence should report this on the appropriate incident form. Some electronic health records also have locations to report exposure to violence on a call. Follow your state laws and department policies to report instances of violence.

Inclusive Workplace Considerations

Cultivating an inclusive workplace is essential for the well-being and effectiveness of EMS teams. In an inclusive environment, all employees feel valued, respected, and able to contribute fully to their roles. Fostering inclusive work environments means no tolerance for discriminatory behaviors, bullying, or harassment. Instead of excluding those who are different, inclusive workplaces value and celebrate differences ensuring that all employees feel respected and supported. As an EMT, you directly contribute to your organizational culture and can help shape it.

Combatting Incivility in the Workplace

Incivility in the workplace refers to a broad range of rude or disrespectful behaviors that can create a hostile or unproductive atmosphere. Incivility can range from dismissive comments, gossip, or exclusionary tactics, to outright bullying. Such behaviors, some of which may be seemingly minor like teasing or practical jokes, can significantly affect team cohesion, communication, and morale. Even the perception of discrimination can weaken morale and motivation and negatively affect the goal of EMS. For EMTs, who rely on seamless collaboration and mutual support to effectively respond to emergencies, incivility can lead to safety concerns, decreased job satisfaction, and increased stress. In EMS, incivility has been linked to higher stress levels and increased likelihood of leaving the profession.[6] It is crucial for

YOU are the EMT

Later that evening, back at the station you find your partner alone in the dorm. You notice his eyes look as though he has been crying. After opening discussion, he tells you that he has been having relationship problems with his family and that his grandfather just passed away last week.

5. Discuss how the last call you went on might be a psychologically traumatizing event for your partner.

6. How can you help your partner?

EMS organizations to foster a culture of respect and professionalism, implementing clear policies and training to address and prevent incivility.

Street Smarts

The IQEE (Interrupt, Question, Educate, Echo) framework serves as a powerful tool to address and dismantle incivility.[43] When a rude or discriminatory comment is made, the process begins with *Interrupt*, where the harmful statement is stopped with a phrase such as, "Excuse me, can I clarify what I think I just heard?" Next is *Question*, which involves asking the person who made the remark to clarify their intention or the underlying meaning of their words. For example, "Tell me what you mean by . . ." *Educate* follows, where factual information is provided to correct misconceptions and promote awareness. You can say something like, "Here's what I know about . . ." Finally, *Echo* is a reminder to reinforce others' actions when you witness them advocating against incivility. This could be a simple expression of thanks for speaking up or sharing an experience. Addressing incivility in a respectful manner with open communication can help avoid defensive responses, where others close themselves off instead of learning.

Sexual Harassment

Sexual harassment is any unwelcome sexual advance, request for sexual favors, or other verbal or physical conduct of a sexual nature when submitting or rejecting is a basis for an employment decision, or such conduct substantially interferes with performance and/or creates a hostile or offensive work environment. There are two types of sexual harassment: quid pro quo, where the harasser requests sexual favors in exchange for something else (eg, a promotion), and hostile work environment, where the harasser engages in inappropriate, unwanted behaviors, such as making jokes, touching or leering, requesting a date, or talking about body parts.

It is important to recognize that the intent of the harasser does not matter. What matters is the perception of the act and the effect the behavior has on someone else. For many years, it was not uncommon to walk into a fire station and see sexually suggestive posters, calendars, or cartoons and to hear sexual jokes or comments. This situation has changed because it is not acceptable professional practice. If you have been harassed, you should report it to your supervisor and/or human resources department and keep notes of what happened and what was said.

Cultural Diversity on the Job

As our society grows more culturally diverse, so do EMS workplaces. You need to be able to work efficiently and effectively with other health care professionals from a variety of different backgrounds and whose beliefs may differ from your own. For many years, EMS and public safety have been disproportionately represented by Caucasian men. Currently 75% of EMS personnel are male and 85% identify as nonminority.[44] Nevertheless, efforts to improve diversity in the EMS workforce are growing. EMTs should expect to work alongside coworkers with varying backgrounds, attitudes, beliefs, and values and to accept their differences.

A diverse EMS workforce brings varied perspectives and cultural competencies, enabling clinicians to better understand and meet the needs of diverse patient populations through improved communication and increased trust. Working with colleagues who have backgrounds different from our own can help improve our **cultural competence**, the ability to deliver care in a way that meets the social, cultural, and linguistic needs of patients. Look at cultural diversity as an asset, and make the most of the differences among people in EMS, thus improving our ability to provide optimum patient care.

Cultural competence exists on a continuum with six stages[44]:

1. **Denial.** Lack of awareness that differences exist among cultures
2. **Defense.** Acknowledgment of differences but continued feelings of superiority for one's own culture
3. **Minimization.** Efforts to downplay the differences among cultures
4. **Acceptance.** Nonjudgmental recognition of cultural differences
5. **Adaptation.** Ability to adapt behavior to cultural differences to work within another culture effectively
6. **Integration.** Ability to move freely and comfortably between a variety of cultures

Cultural humility is an ongoing process in which a person remains curious about others and continuously reflects on their viewpoints with an open mind. This process allows a person to constantly monitor their attitudes toward others, remain aware of their biases, and adapt their viewpoints if needed.

Creating an inclusive workplace in EMS involves addressing incivility and sexual harassment while promoting and celebrating individuals' differences. By implementing clear policies, providing ongoing training, and fostering a culture of respect and inclusion, EMS organizations can ensure a supportive and productive environment for all employees. Inclusive and supportive workplace cultures not only enhance employee well-being but also improve patient care and organizational effectiveness.

YOU are the EMT SUMMARY

1. How can you prepare yourself for this shift?

Making sure you are physically and mentally prepared for a long, busy shift means taking care of your health. In particular, getting adequate sleep of 7 to 9 hours helps ensure that you are able to perform optimally. Nutrition also plays a significant role in your well-being. Consume a balanced meal rich in proteins, healthy fats, and complex carbohydrates beforehand. Also, knowing that you may not get a break for a sit-down meal, it is helpful to pack healthy snacks like fruits, nuts, and whole grains to sustain energy levels throughout the shift. Remember, hydration is equally important, so bring a reusable water bottle to keep with you during the shift. Finally, incorporating relaxation techniques such as deep breathing, mindfulness, or light stretching can help you manage stress and maintain mental equilibrium.

2. What are some strategies you can use to combat fatigue and help you stay safe for the duration of this shift?

Make sure you are alert before beginning this transport. Fatigue countermeasures include physical exercise such as stretching, walking, or jogging in place. Mental exercise such as having a conversation can also help improve alertness. Caffeine can increase alertness, but be mindful of your caffeine consumption, as too much can lead to negative health effects. Finally, a short nap (15 to 20 minutes) can boost alertness. If you do not feel it is safe for you to drive, voice this concern to your partner.

3. How can you prepare yourself psychologically for this call?

Regardless of your years of experience in EMS, you must prepare yourself psychologically and logistically when responding to *every* call. You may experience anxiety during your response to the scene; this is a normal human reaction to a stressful event. The key is to recognize this and to remain focused on the critical tasks that lie ahead. Instead of reacting negatively, channel your anxiety into a positive psychological drive that will make you even more determined to provide the best emergency medical care possible. Consider practicing tactical breathing to help calm your heart rate and keep you alert.

You and your partner should have a plan; clearly delineate each of your roles when you arrive at the scene. Discuss the skills and interventions that may need to be performed, the equipment that will be required, and whether additional resources will be needed. Doing so will help minimize confusion at the scene and the psychological stress it causes.

4. What precautions should you take while cleaning up the scene?

You should always practice standard precautions to avoid coming in content with objects, blood, or body fluids that could lead to exposure. Make sure your PPE is intact as you clean any surfaces or equipment. Handle needles or any other sharp items with extra caution. Make sure to dispose of these in approved, closed, rigid containers. Remember that the surfaces of any equipment that have been exposed, such as the cardiac monitor or electronic devices for documentation, will need to be cleaned. All of your PPE items must be disposed of in a safe manner. Remember your doffing techniques.

5. Discuss how the last call you went on might be a psychologically traumatizing event for your partner.

Any event can be a potentially psychologically traumatizing event. It is the individual's reaction to the event, not the event itself, that makes this determination. Your partner appears to be experiencing a number of serious stressors at home and may not be engaging in techniques to relieve some of this stress. The patient may remind your partner of his recent

YOU are the EMT SUMMARY continued

loss and have a greater psychological effect than if he were to see this same patient at another time.

6. **How can you help your partner?**

Your partner's behavior is consistent with a critical incident stress reaction. If he does not wish to talk, do not force the issue. He needs time to collect his thoughts and to grieve. However, you should reassure your partner that you are willing to listen; some people experience relief just by talking to a coworker, family member, or friend. In other cases, your partner may need to speak to a counselor. You may encourage your partner to speak with a mental health professional and assure him that seeking help is a normal part of rebalancing our well-being and not a sign of weakness.

Prep Kit

Ready for Review

- Your health and wellness are the foundation for your career; without these, you cannot provide care. Wellness includes your mental, physical, and emotional well-being.
- Components of wellness include maintaining proper nutrition; getting sufficient exercise, relaxation, and sleep; refraining from use of tobacco, inappropriate use of drugs, and excessive use of alcohol; protecting yourself from communicable diseases and scene hazards; and taking time to relax, engage with others, and enjoy life.
- Recognizing the signs of stress is important for all EMTs. When signs of stress such as fatigue, anxiety, or anger; feelings of hopelessness, worthlessness, or guilt; and other such indicators are present, mental health problems can develop. Make sure to regularly balance your "stress bucket" with proper nutrition, sleep, relaxation, and time with friends and family, and consider engaging with a counselor or therapist.
- Fatigue has important negative consequences in EMS. Adequate sleep should last between 7 and 9 hours per 24-hour period. When you experience fatigue while working, use tools such as short naps, exercise, mental activities, and judicious caffeine consumption to remain alert.
- Burnout and compassion fatigue are often associated with work in EMS. However, these conditions are not inevitable or permanent. Taking time to rebalance stressors can help prevent or reduce the effects.
- Any event is a potentially psychologically traumatizing event. It is the individual's reaction to the event, not the event itself, that determines whether it is traumatizing. Our reactions are influenced by the stressors we are experiencing at the time.
- Resilience can be built through proper nutrition, exercise, sleep, relaxation, and cultivation of social networks. These practices can reduce the likelihood of PTSD following exposure to traumatic events.
- Every patient encounter should be considered potentially dangerous. It is essential that you take all available precautions to minimize exposure and risk to scene hazards and infectious and communicable diseases.
- A communicable disease is any disease that can be spread from person to person or animal to person.
- Infectious diseases can be transmitted by contact (direct or indirect), or they can be airborne, foodborne, or vector-borne.
- Even if you are exposed to an infectious disease, your risk of becoming ill is small.
- Whether or not an acute infection occurs depends on several factors, including the amount and type of infectious organism and your resistance to that infection.

Prep Kit continued

- You can take several steps to protect yourself against exposure to infectious diseases, including:
  - Keeping up to date with recommended vaccinations
  - Following standard precautions at all times
  - Handling all needles and other sharp objects with great care
- Because it is often impossible to tell which patients have infectious diseases, you should avoid direct contact with the blood and body fluids of all patients.
- You should know what to do if you are exposed to an airborne or bloodborne disease. Your department's designated officer will be able to help you follow the protocol set up in your area.
- Infection control should be an important part of your daily routine. Be sure to follow the proper steps when dealing with potential exposure situations.
- If you think you may have been exposed to an infectious disease, see your physician (or your employer's designated physician) immediately.
- Violent situations can create many hazards for EMS personnel. If you see the potential for violence during a scene size-up, call for additional resources.
- Common workplace issues include incivility and sexual harassment. You should know what to do to address these situations.
- Embracing our diversity, working toward cultural competence, and practicing cultural humility improve our ability to care for patients and improve outcomes.

Vital Vocabulary

aerosol-generating procedure (AGP) Treatments that increase the risk for transmission of infections that are spread through the air or by droplets; CPR is an example.

airborne transmission The spread of an organism via droplets or dust.

bloodborne pathogens Pathogenic microorganisms that are present in human blood and can cause disease in humans. These pathogens include, but are not limited to, hepatitis B virus and human immunodeficiency virus (HIV).

burnout A combination of exhaustion, cynicism, and reduced performance resulting from long-term job stresses in health care and other high-stress professions.

Centers for Disease Control and Prevention (CDC) The primary federal agency that conducts and supports public health activities in the United States. The CDC is part of the US Department of Health and Human Services.

communicable disease A disease that can be spread from one person or species to another.

compassion fatigue A stress disorder characterized by gradual lessening of compassion over time.

contamination The presence of infectious organisms on or in objects such as dressings, water, food, needles, wounds, or a patient's body.

critical incident stress management (CISM) A process that confronts the responses to critical incidents and defuses them, directing the emergency services personnel toward physical and emotional equilibrium.

cultural competence The ability to deliver care in a way that meets the social, cultural, and linguistic needs of patients.

cultural humility An ongoing process in which a person seeks to learn more about others and continuously reflects on their own viewpoints.

designated officer The individual in the department who is charged with the responsibility of managing exposures and infection control issues.

direct contact Exposure or transmission of a communicable disease from one person to another by physical contact.

Prep Kit continued

distress A negative response to a stressor.

exposure A situation in which a person has had contact with blood, body fluids, tissues, or airborne particles in a manner that suggests disease transmission may occur.

foodborne transmission The contamination of food or water with an organism that can cause disease.

hepatitis Inflammation of the liver, usually caused by a viral infection, that causes fever, loss of appetite, jaundice, fatigue, and altered liver function.

host The organism or individual that is attacked by the infecting agent.

human immunodeficiency virus (HIV) Acquired immunodeficiency syndrome (AIDS) is caused by HIV, which damages the cells in the body's immune system so that the body is unable to fight infection or certain cancers.

immune The state of being able to resist the adverse effects of an infectious exposure.

indirect contact Exposure or transmission of disease from one person to another by contact with a contaminated object.

infection The abnormal invasion of a host or host tissues by organisms such as bacteria, viruses, or parasites, with or without signs or symptoms of disease.

infection control Procedures to reduce transmission of infection among patients and health care personnel.

infectious disease A medical condition caused by the growth and spread of small, harmful organisms within the body.

Occupational Safety and Health Administration (OSHA) The federal regulatory compliance agency that develops, publishes, and enforces guidelines concerning safety in the workplace.

pathogen A microorganism that is capable of causing disease in a susceptible host.

personal protective equipment (PPE) Protective equipment that blocks exposure to a pathogen or a hazardous material.

posttraumatic stress disorder (PTSD) A delayed stress reaction to a prior incident. Often the result of one or more unresolved issues concerning the incident, and may relate to an incident that involved physical harm or the threat of physical harm.

potentially psychologically traumatizing event Any incident that deeply affects the mental and emotional well-being of an EMS clinician. These events have the potential to cause posttraumatic stress disorder and other mental health conditions.

resilience The capacity of an individual to cope with and recover from distress.

standard precautions Protective measures that have traditionally been developed by the CDC for use in dealing with objects, blood, body fluids, and other potential exposure risks of communicable disease.

transmission The way in which an infectious disease is spread: contact, airborne, by vehicles, or by vectors.

vector-borne transmission The use of an animal to spread an organism from one person or place to another.

wellness The active pursuit of a state of good health.

References

1. US Departments of Agriculture, US Department of Health and Human Services. *Dietary Guidelines for Americans, 2020–2025.* Dietary Guidelines website. https://www.dietaryguidelines.gov/sites/default/files/2020-12/Dietary_Guidelines_for_Americans_2020-2025.pdf. Published December 2020. Accessed September 4, 2024.
2. American Heart Association (AHA) editorial staff. American Heart Association recommendations for physical activity in adults and kids. AHA website. https://www.heart.org/en/healthy-living/fitness/fitness-basics/aha-recs-for-physical-activity-in-adults. Reviewed January 19, 2024. Accessed September 4, 2024.

Prep Kit continued

3. Chopko BA, Papazoglou K, Schwartz RC. Mindfulness-based psychotherapy approaches for first responders: from research to clinical practice. *Am J Psychother*. 2018;71(2):55–64.
4. UCLA mindful: guided meditations. UCLA Health website. https://www.uclahealth.org/programs/uclamindful/free-guided-meditations/weekly-meditations-talks/guided-meditations. Accessed December 5, 2024.
5. Watson NF, Badr MS, Belenky G, et al. Recommended amount of sleep for a healthy adult: a joint consensus statement of the American Academy of Sleep Medicine and Sleep Research Society. *Sleep*. 2015;38(6):843–844.
6. Cash RE, White-Mills K, Crowe RP, Rivard MK, Panchal AR. Workplace incivility among nationally certified EMS professionals and associations with workforce-reducing factors and organizational culture. *Prehosp Emerg Care*. 2019;23(3):346–355.
7. Sun Q, Ji X, Zhou W, Liu J. Sleep problems in shift nurses: a brief review and recommendations at both individual and institutional levels. *J Nurs Manag*. 2019;27(1):10–18. https://doi.org/10.1111/jonm.12656
8. Patterson PD, Robinson K. *Fatigue in Emergency Medical Services Systems* (Report No. DOT HS 812 767). Washington, DC: National Highway Traffic Safety Administration; August 2019.
9. Brabban A, Turkington D. The search for meaning: detecting congruence between live events, underlying schema and psychotic symptoms. In: Morrison AP, ed. *A Casebook of Cognitive Therapy for Psychosis*. New York, NY: Brunner-Routledge: 2002:59–75.
10. Esser MB, Sherk A, Liu Y, Naimi TS. Deaths from excessive alcohol use—United States, 2016–2021. *MMWR Morb Mortal Wkly Rep*. 2024;73:154–161.
11. Burton R, Sheron N. No level of alcohol consumption improves health. *Lancet*. 2018;392(10152):987–988.
12. Alcohol use and your health. Centers for Disease Control and Prevention website. https://www.cdc.gov/alcohol/about-alcohol-use/?CDC_AAref_Val=https://www.cdc.gov/alcohol/fact-sheets.htm. Published May 15, 2024. Accessed December 5, 2024.
13. Dromgoole D, Remy J. What's not up in smoke: cannabis legalization and its implications for EMS. *JEMS* website. https://www.jems.com/patient-care/whats-not-up-in-smoke-cannabis-legalization-and-its-implications-for-ems/. Published September 15, 2022. Accessed September 4, 2024.
14. Crean RD, Crane NA, Mason BJ. An evidence-based review of acute and long-term effects of cannabis use on executive cognitive functions. *J Addict Med*. 2011 Mar;5(1):1–8.
15. Demerouti E, Bakker AB, Nachreiner F, Schaufeli WB. The job demands-resources model of burnout. *J Appl Psychol*. 2001;86(3):499–512.
16. Crowe RP, Fernandez AR, Pepe PE, et al. The association of job demands and resources with burnout among emergency medical services professionals. *J Am Coll Emerg Physicians Open*. 2020;1(1):6–16.
17. Crowe RP, Bower JK, Cash RE, Panchal AR, Rodriguez SA, Olivo-Marston SE. Association of burnout with workforce-reducing factors among EMS professionals. *Prehosp Emerg Care*. 2018;22(2):229–236.
18. Wynn F. Burnout or compassion fatigue? A comparative concept analysis for nurses caring for patients in high-stakes environments. *Int J Hum Car*. 2020;24(1):59–71. doi:10.20467/1091-5710.24.1.59
19. Renkiewicz GK, Hubble MW. Secondary Traumatic Stress in Emergency Services Systems (STRESS) project: quantifying and predicting compassion fatigue in emergency medical services personnel. *Prehosp Emerg Care*. 2022;26(5):652–663.
20. Norman SB, Maguen S. PTSD: National Center for PTSD: moral injury. US Department of Veterans Affairs website. https://www.ptsd.va.gov/professional/treat/cooccurring/moral_injury.asp. Accessed December 5, 2024.
21. Litz BT, Kerig PK. Introduction to the special issue on moral injury: conceptual challenges, methodological issues, and clinical applications. *J Trauma Stress*. 2019;32(3):341–349.
22. Taigman M, Liebowitz S. *Super-Charge Your Stress Management in the Age of COVID-19*. Vow3 Publishing; 2020.
23. Tedeschi RG, Calhoun LG. The Posttraumatic Growth Inventory: measuring the positive legacy of trauma. *J Trauma Stress*. 1996;9(3):455–471.
24. Grossman D, Christensen LW. *On Combat: The Psychology and Physiology of Deadly Conflict in War and in Peace*. 3rd ed. Human Factor Research Group; 2008.
25. Carson LM, Marsh SM, Brown MM, Elkins KL, Tiesman HM. An analysis of suicides among first responders—findings from the National Violent Death Reporting System, 2015–2017. *J Safety Res*. 2023;85:361–370.
26. Vigil NH, Grant AR, Perez O, et al. Death by suicide—the EMS profession compared to the general public. *Prehosp Emerg Care*. 2019;23(3):340–345.
27. Ali D. Dispelling some common myths about suicide. *Fire Engineering* website. https://digital.fireengineering.com/fireengineering/201809/MobilePagedArticle.action?articleId=1423599#articleId1423599. Published September 2018. Accessed September 4, 2024.
28. Tiesman HM, Elkins KL, Brown M, Marsh S, Carson LM. Suicides among first responders: a call to action. Centers for Disease Control and Prevention website. https://blogs.cdc.gov/niosh-science-blog/2021/04/06/suicides-first-responders/. Updated July 18, 2022. Accessed November 5, 2024.
29. DeGryse D. Chicago Fire Department suicide study. Rosecrance website. https://rosecrance.org/chicago-fire-department-suicide-study/. Accessed September 4, 2024.
30. Bureau of Labor Statistics, US Department of Labor. National census of fatal occupational injuries in 2022.

Prep Kit continued

News Release. USDL-23-2615. Bureau of Labor Statistics website. https://www.bls.gov/news.release/archives/cfoi_12192023.pdf. Published December 19, 2023. Accessed September 4, 2024.

31. National Institute for Occupational Safety and Health. Emergency medical services clinician injury data. CDC website. https://www.cdc.gov/niosh/ems/data/index.html. Published February 16, 2024. Accessed September 4, 2024.
32. Emergency medical services clinician injury data. Centers for Disease Control and Prevention website. https://www.cdc.gov/niosh/ems/data/index.html. Published February 16, 2024. Accessed December 5, 2024.
33. Andrup L, Krogfelt KA, Hansen KS, Madsen AM. Transmission route of rhinovirus, the causative agent for common cold: a systematic review. *Am J Infect Control*. 2023;51(8):938–957.
34. Healthy habits: coughing and sneezing. Centers for Disease Control and Prevention website. https://www.cdc.gov/hygiene/about/coughing-and-sneezing.html. Published April 16, 2024. Accessed September 4, 2024.
35. Glatter KA, Finkelman P. History of the plague: an ancient pandemic for the age of COVID-19. *Am J Med*. 2021;134(2):176–181.
36. Recommendations from the guideline for isolation precautions: preventing transmission of infectious agents in healthcare settings. IV: recommendations. Centers for Disease Control and Prevention website. https://www.cdc.gov/infection-control/hcp/isolation-precautions/recommendations.html. Updated November 22, 2023. Accessed September 4, 2024.
37. C. diff: facts for clinicians. Centers for Disease Control and Prevention website. https://www.cdc.gov/c-diff/hcp/clinical-overview/index.html. Published March 5, 2024. Accessed December 5, 2024.
38. Sands M. Standard number: 1910.134(g)(1)(i)(A), 1910.134(g)(1). Occupational Safety and Health Administration website. https://www.osha.gov/laws-regs/interlinking/standards/1910.134(g)(1)(i)(A)/standard_interpretations. Published May 9, 2016. Accessed September 4, 2024.
39. National Center for Immunization and Respiratory Diseases. Adult immunization schedule by age (addendum updated February 29, 2024). Centers for Disease Control and Prevention website. https://www.cdc.gov/vaccines/schedules/hcp/imz/adult.html. Reviewed February 29, 2024. Accessed September 4, 2024.
40. Clinical testing guidance for tuberculosis: health care personnel. Centers for Disease Control and Prevention website. https://www.cdc.gov/tb-healthcare-settings/hcp/screening-testing/index.html. Published December 15, 2023. Accessed September 4, 2024.
41. Interim guidelines for managing healthcare personnel with SARS-CoV-2 infection or exposure to SARS-CoV-2. Centers for Disease Control and Prevention website. https://www.cdc.gov/covid/hcp/infection-control/guidance-risk-assesment-hcp.html. Published March 18, 2024. Accessed September 4, 2024.
42. Maguire BJ, Browne M, O'Neill BJ, Dealy MT, Clare D, O'Meara P. International survey of violence against EMS personnel: physical violence report. *Prehosp Disaster Med*. 2018;33(5):526–531.
43. Basic strategies. Learning for Justice website. https://www.learningforjustice.org/magazine/publications/speak-up-at-school/in-the-moment/basic-strategies. Accessed September 4, 2024.
44. Khalsa S, Barnes L, Audet R, et al. The impact of cultural humility in prehospital healthcare delivery and education: a position paper from the National Association of EMS Educators (NAEMSE). *Prehosp Emerg Care*. 2020;24(6):839–843.

Additional Resources

Dick T. *People Care: Perspectives and Practices for Professional Caregivers*. 3rd ed. HMP; 2018.

Gormley MA, Crowe RP, Bentley MA, Levine R. A national description of violence toward emergency medical services personnel. *Prehosp Emerg Care*. 2016;20(4):439–447.

Grant L, Kinman G. Emotional resilience in the helping professions and how it can be enhanced: health and social care education. *J Health Soc Care Ed*. 2015;3(1):23–34.

Infection control basics. Centers for Disease Control and Prevention website. https://www.cdc.gov/infection-control/about/index.html. Published April 3, 2024. Accessed September 4, 2024.

National Highway Traffic Safety Administration. *EMS Agenda 2050: A People-Centered Vision for the Future of Emergency Medical Services*; 2019:58. Washington, DC: National Highway Traffic Safety Administration. ems.gov website. https://www.ems.gov/projects/ems-agenda-2050.html. Updated October 18, 2023. Accessed Octcber 4, 2024.

Patterson PD, Higgins JS, Dongen HPAV, et al. Evidence-based guidelines for fatigue risk management in emergency medical services. *Prehosp Emerg Care*. 2018;22(Suppl 1):89–101.

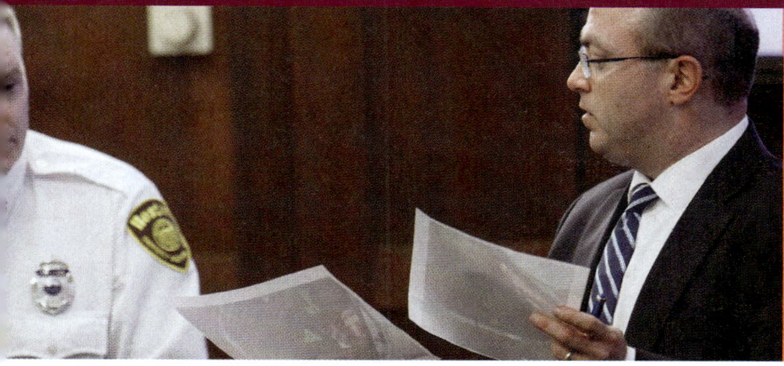

Chapter 3

Medical, Legal, and Ethical Issues

NATIONAL EMS EDUCATION STANDARD COMPETENCIES

Preparatory

Applies knowledge of the emergency medical services (EMS) system, safety/well-being of the emergency medical technician (EMT), medical/legal, and ethical issues to the provision of emergency care.

Medical/Legal and Ethics

- Consent/involuntary consent/refusal of care (pp 62–69)
- Confidentiality (pp 69–71)
- Advance directives (pp 71–73)
- Tort and criminal actions (pp 79–81)
- Evidence preservation (p 84)
- Statutory responsibilities (pp 76–79)
- Mandatory reporting (pp 83–84)
- Ethical principles/moral obligations (pp 86–88)
- End-of-life issues (pp 71–73)
- Patient rights/advocacy (pp 62–69)

KNOWLEDGE OBJECTIVES

1. Define consent and how it relates to decision making. (pp 62–63)
2. Compare expressed consent, implied consent, and involuntary consent. (pp 64–65)
3. Discuss consent by minors for treatment or transport. (pp 65–66)
4. Discuss the conditions when using patient restraints may be indicated. (pp 66–67)
5. Discuss the EMT's role and obligations if a patient refuses treatment or transport. (pp 67–69)
6. Describe the relationship between patient communications, confidentiality, and the Health Insurance Portability and Accountability Act (HIPAA). (pp 69–71)
7. Discuss the importance of do not attempt resuscitation (DNAR) orders and local protocols as they relate to the EMS environment. (pp 71–73)
8. Describe the physical, presumptive, and definitive signs of death. (pp 73–74)
9. Explain how to care for patients who are identified as organ donors. (pp 75–76)
10. Recognize the importance of medical identification devices when treating the patient. (p 76)
11. Discuss the concepts of *scope of practice* and *standards of care*. (pp 76–79)
12. Describe the EMT's legal duty to act. (p 79)
13. Discuss the legal issues of negligence, abandonment, assault and battery, and kidnapping and their implications for the EMT. (pp 79–81)
14. Explain the reporting requirements for special situations, including abuse, drug- or felony-related injuries, childbirth, and crime scenes. (pp 83–84)

15. Describe the roles and responsibilities of the EMT in court. (pp 84–86)
16. Define ethics and morality and their implications for the EMT. (pp 86–88)

SKILLS OBJECTIVES

There are no skills objectives for this chapter.

Introduction

A basic medical, legal, and ethical principle of emergency care is to first do no further harm. As an EMT, you will have the opportunity to do considerably more for your patients than simply preventing further injury. A thorough understanding of medical, legal, and ethical issues related to EMS is essential. EMTs are better positioned to avoid professional legal problems when they act in good faith, follow an appropriate standard of care, and provide compassionate care.

Individual states develop EMS protocols, regulations, and licensing standards and control the scope of practice of EMS clinicians within those states. These state rules are often guided or influenced by a combination of authorities, including the Office of EMS within the National Highway Traffic Safety Administration (NHTSA), a branch of the US Department of Transportation (DOT), and various national EMS-focused organizations such as the National Association of EMS Physicians (NAEMSP) and National Association of State EMS Officials (NASEMSO). Together, these entities create the legal and operational framework for EMS clinicians in each state to follow.

EMS clinicians who provide care on one of the 574 federally recognized American Indian tribal areas may have additional or alternative regulations to follow. These areas are considered sovereign nations and may have laws, rules, and practices that differ from state EMS regulations. Similarly, EMS clinicians in the military may work in many different settings, including field hospitals, battlefields, and various states and countries. They may function with a different and sometimes expanded scope of practice. It is essential that you understand the laws and regulations in the state or jurisdiction where you provide EMS care.

EMTs provide **emergency medical care**—that is, immediate care or treatment—and are often the first link in the chain of prehospital and long-term patient care. As the scope and nature of emergency medical care become more complex, litigation involving participants in EMS systems will likely increase. Providing competent emergency medical care that conforms to the EMT scope of practice and standard of care will help you to avoid both civil and criminal actions.

You must also consider ethical issues. As an EMT, should you stop and treat patients who were involved in an automobile crash while you are en route to another emergency call? Should you begin cardiopulmonary resuscitation (CPR) on a patient who, according to the family, has terminal cancer? Should you begin treatment on a child with obvious signs of death because the parents are begging you to do something? Consider the following situations:

- While transporting a patient to the hospital, he states, "I don't want to go to the hospital anymore. You have to let me out."
- As you begin treating a child you suspect might be the victim of abuse, a parent commands you to stop.
- Your partner takes out his phone to post a comment on his social media account about the last emergency call.

What should you do? Even when emergency medical care is properly rendered, there are still times when you may be sued by a patient who seeks compensation. Administrative action, such as suspension of your state EMT license, may be brought against you for failure to abide by the regulations of your state EMS agency. For these reasons, you must understand the various legal aspects of emergency medical care.

Consent

Typically, consent is required from, or for, every patient before care can be started. A person receiving care must give permission, or **consent**, for treatment. An adult who is conscious, rational, and capable of making informed decisions has a legal right to refuse care, even though this person may be ill or injured. A patient may also consent to some aspects of care and deny consent for others. If the patient refuses care, you may not care for the patient. In fact, doing so may be grounds for both criminal and civil action. Consent can be expressed (actual) or implied.

To provide consent, an individual must have decision-making capacity. **Decision-making capacity** is the ability of a patient to understand the information you are providing, coupled with the ability to process that information and make an informed choice regarding medical care. Additionally, the patient must be capable of communicating their choice. It is important to keep in mind that the law allows patients to make choices that may seem medically unsound and that might endanger their own life. The right of patients who have decision-making capacity to make decisions concerning their health is known as **autonomy**.

Street Smarts

It may be necessary to use creative techniques whenever a language or other communication barrier is present and there is a question about decision-making capacity. Techniques such as using a cell phone translation application, note pad, and yes/no questions can all be helpful in facilitating communication until a medical interpreter is available.

The terms *decision-making capacity* and *competence* are often used interchangeably but there is a distinction: Competence is generally regarded as a legal term; determinations regarding competence are typically made by a court of law. Decision-making capacity is the term more commonly used in health care to determine whether or not a patient is capable of making health care decisions.

The following factors should be considered when determining a patient's decision-making capacity:

- Is the patient's intellectual capacity impaired by mental limitation or any type of dementia?
- Is the patient of legal age (18 years old in most states)?
- Is the patient impaired by alcohol or drug intoxication or serious injury or illness?
- Does the patient appear to be experiencing significant pain?
- Does the patient have a significant injury that could distract them from a more serious injury? (For example, a significant non–life-threatening injury can cause extreme pain and distract the patient from neck pain, which could indicate a potentially more serious problem.)
- Are there any apparent hearing or visual problems?
- Is a language barrier present? Do you and your patient speak the same language?
- Does the patient appear to understand what you are saying? Does the patient ask rational questions that demonstrate an understanding of the information you are trying to share?
- Is the patient oriented to person, place, time, and situation? Establishing this information can be helpful, but it is also possible for a patient to have adequate decision-making capacity despite not knowing the precise day or date. Consider situational factors that might limit a patient's knowledge of such details, such as experiencing homelessness or being a long-term care resident. Conversely, it is possible for a patient to lack decision-making capacity despite being oriented to person, place, time, and situation.

Words of Wisdom

Certain situations such as transport refusal or withholding life support often require a careful, well-documented assessment of a patient's decision-making capacity. This assessment is less critical in situations where the patient is amenable to transport or interventions recommended by EMS clinicians. Your scrutiny of a patient's decision-making capacity should be directly proportional to the gravity of a situation or implications of a decision, especially in situations where a patient's stated decision appears to be contrary to their best interests.

Words of Wisdom

Asking patients, "What do you understand about your current situation?" can be helpful when you are not sure whether they have adequate decision-making capacity. It provides an opportunity to evaluate whether they received important information that you have conveyed to them along with whether they can verbalize the potential implications of consent or refusal of a proposed intervention.

You should be familiar with various types of consent, including expressed consent, implied consent, and involuntary consent.

Expressed Consent

Expressed consent (or actual consent) is the type of consent given when patients specifically acknowledge that they want you to provide care or transport. Expressed consent may be verbal or nonverbal. For example, if you ask a patient if you can check the blood pressure and the patient says yes, that is verbal consent; if the patient nods yes or extends an arm to you, the patient is expressing consent nonverbally.

To be valid, the consent the patient provides must be **informed consent**, which means you explained the nature of the treatment being offered, along with the potential risks, benefits, and alternatives to treatment, as well as potential consequences of refusing treatment. Often, the prehospital environment requires that consent be obtained more quickly than in the hospital setting. Paramedics will often provide additional information if advanced life support (ALS) interventions are necessary. In such cases, there is a greater potential for side effects and other adverse responses associated with drug administration and other forms of advanced care.

Informed consent is valid if given verbally, but it may be difficult to prove at a later point in time. Rarely do EMS clinicians have patients sign a consent form, so it is always advisable to document consent in your patient care report (PCR). Having someone witness the patient's consent may be helpful if the issue of consent is later challenged in court.

Remember, a patient may agree to certain types of emergency medical care but not to others. The patient's right to refuse treatment is discussed later in this chapter.

Street Smarts

Rather than specifically saying, "We would like your consent," the EMT can work the consent into the conversation more casually. For example, the EMT may say, "We're from the ambulance. We're here to take care of you. We would like to check your blood pressure and check you over. Are you okay with that?"

Implied Consent

When individuals are unconscious or otherwise incapable of making a rational, informed decision about care and unable to give consent, the law assumes they would consent to care and transport to a medical facility if they were able to do so. Patients who are intoxicated by drugs or alcohol, mentally impaired, or suffering from certain conditions such as head injury might be included in this category, as would patients who are in cardiac arrest who do not have a legal advance directive. The legal principle that allows treatment under such circumstances is called **implied consent**. Implied consent applies only when a serious medical condition exists and should never be used unless there is a threat to life or limb. For this reason, the principle of implied consent is known as the **emergency doctrine**.

Sometimes what represents a serious threat may be unclear. This may result in legal proceedings and a **medicolegal** judgment, which should be supported by your best efforts to obtain consent and a thoroughly documented PCR. In most instances, the law allows a **surrogate decision maker** to provide consent when the patient does not have

YOU are the EMT

At 1720 hours, you are dispatched to a grocery store at 1175 N. Main Street for a man with a severe headache. You respond to the scene, which is located only a few miles away. The weather is clear, the temperature is 90°F (32°C), and the traffic is heavy.

1. Why is it essential that you obtain consent to treat the patient once you arrive?
2. Should you assess the patient's decision-making capacity once you arrive?

decision-making capacity. A surrogate decision maker is typically a spouse, domestic partner, close relative, or next of kin, often identified in a hierarchy by state laws as a resource when the patient cannot consent to treatment for themselves. You should make every effort to obtain consent from an available relative before treating based on implied consent; however, treatment should never be delayed when the patient has imminently life-threatening injuries.

A variety of states have adopted all or portions of the Uniform Health-Care Decisions Act (UHCDA), a model statute developed by the National Conference of Commissioners on Uniform State Laws. The UHCDA provides a framework and hierarchy that outlines who can consent or refuse proposed treatment on behalf of the patient. Many states have not adopted the UHCDA, and the role of a surrogate decision maker is only minimally referenced in the National Model EMS Clinical Guidelines. It is extremely important that EMS clinicians fully understand state EMS rules related to consent and refusal, particularly in the context of withholding or discontinuing resuscitation efforts.

It is also important to understand that if a patient being treated based on implied consent were to regain consciousness and appear capable of making an informed decision, the doctrine of implied consent would no longer apply. This situation often occurs with calls involving diabetic emergencies, overdoses, episodes of syncope, and seizures.

The theoretical basis of implied consent relies on the idea that patients would likely consent to emergency intervention if they had decision-making capacity and were able to speak for themselves. An ethical dilemma arises when there are obvious signs that a patient would likely refuse a potentially lifesaving intervention. A "do not attempt resuscitation" tattoo on a patient's chest is a classic example of an ethical dilemma that EMS clinicians face when rapid decisions are needed for potentially lifesaving interventions. While the patient may have intended to express their wish not to be resuscitated at the time they obtained the tattoo, the tattoo will likely not be legally recognized because it does not meet all of the key requirements of a DNR: First, a valid DNR can be revoked by the patient at any time; because a tattoo is permanent, it may not be possible for the patient to convey their wish to revoke it. Second, there is likely no witnessed, signed document accompanying the tattoo; this documentation is typically a requirement in state law. Finally, the tattoo does not indicate what type of treatment should be withheld and therefore does not provide sufficient medical guidance.[1] EMS DNAR protocols are designed to facilitate quick decision making but have the potential to put EMS clinicians in ethically challenging situations. When in doubt, consult online medical direction, especially in situations where you are concerned that you might be obligated to perform an unethical intervention in a particular situation.

Involuntary Consent

Assisting patients who are mentally ill, developmentally delayed, or experiencing a behavioral (psychological) crisis, either organic or chemically induced, is complicated. An adult patient who is found legally incompetent is not able to give informed consent. From a legal perspective, this situation is similar to those involving minors. Consent for emergency care should be obtained from someone who is legally responsible for the patient, such as a guardian or conservator. In many cases, however, such permission will not be readily obtainable. Many states have protective custody statutes allowing such a person to be taken to a medical facility. Under certain conditions, law enforcement and prison officials are legally permitted to give consent for any individual who is incarcerated or has been placed under arrest. However, a prisoner who is conscious and capable of making decisions does not necessarily surrender the right to make medical decisions and may refuse care. Know the provisions in your area and involve online medical direction in the process.

Minors and Consent

Because a minor might not have the wisdom, maturity, or judgment to give consent, the law requires that a parent or legal guardian, when available, give consent for treatment or transport (**FIGURE 3-1**). In every state, when a parent cannot be reached to provide consent, health care providers are allowed to give emergency care to a child. In some states, a minor can consent to receive medical care, depending on the minor's age and maturity and the nature of the medical request.

A great deal of confusion surrounds the issue of emancipated minors. An **emancipated minor** is

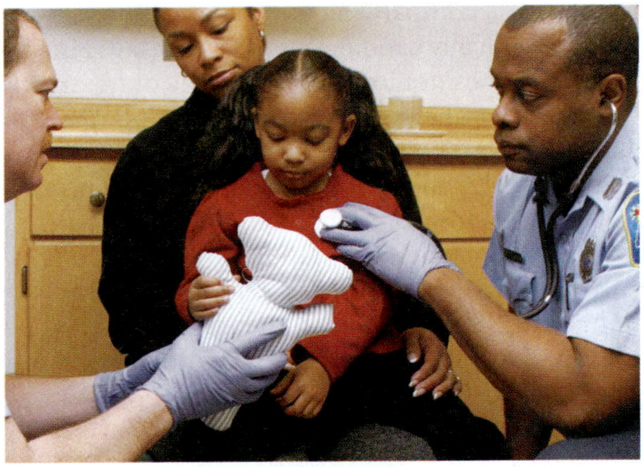

FIGURE 3-1 The law requires that a parent or a legal guardian give consent for treatment or transport of a minor. However, you must never withhold lifesaving care.

a person who, despite being under the legal age in a given state (in most cases, the age is 18 years), can be legally treated as an adult based on certain circumstances. For example, many states consider minors to be emancipated if they are married, if they are members of the armed services, or if they are parents. Minors who are a parent may also give consent for their own child. In addition, minors are usually considered emancipated if living away from and no longer relying on their parents for support. A court may issue an order declaring a minor to be emancipated but this is not commonly seen. You should know your state's laws concerning the issues surrounding emancipation.

If a minor is injured and requires medical treatment in a school or camp setting, teachers and school officials may act **in loco parentis**, which means in the position or place of a parent, and can legally give consent for treatment of the minor if a parent or guardian is not available. You should still attempt to obtain consent from a parent or legal guardian whenever possible; however, if a true emergency exists and the parent or legal guardian is not available, the consent to treat the minor is implied, just as with an adult. You must never withhold lifesaving care for a minor because a person authorized to provide consent is not available.

Some states recognize the concept of a **mature minor**, and give deference to minors who have struggled with chronic or severe illnesses such as cancer. In these states, either the legislature or courts have recognized the **mature minor doctrine**, which provides minors with greater empowerment to consent or refuse various interventions, even if they conflict with parental wishes. These mature minors often have firsthand experience with the pain and suffering involved with longer-term illness or treatment strategies that might be unlikely to be ultimately successful, and have a heightened awareness of the true implications of a proposed treatment.

There may also be additional state laws that allow minors to consent for certain types of treatment themselves without the involvement of a parent or legal guardian. Depending on the state, reproductive services, treatment for a sexually transmitted infection, and even mental health services may not require parental consent for minors. Your EMS agency's treatment guidelines should accurately reflect the laws of your state or jurisdiction.

Despite these exceptions that allow you to care for a minor in the absence of a parent's or guardian's consent, it is important to reach the parents or guardian as soon as possible. In cases where the child has the legal right to consent, their parents would be contacted only with their consent. Even though lifesaving interventions will not be delayed, it is possible that other interventions at the hospital could be delayed until consent is obtained. Follow local protocol or consult medical direction to determine if someone acting in loco parentis will need to accompany the child during transport and be present at the receiving hospital until a parent or guardian arrives.

Forcible Restraint

Forcible restraint is sometimes necessary when you are caring for a patient who is in need of medical treatment and transport but is combative and presents a significant physical risk of danger to self, rescuers, or others (**FIGURE 3-2**). Such behavior may result from an underlying psychiatric or behavioral condition, the effects of drugs or alcohol, or a medical condition such as a head injury or hypoxia. Typically, you should consult medical control for authorization to restrain. In some states, only a police officer may forcibly restrain an individual. In other states, the role of law enforcement in restraining a medical patient is limited. You should be knowledgeable about local laws. Restraint without legal authority or medical justification exposes you

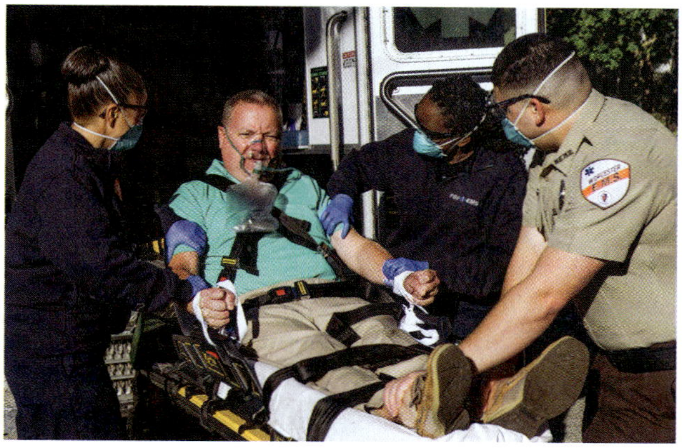

FIGURE 3-2 Know the local laws about forcible restraint of a patient. In some states, only a police officer has the authority to restrain a patient.

to potential civil and criminal penalties. Restraint may be used only in circumstances of risk to the patient or others. When a patient is combative and poses a risk to the rescuer, it is advisable to wait for law enforcement to arrive on scene before attempting to treat the patient. See Chapter 23, *Behavioral Health Emergencies*, for a complete discussion of the use of restraint.

Words of Wisdom

In recent years, two pairs of paramedics have been charged with homicide related to their treatment and monitoring of patients who were forcibly restrained.[2,3] Although the circumstances were substantially different in the two cases, each involved allegations of inadequate assessment and monitoring. In December 2023, two of these paramedics were convicted of criminally negligent homicide, creating a new precedent for the criminal prosecution of EMS clinicians in extreme situations.

Your service should have clearly defined protocols for situations involving restraint. Restraints should be considered only if the patient has a medical condition that appears serious or if the patient suffers from an apparent behavioral disorder that poses a risk to self or others. Verbal de-escalation should always be attempted prior to considering physical restraints. The patient's decision-making capacity should be assessed and thoroughly documented. After restraints are applied, they should not be removed en route unless they pose a risk to the patient, even if the patient promises to behave. Appropriate safe strategies for restraint should be used to minimize the risk of harm to the patient. It is essential that you protect the patient's airway and monitor the patient's respiratory and circulatory status while restrained to avoid asphyxia, aspiration, and other complications. Consider calling for ALS backup to provide pharmacologic sedation, as this may be safer than physical restraint depending on the situation. See Chapter 4, *Communications and Documentation*, for a discussion of performing verbal de-escalation.

The Right to Refuse Treatment

Adults who are conscious, alert, and appear to have decision-making capacity have the right to refuse treatment or withdraw from treatment at any time, which is supported by the principle of autonomy. This is true even if doing so may result in death or serious injury. Such patients present you with a dilemma. Should you provide care against their will? Should you leave them alone? Calls involving refusal of treatment pose a risk of litigation in EMS and require you to proceed cautiously. You must be familiar with local policies regarding refusal of care. In all such cases, you should involve online medical direction and document this consultation. A patient's decision to either accept or refuse treatment should be based on information that you provide. This information should include your assessment of what might be wrong with the patient, a description of the treatment that you think is necessary, any possible risks of treatment, the availability of alternative treatments, and the possible consequences of refusing treatment. Be sure the patient understands everything you say and encourage the patient to ask questions. All of this information should be included in your PCR. Many jurisdictions have preprinted refusal forms to ensure that all of these items are documented or acknowledged. If using a preprinted form, you still must ensure the patient understands what they are signing and the potential risks associated with their decision.

When treatment is refused, you must assess the patient's ability to make an informed decision.

Ask and repeat questions, assess the patient's answers, and observe the patient's behavior. If you determine that the patient has decision-making capacity, consider using an approach called **shared decision making**. Shared decision making is a collaborative process in which the clinician works with the patient to come up with the optimal health care approach, accounting for the patient's unique situation, concerns, and values.[4] This process is helpful when a situation presents more than one reasonable treatment option. In situations where there is only one reasonable treatment or transport option, consider using an approach called **compassionate persuasion**. Compassionate persuasion is similar to informed consent, but it involves guiding a person to accept an offer of treatment that they initially did not want. It may involve a deeper exploration of why an individual (or surrogate decision maker) is resisting a proposed treatment approach, possibly accompanied by negotiating or offering creative solutions to facilitate compromise.

If the patient appears confused or delusional, you cannot assume that the decision to refuse is an informed refusal. Patients who have attempted suicide or conveyed suicidal intent should not be regarded as having normal decision-making capacity. Remember, a single assessment finding usually will not enable you to determine whether the patient is capable of making an informed decision about health care. As with most medical conditions, it is the constellation of findings that will support your conclusion. *When in doubt, providing treatment is usually a much more defensible position than failing to treat a patient.* Contact medical direction when you are unsure. Do not endanger yourself to provide care, and use the assistance of law enforcement if necessary to ensure your own safety.

Before leaving the scene where a patient has refused care, you should again encourage the patient, multiple times if the situation allows, to permit treatment. Remind patients to call 9-1-1 if they change their mind or the condition worsens. Also advise these patients to contact a personal physician as soon as possible. It is essential for you to ask the patient to sign a refusal of treatment form and to thoroughly document all refusals. Your documentation should include any assessment findings that you were able to make and all efforts that you made to obtain consent. Your documentation should also include a description of possible consequences of refusing treatment and transport. The patient's signature should be witnessed by a family member or police officer to help protect you from a later claim for negligence or abandonment. Both of these terms are discussed later in this chapter. A signed patient refusal form does not guarantee your protection against legal action; however, it can help defend you when legal actions arise. Also, it is wise, and often required by local protocol, that you notify medical direction of your actions; medical control can help guide your decisions. In some situations, medical direction can speak directly with the patient to help convince them to permit care and transport.

You may be faced with a situation in which a parent refuses to permit treatment of an ill or injured child. In this situation, you must consider the emotional effect of the emergency on the parent's judgment. As with most cases of refusal, you can usually resolve the situation with patience and calm persuasion. You may need the help of others, such as your supervisor, ALS personnel, medical direction, or law enforcement officials.

When you are not able to persuade the patient, guardian, or parent to proceed with treatment, you must obtain the signature of the individual who is refusing treatment on an official release form that acknowledges refusal. Document any assessment findings, the emergency care that you provided, your efforts to obtain consent, your consultation with medical control, and the responses to your efforts. You should also obtain a signature from a witness to the refusal. Make every effort to have a responsible person, such as a police officer, serve as a witness to these events. Refusal documentation is maintained as part of the patient record. This will be important in the event a legal claim is filed later.

If the patient refuses to sign a release form, inform medical direction and thoroughly document the situation and the refusal. Consider contacting law enforcement or the local child protective services agency if you have a reasonable suspicion of child abuse or neglect. Parent or guardian failure to provide or allow needed medical care for a child could be considered medical neglect. Mandatory child abuse/neglect reporting requirements are discussed later in this chapter. You might be called as a witness in such cases and you must be sure that all documentation is thorough and accurate.

Remember, your safety is your first priority. Act in the best interest of your patient, but do not place yourself in danger attempting to care for a patient who is refusing care.

Words of Wisdom

When a patient, parent, or guardian refuses treatment or transport, protect yourself with both a thorough PCR and official refusal documentation. Have the patient or other refusing party sign the form, document what you have done to ensure an informed refusal, and note the involvement of medical direction in the situation. Be sure to submit the refusal form with your PCR if it is not already part of the PCR.

Confidentiality

Communication between you and the patient is considered confidential and generally cannot be disclosed without permission from the patient or a court order. Confidential information includes the patient history, assessment findings, and treatment provided. Disclosure of such information other than to those clinicians directly involved in the care of the patient without proper authorization may result in liability for **breach of confidentiality**. In most states, records may be released when a legal subpoena is presented or the patient signs a written release. Patient information may also be shared with third-party billing personnel; this is not considered a breach of confidentiality.

Health Insurance Portability and Accountability Act

The Health Insurance Portability and Accountability Act of 1996, abbreviated HIPAA, is a federal law designed to prevent sensitive health care information from being shared without the patient's consent. As related to EMS, the act defines private health care information and safeguards patient confidentiality.[5] It provides guidance on what types of information are protected, the responsibility of health care clinicians regarding that protection, and the penalties for breaching that protection.

HIPAA considers all patient information that you obtain in the course of providing medical treatment to a patient to be **protected health information (PHI)**. This includes not only medical information, but also any information that can be used to identify the patient. As an EMT, you have an obligation to guard all PHI from unlawful disclosure, either written or verbal. Safeguards to protect this information include departmental security measures to prevent HIPAA violations, such as rules to prohibit sharing of passwords or log-in credentials to systems that contain PHI; proper measures to dispose

YOU are the EMT

On arriving at the scene, you find the patient, a 32-year-old man, sitting on the sidewalk outside the grocery store. He is grabbing both sides of his head, but looks up and acknowledges your presence. You begin to assess the patient as your partner opens the jump kit and prepares to take his vital signs.

Recording Time: 0 Minutes	
Appearance	Grabbing both sides of his head; in obvious pain
Level of consciousness	Conscious and alert
Airway	Open; clear of secretions or foreign bodies
Breathing	Increased respiratory rate; adequate depth
Circulation	Radial pulses bilaterally strong and regular; skin baseline color, warm, and dry

Without talking to the patient, your partner begins to take his blood pressure and applies the pulse oximeter to his finger.

3. Are you legally authorized to treat this patient? Why or why not?
4. How does informed consent differ from implied consent?

of documents or other records that contain PHI; and rules to never leave electronic devices or patient reports that contain PHI unattended. PHI must also be maintained when two or more patients, who may or may not be family, are in close proximity of each other, such as in the back of an ambulance.

When an EMT's role provides access to PHI of patients other than those for whom the EMT provided care, those records may be accessed only if there is a legitimate business reason to do so. The records of any other person, whether celebrities, family members, or even oneself, may never be viewed without appropriate permission granted by the department privacy and security officer, as specified in policy.[6]

Words of Wisdom

Do not use a personal electronic device, such as a cell phone, to capture information from a call. Digital images such as photos of a patient's injuries or vehicle, or recordings made by crew members during a patient call, are considered PHI and a confidential part of the patient report. Never post PHI on social media. In health care environments where it is necessary to transmit PHI between health care clinicians for the purpose of patient care, HIPAA-compliant messaging systems are available.

PHI may be disclosed for purposes of treatment, payment, or operations.[7] This means you are permitted to report your assessment findings and treatment to other health care clinicians who are directly involved in the care of the patient. Information may be used for internal quality improvement and training programs, but all identifying information must first be removed. There are also certain situations when you may be legally mandated to report your findings, such as in the case of child abuse or when you receive a subpoena. In most situations, except for treatment purposes, only the minimum amount of information necessary should be released. Failure to abide by the provisions of the HIPAA laws can result in civil and/or criminal action against your response agency and against you personally. Each EMS system is required to have a policy and procedure manual and a privacy officer who can answer questions. You can expect to receive further training on how this act affects your specific response agency.

It cannot be overstated that any sharing of private or protected information, whether it is directly sharing images or recordings or verbally relaying information, is a serious violation of HIPAA and ethical principles, even when done privately. In situations where responders or health care clinicians casually share information, such as in face-to-face conversations at the station or in social media postings, the communications may feel private. The fact remains, however, that private and protected information must remain between the patient and the clinician only. Information about emergency calls may be used under special circumstances for purposes such as education and quality improvement, but all identifying and private information must first be removed.

The general public is often permitted by law to record identifying and protected patient information and images. For example, while it would be unethical and illegal for a responding EMT to take a picture of a severely injured patient while caring for the person at a motor vehicle collision, if the collision takes place on a public road and in public view, members of the general public can, and often will, record the incident. In most of these situations, EMTs, and even law enforcement officers, cannot order members of the public to stop recording, confiscate their phones or cameras, or otherwise interfere with the public.

Street Smarts

Often a polite request made to members of the public to respect patient privacy is sufficient to stop them from filming or photographing at public scenes.

Social Media

Although unauthorized sharing of private and protected patient information is never permitted, sharing personal opinions about work and non–work-related topics via social media is a complex and controversial topic. Whether such sharing is appropriate depends greatly on the nature of the information and the circumstances (eg, who is sharing it, how, when, and where?).

In general, if an EMT uses agency-supplied equipment to record or distribute information, or records or distributes information while in the course of work duties (including volunteering), the agency likely owns the images and information. In many states, the agency must follow requirements to control and store this content and, in some cases, release it to the public on request. Moreover, if EMTs associate themselves with their agency, such as showing a logo, wearing their uniform, or specifically identifying their agency, they may not be able to express their private views in the same way that other members of the general public could. There are no absolute recommendations when it comes to social media, but the following advice may help EMTs avoid serious ethical or legal issues:

- Unless you are operating as an official spokesperson for your agency, avoid logos, uniforms, vehicles, or other markings that associate you with your agency while off duty.
- Conduct yourself online with the same professionalism that you do while on duty.
- Respect your patients, their friends and family, bystanders, your colleagues, and the organization for which you work both in person and online.
- Recognize that free speech does not mean every person has a right to say anything under any circumstances and without repercussions.

Advance Directives

As an EMT, you will respond to calls in which a patient is dying from an illness. When you arrive at the scene, you may find that family members do not want you to try to resuscitate the patient. Without valid written documentation from a physician, such as an advance directive or a **do not attempt resuscitation (DNAR) order** (also known as a do not resuscitate [DNR] order), you may be placed in a very difficult position. Patients with decision-making capacity are able to make rational decisions about their well-being. An **advance directive** is a written document that specifies medical treatment for a patient, should this person become unable to make decisions. Advance directives are most commonly used when a patient becomes comatose, has dementia, or is otherwise unable to meaningfully participate in treatment decisions. An advance directive is often referred to as a living will but may also be referred to as a **health care directive**. Not all advance directives are directions to withhold care. Such care may include nutrition and medication for pain.

DNAR orders give you permission not to attempt resuscitation (**FIGURE 3-3**). Laws differ from state to state, so be familiar with your state's requirements to determine whether the DNAR order will be honored; however, to be valid, DNAR orders must meet the following requirements:

- Signature of the patient or legal guardian
- Signature of one or more physicians or other licensed health care clinicians

In some states, DNAR orders contain an expiration date. DNAR orders with expiration dates must be dated in the preceding 12 months to be valid.

You may also encounter Physician Orders for Life-Sustaining Treatment (POLST) and Medical Orders for Life-Sustaining Treatment (MOLST) forms when caring for patients with serious or terminal illnesses. These explicitly describe acceptable interventions for the patient in the form of medical orders. These forms must be signed by an authorized health care clinician in order to be valid; this may be a physician, physician assistant, or nurse practitioner, and varies by state. If you encounter these documents, follow the guidance of your medical oversight protocols.

Some patients may have named surrogates to make decisions for them regarding their health care in the event that they are incapacitated and unable to make such decisions for themselves. Such designations may be referred to as a **durable power of attorney for health care** or **health care proxy**. There are many different types of powers of attorney and not all are authorized to exercise medical decision making. When presented with a power of attorney at the scene of a medical emergency, you must read it carefully to ascertain its meaning and validity. There may also be surrogate decision makers, discussed earlier, who are authorized by state laws to make health care decisions on behalf of a patient in the event that the patient lacks or loses decision-making capacity and no durable power of attorney for health care or health care proxy is available. In these instances, a specific durable power of attorney or health care proxy form is not required. If there is any question, you should contact online medical direction for assistance. Do not delay emergency care while efforts to interpret the power of

PREHOSPITAL MEDICAL CARE DIRECTIVE
(side one)
IN THE EVENT OF CARDIAC OR RESPIRATORY ARREST, I REFUSE ANY RESUSCITATION MEASURES INCLUDING CARDIAC COMPRESSION, ENDOTRACHEAL INTUBATION AND OTHER ADVANCED AIRWAY MANAGEMENT, ARTIFICIAL VENTILATION, DEFIBRILLATION, ADMINISTRATION OF ADVANCED CARDIAC LIFE SUPPORT DRUGS AND RELATED EMERGENCY MEDICAL PROCEDURES.

Patient: ______________________ Date: __________
(Signature or mark)

Attach recent photograph here or provide all of the following information below:
Date of Birth __________
Sex ______ Race ______
Eye Color __________
Hair Color __________

PHOTO

Hospice Program (if any) __________
Name and telephone number of patient's physician __________

(side two)

I have explained this form and its consequences to the signer and obtained assurance that the signer understands that death may result from any refused care listed above (on reverse side).

______________________ Date__________
(Licensed health care clinician)

I was present when this was signed (or marked). The patient then appeared to be of sound mind and free from duress.

______________________ Date__________
(Witness)

A

Outside the Hospital Do-Not-Resuscitate Identification Card

Patient's Full Name__________

I affirm that I have authorized an Outside the Hospital Do-Not-Resuscitate Order for this patient and have documented the grounds for the order in this patient's medical file.

Attending Physician Signature__________

Attending Physician (print)__________

Address__________ **Phone**__________

Date__________

I, ______________________,
(name)
authorize emergency medical services personnel to withhold or withdraw cardiopulmonary resuscitation from me in the event I suffer cardiac or respiratory arrest.

I understand this means that if my heart stops beating or I stop breathing, no medical procedure to restart heart function or breathing will be instituted.

I understand that I may revoke this order at any time.

Patient or Patient's Representative

Signature__________

Date__________

B

FIGURE 3-3 A. An example of a wallet-size do-not-attempt-resuscitation (DNAR) order. **B.** An example of a pocket-size DNAR order.

attorney are made. Keep in mind that a patient who remains conscious and **competent** does not surrender the right to make medical decisions. The person named in the power of attorney or health care proxy is authorized to make decisions only when the patient is no longer capable of doing so.

Remember, DNAR does not mean "do not treat." Even in the presence of a DNAR order, you are still obligated to provide supportive measures (oxygen, pain relief, and comfort) to a patient who is not in cardiac arrest. These patients may already be receiving **palliative care**, a treatment approach where the focus is on decreasing pain or other symptoms rather than curing the disease or prolonging life. Each agency, in consultation with its medical director and legal counsel, must develop a protocol to follow in these circumstances.

The number of hospice (end-of-life) home health programs is growing, so you may be faced with these situations more often. Specific guidelines vary from state to state, but the following four statements may be considered general guidelines:

1. Patients have the right to refuse treatment, including resuscitation efforts, provided that they are able to communicate their wishes.
2. A written order from a physician is required for DNAR orders to be valid in a health care facility.
3. You should periodically review state and local protocols and legislation regarding advance directives.
4. When you are in doubt or the written orders are not present, and no surrogate decision maker is immediately available, you have an obligation to resuscitate.

When presented with an advance directive, you should never become annoyed with family members and allow yourself to wonder, "Why did they bother to call 9-1-1 if they don't want us to do anything?" The patients, and their families, should be treated with the utmost respect and empathy. If information and support is what they called you for, be sure to provide it. Doing so is part of your job.

Physical Signs of Death

Determination of the cause of death is the medical responsibility of a physician. Other health care professionals may be authorized by state law or organizational policy to make an official pronouncement of death. In most states, EMTs do not have the authority to pronounce a patient dead. If there is any chance that life exists or that the patient can be resuscitated and there are no advance directives, you must make every effort to save the patient at the scene and during transport. If there are obvious signs of death and the decision is made to not begin resuscitation attempts, be sure to not move the body or disrupt the scene. Notify the appropriate authorities based on local protocols and state laws. There are both definitive and presumptive signs of death. In many states, death is defined as the absence of circulatory and respiratory function. Many states have also adopted brain death provisions; these provisions refer to irreversible cessation of all functions of the brain and brainstem. Questions often arise as to whether to begin basic life support. In the absence of physician orders, such as DNAR orders, the general rule is: If the body is still intact and there are no definitive signs of death, initiate emergency medical care.

Hypothermia is a general cooling of the body in which the internal body temperature becomes abnormally low. People have survived hypothermic incidents with temperatures as low as 53.2°F (11.8°C) in a child and 56.7°F (13.7°C) in an adult.[8] In cases of hypothermia, the patient should not be considered dead until the body is warm and lifeless (ie, the patient is "warm and dead") or the body is completely frozen. When the patient's condition is unclear, or if you are unsure if you should initiate care, it is best to begin CPR immediately and contact medical direction for guidance. Remember, not all incidents of hypothermia occur outdoors; for example, an older patient in a home without heat or who has been lying on a cold floor could be hypothermic.

Presumptive Signs of Death

Most medicolegal authorities will consider the presumptive signs of death that are listed in **TABLE 3-1** adequate, particularly when they follow a severe trauma or occur at the end stages of long-term illness such as cancer or other prolonged diseases. More evidence is typically needed in cases of sudden death due to hypothermia, acute poisoning, or cardiac arrest.

YOU are the EMT

Your partner reports that the patient's blood pressure is very high. The patient tells you that he has "blood pressure problems" and experiences a bad headache whenever he does not take his prescribed medication, Prinivil. He does not want to go to the hospital and tells you that the clerk, not he, called 9-1-1.

Recording Time: 4 Minutes	
Respirations	24 breaths/min; regular and unlabored
Pulse	110 beats/min; strong and regular
Skin	Baseline color, warm, and dry
Blood pressure	200/110 mm Hg
Oxygen saturation (Spo_2)	98% (on room air)

5. What should you do when a patient refuses treatment and/or transport?

6. What questions should you ask yourself to help determine whether you can transport this patient against his will?

TABLE 3-1 Presumptive Signs of Death

- Unresponsiveness to painful stimuli
- Lack of a carotid pulse or heartbeat
- Absence of chest rise and fall
- No deep tendon or corneal reflexes
- Absence of pupillary reactivity
- No systolic blood pressure
- Profound cyanosis
- Lowered or decreased body temperature

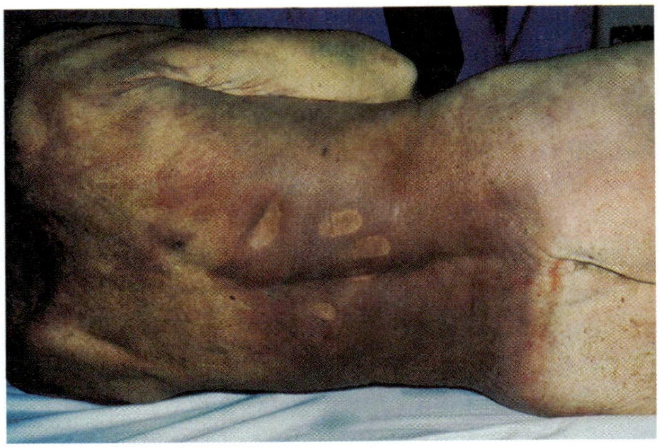

FIGURE 3-4 Dependent lividity is an obvious sign of death caused by discoloration of the body from pooling of the blood to the lower parts of the body.

Definitive Signs of Death

Definitive or conclusive signs of death that are obvious and clear to even nonmedical people include the following:

- Obvious mortal damage, such as decapitation.
- **Putrefaction**. Decomposition of body tissues. Skin may be bloated or ruptured, with or without soft tissue sloughing off. Depending on temperature conditions, this occurs sometime between 40 and 96 hours after death.
- Transection of the torso between the shoulders and hips, with or without severing the spinal column.
- Incineration. Full-thickness burns to more than 90% of body surface area, complete absence of body hair, and charred skin.
- Injuries incompatible with life (massive crush injury, severe displacement of brain matter).
- **Dependent lividity**. Blood settling to the lowest point of the body, causing discoloration of the skin (**FIGURE 3-4**).
- **Rigor mortis**. The stiffening of body muscles caused by chemical changes within muscle tissue. It develops first in the face and jaw, gradually extending downward until the body is in full rigor. The rate of onset is affected by the body's ability to lose heat to its surroundings. The rate of heat loss is greater in someone with less body fat than in someone with more body fat. A body on a tile floor has faster heat loss than a body wrapped up in a blanket in a bed. Rigor mortis occurs sometime between 2 and 12 hours after death.
- **Algor mortis**. The cooling of the body until it matches the ambient temperature

Additionally, the 2022 National Model EMS Clinical Guidelines recommend withholding resuscitation of patients with blunt or penetrating trauma who are apneic and pulseless and who present without other signs of life such as movement, electrocardiographic activity, and pupillary response.

Medical Examiner Cases

Involvement of the medical examiner, or the coroner in some states, depends on the nature and scene of the death. In most states, when trauma is a factor or the death involves suspected criminal or unusual situations such as hanging or poisoning, the medical examiner must be notified (**FIGURE 3-5**). When the medical examiner or coroner assumes responsibility of the scene, that responsibility supersedes all others at the scene, including the family's. The following are a few examples of deaths that may be considered medical examiner cases:

- When the person is dead on arrival (DOA; sometimes referred to as dead on scene [DOS])
- Death without previous medical care or when the physician is unable to state the cause of death
- Suicide
- Violent death
- Poisoning, known or suspected
- Death resulting from unintentional injuries
- Suspicion of a criminal act
- Infant and child deaths

Words of Wisdom

In 1978, Charles B. Gillespie, MD, wrote an EMT Oath that was adopted by the National Association of Emergency Medical Technicians. Statements such as this, including the more recent Code of Ethics for EMS Clinicians endorsed by the EMS Compact, strive to define the key virtues of the EMS profession. The EMT Oath reads as follows[9]:

As an EMS practitioner, I solemnly pledge myself to the following code of professional ethics:

- To conserve life, alleviate suffering, promote health, do no harm, and encourage the quality and equal availability of emergency medical care.
- To provide services based on human need, with compassion and respect for human dignity, unrestricted by consideration of nationality, race, creed, color, or status; to not judge the merits of the patient's request for service, nor allow the patient's socioeconomic status to influence our demeanor or the care that we provide.
- To not use professional knowledge and skills in any enterprise detrimental to the public well being.
- To respect and hold in confidence all information of a confidential nature obtained in the course of professional service unless required by law to divulge such information.
- To use social media in a responsible and professional manner that does not discredit, dishonor, or embarrass an EMS organization, co-workers, other health care practitioners, patients, individuals or the community at large.
- To maintain professional competence, striving always for clinical excellence in the delivery of patient care.
- To assume responsibility in upholding standards of professional practice and education.
- To assume responsibility for individual professional actions and judgment, both in dependent and independent emergency functions, and to know and uphold the laws which affect the practice of EMS.
- To be aware of and participate in matters of legislation and regulation affecting EMS.
- To work cooperatively with EMS associates and other allied health care professionals in the best interest of our patients.
- To refuse participation in unethical procedures, and assume the responsibility to expose incompetence or unethical conduct of others to the appropriate authority in a proper and professional manner.

Code of Ethics. National Association of Emergency Medical Technicians website. https://www.naemt.org/about-ems/code-of-ethics. Revised and adopted June 14, 2023. Accessed August 6, 2024.

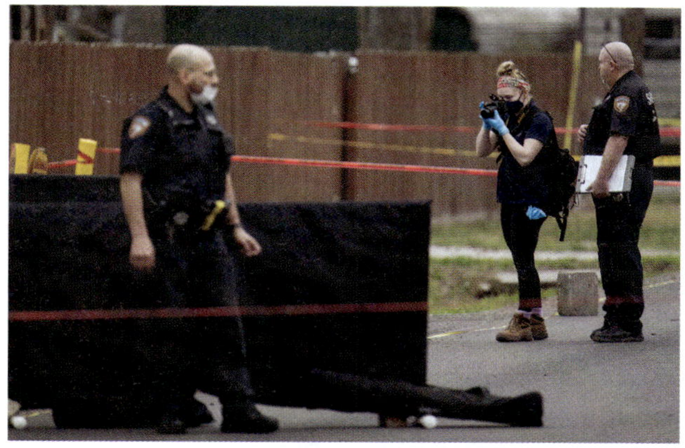

FIGURE 3-5 When trauma is a factor or the death involves an unusual or a suspected criminal situation, the medical examiner must be notified.

You should make every attempt to limit your disturbance of a scene involving a death. Once you have adequately determined death based on local protocols, remove yourself from the scene. This is especially important if there is anything potentially suspicious about the death.

If emergency medical care has been initiated, be sure to keep thorough notes of what was done or found. These records may be important during a subsequent investigation. Leave any supplies used such as an oropharyngeal airway (OPA) or bag-mask device with the body.

In such instances, there is no urgent reason to move the body. The only immediate action that is required of you is to prevent its disturbance. Local protocol will determine your ultimate action in these instances.

Special Situations

Organ Donors

You may be called to a scene involving a potential organ donor. Consent to organ donation is voluntary and knowing. Consent is evidenced by either a donor card or a driver's license indicating that the individual wishes to be a donor (**FIGURE 3-6**). You may need to consult with medical direction when faced with this situation.

In specific circumstances, a patient who is not successfully resuscitated may be a potential organ donor. Certain centers can procure organs,

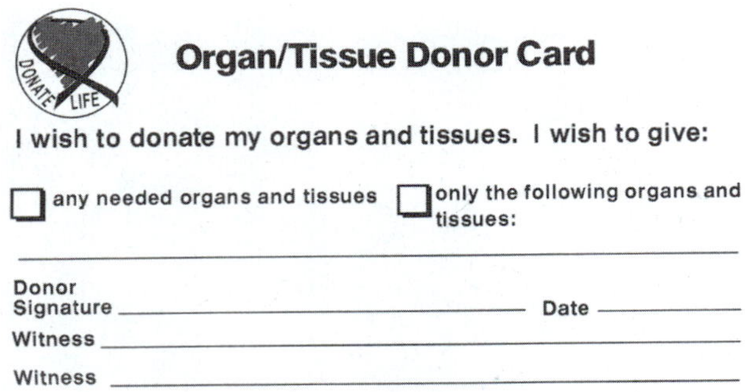
Organ/Tissue Donor Card

I wish to donate my organs and tissues. I wish to give:

☐ any needed organs and tissues ☐ only the following organs and tissues: ______

Donor Signature ______ Date ______

Witness ______

Witness ______

FIGURE 3-6 The patient may be carrying a donor card or driver's license indicating the willingness to be an organ donor.

Courtesy of the U.S. Department of Health and Human Services.

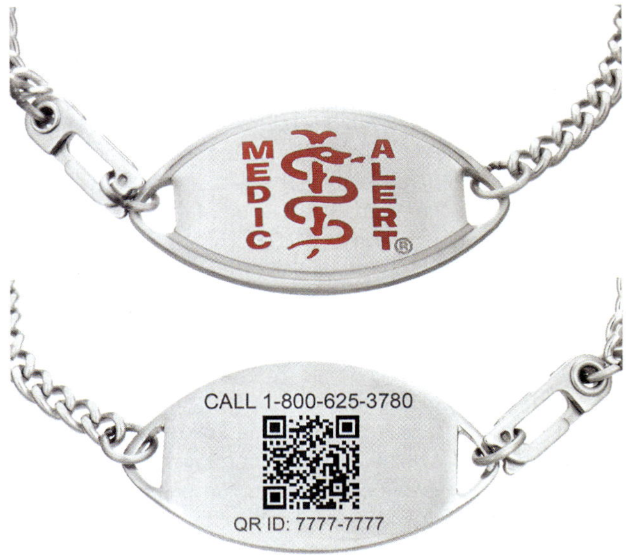

FIGURE 3-7 The patient may be carrying a medical identification card or wearing a bracelet or necklace that indicates important medical information and possible do-not-attempt-resuscitation orders. In the case of MedicAlert, the EMS clinician can obtain stored patient history information from the MedicAlert Foundation.

Used with permission from MedicAlert Foundation.

including the kidneys and liver, in certain situations. These situations typically occur after in-hospital cardiac arrest but may be associated with certain specific out-of-hospital cardiac arrest situations that occur near specialized centers. It is possible to retrieve tissues used for transplant several hours after death.[10] Be aware of your local centers and their protocols and capabilities.

You should treat a potential organ donor in the same way that you would any other patient needing treatment. Use all means necessary to keep the patient alive. Organs that are often donated, such as a kidney, heart, or liver, need oxygen at all times; you must give oxygen to the possible donor or the organs will be damaged and become useless.

Remember, your priority is to save the patient's life. Be sure to learn what the specific protocols are in your area regarding special situations such as organ donation.

Medical Identification Insignia

Many patients will carry important medical identification and information, often in the form of a bracelet, necklace, key chain, or card that identifies patient history information. This may include a DNAR order or information related to medications taken, allergies, diabetes, epilepsy, or some other serious condition (**FIGURE 3-7**). Some patients wear a medical bracelet, which contains pertinent patient information, such as drug interactions, allergies, or emergency contact information. Some of these bracelets, or other forms of identification, include QR codes or USB flash drives.

Scope of Practice

The **scope of practice**, which is most commonly defined by state law, outlines the care you are legally able to provide for the patient. Your medical director further defines the scope of practice by developing protocols and standing orders. The medical director gives you the legal authorization to provide patient care through telephone or radio communication (online) or standing orders and protocols off-line. It is your responsibility as an EMT to know your scope of practice and follow it. You and other EMS personnel have a responsibility to provide proper, consistent patient care and to report problems, such as possible liability or exposure to infectious disease, to your medical director immediately.

If you carry out procedures for which you are not authorized, you are practicing outside your scope of practice, which may be considered negligence or, in some states, even a criminal offense. The scope of practice should not be confused with the standard of care.

Standards of Care

The law generally requires you be concerned about the safety and welfare of others when your behavior

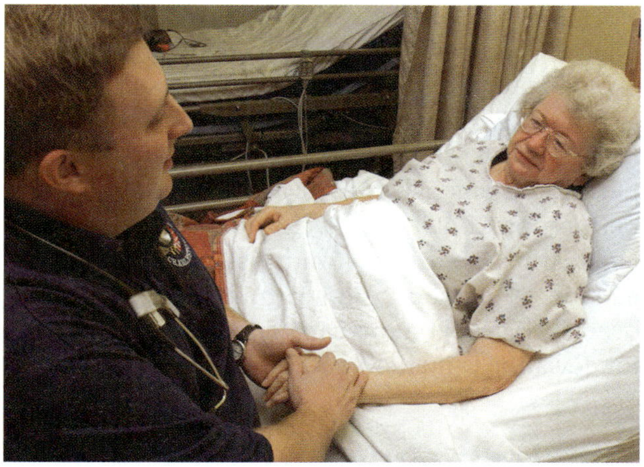

FIGURE 3-8 Act or behave toward others in a way that shows your concern about their safety and welfare.

or activities have the potential for causing others injury or harm (**FIGURE 3-8**). The manner in which you must act or behave as an EMT is called a **standard of care**.

Standard of care is established in many ways, among them local customs, statutes, evidence-based publications, ordinances, protocols, medical literature, textbooks, administrative regulations, and case law. In addition, professional or institutional standards have a bearing on determining the adequacy of your conduct.

Standards Imposed by Local Custom

The standard of care is how a reasonably prudent person with similar training and experience would act under similar circumstances, with similar equipment, and in a similar place. For example, the conduct of an EMT who is employed by an ambulance service is judged in comparison with the expected conduct of other EMTs from comparable ambulance services in the same geographic area. These standards are often based on local protocols.

As an EMT, you will not be held to the same standard of care as physicians or other more highly trained professionals. In addition, your conduct must be judged considering the given emergency situation, taking into account certain factors, including the following:

- Scene safety
- General confusion at the scene of the emergency
- The needs of other patients
- The type of equipment available

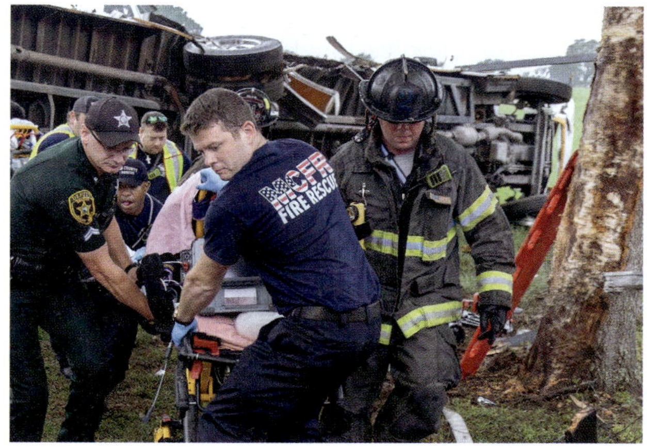

FIGURE 3-9 In emergency situations, you will care for those with potentially life-threatening injuries or illnesses by practicing a standard of care—the accepted level of care expected in your profession for your level of training.

In this context, an **emergency** is a serious situation, such as an injury or an illness that arises suddenly, threatens the life or welfare of a person or group of people, and requires immediate intervention.

Prevailing customs within a community are important elements in determining the standard of emergency care within that community. This means the accepted standard of care can change from one community to another. Examples of prevailing customs can include how hospital destinations are selected, when EMS helicopters are used, and protocols for contacting medical direction (**FIGURE 3-9**).

Standards Imposed by Law

In addition to local customs, standards of emergency medical care may be imposed by statutes, ordinances, administrative regulation, or case law. In many jurisdictions, violating one of these standards is said to create presumptive negligence. Therefore, you must become familiar with the legal standards that may exist in your state. In some states, this may take the form of treatment protocols published by a state agency.[11]

Professional or Institutional Standards

In addition to standards imposed by law, professional or institutional standards may be admitted as evidence in determining the adequacy of an EMT's conduct. Professional standards include recommendations published by organizations and societies that are involved in emergency medical care. Institutional standards include specific rules and procedures of the EMS system, ambulance service, or organization with which you are affiliated.

Two notes of caution: First, you must be familiar with the standards of your organization. Second, if you are involved in formulating standards for a particular agency, they should be reasonable and realistic so that they do not impose an unreasonable burden on EMTs. Regardless, providing the best emergency medical care should be every EMT's goal.

Many standards of care may be imposed on you. State health department regulations usually govern the scope and level of training. Court decisions have resulted in case law defining standards of care. Professional standards are also imposed. For example, the International Liaison Committee on Resuscitation (ILCOR), along with its member the American Heart Association (AHA), updates the standard for basic life support and CPR on a regular basis.

Ordinary care is a minimum standard of care. In general, it is expected that any EMT who offers assistance will exercise reasonable care and act prudently. If you act reasonably, according to the accepted standard, the risk of a civil lawsuit is small. If you apply the standard practices you have been trained to use, you can likely avoid liability. For example, various organizations have defined standards for performing CPR. If you deviate from these standards, you may be liable for civil and possibly criminal prosecution. In addition, state regulatory agencies that oversee EMS operations can sanction EMS personnel for deviating from the standard of care.

Standards Imposed by Textbooks

In the course of a lawsuit, an attorney will often present evidence from a variety of sources in an effort to establish the standard of care in a given situation. Because almost all EMS textbooks follow standards published by the NHTSA, these textbooks are often recognized as contributing to, but not completely defining, the standard of care that is followed by EMTs. However, other sources, such as regulatory standards, primary research sources, national model guidelines, and evidence-based guidelines, are increasingly recognized as higher levels of authority, particularly when there is conflicting information between textbooks.[12] Local protocols or

YOU are the EMT

The patient consents to EMS treatment and transport after you tell him he could be experiencing a serious medical emergency. You place the patient onto the stretcher. While loading the patient in the ambulance, the clerk asks, "What's wrong with him? Did I do the right thing?"

Recording Time: 10 Minutes	
Level of consciousness	Conscious and alert
Respirations	22 breaths/min; regular and unlabored
Pulse	104 beats/min; strong and regular
Skin	Baseline color, warm, and dry
Blood pressure	194/108 mm Hg
Oxygen saturation (Spo_2)	99%

En route to the hospital, you dim the lights in the ambulance, apply a cool compress to the patient's forehead, and ensure that he is in a comfortable position. You then obtain his patient information and medical history.

7. Does HIPAA affect the medical care you provide to your patients? What information are you allowed to discuss with family members, bystanders, the media, and others?

8. How do you respond to the clerk's question in a professional manner without violating HIPAA regulations?

state standards may differ from material presented in textbooks. When such differences occur, you are bound to follow local protocols.

Standards Imposed by States

Medical Practices Act

In some states, EMS personnel are exempt from the licensure requirements of the Medical Practices Act because an EMT is regarded as a nonmedical professional. The practice of medicine is defined as the diagnosis and treatment of disease or illness. EMTs and others in the prehospital care chain assess the need for life support and begin care. Some states, however, have adopted legislation that establishes the scope of practice for EMS clinicians. Therefore, as an EMT you must be aware of the standards established by legislation in your state so you can be sure to provide care that is consistent with those standards.

Certification and Licensure

Most states require initial EMT certification by the National Registry; however, some states provide this initial certification. In all states, after the candidate passes the initial certification exams, they must obtain certification, licensure, or credentialing to practice emergency medical care. Once certified, you are obliged to conform to the competency standards that are generally recognized nationally by various national professional EMS organizations. You must ensure that your certification or licensure remains current and that your knowledge and skill levels are kept up to date. For more information on certification and licensure, see Chapter 1, *EMS Systems and Public Health*.

Duty to Act

Duty to act is an individual's responsibility to provide patient care. Responsibility comes from either statute or function. A bystander is under no obligation to assist a stranger in distress and therefore has no duty to act. For an EMT, there may be a duty to act in certain instances, including the following:

- You are charged with emergency medical response.
- Your service or department's policy states that you must assist in any emergency.

Once your ambulance responds to a call or treatment is begun, you have a legal duty to act. In most cases, if you are off duty and happen to see a motor vehicle crash, you are not legally obligated to stop and assist patients. There may be some circumstances where this is not true, and you should be familiar with the laws and policies that apply in your service area. If you choose to intervene while off duty, you must continue to provide competent care until an equal or higher medical authority assumes care of the patient.

Negligence

Negligence is the failure to provide the same care that a person with similar training would provide in the same or a similar situation. It is deviation from the accepted standard of care that may result in further injury to the patient. Determination of negligence is based on the following four factors:

1. **Duty.** The EMT has an obligation to provide care and to do so in a manner that is consistent with the standard of care established by training and local protocols.
2. **Breach of duty.** There is a breach of duty when the EMT does not act within an expected and reasonable standard of care.
3. **Damages.** There are damages when a patient is physically or psychologically harmed in some noticeable way.
4. **Causation.** There must be a reasonable cause-and-effect relationship between the breach of duty and the damages suffered by the patient. This is often referred to as **proximate causation**, which is derived from the Latin words *proxima*, meaning nearest, and *causa*, meaning cause. An example is dropping the patient during lifting, causing a fracture of the patient's leg. If an EMT has a duty and breaches it, thereby causing harm to a patient, the EMT, the agency, and/or the medical director may be sued for negligence if that breach of duty was the direct cause of the patient's injury.

All four elements must be present for the legal doctrine of liability to apply and for a plaintiff to prevail in a lawsuit against an EMS system or clinician. It is also possible for an EMT or an EMS system to be inferred to be liable even when the plaintiff is unable to clearly demonstrate how an injury occurred, under the theory of **res ipsa loquitur**. In these cases, the prosecution must show that the event was unlikely to have occurred without negligence, that the plaintiff was not at fault, and that the defendant had control over the cause of the harm. An EMT could be held liable under this theory if it can be shown that an injury occurred, that the cause of the injury was in the control of the EMT, and that such injuries generally do not occur unless there is negligence. For example, you and your partner are called to the home of a man with diabetes who has lapsed into unconsciousness. You find the patient lying on a couch with no visible signs of trauma. While loading the patient into the ambulance, your partner slips and the stretcher drops, causing the patient to sustain a facial laceration. The patient later files a lawsuit against you for negligence. Because the patient was unconscious, he is unable to describe exactly how he sustained a facial laceration. Under the theory of res ipsa loquitur, the patient may prevail in his lawsuit by showing that he was under your care, that he suffered an injury, and that his injury would not have occurred unless there was negligence.

In rare cases, the plaintiff may be able to establish liability by using the theory of **negligence per se**. This is a theory that may be used when the conduct of the person being sued is alleged to have occurred in clear violation of a statute. For example, if you were to perform an ALS skill, such as the intravenous administration of a cardiac medication that resulted in injury to a patient, the plaintiff might allege that this was negligence per se. In that case, the plaintiff would not have to establish the circumstances surrounding your conduct. There would be no need to show that the administration of the medication was inappropriate for the patient because you clearly exceeded your scope of practice.

All forms of negligence come under the general category known as **torts**. Torts are simply defined as civil wrongs. They are not within the jurisdiction of US criminal courts. Examples of other tort actions are lawsuits for defamation of character and invasion of privacy.

Abandonment

Abandonment is the unilateral termination of care by the EMT without the patient's consent and without making any provisions for continuing care by a medical professional who is competent to provide care for the patient. Once care is started, you have assumed a duty that must not stop until an equally competent medical provider assumes responsibility. Failure to perform that duty is a serious legal and ethical matter that exposes the patient to harm and can result in civil action against you.

For example, suppose you arrive at the scene of a single-car crash and begin care of two injured patients. A passerby tells you of a two-car crash farther down the road in which five people are injured. You turn over care of the two injured patients from the first crash to the passerby, who is not a trained emergency care provider, and go to the second crash. Abandonment may have occurred because you did not turn care of the patients over to a person who is trained and competent to provide emergency care that meets the needs of the two patients. Consider the following general questions when you must make a decision such as this one:

- What problems may develop from your actions?
- How might the patient's condition worsen if you leave?
- Does the patient need care?
- Are you neglecting your duty to your patient?
- Is the person assuming care capable of providing the level of care needed by the patient?
- Are you abandoning the patient if you leave the scene?
- Are you violating a standard of care?
- Are you acting prudently?

Abandonment may also take place in the emergency department (ED) where you drop off your patient. A part of your obligation as an EMT is to provide appropriate hospital personnel with a report of your assessment findings, the care you provided, and any changes in patient status that occurred during transport to the hospital. The failure to do so could result in a delay in treatment or a misdiagnosis. In such a case, a claim for abandonment could be filed against the EMT who failed to provide the report.

Assault and Battery and Kidnapping

Assault is defined as unlawfully placing a person in fear of immediate bodily harm. Threatening to restrain a patient who does not want to be transported could be considered assault. **Battery** is defined as unlawfully touching a person; this includes providing emergency care without consent. Assault and battery can be either civil or criminal in nature. Civil lawsuits for battery are common in health care. To sustain a criminal case of assault or battery, it is generally necessary to prove the intent to cause harm. The element of intent is rarely present in an EMS clinician's actions; therefore, criminal cases of assault and/or battery are rare. **Kidnapping** is the seizing, confining, abducting, or carrying away of a person by force. In theory, this might include a situation where a patient is transported against their will. In reality, criminal charges of kidnapping are almost unheard of in EMS because the EMT is almost always acting in a good-faith effort to provide care to the patient. It is far more likely that an EMT could be the target of a civil lawsuit for **false imprisonment**. This is defined as the unauthorized confinement of a person that lasts for an appreciable period. Consider a patient who rescinds consent during transport and demands to be let out of the ambulance. If you refuse, you may be accused of false imprisonment.

Serious legal problems may arise in situations in which a patient has not given consent for treatment. Battery could be considered if you apply a physical intervention, such as splinting a fracture or administering an EpiPen, even though it was the correct treatment and the patient had consented to your initial care. Under such circumstances, a patient might file a lawsuit for assault or battery. Criminal charges are possible but far less likely. To protect yourself from these charges, make sure that you obtain expressed consent or that the situation allows for implied consent. It is always wise, if patient can provide expressed consent, to receive continuous verbal consent (eg, "I'm going to apply this splint now. Is that okay?") throughout your care. Consult your medical director or service attorney if you have questions or doubt about a specific situation.

Words of Wisdom

The best way to ensure you make good ethical decisions is to make the welfare of your patient, including their right to autonomy, your top priority.

Defamation

As an EMT, you should also be aware of the laws involving defamation. **Defamation** is the communication of false information that damages the reputation of a person. Defamation that is in writing is referred to as **libel**, and defamation that is spoken is known as **slander**. A legal claim for defamation could arise out of a false statement on a PCR, inappropriate comments made on social media or during "station house" conversations, or sharing "war stories" with friends, relatives, or neighbors. To avoid liability for such a claim and to protect the confidentiality of patients, never communicate information about your patients to nonauthorized people, and be sure that the information contained in your PCRs and other documentation is accurate and relevant. There is never a reason to post information about your patient on social media. You should never comment on your patient's personal information when it is not relevant to your assessment or treatment of the patient.

Good Samaritan Laws and Immunity

All states have adopted **Good Samaritan laws**, which are based on the common law principle that when individuals help another person (ie, act as a Good Samaritan), they should not be liable for errors and omissions that are made in giving good-faith emergency care. These laws are not intended for people who are being compensated for doing a job, however, and do not necessarily protect you from a lawsuit when you are on duty as an EMT. They do apply when you are off duty.

Good Samaritan provisions vary significantly from state to state. Good Samaritan statutes in some jurisdictions provide immunity from a lawsuit, whereas others provide an affirmative defense if you are sued for rendering care. In most cases, they do not prohibit the filing of a lawsuit, nor do they pertain to acts that could be considered wanton, gross, or willful negligence. To be protected by the provisions of a Good Samaritan law, several conditions must generally be met:

1. You had no duty to act.
2. You acted in good faith in rendering care.
3. You rendered care without expectation of compensation.

4. You acted within the scope of your training.
5. You did not act in a grossly negligent manner.

Gross negligence is defined as conduct that constitutes a willful or reckless disregard for a duty or standard of care.

Another group of laws grants immunity from liability to some governmental agencies and sometimes their employees. These laws, which vary widely from state to state, do not provide immunity when injury or damage is caused by gross negligence or willful misconduct. In most cases, immunity statutes apply only to EMS systems that are considered governmental agencies. This concept, known as sovereign or **governmental immunity**, usually provides limitations on liability; immunity is not complete and may depend on the circumstances. For example, in some states, immunity may not protect the clinician when the situation is not deemed to be an emergency or when the EMT is driving the ambulance.[13]

Most states have also adopted specific laws granting special privileges to EMS personnel, authorizing them to perform certain medical procedures. Many states also grant partial immunity to EMTs and physicians and nurses who give emergency instructions to EMS personnel via radio or other forms of communication. Consult your medical director or state EMS agency for more information about the laws in your area.

Records and Reports

Because EMS clinicians are in a position to observe and gather information about diseases, injuries, and emergency events, an obligation to compile such information and report it to certain agencies may be imposed. Even if there is no such requirement, you should compile a complete and accurate record of all incidents in which you have contact with sick or injured patients. A complete and accurate record of an emergency medical incident is an important safeguard against legal complications. The absence of a record, or a substantially incomplete record, increases the likelihood that you may have to testify on memory alone. This can prove to be wholly inadequate and embarrassing in the face of aggressive cross-examination.

You should consider the following two general rules regarding the perception of reports and records in a legal setting:

- If an action or procedure is not recorded on the written report, it was not performed.
- An incomplete or untidy report is evidence of incomplete or inexpert emergency medical care.

YOU are the EMT

While reassessing the patient, he admits to using cocaine. You complete your reassessment and then call in your radio report to the receiving facility. The patient's blood pressure has improved, and he tells you that his headache is not as bad as it was before.

Recording Time: 15 Minutes	
Level of consciousness	Conscious and alert
Respirations	18 breaths/min; regular and unlabored
Pulse	90 beats/min; strong and regular
Skin	Baseline color, warm, and dry
Blood pressure	166/94 mm Hg
Oxygen saturation (Spo_2)	99%

You deliver the patient to the ED and give your oral report to the receiving nurse. After completing your PCR, you and your partner return to service.

9. Should you report the patient's use of illegal substances to law enforcement personnel? Why or why not?
10. Why is it a good idea to have the receiving nurse sign your PCR acknowledging the transfer of care?

You can avoid both of these potentially dangerous presumptions by compiling and maintaining accurate reports and records of all events and patients. PCRs also help the EMS system evaluate individual and service provider performance. These reports are essential to reimbursement for EMS service and are an integral part of most quality assurance programs. Data extraction from PCRs is also used to conduct prehospital emergency care research, which may improve patient outcomes.

The National EMS Information System (NEMSIS) is a tool for the EMS profession. NEMSIS provides the ability to collect, store, and share standardized EMS data throughout the United States. This incredibly useful database can be used to improve the speed and accuracy of data collection. NEMSIS could, for example, provide early warning of a disease outbreak.

Street Smarts

Most lawsuits take years to unfold. If you are called to testify in 2 or 3 years for a case that may have seemed routine, your documentation, particularly how you told the story in the narrative, may provide your only memory of the call when you are on the witness stand.

Special Mandatory Reporting Requirements

Abuse of Children, Older People, and Others

All states have enacted laws to protect abused children, and some have added other protected groups such as the older population and at-risk adults. Most states have a reporting obligation for certain people, ranging from physicians to any person. You must be aware of the requirements of the law in your state. Such statutes frequently grant immunity from liability for libel, slander, or defamation of character to the individual who is obligated to report, even if the reports are subsequently shown to be unfounded, as long as the reports are made in good faith.

Injury During the Commission of a Felony

Many states have laws requiring the reporting of any injury that is likely to have occurred during the commission of a crime, such as gunshot wounds, knife wounds, or poisonings. Again, you must be familiar with the legal requirements of your state.

Drug-Related Injuries

In some instances, drug-related injuries must be reported. These requirements may affect how you approach documenting the care of a patient. However, it should be stressed that the US Supreme Court has held that drug addiction, in contrast to drug possession or sale, is an illness and not a crime. Therefore, an injury that results from a drug overdose may not be within the definition of an injury resulting from a crime.

Some states, by statute, specifically establish confidentiality and excuse certain specified people from reporting drug cases, either to a government agency or to a minor's parents, if, in the opinion of those people, withholding reporting is necessary for the proper treatment of the patient. Once again, you must be familiar with the legal requirements of your state.

Childbirth

Many states require that anyone who attends at a live birth in any place other than a licensed medical facility report the birth. As before, you must be familiar with state requirements.

Other Reporting Requirements

Other reporting requirements may include burns (in children under a certain age), attempted suicides, dog bites, certain communicable diseases, assaults, intimate partner violence, and sexual assault or rape. For discussion of sexual assault and intimate partner violence, see Chapter 35, *Patients With Special Challenges*.

Special Populations

ELDER ABUSE

Elder abuse is as prominent as child abuse in our society. Do not forget to be observant and report any suspicious signs or symptoms to the proper authorities.

Most EMS agencies require that exposures to specific communicable diseases be reported. You may be asked to transport certain patients in restraints, which may also need to be reported. Each of these situations can present significant legal problems. You should learn your local protocols regarding these situations.

Not only do the events that need to be reported vary significantly from state to state, but so do the methods and procedures by which such reporting must take place. For example, although all states require that suspected child abuse be reported, some states require that the report be filed with law enforcement, others with a designated child protection agency, and yet others with the ED. There are often time-sensitive provisions associated with reporting statutes. As has been noted earlier, it is important that you become familiar with reporting requirements of your state. Failure to report may result in disciplinary action, suspension of your privileges to practice as an EMT, a fine, or even criminal prosecution.

Scene of a Crime

If there is evidence at an emergency scene that a crime may have been committed, in most cases you must notify the dispatcher immediately so that law enforcement authorities can respond. Such circumstances should not stop you from providing lifesaving emergency medical care to the patient; however, your safety is a priority, so you must ensure that the scene is safe to enter. At times, you may have to transport the patient to the hospital before law enforcement arrives. While emergency medical care is being provided, you must be careful not to disturb the scene of the crime any more than is absolutely necessary. Notes and drawings should be made of the position of the patient and of the presence and position of any weapon or other objects that may be valuable to the investigating officers. If possible, do not cut through holes in clothing that were caused by weapons or gunshot wounds. Avoid walking through blood, and try to avoid leaving footprints in the dirt or grass at or near a crime scene. When a sexual assault is suspected, try to persuade the victim not to shower or clean themselves. You should confer periodically with local authorities and be aware of their wishes regarding actions you should take at the scene of the crime. It is best if these guidelines can be established by protocol. Many hospitals have specially trained nurses (sexual assault nurse examiners) trained in caring for patients of sexual assault and evidence collection.

Words of Wisdom

State laws vary regarding whether EMS personnel must report rape or sexual assault. In some states, the decision to report these crimes lies with the patient. Note that suspected sexual abuse of children or older adults and domestic abuse must be reported in most states.[14]

The EMT in Court

As an EMT, there are several different circumstances that might cause you to end up in court, either as a witness or a defendant in a civil lawsuit, or as a witness or defendant in a criminal case. Regardless of the circumstances, being in court is often stressful. As a witness in a civil case, you may be called to testify about the condition of the plaintiff when you arrived at the scene of a crash and about the treatment that you provided. In a criminal case, you may be asked to describe a crime scene or the injuries that you found when you examined a crime victim, or to testify concerning any admissions or statements made to you by a criminal defendant.

Whenever you are subpoenaed to testify in any court proceeding, you should immediately notify the director of your service and legal counsel. As a witness you should remain neutral during your testimony. You are simply there to provide the facts as you observed them and not to take sides. Many of the questions that you will be asked likely will be based on the documentation you wrote at the time of the incident. Be sure to review your PCR prior to your court appearance (**FIGURE 3-10**). If you did not document a piece of information, do not try to make up a response.

As a defendant in either a civil or criminal proceeding, your involvement will obviously be far more significant, and the outcome will have far greater personal consequences. In either case, you will definitely require the assistance of an attorney. In a civil lawsuit, where you are being sued in your capacity as an employee or volunteer of an EMS

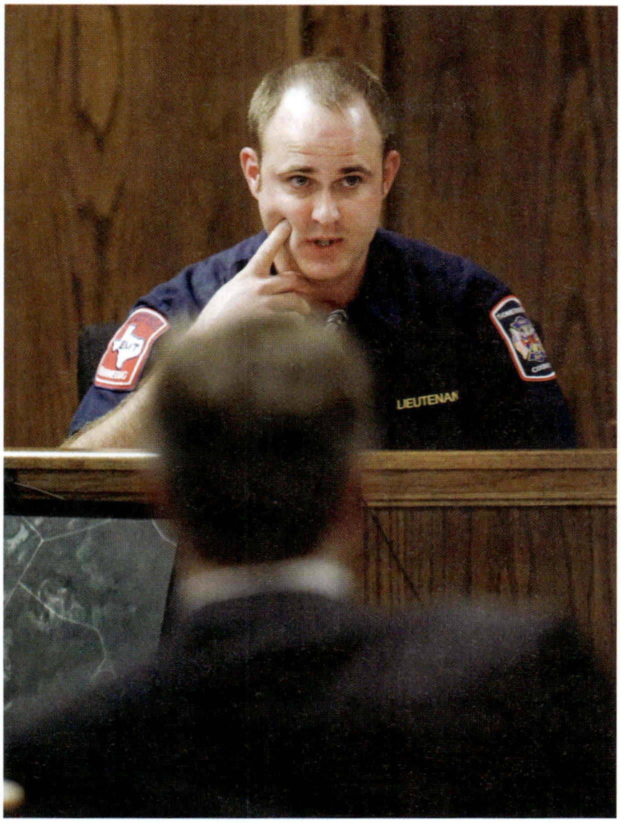

FIGURE 3-10 Court discussions will be based on your documentation. Make sure your documentation is thorough and accurate.

system, your service or its insurance company generally will provide you with legal counsel.

A civil lawsuit begins with the service of a summons and complaint. The complaint sets forth the details of the plaintiff's case and provides the theory on which the plaintiff is relying to recover a judgment against you and your service. If served with a summons, you must bring this to the attention of the head of your service immediately, because the complaint must be responded to within a set time frame, usually within 20 to 30 days. The response to the complaint is called an answer and it will generally deny the claims established in the complaint and set forth one or more defenses on behalf of you and your service. A defense is essentially a reason why the plaintiff should not recover a judgment against you. Depending on the nature of the case filed against you, the type of EMS system that you work for, and the state where you work, there may be multiple possible defense options available to you. These may include statute of limitations, immunity, or contributory negligence.

The **statute of limitations** is the time within which a claim must be initiated. For example, in many states, a claim for negligence must be initiated within 3 years of the discovery of the injury. A case initiated beyond the 3-year period would be barred by the statute of limitations. In such a case, your attorney would include the defense of statute of limitations in the answer that is filed in response to the complaint. In most states the statute of limitations is different for children. States often specify an extended period to file these cases as well as a maximum age by which a claim must be filed. For example, if an injury occurred when a child was 12 years old, the negligence claim would typically not have to be filed until that child's 21st birthday in some states.

Contributory negligence is a legal defense that may be raised when the defendant thinks that the conduct of the plaintiff somehow contributed to any injuries or damages that were sustained by the plaintiff. For example, you are treating a patient with chest pain and you think that the administration of aspirin is indicated. You ask the patient if she is allergic to aspirin and she says no. Shortly after you administer the aspirin, the signs and symptoms of a severe allergic reaction develop in the patient. Later in the hospital, the doctor advises you that the patient's medical chart history indicates that the patient has an allergy to aspirin. The patient states that she forgot she was allergic to aspirin. In this case, the defense of contributory negligence might be raised because it was the patient's forgetfulness and her denial of an aspirin allergy that contributed to the allergic reaction.

The next phase of the case, known as **discovery**, is an opportunity for both sides to obtain information that will enable the attorneys to have a better understanding of the case and assist in negotiating a possible settlement or in preparing for trial. Discovery may include interrogatories, depositions, requests for production of documents, and physical examinations. **Interrogatories** are written questions that each side sends to the other, and **depositions** are oral questions asked of parties and witnesses under oath. On completion of the discovery phase, the parties may try to negotiate a possible settlement. Most cases are settled and do not go to trial. If a settlement is not able to be negotiated, the case will be set for trial. It is not uncommon for a case to take several years to get to trial.

At trial, each side will have an opportunity to present evidence that includes testimony of witnesses and documents such as medical reports and your PCR. Witnesses may include experts such as physicians. Once both sides have concluded presenting evidence, a judge or jury will render a decision or verdict. If a judgment is rendered against you or your service, the plaintiff may be awarded compensatory or punitive damages:

1. **Compensatory damages**. These damages are intended to compensate the plaintiff for the injuries they sustained, including economic damages such as medical bills, damages to personal property, or lost earnings, and non-economic damages such as physical or emotional pain and suffering.
2. **Punitive damages**. Punitive damages are not commonly awarded in negligence cases and are reserved for those cases where the defendant has acted intentionally or with a reckless disregard for the safety of the public.

In most cases, if a judgment is rendered against you, your service or its insurance carrier will pay the judgment.

Street Smarts

When you provide testimony in any phase of a lawsuit, it is best to be brief. Answer only the specific question that is asked based on your review of the patient report or your vivid memories of the incident. Opinions and elaborations subject you to challenges by the attorneys and can make you and your testimony seem less believable to the judge or jury. Also, remember that "I don't know" or "I can't recall" might be the most accurate answer, though these responses could diminish your credibility if not used appropriately. "I don't know" suggests that you were not reasonably expected to know the details in question as part of your job. "I can't recall" suggests that it is reasonable that you do immediately have the information in question but would be able to ascertain it if given the opportunity to review documentation or reflect further.

It is also possible that you could be arrested and charged with a criminal offense arising out of your employment as an EMS clinician. Although these are rare occurrences, EMTs have been charged with crimes, including theft of patient property, physically or sexually assaulting a patient, operating a vehicle while under the influence of drugs or alcohol, manslaughter, and various drug-related offenses. Obviously, any arrest is considered very serious because a conviction could lead to imprisonment, the imposition of fines, and possible loss of the ability to practice as an EMT. Any EMT charged with a criminal offense should immediately secure the services of a highly experienced criminal attorney.

Ethical Responsibilities

In addition to legal duties, you have certain ethical responsibilities as a health care clinician. These responsibilities are to yourself, your patients, your coworkers, and the public.

Words of Wisdom

There is considerable overlap between unethical and illegal or negligent behaviors. In some cases, an EMT may experience a conflict between what is ethical and what is legal. When facing these dilemmas, consider consulting with a supervisor or medical direction to help determine the proper course of action.

Ethics is a person's moral philosophy of right and wrong, and of ideal professional behavior. It is often referred to as the study of morality. **Morality** is a code of conduct that can be defined by society, religion, or a person, affecting character and conscience and the definition of right versus wrong. An entire field of ethics known as **bioethics** has evolved over the past several decades that addresses issues that arise in the practice of health care. Many such issues have drawn national attention, such as those dealing with the termination of life support, rationing of medical resources, and physician-assisted suicide. Ethical issues are present in nearly every EMS incident. As an EMT, you will be expected to conduct yourself in a manner that is consistent with the standards of your profession and to keep the best interests of your patients at the forefront of your conduct and decision making (**FIGURE 3-11**). The manner in which principles of ethics are

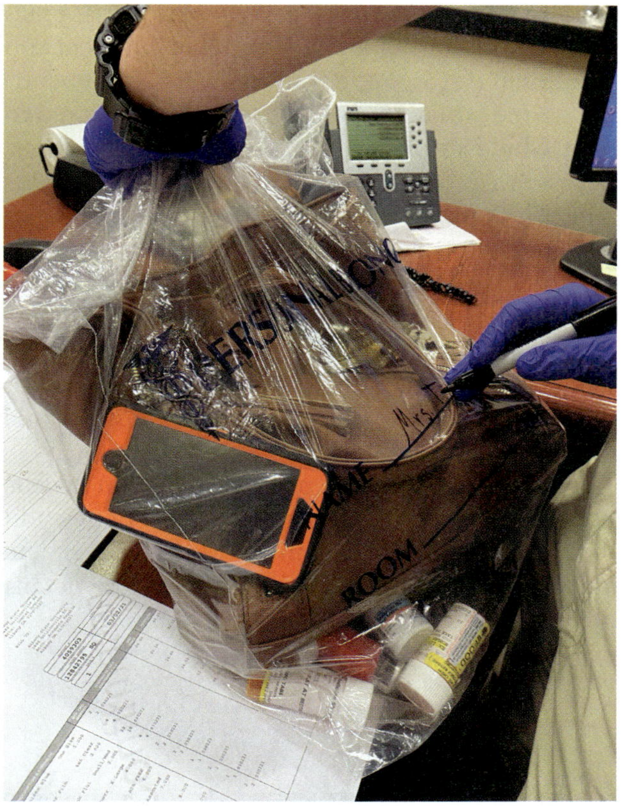

FIGURE 3-11 Your patients trust you not only to provide proper emergency medical care, but also to use sound ethical judgment, which includes safeguarding their possessions.

Courtesy of Rhonda Hunt.

incorporated into professional conduct is known as **applied ethics**.

You will encounter ethical dilemmas in the course of your employment that can be challenging to resolve. Examples might include the following[15]:

- Your partner arrives at work smelling of alcohol.
- You are called to the scene of a belligerent driver who has seriously injured several children after causing a crash while drag racing.
- You are dispatched to a 9-1-1 call for chest pain. Your partner recognizes the address and tells you not to use the lights and siren because this is a "frequent flyer" who constantly calls 9-1-1 to get attention.
- You respond to the home of an older woman in cardiac arrest. One relative hands you DNAR paperwork and states the patient did not want to be resuscitated. Another relative demands that you do everything possible to save the patient.
- One of your coworkers is unable to attend a training session and asks you to sign him in, stating, "You know I would do it for you."

The manner in which you respond to each of these circumstances requires you to evaluate and apply your own moral standards as well as the ethical standards of your profession. Obviously, these choices can be difficult at times, particularly in those cases where your own personal standards of right and wrong do not necessarily agree with the standards of your profession. You know you should report that your partner may be intoxicated while on duty, even if he is a good friend. You might also want to honor the patient's DNAR wishes, but medical direction may order you to initiate care based on the family's request.

Your behavior both on and off the job is a reflection of your personal ethical standards. News stories that depict EMS personnel engaging in any immature or illegal activities serve to lessen the public's confidence in the services that EMTs provide. Illegal drug use or selling drugs, inappropriate use of emergency vehicles, inappropriate visitors entertained at the station, and use of alcohol on duty can have a negative effect on the EMT and on EMS in general and should be strictly forbidden.

If you care about your patients, your coworkers, and the EMS system as a whole, you also may not stand by silently and watch as other EMS clinicians engage in misbehavior. Misconduct should be promptly reported to the appropriate chain of command. Similarly, you are obligated to report medical errors you make or witness to the medical director or another appropriate person as soon as possible.

EMS clinicians should establish their own ethical standards and monitor the ethical behavior of their members. How can you make sure you are acting ethically, especially with all the decisions you have to make in the field? First, you should consider all options available to you and the consequence of each option. Have decisions been made in the past regarding a similar situation? Can an existing policy or rule be applied? How will the consequences of your decision provide the greatest benefit in view of all the alternatives? Involve online medical direction in your decision making (**TABLE 3-2**).

TABLE 3-2 Ethical Decision-Making Checklist

	Yes	No
Is the decision in the best interests of the patient?	❑	❑
Is the decision based on logic and reason rather than emotion?	❑	❑
Does the decision protect the patient's rights?	❑	❑
Would you agree to the same decision if you were the patient?	❑	❑
Would you make the same decision again in similar circumstances?	❑	❑
Can you defend this decision to others?	❑	❑

You must meet your legal and ethical responsibilities while caring for your patients' physical and emotional needs. Patient needs will vary depending on the situation, and you must be prepared to offer whatever physical and emotional support is necessary. In most cases that you will encounter as an EMT, there will be a rule, a law, or a policy that will guide your decision making and your actions. As a professional, you are bound to follow all such policies, rules, and laws even in those rare circumstances where your own personal sense of morals might lead you to a different result. In short, your professional ethics trump personal morals while on duty.

One unquestionable responsibility you have is honest reporting. Remember, absolute honesty in reporting is essential. You must provide a complete and accurate account of the events and the details of all patient care and professional duties.

YOU are the EMT SUMMARY

1. Why is it essential that you obtain consent to treat the patient once you arrive?

Consent is required from every conscious adult before care can be started. The adult patient who is conscious, rational, and capable of making informed decisions has a legal right to refuse care. The patient does not forfeit this right simply because you disagree or because it may not be the best medical decision. The law allows patients to make choices that may seem medically unsound and might even endanger their own life. Failing to honor a competent adult patient's right to refuse care or transport may be grounds for both criminal and civil action against you.

2. Should you assess the patient's decision-making capacity once you arrive?

Your role is to assess the patient's decision-making capacity. Although the terms competence and decision-making capacity are often thought of interchangeably, there is a distinction. Competence is typically determined by a court of law, whereas decision-making capacity refers to whether a patient is capable of making a rational decision. Assessing a patient's decision-making capacity can often be complicated in the prehospital setting, and you may require the assistance of medical direction to make the best decision.

3. Are you legally authorized to treat this patient? Why or why not?

At this point, you have not obtained consent from the patient to begin treating him; in fact, you have not even introduced yourself. Under most circumstances, you may not begin treatment of a mentally competent adult until the person has given you permission, or consent, to do so. If the patient has decision-making capacity, meaning the patient is conscious, alert, not under the influence of drugs or alcohol, and of legal age (18 years in most states), you cannot legally provide care without the patient's consent, even if the patient is obviously sick or injured. Providing care without the patient's consent may be grounds for both criminal and civil action, such as assault and battery.

4. How does informed consent differ from implied consent?

A patient's consent must be informed, which means you have explained the nature of the treatment being

YOU are the EMT SUMMARY continued

offered, including the potential risks, benefits, and alternatives to treatment, as well as any potential consequences of refusing treatment.

Implied consent is based on the legal assumption that a critically ill or injured patient, who is physically unable to give consent (ie, unconscious, under the influence of drugs or alcohol), would consent to EMS treatment and transport if physically able to do so. Consent to treat is also implied when caring for a minor whose parents or caregivers are unable to be located; a minor cannot legally consent to or refuse medical care.

5. What should you do when a patient refuses treatment and/or transport?

When patients refuse treatment and/or transport, it is not unreasonable to ask why they do not wish to be treated. Many people refuse treatment because of financial concerns or the fact that they are scared. In this case, you should explain that his high blood pressure and severe headache could indicate bleeding in the brain or some other potentially life-threatening condition and that only a physician can diagnose his problem. Do not be afraid to advise the patient that his refusal could ultimately result in death if you believe it is true. This is not a scare tactic; it is the truth, and the patient has a right to hear it.

If, despite your best efforts to obtain consent to treat, an adult who has decision-making capacity still refuses, there is little else you can legally do. You should, however, inform medical direction of the situation. In some cases, the physician may wish to speak directly to the patient.

6. What questions should you ask yourself to help determine whether you can transport this patient against his will?

When a patient refuses treatment, you must assess the patient's decision-making capacity. Is the patient's mental condition impaired? Is the patient under the influence of drugs or alcohol? Is the patient of legal age? Is the patient a danger to self or others? These are but a few of the questions that must be answered.

In this case, there is no evidence that has been uncovered thus far that the patient's decision-making capacity is impaired, and although he needs medical attention for his headache and blood pressure, you cannot legally force him to accept it, nor can you transport him against his will.

The best course of action is to ensure that the patient is aware of the potential consequences of his refusal (such as death) and contact medical direction to apprise them of the situation.

7. Does HIPAA affect the medical care you provide to your patients? What information are you allowed to discuss with family members, bystanders, the media, and others?

HIPAA has many aims; however, the section of the act that most directly affects EMS relates to patient privacy. Confidential patient information includes patient history, assessment findings, and treatment details. HIPAA provides guidance on what types of information are protected, the responsibility of health care clinicians regarding that protection, and penalties for breaching that protection. Confidential information can be shared under certain conditions, such as for continuity of care and for billing purposes. You should not allow HIPAA to affect the medical care that you provide to a patient.

You must be very careful about what you discuss with family members, bystanders, the media, and others. You must protect the patient's confidential information. There may be times when this is difficult, especially with concerned family members. When in doubt about what to share, simply provide reassurance that everyone is doing their best for the patient.

8. How do you respond to the clerk's question in a professional manner without violating HIPAA regulations?

This is a great opportunity to praise a conscientious bystander who did the right thing. Thank the clerk, but do not provide him with any confidential patient information. For example, you may say, "You did the right thing during a stressful situation and we appreciate it. We are required to protect the patient's privacy, but I want to reassure you we will take excellent care of the patient from here."

9. Should you report the patient's use of illegal substances to law enforcement personnel? Why or why not?

The patient's use of cocaine is pertinent medical information that may have an effect on the care he receives at the hospital; therefore, it should be included in your PCR and your oral report to the receiving facility. However, the US Supreme Court has held that drug use or addiction (in contrast to possession or sale) is an illness and not a crime. Therefore, you are not legally required to report the patient's admitted use of these substances to law enforcement personnel. If you are in doubt, consult with your EMS

YOU are the EMT SUMMARY continued

medical director. More important, you must be familiar with the reporting requirements of the state in which you function as an EMT.

10. Why is it a good idea to have the receiving nurse sign your PCR acknowledging the transfer of care?

Sign-off is important for several reasons. It ensures that an equal or higher medical authority has accepted care of the patient from you. It also provides a record of who accepted care of the patient in the event there are any questions later. Failure to appropriately transfer care at the receiving hospital may be considered abandonment. Your documentation should show that you have met this obligation.

Prep Kit

Ready for Review

- Under most circumstances, consent is required from every conscious adult before care can be started. The foundation of consent is decision-making capacity.
- You should never withhold lifesaving care unless a valid DNAR order is present.
- Because a minor might not have the wisdom, maturity, or judgment to give consent, the law requires that a parent or legal guardian give consent for treatment or transport.
- Adults who are conscious and alert and who appear to have decision-making capacity have the right to refuse treatment or withdraw from treatment at any time, even if doing so may result in serious injury or death.
- You should include all information pertaining to patient refusals in your PCR.
- Communication between you and the patient is considered confidential and generally cannot be disclosed without permission from the patient or a court order.
- Advance directives, living wills, or health care directives are most commonly used when a patient becomes comatose. Physician Orders for Life-Sustaining Treatment (POLST) and Medical Orders for Life-Sustaining Treatment (MOLST) forms explicitly describe acceptable interventions for the patient in the form of medical orders.
- There are both definitive and presumptive signs of death. In many states, death is defined as the absence of circulatory and respiratory function.
- Consent to organ donation is evidenced by either a donor card or a driver's license indicating that the individual wishes to be a donor.
- Standard of care is established in many ways, among them local customs, statutes, ordinances, protocols, textbooks, administrative regulations, and case law. The scope of practice outlines the care you are able to provide for the patient.
- Once your ambulance responds to a call or treatment is begun, you have a legal duty to act. In most cases, if you are off duty and happen to see a motor vehicle crash, you are not legally obligated to stop and assist patients.
- Determination of negligence is based on the following four factors: duty, breach of duty, damages, and causation. All four elements must be present for the legal doctrine of negligence to apply and for a plaintiff to prevail in a lawsuit against an EMS system or clinician.
- Abandonment is the termination of care without the patient's consent and without making provisions for the transfer of care to a medical professional with skills at the

Prep Kit continued

same level or at a higher level than your own skills. Abandonment is legally and ethically a serious act. Always try to obtain a signature on your PCR from the person accepting transfer of care.
- Assault is defined as unlawfully placing a person in fear of immediate bodily harm. Battery is unlawfully touching a person; this includes providing emergency care without consent. To protect yourself from these charges, be sure to obtain expressed consent whenever possible.
- To avoid liability for defamation, you must only communicate information about your patients to authorized people and you should be sure that the information contained in your PCRs and other documentation is accurate and relevant.
- Good Samaritan laws are based on the common law principle that when you reasonably help another person, you should not be liable for errors and omissions that are made in giving good-faith emergency care.
- Records and reports are important. Compile a complete and accurate record of each incident. The courts consider an action or procedure that was not recorded on the written report as not having been performed, and an incomplete or untidy report is considered evidence of incomplete or inexpert medical care.
- You should know what the special reporting requirements are involving abuse of children, older adults, and others; injuries related to crimes; drug-related injuries; and childbirth.
- You must meet your legal and ethical responsibilities while caring for your patients' physical and emotional needs.
- As an EMT, there are several different circumstances that might cause you to end up in court, either as a witness or a defendant in a civil lawsuit, or as a witness or defendant in a criminal case.

Vital Vocabulary

abandonment Unilateral termination of care by the EMT without the patient's consent and without making provisions for transferring care to another medical professional with the skills and training necessary to meet the needs of the patient.

advance directive Written documentation that specifies medical treatment for a competent patient should the patient become unable to make decisions; also called a living will or health care directive.

algor mortis Cooling of the body after death until it matches the ambient temperature.

applied ethics The manner in which principles of ethics are incorporated into professional conduct.

assault Unlawfully placing a patient in fear of bodily harm.

autonomy The right of a patient to make informed choices regarding health care.

battery Unlawfully touching a patient or providing emergency care without consent.

bioethics The study of ethics related to issues that arise in health care.

breach of confidentiality Disclosure of information without proper authorization.

compassionate persuasion The act of guiding a person to accept an offer of treatment that they initially did not want while respecting patient autonomy.

compensatory damages Damages awarded in a civil lawsuit that are intended to restore the plaintiff to the same condition that they were in prior to the incident.

competent Legally able to make rational decisions about personal well-being.

consent Permission to render care.

contributory negligence A legal defense that may be raised when the defendant thinks that the

Prep Kit continued

conduct of the plaintiff somehow contributed to any injuries or damages that were sustained by the plaintiff.

decision-making capacity Ability to understand and process information and make a choice regarding appropriate medical care.

defamation The communication of false information about a person that is damaging to that person's reputation or standing in the community.

dependent lividity Blood settling to the lowest point of the body, causing discoloration of the skin; a definitive sign of death.

depositions Oral questions asked of parties and witnesses under oath.

discovery The phase of a civil lawsuit where the plaintiff and defense obtain information from each other that will enable the attorneys to have a better understanding of the case and which will assist in negotiating a possible settlement or in preparing for trial. Discovery includes depositions, interrogatories, and demands for production of records.

do not attempt resuscitation (DNAR) order Written documentation by a physician giving permission to medical personnel not to attempt resuscitation in the event of cardiac arrest.

durable power of attorney for health care A type of advance directive executed by a competent adult that appoints another individual to make medical treatment decisions on their behalf, in the event that the person making the appointment loses decision-making capacity.

duty to act A medicolegal term relating to certain personnel who either by statute or by function have a responsibility to provide care.

emancipated minor A person who is under the legal age in a given state but, because of other circumstances, is legally considered an adult.

emergency A serious situation, such as injury or illness that threatens the life or welfare of a person or group of people and requires immediate intervention.

emergency doctrine The principle of law that permits a health care clinician to treat a patient in an emergency situation when the patient is incapable of granting consent because of an altered level of consciousness, disability, the effects of drugs or alcohol, or the patient's age.

emergency medical care Immediate care or treatment.

ethics The philosophy of right and wrong, of moral duties, and of ideal professional behavior.

expressed consent A type of consent in which a patient gives verbal or nonverbal authorization for provision of care or transport.

false imprisonment The confinement of a person without legal authority or the person's consent.

forcible restraint The act of physically preventing an individual from initiating any physical action.

Good Samaritan laws Statutory provisions enacted by many states to protect citizens from liability for errors and omissions in giving good-faith emergency medical care, unless there is wanton, gross, or willful negligence.

governmental immunity Legal doctrine that can protect an EMS clinician from being sued or that may limit the amount of the monetary judgment that the plaintiff may recover; generally applies only to EMS systems that are operated by municipalities or other governmental entities.

gross negligence Conduct that constitutes a willful or reckless disregard for a duty or standard of care.

health care directive A written document that specifies medical treatment for a competent patient, should the individual become unable to make decisions. Also known as an advance directive or a living will.

health care proxy A type of advance directive executed by a competent adult that appoints another individual to make medical treatment

Prep Kit continued

decisions on their behalf in the event that the person making the appointment loses decision-making capacity. Also known as a durable power of attorney for health care.

implied consent Type of consent in which a patient who is unable to give consent is given treatment under the legal assumption that this person would want treatment.

informed consent Permission for treatment given by a competent patient after the potential risks, benefits, and alternatives to treatment have been explained.

in loco parentis Legal authorization for a person or organization to take on some of the functions and responsibilities of a parent.

interrogatories Written questions that the defense and plaintiff send to one another.

kidnapping The seizing, confining, abducting, or carrying away of a person by force, including transporting a competent adult for medical treatment without the individual's consent.

libel False and damaging information about a person that is communicated in writing.

mature minor A child who is of adequate age and maturity to make health care decisions.

mature minor doctrine Legal authorization for certain minors with adequate age and maturity to consent or refuse medical treatment.

medicolegal A term relating to medical jurisprudence (law) or forensic medicine.

morality A code of conduct that can be defined by society, religion, or a person, affecting character, conduct, and conscience.

negligence Failure to provide the same care that a person with similar training would provide.

negligence per se A theory that may be used when the conduct of the person being sued is alleged to have occurred in clear violation of a statute.

palliative care A specialized health care approach focused on treating pain and promoting comfort, rather than attempting to cure a disease or prolong life.

protected health information (PHI) Any information about health status, provision of health care, or payment for health care that can be linked to an individual. This is interpreted rather broadly and includes any part of a patient's medical record or payment history.

proximate causation Proof that a negligent act or lack of action caused an injury or worsened an existing injury.

punitive damages Damages that are sometimes awarded in a civil lawsuit when the conduct of the defendant was intentional or constituted a reckless disregard for the safety of the public.

putrefaction Decomposition of body tissues; a definitive sign of death.

res ipsa loquitur A legal principle stating that a defendant may be held liable without direct evidence if the they had exclusive control over the cause of harm, the injured person played no role in the harm, and the harm would not have occurred without negligent conduct.

rigor mortis Stiffening of the body muscles; a definitive sign of death.

scope of practice A formal definition of the care that the EMT is authorized and expected to provide for a patient; most commonly defined by state law.

shared decision making A collaborative process in which the clinician works with the patient to come up with the optimal health care approach, accounting for the patient's unique situation, concerns and values.

slander False and damaging information about a person that is communicated by spoken word.

standard of care Accepted levels of emergency care expected by reason of training and profession; written by legal or professional organizations so that patients are not exposed to unreasonable risk or harm.

Prep Kit continued

statute of limitations The time within which a case must be commenced.

surrogate decision maker A person authorized to make health care decisions on behalf of a patient when the patient lacks decision-making capacity.

torts Wrongful acts that give rise to a civil lawsuit.

References

1. Vearrier L. Do not resuscitate tattoos: are they valid? ACEP Now website. https://www.acepnow.com/article/do-not-resuscitate-tattoos-are-they-valid/. Published April 10, 2018. Accessed December 9, 2024.
2. Slevin C, Brown M. Paramedics were convicted in Elijah McClain's death. That could make other first responders pause. AP News website https://apnews.com/article/elijah-mcclain-death-officers-trial-acef1eabe02b458f53d30d8fe3bf76a4. Published December 23, 2023. Accessed August 6, 2024.
3. Olsen D. New details emerge in case against EMS workers charged with murder. Illinois Times website. https://www.illinoistimes.com/news-opinion/new-details-emerge-in-case-against-ems-workers-charged-with-murder-16407188. Published February 3, 2023. Accessed August 6, 2024.
4. Probst MA, Kanzaria HK, Schoenfeld EM, et al. Shared decision making in the emergency department: a guiding framework for clinicians. *Ann Emerg Med*. 2017;70(5):688–695.
5. Ogilvie WA, Hawnwan P, Goldstein S. EMS legal and ethical issues. *StatPearls*. National Library of Medicine website. http://www.ncbi.nlm.nih.gov/books/NBK519553/. Updated May 8, 2023. Accessed August 6, 2024.
6. US Department of Health and Human Services. Your rights under HIPAA. HHS.gov website. https://www.hhs.gov/hipaa/for-individuals/guidance-materials-for-consumers/index.html. Reviewed January 19, 2022. Accessed August 6, 2024.
7. Confidentiality. American Medical Association website. https://www.ama-assn.org/delivering-care/ethics/confidentiality. Accessed August 6 2024.
8. Zafren K, Paal P, Brugger H, Lechner R. Induced hypothermia to 4.2°C with neurologically intact survival: a forgotten case series. *Wilderness Environ Med*. 2020;31(3):367–370.
9. Code of Ethics. National Association of Emergency Medical Technicians website. https://www.naemt.org/about-ems/code-of-ethics. Revised and adopted June 14, 2023. Accessed August 6, 2024.
10. What can be donated. Human Resources and Services Administration website. https://www.organdonor.gov/learn/what-can-be-donated. Reviewed February 2024. Accessed August 6, 2024.
11. Kupas DF, Schenk E, Sholl JM, Kamin R. Characteristics of statewide protocols for emergency medical services in the United States. *Prehosp Emerg Care*. 2015 Apr-Jun;19(2):292–301.
12. Gage CB, Terry M, McKenna KD, et al. Consensus standard for evidence integration into EMS education and high-stakes testing. *Prehosp Disaster Med*. 2023;38(3):338–344.
13. Ind. Code § 16-31-6-1. Casetext website. https://casetext.com/statute/indiana-code/title-16-health/article-31-emergency-medical-services/chapter-6-immunity-from-liability/section-16-31-6-1-emergency-medical-services-immunity. Accessed August 6, 2024.
14. Wolfberg D. Pro bono: is reporting rape an EMS obligation? JEMS website. https://www.jems.com/administration-and-leadership/pro-bono-is-reporting-rape-an-ems-obligation/. Published June 15, 2015. Accessed August 6, 2024.
15. American College of Emergency Physicians EMS Committee. *Ethical Questions in Emergency Medical Services: Controversies and Recommendations*. American College of Emergency Physicians website. https://www.acep.org/globalassets/uploads/uploaded-files/acep/clinical-and-practice-management/ems-and-disaster-preparedness/ethical---ems---info-paper.pdf. Published October 2012. Accessed August 6, 2024.

Additional Resources

Advance directive forms. AARP website. http://www.aarp.org/caregiving/financial-legal/free-printable-advance-directives/. Accessed August 6, 2024.

Centers for Medicare and Medicaid Services. Advance directives and long-term care. Medicare.gov website. https://www.medicare.gov/manage-your-health/advance-directives-long-term-care. Accessed August 6, 2024.

Erbay H. Some ethical issues in prehospital emergency medicine. *Turkish J Emerg Med*. 2016;14(4):193–198.

Informed consent. American Medical Association website. https://www.ama-assn.org/delivering-care/ethics/informed-consent. Accessed August 6, 2024.

Prep Kit continued

National Association of State EMS Officials. *National Model EMS Clinical Guidelines: Version 3.0.* https://nasemso.org/wp-content/uploads/National-Model-EMS-Clinical-Guidelines_2022.pdf. Updated March 2022.Accessed January 24, 2024.

Position paper 2024-02: code of conduct. The EMS Compact website. https://www.emscompact.gov/resources/position-statements/position-paper-2024-02-code-of-conduct. Published October 16, 2024. Accessed July 23, 2025.

Privacy in health care. American Medical Association website. https://www.ama-assn.org/delivering-care/ethics/privacy-health-care. Accessed August 6, 2024.

Professionalism in relationships with media. American Medical Association website. https://www.ama-assn.org/delivering-care/ethics/professionalism-relationships-media. Accessed August 6, 2024.

Torabi M, Borhani F, Abbaszadeh A, Atashzadeh-Shoorideh F. Experiences of pre-hospital emergency medical personnel in ethical decision-making: a qualitative study. *BMC Med Ethics*. 2018;19(1):95.

Chapter 4

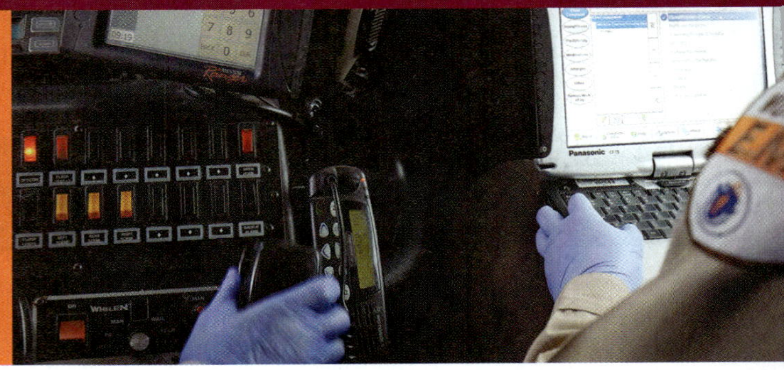

Communications and Documentation

NATIONAL EMS EDUCATION STANDARD COMPETENCIES

Preparatory

Applies knowledge of the emergency medical services (EMS) system, safety/well-being of the emergency medical technician (EMT), and medical/legal and ethical issues to the provision of emergency care.

Therapeutic Communication

- Health care literacy (p 99)
- Interviewing techniques (pp 102–106)
- Verbal defusing strategies (pp 100–101)
- Managing communication challenges (pp 106–112; Chapter 10, *Patient Assessment*)
- Family-centered care (p 109)
- Adjusting communication strategies for age, stage of development, and patients with special needs (pp 109–112; Chapter 10, *Patient Assessment*)
- Nondiscriminatory communication that addresses inherent or unconscious bias, is culturally aware and sensitive, and is intended to improve patient outcome (p 100, p 107)

EMS System Communication

- EMS communication system (pp 129–133)
- Communication with other health care professionals to include cohesive and organized patient handoff (pp 137–138)
- Team communication and dynamics (pp 133–139)
- Telemetric monitoring devices and transmission of clinical data, including video data (pp 131–132)

Documentation

- Recording patient findings (pp 118–129)
- Principles of medical documentation and report writing (pp 118–129)
- Supporting medical necessity (p 124)

Medical Terminology

Uses anatomic and medical terms and abbreviations in written and oral communication with colleagues and other health care professionals.

KNOWLEDGE OBJECTIVES

1. Describe the factors and strategies to consider for therapeutic communication with patients. (pp 98–115)
2. Discuss the techniques of effective verbal communication. (pp 102–106)
3. Discuss special considerations in communicating with older people, children, patients who are hard of hearing, visually impaired patients, and non–English-speaking patients. (pp 107–112)
4. Explain the skills that should be used to communicate with family members, bystanders, people from other agencies, and hospital personnel. (pp 112–114, p 116)

5. Differentiate issues concerning care of the dying patient, death, and the grieving process of family members. (pp 114–118)
6. Recognize the physiologic, physical, and psychological responses to stress. (pp 114–115)
7. Describe the use of written communications and documentation. (p 118)
8. State the purpose of a patient care report (PCR) and the information required to complete it. (pp 118–124)
9. Explain the legal implications of the PCR. (pp 124–129)
10. Describe how to document refusal of care, including the legal implications. (pp 126–129)
11. Discuss state and/or local special reporting requirements, such as for gunshot wounds, dog bites, and abuse. (p 129)
12. Describe the basic principles of the various types of communications equipment used in EMS. (pp 129–133)
13. Describe the use of radio communications, including the proper methods of initiating and terminating a radio call. (pp 133–134)
14. List the correct communication procedures in the following phases of a typical call: initial receipt of call, en route to call, on scene, arrival at hospital (or point of transfer), and return to service. (pp 134–136)
15. List the proper sequence of information to communicate in delivery of a patient report from the ambulance to the receiving health care facility. (pp 137–138)

SKILLS OBJECTIVES

1. Demonstrate the techniques of successful cross-cultural communication. (pp 99–106)
2. Demonstrate completion of a PCR. (pp 118–129)
3. Demonstrate how to make a simulated, concise radio transmission with dispatch. (pp 134–136)

Introduction

Communication is the transmission of information from one person to another. It may be written, verbal, or nonverbal (through body language). Effective communication is an essential part of prehospital care and is critical to achieving a positive relationship with patients, coworkers, and others in the health care industry.

Good verbal communication skills are vital for you as an EMT. Your verbal skills will enable you to gather information from the patient and bystanders. These skills will also make it possible for you to effectively coordinate with the variety of responders who are often present at the scene. Excellent verbal communication is also an integral part of transferring the patient's care to the nurses and physicians at the hospital.

Your nonverbal communication skills can be just as important as your verbal communication skills. The impression you make, including your dress, posture, and demeanor, will have an immediate effect on your relationship with the patient. Throughout the response, the patient and others on scene will continue to interpret your nonverbal cues.

Documentation is the written or electronically recorded portion of your patient care interaction that becomes part of the patient's permanent medical record. It serves many purposes, including describing the care provided on scene and during transport to the hospital. After the call, a review of the documentation can allow others to evaluate the care provided. Documentation also provides an opportunity to communicate the patient's story to others who may participate in the patient's care in the future. Adequate reporting and accurate records ensure the continuity of patient care. Complete patient records also facilitate transfer of care and responsibility, help comply with requirements of health departments and law enforcement agencies, and fulfill your organization's administrative needs. Reporting and record-keeping duties are an essential aspect of patient care, although they are performed only after the patient's condition has been stabilized.

Documentation in the field drives both funding and research for EMS. Seat belts are a prime example. Studies gathered from record keeping in the 1970s showed that patients have a significantly higher survival rate if seat belts are used during motor vehicle crashes. Armed with this information, laws were passed to enforce seat belt usage, and huge amounts of money were spent on educating the public. This, coupled with vehicle design modifications, has resulted in fewer deaths and serious injuries.[1] Fast forward to the present: research has been performed on the data collected in the National Emergency Medical Services Information System (NEMSIS) and on data in other commercial documentation systems that can link prehospital records to hospital discharge outcomes. This research is rapidly expanding the knowledge base about what EMS clinicians actually do on a day-to-day basis and on what treatment measures really make a difference. The findings have dramatically increased EMS clinicians' understanding of which prehospital tools and techniques work best and should be prioritized.

Computer, radio, cell phone, and other electronic communications link you and your team with other members of the EMS, fire, and law enforcement communities. These links help the entire team work together more effectively and provide an important layer of safety and protection for each member. You must know what your communication system can and cannot do, and you must be able to use it efficiently and effectively.

This chapter describes the strategies that you need to be an effective communicator, discusses a variety of effective methods of verbal communication, and provides guidelines for appropriate written documentation of patient care. The chapter concludes by identifying the kinds of communication equipment that are used, along with standard communication procedures and protocols, as well as the role of the Federal Communications Commission in EMS.

Therapeutic Communication

How do we communicate? This simple question can be surprisingly complex, because there are many things to consider during communication. **Therapeutic communication** uses various communication techniques and strategies, both verbal and nonverbal, to encourage patients to express how they are feeling and allow the EMT to listen and understand. These techniques can be used by health care clinicians of any level to gather critical information, defuse tense situations, and achieve a positive relationship with the patient.

Although we focus primarily on using the spoken word to communicate, much of how we communicate, and how others communicate with us, is nonverbal. Nonverbal communication can include the use of gestures or sign language to replace spoken language when, for example, people do not speak the same language or a person is hard of hearing or deaf. However, nonverbal communication is also used to enhance verbal communication, and EMTs need to pay close attention to nonverbal clues to enhance their understanding. For example, a bystander's tone of voice and gestures may indicate a situation that is emotionally charged. A patient's facial expression and posture might indicate physical pain, emotional distress, or anger, even if the person's words say otherwise.

The EMT will also communicate back to the patient using nonverbal communication. Actions such as tapping your foot, rolling your eyes, or folding your arms may send the message you are impatient, are not listening, or just don't care. Also consider the message you send by your posture and proximity to the patient. Consider the effect of towering over a patient versus kneeling down in front of them.

YOU are the EMT

At 0610 hours, your BLS unit is dispatched to 514 E. Bandera Street for a "sick person." You and your partner proceed to the scene, which is approximately 10 minutes away. En route, the dispatcher contacts you and states that she still has the caller on the phone.

1. What information should you ask the dispatcher to obtain from the caller?
2. Why is effective communication between the responding EMS unit and the dispatcher so important?

Health Literacy

An EMT's ability to communicate with and care for a patient is highly dependent on the ability of the patient, their family, caregivers, bystanders, and others to understand and process health information. This is referred to as health literacy. Because of their work in the field, often as the first points of health care contact, EMTs may need to perform tasks that include some social work and health care education.[2] EMTs may be called upon to bring health care information and education directly into the patient's home at the time when the patient, and their loved ones and caregivers, most need it. Often, EMTs educate patients, their families, and caregivers from their own knowledge or from printed and Internet resources made available by agency, regional, and state resources. This information may relate to fall prevention, mental health or addiction assistance, awareness of human trafficking, and other topics relevant to EMS.

Medical Fear

A significant barrier in providing health care is medical fear, or the fear of medicine and medical workers. This condition, which is clinically known as iatrophobia, can be a challenge in any environment but can be especially challenging for EMTs working in the field. Many people have some degree of medical fear, even when they are in good health. This fear is often increased when they become sick or injured. It is up to the EMT to help reassure patients, family, caregivers, and bystanders in ways that do not inadvertently make the medical fear worse. For example, while EMS clinicians may often use humor to defuse a tense situation, this tactic may not be appreciated by people with existing medical fear. Instead, use a calm tone of voice and easy pace to inspire confidence that you can effectively help the patient through this situation. Clear and open communication builds trust, which not only helps dispel medical fear, but also allows for a better patient assessment.

211 Call Line

In some instances, patients may not require transport to the hospital and may not require medical care. The 211 call line is a nationwide resource that connects people with essential community services such as food, housing, and mental health services.[3] When a person calls 211, the referral specialists can access databases of available resources. The callers are matched with private and public health services to help them get the assistance they need.

Age, Culture, and Personal Experience

The thoughts of people are greatly influenced by their personal experiences. For example, an older person who often experiences significant pain may view pain as more of an inconvenience than a problem. A child who has limited experience with pain would likely react much differently. People from various cultures are taught to handle illness, injury, and pain differently. Some cultures encourage people to express their emotions; others see it as a sign of weakness. These social and personal influences will shape how people communicate.

Patients may talk, make gestures, or write a note to express how they are feeling. "I am so sorry to bother you, but my chest hurts a little." "Hey! What took you so long? My chest is killing me!" Both of these messages talk about pain, but they include much more information within them.

The tone, pace, and volume of the language will tell you about the mood of the person who is communicating. These clues also provide some insight into the perceived importance of the message. For example, the patient who is yelling at you may be angry, scared, or both. Take note not only of the words being spoken, but how they are said.

Body language and eye contact are often greatly affected by culture. In some cultures, direct eye contact is viewed as impolite, whereas in other cultures it is impolite to look away while speaking. For example, in the United States and most European countries, direct eye contact conveys honesty and respect. Conversely, in some Latin American, Asian, and African cultures, direct eye contact conveys hostility and confrontation.

People tend to translate the messages they receive using their own worldview. **Ethnocentrism** occurs when you consider your own cultural values as more important when you are interacting with people of a different culture. If you are North American, for example, you might think that a patient is hiding something, afraid, or untrustworthy if the patient looks away from you while you are talking. These conclusions may be true if the two people are communicating from the perspective of a North American culture. All aspects of communication—eye contact, social distances, body language, and even touching—have a cultural foundation. In Thailand, for example, touching another person's head is reserved for those who are very intimate. If you were performing a physical examination on a person from Thailand, and they pulled back when you touched their head, it would be a good idea to ask them why they reacted in that manner. Once you determine their objection, explain why this part of the examination is important and reestablish the person's permission before touching their head. You do not have to know the cultural conventions of every patient, but you should remain curious and ask when you encounter this type of situation. However, you should educate yourself on specific cultures you are likely to encounter in your work and need to be aware that cultures may differ greatly from your own.

The best way to avoid ethnocentrism is to practice **cultural humility**. Individuals with cultural humility are curious about others and keep an open mind when interacting with people from cultures that are unfamiliar to them so they can reflect and learn from those experiences.[4] Even during life-threatening emergencies, it is important to recognize and respect others' cultures. Further, EMS clinicians must be aware of their personal biases. All people have biases; however, they are often unaware of how their biases affect their interactions with others, a condition referred to as **unconscious bias**, or implicit bias. While unconscious biases are natural and normal, they may cause clinicians to make a snap judgment about a patient that can negatively affect patient care. EMS clinicians must work to acknowledge their biases and prevent them from affecting the care they provide to their patients.

Cultural imposition takes this idea to an extreme. Some health care clinicians may consciously or subconsciously force their cultural values onto their patient because they believe their values are better. For example, consider a child who is brought to the emergency department (ED) with red marks on his back from coining, a traditional Asian healing practice in which hot coins are rubbed on the person's back to relieve illness. The parents explain to the physician that the coining helped for a short time, but now the child seems to be getting sicker. The physician responds angrily to the parents, accusing them of potential abuse and insisting that their practices are harmful (although they are not). This accusation reflects cultural imposition.

Words of Wisdom

There is an increasing body of research showing how bias can affect out-of-hospital care. Studies have shown that among other problems, women are less likely than men to receive cardiopulmonary resuscitation (CPR) or defibrillation, that Black patients are less likely than others to receive appropriate pain management for long bone fractures, and that incorrect diagnosis for stroke and heart attack is more likely in women.[5–8] Unconscious bias is likely a factor in these health care inequities.

Nonverbal Communication

Facial Expressions, Body Language, and Eye Contact

Eye contact and body language are powerful communication tools. The body language we consciously or subconsciously choose provides more information than words alone. Consider the images in **FIGURE 4-1**. Without any words, the mood of each of these people should be clear.

Patients can become hostile toward EMS clinicians. Signs that a patient may become an aggressor can be remembered with the mnemonic STAMP: Staring, Tone of voice, Anxiety, Mumbling, and Pacing. However, remember that signs of impending hostility can vary widely among individuals and may be extremely subtle or prone to rapid change. Communication methods to de-escalate a situation (sometimes referred to as defusing) include the following[9,10]:

- Make sure you have sufficient backup to ensure the safety of the patient and your crew.
- Minimize distractions such as bright or flashing lights, loud noise or conversations, or other individuals the patient may see as aggressive or threatening.
- One clinician engages in de-escalation early.
- Speak clearly, concisely, and calmly, in a nonconfrontational manner.
- Determine what the patient wants and needs.

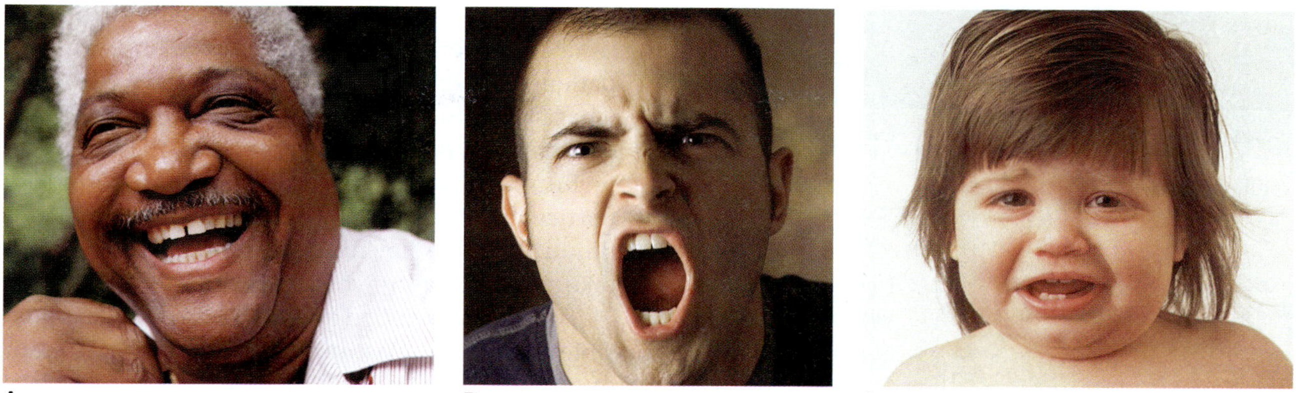

A B C

FIGURE 4-1 The effectiveness of body language. **A.** Happy. **B.** Angry. **C.** Sad.

A, C: © Photodisc; **B:** © Photodisc/Thinkstock.

- Use nonthreatening body language when communicating with the patient.
- Attempt to understand the patient's fears and concerns, even if you do not agree with them. Agree and accept them when you can.
- Be empathetic and professional.
- Set limits on patient behavior that may be destructive or injurious.
- Carefully choose and make clear what you can negotiate with the patient and what is nonnegotiable. Choice may give the patient some sense of internal control.
- Allow time for the patient to think and respond.
- Do not threaten the patient.

If you are interacting with an angry patient, you must stay calm and try to defuse the situation before it escalates.

Remember, it is important for you to be attentive to facial expressions, body language, and eye contact—your own and your patient's. These physical cues will help you and your patient to truly understand the message being sent. Additional techniques you can use to calm a patient and establish a therapeutic rapport will be discussed later in this chapter.

Physical Factors

Various physical factors affect communication; these factors are referred to as noise. **Noise** is anything that makes it difficult to understand the meaning of the message. Literal noise, or sounds in the environment, can make it difficult to understand the patient or for the patient to understand you. Lighting, distance, or physical obstacles are other factors that may affect your communication. Control these factors when possible by moving the patient, removing others from the area, turning off loud equipment, or adjusting the ambient light.

Cultural norms often dictate the amount of space, or proximity, between people when communicating (**TABLE 4-1**). The degree to which people feel comfortable depends on the person with whom they are communicating. As a person gets closer, a greater sense of trust must be established. When you finally enter someone's intimate space, there must be a high sense of trust.

Understanding how communication works and the importance of effective communication is important when gathering information from the patient. Your communication skills will be put to the test when you communicate with patients and/or families in emergency situations. Remember that someone who is sick or injured is scared and might not understand what you are doing or saying.

Street Smarts

It is tempting to match an agitated patient's voice tone and loud volume. Doing so is unwise and often escalates the situation. You must consciously moderate your voice so that it remains calm, neutral, and at a normal volume even when you feel anxious inside. Because people tend to match the other person's tone of speech, your calm demeanor can go a long way toward de-escalating the situation.

TABLE 4-1 Guidelines for Personal Space in the United States

Space	Distance	Description
Intimate	Less than 18 in. (46 cm)	Whispering, touching; must be invited
Personal	18 in. to 4 ft (46 cm–1.2 m)	Conversations with close friends or family
Social	4 to 10 ft (1.2 m–3.0 m)	Conversations with acquaintances
Public	10 to 25 ft (3.0–7.6 m)	nteracting with strangers

Therefore, your gestures, body movements, and attitude toward the patient are crucial in gaining the trust of both the patient and their family.

Verbal Communication

As an EMT, you must master many communication skills, including those associated with radio operations and written communications. Skilled verbal communication with the patient and family, bystanders, and the rest of the health care team is an essential part of high-quality patient care and transport. You must be able to listen effectively to fully understand the nature of the scene and the patient's problem. You must also be able to organize your thoughts to quickly and accurately verbalize instructions to the patient, bystanders, and other health care professionals.

One of the most fundamental aspects of what EMTs do is to ask patients questions. There are two types of questions: **open-ended questions** are ones in which a patient needs to provide some level of detail to give an answer, whereas **closed-ended questions** can be answered in short or single-word responses. When first approaching your patient, you should use open-ended questions. "What seems to be bothering you today?" or "How can I help you today?" Open-ended questions allow a free flow of conversation. They let the patient direct you to their concerns.

Closed-ended questions are important to use when patients are unable to provide long or complete answers to questions. Perhaps the patient is having severe breathing problems, or maybe the patient is a child who is scared and does not know what to say. In situations for which thoughtful answers are not possible, closed-ended questions that invite a "yes" or "no" answer are appropriate and are particularly useful when assessing a patient's condition. "Are you having trouble breathing? Do you take medications for your heart?"

With closed-ended questions, however, it is possible for you to miss important issues if pertinent questions are not asked. Imagine how many ways a person can be sick or injured. Now imagine trying to come up with a single yes/no question for each sickness or injury. Closed-ended questions typically provide limited information, and you should consider the answers to these questions as only a starting point toward understanding the patient's condition.

Street Smarts

Whether using open-ended or closed-ended questions, avoid leading the patient toward an answer you expect or wish to hear. Leading questions have a built-in answer. For example, the question "You don't take any medications, right?" encourages the patient to simply agree with the answer you provided. A better question would be, "Do you take any medications?"

Before beginning your interview with the patient, determine which clinician will lead the interview. This will ensure that you and your partner do not ask questions at the same time or ask repetitive questions. When you are asking questions of the patient, be conscious of how many questions you are asking. "How are you doing today? Have you been feeling ill?" This common approach actually asks the patient two kinds of questions, one open-ended and one closed-ended. Often the patient will respond with a simple "yes." To avoid this situation, it is best to ask a single question, wait for an answer, and then proceed to another question.

There are many powerful communication tools you can use when trying to obtain information from patients. Sometimes patients will hide information, either consciously or unconsciously, due to fear or confusion. The techniques in **TABLE 4-2** provide

TABLE 4-2 Therapeutic Communication Techniques

Communication Technique	Definition	Example
Facilitation	Encourage the patient to talk more or provide more information.	EMT: "I am listening to you. Can you tell me more about that?" or "Go on."
Pause	Do not speak.	Give the patient space and time to think and respond, especially if the individual is having a hard time speaking.
Reflection	Restating a patient's statement made to you to confirm your understanding.	Patient: "I am so depressed that I could die." EMT: "I understand that you are feeling depressed."
Empathy	Be sensitive to the patient's feelings and thoughts.	Use eye contact and, if appropriate, touching to reinforce communication; adjust tone of voice and pace to allow for open communication.
Clarification	Ask the patient to explain what was meant by an answer.	Patient: "I just feel sick." EMT: "Can you tell me how you are feeling sick? What feels wrong?"
Confrontation	Make the patient who is in denial or in a mental state of shock focus on urgent and life-critical issues.	Patient: "I am having pain in my chest, my back has been hurting me, and I ran out of my blood pressure medication." EMT: "We will talk about your medicines in a moment. Please tell me about your chest pain."
Interpretation	Restate the patient's complaint to confirm your understanding.	EMT: "If I understand correctly, you have been feeling pain for the past 3 days, and it has gotten worse today. Is that correct?" Patient: "That's right."
Explanation	Provide factual information to support a conversation.	Patient: "I do not understand what is happening." EMT: "We have checked your blood sugar and blood pressure and don't see anything we need to immediately treat."
Summarization	Provide a brief summary of what the patient or family member has told you.	EMT: "So I heard you say that you had indigestion that began last night. This morning you felt chest pain that is moving to your back and nothing you have done makes you feel better."

you with strategies that will assist you in gathering patient information. They can be helpful to use not only with patients who are willing to share, but with those who are resistant to sharing information.

When you interview the patient, consider using touch to communicate caring and compassion. While touch is a powerful tool, keep in mind that it should be used consciously and sparingly (**FIGURE 4-2**). Many people will be uncomfortable with a stranger touching them suddenly. If you are going to touch the patient, approach slowly and touch the patient's shoulder or arm respectfully. You can consider holding the patient's hand. This allows you to touch the patient, showing you care about what the person is telling you, and allows you to remain at a slight distance.

Avoid touching the patient's torso, chest, or face simply as a means of communication, because these areas are often viewed as intimate. Also, to touch these areas, you will need to get closer to the patient, potentially invading the patient's intimate space. **TABLE 4-3** provides other tips on what to avoid when communicating with patients.

The presence of family, friends, and bystanders during your interview of the patient can be valuable. Sometimes, however, well-meaning family members will speak for the patient, and, at times, you may need to ask the family member to allow the patient to answer. Ultimately, you will need to assess the situation and determine whether the additional people are helping you care for the patient or hindering your efforts. Do not be afraid to ask others to step outside or step aside for a moment while you talk with the patient. It is generally best to keep families together, but in cases where a family member is not helpful, consider giving the person a task to do, such as gathering medications or clothing. This task can transform the person from

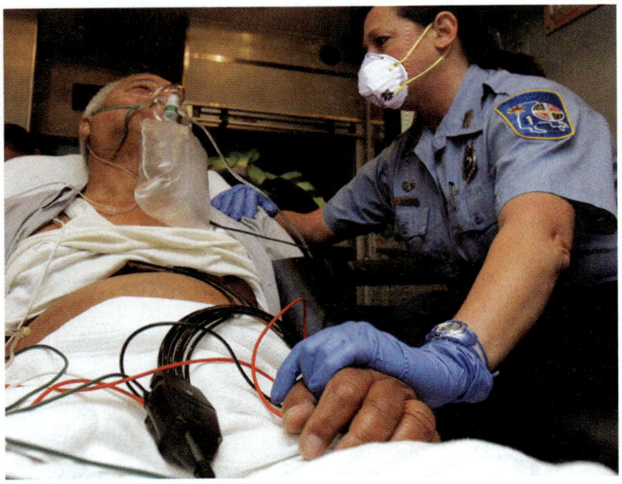

FIGURE 4-2 Using touch conveys a sense of caring and compassion.

Safety Tips

Everything you do, whether consciously or unconsciously, communicates something. As a health care professional, you need to ensure that your body language reflects your words. Remember, people call 9-1-1 because they are in crisis. Part of being a good EMT is being able to project calm and control into a chaotic environment. You may not feel calm, but a good EMT will "never let them see you sweat."

TABLE 4-3 Interview Techniques to Avoid

Improper Technique	Example of What *Not* to Say	Rationale
Providing false hope or reassurance	EMT: "It will be okay." "This is nothing to worry about."	You do not know that everything will be okay.
Giving unsolicited advice	EMT: "Well, if I were you, I wouldn't have called the ambulance at all."	This demeans the patient and makes you seem arrogant, rather than helpful.
Asking leading or biased questions	EMT: "You probably don't want to go to the ED because you don't have any insurance, right?"	Your patient deserves respectful communication. It is inappropriate for you to suggest to the patient that an ambulance was not needed, even if that is what you believe.
Interrupting the patient	Patient: "Well, I was having trouble breathing last month and—" EMT: "Can we move on to how you are feeling now?"	You may seem bored or annoyed that the patient is taking up your time.
Speaking in professional jargon	EMT: "I think we need to take you to the ED stat. We will give you ASA and NTG en route. Any questions?"	This type of communication confuses the patient. Most patients do not understand medical jargon. (Consider, however, the need for precision. If the scene allows, you may be able to use the medical term, then immediately translate it for the patient.)

a hindrance into a valuable aide. Consider how the patient will feel without loved ones nearby. Separating them may make the patient more anxious.

These 10 Golden Rules will help you to calm and reassure your patient and provide a therapeutic rapport:

1. **If it is culturally appropriate, make eye contact with your patient.** Give patients your undivided attention. This will let them know they are your top priority. Look the patient straight in the eye to establish a **rapport**. Establishing a rapport is building a trusting relationship with your patient. This will make caring for the patient much easier.
2. **Provide your name and use the patient's proper name.** Introduce yourself and your partner. If your department provides you with a name tag, wear it. Ask patients what they wish to be called. Avoid using terms such as "honey" or "dear." Use a patient's first name only if the patient is a child or the patient asks you to use their first name. Unless the patient tells you otherwise, use a courtesy title, such as "Mr. Peters," "Mrs. Smith," or "Ms. Butler." If you do not know the patient's name, refer to the patient as "sir" or "ma'am." (As discussed later, always be careful when using gender-specific terms so that you do not address the person incorrectly.)
3. **Tell the patient the truth.** Even if you have to say something unpleasant, telling the truth is better than lying. Lying will destroy the patient's trust in you and decrease your own confidence. You might not always tell the patient everything, but if the patient or a family member asks a specific question, you should answer truthfully. A direct question deserves a direct answer. If you do not know the answer to a patient's question, say so. For example, a patient may ask, "Am I having a heart attack?" To which you would answer, "I don't know, but we will certainly get more information at the hospital. Right now, I am caring for you and want you to be comfortable."
4. **Use language that the patient can understand.** Do not talk up or down to the patient in any way. Never use "baby talk" with older patients or with anyone other than infants. Avoid technical medical terms that the patient might not understand. For example, ask whether the patient has a history of "heart conditions." This will usually result in more accurate information than if you ask about "previous episodes of myocardial infarction" or a "history of cardiomyopathy."
5. **Be careful what you say about the patient to others.** You need to understand the relationship between the person you are talking with (such as a bystander) and the patient. Ask the patient if it is okay for you to talk with this person. While speaking to others, ensure that you leave the general area of the patient if you must have a confidential conversation. Be mindful that sharing patient information may be a Health Insurance Portability and Accountability Act (HIPAA) violation. Do not talk about patients in their presence as if they are not there; doing so gives the impression they have no choice in their own medical care. This is easy to forget when the patient has impaired cognitive (thought) processes or has difficulty communicating.
6. **Be aware of your body language.** Nonverbal communication is extremely important in dealing with patients (**FIGURE 4-3**). In stressful situations, patients may misinterpret your gestures and movements. Be particularly careful not to appear frustrated or threatening. Instead, position yourself at the same level or at a lower level than the patient when practical. Remember that you should always conduct yourself in a calm, professional manner.

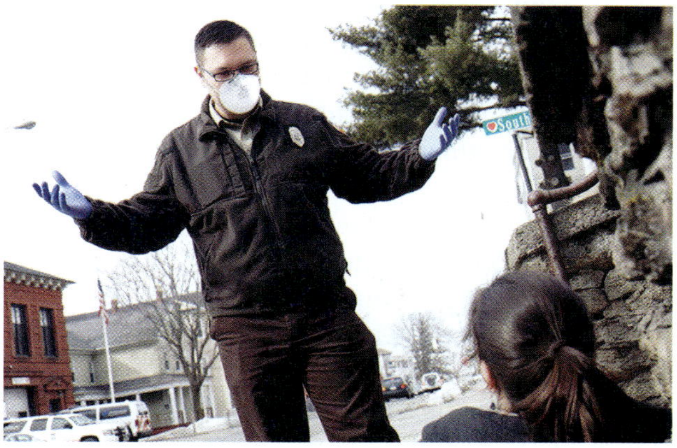

FIGURE 4-3 Watch your body language, because patients may misinterpret your gestures, movements, and stance.

7. **Always speak slowly, clearly, and distinctly.** Pay close attention to your tone of voice.
8. **If the patient is hard of hearing, face the person to allow lip-reading.** Try lowering or raising the tone of your voice; some people who are hard of hearing can hear certain pitches better than others. Do not shout at a person who is hard of hearing. Shouting will make it harder for the patient to hear you and may frighten the patient. Never assume that an older patient is hard of hearing or otherwise unable to understand you. Also, if you are unable to communicate with the patient, have your partner try. Another technique is to have patients put the stethoscope in their ears while you speak softly into the diaphragm to help amplify the sound.
9. **Allow time for the patient to answer or respond to your questions.** Do not rush a patient unless there is immediate danger. Sick and injured people may not be thinking clearly and may need time to answer even simple questions. This is especially true when treating older patients.
10. **Act and speak in a calm, confident manner while caring for the patient.** Make sure you attend to the patient's comfort and needs. Try to make the patient physically comfortable and relaxed. Find out whether the patient is more comfortable sitting or lying down. Is the patient cold or hot? Does the patient want a friend or relative nearby?

Patients literally place their lives in your hands. They deserve to know that you can provide medical care and that you are concerned about their well-being. These 10 Golden Rules will help provide a good foundation and will make it easier to gather information when the patient wants to talk.

Sometimes, you need to gather information from a reluctant audience. Patients may be defensive about their problems and may not want to talk about them because they are embarrassed. They may direct the conversation away from the true problem. With these patients, start the conversation as usual. Introduce yourself. Be open and compassionate. If you find yourself not getting any real answers, then consider using one of the techniques described earlier in Table 4-2.

Interpersonal Skills

Emotional Intelligence

Emotional intelligence is the ability to understand and manage your own emotions and properly respond to others' emotions. Sometimes referred to as people skills, emotional intelligence can help EMTs defuse conflict, build a rapport, communicate more effectively, and manage difficult situations.[11,12] Emotional intelligence is commonly understood to have five attributes.

1. **Self-awareness.** The ability to recognize your own emotions and how they affect your thoughts and behavior.
2. **Self-regulation.** The ability to control impulsive emotions and behaviors and to manage emotions in positive ways.
3. **Motivation.** The ability to motivate yourself and others in a positive direction, often deferring short-term rewards for long-term success.
4. **Empathy.** The ability to understand the concerns, emotions, and needs of others by picking up on communication and social cues and clues.
5. **Social skills.** The ability to develop and maintain positive rapport and relationships through effective communications.

Think of people in your life whom you consider kind, caring, and exceptional listeners. These are people with high emotional intelligence. They can identify, understand, and manage their own emotions and the emotions of others.

As an EMT, you should seek to understand and improve your own emotional intelligence. Consider the following tips:

- Assess how you react to stressful situations. Do you become upset by every little frustration, such as delays, people not performing tasks correctly, or things not going your way? Try to manage your frustration, and work on staying calm and in control when faced with minor irritations.
- Practice mindfulness. Purposely focus your attention on the current moment, without blame and judgment of yourself or others. Doing so can help calm and focus you and make you more aware of the situation around you.
- Take responsibility for your actions. Don't be quick to immediately blame or attack others

if things don't go your way. Acknowledge your own role in the situation.

- Consider how your actions will affect others before you take those actions. Think about how your words and actions will make others feel.

When communicating in difficult situations, especially when high levels of emotion are involved, a communication method known as the behavioral change stairway model may be helpful.[13] This five-step model was developed by the Federal Bureau of Investigation to manage hostage negotiations quickly and effectively. It can be adapted to most crisis communications. Each step should be followed in order, as each step builds on the previous step or steps to help improve communications, build rapport, and de-escalate crisis situations.

1. **Employ active listening.** Carefully listen to what the other person has to say, and let the person know you are doing so. Acknowledge what the person is saying, and do not interrupt, disagree, or give commands.
2. **Display empathy.** Use your emotional intelligence to understand the patient's perspective. You do not have to agree with the person's beliefs or actions, but you have to understand where the person is coming from and what the person wants.
3. **Build a rapport.** Once you have listened to and empathized with the person, it is much easier, especially in a crisis, to "speak the person's language."
4. **Exert influence.** Look at realistic solutions to move the situation forward in a positive way. Understanding the person's perspective along with your own needs, consider how you can move forward in a way the person will understand.
5. **Initiate behavior change**: Propose a solution that makes sense to the other person and is acceptable to you.

Person-First Language

The language we use to describe our patients greatly influences how we think about our patients. For example, referring to someone as a "diabetic" may cause us to think of the person as more of a disease than a person; moreover, it may cause us to assume that any medical complaint the person is experiencing relates to diabetes, despite having not performed a complete and open-minded interview and assessment. Failing to use person-first language has been shown to negatively affect patient–clinician relationships as well as patient outcomes.[14] Instead of a "diabetic," the person should be referred to as a "patient with diabetes."

Like other medical terminology, terminology related to sex, gender identity, and sexual orientation can be complicated. Here, again, your use of language can strengthen or hinder your relationship with the patient and ability to provide proper care. If unsure what terminology to use, it is best to simply ask the patient their preference, just as you may ask what name they prefer to be called.[15] If the patient says his legal name is Robert but you can call him Bob, he may not appreciate if you keep calling him Robert. If you are unsure of the patient's gender, avoid gender-specific terminology; for example, you may refer to an individual using gender-neutral terms, such as "the patient" or "they." In addition, never assume a man has a wife and a woman has a husband. Ask the patient if they have a partner or a spouse.

Communicating With Older Patients

In 2022, about 58 million people, representing more than 17% of the US population, were older than 65 years; this population is expected to reach 22% by 2050.[16] Thus, EMS clinicians can expect an ever-increasing number of encounters with people in this age category. However, a person's actual age might not be the most important factor in classifying a person as geriatric. It is more important to determine a person's functional age. The functional age relates to the person's ability to function in daily activities, mental state, health status, and activity pattern.

As an EMS clinician, when you enter a scene to care for an older patient, you have been called because a person needs help. What you say and how you say it has an effect on the patient's perception of the call. You should present yourself as competent, confident, and caring. You must take charge of the situation, but do so with compassion. You are there to listen and act on what you learn. Do not limit your assessment to the obvious problem. Often, older patients who express that they are not well, or who are overly concerned about their health or general condition, are at risk for a serious decline in their physical, emotional, or psychological state.

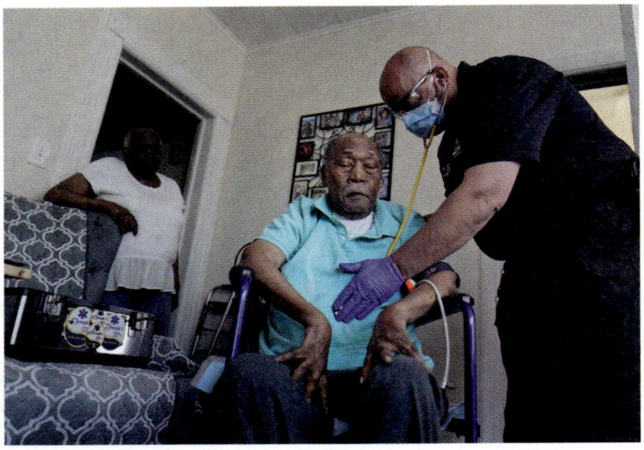

FIGURE 4-4 You need a great deal of compassion and patience when caring for some older patients. Do not assume that a patient has dementia or is confused simply because they are older.

In general, older people think clearly, can give you a clear medical history, and are able to answer your questions appropriately (**FIGURE 4-4**). Do not assume that a patient has dementia or is likely to be confused simply because they are older. Conversely, communicating with some older patients is extremely difficult, and you may encounter hostility, irritability, and in some cases, confusion. Do not assume this to be normal behavior for an older patient. These signs may be caused by lack of oxygen (hypoxia); brain injury, including stroke; unintentional drug overdose; infection; abnormal blood glucose level; or even insufficient perfusion (circulation of blood and, therefore, nutrients to the cells). Never attribute altered mental status to old age. In addition, your older patients may have difficulty hearing or seeing you. Therefore, you need great patience and compassion when you are called on to care for such a patient. Think of the patient as someone's grandmother or grandfather, or even as yourself when you reach that age.

Words of Wisdom

Remember that most older patients are not cognitively impaired. Be careful to assess each patient's individual abilities.

Approach an older patient slowly and calmly. Allow plenty of time for the patient to respond to your questions. Watch for signs of confusion, anxiety, or impaired hearing or vision. Patients should feel confident that everything possible is being done for them.

If appropriate, help the patient pack a few personal items before leaving for the hospital. Be sure

YOU are the EMT

You arrive at the scene and find the patient, an 83-year-old woman, sitting on the couch in her living room. She is conscious and alert and tells you that she started having light-headedness and nausea about an hour ago. As you begin your assessment, you note that she has hearing aids in both ears.

Recording Time: 0 Minutes	
Appearance	Calm; no obvious distress
Level of consciousness	Conscious and alert
Airway	Open; clear of secretions or foreign bodies
Breathing	Normal rate and depth; regular
Circulation	Radial pulses strong and regular; skin circulation assessed as adequate by examination of mucous membranes inside the inner lower eyelid and capillary refill with skin warm and dry

3. How can you maximize successful communication with a patient who is hard of hearing?

4. Should your general approach to the assessment process be any different for this patient versus a younger patient? Why or why not?

to locate hearing aids, eyeglasses, or dentures before departure if such items will significantly improve the patient's stay. If you do so, you should document on the patient care report (PCR) that these items accompanied the patient to the hospital and the person to whom they were given in the ED. Older patients are often worried about the safety of their home, valuable items, and pets. Take the time to share these concerns with the person assuming care of the patient at the hospital.

Street Smarts

The role of **family-centered care** in all health care interactions, including EMS, is increasingly understood to benefit not just the patient but their family or other caregivers. In family-centered care, patients of all ages and other stakeholders in the patient's well-being, often family members, are treated with respect and inclusion regarding the care of the patient. Their involvement has been shown to improve quality of care and reduce errors.[17–19] For example, their knowledge of the patient may improve history gathering or may help inform medication decisions. Their presence during procedures and transport may help calm the patient. Beyond the emergency response, allowing them to share their thoughts and values can help shape agency policy.

Encouraging and effectively using the family's assistance requires training and practice. Agencies are encouraged to develop guidelines, such as determining which individuals may ride in the patient compartment and how they will be secured, so that clinicians will not have to make difficult decisions, with possible legal implications, in the moment.

Communicating With Children

Everyone who is thrust into an emergency becomes frightened to some degree. However, fear is probably most obvious and severe in children. Children may be frightened by your uniform, the ambulance, and the number of people who have suddenly gathered around. Even a child who says little may be very much aware of all that is going on.

Familiar faces and objects will help to reduce this fright. Let a child keep a favorite toy, doll, or security blanket to give the child some sense of control and comfort. Having a family member or friend nearby is also helpful. When not impractical due to the child's condition, it is often helpful to let the parent or a guardian hold the child during your evaluation and treatment. However, you will have to make sure this person will not upset the child or prevent the child from telling you important information. Sometimes, adult family members are not helpful because they become too upset by what has happened, or the child will not share important information in front of them. An overly anxious parent or relative can make things worse. Be careful about selecting the proper adult for this role. Remember, caring for an infant or child often means caring for the parents or caregivers, and family members often need emotional support. Make sure you are calm, efficient, professional, and sensitive as you care for pediatric patients and their families.

A child may not be able to communicate verbally, but the child's appropriate or inappropriate reaction to the environment or situation can communicate a great deal of information about their level of consciousness and condition.

Street Smarts

Children often take cues from their parents or caregivers. A calm caregiver usually results in a calm child. An agitated caregiver can mean an agitated child. Measures that calm the caregivers will often reassure and calm the child in turn.

Children can easily see through lies or deceptions, so you must always be honest with them. Explain to the child as often as necessary why certain things are happening. If treatment will hurt, such as applying a splint, tell the child ahead of time.

Respect a child's modesty. Children school-age and older are often embarrassed if they have to undress or be undressed in front of strangers. This anxiety often intensifies during adolescence. When a wound or site of injury has to be exposed, try to do so out of the sight of strangers, and when appropriate be sure to have a parent or guardian present. Again, it is extremely important to tell the child what you are doing and why you are doing it.

You should speak to a child in a professional, yet friendly way. When speaking to a child, make

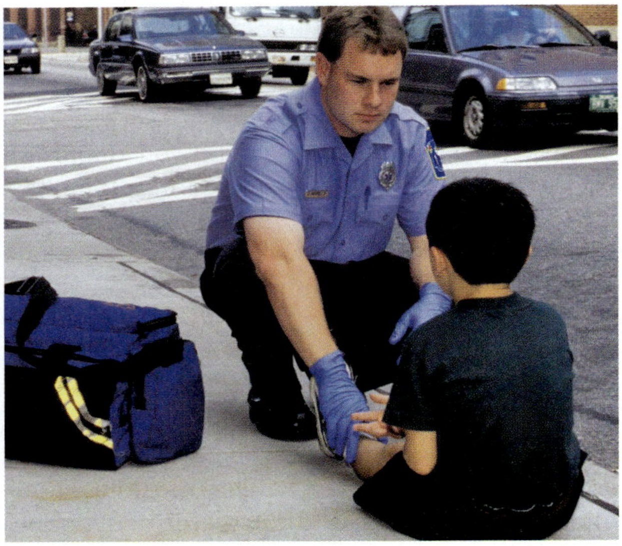

FIGURE 4-5 Maintain eye contact with a child to let the child know that you are there to help and that you can be trusted.

sure to use an appropriate tone and vocabulary. Use the child's name when speaking to them or to their caregivers. A child should feel reassured that you are there to help in every way possible. Maintain eye contact with a child, as you would with an adult, to let the child know that you are there to help and that you can be trusted (**FIGURE 4-5**). It is helpful to position yourself at the child's eye level so you do not appear to tower above the child.

Special Populations

REASSURING A CHILD ON SCENE

A man has fallen and hurt his ankle. The injury is not severe, so a splint is placed on his leg and he is moved to the ambulance. All this time, his 4-year-old daughter is watching. Suddenly she runs to the other side of the room and begins to cry. She watched the EMTs take her daddy away. What should you do?

Talk to the child. Have her come over to the ambulance cot and see that her daddy is okay. Tell her about the splint and how it will make her daddy's leg better. Let her touch her daddy and say goodbye. Let her daddy tell her that he will be home soon. Sometimes the obvious patient is not always the only patient.

Communicating With Patients Who Are Deaf or Hard of Hearing

You must be able to communicate with patients who are hard of hearing so you can provide necessary or even lifesaving care. Most patients who are hard of hearing have normal intelligence and can easily understand what is going on around them, provided you can successfully communicate with them. Many patients who are hard of hearing can read lips to some extent. Therefore, you should place yourself in a position so the patient can see your lips. Many patients who are hard of hearing have hearing aids to help them communicate. Be careful that hearing aids are not lost during an accident or fall. Hearing aids may also be forgotten if the patient is confused or ill. Look around for one in the immediate area, or ask the patient or the family about use of a hearing aid.

Remember the following five steps to efficiently communicate with patients who are hard of hearing:

1. **Have paper and a pen available.** This way, you can write down questions and the patient can write down answers, if necessary. Be sure to print so that your handwriting is not a communication barrier.
2. **If the patient can read lips, you should face the patient and speak distinctly at a normal pace.** Do not cover your mouth or mumble. If it is dark, consider shining a light on your face.
3. **Never shout.** Shouting will not help the patient hear you and may frighten the patient.
4. **Listen carefully, ask short questions, and give short answers.** Remember that although many patients who are hard of hearing can speak distinctly, some cannot.
5. **Learn some simple phrases in sign language.** For example, knowing the signs for "sick," "hurt," and "help" may be useful if you cannot communicate in any other way (**FIGURE 4-6**).

Communicating With Visually Impaired Patients

Like patients who are hard of hearing, visually impaired and blind patients have usually accepted and learned to deal with their disability. Of course, visually impaired patients are not necessarily completely blind. Many can perceive light and dark or can see shadows or movement. Ask these patients

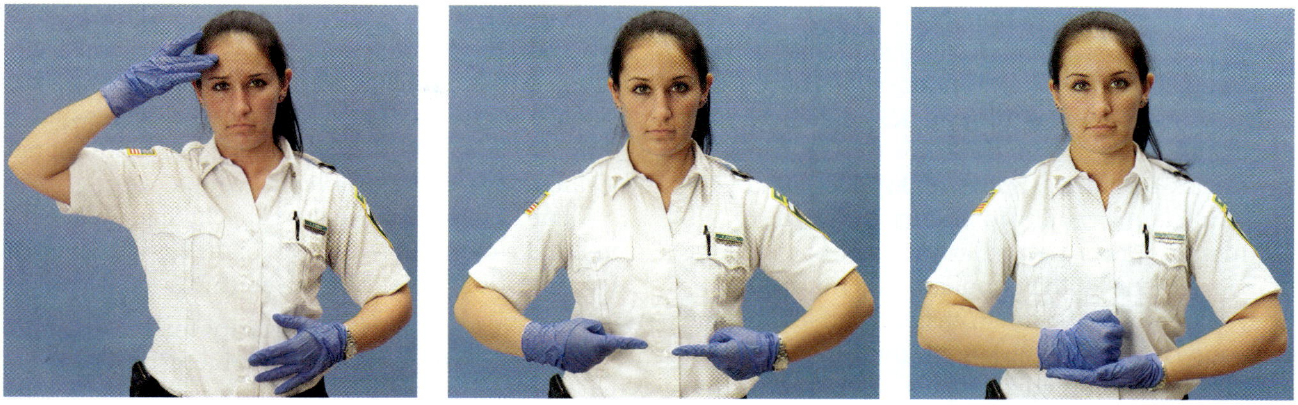

A B C

FIGURE 4-6 Learn simple phrases in sign language. Signing requires movement and is best learned by attending a sign language class. **A.** Sick. **B.** Hurt. **C.** Help.

whether they can see at all. Also remember, as with other patients who have disabilities, you should expect visually impaired patients to have normal intelligence.

As you begin caring for a visually impaired patient, explain everything you are doing in detail as you are doing it. Be sure to stay in physical contact with the patient as you begin your care. Place your hand lightly on the patient's shoulder or arm and try to avoid sudden movements. Guide patients who can walk to the ambulance by placing their hand on your arm, taking care not to rush. Transport eyeglasses and any mobility aids, such as a cane, with the patient to the hospital.

A visually impaired person may have a guide dog. Guide dogs are easily identified by their special harnesses (**FIGURE 4-7**). Guide dogs are trained to not leave their owners and to not respond to strangers. A visually impaired patient who is conscious can tell you about the dog and give instructions for its care. If the patient is stable, bring the guide dog to the hospital in the back of the ambulance with the patient because it will help to alleviate some of the stress for both the patient and the dog. If the patient is unstable, the dog is injured or unruly, or for other safety or patient care reasons it is inappropriate to transport the dog, then you should arrange for the dog's care. Contact your supervisor for assistance. The exact method for managing a patient with a guide dog (or other medical care animal) will be outlined in your department's policies and procedures. Follow your local protocols.

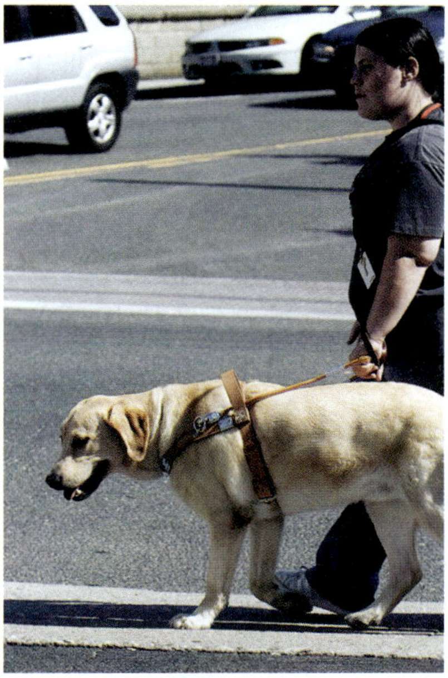

FIGURE 4-7 A guide dog is easily identified by its special harness.

Communicating With Non–English-Speaking Patients

Part of patient care includes obtaining a medical history from the patient. You cannot skip this step simply because the patient does not speak English. Most patients who do not speak English fluently will still know certain important words or phrases.

Your first step is to find out how much English the patient can speak. Use short, simple questions and simple words whenever possible, and avoid difficult medical terms. You can help patients better understand if you point to specific parts of the body as you ask questions. Speaking louder will not increase a patient's ability to understand you.

In many areas, particularly large urban centers, major segments of the population do not speak English. Your job will be much easier if you learn some common words and phrases in their language, especially common medical terms. Pocket cards that show the pronunciation of these terms are available. If the patient does not speak any English, use a smartphone app or website to help you translate, or find an interpreter. In an emergency, it may be necessary to have a family member or friend translate until a professional interpreter is located. Also, remember to request a translator at the hospital while providing the radio report if the patient's language is known. Hospitals must have professional foreign language interpreters in-house or on-call for this purpose.

Street Smarts

When communicating with the help of an interpreter, look at the patient as you ask questions and listen to the interpreter's answers. Keeping your eyes on the patient allows you and the patient to interpret body language that accompanies verbal communication and maintains the relationship with the patient.

Mission-Critical Communications

Mission-critical communications are any communications where disruption will result in the failure of the task at hand. Although mission-critical communications will change from industry to industry, many of the problems encountered as well as recommendations to help avoid errors and improve effectiveness can be employed by EMS clinicians.

A concept central to mission-critical communications is the shared **mental model**. A mental model is the picture individuals have in their head of "what's going on." Even though individuals on a team may be in different roles, seeing different things from different perspectives, for any team to work effectively together, all members must share a mental model. The goal of mission-critical communications is an efficient, effective, and error-free transfer of the mental model. When clinicians have different ideas of "what's going on," situational awareness fails and problems begin.

For an individual health care clinician or a team to build a mental model, the following sequence of four questions must be answered:

1. What is the focused priority for the patient? (What is the crux of the problem?)
2. What is the history of prior care? (What got us to this point?)
3. What is the patient's current state? (Where are we right now?)
4. What are the patient's immediate needs? (What is the very next thing that needs to happen?)

Answering these four questions quickly and efficiently will not just help avoid errors and misunderstandings but will provide a handoff that allows receiving clinicians to continue forward progress in patient care rather than spend time with unnecessary questions and clarifications or, even worse, begin the patient interview and assessment essentially from scratch.

Patient Care Handoff

Patient care is a coordinated effort among numerous providers, from bystanders and first responders to paramedics, from primary care physicians to ED nurses, and beyond. Effective communication between the EMT and other health care professionals is a cornerstone of efficient, effective, and appropriate patient care. Nowhere is communication more important than during patient care **handoff**, often called handover. Patient care handoff is the transfer of pertinent patient information and the responsibility for the patient's care. It often involves the physical movement of the patient and associated equipment from the ambulance stretcher to the hospital bed.

Even on a single emergency call, an EMT may be involved in numerous patient care handoffs. For example, a first responder or primary-care medical clinician may hand over patient care on arrival of an EMT, the EMT may hand over care on arrival of a paramedic, and the EMT–paramedic team may hand over care to the ED staff. As common as this occurrence may be, it is a hazardous one. The

American College of Emergency Physicians has called patient handoff "the most dangerous point in a patient's ED journey," and the World Health Organization has identified communication during patient handoff as a critical failure point that can cause "serious breakdowns in the continuity of care, inappropriate treatment, and potential harm to the patient." Furthermore, communication failures between reporting clinicians and receiving clinicians are a major source of medical liability for clinicians and organizations, accounting for a significant proportion of malpractice claims in all health care sectors, including EMS.

Although the degree of control that EMTs may have over the system in which they work will vary, a five-point method can be used by clinicians both when giving and when receiving the handoff report in virtually all situations.

Giving the Handoff Report

1. **Initiate eye contact.** When handing over patient care, responsibility, and information, it is critical to begin by making eye contact with the person to whom the patient is being transferred. Eye contact helps identify that the handoff is beginning, and which individuals are reporting and receiving. It sends the message, "We are communicating now, you and I."
2. **Manage the environment.** Whenever possible, try to minimize noise, interruptions, and distractions by, for example, momentarily turning down a radio, stopping nonpriority activities, or moving to a quieter area to give the report. Avoid moving the patient during the handoff report so that the attention of both you and the person receiving the report is focused on the patient information.
3. **Ensure the ABCs.** If there is priority critical care that must be initiated or continued, it must be immediately conveyed and addressed by the receiving clinician or team (ie, the doctor, nurse, or whomever will be taking responsibility for the patient). Such care includes lifesaving interventions that are either needed immediately (eg, the placement of an endotracheal tube) or that must be continued (eg, CPR) for the patient to survive. The full handoff report may be delayed until after the immediate life threat is addressed.
4. **Provide a structured report.** Research on mission-critical communications has shown that the use of a structured format greatly improves efficiency and reduces errors. Numerous standardized report formats exist. Although not inherently superior to other structured formats, SBAR (which stands for situation, background, assessment, and recap/Rx) is widely used in hospitals and is likely to be well understood by a variety of health care clinicians. The mnemonic is sometimes modified slightly to SBAT when used in EMS:
   - Situation (a concise statement of the problem)
   - Background (relevant, brief information about the patient situation)
   - Assessment (your assessment findings and what you think)
   - Treatment (care that has been provided to the patient)
5. **Provide documentation.** The verbal report should consist of the patient's priority conditions, prior care, current state, and immediate needs. The numerous other patient details should be transferred via a paper or electronic report. Avoid clouding the handoff with information that is not immediately necessary.

Consider the following example of a structured report that uses the SBAT format to focus on priority issues, prior care, current state, and immediate needs (**FIGURE 4-8**):

S This is a trauma alert. We have a hypotensive 28-year-old female involved in a motor vehicle collision with an unstable pelvis and right-side open tibia/fibula fracture.

B Patient was struck by a motor vehicle at approximately 35 mph approximately 20 minutes ago.

A She is conscious and alert but slow to respond. Vital signs are BP, 88/48; pulse, 124 and irregular; respirations, 24; and Sao_2, 96%. Head to toe finds injuries to the pelvis and the left leg as well as minor abrasions, but no other significant findings. Her only significant medical history is asthma.

T We applied oxygen and stabilized her pelvis and left leg, and both have good distal PMS. Do you have any questions?

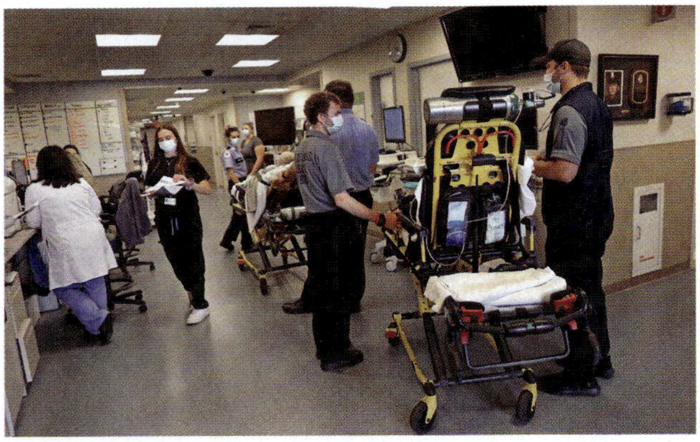

FIGURE 4-8 Once you arrive at the hospital, a staff member will take a patient handoff report and responsibility for the patient from you.

Receiving the Handoff Report

1. **Maintain eye contact.**
2. **Manage the environment.** Many hospitals now establish a moment of silence during trauma, cardiac, stroke, sepsis, and other alerts and critical patient situations. Although this is not always possible for the EMT receiving the handoff in the field, attempt to pause during the report so you can focus on key information.
3. **Ensure understanding.** Once you have received the handoff report, ask questions as necessary to clarify and correct any issues.
4. **Summarize.** This is *not* a repeat of the entire handoff report, but a summary of the receiving clinician's mental model. This mental model summary is stated aloud so that the reporting clinician and members of the receiving team can ask questions or correct any errors to ensure the shared mental model is correct.
5. **Gather supplementary patient documentation.**

Communicating With Critically Ill and Injured Patients

When you are caring for a critically ill or injured patient, the patient needs to know who you are and what you are doing. Let the patient know you are attending to their immediate needs and these are your primary concerns at this moment. As soon as possible, explain to the patient what is going on. Confusion, anxiety, and other feelings of helplessness will be decreased if you keep the patient informed from the start. Never assume a patient cannot hear you. Avoid making unprofessional comments during resuscitation, and treat all patients with dignity and respect.

Saying the wrong thing to a patient who is dying may increase the distress of the patient or their family. Knowing how to effectively communicate in these situations can bring the patient needed comfort, which may in turn allow you to provide better care.

Avoid Sad and Grim Comments

EMTs, other safety personnel, family members, and bystanders must avoid making grim comments about a patient's condition. Remarks such as "This is a bad one" or "The leg is badly damaged. I think he'll lose it" are inappropriate. These remarks may upset or increase the patient's anxiety and compromise possible recovery outcomes. This is especially true for a patient who may be able to hear but cannot respond.

Street Smarts

When communicating at the scene of an emergency, be mindful that you are often being recorded. Family, bystanders, law enforcement, or even the patient may be recording the entire emergency encounter on their cell phone or other electronic device. Choose your words carefully so your communications are professional and will not later be misinterpreted.

Orient the Patient

A patient may be disoriented in an emergency situation. The aura of the emergency situation—lights, sirens, smells, and strangers—is intense. The seriousness and the effect of injuries or acute illness may cause the patient to be confused or unsettled. It is important for you to orient the patient to their surroundings. Use concise statements such as, "Mr. Rosa, you've had a vehicle crash, and I'm now splinting your arm. I'm EMT Short of Ridgefield EMS. I'll be caring for you."

Be Honest

When approaching any patient, you must decide how much information each patient is able to understand and accept. You should be honest without further alarming the patient or giving unnecessary information or information that may not be understood. Simply explain what you are doing and allow the patient to be part of the care being given; this can relieve feelings of helplessness as well as some of the fear.

Allow for Hope

In trauma and acute medical conditions, patients may ask you whether they are going to die. At these times, you may feel at a loss for words. You may also know, on the basis of past experience or in view of the seriousness of the current situation, that the prognosis is poor. However, it is not your responsibility to tell the patient they are dying. If there is the slightest chance of hope remaining, you want that message transmitted in your attitude and in the statements you make to the patient. Convey to them that you will provide the best care that you possibly can.

Help Locate and Notify Family Members

Many patients will be concerned and ask you to notify their family or others close to them. The patient may not be able to assist you in doing this. In these cases, you should make sure an appropriate and responsible person makes an effort to locate the desired persons. Assuring the patient that someone is going to make these notifications may be an important aspect of the patient's care because it will help to calm the patient.

Death and Dying

Everyone working as an EMT will experience grief at one time or another. Death can occur in any setting and can occur either quite suddenly or after a prolonged illness. For some EMTs, it may be an infrequent occurrence. Others, in urban settings, may see death many times in responding to motor vehicle crashes, drug overdoses, suicides, or homicides. Moreover, any area can experience a mass-casualty incident, such as an airplane crash, a hazardous materials incident, or a natural disaster. In all of these situations, coming to grips with your thoughts, understanding, and adjustment to death is not only important personally, but also a function of delivering emergency medical care.

The Grieving Process

This section discusses how to care for a grieving patient, as well as how to cope with your own grief that may result from a difficult call. Keep in mind, the grieving process may begin even before the loss of life. The patient and their family will sometimes know the patient is dying, regardless of anyone's interventions. In these situations, you may need to provide reassurance and emotional care.

The death of a human being is one of the most difficult events for another human being to accept. For a relative or close friend of the deceased, it is even more difficult. Emotional responses to the loss of a loved one or friend are appropriate and should be expected. In fact, it is expected you will feel emotional about the death of a patient. Feelings and emotions are part of the grieving process. All of us experience these feelings after a stressful situation that causes us personal pain.

In 1969, Dr. Elisabeth Kübler-Ross published *On Death and Dying*, which revealed her theory on the stages of grief people go through. They are as follows:

1. **Denial.** Refusing to accept diagnosis or care, unrealistic demands for miracles, or persistent failure to understand why there is no improvement.
2. **Anger, hostility.** Projecting bad news onto the environment and commonly in all directions, at times almost at random. The person lashes out. Someone must be blamed, and those who are responsible must be punished. This is usually an ugly phase, and it may even be inappropriately directed toward the EMT.
3. **Bargaining.** Attempting to negotiate a favorable outcome for good behavior or promising to change. "I promise to be a 'perfect patient' if only I can live until 'x' event."
4. **Depression.** Internalizing anger, hopelessness, and the desire to die. It rarely involves suicidal threats, complete withdrawal, or giving up long before the illness seems terminal. The patient is usually silent.
5. **Acceptance.** Accepting the impending death of the patient, or accepting the death of a loved one.

There is no right or wrong way to grieve. Each person will experience grief and respond to it in their own way. The stages of grief may follow one another, they may occur simultaneously, or a person may jump back and forth between stages. The stages may last different amounts of time.

Conveying the News of Death

There will be times when you must tell a person that their loved one has died. This conversation is never easy, especially when you are new to the profession. Learning to use a structured notification process can make these conversations easier for both the patient's loved ones and for you. The GRIEV_ING process is widely recognized as an effective strategy for conveying this news.[20] If possible, practice using this tool before you must employ it on a real call.

Gather. Gather the family; ensure that all members are present.

Resources. Call for support resources available to assist the family with their grief (ie, chaplain services, ministers, family, friends).

Identify. Identify yourself, identify the deceased or injured patient by name, and identify the state of knowledge of the family relative to the events of the day.

Educate. Briefly educate the family as to the events that have occurred; educate them about the current state of their loved one.

Verify. Verify that their family member has died. Be clear: Use the words "dead" or "died."

[Space] Give the family personal space and time for an emotional moment; allow the family time to absorb the information.

Inquire. Ask if there are any questions, and answer them all.

Nuts and bolts. Inquire about organ donation, funeral services, and personal belongings. Offer the family the opportunity to view the body, if appropriate.

Give. Give them your card and access information. Offer to answer any questions that may arise later. Always return their call.

The EMT's Role During Death and Dying

As patients and bystanders are grieving, you can do helpful things and make simple suggestions. Provide gentle and caring support. Family members may express a range of emotions, from rage, to anger, to despair. Many people will be rational and cooperative. Their concerns will usually be relieved by your calm, efficient manner. Your actions and words, even a simple touch, can communicate caring.

> **Street Smarts**
>
> Although you must treat all patients with respect and dignity, use special care with dying patients and their families. Be concerned about their privacy and their wishes, and let them know you take their concerns seriously. However, it is best to be honest with patients and their families; do not give them false hope.

Reinforcing the reality of the situation is important. This can be accomplished by merely saying to a grieving person, "I am so sorry for your loss." Being honest and sincere is important. The following statements are usually regarded as sincere and thoughtful expressions of your empathy for the person's loss:

- I'm sorry for your loss.
- It is okay to be angry.
- It must be hard to accept.
- That must be painful for you.
- Tell me how you are feeling.
- If you want to cry, it's okay.

Some statements of consolation tend to be trite. Saying something like "They are in a better place now" is not helpful and makes assumptions about a grieving person's beliefs. Although such statements may be said with the intention of making the person feel better about a situation, they can also be viewed as an attempt to diminish the person's grief. Each person's beliefs about death and dying are different and may not mirror your own. The grieving person needs to be validated. Avoid statements that do not convey a true understanding of the person's feelings. If you have not experienced a death, it is okay to say so; do not pretend you have.

Similarly, do not attempt to bring closure or otherwise direct a person's grief. People may be offended by advice or explanations about their feelings. Statements such as "Oh, you shouldn't feel that way" are judgmental. If you judge what the grieving person is feeling, they will likely stop talking with you. People feel what they feel. Remember, anger is a stage of grieving. The anger may be directed at you. The anger seems irrational to everyone except the person grieving; therefore, it is necessary that you maintain a professional attitude and let the person grieve in their own way.

Cultural Implications of Death and Dying

Religious and cultural traditions may have a large impact on how patients and their loved ones respond to critical illness or death. Their emotional reactions and actions during the dying process or after death may vary substantially from yours. Ethnic and cultural traditions may impact how the patient and family view suffering, death, or health care. It is important to respect these differences and to remain curious, asking questions if you do not understand their actions or responses to the situation. You should be careful not to make statements that impose your own beliefs on others who are grieving.

Death and Dying of a Child

The death or life-threatening emergency of a child is a tragic and dreaded event. It will not be unusual for you to think about the fact that the dead or dying child still has a lot more to do in life and should have many more years to live. In our society, we often assume only older people are supposed to die. Many people are unprepared for what they will feel when a child dies. You may think about your own children and other children you know.

One of your responsibilities may be to help the family during the resuscitation or in the initial period after the death. As an EMT, until more definitive and professional help can be arranged, you may be in the best position to help the family begin to cope with their loss. How a family initially deals with the death of a child will affect its stability and endurance. You can help a family through their initial period of grief and provide information about follow-up counseling and support services that are available.

Caring for a family whose child has died is typically a profoundly emotional experience for both the family and the EMS clinicians involved. There are no perfect strategies to lessen the emotional impact of these situations; however, parents of children who died in an out-of-hospital setting have indicated three strategies used by prehospital clinicians that helped them cope with the death of their child[21]:

- Excellent, fast, coordinated care
- Family presence during the attempted resuscitation
- Continuous communication regarding what was happening

Often, the parents cannot believe the death is real, even if they have been preparing for it, as in the case of a terminal illness such as leukemia. If it is possible and appropriate, find a place where the mother and father can hold or touch the child. This is important in the parents' grieving process; it helps to lessen the sense of disbelief and makes the death real. Even if the parents do not ask to see the child, you should consider telling them that they may do so. However, use discretion. Certain circumstances, such as a crime scene or a traumatic death in which there is significant disfigurement of the body, may require a delay until support services can arrive or the family physician or others who can help the parents through this difficult situation can be contacted. This situation may also involve preparing the parents for what they will see and the changes brought on by rigor mortis or asphyxiation, for example.

Sometimes, you do not need to say much. In fact, silence can sometimes be more comforting than words. You can express your own sorrow, but do not overload grieving parents with a lot of information. At this point, they cannot handle it. Nonverbal communication, such as holding a hand or touching a shoulder, may be more valuable. Let the family's actions be your guide to what is appropriate. If you sense the parents want to talk, it is important for you to encourage them to talk about their feelings.

Street Smarts

Patients don't care what you know until they know that you care.

Often, the emotional impact of a child's death is significant. In these cases, take appropriate measures to seek care for yourself after the call has concluded. This may include attending a structured debriefing, participating in peer support, using employee assistance programs, or seeking mental health support or counseling. For further discussion of the EMT's mental health, see Chapter 2, *Workforce Safety and Wellness*.

Written Communications and Documentation

The **patient care report (PCR)**, also known as a prehospital care report, is the legal document used to record all aspects of the care your patient received, from initial dispatch to arrival at the hospital. Either term can be used, and both are acceptable. You may be able to complete the report en route to the hospital if the trip is long enough and the patient needs minimal care. Usually, you will finish the report after you have transferred care of the patient to an ED staff member. PCRs may be written or electronic (ePCRs), which will be discussed later in this chapter.

The information you collect during a call becomes part of the PCR, and that information is ultimately entered into a data pool. NEMSIS has been collecting prehospital care information for research purposes since the early 1970s. NEMSIS has identified specific data points (uniform components) needed to enable communication and comparison of EMS runs between agencies, regions, and states. The minimum data set includes both narrative components and checkboxes (**FIGURE 4-9**). The NEMSIS website (http://nemsis.org) provides the national data set and interesting facts about delivery of EMS within the United States.

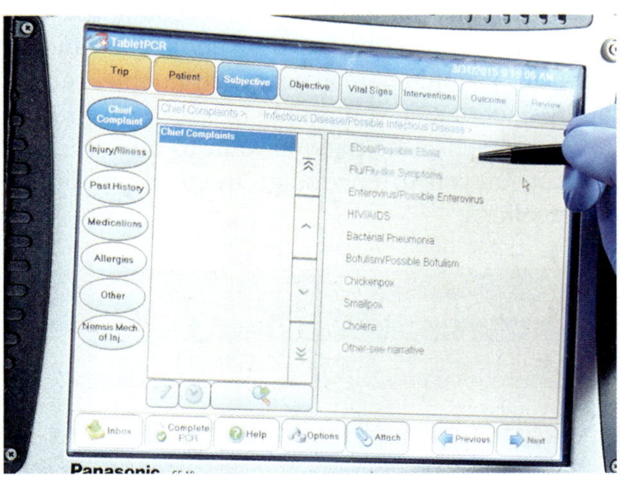

FIGURE 4-9 The minimum data set includes patient and administrative information, including narrative components and checkboxes.

Because EMS systems track their own time, make sure your watch is synchronized with your documentation device and dispatch time at the beginning of the shift. Another way you can manage this information is to contact the dispatcher and request the time. Either way, it is important to be able to keep close track of time. Accurate documentation will depend on it.

You will begin gathering patient information as soon as you reach the patient. Continue collecting information as you provide care until you arrive at the hospital.

Patient Care Report

As discussed, a PCR helps ensure efficient continuity of patient care. This report describes the nature of the patient's injuries or illness at the scene and the initial treatment you provide. Although this report might not be read immediately at the hospital, it may be referred to later for important information. The report serves the following six functions:

1. Transfer of information and continuity of care
2. Compliance and legal documentation
3. Administrative information
4. Reimbursement
5. Education
6. Data collection for quality improvement and research

A good PCR documents any changes in the patient's condition on arrival at the hospital. It is critical that you document everything in the clearest manner possible. The information in the report will help to prove that you have provided a standard of care and, in some instances, shows you have properly handled unusual or uncommon situations. Both objective and subjective information is included in this report.

The following are examples of information collected on a PCR:

- Chief complaint or chief concern
- Mechanism of injury or nature of illness
- Level of responsiveness (according to the AVPU [Awake and alert, responsive to Verbal stimuli, responsive to Pain, Unresponsive] scale)

- Level of consciousness and orientation (person, place, time, and events)
- Vital signs
- Initial and ongoing assessment
- Patient demographics (age, sex, ethnic background)
- Transport information (how the patient was moved, reason for destination choice)

Should you ever be called on to provide testimony concerning patient care, both you and your PCR will be used to present evidence. As with your personal appearance, your PCR will reflect a professional or a nonprofessional image. A neat, concise, well-written document, including correct spelling and grammar, will reflect good patient care. Consider the adage, "If the report looks sloppy, the patient care was also sloppy." The legal implications of your documentation are discussed further in Chapter 3, *Medical, Legal, and Ethical Issues*.

These reports also provide valuable administrative information, such as that used for patient billing. Information included in PCRs can be used to evaluate response times, mileage, time on scene, equipment usage, appropriateness of patient care and transport, and other areas of administrative responsibility. The following are examples of administrative information gathered from a PCR:

- Time the incident was reported
- Time the EMS unit was notified
- Time the EMS unit arrived at the scene
- Time the EMS crew made contact with the patient
- Time the EMS unit left the scene
- Time the EMS unit arrived at the receiving facility
- Time the patient care was transferred
- Time the EMS unit was back in service

It is standard procedure to use military time in EMS documentation. With military time, each time is unique; for example, 12 noon cannot be confused with 12 midnight. Military times are shown in **TABLE 4-4**. Military time is spoken in "hundred hours." For example, 1300, which is 1:00 PM, is spoken as "thirteen hundred hours," and 0100, which is 1:00 AM, is spoken as "zero one hundred hours."

Data may be obtained from the PCR to analyze causes, severity, and types of illness or injury requiring emergency medical care. These reports may also be used in an ongoing program for evaluation of the quality of patient care. All reports are

TABLE 4-4 Military Times

Regular Time	Military Time	Regular Time	Military Time
Midnight	0000	Noon	1200
1:00 AM	0100	1:00 PM	1300
2:00 AM	0200	2:00 PM	1400
3:00 AM	0300	3:00 PM	1500
4:00 AM	0400	4:00 PM	1600
5:00 AM	0500	5:00 PM	1700
6:00 AM	0600	6:00 PM	1800
7:00 AM	0700	7:00 PM	1900
8:00 AM	0800	8:00 PM	2000
9:00 AM	0900	9:00 PM	2100
10:00 AM	1000	10:00 PM	2200
11:00 AM	1100	11:00 PM	2300

periodically reviewed by your system to make sure trauma triage and/or other prehospital care criteria have been met.

There are many requirements of a PCR (**TABLE 4-5**). Often, these requirements vary from jurisdiction to jurisdiction, mainly because different agencies obtain information from them. Although no universally accepted form exists, certain uniform data points are common in all areas. The benefits of collecting such information are significant, one being that national and local trends can be detected. For example, a local EMS agency may discover that approximately 15% of their local EMS calls involve children ages birth to 9 years. Of those patients, 3% have a respiratory complaint. Such information is invaluable to plan for training and equipment. National trends can be identified using the NEMSIS data base. These data can drive EMS initiatives on a national level.

Finally, PCRs are used by individual agencies to determine patterns of EMS responses. Busy times and high call-volume areas can be predictive, and a thorough review of PCRs can set the stage for scheduling shifts and for system status management, including where units are placed or where new stations should be built.

Types of Forms

Most PCRs are completed in an electronic format often referred to as an ePCR (**FIGURE 4-10**). Although the features of ePCR software and services vary greatly, virtually all are designed to comply with NEMSIS data collection requirements. Some ePCRs will be initially completed on a computer, tablet, or other device and then uploaded to a local or state database, whereas other ePCRs collect and record each page or even each data field as it is entered. Electronic PCRs have several advantages over the written forms. For example, ePCRs allow you to transmit patient information directly to hospital computers for review by the physician, pharmacy,

TABLE 4-5 Sample Uniform Components of a Patient Care Report

- Patient's name, sex, date of birth, and address
- Dispatched as (When was the ambulance called? What was the nature of the call as reported by the dispatcher?)
- Chief complaint or chief concern
- Location of the patient when first seen (including specific details, especially if the incident is a car crash or when criminal activity is suspected)
- Rescue and treatment given before your arrival
- Signs and symptoms found during your patient assessment
- Care and treatment given by you at the site and during transport
- Response to treatment
- Vital signs
- SAMPLE history (Signs and symptoms, Allergies, Medications, Pertinent past medical history, Last oral intake, Events leading up to the illness or injury)
- Changes in vital signs and condition
- Additional orders received from the hospital
- Name of person receiving the patient report
- Date of the call
- Time of the call
- Location of the call
- Time of dispatch
- Time of arrival at the scene
- Time of leaving the scene
- Time of arrival at the hospital
- Patient's insurance information
- Names and/or certification numbers of the EMTs who responded to the call
- Name of the transport destination
- Type of response to the scene and type of transport: emergency or routine

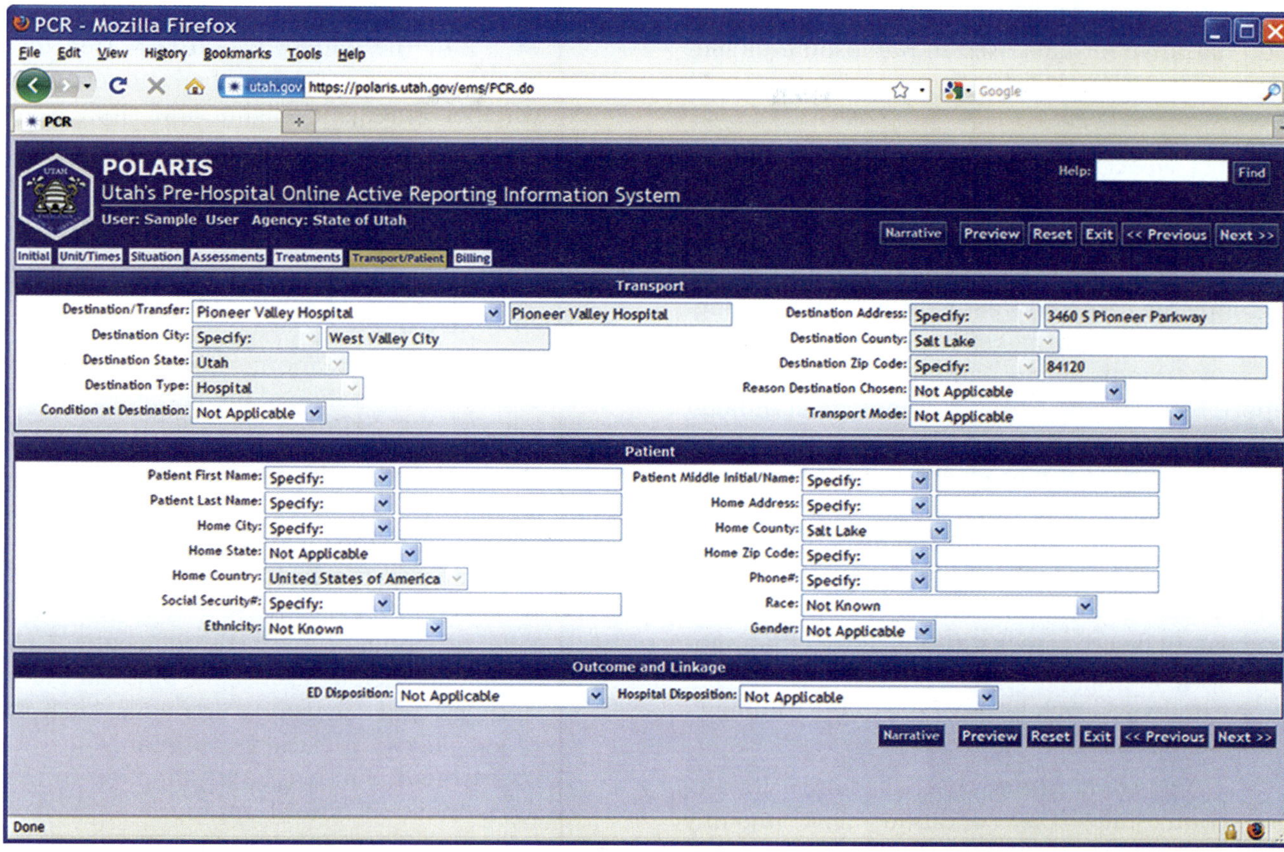

FIGURE 4-10 An electronic PCR (ePCR).

Courtesy of the Utah Department of Health.

and other professionals providing patient care and may be directly integrated with the patient's electronic medical record.

In cases where there is a temporary failure of Internet connectivity or where ePCRs have not yet been fully implemented, the PCR may be completed on a paper form, which can be uploaded later. When using paper forms, fill in the boxes completely and avoid making stray marks on the sheet.

The narrative section of the PCR is arguably the most important portion. Here you will describe all of the facts related to the EMS call. The narrative should tell the story and present a clear, detailed picture of what you found, what you did, and how it affected the patient's condition. Be sure to include significant negative findings and important observations about the scene. Make sure what you write is not an opinion, but is factually based on findings. For example, you may write, "The patient admits to drinking today" or "The patient smelled of alcohol." These are clear descriptions that do not make any judgments about the patient's condition. However, stating "the patient was drunk" is a personal judgment that may not be supportable. Choose your words carefully and thoughtfully. Your job is to reproduce the important facts of the EMS call in writing. Although some ePCRs can automatically generate narratives from previously entered data, such automatically generated documentation is virtually always a starting point only and should not be considered complete or substitute for a fully written narrative.

Standardized Narrative Formats

Many EMS systems require the use of a standardized format to document care. While many different formats have been developed, they are all designed to ensure that important information is not omitted. Further, the standardized format allows others who consult your patient report, such as physicians, billing clerks, or administrators, to find information within it quickly. Historically, the two most common narrative formats used in prehospital patient care are CHART and SOAP.

CHART Method

CHART stands for Chief complaint, History and physical examination, Assessment, Treatment (Rx), and Transport. This method's strength is that it groups the care and treatment into smaller, logical sections, which makes it easier to locate specific assessments or care without reading the entire report. Its weakness is that it is somewhat difficult to learn.

To document a narrative using CHART, begin with the dispatch information. For example, your report may open with, "Unit 4 dispatched from headquarters for [dispatch code] to a [location]." Use a specific location type, such as residence, roadway, or health care institution, rather than simply saying "scene."

Next, review each letter of the CHART abbreviation, as follows:

- **C Chief complaint or chief concern.** This section states the condition most urgently requiring EMS intervention. It may be the patient's reported problem or your professional judgment of the most immediate threat to the patient. For example, a patient may complain of a headache (chief complaint), but you are most concerned because it is evident the person has signs of possible stroke, such as paralysis on one side (chief concern).
- **H History.** The history includes details relating to the current event (history of present illness, or HPI) and the patient's medical history prior to this event (past medical history, or PMH). These details come from the patient or others on scene, from dispatch, or from the patient record.
- **A Assessments.** Describe all assessments you perform on the patient, including vital signs and the physical examination.
- **R Treatments (Rx).** The *R* in CHART comes from the medical abbreviation for treatment. This section details all interventions that were performed. The patient's response to the treatment should also be documented.
- **T Transport.** This final section explains how the patient was moved to the ambulance and possibly why the person was moved in that way; how the patient was transported (eg, how the person was positioned and secured); whether emergency lights and siren were used; where the patient was taken, including the room number; and the person to whom the report was given and care was transferred (eg, nurse Jones).

SOAP Method

The SOAP framework is another common method to structure documentation of the narrative.

- **S Subjective.** This section includes information provided by the patient or others on the scene, such as the chief complaint, events leading up to the incident, mechanism of injury, and past medical history.
- **O Objective.** The objective section includes details you gather primarily through patient assessment, such as vital signs, physical exam findings, and other measurements, such as blood glucose or oxygen saturation.
- **A Assessment.** Summarize key findings in the assessment section. If appropriate, provide your impression of what the patient's problem might be (eg, possible fractured lower leg or possible stroke).
- **P Plan.** Within the plan area, document treatment provided for the patient.

The SOAP method is fairly simple to learn, and when it is completed, it provides a means for the reader to review the assessment and management.

Regardless of the method used, the PCR's narrative section should include the following information:

- Time of events
- Assessment findings
- Emergency medical care provided
- Changes in the patient after treatment
- Observations at the scene
- Final patient disposition
- Refusal of care (if relevant)
- Staff person who continued care

In written documentation, avoid radio codes and abbreviations. Remember, EMS personnel are not the only people who will be reading this document. Other hospital and billing personnel will need to read the document and note the source of the information. Be sure to spell words correctly, especially medical terms. If you do not know the correct spelling of a particular word, find out how to spell it or use another word. Be sure to record the time with all assessment findings. **TABLE 4-6** provides guidelines on how to write the narrative portion of your report. Whether you completed a medical or trauma assessment, the assessment-based

TABLE 4-6 How to Write a Narrative Report

Standard precautions	Were standard precautions initiated? If so, state which precautions were used and why.
Scene safety	Did you have to make your scene safe? If so, what did you do and why did you do it? Did this create a delay in patient care?
NOI/MOI	Describe the primary medical condition (nature of their illness) or the cause of the traumatic injury (mechanism of injury).
Number of patients	Record only when more than one patient is present; "This is patient 2 of 3."
Additional help	Did you call for help? If so, state why, at what time, and what time the help arrived. Was transport delayed?
Initial general impression	Simply record, if not already documented on the PCR.
Level of consciousness	Describe the patient's level of consciousness and any changes during treatment and transport.
Chief complaint	Note pertinent statements made by the patient and/or bystanders. This includes any pertinent denials (eg, *Patient denies chest pain.*). If documenting a person's exact words, use quotation marks (eg, *The patient stated, "I have a stabbing pain in my chest."*).
Life threats	Describe all interventions and how the patient responded. Example: *Assisted ventilations with O_2 (15 L/min) at 20 BPM with no change in LOC.*
ABCs	Document what you found, and again, any interventions performed.
Oxygen	Record if oxygen was used, how it was applied, and how much was administered.
Primary, secondary, patient history, or reassessment	State the type of assessment used and any pertinent findings. Example: *Secondary assessment revealed unequal pupils, crepitus to right ribs, and deformity of left tibia.*
SAMPLE/OPQRST	Note and quote any pertinent answers. Describe patient's past medical history as appropriate. Include prescription medications.
Vital signs	Your service may want you to record vital signs in the narrative portion, as well as other places in the PCR. Typically, at least two sets of vital signs are documented.
Medical direction	Quote any orders given to you by medical direction and the name and title of the authorized individual who gave them.
Management of secondary injuries/treatment for shock	Report all patient interventions, at what time they were completed, and how the patient responded.
Receiving facility	Document the name of the facility, the area of the facility where the patient was delivered, and the room number (if known).
Transfer of care	Record the name of the staff person who received your report and took over patient care, as well as the time.

Abbreviations: ABCs, airway, breathing, and circulation; LOC, level of consciousness; MOI, mechanism of injury; NOI, nature of illness; OPQRST, mnemonic used to facilitate the evaluation of a patient's pain: Onset, Provocation or palliation, Quality, Region/radiation, Severity, and Timing of pain; PCR, patient care report; SAMPLE, mnemonic used to determine Signs and symptoms, Allergies, Medications, Pertinent past history, Last oral intake, and Events leading up to the injury or illness.

Courtesy of Jay C. Keefauver.

approach follows each step of the assessment or assessments as a guideline to narrative writing.

Remember that the report form itself, and all the information in it, is considered a confidential document, as are all formal and informal notes that contain protected patient information. Be sure you are familiar with federal, state, and local laws concerning confidentiality. All prehospital forms must be handled with care and stored in an appropriate manner once you have completed them. After you have completed a report, distribute copies to the appropriate locations, according to state and local protocol. In most instances, a copy of the report will remain at the hospital and will become part of the patient's medical record.

Depending on the requirements of the EMS system in which you work, you may not have the time to complete the full PCR while at the hospital; some EMS systems allow for shorter handoff notes to be left at the hospital. The full report can then be completed at the station or transmitted electronically.

Street Smarts

When using an electronic documentation system, be sure to review your report before submitting it. EMTs often click through the checkboxes and drop-down menus quickly, but it is essential that what is documented in this part of the ePCR matches what is documented in the narrative. The checkboxes should not indicate the patient is awake and alert to person, place, time, and location when you have documented in the narrative that the patient is confused and does not know the present location. This is an easy error to make but is usually caught by performing a brief review of the report.

Documenting Medical Necessity

Medicare and Medicaid payers will reimburse for ambulance transport only if the services are documented as being medically necessary.[22] *Medically necessary* means it would have been unsafe or impossible to transport the patient by any other means.

The following scenarios constitute medical necessity:

- The patient was transported in an emergency situation (eg, as a result of an accident, injury, or acute illness) and could not be transported by other means.
- The patient needed to be restrained to prevent injury to self or others.
- The patient required oxygen (and did not have their own portable tank) or other emergency treatment during transport to the nearest appropriate facility.
- The patient was unconscious or in shock.
- The patient exhibited signs and symptoms of acute respiratory distress or cardiac distress such as shortness of breath or chest pain.
- The patient exhibited signs and symptoms that indicated the possibility of acute stroke.
- The patient needed to remain immobile because of a fracture that had not been stabilized or the possibility of a fracture.
- The patient experienced severe hemorrhage.
- The patient was confined to a bed before and after the ambulance trip. For a patient to be considered bed-confined, the person must be unable to get up from bed without assistance, unable to ambulate, and unable to sit in a chair or a wheelchair.

Medical necessity also applies to the level of care provided for the patient. For example, it would be inappropriate to document that advanced life support interventions were provided to a patient who did not need them. It is therefore crucial to clearly document the patient's dispatch-reported condition, the actual patient condition the EMT found on scene, EMS treatments and services rendered and the patient's response to those treatments, and an objective report of the patient's appearance and mental status.

Another essential element to ensure your EMS agency is appropriately reimbursed for services provided is signatures. Every attempt should be made to obtain appropriate signatures from the patient or guardian.

Words of Wisdom

Documentation is usually an EMT's least favorite EMS activity, particularly as it relates to the details needed for billing. Yet, the budget of most EMS agencies relies heavily, or in some cases entirely, on collections from bills for patient care. Attention to detail in this EMT role can have a huge effect on the operating funds of your agency.

Health Information Exchanges

Some EMS systems use a **health information exchange (HIE)** (sometimes referred to as a health data exchange [HDE]) to improve sharing of data between EMS and other health care clinicians. HIEs allow EMS clinicians to access relevant health data (eg, past medical problems, medications, allergies, end-of-life decisions), avoid unnecessary duplication of effort in data entry, and view patient outcomes related to hospital care. HIEs allow EMTs to contribute to and access electronic health information on both a regular basis and during times of disaster, when accurate patient medical records may be destroyed or difficult to obtain. In some systems, the HIE allows designated personnel at an EMS agency the ability to access the patient's hospital diagnosis. This allows the EMT to reflect on their assessment of the patient and determine if their clinical judgments and treatment plans were appropriate.

Most HIEs follow the SAFR framework to improve patient care by giving health care clinicians rapid and universal access to accurate patient medical information. The SAFR mnemonic is described as follows[23,24]:

- **S Search.** EMS clinicians in the field can search for hospital and other records that will help them make treatment and transport decisions.
- **A Alert.** Hospitals are notified of incoming EMS patients with automated systems that populate ED dashboards with information entered by EMS in the field.
- **F File.** The data in EMS electronic patient care reports are incorporated directly into patients' longitudinal health records.
- **R Reconcile.** Feedback on outcomes and other hospital data are provided to EMS agencies for billing and quality improvement.

Reporting Errors

Everyone makes mistakes. If you leave something out of a report or record information incorrectly, do not try to cover it up. Rather, write down what did or did not happen and the steps that were taken to correct the situation. Falsifying information on the PCR may result in suspension and/or revocation of your certification or license, and may have legal implications. More important, falsifying information results in poor patient care, because other health care clinicians have a false impression of assessment findings or the treatment given. For example, if you did not give the patient oxygen, do not document that the patient was given oxygen.

Document only the vital signs that were obtained. Failure to include pertinent information in the original documentation means someone (perhaps a court of law) must later take the clinician's word for it, if the clinician even remembers such details when the time comes.

What if the wrong drug or the wrong dose is given to a patient? What if the patient is accidentally dropped? Unfortunately, these things can and do happen. It is important that you document the event. Do not lie or cover it up by withholding the information. In your narrative, provide a factual account of what happened. For example: "Ordered: one sublingual nitroglycerin. Given: two sublingual nitroglycerin. Patient blood pressure checked following administration. No changes noted" or "While loading the patient into the ambulance, the patient was dropped. Patient was on the ambulance cot when it fell a total of 4 feet. Patient was not thrown off cot. Patient was assessed after being dropped and reported feeling scared and having neck pain. Hospital advised."

Words of Wisdom

Additional details regarding any incident or error are documented in a separate departmental incident report. For example, in the scenario of a patient who was dropped, the EMT will document specific additional information, such as "a large crack in the sidewalk that was not seen due to very dark conditions."

If you discover an error as you are completing a handwritten report, draw a single horizontal line through the error, initial it, and write the correct information next to it (**FIGURE 4-11**). Do not try to erase or cover the error with correction fluid. This may be interpreted as an attempt to cover up a mistake.

If an error is discovered after you submit your report, follow the same process. Make sure to add a note with the correct information. If you

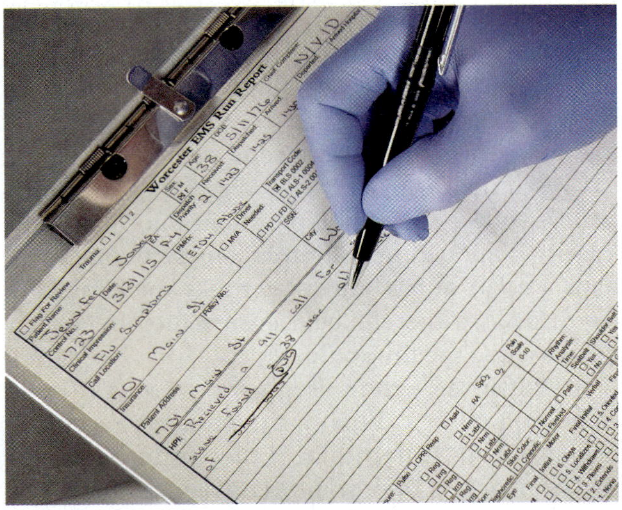

FIGURE 4-11 If you make a mistake on a handwritten report, the proper way to correct it is to draw a single horizontal line through the error, initial it, and write the correct information next to it.

accidentally left out information, begin the new section with the word "addendum," add the new information, and then add the date and your initials. When using a paper system, you may be able to add addendums using specific addendum forms. If you are using an electronic documentation system, refer to the system's direction regarding how to make an amendment to the original document. Most electronic systems will allow for amendments that are date stamped but will prevent erasure in a completed document.

Documenting Refusal of Care

Refusal of care is an important potential source of litigation in EMS; therefore, thorough documentation is crucial. Adult patients with decision-making capacity have the right to refuse treatment and, in fact, must specifically provide permission for treatment to be initiated. If you are not able to persuade the patient to proceed with treatment, document any patient assessment findings, emergency medical care given, your efforts to obtain consent, and the patient's response to your efforts. Have the patient sign a refusal form (**FIGURE 4-12**). You should also have a family member, police officer, or bystander sign the form as a witness. If the patient refuses to sign the refusal form, have a family member, police officer, or bystander sign the form verifying that the patient refused to sign. Inform online medical direction when patients refuse care. For further discussion of decision-making capacity and the right to refuse care, see Chapter 3, *Medical, Legal, and Ethical Issues.*

Even if a patient refuses care, you must complete the PCR. You will need to document the advice you gave regarding the risks associated with refusal of care. Report clinical information, such as the level of consciousness (LOC), showing the decision-making capacity of the person refusing care. Note pertinent patient comments and any medical advice given to the patient by the physician or medical direction through phone or radio. Also include a description of the care that you wished to provide for the patient. There are many local variations of requirements for patient refusals. Items that are typically included within the PCR of a patient refusal include the following:

- Complete assessment
- Evidence the patient has the decision-making capacity to make a rational, informed decision
- Discussion with the patient as to what care/transportation EMS recommends
- Discussion with the patient as to what may happen if the patient does not allow care or transport. Typically, these consequences should be listed and clear to include the possibility of severe illness/injury or death if care or transport is refused.
- Discussion with family/friend/bystanders to try to encourage the patient to allow care
- Discussion with medical direction according to local protocol
- Presentation of alternatives to EMS care, such as visiting a family doctor or being transported to the hospital by a family member
- Willingness of EMS to return if the patient changes their mind
- Signatures. Have a family member, police officer, or bystander sign the form as a witness. If the patient refuses to sign the refusal form, have a family member, police officer, or bystander sign the form verifying that the patient refused to sign.

If the patient refused care or did not allow a complete assessment, document that the patient did not allow for proper assessment, and document whatever assessments were completed.

Patient Initiated Refusal of EMS

Patient Name: Doe, John	Primary Care Giver: John Smith, NREMT-P	
Agency: BALTIMORE COUNTY FIRE DEPARTMENT	Incident#: 1122141	eMEDS#: 00314105399
Unit #: Medic 14	Inc Date Entered: 11/22/2025	Inc Time Entered: 1824 hrs

I (or my guardian) have been informed regarding the state of my present physical condition to the extent I allowed an examination, and I (or my guardian) hereby refuse to accept such medical care and/or transportation as recommended by representatives of the EMS System above.

I (or my guardian) do hereby for myself, my heirs, executors, and administrators and assigns forever release and fully discharge said EMS system, its officers, employees, medical consultants, hospitals, borrowed servants or agents from any and all conceivable liability that might arise from this refusal of care and/or transportation, and I (and my guardian) therefore agree to hold them completely harmless. I (or my guardian) have been informed that a refusal of care and/or transportation for an evaluation may cause me to suffer PAIN, DISABILITY, LOSS of FUNCTION, WORSENING of my CONDITION, or even DEATH as a result of my illness/injury. As a competent adult, I (or my guardian) fully understand all of the above, and am/is capable of determining a rational decision on my own behalf.

Providers: When encountering a patient who is attempting to refuse EMS treatment or transport, access his or her condition, and record whether the patient screening reveals any lack of medical decision-making capability (1-3,4a or b) or high risk criteria (5-8).

1) Medical Capacity: Was the patient disoriented to person? If yes, transport	☐ Yes ☑ No
2) Medical Capacity: Was the patient disoriented to place? If yes, transport	☐ Yes ☑ No
3) Medical Capacity: Was the patient disoriented to time? If yes, transport	☐ Yes ☑ No
4) Medical Capacity: Was the patient disoriented to situation? If yes, transport	☐ Yes ☑ No
5) Medical Capacity: Did the patient show altered level of consciousness? If yes, transport	☐ Yes ☑ No
6) Medical Capacity: Alcohol or drug ingestion by history or exam with slurred speech? If yes, transport	☐ Yes ☑ No
7) Medical Capacity: Alcohol or drug ingestion by history or exam with unsteady gait? If yes, transport	☐ Yes ☑ No
8) Medical Capacity: Patient does not understand the nature of illness and potential for bad outcome? If yes, transport	☐ Yes ☑ No
9) At Risk Criteria (Abnormal vital signs): For adults. Pulse greater than 120 or less than 60? If yes, consult	☐ Yes ☑ No
10) At Risk Criteria (Abnormal vital signs): For adults. Systolic BP less than 90? If yes, consult	☐ Yes ☑ No
11) At Risk Criteria (Abnormal vital signs): For adults. Respirations greater than 30 or less than 10? If yes, consult	☐ Yes ☑ No
12) At Risk Criteria (Abnormal vital signs): For minor/pediatric patients. Age inappropriate HR? If yes, consult	☐ Yes ☑ No
13) At Risk Criteria (Abnormal vital signs): For minor/pediatric patients. Age inappropriate RR? If yes, consult	☐ Yes ☑ No
14) At Risk Criteria (Abnormal vital signs): For minor/pediatric patients. Age inappropriate BP? If yes, consult	☐ Yes ☑ No
15) At Risk Criteria: Serious chief complaint (chest pain, SOB, syncope)? If yes, consult	☐ Yes ☑ No
16) At Risk Criteria: Head injury with history of loss of consciousness? If yes, consult	☐ Yes ☑ No
17) At Risk Criteria: Significant MOI or high suspicion of injury? If yes, consult	☐ Yes ☑ No

Inc. Date: 11/22/2025 Patient Name: Doe, John BALTIMORE COUNTY FIRE DEPARTMENT Page: 1
Incident #: 1122141 Date Printed: 11/24/2025 18:24

FIGURE 4-12 Even though adult patients with decision-making capacity have the right to refuse medical treatment, ask them if they would be willing to sign a refusal form to document their informed refusal.

18) At Risk Criteria: For minor/pediatric patients. ALTE, significant past medical history, or suspected intentional injury? If yes, consult	☐ Yes ☑ No
19) At Risk Criteria: Provider impression is that the patient requires hospital evaluation? If yes, consult	☐ Yes ☑ No
20) Providers: Did you perform an assessment (including exam) on this patient? If yes to # 20, skip to # 22	☐ Yes ☑ No
21) Providers: If unable to examine, did you attempt vital signs?	☐ Yes ☑ No
22) Providers: Did you attempt to convince the patient or guardian to accept transport?	☐ Yes ☑ No
23) Providers: Did you contact medical direction for patient still refusing service?	☑ Yes ☐ No
24) Patient: The patient or his or her representative refuses EMS examination.	☐ Yes ☑ No
25) Patient: The patient or his or her representative refuses EMS treatment.	☐ Yes ☑ No
26) Patient: The patient or his or her representative refuses EMS transport.	☑ Yes ☐ No

Patient Signature: **Printed Name:**

Patient Phone: **Date:** 18:24 11/24/2025

Patient Address:

Initial Disposition

Patient Refused Exam ☑	Patient Refused Treatment ☑	Patient Refused Transport ☑
Patient Accepted Exam ☐	Patient Accepted Treatment ☐	Patient Accepted Transport ☐
Auth. Decision Maker (ADM) Refused Exam ☐	Auth. Decision Maker (ADM) Refused Treatment ☐	Auth. Decision Maker (ADM) Refused Transport ☐

Intervention

Attempt to Convince Patient ☑ Attempt to Convince Family Member/Auth. Decision Maker (ADM) ☐ Contact Medical Direction ☑ Contact Law Enforcement ☐ None of the Above Available ☐

AMA Contact Medical Direction Facility St Elsewhere Hospital

Final Disposition

Patient Refused Exam ☐	Patient Refused Treatment ☐	Patient Refused Transport ☑
Patient Accepted Exam ☑	Patient Accepted Treatment ☑	Patient Accepted Transport ☐
Auth. Decision Maker (ADM) Refused Exam ☐	Auth. Decision Maker (ADM) Refused Treatment ☐	Auth. Decision Maker (ADM) Refused Transport ☐

Provide in the patient's own words why he/she refused the above care/service:

"Patient reports that despite the damage to his vehicle, he has only a small laceration on his finger and no other symptoms. He eventually agreed to allow EMS to evaluate him and provide a bandage for a small finger laceration (index finger, right hand). He agreed to follow up with his primary care MD later today. When offered transport to the hospital he indicated, "No. thanks. I will be fine." Discussed plan with Dr Smith at St Elsewhere ED who agreed with plan and recommended reiterating to Mr Smith the importance of close follow-up with his primary care MD for tetanus prophylaxis and consideration of laceration care to include sutures.

Inc. Date: 11/22/2025 Patient Name: Doe, John BALTIMORE COUNTY FIRE DEPARTMENT Page: 2

Incident #: 1122141 Date Printed: 11/24/2025 18:24

FIGURE 4-12 *(Continued)*

Refusal of care pertains not only to patients who do not wish to be transported to the hospital, but also to those who refuse a certain aspect of care. For example, a patient involved in a car crash who has neck pain may wish to be treated and transported but refuses to allow you to apply a cervical collar. In these instances, you should carry out all other medical care and document that the patient refused application of a cervical collar. Just because the patient refuses a cervical collar is no reason to deny oxygen. Any time a patient refuses any part of the standard treatment, it needs to be documented in the PCR.

Special Reporting Situations

In some situations, you may be required to file special reports with appropriate authorities. These situations may involve gunshot wounds, dog bites, certain infectious diseases, or suspected physical or sexual abuse. Learn your local requirements for reporting these incidents. Failure to report them may have legal consequences. It is important that the report be accurate, complete, objective, and submitted in a timely manner.

A voluntary, anonymous tool for reporting incidents that may have resulted in injury to a patient or clinician is the EMS Voluntary Event Notification Tool (EVENT).[25] This tool is designed to help understand and correct potential safety issues that clinicians may otherwise be afraid to discuss openly. Events that should be reported include near-miss events, unsafe conditions, and violence directed at EMS clinicians. Such events should be reported regardless of whether actual harm resulted.

Another special reporting situation is a mass-casualty incident (MCI). The local MCI plan should have some means of temporarily recording important medical information (such as a triage tag that can be used later to complete the form). The standard for completing the form in an MCI is not the same as for a typical call. Your local plan should have specific guidelines. MCIs are discussed in Chapter 38, *Incident Management*.

Communications Systems and Equipment

Radio and telephone communications link you and your team with the hospital and other members of the EMS, fire, and law enforcement communities. This link helps the entire team to work together more effectively and provides an important layer of safety and protection for each member of the team. You must know what your system can and cannot do, and you must be able to use your system efficiently and effectively. You must be able to send precise, accurate reports about the scene, the patient's condition, and the treatment that you provide.

As an EMT, you must be familiar with two-way radio communications and have a working knowledge of the mobile and handheld portable radios and cell phones that are used in your agency.

YOU are the EMT

As your partner takes the patient's vital signs, you ask the patient further questions regarding her chief complaint. She denies any other complaints or past medical history and tells you that she only takes a multivitamin supplement. Her blood glucose level is obtained at 112 mg/dL.

Recording Time: 5 Minutes	
Respirations	20 breaths/min; regular and unlabored
Pulse	68 beats/min; strong and regular
Skin	Adequate circulation; warm and dry
Blood pressure	122/62 mm Hg
Oxygen saturation (Spo_2)	98% (on room air)

5. What techniques can facilitate the process of interviewing an older patient?

Base Station Radios

The dispatcher usually communicates with field units by transmitting through a fixed radio base station that is controlled from the dispatch center. A **base station** is any radio hardware containing a transmitter and receiver that is located in a fixed place. The base station may be used by an operator speaking into a microphone that is connected directly to the equipment. It also works remotely through telephone lines or by radio from a communications center. Base stations may include dispatch centers, fire stations, ambulance bases, or hospitals.

A two-way radio consists of two units: a transmitter and a receiver. Some base stations may have more than one transmitter and/or more than one receiver. They may also be equipped with one multichannel transmitter and several single-channel receivers. A **channel** is an assigned frequency or frequencies used to carry voice and/or data communications. Regardless of the number of transmitters and receivers, they are commonly called *base radios* or *stations*. Base stations usually have more power (often 100 watts or more) and higher, more efficient antenna systems than mobile or portable radios. This increased broadcasting range allows the base station operator to communicate with field units and other stations at much greater distances.

The base radio must be physically close to its antenna. Therefore, the actual base station cabinet and hardware are commonly found on the roof of a tall building or at the bottom of an antenna tower. The base station operator may be miles away in a dispatch center or hospital, communicating with the base station radio by dedicated lines or special radio links. A **dedicated line**, also known as a *hotline*, is used for specific point-to-point contact. This type of phone, typically located within an ED, is not on the main switchboard. EMS personnel are able to call the number directly without being placed on hold or transferred. This type of line makes recording medical command conversations much easier.

Mobile and Portable Radios

In the ambulance, you will use both mobile and portable radios to communicate with the dispatcher, other emergency personnel, and/or medical direction. An ambulance will often have more than one mobile radio, each on a different frequency (**FIGURE 4-13**). One radio may be used to communicate with the dispatcher or other public safety agencies. A second radio is often used for communicating patient information to medical direction.

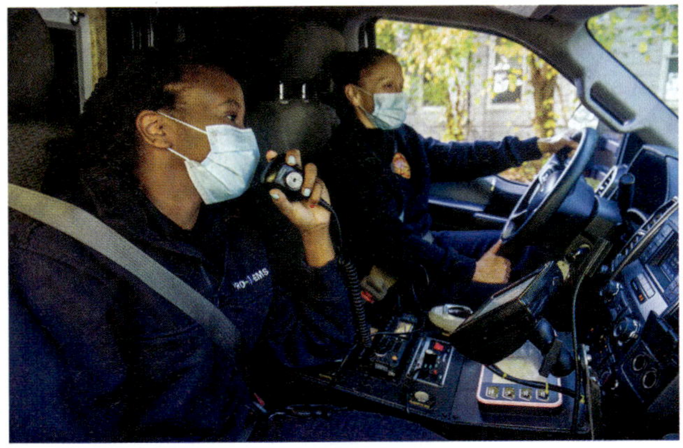

FIGURE 4-13 Some ambulances have more than one mobile radio to allow communications with hospitals, mutual aid jurisdictions, and other agencies.

A mobile radio is installed in a vehicle and usually operates at lower power than a base station. Most **VHF (very high frequency)** mobile radios operate between 30 and 300 megahertz (MHz). **UHF (ultra-high frequency)** mobile radios operate between 300 MHz and 3,000 MHz. Radios that operate at 800 MHz are increasingly common in EMS systems. These systems provide a great amount of system flexibility without the need for vast numbers of frequencies. What was once accomplished with 30 separate frequencies can be done with fewer than 10. Mobile antennas are much closer to the ground than base station antennas, so communications from the unit are typically limited to 10 to 15 miles over average terrain.

Portable radios are handheld devices that operate at 1 to 5 watts of power. Because the entire radio can be held in your hand, when in use, the antenna is often no taller than you. The transmission range of a portable radio is more limited than that of mobile or base station radios. Portable radios are essential in helping to coordinate EMS activities at the scene of an MCI. They are also helpful when you are away from the ambulance and need to communicate with dispatch, another unit, or medical direction (**FIGURE 4-14**).

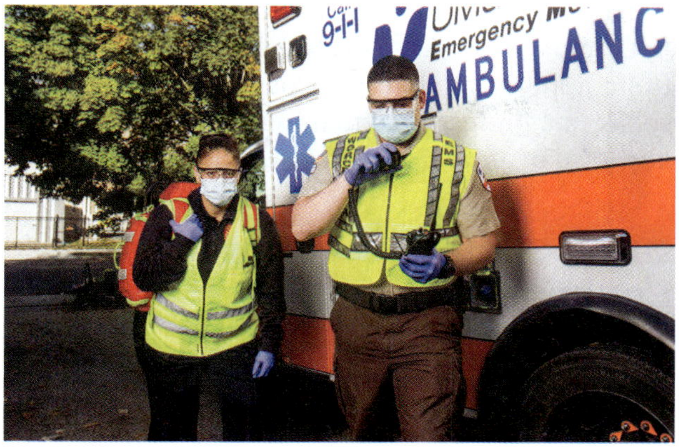

FIGURE 4-14 A portable radio is essential if you need to communicate with the dispatcher or medical direction when you are away from the ambulance.

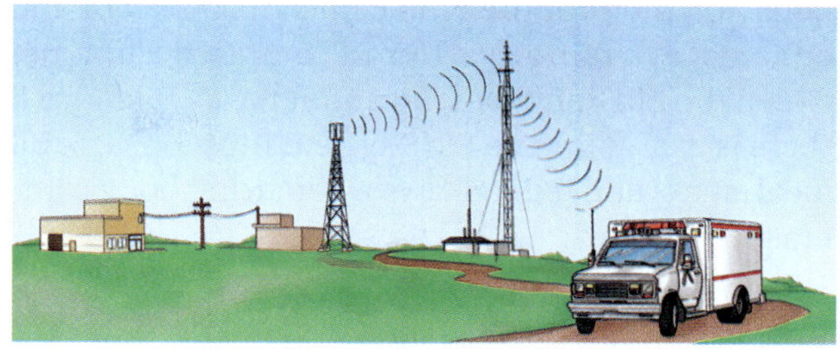

FIGURE 4-15 A message is sent from the control center to the transmitter by a landline. The radio carrier wave is picked up by the repeater for rebroadcast to outlying units. Return radio traffic is picked up by the repeater and rebroadcast to the control center.

Repeater-Based Systems

A **repeater** is a special base station radio that receives messages and signals on one frequency and then automatically retransmits them on a second frequency. Because a repeater is a base station (with a large antenna), it is able to receive lower power signals, such as those from a portable radio, from a long distance away. The signal is then rebroadcast with all the power of the base station (**FIGURE 4-15**). EMS systems that use repeaters usually have outstanding systemwide communications and are able to get the best signal from portable radios. There are also mobile repeaters that may be found in ambulances or placed in various areas around an EMS system area.

At times, you may be able to communicate with a base station radio, but you will not be able to hear or transmit to another mobile unit that is also communicating with that base. Repeater base stations eliminate such problems. They allow two mobile or portable units that cannot reach each other directly to communicate through the repeater, using its greater power and antenna.

Digital Equipment

Although most people think of voice communications when they think of two-way radios, digital signals are also a part of EMS communications. With **telemetry**, electronic signals are converted into coded, audible signals. These signals can then be transmitted by radio or telephone to a receiver with a decoder at the hospital. The decoder converts the signals back into electronic impulses that can be displayed on a screen or printed. New technology also allows for digital telemetry. For example, data from cardiac monitors can be transmitted via Bluetooth-enabled mobile devices to a monitoring center, where physicians can review the data and quickly contact patients, if needed. Rhythm strips and 12-lead electrocardiograms (ECGs) are transmitted to the hospital to identify abnormal heart rhythms and critical cardiac information such as ST-segment elevation myocardial infarction (STEMI) alerts, allowing informed treatment decisions to be made during the prehospital phase. Digital signals are also used in some types of paging and tone alerting systems because they transmit faster than spoken words and allow more choices and flexibility.

Increasingly, EMS systems are using other telemedicine tools to exchange information or consult with other health care entities. New communication platforms permit EMTs to notify the hospital of an incoming patient's details electronically by tapping a button. Telemonitoring systems may also permit direct transmission of electronic patient data such as ECGs, vital signs, and in some cases even patient video images to the receiving facility. In other cases, video consultation has been implemented so that medical direction or other health specialists can conduct a video interview with the patient using a tablet or other mobile device. This can result in a decision that the patient does not require transport, or in other cases, that care in a specialty facility is urgently needed.[26]

Body cameras are also being used in some EMS agencies to document the patient's condition and behavior, monitor the EMS clinician's behavior and adherence to protocols, record communication between the EMT and patient, and serve as evidence if there is a lawsuit. The EMS system must observe all local, state, and federal laws when using body camera technology.[27]

Cellular/Satellite Telephones

Whereas dispatchers communicate with field units by transmitting through a fixed radio base station, it is common for EMTs to communicate with receiving facilities by **cellular telephone**. These telephones are effectively low-power portable radios that communicate through a series of interconnected repeater stations called *cells* (hence the name network). Another option is a satellite phone, or satphone. These phones use a satellite, instead of a cell, to receive and relay the signals.

Many cellular systems make equipment and air time available to EMS systems at little or no cost as a public service. The public is often able to call 9-1-1 or other emergency numbers on a cellular telephone free of charge. However, this easy access may result in overloading and jamming of cellular systems in mass-casualty and disaster situations. To overcome this problem, the federal government funded the FirstNet program. States that participate in this program have priority access to secure, priority high-speed broadband cellular data transmission during high-use events.[28]

When using these systems, ensure that a reference of commonly called numbers is available. Local hospitals, poison control, police services, and the number to the dispatcher should be readily available. Cellular and satellite systems also have areas of bad reception. As an EMT, it is important to be aware of any areas in which your equipment will not work.

As with all repeater-based systems, a cellular or satellite telephone is useless if the equipment fails, if there is a loss of power, or if it is damaged by severe weather or other circumstances.

A **scanner** is a radio receiver that searches or scans across several frequencies, stops whenever it receives a radio broadcast on that frequency, and continues once the message is complete. Although cellular and satellite telephones are more private than most other forms of radio communications, keep in mind that these telephones use digital signals, which makes eavesdropping difficult but not impossible. Therefore, you must always be careful to appropriately respect patient privacy and to speak in a professional manner every time you use any form of an EMS communications system.

Other Communications Equipment

Ambulances and other field units are usually equipped with an external public address system. This system may be a part of the siren or the mobile radio. The intercom between the cab and the patient compartment may also be a part of the mobile radio. These components do not involve radio wave transmission, but you must understand how they work and practice using them before you really need them.

EMS systems may use a variety of two-way radio hardware. Some systems operate VHF equipment in the **simplex** (push to talk, release to listen) mode. In this mode, radio transmissions can occur in either direction but not simultaneously. When one party transmits, the other can only receive. Once one party finishes transmitting, the other party can then reply. Other systems conduct **duplex** (simultaneous talk–listen) communications on UHF frequencies and cellular telephones. In the full duplex mode, radios can simultaneously transmit and receive communications on one channel. This is sometimes called paired frequencies. A third possible configuration for a communications system is **multiplex**. This design utilizes two or more frequencies, which enables more than one transmission to occur simultaneously and provides for the transmission of both audio and data signals via separate channels. This type of system is what allows paramedics to transmit a patient's ECG to the hospital from the scene or back of the ambulance. Many VHF and UHF channels, commonly called **MED channels**, are reserved exclusively for EMS use. However, hundreds of other commercial, local government, and fire services frequencies are also used for EMS communications.

Trunking, or 800-MHz, systems take advantage of the latest technologies in communications. Instead of being assigned to one or two frequencies, in a trunking system, many frequencies are assigned to a group. As the radio conversation begins, a computer selects the next open frequency and you begin talking. When you speak a second time, you will likely be speaking on a different frequency because the computer is constantly monitoring for frequency load and reassigning transmissions to unused frequencies. These systems allow for greater traffic without greater numbers of frequencies. Therefore, you do not need to worry about being able to transmit or receive. In a trunking system, the computer will switch you to another channel without you being aware and you will operate the radio as you normally do.

Any large-scale emergency requires cooperative efforts from several agencies, such as law enforcement, fire departments, and EMS. At times, more than one jurisdiction is involved and effective communication between all of those involved becomes challenging. An **interoperable communications system** allows all agencies involved to share valuable information with each other in real time. This system utilizes a voice-over-Internet protocol (VoIP) format to connect landlines, cell phones, and computers to create a seamless, reliable exchange of information between all parties.

Another type of communication system is a **mobile data terminal (MDT)** (**FIGURE 4-16**). An MDT is a small computer terminal inside the ambulance or other vehicle that directly receives data from the dispatch center. MDTs allow for greatly expanded communication capabilities. Instead of asking the dispatcher to confirm whether they said 11345 Main Street or 11354 Main Street, you look at the terminal where the address is displayed. Satellite communications can track your progress to the scene and can provide important scene information, such as

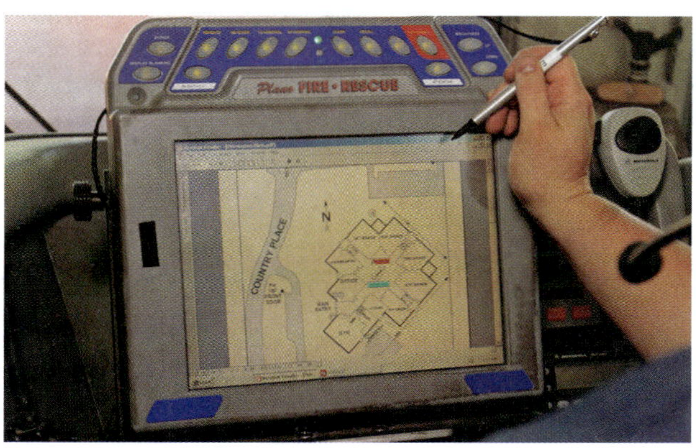

FIGURE 4-16 A mobile data terminal.

known violent calls to this address, the nature of those calls, and the number of times the ambulance has been called.

Your ability to effectively communicate with other units or medical direction depends on how well the weaker radio can talk back. Base and repeater station radios often have higher antennas and much greater power than mobile or portable units do. This increased power ensures that signals are generally heard and understood from a far greater distance than the signal produced from a mobile unit. Remember, when you are at the scene, you may be able to clearly hear the dispatcher or hospital on your radio, but you may not be heard or understood when you transmit.

Even small changes in your location can significantly affect the quality of your transmission. Also, remember that the location of the antenna is critical for clear transmission. Commercial aircraft flying at 37,000 feet can transmit and receive signals over hundreds of miles, yet their radios have only a few watts of power. The power comes from their antenna positioned at 37,000 feet.

The success of communications depends on the efficiency of your equipment. A damaged antenna or microphone often prevents high-quality communications. Check the condition and status of your equipment at the start of each shift, and then correct or report any problems.

Radio Communications

All radio operations in the United States, including those used in EMS systems, are regulated by the **Federal Communications Commission (FCC)**. The FCC has jurisdiction over interstate and international telephone and telegraph services and satellite communications, all of which may involve EMS activity.

The FCC has five principal EMS-related responsibilities:

1. **Allocate specific radio frequencies for use by EMS clinicians.** Modern EMS communications began in 1974. At that time, the FCC assigned 10 MED channels in the 460- to 470-MHz (UHF) band to be used by EMS clinicians. These UHF channels were added to the several VHF frequencies that were already available for EMS systems. However, these VHF frequencies had to be shared with other

special emergencies uses, including school buses and veterinarians.

2. **License base stations and assign appropriate radio call signs for those stations.** An FCC license is usually issued for 5 years, after which time it must be renewed. Each FCC license is granted only for a specific operating group. Often, the longitude and latitude (locations) of the antenna and the address of the base station determine the call signs.
3. **Establish licensing standards and operating specifications for radio equipment used by EMS clinicians.** Before it can be licensed, each piece of radio equipment must be submitted to the FCC by its manufacturer for type acceptance, based on established operating specifications and regulations.
4. **Establish limitations for transmitter power output.** The FCC regulates broadcasting power to reduce radio interference between neighboring communications systems.
5. **Monitor radio operations.** This includes making spot field checks to help ensure compliance with FCC rules and regulations.

The FCC's rules and regulations are written in technical and legal language and fill many volumes. Only small sections deal with EMS communication issues such as interoperable communications on the 700-MHz spectrum, 800-MHz spectrum, and VHF/UHF systems; 9-1-1 and E9-1-1; emergency alert systems; and disaster communications.[29] You are not responsible for reading these documents. For appropriate guidance on technical issues, contact your EMS system supervisor. In fact, many EMS systems look to radio and telephone communications experts for advice on technical issues.

Responding to the Scene

EMS communication systems may operate on several frequencies and use different frequency bands and channels of communication, including MDTs. However, all EMS systems depend on effective communication between the EMTs in the field and the dispatch center. Call takers collect emergency information from 9-1-1 calls and other communication channels. Dispatchers then send appropriate resources. In some cases, a single person takes on the roles of both call taker and dispatcher.

Call takers and dispatchers have several important responsibilities during the alert and dispatch phase of EMS communications. They must do all of the following:

- Properly screen and assign priority to each call (according to predetermined protocols).

YOU are the EMT

The patient wishes to be evaluated at the hospital and agrees to EMS transport, is placed on the stretcher, and is loaded into the ambulance. You cover her with a blanket to keep her warm and proceed to a hospital located 15 miles away. En route, you reassess her condition.

Recording Time: 11 Minutes	
Level of consciousness	Conscious and alert
Respirations	20 breaths/min; regular and unlabored
Pulse	74 beats/min; strong and regular
Skin	Warm and dry
Blood pressure	118/60 mm Hg
Oxygen saturation (Spo_2)	98% (on room air)

The patient's condition remains unchanged since your initial encounter. You contact the receiving facility and provide them with a radio report.

6. What are the components of a radio report to the hospital?
7. How does the handoff report differ from the radio report?

- Select and alert the appropriate EMS response unit or units.
- Dispatch and direct EMS response unit or units to the correct location.
- Coordinate the EMS response unit or units with other public safety services until the incident is over.
- Provide emergency medical instructions to the telephone caller (according to predetermined protocols) so that essential care (eg, CPR) may begin before the EMTs arrive.

When the first call to 9-1-1 comes in, the call taker or dispatcher must judge its relative importance to begin the appropriate EMS response using emergency medical dispatch protocols. First, the call taker must find out the exact location of the patient and the nature and severity of the problem. The call taker asks for the caller's telephone number, the patient's name and age, and other information, as directed by local protocol. Next, the call taker asks for some description of the scene, such as the number of patients or special environmental hazards.

Using this information, the dispatcher will assign the appropriate EMS response unit or units based on local protocols and the following factors:

- Dispatcher's determination of the nature and severity of the problem (Many emergency medical dispatch systems will determine this automatically based on a caller's answers to a defined series of questions.)
- Roles (EMR, EMT, AEMT, paramedic) of available EMS response unit or units
- Anticipated response time to the scene
- Need for additional specialty EMS units, fire suppression, rescue, hazardous materials team, air medical support, or law enforcement

The dispatcher's next step is to alert the appropriate EMS response unit or units (**FIGURE 4-17**). Alerting these units may be done in a variety of ways. The dispatcher may use the dispatch radios, MDTs, pagers, cell phones, or other devices to contact units. Dedicated lines (hotlines) between the control center and the EMS station may also be used.

The dispatcher may also page EMS personnel. Pagers are commonly used in EMS operations to alert on-duty and off-duty personnel. **Paging** involves the use of a coded tone or digital radio signal and a voice or display message that is transmitted to pagers (beepers) or desktop monitor radios. Paging signals may be sent to alert specific personnel or may be blanket signals that activate all pagers in the EMS service. Pagers and monitor radios are convenient because they are usually silent until their specific paging code is received. Alerted personnel contact the dispatcher to confirm the message and receive details of their assignments.

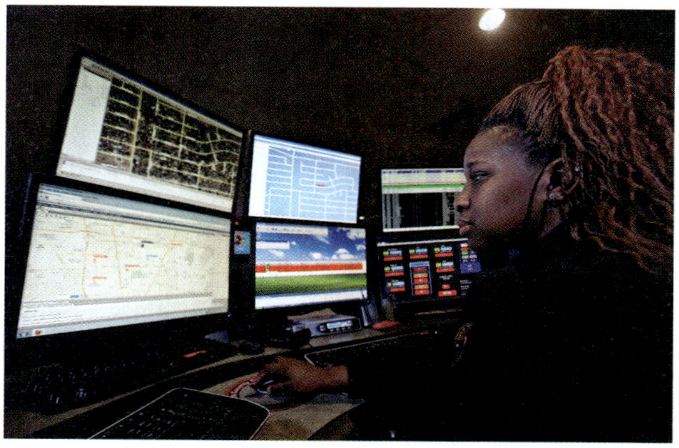

FIGURE 4-17 You will be assigned to a call by the dispatcher.

Once EMS personnel have been alerted, they must be properly dispatched and sent to the incident. Every EMS system should use a standard dispatching procedure. The dispatcher should give the responding unit or units the following information:

- Nature and severity of the injury, illness, or incident
- Exact location of the incident
- Number of patients
- Responses by other public safety agencies
- Special directions or advisories, such as adverse road or traffic conditions, severe weather reports, or potential scene hazards
- Time at which the unit or units are dispatched

Your unit must confirm with the dispatcher that you have received the information and are en route to the scene. Local protocol will dictate whether it is the job of the dispatcher or your unit to notify other public safety agencies that you are responding to an emergency. In some areas, the ED is also notified when an ambulance responds to an emergency.

You should report any problems during your response to the dispatcher. You should also inform the dispatcher when you have arrived at the scene. The arrival report to the dispatcher should include any obvious details that you see during scene size-up. For example, you might say, "Dispatch, BLS Unit Two is on scene at 4 Locust Lane. It is a gray house with street-side parking." This information is particularly useful if additional units are responding to the same scene.

All radio communications during dispatch, as well as during other phases of operations, must be brief and easily understood. Speak in plain English and do not use code words in your transmissions. The use of 10-codes is specifically discouraged because their meanings vary by jurisdiction, which increases the possibility for misunderstanding a transmission. Your tone and pace should be slow, relaxed, and clear. **TABLE 4-7** lists common instances for which EMS clinicians will need to use the radio to communicate with dispatch. Some of these notifications may be done electronically using preprogrammed features on the MDT (eg, to indicate arrival on scene).

TABLE 4-8 lists tips for using the radio. Although these may change slightly from department to department, they provide a good foundation from which to begin.

TABLE 4-7 Typical EMS Communications With Dispatch

Phase of EMS Call	EMS Unit Communication
Initial receipt of call	Acknowledge call. Respond to the call.
En route to call	Request assistance with directions, if needed. Request additional information, if needed. Request additional resources, if needed.
On scene	Report arrival at scene. Check in; often a system will require EMS units to transmit every 10–20 minutes as a safety measure. Request additional resources, if needed.
Beginning of transport	Notify dispatch when transport begins, and state destination hospital and mode of transport (lights and siren or nonemergent).
Arrival at hospital (or point of transfer)	Notify dispatch of arrival at point of transfer.
Return to service	Notify dispatch when the unit is available for another call. (If an ambulance transports to an out-of-district hospital, the crew will also need to tell dispatch when they are back in district.)
Miscellaneous	Some systems require EMS units to notify dispatch any time they are not in station, and their location.

TABLE 4-8 Tips When Using EMS Radio Communications

To speak, press the "talk" button, and wait a moment before speaking.
Hold the microphone 2 to 3 in. (5–8 cm) from your mouth.
Keep the transmission brief.
Use plain language. Avoid the use of codes or agency-specific terms.
When transmitting numbers, such as an address, provide both the number and the individual digits (ie, "Respond to 1381, 1-3-8-1, Main Street").
Remember that the airwaves are public and the use of scanners is popular.
Use the words "affirmative" and "negative" instead of "yes" or "no."
Use EMS frequencies only for EMS communications.
Be aware of background noise when you are transmitting.

Communicating With Medical Direction and Hospitals

The principal reason for radio communication is to facilitate communication between you and medical direction (and the hospital). Medical direction may be located at the receiving hospital, at another facility, or sometimes even in another city or state. You must, however, consult with medical direction to notify the hospital of an incoming patient, request advice or receive orders, or advise the hospital of special situations.

It is important to plan and organize your radio communication before you push the transmit button. Remember, a concise, well-organized report is the best method of accurately and thoroughly describing the patient and medical condition to the clinicians who will be receiving the patient. It also demonstrates your competence and professionalism to all who hear your report. Well-organized radio communications with the hospital will engender confidence in the receiving facility's physicians and nurses, as well as others who are listening. In addition, the patient and family will be comforted by your professionalism and ability to communicate clearly. A well-delivered radio report puts you in control of the information, which is correct procedure.

Hospital notification is the most common type of communication between you and the hospital. The purpose of these calls is to notify the receiving facility of the patient's chief complaint and condition (**FIGURE 4-18**). On the basis of this information, the ED is able to appropriately prepare staff and equipment to receive the patient. This is primarily a one-way form of communication. You are telling the ED what to expect. You are not asking for advice or orders; you are simply notifying them.

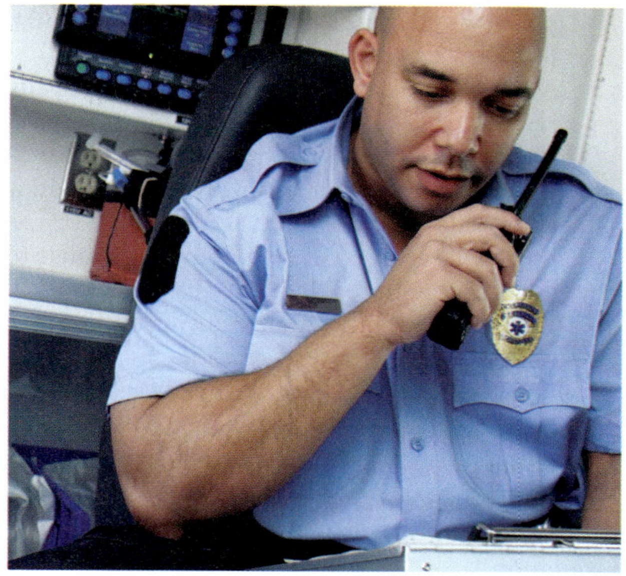

FIGURE 4-18 The patient report should be given in an objective, accurate, and professional manner.

Giving the Patient Report

The patient report should follow a standard format established by your EMS system. The report commonly includes the following 10 elements:

1. Your unit identification and level of services. Example: "Ridgefield Medic 2."
2. Any special "alert" indicated by the patient's status or care. For example, a patient suffering from a severe traumatic injury will be a "trauma alert," or a heart attack may call for a "cardiac alert."
3. The receiving hospital and your estimated time of arrival. Example: "Ridgefield Community Hospital, ETA 10 minutes," or other patient status information according to local protocols.
4. The patient's age and sex. Example: "An 86-year-old female." The patient's name should not be given over the radio because it may be overheard. This would be a violation of the patient's privacy.
5. The patient's chief complaint or your chief concern regarding the patient's problem and its severity. Example: "Patient reports severe pelvic and neck pain."
6. A brief history of the patient's current problem. Example: "Patient fell into bathtub at 0300 this morning and wasn't able to get out." Other important history information that may pertain to the current problem should also be included, such as "The patient has diabetes and takes insulin."
7. A brief report of physical findings. This report should include level of consciousness, the patient's general appearance, pertinent abnormalities noted, and vital signs. Example: "The patient is alert and oriented, has adequate circulation based on examination of mucous membranes inside the inner lower eyelid, and is cold to the touch. We noted crepitus in the

pelvic girdle. Her blood pressure is 112/84, pulse is 72, and respirations 14."

8. A brief summary of the care given and any patient response. Example: "We have applied a cervical collar. She still has pulse, motor, and sensory function distally in all four extremities."
9. A brief description of the patient's response to the treatment provided.
10. Determine whether the receiving facility has any additional questions or orders.

Be sure you report all patient information in an objective, accurate, and professional manner. Remember that people with scanners are listening. You could be successfully sued for slander if you describe a patient in a way that injures the patient's reputation.

Words of Wisdom

Some EMS systems assign roles in their units: a primary person to speak on the radio and a primary person to administer patient care. In these systems, all members of the crew must communicate closely to make this process work. EMTs are involved in every role, but the partial division of responsibilities can be efficient and effective. This approach is most common in systems that use extensive online medical direction.

Calling Medical Direction

You can use the radio in your unit or a portable radio to call medical direction. Increasingly, cellular telephones are used. Regardless of the type of communication, you should use a channel that is relatively free of other radio traffic and interference and one that is recorded. Medical direction communications create medicolegal considerations, requiring that such conversations be recorded. There are several ways to control access on ambulance-to-hospital channels. In some EMS systems, the dispatcher monitors and assigns appropriate, clear medical direction channels. Other EMS systems rely on special communications operations, such as centralized medical emergency dispatch or resource coordination centers, to monitor and allocate the medical direction channels.

Because of the large number of EMS calls to medical direction, your radio report must be concise and well organized and must contain only important information. In addition, because you need specific directions on patient care, the information that you provide to medical direction must be accurate. Remember, the physician on the other end bases the instructions provided on the information you offer.

As discussed earlier, you should use proper medical terminology when giving your report. Never use codes when communicating with medical direction

YOU are the EMT

With an estimated time of arrival at the hospital of 20 minutes, you reassess the patient and note that her condition has remained unchanged.

Recording Time: 16 Minutes	
Level of consciousness	Conscious and alert
Respirations	18 breaths/min; regular and unlabored
Pulse	72 beats/min; strong and regular
Skin	Warm and dry
Blood pressure	120/60 mm Hg
Oxygen saturation (Spo_2)	99% (on room air)

You arrive at the hospital and give your handoff report to the charge nurse. After answering the nurse's questions, you complete your PCR and return to service.

8. What functions does the PCR serve?

Words of Wisdom

Orders that are unclear or seem inappropriate or incorrect should be respectfully questioned. Do not blindly follow an order that does not make sense to you.

unless you are directed by local protocol to do so. Most medical oversight systems handle many EMS agencies and will most likely not know your unit's special codes or signals.

To ensure complete understanding, once you receive an order from medical direction, such as an order for a medication or the denial of a request for a particular treatment, you must repeat the order back, word for word, and then receive confirmation. This helps to eliminate confusion and the possibility of poor patient care. Orders that are unclear or seem inappropriate or incorrect should be questioned. Do not blindly follow an order that does not make sense to you. The physician may have misunderstood or may have missed part of your report. In that case, the physician may not be able to respond appropriately to the patient's needs. The role of medical oversight will be discussed further in Chapter 12, *Principles of Pharmacology and Medication Administration*.

Words of Wisdom

In some EMS systems, the physician medical director delegates some medical oversight functions to specially trained physician assistants or nurse practitioners. Sometimes, the EMT may be speaking to these clinicians when calling to consult about patient care or transport.[30]

Information About Special Situations

Depending on your system's procedures, you may initiate communication with one or more hospitals to advise them of an extraordinary call or situation. For instance, a small rural hospital may be better able to respond to multiple victims of a highway crash if it is notified when the ambulance is first responding. At the other extreme, an entire hospital system must be notified of any disaster, such as a plane or train crash, as early as possible to enable activation of its staff call-in system. These special situations may also include hazardous materials situations, rescues in progress, MCIs, or any other situation that could require special preparation on the part of the hospital. In some areas, mutual aid frequencies may be designated in MCIs so that responding agencies can communicate with one another on a common frequency.

When notifying the hospital of any special situations, keep the following in mind: The earlier the notification, the better. You should ask to speak to the charge nurse or physician in charge, as this person is best able to mobilize the resources necessary to respond. Also, whenever possible, provide an estimate of the number of people who may be transported to the facility. Be sure to identify any conditions the patient or patients may have that require special needs, such as burns or hazardous materials exposure, to assist the hospital in preparation. In many cases, hospital notification is part of a larger disaster or hazardous materials plan. Follow the plan for your system.

Maintenance of Radio Equipment

Similar to all other EMS equipment, radio and cellular communication equipment must be serviced by properly trained and equipped personnel. Remember that they are your lifeline to other public safety agencies (which function to protect you), as well as to medical direction, and it must perform under emergency conditions. Equipment that is operating properly should be serviced at least once per year. Any equipment that is not working properly should be immediately removed from service and sent for repair. Outdated equipment should be removed from service as new equipment becomes available.

When you are beginning your shift, it is typical to check the ambulance to ensure that it is ready to go. You cannot assume that the crew before you left the ambulance well stocked and in operational readiness. Your communication equipment is an important component that needs to be checked to ensure that it is operating correctly and using the correct frequency.

Sometimes, communication equipment will stop working during a run. Your EMS system must have several backup plans and options for this scenario. The goal of a backup plan is to make sure you can maintain contact when the usual procedures do not work. Fortunately, there are quite a few options.

The simplest backup plan relies on written standing orders. **Standing orders** are written documents that have been signed by the EMS system's medical director. These orders outline specific directions, permissions, and sometimes prohibitions regarding patient care. By their very nature, standing orders do not require direct communication with medical direction. When properly followed, standing orders or formal protocols have the same authority and legal status as orders given over the radio. They exist to one extent or another in every EMS system and can be applied to all levels of EMS clinicians. Other backup plans can involve using a cell phone and calling the ED directly. The problem with this approach is that the conversation may not be recorded. Medical direction conversations are often recorded for the purpose of quality improvement.

YOU are the EMT SUMMARY

1. What information should you ask the dispatcher to obtain from the caller?

A "sick person" could be anyone from a patient with the flu to a patient in cardiac arrest. What you do when you arrive at the scene, such as donning appropriate personal protective equipment, may be modified by information from the caller if there is a potential of significant infectious disease. You may also need to delay entry to the scene if there are environmental concerns such as an unusual odor or the possibility of carbon monoxide that would need a fire department dispatch. For all you know, the patient could be experiencing a psychiatric crisis with a potential for violence, in which case law enforcement should be dispatched to secure the scene before your arrival.

After determining the nature of the patient's illness and gathering information that will maximize your own safety, your next priority is to determine if the patient is conscious and breathing adequately or if respirations may be compromised. Try to ascertain the patient's age and sex, if possible. Although you will truly not know what you are dealing with until you arrive at the scene and assess the patient, you should capitalize on the fact that the dispatcher still has the caller on the phone. The more information you obtain prior to arrival at the scene, the better prepared you will be to care for the patient.

2. Why is effective communication between the responding EMS unit and the dispatcher so important?

Effective communication between the dispatcher and the EMS unit is important because accurate, thorough communication results in quicker and more effective care for the patient at the scene. Once you respond to a scene, you will confirm with the dispatcher that you are en route. Should there be any delay in your unit's response, your communication with the dispatcher allows adjustments to the response as needed.

During an emergency call, you will communicate with the dispatcher regarding any problems. Depending on your local protocol, the dispatcher will inform other public agencies that you are responding, and coordinate efforts with them to ensure that needed resources are mobilized.

If the dispatcher remains on the line with the caller, additional information about changes in the patient's condition may be available while you are responding. The dispatcher can also relay any information from other responders that arrive before your unit related to the patient's condition or scene concerns.

3. How can you maximize successful communication with a patient who is hard of hearing?

First, determine the degree of the patient's hearing loss; her hearing aids may allow her to hear normally. Do not assume she is totally deaf. Remember, most patients who are hard of hearing have a normal intelligence level. Provided you successfully communicate with them, they usually understand what is going on around them. In some cases, placing a stethoscope in the patient's ears and talking slowly and precisely into the diaphragm of the stethoscope may amplify the sound enough if a hearing aid is not working or is not available.

Many patients who are hard of hearing can read lips to some extent; therefore, you should position yourself where the patient can see your lips. Even if they do not read lips, they can receive communication clues from your facial expressions or head motions. Never shout in the ear of a patient who is hard of hearing. Listen carefully, ask short questions, and give short answers whenever possible.

If your efforts to verbally communicate with the patient are unsuccessful, write down your questions on paper and ask the patient to write down her response. Print legibly, so your handwriting is not a communication barrier.

YOU are the EMT SUMMARY continued

You can ask a family member or friend at the scene to interpret if this individual knows sign language. Learn some simple phrases in sign language, such as "hurt," "sick," and "help" in case you cannot communicate in any other way.

4. Should your general approach to the assessment process be any different for this patient versus a younger patient? Why or why not?

As a result of the natural process of aging, some older patients may not react to pain the same as younger patients. An older person who has fallen, for example, may not report any pain, despite the presence of an obvious injury.

Assess the patient just as you would a younger patient; however, you may need to allow extra time for her to answer your questions. As with any patient, she should feel confident that everything possible is being done for her. If the patient seems confused or has difficulty communicating, you should not assume that the cause is age-related. A change from the patient's normal status may be due to a medical cause such as a low oxygen or low blood glucose level.

5. What techniques can facilitate the process of interviewing an older patient?

Many of the same techniques used to interview younger patients can be used effectively to interview older patients. When interviewing an older patient, however, patience is even more important. Identify yourself; do not assume that an older person, or any person for that matter, knows who you are. Remain aware of how you present yourself; frustration and impatience can be conveyed through body language.

Look directly at an older patient and speak slowly and distinctly. Do not increase the volume of your voice based on the assumption that the patient is hard of hearing. After asking the patient a question, allow her ample time to answer it and then actively listen to her response. As with any patient, show respect. Refer to her as Mrs. or Ms. unless she asks to be addressed otherwise.

Do not talk about the patient in front of her; doing so gives the impression that she has no choice in her medical care. This may escalate her fear of losing independence.

6. What are the components of a radio report to the hospital?

The purpose of the radio report is to inform the receiving facility that you are transporting to its location and to provide an overview of the patient's condition so it can adequately prepare to receive the patient. Your radio report to the receiving hospital should be concise: brief in length, yet comprehensive in scope. Identify your EMS system and unit number and then advise the nurse or physician that you are prepared to give a radio report with any appropriate alerts. After this person confirms being able to hear you, begin your radio report with the patient's age, sex, chief complaint, or chief concern, and level of consciousness. Next, provide a brief elaboration of the patient's chief complaint (eg, the history of present illness), your assessment findings, pertinent history, initial vital signs, and the most recent set of vital signs. Summarize any treatment that you provided and the patient's response, if any, to your treatment, or any other changes in the patient's condition since you made contact. Finally, give the hospital your estimated time of arrival and transport mode.

7. How does the handoff report differ from the radio report?

Patient care transfer occurs during your handoff report, not your radio report. Once a hospital staff member is ready to take responsibility for the patient, you should provide that person with a formal oral report of the patient's condition.

The following components may be included in your handoff report, depending on the process at the receiving hospital:

- **Situation.** The patient's name and the chief complaint or chief concern
- **Background.** A brief description of the nature of the problem and pertinent history
- **Assessment.** Key assessment findings and any changes in the patient's condition
- **Treatment.** Treatment provided to the patient prior to arrival

8. What functions does the PCR serve?

In addition to your radio and handoff reports, you should complete a formal PCR before you leave the hospital or shortly thereafter depending on your local jurisdictional protocol. There are two types of PCRs: written and electronic. A copy of the report, whether written or transmitted electronically, must be left at the hospital at some point.

The PCR describes the nature of the patient's injuries or illness at the scene, the treatment you provided initially and en route, vital signs, and the patient's condition on arrival at the hospital. The PCR serves the following functions:

1. Transfer of information and continuity of care
2. Compliance and legal documentation

YOU are the EMT SUMMARY continued

3. Administrative information
4. Reimbursement
5. Education
6. Data collection for quality improvement and research

The information in the PCR confirms that you provided proper patient care. In some cases, it also shows that you properly handled unusual or uncommon situations. You should include both objective (what you find) and subjective (what the patient tells you) information in the PCR. A well-written, neat, and concise PCR, including correct spelling and grammar, reflects good patient care. If the report looks sloppy, the care you provided may be assumed to have been the same.

EMS Patient Care Report (PCR)					
Date: 2/16/2025	**Incident No.:** 030109	**Nature of Call:** Sick person		**Location:** 514 E. Bandera St.	
Dispatched: 0610	**En Route:** 0610	**At Scene:** 0616	**Transport:** 0627	**At Hospital:** 0650	**In Service:** 0705

Patient Information	
Age: 83 **Sex:** F **Weight (in kg [lb]):** 50 kg (110 lb)	**Allergies:** None **Medications:** Vitamins **Past Medical History:** None **Chief Complaint:** Light-headedness and nausea

Vital Signs				
Time: 0621	**BP:** 122/62	**Pulse:** 68	**Respirations:** 20	**Spo_2:** 98%
Time: 0627	**BP:** 118/60	**Pulse:** 74	**Respirations:** 20	**Spo_2:** 98%
Time: 0632	**BP:** 120/60	**Pulse:** 72	**Respirations:** 18	**Spo_2:** 99%

EMS Treatment (circle all that apply)				
Oxygen @ ___ L/min via: **NC NRM Bag mask**		**Assisted Ventilation**	**Airway Adjunct**	**CPR**
Defibrillation	**Bleeding Control**	**Bandaging**	**Splinting**	**Other:** Blood glucose assessment, blanket for warmth

Narrative

Dispatched for a "sick person."

Chief complaint: Light-headedness and nausea

History: Only medications are vitamins; no prescribed medications or known drug allergies. The patient reported light-headedness and nausea that had started approximately 1 hour earlier. Patient denied chest pain, shortness of breath, abdominal pain, headache, or significant medical problems.

Assessment: Arrived on scene to find the patient, an 83-year-old woman, sitting on the couch in her living room. She was conscious and alert; her airway was patent and her breathing was adequate. Assessment did not reveal any gross abnormalities. Her blood glucose level was 112 mg/dL. Obtained vital signs.

Treatment (Rx): Prepared patient for transport. Patient was assisted to sit on the ambulance cot for movement to the ambulance. Applied blanket because the patient stated she was cold.

Transport: Began transport and monitored patient's mental status and vital signs en route. Her condition remained unchanged. The patient wears hearing aids in both ears but was easy to communicate with. Arrived at the hospital and transferred patient care without incident. Oral report was given to staff nurse Duckworth. Returned to service at 0705.

End of report

Prep Kit

Ready for Review

- Many verbal and nonverbal factors and strategies are necessary for therapeutic communication.
- Excellent communication skills are crucial in relaying pertinent information to the hospital before arrival.
- Remember that people who are sick or injured may not understand what you are doing or saying. Therefore, your body language and attitude are important in gaining the trust of both the patient and family. You must also take special care of people such as children, older adults, patients who are hard of hearing, patients who are visually impaired, and non–English-speaking patients.
- As an EMT, you must have excellent verbal communication skills. You should be able to interact with the patient and any family members, friends, or bystanders.
- Part of the EMT's role is caring for critically ill and injured patients. Effective and compassionate communication in these situations will help you provide optimal patient care while meeting the emotional needs of your patients and their families.
- You will encounter death and dying in your work as an EMT. Your ability to help others as they grieve can have a lasting effect on their emotional well-being.
- You must aim to complete a patient care report before you leave the hospital. This is a vital part of providing emergency medical care and ensuring the continuity of patient care. This information guarantees the proper transfer of responsibility, complies with the requirements of health departments and law enforcement agencies, and fulfills your agency's administrative needs.
- Radio and telephone communications link you and other members of the EMS, fire, and law enforcement communities. This enables your entire team to work together more effectively.
- Understand and be able to use different forms of communication. Be familiar with two-way radio communications and have a working knowledge of mobile and handheld portable radios. You must know when to use them and what type of information you can transmit.
- Know what your communication system can and cannot handle. You must be able to communicate effectively by sending precise, accurate reports about the scene, the patient's condition, and the treatment that you provide.
- Remember, the lines of communication are not always exclusive; therefore, speak in a professional manner at all times and protect patient privacy.
- Your reporting and record-keeping duties are essential, but they should never come before the care of a patient.

Vital Vocabulary

base station Any radio hardware containing a transmitter and receiver that is located in a fixed place.

cellular telephone A low-power portable radio that communicates through an interconnected series of repeater stations called cells.

channel An assigned frequency or frequencies that are used to carry voice and/or data communications.

chief complaint The reason a patient called for help; also, the patient's response to questions such as "What's wrong?" or "What happened?"

chief concern The condition requiring the most urgent intervention as determined by the clinician's assessment of the patient; it is not always the same as the chief complaint.

closed-ended questions Questions that can be answered in short or single-word responses.

communication The transmission of information to another person—verbally or through body language.

cultural humility The attribute of being curious about others and keeping an open mind when

Prep Kit continued

interacting with people from an unfamiliar culture.

cultural imposition A type of bias in which individuals impose their beliefs, values, and practices on others because they believe their ideals are superior.

dedicated line A special telephone line that is used for specific point-to-point communications; also known as a *hotline*.

documentation The recorded portion of the EMT's patient interaction, either written or electronic. This becomes part of the patient's permanent medical record.

duplex The ability to transmit and receive simultaneously.

emotional intelligence The ability to understand and manage one's own emotions and properly respond to the emotions of others.

ethnocentrism A type of bias in which individuals consider their own cultural values as more important when interacting with people of a different culture.

family-centered care An approach to health care in which patients of all ages and other stakeholders in the patient's well-being, often family members, are treated with respect and inclusion regarding the care of the patient.

Federal Communications Commission (FCC) The federal agency that has jurisdiction over interstate and international telephone and telegraph services and satellite communications, all of which may involve EMS activity.

handoff The transfer of pertinent patient information and the responsibility for the patient's care; often involves the physical movement of the patient and associated equipment; also known as handover.

health information exchange (HIE) A system that allows EMS clinicians to access relevant health data (eg, past medical problems, medications, allergies, end-of-life decisions), avoid unnecessary duplication of effort in data entry, and view patient outcomes related to hospital care.

interoperable communications system A communication system that uses voice-over-Internet protocol (VoIP) technology to allow multiple agencies to communicate and transmit data.

MED channels VHF and UHF channels that the Federal Communications Commission has designated exclusively for EMS use.

mental model A person's perception of "what's going on" in a given situation.

mission-critical communications Any communications where disruption will result in the failure of the mission at hand.

mobile data terminal (MDT) A small computer terminal inside the ambulance that directly receives data from the dispatch center.

multiplex The ability to transmit audio and data signals through the use of more than one communications channel.

noise Anything that dampens or obscures the true meaning of a message.

open-ended questions Questions for which the patient must provide detail to give an answer.

paging The use of a radio signal and a voice or digital message that is transmitted to pagers ("beepers") or desktop monitor radios.

patient care report (PCR) The legal document used to record all patient care activities. This report has direct patient care functions but also administrative and quality control functions. PCRs are also known as *prehospital care reports*.

rapport A trusting relationship that clinicians build with their patients.

repeater A special base station radio that receives messages and signals on one frequency and then automatically retransmits them on a second frequency.

scanner A radio receiver that searches or scans across several frequencies until the message is completed; the process is then repeated.

simplex Single-frequency radio; transmissions can occur in either direction but not simultaneously; when one party transmits, the other can

Prep Kit continued

only receive, and the party that is transmitting is unable to receive.

standing orders Written documents, signed by the EMS system's medical director, that outline specific directions, permissions, and sometimes prohibitions regarding patient care; also called *protocols.*

telemetry A process in which electronic signals are converted into coded, audible signals; these signals can then be transmitted by radio or telephone to a receiver with a decoder at the hospital.

therapeutic communication Verbal and nonverbal communication techniques that encourage patients to express their feelings and to achieve a positive relationship.

trunking Telecommunication systems that allow a computer to maximize use of a group of frequencies.

UHF (ultra-high frequency) Radio frequencies between 300 and 3,000 MHz.

unconscious bias Beliefs that a person holds about others that are not based on fact or objectively analyzed experiences and that the person is not consciously aware of holding.

VHF (very high frequency) Radio frequencies between 30 and 300 MHz; the VHF spectrum is further divided into high and low bands.

References

1. Seat belts. National Highway Traffic Safety Administration website. https://www.nhtsa.gov/vehicle-safety/seat-belts. Accessed November 7, 2024.
2. Davies J. Exploring health literacy: improving patient outcomes and reducing resources. EMS.Aware website. https://www.emsaware.org/articlesforthepublic/exploring-health-literacy-improving-patient-outcomes-amp-reducing-resources. Published January 15, 2024. Accessed November 7, 2024.
3. Dial 211 for essential community services. Federal Communications Commission website. https://www.fcc.gov/sites/default/files/dial_211_for_essential_community_services.pdf. Reviewed April 18, 2024. Accessed November 7, 2024.
4. Khalsa S, Barnes L, Audet R, et al. The impact of cultural humility in prehospital healthcare delivery and education: a position paper from the National Association of EMS Educators (NAEMSE). *Prehosp Emerg Care.* 2020;24(6):839–843.
5. Blewer AL, Starks MA, Malta-Hansen C, et al. Sex differences in receipt of bystander cardiopulmonary resuscitation considering neighborhood racial and ethnic composition. *J Am Heart Assoc.* 2024;13(5):e031113. doi:10.1161/JAHA.123.031113
6. Crowe RP, Kennel J, Fernandez AR, et al. Racial, ethnic, and socioeconomic disparities in out-of-hospital pain management for patients with long bone fractures. *Ann Emerg Med.* 2023;82(5):535–545.
7. Farcas AM, Joiner AP, Rudman JS, et al. Disparities in emergency medical services care delivery in the United States: a scoping review. *Prehosp Emerg Care.* 2023;27(8):1058–1071.
8. Robinson AE, Driver BE, Cole JB, et al. Factors associated with physical restraint in an urban emergency department. *Ann Emerg Med.* 2024;83(2):91–99.
9. Quick safety: de-escalation in health care. The Joint Commission website. https://www.jointcommission.org/resources/news-and-multimedia/newsletters/newsletters/quick-safety/quick-safety-47-deescalation-in-health-care/. Published January 2019. Accessed November 7, 2024.
10. Lamont S, Brunero S. Managing challenging behaviour and workplace violence. In: Roberts L, Hains D, eds. *Mental Health and Mental Illness in Paramedic Practice*. Elsevier; 2020:355–379.
11. Codier E, Codier D. A model for the role of emotional intelligence in patient safety. *Asia-Pacific Oncol Nurs.* 2015;2(2):112–117.
12. Goleman D. (2020). *Emotional Intelligence: Why It Can Matter More than IQ*. Bloomsbury Publishing; 2020.
13. Duckworth R. How to use the FBI's Behavioral Change Stairway Model to influence like a pro. *EMS1.com* website. https://www.ems1.com/ems-training/articles/how-to-use-the-fbis-behavioral-change-stairway-model-to-influence-like-a-pro-c5W8CNGj5tuZZ0Av/. Published May 14, 2018. Accessed November 7, 2024.
14. Johnson Dawkins D, Daum DN. Person-first language in healthcare: the missing link in healthcare simulation training. *Clin Simulat Nurs.* 2022;71:135–140.
15. Respecting patient pronouns and using gender-affirming language in medical care. University of Texas Arlington website. https://academicpartnerships.uta.edu/healthcare-nursing-online-programs/rn-to-bsn/respecting-patient-pronouns-medical-care/. Published July 6, 2022. Accessed November 7, 2024.
16. United Health Foundation. Population—adults ages 65+ in the United States. America's Health Rankings website. https://www.americashealthrankings.org/explore/measures/pct_65plus#. Published 2024. Accessed November 7, 2024.

Prep Kit continued

17. Dudley N, Ackerman A, Brown KM, et al. Patient- and family-centered care of children in the emergency department. *Pediatrics*. 2015;135(1):e255–e272. doi:10.1542/peds.2014-3424
18. O'Malley PJ, Brown K, Krug SE; Committee on Pediatric Emergency Medicine. Patient- and family-centered care of children in the emergency department. *Pediatrics*. 2008;122(2):e511–e521. doi:10.1542/peds.2008-1569
19. Loyacono TR. Family-centered prehospital care. *Emerg Med Serv*. 2001;30(6):64–83.
20. Hobgood C, Mathew D, Woodyard DJ, Shofer FS, Brice JH. Death in the field: teaching paramedics to deliver effective death notifications using the educational intervention "GRIEV_ING". *Prehosp Emerg Care*. 2013;17(4):501–510.
21. Fallat ME, Barbee AP, Forest R, McClure ME, Henry K, Cunningham MR. Perceptions by families of emergency medical service interventions during imminent pediatric out-of-hospital death. *Prehosp Emerg Care*. 2019;23(2):241–248.
22. Centers for Medicare and Medicaid Services. *Provider Compliance Tips for Ambulance Services*. US Department of Health and Human Services website. https://www.hhs.gov/guidance/document/provider-compliance-tips-ambulance-services-1. Issued March 18, 2021. Accessed November 7, 2024.
23. *Emergency Medical Services (EMS) Data Integration to Optimize Patient Care*. The Office of the National Coordinator for Health Information Technology website. https://www.healthit.gov/sites/default/files/emr_safer_knowledge_product_final.pdf. Published January 2017. Accessed November 7, 2024.
24. Health information exchange. California Emergency Services Authority website. https://emsa.ca.gov/hie/. Accessed November 7, 2024.
25. EVENT: An EMS Voluntary Event Notification Tool from EMSForward. Center for Patient Safety website. https://www.emsforward.org/event. Accessed November 7, 2024.
26. Su JS, Quinn E. EMS telemedicine in the prehospital setting. *StatPearls*. National Library of Medicine website. https://www.ncbi.nlm.nih.gov/books/NBK597357/. Updated November 2, 2024. Accessed November 7, 2024.
27. EMS body-worn camera quickstart guide: legal considerations of EMS agencies. Version 1.0. NEMSIS website. https://nemsis.org/wp-content/uploads/2021/06/EMS-Body-worn-Camera-Quickstart-Guide_Legal-Considerations_06.2021.pdf. Accessed November 7, 2024.
28. Emergency medical services (EMS). FirstNet website. https://www.firstnet.com/industry-solutions/ems.html. Accessed November 7, 2024.
29. Emergency communications. Federal Communications Commission website. https://www.fcc.gov/general/emergency-communications. Updated November 30, 2015. Accessed November 7, 2024.
30. Wright D, Baker T, Muthersbaugh H, Platt T, Kerr R, Miller J. Position statement: the role of the EMS physician assistant (PA) and nurse practitioner (NP) in EMS systems. *Prehosp Emerg Care*. Published online November 5, 2021. doi:10.1080/10903127.2021.1977878

Additional Resources

Bonvillain N. *Language, Culture, and Communication: The Meaning of Messages*. Rowman & Littlefield; 2019

Dick T. Ease patient's fear for better care. *JEMS* website. https://www.jems.com/operations/ease-patient-s-fear-better-car/. Published July 31, 2010. Accessed November 7, 2024.

Duckworth R. Five ways to perfect the patient handoff. *EMS World* website. https://www.hmpgloballearningnetwork.com/site/emsworld/214306/ce-article-five-ways-perfect-patient-handoff. Published November, 2016. Accessed November 7, 2024.

Duckworth R. Hard times for soft skills. *Rescue Digest* website. http://www.rescuedigest.com/2015/06/15/hard-times-for-soft-skills/. Published June 15, 2015. Accessed November 7, 2024.

Fitzpatrick D, McKenna M, Duncan EAS, Laird C, Lyon R, Corfield A. Critcomms: a national cross-sectional questionnaire based study to investigate prehospital handover practices between ambulance clinicians and specialist prehospital teams in Scotland. *Scand J Trauma Resusc Emer Med.* 2018;26(1):45.

General Devices. Patient handoffs continue to present challenges and risk to hospitals. General Devices website. https://blog.general-devices.com/patient-handoffs. Published April 16, 2018. Accessed November 7, 2024.

Implicit Association Test (IAT). Harvard University website. https://edib.harvard.edu/implicit-association-test-iat. Accessed December 17, 2024.

James MK, Clarke LA, Simpson RM, et al. Accuracy of pre-hospital trauma notification calls. *Am J Emerg Med*. 2019;37(4):620–626.

The EMS-ED handoff: a critical moment in patient care. NAEMSP National Association of EMS Physicians website. https://naemsp.org/2017-7-27-the-ems-ed-handoff-a-critical-moment-in-patient-care/. Published July 27, 2017. Accessed November 7, 2024.

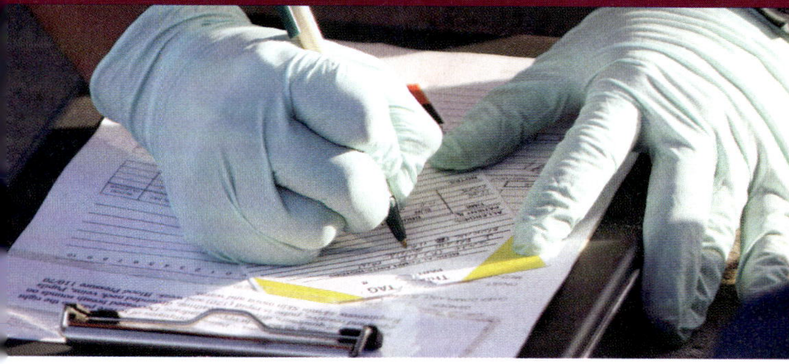

Chapter 5

Medical Terminology

NATIONAL EMS EDUCATION STANDARD COMPETENCIES

Medical Terminology

Uses anatomic and medical terms and abbreviations in written and oral communication with colleagues and other health care professionals.

KNOWLEDGE OBJECTIVES

1. Explain the purpose of medical terminology. (p 148)
2. Identify the four components of a medical term. (p 148)
3. Describe the following directional terms: anterior (ventral), posterior (dorsal), right, left, superior, inferior, proximal, distal, medial, lateral, superficial, and deep. (pp 151–154)
4. Describe the prone, supine, Fowler, and semi-Fowler positions of the body. (pp 154–155)
5. Break down the meaning of a medical term based on the components of the term. (p 155)
6. Identify error-prone medical abbreviations and symbols. (pp 155–157)
7. Interpret selected medical abbreviations and symbols. (pp 157–169)

SKILLS OBJECTIVES

There are no skills objectives for this chapter.

Introduction

As an EMT, it is essential that you have a strong working knowledge of medical terminology. Understanding key terms, abbreviations, and symbols is important for effective communication, data interpretation, and documentation. Understanding how terms are formed and the definitions for the various parts of a medical term will help you determine the meaning of an unknown term by breaking the word apart. Once you understand medical terminology, you will be able to communicate more effectively with other members of the EMS, health care, and public safety systems.

Street Smarts

Although medical terminology is effective and necessary when speaking to members of the health care team, it may confuse patients. Use simple, straightforward language without medical terms when teaching in the community or providing patient care.

Anatomy of a Medical Term

Medical terms are composed of distinct parts that perform specific functions. Changing or deleting any of those parts can significantly change the function (or meaning) of a word. Components of medical terms include the following:

- **Word root**—the foundation of the word
- **Prefix**—a word part that occurs before the word root
- **Suffix**—a word part that occurs after the word root
- **Combining vowel**—a vowel that joins one or more word roots to other components of a term

The meaning of each part and the manner in which the parts come together determine the word's meaning. Changing or deleting any portion of a term can significantly alter its content.

Beyond the discussion that follows, master tables at the end of this chapter list medical terminology, including prefixes, suffixes, word roots, and abbreviations, that you will often use in your work.

Word Roots

The main part or stem of a word is called a word root, sometimes referred to as a root word. A word root conveys the essential meaning of the word and frequently indicates a body part, organ, or organ system. Some word roots constitute a complete term in themselves, and some terms consist of more than one word root. For example, *cardiopulmonary* combines the roots *cardio*, meaning heart, and *pulmon*, meaning lungs, to represent the association of these two body systems. In the case of the term *geriatrics*, the root *geras* is derived from a Greek word meaning old age, and the suffix *iatric* refers to physician or medicine. Geriatrics is the study of older adults.[1]

Prefixes

A prefix is the part of a term that appears at the beginning of a word. It generally describes location, number, amount, color, or intensity. Prefixes are found in general language (eg, *auto*pilot, *sub*marine, *tri*cycle), as well as in medical and scientific terminology. Not all medical terms have prefixes.

A prefix gives the word root a specific meaning. When a medical word contains a prefix, the meaning of the word is altered. For example, *pnea* is the word root for breathing. Adding the prefix *a-* (without), *brady-* (slow), or *tachy-* (rapid) to a word creates three very different terms:

- a/pnea—without breathing
- brady/pnea—slow breathing
- tachy/pnea—rapid breathing

By learning to recognize a few of the more commonly used medical prefixes, you can figure out the meaning of terms that may not be immediately familiar to you.

Suffixes

Suffixes are placed at the end of words and usually indicate a process or procedure, condition, disease, amount, or part of speech. An example of a commonly used suffix is *-itis*, which means inflammation. When this suffix is paired with the word root *arthro-*, meaning joint, the resulting word is *arthritis*, an inflammation of the joints.

Combining Vowels

A combining vowel is the part of a term that connects a word root to a suffix or another word root. In most cases, the combining vowel is an *o*; however, it may also be an *i* or an *e*. A combining vowel is usually used when joining a suffix that begins with a consonant or when joining another word root. For example, take the term *gastroenterology*, the study of diseases of the stomach and small intestines:

- gastr/o + enter/o + logy
- stomach + small intestines + the study of

In this term, *gastr* and *enter* are both word roots, -*logy* is the suffix, and *o* is the combining vowel (used twice). The combining vowel helps ease the pronunciation of the term. Without the vowel, the term would be rather difficult to pronounce: *gastrenterlogy.*

Word Building Rules

When building or taking apart a medical term, it is helpful to understand some basic rules. The following summarizes the rules covered thus far:

1. The prefix, if included in a term, is always at the beginning of the term.
2. The suffix, if included in a term, is always at the end.
3. A combining vowel may be used between word parts to aid in pronunciation.

Plural Endings

To change a term from a singular to plural form, certain rules apply. In some cases, you simply add an *s* to the word (lung becomes lungs). However, for some medical terms, making the plural form is more complicated. You may encounter the following rules when converting terms from singular to plural:

1. Singular words that end in *a* often change to *ae* when plural.
   - Example: vertebra becomes vertebrae.
2. Singular words that end in *is* change to *es* when plural.
   - Example: diagnosis becomes diagnoses.
3. Singular words that end in *ex* or *ix* change to *ices.*
   - Example: apex becomes apices.
4. Singular words that end in *on* or *um* change to *a.*
   - Examples: ganglion becomes ganglia, ovum becomes ova.
5. Singular words that end in *us* change to *i.*
   - Example: bronchus becomes bronchi.

Special Word Parts

As already described, prefixes appear at the beginning of a word, before the word root. Prefixes used to indicate numbers, colors, and directions are described in the following sections. Look at the prefixes, meanings, and examples. Can you think of other terms using the same prefix with another root? Do you see how it changes the meaning?

Numbers

Several prefixes are used to indicate if a term involves a number such as one-half, or one or two or more parts or sides. Common prefixes for numbers are listed in **TABLE 5-1**.

YOU are the EMT

It is almost the end of your shift when you get a call for a routine transfer from the nursing home to the hospital for a 79-year-old patient with constipation and abdominal pain at the request of her gerontologist. The patient has not had any cardiovascular or gastrointestinal symptoms. On your arrival, you are met by a nurse who informs you the patient is new to the geriatric facility and that the most recent vital signs reveal hypotension, tachycardia, and tachypnea.

Your patient's skin is pale, compared to its baseline tone, and wet. When you gently palpate the abdomen, you feel a pulsating mass in the area of the umbilicus. Your partner has placed a nonrebreathing oxygen mask on the patient at 12 L/min and obtained vital signs.

1. What can you determine about the patient's medical history based on the medical terms used in the dispatch information?
2. What do the vital signs the nurse reported suggest about the patient's blood pressure, heart rate, and breathing rate?

Colors

Several word roots are used to describe color. The most common include those listed in **TABLE 5-2**.

Positions and Directions

Prefixes can also be used to describe a position, direction, or location. The most common include those listed in **TABLE 5-3**.

TABLE 5-1 Common Number Prefixes

Prefix	Meaning	Example	Definition of Example
uni-	one	unilateral	one side
dipl-	two; double	diplopia	double vision
null-	none	nullipara	never given birth
primi-	first	primigravida	pregnant for the first time
multi-	many	multiparous	having given birth to more than one offspring
bi-	two	bilateral	pertaining to both sides
tri-	three	trigeminy	irregular heartbeat of two normal beats followed by one premature beat
quad-	four	quadriplegic	paralysis of all four extremities
tetra-	four	tetralogy of Fallot	congenital defect involving four anatomic abnormalities of the heart
deca-	ten	decagram	measurement of 10 grams
semi-	half; partial	semiconscious	partially conscious
hemi-	half; one sided	hemiplegia	paralysis on one side of the body
pan-	all, entire	pandemic	a worldwide epidemic

TABLE 5-2 Word Roots That Describe Color

Root	Meaning	Example	Definition of Example
cyan/o	blue	cyanosis	blue discoloration of the skin or mucous membranes
leuk/o	white	leukocyte	white blood cells that fight infection
erythr/o	red	erythrocyte	red blood cells that contain hemoglobin to carry oxygen
cirrh/o	yellow-orange	cirrhosis	inflammation of the liver causing yellow-orange pigmentation of the skin and/or eyes
melan/o	black	melena	black, tarry stool typically caused by upper gastrointestinal bleeding
poli/o	gray	poliomyelitis	acute viral disease that attacks the motor neurons of the central nervous system (brain and spinal cord)
alb	white	albumin	a protein found in blood plasma or serum (the word root *albumen* is Latin for egg white, a source of this protein, and the suffix *-in* indicates protein)

TABLE 5-3 Prefixes That Describe Position

Prefix	Meaning	Example	Definition of Example
To/From			
ab-	away from	abduction	away from the point of reference
ad-	to, toward	adduction	toward the center
Above/Below/Around			
de-	down, from, away	decontaminate	to remove contaminants from
circum-	around, about	circumferential burn	a burn around an entire area (arm, chest, abdomen, etc)
peri-	around	pericardium	sac around the heart
trans-	across, through, beyond	transplant	tissue moved from one person to another
epi-	above, upon, on	epigastric	above or over the stomach
supra-	above, over	suprasternal notch	top of the sternum
retro-	behind	retroperitoneal	area behind the peritoneum
sub-	under, beneath	subcutaneous	beneath the skin
infra-	below, under	infraclavicular	below the clavicle
para-	near, beside, beyond, apart from	parasternal	beside the sternum
contra-	against, opposite	contraindicated	something that is not indicated
Outside/Inside			
ecto-	out, outside	ectopic pregnancy	pregnancy where the embryo attaches outside of the uterus
endo-	within	endoscopy	procedure used to examine inside the body (with an endoscope)
extra-	outside, in addition	extraneous	outside the organism and not belonging to it
intra-	inside, within	intrauterine	within the uterus
ipsi-	same	ipsilateral	on or affecting the same side

Common Direction, Movement, and Position Terms

Directional Terms

When discussing where an injury is located or how pain radiates in the body, you need to know the correct directional terms (**FIGURE 5-1**). **TABLE 5-4** provides the basic terms used in medicine. Notice how directional terms are paired as opposites.

Right and Left

The terms *right* and *left* refer to the patient's right and left sides, not to your right and left sides.

Superior and Inferior

The **superior** part of the body, or any body part, is the portion nearer to the head from a specific reference point. The part nearer to the feet is the **inferior** portion. These terms are also used to describe the relationship of one structure to another when both

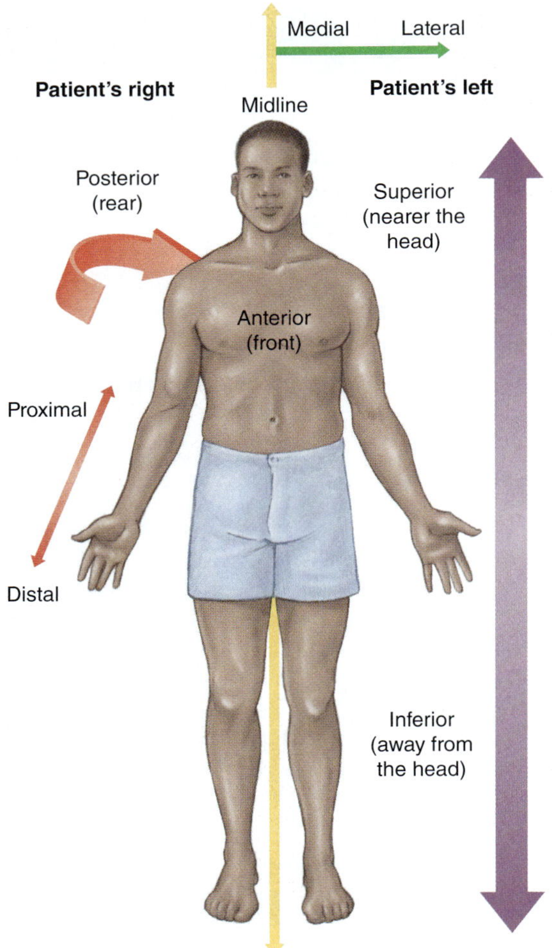

FIGURE 5-1 Directional terms indicate distance and direction from the midline.

TABLE 5-4 Directional Terms

Common Term	Directional Term	Definition
Front	Anterior (ventral)	The front surface of the body
Back	Posterior (dorsal)	The back surface of the body
Right	Right	The patient's right
Left	Left	The patient's left
Top	Superior	Closest to the head
Bottom	Inferior	Closest to the feet
Closest	Proximal	Closest to the point of attachment
Farthest	Distal	Farthest from the point of attachment
Middle	Medial	Closest to the midline
Side	Lateral	Farthest from the midline
In	Deep	Farthest from the surface of the skin
Out	Superficial	Closest to the surface of the skin

structures are part of the trunk or head. For example, the xyphoid is superior to the umbilicus and inferior to the mandible (lower jaw).

Lateral and Medial

Parts of the body that lie farther from the midline are called **lateral** (outer) structures. The parts that lie closer to the midline are called **medial** (inner) structures. For example, the thigh has medial (inner) and lateral (outer) surfaces. In general terms, *lateral* means side. For example, lying on the left side is called left lateral recumbent. Something that occurs on both sides is referred to as *bilateral*. When describing the location of an injury, the terms *medial* and *lateral* help pinpoint an exact location. For example, the patient has a 2-inch (5-cm) laceration on the medial aspect of the thigh (toward the inside).

Proximal and Distal

The terms *proximal* and *distal* are used to describe the relationship of any two structures on an extremity. **Proximal** describes structures that are closer to the trunk. **Distal** describes structures that are farther from the trunk or nearer to the free end of the extremity. For example, the elbow is distal to the shoulder and proximal to the wrist and hand.

Superficial and Deep

Superficial means closer to or on the skin. **Deep** means farther inside the body or tissue and away from the skin. For example, a superficial burn involves only the top layer of skin, similar to a sunburn. An abrasion is a superficial wound, similar to scraping your knee, whereas a deep laceration involves a cut deeper into the tissue such as with a knife.

Ventral and Dorsal

Ventral refers to the belly side of the body, or the anterior surface of the body. **Dorsal** refers to the spinal side of the body, or the posterior surface of the body, including the back of the hand. Dorsal and ventral are used less frequently than the terms **anterior** (the front surface of the body) and **posterior** (the back surface of the body).

> **Street Smarts**
>
> It's easy to recall *dorsal* if you think of a fish's dorsal fin, which is on its back.

Palmar and Plantar

The anterior region of the hand (palm) is referred to as the **palmar** surface. The bottom of the foot (sole) is referred to as the **plantar** surface.

Apex

The **apex** (plural: apices) is the tip of a structure. For example, the apex of the heart is the bottom (inferior portion) of the ventricles in the left side of the chest.

Movement Terms

The following terms relate to movement (**FIGURE 5-2**):

- **Flexion**, in regard to limbs, means decreasing the angle of the joint; in regard to the spine, it means bending the spine forward.
- **Extension**, in regard to limbs, means increasing the angle of the joint; in regard to the spine, it means arching the spine backward.
- **Adduction** is motion toward the midline.
- **Abduction** is motion away from the midline.

> **Words of Wisdom**
>
> Using the correct anatomic terminology in your patient care report improves patient care by making the report more useful to hospital personnel and enhances your professional image as an EMT.

Other Directional Terms

Many structures of the body occur bilaterally. A body part that appears on both sides of the midline is **bilateral**. For example, the eyes, ears, hands, and feet are bilateral structures, meaning there is one on each side of the midline. This is also true for structures inside the body, such as the lungs and kidneys. Something that appears on only one side of the body is said to occur *unilaterally*. For example, unilateral chest expansion means that only one lung is expanding with inhalation (such as with a pneumothorax). Pain that occurs on only one side of the body could be called unilateral pain.

As part of the assessment process, you will palpate the abdomen and report findings. Therefore, it is important that you are able to describe the exact location of areas of the abdomen. The way

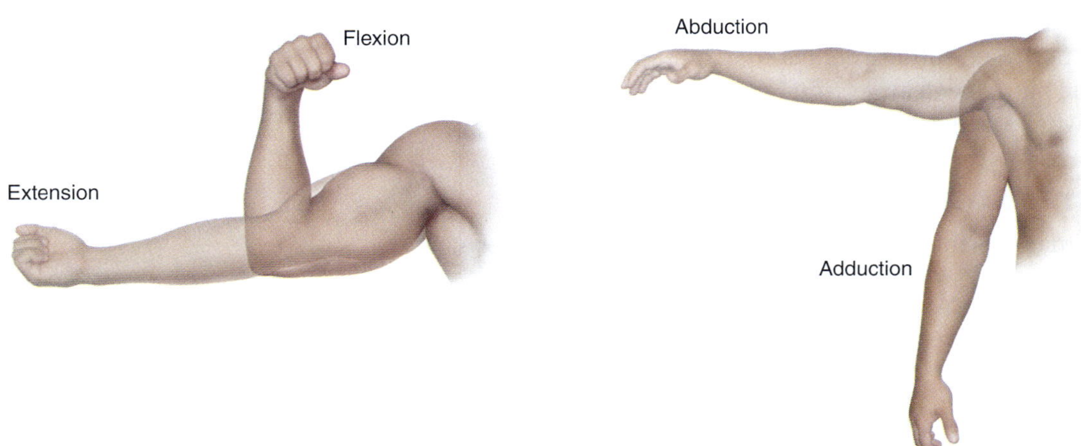

A B

FIGURE 5-2 A. Flexion and extension at the elbow. **B.** Adduction and abduction at the shoulder.

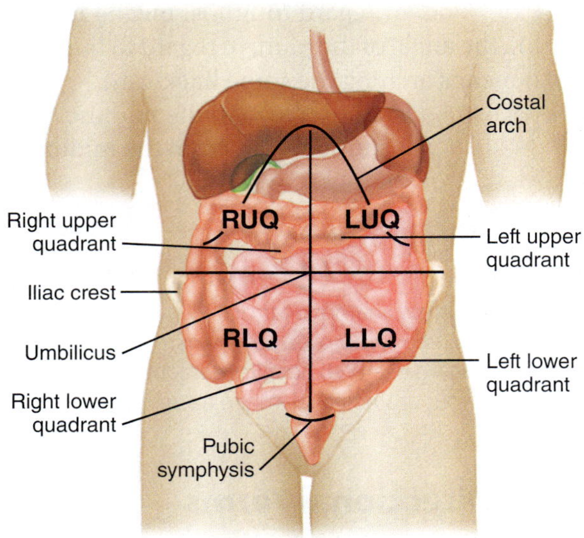

FIGURE 5-3 The abdomen is divided into four quadrants. LLQ, left lower quadrant; LUQ, left upper quadrant; RLQ, right lower quadrant; RUQ, right upper quadrant.

to describe the sections of the abdominal cavity is by **quadrants**. Imagine two lines intersecting at the umbilicus, dividing the abdomen into four equal areas (**FIGURE 5-3**). These are referred to as the right upper quadrant, left upper quadrant, right lower quadrant, and left lower quadrant. Remember that here, too, right and left refer to the patient's right and left, not yours.

It is important to learn all of these terms and concepts so you can describe the location of any injury or assessment findings. When you use these terms properly, any other medical personnel who care for the patient will know immediately where to look and what to expect.

Anatomic Positions

There are many terms used to describe the position of the patient on your arrival or during transport to the emergency department (**FIGURE 5-4**).

Prone and Supine

These terms describe the position of the body. The body is in the **prone** position when lying facedown; the body is in the **supine** position when lying faceup.

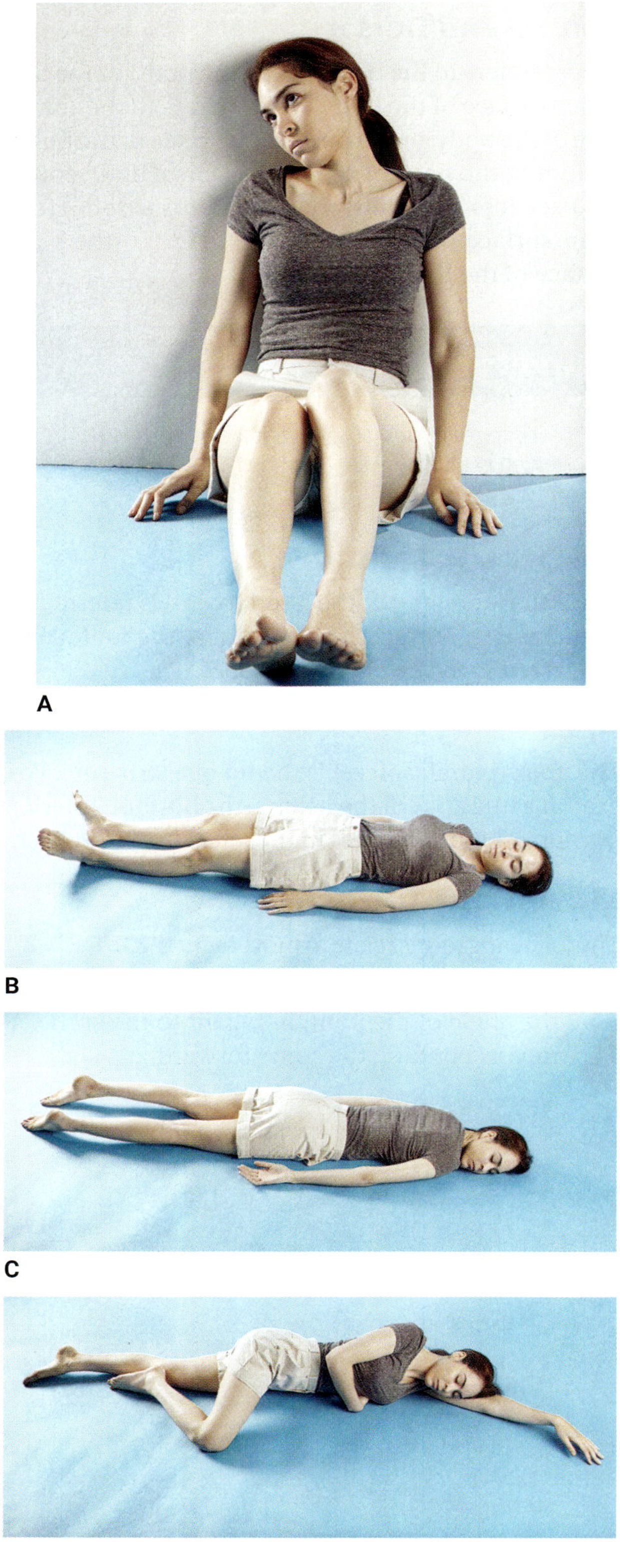

A

B

C

D

FIGURE 5-4 **A.** Fowler position. **B.** Supine. **C.** Prone. **D.** Recovery position.

Fowler Position

The **Fowler position** was named after a US surgeon, George R. Fowler, MD, at the end of the 19th century. Dr. Fowler placed his patients in a semi-reclining position with the head elevated to help them breathe easier and to control the airway. A patient who is sitting upright is therefore said to be in the Fowler position. Some refer to semi-Fowler position as sitting with the back of the stretcher at a 45° angle and high-Fowler position as sitting at a 90° angle.

Breaking Terms Apart

Just as you use parts of terms to build new words, you can use knowledge of the meaning of parts to decipher the meaning of a term. When trying to define a term, begin with the suffix and work backward. If the term also contains a prefix, define the suffix, then the prefix, and then the word root. Here are some examples:

- nephropathy
  - nephr/o/pathy
  - -pathy (suffix meaning disease)
  - o (combining vowel)
  - nephr (word root meaning kidney)
  - nephropathy = disease of the kidney
- dysuria
  - dys/ur/ia
  - -ia (suffix meaning condition of)
  - dys- (prefix meaning difficult, painful, or abnormal)
  - ur (word root meaning urine)
  - dysuria = painful urination (pain when urinating) or difficulty urinating

Words of Wisdom

Accurate spelling is essential in medical terminology. For example, the suffix *-phasia* means speaking, whereas *-phagia* means eating or swallowing. The prefix *dys-* means difficult or painful. Combining these word parts, *dysphasia* means difficulty speaking, while *dysphagia* means difficulty eating or swallowing. Thus, while these terms are spelled and pronounced similarly, they have very different meanings. Likewise, the terms *ilium* and *ileum* are pronounced exactly the same, but refer to different anatomic parts. The ilium is the largest bone of the pelvis, and the ileum is the last part of the small intestine. Knowing anatomy and the context of how these words are used will help you correctly determine (and spell) the term in a given situation.

- hyperemesis
  - hyper/emesis
  - hyper- (prefix meaning excessive)
  - emesis (word root meaning vomiting)
  - hyperemesis = excessive vomiting
- analgesic
  - an/alges/ic
  - -ic (suffix meaning pertaining to)
  - an- (prefix meaning without or absence of)
  - alges (word root meaning pain)
  - analgesic = pertaining to no pain

Abbreviations and Symbols

Medical abbreviations and symbols are a type of shorthand used to communicate in the medical world. They came about for the same reason that people send text messages and tweets using text shorthand: you can communicate faster using this method. Similarly, medical abbreviations and symbols, though somewhat standardized, can have different meanings to different providers in different contexts. Use only commonly understood abbreviations to minimize misinterpretations and errors. The Institute for Safe Medication Practices provides lists of abbreviations that can lead to errors.[2] The Joint Commission's do-not-use list specifies abbreviations that should not be used (**TABLE 5-5**).[3,4]

Abbreviations

Abbreviation is an umbrella term for any word or phrase that has been shortened so that it may be spoken or written more concisely. You will encounter various types of abbreviations in the health care field. The simplest type is the omission of a portion of the word or phrase, such as when someone says "prep" instead of "prepare" or "cath lab" instead of "catheter laboratory." Other common types of abbreviations are initialisms and acronyms. When you shorten a word or phrase using an initialism, you pick representative letters from the full term and pronounce each letter separately. For example, *emergency medical technician* becomes *EMT*, pronounced "E-M-T." When you use an acronym, you are shortening several words, usually using the first letter of each word, to make a shorter term that is pronounced as its own word. For example, the SAMPLE acronym represents several words that are pronounced as a single word, "sample." Other types of abbreviations have unique pronunciations.

TABLE 5-5 The Joint Commission's List of Prohibited Abbreviations[a]

Do Not Use	Potential Problem	Use Instead
U, u (unit)	Mistaken for the number 0 (zero), the number 4 (four), or *cc*	Write *unit*.
IU (International Unit)	Mistaken for IV (intravenous) or the number 10 (ten)	Write *international unit*.
Q.D., QD, q.d., qd (daily) Q.O.D., QOD, q.o.d., qod (every other day)	Mistaken for one another Period after the *Q* mistaken for *I* and the *O* mistaken for *I*	Write *daily*; write *every other day*.
Trailing zero (X.0 mg)[b] Lack of leading zero (.X mg)	Decimal point is missed	Write *X mg*. Write *0.X mg*.
MS	Can mean morphine sulfate or magnesium sulfate	Write *morphine sulfate*.
MSO_4 and $MgSO_4$	Confused for one another	Write *magnesium sulfate*.

[a]Applies to all orders and all medication-related documentation that is handwritten or electronic.

[b]Exception: A "trailing zero" may be used in reporting laboratory results, imaging studies that report size of lesions, or catheter/tube sizes. It should not be used in medication orders, as it may result in a 10-fold dose of a drug.

For example, USAR (which stands for urban search and rescue) is pronounced "U-sar."

When using abbreviations on patient care reports, remember to use only standard, accepted abbreviations to avoid confusion and errors. Misunderstandings will occur if not everyone involved in the emergency care of a patient understands the meaning of abbreviations. The use of some symbols and abbreviations has been associated with medical errors. For this reason, some states or agencies limit the use of abbreviations. To reduce the risk of error related to abbreviations, avoid drug name abbreviations (eg, nitro may be interpreted as nitroglycerin or sodium nitroprusside). In fact, using MS or MSO_4 to abbreviate the drug morphine is prohibited by the Joint Commission because of the high risks associated with it. Using a single letter to indicate a body part (eg, H for hand, L for lung) should also be avoided.[5]

The tables at the end of this chapter include a list of commonly used abbreviations related to medication administration, medicine in general, and EMS/public safety. Electronic patient care reports have reduced the need to use abbreviations. When possible, the EMT should write the word out. This list is intended to help you decipher documents written by other health care professionals. Before using any abbreviations in your own reports, be familiar with accepted use of abbreviations in your local jurisdiction or service area.

YOU are the EMT

Advanced life support (ALS) assistance is 30 minutes away, so after administering oxygen and assessing vital signs, you prepare the patient for transport and glance over the patient's history in the transfer record. It states: Patient Hx: AAA, CHF, AMI in 2015, GERD, and type 1 DM.

3. What additional important information do the abbreviations in the transfer documents reveal?
4. How might that information influence your treatment or transport?

Words of Wisdom

Medical professionals use many medical terms, abbreviations, and symbols. The material in this chapter provides only a small sample. You may find it helpful to invest in a phone app or pocket reference guide to assist you when you encounter unfamiliar terms.

Symbols

Like abbreviations, symbols are sometimes used as a shortcut in communication and documentation. As with abbreviations, it is important to use only the symbols that are widely understood and accepted (**TABLE 5-6**). The number of symbols used in EMS is declining because some are associated with an increased risk of medical errors.

Master Tables

TABLES 5-7 through **5-11** provide a thorough reference list of common word roots, combining forms, prefixes, suffixes, and abbreviations.

Street Smarts

When reading patient transfer records, ask about terms or abbreviations that you do not understand. Do not use abbreviations that you are unfamiliar with in your own documentation or written communications as the risk of miscommunication is high.

TABLE 5-6 Common Symbols

Symbol	Meaning
°	degree
↑	increase(d)[a]
↓	decrease(d)[a]
Ⓡ	right
Ⓛ	left
μ	micro
α	alpha
β	beta
~	approximately
N	normal
×2	times two
/	per
≠	not equal
>	greater than[a]
<	less than[a]
?	questionable, possible
Δ	change
–	negative
♀	female
♂	male

[a]Some sources caution that these symbols may be associated with errors when used in medical communications. It is suggested that words be used instead of these symbols.

YOU are the EMT

En route to the hospital, you call with a report: "EMT 123 to Regional Medical Center. We are en route to your facility with a 79-year-old patient reporting abdominal pain that started 2 hours ago. History of abdominal aortic aneurysm, hypertension, congestive heart failure, acute myocardial infarction in 2015, gastroesophageal reflux disease, and type 1 diabetes. Patient's skin is pale compared with baseline and wet and there is a pulsating mass in the periumbilical area and the pedal pulses are absent on the left. BP is 80/50 mm Hg; pulse is 108 beats/min; respirations are 24 breaths/min. Patient is on NRB mask at 12 L/min. Our ETA is 10 minutes."

5. How could a misunderstanding of the medical terminology or abbreviations affect this patient's care on arrival to the hospital?
6. What do the abbreviations used in the verbal report to the hospital mean?

TABLE 5-7 Common Word Roots and Combining Forms

Root	Meaning	Root	Meaning
abdomin/o	abdomen	bi/o	life
acou/o	hear	bil/i	bile
aden/o	gland	blast/o	germ, bud, developing cell
adip/o	fat	blephar/o	eyelid
alb/o	white	brachi/o	arm
alges/o	pain	bronch/i	airway, bronchus
andr/o	man, male	bucc/o	cheek
angi/o	vessel	burs/o	pouch or sac
angin/o	blood vessel	calc/i	calcium
ankyl/o	fused, stiff	capn/o	carbon dioxide
anter/o	front	carcin/o	cancer
aort/o	aorta	cardi/o	heart
append/o	appendix	carp/o	wrist
arteri/o	artery	cartil/o	cartilage, gristle
arthr/o	joint	caud/o	tail
asthen/o	weak	cec/o	blind intestine, cecum
atel/o	incomplete	cel/o	hernia, protrusion
ather/o	fat	cent/e	to puncture (a body cavity)
atri/o	atrium	cent/i	one-hundredth or 100
audi/o	to hear	cephal/o	head
aur/o	ear	cerebr/o	brain, cerebrum
aut/o	self	cervic/o	neck
bacteri/o	bacteria	chol/e	bile
bi	two	chondr/o	cartilage

YOU are the EMT

Within 30 minutes of arriving at the hospital, your patient undergoes CT scanning that confirms a diagnosis of ruptured abdominal aortic aneurysm (AAA), and the patient undergoes surgery immediately.

Knowing that the abbreviations related to the patient's history pointed to severe cardiovascular disease and a condition that may require urgent surgery helped direct the assessment and subsequent field impression to AAA. This allowed the hospital to be prepared with the right personnel and resources. In your communications, you were careful to avoid excessive or inappropriate use of abbreviations, which could have led to confusion and errors.

Root	Meaning	Root	Meaning
chrom/o	color	emesis	vomit
chron/o	time	emmetr/o	according to measure
cirrh/o	yellow-orange	encephal/o	brain
cleid/o	clavicle	enter/o	small intestine
col/o	colon	episi/o	vulva
colp/o	vagina	erythr/o	red
condyl/o	knuckle of a joint	esthesi	sensation or perception
cor/o	pupil	febr	fever
corne/o	cornea	flex	bend
cost/o	rib	foramen	opening
crani/o	cranium, skull	fract	break
cubitus	elbow	gastr/o	stomach
cutane/o	skin	ger(ont)/o	older adult
cyan/o	blue	gest	carry, produce, congestion
cycl/o	circle or cycle	glyc/o	sugar, sweet
cyst/o	bladder	gno	know
cyt/o	cell	gyn/o	woman, female
derm(at)/o	skin	hem(at)/o	blood
digit	finger or toe	hepat/o	liver
dipl/o	two, double	heter/o	other, different
dips/o	thirst	hom/o	the same
disk/o	flat shape, intervertebral disk	hydr/o	water
dist/o	distant, away	idi/o	person, self
diverticul/o	diverticulum, a small blind pouch	lact/o	milk
dors/o	back	leuk/o	white
duct/o	lead, move	lingu/o	tongue
duoden/o	duodenum	mal/o	abnormal, bad
ech/o	to bounce, sound	medi/o	middle
ede	swelling	melan/o	black, dark
elast/o	change shape	men/o	month, menstruation
electr/o	electricity	mening/o	usually refers to the meninges
embol/o	a plug	myel/o	marrow or spinal cord
embry/o	embryo	my/o	muscle

(*continues*)

TABLE 5-7 Common Word Roots and Combining Forms (*continued*)

Root	Meaning	Root	Meaning
nephr/o	kidney	pyr/o	fire, heat
neur/o	nerve	quadr/o; quar	four
ocul/o	eye	ren/o	kidney
ophthalm/o	eye	rhin/o	nose
oste/o	bone	sangui(n)	blood
ot/o	ear	scler/o	hard
ov/o	egg	sebum	fatty secretion of the sebaceous glands
palpate	to examine by touch	sect/o	cut
path/o	disease	sept/o	wall, divider; also seven
ped/o	child or foot	serum	clear portion of blood
percuss	to examine by tapping sharply	sinus	cavity, channel, or hollow space
phag/o	eat	som(at)	body
pharyng/o	throat	spir/o	coil, to breathe
phot/o	light	stern/o	sternum (breastbone)
phylaxis	protection, immunity	stomat/o	mouth
pleur/o	rib, side	thorac/o	chest
pneum(at)/o	lungs, air	tom/o	cut
pneumo(n)/o	lung	toxic/o	poisonous
pod(i)	foot	trich/o	hair
poli/o	gray	ur/o	urine
pseud/o	false	uter/o	uterus, womb
psych/o	mind	varic/o	dilated vein
pto	fall	vas/o	blood vessel
ptyal/o	saliva	viscer/o	internal organs
pulmon/o	lungs	xen/o	foreign (material)
pur, py	pus	xer/o	dry

TABLE 5-8 Common Prefixes

Prefix	Meaning	Prefix	Meaning
a-	without, lack of	mega-	large
ab-	away from	meta-	after, change
ad-	to, toward	micro-	small
an-	without, lack of	mono-	one, single
ana-	up, back, again	multi-	many
ante-	before, forward	neo-	new
anti-	against, opposed to	noct-	night
auto-	self	nulli-	none
bi-	two	olig(o)-	little, deficient
brady-	slow	ortho-	straight or normal
circum-	around, about	pan-	all, entire
contra-	against, opposite	para-	near, beside, beyond, apart from
de-	down from, away	per-	through
di-	twice, double	peri-	around
dia-	through, completely	poly-	many
dys-	difficult, painful, abnormal	post-	after, behind
ect(o)-	out, outside	pre-	before
end(o)-	within	primi-	first
epi-	upon, over, above	pro-	before, in front of
eu-	easy, good, normal	quadr(i)-	four
ex(o)-	outside, away from	re-	back
extra-	outside, in addition	retro-	backward, behind
hemi-	half	semi-	half, partial
hyper-	over, excessive, high	sub-	under, below
hypo-	under, below normal	super-	above, excessive, or more than normal
in-	in, into, not, without	supra-	above, upper
infra-	below, under	sym-	together, joined
inter-	between	syn-	together, joined
intra-	inside, within	tachy-	rapid, fast
ipsi-	same	tetra-	four
iso-	equal	trans-	across, through, beyond
macro-	large	tri-	three
mal-	bad or abnormal	uni-	one

TABLE 5-9 Common Suffixes

Suffix	Meaning	Suffix	Meaning
-al	pertaining to	-oma	tumor
-algia	pertaining to pain	-osis	pertaining to a disease process (*see also* -sis)
-asthenia	weakness	-ostomy	surgical creation of an opening
-blast	immature cell	-pathy	disease or a system for treating disease
-cele	pertaining to a tumor or swelling	-phagia	pertaining to eating or swallowing
-centesis	pertaining to puncturing an organ or body cavity, often to drain excess fluid or obtain a sample for analysis	-phasia	pertaining to speech
-cyte	cell	-phobia	pertaining to an irrational fear
-ectomy	surgical removal of	-plasty	plastic surgery
-emesis	vomiting	-plegia	paralysis
-emia	pertaining to the presence of a substance in the blood	-pnea	pertaining to breathing
-esthesia	pertaining to sensation or perception	-ptosis	drooping
-genic	causing	-rrhage	abnormal or excessive flow or discharge
-gram	record	-rrhagia	abnormal or excessive flow or discharge
-graph	a record or the instrument used to create the record	-rrhaphy	suture of; repair of
-ia	condition of	-rrhea	flow or discharge
-ic	pertaining to	-scope	instrument for examination
-itis	inflammation	-scopy	examination with an instrument
-lysis	decline, disintegration, or destruction	-sis	a process, action, or condition (*see also* -osis)
-megaly	enlargement of	-stasis	slowing or stopping of the normal flow of a fluid, such as blood
-meter	measuring instrument	-taxis	order, arrangement of
-ology	science or study of	-trophic	pertaining to nutrition

TABLE 5-10 Common EMS and Public Safety Abbreviations[a]

Abbreviation	Meaning	Abbreviation	Meaning
ACLS	advanced cardiac life support	CDC	Centers for Disease Control and Prevention
ADA	Americans With Disabilities Act	CHARTE	Chief complaint, History, Assessment, Treatment (Rx), Transport, Exceptions
AEIOUTIPS	Alcohol; Epilepsy, endocrine, electrolytes; Insulin; Opiates and other drugs; Uremia (kidney failure); Trauma, temperature; Infection; Poisoning, psychogenic causes; Shock, stroke, seizure, syncope, space-occupying lesion, subarachnoid hemorrhage	CHEMTREC	Chemical Transportation Emergency Center
ALS	advanced life support	CHF	congestive heart failure
AED	automated external defibrillator	CISM	critical incident stress management
AEMT	advanced EMT	CO_2	carbon dioxide
AICD	automated implantable cardioverter defibrillator	COASTMAP	Consciousness, Orientation, Activity, Speech, Thought, Memory, Affect, Perception, Cranial nerves, Motor system, Reflexes, Sensory system
ALTE	apparent life-threatening event (preferred term is now BRUE)	COPD	chronic obstructive pulmonary disease
AMA	against medical advice	COVID-19	coronavirus disease 2019
APGAR	appearance, pulse, grimace, activity, respirations	CPAP	continuous positive airway pressure
ATV	automatic transport ventilator	CPR	cardiopulmonary resuscitation
AVPU	Awake and alert, responsive to Verbal stimuli, responsive to Pain, Unresponsive	CQI	continuous quality improvement
BGL	blood glucose level	CRM	crew resource management
BLS	basic life support	CSF	cerebrospinal fluid
BP	blood pressure	DCAP-BTLS	Deformities, Contusions, Abrasions, Punctures/penetrations, Burns, Tenderness, Lacerations, Swelling
BPAP	bilevel positive airway pressure	DNR/DNAR	do not resuscitate/do not attempt resuscitation
BRUE	brief resolved unexplained event	DOA	dead on arrival
BSA	body surface area	EBM	evidence-based medicine
BSI	body substance isolation	ECG	electrocardiogram
BVM	bag-valve mask	EMR	emergency medical responder
C-spine	cervical spine	EMT	emergency medical technician

(*continues*)

TABLE 5-10 Common EMS and Public Safety Abbreviations[a] *(continued)*

Abbreviation	Meaning	Abbreviation	Meaning
EOC	Emergency Operations Center	LVAD	left ventricular assist device
ERG	*Emergency Response Guidebook*	MCI	mass-casualty incident
ESRD	end-stage renal disease	MICU	mobile intensive care unit, medical intensive care unit
ET	endotracheal	MIH/MIHC	mobile integrated health care
ETA	estimated time of arrival	MOI	mechanism of injury
$ETCO_2$	end-tidal carbon dioxide	MVA	motor vehicle accident
ETOH	ethyl alcohol	MVC	motor vehicle crash
ETT	endotracheal tube	NKA	no known allergies
FB	foreign body	NKDA	no known drug allergies
FBAO	foreign body airway obstruction	NPA	nasopharyngeal airway
GCS	Glasgow Coma Scale	OPQRST	Onset, Provocation/palliation, Quality, Region/radiation, Severity, Timing
GSW	gunshot wound	PAPR	powered air-purifying respirator
H&P	history and physical	PCR	patient care report
hazmat	hazardous materials	PMS	pulse, motor function, sensation
HF	heart failure	POLST	physician orders for life-sustaining treatment (or portable medical order)
Hg	mercury	ppm	parts per million
HIE	health information exchange	PTSD	posttraumatic stress disorder
HIPAA	Health Insurance Portability and Accountability Act	QA	quality assurance
HR	heart rate	QI	quality improvement
IC	incident commander	RICES	Rest, Ice, Compression, Elevation, Splinting
ICS	incident command system, intercostal space	SAMPLE	Signs and symptoms, Allergies, Medications, Pertinent past medical history, Last oral intake, Events leading up to the illness or injury
IMS	incident management system	SDS	safety data sheet(s)
ITD	impedance threshold device	SG	supraglottic
J	joule	SGA	supraglottic airway
LDB	load distributing band	SIDS	sudden infant death syndrome
LSV	life support vehicle	SLUDGE	Salivation, Lacrimation, Urination, Defecation, Gastrointestinal upset, Emesis

Abbreviation	Meaning	Abbreviation	Meaning
SMR	spinal motion restriction	Spo_2	Saturated pressure of oxygen as measured by pulse oximeter
SOAP	Subjective, Objective, Assessment, Plan	TCP	transcutaneous pacing
Spco	saturated pressure of carbon monoxide	WMD	weapon of mass destruction
SpMet	saturated pressure of methemoglobin		

[a] Abbreviations are sometimes written with periods (eg, abd., a.c.), and different capitalization might be used that may convey a different meaning. This table does not include all possible meanings. If you are uncertain, always ask the person using the abbreviation.

TABLE 5-11 Common Medical Abbreviations[a]

Abbreviation	Meaning	Abbreviation	Meaning
ā	before	AO × 4, A/O × 4	alert and oriented to person, place, time, and self
AAA	abdominal aortic aneurysm	AP	anteroposterior
abd	abdomen	ARDS	adult respiratory distress syndrome
ABC, ABCs	airway, breathing, circulation	ASA	aspirin
ABG	arterial blood gas	ASD	autism spectrum disorder
AC	acromioclavicular	ASHD	arteriosclerotic or atherosclerotic heart disease
Ac	before meals	ATP	adenosine triphosphate
ACS	acute coronary syndrome	AV	atrioventricular
ADL, ADLs	activity/activities of daily living	bid/b.i.d./BID	twice daily
AF, A-fib	atrial fibrillation	BKA	below-the-knee (transtibial) amputation
AICD	automated implantable cardioverter defibrillator	BM	bowel movement
AIDS	acquired immunodeficiency syndrome	BPM	beats per minute
AGP	aerosol-generating procedure	BRUE	brief resolved unexplained event
AK	above the knee	BS	blood sugar, breath sounds, bowel sounds, bachelor of science (degree)
AKA	above-the-knee (transfemoral) amputation	bx	biopsy
AMI	acute myocardial infarction	c̄	with
ant	anterior	°C	degrees Celsius (centigrade)

(*continues*)

TABLE 5-11 Common Medical Abbreviations[a] (*continued*)

Abbreviation	Meaning	Abbreviation	Meaning
CABG	coronary artery bypass graft	EEG	electroencephalogram
CAD	coronary artery disease	ENT	ears, nose, and throat
CBC	complete blood cell count	EPAP	expiratory positive airway pressure
CC or C/C	chief complaint	ER	emergency room
CCU	coronary care unit	°F	degrees Fahrenheit
C diff	*Clostridioides difficile*	FIO_2	fraction of inspired oxygen
CHF	congestive heart failure	FBS	fasting blood sugar
CKD	chronic kidney disease	Fe	iron
cm[b]	centimeter	FHR	fetal heart rate
CN	cyanide	FHx	family history
CNS	central nervous system	fl., fld	fluid
c/o	complaining of	fx	fracture
CO	cardiac output, carbon monoxide	g	gram
COLD	chronic obstructive lung disease	GB	gallbladder
CA	cancer, cardiac arrest, chronologic age, coronary artery	GERD	gastroesophageal reflux disease
CP	chest pain, chemically pure, cerebral palsy	GI	gastrointestinal
CRT	capillary refill time	GTT	glucose tolerance test
CSF	cerebrospinal fluid	GU	genitourinary
CT	computed tomography	gyn	gynecologic
CVA	cerebrovascular accident (now called stroke)	h	hour
D_5W	5% dextrose in water solution	HA, H/A	headache
DKA	diabetic ketoacidosis	Hb, Hgb	hemoglobin
DM	diabetes mellitus	HBV	hepatitis B virus
DOE	dyspnea on exertion	Hct	hematocrit
DTs	delirium tremens	HCV	hepatitis C virus
DVT	deep vein thrombosis	HIV	human immunodeficiency virus
Dx	diagnosis	H_2O	water
ED	emergency department, erectile dysfunction	HPI	history of present illness
EDC	estimated date of confinement (due date)	HR	heart rate

Abbreviation	Meaning
hr	hour/hours
HTN	hypertension
Hx	history
I&O	intake and output
ICP	intracranial pressure
ICU	intensive care unit
IM	intramuscular
IN[c]	intranasal
IO	intraosseous
IPAP	inspiratory positive airway pressure
IUD	intrauterine device (contraceptive)
IV	intravenous
JVD	jugular venous distention
kg	kilogram
L	liter
LE	lower extremity, lupus erythematosus
LKW	last (time) known well
LLL	left lower lobe of the lung
LLQ	left lower quadrant of the abdomen
L/m, LPM	liters per minute
LMP	last menstrual period
LOC	level of consciousness, loss of consciousness
LR	lactated Ringer solution
LUL	left upper lobe of the lung
LUQ	left upper quadrant of the abdomen
LVO	large vessel occlusion
MAE	moves all extremities
MAEW	moves all extremities well
MAP	mean arterial pressure
MDI	metered-dose inhaler
mg	milligram
MI	myocardial infarction
mL	milliliter
mm	millimeter
mm Hg	millimeters of mercury
MRI	magnetic resonance imaging
MRSA	methicillin-resistant *Staphylococcus aureus*
NA, N/A	not applicable
NAD	no apparent distress, no appreciable disease
NAS	intranasal
NC	nasal cannula
NG	nasogastric
NICU	neonatal intensive care unit
NIPPV (NPPV)	noninvasive positive-pressure ventilation
NIV	noninvasive ventilation
NP	nurse practitioner
npo	nil per os (nothing by mouth)[b]
NRB, NRBM	nonrebreathing mask
NS	normal saline
NSAID	nonsteroidal anti-inflammatory drug
NSR	normal sinus rhythm
N/V	nausea and vomiting
N/V/D	nausea, vomiting, and diarrhea
O_2	oxygen
OB	obstetrics
OBS	organic brain syndrome
OD	overdose, right eye[c]
OG	orogastric
OP	outpatient
OPA	oropharyngeal airway
OR	operating room
OTC	over-the-counter

(*continues*)

TABLE 5-11 Common Medical Abbreviations[a] (*continued*)

Abbreviation	Meaning	Abbreviation	Meaning
oz	ounce	PTT	partial thromboplastin time
p	after	PVC	premature ventricular contraction, polyvinyl chloride
PA	physician assistant; posteroanterior	PVD	peripheral vascular disease
$Paco_2$	partial pressure of carbon dioxide (arterial blood)	q	every[c]
Pao_2	partial pressure of oxygen (arterial blood)	RA	rheumatoid arthritis, right atrium
para	number of births after 20 weeks' gestation	RAD	reactive airway disease
pc	after meals	RBC	red blood cell
PE	pulmonary embolism, physical examination	RLL	right lower lobe of the lung
PEARL or PERL	pupils equal and reactive to light	RLQ	right lower quadrant of the abdomen
PEARRL	pupils equal and round, regular in size, react to light	RN	registered nurse
ped or peds	pediatric	R/O	rule out
PEEP	positive end-expiratory pressure	ROM	range of motion, rupture of membranes
PERRL	pupils equal, round, and reactive to light	RUL	right upper lobe of the lung
PERRLA	pupils equal, round, and reactive to light and accommodation	RUQ	right upper quadrant of the abdomen
PID	pelvic inflammatory disease	Rx	prescription
PMH	past medical history	s̄	without
PND	paroxysmal nocturnal dyspnea	Sao_2	oxygen saturation
PO, po	orally (by mouth)[b]	SG	supraglottic
PPE	personal protective equipment	SICU	surgical intensive care unit
prn	when required (as needed)[b]	SIRS	systemic inflammatory response syndrome
psi	pounds per square inch	SL	sublingual
PSVT	paroxysmal supraventricular tachycardia	SOB	shortness of breath
pt	patient	S/S, S&S	signs and symptoms
PT	physical therapy, prothrombin time	stat	immediately

Abbreviation	Meaning	Abbreviation	Meaning
STEMI	ST-segment elevation myocardial infarction	Tx	treatment
STI	sexually transmitted infection	UA	unstable angina, urinalysis
subcut/SUBQ	subcutaneous	UE	upper extremity
SUD	substance use disorder	URI	upper respiratory infection
SVT	supraventricular tachycardia	US	ultrasonography
Sx	symptoms	UTI	urinary tract infection
T	temperature	VD	venereal disease
tab	tablet	VF/V-fib	ventricular fibrillation
TB	tuberculosis	VRE	vancomycin-resistant *Enterococcus*
TBA	to be admitted, to be announced	VS	vital signs
TBI	traumatic brain injury	VT/V tach	ventricular tachycardia
TBSA	total body surface area	WBC	white blood cell
tech	technician, technologist	WNL	within normal limits
TIA	transient ischemic attack	W/O	without
tid/t.i.d./TID	three times per day	wt	weight
TKO	to keep open	yo; y/o	year old

[a] Abbreviations are sometimes written with periods (eg, abd., a.c.), and different capitalization might be used that may convey a different meaning. This table does not include all possible meanings. If you are uncertain, always ask the person using the abbreviation.

[b] Note that an *s* is not added to abbreviations for units of measure (eg, cm, h, mg) to distinguish plural from singular.

[c] Some sources caution that these abbreviations may be associated with errors when used in medical communications. It is suggested that words be used instead of these abbreviations.

YOU are the EMT SUMMARY

1. What can you determine about the patient's medical history based on the medical terms used in the dispatch information?

This very limited information suggests there are no reported signs of cardiovascular disease such as chest pain and no reported signs or symptoms of gastrointestinal illness such as nausea, vomiting, or diarrhea reported to dispatch. Word roots in this case include *gastro* (stomach) and *entero* (intestine), which are combined with the suffix *itis* (inflammation) in the word *gastroenteritis*. Additionally, *cardio* (heart) and *vas* (blood vessel) are word roots in the word *cardiovascular*. Some of the prefixes used in this case included *hypo* (low) in the word *hypotension* (relating to the blood pressure) and *tachy* (fast) in the words *tachycardia* (relating to the heart rate) and *tachypnea* (relating to the respiratory rate).

2. What do the vital signs the nurse reported suggest about the patient's blood pressure, heart rate, and breathing rate?

The nurse's report suggests that the patient's blood pressure is low and that the heart and breathing rates are fast.

YOU are the EMT SUMMARY continued

3. What additional important information do the abbreviations in the transfer documents reveal?

The record indicates the patient has a history of an abdominal aortic aneurysm, hypertension, congestive heart failure, acute myocardial infarction (heart attack), gastroesophageal reflux disease, and type 1 diabetes.

4. How might that information influence your treatment or transport?

Failure to recognize key information conveyed in abbreviations or medication terminology could result in failure to look for specific signs and symptoms that could influence your patient care, or result in transport to an inappropriate hospital.

5. How could a misunderstanding of the medical terminology or abbreviations affect this patient's care on arrival to the hospital?

In this case, knowing that the patient has abnormal vital signs and a history of AAA will allow the hospital to alert specialized teams to prepare for blood administration and possibly surgery. In addition, passing this history along in the report may allow them time to divert your ambulance to a facility that can more appropriately care for your patient.

6. What do the abbreviations used in the verbal report to the hospital mean?

The abbreviations in the report are EMT, emergency medical technician; BP, blood pressure; NRB, nonrebreathing; L/min, liters per minute (could also use LPM); and, ETA, estimated time of arrival.

Prep Kit

Ready for Review

- Knowledge of medical terminology is essential for health care team members to effectively communicate and document calls.
- Understanding how terms are formed, and the definitions for the various parts of a medical term, will help you determine the meaning of an unknown term.
- Parts that can make up a word include the word root, prefix, suffix, and combining vowels. Not every part is included in every word. Each part can significantly change the meaning of a word.
- The word root is the stem of the word and conveys the core meaning. It frequently indicates a body part. Terms may include more than one word root.
- A prefix and/or suffix can be added to the word root to create a term. Changing the prefix or suffix will change the meaning of the term.
- A prefix is the part of a term that appears at the beginning of a word. It generally describes location and intensity but may also indicate numbers, colors, or direction.
- A suffix is placed at the end of a word to change the original meaning. In medical terminology, a suffix usually indicates a procedure, condition, disease, or part of speech.
- A combining vowel is used in some terms to connect one part of a word to another to make the word easier to pronounce.
- Usually, to make a term plural, an *s* is added at the end. For some terms, a different approach is used to create the plural form.
- Directional terms indicate distance and direction from the midline. These include right, left, superior, inferior, lateral, medial, proximal, distal, superficial, deep, ventral, dorsal, palmar, plantar, and apex.

Prep Kit continued

- Terms related to movement include flexion, extension, adduction, and abduction.
- Anatomic position refers to the position of the body, such as the position the patient is in when you arrive on scene. Anatomic positions include prone, supine, and Fowler.
- Abbreviations and symbols are used as shorthand to communicate and document in a concise manner. To avoid potentially dangerous misinterpretation of your documentation, be sure to use only abbreviations that are commonly understood; avoid using abbreviations that are not recommended.

Vital Vocabulary

abduction Motion of a limb away from the midline.

adduction Motion of a limb toward the midline.

anterior The front surface of the body; the side facing you in the standard anatomic position.

apex The pointed extremity of a conical structure; plural form: *apices*.

bilateral A body part or condition that appears on both sides of the midline.

combining vowel The vowel used to combine two word roots or a word root and suffix.

deep Farther inside the body and away from the skin.

distal Farther from the trunk or nearer to the free end of the extremity.

dorsal The posterior surface of the body, including the back of the hand.

extension The straightening of a joint or backward bending of the spine.

flexion The bending of a joint or forward bending of the spine.

Fowler position An inclined position in which the head of the bed is raised.

inferior Below a body part or nearer to the feet.

lateral Parts of the body that lie farther from the midline; also called outer structures.

medial Parts of the body that lie closer to the midline; also called inner structures.

palmar The anterior region of the hand (palm).

plantar The bottom surface of the foot.

posterior The back surface of the body; the side away from you in the standard anatomic position.

prefix The part of a term that appears before a word root, changing the meaning of the term.

prone Lying facedown.

proximal Closer to the trunk.

quadrants The sections of the abdominal cavity; a descriptive tool in which two imaginary lines intersect at the umbilicus, dividing the abdomen into four equal areas.

suffix The part of a term that comes after the word root, at the end of the term.

superficial Closer to or on the skin.

superior Above a body part or nearer to the head.

supine Lying faceup.

ventral The anterior surface of the body.

word root The main part of a term that contains the primary meaning.

Prep Kit continued

References

1. Forciea MA. Geriatric medicine: history of a young specialty. *AMA Journal of Ethics* website. https://journalofethics.ama-assn.org/article/geriatric-medicine-history-young-specialty/2014-05. Published May 2014. Accessed August 28, 2024.
2. Institute for Safe Medication Practices (ISMP). *ISMP list of error-prone abbreviations, symbols, and dose designations*. ISMP; 2021.
3. Do not use list fact sheet. The Joint Commission website. https://www.jointcommission.org/resources/news-and-multimedia/fact-sheets/facts-about-do-not-use-list/. Accessed August 28, 2024.
4. Managing health information: use of abbreviations, acronyms, symbols and dose designations—understanding the requirements. The Joint Commission website. https://www.jointcommission.org/standards/standard-faqs/ambulatory/information-management-im/000001457/. Updated December 6, 2022. Accessed August 28, 2024.
5. Davis NM. Medical abbreviations with multiple meanings: a prescription for disaster. *Med Writ*. 2020;29(4):16–19.

Additional Resources

Cimino JJ, Clayton PD, Hripcsak G, Johnson SB. Knowledge-based approaches to the maintenance of a large controlled medical terminology. *J Am Med Inform Assoc*. 1994;1(1):35–50.

Hamiel U, Hecht I, Nemet A, et al. Frequency, comprehension and attitudes of physicians towards abbreviations in the medical record. *Postgrad Med J*. 2018;94(1111):254–258.

Medical abbreviations. Taber's Online website. https://www.tabers.com/tabersonline/view/Tabers-Dictionary/767492/all/MedicalAbbreviations. Accessed February 16, 2024.

Thompson CL, Pledger LM. Doctor–patient communication: is patient knowledge of medical terminology improving? *Health Commun*. 1993;5(2):89–97.

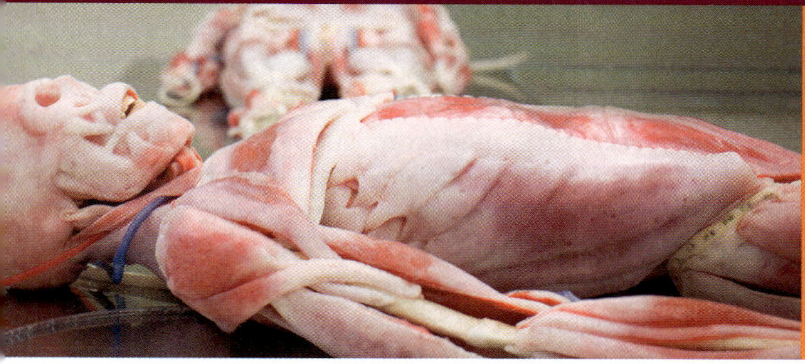

Chapter 6

The Human Body

NATIONAL EMS EDUCATION STANDARD COMPETENCIES

Preparatory

Applies knowledge of the emergency medical services (EMS) system, safety/well-being of the emergency medical technician (EMT), and medical/legal and ethical issues to the provision of emergency care.

Anatomy and Physiology

Applies knowledge of the anatomy and function of all human systems to the practice of EMS.

Pathophysiology

Applies knowledge of the pathophysiology of respiration and perfusion to patient assessment and management.

Special Patient Populations

Applies knowledge of growth, development, and aging and assessment findings to provide basic emergency care and transportation for a patient with special needs.

KNOWLEDGE OBJECTIVES

1. Identify the body's topographic anatomy, including the anatomic position and the planes of the body. (pp 174–175)
2. Identify the anatomy and physiology of the skeletal system. (pp 175–181)
3. Describe the anatomy and physiology of the musculoskeletal system. (pp 181–184)
4. Discuss the anatomy and physiology of the respiratory system. (pp 184–191)
5. Discuss the anatomy and physiology of the circulatory system. (pp 191–201)
6. Discuss the anatomy and physiology of the nervous system. (pp 201–205)
7. Describe the anatomy and the physiology of the integumentary system. (pp 205–206)
8. Explain the anatomy and physiology of the digestive system. (pp 206–211)
9. Describe the anatomy and physiology of the lymphatic system. (p 211)
10. Discuss the anatomy and physiology of the endocrine system. (pp 211–213)
11. Describe the anatomy and physiology of the urinary system. (pp 213–214)
12. Discuss the anatomy and physiology of the genital system. (pp 214–215)
13. Describe the life support chain, aerobic metabolism, and anaerobic metabolism. (pp 215–217)
14. Define pathophysiology. (p 217)

SKILLS OBJECTIVES

There are no skills objectives for this chapter.

Introduction

As an EMT, having a clear understanding of human anatomy, physiology, and pathophysiology is essential. **Anatomy** is a field of study that focuses on the physical *structure* of the body and its systems. **Physiology** goes a step further, examining the normal *functions and activities* of these biologic components. **Pathophysiology** is the study of functional *changes* that accompany a particular disease or syndrome. This chapter provides basic information about the many structures and functions of the body and its parts.

Topographic Anatomy

Many anatomic landmarks on the surface of the body are easy to identify. It is not too difficult to find the **umbilicus** (navel) or the lower tip of the sternum (breastbone). In much the same way that "X marks the spot" on a map where something hidden can be found, these surface structures—the body's **topographic anatomy**—help guide the EMT to the locations of internal features that lie beneath. Understanding these external-to-internal relationships is fundamental to an effective patient assessment.

Directional terminology ensures consistency and clarity of communication between clinicians. Imagine being on scene with a trauma patient and calling the emergency department to report your findings. When the nurse answers the phone, you need to relay the specific location of your patient's injury as clearly and concisely as possible. And the nurse, in turn, must be able to quickly and accurately interpret your description, virtually "seeing" what *you* see. How will you accomplish this task?

Begin by imagining the patient standing in the **anatomic position**, with palms and toes facing toward you. This position is a frame of reference used by all health care clinicians. In addition, directional terms are always presented from the patient's perspective (eg, the *patient's* right leg), as opposed to the EMT's point of view. To illustrate, imagine you are face to face with a patient complaining of pain in his left arm. From your point of view, the affected arm is on the right; but from the patient's point of view, the arm is on the left. Both perspectives are accurate, but when reporting the information to another health care clinician, you would refer to the affected limb as "the *patient's* left arm."

The Planes of the Body

Another approach used when describing a particular location on the patient's body is to divide the body into anatomic planes. These imaginary straight-line divisions begin with three main axes (**FIGURE 6-1**). The **coronal (frontal) plane** runs

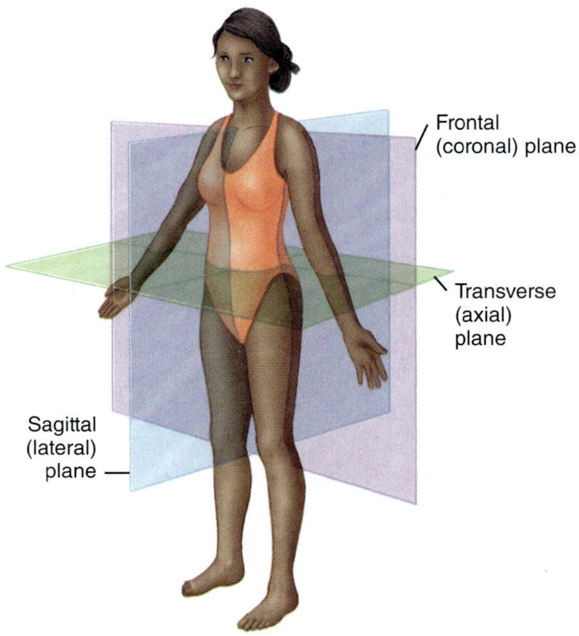

FIGURE 6-1 Anatomic planes of the body.

YOU are the EMT

At 1740 hours, you are dispatched to 4616 84th Street for a 60-year-old man with severe abdominal pain. The weather is overcast, the traffic is heavy, and your response time to the scene is approximately 6 minutes.

1. How will knowledge of anatomy and physiology help you provide appropriate patient care?

TABLE 6-1 Planes of the Body

Plane of the Body	Description
Coronal (frontal)	Front and back
Sagittal (lateral)	Left and right
Midsagittal (midline)	Left and right (equal halves)
Transverse (axial)	Top and bottom

vertically through the body and divides it into front and back sections. The **sagittal (lateral) plane** also runs vertically, but divides the body into left and right sections. It is worth noting that these sections do not necessarily need to be divided equally in each plane; however, a subtype of the sagittal plane, the **midsagittal (midline) plane**, divides the body into equal left and right halves. Your nose and umbilicus are found along this midline. Last, the **transverse (axial) plane** divides the body horizontally into top and bottom sections. These planes help you to identify the location of internal structures and understand the relationships between and among the organs (**TABLE 6-1**).

From Cells to Systems

Cells are the foundation of the human body. Trillions of cells compose the human body.[1] Every organ, every body part, and every structure can be reduced to individual cells. Cells that share a common function grow close to each other, forming tissues. Groups of tissues that perform similar or interrelated jobs form **organs**. Organs with similar functions work together to comprise the different body systems discussed in this chapter.

The Skeletal System: Anatomy

The **skeletal system** serves many functions, but some of the most obvious are to (1) provide structural support to bear the body's weight, (2) establish a framework to attach soft tissues and internal organs, and (3) protect vital organs such as the brain, heart, and lungs. In addition, the red marrow found within the internal cavities of many bones produces red blood cells.

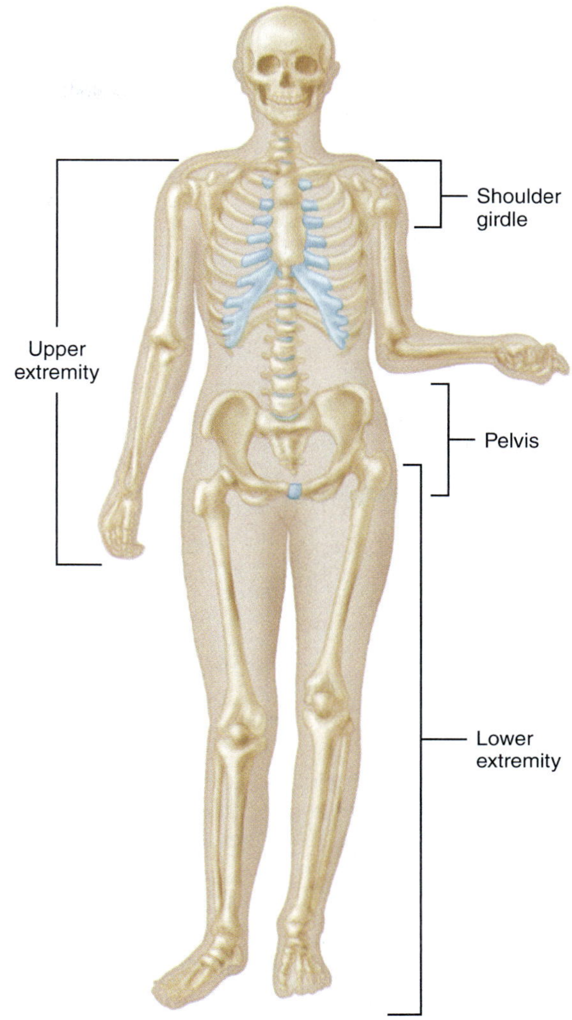

FIGURE 6-2 The 206 bones of the skeleton give the body its form, protect the vital organs, and allow the body to move. The axial skeleton runs in a straight line from the skull to the base of the spine (ie, the coccyx). The appendicular skeleton is made up of the arms and legs and their points of attachment to the axial skeleton (ie, the shoulder and pelvis).

Bones

The 206 bones that compose the skeletal system in most people are divided between the axial and appendicular skeletons (**FIGURE 6-2**).[2] The **axial skeleton** forms the longitudinal axis of the body, from the skull to the tailbone (coccyx). It includes the skull, facial bones, **thoracic cage**, and vertebral column. The **appendicular skeleton** comprises the upper and lower extremities (ie, arms and legs) and

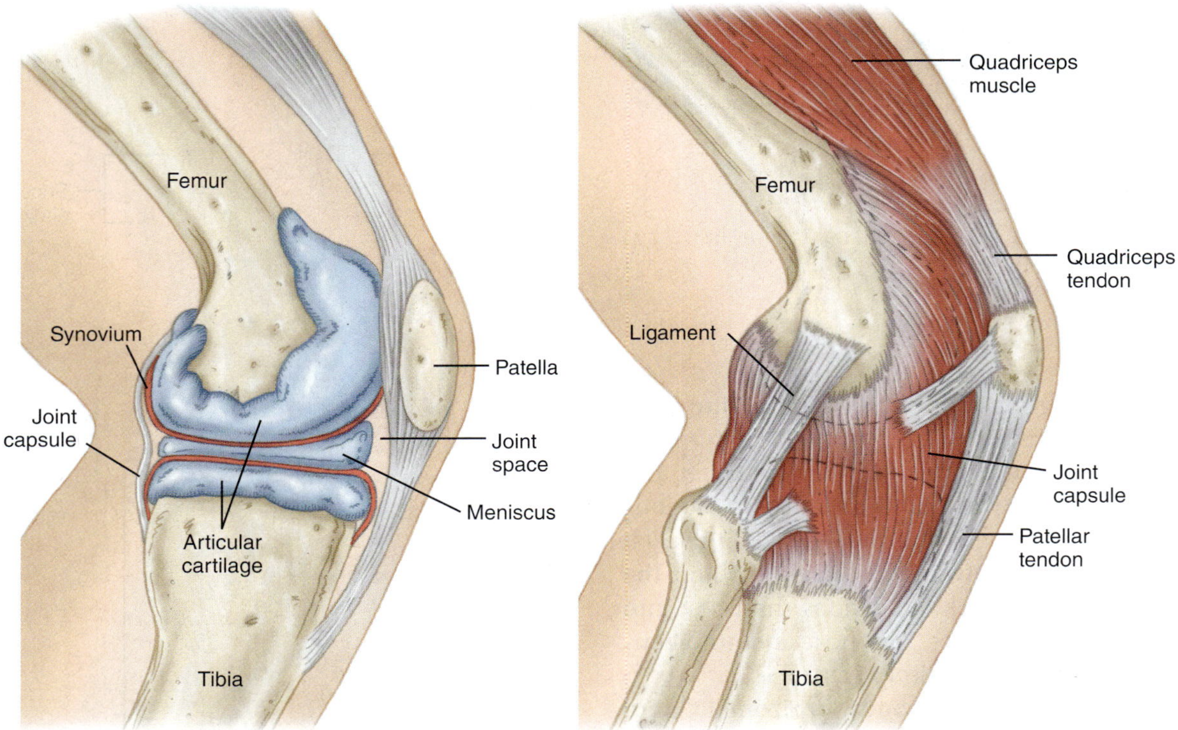

FIGURE 6-3 Most joints consist of bone ends, a fibrous joirt capsule, synovial membranes, and ligaments. The degree to which a joint can move is determined by how the ligaments hold the bone ends and by the configuration of the bones themselves.

the points by which they connect with the axial skeleton (eg, the shoulder). The pelvis includes portions from both the axial and appendicular skeletons.

Joints

A **joint** is where two bones meet (**FIGURE 6-3**). The names of most joints are often formulated by combining the names of these adjoining bones. For example, the sternoclavicular joint is the articulation between the sternum and the clavicle.

The fibrous tissues that connect bone to bone, helping to stabilize these joints, are called **ligaments**. The semirigid yet flexible tissue that covers and cushions the ends of articulating bones is called **cartilage**. Aided by the body's muscles, most joints permit a broad range of motion (eg, bending at the knee). The tissues that attach bone to muscle are called **tendons** (**TABLE 6-2**). In other joints, called **symphyses**, such as joints that connect the pubic bones at the front of the pelvis, only slight motion is possible. Last, some joints are fused to create solid, immobile, bony structures (eg, the fibrous joints between the cranial bones of the adult skull).

TABLE 6-2 Support Structures Within the Skeletal System

Name	Function
Ligament	Connects bone to bone
Tendon	Connects muscle to bone
Cartilage	Provides cushion between bones

The bone ends of most joints are held together by a fibrous sac called the **joint capsule**. This sac is composed of connective tissue (connecting bone to bone). At certain points around the joint, the capsule is lax and thin, permitting movement. In other areas, it is thick and resists stretching and bending. For example, while a joint such as the **sacroiliac joint** is virtually surrounded by tough, thick ligaments and will therefore have little motion, the shoulder, having more elastic ligaments, is free to move in almost any direction (and will, as a result, be more susceptible to dislocation).[3] In moving joints, the ends of the bones are covered with a thin layer of cartilage known as **articular cartilage**. This cartilage is a pearly white substance that allows the ends of the bones to glide easily. On the inner lining of the joint capsule is the **synovial membrane**. This special tissue is responsible for making a thick lubricant called **synovial fluid**. This lubricating substance allows the ends of the bones to glide over each other as opposed to rubbing and grating over each other.

The degree to which a joint can move is determined by the extent to which the ligaments hold the bone ends together and also by the configuration of the bone ends themselves. The shoulder and hip joints are **ball-and-socket joints**, which allow rotation and bending (**FIGURE 6-4**). The finger joints, elbow, and knee are **hinge joints**, with motion restricted to **flexion** (bending) and **extension** (straightening) (**FIGURE 6-5**). Rotation is not possible because of the shape of the joint surfaces and the strong restraining ligaments on both sides of the joint. Although the amount of motion varies from joint to joint, all joints have a definite limit beyond which motion cannot occur. When a joint is forced beyond this limit, damage to some structure must occur. Either the bones that form the joint will break, or the supporting capsule and ligaments will be disrupted.

The Axial Skeleton

The Skull

The skull consists of 28 bones divided into three groups: the cranium and the facial bones (22), and three small bones in each ear. The **cranium** comprises the **frontal bones**, **temporal bones**, **parietal bones**, **occipital bone**, **ethmoid bone**, and **sphenoid bone**. Fused together, these bones encase and protect the brain (**FIGURE 6-6**).

At the base of the cranium, a large opening called the **foramen magnum** (Latin for "great opening") serves as the passageway for the spinal cord to connect with the brain and descend into the spinal, or vertebral, column.

The 14 facial bones include the upper jawbones (**maxillae**), the lower jawbone (**mandible**), and the cheek bones (**zygomas**). The **orbit**, or eye socket, is not a bone itself; it is a cavity formed by the joining of multiple facial bones. The upper third of the nose is made up of the very short *nasal bones* that form the bridge of the nose; the remaining two-thirds consist of flexible cartilage.

The Spinal Column

The **vertebral column** (or spinal column) consists of 33 **vertebrae**. The vertebrae can be divided into five sections, with each vertebra labeled according to its respective section and numbered from the top down (**FIGURE 6-7**).

- **Cervical spine**. The first seven vertebrae (C1 through C7) in the neck form the cervical spine. The skull rests on and attaches to both the first cervical vertebra (the atlas) and the

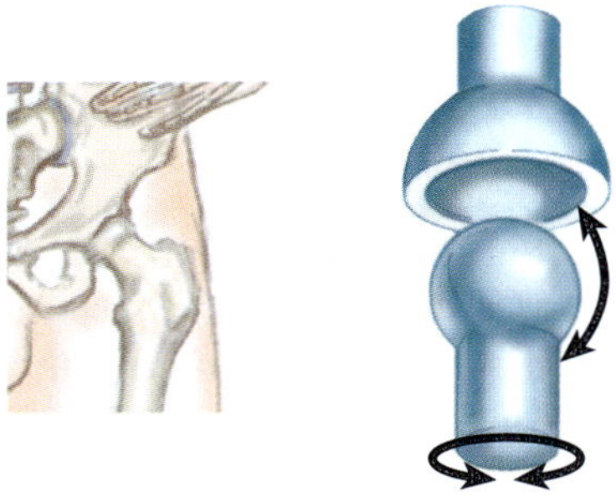

FIGURE 6-4 The hip is an example of a ball-and-socket joint.

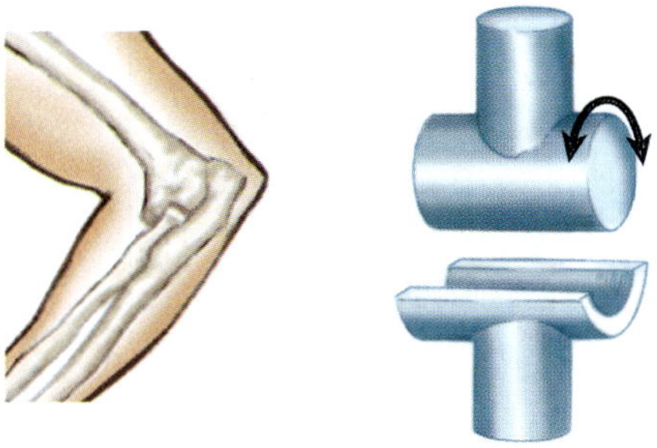

FIGURE 6-5 The elbow joints are hinge joints, which allow motion in only one plane (flexion and extension).

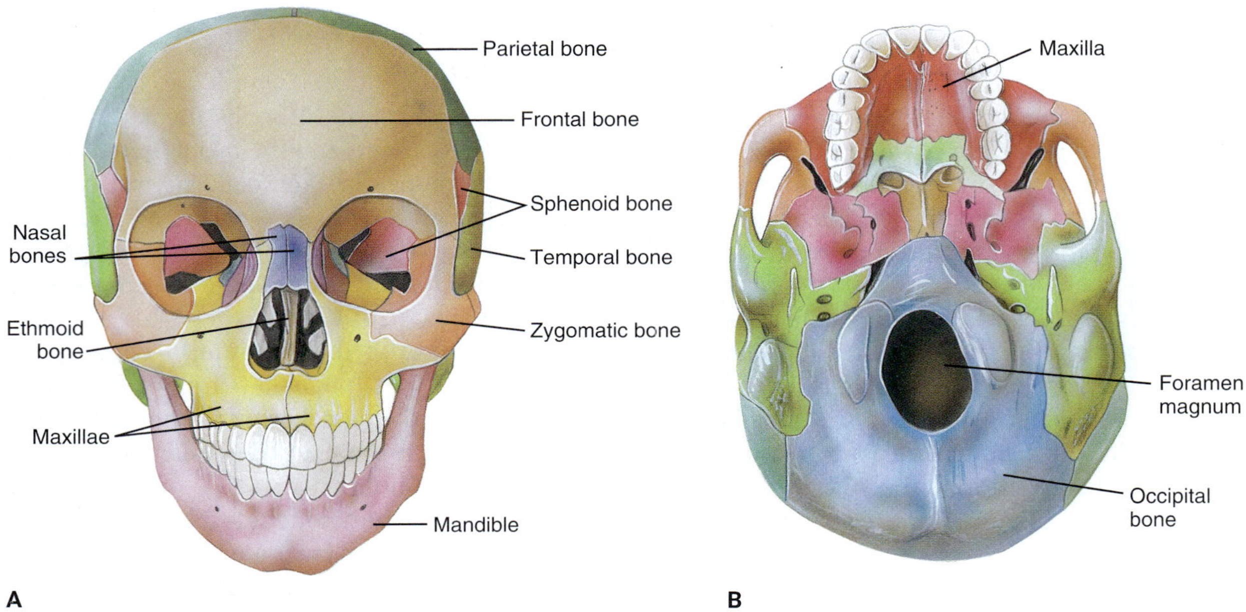

FIGURE 6-6 The skull. **A.** Anterior view. **B.** Inferior view.

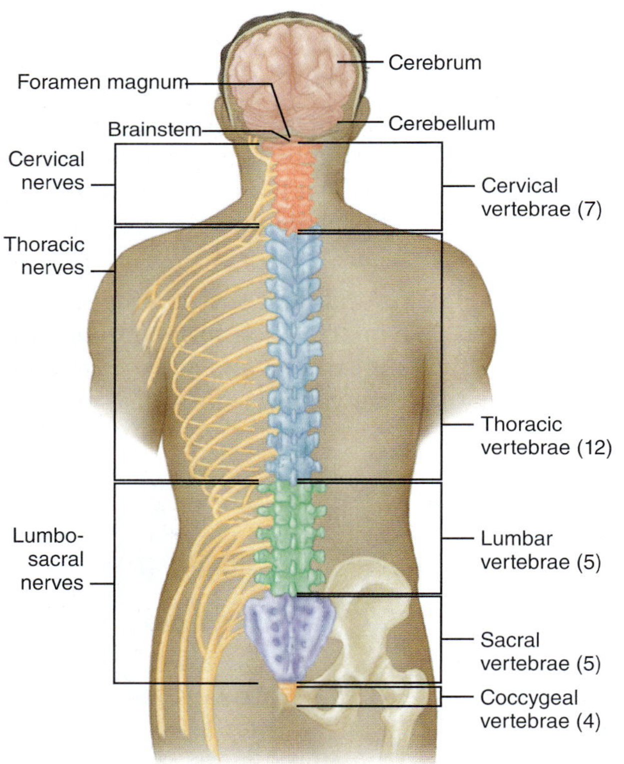

FIGURE 6-7 The vertebral column is composed of 33 bones divided into five sections.

second cervical vertebra (the axis). The vertebrae fit together but move separately, allowing the head to turn in multiple directions.

- **Thoracic spine**. The next 12 vertebrae make up the thoracic spine. One pair of ribs is attached to each of the thoracic vertebrae.
- **Lumbar spine**. The next five vertebrae form the lumbar spine.
- **Sacrum**. The five sacral vertebrae are fused together to form one bone called the sacrum. The sacrum joins the iliac bones of the pelvis via strong ligaments at the sacroiliac joints.
- **Coccyx**. The last four vertebrae, also fused together, form the coccyx, commonly referred to as the tailbone.

The vertebrae are connected by ligaments, and the gaps between the vertebrae are occupied by cushioning, shock-absorbing structures called **intervertebral disks**. These ligaments and disks permit a limited degree of motion, while preventing any extreme movement that might harm the spinal cord. An injury to the vertebrae or the tissues between them has the potential to cause spinal cord damage.

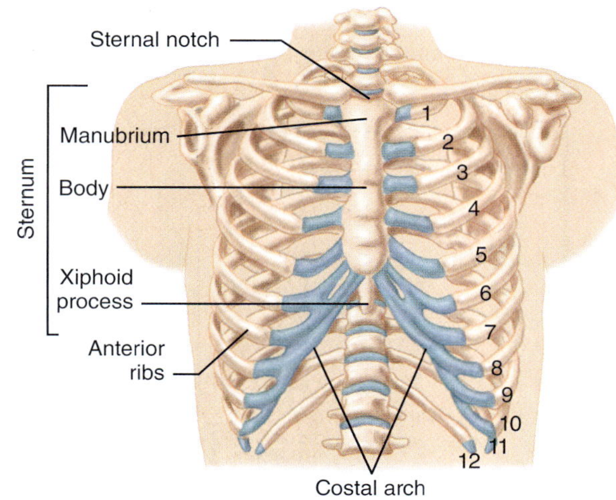

FIGURE 6-8 The thorax.

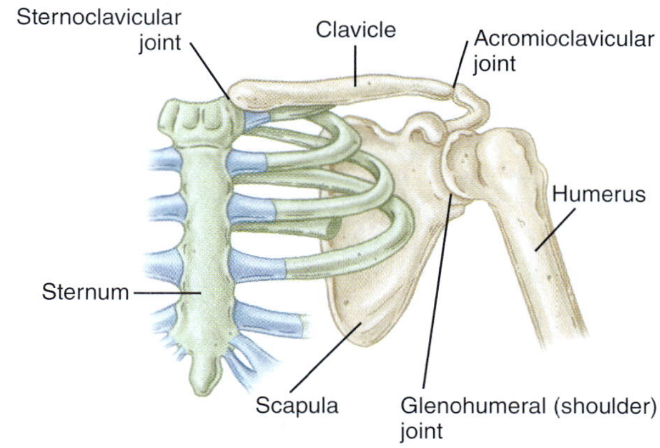

FIGURE 6-9 The bones of the shoulder girdle include the clavicle and scapula.

The Thorax

The **thorax** (chest) contains the heart, lungs, esophagus, and great vessels (the aorta and the superior and inferior venae cavae). It is formed by the 12 thoracic vertebrae (T1 through T12) and their 12 pairs of ribs.

Midline on the anterior surface of the chest is the **sternum** (breastbone). The sternum has three main parts: the manubrium, the body, and the xiphoid process. The **manubrium** is the uppermost section. The superior edge of the manubrium forms a landmark called the *sternal notch.* Immediately inferior to the manubrium is the sternal *body*, the largest bony section of the sternum. Last, the inferior tip of the sternum is formed by a narrow, cartilaginous structure called the **xiphoid process** (**FIGURE 6-8**).

The Appendicular Skeleton

Upper Extremities

The upper extremities (ie, arms) extend distally from the **pectoral girdle** (shoulder), which comprises the **clavicle** (collarbone) and the **scapula** (shoulder blade) (**FIGURE 6-9**). The medial end of the clavicle articulates with the manubrium of the sternum; this is the only joint that directly connects the shoulder girdle and the axial skeleton. The clavicle's lateral end articulates with the scapula. The scapula is supported and positioned by skeletal muscles and has no bony or ligamentous connections to the thoracic cage.

The scapula articulates with the proximal head of the **humerus**, the single bone of the upper arm. Distally, the humerus articulates with the two bones that make up the forearm: the **radius** on the lateral, or thumb, side and the **ulna** on the medial, or little finger, side.

At their distal ends, the radius and ulna articulate with the proximal row of wrist bones, via a modified ball-and-socket joint (**FIGURE 6-10**). The eight bones that form the wrist are called **carpals**. Extending from the carpals are five **metacarpals**, which form the palm of the hand. The metacarpals in turn articulate with the bones of the fingers, or **phalanges**. The thumb is composed of two phalanges (proximal and distal); the remaining four digits each contain three phalanges (proximal, middle, and distal).

The Pelvis

The **pelvic girdle** consists of two large hip bones called the **coxae**, the sacrum, and the coccyx (**FIGURE 6-11**). Each coxa is formed by the fusion of three bones: the **ilium**, the **ischium**, and the **pubis**. Joining the left and right pubic bones is a cartilaginous articulation that limits movement between these two bones; this structure is called the **pubic symphysis**. The pelvis articulates with the femur bone of the leg at the hip joint, or **acetabulum**. The female pelvis is wider than the male pelvis and has other structural differences to permit childbirth.

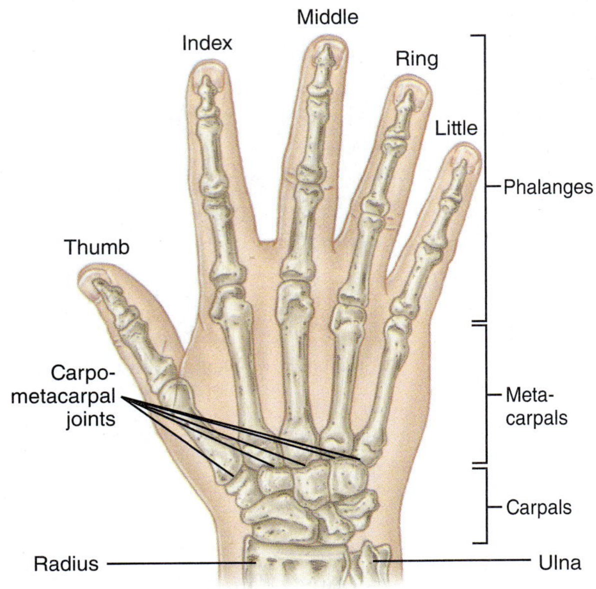

FIGURE 6-10 The major bones in the wrist and hand include the carpals, the metacarpals, and the phalanges.

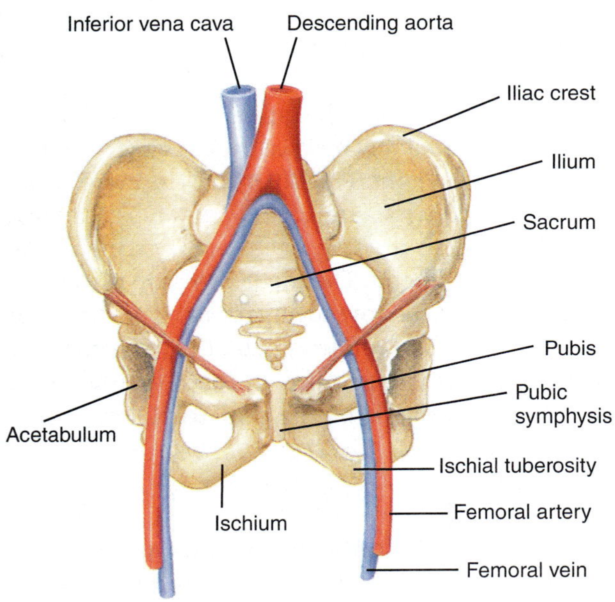

FIGURE 6-11 The pelvis is a closed, bony ring that consists of the sacrum, ilium, ischium, pubis, acetabulum, and pubic symphysis.

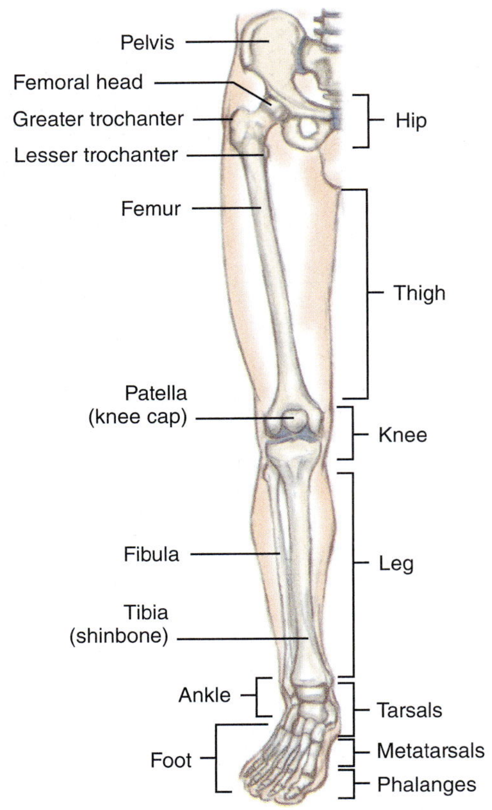

FIGURE 6-12 The major parts of the lower extremities include the femur, femoral head, greater and lesser trochanters, patella, tibia, and fibula.

The Lower Extremities

The **femur** (thighbone) is the longest and one of the strongest bones in the body. The femur's rounded superior end is referred to as the **femoral head**. The femoral head articulates with the acetabulum of the pelvic girdle by a ball-and-socket joint. Immediately inferior and lateral to the head is the narrowed femoral neck. A projection called the **greater trochanter** is located proximal to the femoral head and neck on the lateral side of the femur. A second projection, called the **lesser trochanter**, is found on the medial side of the femur, just inferior to the femoral neck (**FIGURE 6-12**). Both trochanters serve as anchor points for the major muscles of the thigh.

At the inferior end of the femur, a hinge joint commonly referred to as the knee connects the femur to the bones of the lower leg. The anterior side of the knee is covered by a specialized bone called the **patella** (kneecap). The lower leg comprises two bones: the tibia and the fibula. The larger of the two, the **tibia** (shinbone), articulates with the inferior end of the femur at the knee joint. It is positioned on the medial side of the lower leg and can be palpated along its entire length on the anterior surface of the leg, just beneath the skin. The smaller **fibula** lies on the lateral side of the lower leg. The ankle joint includes protrusions from the broadened distal ends of the tibia and fibula. On the lateral side, the fibula's lateral **malleolus** can be palpated. On the medial side, the prominence from the distal tibia is called the medial malleolus.

Ankle and Foot

The foot comprises the **tarsals**, **metatarsals**, and phalanges. The seven tarsals include the large **calcaneus**, or heel bone, and the **talus** (**FIGURE 6-13**). The distal ends of the tibia and fibula articulate with the talus to form the ankle. The hinge joint of the ankle allows flexion and extension of the foot.

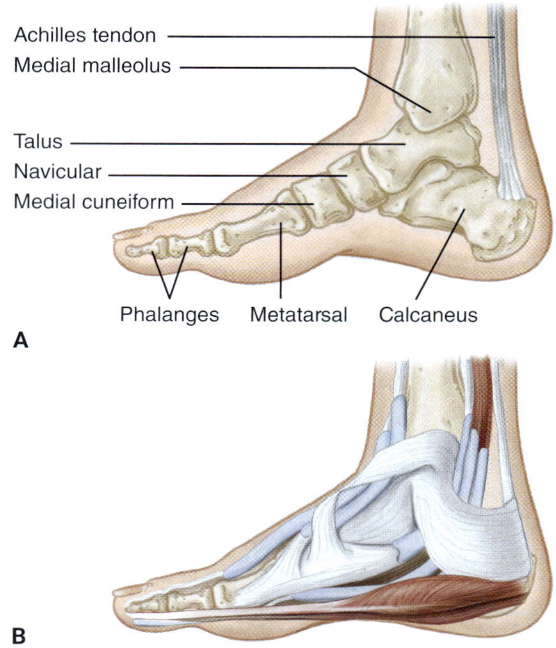

FIGURE 6-13 A. The surface landmarks of the foot, including the talus, the calcaneus, and the phalanges. **B.** Soft tissue of the ankle.

> **Words of Wisdom**
>
> As you gain a better understanding of the anatomy and physiology of the body, remember that these systems work together, not in isolation. A person who falls and breaks a leg may appear to have an isolated bone injury. But is there bleeding inside the leg? Is there damage to the nerves, tendons, or ligaments? Has the injury disrupted the skin, creating a risk for infection? A seemingly simple illness or injury can involve several body systems, not all of which are obvious at first glance. Always perform a thorough patient assessment.

The five metatarsal bones form the middle of the foot. The bottom surface of the foot is referred to as the plantar surface, while the top of the foot is described as the dorsum or dorsal surface. The five toes of each foot are formed by 14 phalanges, with 2 in the great toe and 3 in each of the remaining toes.

The Skeletal System: Physiology

The skeletal system is responsible for several functions: It gives the body shape, provides protection of fragile organs, and allows for movement. Another function of the skeletal system is the storage of calcium. Associated with and in reaction to the normal stress from daily activity, the bones are continually rebuilding and growing. Calcium is essential to the formation of hard, resilient bones. It is also vital to the function and well-being of other body systems. The heart, muscles, and nervous system are a few examples.

The skeletal system also plays a crucial role in the creation of various types of blood cells and components. Specialized cells present in the bone marrow are transformed into red blood cells, white blood cells, and platelets. This transformation occurs continuously to replace existing blood cells that die normally; however, the speed of production increases when the need arises. For example, hypoxia increases the rate of red blood cell production; infection or tissue damage increases white blood cell formation; and bleeding speeds up platelet creation.

The Musculoskeletal System: Anatomy

Muscle is a form of tissue that facilitates movement. The human body contains three types of muscle: skeletal, smooth, and cardiac (**FIGURE 6-14**).

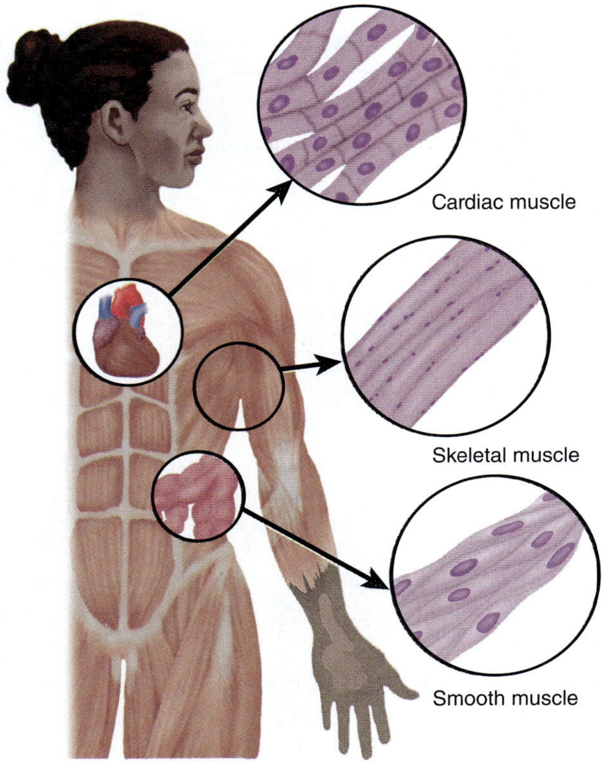

FIGURE 6-14 The three types of muscle are skeletal, smooth, and cardiac.

Skeletal muscle, so named because it attaches to the bones of the skeleton, accounts for the bulk of human muscle mass. Because of its characteristic striped appearance, skeletal muscle is often referred to as *striated* muscle. It is also known as **voluntary muscle** because its movements are under our conscious control. For example, highlighting a sentence in your textbook requires you to consciously control the voluntary muscles involved in this action.

By contrast, the activities of smooth muscle and cardiac muscle do not require conscious thought. For example, you do not need to consciously control the muscles involved in making your heart beat. For this reason, smooth and cardiac muscle are recognized as **involuntary muscle**.

Smooth muscle is found within blood vessels and the intestines. When you hear your stomach growling, you are in fact hearing the rhythmic smooth muscle contractions of the intestines. **Cardiac muscle** is unique from other muscle types in that it can generate its own electrical impulses.

Skeletal Muscle

As the name implies, *musculoskeletal* is a term that refers to a partnership between bone and muscle. Thus, whenever we discuss the **musculoskeletal system**, we acknowledge this relationship. Voluntary movements, such as walking, raising your hand, and nodding your head, would not be possible otherwise.

In most instances, a given motion, no matter how small, requires the simultaneous participation of multiple muscles. Skeletal muscles often function in *antagonistic pairs*. The muscles of the upper arm include the **biceps** muscle, which is located on the anterior aspect of the humerus. This muscle bends the elbow by moving the lower part of the arm toward the head. If the muscle were working alone, you would have little control over the speed of that movement. The way the body achieves control and fine movement is to have the biceps compete against another muscle group. The biceps competes with the **triceps** muscle, which is the three-headed muscle of the back of the arm that functions to straighten the elbow. Without the triceps, you would slap yourself in the face every time you bend your arm. Conversely, the biceps works to slow the movement of the triceps as the arm is extended.

There are more than 600 muscles in the musculoskeletal system. **FIGURE 6-15** and **TABLE 6-3** show the major muscles, their locations, and their functions.

The Musculoskeletal System: Physiology

Although the primary functions of the musculoskeletal system are movement and postural maintenance, this system has several other functions. One of these is the production of heat. When a person is cold, shivering begins. This involuntary shaking of the muscles generates heat, thereby maintaining *homeostasis* (the body's self-regulating process for preserving internal balance, or equilibrium, in order to survive). Muscles also protect underlying structures, such as the internal organs. For example, the intestines are protected by the rectus abdominus muscles.

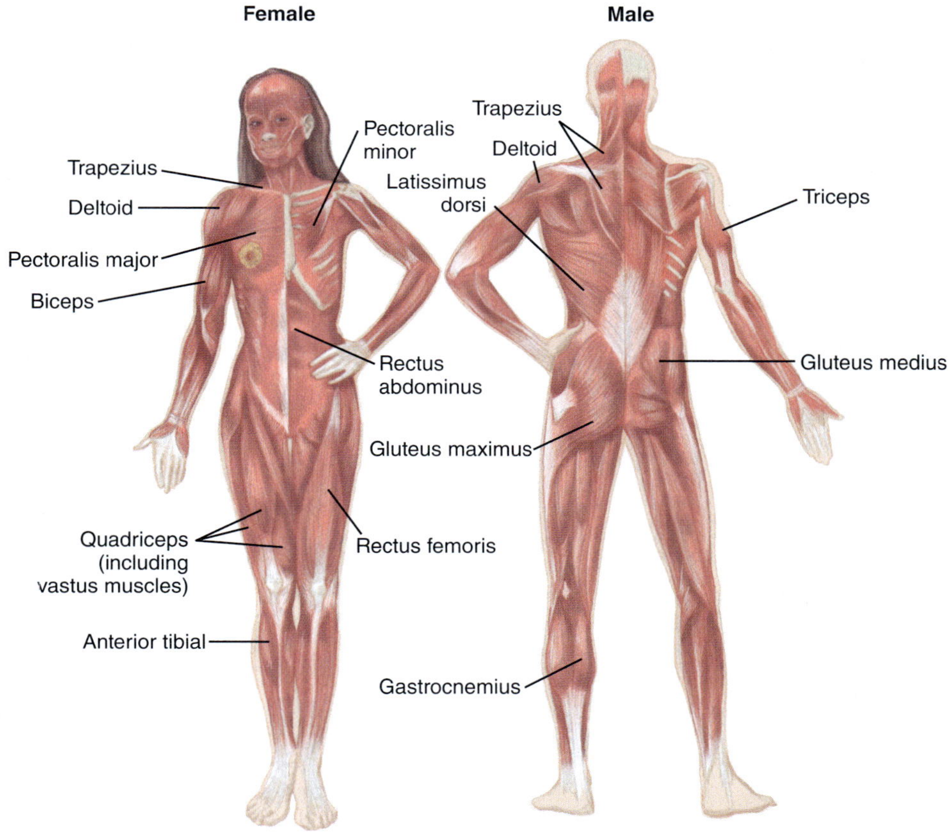

FIGURE 6-15 The major muscle groups.

TABLE 6-3 Muscles: Locations and Functions

Muscle Name	Location	Function
Biceps	Anterior, humerus	Flexes lower arm
Deltoid	Shoulder joint	Flexes and extends to allow arm to move to the front and back; abducts to raise arm away from body
Triceps	Posterior, humerus	Extends lower arm
Pectoralis	Anterior, thorax	Flexes and rotates arm
Latissimus dorsi	Posterior, thorax	Extends and rotates arm
Rectus abdominis	Anterior, abdomen	Flexes and rotates spine
Tibialis anterior	Anterior, tibia	Points foot toward head
Gastrocnemius	Posterior, tibia	Points foot away from head
Quadriceps (four separate muscles)	Anterior, femur	Extends knee and flexes hip
Biceps femoris	Posterior, femur	Bends knee and extends hip
Gluteus (three separate muscles)	Posterior, pelvis/buttocks	Extends and rotates thigh

Special Populations

THE MUSCULOSKELETAL SYSTEM IN CHILDREN

A child's bones are softer than those of an adult. The skeletal system contains open growth plates at the ends of long bones, which enable these bones to grow during childhood. As a result of the active growth plates, children's bones are weaker and more flexible, making them susceptible to fracture with stress. Untreated injuries involving the growth plate can lead to a risk of length discrepancies. Be especially careful to stabilize extremities with suspected sprains or strains because they may be fractures through growth plates.

The bones of the infant's head are flexible and soft. The joints between each cranial bone are called **sutures** and are not fused together before birth. This allows more flexibility for the bones of the skull to move slightly to permit the head to be delivered through the narrow birth canal and allows the growth of the brain during fetal and early infant development. Located on the front (anterior) and back (posterior) portions of the head are soft spots known as **fontanelles**. Each closes as the sutures fuse the bones of the cranium together at specific stages of development: 18 months for the anterior fontanelle and 6 months for the posterior fontanelle (**FIGURE 6-16**). It is important to note that when the anterior fontanelle is still open it may curve out or bulge at times. Some bulging is a normal assessment finding when the infant is either crying, coughing, or lying on the back or stomach. However, the fontanelles of an infant can be a useful assessment tool for such issues as increased intracranial pressure (bulging with a noncrying infant) or dehydration (a sunken appearance).

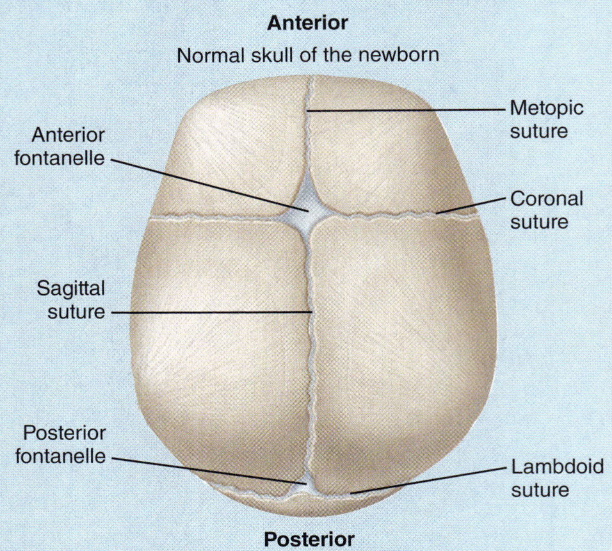

FIGURE 6-16 The sutures of the skull of a newborn.

The thoracic cage in young children is highly elastic and flexible because it is primarily composed of cartilaginous connective tissue. The ribs and vital organs are less protected by muscle and fat. The ribs do not extend as far down on infants and young children, making the liver and spleen more susceptible to injury. The highly flexible ribs mean that fractures in pediatric patients are rare, unless a high-energy impact to the chest wall is encountered, such as during a motor vehicle crash. However, underlying damage, especially to the lungs, may still exist within the thoracic cavity without any exterior markings.

The Respiratory System: Anatomy

The **respiratory system** is the set of organs responsible for breathing, or respiration, and the exchange of oxygen and carbon dioxide that occurs within the lungs (**FIGURE 6-17**). It includes the nose, mouth, pharynx, larynx, trachea, bronchi, and bronchioles, which are all air passages or airways. The system also includes the lungs, where oxygen is passed into the blood and carbon dioxide removed. Finally, the respiratory system includes the diaphragm, the muscles of the chest wall, and accessory muscles of breathing, which permit normal respiratory movement. In this text, "airway" usually refers to the upper airway or the respiratory passage above the larynx (voice box). These structures are divided between the upper airway and lower airway.

The Upper Airway

The structures of the upper airway are located anteriorly at the midline. In descending order, they include the following:

- **Nasopharynx**. Upper section of the pharynx that connects with the nasal cavity above the soft palate
- Oropharynx. Section of the pharynx at the back of the throat, from the soft palate to the U-shaped hyoid bone near the base of the tongue

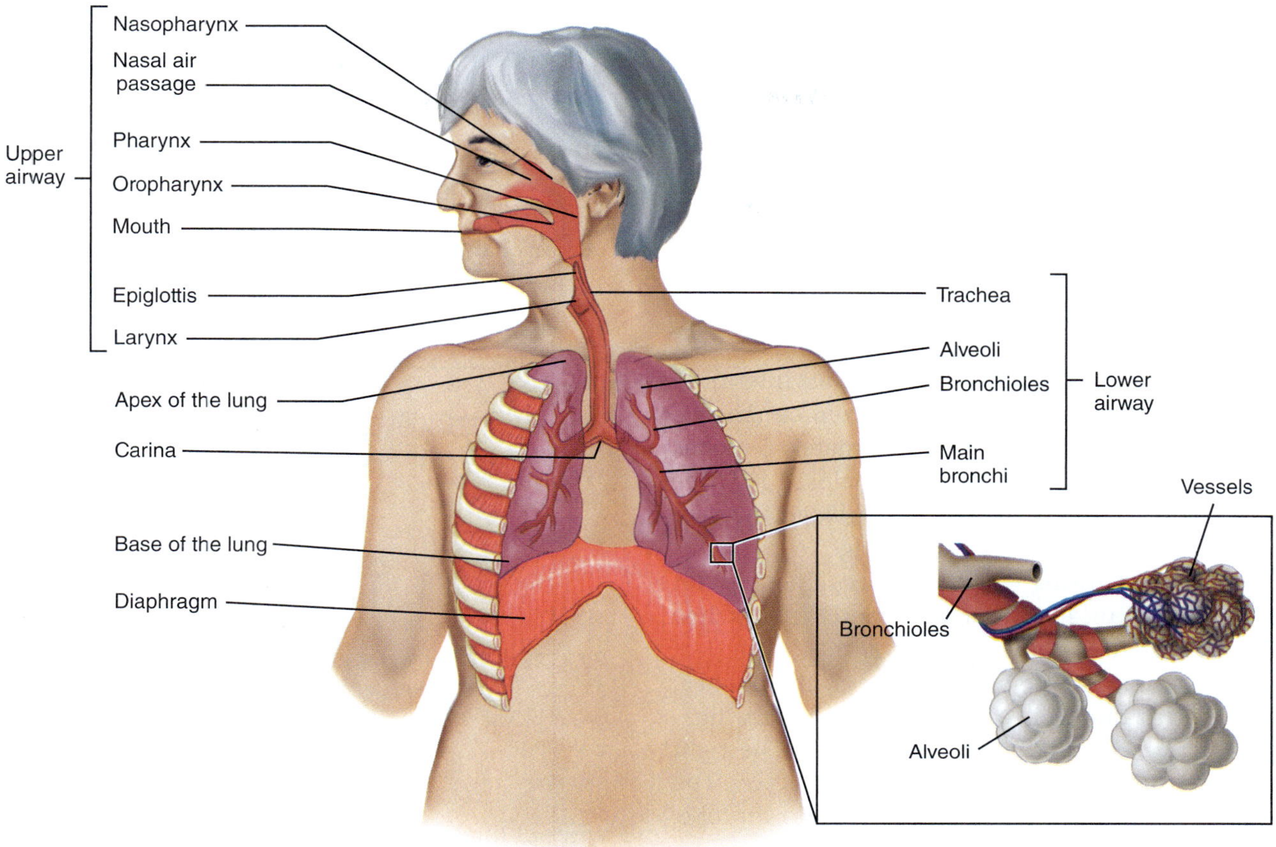

FIGURE 6-17 The respiratory system consists of all structures of the body that contribute to the process of breathing.

- Laryngopharynx. Lowest part of the pharynx, where it divides into the esophagus and the larynx
- Larynx (voice box)

At the base of the larynx, the vocal cords (ie, glottis) mark the transition point from the upper airway to the lower airway.

The nose and mouth lead to the oropharynx. The **pharynx** (throat) is composed of the nasopharynx, oropharynx, and the laryngopharynx. The nostrils lead to the nasopharynx (above the roof of the mouth and soft palate), and the mouth leads to the oropharynx. The nasal passages and nasopharynx warm, filter, and humidify air as you inhale. Air enters through the mouth more rapidly and directly. As a result, it is less moist than air that enters through the nose.

Food, liquids, and air all can travel through the oropharynx, but on reaching the laryngopharynx they must diverge, with food/liquids continuing posteriorly into the esophagus, while air proceeds to the anteriorly positioned larynx (voice box) and **trachea** (windpipe). The larynx does not tolerate any solid or liquid material, and any contact will result in a violent episode of coughing and spasm of the vocal cords. To help keep food and liquid out of the trachea while permitting air to pass, a thin, leaf-shaped flap (the **epiglottis**) covers the larynx during swallowing and then lifts open to allow for air passage during breathing.

The Lower Airway

Structures of the lower airway include the trachea, the bronchial tree (main stem bronchi and bronchioles), the alveoli, and the lungs themselves.

The **thyroid cartilage** (Adam's apple), which tends to be more visible in men, is in the anterior midline portion of the neck. This cartilage is the anterior part of the larynx. Tiny muscles open and close the vocal cords and control tension on them.

Sounds are created as air is forced past the vocal cords, making them vibrate. The pitch of the sound changes as the cords open and close. You can feel the vibrations if you place your fingers lightly on the larynx as you speak or sing. The vibrations of air are shaped by the tongue and muscles of the mouth to form understandable sounds. Immediately below the thyroid cartilage is the palpable **cricoid cartilage**.

Between the thyroid and cricoid cartilage lies the **cricothyroid membrane**, which can be felt as a depression in the midline of the neck just inferior to the thyroid cartilage. Below the cricoid cartilage is the trachea. The trachea is approximately 5 inches (13 cm) long and is a semirigid, enclosed air tube made up of C-shaped rings of cartilage that are open in the back. The rings of cartilage keep the trachea from collapsing when air moves into and out of the lungs. Air and other gases enter the trachea and proceed to the lungs.

The two lungs are held in place by the trachea, the arteries and veins, and the pulmonary ligaments. Each lung is divided into lobes. The right lung has three lobes: upper, middle, and lower. The left lung has two: an upper lobe and a lower lobe. Each lobe is divided further into segments

The lungs are supplied air by the right and left main stem **bronchi**, which are two tubes that branch from the trachea at a structure called the **carina** (see Figure 6-17). Each bronchus enters its respective lung and branches into smaller and smaller airways called **bronchioles**. The bronchioles end in about 700 million tiny, grapelike clusters of air sacs called **alveoli**. It is within these alveolar sacs that oxygen and carbon dioxide are exchanged between the lungs and the bloodstream (**FIGURE 6-18**).

The respiratory structures covered thus far serve as a pathway by which air can reach the alveoli. The alveoli are referred to as the functional units of the respiratory system. The walls of the alveoli contain a network of tiny blood vessels (pulmonary capillaries) that carry carbon dioxide from the body to the lungs (for removal through exhalation) and oxygen from the lungs to the body.

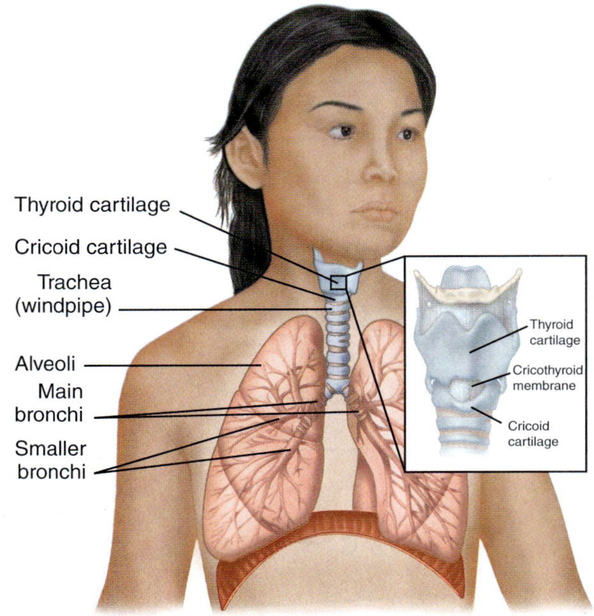

FIGURE 6-18 The lungs contain hundreds of millions of air sacs (alveoli), which lie at the ends of air passages. Small blood vessels surround the alveoli, allowing for gas exchange.

Mechanics of Breathing

For air to flow in and out of the lungs, the lungs must be able to expand and relax. The lungs cannot accomplish this on their own, because they are without muscle tissue. However, an effective mechanism is in place to ensure that the lungs follow the motion of the chest wall, expanding and contracting with it. Covering each lung is a layer of smooth, glistening tissue called **pleura** (**FIGURE 6-19**). Another layer of pleura lines the inside of the chest cavity. The two layers are called visceral pleura (covering the lungs) and parietal pleura (lining the chest wall). Between these two layers is a small amount of fluid that permits smooth gliding of the tissues.

Between the parietal pleura and the visceral pleura is the **pleural space**, called a potential space because the space does not exist under normal conditions. These two layers are usually sealed tightly to one another by a thin film of fluid. When the chest wall expands, the lung is pulled with it and made to expand by the force exerted through these closely applied pleural surfaces. When blood or air leaks into the pleural space, however, the surfaces separate.

Muscles of Breathing

There are several muscles involved in making the lungs expand and contract. The primary muscle of breathing is the **diaphragm**, a dome-shaped muscle

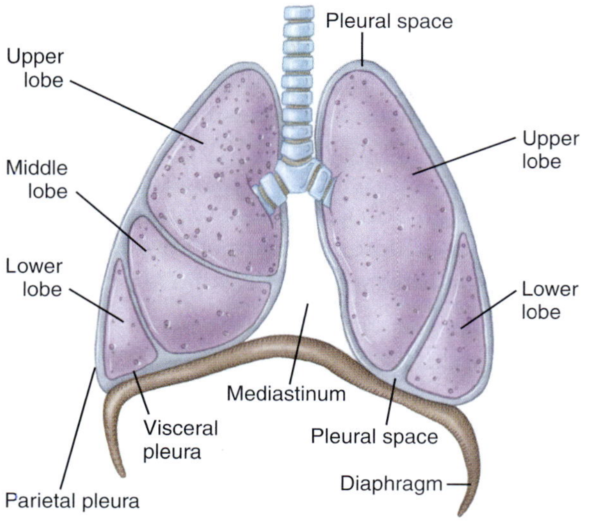

FIGURE 6-19 The pleura lining the chest wall and covering the lungs is an essential part of the breathing mechanism. The pleural space is not an actual space until blood or air leaks into it, causing the pleural surfaces to separate.

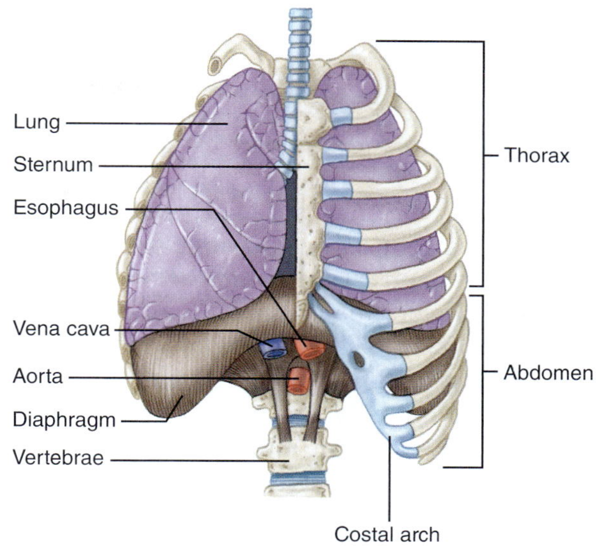

FIGURE 6-20 The dome-shaped diaphragm divides the thorax from the abdomen. It is pierced by the great vessels and the esophagus.

that divides the thorax from the abdomen and that is pierced by the great vessels and the esophagus (**FIGURE 6-20**).

The diaphragm is unique because it has characteristics of both voluntary (skeletal) and involuntary (smooth) muscles. Voluntary functions allow you to control the diaphragm if, for example, you choose to take a deep breath, cough, or hold your breath. Involuntary functions ensure that you continue to breathe without having to attend to this vital function at all times. Even though you can hold your breath or temporarily breathe faster or slower (voluntary functions), you cannot continue these variations in breathing pattern indefinitely. When

YOU are the EMT

When you arrive at the scene, you find the patient lying on his side on the floor of his bedroom. His knees are drawn up to his abdomen, and he is in severe pain. He also says he is nauseous. As you assess the patient, your partner opens the jump kit and prepares to obtain vital signs.

Recording Time: 0 Minutes	
Appearance	Restless; diaphoretic; in severe pain
Level of consciousness	Conscious and alert
Airway	Open; clear of secretions and foreign bodies
Breathing	Increased rate; adequate depth
Circulation	Radial pulses present and strong; skin cool and clammy

The patient tells you that the pain is in the right upper side of his abdomen and that it began suddenly about 20 minutes ago.

2. On the sole basis of the patient's chief complaint, which organs should you suspect are the cause of his condition?

3. What additional questions should you ask to gather more information about his chief complaint?

the concentration of carbon dioxide becomes too high, automatic regulation of breathing resumes. Therefore, although the diaphragm looks like voluntary skeletal muscle and is attached to the skeleton, it behaves, for the most part, like an involuntary muscle.

The other muscles involved in breathing are the neck (cervical) muscles, the intercostal muscles, the abdominal muscles, and the pectoral muscles. During inhalation, the diaphragm and intercostal muscles contract. When the diaphragm contracts, it moves down slightly, enlarging the thoracic cage from top to bottom. When the intercostal muscles contract, they move the ribs up and out. These actions combine to enlarge the chest cavity in all dimensions. As the volume of the chest cavity increases, pressure in the cavity falls and air rushes into the lungs. This is referred to as negative-pressure breathing because air is essentially sucked into the lungs. This part of the cycle is active, requiring the muscles to contract.

During exhalation, the diaphragm and the intercostal muscles relax. Unlike inhalation, exhalation does not normally require muscular effort. As these muscles relax, all dimensions of the thorax decrease, and the ribs and muscles assume a normal resting position. When the volume of the chest cavity decreases, air in the lungs is compressed into a smaller space. Pressure is increased, and air is pushed out through the trachea. This phase of the cycle is passive.

Words of Wisdom

When you assess a patient, make sure you assess both sides of the patient. It may seem like a waste of time to assess the left arm when the right arm is the one that is injured. However, you need to compare the sides to see whether there are differences. An abnormality on one arm may be normal if the same abnormality is found on the other arm. This idea of comparing sides applies to the respiratory system as well. You need to listen to both sides of the chest to evaluate the patient's lung sounds. Lung sounds can change on only one side of the chest, or they can change on both sides of the chest. Use all information you obtain from both sides of the body to help you make your patient care decisions.

The process of breathing is typically easy and requires little muscular effort. But, now imagine breathing through a straw and suddenly the diameter of the straw decreases. The smaller the diameter of the straw, the more effort you will have to exert to move air. As the resistance in the airway increases, you will begin to use accessory muscle groups, namely your abdominal and pectoral muscles, to assist the diaphragm in moving that air.

The Respiratory System: Physiology

The function of the respiratory system is to provide the body with oxygen and eliminate carbon dioxide. The exchange of oxygen and carbon dioxide takes place in the lungs and in the tissues. It is a complicated process that occurs automatically unless the airways or the lungs become diseased or damaged. There are two separate yet interdependent overall functions of the respiratory system: ventilation and respiration.

Ventilation is simply the movement of air between the lungs and the environment. It requires chest rise and fall. You are providing artificial ventilation when you assist a patient who is not breathing with a bag-mask device: a large bag filled with air that, when squeezed, pushes air out one end. The typical device holds approximately 1,000 to 1,200 mL of air. Bag-mask devices are designed to rapidly reinflate and allow you to control the amount of air that is moved to achieve chest rise and fall in any given patient. Artificial ventilation uses positive-pressure ventilation to provide oxygen to the lungs and to remove carbon dioxide from them until the patient is able to resume normal ventilation. **Respiration** is the process of gas exchange at the cellular level. Respiration provides the much-needed oxygen to cells and removes the waste product carbon dioxide. This exchange of gases also helps to control the pH level of the blood.

Respiration

As blood travels through the body, it delivers oxygen and nutrients to cells. At the capillaries, the oxygen is off-loaded from red blood cells. It passes through the thin capillary wall and enters the tissue cells, where it is used to produce energy. Carbon dioxide and cell wastes are transported in the reverse,

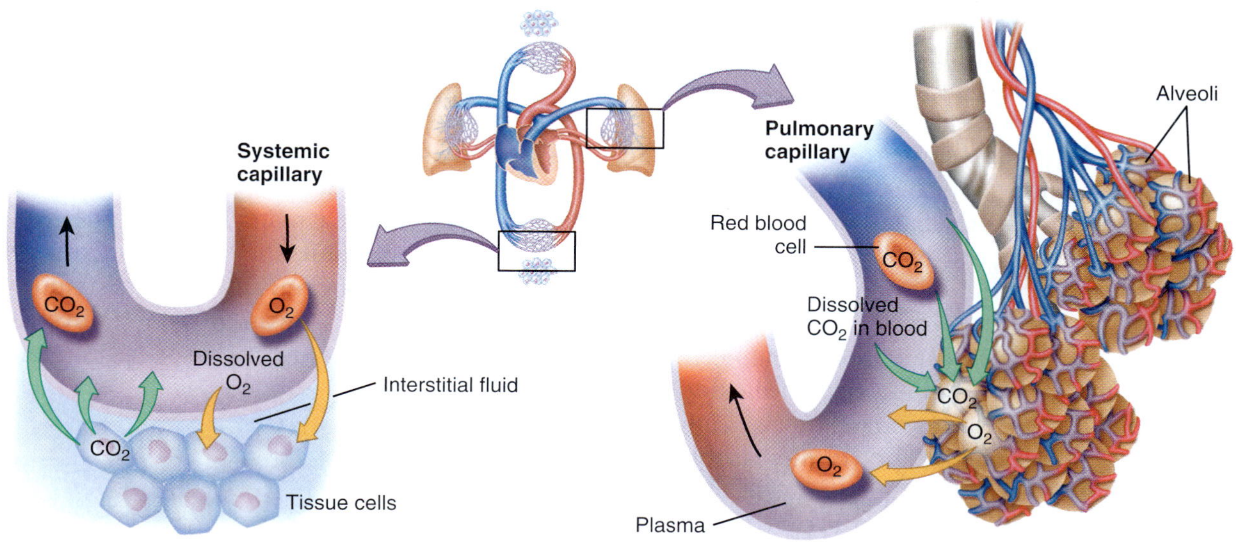

FIGURE 6-21 In the capillaries, oxygen (O_2) passes from the blood to the tissue cells, and carbon dioxide (CO_2) and waste pass from the tissue cells to the blood.

leaving the cells, crossing the capillary walls, and entering the bloodstream (**FIGURE 6-21**).

Room air is composed mostly of nitrogen, with oxygen contributing the next largest portion (about 21%) and carbon dioxide contributing less than 0.04%. Each time you take a breath, the alveoli receive a supply of oxygen-rich air. Recall that the oxygen then passes into a network of pulmonary capillaries, which are located in the walls of the alveoli. The walls of the capillaries and the alveoli are extremely thin. Thus, air in the alveoli and blood in the capillaries are only separated by two thin layers of tissue.

Oxygen and carbon dioxide pass rapidly across these thin tissue layers by diffusion. **Diffusion** is a passive process in which molecules move from an area with a higher concentration of molecules (oxygen in the air) to an area of lower concentration (oxygen in the bloodstream). There are more oxygen molecules in the alveoli than in the blood. Therefore, the oxygen molecules move from the alveoli into the blood. Because there are more carbon dioxide molecules in the blood than in the inhaled air, carbon dioxide moves from the blood into the alveoli. This process is completely passive; nature does all the work.

The blood does not use all the inhaled oxygen as it passes through the body. Exhaled air contains 16% oxygen and 3% to 5% carbon dioxide; the rest is nitrogen (**FIGURE 6-22**).

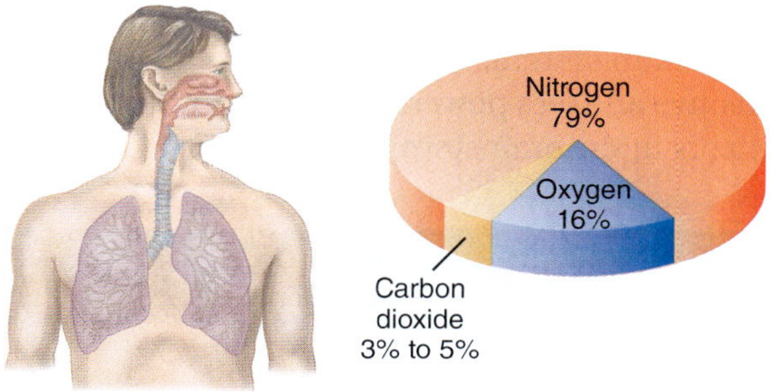

FIGURE 6-22 The components of exhaled air include oxygen, carbon dioxide, and nitrogen.

The Chemical Control of Breathing

The brain—specifically, the brainstem—controls breathing. The nerves in this area act as sensors for the level of carbon dioxide in the blood and subsequently the spinal fluid. The brain automatically controls breathing if the level of carbon dioxide or oxygen in the arterial blood is too high or too low. In fact, adjustments can be made in just one breath. For these reasons, you cannot hold your breath indefinitely or breathe rapidly and deeply indefinitely.

Breathing occurs as the result of a buildup of carbon dioxide, which causes the pH level to decrease in the **cerebrospinal fluid (CSF)**. CSF is a colorless fluid in and around the brain and spinal cord that cushions these structures and filters out impurities and toxins. The cells are constantly working to eliminate carbon dioxide to regulate the acid–alkaline balance of the body. When the level of carbon dioxide becomes too high, a slight change occurs in the pH (the measure of acidity) of the CSF. The medulla oblongata (a portion of the brainstem), which is sensitive to pH changes, stimulates the **phrenic nerve**, sending a signal to the diaphragm to increase its rate of contraction. As the diaphragm becomes more active, the respiratory rate and tidal volume increase (discussed later in this chapter). As minute volume increases, more carbon dioxide is exhaled. The primary reason you breathe is to lower your level of carbon dioxide, not to increase your level of oxygen.

The body also has a backup system to control respiration called the **hypoxic drive**. When the oxygen level falls, this system will also stimulate breathing. There are areas in the brain, the walls of the aorta, and the carotid arteries that act as oxygen sensors. These sensors are easily satisfied by minimal levels of oxygen in the arterial blood. Therefore, the backup system, the hypoxic drive, is much less sensitive and less powerful than the carbon dioxide sensors in the brainstem.

Special Populations

THE AIRWAY IN CHILDREN

The anatomy of a child's airway differs from that of an adult in several ways. The back of the infant's or young child's head is larger. The tongue is proportionately larger and is located more anterior in the mouth. The trachea is smaller in diameter and more flexible. The airway itself is lower and narrower (funnel-shaped). See Chapter 16, *Respiratory Emergencies*, for a more detailed discussion of the child's airway.

The Nervous System Control of Breathing

The exact way breathing occurs is complicated and also poorly understood by science. It is known that the medulla oblongata is primarily responsible for initiating the ventilation cycle and is primarily stimulated by high carbon dioxide levels in the blood and CSF. The function of the medulla is to keep you breathing without having to think about it. The medulla helps control the rhythm of breathing, initiates inspiration, sets the base pattern for respirations, and sends signals down the phrenic nerve to the diaphragm, triggering it to contract.

The pons, another area within the brainstem, has two areas, both of which help augment respirations during emotional or physical stress. The pons is involved in changing the depth of inspiration, expiration, or both. The medulla and the pons work together to help you get the right amount of air when you need it. The anatomy and physiology of the nervous system are discussed in more detail later in this chapter.

Special Populations

RESPIRATORY RATES OF CHILDREN

An infant needs to breathe faster than an older child. A respiratory rate of 30 to 60 breaths/min is normal for the newborn, whereas the adolescent is expected to have rates closer to the adult range (12 to 20 breaths/min). For a detailed discussion of normal pediatric breathing and respiratory demands, see Chapter 16, *Respiratory Emergencies*.

Ventilation

A substantial amount of air can be moved within the respiratory system. **FIGURE 6-23** shows the typical volumes. An adult man has a total lung capacity of 6,000 mL (equivalent to three 2-liter

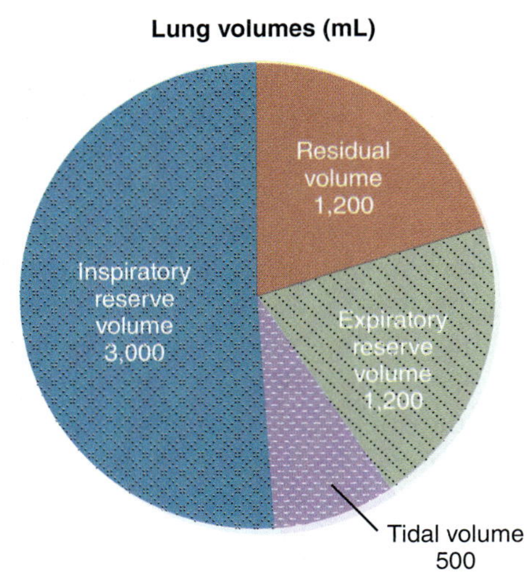

FIGURE 6-23 Lung volumes, in milliliters.

bottles of soda). An adult woman has about one-third less total capacity because the lung size is smaller.

Tidal volume is the amount of air that is moved into or out of the lungs during a single breath, generally 500 mL in an adult. **Inspiratory reserve volume** is the deepest breath you can take after a normal breath. Conversely, **expiratory reserve volume** is the maximum amount of air that you can forcibly breathe out after a normal breath. Gas remains in the lungs after exhalation simply to keep the lungs open. This is the **residual volume**. A loss of residual volume occurs when a direct impact to the chest "knocks the wind out" of a person.

Dead space is the portion of the respiratory system that has no alveoli, and, therefore, little or no exchange of gas between air and blood occurs. The mouth, trachea, bronchi, and bronchioles are all considered dead space.

Minute volume is another measure used to assess ventilation; it is the amount of air that moves in and out of the lungs in 1 minute.

$$\text{Minute volume} = \text{Respiratory rate} \times \text{Tidal volume}$$

This calculation helps you to determine if a patient is breathing adequately. While riding in the ambulance it will be difficult to determine the patient's exact tidal volume, but you will be able to estimate it. Consider the scenario of a patient who is breathing at a normal rate of 20 breaths/min. Yet, when you look at the patient's chest, it is barely moving. When you feel for air movement out of the mouth, you find very little movement. The patient is in trouble and needs your assistance now! Even though the patient's respiratory rate is normal, the amount of air being moved is inadequate. The minute volume is too low, and the patient needs ventilatory assistance. Always evaluate the amount of air being moved with each breath when assessing a patient's respirations.

Characteristics of Normal Breathing

You can think of a normal breathing pattern as a bellows system. Normal breathing should appear easy, not labored. As with a bellows that is used to move air to start a fire, breathing should be a smooth flow of air moving into and out of the lungs.

Normal breathing has the following characteristics:

- A normal rate and depth (tidal volume)
- A regular rhythm or pattern of inhalation and exhalation
- Clear, audible breath sounds on both sides of the chest
- Regular rise and fall movement on both sides of the chest

The Circulatory System: Anatomy

The **circulatory system** is a complex arrangement of connected tubes, including the arteries, arterioles, capillaries, venules, and veins (**FIGURE 6-24**). Another name for this system is the cardiovascular (heart/blood vessels) system. The circulatory system is entirely closed, with capillaries connecting arterioles and venules. There are two circuits in the body: the **systemic circulation** in the body and the **pulmonary circulation** in the lungs. The systemic circulation, the circuit in the body, carries oxygen-rich blood from the left ventricle through the body and back to the right atrium. In the systemic circulation, as blood passes through the tissues and organs, it gives up oxygen and nutrients and absorbs cellular wastes and carbon dioxide. Many cellular wastes are eliminated in passages through the liver and kidneys. The pulmonary circulation, the circuit in the lungs, carries oxygen-poor blood from the right ventricle through the lungs and back to the left atrium. In the pulmonary circulation, as blood passes through the lungs, it is refreshed with oxygen and gives up carbon dioxide.

The Heart

The **heart** is a hollow muscular organ approximately the size of a clenched fist. It is made of a specialized muscle tissue called cardiac muscle or **myocardium** and works as two paired pumps; the left side is more muscular. A wall called the septum divides the heart down the middle into right and left sides. Each side of the heart is divided again into an upper chamber (**atrium**) and a lower chamber (**ventricle**). The left side of the heart, which pumps blood to the body, is a high-pressure pump; the right side supplies blood to the lungs and is a low-pressure pump.

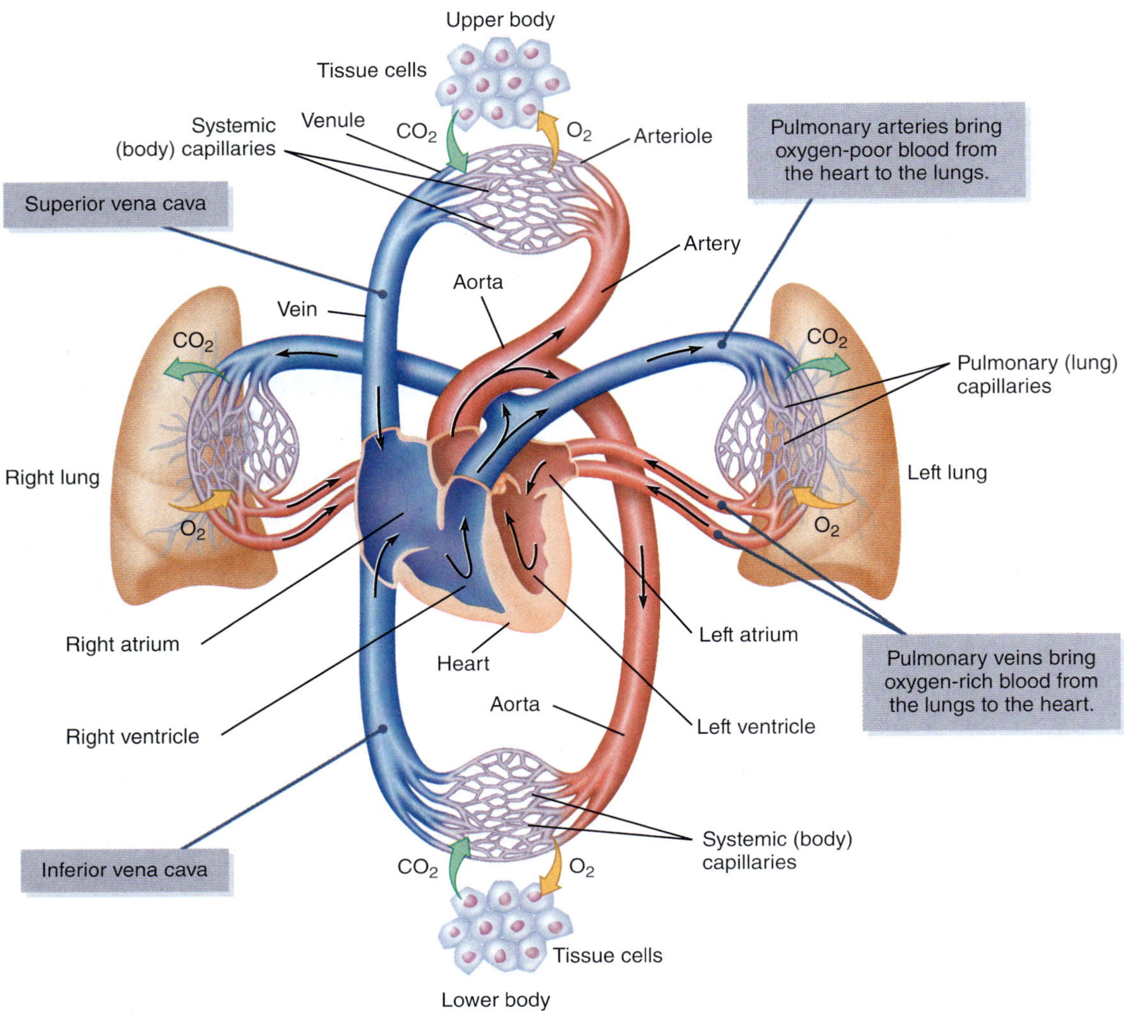

FIGURE 6-24 The circulatory system includes the heart, arteries, veins, and interconnecting capillaries. The capillaries are the smallest vessels and connect venules and arterioles. At the center of the system, and providing its driving force, is the heart. Blood circulates through the body under pressure generated by the two sides of the heart.

The heart is an involuntary muscle. As such, it is under the control of the autonomic nervous system. However, it has its own electrical system and continues to function even without its central nervous system control. It is also unlike skeletal and smooth muscle in its requirement for a continuous supply of oxygen and nutrients, as it cannot function on anaerobic metabolism.

The heart must function continuously from birth to death and has developed special adaptations to meet the needs of this continuous function. It can tolerate a serious interruption of its own blood supply for only a few seconds before the signs of a heart attack develop. Thus, its blood supply is rich and well distributed.

Circulation

The heart muscle's blood supply comes from the root of the aorta as it emerges from the heart.[4] The aorta has two branches at its base that form the left and right coronary arteries. These arteries supply the heart muscle with oxygenated blood.

The right side of the heart receives blood from the veins of the body (**FIGURE 6-25A**). The blood enters from the superior and inferior venae cavae

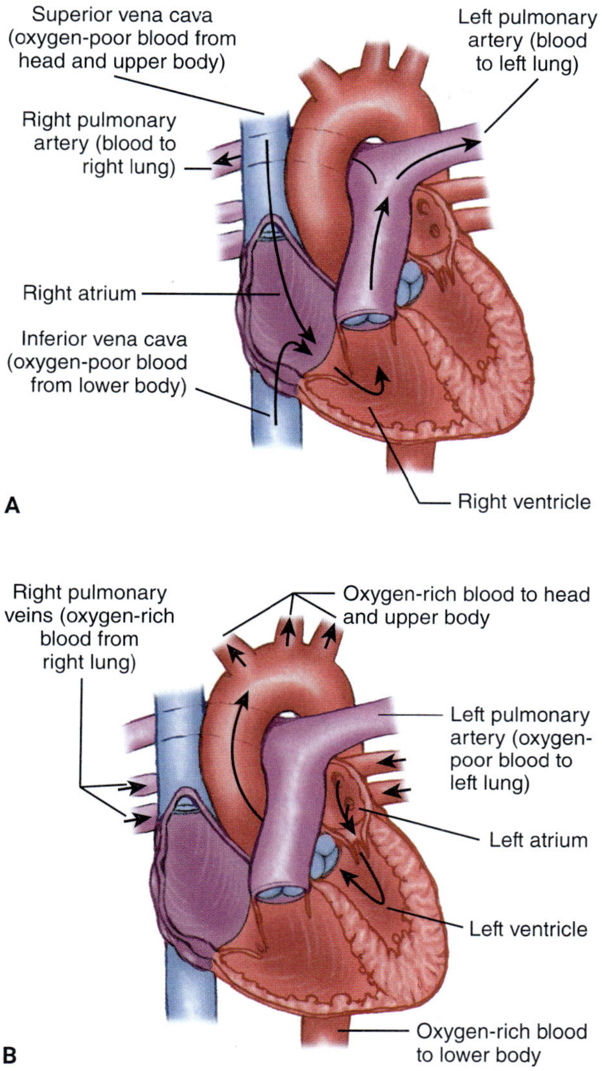

FIGURE 6-25 A. The right (lower pressure) side of the heart pumps blood from the body through the lungs. **B.** The left (higher pressure) side of the heart pumps oxygen-rich blood to the rest of the body.

into the right atrium and then passes through the tricuspid valve to fill the right ventricle. After the right ventricle is filled, the tricuspid valve closes to prevent backflow as the right ventricular muscle contracts. Contraction of the right ventricle causes blood to flow through the pulmonic valve into the pulmonary artery and the pulmonary circulation.

The left side receives oxygenated blood from the lungs through the **pulmonary veins** into the left atrium, where the blood passes through the mitral valve into the left ventricle (**FIGURE 6-25B**). Contraction of this most muscular of the pumping chambers pumps the blood through the aortic valve into the aorta and then to the arteries of the body.

The flow of blood through the four heart chambers is governed by one-way valves. The valves prevent the backflow of blood and keep it moving through the circulatory system in the proper direction. The **chordae tendineae** are thin bands of fibrous tissue that attach to the valves in the heart and prevent them from inverting. When a valve controlling the filling of a heart chamber is open, the other valve allowing it to empty is shut, and vice versa. Normally, blood moves in only one direction through the entire system.

Normal Heartbeat

In the normal adult, the resting heartbeat may range from 60 to 100 beats/min. A well-conditioned athlete may have a normal resting **heart rate (HR)** of 45 to 60 beats/min. During vigorous physical activity, the heart rate may rise to as fast as 180 beats/min until the activity stops. At each beat, 70 to 80 mL of blood is ejected from the adult heart. The amount of blood moved in one beat is called the **stroke volume (SV)**. In 1 minute, the entire blood volume of 5 L is circulated through all the vessels. The amount of blood moved in 1 minute is called the **cardiac output (CO)**. Cardiac output is equal to heart rate times stroke volume. Mathematically, cardiac output can be expressed as follows:

$$CO = HR \times SV$$

For example: 70 beats/min × 75 mL/beat = 5,250 mL/min or 5.25 L/min.

Electrical Conduction System

A network of specialized tissue with the capacity to conduct electrical current runs throughout the heart. The flow of electrical current through this network causes smooth, coordinated contractions of the heart. These contractions produce the pumping action of the heart. Each mechanical contraction of the heart is associated with two electrical processes. The first is depolarization, during which the electrical charges on the surface of the muscle cell change from positive to negative. The second is repolarization, during which the heart returns to its resting state and the positive charge is restored to the surface.

When the heart is working normally, the electrical impulse begins high in the atria at the sinoatrial node, then travels to the atrioventricular node and bundle of His, and moves through the Purkinje fibers to the ventricles. This movement produces a smooth flow of electricity through the heart, which depolarizes the muscle and produces a coordinated pumping contraction. Just as the walls of the heart can be injured when deprived of blood flow and oxygen, if areas of the heart's conduction system are deprived of blood flow and oxygen, serious abnormalities of the heart's rate, rhythm, and coordinated contraction can occur. Simply put, when the conduction system is injured, the heart will not beat properly. This may lead to dangerously low blood pressure, which, if untreated, can result in the patient experiencing a loss of consciousness or cardiac arrest. Blood pressure is discussed later in the chapter.

Words of Wisdom

Many of the abnormal cardiac rhythms associated with cardiac arrest can be effectively treated with defibrillation. Therefore, any patient in cardiac arrest should have an automated external defibrillator (AED) applied as soon as possible.

Arteries

The arteries carry blood from the heart to all body tissues. They branch into smaller arteries and then into arterioles. The arterioles, in turn, branch into the vast network of capillaries. The walls of an artery are made of fine, circular muscle tissue. Some arteries are made of fine circular muscle and elastic tissue. See Chapter 17, *Cardiovascular Emergencies*, for an illustration of the body's major arteries and veins.

Arteries contract to accommodate loss of blood volume and increase blood pressure. Blood is supplied to tissues as they need it. For example, the digestive system is supplied with more blood after you eat a meal. The leg muscles are more heavily supplied when jogging. Some tissues need a constant blood supply, especially the heart, kidneys, and brain. Other tissues, such as the muscles in the extremities, the skin, and intestines, can function with less blood when at rest. The ability to respond to the needs of the body is possible because of the way arteries are constructed. The middle layer of the artery is the **tunica media**, formed from smooth muscles that can contract and dilate to change the diameter of the blood vessel.

The **aorta** is the main artery leaving the back left side of the heart; it carries freshly oxygenated blood to the body. This blood vessel is found just in front of the spine in the chest and abdominal cavities. The aorta has many branches that supply the body's vital organs. The coronary arteries supply the heart; the carotid arteries supply the head; the hepatic arteries supply the liver; the renal arteries supply the kidneys; and the mesenteric arteries supply the digestive system. The aorta divides at the level of the umbilicus into the two common iliac arteries that lead to the lower extremities. All branches of the aorta ultimately become arterioles leading into the body's capillary network.

The **pulmonary artery** begins at the right side of the heart and carries oxygen-depleted blood to the lungs. It divides into finer and finer branches until it meets with the pulmonary capillary system located in the thin walls of the alveoli. These arteries are the only ones in the body that carry oxygen-depleted blood.

Arteries branch into smaller arteries and then into arterioles. **Arterioles** are the smallest branches of an artery leading to the vast network of capillaries.

The **pulse**, which is palpated most easily at the neck, wrist, or groin, is created by the forceful pumping of blood out of the left ventricle and into the major arteries. It is present throughout the entire arterial system. It can be felt most easily where the larger arteries near the skin can be pushed against a solid structure, such as a bone or large muscle (**FIGURE 6-26**). Pulses and their locations are listed in **TABLE 6-4**.

Capillaries

In the body, there are billions of cells and billions of capillaries. **Capillary vessels** are fragile divisions of the arterial system that allow contact between the blood and the cells of the tissues. Oxygen and other nutrients pass from blood cells and plasma in the capillaries to the individual tissue cells through the thin wall of the capillary. Carbon dioxide and other metabolic waste products pass in a reverse direction from the tissue cells to the blood to be carried away. Blood in arteries is characteristically bright red, because its hemoglobin is rich in oxygen. Blood in the veins is dark blue-red, because it has passed through a capillary bed and given up its oxygen to the cells. Capillaries connect directly at one end with the flow-regulating arterioles and at the other with the venules.

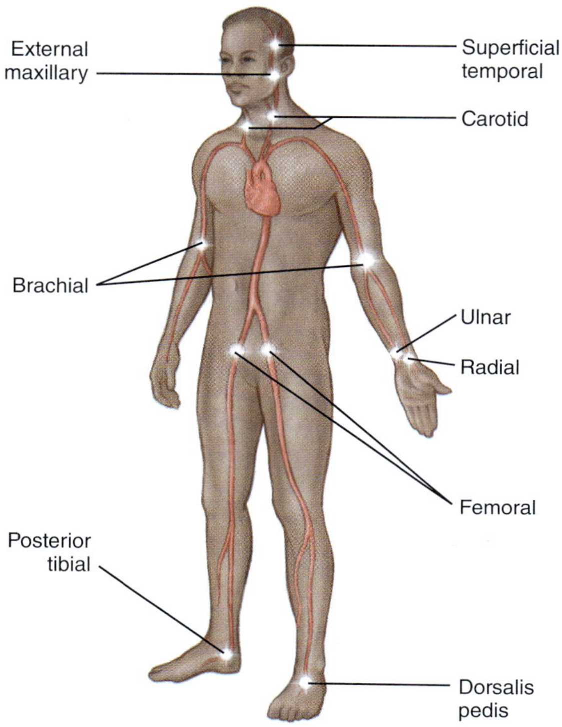

FIGURE 6-26 The central and peripheral pulses can be felt where the large arteries are near the skin.

Capillaries allow blood to move through them a single cell at a time.

Veins

Once oxygen-depleted blood passes through the network of capillaries, it moves to the venules, which are the smallest branches of the veins. The blood returns to the heart via a network of larger and larger veins. Veins have much thinner walls than arteries and are generally larger in diameter. The veins become larger and larger and ultimately form two major vessels, called the superior and inferior venae cavae. These two veins lie just to the right of the spine and collect blood just before it enters the heart. Because pressure generated by the heart dissipates as blood passes through the capillaries, venous blood flow is assisted by gravity, skeletal muscle contraction, and intrathoracic pressure changes from breathing. One-way flow in the veins is governed by valves within the veins.

The **superior vena cava** carries blood returning from the head, neck, shoulders, and upper extremities. Blood from the abdomen, pelvis, and lower extremities passes through the **inferior vena cava**. The superior and inferior venae cavae join at the right atrium of the heart. The right ventricle receives blood from the right atrium and pumps it through the pulmonary arteries into the lungs. The venae cavae, aorta, and pulmonary arteries and veins are collectively known as the **great vessels**.

Recall that the body's ability to adjust blood flow to meet the body's needs is critical to survival.

TABLE 6-4 Pulse Locations

Central Versus Peripheral	Pulse Name	Location Where Felt
Central pulses	**Carotid artery** pulse	At the upper portion of the neck
	Femoral artery pulse	In the groin
Peripheral pulses	**Radial artery** pulse	At the wrist at the base of the thumb
	Brachial artery pulse	On the medial aspect of the arm, on the anterior surface of the elbow joint (adults and older children); midway between the elbow and shoulder (infants and small children)
	Posterior tibial artery pulse	Posterior to the medial malleolus
	Dorsalis pedis artery pulse	On the top of the foot

TABLE 6-5 Effects of Blood Vessel Diameter on Blood

State	Effects
Constricted blood vessel	Decreased size of container Increased pressure within container
Normal diameter	Balance of size and pressure
Dilated blood vessel	Increased size of container Decreased pressure within container

The body constricts blood vessels to change the size of the total blood volume container. A smaller container that has the same amount of liquid as the original container means a higher liquid pressure.

The state of the blood vessels (ie, how dilated or constricted they are) is referred to as the **systemic vascular resistance (SVR)**. SVR is the resistance to blood flow within all blood vessels except the pulmonary vessels. The pathophysiology section of this chapter will discuss how various types of shock affect container size. In some types of shock, blood vessels dilate, the container becomes too large, and the patient's blood pressure falls dramatically (**TABLE 6-5**).

Blood Composition

Blood is composed of plasma, red blood cells, white blood cells, platelets, and protein molecules. **Red blood cells**, or erythrocytes, contain **hemoglobin**, a protein responsible for carrying oxygen. Most carbon dioxide is carried in the form of bicarbonate dissolved in the plasma, while a tiny amount of carbon dioxide is carried by hemoglobin. **White blood cells**, or leukocytes, play an important role in the body's immune defense against infection. **Platelets** are tiny, irregular, disc-shaped elements that are much smaller than the cells. They are essential in the initial formation of a blood clot, the mechanism that stops bleeding.

Plasma is the liquid portion of the blood that carries the blood cells, hormones, and nutrients. About 99% of its composition is water and proteins. Its composition can be broken down as follows:

- **Water.** Constitutes 92% of plasma.
- **Proteins.** Constitute 7% of the plasma. The majority of this protein is albumin, which has a role in controlling the movement of water into and out of the circulation. Also include clotting factors, enzymes, and some hormones.
- **Oxygen.** Very little oxygen is dissolved in the plasma; most is bound to the hemoglobin found in red blood cells.
- **Carbon dioxide.** Transported as bicarbonate in the plasma.
- **Nitrogen.** Accounting for roughly 78% of the air we breathe, this gas is dissolved within the plasma.
- **Nutrients.** Fuel for the cells.
- **Cellular wastes.** Lactic acid, carbon dioxide, etc.
- **Others.** Hormones, other cellular products.

The Spleen

The **spleen** is a solid organ located under the rib cage in the left upper quadrant of the abdomen. Although it is a lymphatic organ, it plays an important supportive role for the circulatory system. Red blood cells have a life span of about 120 days. As they age and degrade, they are filtered from the bloodstream and digested in the spleen and liver. Hemoglobin is then recycled.

Because its tissue is delicate and due to its position directly under flexible ribs (with very little soft tissue to cushion it), the spleen is one of the most frequently injured abdominal organs after blunt trauma. And because it is so highly vascular, an injured spleen can produce significant internal bleeding.

The Circulatory System: Physiology

Blood pressure (BP) is the force of circulating blood against the walls of the arteries. This pressure wave keeps the blood moving through the body. When the left ventricle of the heart contracts, it pumps blood into the aorta. This phase in the cardiac cycle is called **systole**. The pressure inside the arteries during this time is referred to as the systolic blood pressure. The time between contractions when the ventricle is relaxed and refilling with blood is called **diastole**. The resting pressure in the arteries during this phase is the diastolic blood pressure. The values of the systolic and diastolic pressures are measured with a **sphygmomanometer** (blood pressure

TABLE 6-6 Cardiovascular Values

Name	Description	Comments/Notes
Systolic blood pressure	Pressure within the arteries when the heart is contracting; left ventricular force	Indicates heart pumping effectiveness Indicates blood available to the heart
Diastolic blood pressure	Pressure within the arteries when the heart is at rest	Indicates adequate cardiac relaxation and pressure in the arteries between heartbeats
Pulse pressure	Difference between systolic blood pressure and diastolic blood pressure	Relationship between systolic and diastolic pressures; increases with age; may decrease with some cardiac conditions
Preload	Amount of blood returning to the heart	Too little preload and blood pressure falls Too high preload and fluid may be forced into the alveoli
Afterload	Pressure to be overcome when left ventricle contracts (pressure within the aorta)	Diastolic pressure is an indirect indicator of afterload
Stroke volume (SV)	Amount of blood moved with one contraction of the heart (left ventricle)	Weak left ventricle moves less blood per beat than a strong left ventricle
Cardiac output (CO)	Amount of blood moved in 1 minute	$CO = SV \times HR$
Systemic vascular resistance (SVR)	Resistance to blood flow within all of the blood vessels (excluding the pulmonary vessels)	The higher the SVR, the smaller the container; therefore, the higher the pressure of blood within the vessel
Mean arterial pressure (MAP)	Average arterial pressure during systole and diastole	$MAP = CO \times SVR$

cuff) and are expressed numerically in millimeters of mercury (mm Hg). Blood pressure is displayed as the systolic number over the diastolic number. Additional cardiovascular values of importance are shown in **TABLE 6-6**.

The average adult has approximately 5 L of blood. Children have 2 to 3 L, depending on age and size. Infants have approximately 300 mL. Thus, while the loss of a relatively small amount of blood might be insignificant for an adult, an equal amount of blood loss in an infant could be fatal.

Normal Circulation in Adults

In all healthy people, the circulatory system is automatically adjusted and readjusted constantly so that 100% of the capacity of the arteries, veins, and capillaries holds 100% of the blood at that moment. All of the vessels are never fully dilated or constricted. The size of arteries and veins is controlled by the nervous system, according to the amount of blood that is available and many other factors, to keep blood pressure normal at all times. Under the condition of normal pressure, with a system that can hold just 100% of the blood available, all parts of the system will have adequate blood supply all the time.

Perfusion is the circulation of blood in an organ or tissue. When perfusion is adequate, the cells' metabolic needs are met. Blood enters an organ or tissue through the arteries and leaves it through the veins. Loss of normal blood pressure is an indication that blood is no longer circulating efficiently to every organ in the body. (However, a "good blood pressure" does not necessarily indicate that blood is reaching all parts of the body.) There are many reasons for loss of blood pressure. The result in each case is the same: Organs, tissues, and cells are no longer adequately perfused or supplied with oxygen and fuel, and wastes accumulate. Under these conditions, cells, tissues, and whole organs may die. **Hypoperfusion** (inadequate perfusion) affecting the entire body is called **shock**.

Words of Wisdom

When multiple systems are affected (ie, systemic), the terms *shock* and *hypoperfusion* may be used interchangeably. However, hypoperfusion can also be limited to a specific region of the body, such as an arm, perhaps from an arterial occlusion (blockage). By contrast, shock is always systemic. In short, shock is a state of *systemic* hypoperfusion. The entire body is not receiving the oxygenated blood it needs for normal function.

Inadequate Circulation in Adults

When a patient has a small amount of blood loss, the arteries, veins, and heart automatically adjust to the smaller volume. The adjustment occurs to maintain adequate pressure throughout the circulatory system and maintain circulation for every organ. The adjustment occurs rapidly after the loss, usually within minutes. Specifically, the vessels constrict to provide a smaller bed for the reduced volume of blood to fill, and the heart pumps more rapidly to circulate the remaining blood more efficiently. As the blood pressure falls, the pulse increases to keep the cardiac output constant at 5 to 6 L per minute. If the loss of blood is too great, the adjustment fails, and the patient goes into shock. **FIGURE 6-27** illustrates this formula.

Special Populations

PULSE RANGES OF CHILDREN

It is important to know the normal pulse ranges when evaluating children. An infant's heart can beat as many as 160 times per minute or more if the body needs to compensate for injury or illness. This is the primary method the infant's body uses to compensate for decreased perfusion. See Chapter 10, *Patient Assessment*, for a review of the normal pulse rates in children and warning signs of decompensation.

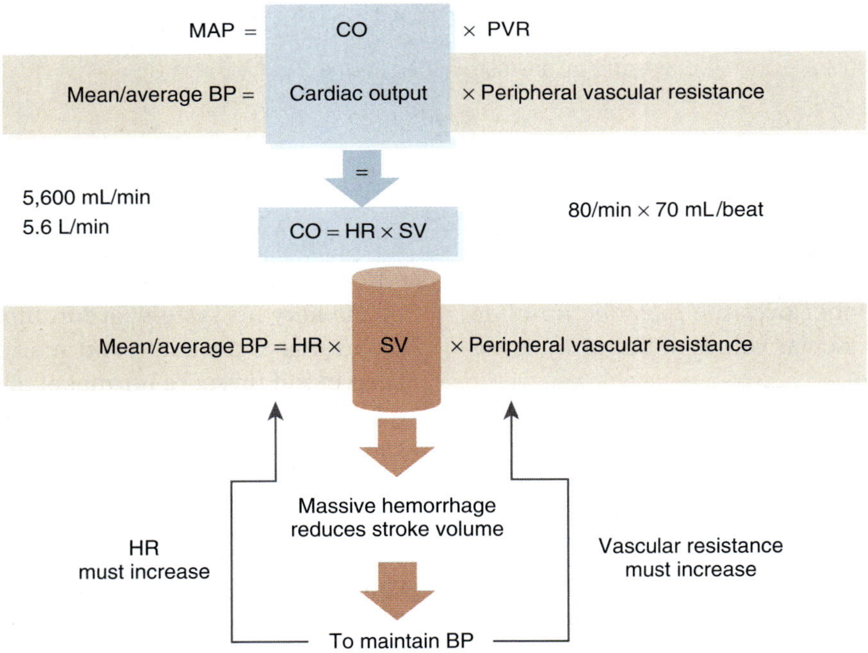

FIGURE 6-27 Significant blood loss results in reduced stroke volume (SV). To compensate, the body increases both heart rate (HR) and systemic vascular resistance to maintain mean arterial pressure (MAP).

Abbreviation: BP, blood pressure

The Function of Blood

Most blood is unevenly distributed throughout the body. Approximately 30% of blood is found within the heart, arteries, and capillaries. Seventy percent of blood is found within the veins and venules. This may seem confusing, but if you remember that the heart and arteries are high-pressure systems and veins are low-pressure systems, it becomes clearer. As blood pressure falls, blood flow slows down and there is more blood in the veins. The blood flows away from the left ventricle and moves back to the right atria.

Consider the movement of blood and its ultimate function of perfusion. You know that capillaries are the smallest portions of the circulatory system, where materials are able to exit and enter the bloodstream. Nutrients move from the capillaries into the **interstitial space** (space between the cells) and into the **intracellular space** (within the cell). Wastes move from the cells through the interstitial space and into the capillaries.

Inside the capillary, two main forces are at work: hydrostatic pressure and oncotic pressure. **Hydrostatic pressure** occurs as fluid pushes against the vessel walls to force fluid out of the capillary. **Oncotic pressure** is the opposing force and occurs because proteins in the blood plasma cause water to be pulled into the capillary by diffusion.

The movement of fluid into and out of the capillaries occurs as follows. Blood flows into the arterial side of the capillary. Water is forced out because the pressure is high. At the same time, water is trying to enter the capillary. Pressure on the arterial side is higher, so the hydrostatic pressure is also higher, and water, carrying nutrients, leaves the capillary and enters the interstitial space. However, the hydrostatic pressure is greatly diminished by the time the fluid reaches the venous side because the venous side of the circulatory system has much lower pressure. This decrease in pressure allows oncotic pressure to pull fluid into the capillary because that pressure is now higher than the capillary hydrostatic pressure. Water, along with all of the wastes from the cells, enters the venous side of the capillary. These wastes are then carried away (**FIGURE 6-28**).

Another function of blood is the ability to clot. Coagulation, or clotting, occurs as the result of a complex chemical process that creates small fibers near the injured blood vessel, trapping red blood cells. This chemical process involves platelets and clotting factors that are in the bloodstream. **TABLE 6-7** outlines the major functions of the blood.

Blood under pressure will gush or spurt intermittently from an artery. When blood comes from a vein, it flows in a steady stream, sometimes very rapidly if it is a large vein. From capillaries, blood

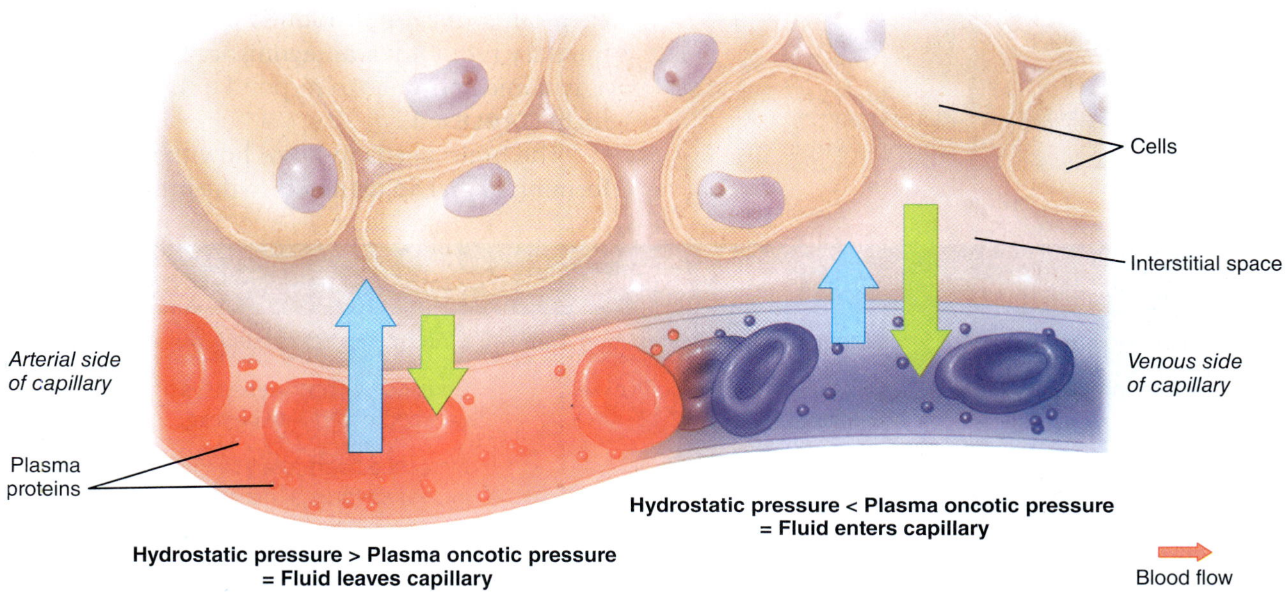

FIGURE 6-28 Fluid movement from capillaries to interstitial space and back.

will ooze at many tiny individual points. Clotting after venous or capillary bleeding normally takes from 6 to 10 minutes.

Nervous System Control of the Cardiovascular System

The nervous system, discussed next, has direct effects on the cardiovascular system. When the body is stressed, the sympathetic nervous system sends commands to the adrenal glands (which sit atop the kidneys) where two hormones, **epinephrine** (also known as adrenaline) and **norepinephrine** (also known as noradrenaline), are secreted to stimulate the heart and blood vessels. The release of epinephrine and norepinephrine affects receptors within the heart and blood vessels and improves the ability to cope with stress, known as the fight-or-flight reaction. Two types of receptors within the heart and blood vessels will be discussed next so you can understand how the nervous system controls the circulatory system.

The heart and blood vessels have **alpha-adrenergic receptors** and **beta-adrenergic receptors** within them. **Adrenergic** simply means related to the adrenal gland, where epinephrine and norepinephrine are made. The alpha-adrenergic receptors are found in the blood vessels. When stimulated, the blood vessels constrict, thereby increasing blood pressure. The beta-adrenergic receptors are found in the heart and lungs. When beta-1 receptors are stimulated, they cause the heart to increase its rate and also squeeze harder with each contraction. This increases cardiac output. When beta-2 receptors are stimulated, the bronchi in the lungs dilate. This allows more air to be inhaled and exhaled; therefore, more oxygen reaches the alveoli and is available to the cells of the body. Together, the alpha- and beta-adrenergic receptors prepare the body for fight or flight.

The parasympathetic nervous system also has effects on the cardiovascular system. When stimulated, this system causes the heart to slow and beat more weakly. Although the sympathetic and parasympathetic divisions function in opposition to each other, this opposition is considered complementary rather than antagonistic. The net effect is a dynamic body able to respond quickly for fight or flight (**TABLE 6-8**).

The brain needs to know how the body is performing so that adjustments in the pressure exerted

TABLE 6-7 Functions of the Blood and the Components of Blood in Use

Function	Component of the Blood in Use
Fights infection	White blood cells
Transports oxygen	Red blood cells (hemoglobin)
Transports carbon dioxide	Plasma
Controls (buffers) pH	Chemicals within the plasma
Transports wastes and nutrients	Plasma (water)
Clotting (coagulation)	Platelets and clotting factors in the plasma

TABLE 6-8 Nervous System Effects on the Cardiovascular System

Portion of Nervous System	Receptor	Stimulation Area	Effect When Stimulated
Sympathetic nervous system	Alpha-1	Blood vessels	Constricted blood vessels; skin becomes pale compared with baseline, cool, clammy
	Beta-1	Heart	Increased heart rate Increased force of heart contraction
	Beta-2	Lungs	Bronchodilation
Parasympathetic nervous system	Muscarinic	Heart	Decreased heart rate Decreased force of contraction

by circulating blood can be made. How is the brain alerted to what is happening at the feet, the liver, or the heart? Signals are sent through the nervous system from special pressure sensors (baroreceptors) spread throughout the body, which allow the brain to receive information about blood pressure. Remember, the main function of the cardiovascular system is to perfuse blood throughout the body. The main locations for these pressure receptors are found in the arch of the aorta and the carotid arteries. By measuring the pressure in these two locations, the body can ensure that the most vulnerable and most important cells get oxygen.

With this information, the brain is able to act to maintain perfusion. To see the system in action, consider what happens when a healthy person kneels down to the floor then jumps up as fast as they can. Are they likely to pass out? Most likely not, because these systems with their pressure sensors are designed to maintain perfusion.

When you jumped up quickly, gravity was relocating the blood out of your brain. The baroreceptors detected the decrease in blood pressure at the carotid arteries. A signal was sent to the brain. The brain understood the implication of low blood pressure and immediately turned on the sympathetic nervous system. The blood vessels contracted, and the heart rate increased. The heart pumped harder. Your blood pressure returned to normal and may even have gone slightly high. Again, the baroreceptors detected this change. Signals were sent to the brain. The sympathetic nervous system was turned off. The parasympathetic nervous system was turned on. The heart rate slowed, and the force of the heart's contractions weakened. All of this happened in a fraction of a second. That is how responsive the cardiovascular system can be.

Special Populations

BARORECEPTORS IN OLDER ADULTS

These pressure receptors and their responses are less effective in some older adults, particularly those who take medications to control blood pressure. As a result, these individuals may feel light-headed or may faint (have a syncopal episode) if they stand quickly, particularly when moving from a lying position.

The Nervous System: Anatomy and Physiology

The **nervous system** is perhaps the most complex organ system within the human body. It comprises the brain, spinal cord, and thousands of nerves spread throughout the body. This system has many functions, such as the control of breathing, heart rate, and blood pressure. However, what makes the nervous system so special is that it allows the performance of higher-level activity. Reading a good book, enjoying music, having a discussion with a friend, and even watching television require the brain to engage memory, understanding, and thought. This is where the true complexity of the nervous system is revealed.

The nervous system is divided into two main portions: the **central nervous system (CNS)** (the brain and spinal cord) and the **peripheral nervous system (PNS)** (the nerves outside of the brain and spinal cord that link the CNS to various organs throughout the body).

The PNS can be further divided into the somatic and autonomic nervous systems. The **somatic nervous system** regulates activities over which we have voluntary control, such as walking, talking, and writing. The **autonomic nervous system** controls those functions that occur autonomously (ie, automatically), including digestion, dilation and constriction of blood vessels, sweating, and other involuntary actions (**FIGURE 6-29**).

The Central Nervous System

Brain

The **brain** controls all functions of the body, and it assembles and interprets the information received through the body's various senses. It stores information in memory; it controls thought, speech, movement of skeletal muscle, and involuntary processes such as heart and breathing rates. The brain is subdivided into several components, all of which have specific roles. Three major subdivisions of the brain are the cerebrum, the cerebellum, and the brainstem (see Figure 6-30).

The **cerebrum** accounts for the largest portion of the brain (about three-fourths). Its surface, the cortex, is made up of **neurons** (nerve cells), which give it a gray-brown color (thus the reason why the cerebrum is sometimes called the gray matter).

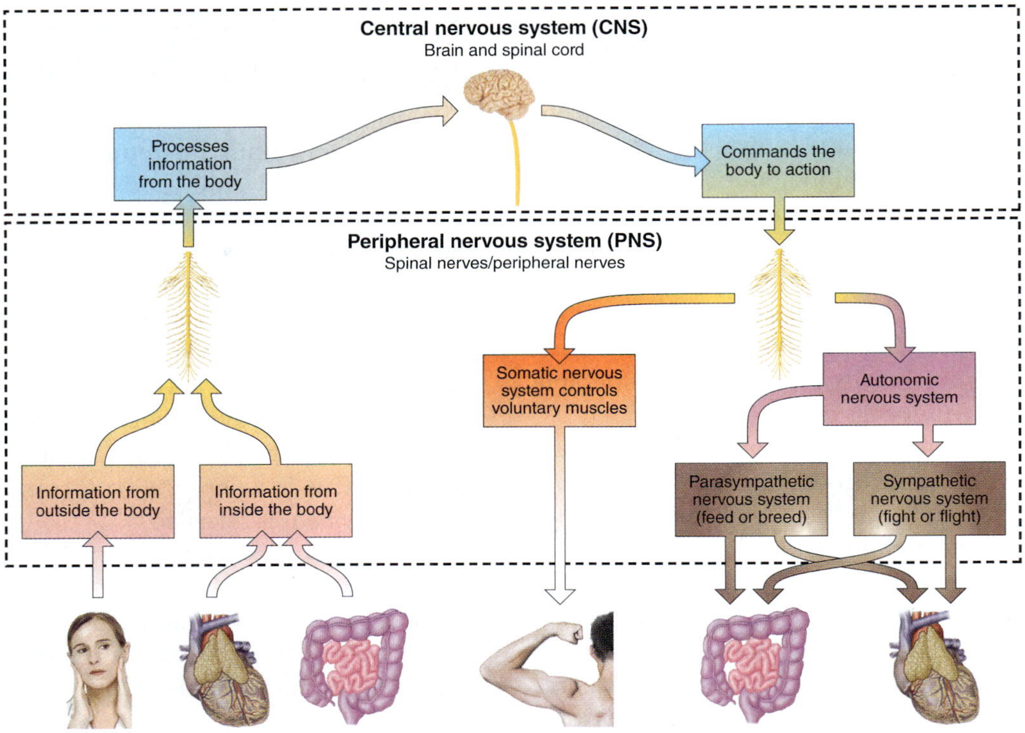

FIGURE 6-29 The basic configuration of the nervous system.

The cerebrum is responsible for higher brain functions, such as interpreting what we see, hear, or feel; encoding and decoding speech; reasoning and learning; controlling precise muscle movements (ie, fine motor control); and managing emotions.

The cerebrum can be divided into right and left halves, or hemispheres. These hemispheres can be further divided into lobes. In general, control of one side of the body belongs to the hemisphere on the opposite side (eg, the left hemisphere controls the movements of the right leg). Each hemisphere has four lobes: frontal, parietal, temporal, and occipital. No single lobe operates entirely on its own; complex relationships exist between them and with other parts of the brain. However, each lobe has a certain set of duties for which it is recognized as having the greatest degree of control. For example, personality, judgment, planning, problem solving, concentration, and self-awareness all are attributed to the **frontal lobe**. The **parietal lobe** controls our recognition of spatial relationships and it integrates sensory information received from the body to form our perception of the world around us. The **occipital lobe** is responsible for vision. Taste, hearing, and our ability to understand words all are functions of the **temporal lobe**.

Located beneath the cerebrum is the **cerebellum**, a structure that controls balance, muscle coordination, and posture. Without the cerebellum, highly specialized muscular activities such as writing would be impossible.

Deep within the cranium, the well-protected **brainstem** acts as a relay center connecting the cerebrum and cerebellum to the spinal cord. It is the most primitive part of the CNS, controlling virtually all involuntary, life-sustaining functions, such as heart rate, breathing, temperature regulation, digestion, vomiting, swallowing, coughing, and the wake/sleep cycle. The brainstem comprises the **midbrain**, the **pons**, and the **medulla oblongata**.

One noteworthy feature within the brainstem is a network of neurons called the **reticular activating system (RAS)**. One of its functions is to regulate consciousness. When stimulated, it wakes the cerebral cortex. Without the RAS, wakefulness and awareness would not be possible. When someone experiences a concussion from a head injury, the immediate loss of consciousness is due to a momentary interruption in the RAS. Much like a computer having to reboot, the RAS must "reboot" for the patient to regain conscious awareness.

The brain has many other anatomic elements, all of which have important functions. **TABLE 6-9** summarizes several key components of the nervous system and their functions.

Cerebrospinal Fluid

In addition to filtering out impurities and toxins, CSF absorbs shocks. When significant forces are applied to the head, CSF allows the brain to shift inside the skull without being damaged. Some skull fractures may allow the clear, colorless CSF to leak from the ears or nose. This is considered a significant finding. Refer to Chapter 28, *Head and Spine Injuries*, for more information.

Circulation in the Head

The brain requires a constant flow of oxygenated blood. Blood is supplied to the head through the carotid arteries, which can be palpated on either side of the neck. Deoxygenated blood drains from the head via the internal and external jugular veins.

TABLE 6-9 Structures of the Nervous System and General Functions

System	Major Structure	Subdivision	General Function
Central nervous system	Brain	Occipital lobe	Vision and storage of visual memories
		Parietal lobe	Sense of touch and texture; storage of those memories
		Temporal lobe	Hearing, smell, and language; storage of sound and odor memories
		Frontal lobe	Voluntary muscle control and storage of those memories
		Prefrontal area	Judgment and predicting consequences of actions, abstract intellectual functions
		Limbic system	Basic emotions, basic reflexes (eg, chewing, swallowing)
		Diencephalon (thalamus)	Relay center; filters important signals from routine signals
		Diencephalon (hypothalamus)	Emotions, temperature control, interface with endocrine system (hormone control)
	Brainstem	Midbrain	Level of consciousness, reticular activating system, muscle tone, and posture
		Pons	Respiratory patterning and depth
		Medulla oblongata	Heart rate, blood pressure, respiratory rate
	Spinal cord		Reflexes, relays information to and from body and the brain
Peripheral nervous system	Cranial nerves		Brainstem to head and neck; special peripheral nerves that connect directly to body parts
	Peripheral nerves		Brain to spinal cord to body part; receive stimulus from body, send commands to body

Spinal Cord

The **spinal cord** is an extension of the brainstem (**FIGURE 6-30**). The opening at the base of the cranium, which allows the brain and cord to connect, is called the foramen magnum. The spinal cord then travels downward, encased within the vertebral column, through a passageway called the spinal canal. The spinal canal is formed by the openings that run vertically through the middle of adjoining vertebrae. The cord terminates at the level of the second lumbar vertebra (L2).

The cord contains nerve cell bodies, but most of the spinal cord's volume is composed of extensions from those bodies (called axons) that facilitate communication between neurons. Before connecting with the brain, nerve fibers from the spinal cord cross over from one side to the other. This accounts for the fact that many actions taking place on one side of the body are controlled by the cerebral hemisphere on the opposite side. The primary function of the spinal cord is to transmit messages between the brain and the body. These messages are passed along the nerve fibers as electrical impulses, moving quickly from one nerve to the next.

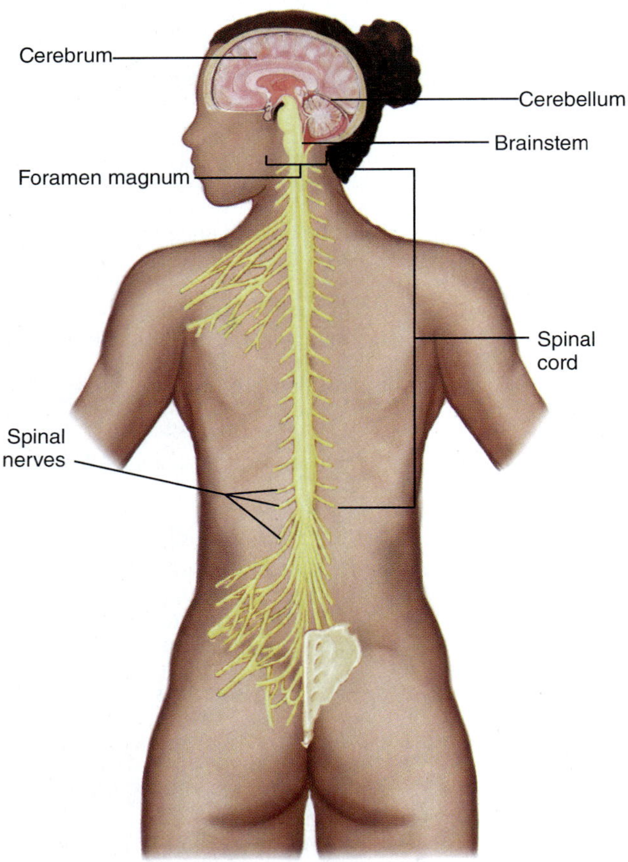

FIGURE 6-30 The brain lies well protected within the skull. Its major subdivisions are the cerebrum, the cerebellum, and the brainstem. The spinal cord is a continuation of the brainstem. It exits the skull at the foramen magnum and extends down to the level of the second lumbar vertebra.

The Peripheral Nervous System

The PNS is divided into the somatic nervous system and the autonomic nervous system. The autonomic nervous system, in turn, is divided between the sympathetic and parasympathetic nervous systems. The **sympathetic nervous system** is responsible for the fight-or-flight reaction that enables us to respond under stress. This reaction generally increases activity within the body. When stimulated, the sympathetic nervous system increases blood flow to the skeletal muscles, increases heart and respiratory rates, dilates the pupils, increases production and use of energy, dilates respiratory passageways, and causes sweating.

By contrast, the **parasympathetic nervous system** tends to slow the body's activities or return the body to its resting state. Effects include pupil constriction, promotion of digestive system activities, constriction of airway passages, and reduction of heart rate and force of contraction.

There are two types of nerves used in the PNS: sensory nerves and motor nerves.

Sensory Nerves

Sensory nerves are complex. They can be found in the eyes, ears, skin, muscles, joints, lungs, and other organs. When a sensory cell is stimulated, it transmits a message to the brain. There are many different kinds of sensory nerves. Some detect heat or cold, whereas others relay information about position, motion, pressure, pain, balance, light, taste, smell, or some other sensation. Every sensory nerve uses specialized nerve endings unique to its type, so that it perceives and communicates information about a single type of sensation. Most sensory nerves must carry information to the brain via the spinal cord. Others take information to the brain directly, without having to go through the spinal cord first.

One example of a nerve with a direct line of communication with the brain that bypasses the spinal cord is the optic nerve. Its nerve endings are found in the retina of the eye. When stimulated by light, the optic nerve carries visual information from the eye straight to the occipital lobe of the brain, where it is interpreted. It does not pass through the spinal cord.

By contrast, when sensory nerve endings in the extremities are stimulated, they transmit the impulses along a peripheral nerve to the spinal cord. The information is then conducted up the spinal cord, passing from one neuron to the next, until it reaches the parietal lobe of the cerebrum.

In many cases, sensory information cannot be acted on until the brain has received and decoded the message sent by the sensory nerves. The brain must then reply with a command, telling the body how to respond. In other cases, certain stimuli can evoke a physical response even before the message reaches the brain. In such instances, the impulse is intercepted by a nearby motor nerve, which promptly initiates physical movement. For example, imagine accidentally placing your hand on a hot stove. Technically, you will withdraw your hand *before* you feel the heat. Such withdrawal reflexes exist to limit damage to the body.

Motor Nerves

Every skeletal muscle in the body has its own motor nerve. Whereas sensory nerves carry information *to* the brain, **motor nerves** carry information *from* the brain to the muscles. Motor neuron cell bodies reside in the spinal cord. From these cell bodies, **axons** extend to skeletal muscles. When an electrical impulse is generated by the cerebral cortex, it travels down the nerve to the muscle that neuron controls. In response, the muscle contracts.

The Integumentary System (Skin): Anatomy

The cutaneous membrane, or skin, is the largest single organ in the body. It has two major components: the epidermis and the dermis. Beneath these layers is **subcutaneous tissue**. See Chapter 26, *Soft-Tissue Injuries,* for a detailed illustration of the skin's anatomy.

The outermost layers that make up the skin's surface are known collectively as the **epidermis** (*epi-* is a prefix meaning "above"). The epidermis forms a watertight barrier that provides considerable protection, keeping microorganisms from getting inside the body while preventing fluid from escaping. Its thickness varies depending on its location on the body. On the soles of the feet and the palms of the hands, the back, and the **scalp**, the skin is quite thick, while in other areas it is only two or three cells thick.

Epidermal cells are arranged in multiple layers. The innermost layer, called the **germinal layer**, continuously produces new cells that gradually ascend through the other skin layers. The germinal layer also contains cells that produce pigment granules, which give the skin its color. In time, germinal layers reach the exposed surface layer, called the **stratum corneum**. Whereas the germinal layer is supplied with blood, the stratum corneum is not. Thus, the cells of the corneum are dead and are continually shed and replaced by new cells arriving from the layers below. The journey from the germinal layer to the surface takes about 4 weeks.

Located beneath the epidermis, the **dermis** is home to the **sweat glands**, sebaceous (oil) glands, hair follicles, blood vessels, and nerve endings. Sweat reaches the surface of the skin by way of small pores, or ducts, that pass from sweat glands in the dermis and up through the epidermis. Sweat helps to cool the body.

Hair follicles are small organs that produce hair. As hair grows, it passes along a shaft, ultimately reaching and emerging from the epidermal surface. Connected to the hair is a small muscle that pulls the hair into an erect position when triggered by certain stimuli (eg, cold air or fright). Hairs grow and are shed according to a hair growth cycle. Adjacent to hair follicles, **sebaceous glands** secrete an oily substance called sebum along the hair follicles to the skin surface. Sebum seals the surface, waterproofing the skin and preventing it from drying and cracking.

Blood vessels provide nutrients and oxygen to the skin. The blood vessels lie in the dermis. A complex array of nerve endings also lies in the dermis. These specialized nerve endings are sensitive to environmental stimuli; they respond to these stimuli and send impulses along the nerves to the brain.

Beneath the skin, immediately under the dermis and attached to it, lies the subcutaneous tissue. The subcutaneous tissue is composed largely of fat, which serves as an insulator for the body and a reservoir that stores energy. The amount of subcutaneous tissue varies greatly from individual to individual. The subcutaneous layer helps to anchor the skin to the structures below (eg, the muscles and skeleton). As you age, the loss of subcutaneous tissue, coupled with a decrease in skin elasticity, causes a reduction in support for the skin, resulting in wrinkles.

While skin covers the entire external surface of the body, it does not cover the inner surface of various openings to the body such as the mouth, nose, anus, and vagina. Instead, these structures are lined with mucous membranes. **Mucous membranes** are quite similar to skin in that they provide a protective barrier against bacterial invasion. However, they differ from skin in that they secrete **mucus**, a watery substance that lubricates and keeps them moist. A continuous mucous membrane lines the entire length of the gastrointestinal tract, from mouth to anus.

The Integumentary System (Skin): Physiology

The skin serves multiple functions. Chief among these are to (1) protect the body from the environment, (2) maintain normal body temperature, and (3) transmit sensory information (ie, touch, pain, pressure, and temperature) from the environment to the brain.

The protective functions of the skin are numerous. Water makes up a large portion of the body. This water contains a delicate balance of chemical substances in solution. The skin is watertight and serves to keep this balanced internal solution intact. The skin also protects the body from the invasion of infectious organisms: bacteria, viruses, and fungi. These organisms are everywhere and are routinely found lying on the skin surface. However, they typically do not penetrate the skin unless it is broken by injury; thus, the skin provides a constant protection against outside invaders.

The major organ for regulation of body temperature is the skin. Blood vessels in the skin constrict when the body is in a cold environment and dilate when the body is in a warm environment. In a cold environment, constriction of the blood vessels shunts the blood away from the skin to decrease the amount of heat radiated from the body surface. When the outside environment is hot, the vessels in the skin dilate, bringing blood closer to the surface. The skin becomes flushed (red), and heat radiates from the body surface.

Also, in a hot environment, sweat is secreted to the skin surface from the sweat glands. Evaporation of the sweat causes the body temperature to fall because water absorbs heat as it evaporates. Sweating alone is not as effective in reducing body temperature; evaporation of the sweat must also occur, meaning that cooling is less efficient in humid conditions.

Information from the environment is carried to the brain through a rich supply of sensory nerves that originate in the skin. Nerve endings that lie in the skin are adapted to perceive and transmit information about heat, cold, external pressure, pain, and the position of the body in space. The skin thus recognizes any changes in the environment. The skin also reacts to pressure, pain, and pleasurable stimuli.

Special Populations

THE INTEGUMENTARY SYSTEM OF CHILDREN

The integumentary system of the child differs from that of the adult in several ways. The child's skin is thinner, with less subcutaneous fat; thus, it tends to burn more deeply and easily than that of an adult, as in the case of a sunburn. Infants and children also have a larger ratio of body surface area to body mass, which can lead to significant fluid and heat losses. These differences make them more likely than adults to suffer heat- and cold-related emergencies.

The Digestive System: Anatomy

The digestive system, also called the gastrointestinal system, is composed of the gastrointestinal tract (stomach and intestines), mouth, salivary glands, pharynx, esophagus, liver, gallbladder, pancreas, rectum, and anus. The function of this system is **digestion**: the processing of food that nourishes the individual cells of the body. Most of the organs of this system are found within the abdomen.

The Abdomen

The **abdomen** is the second major body cavity; it contains the major organs of digestion and excretion. The diaphragm separates the thorax from the abdominal cavity. Anteriorly and posteriorly, thick muscular abdominal walls create the boundaries of this space. Inferiorly, the abdomen is separated from the pelvis by an imaginary plane that extends from the pubic symphysis through the sacrum (**FIGURE 6-31**). Some organs lie in the abdomen and the pelvis, depending on the posture of the patient.

The simplest and most common method of describing the portions of the abdomen is by quadrants, the four equal areas formed by two imaginary lines that intersect at right angles at the umbilicus. On the anterior abdominal wall, the quadrants thus formed are the right upper, right lower, left upper, and left lower (**FIGURE 6-32**). Pain or injury in a given quadrant usually arises from or involves the organs that lie in that quadrant. This simple means of designation will allow

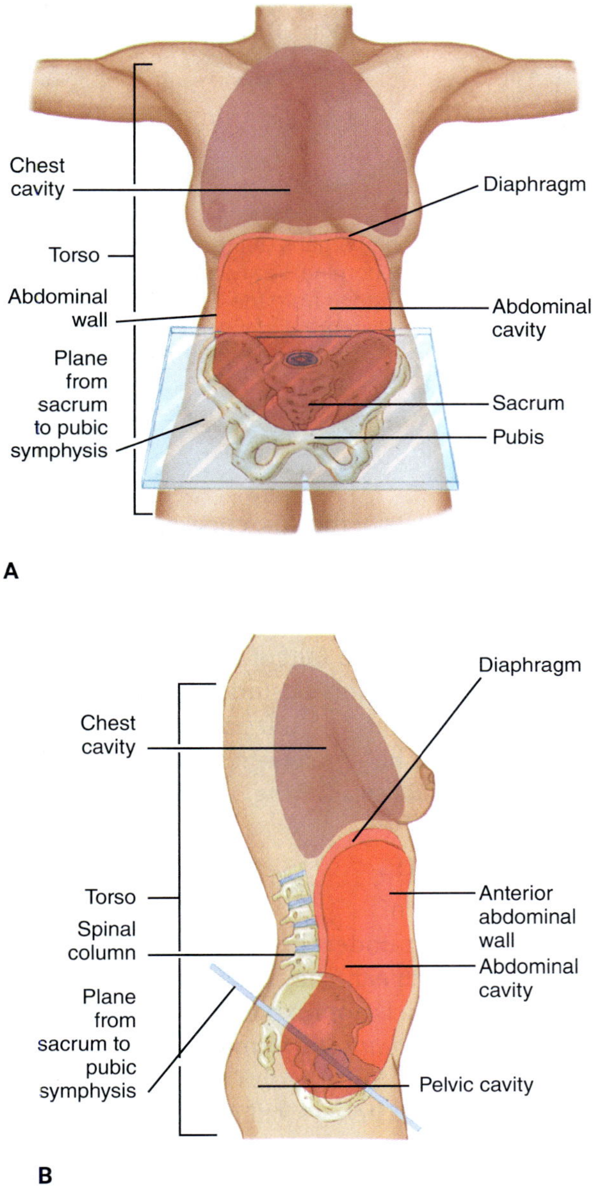

FIGURE 6-31 The boundaries of the abdomen are the anterior and posterior abdominal cavity walls, the diaphragm, and an imaginary plane from the pubic symphysis to the sacrum. The region below the plane is called the pelvic cavity. **A.** Anterior view. **B.** Lateral view.

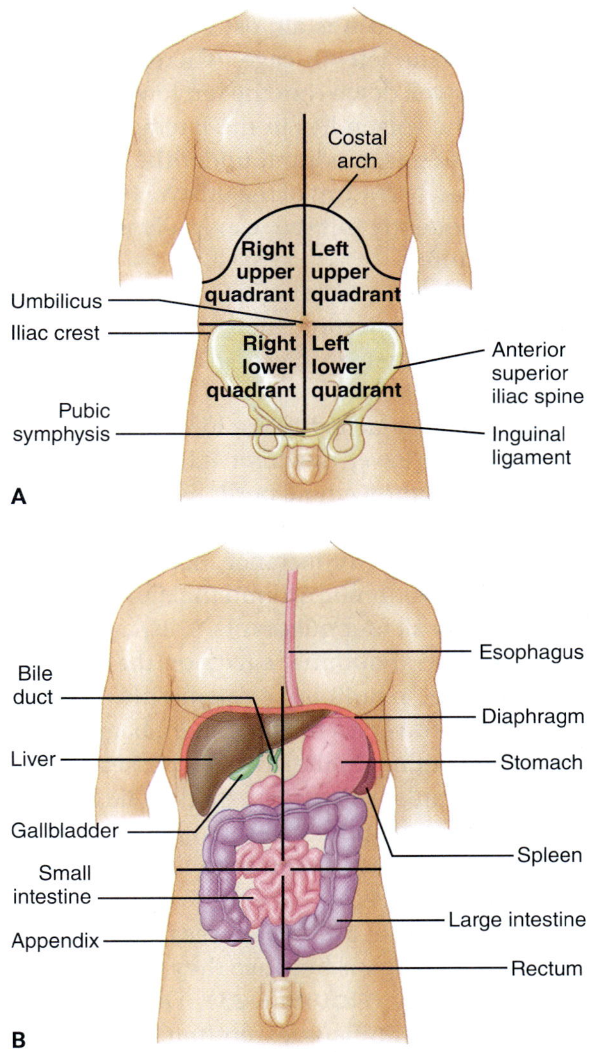

FIGURE 6-32 **A.** In the abdomen, quadrants are the easiest system for identifying areas. Major bony landmarks are also shown. **B.** Several of the organs in the abdomen lie in more than one quadrant.

you to identify injured or diseased organs that require emergency attention.

Organs and Vascular Structures

In the right upper quadrant (RUQ), the major organs are the liver, the gallbladder, and a portion of the colon. Most of the liver lies in this quadrant, almost entirely under the protection of the 8th to 12th ribs. The liver fills the entire anteroposterior depth of the abdomen in this quadrant. Therefore, the liver is at risk for injuries in this area.

In the left upper quadrant (LUQ), the major organs are the stomach, the spleen, and a portion of the colon. The spleen is almost entirely under the protection of the left rib cage, whereas the stomach may sag well down into the left lower quadrant when full. The spleen lies in the lateral and posterior portion of this quadrant, under the diaphragm and immediately in front of the 9th to 11th ribs. The spleen is frequently injured, especially when these ribs are fractured.

The right lower quadrant (RLQ) contains two portions of the large intestine: the **cecum**, the first portion into which the small intestine (ileum) opens, and the ascending colon. The **appendix** is a small, tubular structure that is attached to the lower border of the cecum. The left lower quadrant (LLQ) contains the descending and the sigmoid portions of the colon.

Several organs lie in more than one quadrant. The small intestine, for instance, occupies the central part of the abdomen around the umbilicus, and parts of it lie in all four quadrants. The pancreas lies just behind the abdominal cavity on the posterior abdominal wall in both upper quadrants. The large intestine also traverses the abdomen, beginning in the RLQ and ending in the LLQ as it passes through all four quadrants. The urinary bladder lies just behind the pubic symphysis in the middle of the abdomen and, therefore, lies in both lower quadrants and also in the pelvis.

The kidneys and pancreas are called **retroperitoneal** organs because they lie behind the abdominal cavity (**FIGURE 6-33**). They are above the level of the umbilicus, extending from the 11th rib to the 3rd lumbar vertebra on each side. The kidneys are approximately 5 inches (13 cm) long and lie just anterior to the costovertebral angle, which is the junction between the posterior aspect of the lower portion of the rib cage and the spine.

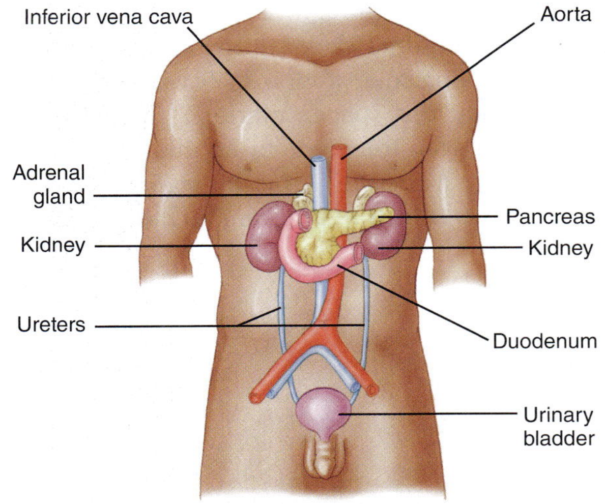

FIGURE 6-33 The major organs of the retroperitoneal space lie behind the abdominal cavity, above the level of the umbilicus, and extend from the 11th rib to the 3rd lumbar vertebra. The bladder, inferior vena cava, and aorta also lie in this space.

Mouth

The mouth consists of the lips, cheeks, gums, teeth, and tongue. A mucous membrane lines the mouth. The roof of the mouth is formed by the hard and soft palates. The hard palate is a bony plate lying anteriorly; the soft palate is a fold of mucous membrane and muscle that extends posteriorly from the hard palate into the throat. The soft palate is designed to hold food that is being chewed within the mouth and to help initiate swallowing.

Salivary Glands

There are two sets of **salivary glands**, one set on each side of the mouth under the tongue, and the other set in front of each ear. They produce 0.5 to 1.5 L of saliva daily.[5] Saliva is approximately 98% water. The remaining 2% is composed of mucus, salts, and organic compounds. Saliva serves as a binder for the chewed food that is being swallowed and as a lubricant within the mouth. Saliva also contains certain digestive enzymes.

Oropharynx

The **oropharynx** is a tubular structure that extends vertically from the back of the mouth to the esophagus and trachea. An automatic movement of the pharynx during swallowing lifts the larynx to permit the epiglottis to close over it so that liquids and solids are moved into the esophagus and away from the trachea.

Esophagus

The **esophagus** is a collapsible tube about 10 inches (25 cm) long that extends from the end of the pharynx to the stomach and lies just anterior to the spinal column in the chest. Contractions of the muscle in the wall of the esophagus propel food through it to the stomach. Liquids pass with very little assistance.

Stomach

The stomach is a hollow organ located in the left upper quadrant of the abdominal cavity, largely protected by the lower left ribs. Muscular contractions in the wall of the stomach and gastric juice, which contains a lot of mucus, convert ingested food to a thoroughly mixed semisolid mass, called **chyme**. The stomach produces approximately 1.5 L of gastric juice daily for this process. The primary function of the stomach is to receive food in large quantities intermittently, store it, and provide for its movement into the small bowel in regular, small amounts. In 1 to 3 hours, the semisolid food mass derived from one meal is propelled by muscular contraction into the duodenum, the first part of the small intestine.

Pancreas

The **pancreas**, a flat, solid organ, lies below and behind the liver and stomach and behind the peritoneum. It is firmly fixed in position, deep within the abdomen, and is not easily damaged. It contains two kinds of glands, and the two portions of the pancreas are intertwined. One portion is exocrine, and it secretes nearly 2 L of pancreatic juice daily. This juice contains many enzymes that aid in the digestion of fat, starch, and protein. Pancreatic juice flows directly into the duodenum through the pancreatic ducts. The other portion of the gland, the islets of Langerhans, is endocrine. These islets are where insulin and glucagon (hormones) are produced. Insulin and glucagon regulate the amount of glucose in the blood.

Liver

The **liver** is a large, solid organ that takes up most of the area immediately beneath the diaphragm in the right upper quadrant and also extends into the left upper quadrant. It is the largest solid organ in the abdomen and has several functions. Poisonous substances produced by digestion are brought to the liver and rendered harmless. Factors that are necessary for blood clotting and for the production of normal plasma are formed here. Between 0.5 and 1 L of bile is made by the liver daily to assist in the normal digestion of fat. The liver is the primary organ for the storage of sugar or starch for immediate

YOU are the EMT

Your partner obtains and records the patient's vital signs and then gives him supplemental oxygen while you complete your assessment. The patient tells you he has a history of gallbladder problems. Based on your assessment and the patient's medical history, you suspect that the gallbladder is the origin of his pain.

Recording Time: 2 Minutes	
Respirations	24 breaths/min; adequate depth
Pulse	110 beats/min; strong and regular
Skin	Baseline color, warm, and moist
Blood pressure	142/82 mm Hg
Oxygen saturation (Spo_2)	98% on oxygen

4. What additional symptoms would you expect the patient to experience based on the function of the gallbladder?

use by the body for energy. It also produces many of the factors that aid in the proper regulation of immune responses. The liver is fragile and, because of its size, relatively easily injured. Blood flow in the liver is high, because all of the blood that is pumped to the gastrointestinal tract passes into the liver, through the portal vein, before it returns to the heart. In addition, the liver has a generous arterial blood supply of its own. Ordinarily, approximately 25% of the cardiac output of blood (1.5 L) passes through the liver each minute.

Bile Ducts

The liver connects with the intestine by way of the **bile ducts**. The **gallbladder** is a small pouch extending from the bile ducts that serves as a reservoir and concentrating organ for bile produced in the liver. Together, the bile ducts and the gallbladder form the biliary system. The gallbladder discharges stored and concentrated bile into the duodenum through the common bile duct. The presence of food in the duodenum triggers a contraction of the gallbladder to empty it. The gallbladder usually contains about 60 to 90 mL of bile.

Small Intestine

The **small intestine** is the major hollow organ of the abdomen. The cells lining the small intestine produce enzymes and mucus to aid in digestion. Enzymes from the pancreas and the small intestine carry out the final processes of digestion. More than 90% of the products of digestion (amino acids, fatty acids, and simple sugars), together with water, ingested vitamins, and minerals, are absorbed across the wall of the lower end of the small intestine into veins to be transported to the liver. The small intestine is composed of the duodenum, the jejunum, and the ileum. The duodenum, which is about 12 inches (30 cm) long, is the part of the small intestine that receives food from the stomach. Here, food is mixed with secretions from the pancreas and liver for further digestion. Bile, produced by the liver and stored in the gallbladder, is emptied as needed into the duodenum. Bile is green-black, but through changes during digestion, it gives feces its typical brown color. Its major function is in the digestion of fat. The jejunum and ileum together measure more than 20 feet (6 m) on average to make up the rest of the small intestine.

Large Intestine

The **large intestine**, another major hollow organ, consists of the cecum, the colon, and the rectum. About 5 feet (1.5 m) long, it encircles the outer border of the abdomen around the small bowel. The major function of the colon, the portion of the large intestine that extends from the cecum to the rectum, is to absorb the final 5% to 10% of digested food and water from the intestine to form solid stool, which is stored in the rectum and passed out of the body through the anus.

Appendix

Recall that the appendix is a tube that opens into the cecum (the first part of the large intestine) in the right lower quadrant of the abdomen. It is 3 to 4 inches (8 to 10 cm) long and may easily become obstructed and, as a result, inflamed and infected. Appendicitis, which is the term for this inflammation, is one of the major causes of severe abdominal distress.

Rectum

The lowermost end of the colon is the **rectum**. It is a large, hollow organ that is adapted to store quantities of feces until it is expelled. At its terminal end is the anus, a 2-inch (5-cm) canal lined with skin. The rectum and anus are supplied with a complex series of circular muscles, called **sphincters**, that control, voluntarily and automatically, the escape of liquids, gases, and solids from the digestive tract. **TABLE 6-10** provides a summary of the organs and functions of the digestive system.

The Digestive System: Physiology

Digestion of food, from the moment it is taken into the mouth until essential compounds are extracted and delivered by the circulatory system to nourish all cells in the body, is a complicated chemical process. In succession, different secretions, primarily **enzymes**, are added to the food by the salivary glands, the stomach, the liver, the pancreas, and the small intestine to convert the food into basic sugars, fatty acids, and amino acids. These basic products of digestion are carried across the wall of the intestine and transported through the

TABLE 6-10 Digestive Organs and Functions

Organ/Structure	Function
Mouth	Mechanically breaks down food; begins chemical breakdown with saliva
Esophagus	Moves food from the mouth to the stomach; muscular and vascular structure
Stomach	Performs mechanical and chemical breakdown of food: food in, chyme out
Small intestine: duodenum, jejunum, and ileum	Major site for chemical breakdown of food; major absorption of water, fats, proteins, carbohydrates, and vitamins
Large intestine	Water absorption; formation of feces; bacterial digestion of food
Anus/rectum	Last portion of large intestine; sphincter to control release of feces
Liver	Production of bile; assists with carbohydrate, protein, and fat metabolism of nutrients within the bloodstream; manufactures proteins for immune regulation and clotting; detoxification of blood; elimination of waste
Pancreas	**Exocrine**: produces enzymes for protein, carbohydrate, and fat breakdown within the duodenum **Endocrine**: produces insulin and glucagon
Gallbladder	Storage of bile

portal vein to the liver. In the liver, the products are processed further and stored or transported to the heart through veins draining the liver. The heart then pumps the blood with these nutrients throughout the arteries to the capillaries, where the nutrients pass through the capillary walls to nourish the body's individual cells.

In normal routine activity, without any food or fluid ingestion at all, between 8 and 10 L of fluid is secreted daily into the gastrointestinal tract. This fluid comes from the salivary glands, stomach, liver, pancreas, and small intestine. In a healthy adult, about 7% of the body weight is delivered as fluid daily to the gastrointestinal tract. If significant vomiting or diarrhea occurs for more than 2 or 3 days, the person will experience a substantial alteration of body composition and become severely ill.

The Lymphatic System: Anatomy and Physiology

The lymphatic system includes the spleen, lymph nodes, lymph, lymph vessels, thymus gland, and other components. It supports both the circulatory system and the immune system. Unlike the circulatory system, the lymphatic system has no pump and relies on muscle contractions and movements of the body for lymph to flow.

Lymph is a thin, straw-colored fluid that transports materials from the lymph tissue into the central venous circulation via the thoracic ducts. Lymph vessels form a network throughout the body. **Lymph nodes** are located in various places along the lymph vessels in the body. These tiny, oval-shaped structures filter lymph.

Together with the circulatory system, the lymphatic system helps to rid the body of toxins and other harmful materials. The spleen also plays an important role in the body's immune function. It houses immune cells that help eliminate infectious agents.

The Endocrine System: Anatomy and Physiology

The brain controls the body through the nervous system using electrical impulses, and the endocrine system using hormones. The **endocrine system** is a complex message and control system that integrates many body functions. Endocrine glands release their hormones directly into the bloodstream (**FIGURE 6-34**). Epinephrine, norepinephrine, and

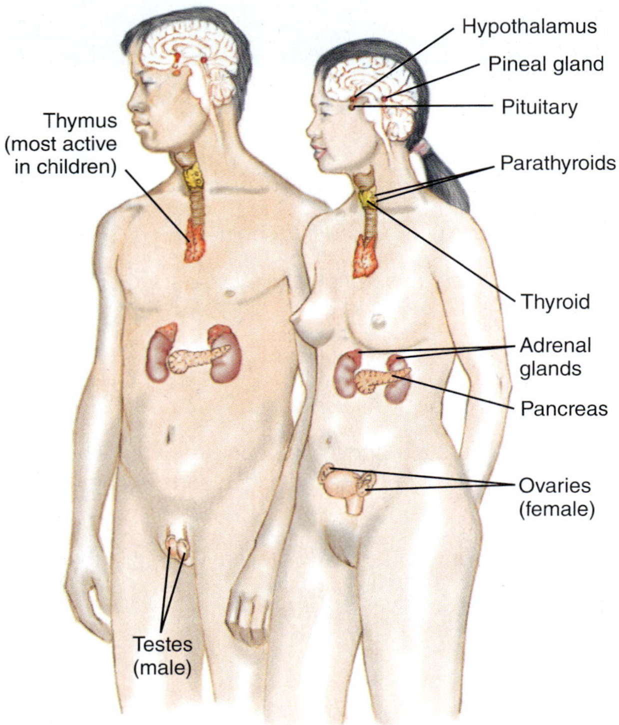

FIGURE 6-34 The endocrine system controls the production and release of hormones in the body.

insulin are examples of hormones. Each endocrine gland produces one or more hormones. Each hormone has a specific effect on some organ, tissue, or process (**TABLE 6-11**). The brain controls the release of hormones by the endocrine glands. **Hormones** can have a stimulating or an inhibiting effect on the body's organs and systems. For example, when you are frightened, your brain stimulates the adrenal gland through a hormone to release epinephrine and norepinephrine. This increases your blood pressure and heart rate. The resulting increase in blood pressure and heart rate decreases the amount of hormone released by the adrenal gland. The brain then reduces the amount of stimulation to the **adrenal glands**. Thus, a new steady state is achieved at heightened levels of alertness. This cycle is known as a feedback loop, and it helps keep the body's systems and functions in balance (**FIGURE 6-35**).

Excesses or deficiencies in hormone levels cause various endocrine diseases. One example is diabetes mellitus, an illness in which insulin production is deficient, causing a rise in blood glucose. If untreated, diabetes can lead to serious illness or death. See Chapter 20, *Endocrine and Hematologic Emergencies*, for further discussion.

TABLE 6-11 Endocrine Glands

Gland	Location	Function	Hormones Produced
Adrenal	Above the kidneys	Stress response, fight-or-flight reaction	Epinephrine, norepinephrine, cortisol, and others
Ovaries	Female pelvis (two glands)	Regulate sexual function, characteristics, and reproduction	Estrogen and others
Pancreas	Retroperitoneal space	Regulates glucose metabolism and other functions	Insulin, glucagon, and others
Parathyroid	Neck (behind and beside the thyroid) (three to five glands)	Regulates serum calcium	Parathyroid hormone
Pituitary	Base of skull	Regulates all other endocrine glands	Multiple, controls other endocrine glands
Testes	Male scrotum (two glands)	Regulate sexual function, characteristics, and reproduction	Testosterone and others
Thyroid	Neck (over the larynx)	Regulates metabolism	Thyroxine and others

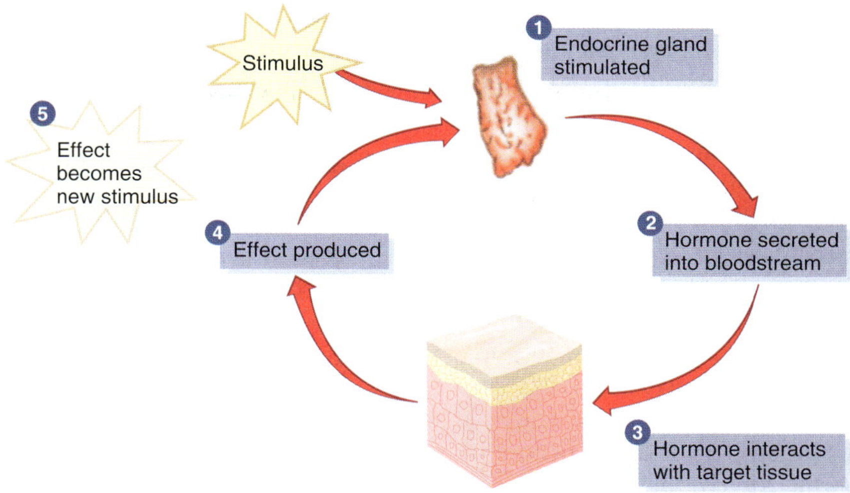

FIGURE 6-35 The endocrine system is tightly controlled with primary and secondary feedback loops to keep body systems in balance.

The Urinary System: Anatomy and Physiology

The **urinary system** controls the discharge of certain waste materials filtered from the blood by the kidneys. In the urinary system, the kidneys are solid organs; the ureters, bladder, and urethra are hollow organs. The main functions of the urinary system are (1) to control fluid balance in the body, (2) to filter and eliminate wastes, and (3) to control pH balance.

The body has two **kidneys** that lie on the posterior muscular wall of the abdomen behind the peritoneum in the retroperitoneal space. These organs rid the blood of toxic waste products and control its balance of water and salts. Blood flow in the kidneys is high. Nearly 20% of the output of blood from the heart passes through the kidneys each minute. Large vessels attach the kidneys directly to the aorta and the inferior vena cava. Waste products and water are constantly filtered from the blood to form urine.

YOU are the EMT

You prepare the patient for transport. He remains conscious and alert, but is still experiencing severe pain. Shortly after loading him into the ambulance and departing the scene, you perform a reassessment.

Recording Time: 12 Minutes	
Level of consciousness	Conscious and alert
Respirations	24 breaths/min; adequate depth
Pulse	112 beats/min; strong and regular
Skin	Baseline color, warm, and moist
Blood pressure	138/88 mm Hg
Oxygen saturation (Spo_2)	97% on oxygen

You allow the patient to assume a position of comfort, which seems to help with his pain. With an estimated time of arrival at the hospital of 10 minutes, you call in your radio report.

5. How does knowledge of anatomy, physiology, and medical terminology facilitate communication with other health care professionals?

The kidneys continuously concentrate this filtered urine by reabsorbing the water as it passes through a system of specialized tubes within them. The tubes finally unite to form the **renal pelvis**, a cone-shaped area within the kidney that collects urine and funnels it through the ureter into the bladder. Normally, each kidney drains its urine into one ureter through which the urine passes to the bladder.

A **ureter** passes from the renal pelvis of each kidney along the surface of the posterior abdominal wall behind the peritoneum to drain into the urinary bladder. The ureters are small (0.2 inch [0.5 cm] in diameter), hollow, muscular tubes. **Peristalsis**, a wavelike contraction of smooth muscle, occurs in these tubes to move the urine to the bladder.

The **urinary bladder** is located immediately behind the pubic symphysis in the pelvic cavity and is composed of smooth muscle with a specialized lining membrane. The two ureters enter posteriorly at its base on either side. The bladder empties to the outside of the body through the **urethra**. In a man, the urethra passes from the anterior base of the bladder through the penis. In a woman, the urethra opens in front of the vagina. A healthy adult forms 1.5 to 2 L of urine every day. This waste is extracted and concentrated from the 1,500 L of blood that circulates through the kidneys daily.

The Genital System: Anatomy and Physiology

The **genital system** controls the reproductive processes. The male genitalia, except for the **prostate gland** and the **seminal vesicles**, lie outside the pelvic cavity. The female genitalia, with the exception of the clitoris and labia, are contained entirely within the pelvis. The male and female reproductive organs have certain similarities and, of course, basic differences. They produce sperm and egg cells and reproductive hormones and play a significant role in sexual intercourse and reproduction.

The Male Reproductive System and Organs

The male reproductive system consists of the testicles, epididymis, vasa deferentia, prostate gland, seminal vesicles, and penis (**FIGURE 6-36**). Each

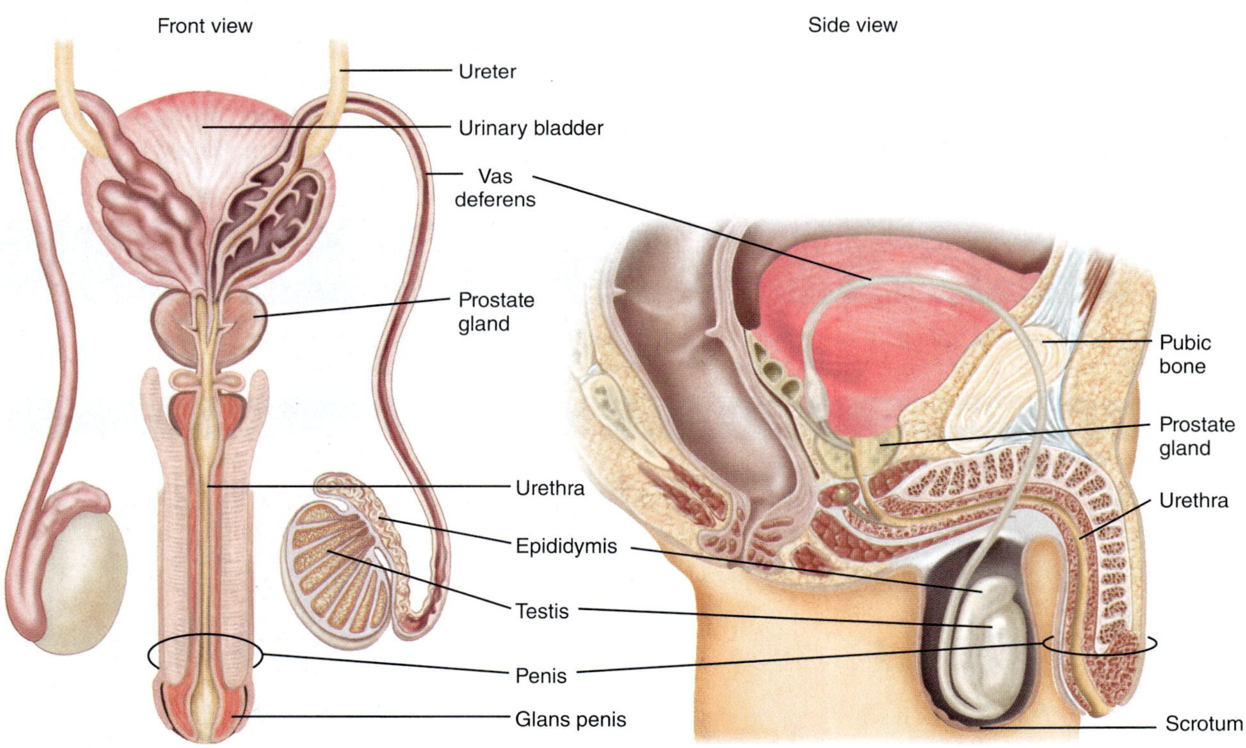

FIGURE 6-36 The male reproductive system consists of the testicles, epididymis, vasa deferentia, prostate gland, seminal vesicles, and penis.

testicle contains specialized cells and ducts; some of these produce male hormones, and others develop sperm. The hormones are absorbed directly into the bloodstream from the testicles. The sperm are immature and are moved from the testicles to the epididymis so they can develop. The sperm are carried through vasa deferentia (singular: vas deferens) to the seminal vesicles, where they are stored. During ejaculation, they are passed through the urethra.

The function of the reproductive system is to reproduce. Sperm are able to join with an egg to form an embryo. In addition to reproduction, this system is responsible for the production of sex hormones. Many of the physical characteristics of men, such as increased muscle mass, body hair, and deep voice, are attributed to the powerful effects of the hormones (chiefly testosterone) released by the testes. Finally, the penis, though part of the reproductive system, is also part of the urinary system. Any damage or infection to the penis can cause problems within the urinary bladder and/or the kidneys.

The Female Reproductive System and Organs

The female reproductive organs include the ovaries, fallopian tubes, uterus, cervix, and vagina (**FIGURE 6-37**). The **ovaries**, like the testicles, produce sex hormones and specialized cells for reproduction. The female sex hormones are absorbed directly into the bloodstream. A specialized ovum, or egg cell, matures and is released regularly during the adult woman's reproductive years. The ovaries release a mature egg approximately every 28 days. This egg travels through the fallopian tube, where fertilization normally occurs. The fallopian tubes exit into the uterus.

The **fallopian tubes** (sometimes called uterine tubes) connect with the uterus and carry the ovum into the cavity of this organ. The uterus is pear-shaped and hollow, with muscular walls. The narrow opening from the uterus to the vagina is the cervix. The **vagina** (birth canal) is a muscular, distensible tube that connects the uterus with the vulva (the external female genitalia). The vagina receives the penis during sexual intercourse, when **semen** is deposited in it. The sperm in the semen may pass through the uterus and fertilize an egg, typically in the fallopian tube, resulting in pregnancy. Should the pregnancy come to completion at about 40 weeks, the newborn will pass through the vagina and be born. The vagina also channels the menstrual flow from the uterus out of the body.

The functions of the female reproductive system are similar to those of the male reproductive system: reproduction and hormone balance.

Life Support Chain

To perform their job, the body's cells, tissues, and organs, regardless of their function, all depend on the reliable supply of oxygen and nutrients and the

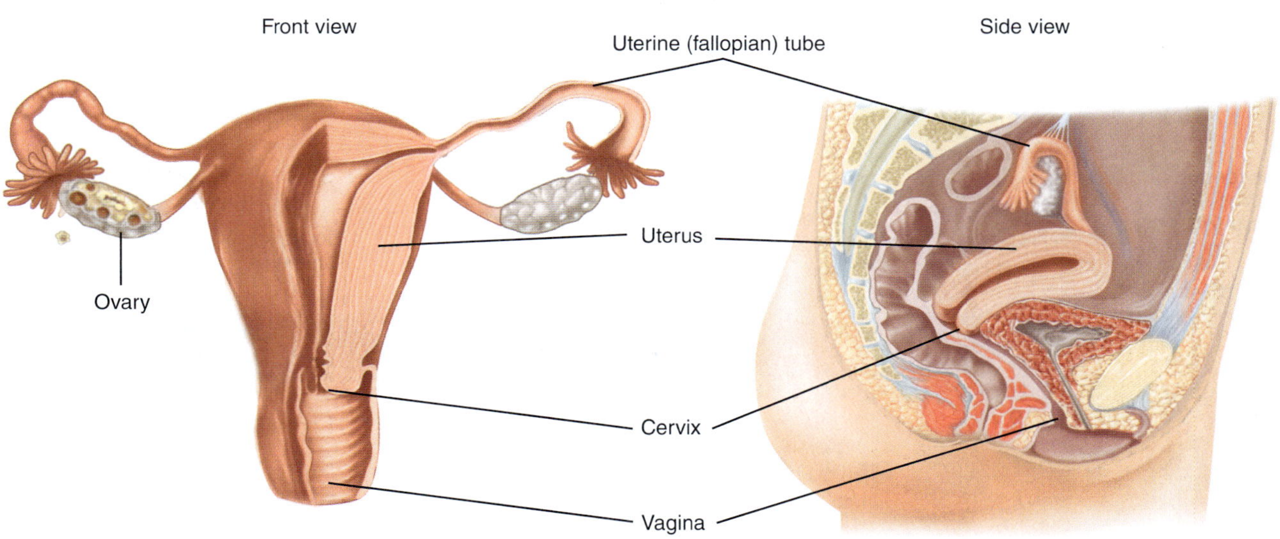

FIGURE 6-37 The female reproductive system consists of the ovaries, fallopian tubes, uterus, cervix, and vagina.

removal of wastes. Oxygen is brought to the cells via the respiratory and circulatory systems. Nutrients are derived from the food we eat after the digestive system breaks it down into, among other things, glucose. The circulatory system then delivers these supplies while picking up and carrying away wastes through the process of perfusion. If interference occurs in this delivery system, cells will become damaged or die.

Cells use oxygen to turn available nutrients into chemical energy through the biochemical process of **metabolism**. **Adenosine triphosphate (ATP)** is used in energy metabolism and storage. Cells create ATP, or energy, optimally when oxygen is present, referred to as **aerobic metabolism** (meaning "with air"), as doing so provides the cells with about 16 times more ATP than is possible without oxygen.[6] The waste products of aerobic metabolism are carbon dioxide and water.

In the absence of oxygen, most cells turn to a faster yet less efficient means of producing ATP called **anaerobic metabolism** (without air). The most well-known by-product of anaerobic metabolism is **lactic acid**. Most cells can tolerate anaerobic metabolism for longer than a few minutes. Some specialized cells (such as the heart and brain) are unable to survive without a constant supply of oxygen. Brain cells, for example, begin to die after only 4 to 6 minutes without oxygen.

As lactic acid and other wastes accumulate around the cells, the area becomes toxic. Cells subjected to this toxic waste may die. Given enough time and a large enough number of affected cells, tissues and even whole organs may fail.

The main force enabling all of this movement of materials, including oxygen, waste, and nutrients, is diffusion. Recall that when you breathe, oxygen moves from an area of higher concentration to one of lower concentration.

Words of Wisdom

Remember the key differences between aerobic and anaerobic metabolism:

- When cells function with oxygen, they use aerobic metabolism. They generate large amounts of ATP (cellular energy) and produce carbon dioxide and water as waste products.
- When cells function without oxygen, they use anaerobic metabolism. They generate small amounts of ATP (cellular energy) and produce lactic acid as waste.

Cells are surrounded by fluid that allows for easy movement of nutrients and wastes. A physical property of this fluid that is a critical factor for cell survival is pH, which is the measure of acidity or alkalinity in a solution. Solutions that are high in pH (>7.0) are considered alkaline. A common example is soap. Solutions that are low in pH (<7.0) are considered acidic. Sulfuric acid in automotive batteries is one example. A solution that is neither acidic nor alkaline is considered neutral (pH 7.0). The body's cells want to exist in a near-neutral environment (**FIGURE 6-38**).

Your body works to maintain a pH of 7.35 to 7.45, which is normal for the human body. Carbon

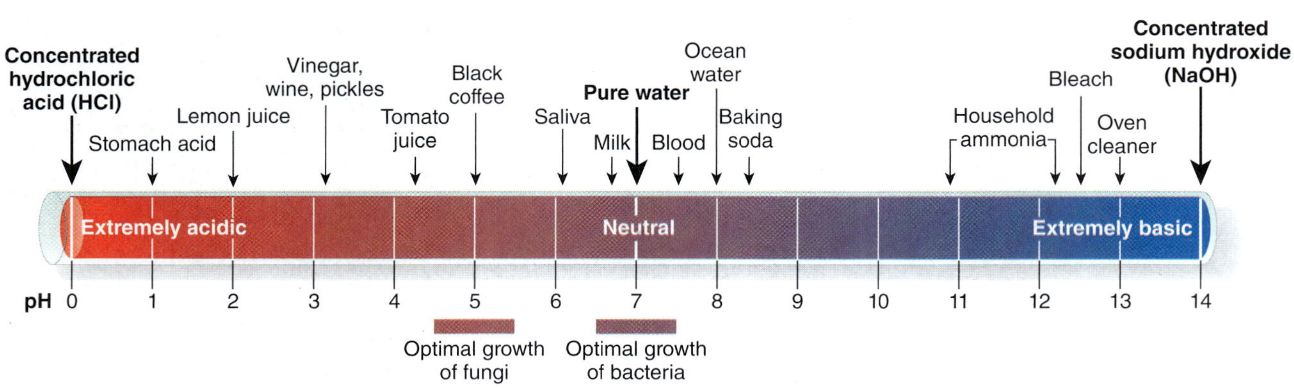

FIGURE 6-38 The human body is typically near neutral (approximately 7.4) on the pH scale.

dioxide, a waste product of metabolism, is transported by combining with water to create *carbonic acid*, which is more soluble in the plasma and less acidic than carbon dioxide would be alone. The plasma also contains sodium bicarbonate, which is alkaline and helps to buffer or neutralize the acidic waste products of cells to protect the blood vessels. The carbonic acid is transported to the lungs where it dissociates back into water and carbon dioxide and is exhaled.

The blood and lungs interact continuously to help maintain the pH level in the body by controlling the level of carbon dioxide, and therefore the level of carbonic acid, in the blood. If the blood becomes acidic, the respiratory centers in the brainstem will increase breathing to "blow off" more carbon dioxide. If too much carbon dioxide is blown off, then the body can become too alkaline, which is what happens during hyperventilation.

Pathophysiology

As mentioned previously, pathophysiology is the study of how normal physiologic processes are affected by disease. Many diseases can occur in patients and will result in calls to EMS. Some examples are diabetes (a disease of the pancreas), pneumonia (a disease of the lungs), and stroke (resulting from disease of the brain). Pathophysiologic changes that occur with specific diseases and trauma, respectively, are discussed in the chapters of Section 6, *Medical*, and Section 7, *Trauma*.

Respiratory compromise and shock are two common emergencies that you will likely encounter in your work as an EMT. This section provides an overview of respiratory compromise, shock, and alteration of cell metabolism as background for how the body responds to disease or injury.

Respiratory Compromise

Respiratory compromise is the inability of the body to move gas effectively, which can result in a decreased level of oxygen in the body (**hypoxia**), an elevated level of carbon dioxide in the body (**hypercapnia**), or both. Recall the two concepts of breathing: ventilation and respiration. Ventilation is the movement of air between the lungs and environment, whereas respiration is the process of gas exchange. Respiratory compromise results when one of these functions is impaired.

Factors That Impair Ventilation

The ability to move gas back and forth can be impaired in a variety of ways. A blocked airway is one example. Choking while eating will partially or completely block the movement of air through the trachea.

Impairment of the muscles of breathing will impair the movement of gas into and out of the lungs. Neuromuscular diseases, such as cerebral palsy, can interfere with the ability of the brain to send signals to the diaphragm. If a patient's level of consciousness is too low, ventilatory problems can occur. This means that any condition that results in a loss of consciousness can have a direct effect on ventilation.

Ventilation can also be impaired when the lower airway is obstructed, such as during an asthma attack. In asthma, contraction of smooth muscle in the bronchi in the lower airways prevents effective ventilation. Early in an asthma attack, hyperventilation results in a decrease in the amount of carbon dioxide in the blood. As the patient fatigues, the level of carbon dioxide increases.

Ventilation can also be impaired by numerous other factors, including drug overdose (which depresses the CNS), trauma to the chest wall, and allergic reactions. These emergencies are discussed further in their respective chapters.

Factors That Impair Respiration

Impairment of respiration (movement of gas at the cellular level) can also cause respiratory compromise.

Respiration can be impaired at high altitudes. At high altitudes, gas pressures change. The low atmospheric pressure of oxygen at high altitudes can impair oxygen movement into the blood.

Respiration can also become compromised when movement of the gas across the cell membrane is impaired. If the patient has fluid in the alveoli, this fluid may prevent or hinder gas exchange. In pneumonia, mucus and pus form a barrier, preventing gas from accessing the alveoli. If one of the blood vessels bringing blood to the lungs is clogged, this will also affect the amount of gas that diffuses into and out of the blood.

> **Words of Wisdom**
>
> There are two ways to express the amount of oxygen in the air: as a straight percentage or as a fraction of the inspired oxygen (FIO_2). FIO_2 is expressed as the decimal equivalent of the percentage of oxygen being delivered. Therefore, because oxygen makes up 21% of ambient room air, the FIO_2 of ambient room air is 0.21. The oxygen from a nonrebreathing mask at 15 L/min is approximately 95%; therefore, the FIO_2 of the air from a nonrebreathing mask at 15 L/min is approximately 0.9 to 0.95.

Ventilation/Perfusion Mismatch

One way to describe respiratory function, and therefore to understand respiratory compromise, is the ventilation/perfusion ratio, abbreviated **$\dot{V}/\dot{Q}$ ratio**. This concept describes how much gas is being moved effectively (ventilation) through the lungs and how much blood is flowing around the alveoli where gas exchange (perfusion) occurs. A mismatch occurs when one of those two variables is abnormal.

For example, in a patient with pulmonary embolism, a blood clot breaks off from a large vein and creates a sudden clog in one of the branches of the pulmonary arteries, preventing blood flow to the alveoli in part of the lung. A ventilated segment of that part of the lung does not receive blood, and therefore gas is not exchanged. This results in a ventilation/perfusion mismatch, expressed as a change in the $\dot{V}/\dot{Q}$ ratio.

Another example is edema caused by pulmonary contusion, in which gas is unable to move effectively through the alveoli in a portion of the lung. Due to fluid leak into bruised tissues in a portion of the lung, blood passing through that portion does not undergo air exchange because there is no ventilation occurring in that portion of the lung. Therefore the "V" portion of the $\dot{V}/\dot{Q}$ ratio is impacted.

When either the "V" or the "Q" is impacted, respiratory compromise can occur.

Effects of Respiratory Compromise on the Body

Regardless of the cause of impaired ventilation or respiration, the overall effect of respiratory compromise is the same.

- Oxygen levels throughout the body fall and carbon dioxide levels rise.
- The brain detects an increase in carbon dioxide levels.
- The body increases its respiratory rate to return the carbon dioxide levels to normal.
- If increased respiration does not occur or is not effective in returning the carbon dioxide levels to normal, the blood will become more acidic.
- Similarly, blood oxygen levels will begin to fall. This will cause the brain to issue further commands to breathe.

Decreased oxygen levels will force cells to move from aerobic metabolism to anaerobic metabolism. Remember, heart and brain cells cannot survive without a constant supply of oxygen and will die in minutes. Anaerobic metabolism generates a fraction of the needed energy, and cellular functions will be impaired. Recall that a by-product of anaerobic metabolism is lactic acid. If too much of this acid is created, the pH of the blood will drop further. If the pH becomes too low, cells will die (**TABLE 6-12**).

Shock

Recall that shock (systemic hypoperfusion) is a condition in which organs and tissues receive an inadequate supply of blood and oxygen; in other words, they are poorly perfused. It can occur due to inadequacy of the central circulation (insufficient blood volume, or a heart that does not pump effectively) or of the peripheral circulation (inability of the body to control the size of the blood vessels). Shock is categorized into several types depending on the cause. These types, as well as the body's compensatory mechanisms, are described in detail in Chapter 13, *Shock*.

Oxygen delivery is directly related to the concentration of red blood cells (and their hemoglobin concentration), the amount of oxygen being carried by the blood (oxygen saturation), and the pumping ability of the heart (cardiac output). Impairment in any one of these three areas will lead to impaired oxygen delivery and shock. Impaired oxygen delivery causes cellular hypoxia (decreased amount of oxygen delivered to the cells), which leads to anaerobic metabolism, lactic acid production, and organ dysfunction.

TABLE 6-12 Summary of Respiratory Compromise

Category	Problem	Effect
Ventilation	Damage to the regulatory centers of the brain	Erratic, absent, or slow breathing pattern and rate
	Inability to exhale effectively	Carbon dioxide builds up in blood
	Inability to inhale effectively	Oxygen levels in the blood decrease
	Injury to chest	Breathing depth decreases
	Obstruction of the airway	Decreased or absent movement of air
	Overdose/toxic exposure	Decreased level of consciousness leading to decreased breathing rate and depth
	Loss of consciousness	Breathing depth decreases
	Weakened respiratory muscles	Breathing depth decreases
Respiration	Fluid within the alveoli (pulmonary edema)	Prevents gas from entering the alveoli
	Mucus or infectious wastes	Prevent gas from entering the alveoli
	Impaired blood flow to the lungs (pulmonary embolism)	Affects blood flow to lung tissue where gas exchange occurs
Oxygenation	Decreased oxygen in the air breathed	Affects diffusion of gas
	Increased carbon dioxide in the air breathed	Affects diffusion of gas
	Toxins in the air breathed	Affect ability of oxygen to be carried effectively in blood

YOU are the EMT

Shortly before arriving at the hospital, you reassess the patient. He remains conscious and alert and tells you that his pain is less severe than before. After transferring patient care to the attending physician, you later learn that the patient had an inflamed gallbladder, which was surgically removed.

Recording Time: 20 Minutes	
Level of consciousness	Conscious and alert
Respirations	20 breaths/min; adequate depth
Pulse	90 beats/min; strong and regular
Skin	Baseline color, warm, and moist
Blood pressure	132/80 mm Hg
Oxygen saturation (Spo_2)	98% on oxygen

6. Should your documentation of an EMS call differ from your verbal communication with other health care professionals? Why or why not?

The effects of inadequate perfusion on the body are similar to those of respiratory compromise. The level of oxygen supplied to the tissues falls. This causes the cells to engage in anaerobic metabolism, which results in increased lactic acid production. A severe metabolic acidosis ensues, leading to increased levels of carbonic acid within the blood. Patients who can compensate increase their breathing rate and depth, thereby increasing their minute volume.

Baroreceptors detect the decreased blood pressure and initiate the release of epinephrine and norepinephrine. The heart rate will increase, the heart will beat more forcefully, and the blood vessels will constrict. The body's goal is to maintain blood pressure to the areas of the body that are unable to survive without oxygen: the brain and the heart.

Another compensatory mechanism is the movement of fluid outside of the cells and outside of the blood vessels (interstitial fluid) into the capillaries. This helps refill the blood vessels and restore some fluid volume so the heart has enough liquid to pump.

Ultimately the effect of all types of shock is decreased availability of fuel for the cells and impairment of cellular metabolism. Once a certain level of tissue hypoperfusion is reached, cell damage proceeds in a similar manner regardless of the underlying cause of the shock.

Alteration of Cellular Metabolism

Impairment of **cellular metabolism** results in the inability to properly use oxygen and glucose at the cellular level.

As discussed, when there is poor perfusion of oxygenated blood or inadequate oxygen, cells will create energy through anaerobic metabolism. Anaerobic metabolism serves as a temporary backup system to allow cells to function at low energy levels for a short time. Most cells are able to function to help bridge the gap until their normal oxygen supply is restored.

However, anaerobic metabolism has some important drawbacks. Recall that metabolism without sufficient oxygen results in a buildup of lactic acid, which ultimately can result in metabolic acidosis. The acidity resulting from anaerobic metabolism decreases hemoglobin's ability to bind to oxygen, thus reducing the amount of oxygen carried to the cells. The process of anaerobic metabolism also produces less energy in the form of ATP, making it difficult for cells to function normally, and eventually resulting in cellular injury.

Cellular injury may, up to a point, be repairable if normal tissue perfusion is restored. When irreversible injury occurs, however, no treatment will help. Cell death is followed by necrosis, a process in which the cell breaks down. The cell membrane becomes abnormally permeable, leading to an influx of electrolytes and fluids. The cell and its components (organelles) swell and are ultimately destroyed, resulting in cell death.

Therefore, when perfusion is ineffective, it needs to be restored so that cells can return to a state of aerobic metabolism and life can continue. Many interventions you will perform as an EMT are aimed at improving conditions that can result in impaired perfusion.

YOU are the EMT SUMMARY

1. How will knowledge of anatomy and physiology help you provide appropriate patient care?

Knowledge of anatomy and physiology is important for anyone who provides patient care, emergency or otherwise. When a patient reports pain to any part of the body, your knowledge of human anatomy will help you form a logical field impression (that is, what you believe to be the primary problem) regarding which organ or organs may be affected. Your knowledge of physiology will also help you predict the negative effects the patient may experience based on the organ or organs affected. From this information, an appropriate treatment plan can be formulated and implemented.

Although you are not expected to diagnose a patient's condition, a strong fundamental knowledge of anatomy, physiology, and medical terminology will help you communicate the correct information to the emergency department physician or nurse.

2. On the sole basis of the patient's chief complaint, which organs should you suspect are the cause of his condition?

The major organs in the right upper quadrant (RUQ) are the liver, gallbladder, and a portion of the large intestine (colon). Although your initial thoughts should focus on dysfunction of one or more of

YOU are the EMT SUMMARY continued

these organs, the patient's true problem may exist elsewhere in his abdomen and the pain just happens to be manifesting in his RUQ. Although your objectives are to recognize that the patient has an acute abdominal problem and to find and treat life-threatening conditions, you will need to ask additional questions to clarify his complaint. His answers to your questions will help you formulate a field impression.

3. What additional questions should you ask to gather more information about his chief complaint?

After determining why the patient called 9-1-1, ask the patient to elaborate on the complaint; this is called the history of present illness. The OPQRST mnemonic is a useful tool for this purpose.

The patient has already told you that his pain began suddenly 20 minutes ago, so the "O" and "T" in the OPQRST have been established. Ask him if anything makes his pain better or worse; patients with abdominal pain often draw their knees into their abdomen to take pressure off the abdominal muscles, which may provide them with slight relief from their pain. Ask the patient if the pain stays in the RUQ of his abdomen or moves/travels somewhere else; determine if he has referred pain by asking if he hurts anywhere else in addition to his RUQ. Assess the severity of his pain by using a 0 to 10 scale, with 0 being no pain and 10 being the worst pain ever experienced. Pain severity should be assessed frequently, especially after any interventions have been performed. Although chronic pain can indicate a serious underlying problem, you should be especially concerned that his pain began acutely.

Other questions to ask the patient should focus on common symptoms associated with abdominal pain, such as nausea and/or vomiting, diarrhea, and urinary difficulty, among others. When possible, try not to ask leading questions (ie, "Are you nauseated?"); instead, simply ask him if he has any other symptoms.

4. What additional symptoms would you expect the patient to experience based on the function of the gallbladder?

The gallbladder contracts only when food enters the duodenum; patients with inflammation of the gallbladder (cholecystitis) typically have pain in the RUQ within 1 hour or so after eating a meal. In many cases, the patient also reports referred pain to the right shoulder. Other symptoms of gallbladder disease include nausea, vomiting, and heartburn.

Most cases of cholecystitis occur when gallstones form and block the outlet of the gallbladder. In some cases, the gallstones spontaneously pass; however, if they do not, the patient experiences pain of varying intensity.

5. How does knowledge of anatomy, physiology, and medical terminology facilitate communication with other health care professionals?

As part of the health care team, everything you do should benefit the patient. An integral part of patient care is effective communication with other health care professionals. Your ability to speak the language of medicine will minimize communication barriers between you and other members of the health care team and therefore will directly benefit your patient.

Whether you are calling in your radio report from the ambulance or giving a verbal report at the hospital, the use of appropriate medical terminology ensures that the information you pass along is relevant and accurate.

Review human anatomy and physiology and medical terminology on a regular basis. Although the structure and function of the body and the terms used to describe it do not change, your ability to recall the information can deteriorate over time.

6. Should your documentation of an EMS call differ from your verbal communication with other health care professionals? Why or why not?

In general, your verbal communication and the patient care report (PCR) should reflect the same relevant and accurate information, although you may expand on some of the details in your written report. For example, a verbal report will likely only indicate one set of vital signs or any significant changes in the vital signs, whereas your PCR will usually have several sets of vital signs.

Similarly, your written report may expand on the list of medications or contain data on time that would not be included in a verbal report. However, both reports should contain any significant information about the patient, his condition, symptoms and history, treatments given, and any changes during the call. When possible, use proper medical terminology when documenting the patient's complaint, history of present illness, medical history, and any treatment provided in the prehospital setting. If you are unsure of the correct medical term

YOU are the EMT SUMMARY continued

to accurately describe a particular aspect of the patient's complaint or physical examination, use plain English.

The PCR is read by the personnel who assume patient care from you and may have a direct effect on future care that the patient receives. It also becomes part of the patient's permanent medical record. The use of proper medical terminology, coupled with an accurate depiction of the care you provided, will facilitate continuity of the patient's care.

Prep Kit

Ready for Review

- To properly care for your patients, you must have a thorough understanding of human anatomy and physiology so you can assess your patients' condition and communicate with hospital personnel and other health care clinicians.
- You must be able to identify superficial landmarks of the body and know what lies underneath the skin so that you can perform an accurate patient assessment.
- The skeleton gives the body its recognizable human form through a collection of bones, ligaments, tendons, and cartilage.
- The skeletal system provides protection for fragile organs, allows for movement, and gives the body its shape.
- The contraction and relaxation of the musculoskeletal system gives the body its ability to move.
- The respiratory system consists of all the structures of the body that contribute to the process of breathing. It includes the nose, mouth, throat, larynx, trachea, bronchi, and bronchioles.
- The function of the respiratory system is to provide the body with oxygen and eliminate carbon dioxide.
- The circulatory system is a complex arrangement of connected tubes, including the arteries, arterioles, capillaries, venules, and veins.
- The nervous system is perhaps the most complex organ system within the human body. It consists of the brain, spinal cord, and nerves.
- The skin is divided into two parts: the superficial epidermis, which is composed of several layers of cells, and the deeper dermis, which contains the specialized skin structures.
- The skin, the largest single organ in the body, has multiple functions, chiefly to protect the body in the environment, to regulate the temperature of the body, and to transmit information from the environment to the brain.
- The digestive system is composed of the gastrointestinal tract (stomach and intestines), mouth, salivary glands, pharynx, esophagus, liver, gallbladder, pancreas, rectum, and anus.
- Digestion of food, from the moment it is taken into the mouth until essential compounds are extracted and delivered by the circulatory system to nourish all cells in the body, is a complicated chemical process.
- The lymphatic system is composed of the spleen, lymph nodes, lymph, lymph vessels, thymus gland, and other components. It supports the circulatory system and the immune system, and relies on muscle contractions and movements of the body for lymph to flow.
- The endocrine system is a complex message and control system that integrates many body functions.
- The urinary system controls the discharge of certain waste materials filtered from the blood by the kidneys.

Prep Kit continued

- The genital system controls the reproductive processes by which life is created.
- Solutions that have a high pH level (>7.0) are considered alkaline. Solutions that have a low pH level (<7.0) are considered acidic. A solution that is neither acidic nor alkaline is considered neutral (pH 7.0). Normal body pH is 7.35 to 7.45.
- Pathophysiology is the study of how normal physiologic processes are affected by disease.
- Respiratory compromise is the inability of the body to move gas effectively. Respiratory compromise results when either ventilation or respiration is impaired.
- Shock is a condition in which organs and tissue receive an inadequate flow of blood and oxygen, or perfusion. Impaired oxygen delivery causes cellular hypoxia, which in turn leads to anaerobic metabolism, lactic acid production, and organ dysfunction.
- Impairment of cellular metabolism results in the inability to properly use oxygen and glucose at the cellular level. When irreversible cellular injury occurs, no treatment will help. Therefore, when perfusion is ineffective, it needs to be restored quickly.

Vital Vocabulary

abdomen The body cavity that contains many of the major organs of digestion and excretion. It is located below the diaphragm and above the pelvis.

acetabulum The depression on the lateral pelvis where its three component bones join, in which the femoral head fits snugly.

adenosine triphosphate (ATP) The nucleotide involved in energy metabolism; used to store energy.

adrenal glands Endocrine glands located on top of the kidneys that release adrenaline when stimulated by the sympathetic nervous system.

adrenergic Pertaining to nerves that release the neurotransmitter norepinephrine, or noradrenaline (eg, adrenergic nerves, adrenergic response); also pertains to the receptors acted on by norepinephrine.

aerobic metabolism Metabolism that can proceed only in the presence of oxygen.

alpha-adrenergic receptors Portions of the nervous system that, when stimulated, can cause constriction of blood vessels.

alveoli The air sacs of the lungs in which the exchange of oxygen and carbon dioxide takes place.

anaerobic metabolism Metabolism that takes place in the absence of oxygen; the main by-product is lactic acid.

anatomic position The position of reference in which the patient stands facing forward, arms at the side, with the palms of the hands forward.

anatomy The study of the physical structure of the body and its components.

aorta The main artery leaving the left side of the heart and carrying freshly oxygenated blood to the body.

appendicular skeleton The portion of the skeletal system that comprises the arms, legs, pelvis, and shoulder girdle.

appendix A small, tubular structure that is attached to the lower border of the cecum in the lower right quadrant of the abdomen.

arterioles The smallest branches of arteries leading to the vast network of capillaries.

articular cartilage A pearly layer of specialized cartilage covering the articular surfaces (contact surfaces on the ends) of bones in synovial joints.

atrium One of the two upper chambers of the heart.

autonomic nervous system The part of the nervous system that regulates functions, such as

Prep Kit continued

digestion and sweating, that are not controlled voluntarily.

axial skeleton The part of the skeleton comprising the skull, vertebral column, and rib cage.

axons Extensions of a neuron that carry impulses away from the nerve cell body to the dendrites (receivers) of another neuron.

ball-and-socket joints Joints that allow internal and external rotation, as well as bending.

beta-adrenergic receptors Portions of the nervous system that, when stimulated, can cause an increase in the force of contraction of the heart, an increased heart rate, and bronchial dilation.

biceps The large muscle that covers the front of the humerus.

bile ducts The ducts that convey bile between the liver and the intestine.

blood pressure (BP) The pressure that the blood exerts against the walls of the arteries as it passes through them.

brachial artery The major vessel in the upper extremities that supplies blood to the arm.

brain The controlling organ of the body and center of consciousness; functions include perception, control of reactions to the environment, emotional responses, and judgment.

brainstem The area of the brain between the spinal cord and cerebrum, surrounded by the cerebellum; controls functions that are necessary for life, such as respiration.

bronchi Hollow airway passages that branch to the right and left from the trachea and divide into smaller bronchioles.

bronchioles Small branches of bronchi that terminate at alveoli.

calcaneus A large bone that forms the heel of the foot; also called the heel bone.

capillary vessels The tiny blood vessels between the arterioles and venules that permit transfer of oxygen, carbon dioxide, nutrients, and waste between body tissues and the blood.

cardiac muscle The heart muscle.

cardiac output (CO) A measure of the volume of blood circulated by the heart in 1 minute, calculated by multiplying the stroke volume by the heart rate.

carina The structure at which the trachea divides into the left and right main stem bronchi.

carotid artery The major artery that supplies blood to the head and brain.

carpals Small bones that compose the wrist.

cartilage The smooth connective tissue that forms the support structure of the skeletal system and provides cushioning between bones; also forms the nasal septum and portions of the outer ear.

cecum The first part of the large intestine, into which the ileum opens.

cells The fundamental units of the human body.

cellular metabolism A set of chemical reactions that supplies cells with energy. Includes both anaerobic and aerobic metabolism.

central nervous system (CNS) The brain and spinal cord.

cerebellum One of the three major subdivisions of the brain, sometimes called the little brain; coordinates the various activities of the brain, particularly fine body movements.

cerebrospinal fluid (CSF) Fluid produced in the ventricles of the brain that flows in the subarachnoid space and bathes the meninges.

cerebrum The largest part of the three subdivisions of the brain, sometimes called the gray matter; made up of several lobes that control movement, hearing, balance, speech, visual perception, emotions, and personality.

cervical spine The portion of the vertebral column consisting of the first seven vertebrae that lie in the neck.

chordae tendineae Thin bands of fibrous tissue that attach to the valves in the heart and prevent them from inverting.

Prep Kit continued

chyme The substance that leaves the stomach. It is a combination of all of the eaten foods with added stomach acids.

circulatory system The complex arrangement of connected tubes, including the arteries, arterioles, capillaries, venules, and veins, that moves blood, oxygen, nutrients, carbon dioxide, and cellular waste throughout the body.

clavicle The collarbone; it is lateral to the sternum and anterior to the scapula.

coccyx The last three or four vertebrae of the spine; the tail bone.

coronal (frontal) plane An imaginary plane where the body is divided into front and back parts.

coxae The hip bones (singular: coxa).

cranium The part of the skull that encloses the brain and is composed of eight bones.

cricoid cartilage A firm ridge of cartilage that forms the lower part of the larynx.

cricothyroid membrane A thin sheet of fascia that connects the thyroid and cricoid cartilages that make up the larynx.

dead space Any portion of the airway that does contain air and cannot participate in gas exchange, such as the trachea and bronchi.

dermis The inner layer of the skin, containing hair follicles, sweat glands, nerve endings, and blood vessels.

diaphragm A muscular dome that forms the undersurface of the thorax, separating the chest from the abdominal cavity. Contraction of the diaphragm (and the chest wall muscles) brings air into the lungs. Relaxation allows air to be expelled from the lungs.

diastole The relaxation, or period of relaxation, of the heart, especially of the ventricles.

diffusion Movement of a gas from an area of higher concentration to an area of lower concentration.

digestion The processing of food that nourishes the individual cells of the body.

dorsalis pedis artery The artery on the anterior surface of the foot between the first and second metatarsals.

endocrine A type of pancreatic gland that produces insulin and glucagon.

endocrine system The complex message and control system that integrates many body functions, including the release of hormones.

enzymes Substances designed to speed up the rate of specific biochemical reactions.

epidermis The outer layer of skin, which is made up of cells that are sealed together to form a watertight protective covering for the body.

epiglottis A thin, leaf-shaped valve that allows air to pass into the trachea but prevents food and liquid from entering.

epinephrine A hormone produced by the body (commonly called adrenaline) and a drug produced by pharmaceutical companies that increases pulse rate and blood pressure; the drug of choice for an anaphylactic reaction.

esophagus A collapsible tube that extends from the pharynx to the stomach; muscle contractions propel food and liquids through it to the stomach.

ethmoid bone A bone in the skull that separates the nasal cavity from the brain.

exocrine A type of gland, such as those in the pancreas, that produces enzymes for protein, carbohydrate, and fat breakdown within the duodenum.

expiratory reserve volume The amount of air that can be exhaled following a normal exhalation.

extension The straightening of a joint.

fallopian tubes The tubes that connect each ovary with the uterus and are the primary location for fertilization of the ovum.

femoral artery The major artery of the thigh, a continuation of the external iliac artery. It supplies blood to the lower abdominal wall, external genitalia, and legs. It can be palpated in the groin area.

Prep Kit continued

femoral head The proximal end of the femur, articulating with the acetabulum to form the hip joint.

femur The thighbone; the longest and one of the strongest bones in the body.

fibula The smaller of the two bones that form the lower leg, located on the lateral side.

flexion The bending of a joint.

fontanelles Areas where the newborn's or infant's skull has not fused together; usually disappear by approximately 18 months of age.

foramen magnum A large opening at the base of the skull through which the brain connects to the spinal cord.

frontal bones The bones of the cranium that form the forehead.

frontal lobe The brain area primarily responsible for personality, judgment, planning, problem solving, concentration, and self-awareness.

gallbladder A sac on the undersurface of the liver that collects bile from the liver and discharges it into the duodenum through the common bile duct.

genital system The reproductive system in men and women.

germinal layer The deepest layer of the epidermis where new skin cells are formed.

greater trochanter A bony prominence on the proximal lateral side of the thigh, just below the hip joint.

great vessels The collective term for the venae cavae, aorta, and pulmonary arteries and veins.

hair follicles The small organs that produce hair.

heart A hollow muscular organ that pumps blood throughout the body.

heart rate (HR) The number of heartbeats during a specific time (usually 1 minute).

hemoglobin An oxygen-carrying protein found in red blood cells.

hinge joints Joints that can bend and straighten but cannot rotate; they restrict motion to one plane.

hormones Substances formed in specialized organs or glands and carried to another organ or group of cells in the same organism; they regulate many body functions, including metabolism, growth, and body temperature.

humerus The supporting bone of the upper arm.

hydrostatic pressure The pressure that a fluid exerts against the walls of its container.

hypercapnia An abnormally high level of carbon dioxide in the bloodstream.

hypoperfusion A condition in which the circulatory system fails to provide sufficient circulation to maintain normal cellular function; also called shock.

hypoxia Deficient oxygen concentration in the tissues.

hypoxic drive A "backup system" to control respiration; senses drops in the oxygen level in the blood.

ilium One of three bones that fuse to form the pelvic ring.

inferior vena cava One of the two largest veins in the body; carries blood from the lower extremities and the pelvis and the abdominal organs to the heart.

inspiratory reserve volume The amount of air that can be inhaled after a normal inhalation; the amount of air that can be inhaled in addition to the normal tidal volume.

interstitial space The space in between the cells.

intervertebral disks Tough, elastic structures between adjoining vertebrae that act as shock absorbers.

intracellular space The space within a cell or cells.

involuntary muscle Muscle over which a person has no conscious control. It is found in many automatic regulating systems of the body.

Prep Kit continued

ischium One of three bones that fuse to form the pelvic ring.

joint The place where two bones come into contact; also called an articulation.

joint capsule The fibrous sac that encloses a joint.

kidneys Two retroperitoneal organs that excrete the end products of metabolism as urine and regulate the body's salt and water content.

lactic acid A metabolic by-product of the breakdown of glucose that accumulates when metabolism proceeds in the absence of oxygen (anaerobic metabolism).

large intestine The portion of the digestive tube that encircles the abdomen around the small bowel, consisting of the cecum, the colon, and the rectum. It helps regulate water balance and eliminate solid waste.

lesser trochanter The projection on the medial/superior portion of the femur.

ligaments Bands of fibrous tissue that connect bones to bones. Ligaments support and strengthen a joint.

liver A large, solid organ that lies in the right upper quadrant immediately below the diaphragm; it produces bile, stores glucose for immediate use by the body, and produces many substances that help regulate immune responses.

lumbar spine The lower part of the back, formed by the lowest five nonfused vertebrae; also called the dorsal spine.

lymph A thin, straw-colored fluid that carries oxygen, nutrients, and hormones to the cells and carries waste products of metabolism away from the cells and back into the capillaries so that they may be excreted.

lymph nodes Tiny, oval-shaped structures located in various places along the lymph vessels that filter lymph.

malleolus A rounded bony prominence on either side of the ankle; also called the ankle bone.

mandible The bone of the lower jaw.

manubrium The upper quarter of the sternum.

maxillae The upper jawbones that assist in the formation of the orbit, the nasal cavity, and the palate and hold the upper teeth.

medulla oblongata Nerve tissue that is continuous inferiorly with the spinal cord; serves as a conduction pathway for ascending and descending nerve tracts; coordinates heart rate, blood vessel diameter, breathing, swallowing, vomiting, coughing, and sneezing.

metabolism The biochemical processes that result in production of energy from nutrients within cells.

metacarpals Bones of the hand, situated between the carpals and phalanges.

metatarsals Bones of the foot, situated between the tarsals and phalanges.

midbrain The part of the brain that is responsible for helping to regulate the level of consciousness.

midsagittal (midline) plane An imaginary vertical line drawn from the middle of the forehead through the nose and the umbilicus (navel) to the floor, dividing the body into equal left and right halves.

minute volume The volume of air that moves in and out of the lungs per minute; calculated by multiplying the tidal volume and respiratory rate; also called minute ventilation.

motor nerves Nerves that carry information from the central nervous system to the muscles of the body.

mucous membranes The lining of body cavities and passages that communicate directly or indirectly with the environment outside the body.

mucus The watery secretion of the mucous membranes that lubricates the body openings.

musculoskeletal system The bones and voluntary muscles of the body.

myocardium The heart muscle.

nasopharynx The part of the pharynx that lies above the level of the roof of the mouth, or palate.

Prep Kit continued

nervous system The system that controls virtually all activities of the body, both voluntary and involuntary.

neurons The functional units of the nervous system; also called nerve cells.

norepinephrine A hormone produced by the body and a drug sometimes used in the treatment of shock; produces vasoconstriction through its alpha-stimulator properties.

occipital bone The most posterior bone of the cranium.

occipital lobe The brain area primarily responsible for vision.

oncotic pressure The pressure of water to move, typically into the capillary, as the result of the presence of plasma proteins.

orbit The eye socket, made up of the maxilla and zygoma.

organs Groups of tissues that perform similar or interrelated jobs.

oropharynx A tubular structure that extends vertically from the back of the mouth to the esophagus and trachea.

ovaries The primary female reproductive organs that produce an ovum, or egg, that, if fertilized, will develop into a fetus.

pancreas A flat, solid organ that lies below the liver and the stomach; it is a major source of digestive enzymes and produces the hormone insulin.

parasympathetic nervous system A subdivision of the autonomic nervous system, involved in control of involuntary functions, mediated largely by the vagus nerve through the chemical acetylcholine.

parietal bones The bones that lie between the temporal and occipital regions of the cranium.

parietal lobe The brain area primarily responsible for processing sensory and spatial information.

patella The kneecap; a specialized bone that lies within the tendon of the quadriceps muscle.

pathophysiology The study of how normal physiologic processes are affected by disease.

pectoral girdle The supporting structure for the arms, which attaches the arms to the axial skeleton. It comprises the clavicles and scapulae; also called the shoulder girdle.

pelvic girdle The supporting structure for the legs, which serves to connect the legs to the axial skeleton.

perfusion The circulation of oxygenated blood within an organ or tissue in adequate amounts to meet the current needs of the cells.

peripheral nervous system (PNS) The part of the nervous system that consists of 31 pairs of spinal nerves and 12 pairs of cranial nerves; these may be sensory nerves, motor nerves, or connecting nerves.

peristalsis The wavelike contraction of smooth muscle by which the ureters or other tubular organs propel their contents.

phalanges The bones of the fingers and toes.

pharynx A muscular tube that allows air, liquid, and food to pass from the nose or mouth to the lower airways and esophagus; composed of the nasopharynx, oropharynx, and the laryngopharynx; commonly referred to as the throat.

phrenic nerve A nerve that controls the diaphragm and is necessary for adequate breathing.

physiology The study of the normal functions of living organisms and their parts.

plasma A sticky, yellow fluid that carries the blood cells and nutrients and transports cellular waste material to the organs of excretion.

platelets Tiny, disc-shaped elements that are much smaller than the cells; they are essential in the initial formation of a blood clot, the mechanism that stops bleeding.

pleura The serous membranes covering the lungs and lining the thorax, completely enclosing a potential space known as the pleural space.

pleural space The potential space between the parietal pleura and the visceral pleura; described

Prep Kit continued

as "potential" because under normal conditions, the space does not exist.

pons An organ that lies below the midbrain and above the medulla and contains numerous important nerve fibers, including those for sleep, respiration, and the medullary respiratory center.

posterior tibial artery The artery just behind the medial malleolus; supplies blood to the foot.

prostate gland A small gland that surrounds the male urethra where it emerges from the urinary bladder; it secretes a fluid that is part of the ejaculatory fluid.

pubic symphysis A hard, bony, and cartilaginous prominence found at the midline in the lowermost portion of the abdomen where the two halves of the pelvic ring are joined by cartilage at a joint with minimal motion.

pubis One of three bones that fuse to form the pelvic ring.

pulmonary artery The major artery leading from the right ventricle of the heart to the lungs; carries oxygen-poor blood.

pulmonary circulation The flow of blood from the right ventricle through the pulmonary arteries and all of their branches and capillaries in the lungs and back to the left atrium through the venules and pulmonary veins; also called the lesser circulation.

pulmonary veins The four veins that return oxygenated blood from the lungs to the left atrium of the heart.

pulse The wave of pressure created as the heart contracts and forces blood out the left ventricle and into the major arteries.

radial artery The major artery in the forearm; it is palpable at the wrist on the thumb side.

radius The bone on the thumb side of the forearm.

rectum The lowermost end of the colon.

red blood cells Cells that carry oxygen to the body's tissues; also called erythrocytes.

renal pelvis A cone-shaped area that collects urine from the kidneys and funnels it through the ureter into the bladder.

residual volume The air that remains in the lungs after maximal expiration.

respiration The inhaling and exhaling of air; the physiologic process that exchanges carbon dioxide from fresh air.

respiratory compromise The inability of the body to move gas effectively.

respiratory system All the structures of the body that contribute to the process of breathing, consisting of the upper and lower airways and their component parts.

reticular activating system (RAS) Located in the upper brainstem; responsible for maintenance of consciousness, specifically one's level of arousal.

retroperitoneal Behind the abdominal cavity.

sacroiliac joint The connection point between the pelvis and the vertebral column.

sacrum One of three bones (the others being the two pelvic bones) that make up the pelvic ring; consists of five fused sacral vertebrae.

sagittal (lateral) plane An imaginary line where the body is divided into left and right parts.

salivary glands The glands that produce saliva to keep the mouth and pharynx moist.

scalp The thick skin covering the cranium, which usually bears hair.

scapula The shoulder blade.

sebaceous glands Glands that produce an oily substance called sebum, which discharges along the shafts of the hairs.

semen Fluid ejaculated from the penis and containing sperm.

seminal vesicles Storage sacs for sperm and seminal fluid, which empty into the urethra at the prostate.

sensory nerves The nerves that carry sensations such as touch, taste, smell, heat, cold, and pain from the body to the central nervous system.

Prep Kit continued

shock A condition in which the circulatory system fails to provide sufficient circulation to maintain normal cellular functions; also called hypoperfusion.

skeletal muscle Muscle that is attached to bones and usually crosses at least one joint; striated, or voluntary, muscle.

skeletal system The framework of the body, composed of bones and other connective tissues, that supports and protects internal organs and other body tissues.

small intestine The portion of the digestive tube between the stomach and the cecum, consisting of the duodenum, jejunum, and ileum.

smooth muscle Involuntary muscle; it constitutes the bulk of the gastrointestinal tract and is present in nearly every organ to regulate automatic activity.

somatic nervous system The part of the nervous system that regulates activities over which there is voluntary control.

sphenoid bone A bone in the skull that helps connect the neurocranium (the portion of the skull that protects the brain and sensory organs) to the facial skeleton.

sphincters Muscles arranged in circles that are able to decrease the diameter of tubes. Examples are found within the rectum, bladder, and blood vessels.

sphygmomanometer A device used to measure blood pressure.

spinal cord An extension of the brain, composed of virtually all the nerves carrying messages between the brain and the rest of the body. It lies inside of and is protected by the spinal canal.

spleen A solid lymphatic organ located in the left upper quadrant of the abdomen.

sternum The breast bone.

stratum corneum The outermost or dead layer of the skin.

stroke volume (SV) The volume of blood pumped forward with each ventricular contraction.

subcutaneous tissue Tissue, largely fat, that lies directly under the dermis and serves as an insulator of the body.

superior vena cava One of the two largest veins in the body; carries blood from the upper extremities, head, neck, and chest into the heart.

sutures Fibrous joints that connect the unfused cranial bones after birth.

sweat glands The glands that secrete sweat, located in the dermal layer of the skin.

sympathetic nervous system The adrenergic part of the autonomic peripheral nervous system responsible for the fight-or-flight response.

symphyses Joints that have grown together to form a very stable connection.

synovial fluid The small amount of liquid within a joint used as lubrication.

synovial membrane The lining of a joint that secretes synovial fluid into the joint space.

systemic circulation The portion of the circulatory system outside of the heart and lungs.

systemic vascular resistance (SVR) The resistance that blood must overcome to be able to move within the blood vessels; related to the amount of dilation or constriction in the blood vessel.

systole The contraction, or period of contraction, of the heart, especially that of the ventricles.

talus The bone that forms the lower portion of the ankle.

tarsals The group of bones situated between the lower leg bones (ie, tibia and fibula) and the metatarsal bones of the foot.

temporal bones The lateral bones on each side of the cranium; the temples.

temporal lobe The brain area primarily responsible for taste, hearing, and the ability to understand words.

Prep Kit continued

tendons The fibrous connective tissues that attach muscle to bone.

testicle A male genital gland that contains specialized cells that produce hormones and sperm.

thoracic cage The chest or rib cage.

thoracic spine The 12 vertebrae that lie between the cervical vertebrae and the lumbar vertebrae. One pair of ribs is attached to each of these vertebrae.

thorax The chest cavity that contains the heart, lungs, esophagus, and great vessels.

thyroid cartilage A firm prominence of cartilage that forms the upper part of the larynx; the Adam's apple.

tibia The shinbone; the larger of the two bones of the lower leg.

tidal volume The amount of air moved in and out of the lungs in one relaxed breath; about 500 mL for an adult.

topographic anatomy The superficial landmarks of the body that serve as guides to the structures that lie beneath them.

trachea The windpipe; the main trunk for air passing to and from the lungs.

transverse (axial) plane An imaginary line where the body is divided into top and bottom parts.

triceps The muscle in the back of the upper arm.

tunica media The middle and thickest layer of tissue of a blood vessel wall, composed of elastic tissue and smooth muscle cells that allow the vessel to expand or contract in response to changes in blood pressure and tissue demand.

ulna The inner bone of the forearm, on the side opposite the thumb.

umbilicus The navel; also called the belly button.

ureter A small, hollow tube that carries urine from the kidneys to the bladder.

urethra The canal that conveys urine from the bladder to outside the body.

urinary bladder A sac behind the pubic symphysis made of smooth muscle that collects and stores urine.

urinary system The organs that control the discharge of certain waste materials filtered from the blood and excreted as urine.

vagina The outermost cavity of a woman's reproductive tract; the lower part of the birth canal.

ventilation The movement of air between the lungs and the environment.

ventricle One of two lower chambers of the heart.

vertebrae The bones of the vertebral column.

vertebral column The structure formed by the 33 vertebrae, separated by intervertebral disks. It houses and protects the spinal cord; also called the spinal column.

voluntary muscle Muscle that is under direct voluntary control of the brain and can be contracted or relaxed at will; skeletal, or striated, muscle.

$\dot{V}/\dot{Q}$ ratio A measurement that examines how much gas is being moved effectively and how much blood is flowing around the alveoli where gas exchange (perfusion) occurs.

white blood cells Blood cells that have a role in the body's immune defense mechanisms against infection; also called leukocytes.

xiphoid process The narrow, cartilaginous lower tip of the sternum.

zygomas The quadrangular bones of the cheek, articulating with the frontal bone, the maxillae, the zygomatic processes of the temporal bone, and the great wings of the sphenoid bone.

Prep Kit continued

References

1. Hatton IA, Galbraith ED, Merleau NSC, Miettinen TP, Smith BM, Shander JA. The human cell count and size distribution. *Proc Natl Acad Sci USA*. 2023;120(39): e2303077120. doi:10.1073/pnas.2303077120
2. Cowan PT, Launico MV, Kahai P. Anatomy, bones. *StatPearls*. National Library of Medicine website. https://www.ncbi.nlm.nih.gov/books/NBK537199/. Updated April 21, 2024. Accessed January 13, 2025.
3. Shoulder ligaments. Shoulderdoc.co.uk website. https://www.shoulderdoc.co.uk/article/1179. Accessed January 13, 2025.
4. Ogobuiro I, Wehrle CJ, Tuma F. Anatomy, thorax, heart coronary arteries. *StatPearls*. National Library of Medicine website. https://www.ncbi.nlm.nih.gov/books/NBK534790/#. Updated July 24, 2023. Accessed January 13, 2025.
5. Iorgulescu G. Saliva between normal and pathological. Important factors in determining systemic and oral health. *J Med Life*. 2009;2(3):303–307.
6. Chaudhry R, Varacallo MA. Biochemistry, glycolysis. *StatPearls*. National Library of Medicine website. https://www.ncbi.nlm.nih.gov/books/NBK482303/. Updated August 8, 2023. Accessed January 13, 2025.

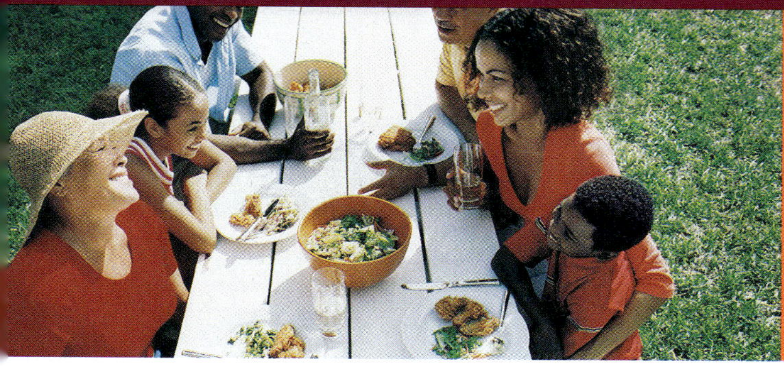

Chapter 7

Life Span Development

NATIONAL EMS EDUCATION STANDARD COMPETENCIES

Preparatory

Applies knowledge of the emergency medical services (EMS) system, safety/well-being of the emergency medical technician (EMT), medical/legal, and ethical issues to the provision of emergency care.

Life Span Development

Applies knowledge of life span development to patient assessment and management.

KNOWLEDGE OBJECTIVES

1. Describe special assessment considerations relating to the anatomy and physiology of the pediatric patient compared to the adult patient and the implications for EMTs. (pp 234–235)
2. Explain the terms used to designate the following stages of life: infants, toddlers and preschoolers, school-age children, adolescents (teenagers), early adults, middle adults, and older adults. (p 234)
3. Discuss the physical and cognitive developmental stages of newborns and infants, including health risks, signs that may indicate illness, and patient assessment. (pp 235–239)
4. Discuss the physical and cognitive developmental stages of a toddler, including health risks, signs that may indicate illness, and patient assessment. (pp 239–242)
5. Discuss the physical and cognitive developmental stages of a preschool-age child, including health risks, signs that may indicate illness, and patient assessment. (pp 239–242)
6. Discuss the physical and cognitive developmental stages of a school-age child, including health risks, signs that may indicate illness, and patient assessment. (pp 242–243)
7. Discuss the physical and cognitive developmental stages of an adolescent, including health risks, patient assessment, and privacy issues. (pp 243–246)
8. Describe the major physical and psychosocial characteristics of an early adult's life. (p 246)
9. Describe the major physical and psychosocial characteristics of a middle adult's life. (pp 246–247)
10. Describe the major physical and psychosocial characteristics of an older adult's life. (pp 247–252)

SKILLS OBJECTIVES

There are no skills objectives for this chapter.

Introduction

As an EMT, you must be aware of the obvious and not-so-obvious changes a person undergoes physically, behaviorally, and mentally at various stages of life. Your understanding of these changes will help guide your assessment of the patient's condition and, subsequently, the care you provide.

Vital Signs

In general, the younger the person, the faster the pulse and respiratory rates should be. Finding a pulse rate of 140 beats/min and a respiratory rate of 40 breaths/min is usually normal for an infant. However, for a 30-year-old adult, the same values would likely signal the presence of a life-threatening condition. Normal blood pressure values also vary widely between different age groups, but unlike pulse and respiratory rates, blood pressure values tend to *increase* with age. **TABLE 7-1** lists approximate normal vital signs for various age groups.

Special Populations

ASSESSMENT CONSIDERATIONS IN THE PEDIATRIC PATIENT

Children differ anatomically, physically, and emotionally from adults. The illnesses and injuries that children sustain, and their responses to them, vary based on age or developmental level. Children are not small adults; therefore, you must tailor your approach to accommodate their unique needs. A young child may not be able to tell you what is wrong. Fear of EMS providers and pain can make the child difficult to assess. In addition, the child's parents or primary caregivers may be stressed, frightened, or behaving irrationally. For these reasons, **pediatrics**, the specialized medical practice devoted to the care of young patients, can be extremely challenging.

Whereas each child is unique, the thoughts and behaviors of children are often grouped into six stages: newborn, infancy, the toddler years, preschool years, school-age years, and adolescence. Children in each stage grapple with different developmental issues. Even though there are specific issues that are important to different age groups, there are also some general rules that apply when you care for children of any age.

TABLE 7-1 Vital Signs at Various Ages[a]

Age	Pulse Rate (beats/min)[b]	Respiratory Rate (breaths/min)	Systolic Blood Pressure (mm Hg)	Temperature Normal 98.6°F (37°C)
Newborn (0 to 1 month)	100 to 205	30 to 60	67 to 84	97°F to 100.4°F (36°C to 38°C)
Infant (1 month to 1 year)	100 to 180	30 to 53	72 to 104	97°F to 100.4°F (36°C to 38°C)
Toddler (1 to 3 years)	98 to 140	22 to 27	86 to 106	97°F to 100.4°F (36°C to 98°C)
Preschool age (3 to 6 years)	97 to 118	20 to 28	89 to 112	97°F to 100.4°F (36°C to 98°C)
School age (6 to 12 years)	75 to 118	18 to 25	97 to 115	97°F to 100.4°F (36°C to 98°C)
Adolescent (12 to 18 years)	60 to 100	12 to 20	110 to <120	98.6°F (37°C)
Adult (18 years and older)	60 to 100	12 to 20	90 to 120	98.6°F (37°C)

[a]Vital signs and age ranges may vary in different sources.

[b]Pulse rate may be slightly slower when children are sleeping.

Newborns (Birth to 1 Month) and Infants (1 Month to 1 Year)

Unmatched by any other phase of life, the list of developmental changes occurring in the first year is long and substantial. These 12 months are often divided into two stages: newborn and infant. From birth to 1 month of age, a person is called a **newborn**. From 1 month to 1 year of age, a person is identified as an **infant** (**FIGURE 7-1**). An in-depth discussion of the neonatal period is included in Chapter 34, *Obstetrics and Neonatal Care.*

Physical Changes

Weight

At birth, a newborn usually weighs between 6 and 8 pounds (3 to 3.5 kg). The head accounts for approximately 25% of this weight. During the first week, a newborn's body weight decreases by 5% to 10%, due to fluid loss. By the second week, the newborn begins to gain weight. From there on, infants grow at a rate of approximately 1 ounce (30 g) per day, doubling their weight within 4 to 6 months and tripling it by the end of the first year.

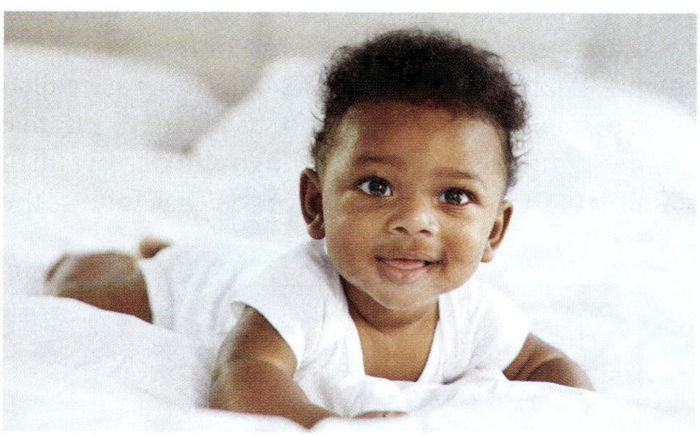

FIGURE 7-1 An infant is 1 month to 1 year of age.

> **Special Populations**
>
> **RISK OF HEAD INJURY IN YOUNG CHILDREN**
>
> Because their heads account for 25% of their total body weight, newborns and infants often land headfirst when they fall. The risk of head injury is further increased due to their inability to extend their arms to cushion or slow their fall. Keep these characteristics in mind when considering the possibility of head and spinal trauma in this age group.

Cardiovascular System

Prior to birth, fetal blood is circulated through the umbilical cord and placenta, where oxygen and waste are transferred between mother and baby. Mother and baby do not share blood. During the birthing process, hormones and pressure changes help the newborn make the transition from fetal circulation to extrauterine circulation. See Chapter 34, *Obstetrics and Neonatal Care*, for more information on fetal circulation.

Pulmonary System

Prior to taking the first breath, a newborn's lungs have never been filled with air. As such, a newborn's first breath is forceful and is facilitated in part by the chest's passage through the birth canal and the subsequent increase in intrathoracic pressure.

Newborns are primarily nose breathers. Infants younger than 6 months are particularly susceptible to nasal congestion, which can lead to viral upper respiratory infections. If you respond to a call for a baby with difficulty breathing, make sure the nasal passages are clear of mucus and other obstructions.

An infant's upper airway is quite different from that of an adult. The infant's tongue is larger in proportion to the size of the oral cavity, and the airway is proportionally shorter and narrower. As a result,

> **YOU are the EMT**
>
> At 1310 hours, you respond to 8601 Douglas Avenue for a 65-year-old man who reports dizziness while shopping for groceries. Dispatch alerts you the location is a large grocery store and the patient will be at the customer service desk right inside the store.
>
> 1. How does a patient's age affect your assessment?
> 2. What are some physical differences between middle adults and older adults?

airway obstruction is more common in infants than in older children and adults. Due to factors such as the proportionally oversized occiput, the increased flexibility of the trachea, and the infant's limited or absent ability to change positions, it is crucial that the EMT preserve the airway's patency through proper positioning. Hyperextending or hyperflexing the infant's head and neck can easily produce an airway obstruction.

The rib cage of an infant is less rigid and the ribs sit horizontally. This explains the distinctive diaphragmatic breathing (belly breathing) typically seen in infants.

When providing bag-mask ventilations to an infant, be aware that the infant's lungs are fragile. Forceful ventilations and overinflation increase pressure in the lungs and are more likely to result in pressure-induced trauma, referred to as **barotrauma**.

The muscles that infants use to breathe are immature, and the number of alveoli in their lungs is relatively low. Fortunately, the amount of oxygen they need is also relatively low for the first few minutes of life. When stressed, however, their respiratory system's ability to compensate is limited. They can hold out for a short time, but without expedient support, infants struggling to breathe can quickly tire and become overheated and dehydrated. Thus, respiratory problems in the very young can quickly turn life threatening.

Words of Wisdom

When you are counting breaths in an infant, count the number of times the abdomen rises instead of concentrating solely on the chest rise.

Nervous System

Although the human nervous system is remarkably well established at birth, it has yet to fully mature. However, in a healthy, term infant, certain reflexes are present at birth. The **Moro reflex** (commonly called the startle reflex) is illustrated when newborns are caught off guard and startled, at which time they open their arms wide, spread their fingers, and appear to be grabbing for something. The **palmar grasp reflex** occurs when an object is placed into a newborn's palm and the hand instinctively closes around the object. Two other reflexes play an important role in feeding. The **rooting reflex** is displayed when something touches the newborn's cheek and the head intuitively turns in the direction of the touch. The **sucking reflex** is illustrated when breastfeeding mothers stroke the baby's lips with their nipple, prompting the child to latch on. Most of these reflexes disappear by 1 year of age.

At birth, the bones of the cranium are not yet fully developed or fused together. Instead, the gaps between these bones are connected by relatively flexible fibrous tissue. These areas, called **fontanelles**, allow the newborn's head to change shape slightly as it passes through the narrow birth canal (**FIGURE 7-2**). In the months that follow, the

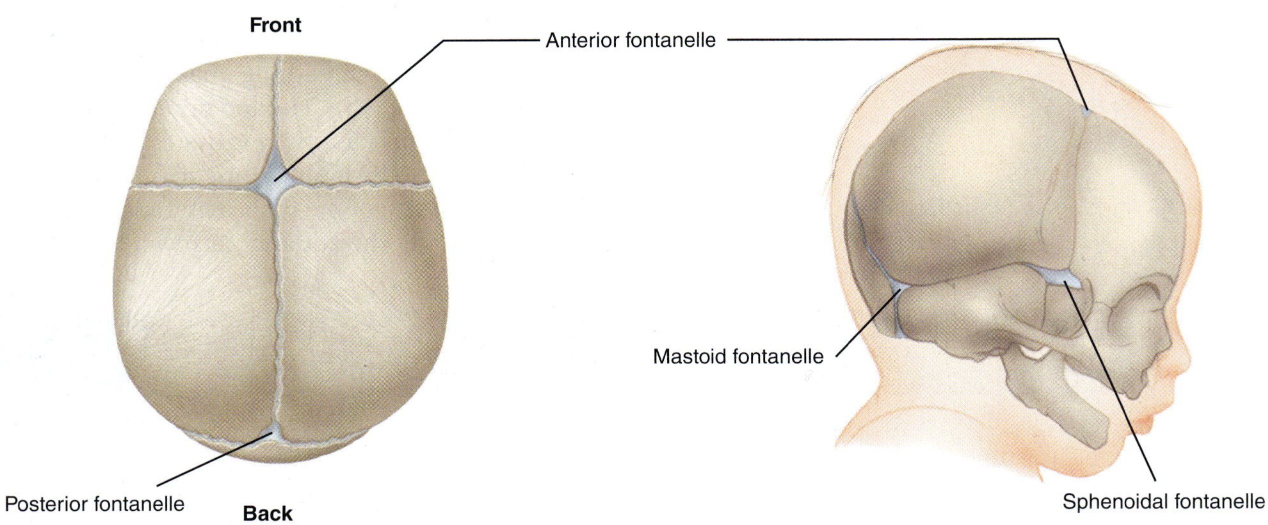

FIGURE 7-2 Fontanelles.

fontanelles begin to shrink as the cranial bones grow together and fuse, forming a unified, rigid structure. The posterior fontanelle normally closes by the third month. The anterior fontanelle closes between 9 and 18 months. When present, the fontanelles can provide the EMT with valuable information about the child's condition. For example, a depressed fontanelle may indicate dehydration, whereas a bulging fontanelle is often a sign that pressure inside the cranium has increased. Information on intracranial pressure is presented in Chapter 28, *Head and Spine Injuries*.

At birth, newborns are unable to do much without assistance. They cannot roll from their backs onto their abdomens, and their eyes are incapable of focusing on objects beyond a very short distance. Head control is limited, but infants can turn their heads toward faces. By 2 months of age, infants can track objects with their eyes and recognize familiar faces. At 6 months, they can sit upright, and they begin to make cooing and babbling sounds. They may follow a bright light or toy with their eyes or turn their heads toward a loud sound or a familiar voice. By the time infants are 12 months of age, they usually have begun to walk, point, and talk.[1]

Immune System

While still in the womb, the newborn's immune system is supported by the mother's antibodies, delivered through the placenta. Infants continue to carry some of this immunity. This passive immunity is further strengthened by antibodies contained in breast milk.

Words of Wisdom

Another development that occurs during infancy is the emergence of baby teeth. Teething (teeth breaking through the gums) can be painful and is sometimes accompanied by a low-grade fever.

Psychosocial Changes

An infant's psychosocial development begins at birth and continues to advance as the infant interacts with, and reacts to, the environment. **TABLE 7-2** outlines typical ages at which major psychosocial changes are noticed.

TABLE 7-2 Noticeable Characteristics at Various Ages

Age	Characteristic
2 months	Recognizes familiar faces; uses eyes to track objects and people
3 months	Brings objects to the mouth; smiles and frowns
4 months	Reaches arms out to people; drools
5 months	Sleeps throughout the night; distinguishes family members from strangers
6 months	Begins teething; sits upright; speaks one-syllable words
7 months	Afraid of strangers; displays mood swings
8 months	Responds to "no"; can sit alone; plays peek-a-boo
9 months	Pulls self up to stand; explores objects by placing them in the mouth
10 months	Responds to name; crawls efficiently
11 months	Begins to walk without assistance; becomes frustrated by restrictions
12 months	Identifies with name; walks

Other than crying, early infants (ie, 2 months or younger) have a limited ability to communicate pain or discomfort. Infants may cry if certain basic physical needs must be met, such as food, warmth, and comfort. Parents are often able to discern the reason for their child's crying by simply listening to the tone of those cries. They can distinguish between a cry of anger and one motivated by frustration, pain, fear, hunger, discomfort, or sleepiness. Another distinctive cry is one of distress, prompted by some unexpected event that has caused a situational crisis for the child.

Soothing an infant should be relatively easy for the parent or caregiver, such as by holding, cuddling, or rocking the infant. Hearing is generally well developed at birth, so calm and reassuring talk is often helpful as well. Every reasonable attempt should be made to identify why the infant is crying. If all obvious needs have been addressed and the infant is still inconsolable, then this could be a sign of significant illness.

At 2 to 6 months, the infant has an increased awareness of their environment and will use both hands to examine objects and explore the world. Infants experience fewer sleep interruptions at night, but sleep and nap schedules remain variable at this age.[2] At this point in development, infants will begin to roll over. As with younger infants, persistent crying and irritability can be an indicator of serious illness. A lack of eye contact in a sick infant can also be a sign of significant illness, depressed mental status, or a delay in development.

At 6 to 12 months, infants begin to babble, and by their first year, they can say their first word. At this age, most infants are able to sleep through the night without major interruptions.[2] They are teething and tend to explore their world by picking things up and placing them in their mouths. This behavior increases the risk for choking and poisonings from toxic substances.

Children develop relationships with their parents and caregivers early in their lives. *Bonding*, the formation of a close, personal relationship, is generally fostered by a *secure attachment*, which results when infants understand that their parents/caregivers will respond to their needs. Having this sense of a "safety net" inspires the child to venture out and explore.

By contrast, *anxious-avoidant attachment* is the result of recurring rejection. Infants who acquire this form of attachment show little emotional response to their parents/caregivers and treat them as they would a stranger. These children may compensate by developing an isolated lifestyle wherein they avoid having to depend on the support and care of others.

In older infants, *separation anxiety* is common and is characterized by clingy behavior and fear of unfamiliar places and people. Crying as a means of protest is normal at this age. As they grow accustomed to their homes and families, infants have an inherent need for a secure, stable environment. An environment that is too unpredictable may trigger feelings of despair, causing the child to become withdrawn. This experience may even lead to trust issues later in life.

Trust versus mistrust refers to the stage of psychosocial development beginning at birth and concluding at approximately 18 months of age. As the name implies, it is a time when children learn whether they can trust the people around them. Because infants depend entirely on their parents/caregivers, a crucial element in the formation of this trust is the quality of care the infant receives from them. When their needs are met consistently in a stable environment, children learn to trust those responsible for their well-being. Conversely, if their parents/caregivers are inconsistent, emotionally unavailable, or rejecting, children may develop a sense of mistrust.

Street Smarts

When caring for the very young, try to preserve as much of their routine as is reasonable. An easy way to achieve this is to keep family and familiar items nearby and conduct your assessment with the family member holding the infant.

Assessment Considerations for Newborns and Infants

Begin your assessment by observing the infant from a distance, preferably in a parent's or caregiver's arms (**FIGURE 7-3**). This will avoid separation anxiety, making the assessment easier. As with the younger infants, persistent crying or irritability can be a symptom of serious illness.

Provide as much sensory comfort as you can: Warm your hands and the end of the stethoscope and offer a pacifier if the parent or caregiver allows it. If possible, have a parent or caregiver hold the infant during all procedures or allow this person to stay close to the infant. If possible, plan to do any painful or uncomfortable procedures at the end of

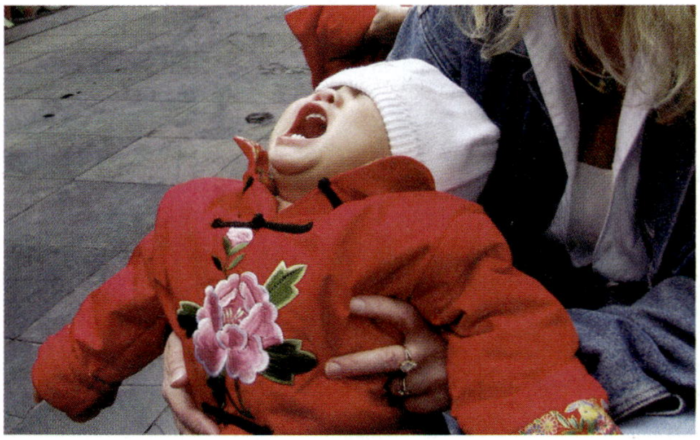

FIGURE 7-3 Infants are usually not afraid of strangers, but as they reach 6 months to 1 year, they may become irritable or cry if separated from their parents or caregivers.

the assessment process, so that the infant does not become agitated while you are trying to perform a physical examination. Infants between ages 2 and 6 months are more active, which makes them easier to evaluate.

Complete each procedure efficiently and avoid interruptions. Explain each procedure to the parent or caregiver before you perform it, because the procedure and the infant's reaction to it may be upsetting.

Infants have poor thermoregulation (the body's ability to maintain normal temperature). Their heads also have a relatively large surface area. These factors predispose them to hypothermia, so parents or caregivers will often bundle infants to keep them warm. Therefore, it is often necessary to unbundle the infant during your assessment.

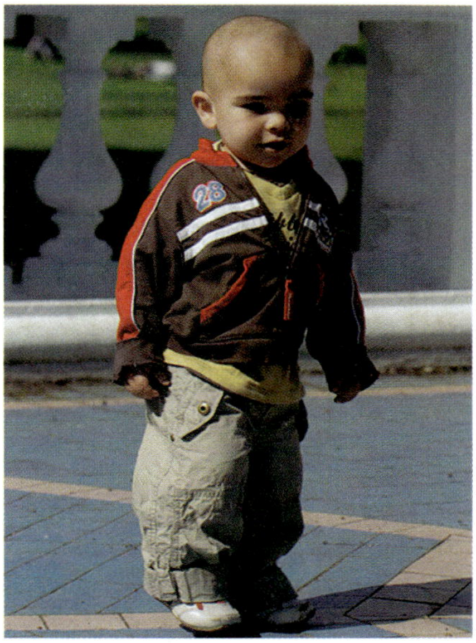

FIGURE 7-4 A toddler is 1 to 3 years of age.

Toddlers (1 to 3 Years) and Preschoolers (3 to 6 Years)

After infancy, until approximately age 3 years, a child is called a **toddler**. A child age 3 to 6 years is considered a **preschooler**. Children in these age groups experience rapid changes in growth and development.

Physical Changes

The cardiovascular system of a toddler (**FIGURE 7-4**) or preschooler (**FIGURE 7-5**) is not dramatically different from that of an adult. Their lungs continue to develop more terminal bronchioles and alveoli to meet the ever-increasing oxygen demands of their growing bodies. However, the musculature of their lungs is not well developed. This anomaly prevents them from sustaining deep or rapid respirations for an extended period.

Between 6 months and 1 year of age, infants have lost passive immunity, those antibodies they received from the mother in utero. This makes toddlers much more susceptible to infection. As toddlers spend more time around other children, they are exposed to a variety of viruses and bacteria.

YOU are the EMT

As you begin your assessment, the patient tells you he has been stressed lately and has had several episodes of lightheadedness over the past few days. He denies having chest pain, shortness of breath, or any other symptoms. As you are assessing the patient, your partner prepares to take his vital signs.

Recording Time: 0 Minutes	
Appearance	Calm
Level of consciousness	Conscious and alert
Airway	Open; clear of secretions or foreign bodies
Breathing	Normal rate; adequate depth
Circulation	Radial pulses strong and regular; skin normal for baseline, warm, and dry

3. What are some common psychosocial concerns experienced by older adults?

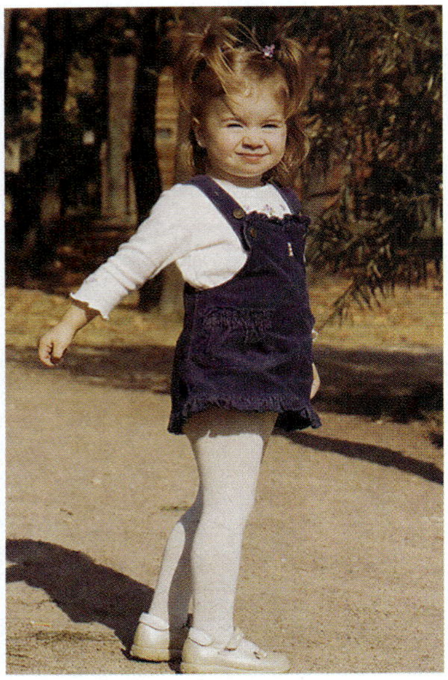

FIGURE 7-5 A preschooler is 3 to 6 years of age.

Viral infections (colds) develop frequently, often manifesting with gastrointestinal distress or upper respiratory symptoms. In the process, however, these exposures initiate the development of antibodies, resulting in acquired immunity.

Neuromuscular growth also makes considerable progress at this age. By performing activities such as walking, running, jumping, and playing catch, toddlers and preschoolers learn to use their muscles and expansive nervous system. This boost in physical activity supports an increase in muscle mass and bone density. The progression in how they play at this age demonstrates their transition from exclusively gross motor activity (eg, grabbing an object using the entire palm) to including fine motor skills (eg, picking up a crayon using only the thumb and forefinger). Remember, children build motor skills by exploration, which means in the process of learning to walk and run, they also fall down often. By the end of this stage, the weight of a preschooler's brain is roughly 90% of the adult brain's weight.

Another milestone during this stage is the maturation of the renal system and the establishing of elimination patterns (ie, toilet training). Physiologically, by 12 to 15 months of age, toddlers possess the neuromuscular capability to control the bladder. However, many are not psychologically prepared until approximately 18 to 30 months of age. The mean age when toddlers complete toilet training is 28 months.

The risk of foreign body airway obstruction continues to be high at this age. Because of a lack of molars, toddlers may not be able to fully chew their food before swallowing, leading to an increased risk of choking.

Psychosocial Changes

The psychosocial challenge for the toddler age group is sometimes referred to as autonomy versus shame and doubt. Caregivers play an important role in this stage. By encouraging a toddler's attempts at self-sufficiency, caregivers can help them develop a sense of autonomy. Conversely, by being overly critical or restrictive, they may cause the toddler to feel shame and doubt in their abilities. Through milestones such as speech development and toilet training, the child begins to attain a measure of self-sufficiency.

At 12 to 18 months, toddlers begin to walk and to explore their environment. They are able to open doors, drawers, boxes, and bottles. Because they are explorers by nature and are not afraid, injuries in this age group increase. At this age, toddlers begin to imitate the behaviors of older children and parents and may express a desire to dress like their mommies or daddies. Despite becoming more independent, they are nevertheless very attached to their parents, deriving feelings of safety and security from their presence. Separation anxiety typically peaks between 10 and 18 months of age.

By 2 years of age, most children are speaking and can put together words in two- to three-word sentences. When you point to a common object, they should be able to name it. By 36 months of age, most children have mastered basic language skills, understanding full sentences by the time they are 3 or 4 years of age. As they progress further through this stage, they make a transition from using language solely for the purpose of communicating what they want, to using it creatively and playfully.

Around age 18 to 36 months, toddlers become more socially interactive with other children and begin to understand the concept of cause and effect. These developments allow them to play games and, as a result, learn to control their own behavior, follow rules, and be competitive. The toddler's balance and gait also improve rapidly during this period. Running and climbing are two skills that develop. Significant learning and development occur as the child observes other children. By observing their role models, they also learn to recognize gender differences.

Preschool-age children (age, 3 to 6 years) are able to use simple language effectively. The most rapid increase in language occurs during this stage. These children can walk and run well and begin throwing, catching, and kicking during play. Toilet training is mastered at this stage.

During the preschool period, children are learning which behaviors are appropriate and which behaviors will lead to a "time out." Tantrums may occur when preschool-age children feel they cannot control a situation or its outcomes.

Street Smarts

When responding to a severely sick or injured child, you may find a secondary patient on scene: a parent. For some, the sudden stress, fear, and uncertainty will be overwhelming, causing panic. The parent's distress can add to an already intense situation and can cause the child to be similarly anxious.

Assessment Considerations for Toddlers

Stranger anxiety may still develop early in this period. Toddlers may resist separation from parents or caregivers and be afraid to let others come near them. Allow the toddler to hold any special object that brings the toddler comfort ("Would you like to hold your blankie while I listen to your tummy?"). When possible, demonstrate the assessment on a doll or stuffed animal first, which may limit the toddler's anxiety and make it easier to perform the assessment. Because of their newfound independence, they may also be unhappy about being restrained or held for procedures. Two-year-olds have a well-deserved reputation for having their own ideas about almost everything, which is why these years are often called the "terrible twos."

Toddlers have trouble describing or localizing pain because they do not have the verbal ability to be precise. Pain in the abdomen may be expressed as "My tummy hurts," and the physical examination may reveal tenderness throughout the body. However, they should be able to identify and name major body parts such as the ears, arms, and legs. Thus, do not assume they cannot contribute to your assessment. Use of visual clues and the Wong-Baker FACES pain rating scale can be helpful with this age group. The Wong-Baker FACES pain scale is shown in Chapter 10, *Patient Assessment.*

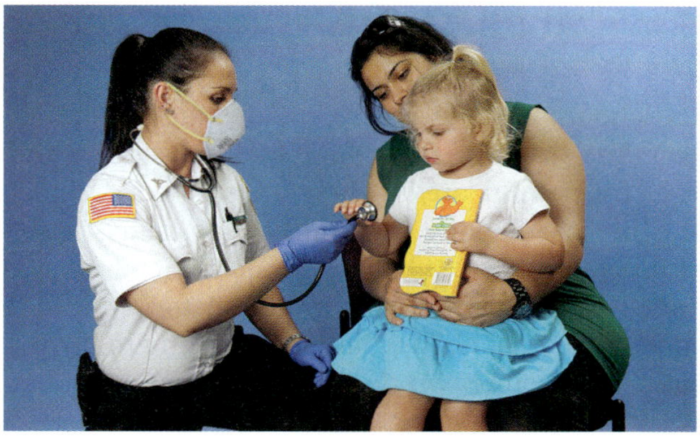

FIGURE 7-6 Allow a toddler to sit on the parent's or caregiver's lap during your assessment, and use a toy to distract the child.

Toddlers can be curious and adventuresome, so you may be able to distract them (**FIGURE 7-6**). For example, you might allow the toddler to play with a tongue depressor while you assess the vital signs. Restrain the toddler for as short a time as possible, and allow the child to be comforted by the parent or caregiver immediately after a painful procedure. If the primary assessment reveals no life threats, begin your assessment at the feet or far from the location of any pain to keep from upsetting the toddler.

As with infants, persistent crying or irritability in a toddler can be a symptom of serious illness or injury. Painful procedures make a lasting impression at this stage. Older toddlers may remember negative experiences with physicians or nurses, such as vaccinations or stitches, and fear treatment. Remember to involve the parent or caregiver in any procedures. This not only provides you with an extra set of hands, but the presence of the parent or caregiver will comfort the toddler. If a parent or caregiver is unavailable, reassure the toddler using simple words and a calm, soothing voice.

Street Smart

Toddlers tend to cling to their parents or caregivers and often have a special object such as a blanket or teddy bear that comforts them when they are separated. Be sure to use any comforting objects when available to help calm the toddler.

Assessment Considerations for Preschoolers

Preschool-age children can understand directions, be more specific in describing their sensations, and identify painful areas when questioned. Despite the increased ability to communicate, much of the child's history will still be obtained from parents or caregivers. Remember to communicate simply and directly. Tell the child what you are going to do immediately before you do it; this way, the child has no time to develop frightening fantasies. Also keep in mind that the preschool-age child can be very literal. Asking if you may "take" the blood pressure may lead the child to believe that you will not give it back. Use plain language and provide plenty of reassurance. In this example, it would be better to say you will "measure" their blood pressure.

At this age, preschool-age children are easily distracted with counting games, small toys, or conversation (**FIGURE 7-7**). They have a rich imagination, which can make them particularly fearful about pain and change involving their bodies. Appealing to their imaginative thinking may allow treatment to go a bit smoother. For example, have the child pretend to be a superhero inhaling special powers while breathing in oxygen. Be sure to adjust the level of the game to the developmental level of the child.

At this age, children often believe that their thoughts or wishes can cause injury or harm to themselves or to others. They may also believe that an injury is the result of a bad deed they did earlier in the day. Do not assume that preschool-age children have an accurate understanding of the situation or know more than they actually do.

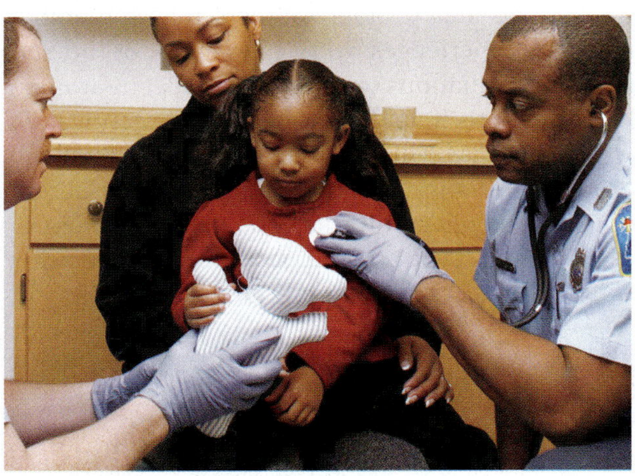

FIGURE 7-7 A preschool-age child can be easily distracted by games or conversation.

While caring for this age group and others within the pediatric population, never lie to the patient. Once you have lost your pediatric patient's trust, it will be a challenge to regain it.

Begin your assessment with the feet and move toward the head, similar to assessing a toddler. Use adhesive bandages to cover the site of an injection or other small wound, because the preschool-age child might be worried about their body being broken, like a toy that gets thrown away. They may not understand the concept of healing. Keep in mind that modesty is developing at this age, so keep the child covered when possible.

Street Smarts

Look at the world through the eyes of your patient. To a toddler or young child, you are a giant carrying unfamiliar and scary objects. One way to gain young patients' trust is to get down on their level. Kneel down so you can look the patient in the eyes. Enabling children to see and speak with you from their perspective can go a long way in providing effective care.

School-Age Children (6 to 12 Years)

A child who is **school age** (age, 6 to 12 years) is beginning to act more like an adult (**FIGURE 7-8**). These children can think in concrete terms, respond sensibly to direct questions, and help take care of themselves. School is important at this stage and concerns about popularity and peer pressure occupy a great deal of time and energy. Children with chronic illness or disabilities can become self-conscious because of concerns about fitting in with their peers.

Physical Changes

A school-age child's physical traits and functions continue to mature at a relatively rapid pace. Most gain approximately 4 pounds (2 kg) and grow 2.5 inches (6 cm) each year. Baby teeth are replaced by permanent teeth, and brain activity in both

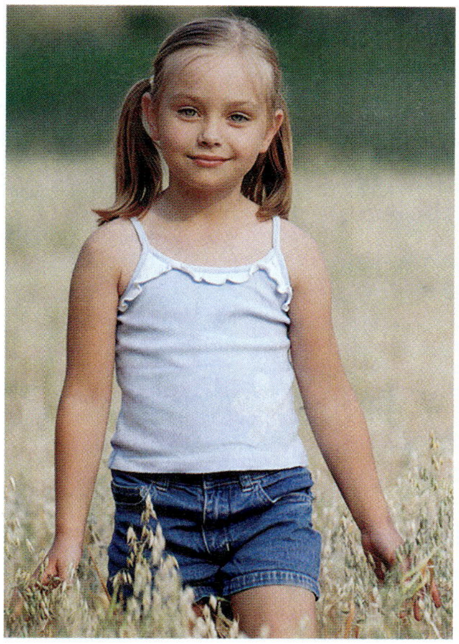

FIGURE 7-8 A school-age child is 6 to 12 years of age.

hemispheres increases significantly. Schooling for these children typically spans from kindergarten through fifth or sixth grade.

Psychosocial Changes

School-age children experience substantial psychosocial growth. During this critical time in human development, children learn various types of reasoning. With **preconventional reasoning**, the child's moral compass is directed by external forces, such as parental discipline. For younger school-age children, whether a behavior is right or wrong is judged by its consequences: punishment or incentive. When children reach the level of **conventional reasoning**, their behavior is more motivated by the approval of peers, community, and society. They still accept the rules set by authority figures, but now they do so primarily because they perceive those rules as necessary for positive relationships and acceptance. For children who reach the third level, **postconventional reasoning**, moral judgments are more abstract, with the individual beginning to follow an internalized moral compass (ie, conscience). This form of reasoning typically develops further during adolescence.

During this stage, school-age children begin to develop their self-concept and self-esteem. *Self-concept* is our perception of ourselves; *self-esteem* is how we feel about ourselves and how we fit in with our peers.

Assessment Considerations for School-Age Children

Your assessment begins to be more like an adult assessment; talk to the child, not just the parent or caregiver, while taking the medical history. Doing so will help you gain the patient's trust. At this stage, the child is usually familiar with the process of physical examination through check-ups and immunizations. This may make your job easier or more difficult, depending on whether the child's prior health care experiences have been positive or negative. Begin your assessment at the head and move toward the feet, similar to assessing an adult.

Whenever possible, give the school-age child simple, appropriate choices, such as "Would you like to sit up or lie down?" or "Would you like to take off your clothes yourself?" Only ask the type of questions that let you control the answer and do not bargain or debate with the patient. For example, ask the child if you may find out the blood pressure on the child's right or left arm. Presenting a choice allows you to obtain assessment information and gives the child some control in a frightening situation. Encourage cooperation by allowing children to listen to their own heartbeat through the stethoscope. Respect the patient's modesty during the examination.

At this stage, children begin to understand that death is final, but their understanding of what death is and why it occurs is still unrealistic. This may increase their anxieties about illness or injury.

Adolescents (12 to 18 Years)

An **adolescent** (age, 12 to 18 years) is able to think abstractly and can participate in decision making (**FIGURE 7-9**). This is also the stage when personal morals begin to develop. Adolescents can discriminate between right and wrong. They are now able to incorporate their own values and beliefs into their daily decision-making process. Even though this age group is physically similar to adults, adolescents are still children on an emotional level. They gradually shift from relying on family for emotional psychological support, social development, and acceptance to relying on friends and peers. Interest in romantic

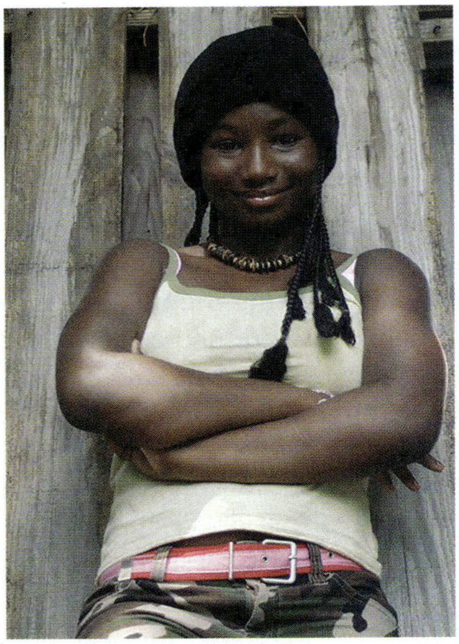

FIGURE 7-9 An adolescent is 12 to 18 years of age.

relationships begins. Schooling for these children typically spans from 6th through 12th grades.

Physical Changes

Vital signs for adolescents begin to level off within the adult ranges, with a systolic blood pressure generally between 90 and 110 mm Hg, a pulse rate between 60 and 100 beats/min, and respiratory rate of 12 to 20 breaths/min.

During the adolescent period, teens experience a 2- to 3-year growth spurt (ie, an increase in muscle and bone growth). Growth begins with the hands and feet, then moves to the long bones of the extremities, and finishes with growth of the torso. At the conclusion of the growth spurt, muscle mass and bone density have nearly reached adult levels. Girls tend to experience this growth at an earlier age than boys, finishing by approximately 16 years of age. Boys typically reach their growth peak by 18 years.

Another important milestone of adolescence is the maturation of the endocrine and reproductive systems. Secondary sexual development begins, along with enlargement of the external reproductive organs. Pubic and axillary hair appear. Vocal sound changes in range and depth.

In girls, the deposit of adipose (fat) tissue causes the breasts and thighs to increase in size. Menstruation begins with *menarche*, the first menstrual bleeding; however, it is not uncommon for some

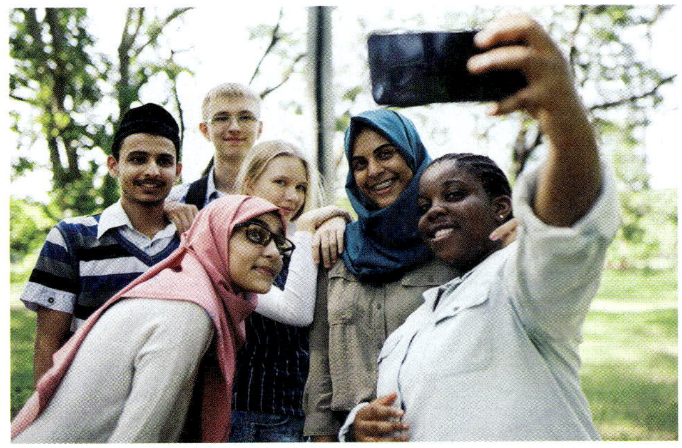

FIGURE 7-10 Adolescents want to fit in and may struggle to create their identities.

girls to begin menstruation prior to adolescence. Along with these changes comes the capacity for reproduction. By the middle of adolescence, the male body can produce sperm, and the female body produces eggs (oocytes).

Psychosocial Changes

During this phase, adolescents are seeking independence but are very much still dependent on parents and the community. In seeking to express their independence, adolescents may begin to distance themselves from parents and siblings, desiring privacy and personal space. Most begin spending more time with friends and struggling to create a sense of identity (**FIGURE 7-10**). While "trying on" different personas, they may begin dressing in a certain style of clothing that fits their desired personality. Self-consciousness increases, as both sexes become more concerned with their physical appearance and how they are perceived by peers. **Sexual orientation**, a person's emotional, romantic, or sexual attraction to other people, and **gender identity**, one's innermost concept of self, are also developing during this period. They may feel confused about how they feel and who they are attracted to, especially if their feelings conflict with family and social norms. Not knowing how to express or manage these feelings may result in suicidal thoughts and actions.[3]

At times, adolescence can be intensely emotional. Teenagers often find themselves caught between two worlds; they want to be treated like adults, yet they continue to want and need their parents' support. Rebellious behavior and experimentation are common. Adolescents often feel that they are free from danger and "indestructible." Smoking, illicit drug use, unsafe driving, unprotected sex, and other high-risk behaviors tend to peak at around age 14 to 16 years, along with antisocial behavior and peer pressure. Some of the risks that adolescents take can ultimately facilitate development and judgment and help to shape their identity as an adult. However, unintended consequences, such as trauma, drug and/or alcohol misadventure, sexually transmitted infection, and pregnancy, may occur.

Even without these particular manifestations, the adolescent's struggle toward independence can have devastating setbacks. Patience and support from family and friends are essential in assisting a young person's transition into adulthood.

At this age, young people develop a code of personal ethics, influenced in part by their parents' ethics and values and partly by their peers and personal experience.

Street Smarts

When you interview adolescents in the presence of their family, they may withhold certain information or even lie to protect their privacy or image. For this reason, you should attempt to ask more sensitive questions privately, where adolescents feel they can answer without constraint.

Assessment Considerations for Adolescents

Adolescents can often understand complex concepts and treatment options; provide them with information when they request it (**FIGURE 7-11**). When the adolescent's condition is stable, discuss the situation and allow the adolescent to be involved. Provide adolescents with choices regarding their health, while also lending guidance if needed. You will find adolescents to be more helpful and understanding of necessary procedures than younger patients.

Body image and physical modesty are important considerations when assessing an adolescent.

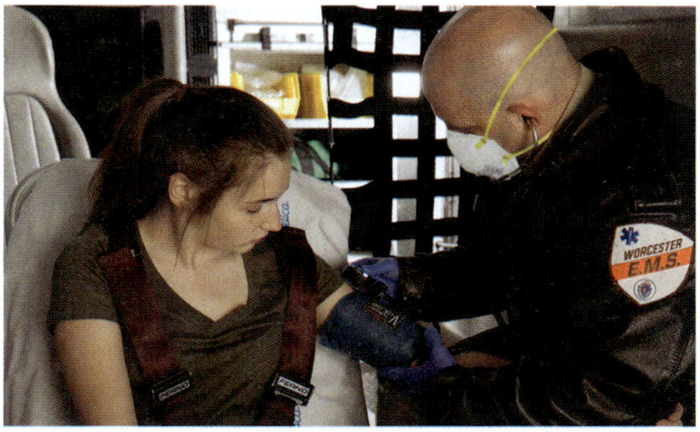

FIGURE 7-11 Respect the adolescent's privacy at all times; share any requested information with the patient.

YOU are the EMT

As your partner takes the patient's vital signs, he tells you he recently had a close friend pass away, which has been difficult for him and his wife. He tells you this loss has made him unsure about the future and has raised fears of his own mortality. He is still light-headed and now reports a headache. You advise him he should be transported to the hospital via EMS, but he tells you he would rather drive himself.

Recording Time: 5 Minutes	
Respirations	14 breaths/min; regular and adequate
Pulse	76 beats/min; strong and regular
Skin	Baseline color, warm, and dry
Blood pressure	174/98 mm Hg
Oxygen saturation (Spo_2)	98% (on room air)

4. Are the patient's vital signs consistent with his age?
5. Why should you transport this patient to the hospital?

This patient may exaggerate or understate simple injuries or illnesses due to anxiety about body image or fear of disfigurement. If assessment of an adolescent requires exposure or partial exposure, take every measure to respect the patient's privacy. If an EMT of the same gender is available to perform the physical examination, it may lessen the stress of the event. Allow the adolescent to speak openly about any thoughts and concerns.

Be aware that female adolescents may be pregnant, so privately ask, "Is there a chance you could be pregnant?" Communicate the patient's answer to the receiving facility and note it on your patient care report. The adolescent might not want this information known to parents or caregivers and may fear the consequences. If you suspect that the patient might want to tell you something, but is silent in front of a parent or caregiver, try to interview the adolescent without the parent or caregiver present.

Adolescents have a clear understanding of the purpose and meaning of pain. Whenever possible, explain any necessary procedures well in advance. Assess their level of pain by observing facial and body expression as well as by asking questions; adolescents can be reserved and may not request pain relief even when they need it. To distract them, find out some of their interests, such as sports or movies, and get them talking.

Street Smarts

Keep in mind that adolescents may have mood swings or depression and when ill or injured, may act younger than their age.

Early Adults (18 to 40 Years)

Physical Changes

Following adolescence, a person is classified as an **early adult** (age, 18 to 40 years) (**FIGURE 7-12**). The vital signs of early adults do not vary greatly from those seen throughout adulthood. Ideally, the typical early adult pulse rate is approximately 70 beats/min, the respiratory rate will stay in the range of 12 to 20 breaths/min, and the systolic blood pressure will be approximately between 90 and 120 mm Hg.

From approximately 18 to 25 years of age, men and women typically reach their physical peak. Lifelong habits and routines are established, whether healthy or unhealthy (eg, diet, exercise, tobacco use).

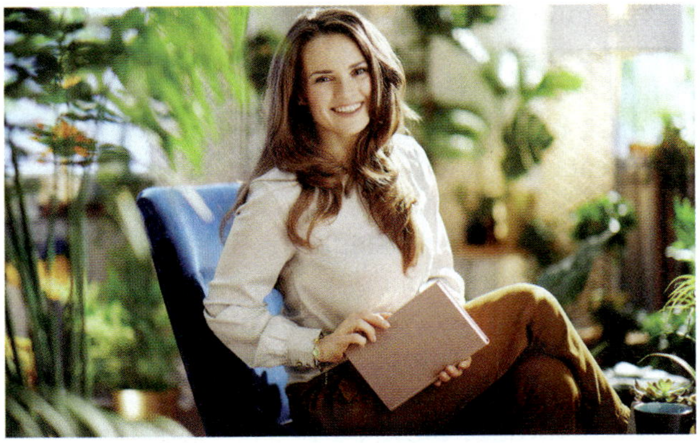

FIGURE 7-12 An early adult is 18 to 40 years of age.

In the latter years of early adulthood, the effects of aging gradually become evident (ie, subtle wear and tear). Muscle strength decreases, and reflexes slow. The disks between vertebrae begin to settle, sometimes producing a decrease in height. Metabolism also decreases, while fatty tissue increases. Thus, without adjusting their diet and level of activity accordingly, the early adult may experience unwanted weight gain, while simultaneously finding it more difficult to lose weight than in previous years.

Psychosocial Changes

Most early adults spend these years focusing on family and career: "settling down," getting married, starting a family, and striving for career achievement. Although immensely rewarding, these life events also bring about significant stress. Interestingly, despite the amount of stress and change, this age group enjoys one of the more stable periods of life psychologically.

Middle Adults (40 to 65 Years)

Physical Changes

For a **middle adult** (age, 40 to 65 years) (**FIGURE 7-13**), the aging process continues to take its toll. Middle adults become more susceptible to vision and hearing loss, cardiovascular health becomes a growing concern, and the incidence of cancer increases. Women in their late 40s to early 50s enter menopause: the end of menstruation and the ability to reproduce.

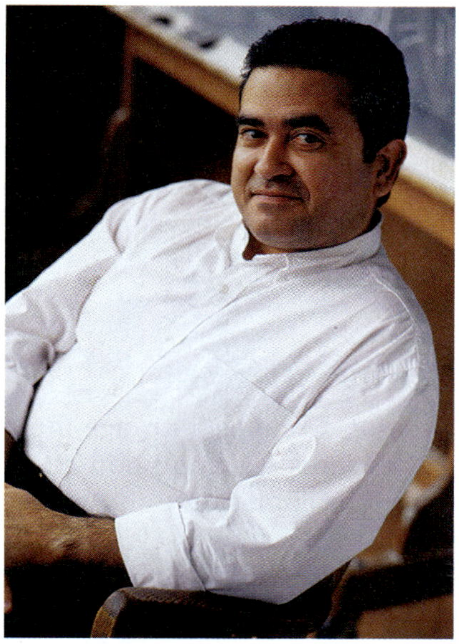

FIGURE 7-13 A middle adult is 40 to 65 years of age.

Middle adults may experience increased cholesterol levels, decreased cardiac efficiency, and difficulties with weight control. However, many of the effects of aging can be diminished with proper exercise and a healthy diet.

Middle adults may also have conditions of which they are unaware, including diabetes and hypertension. In the United States, medical conditions, rather than injury, become the leading cause of morbidity for this age group. Whereas the leading cause of death in 2021 for all age groups 1 to 45 years was unintentional injury, including poisoning, motor vehicle crashes, falls, and drowning, the leading causes of death for middle adults were cancer, heart disease, and coronavirus disease 2019 (COVID-19).[4]

Psychosocial Changes

The pressure to accomplish their professional and relational goals, the need to adjust after their adult children leave the home (ie, empty nest syndrome), and the worries that come with assessing whether they will have the financial means to retire are among the many psychosocial challenges facing the middle adult. However, they have the physical, emotional, and spiritual reserves needed to overcome these challenges, and their health is generally stable.

By this time, the parents of middle adults have become *older adults* (discussed in the next section), many of whom will require care and assistance in completing routine tasks of daily life. In the United States, many of these older adults receive such care at home, from family members. Therefore, in addition to supporting children departing for college, middle adults may experience an overlapping period during which they must also care for their aging parents.

Older Adults (65 Years and Older)

Geriatrics is the assessment and treatment of disease in an **older adult**. In this chapter, 65 years is used as the threshold age for older adulthood; this is consistent with the definition used by many other medical groups and governmental agencies. How fast one ages, though, is a function of genetics, lifestyle, and, perhaps, attitude.

Geriatric patients present a unique challenge for health care providers because the classic presentations of injuries and illness are often altered by chronic conditions, multiple medications, and the physiology of aging. To provide effective treatment for this growing population, you must understand the issues related to aging and modify some of your assessment and treatment approaches accordingly.

Words of Wisdom

The concept of chronologic age versus functional or biologic age is gaining wide acceptance. Chronologic ages refer to the number of years a person has been alive. Functional age is based on genetics, lifestyle, and the number of health problems a person has experienced over their lifetime that may interfere with their ability to perform normal tasks and increase their risk of illness or injury.[5] Cognitive and physical health varies widely among older adults. Each person is unique and must be assessed with that assumption.

Generational Considerations

It is important to understand and appreciate how the life of an older person might differ from yours. You will see older people who have recently lost a spouse and are struggling to fill the spouse's role, such as by managing the finances or doing the housework. Many older people also live on a fixed income, which can be challenging. Some older people may

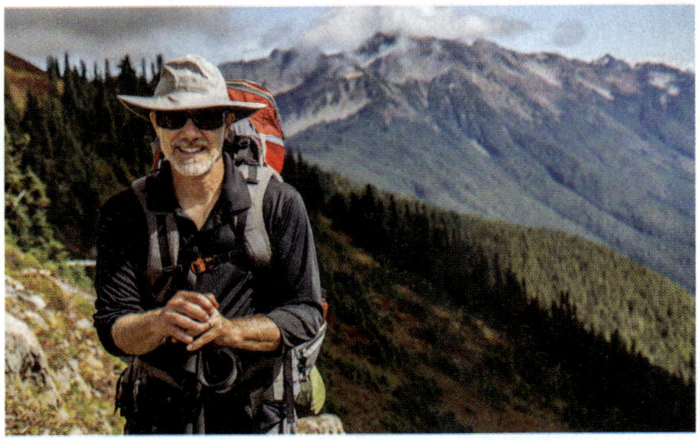

FIGURE 7-14 An older adult is 65 years or older. Physical activity can help older people reduce their risk of illness and injury.

not take all of their medications in an effort to save money. Others fear losing their independence and not being able to live in their own home.

Sometimes, it takes time and patience to interact with an older person. Always treat the patient with respect. Make every attempt to avoid **ageism**, which is a stereotyping of older people that can lead to poor patient assessment and care. Common stereotypes include assuming that the patient has dementia, is hard of hearing, has a sedentary lifestyle, or is immobile. Older people can stay fit and be active, even though they are not able to perform at the same level as they did in their youth (**FIGURE 7-14**).

Physical Changes

Life expectancy is continually changing. In the early 1900s, the mean human life expectancy was 47 years of age. In more modern times, that number has increased to approximately 76 years, with a maximum life expectancy of approximately 120 years.[6] As a result, more and more people will live to become an older adult. How long an individual lives is determined by many factors, including the person's birth year and country of residence. These two factors correlate with advances in public health, enhanced awareness of healthy eating habits, improved attitudes toward exercise, and access to ever-advancing medical care. Currently, older adults are staying active longer than their ancestors. Thanks to medical advances, they are often able to overcome numerous medical conditions, but may need multiple medications to do so.

> **Street Smarts**
>
> Some older patients have physical, cognitive, and psychological barriers that impede their ability to communicate effectively. Proper assessment and care for this population will often depend on your ability to use patience when interviewing them.

Cardiovascular System

Cardiac function declines with age, due in large part to atherosclerosis, a condition characterized by the buildup of cholesterol and calcium along the inner walls of blood vessels, resulting in the formation of plaque. As plaque accumulates, the flow of blood through the affected vessels becomes restricted or blocked entirely. This results in an increased risk of heart attack, stroke, and other vascular illnesses. In the United States, approximately one-half of adults older than 45 years have atherosclerotic disease, with the risk increasing with advanced age.[7]

Additional cardiovascular effects of aging include increased incidence of bradycardia and other abnormal heart rhythms, an increased risk for hypertension, and diminished ability of the heart to increase cardiac output to meet the body's demands. These changes translate into a heart that is less able to cope with exercise or disease. In the event of a life-threatening illness, the body typically preserves blood pressure by increasing the heart rate.

Because the vascular system of the older adult becomes stiff, blood vessels are unable to dilate and contract as effectively. As a result, the diastolic blood pressure increases and the heart must work harder to overcome vascular resistance to move blood throughout the body. Over time, the increase in workload can be detrimental to the heart, resulting in heart failure.

Human blood cells originate within bone marrow. But with advancing age, bone marrow is replaced by fatty tissue. Consequently, the loss of marrow equals a reduction in the body's capability to manufacture new blood cells. Alone, this change is not cause for alarm. However, in the presence of traumatic injury in which a relatively large volume of blood is lost quickly, the impeded capability to replace lost cells can have devastating effects.

Respiratory System

In older adults, respiratory function gradually declines. The surface area of the alveoli decreases, as do the elasticity of the lungs and the strength of the intercostal muscles and diaphragm. Together, these factors make breathing more laborious for older adults. By the time older adults are 75 years old, their vital capacity (the volume of air moved during the deepest inspiration and expiration) has declined to approximately 50% of that of a young adult. In addition, their normal oxygen saturation level declines to approximately 95%.[8]

The chest becomes more rigid, yet more fragile. Instead of bending and flexing under stress, the calcified rib case is more susceptible to fracture. Normally, these changes in the respiratory system are gradual, often going unnoticed until the onset of a severe, life-threatening condition, in which case the lack of respiratory reserve becomes more pronounced.

As the patient ages, the structures protecting the upper airway decrease in function. Cough and gag reflexes diminish along with the ability to clear secretions. The cilia that line the airway dwindle, and sensation within the airway declines, making it more difficult for the older adult to maintain upper airway patency. Thus, older adults are at greater risk of aspiration and airway obstruction.

When a younger patient inhales, the airway maintains its shape, allowing air to enter. As the smooth muscles of the lower airway weaken with age, strong inhalation can cause the walls of the airway to collapse inward, producing inspiratory wheezing, lower flow rates, and air trapping in the alveoli (incomplete expiration). Because of these reductions in function, and because the white blood cells of the airway are less aggressive toward invading organisms, the older patient is more susceptible to lung infections.

Endocrine System

Endocrine function also declines with age. Glucose metabolism slows, while insulin production decreases. Sexually, men often continue to produce sperm long into their 80s (although the rigidity of the penis typically diminishes over time). The size of a woman's uterus and vagina decreases. Hormone production in both sexes gradually declines, and although sexual desire may lessen, it does not ordinarily cease entirely.

Digestive System

Age-related changes in gastric and intestinal functions may inhibit nutritional intake and utilization. Tooth loss can make chewing more difficult; taste

YOU are the EMT

After expressing your concern about the patient's condition and advising him that driving himself to the hospital would not be safe, he agrees to be transported via EMS. You place the patient onto the stretcher, load him into the ambulance, and begin transport to a hospital located a short distance away. En route, you reassess his vital signs; assess his blood glucose level, which reads 100 mg/dL; and then call your radio report to the hospital.

Recording Time: 11 Minutes	
Level of consciousness	Conscious and alert
Respirations	14 breaths/min; regular and adequate
Pulse	80 beats/min; strong and regular
Skin	Baseline color, warm, and dry
Blood pressure	180/102 mm Hg
Oxygen saturation (Spo_2)	99% (on room air)

6. What additional treatment, if any, does this patient require?

buds become less sensitive to salty and sweet foods; and food in general may be perceived as bland and flavorless, as the senses of smell and taste response begin to fade. A decrease in saliva secretion impairs the body's ability to break down complex carbohydrates. Similarly, gastric acid secretion diminishes. Peristalsis (the process by which intestinal contractions move food along the digestive tract) slows with age, sometimes resulting in constipation and/or suppressed feelings of hunger. Because blood flow to the intestines can drop by as much as 50%, the extraction of vitamins and minerals from digested food can also wane. Gallstones become increasingly common, and changes in the elasticity of the anal sphincter can lead to fecal incontinence.

Renal System

Between the ages of 18 and 75 years, the kidneys will lose almost one-half of their functional units (the nephrons), and their filtration capabilities will decline significantly.[9] This is due in part to a decrease in blood supply to the nephrons of the kidneys. Nephrons filter blood within the kidney. As a result of the changes, the renal system's ability to remove waste from the body declines, as does its ability to conserve fluids when needed.

Nervous System

By the time a person is 70 years of age, the brain has decreased in weight by as much as 11%.[10] Motor and sensory neural networks are slower and less responsive. However, the brain's metabolic rate and oxygen consumption remain unchanged. Although it is generally true that the infant brain has a larger number of neurons than its adult counterpart, the adult brain is much more flexible. This is because the number of interconnections between neurons increases with age. These connections produce redundancies within the brain that permit the loss of neurons without a loss of knowledge or skill. However, although cognitive function remains intact throughout most of older adulthood, mental function often declines in the 5 years immediately preceding death.

One consequence of the reduced number of neurons is the alteration of sleep patterns. Instead of sleeping through the night, the older adult may take a nap during the day and be awake late at night. It is not uncommon for older adults to develop a biphasic (two-phased) sleep cycle (eg, sleeping from 0100 to 0600 hours and then taking a nap from 1200 to 1500 hours).

Throughout life, the cranial vault is almost entirely occupied by the brain, the meningeal layers, and the cerebrospinal fluid between these layers. As such, there is virtually no empty space. However, in older adults, the age-related shrinkage of the brain creates a void between the brain and the outermost layer of the meninges. The resulting space gives the brain room to move inside the cranium (**FIGURE 7-15**). As such, any mechanism that causes a rapid or forceful shifting of the brain has the potential to result in the tearing of bridging veins. Subsequent slow venous bleeding into the open space may go unnoticed for some time.

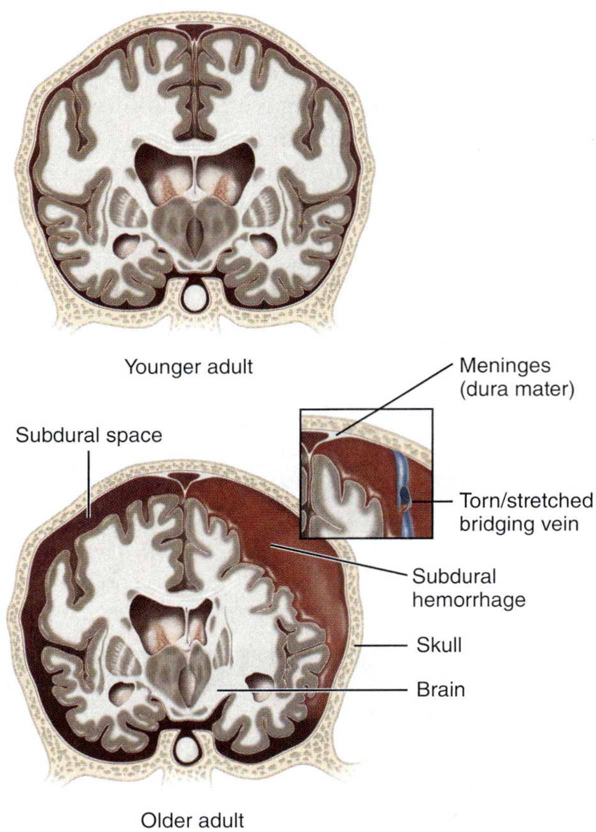

FIGURE 7-15 Age-related atrophy or shrinkage of the brain creates space between the brain and dura mater (subdural space). When the bridging veins are stretched and torn, blood may accumulate in this area.

The functioning of the peripheral nervous system slows with age. Sensations become diminished and may be misinterpreted. Nerve endings deteriorate, and the ability of the skin to sense the surroundings becomes hindered. Hot, cold, sharp, and wet objects all can create dangerous situations because the body cannot sense them quickly enough. Combined with prolonged reaction time and slower reflexes, these sensory alterations may contribute to the higher incidence of falls and trauma in older adults.

Street Smarts

Some of your geriatric patients will present with confusion. The confusion may be the result of long-standing dementia, such as Alzheimer disease. At other times, it may be new and sudden, resulting from a reversible cause such as infection. In this case, the confusion is referred to as delirium. In either situation, you may find the patient unable to answer your questions. If the patient cannot answer your questions, you must determine how to obtain the information you need. Never assume confusion is a normal part of aging. Look for possible causes of the altered mental status.

Sensory Changes

Pupillary reaction and ocular movements become more restricted with age. The pupils are generally smaller in older patients, and the opacity of the eye's lens diminishes visual acuity and causes the pupils to be sluggish in their reaction to light. Visual distortions are also common in older people. Thickening of the lens makes it more difficult for the eye to focus, especially at close range. Peripheral fields of vision narrow, and increased sensitivity to glare constricts the visual field.

Hearing difficulty is found in nearly one-half of adults older than 75 years.[11] Uncorrected hearing loss contributes to social isolation, cognitive decline, and decreased mobility. Changes in several hearing-related structures may lead to a loss of high-frequency hearing or even deafness. Even so, although it is often assumed that all older adults have difficulty hearing and seeing, many older adults have remarkably good vision and hearing. Some may need eyeglasses or hearing aids, but this does not mean they are almost deaf or nearly blind.

Psychosocial Changes

Many older Americans live at home and may have the assistance of family, friends, or home health care, but they are shown to be relatively healthy, active, and independent. The increasing number of older adults in the United States as a result of the baby boom of the 1940s through the 1960s has produced a need for additional assisted living facilities. These facilities allow older adults to live in campus-based communities with people in their own age group, while enjoying the independence and privacy of their own apartment and the security of nursing care, maintenance, and food preparation, if desired (**FIGURE 7-16**). Unfortunately, availability of these facilities is limited, and they can be expensive.

An additional and important consequence of congregate living facilities is the proximity of the residents to one another. Although having people close to each other is advantageous from a social interaction standpoint, it limits the natural social distancing that occurs when people live completely independently. Residents of these communities interact with one another and with caregivers on a close, regular basis, which has the disadvantage of enhancing the spread of contagious diseases such as the flu and COVID-19. Furthermore, residents of these facilities are necessarily more susceptible to the consequences of these diseases. This helps explain the disproportionate effect that epidemics and pandemics associated with these diseases have on older adults living in continuing care, assisted living, and nursing home communities.

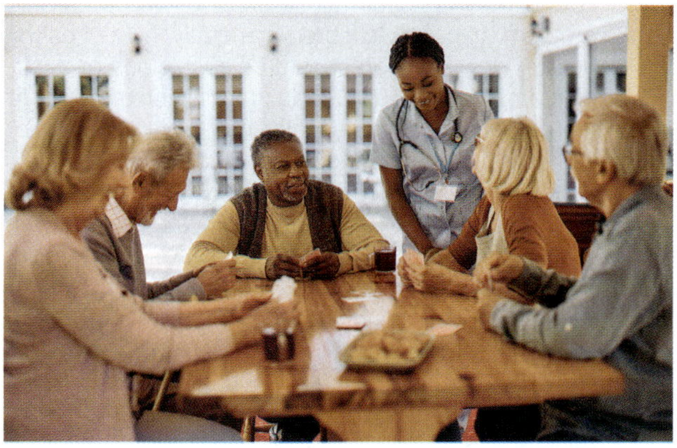

FIGURE 7-16 A small percentage of older adults live in assisted living facilities.

Few things in life cause more worry and stress than money problems. Older adults, in particular, may worry about the rising cost of health care. At times, some may have to choose between paying for groceries or paying for medications. In the United States, poverty is of particular concern for single and minority older women.[12] The financial struggle is compounded by the fact that currently, compared to past generations, families of older adults are less likely to assume responsibility for their aging family members.

One challenge facing older adults is the growing realization of their mortality. Everyone dies; but for younger people, the concept of death is little more than an intellectual exercise with a distant connection to reality. By contrast, the death of a spouse, close friend, or other loved one with whom the older adult may have shared 50 years or more of their life, can be a strong reminder that death is not only inevitable, but close by.

For some, the loss of loved ones leaves the older adult without a source of social support, and this places them at greater risk of isolation and depression. Fortunately, many older adults are happy and actively participating in life. With good financial resources and a good support system of family and friends, adults in their 80s and beyond can enjoy life and continue to feel productive.

YOU are the EMT SUMMARY

1. How does a patient's age affect your assessment?

The fundamental concepts of patient assessment are the same for all age groups. However, factors such as physical development, communication skills, behavior, and vital sign values vary with age.

Communication with the patient is an integral part of the patient assessment process, especially the history-taking phase. Depending on the patient's age, communication can be relatively easy or extremely difficult.

Certain medical conditions that are common in one age group are uncommon in others. Determining a patient's risk factors for disease is an important part of the history-taking process and affects your index of suspicion. For example, it is rare, although not impossible, for an otherwise healthy 8-year-old child with chest pain to be experiencing a cardiac problem because children generally have healthy hearts. However, you should be suspicious of a cardiac problem if a 55-year-old patient with a history of high blood pressure, a major risk factor for cardiovascular disease, has the same symptoms.

Older patients are more likely to have one or more chronic diseases that can be the origin of the current problem (eg, chronic lung disease exacerbation), complicate the current problem (eg, respiratory infection in a patient with a history of asthma or chronic lung disease), or make the assessment process more difficult (eg, obtaining history in a patient with a medical problem who has dementia). Older patients also frequently take medications that can affect assessment (eg, blood pressure medications that may keep pulses lower than would normally occur in response to disease or injury) or exacerbate symptoms (eg, too much insulin for the amount of food intake).

Understanding which illnesses are common in various age groups will help you formulate a plausible field impression—that is, what you believe is wrong with the patient based on your assessment findings and the patient's history.

2. What are the physical differences between middle adults and older adults?

Middle adults (40 to 65 years of age) have reached the halfway point in human life expectancy. However, provided they are otherwise healthy, their vital signs and physical abilities usually remain consistent with those of early adults. Their average pulse rate is 70 beats/min, their respiratory rate is between 12 and 20 breaths/min, and their systolic blood pressure is between 90 and 120 mm Hg.

The age-related physical changes that occur in older adults (65 years of age and older) are more pronounced than they are in middle adults and affect nearly every organ and organ system in the body.

The vital signs of older adults depend largely on their underlying health and are often affected by medications taken. In general, however, age-related vital sign changes include a decrease in heart rate during exertion and an increase in diastolic blood pressure. The elasticity of the lungs also decreases, forcing this group to rely more on their intercostal muscles to breathe. In addition, the ribs become more rigid due to calcification, which adds to breathing difficulty.

YOU are the EMT SUMMARY continued

Other physical changes that occur during late adulthood include a decrease in metabolism and insulin production, which can lead to diabetes, decreased gastrointestinal function, decreased taste bud sensation, decreased kidney size and filtration (kidney function declines by 50% from age 20 to age 90 years), nervous system changes (including a 10% to 20% decrease in brain weight by 80 years of age) and sensory and motor nerve deterioration, and vision and hearing loss, among others. Additionally, decreased muscle mass and strength in older adults may alter body temperature regulation or cause problems with balance, leading to a higher risk of falls as compared with middle adults. Thinning bones due to osteoporosis also increase the risk of bone fractures in late adulthood.

The anatomic and physiologic changes that occur between middle and late adulthood must be taken into consideration during your assessment.

Keep in mind, however, that compared with middle adults, older adults often have fewer classic signs and symptoms of a wide variety of medical conditions. For example, pain sensation may be diminished due to nervous system decrease, fever may be less likely in infection due to diminished immune system function, or increased heart rate in response to a medical problem or trauma may not occur due to diminished heart function or medications being taken by older adults.

3. What are some common psychosocial concerns experienced by middle adults?

During middle adulthood, many people's concerns center on finances. This often causes stress and uncertainty.

A unique psychosocial concern in middle adults relates to their children and their parents. As their children move away from home, which forces them to readjust their lifestyle (empty nest syndrome), their own parents are getting older and now need care. Most middle adults prefer to care for their parents in their own home or in their parents' home; however, this often increases the stress and anxiety they are already experiencing from other factors such as finances or retirement.

4. Are the patient's vital signs consistent with his age?

The patient's heart rate and respiratory rate are consistent with his age. However, his blood pressure is not. A typical middle adult's systolic blood pressure ranges between 90 and 120 mm Hg; the diastolic blood pressure usually ranges between 70 and 80 mm Hg.

Ask the patient if he keeps a journal of his vital signs or if he has had his vital signs recently taken. If he knows, ask him what his blood pressure typically reads; clearly, hypertension cannot be diagnosed based on a single blood pressure reading. If he tells you his current blood pressure is consistent with what it normally reads, ask him if he is under a physician's care or being treated with any medication. If he is not, you should advise him to be evaluated by a physician; he may have hypertension and not be aware of it. Hypertension is often referred to as the silent killer, and a blood pressure of 174/98 mm Hg is abnormal at any age.

5. Why should you transport this patient to the hospital?

This patient should *not* drive himself to the hospital. He experienced a near-syncopal episode, which could indicate a variety of underlying medical conditions, some of them potentially life threatening. The patient is light-headed, reports a headache, and is hypertensive. He should be informed that if he drives himself to the hospital, he could experience worsening of his light-headedness or even a syncopal episode while driving; this would jeopardize not only his own safety but also the safety of other motorists.

Although the patient is of legal age and has the decision-making capacity to legally refuse EMS transport, you should make *every effort* to convince him to agree to EMS transport and advise him that his refusal could potentially result in death.

6. What additional treatment, if any, does this patient require?

Further treatment of this patient should be investigatory into the cause of the patient's dizziness and headache. Continue to monitor his mental status and ABCs (Airway, Breathing, Circulation) and make him comfortable. The patient should be assessed using a prehospital stroke test, and a 12-lead electrocardiogram should be obtained and transmitted to the hospital for interpretation or interpreted by ALS as directed by local protocol. Additionally, dimming the lights in the back of the ambulance may provide him with some relief from his headache.

Remain alert for any changes in his neurologic status, such as slurred speech, unilateral weakness (weakness to one side of the body), or confusion, and contact the receiving facility if any changes are noted.

Prep Kit

Ready for Review

- Each developmental stage is marked by different physical and psychosocial changes and characteristics; infants (1 month to 1 year) develop at a surprising rate.
- The vital signs of toddlers (age, 1 to 3 years) and preschoolers (age, 3 to 6 years) differ somewhat from those of an infant. During this stage, children learn to speak and express themselves.
- From ages 6 to 12 years, the school-age child's vital signs and body gradually approach those observed in adulthood. During this stage, children develop self-esteem.
- The vital signs of adolescents (age, 12 to 18 years) begin to level off within the adult ranges. Adolescents focus on creating their self-image.
- Early adults, ages 18 to 40 years, typically focus on work and family. Despite their many responsibilities, this is usually a healthy and psychologically stable period of life.
- Middle adults, ages 40 to 65 years, typically focus on achieving life goals. They may need to balance work responsibilities with the responsibility of caring for both their children and their aging parents.
- Older adults, ages 65 years and older, often maintain their independence and enjoy happy, active lives. They typically become more concerned with their mortality and the mortality of friends and loved ones.
- Vital signs do not vary greatly throughout adulthood.

Vital Vocabulary

adolescent A young person age 12 to 18 years.

ageism The assumption that older people are less healthy or capable; can lead to poor patient assessment and care.

barotrauma Injury caused by pressure to enclosed body surfaces, for example, from too much pressure in the lungs.

conventional reasoning A type of reasoning in which a child looks for approval from peers and society.

early adult A young adult age 18 to 40 years.

fontanelles Areas where the newborn's or infant's skull has not fused together; usually disappear at approximately 18 months of age.

gender identity A personal sense of oneself as male or female (or, less commonly, both or neither).

geriatrics The assessment and treatment of disease in someone who is age 65 years or older.

infant A young child age 1 month to 1 year.

life expectancy The average number of years a person can be expected to live.

middle adult An adult age 40 to 65 years.

Moro reflex An infant reflex in which, when an infant is caught off guard, the infant opens their arms wide, spreads the fingers, and seems to grab at things.

newborn A person age birth to 1 month.

older adult An adult age 65 years or older.

palmar grasp reflex An infant reflex that occurs when something is placed in the infant's palm; the infant grasps the object.

pediatrics A specialized medical practice devoted to the care of the young.

postconventional reasoning A type of reasoning in which a child bases decisions on their conscience.

preconventional reasoning A type of reasoning in which a child acts almost purely to avoid punishment or to get what they want.

preschooler A child age 3 to 6 years.

rooting reflex An infant reflex that occurs when something touches an infant's cheek, and the infant instinctively turns their head toward the touch.

Prep Kit continued

school age A person who is 6 to 12 years of age.

sexual orientation A person's emotional, romantic, or sexual attraction to other people.

sucking reflex An infant reflex in which the infant starts sucking when their lips are stroked.

toddler A child age 1 to 3 years.

trust versus mistrust The stage of development from birth to approximately 18 months of age, during which infants gain trust in their parents or caregivers if their world is planned, organized, and routine.

References

1. Moore C, Dailey S, Garrison H, Amatuni A, Bergelson E. Point, walk, talk: links between three early milestones, from observation and parental report. *Dev Psychol*. 2019;55(8):157–1593.
2. Bruni O, Baumgartner E, Sette S, et al. Longitudinal study of sleep behavior in normal infants during the first year of life. *J Clin Sleep Med*. 2014;10(10):1119–1127.
3. Russell ST, Joyner K. Adolescent sexual orientation and suicide risk: evidence from a national study. *Am J Public Health*. 2001;91(8):1276–1281.
4. Web-based Injury Statistics Query and Reporting System (WISQARS). Ten leading causes of death, United States—2021. Centers for Disease Control and Prevention website. https://wisqars.cdc.gov/lcd/?o=LCD&y1=2021&y2=2021&ct=10&cc=ALL&g=00&s=0&r=0&ry=0&e=0&ar=lcd1age&at=groups&ag=lcd1age&a1=0&a2=199. Reviewed November 8, 2023. Accessed October 3, 2024.
5. Lopez-Jimenez F. Understanding the difference between biological age and chronological age. Mayo Clinic website. https://mcpress.mayoclinic.org/healthy-aging/understanding-the-difference-between-biological-age-and-chronological-age/. Published July 25, 2024. Accessed October 3, 2024.
6. National Center for Health Statistics. Life expectancy. Centers for Disease Control and Prevention website. https://www.cdc.gov/nchs/fastats/life-expectancy.htm. Reviewed February 7, 2023. Accessed October 3, 2024.
7. National Heart, Lung, and Blood Institute Atherosclerosis: what is atherosclerosis? National Institutes of Health website. https://www.nhlbi.nih.gov/health/atherosclerosis. Updated March 24, 2022. Accessed October 3, 2024.
8. Shaikh J, What are blood oxygen levels? MedicineNet website. medicinenet.com/what_are_blood_oxygen_levels/article.htm. Reviewed December 21, 2022. Accessed October 3, 2024.
9. van der Burgh AC, Rizopoulos D, Ikram MA, Hoorn EJ, Chaker L. Determinants of the evolution of kidney function with age. *Kidney Int Rep*. 2021;6(12):3054–3063.
10. Mauk K. *Gerontological Nursing*. 4th ed. Burlington, MA: Jones & Bartlett Learning; 2018.
11. Age-related hearing loss (presbycusis). National Institute on Deafness and Other Communication Disorders website. https://www.nidcd.nih.gov/health/age-related-hearing-loss. Updated March 17, 2023. Accessed October 3, 2024.
12. Older women and poverty: single and minority women. Women's Institute for a Secure Retirement website. https://wiserwomen.org/fact-sheets/facts-and-solutions/older-women-and-poverty-single-minority-women/. Accessed October 3, 2024.

Additional Resources

American Heart Association (AHA). *Pediatric Advanced Life Support Provider Manual*. Dallas, TX: AHA; 2020.

National Highway Traffic Safety Administration. *National Emergency Medical Services Education Standards*. https://www.ems.gov/assets/EMS_Education-Standards_2021_FNL.pdf. EMS.gov website. Published January 2021. Accessed October 3, 2024.

National Association of State EMS Officials. *National Model EMS Clinical Guidelines: Version 3.0*. https://nasemso.org/wp-content/uploads/National-Model-EMS-Clinical-Guidelines_2022.pdf. Updated March 2022. Accessed October 3, 2024.

Wyckoff AS. Thermometer use 101. *AAP News*. 2009;30(11):29.

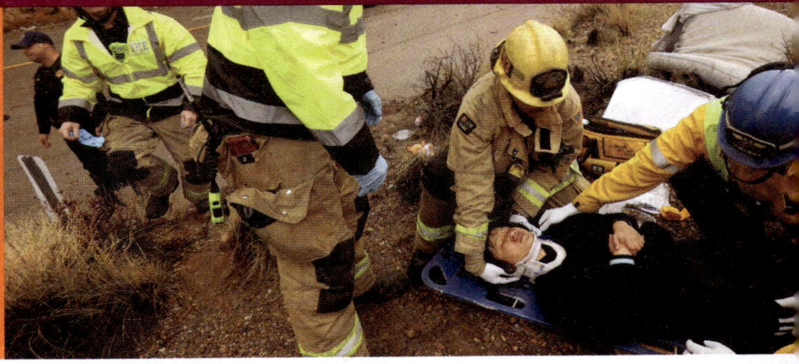

Chapter 8

Lifting and Moving Patients

NATIONAL EMS EDUCATION STANDARD COMPETENCIES

Preparatory

Applies knowledge of the emergency medical services (EMS) system, safety/well-being of the emergency medical technician (EMT), medical/legal, and ethical issues to the provision of emergency care.

Workforce Safety and Wellness

- Standard safety precautions (see Chapter 2, *Workforce Safety and Wellness*)
- Personal protective equipment (see Chapter 2, *Workforce Safety and Wellness*)
- Lifting and moving patients (pp 257–294)
- Crew resource management (see Chapter 9, *The Team Approach to Health Care*)
- Stress management (see Chapter 2, *Workforce Safety and Wellness*)
- Prevention of work-related injuries and illnesses (pp 258–265)
- Responder mental health, resilience, and suicide prevention (see Chapter 2, *Workforce Safety and Wellness*)
- Wellness principles (see Chapter 2, *Workforce Safety and Wellness*)
- Disease transmission (see Chapter 2, *Workforce Safety and Wellness*)

KNOWLEDGE OBJECTIVES

1. Explain the technical skills and general considerations required of EMTs during patient packaging and patient handling. (pp 257–265)
2. Define the term *body mechanics*. (pp 258–265)
3. Explain the special considerations and guidelines related to moving and transporting geriatric patients. (p 262)
4. Explain the special considerations and guidelines related to moving and transporting pediatric patients. (p 262)
5. Discuss how following proper patient lifting and moving techniques can help prevent work-related injuries. (pp 259–265)
6. Identify how to avoid common mistakes when lifting and carrying a patient. (pp 260–265)
7. Explain the general considerations required of EMTs to safely move patients without causing the patient further harm and while protecting themselves from injury. (pp 265–267)
8. Explain the importance of effective team communication when moving a patient. (pp 265–266)
9. Describe the context in which you may perform an emergency patient move. (pp 267–270)
10. Describe the different methods of performing an emergency patient move. (pp 270–276)
11. Describe specific situations in which a nonurgent move may be necessary to move a patient. (pp 275–276)

12. Explain the need for and use of the most common patient-moving equipment. (pp 276–294)
13. Explain the purpose and use of a wheeled ambulance stretcher. (pp 276–284)
14. Discuss the guidelines for lifting and moving bariatric patients. (p 278)
15. Explain the purpose and use of a backboard. (p 284)
16. Explain the purpose and use of a scoop stretcher. (pp 284–285)
17. Explain the purpose and use of a vacuum mattress. (pp 284–285)
18. Explain the purpose and use of a stair chair. (pp 288–290)
19. Explain the purpose and use of a neonatal isolette. (pp 290–291)
20. Explain the purpose and use of common transfer devices, including the Binder Lift and Slipp patient mover. (p 291)
21. Explain the purpose and use of alternative stretchers, including the portable/folding stretcher, flexible stretcher, and basket stretcher. (pp 291–293)
22. Explain the importance of decontaminating equipment in the prevention of disease transmission. (p 294)

SKILLS OBJECTIVES

1. Perform a power lift to lift a patient. (pp 260–261, Skill Drill 8-1)
2. Demonstrate a power grip. (p 262)
3. Demonstrate the body mechanics and principles required for safe reaching and pulling, including the technique used for performing log rolls. (pp 263–265)
4. Demonstrate how to perform an emergency or urgent move. (pp 267–275)
5. Perform the rapid extrication technique to move a patient from a vehicle. (pp 272–273, Skill Drill 8-2)
6. Perform the extremity lift to move a patient. (pp 275–276, Skill Drill 8-3)
7. Demonstrate how to use the draw sheet method to transfer a patient onto a stretcher. (pp 278–279)
8. Demonstrate how to log roll a patient on the ground (pp 279–280, Skill Drill 8-4)
9. Demonstrate how to load a stretcher into an ambulance. (pp 282–284, Skill Drill 8-5)
10. Use a scoop stretcher to move a patient. (pp 284–285, Skill Drill 8-6)
11. Perform the diamond carry to move a patient. (pp 285–286, Skill Drill 8-7)
12. Perform the one-handed carry to move a patient. (p 287, Skill Drill 8-8)
13. Perform a patient carry to move a patient down the stairs on a backboard. (p 289, Skill Drill 8-9)
14. Perform a patient carry using a stair chair to move a patient down the stairs. (pp 289–290, Skill Drill 8-10)

Introduction

In the course of a typical call, you will have to move the patient several times to provide emergency medical care and transport. Once you have assessed the patient and provided emergency care, the patient is generally moved onto a stretcher. You will need to determine if the patient is able to ambulate and whether ambulation is appropriate given the patient's condition. In some cases, you will have to lift and carry the patient to the stretcher. Once the patient is on the stretcher, you will safely secure the patient using the stretcher's securing devices, move the stretcher to the ambulance, and load the stretcher into the patient compartment. On arrival at the hospital, the patient must be removed from the ambulance, wheeled into the emergency department (ED), and transferred to the ED bed.

Every year, a significant number of EMTs are injured when they attempt to lift and move patients.[1] Back injuries are the leading cause of injury that forces EMTs and paramedics to leave the profession.[2] To avoid injury to the patient, yourself, or your team, you need to learn how to lift and carry a patient properly, using proper body mechanics. To move a patient safely in the various situations that you may encounter in the field, it is necessary to learn how to perform emergency body drags and lifts, rapidly extricate a patient from a vehicle onto the stretcher, assist a patient from a chair or bed onto the stretcher, lift a patient from the floor onto the stretcher, and manually carry a patient up or down stairs. You and your team should know how to ensure spinal motion restriction for a patient with a suspected spinal injury and how to package patients with and without suspected spinal injury. You also need to know how to properly use patient-moving devices, such as a stretcher, stair chair, backboard, scoop stretcher, flexible stretcher, and any other equipment your service may carry. You must know which device or combination of devices is appropriate for the current situation.

At times, you and your team may need to move a patient who is very heavy or carry a patient on a trail or across rugged terrain. You will be introduced to various types of equipment that can be used in these situations along with special techniques for loading and unloading the stretcher and transferring the patient from the stretcher to a bed in the ED.

Always be mindful that lifting and carrying are dynamic processes. Performing these actions safely requires an understanding of anatomy, body mechanics, team dynamics, and patient positioning. This chapter begins by explaining these basic principles, then applies these principles to the specific techniques and equipment you will use in the field.

Principles of Moving and Positioning the Patient

Patient packaging and handling are technical skills that you will learn and perfect through repeated training and practice. Even when you are lifting, moving, or transferring relatively lightweight patients, the need for proper body mechanics should remain paramount. Occasionally, injuries occur when proper lifting techniques are used; however, using proper body mechanics and maintaining physical fitness greatly reduces the risk of injury.

Moving a patient should be done in an orderly, planned, and unhurried manner. This approach will protect you, your team, and the patient from further injury and reduce the risk of worsening the patient's condition when they are moved. Therefore, practice each technique with your team often so that when you must move a patient, you can perform the move quickly, safely, and efficiently. You must also master the skills necessary for the use of all equipment and understand the advantages and limitations of each device before you use it in the field. After each patient transfer, you and your team should evaluate the appropriateness of the technique that you used, as well as your technical skill in completing the transfer. You must also be sure to maintain your equipment according to the manufacturer's instructions. Using clean, well-maintained equipment is a critical part of providing high-quality patient care.

After transferring the patient to the ED, you and your team must begin preparation for your next call by reviewing the positive points about the transport and discussing changes that would improve the next run. This process of evaluation should help you identify the following:

- Procedures that need more practice
- Equipment that needs to be cleaned or serviced
- Skills that you need to review or acquire

Anatomy and Body Mechanics

The shoulder girdle rests on the rib cage and is supported by the vertebrae that lie inferior to it. The arms are connected to and hang from the shoulder

YOU are the EMT

You are dispatched to a motor vehicle crash with an overturned vehicle. You arrive on scene to find a four-door sedan lying on the passenger side in a deep ditch. The vehicle is resting on a concrete pipe and a metal signpost. There are two patients, neither of whom appear to be restrained. The driver is an older man who is unresponsive. You note that his skin is ashen with cyanosis around his lips. He is crumpled in a semi-supine position over the second patient. Only the top of the head of the passenger is visible, but she is alert and able to speak with you.

1. What immediate challenges do you face?
2. Why is knowledge of body mechanics important when lifting and moving a patient?
3. What other resources are needed?

girdle. When a person stands upright, the individual weight-bearing vertebrae are stacked on top of each other and aligned over the sacrum. The sacrum is both the mechanical weight-bearing base of the spinal column and the fused central posterior section of the pelvic girdle. **Body mechanics** is the relationship between the body's anatomic structures and the physical forces associated with lifting, moving, and carrying; in other words, it refers to the ways in which the body moves to achieve a specific action. Maintaining proper posture and body movement during daily activities is applying the use of body mechanics. Using good body mechanics while lifting and moving patients reduces your risk of injury.

When a person stands upright, the weight of anything being lifted and carried in the hands is reflected onto the shoulder girdle, the spinal column inferior to it, the pelvis, and then the legs (**FIGURE 8-1**). In lifting, if the shoulder girdle is aligned over the pelvis and the hands are held close to the legs, the force that is exerted against the spine occurs in an essentially straight line down the vertebrae in the spinal column. Therefore, with the back properly maintained in an upright position, little strain occurs against the muscles and ligaments that keep the spinal column in alignment, and significant weight can be lifted and carried without injury to the back (**FIGURE 8-2**). However, injuries may occur if you lift while leaning forward, or even if you lift while the back is straight, while you are bent forward at the hips. When the shoulder girdle lies significantly anterior to the pelvis the force of lifting is exerted primarily across, rather than down, the spinal column. When this occurs, the weight is supported by the muscles of the back and ligaments that run from the base of the skull to the pelvis, rather than by each vertebral body and disk resting on those aligned below it. In addition, the upper spine and torso serve as a lever so that the force that is exerted against the muscles and ligaments in

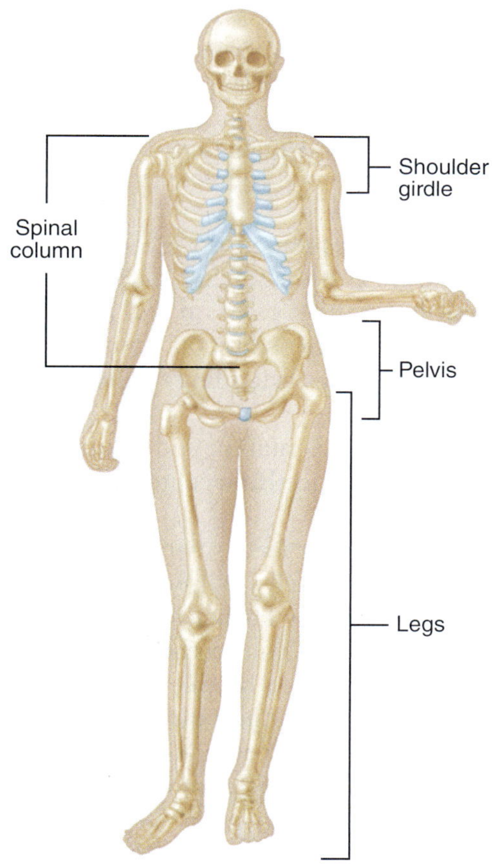

FIGURE 8-1 When you stand upright, the weight of anything that you lift and carry in your hands is borne by the shoulder girdle, the spinal column, the pelvis, and the legs.

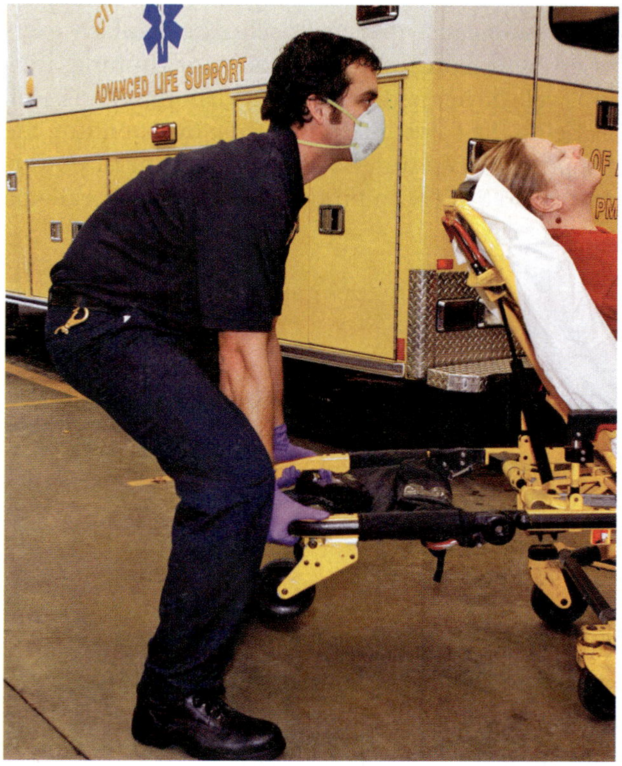

FIGURE 8-2 If your body is properly aligned when you lift, the line of force exerted against the spine occurs in an essentially straight line down the vertebrae. In this way, the vertebrae support the lift.

the lumbar and sacral regions, as a result of the mechanical advantage produced, is many times that of the combined weight of your upper body and the object you are lifting. Therefore, the first key rule of lifting is to always keep your back in a straight, upright (vertical) position, and lift without twisting. Always face the patient and point your feet in the same direction. After lifting the patient, change the direction of your feet as opposed to twisting or turning from the waist.

When lifting, spread your legs approximately shoulder width apart, and place your feet so that your center of gravity is properly balanced between them. Your weight should be balanced on the balls of your feet and heels, not your toes. Then, with the back held upright, bring your upper body down by bending the legs. Once you have properly grasped the patient or stretcher and made any necessary adjustments in the location of your feet, lift by straightening your legs until you are in a standing position and then curling your arms up to waist height. If you still have not reached the desired height, reposition your legs so they are closer together and repeat the process. Because the leg muscles are regularly exercised by walking, climbing stairs, or running, they are well developed and strong. Therefore, as well as being the safest method, lifting by extending the properly placed flexed legs is also the most powerful way to lift. This method is appropriately called a **power lift**.

Words of Wisdom

The stretcher is designed so that the patient's head is slightly higher than the feet. Always position the tallest EMS clinician at the head of the stretcher when lifting to offset this difference in the height of the stretcher.

One mistake to avoid is lifting a patient or other heavy object with your arms outstretched. Even if your back is held properly upright, adverse forces across the spinal column and leverage against the low back will occur if your hands are significantly anterior to the plane described by the front of the torso (the plane consists of the anterior torso and imaginary lines extended vertically above and below it). Whenever you lift or carry a patient, be sure to hold your arms so that your hands are almost adjacent to the plane described by your anterior torso, and always keep the weight that you are lifting as close to your body as possible.

Another rule to remember when lifting is to avoid placing lateral force across the spine and sideways leverage against the low back. If you lift with only one arm or with the arms extended more to one side than the other, more force will be exerted against one side of the shoulder girdle than the other, causing lateral force to be exerted across the spinal column. To prevent this, keep your arms approximately the same distance apart as when hanging at each side of the body, with the weight distributed equally and properly centered between them. If the weight is not balanced between both arms or properly centered between the shoulders when you are preparing to lift, turn and/or move to the left or right until the weight is properly balanced and centered. To lift safely and produce the maximal power lift, take the following steps (**SKILL DRILL 8-1**):

1. Tighten your back in its normal upright position, and use your abdominal core muscles to lock it in.
2. Spread your legs apart approximately 15 inches (38 cm), and bend your legs to lower your torso and arms.
3. With arms extended down each side of the body, grasp the stretcher or backboard with your hands held palm up and just in front of the plane described by the anterior torso and imaginary lines extending vertically from it to the ground.
4. Adjust your orientation and position until the weight is balanced and centered between both arms (**Step 1**).
5. Reposition your feet as necessary so that they are approximately 15 inches (38 cm) apart with one slightly farther forward and rotated so that you and your center of gravity will be properly balanced between them. Be sure to keep your feet flat and distribute your weight to the balls of the feet or just behind them. The knees should not bend more than 90°, nor extend past the toes.
6. With the arms extended downward, lift by straightening your legs until you are fully standing. Make sure your back is held upright and that your upper body comes up before your hips (**Step 2**).

Skill Drill 8-1 Performing the Power Lift

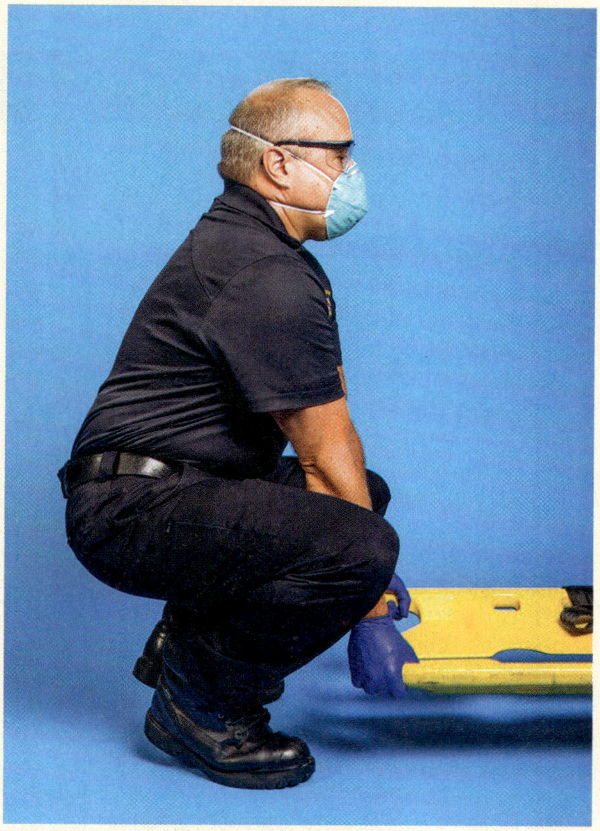

Step 1

Lock your back using your abdominal muscles. Spread and bend your legs. Grasp the backboard, palms up and just in front of you. Balance and center the weight between your arms.

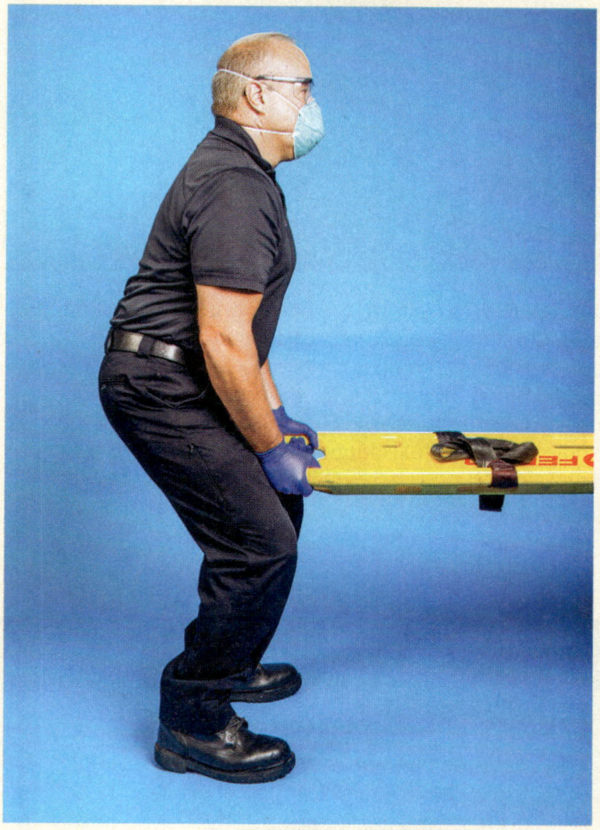

Step 2

Position your feet and distribute your weight evenly. Lift by straightening your legs, keeping your back locked in.

Reverse these steps whenever you are lowering the stretcher. Always remember to avoid bending at the waist or twisting as you stand.

Your safety, as well as that of the other EMS clinicians and the patient, depends on the use of proper lifting techniques and maintaining a proper hold when lifting or carrying a patient. If you do not have proper hold of the stretcher or of the patient in a body lift, you will not be able to bear a proper share of the weight, and there is an increased risk that you might suddenly lose your grasp with one or both hands. If you temporarily lose your grasp, the position and weight distribution of the stretcher will change suddenly, and the other team members must quickly overextend beyond a safe distance to avoid dropping the patient. As a result, sudden excessive force may be placed across each one's spine, causing low back injury.

You should use the **power grip** to get the maximum force from your hands and arms whenever you are lifting a patient (**FIGURE 8-3**). The arm and hand have their greatest lifting strength when

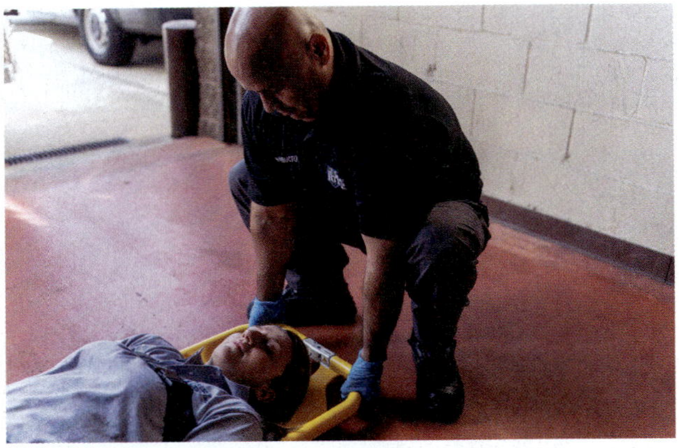

FIGURE 8-3 To perform the power grip, grasp the handle of the stretcher or backboard with your palms up and your thumbs extending up. Make sure your hands are approximately 10 inches (25 cm) apart and that your fingers are all at the same angle. The underside of the handle should be fully supported by the palms of your hands.

Courtesy of Aura Prep/Rescue Training International.

Special Populations

GERIATRIC CONSIDERATIONS

Most patients transported by EMS are older adults (geriatric patients). These patients will need to be moved, lifted, and carried frequently. The aging process is associated with multiple changes in the body, including the musculoskeletal system and the integumentary system (ie, the skin). As people age, they may become less flexible, and bones become more brittle. Using the extremities to move or carry a geriatric patient may cause the person a significant amount of pain or discomfort. In some older patients, pulling an arm or leg may cause a dislocation or fracture. The skin of a geriatric patient is thinner and more susceptible to tears and bruising. Be careful not to cause a skin tear when gripping an arm or leg. Chronic medical conditions such as rheumatoid arthritis may limit the patient's movement and are associated with pain. Some older patients cannot lie flat or straighten their arms. Usual moving and packaging techniques may not be appropriate for some patients with spinal deformations (eg, kyphosis). Extra padding and support may be necessary to transport some patients comfortably. EMTs must keep these considerations in mind as they prepare to move, lift, and carry geriatric patients. Do not cause additional injury or pain to your patient.

facing palm up. Whenever you grasp a stretcher or backboard, your hands should be at least 10 inches (25 cm) apart. Each hand should be inserted under the handle with the palm facing up and the thumb

Special Populations

PEDIATRIC CONSIDERATIONS

Transporting pediatric patients can present a variety of challenges for the EMT. First, small children (ie, children whose height is less than a length-based resuscitation tape[3]) do not fit safely on adult transport devices. For example, strap locations are designed for adult patients. The safest way to transport a child is by using a device made for the transport of children (**FIGURE 8-4**).[4] Pediatric transport devices are available that include five-point harnesses that can be secured to the ambulance stretcher. Many of these devices are designed to integrate onto wheeled stretchers.

An additional consideration is transport of the parent or caretaker with the child. Some agencies have policies stating all riders must be safely restrained in the front seat, but separation of the parent and child may cause further anxiety to an already frightened child. If the parent or caretaker is allowed to ride in the back of the ambulance with the child, the EMT must make certain the adult caregiver is safely restrained as well. Infants and children should not be transported in the arms of an adult. See Chapter 36, *Transport Operations*, for further discussion of transport considerations.

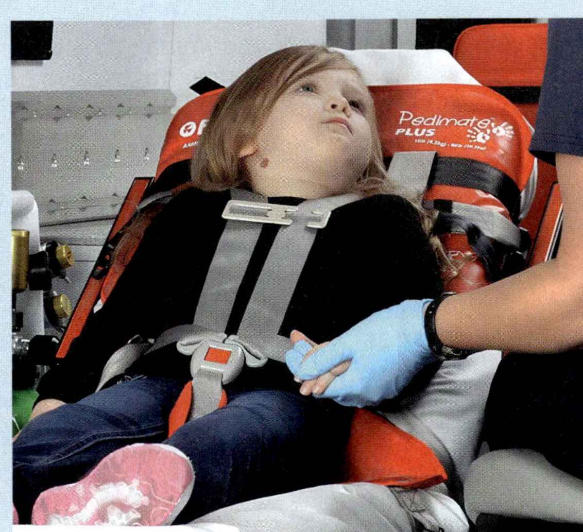

FIGURE 8-4 Transport small children using a device designed to accommodate their size.

Courtesy of Ferno-Washington, Inc. www.ferno.com.

extended upward. Next, advance the hand until the thumb prevents further insertion and the cylindrical handle lies firmly in the crease of your curved palm. Curl your fingers and thumb tightly over the top of the handle. All your fingers should be at the same angle. To have the proper power grip, make sure that the underside of the handle is fully supported on your curved palm with only the fingers and thumb preventing it from being pulled sideways or upward out of the palm.

If you must lift the object higher once you have lifted by extending your legs, you will be able to "curl" the object higher by using your biceps to flex the arms while maintaining the power grip and weight supported in the palms.

Never grasp a stretcher or backboard with the hand placed palm down over the handle. When you are lifting with the palm down, the weight is supported by the fingers rather than the palm. This hand orientation places the tips of the fingers and thumb under the handle. If the weight forces them apart, your grasp on the handle will be lost.

Safe Reaching and Pulling

The same basic body mechanics and principles apply to moving, lifting, and carrying a patient.

When you use a body drag to move a patient, your back should always be locked in by tightening your abdominal muscles, not curved laterally or bent laterally. It should be held in its normal upright position. Avoid any twisting so that the vertebrae remain in their normal alignment. When you reach overhead, avoid hyperextending your back. When you pull a patient who is on the ground, always kneel to minimize the distance that you will have to lean over (**FIGURE 8-5A**). To keep your reach within the recommended distance, reach forward and grasp the patient so that your elbows are just beyond the anterior torso (**FIGURE 8-5B**). When you pull a patient who is at a different height from you, bend your knees until your hips are just below the height of the plane across which you will be pulling the patient. During pulling, extend your arms no more than approximately 15 to 20 inches (38 to 50 cm) in front of your torso. Reposition your feet (or knees, if kneeling) so that the force of pull will be balanced equally between both arms and the line of pull will be centered between them. Pull the patient by slowly flexing your arms. When you can pull no farther because your hands have reached the front of your torso, stop and move back another 15 to 20 inches (38 to 50 cm). Then, when properly positioned, repeat the steps. Alternate between pulling the patient by flexing your arms and then repositioning yourself so that your arms are again extended with your hands approximately 15 inches (38 cm) in front of your torso. By not moving yourself and the patient simultaneously, you will prevent undesirable jostling of the patient and the risk that sudden force will occur across your spine. You should also try to prevent injury to yourself by avoiding situations that involve strenuous effort lasting longer than 1 minute.

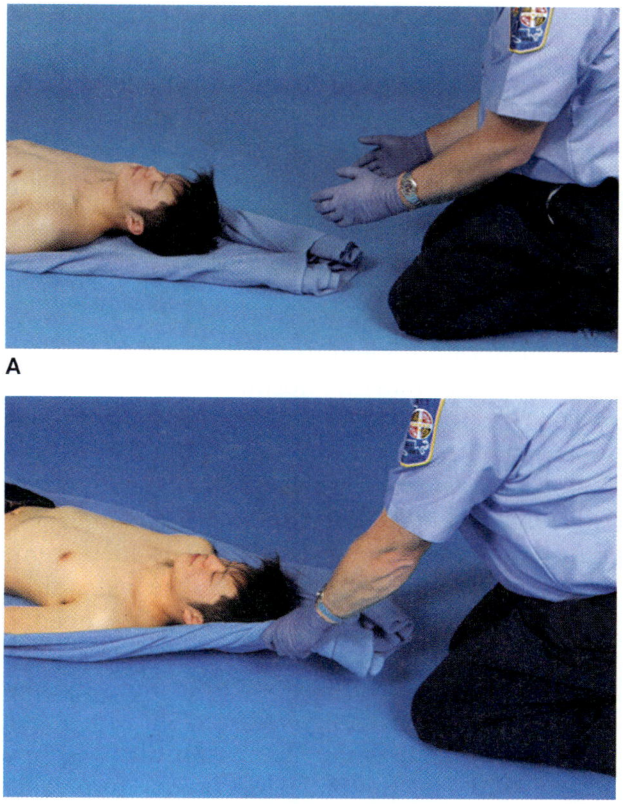

A

B

FIGURE 8-5 Reaching and pulling safely. **A.** Kneel to pull a patient who is on the ground. **B.** When pulling, your elbows should only extend just beyond the anterior torso.

If you must drag a patient across a bed, kneel on the bed to avoid reaching beyond the recommended distance. Then follow the steps described previously until the patient is within 15 to 20 inches (38 to 50 cm) of the bed's edge (see Figure 8-5). You can then complete the drag while standing at the side of the bed. Rather than dragging the patient by their clothing, use the sheet or blanket under the patient for this purpose. You can roll the bedding under the patient until it is approximately 6 inches (15 cm) wider than the patient. Pull on the rolled bedding smoothly and evenly to glide the patient to the bedside. If available, use a commercial transfer device, such as a Smooth-Mover or Slipp transfer mover, or a flexible stretcher. Always follow the manufacturer's instructions.

Transfer the patient from the stretcher to a bed in the ED or the patient's hospital room with a body drag. With the stretcher at the same height as the bed or slightly higher and held firmly against the bed's side, you and another EMS clinician should kneel on the hospital bed and, in the manner previously described, drag the patient in increments until they are properly centered on the bed. A third person may need to take both sides of the head to move the patient safely.

Sometimes during a body drag, you and another EMT may have to pull the patient with one of you on either side of the patient (**FIGURE 8-6**). You will have to alter the pulling technique to prevent pulling sideways and producing adverse lateral leverage against your lower back. Position yourself by kneeling just beyond the patient's shoulder and facing toward the groin. By extending one arm across and in front of your chest, you can grasp the armpit and, with your other arm extended in front and to the side of the patient's torso, the patient's belt. Then, by raising your elbows and flexing your arms, you can pull the patient with the line of force at the minimum angle possible.

Words of Wisdom

When moving a patient, you may grab the patient's belt to assist with the move. Never grab belt loops or pockets, which can easily rip with the patient's weight.

Generally, when log rolling a patient onto their side, you will initially have to reach farther than 18 inches (46 cm) (**FIGURE 8-7**). To minimize this distance, kneel as close to the patient's side as possible, leaving only enough room so that your knees will not prevent the patient from being rolled. When you lean forward, keep your back straight and lean

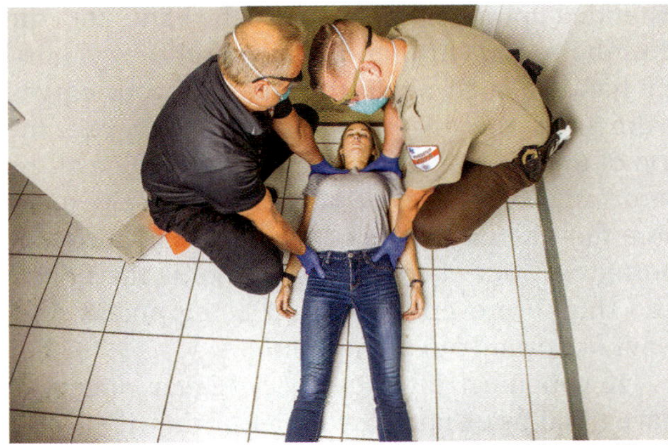

FIGURE 8-6 A body drag with an EMT on each side of the patient.

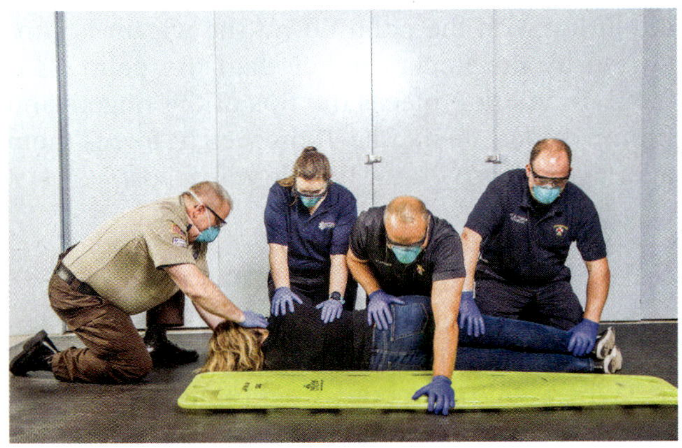

FIGURE 8-7 Placing a patient onto a backboard.

solely from the hips. Be sure to use your shoulder muscles to help with the roll. To minimize the amount of time you are extended like this and to support the patient's weight, roll the patient without stopping until the patient is resting on their side and braced against your thighs. Pulling toward you

Words of Wisdom

You will often be called on to lift a patient in coordination with someone you have never worked with before. Pay attention to what each person is doing, and verbalize your actions to decrease the risk of dropping the patient or hurting one another. If you have the chance to practice lifts with a new partner prior to your first call together, do so.

allows your legs to prevent the patient from rolling over completely and from rolling beyond the intended distance.

Safe Lifting and Carrying

Whenever possible, use a device that can be rolled to move a patient. However, in a situation where a wheeled device is not available or appropriate, you must understand and follow certain guidelines for carrying a patient on a patient-moving device. **TABLE 8-1** presents the guidelines.

Patient Weight

You should estimate how much the patient weighs before you attempt to lift. In the United States, the average weight for a male adult is approximately 200 pounds (91 kg), and the average weight for a female adult is approximately 170 pounds (77 kg).[5] Depending on your individual strength, you and another EMS clinician may be able to safely lift a patient; however, due to safety concerns, consider using four clinicians to lift when possible. There is more stability with a four-person carry, and the carry requires less strength. You should know how much you can comfortably and safely lift, and should not attempt to lift a proportional weight (the share of the weight that you will bear) that exceeds this amount. If you find that lifting the patient places a strain on you, stop the lift and lower the patient. You should then obtain additional help before again attempting to lift the patient. Be sure to communicate clearly and frequently with your partner and other clinicians whenever you are lifting a patient.

Protocols should include a method to rapidly summon additional help to lift and carry a heavy patient or, as in the case of a cardiac arrest, provide and maintain the necessary care in the field. In addition, you must know, or be able to find out, the weight limitations of the equipment you are using and how to handle patients who exceed those weight limitations. Special bariatric techniques, equipment, and resources are generally required to move any patient who weighs more than 350 pounds (159 kg) to the ambulance (discussed later in the chapter). These resources should be called for when you arrive on scene and have assessed the situation.

TABLE 8-1 Guidelines for Carrying a Patient on a Patient-Moving Device

- Estimate the weight of both the patient and the associated equipment to be lifted, and gauge the limitations of your team's abilities.
- Coordinate your movements with those of the other team members while constantly communicating with them.
- Do not twist your body as you are carrying the patient.
- Keep the weight that you are carrying as close to your body as possible while keeping your back in a locked-in position.
- Do not bend at the waist; doing so could hyperextend your back. Instead, flex at the hips, and bend at the knees.

Directions and Commands

To safely lift and carry a patient, you and your team must anticipate and understand every move, and each move must be executed in a coordinated manner. Before any lifting is initiated, the team leader should indicate where each team member is to be located and rapidly describe the sequence of steps that will be performed to ensure the team knows what is expected. If you must lift and move the patient through a number of separate stages, the team leader should first give an abbreviated overview of the stages, followed by a more detailed explanation of each stage just before it will occur.

Orders that will initiate the actual lifting or moving or any significant changes in movement should be given in two parts: a preparatory command and a command of execution. For example, if the team leader says, "All ready to stop. STOP!," the phrase "All ready to stop" will get your attention, identify who should act, and prepare you to act; the declarative "STOP!" will indicate the exact moment of execution. Commands of execution should be delivered in a louder voice. Often, a countdown is helpful when you need to lift a patient. To avoid confusion in using a countdown, the leader should always clarify whether "three" is to be a part of the preparatory command or whether it is to serve as the order to execute. The leader can say, "We're going to lift on three. One, two, THREE!" or "I'm going to count to three, and then we're going to lift. One, two, three, LIFT!"

Safety Tips

Choose one clinician to be the team leader and direct all movements to prevent confusion. The leader is typically the clinician closest to the head of the patient, which allows the best view of the operation. This person should explain the procedure in advance and verbalize instructions such as "We will lift on three" or "We will count to three and then lift."

You should carefully plan ahead and select the methods that will involve the least amount of lifting and carrying. Remember to always consider whether there is an option that will cause less strain to you and the other clinicians.

Patient Positioning

When treating patients, they must be properly positioned based on the chief complaint. Certain conditions, such as head injury, shock, spinal injury,

YOU are the EMT

Due to the critical condition of the driver, you immediately request paramedic backup. Because of the position of the vehicle and the patients, you determine that the patients are entrapped and that the vehicle is potentially unstable. You ask dispatch to send a rescue unit to assist with stabilizing the vehicle and extricating the victims. You are able to look through the door and perform a primary assessment on the patients while waiting for further assistance.

Patient 1 (the driver)

Recording Time: 0 Minutes	
Appearance	Motionless; ashen skin with cyanosis around the mouth
Level of consciousness	Unresponsive
Airway	Snoring respirations
Breathing	Increased rate; shallow depth
Circulation	Unable to reach patient to feel for pulse; no obvious bleeding

Patient 2 (the passenger)

Recording Time: 0 Minutes	
Appearance	Unable to visualize due to patient's position, but she is anxious and reports some pain to her back and right side
Level of consciousness	Alert and oriented
Airway	Open; clear of secretions and foreign bodies
Breathing	Unable to assess, but talking in complete sentences with no sounds of distress and she denies any dyspnea
Circulation	Unable to assess due to patient's position

The passenger tells you that the driver, her husband, is normally on oxygen and the tube was pulled off during the crash. She thinks she may be sitting on the portable oxygen machine. She also thinks that she may have "cracked a rib or two" when she was thrown against the door. She begs you to please help her husband before it is too late.

4. Do you consider the driver to be in stable or unstable condition? Should you wait for further assistance or proceed to gain access to him?
5. Once you are able to gain access, what are your concerns for the use of proper body mechanics while removing these patients?

Words of Wisdom

Remember that moving a patient is a dynamic process, and the team leader must be prepared to alter the sequence of moves as needed. Any alteration in the original established plan must be clearly vocalized to all EMS clinicians involved in the move.

pregnancy, and obesity, call for special lifting and moving techniques. Special considerations include the following:

- Although patients with a potential spinal injury should be secured to restrict movement of the spine, patients with no suspected injury reporting chest pain or respiratory distress should be placed in a position of comfort—typically a Fowler or semi-Fowler position—unless they are hypotensive.
- Patients who are in shock should be packaged and placed in a supine position.
- Patients in late stages of pregnancy should be positioned and transported on their left side if they are supine.
- Place an unresponsive patient with no suspected spinal, hip, or pelvic injury into the recovery position by rolling the patient onto the side without twisting the body.
- Transport a patient who is nauseated or vomiting in a position of comfort, but ensure that you are positioned appropriately to manage and maintain a patent airway.

Always remember to treat the patient with respect and preserve their dignity regardless of how they are transported.

Words of Wisdom

Restraints should never be punitive and should be applied only if the patient poses a threat to you, your team members, themselves, or bystanders. Follow local protocols for the use of restraints. Once restraints have been applied, never remove them until you arrive at the hospital and are requested to remove them by the hospital staff. See Chapter 23, *Behavioral Health Emergencies*, for further discussion of emergencies that may involve patient restraint.

Safety Tips

Follow these rules to keep you and your patient safe:

- Minimize the number of total body lifts you have to perform.
- Coordinate every lift in advance.
- Minimize the total amount of weight you have to lift.
- *Never* lift with your back.
- Do not carry what you can put on wheels.
- Ask for help when you think it will be needed.

Personnel Considerations

As an EMT, you will be required to assist in the movement of patients. To minimize injuries, before moving any patient, teams should develop a complete plan. Some questions to ask are as follows:

- Am I physically strong enough to lift and move this patient?
- Is there adequate room to get the proper stance to lift the patient?
- Do I need additional clinicians for lifting assistance?

The answers to these questions need to be evaluated prior to moving your patient. Remember that injured EMTs cannot help anyone.

Street Smarts

Lifting and moving patients is a large part of the job when working as an EMS clinician. It is important that you work to keep yourself in good physical shape. Weight training and stretching in addition to eating well and getting enough sleep will help you remain active and effective in the field.

Emergency Moves

When there is a potential for danger to you or the patient, use an **emergency move** to drag or pull a patient to a safe place before assessment and care are provided. The risk of serious harm or death due to fire, explosives, or hazardous materials; your inability to protect the patient from other hazards; or your inability to gain access to others in a vehicle who need lifesaving care all are situations in which you should use an emergency move. In such conditions, protecting the cervical spine is secondary to rapidly getting your patient to safety.

The only other time you should use an emergency move is if you cannot properly assess the patient or provide critical emergency care because of the patient's location or position.

If you are alone and danger at the scene makes it necessary for you to use an emergency move, regardless of a patient's injuries, you should use a drag to pull the patient along the long axis of the body. Remember that it is impossible to remove a patient quickly from a vehicle while properly applying spinal motion restriction techniques. However, if you follow certain guidelines, you can usually remove a patient from a life-threatening situation without causing further injury to the patient.

You can move a patient on their back along the floor or ground by using one of the following methods:

- Pull on the patient's clothing in the neck and shoulder area (**FIGURE 8-8A**).
- If the shirt has buttons, the top two should be undone to prevent the patient from choking.
- Place the patient onto a blanket, coat, or other item that can be pulled (**FIGURE 8-8B**).
- Place your arms under the patient's shoulders and through the armpits, and, while grasping your opposite wrist, drag the patient backward (**FIGURE 8-8C**).

If you are alone and must remove an unresponsive patient from a vehicle, first move the patient's legs so they are clear of the pedals and are against the seat. Then rotate the patient so that their back is positioned toward the open vehicle door. Next, place your arms through the armpits and support the patient's head against your body (**FIGURE 8-9A**). While supporting the patient's weight, drag the patient from the seat. If the legs and feet clear the vehicle easily, you can rapidly drag the patient to a safe location by continuing this method (**FIGURE 8-9B**). If the legs and feet do not clear the vehicle easily, you can slowly lower the patient until they are lying on their back next to the vehicle, clear the legs

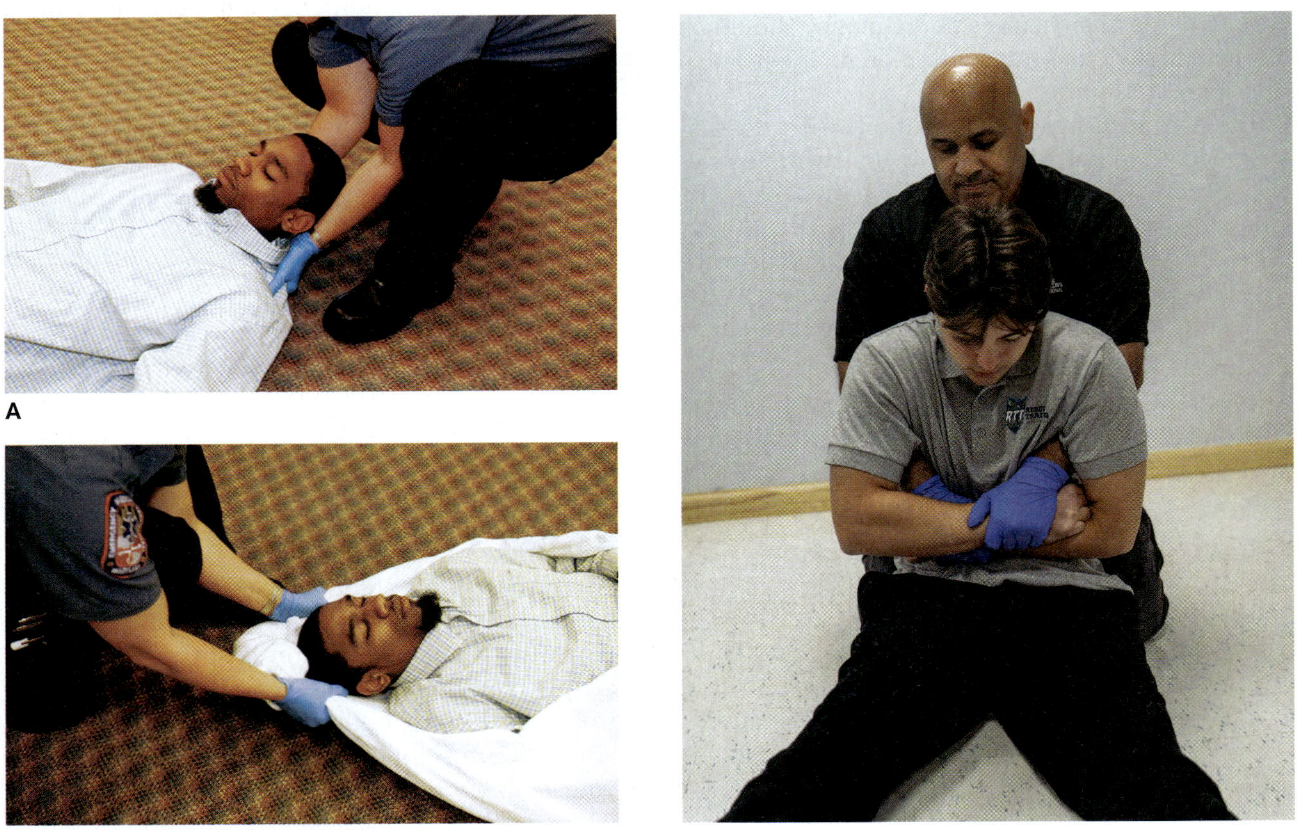

A

B

C

FIGURE 8-8 Dragging methods. **A.** Emergency clothes drag. **B.** Blanket drag. **C.** Arm-to-arm drag.

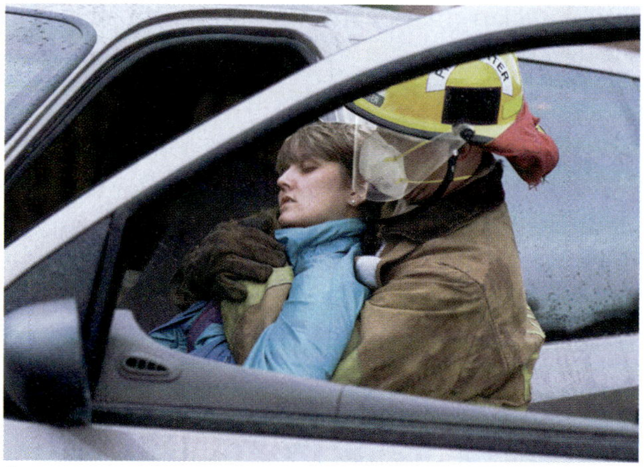
A

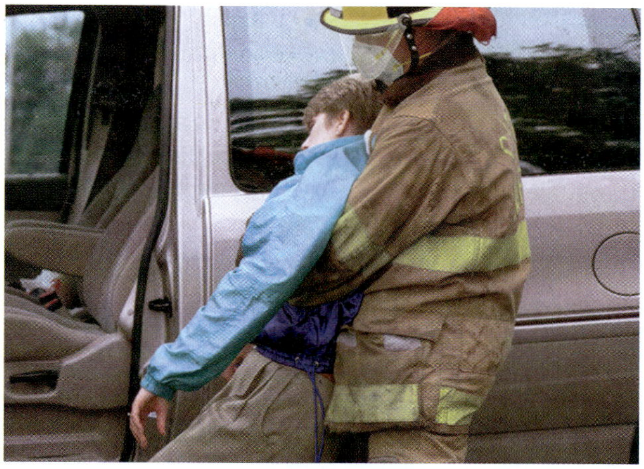
B

FIGURE 8-9 One-person technique for moving an unresponsive patient from a vehicle. **A.** Grasp the patient under the arms. **B.** Lower the patient down into a supine position.

YOU are the EMT

Once the vehicle has been stabilized, you are able to gain access through the rear driver's-side door that is about halfway open. The vehicle is still positioned on the passenger's side. A paramedic unit is standing by, awaiting removal of the driver. You are able to wedge half of a backboard through the doorway with a firefighter holding the other end, but there is no room inside for additional clinicians.

Patient 1 (the driver)

Recording Time: 5 Minutes	
Appearance	Motionless; ashen skin with cyanosis around the mouth
Level of consciousness	Unresponsive
Airway	Snoring respirations
Breathing	Increased rate; shallow depth
Circulation	Weak and rapid radial pulse; no obvious bleeding

Patient 2 (the passenger)

Recording Time: 5 Minutes	
Respirations	Seem to be a little rapid, but still unable to visualize patient
Pulse	Unable to assess due to patient's position
Skin	Baseline color where visualized
Blood pressure	Unable to assess
Oxygen saturation (Spo_2)	Unable to assess

6. What type of move is best for removing the driver?
7. What steps can you take to maximize safety while lifting a patient?

from the vehicle, and, as previously described, use a long-axis body drag to move the patient a safe distance from the vehicle.

You should use one-person techniques to move a patient only if an immediately life-threatening danger exists and you are alone or, because of the pressing nature of the danger, your partner is moving a second patient simultaneously. Additional one-clinician drags, carries, and lifts are shown in **FIGURE 8-10**.

Urgent Moves

An urgent move may be necessary to move a patient with an altered level of consciousness, inadequate ventilation, shock (hypoperfusion), or

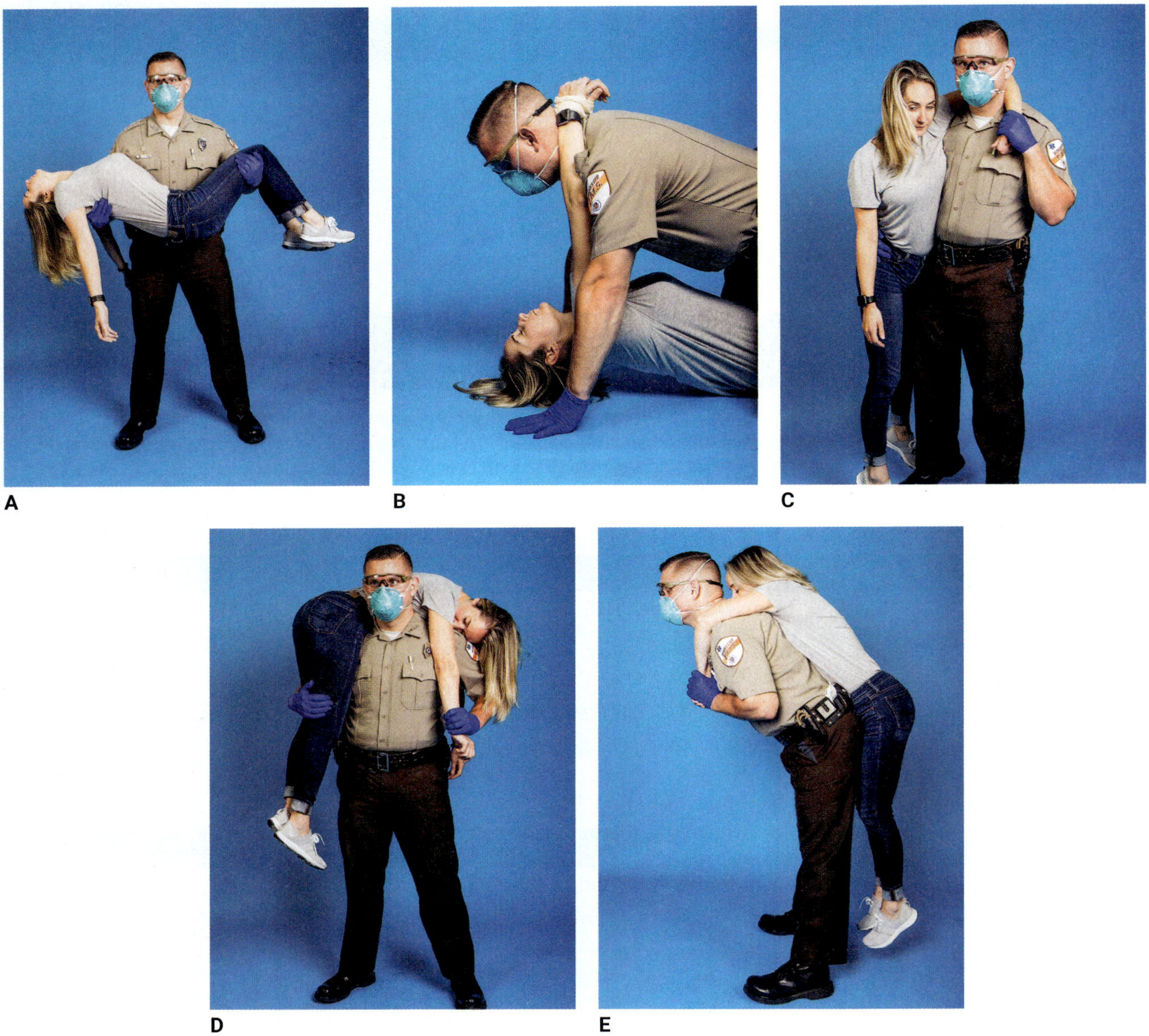

FIGURE 8-10 One-person drags, carries, and lifts. **A.** Front cradle. **B.** Firefighter's drag. **C.** One-person walking assist. **D.** Firefighter's carry. **E.** Pack-strap carry.

cardiac arrest. An extreme weather condition may also make an urgent move necessary. In some cases, patients must be urgently moved from the location or position in which they are found. When a patient who is sitting in a vehicle must be urgently moved, use the rapid extrication technique.

Rapid Extrication (Lift-and-Slide) Technique From a Vehicle

An alert, stable patient suspected of having a spinal injury may be allowed to self-extricate from a vehicle to a nearby transfer device or stretcher after a cervical collar is applied. If the patient and the scene are stable but the patient is not able to self-extricate, you might use an extrication-type vest to remove the patient from the vehicle. However, proper placement of either of these devices on the patient usually requires between 6 and 8 minutes, and in some cases, even longer.

If the patient is not able to self-extricate because of serious injuries, responders can use the **rapid extrication technique** (sometimes referred to as the lift-and-slide technique) to move the patient from a seated position in the vehicle to a supine position on a backboard very quickly if needed.[6] The rapid nature of this type of extrication can increase the risk of harm if the patient has a spinal injury. As such, it is important to perform the skill carefully and with good team communication. Situations in which this technique may be used when the patient cannot self-extricate include the following:

- The vehicle or scene is unsafe.
- Explosives or other hazardous materials are on the scene.
- There is a fire or a danger of fire.
- The patient cannot be properly assessed before being removed from the vehicle.
- The patient has a life-threatening condition.
- The patient blocks your access to another seriously injured patient.

Because of the increased risk, do not use this technique if no urgency exists. If the patient can stand and pivot to the stretcher, it is safer to have them do so.

The rapid extrication technique requires a team of three clinicians who are knowledgeable and practiced in the procedure. Take the following steps when using the rapid extrication technique (**SKILL DRILL 8-2**). Whether a backboard is used for this skill will depend on your local protocols. Here, use of a backboard is included. Note that backboards are discussed in greater detail later in this chapter.

1. The first clinician applies manual in-line support of the patient's head and cervical spine from behind. Support may be applied from the side, if necessary, by reaching through the driver's-side doorway (**Step 1**).
2. The second clinician serves as team leader and, as such, gives the commands until the patient is supine on the backboard. Because the second clinician lifts and turns the patient's torso, they must be physically capable of moving the patient. The second clinician works from the driver's-side doorway. If the first clinician is also working from that doorway, the second clinician should stand closer to the door hinges toward the front of the vehicle. The second clinician applies a cervical collar and may perform the primary assessment (**Step 2**).
3. The second clinician continuously supports the patient's torso until the patient is supine on the backboard. Once the second clinician takes control of the patient's torso, usually in the form of a body hug, they should not let go of the patient for any reason. Some type of cross-chest shoulder hug usually works well, but you will have to decide what method works best for any given patient. You must remember that you cannot simply reach into the vehicle and grab the patient; this will only twist the patient's torso. You must rotate the patient as a complete unit.
4. The third clinician works from the front passenger's seat and is responsible for rotating the patient's legs and feet as the torso is turned, ensuring that they are free of the pedals and any other obstruction. With care, the third clinician should first move the patient's nearer leg laterally without rotating the patient's pelvis and lower spine. The pelvis and lower spine rotate only as the third clinician moves the patient's second leg during the next step. Moving the nearer leg early makes it much easier to move the second leg in concert with the rest of the body. After the third clinician moves the legs together, they should be moved as a unit (**Step 3**).

Skill Drill 8-2 Performing the Rapid Extrication Technique

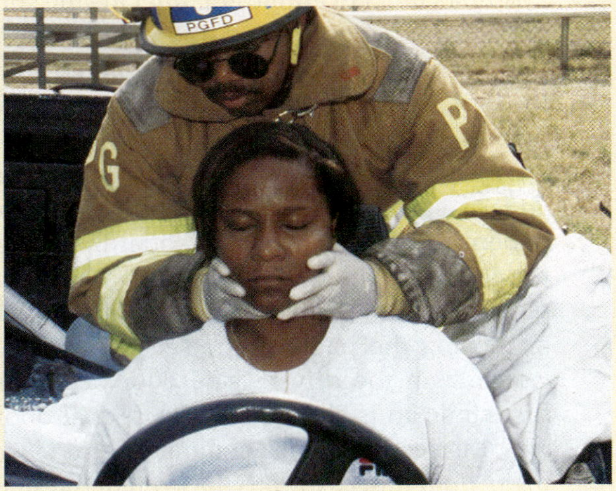

Step 1

The first clinician provides in-line manual support of the head and cervical spine.

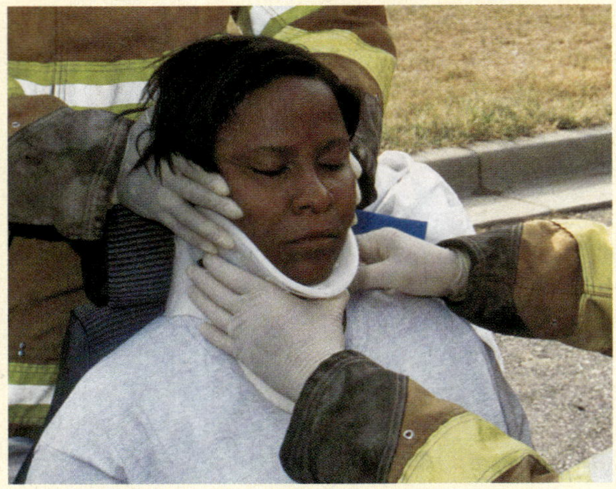

Step 2

The second clinician gives commands, applies a cervical collar, and performs the primary assessment.

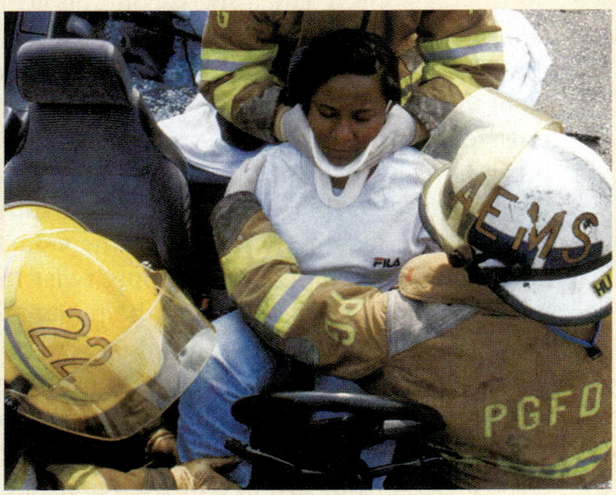

Step 3

The second clinician supports the torso. The third clinician frees the patient's legs from the pedals and moves the legs together, without moving the pelvis or spine.

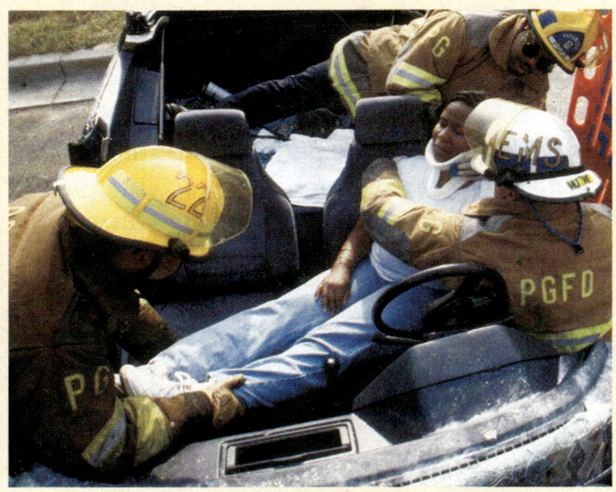

Step 4

The second clinician and the third clinician rotate the patient as a unit in several short, coordinated moves. The first clinician (relieved by the fourth clinician as needed) supports the patient's head and neck during rotation (and later steps).

Skill Drill 8-2 Performing the Rapid Extrication Technique

continued

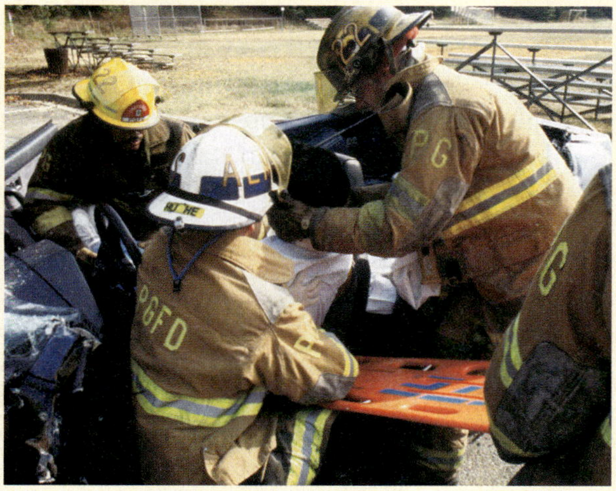

Step 5

The first (or fourth) clinician places the backboard on the seat against the patient's buttocks. (Use of a backboard may depend on local protocols.)

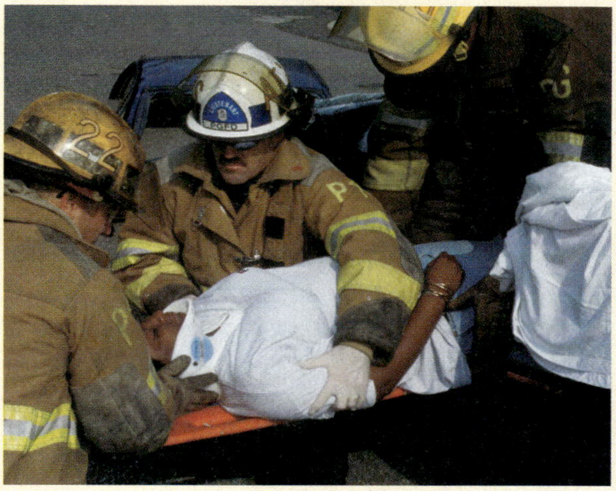

Step 6

The third clinician moves to an effective position for sliding the patient. The second and the third clinicians slide the patient along the backboard in coordinated 8- to 12-inch (20- to 30-cm) moves until the patient's hips rest on the backboard.

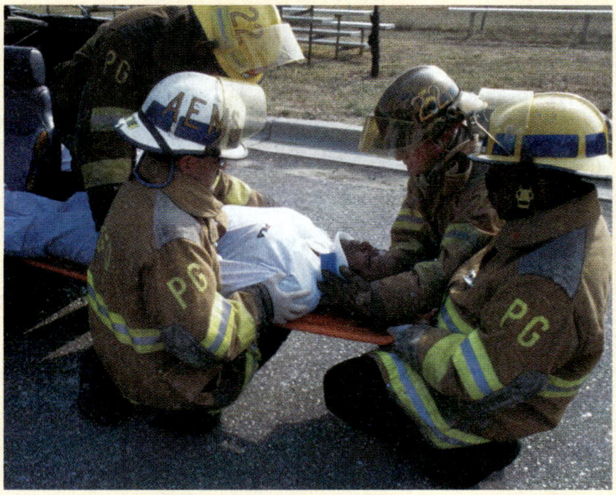

Step 7

The third clinician exits the vehicle and moves to the backboard opposite the second clinician. They continue to slide the patient until the patient is fully on the backboard.

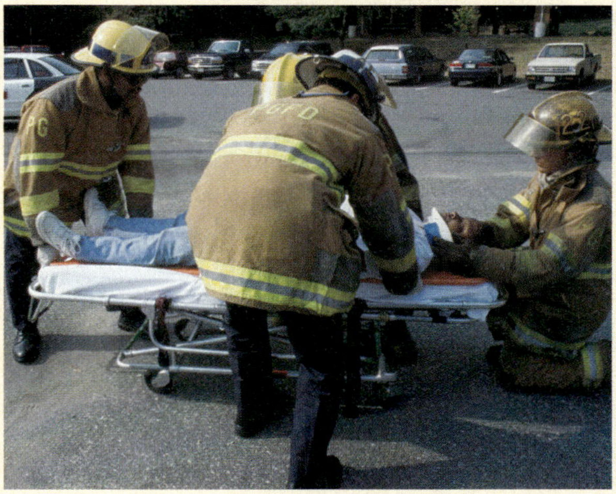

Step 8

The first (or fourth) clinician continues to stabilize the head and neck while the second clinician and the third clinician carry the patient away from the vehicle and onto the prepared stretcher.

5. These initial steps of the rapid extrication technique direct the team to its starting positions and responsibilities. The first clinician applies in-line support and stabilization of the head and neck. The second clinician gives orders and supports the torso. The third clinician moves and supports the patient's legs. The team is now ready to move the patient.
6. The patient is rotated 90° so their back is facing out the driver's door and their feet are on the front passenger's seat. This coordinated movement is done in three or four short, quick "eighth turns." The second clinician directs each quick turn by saying, "Ready, turn," or "Ready, move." Hand position changes should be made between moves.
7. In most cases, the first clinician will be working from the backseat and will have removed the headrest (if possible). At some point, the first clinician will be unable to follow the torso rotation, either because the doorpost is in the way or because they cannot reach farther from the backseat. At that time, the third clinician should assume temporary in-line support of the head and neck until the first clinician can regain control of the head from outside the vehicle. If a fourth clinician is present, this person stands next to the second clinician. The fourth clinician takes control of the patient's head and neck from outside the vehicle without involving the third clinician. As soon as the change has been made, the rotation can continue (**Step 4**).
8. Once the patient has been fully rotated, the backboard should be placed against the patient's buttocks on the seat. Do not try to wedge the backboard under the patient. If only three clinicians are present, be sure to place the backboard within arm's reach of the driver's door before the move so that the backboard can be pulled into place when needed. In such cases, the far end of the backboard can be left on the ground. When a fourth clinician is available, the first clinician exits the backseat of the vehicle, places the backboard against the patient's buttocks, and maintains pressure toward the interior of the vehicle from the far end of the backboard. (Note: When the door opening allows, some clinicians prefer to insert the backboard onto the seat before the patient is rotated.)
9. As soon as the patient has been rotated and the backboard is in place, the second clinician and the third clinician lower the patient onto the backboard while supporting the head and torso so that neutral alignment is maintained. The first clinician holds the backboard until the patient is secured (**Step 5**).
10. Next, the third clinician must move across the front seat to be in position at the patient's hips. If the third clinician stays at the patient's knees or feet, they will be ineffective in helping to move the body's weight. The knees and feet follow the hips.
11. The fourth clinician maintains manual in-line support of the head and now takes over giving the commands. The second clinician maintains the direction of the extrication. The second clinician stands with their back to the door, facing the rear of the vehicle. The backboard should be immediately in front of the third clinician. The second clinician grasps the patient's shoulders or armpits. Then, on command, the second clinician and the third clinician slide the patient 8 to 12 inches (20 to 30 cm) along the backboard, repeating this slide until the patient's hips are firmly on the backboard (**Step 6**).
12. At that time, the third clinician gets out of the vehicle and moves to the opposite side of the backboard, across from the second clinician. The third clinician now takes control at the shoulders, and the second clinician moves back to take control of the hips. On command, these two clinicians move the patient along the backboard in 8- to 12-inch (20- to 30-cm) slides until the patient is placed fully on the backboard (**Step 7**).
13. The first (or fourth) clinician continues to maintain manual in-line support of the patient's head. The second clinician and the third clinician now grasp their side of the backboard and then carry it and the patient away from the vehicle onto the prepared stretcher nearby (**Step 8**).

When possible, place the wheeled stretcher underneath the backboard. Once the backboard and patient have been placed on the stretcher, begin lifesaving treatment immediately. If you used the rapid extrication technique because the scene was dangerous, you and your team should immediately move the stretcher a safe distance away from the scene before you assess or treat the patient. The long spine board is then removed unless its use is indicated by multiple extremity injuries, or removing it will delay immediate transport or other urgent treatment.[6]

See Chapter 37, *Vehicle Extrication and Special Rescue*, for further discussion of vehicle extrication techniques.

Nonurgent Moves

When both the scene and the patient are stable, carefully plan how to move the patient. If your patient move is rushed or poorly planned, it may result in discomfort or injury to the patient, you, and/or your team. Before you attempt any move, the team leader must be sure that there are enough clinicians, any obstacles have been identified or removed, the proper equipment is available, and the procedure and path to be followed have been clearly identified and discussed. Remember, communication is the key to success.

In nonurgent situations, you and your team may choose one of several methods for lifting and carrying a patient and should coordinate your movements through direct verbal commands. You may adapt these procedures to meet your needs on a case-by-case basis.

Extremity Lift

The **extremity lift** may be used for patients with no suspected extremity or spinal injuries who are supine or in a sitting position. The extremity lift may be especially helpful when the patient is in a very narrow space or there is not enough room for the patient and several clinicians to stand side by side. Perform the extremity lift as follows (**SKILL DRILL 8-3**):

1. Kneel behind the patient's head as your partner kneels at the patient's feet. You and your partner should be facing each other.
2. The patient's hands should be crossed over the chest.
3. Place one hand under each of the patient's armpits. Grasp the patient's wrists or forearms

YOU are the EMT

There is no easy way to remove the driver, but by bracing yourself through the seats you are able to grab his belt and pull him toward you. Once you get the patient's head and shoulders between the headrests, the firefighter helps pull him onto the backboard. As soon as he is secured on the backboard, several other clinicians help the firefighter pull the backboard out of the vehicle and transfer him to the waiting paramedic unit for evaluation, treatment, and transport. You now have access to the passenger, who is sitting waist-deep in water and still reporting pain in her back and right side. She tells you that she has a history of back pain and thinks she can move a little with help.

Patient 2 (the passenger)

Recording Time: 20 Minutes	
Level of consciousness	Alert and oriented
Respirations	20 breaths/min; adequate depth
Pulse	112 beats/min; strong and regular
Skin	Baseline color, cool, and moist
Blood pressure	148/92 mm Hg
Oxygen saturation (Spo_2)	99% (on room air)

8. How is a patient's weight distributed when on a carrying device? Why is it important to know this?
9. Considering her complaints and the fact that her condition is stable, what are your best options for removing the passenger?

Skill Drill 8-3 Performing the Extremity Lift

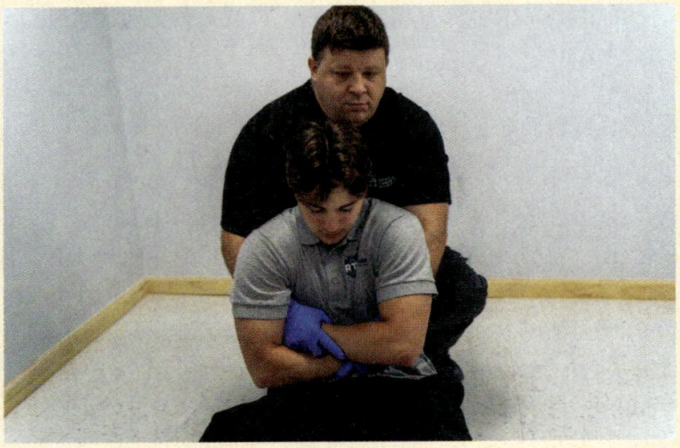

Step 1

The patient's hands are crossed over the chest. Grasp the patient's wrists or forearms and pull the patient to a sitting position.

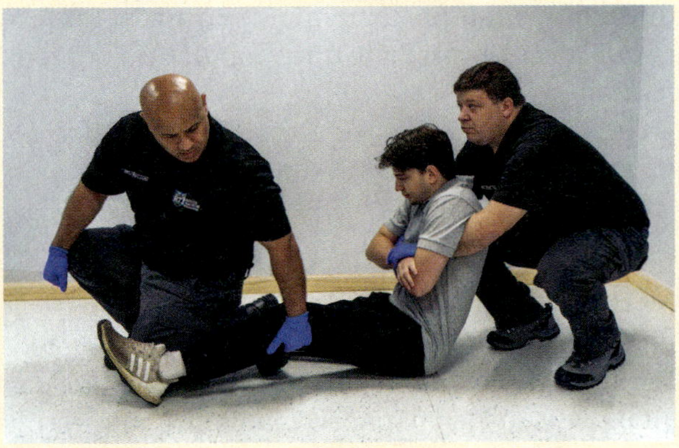

Step 2

Your partner moves to a position between the patient's legs, facing in the same direction as the patient, and places their hands under the knees.

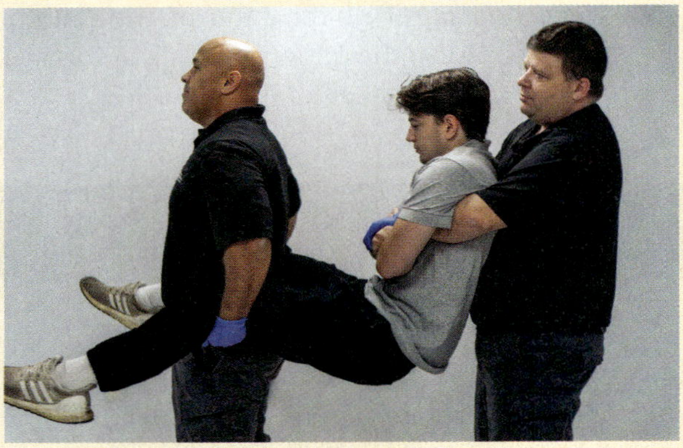

Step 3

Rise to a crouching position. On command, lift and begin to move.

Courtesy of Aura Prep/Rescue Training International.

and pull the upper torso until the patient is in a sitting position (**Step 1**).

4. Your partner moves to a position between the patient's legs, facing in the same direction as the patient, and slips their hands under the patient's knees (**Step 2**).
5. As you give the command, stand fully upright and move the patient to the stretcher (**Step 3**).

You will be less likely to injure yourself if you bend at the hips and knees and use your legs for lifting. However, this lift and carry method increases pressure on the patient's chest, so the patient may be uncomfortable in this position.

Equipment for Lifting and Moving Patients

The Wheeled Ambulance Stretcher

The **wheeled ambulance stretcher** (also called an ambulance stretcher, gurney, litter, or cot) is the most commonly used device to transport patients. The wheeled ambulance stretcher is a specially designed stretcher that can be rolled along the ground and typically weighs between 110 and 165 pounds (50 and 75 kg), depending on its design and features (**FIGURE 8-11**). Because of its weight, it is generally

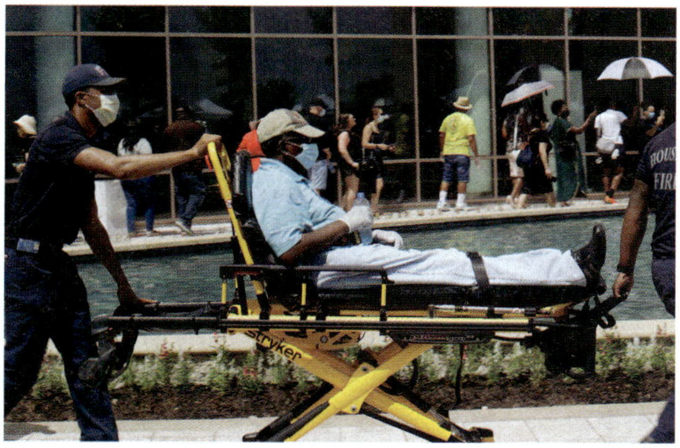

FIGURE 8-11 The wheeled ambulance stretcher is specially designed to roll along the ground.

© Eric Gay/AP Photo.

not taken up or down stairs or to other locations where the patient must be carried for any significant distance.

The modern stretcher is available in a number of different models, which may include varying features. During your training, familiarize yourself with the specific features of the stretchers that your ambulance service carries. You must know where to locate the controls to adjust and lock each feature and how each one works.

The stretcher has a specific head end and foot end. It has a strong, rectangular, tubular metal main frame to which all of its other parts are attached. The stretcher should be pulled, pushed, and lifted only by its main frame or handles, which are attached to the frame specifically for this purpose.

A retractable siderail is attached along the central portion of the main frame of the stretcher at each side. One siderail is lowered out of the way when a patient is being loaded onto the stretcher. Once the patient has been properly placed on the stretcher, the siderail is drawn up and locked in an elevated position perpendicular to the surface of the stretcher. The siderail can be lowered only if its locking mechanism is released. The use of siderails is important, as these devices help prevent patients from rolling off the stretcher and provide a gripping area that aids in adjusting their position. Nevertheless, the siderails do not secure the patient and may not prevent the patient from falling off the stretcher.

The underside of the main frame of the stretcher is supported on a folding undercarriage that has a smaller, horizontal, rectangular frame and four large rubber casters. The folding undercarriage is designed so that the stretcher bed can be adjusted to any height from approximately 12 inches (30 cm) above the ground, which is the desired height when the stretcher is secured in the ambulance, to 32 to 36 inches (81 to 91 cm) above the ground, which is the desired height when the stretcher is being rolled. Because the stretcher can be locked at set heights between its lowest height and its fully extended height, it can be locked at the same height as any bed or examining table to allow the patient to sit or be slid from one to the other. This permits you to transfer the patient without the need for additional lifting. The controls for folding the undercarriage are designed so that the stretcher remains locked at its current height when the controls are not being activated. As an additional safety feature on most stretchers, the main frame must be slightly lifted to remove all weight from the undercarriage before it will fold, even if the control is pulled. Therefore, if the handle is accidentally pulled, the elevated stretcher will not suddenly drop. Controls for elevating and lowering most stretchers are located at the foot end. You and your partner must use the proper lifting mechanics to lift the wheeled ambulance stretcher.

In an effort to decrease the potential for back injuries to EMS clinicians, manufacturers have developed pneumatic and electronic stretchers. Similar in appearance to conventional wheeled stretchers, electronic stretchers are battery operated and have electronic controls to facilitate raising and lowering of the undercarriage at the touch of a button (**FIGURE 8-12**). Some of these wheeled stretchers also have the ability to be loaded and unloaded from the ambulance by motor and thus require only one clinician to control the equipment during loading. These devices limit the risk of injury to clinicians and to the patient by removing the physical strain of the task. Due to the electronic controls and associated equipment, the weight of these devices may be increased compared to conventional wheeled stretchers. Particular caution should be exercised when transporting the patient on uneven terrain or down one or two steps with these devices to avoid tipping or falling.

The mattress on a stretcher is fluid resistant so that it does not absorb any type of potentially infectious material, including water, blood, or other body fluid. This material also allows for easy cleaning and disinfecting.

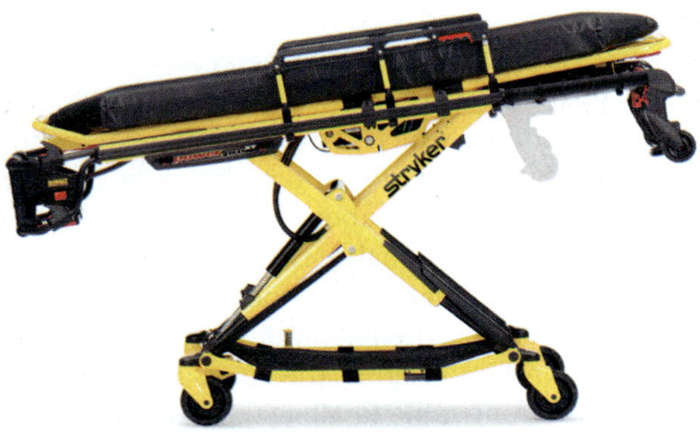

FIGURE 8-12 An electronic stretcher.

Courtesy of Stryker Medical, a division of Stryker Corporation.

Transferring the Patient Onto a Stretcher

There are several ways to transfer the patient from a bed onto the stretcher. The preferred method is to use a draw sheet or commercial patient transfer device.

To move the patient from a bed onto a stretcher, or vice versa, use the draw sheet method. Place the stretcher next to the bed, making sure it is at the same height or slightly lower than the bed and that the rails are lowered and straps are unbuckled. Be sure to hold or secure the stretcher to keep it from moving. Loosen the bottom sheet

Special Populations

BARIATRIC CONSIDERATIONS

In the United States, 41.9% of adults (more than 100 million people) are considered to have obesity.[7] The incidence of obesity is higher among adults aged 40 to 59 years (almost 45%) than among adults aged 20 to 39 years (40%) or adults 61 years or older (almost 42%). The incidence among children is also alarming; approximately 20% of all children and adolescents in the United States are considered to have obesity.[8] The obesity rate has tripled compared to just one generation ago and continues to increase. In 2019, the estimated annual cost of medical care for patients with obesity in the United States was $173 billion, or approximately $1,861 higher for a person with obesity than for a person of healthy weight.[7] Obesity has reached epidemic proportions in the United States, and many programs are now aimed at teaching people from a young age the importance of exercise and a healthy diet.

Bariatrics is the branch of medicine concerned with the management (prevention or control) of obesity and allied diseases. The term comes from the Greek words *baros*, meaning weight, and *iatreia*, meaning medical treatment. There is a direct correlation between the degree of obesity and the frequency and severity of health problems; therefore, the larger the patient, the more likely the person will need emergency treatment and transport.

Because of the increased weight and large girth of bariatric patients, they may not fit comfortably or safely on the standard wheeled stretcher. As a result, a specialized type of wheeled stretcher has been developed, called a bariatric stretcher (**FIGURE 8-13**). This type of stretcher is similar in design to the common wheeled stretcher; however, it has several differences. Bariatric stretchers typically have a wider patient surface area to allow for increased comfort, and in addition, ensure the patient's dignity is maintained during transport. Bariatric stretchers also have a wider wheelbase, allowing for increased stability when rolling the patient over uneven terrain. Bariatric stretchers are sometimes equipped with optional features such as a tow package, which allows an ambulance-mounted winch to assist in loading the patient into the ambulance, decreasing the risk of back injuries for EMS clinicians. Another optional feature is telescoping side lift handles, which provide increased leverage when lifting with multiple clinicians. However, the most important feature of the bariatric stretcher is the increased weight-lifting capacity. Typical wheeled ambulance stretchers, depending on manufacturer ratings, allow for a maximum weight of 650 pounds (295 kg). Bariatric stretchers are usually able to support maximum weights as high as 1,600 pounds (725 kg) when rolled in the lowest position.

Bariatric stretchers and ambulances are not always readily available. If there is a bariatric ambulance available for your system or in another agency of your region, you will most likely need to request its response. Similar to requesting other services, the sooner the request is made to dispatch, the sooner the specialty vehicle will arrive.

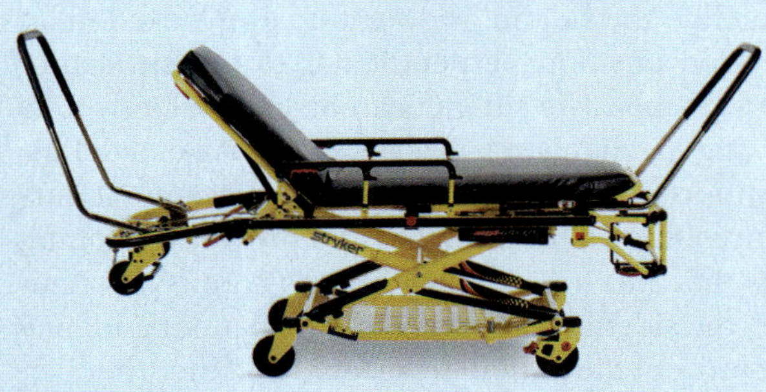

FIGURE 8-13 A bariatric stretcher.

Courtesy of Stryker Medical, a division of Stryker Corporation.

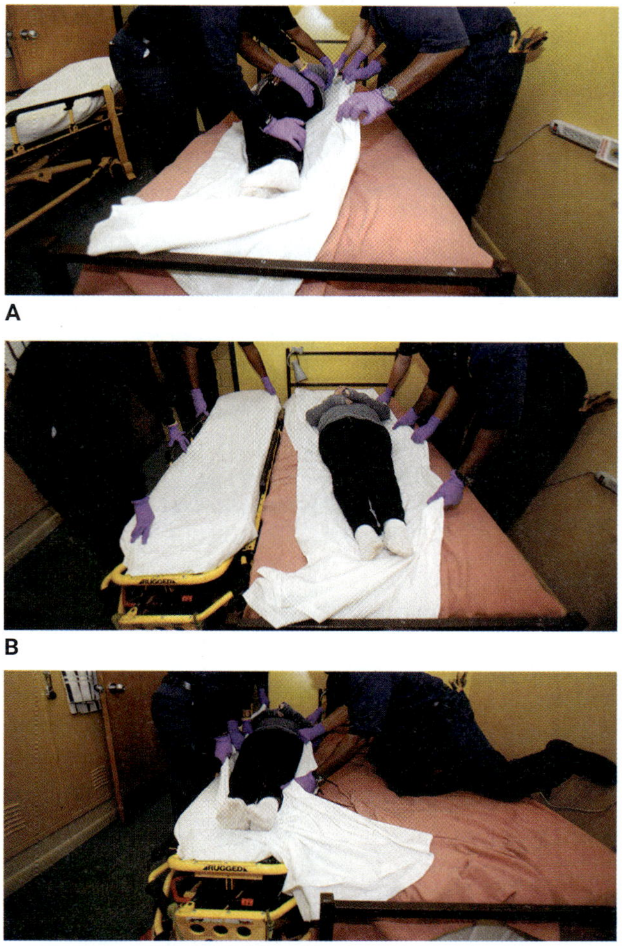

FIGURE 8-14 The draw sheet method. **A.** Log roll the patient onto a sheet or blanket. **B.** Place the stretcher parallel to the bed. Secure the stretcher. Gently pull the patient to the edge of the bed. **C.** Transfer the patient to the stretcher.

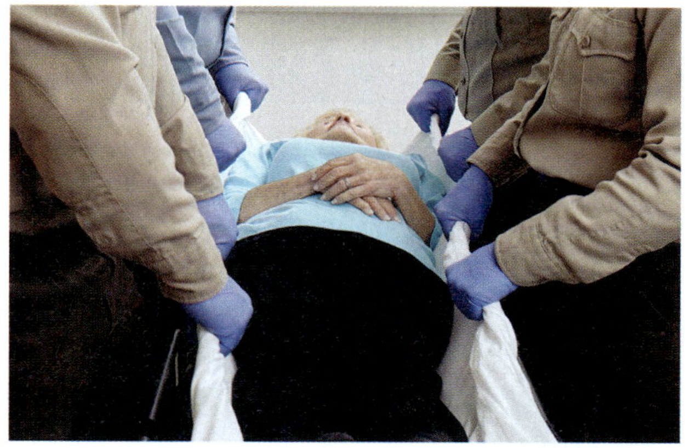

FIGURE 8-15 When lifting a patient by a bed sheet, center the patient on the sheet and tightly roll up the excess fabric on each side. This produces a cylindrical handle that provides a strong way to grasp the fabric.

Safety Tips

A flexible stretcher or patient mover device may be used to move patients from a bed onto a stretcher.

underneath the patient, or log roll the patient onto a blanket or transfer device (**FIGURE 8-14A**). Reach across the stretcher, and grasp the sheet or blanket firmly at the patient's head, chest, hips, and knees (**FIGURE 8-14B**). Gently slide the patient onto the stretcher (**FIGURE 8-14C**).

When lifting a patient by a sheet or blanket, center the patient on the sheet and tightly roll up the excess fabric on each side. This produces a cylindrical handle that provides a strong, secure way to grasp the fabric (**FIGURE 8-15**). Although sliding boards or other devices may not be carried on your ambulance, you may have access to these items in the hospital or at nursing homes that will assist you in sliding the patient from bed to stretcher or stretcher to bed with minimal effort.

Another option to move a patient from a bed to the stretcher is to assist the person to the edge of the bed, if the patient is physically able, and place the patient's legs over the side, helping the patient to sit up. Move the stretcher so that its foot end touches the bed near the patient. Help the patient to stand and rotate so that they can sit down on the center of the stretcher. Lift the patient's legs, and rotate them onto the stretcher while your partner lowers the patient's torso onto the stretcher.

To move a patient from the ground or the floor onto the stretcher, use one of the following methods:

- Use a log roll or long-axis drag to place the patient onto a backboard, and then lift and carry the backboard to the stretcher. Place both the backboard and the patient onto the stretcher.
- Use a scoop stretcher.
- Log roll the patient onto a blanket, centering the patient on the blanket and rolling up the excess material on each side (**SKILL DRILL 8-4**). Lift the patient by the blanket, and then to the nearby wheeled stretcher.

Skill Drill 8-4 Log Rolling a Patient on the Ground

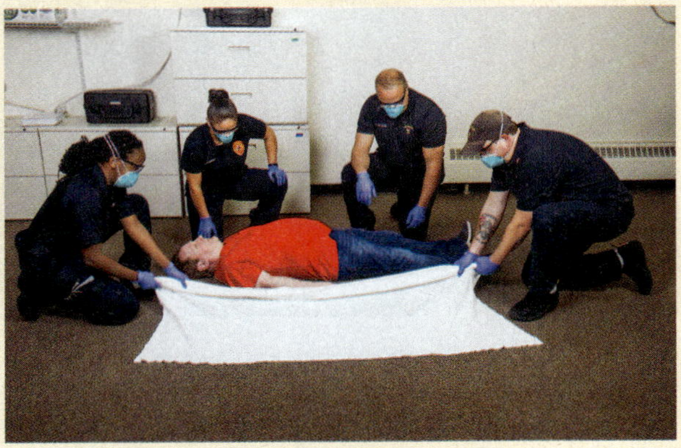

Step 1

Prepare the blanket by rolling it up by half.

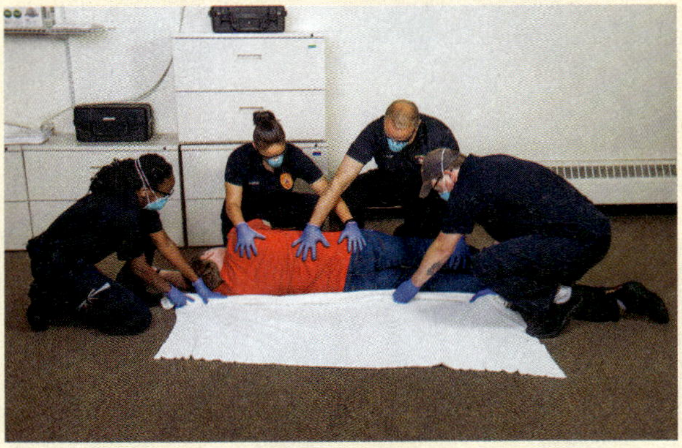

Step 2

Log roll the patient.

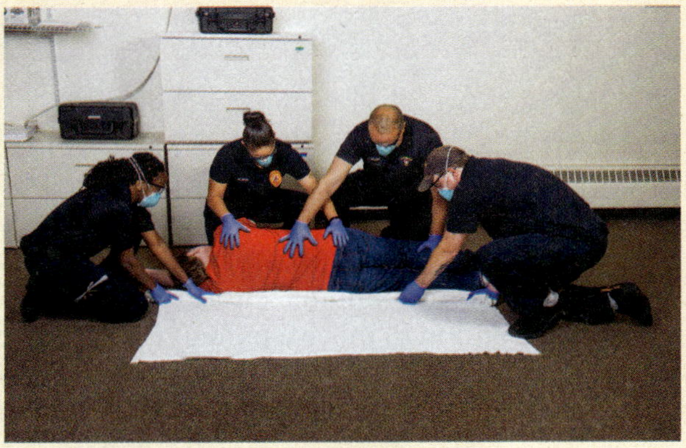

Step 3

Position the blanket underneath the patient. Lower the patient onto the blanket and then log roll the patient in the opposite direction to unroll the blanket.

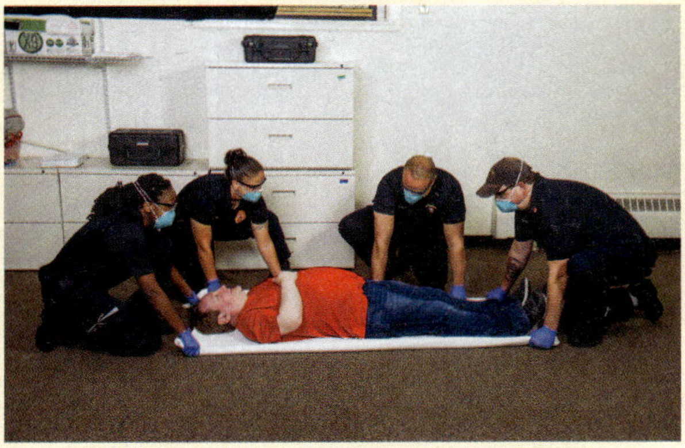

Step 4

Lift the blanket and transfer the patient to the stretcher.

Words of Wisdom

Ensure a thorough patient care report by including details of how you moved the patient and why assistance in moving was needed. For example: "Moved patient to stretcher with draw sheet lift due to unresponsiveness."

Pushing a Wheeled Stretcher

When you are rolling the wheeled ambulance stretcher, make sure it is in the fully elevated position. In most instances, one clinician pushes the head of the stretcher while another clinician guides the foot of the stretcher, with the patient facing in the direction of the stretcher movement until it is ready to load in the ambulance. If you are guiding the stretcher from the foot end, make sure your arms are held close to your body, and be careful to avoid reaching significantly behind you or hyperextending your back (**FIGURE 8-16**). Recall that your back should be locked, straight, and untwisted. While you are walking and guiding the stretcher, bend slightly forward at the hips. As you walk, your legs are pulled back with your feet on the ground, your pelvis is moved forward, and the movement of the pelvis is transferred to the stretcher through your straight torso and firmly held arms. Try to keep the line of the pull through the center of your body by bending your knees.

If you are controlling the head end, you should assist your partner by pushing with your elbows bent so that the hands are approximately 12 to 15 inches (30 to 38 cm) in front of the torso. To protect your elbows from injury, never push an object with your arms fully extended in a straight line and the elbows locked. When you push with the elbow bent but firmly held from bending further, the strong muscles of the arm serve as a shock absorber if the wheels or foot end of the stretcher strikes an obstacle that causes its progress to be suddenly slowed or stopped. Be sure that you push from the area of your body that is between the waist and shoulder. If the weight you are pushing is lower than your waist, push from a kneeling position. Remember not to push or pull from an overhead position.

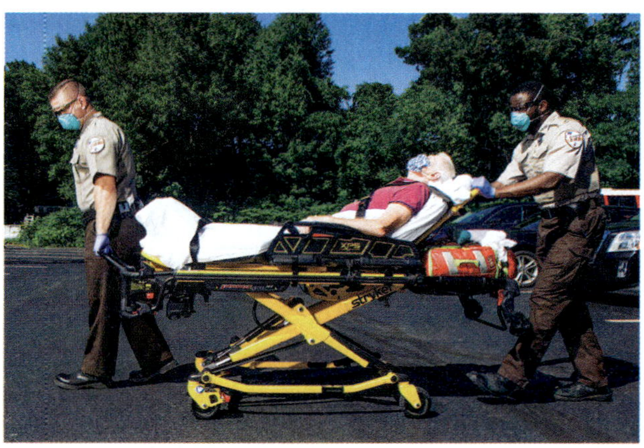

FIGURE 8-16 Push the stretcher from the head end. If you are guiding the stretcher from the foot end, make sure your arms are held close to your body, and be careful to avoid reaching significantly behind you or hyperextending your back. Your back should be locked, straight, and untwisted.

Patients must always be secured with all of the straps on the stretcher. In the event of a crash while en route to the hospital, the straps help to protect the patient from further injury. Secure the patient to the wheeled ambulance stretcher as follows:

1. Secure the stretcher's safety belts over the patient's shoulders and around the patient's chest in a four-point harness fashion. The belts should be tight enough to keep the patient secured on the stretcher but not limit breathing.
2. Secure the stretcher's safety belt over the patient's hips.
3. Secure the stretcher's safety belt over the patient's thighs.
4. Secure the stretcher's safety belt over the patient's ankles.

Because stretcher designs vary, follow the manufacturer's directions.

The stretcher is designed to be rolled on flat surfaces. Ensure the intended travel path is free from debris and potential obstacles. If the patient must be moved over a lawn or other irregular surface, you must lift and carry the stretcher over the terrain. A four-person carry is much safer if the stretcher must be moved over rough ground.

If the loaded stretcher must be carried down a short flight of steps, be sure to first retract or raise the undercarriage; however, doing so is not necessary when the stretcher must be lifted over a curb, a single step, or an obstacle of a similar height (**FIGURE 8-17**).

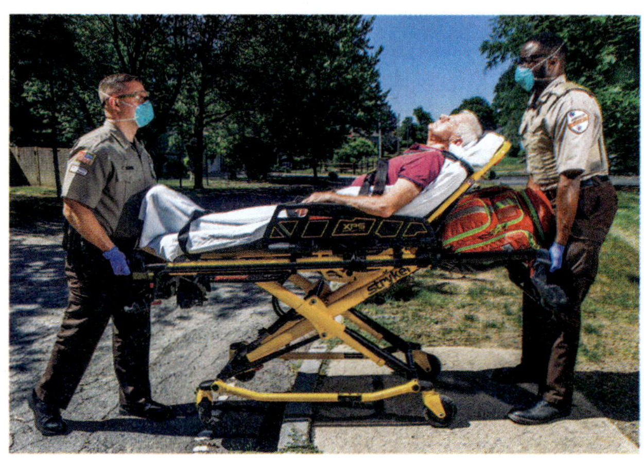

FIGURE 8-17 You do not need to retract the undercarriage of the stretcher when lifting it over a curb, a single step, or an obstacle of similar height.

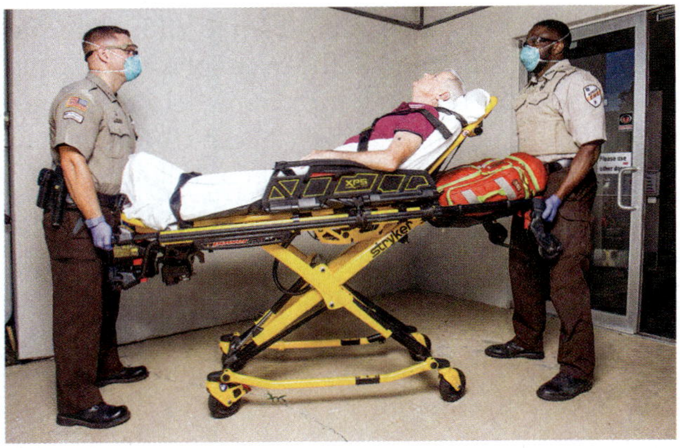

FIGURE 8-18 Hold the main frame of the stretcher when it is elevated so that even if the patient moves, the stretcher does not tip over.

Loading a Wheeled Stretcher Into an Ambulance

Whenever a patient has been placed onto the stretcher, one clinician must hold the main frame to prevent movement. When the stretcher is elevated, the main frame and the patient extend considerably beyond the wheels at both the head end and the foot end of the stretcher. Therefore, whenever a patient is on an elevated stretcher, you must ensure that it is held firmly between two hands at all times so that even if the patient moves, the stretcher cannot tip (**FIGURE 8-18**).

Inside the ambulance are strong clamps that fasten around the undercarriage when the stretcher is pushed into them. The clamps are located in a rack on the floor or side of the patient compartment, or through a center-mounted track system, and will hold the stretcher in place until they are released at the hospital. You can control and release the clamps with a single handle when standing on the ground at the open back doors of the ambulance when the stretcher is to be unloaded.

When you reach the back of the ambulance, you and your partner will roll the front wheels onto the floor in the back of the ambulance, advancing the stretcher until the safety hook catches the stretcher. The clinician at the foot of the stretcher then lifts and releases the undercarriage. The second clinician lifts the undercarriage with the wheels up to the level of the ambulance floor. Again, use of proper lifting mechanics is paramount to avoid the risk of back injury. Both clinicians then guide the stretcher into the locking mechanism in the back of the ambulance. As described previously, often the raising and lowering of the stretcher is done with a battery-powered motor; however, it is still important for you to maintain a firm grip on the stretcher. Newer automatically loading stretchers will manage the entire loading and unloading of the stretcher and only require the clinician to operate the buttons on the stretcher.

Safety Tips

Always follow these guidelines to load the stretcher into the ambulance:

- Make sure there are enough clinicians for sufficient lifting power.
- Follow the manufacturer's directions for safe and proper use of the stretcher.
- Make sure all stretchers and patients are fully secured before the ambulance is moved.

An intravenous (IV) pole is attached to many stretchers. The IV pole can be unfolded or extended above the main frame to hold an IV bag above the patient while you move the stretcher to the ambulance. Some wheeled ambulance stretchers even include a carrier to hold a cardiac monitor or automated external defibrillator and portable oxygen unit. If the model you use does not include these features, you will have to secure the portable oxygen unit and cardiac monitor or automated external defibrillator to the top surface of the stretcher mattress at the patient's legs. If possible, remove these items before lifting the stretcher to avoid the excess weight. These items must be secured in the ambulance prior to departing the scene.

Follow these steps to load the stretcher into an ambulance (**SKILL DRILL 8-5**).

1. Tilt the head end of the main frame upward, and place it into the patient compartment with the wheels on the floor. The two additional wheels that extend just below the head end are attached to the main frame and will enable this movement. Ensure that the safety bar under the head of the stretcher catches on the hook prior to lifting the stretcher (**Step 1**).

Skill Drill 8-5 Loading a Stretcher Into an Ambulance

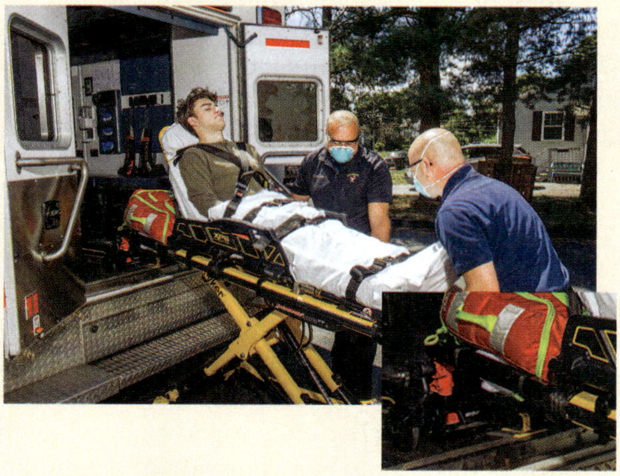

Step 1

Lift the stretcher into the load position, and place it into the patient compartment with the wheels on the floor and the safety bar latched on the hook.

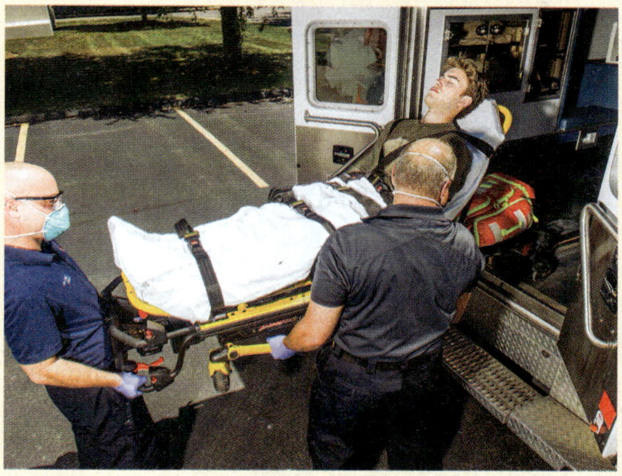

Step 2

The second clinician on the side of the stretcher releases the undercarriage lock and lifts the undercarriage. Some newer powered stretchers lift the undercarriage with the push of a button.

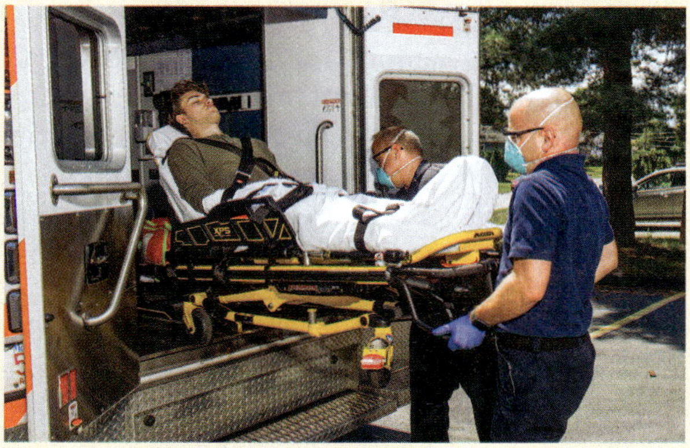

Step 3

Roll the stretcher into the back of the ambulance.

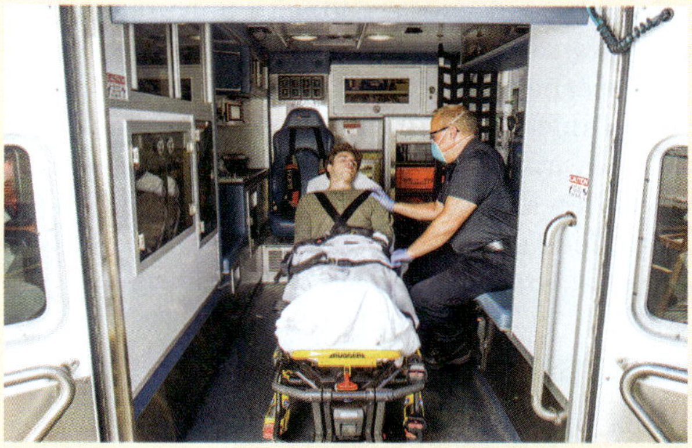

Step 4

Secure the stretcher to the clamps mounted in the ambulance.

2. With the patient's weight supported by these two head-end wheels and the EMT at the foot end of the stretcher, move to the side of the main frame and release the undercarriage lock to lift the undercarriage up to its fully retracted position. The wheels of the undercarriage and the two on the head end of the main frame will now be on the same level (**Step 2**).
3. Simply roll the stretcher the rest of the way into the back of the ambulance, where it will rest on all six wheels (**Step 3**).

4. Secure the stretcher in the ambulance with the strong clamps that fasten around the undercarriage when the stretcher is pushed into them. The clamps are located in a rack on the floor or side of the patient compartment (**Step 4**).

Backboards

A **backboard** is a long, flat board made of rigid, rectangular material (**FIGURE 8-19**). Backboards are also called long backboards, spine boards, trauma boards, or longboards. A backboard is sometimes used to move patients out of awkward places.

Backboards are 6 to 7 feet long (approximately 2 m). Parallel to the sides and ends of the backboard are a number of long holes that are approximately 0.5 to 1 inch (1 to 2.5 cm) from the outer edge. These holes form handles and handholds so that the board can be easily grasped, lifted, and carried. The handles and adjacent holes also allow the patient to be secured to the board using straps located at each side and end of the backboard.

For many years, backboards were made of thick marine plywood and sealed with polyurethane or marine varnish. Newer backboards are made of lighter plastic materials that will not absorb blood or other infectious substances. Some services are moving away from backboard use due to injuries patients can receive after being secured to them for long periods and are instead using other devices, such as vacuum mattresses.

Scoop Stretchers

Another option when moving a patient is to use a **scoop stretcher**. With a scoop stretcher, the two halves of the device are inserted under each side of the patient, and the two sides are fastened together. Then the patient is lifted and carried to the nearby wheeled stretcher. Scoop stretchers can be used to lift a patient at risk for a spine injury (with cervical collar) or with an unstable pelvis or other injury that would prevent rolling the patient. To use a scoop stretcher, follow the steps in **SKILL DRILL 8-6**.

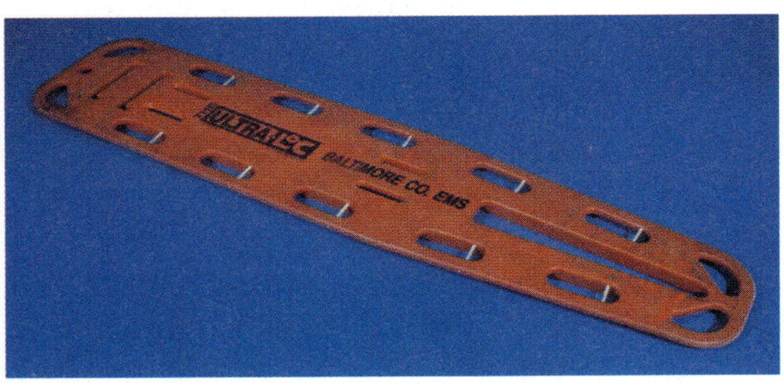

FIGURE 8-19 A backboard is one device used to transfer patients who must be moved in a supine position.

1. With the scoop stretcher separated, measure the length of the patient and adjust to the proper length (**Step 1**).
2. Position the stretcher, one side at a time. Lift the patient's side slightly by pulling on the far hip and upper arm, while your partner slides the stretcher into place (**Step 2**).
3. Lock the stretcher ends together by engaging their locking mechanisms one at a time and continue to lift the patient slightly as needed to avoid pinching (**Step 3**).
4. Apply and tighten straps to secure the patient to the scoop stretcher before transferring to the wheeled stretcher (**Step 4**).

Vacuum Mattresses

When using a vacuum mattress, the patient is placed on the mattress and the air is removed from the device, allowing it to mold around the patient (**FIGURE 8-20**). Vacuum mattresses fit snugly to the curvatures and contours of the body and limit pressure-point tenderness. Padding may be used for tender areas but is not required for most patients. The vacuum mattress is seen as equivalent to padding to secure the patient's neck and spine and is more comfortable for the patient than the backboard. See Chapter 28, *Head and Spine Injuries*, for more information about the vacuum mattress.

Lifting and Carrying a Patient on a Backboard or Similar Transport Device

If a patient is supine on a backboard or is lying in a semi-Fowler position on the stretcher, their weight is not equally distributed between the two ends of the device. For a patient in a horizontal position, between 68% and 78% of the body weight is in the torso. Therefore, more of the patient's weight rests on the head half of the device than on the foot half.

Skill Drill 8-6 Using a Scoop Stretcher

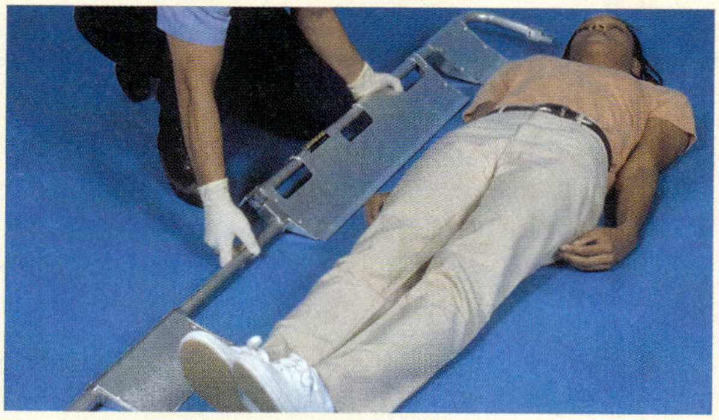

Step 1

Adjust the length of the stretcher.

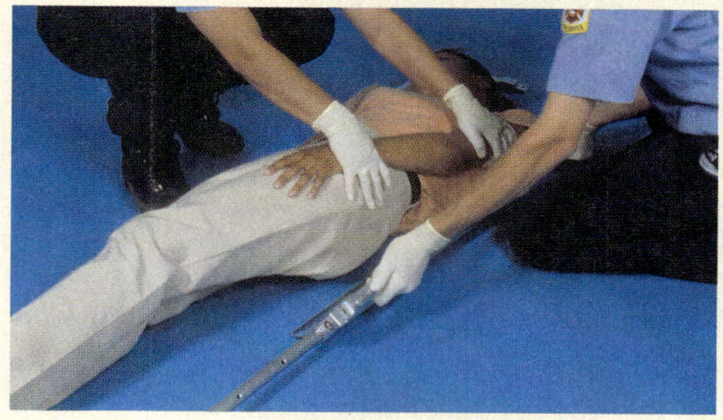

Step 2

Lift the patient slightly and slide the stretcher into place, one side at a time.

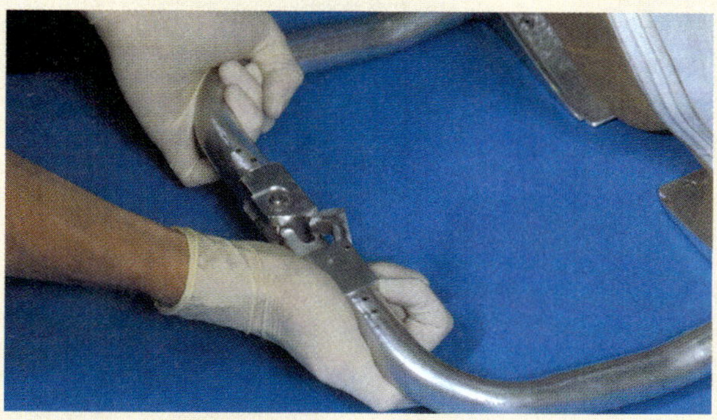

Step 3

Lock the stretcher ends together, and avoid pinching both the patient and your fingers!

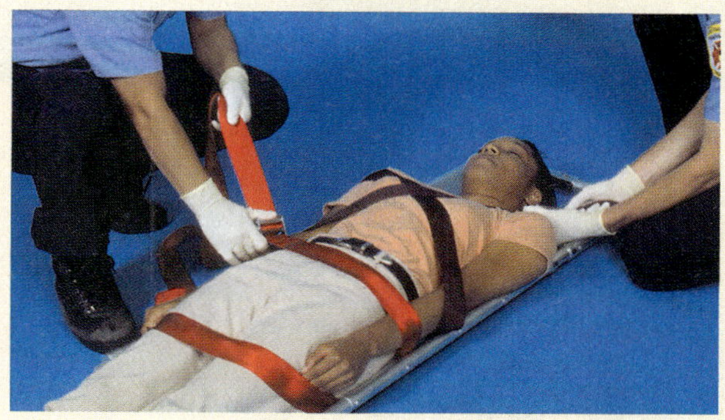

Step 4

Secure the patient to the scoop stretcher, and transfer to the stretcher.

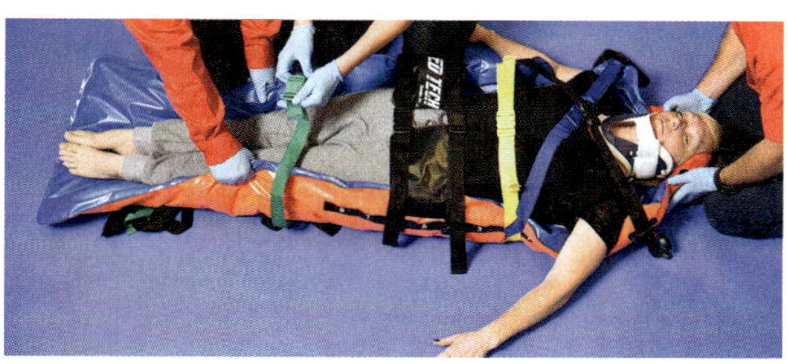

FIGURE 8-20 The vacuum mattress fits snugly to the curvatures and contours of the body and limits pressure-point tenderness.

A patient on a backboard or similar device can be lifted and carried by four clinicians in a **diamond carry**, with one clinician at the head end of the device, one at the foot end, and one at each side of the patient's torso (**FIGURE 8-21**). Follow these steps to perform the diamond carry (**SKILL DRILL 8-7**):

1. To best balance the weight, the clinicians at each side should be located so that they are able to grasp the backboard or stretcher with one hand distal to the patient's waist and the other hand located midthorax. While facing

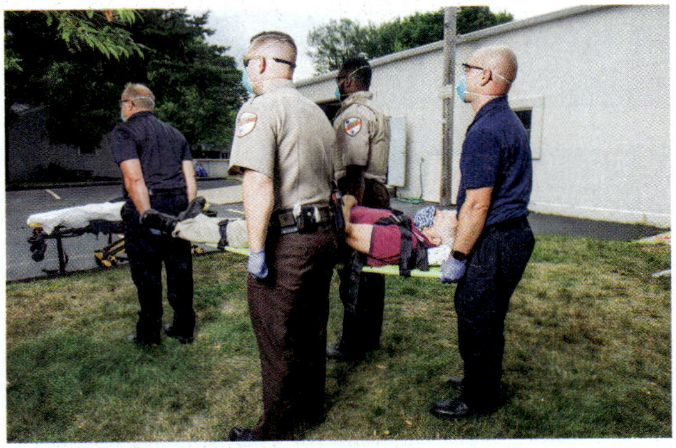

FIGURE 8-21 The diamond carry requires four clinicians: one at the head of the backboard, one at the foot end, and one at each side of the patient's torso.

the patient, all four clinicians lift the device to carrying height using correct lifting techniques, including a locked-in back (**Step 1**).

2. The clinicians at each side should turn the hand that is closer to the patient's head so the palm is facing their own body, then release the other hand (**Step 2**).
3. The clinicians at each side turn toward the patient's feet. The clinician at the foot end turns to face forward. All four clinicians should face the same direction and walk forward when carrying the patient (**Step 3**).

A patient on a backboard should be carried feetfirst to place the lightest load on the clinician at the patient's feet, who, to walk forward, must turn and grasp the handles with their back to the device.

Skill Drill 8-7 Performing the Diamond Carry

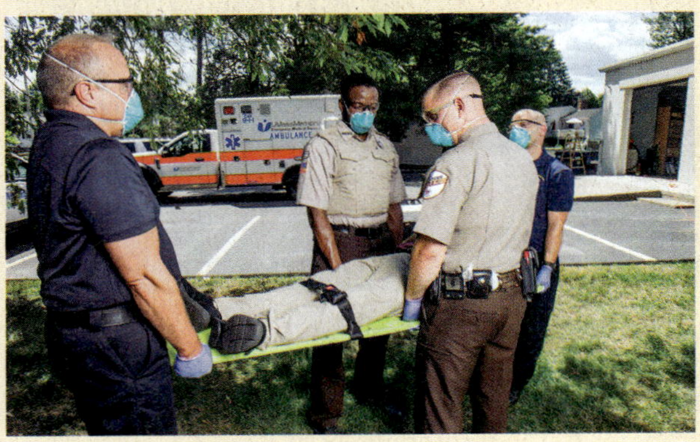

Step 1

All four clinicians lift the device while facing the patient.

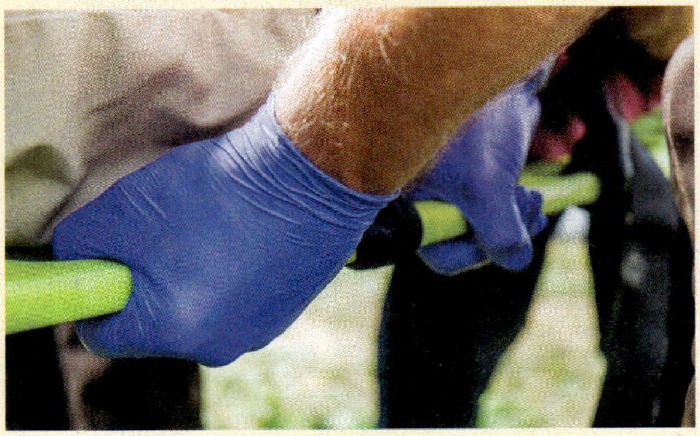

Step 2

The clinicians at each side turn the hand closest to the patient's head so the palm is facing themselves, then release the other hand.

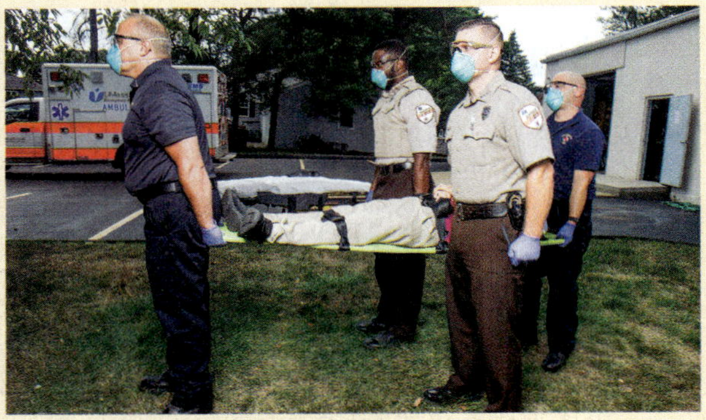

Step 3

The clinicians at each side turn toward the foot end. The clinician at the foot end turns to face forward.

Carrying the patient feetfirst will also allow an alert patient to see in the direction of movement, which may reduce anxiety.

Another method of lifting and carrying a patient on a backboard is the one-handed carry. With this method, four or more clinicians each use one hand to support the backboard so that they are able to face forward as they are walking. To perform the one-handed carry, follow the steps in **SKILL DRILL 8-8**:

1. Before lifting the backboard, clinicians position themselves so there are two on each side of the backboard facing across from each other. The clinicians grip the backboard with both hands (**Step 1**).
2. The clinicians lift the backboard to carrying height using correct lifting techniques, including a locked-in back (**Step 2**).
3. The clinicians turn in the direction they will be walking and switch to using one hand, with the palm facing their own body (**Step 3**).

Be sure to pick up and carry the backboard with your back in the upright position. If you need to lean to either side to compensate for a weight imbalance, you have probably exceeded your weight-carrying limit. If this occurs, reevaluate the carry; additional clinicians may be needed to avoid injuring yourself or dropping the patient.

While a four-clinician method is ideal when the patient must be carried, if only two clinicians are available, or if space is limited, a two-person method may be necessary. In a two-person carry, the two clinicians should stand facing each other, with one person at the head end of the lifting device and the other at the foot end. With this type of carry, one clinician will have to walk backward.

Skill Drill 8-8 Performing the One-Handed Carry

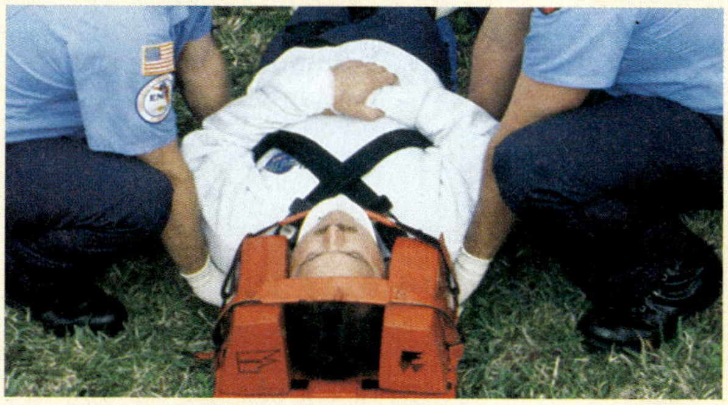

Step 1

With two clinicians facing each other on each side of the backboard, the clinicians grip the backboard with both hands.

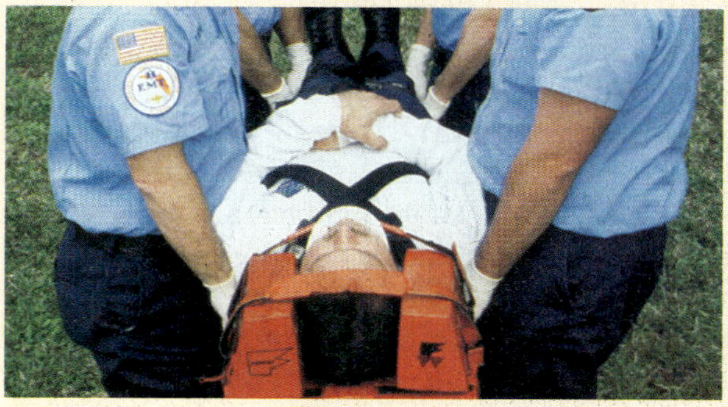

Step 2

The team lifts the backboard to carrying height.

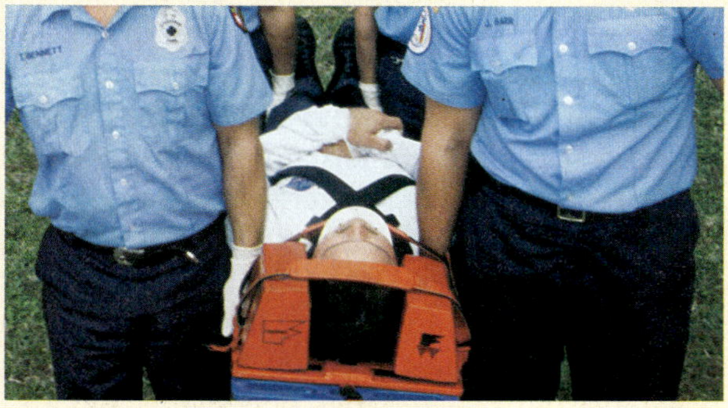

Step 3

Clinicians turn in the direction they will walk and switch to using one hand.

Moving a Patient on Stairs Using a Backboard or Similar Transport Device

When a patient is unresponsive or must be moved in a supine position, such as when spinal motion restriction is required, secure the patient onto a flexible stretcher, backboard, or vacuum mattress. Be sure that the patient is anatomically secured to the device so that they cannot slide. Carry the patient on the backboard down the stairs to the wheeled stretcher. When carrying the patient down stairs or an incline, the patient should be carried feetfirst so that the head end is elevated higher than the foot end.

When moving on stairs, as usual, the head end of the device will bear the greatest proportion of the patient's weight, so make sure the strongest clinician is positioned at the head end. (Even with four or more clinicians carrying the patient, the strain on the clinician at the head end will be increased when you must negotiate a narrow flight of stairs.) However, keep in mind that a proportionally greater weight will also be distributed to the clinician at the lower end when the device becomes angled (because of gravity). You should anticipate this and make sure the two strongest clinicians are positioned at each end of the device. Because of the incline of the stairway, if one of the two strongest clinicians is considerably taller than the other, it will be easier if the shorter clinician is at the upper end and the taller clinician is at the lower end. This minimizes bending while lifting and moving the patient. Once you reach the stretcher, place both the device and the patient on the stretcher; then secure both to the stretcher using additional straps.

Words of Wisdom

You will often have to perform several additional steps to place the patient onto a backboard and/or carry the patient down a flight of stairs. You will also have to add a stop at the top of the stairway so that everyone can reposition before carrying the patient down the stairs. Repositioning usually requires lowering the backboard to the ground and lifting it again when all clinicians are in their proper places. If you are carrying the patient in a stair chair, the additional step occurs after you have descended the stairs and reached the stretcher. At that point, you will have to assist or lift the patient from the stair chair onto the stretcher.

To carry a patient on stairs on a backboard or a vacuum mattress, follow the steps in **SKILL DRILL 8-9**:

1. Apply the straps to pass tightly across the upper torso over the shoulder and across the patient's chest, but not over the arms, to hold the patient in place while leaving the arms free. The strap is secured to the handles at both sides of the backboard or vacuum mattress so that it cannot slide toward the foot end of the device. Strap the patient securely to the device (**Step 1**).
2. When carrying the patient down stairs or an incline, make sure the backboard or vacuum mattress is carried with the foot end first so that the head end is elevated higher than the foot end. The straps will prevent the patient from sliding down or off the device (**Step 2**).

Street Smarts

Patients are commonly uneasy and scared as they are being carried, especially when they are being carried up or down stairs. Remember to talk with your patient continually while the move is taking place. Ask the patient to help by keeping arms in and holding still, and offer reassurance that the EMS team is working safely.

Stair Chairs

When you must carry an alert patient up or down a flight of stairs or other significant incline, use a stair chair if the patient's condition allows them to be placed in a sitting position. A **stair chair** is a lightweight folding chair with a molded seat, adjustable safety straps, and fold-out handles at both the head and foot ends (**FIGURE 8-22**). Most models have rubber wheels in the back with casters in front so that they can roll along the floor and make turns. Some have a specially designed track to facilitate movement down steps with little lifting required. Powered stair chair models are motorized to assist rescuers when moving patients up or down stairs. Stair chairs serve as an adjunct for moving a patient up or down stairs to the ground floor, where the prepared wheeled ambulance stretcher is waiting. You can roll the stair chair on the floor until you reach the stairwell, and then both clinicians carry it

Skill Drill 8-9 Carrying a Patient on Stairs Using a Backboard or Similar Transport Device

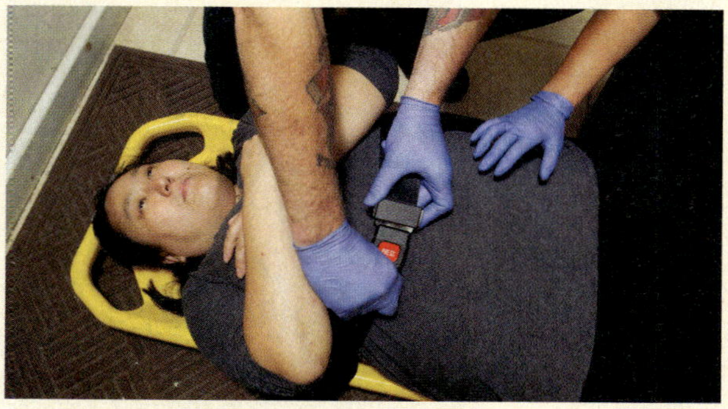

Step 1

Strap the patient securely. Make sure one strap is tight across the upper torso, under the arms, and secured to the handles to prevent the patient from sliding.

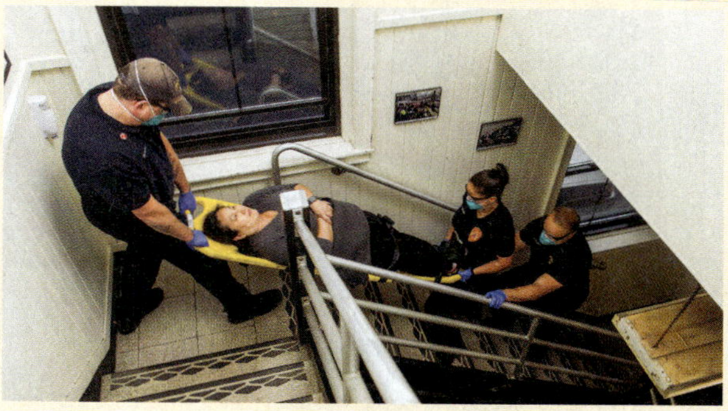

Step 2

Carry a patient down stairs with the foot end first, always keeping the head elevated. Unless the patient is completely alert and cooperative, hands need to be secured for safety and to prevent the patient from grabbing onto the railing of the stairs or the patient's hands from falling off the side of the board.

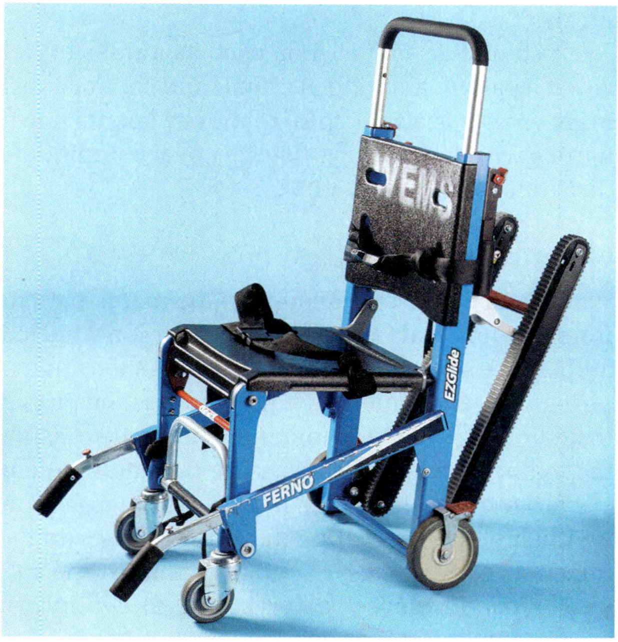

FIGURE 8-22 A wheeled stair chair can be used to transfer an alert patient up or down a flight of stairs.

(rather than roll and bump it) up or down the stairs. You will find this is one of the most useful tools for moving a patient.

When the patient is upstairs, you should take the wheeled ambulance stretcher to the ground floor landing and prepare it for the patient. Place it at the proper height, lower the side rails, turn down the cover sheet, and remove any equipment that you may have secured on the top. You should then take the stair chair upstairs and load the patient into it. Once reaching the bottom of the stairs, transfer the patient from the stair chair onto the stretcher.

Follow these steps to use a stair chair without tracks (**SKILL DRILL 8-10**):

1. Secure the patient to the stair chair with straps. At a minimum, use a lap belt at the hips and two straps around the chest. You will need to coach the patient to hold on to the chest straps tightly to prevent the patient from grabbing onto the stair well or rails and throwing the team off balance.

Skill Drill 8-10 Using a Stair Chair

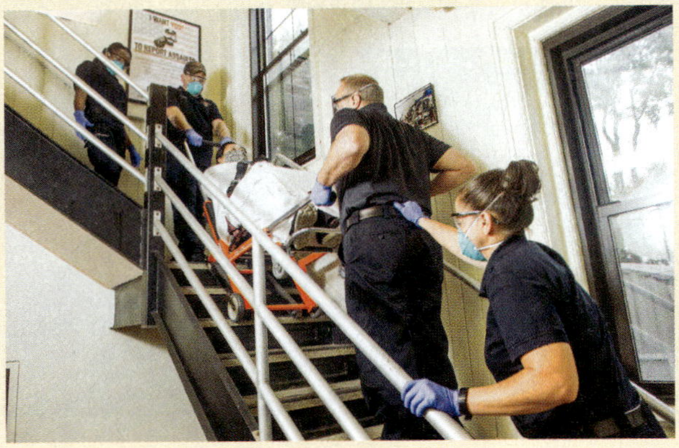

Step 1

Position and secure the patient on the chair with straps. Take your places at the head and foot of the chair.

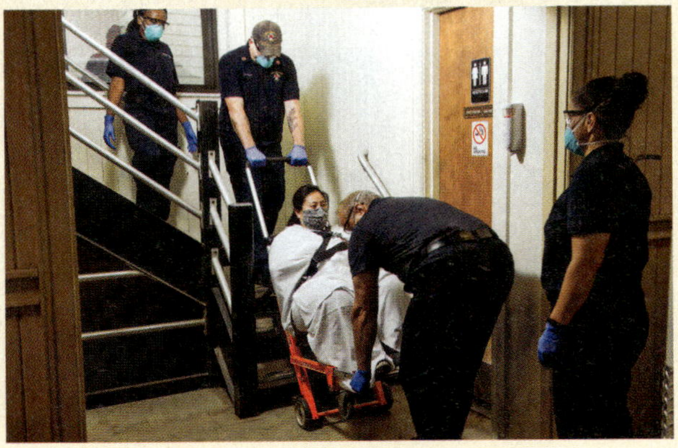

Step 2

Lower the chair to roll on landings and for transfer to the stretcher.

2. Take your places around the patient seated on the chair: one clinician at the head end and one at the foot end (**Step 1**). The clinician at the head will give directions to coordinate the lift and movement. If a third clinician is on scene, this person may precede the clinician who is at the patient's feet, keeping a hand on their back and assisting by opening doors and providing guidance and support. For lengthy carries, a third clinician can also rotate into the carrying team to provide breaks for the other two.
3. When reaching landings and other flat intervals in the move, lower the chair to the ground and roll the chair to the next position. On reaching the ground level where the stretcher awaits, roll the chair into position next to the stretcher in preparation for transferring the patient (**Step 2**).

As with other carries, always remember to keep your back in a locked-in position and to flex at the hips, not the waist. Bend at the knees and keep the patient's weight and your arms as close to your body as possible. Twisting while carrying or moving a patient will increase your risk of injury.

A stair chair can also be used as a transfer device if a patient is sitting in a chair and cannot assist in moving. It is also helpful to move patients down narrow winding hallways that do not accommodate the stretcher. (**FIGURE 8-23**).

Neonatal Isolettes

When you need to transport a neonatal patient from one hospital to another, the common wheeled ambulance stretcher will not suffice. To safely transport a neonatal patient, the patient must be placed inside of an isolette, sometimes referred to as an incubator. The isolette keeps the neonatal patient warm with moistened air in a clean environment and helps to protect the infant from noise, drafts, infection, and excess handling. These specialized transport devices come in one of two forms: an isolette that is placed directly on top of the wheeled stretcher and secured with seat belts or a free-standing isolette that is secured into the back

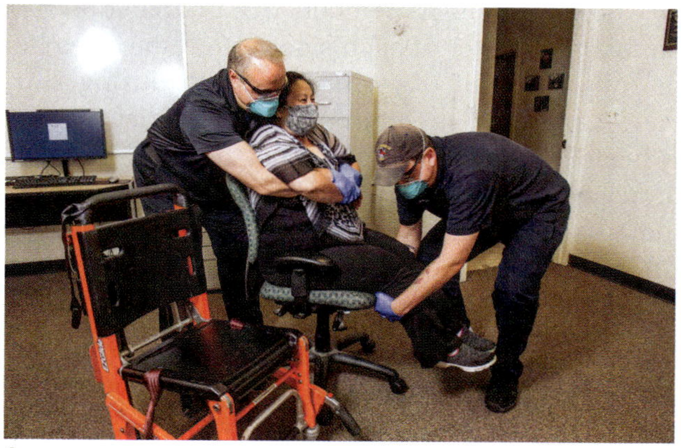

A

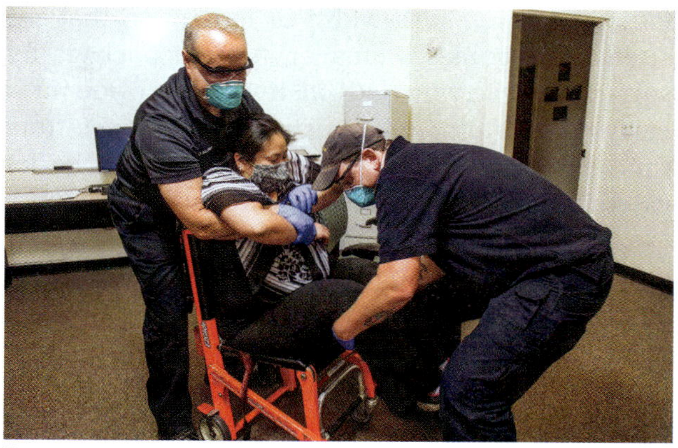

B

FIGURE 8-23 Moving a patient from a chair to a stair chair. **A.** If present, any removable side pieces on the chair should be removed or placed in a position so they will not interfere. Slide your arms through the patient's armpits, and grasp the patient's crossed forearms. Your partner grasps the patient's legs at the knees. **B.** Gently lift the patient into the locked stair chair.

of the ambulance, taking the place of the standard stretcher (**FIGURE 8-24**).

Binder Lifts

A Binder Lift gives EMS clinicians another safe way to lift patients as a team to help prevent injuries. It is used only for patients with nontraumatic injuries who do not require spinal motion restriction. The binder is wrapped around the patient's torso. It has 24 to 32 handles for clinicians to use during the patient lift before moving the patient to a stair chair or stretcher. The design allows for application even

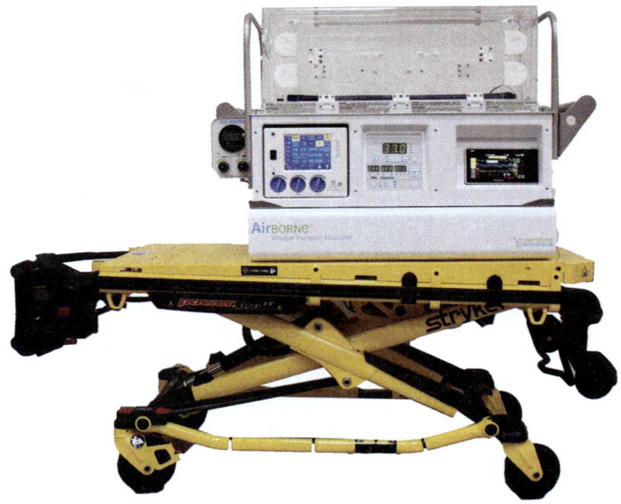

FIGURE 8-24 Neonatal isolette.

in confined spaces, such as a bathroom. It may also be used to assist patients into a standing position when they have slid down onto the floor and simply need assistance getting up.

Slipp Patient Movers

A Slipp patient mover is a device that can be used to transfer patients of any weight from one surface to another. The Slipp is composed of a smooth material that seals in a thin layer of fluid. This design reduces friction between the patient and the surface on which they are lying. The patient is rolled onto their side and the Slipp, along with a draw sheet on top, is positioned under the patient. The patient is then rolled back onto the Slipp and pulled by the draw sheet across the Slipp and onto the stretcher, hospital bed, or other location. It is essential that both the bed and the stretcher are locked during this type of move to prevent them from separating.

Portable/Folding Stretchers

A **portable stretcher** is a stretcher with a strong, rectangular, tubular metal frame and rigid fabric stretched across it (**FIGURE 8-25**). Portable stretchers do not have a second multipositioning frame or adjustable undercarriage. Some models have two wheels that fold down approximately 4 inches

(10 cm) underneath the foot end of the frame and legs of a similar length that fold down from the head end at each side. The wheels make it easier to move the loaded stretcher. The legs should not be used as handles.

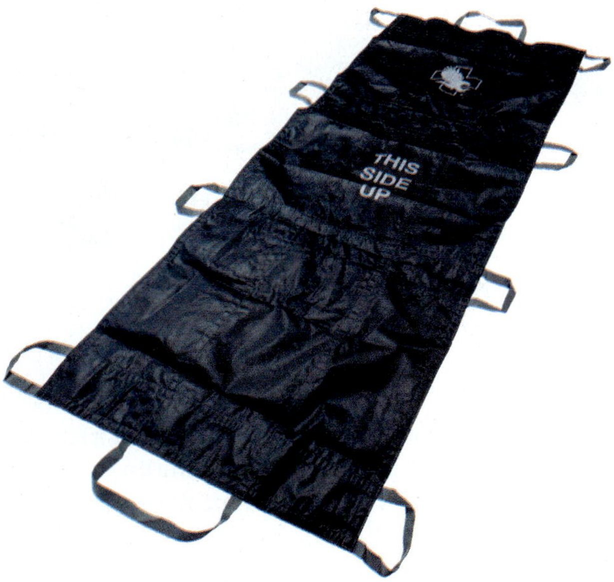

FIGURE 8-25 A portable stretcher.

Used with permission from North American Rescue.

Some portable stretchers can be folded in half across the center of each side so that the stretcher is only one-half of its usual length during storage. A portable stretcher weighs much less than a wheeled stretcher and does not have a bulky undercarriage. However, because most models do not have wheels, you and your team must support all of the patient's weight and any equipment along with the weight of the stretcher.

Flexible Stretchers

Several types of flexible (also referred to as soft) stretchers are available and can be rolled up across either the stretcher's width or length, so that the stretcher becomes a smaller, tubular package for storage and carrying (**FIGURE 8-26**). When you must carry the equipment a considerable distance from the nearest place that the ambulance can be located, this is an important consideration. A **flexible stretcher** conforms around the patient's sides and does not extend beyond them. When these stretchers are extended, they are particularly useful when you must remove a patient from or through a confined space or when moving cardiac arrest patients from the ground to the stretcher. Certain flexible stretchers can also be used if the patient must be belayed or rappelled by ropes.

YOU are the EMT

A cervical collar and an extrication vest are applied. You are then able to remove the passenger from the wreckage and onto a backboard. After loading her into the ambulance, you perform a complete assessment and transport her to the local trauma center for evaluation.

Recording Time: 27 Minutes	
Level of consciousness	Alert and oriented
Respirations	16 breaths/min; adequate depth
Pulse	110 beats/min; strong and regular
Skin	Baseline color, warm, and moist
Blood pressure	148/72 mm Hg
Oxygen saturation (Spo_2)	100% (on room air)

On arrival at the hospital, the patient tells you that she is still experiencing pain in the passenger back, although it is not as severe and feels like "a pulled muscle." After moving her from the wheeled stretcher to the hospital bed, you give your verbal report to the staff nurse and return to service.

10. How can you minimize the risk of injury while moving a patient on a wheeled ambulance stretcher?

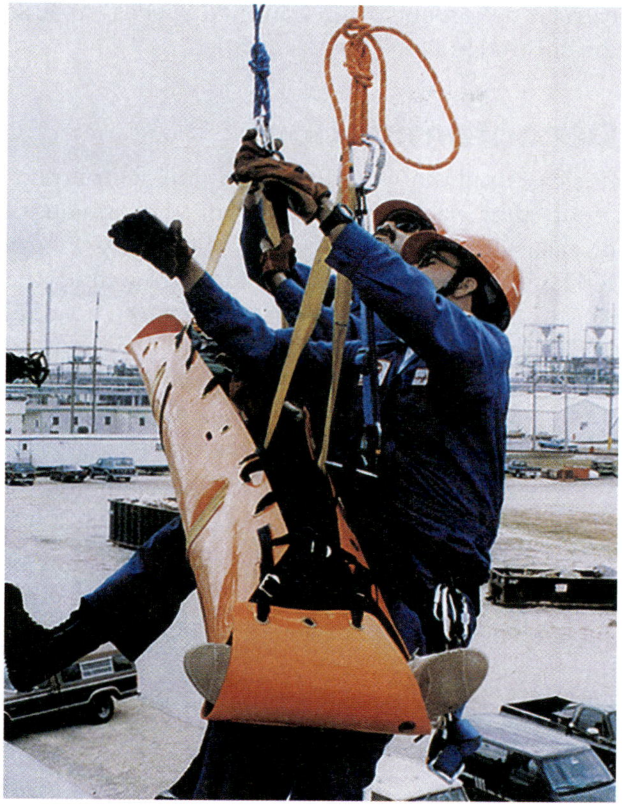

FIGURE 8-26 A flexible stretcher.

> **Words of Wisdom**
>
> When you encounter a patient in a confined space, such as a bathroom, it can pose a unique set of problems. Prior to moving a patient in a confined space, it is important to discuss the process with your fellow team members. Ensure that everyone agrees with the extrication plan and understands their role. Consider whether an assistive lifting device would be helpful. Remember that communication with the crew, as well as the patient, will assist in minimizing potential problems.

Basket Stretchers

Use a rigid **basket stretcher**, also called a Stokes basket or litter, to carry a patient across uneven terrain from a remote location that is inaccessible by ambulance or other vehicle (**FIGURE 8-27**). If you suspect that the patient has a spinal injury, first secure the person on a backboard and then place the backboard into the basket stretcher. Once you have

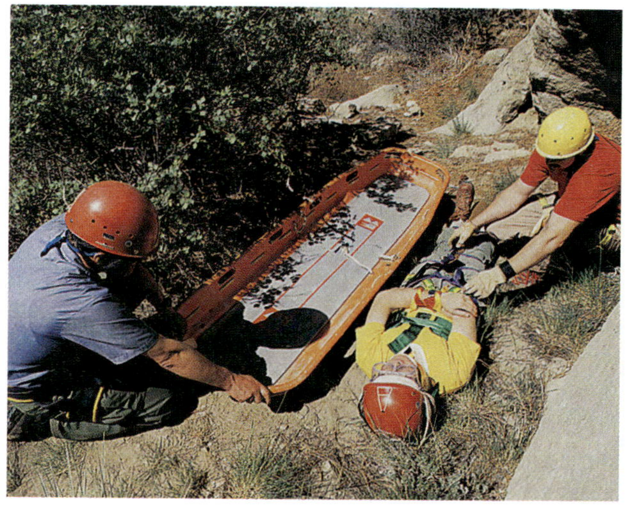

FIGURE 8-27 A basket stretcher.

reached the ambulance and wheeled ambulance stretcher, you can remove the patient secured to the backboard from the basket stretcher and place the patient on the stretcher.

Basket stretchers are made of plastic with an aluminum frame or have a full steel frame that is connected by a woven wire mesh. The wire basket is uncomfortable for the patient unless the wire is padded. Either type can be used to carry a patient across fields, rough terrain, or trails, or on a toboggan, boat, or all-terrain vehicle. Basket stretchers are also used for technical rope rescues and some water rescues. Not all basket stretchers are rated or appropriate for each of these specialized rescue uses.

Short Backboards

Until you can perform spinal motion restriction with another device, you can use a short (or half-spine) backboard to stabilize the torso, head, and neck of an alert, seated patient with no life-threatening injuries who is unable to self-extricate and has only a suspected spinal injury. Short backboards are 3 to 4 feet long (approximately 1 m). The wooden short backboard has largely been replaced with a more secure vest-type device, such as the Kendrick extrication device (KED), that is specifically designed to stabilize the patient until they are moved from a sitting position to a supine position on a backboard (**FIGURE 8-28**). However, with the advent of new spinal motion restriction guidelines, vest-type devices are rarely used. They can be helpful when

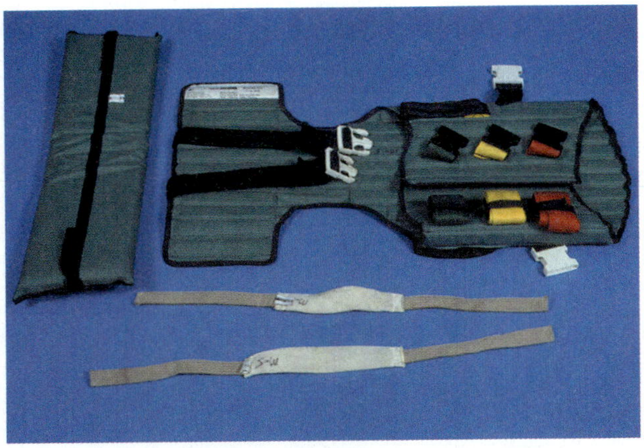

FIGURE 8-28 The Kendrick extrication device (KED) is a vest-type stabilization device.

extricating patients from confined spaces, such as the covered hull of a boat.

Decontamination

It is essential that you decontaminate your equipment after each use to prevent the spread of disease—for your own safety, the safety of the EMTs using the equipment after you, and the safety of your patients. Just as you expect a hospital bed to be disinfected after the previous patient, so too with your stretcher and other transport equipment. Know and follow your local standard operating procedures for disinfecting equipment after each call. For further discussion of equipment decontamination, see Chapter 2, *Workforce Safety and Wellness.*

YOU are the EMT SUMMARY

1. What immediate challenges do you face?

Your first concern is for the stability and safety of the vehicle. Prior to attempting to physically access the patients, safety measures must be taken to stabilize the vehicle and prevent further rollover or collapse during the extrication process.

If the patients are not trapped, the vehicle is stabilized, and you decide to remove a patient yourself, the next consideration is the size of the patient. Does the patient weigh more than you and your partner can safely lift? There is also the consideration of working in an enclosed space that may not allow for additional clinicians to help with the initial movement of a patient.

Additionally, there are two patients and at least one is in critical condition. This further increases the stress on you and may lead to injury if the lift is not adequately planned. While your intention to help the patient is admirable, you must remember that you will be useless to the team and the patient if you are injured in the process.

2. Why is knowledge of body mechanics important when lifting and moving a patient?

Body mechanics describes the way you move your body. Posture is an important component in body mechanics. Good posture means the spine is in a neutral position. Knowing how your body moves will minimize the risk of a back injury when you are lifting or moving a patient. Always keep your back in a straight and upright position and lift without twisting.

3. What other resources are needed?

You already know the driver is unresponsive and showing signs of dyspnea with cyanosis. You also know that both patients are entrapped in the overturned vehicle, and extrication will be required. Therefore, immediately call for paramedic backup and a rescue unit, as well as lifting assistance. There will be a delay in care as the patients are extricated. Having advanced units standing by will decrease the time to definitive care. You will likely need a second ambulance, or if you are a long distance from a Level I trauma center, consider the use of air transport, if available. Ask the dispatcher for a fire or rescue response if it is not already on scene or en route to the scene. The rescuers can disconnect batteries and stabilize the vehicle, and they may be needed to help extricate the patients.

Law enforcement should be dispatched for crowd control and to help with directing traffic around the scene to make it safe for everyone to work. Each agency has its own job to do, and the sooner each agency is dispatched, the quicker the patient will receive optimal care.

4. Do you consider the driver to be in stable or unstable condition? Should you wait for further assistance or proceed to gain access to him?

The condition of the driver is unstable due to his altered level of consciousness and cyanosis. Regardless, you must never enter a scene that is not safe. With the vehicle lying on its side in such a precarious

YOU are the EMT SUMMARY continued

position, any weight added could cause it to roll over and crush you or cause further injury to the patients. If you enter the vehicle in such a situation, you risk making the situation even more hazardous to vehicle occupants and to the rest of the rescue team. The vehicle must be stabilized prior to gaining access to the patients. Safety of the crew is paramount before any patient care is provided.

If the passenger is able to lift her arms and the tubing is long enough, it may be possible to toss a nonrebreathing mask into the vehicle and have her place and hold the mask over the face of her husband to provide him with oxygen before further treatment begins. Any further care will have to be postponed until the vehicle has been stabilized.

5. Once you are able to gain access, what are your concerns for the use of proper body mechanics while removing these patients?

The overturned vehicle is a confined space that allows for access by only one EMT. This means that you must consider your lifting limits and think through what type of equipment may be utilized to place the least amount of physical stress on you. The patients may have to be moved in carefully planned stages. Try to use your legs to do most of the lifting, and try to keep your back as straight as possible within the limitations imposed.

6. What type of move is best for removing the driver?

Due to the unstable condition of the patient, it is necessary to move him as quickly and safely as possible. Unfortunately, with such a confined space there is no way to utilize additional help to maintain spinal alignment. If the rescue team is able to wedge a backboard through the open door of the vehicle, it will give you a platform to stand or kneel on, as well as something on which to move the patient. The best options for moving the driver likely would be to use a clothes drag or to grab underneath his arms and pull him upward if you are able to reach that far. If the passenger is able to use her arms, she may be able to help push upward from his hips to assist you in moving him. He will have to be pulled between the headrests if there is no other access. In some vehicles, it may be possible to remove the headrests. Make sure he is moved in small increments, using your arms to "curl" and repositioning often to protect your back. After his head and shoulders have been pulled though the seats, a second clinician can possibly reach through far enough to help pull him onto the backboard and then assist in removing him and the backboard from the vehicle.

7. What steps can you take to maximize safety while lifting a patient?

To safely lift and carry a patient, you and your team must anticipate and understand every move, and each move must be coordinated. To avoid confusion, which may result in one or more clinicians suddenly bearing an unexpected amount of weight, the team leader (typically the clinician closest to the head of the patient) should call out all of the lifting commands.

The following general guidelines should be followed to maximize safety when lifting any patient:

- Keep your legs shoulder width apart.
- Keep your back in a straight, locked-in position.
- Keep the patient's weight as close to your body as possible.
- Bend at the knees, not the waist, when lifting.
- Avoid lifting and reaching at the same time.
- Avoid twisting your body as you are lifting.
- Lift with your palms facing up (power grip).
- Communicate with your partner (or team) at all times.

8. How is a patient's weight distributed when on a carrying device? Why is it important to know this?

To position your team accordingly, and thus minimize the potential for injury, it is important to know how a patient's weight is distributed when secured to the carrying device.

If a patient is supine on a backboard or a scoop stretcher or is in a semi-sitting position on an ambulance stretcher, weight is not equally distributed between the two ends of the device. When a patient is in a horizontal position, between 68% and 78% of their weight is in the torso. Therefore, the strongest clinician or clinicians should be positioned at the head end of the carrying device. However, you should still position the remaining clinicians so that each one, including the clinician or clinicians at the patient's head, bears an equal amount of the patient's weight.

9. Considering her complaints and the fact that her condition is stable, what are your best options for removing the passenger?

An urgent move is not required because the patient's condition is stable. Think through the possibilities while you provide reassurance to the patient. She has the potential for spinal injuries because of the mechanism of injury and because she is reporting back pain. For a stable patient who cannot self-extricate and is reporting neck or

YOU are the EMT SUMMARY continued

back pain, a short vest-type device, such as the KED, may be used. Apply a cervical collar to the patient and then position the vest device behind the patient and have her thread the leg straps underneath her legs. Continuously remind the patient to hold her head still and try to move as little as possible because there is no room for another clinician to hold cervical spine control. Once the device is positioned, you will have to lean through the seats to attach and secure the straps. Once secured, the patient can be moved as a unit. Pull her through the seats and onto the waiting backboard, where you will have additional assistance to remove her from the vehicle and transfer her onto the ambulance stretcher.

10. How can you minimize the risk of injury while moving a patient on a wheeled ambulance stretcher?

When you move a patient on a wheeled ambulance stretcher, make sure it is elevated whenever possible, not lowered to the ground. If the stretcher is lowered to the ground, you will have to bend down and move the patient at the same time; this increases the potential for a back injury.

When the stretcher is elevated, the main frame and the patient are considerably higher than the wheels; this makes the stretcher top-heavy. Therefore, when you are moving a patient on an elevated stretcher, ensure that you hold the frame firmly between both of your hands at all times so that if the patient moves, the stretcher will not tip over.

If you are guiding the stretcher from the foot end, make sure your arms are held close to your body, and avoid reaching a great distance behind you or hyperextending your back. Your back should be locked, straight, and untwisted. To avoid hyperextending your elbows or injuring your shoulder, keep your elbows slightly flexed and use the muscles of your arms to pull.

If you are guiding the stretcher from the head end, push with your arms and bend your elbows so that your hands are approximately 12 to 15 inches (30 to 38 cm) in front of your torso. To protect your elbows from injury, avoid pushing the stretcher with your arms fully extended and your elbows locked. When you push with your elbows bent but firmly held from bending further, the strong muscles of your arms serve as a shock absorber if the wheels of the stretcher strike an obstacle, causing the stretcher to come to an abrupt stop.

Prep Kit

Ready for Review

- The safety of you, your team, and the patient depends on the use of proper lifting techniques and maintaining a proper hold when lifting or carrying a patient. You must practice each technique with your team often so that you are able to perform the move quickly, safely, and efficiently.
- Some patients, including geriatric, pediatric, and bariatric patients, present unique packaging and transport considerations that you must understand for their and your crew's safety.
- Good body mechanics are important to prevent injuries, but are not always sufficient. Special devices and technology should be used when possible to further decrease your risk of injury.
- The key rule of lifting is to always keep your back in an upright position and lift without twisting. You can lift and carry significant weight without injury as long as your back is in the proper upright position.
- Know how much you can comfortably and safely lift, and do not attempt to lift more than this amount. Rapidly summon additional help to lift and carry a weight that is greater than you are able to lift.
- If you do not have a proper hold, you will not be able to bear your share of the weight, or you may lose your grasp with one or both hands and possibly cause a low back injury to one or more clinicians.
- When working as a team to move a patient, the team leader is responsible for

Prep Kit continued

coordinating the moves. Directions and commands are important parts of safe lifting and carrying.

- You and your team must anticipate and understand every move and execute it in a coordinated manner.
- Normally, you should move a patient with nonurgent moves, in an orderly, planned, and unhurried manner, selecting methods that involve the least amount of lifting and carrying.
- At times, you may have to use an emergency move to maneuver a patient before providing assessment and care. Perform an urgent move if a patient has an altered level of consciousness or inadequate ventilation, if the patient is in shock, or during extreme weather conditions.
- The devices most commonly used to move and transport patients include the wheeled ambulance stretcher, the backboard, the vacuum mattress, and the scoop stretcher.
- It is best to move a patient on a device that can be rolled. However, if a wheeled device is not available, you must understand and follow certain guidelines for carrying a patient on a backboard or other patient-moving device.
- When you must carry a patient up or down a flight of stairs or other significant incline, use a stair chair. The exception to this is when the patient is in cardiac arrest, must be moved in a supine position, or must receive spinal motion restriction during transport, in which case the patient will be moved on the stairs on a backboard.
- If you must carry a loaded backboard or stretcher up or down stairs or other inclines, be sure that the patient is tightly secured to the device to prevent sliding. Carry the backboard or stretcher foot end first so that the patient's head is elevated higher than the feet.
- Other devices that are used to lift and carry patients include bariatric stretchers, binder lifts, Slipp patient movers, flexible stretchers, short backboards, basket stretchers (Stokes litters), and neonatal isolettes.
- You will learn the technical skills of patient packaging and handling through practice and training.

Vital Vocabulary

backboard A long, flat board made of rigid, rectangular material that is used to provide support to a patient who is suspected of having a hip, pelvic, spinal, or lower extremity injury; also called a spine board, trauma board, and longboard.

bariatrics A branch of medicine concerned with the management (prevention or control) of obesity and allied diseases.

basket stretcher A rigid stretcher commonly used in technical and water rescues that surrounds and supports the patient yet allows water to drain through holes in the bottom; also called a Stokes basket or litter.

body mechanics The relationship between the body's anatomic structures and the physical forces associated with lifting, moving, and carrying; the ways in which the body moves to achieve a specific action.

diamond carry A carrying technique in which one clinician is located at the head end of the stretcher or backboard, one at the foot end, and one at each side of the patient; each of the two clinicians at the sides uses one hand to support the stretcher or backboard so that all are able to face forward as they walk.

emergency move A move in which the patient is dragged or pulled from a dangerous scene before assessment and care are provided.

extremity lift A lifting technique that is used for patients who are supine or in a sitting position with no suspected extremity or spinal injuries.

flexible stretcher A stretcher that is a rigid carrying device when secured around a patient but can be folded or rolled when not in use; also called a soft stretcher.

Prep Kit continued

portable stretcher A stretcher with a strong, rectangular, tubular metal frame and rigid fabric stretched across it.

power grip A technique in which the stretcher or backboard is gripped by inserting each hand under the handle with the palm facing up and the thumb extended, fully supporting the underside of the handle on the curved palm with the fingers and thumb.

power lift A lifting technique in which the EMT's back is held upright, with legs bent, and the patient is lifted when the EMT straightens the legs to raise the upper body and arms.

rapid extrication technique A technique to move a patient from a sitting position inside a vehicle to supine on a backboard in less than 1 minute when conditions do not allow for standard methods of spinal motion restriction.

scoop stretcher A stretcher that is designed to be split into two or four sections that can be fitted around a patient who is lying on the ground or other relatively flat surface.

stair chair A lightweight folding device that is used to carry an alert, seated patient up or down stairs.

wheeled ambulance stretcher A specially designed stretcher that can be rolled along the ground. A collapsible undercarriage allows it to be loaded into the ambulance; also called an ambulance stretcher.

References

1. Reichard AA, Marsh SM, Tonozzi TR, Konda S, Gormley MA. Occupational injuries and exposures among emergency medical services workers. *Prehosp Emerg Care*. 2017;21(4):420–431.
2. Friedenberg R, Kalichman L, Ezra D, Wacht O, Alperovitch-Najenson D. Work-related musculoskeletal disorders and injuries among emergency medical technicians and paramedics: A comprehensive narrative review. *Arch Environ Occup Health*. 2022;77(1):9–17.
3. Pediatric transportation. New Hampshire Department of Safety, Division of Fire Standards and Training and Emergency Medical Services website. https://media.emscimprovement.center/documents/NH_PediTransport_Protocol.pdf. Published 2020. Accessed November 22, 2024.
4. Lyng J, Adelgais K, Alter R, et al. Recommended essential equipment for basic life support and advanced life support ground ambulances 2020: a joint position statement. *Prehosp Emerg Care*. 2021;25(3):451–459.
5. Body measurements. Centers for Disease Control and Prevention website. https://www.cdc.gov/nchs/fastats/body-measurements.htm. Reviewed September 10, 2021. Accessed February 18, 2025.
6. National Association of State EMS Officials. *National Model EMS Clinical Guidelines: Version 3.0*. https://nasemso.org/wp-content/uploads/National-Model-EMS-Clinical-Guidelines_2022.pdf. Updated March 2022. Accessed November 22, 2024.
7. Adult obesity facts. Centers for Disease Control and Prevention website. https://www.cdc.gov/obesity/adult-obesity-facts/index.html. Published May 14, 2024. Accessed November 22, 2024.
8. Childhood obesity facts. Centers for Disease Control and Prevention website. https://www.cdc.gov/obesity/childhood-obesity-facts/childhood-obesity-facts.html. Published April 2, 2024. Accessed November 22, 2024.

Additional Resources

National Highway Traffic Safety Administration. *National Emergency Medical Services Education Standards*. https://www.ems.gov/assets/EMS_Education-Standards_2021_FNL.pdf. EMS.gov website. Published January 2021. Accessed November 22, 2024.

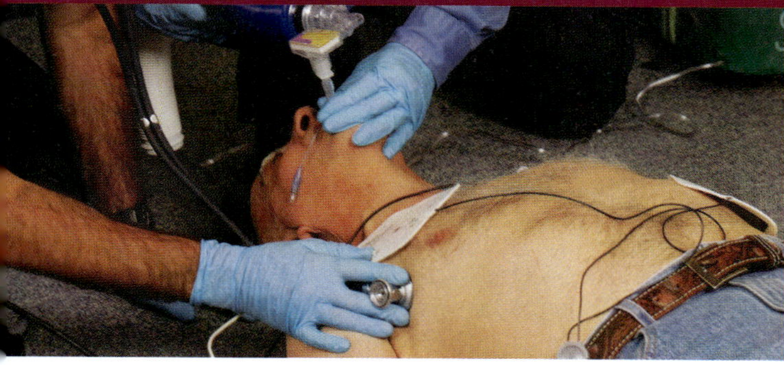

Chapter 9

The Team Approach to Health Care

NATIONAL EMS EDUCATION STANDARD COMPETENCIES

Preparatory

Applies knowledge of the emergency medical services (EMS) system, safety/well-being of the emergency medical technician (EMT), medical/legal, and ethical issues to the provision of emergency care.

EMS System Communication

- EMS communication system (Chapter 4, *Communications and Documentation*)
- Communication with other health care professionals to include cohesive and organized patient handoff (pp 308–309)
- Team communication and dynamics (pp 301–312)
- Telemetric monitoring devices and transmission of clinical data, including video data (Chapter 4, *Communications and Documentation*)

KNOWLEDGE OBJECTIVES

1. Define continuum of care. (p 301)
2. List the five essential elements of a group. (p 303)
3. Explain the advantages of a team over a group; include the advantages of regularly training and practicing together. (pp 301–308)
4. Describe the attributes of effective team leaders and members. (pp 305–306)
5. Explain how crew resource management (CRM) can be useful in the prehospital environment. (pp 306–308)
6. List the key guidelines to ensure effective transfer of patient care from one health care clinician to another. (pp 308–309)
7. List the steps a receiving health care clinician should perform when taking a patient care report. (p 309)
8. Explain the stages of effective decision making. (pp 310–312)
9. Describe decision traps that can lead to decision-making errors. (p 312)
10. Describe the steps EMTs can take to troubleshoot interpersonal conflicts. (pp 312–313)

SKILLS OBJECTIVES

There are no skills objectives for this chapter.

Introduction

As an EMT, you are a critical member of the emergency health care team. A **team** consists of a group of health care clinicians who are assigned specific roles and are working interdependently in a coordinated manner under a designated leader. It includes not only first responders, paramedics, and other EMTs, but also physicians, nurses, and other personnel who will help care for patients throughout the duration of their injury or illness (**FIGURE 9-1**). You play a pivotal role by bringing emergency medicine into patients' homes, assisting with advanced patient care skills, and ensuring the effective transfer of patient care to emergency department (ED) staff when you arrive at the hospital.

Increasingly, some EMTs work in health care settings such as hospital EDs, urgent care centers, or other outpatient areas.[1] In those settings, the role of the EMT may vary widely. Regardless of the setting, the EMT's ability to function effectively as part of a team is critical to the safety and outcomes of the patient, the efficiency and effectiveness of the team, and the well-being of the EMT and other team members.[2]

This chapter will provide an overview of the team health care approach and discuss how diversity among clinicians' backgrounds, skills, and abilities can strengthen a team. The chapter will also discuss how to assist with advanced skills and manage interpersonal conflict.

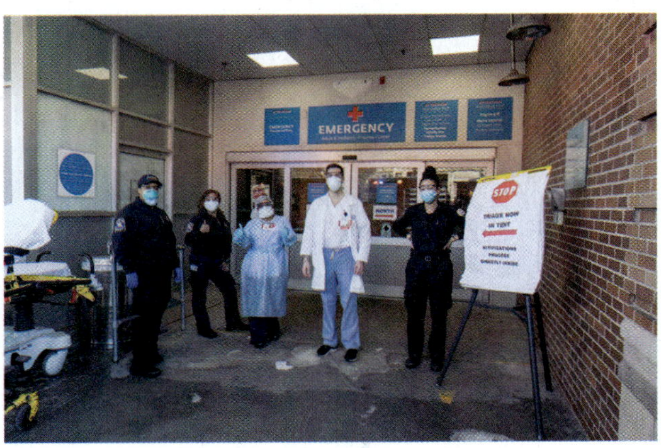

FIGURE 9-1 As an EMT, you will work with various health care clinicians along the continuum of care.

Words of Wisdom

The benefit of effective teamwork on the delivery of health care is highlighted by programs such as the World Health Organization's *Being a Team Player* and the Agency for Healthcare Research and Quality's *TeamSTEPPS*.[3,4]

The Culture of Safety in EMS

One of the key goals of EMS Agenda 2050 is EMS systems that are designed to be inherently safe to minimize patient, EMS clinician, and public exposure to injury, infections, illness, or stress during patient response and care delivery. As part of this effort, decisions should be made with the safety of all as a priority. In other words, EMS should have a culture of safety.[5] A culture of safety within an EMS system is linked to a decreased number of errors and near misses.[6] Several common elements lead to both positive and negative safety cultures (**TABLE 9-1**). Underpinning such a culture are elements such as data collection, just culture, coordinated support and resources, EMS education initiatives, EMS safety standards, and reporting and investigation of errors and near misses.

Just Culture

Just culture is an approach to leadership in organizations that balances fairness and accountability and encourages people to report errors and

TABLE 9-1 Positive and Negative Attributes Contributing to a Culture of Safety

Positive	Negative
Trust	Lack of communication
Teamwork	Taking shortcuts
Communication	Punishment
Sensitivity	Poor teamwork
Mutual support	Freelancing

near misses. It focuses on risk management—that is, proactively identifying problems in the system that could lead to error or opportunities to improve safety. In a just culture, both the EMS system and individual clinicians are held accountable for overall safety.

In a just culture, behaviors associated with error or risk are categorized as human error, at-risk behavior, or reckless behavior. The EMS system considers human error to be a function of three factors: (1) a person intended to do the right thing but somehow committed an error, such as choosing the wrong treatment; (2) a person performed a skill incorrectly; or (3) a person meant to do something but did not follow through. In a just culture, the reasons for the error are investigated and the individual who committed the error is counseled or educated. At-risk behavior is conceptually different than this description of human error. At-risk behavior is when an EMT actively makes a choice to take a risk, believing that the potential adverse outcome is insignificant or that it was justified in the moment (the potential benefit outweighed the risk). An example of at-risk behavior would be failing to complete the beginning-of-shift checklist for the ambulance equipment and discovering there was no blood glucose monitor. This situation typically requires coaching and increased awareness. Reckless behavior involves a conscious disregard for a significant and unjustified risk, and it usually results in disciplinary action. An example of reckless behavior would an administering an intravenous medication, even though doing so is not within the EMT's scope of practice.[7,8]

Words of Wisdom

When procedures that are established to promote safety are routinely ignored, noncompliance with the procedure becomes the norm in the EMS system. This process, known as normalization of deviance, increases risk to both patients and those working within the system.[9–11] Examples include routine failure to wear appropriate eye protection when performing airway procedures that risk splash or spray of body fluids and failure to follow checklists during procedures.

Interdisciplinary Collaboration

As an EMT, you will need to do more than just acquire clinical knowledge and master necessary skills. You must also learn to be an effective team member. Essentially, this means communicating and collaborating with others from other public safety or health care entities who may have different backgrounds and levels of expertise than you have. By working as a team, emergency health care clinicians, from the first responders in the field to the physicians in the hospital, can improve patient and clinician safety and deliver quality patient care. For public safety, hospital, basic life support (BLS), and advanced life support (ALS) clinicians to perform well together, each team member must share a common goal and demonstrate excellent communication skills.

An Era of Team Health Care

Currently, it is understood that for the delivery of EMS to be effective, health care clinicians must work together toward a unified goal of quality patient care. Historically, however, this was not always the case. Previous models of emergency care often consisted of clinicians who worked independently, passing the patient from one individual or group to the next. Gradually, emergency health care clinicians recognized that by working as a unified team from first patient contact to patient discharge, it was possible to improve individual and team performance, patient and clinician safety, and, ultimately, patient outcomes. This concept is known as the **continuum of care**.

To illustrate the continuum of care, suppose you and your partner transport a multisystem trauma patient to the hospital. You must accurately deliver a handoff report to the hospital clinicians and work with that team to safely transition the patient's care. The team meeting you at the hospital for a critically ill trauma patient often includes an emergency room nurse and physician, surgeon, radiology technician, phlebotomist, registration clerk, and perhaps a multitude of students from each of these specialties. The team will use what you share to continue care for the patient and may ask for additional scene clues or photos to predict the patient's injuries. Similarly, as a member of the continuum of care, you may receive updates on the patient's condition and the ultimate outcome of the patient.

Community Paramedicine and Mobile Integrated Healthcare Teams

Community paramedicine and **mobile integrated healthcare (MIH)** teams may be the best examples of the team concept of continuum of care. Recall that in the MIH model, health care is provided within the community rather than at a physician's office or hospital. The success of MIH programs has shown that EMS clinicians, working as a unified team with in-hospital and other community health care clinicians, can improve patient outcomes, increase patient satisfaction, and reduce health care costs. See Chapter 1, *EMS Systems and Public Health*, for more detail about the MIH model.

Differences Among Teams

The structure and effectiveness of emergency health care teams differ from system to system. EMS clinicians may be trained as emergency medical responders (EMRs) or may be BLS- or ALS-certified. They may be volunteers, part-time employees, or full-time employees, and they may be based in police or fire departments, hospitals, or private agency settings. Multiple EMS agencies across different regions or response districts may respond to the same 9-1-1 call. Because of the variety of clinicians, agencies, and systems involved in each call, it may be difficult for all first responders to function as one unified team. For instance, you may find it challenging to share patient assessment information and integrate newly arriving public safety personnel into ongoing care. Such challenges can be overcome by ensuring effective communication and mutual respect. In this case, as new clinicians arrive, it is helpful to think of them as "joining the team" as opposed to "taking over."

Types of Teams

Depending on the EMS system in which you work, you may consistently interact with the same team members. Other systems, especially those that rely on a large volunteer workforce, may require emergency health care clinicians to assemble their teams "on the fly" for each individual call.

Regular Teams

Some EMS systems rely on regular teams. In this model, EMTs consistently interact with the same partner or team and often develop a rapport with the other emergency responders and hospital staff with whom they frequently interact. Regular teams often train together. Team members who frequently train and work together are more likely to move smoothly from one step in the procedure to the next, performing as one seamless unit. By contrast, team members who train and work together less often may need more explicit verbal direction to accomplish their tasks, which can potentially lead to conflict or patient care delays.

Temporary Teams

In this model, EMTs work with clinicians with whom they do not regularly interact or may not even know. This situation, which may occur at a large event or disaster involving clinicians from other agencies or states, creates a special challenge. For a temporary team to function effectively, clinicians must work within an environment that supports and promotes collaboration rather than competition. It is crucial to have a clear understanding of the roles, responsibilities, and capabilities of each team member. One of the best ways to accomplish this is to train together when possible.

Special Teams

Some EMS systems form special teams whose members have particular knowledge, skills, abilities, equipment, and/or training to serve a specialized role within the larger emergency health care team. Examples include the following:

- Fire Team
- Rescue Team
- Critical Care Team
- Hazardous Materials (Hazmat) Team
- Tactical EMS Team
- Special Event EMS Team
- EMS Bike Team
- In-Hospital Patient Care Technicians
- Mobile Integrated Healthcare (MIH) Technicians

Principles of Effective Team Performance

Do not assume that any gathering of EMS clinicians responding to a call is a team. True emergency response teams have better interaction, performance, and patient outcomes than groups of health care clinicians who do not share a team dynamic.

In 1945, the Research Center for Group Dynamics first defined the five essential elements of a group that people must share[12]:

1. A common goal
2. An image of themselves as "a group"
3. A sense of continuity of the group (an understanding that the group may work together more than once, even in a slightly different configuration)
4. A set of shared values (how the group wants to get things done)
5. Different roles within the group (often self-assigned)

While these elements will allow clinicians to function as a group, they should be considered only a starting point toward building a high-performing emergency response team. The following discussion explains the principles that underlie optimal team performance.

A Shared Goal

Every health care clinician on the team, from EMT to paramedic to emergency physician, must be committed to a common goal: typically, the best possible patient outcome. Although this may seem like common sense, evidence of clinicians not working as a team can be heard in such alarming phrases as "Why take the time to splint the patient if they're only going to undo it in the ED?" and "The patient doesn't need aspirin right now. We're close to the hospital. They can do it there."

Clear Roles and Responsibilities

To achieve a common goal, each first responder must know what needs to be done and what is expected of them. An excellent example of this is the pit crew approach to CPR for cardiac arrest situations (**FIGURE 9-2**). The term originated in motor racing, in which teams of technicians rapidly assess and repair vehicles in a matter of seconds. Similarly, pit crew CPR consists of defining each intervention that needs to be addressed during cardiac arrest (compressions, defibrillation, airway management, vascular access, medications) and training clinicians *before* the call to rapidly identify, prioritize, and take over any areas that are not being addressed as soon as they arrive on scene. The effectiveness of pit crew CPR depends on defining clear roles and responsibilities among team members. Tasks are divided among team members based on their training and experience so that each person has a clearly defined job. It is an outstanding example of how training together can allow clinicians with different certifications from various agencies to rapidly come together as a team to improve outcomes for critically ill patients. It is important to note that not all EMS agencies use the pit crew approach and that the configuration will change based on the number of available first responders.

Diverse and Competent Skill Sets

As discussed, EMS clinicians often have varying levels of certification or licensure. Think of these diverse backgrounds and skill sets not as obstacles, but as opportunities to fill roles and responsibilities within a high-performing team. Again, the best way for a team to be effective during an emergency call

YOU are the EMT

At 0905 hours, you are dispatched to a private home at 6 Catoonah Street for a 72-year-old man who is unresponsive. The dispatcher has no additional information to provide. An EMR crew from the fire department has been dispatched and will likely arrive before you. The weather is clear and sunny, the temperature is 82°F (27.8°C), and the traffic is light. Your response time to the scene is approximately 6 minutes.

1. How will you work together as a team with the EMRs?
2. How will members of this team decide who will perform each role?

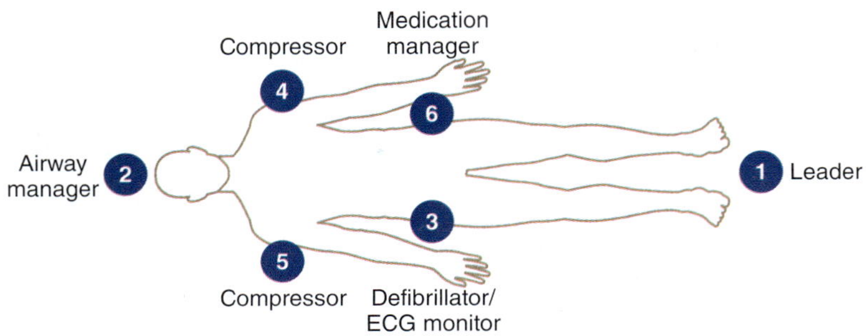

FIGURE 9-2 Example of a six-person pit crew that includes both BLS clinicians and ALS clinicians. Although this example does not explicitly describe the pit crew model presented in the text, the same concepts can be applied to a BLS-only arrest. BLS clinicians may be in charge of running the arrest or may otherwise participate in the arrest. Teamwork-oriented resuscitation can improve patient outcomes by minimizing the chance for error and improving team speed and efficiency.

Abbreviation: ECG, electrocardiograph

is to practice with one another and become familiar with each other's tools, techniques, capabilities, and preferences, so that each team member is competent *before* the call comes in.

Effective Collaboration and Communication

For team members to collaborate successfully, you must communicate effectively with one another. Four important elements of team communication include the following:

- **A clear message.** Speak calmly, confidently, and concisely so that the information delivered or the action requested is clear to your listeners. Be clear who you are speaking to by using names or ranks when giving direction, as opposed to just asking "someone" to do a task.

YOU are the EMT

When you arrive on scene, a frantic bystander waves you inside. She tells you, "It's my husband! He isn't breathing!" As you walk to the front door, the fire officer meets you and tells you that two EMRs are already inside caring for the patient. The scene is safe. As you enter the residence you find the patient, an older man, lying in a supine position on the floor of the living room. He is being ventilated with a bag-mask device by one EMR as another EMR performs a reassessment. As you approach the patient with your equipment bag, airway kit, and automated external defibrillator (AED), the EMR performing the reassessment looks up and tells you, "We've lost a pulse." The EMR immediately starts chest compressions while you prepare the AED.

Recording Time: 2 Minutes	
Appearance	Motionless
Level of consciousness	Unconscious and unresponsive
Airway	Open; maintained by fire department EMRs
Breathing	Absent; bag-mask ventilations at a rate of 1 breath every 5 seconds
Circulation	No pulse; skin cool and pale (compared to baseline color); CPR has been started

3. Which roles will need to be assigned to perform cardiac arrest resuscitation?
4. The AED analyzes the patient's heart rhythm and advises you whether to deliver a shock. How can your team maximize patient perfusion and minimize "hands-off" time during this part of the cardiac arrest?

- **Closed-loop communication.** When a team member speaks, you should repeat the message back to them. This technique helps confirm that you heard and understand the message, and will act on it.
- **Courtesy.** All team members expect and deserve to be spoken to politely. "Please" and "thank you" do not take that much time.
- **Constructive intervention.** Sometimes it is necessary for you to respectfully question or correct team members (or the team leader) if you believe a mistake has been or is about to be made. Doing so is not only allowed and encouraged, it is essential for effective team performance and is a fundamental part of **crew resource management (CRM)**, a concept discussed later in this chapter.

Street Smarts

Make an effort to learn the names of public safety or other health care clinicians with whom you routinely interact on calls. Addressing a person by name can immediately break down barriers during stressful interactions.

Supportive and Coordinated Leadership

The **team leader** is the team member who provides role assignments, coordination, oversight, centralized decision making, and support for the team to accomplish their goals and achieve desired results. Team leaders are often defined by policy, procedure, or statute. They may be the most senior clinician in the group or the person with the highest level of certification. Team leaders who simply command others are not leading a team; they are simply directing a group in which each individual is told what to do, and often, how to do it, leaving the group members to rely on the leader for task assignment, troubleshooting, and almost all decisions. This type of leadership limits the group's ability to adapt and deliver critical medical care in an uncontrolled field environment.

The team leader must decide the following[13]:

- Which actions are needed to ensure the team goals are achieved
- Which team needs must be addressed to accomplish team goals
- Which skills are needed to collaborate and effectively perform those actions

An effective team leader helps the individual team members to do their jobs not only by providing support, but also by working together with them and sharing knowledge to facilitate coordination. In this way, a team leader helps the team produce a better outcome. Team leaders also foster communication and team dynamics using concepts such as CRM and team **situational awareness** (the knowledge and understanding of one's surroundings and the ability to recognize potential threats to safety).

Words of Wisdom

On most EMS calls, the team leader, with help from the other team members, is responsible for assessing and treating the patient. This responsibility involves the following tasks[14]:

1. Formulating a field impression
2. Directing treatment
3. Determining how sick the patient is (acuity)
4. Selecting the appropriate patient disposition (ie, treat on scene or transport destination)
5. Delegating responsibility
6. Helping to move the patient in the safest, most appropriate manner

Effective Team Membership

A team leader cannot manage an emergency call alone. Skilled team members are needed to ensure that critical calls are managed safely and effectively. Good team members communicate effectively; accept feedback; are good followers; have confidence, compassion, and maturity; maintain situational awareness; and use appreciative, or positive, inquiry to approach organization change. They use closed-loop communication, perform tasks accurately and in a timely manner, and then report progress on those tasks to the team leader. Good team members treat their fellow team members with respect, regardless of their rank or experience. It is a team member's responsibility to speak up immediately and suggest a corrective action if a harmful action is ordered or performed by others or if a procedure is not being performed but is indicated. Each person on the team is accountable for the safety and well-being of the patient and other crew members.

Street Smarts

An essential component of teamwork is trust. Team members must be able to trust each other to do their best, do what is correct, and watch out for each other. Trust must be earned. As a team member, you must continually be diligent to maintain a good attitude, skill proficiency, and current knowledge.

Crew Resource Management

CRM is a way for team members to work together with the team leader to develop and maintain a shared understanding of the emergency situation. CRM arose in the aviation industry in the 1980s due to a rise in the number of plane crashes.[15] Several examples of aviation mishaps, including collisions and jets running out of fuel, prompted the adoption of this passenger-centered approach where everyone's job, regardless of hierarchy, is to get the passengers to their destination safely.

Just like in aviation, CRM allows first responders with different skill sets to collaborate and communicate, fulfill their roles and responsibilities, and achieve the shared goal of the best possible patient outcome (**FIGURE 9-3**). Using CRM strategies can help resolve conflict, improve team communication, allow for productive feedback, help manage workload, and lead to improved clinical decision making. The concept of CRM says that each member is responsible for maintaining awareness of the current patient situation and sharing any critical information with the team leader. Likewise, the team leader is responsible for listening to any critical information provided by you or other team members, and incorporating it during decision making.

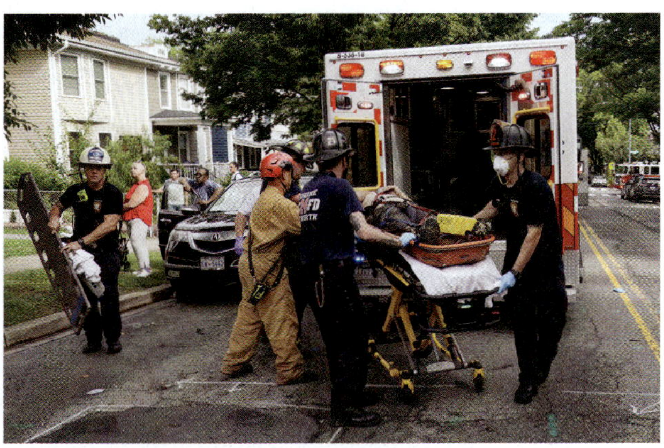

FIGURE 9-3 Collaboration and communication are crucial aspects of crew resource management.

In the noisy and often distracting environment in which EMS clinicians work, it is easy for errors to occur. Misunderstandings and misinterpretations may occur due to situational awareness failures. These failures are more likely when one or more emergency responders do not accurately perceive what is happening, such as when there is a lack of information. For example, on some calls, clinicians may not know crucial details of the patient's medical history, data may be hard to detect or interpret (eg, trying to hear lung sounds when it is noisy), or clinicians may fail to monitor data, such as forgetting to put on the pulse oximeter to measure the oxygen level.

Errors and miscommunication can occur when an EMT sends or receives a message. To reduce the incidence of errors on either end of the communication chain, clinicians should use closed-loop communication. In this system, each member confirms that a message has been received correctly so both parties know they share the same understanding. Here is an example of closed-loop communication: An EMT says, "Let's go with 2 liters of oxygen." Their partner replies, "Got it. I'll put the patient on 10 liters of oxygen." The EMT recognizes immediately that their partner did not receive the intended message and responds, "No, not 10 liters. We need to go with 2 liters." Their partner then replies, "Got it. I'll put the patient on 2 liters of oxygen."

There are times when even the most seasoned EMS crew members lose situational awareness or make an error. It is essential to speak up when there is an error of omission (something not being done) or commission (something being done incorrectly or inappropriately). When you believe there is an immediate or potential problem that must be brought to the attention of the team leader, first, get the attention of the crew member, preferably by

Words of Wisdom

The concept of CRM is often described as using communication, teamwork, and redundancy to reduce risk. If you think of Swiss cheese, the holes are opportunities for a failure to occur. Failures may be latent, in which case there is a preexisting flaw in the system design or processes that makes it easier for an error to occur, or active, in which case a person or team performs in an unsafe manner (**FIGURE 9-4**). CRM employs tactics to block those holes and prevent a bad outcome. For example, if something is not stocked properly on your ambulance and you arrive to a call without it, the patient may potentially not receive appropriate care. However, using a checklist ensures the ambulance is fully stocked, thus preventing a potential bad outcome.

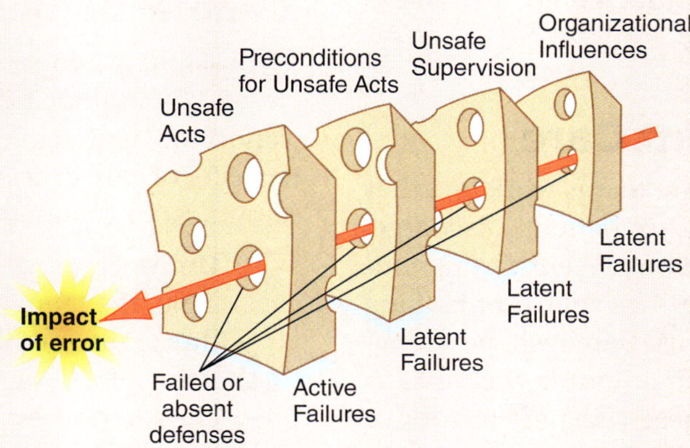

FIGURE 9-4 The Swiss cheese model of error.

Reproduced from Reason J. Human error: models and management. *BMJ*. March 18, 2000;320:768–770 with permission from BMJ Publishing Group Ltd.

addressing them by name or rank, and then use the PACE mnemonic:

- **P Probe.** Look or ask to confirm the problem or make sense of the situation. For example, your team leader has suggested that you both lift a patient from the floor. The patient is stable and has morbid obesity. You say, "Lieutenant, you indicated that you and I should lift this patient from the floor?" If the team leader confirms that you have understood the instruction, proceed to the next step.
- **A Alert.** Communicate the problem to the team leader: "Lieutenant, do you think it's safe for us to lift this patient by ourselves?"
- **C Challenge.** If the issue is not corrected, then clearly challenge the team's current course of action that is leading to the problem and suggest an alternative plan: "Lieutenant, I think we could injure our backs if we lift this patient alone. Should we wait for help to arrive?"
- **E Emergency.** If the problem is clear and critical (such as an immediate safety issue), then immediately communicate the emergency to the entire team. This is used when there is an imminent and serious danger: "Lieutenant, I am unable to help you lift this patient without additional help. I will call for assistance now."

If the other team member agrees that the original plan should be altered, it is essential for the leader to communicate the change to everyone else on the team.

The CRM concept does not mean you are free to ignore the chain of command within your department or the incident command system or National Incident Management System structure. It means you are empowered to provide the team leader and other team members with immediate feedback in the event of a potential threat to patient or crew safety. It means the team, as a whole, recognizes the importance of every individual's input and that the team is committed to creating open lines of

Words of Wisdom

It is important to avoid side conversations and commentary when caring for a patient. Nonessential conversation can be distracting, creates unnecessary noise, causes lapses in situational awareness, and can lead to errors in patient care.

communication. CRM empowers people to speak clearly and concisely when they detect a problem or potential problem.

Transfer of Patient Care

Although effective health care teams work together from first patient contact to patient discharge, clearly not all clinicians will be present throughout the entire continuum of care. At several points along the continuum, the patient's care will be transferred, or "handed off," from one unit of clinicians on the team to another. These transfers introduce the possibility of critical patient care errors, especially when they occur several times and in different settings. Effective teams minimize the number of transfers during patient care, and adhere to strict and careful guidelines when they are needed.

Just like in a relay race, a proper transfer of patient care will allow the team to keep moving forward with patient care. When incorrect information is handed off, information is omitted, or care is interrupted, errors or delays in patient care can result. For this reason, it is important for you to trust other team members, even those who work at different levels or for various agencies. For example, if an EMR reports a patient had a syncopal episode, but the patient is now alert, then do not assume the EMR's information is incorrect.

General Guidelines

If possible, a single person (ie, the team leader) should coordinate the patient's transfer of care and report the patient information. Whenever the verbal transfer of care occurs, all team members should do their best to ensure the following:

- **Uninterrupted critical care.** Whenever possible, the team member giving the report and the team member taking the report should hand off lifesaving care (such as performing chest compressions) to another team member, allowing them to focus on the transfer of care.
- **Minimal interference.** The transfer of patient care should occur in a location with the least interference possible. If the transfer takes place at the patient's side, it should not occur while the patient is being moved.

YOU are the EMT

After the AED reanalyzes and advises a shock, you clear the patient and deliver the defibrillation, quickly directing the two EMRs to rotate compressors and continue CPR. As the EMRs continue compressions and bag-mask ventilations, the paramedics arrive.

Recording Time: 12 Minutes	
Respirations	Absent; ventilations are being assisted
Pulse	Absent; fire department EMR performing CPR
Skin	Cool and cyanotic
Blood pressure	Pulses are felt during compressions
Oxygen saturation (Spo_2)	85%

While your partner gathers a medical history from the patient's wife and the fire officer collects the patient's medications, one of the paramedics asks you to assist setting up to intubate the patient.

5. When should you give the patient's medical history and medication list to the paramedic?
6. How should you respond if you notice that the EMR doing CPR is compressing at an inappropriate rate?

- **Respectful interaction.** Each team member involved in the transfer must be respectful of members' different roles and recognize the importance of each role. Verbal and nonverbal communication should convey respect and attention between clinicians.
- **Common priorities.** Both the team member giving the report and the team member taking the report must focus on their common priorities (critical assessment findings and patient care) vital for the best possible patient outcome.
- **Common language or system.** Whenever possible, a mutually agreed-on and standardized patient handoff format should be used.

See Chapter 4, *Communications and Documentation*, for information on verbal and written patient care reports.

Words of Wisdom

Whether it be from a bystander, an EMR, or a fellow EMT, when taking a patient handoff report, the receiving care clinician should do the following:

- **Maintain eye contact.** Make eye contact with the individual giving a report. This helps both clinicians to stop other noncritical work and focus on the transfer of information and patient care.
- **Consider the environment.** The very nature of EMS means clinicians do not have the level of control over the environment that they would like. However, when taking a report, you should make every effort to create or move to an environment that is quieter and less distracting.
- **Ensure understanding.** Ask any questions to ensure you understand what was reported.
- **Sum up.** Quickly summarize the critical components of the handoff to allow the reporting team member to correct any misunderstandings and to reinforce the information to the new team members taking over patient care.
- **Supplement.** Obtain any relevant paperwork or other materials that will be helpful for communicating information to the next set of health care clinicians.

BLS and ALS Clinicians Working Together

In the world of prehospital emergency care, BLS and ALS care cannot exist independently of each other. EMS system staffing varies widely. In some EMS systems, the ambulance is staffed by only paramedics; in other cases, only by EMTs, or by a combination of licensure levels. In situations where there are two EMTs staffing the ambulance, one will assume team leadership and the other team membership on each call.

ALS Assist

When an EMT is treating a patient and ALS clinicians are on scene, a critical part of the EMT's team member role will be **ALS assist**. When providing an ALS assist, the EMT, while remaining within the EMT scope of practice, supports the ALS clinician in performing advanced-level skills and procedures. When AEMT or paramedic skills are indicated, the EMT should anticipate what equipment or non-ALS patient preparation is needed to be ready to intervene.

As an EMT, there are many different ALS skills with which you may be able to assist. The exact list of ALS procedures and how they are performed varies from system to system. In general, assisting follows a four-step process: (1) preparing the patient, (2) setting up equipment, (3) assisting the ALS clinician who is performing the procedure, and (4) continuing care. For example, electrocardiogram (ECG) interpretation is within the scope of practice of the paramedic, but not the EMT.[16] However, the EMT can place the ECG electrodes on the patient, turn on the monitor, and transmit the data to the ED, allowing the paramedic to focus on other aspects of the patient's care. Specific steps to assist with advanced airway skills and vascular access are discussed in subsequent chapters.

The ALS assist role does not diminish the EMT's role in other important functions. For example, if a patient experiences sudden cardiac arrest, then BLS care (high-quality CPR and defibrillation) are the core interventions around which ALS clinicians build their resuscitative efforts. It would be a mistake to think of BLS care as only the first steps of ALS care. As an EMT, you may begin BLS efforts early, but keep in mind that BLS efforts must continue throughout the continuum of care. To successfully stabilize and treat the patient's condition, you must carefully coordinate your efforts with the advanced tools and techniques used by ALS clinicians and assist them to perform their ALS skills. Remember, excellent communication skills and teamwork are essential elements of emergency medicine. Each member of the EMS team must work in harmony with one goal in mind: high-quality patient care.

As mentioned previously, all team members, regardless of their level of licensure, are responsible for the safety of the patient, crew, and bystanders on an EMS call. The skilled EMT may recognize a dangerous situation or possible error that others on scene have not noticed, even higher-level clinicians. It is essential for the EMT to speak up in such instances. In an effective EMS system, all members have the confidence to voice concerns, and all members have the professionalism to listen.

Where BLS Care Ends and ALS Care Begins

Many patient care skills can be considered advanced; however, the tools and techniques that you can use as an EMT versus those that are reserved for ALS clinicians vary from system to system. What may be a paramedic-only skill in your EMS system may be common for an AEMT or EMT to perform in another.

It is your responsibility to understand what is allowed by the scope of practice, standard of care, and local protocols where you work. If you work outside these bounds, such as performing a skill for which you are not authorized, then you risk legal liability. This liability is not reduced because you were unaware you were "not supposed to do that." Scope of practice, standard of care, and local protocols are discussed in greater detail in Chapter 3, *Medical, Legal, and Ethical Issues*.

For an EMS team to effectively perform an advanced skill, its members should train and practice together. Although good EMTs know what they are allowed to do in assisting with an advanced procedure, great EMTs have the foundational knowledge to understand the procedure. Most important, EMTs must understand that when using any advanced tool or technique, the focus is always on achieving a goal (solving a clinical problem) rather than simply completing a procedure.

Critical Thinking and Clinical Decision Making in EMS

EMTs in some systems work with an EMT partner and are the primary decision makers on the ambulance. When a life threat occurs, the EMT must make critical decisions (often many) that can affect the patient's outcome. Effective decisions are based on sound, up-to-date knowledge and the information provided from the patient, the patient's history, and physical examination. EMTs must use a series of steps to ensure the proper course of action is chosen. These steps occur in continuous cycles throughout each phase of the call.

The strategies the team leader uses to make decisions depend on the nature of the situation (**FIGURE 9-5**). The team leader must do the following[17]:

1. **Gather data (cues).** This begins with the dispatch information and continues when the EMT gathers the patient history and completes the physical examination. A thorough assessment is at the heart of good clinical decision making. (Chapter 10, *Patient Assessment*, describes this process in detail.)
2. **Interpret the data.** The team leader must decide what the cues mean. Is there a clear pattern? Is more information needed?
3. **Decide what the problem is (ie, form a hypothesis, or field impression).** Based on the cues and their interpretation, the team leader defines the problem that must be addressed.
4. **Develop a plan.** The EMT determines what treatment is needed to solve the patient's immediate problems based on the information at hand.
5. **Communicate the plan to the team, and take the appropriate actions to implement it.** During this time, the team leader reflects on whether it is the right choice and invites feedback from the team.
6. **Evaluate the effect of the decision.** During this phase, the patient and situation are reassessed. Based on this reevaluation, the team either continues with the plan or adjusts it. For example, an EMT crew treating a patient with chest discomfort, possibly experiencing a heart attack, may make an initial determination to not administer oxygen because the patient is not short of breath. Reassessment reveals the patient is now experiencing mild shortness of breath. The EMT crew should change the initial treatment plan and administer oxygen.

Assessments at each phase of the call must take into account specific cues from the patient (eg, age, sex/gender) and environmental cues (eg, weather,

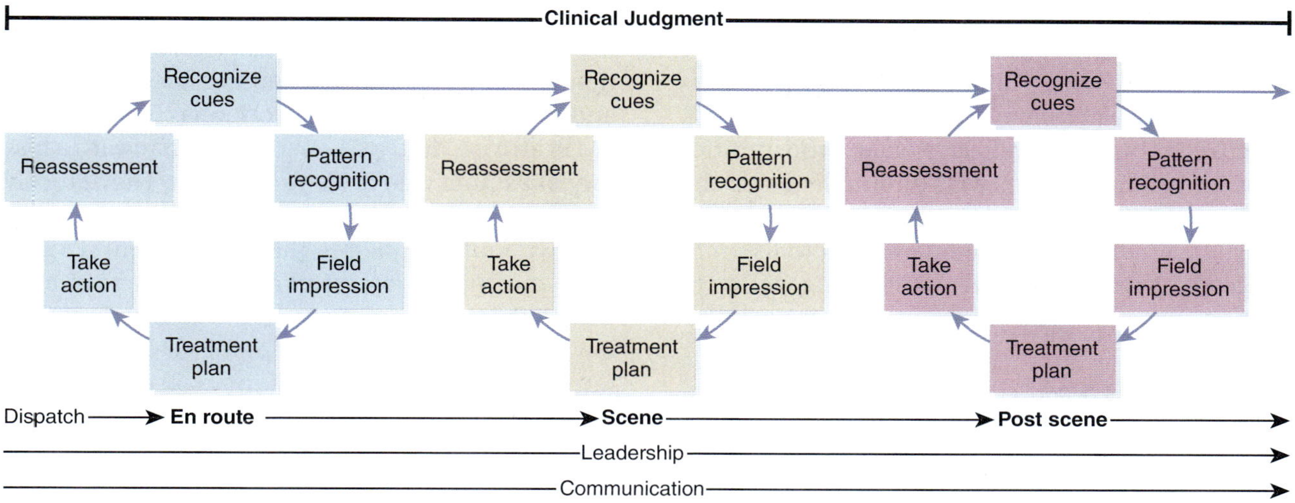

FIGURE 9-5 The EMT must gather cues, form a field impression and action plan, communicate clearly with other team members, and evaluate the effect of actions taken.

hazards). The success of the call also depends on the EMT's abilities and knowledge regarding the problem at hand and factors such as fatigue or stress.

Throughout the call, the leadership and communication skills previously described are critical to the mission's success.

Stages of the Decision-Making Process

Prearrival

The decision-making process on many calls begins when the initial dispatch information is received. Knowing the nature of the emergency, especially when the call is low frequency and high risk, can help the EMT prepare, even before arriving on the scene. En route to the call, the EMT should mentally rehearse the steps in the care that may be needed. A leader should be clearly designated. Crew members can discuss their roles, what additional help may be needed, what equipment should be taken in, and what transport destination should be considered. For example, if the call is for a pediatric cardiac arrest, consider the ratio of compressions to ventilations needed and the size of equipment, such as the bag-mask device that will be used.

Arrival

Provide the scene size-up and request additional resources as soon as possible. Position equipment in a standard location when possible so other responders can anticipate where to find supplies when needed. Assess and intervene for life threats immediately. This initial size-up and patient assessment often cause adjustments to the plan. These adjustments will need to be determined by the team leader in collaboration with their team.

The EMT must first consider and treat life threats. When given information about the patient, EMTs should first rule out the worst-case scenario. The acronym ROWS (*R*ule *O*ut *W*orst-case *S*cenario) is sometimes used to remember this step.[18]

During the Call

Although the overall goals of the scene are to find and treat life threats and transport the patient to the appropriate facility, often many other small, short-term goals have to be achieved to accomplish these overall goals.

After the Call

After a stressful or complicated call, it is important to debrief and talk about what happened. If the team consists of an EMT and partner, that discussion can be informal and happen during the cleanup after the call. Sometimes this is called a back-step debrief. For complex calls, a department may assemble the entire team to talk about the call. Formal debriefings may include the medical director, supervisory staff, and personnel from other departments. These should be structured to help everyone gain an understanding of what happened on the call (not everyone has the same perspective), what went well, and what opportunities exist for improvement. EMTs should listen to the feedback with an open mind. Moving from novice to expert practice means being willing to listen to suggestions for improvement and being willing to change.

Decision Traps

Because EMTs are human, they are subject to mental blocks that can lead to errors in decision making. Although decision traps may come in many forms, they typically fall into two categories: those that cause the EMT to either overestimate or underestimate the probability of disease or injury and those that result in failure to consider all reasonable possibilities.

Common Decision Traps in EMS

Traps that frequently lead to decision-making errors in EMS are bias, anchoring, and overconfidence.[18]

Everyone has biases. **Biases** are fixed beliefs about something. Once established, they are hard to rethink. It can be harmful when an EMT remains locked into the bias and considers only one possible idea, ignoring or not seeking other data. For example, suppose a patient has fallen and has an altered level of consciousness. This patient is known to have alcohol use disorder and has an odor resembling alcohol on their breath. The EMT assumes the patient is intoxicated and that their slurred speech is related to their alcohol ingestion; as a result, while gathering their history, the EMT asks only questions that follow that path. As a result, the EMT fails to ask detailed questions about the nature of the fall or the patient's medical history or other signs and symptoms and misses the fact that the patient has sustained a head injury.

Street Smarts

Many biases are unconscious, meaning the individual does not even realize they have them. These biases contribute to well-documented inequities in patient care.

Another type of error, **anchoring**, occurs when the EMT settles on one possible cause of the patient's problems early (sometimes before the call) and fails to consider other options. For example, EMTs arrive to find a 24-year-old woman with a history of asthma who is short of breath. They quickly administer a breathing treatment and begin transport without completing their assessment. Due to their incomplete assessment, they fail to realize that, although the patient does have asthma, today she is having a life-threatening allergic reaction (anaphylaxis), and her condition worsens en route to the hospital.

Overconfidence is another decision trap that some EMTs fall into. It occurs when the EMT overestimates their ability. In this case, ability may apply to skills such as emergency driving, assessment, splinting, or decision making. Overconfidence may cause the EMT to choose the wrong treatment path or to ignore others when they disagree with a decision, resulting in actions that harm either the patient, the crew, or the public.

Avoiding Decision Traps

The first step toward avoiding errors related to bias is developing a solid knowledge base and an organized approach to patient care that is consistent and thorough. EMTs must also recognize their blind spots: areas where they know biases exist, such as those related to intoxicated patients, patients with obesity, or older adults. Knowing those biases exist should set off an alarm on those calls, signaling the need to take extra care not to fall into a decision trap.

Troubleshooting Team Conflicts

As outlined in this chapter, applying the principles of effective emergency health care teams will help to minimize interpersonal conflicts. However, because most emergency health care teams consist of highly trained, enthusiastic, and dedicated people, it is inevitable that conflict will arise from time to time. When conflict occurs, keep in mind the following five principles:

- **The patient comes first.** Regardless of interpersonal conflicts that may arise, the patient's needs must always come first.
- **Do not engage.** If the problem causing the conflict does not directly and immediately

affect patient care, then do not engage. Have the discussion after the call, when more positive communication may be possible.

- **Keep your cool.** Maintain your composure. If you feel that the conflict is over a critical component of patient care, then follow the PACE mnemonic discussed previously. If it is not, then begin by taking a deep breath and slowly counting to 10.
- **Separate the person from the issue.** If the conflict arises from the behavior of another team member and the conflict cannot be delayed or avoided, then focus on the behavior itself rather than the individual.
- **Choose your battles.** Remember, there is strength in the diversity of team members. Not everyone will work in exactly the same way, and that is a good thing. Avoid engaging in conflict over minor issues in patient care that center around one clinician's "style" over another.

The Team Approach to Behavioral and Mental Health Calls

Behavioral health calls, by their unpredictable and emotionally charged nature, can be very complex and stressful for both the patient and the first responders. Difficulties in finding appropriate in- or outpatient care for these patients and the potential for the patient's negative behaviors to escalate if law enforcement or other first responders arrive on the scene can further complicate the successful care and disposition of these patients.

Increasingly, communities are implementing a team approach so that appropriate, safe, and timely care is provided to a behavioral health patient in crisis. The successful team may include EMS, police who have taken crisis intervention training classes, and mental health or social service professionals. Preplanning and rehearsal with this team is ideal to clearly delineate responsibilities of each role, maintain safety for all involved, and avoid conflict during patient care.[19]

Police can provide the initial assessment of scene safety; mental health and social service workers, who in some cases respond with law enforcement, may identify an appropriate disposition or resources for the patient; or EMS may facilitate a telemedicine visit with mental health professionals from the scene of the emergency after assessing the patient. For a successful outcome, team members must use the teamwork approaches described in this chapter to maintain situational awareness, communicate using the principles of CRM, and focus on the goal of a good patient outcome.[20]

YOU are the EMT

The patient is intubated and has an intravenous (IV) line established. Before any medications are administered, the patient regains a pulse, even though he remains unconscious. You transport the patient to the local hospital, which is only a few minutes away. The paramedic gives a radio report while en route.

Recording Time: 24 Minutes	
Level of consciousness	Unconscious and unresponsive
Respirations	6 breaths/min (baseline); ventilations are being assisted
Pulse	104 beats/min
Skin	Pale and cyanotic compared with baseline
Blood pressure	104/80 mm Hg
Oxygen saturation (Spo_2)	92% (with assisted ventilation)

On arrival, you bring the patient into the resuscitation room, where the ED team members await.

7. In the ED, if the paramedic is giving the handoff report, then who will ensure that patient care is continued during the transfer of care?
8. During the transfer of patient care, at what point is the EMS unit of the team relieved of responsibility for caring for the patient?

YOU are the EMT SUMMARY

1. How will you work together as a team with the EMRs?

Because the EMRs will arrive at the scene before you, they will have begun patient care. When you arrive, begin by making contact with the EMR in charge while your partner assists the other EMRs. Gather information about the patient's current condition as well as the care that has already been provided, so you understand the patient care priorities as well as which roles need to be filled and what tasks need to be completed. This information-gathering step will allow you to seamlessly integrate into the patient care team for the call already in progress.

2. How will members of this team decide who will perform each role?

Throughout the emergency call, clinician roles and responsibilities will change as patient needs and available resources change. In some cases, certain roles will need to be filled by clinicians with specific levels of expertise or advanced certifications. In other cases, local protocol will require the highest-certified or most senior clinician to be the team leader. It will not always be necessary (and may even set the team back) for an arriving responder to take over simply because they have a higher certification. For example, if you arrive on this scene to find the patient in respiratory arrest with an EMR already providing ventilations, then it may not be helpful to have the EMR stop and hand over the procedure. The most helpful way, assuming there are no higher patient priorities at that time, would be for you to step into another necessary but unfilled role or to verify that the ventilations by the EMR are adequately done and then focus on other procedures that need to be accomplished. In this case, you can check that compressions are being done correctly while you are applying the AED.

3. Which roles will need to be assigned to perform cardiac arrest resuscitation?

Depending on local protocol, the next role is to manage the patient's airway and breathing. If the person filling this role is a BLS clinician, then they will utilize a bag-mask device, oxygen, and airway adjuncts as allowed by local protocol. If an ALS clinician arrives, then they may assume this role from a BLS clinician. In this scenario, this role has already been filled by the second EMR, but a paramedic may intubate or utilize another advanced airway. That paramedic may take over ventilations, but in most cases will have an EMT or EMR resume ventilation through the endotracheal tube or advanced airway. If advanced clinicians are available, the next function in a cardiac arrest would be to gain vascular access and administer medication. In this situation, one of the paramedics would fulfill this role.

If enough clinicians are available, then a fifth role is that of team leader, who directs the care given. The team leader's tasks include gathering patient history and assessment information from the family, bystanders, or the first responders, formulating a resuscitation plan, and coordinating all of the other roles. In some cases, the team leader will change. In this case, you or your partner may have been the team leader making decisions about the resuscitation until ALS arrived. Often in medical situations, the paramedic assumes the team leader role after receiving the assessment, history, and treatment information already gathered by the previous clinicians on the scene. Other times, such as at trauma scenes, hazmat scenes, or mass-casualty incidents, a fire officer can fulfill this role for management of the overall situation until the patient is transported, when team leadership would likely be taken over by one of the transporting clinicians.

4. The AED analyzes the patient's heart rhythm and advises you whether to deliver a shock. How can your team maximize patient perfusion and minimize "hands-off" time during this part of the cardiac arrest?

The EMR performing CPR should resume compressions immediately after the shock is delivered, without having to be directed to do so by the team leader.

In general, methods for minimizing hands-off time will depend greatly on the amount of training and practice the clinicians on the resuscitation team have had prior to the call. After any defibrillation, CPR should resume immediately after the shock is delivered, regardless of the patient's cardiac rhythm, unless the patient has obvious signs of circulation (such as movement, breathing, or speaking). In a well-coordinated team, everyone should understand this priority, even if the team members hold different levels of certification or are from different organizations. However, team members who have not practiced or worked together before may wait until the team leader gives them specific direction because they do not know what to expect next. In cardiac resuscitation, this can lead to delays in the resumption of CPR, which negatively affects the patient's chances of successful resuscitation.

5. When should you give the patient's medical history and medication list to the paramedic?

As a single ALS clinician arriving on scene of a cardiac resuscitation, the paramedic will have multiple

YOU are the EMT SUMMARY continued

roles to fill. The most obvious role is that of team leader. However, a dilemma the paramedic may face is that they may be the only one able to complete certain ALS-level tasks such as cardiac rhythm interpretation, obtaining vascular access, and medication administration.

As a result, the exact answer to this question will depend on the specifics of the situation. Generally, most ALS clinicians assuming the role of team leader on arrival will want an immediate verbal report of priority patient concerns, priority assessment, medical history, and key interventions that have been performed. Therefore, in this case, you should provide a verbal report to the paramedic as soon as possible on arrival.

When it is possible, the full patient demographics, medical history, medication list, and other pertinent information should be written down in a clear format and turned over to the paramedic team leader for additional reference, and then given to the team members on arrival at the ED.

6. How should you respond if you notice that the EMR doing CPR is compressing at an inappropriate rate?

If you notice that a member of the patient care team is not completing a task correctly, you have an obligation to speak up. It is inappropriate to allow known and witnessed errors to occur during a patient care event without offering input for correction. The CRM techniques discussed in this chapter provide a format for team members to appropriately and professionally interact to ensure the best patient care is being performed. Gain the attention of the person doing CPR or the team leader. State the concern as you see it: "I believe the rate of compressions should be faster. Do you agree?" This allows team members to reflect on action and make corrections without placing blame or criticism.

7. In the ED, if the paramedic is giving the handoff report, then who will ensure that patient care is continued during the transfer of care?

It is important for other team members to avoid interrupting or causing interference with the handoff report. It is just as important for team members to ensure that priority treatments (think ABCs) are continued during the transfer of care until treatments are assumed by the receiving team members.

It is for this reason that many team-focused patient handoff protocols specify that all priority treatments must be completely taken over by the receiving team before the handoff report is given. This ensures that the team's complete attention can be given to the person (in this case, the paramedic) providing the report. Many protocols even include a specific, so-called moment of silence to ensure that the report is given only once and that all team members received the information. This is especially important during critical care handoffs such as this cardiac arrest, but this concept can also apply to severe trauma and "alert" situations such as a heart attack, stroke, and sepsis.

8. During the transfer of patient care, at what point is the EMS unit of the team relieved of responsibility for caring for the patient?

It is crucial for team members to ensure that patient care continues through any transition of team members, from the time you arrive on scene to join the team to the moment you hand off care to your team members in the ED.

Once the handoff is complete, it is important for you to ask if your team members in the ED have any remaining questions or need anything else from you. Do not make assumptions. Ask explicit questions aloud, such as "Do you have any questions?" and "Is there anything else that you need from me?" You should receive a clear response from the team members to whom you are handing off patient care.

Prep Kit

Ready for Review

- Just culture is an approach to leadership in organizations that balances fairness and accountability and encourages people to report errors and near misses. It focuses on risk management.
- Emergency health care clinicians must know how to work effectively as a unified team, from first patient contact to patient discharge. Ensuring consistent patient care across all

Prep Kit continued

team members is known as the continuum of care.

- Although some EMS systems allow EMTs to work together in regular teams, others require clinicians to assemble their teams "on the fly" for each call (temporary teams). It is especially important for team members to train and practice together if they are from different organizations.
- An effective team must work interdependently toward a shared goal (best possible patient outcome) instead of focusing on individual, task-based goals (such as splinting an arm or starting an IV line).
- An effective team must have clearly defined roles and responsibilities. The diverse and highly competent team members must communicate and collaborate efficiently under supported and coordinated leadership.
- An effective team must have a team leader to coordinate and guide decision making. For this system to work, every member must be responsible for maintaining individual situational awareness and conveying critical information to each other and to the team leader.
- For all emergency health care clinicians to work together successfully, they must be well versed in efficient patient handoff techniques.
- The ALS skills with which you may assist will vary from EMS system to EMS system, but you will generally follow a four-step process: (1) preparing the patient, (2) setting up equipment, (3) performing the procedure, and (4) continuing care.
- Effective decision making is an ongoing process that may be broken down into stages, according to factors that should be considered before arrival, on arrival, during the call, and after the call.
- EMTs must be aware of and avoid decision traps, such as bias, anchoring, and overconfidence, which can lead to decision-making errors.

Vital Vocabulary

ALS assist An intervention in which a clinician trained in basic life support provides assistance, while remaining within their scope of practice, to a clinician who is performing an advanced life support (ALS) procedure.

anchoring A decision-making error in which the clinician settles on one possible cause of the patient's problems early and fails to consider other options.

biases Fixed beliefs that are not based on objective knowledge.

community paramedicine A health care model in which experienced paramedics receive advanced training to equip them to provide additional services in the prehospital environment, such as health evaluations, monitoring of chronic illnesses or conditions, and patient advocacy.

continuum of care The concept of consistent patient care across the entire health care team from first patient contact to patient discharge; working together with a unified goal results in improved individual and team performance, better patient and clinician safety, and improved patient outcome.

crew resource management (CRM) A set of procedures for use in environments where human error can have disastrous consequences. It empowers people within a team to communicate effectively with one another with a goal of improving team situational awareness, patient and crew safety, and overall communication.

mobile integrated healthcare (MIH) A method of delivering health care that involves providing health care within the community rather than at a physician's office or hospital.

Prep Kit continued

overconfidence A decision-making error in which the clinician overestimates their ability and chooses the wrong treatment path or ignores others' input, resulting in harmful actions.

situational awareness A state of sustained knowledge and understanding of one's surroundings and of potential risks to the safety of the patient or EMS team.

team In the context of EMS, a group of health care clinicians who are assigned specific roles and are working interdependently in a coordinated manner under a designated leader.

team leader The team member who provides role assignments, coordination, oversight, centralized decision making, and support for the team to accomplish their goals and achieve desired results.

References

1. National Association of State EMS Officials. *National EMS Scope of Practice Model 2019.* Washington, DC: National Highway Traffic Safety Administration; February 2019. Report No. DOT HS 812-666. https://www.ems.gov/assets/National_EMS_Scope_of_Practice_Model_2019.pdf. Accessed September 27, 2024.
2. Rosen MA, DiazGranados D, Dietz AS, et al. Teamwork in healthcare: key discoveries enabling safer, high-quality care. *Am Psychol.* 2018 May-Jun;73(4):433–450.
3. Course: To Err Is Human. Topic: Being an Effective Team Player. World Health Organization website. https://cdn.who.int/media/docs/default-source/patient-safety/curriculum-guide/resources/ps-curr-handouts/course04_handout_being-an-effective-team-player-.pdf?sfvrsn=50aecf5a_9&download=true. Published 2021. Accessed September 27, 2024.
4. TeamSTEPPS 3.0. Agency for Healthcare Research and Quality website. https://www.ahrq.gov/teamstepps-program/index.html. Accessed September 27, 2024.
5. A culture of safety in EMS systems. American College of Emergency Physicians website. https://www.acep.org/siteassets/new-pdfs/policy-statements/a-culture-of-safety-in-ems-systems.pdf. Published 2021. Accessed September 27, 2024.
6. Weaver MD, Wang HE, Fairbanks RJ, Patterson D. The association between EMS workplace safety culture and safety outcomes. *Prehosp Emerg Care.* 2012;16(1):43–52.
7. Boysen PG 2nd. Just culture: a foundation for balanced accountability and patient safety. *Ochsner J.* 2013;13(3):400–406.
8. Marx DA. *Patient Safety and the "Just Culture": A Primer for Health Care Executives.* Trustees of Columbia University; 2001.
9. Banja J. The normalization of deviance in healthcare delivery. *Bus Horiz.* 2010;53(2):139.
10. Sedlar N, Irwin A, Martin D, Roberts R. A qualitative systematic review on the application of the normalization of deviance phenomenon within high-risk industries. *J Safety Res.* 2023;84:290–305.
11. Wright I. Normalization of deviance is contrary to the principles of high reliability. *AORN J.* 2023;117(4):231–238.
12. Institute for Social Research. University of Michigan, Research Center for Group website. https://rcgd.isr.umich.edu/. Accessed September 27, 2024.
13. Breaux P. How to achieve effective teamwork in EMS. EMS World website. https://www.hmpgloballearningnetwork.com/site/emsworld/article/10613600/how-achieve-effective-teamwork-ems. Published January 12, 2012. Accessed September 27, 2024.
14. Paramedic Psychomotor Competency Portfolio (PPCP). National Registry of Emergency Medical Technicians website. https://content.nremt.org/static/documents/Paramedic_Psychomotor_Competency_Portfolio_Manual_v4.pdf. Published 2015. Accessed September 27, 2024.
15. Helmreich RL, Merritt AC, Wilhelm JA. The evolution of Crew Resource Management training in commercial aviation. *Int J Aviat Psychol.* 1999;9(1):19–32.
16. National Association of State EMS Officials. (2021, August). National EMS scope of practice model 2019: Including change notices 1.0 and 2.0 (Report No. DOT HS 813 151). National Highway Traffic Safety Administration. https://www.ems.gov/assets/National_EMS_Scope_of_Practice_Model_2019_Change_Notices_August_2021.pdf
17. Gugiu MR, McKenna KD, Platt TE, Panchal AR; National Registry of Emergency Medical Technicians. A proposed theoretical framework for clinical judgment in EMS. *Prehosp Emerg Care.* 2023;27(4):427–431.
18. Croskerry P. Achieving quality in clinical decision making: cognitive strategies and detection of bias. *Acad Emerg Med.* 2002;9(11):1184–1204.

Prep Kit continued

19. Levy MK, Tan DK, McArdle DQ, et al. Consensus statement of the National Association of EMS Physicians, International Association of Fire Chiefs, and the International Association of Chiefs of Police: best practices for collaboration between law enforcement and emergency medical services during acute behavioral emergencies. *Prehosp Emerg Care*. Published online September 12, 2024. doi:10.1080/10903127.2024.2402530
20. Ding ML, Gerberi DJ, McCoy RG. Engaging emergency medical services to improve postacute management of behavioural health emergency calls: a protocol of a scoping literature review. *BMJ Open*. 2023;13(3):e067272. doi:10.1136/bmjopen-2022-067272

Additional Resources

EMS Agenda 2050 Technical Expert Panel. *EMS Agenda 2050: A People-Centered Vision for the Future of Emergency Medical Services* (Report No. DOT HS 812 664). Washington, DC: National Highway Traffic Safety Administration; January 2019.

National Association of State EMS Officials. National Model EMS Clinical Guidelines: Version 3.0. https://nasemso.org/wp-content/uploads/National-Model-EMS-Clinical-Guidelines_2022.pdf. Updated March, 2022. Accessed September 27, 2024.

National Highway Traffic Safety Administration. *National Emergency Medical Services Education Standards 2021*. https://www.ems.gov/assets/EMS_Education-Standards_2021_FNL.pdf. Published December 2021. Accessed September 27, 2024.

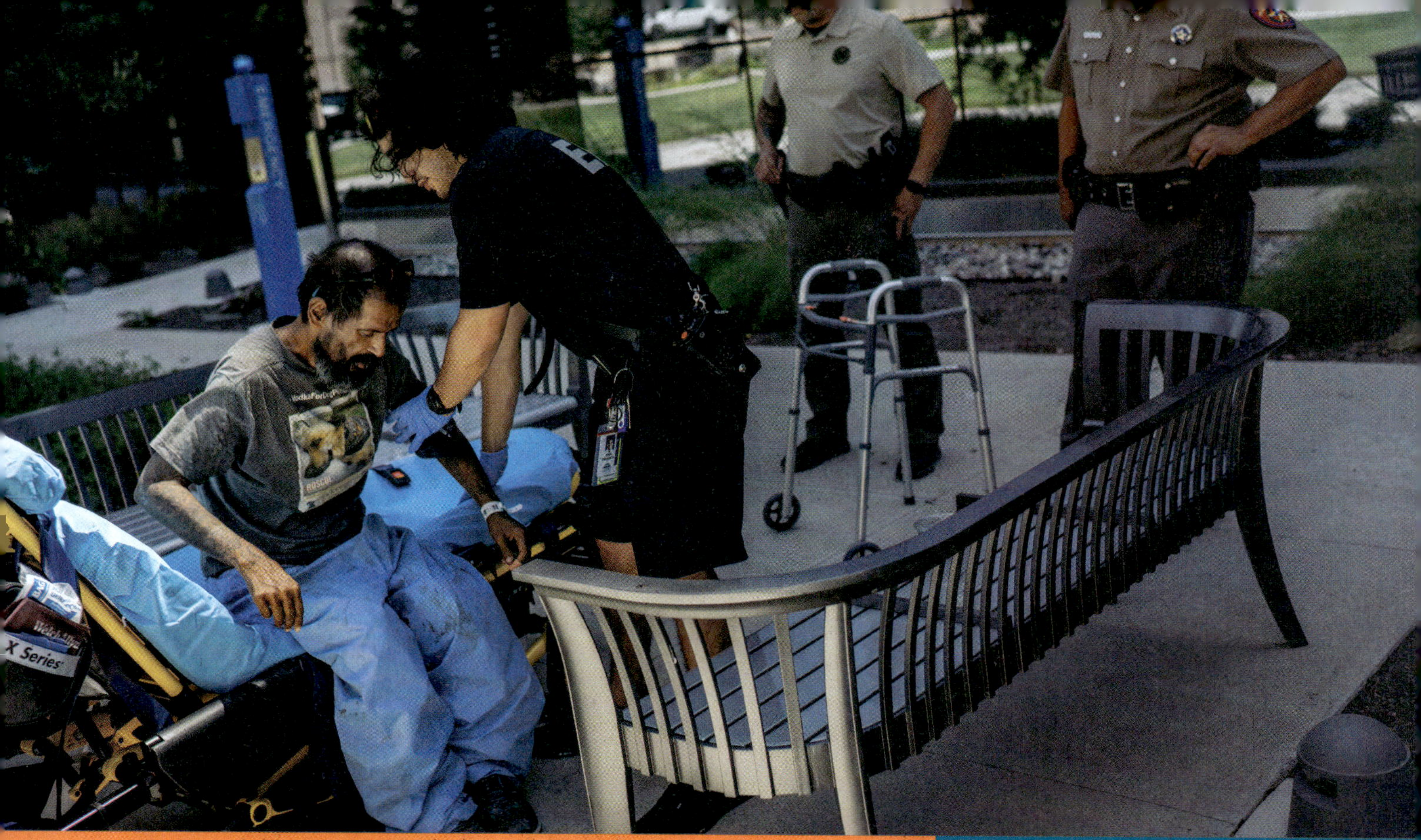

Patient Assessment

SECTION

2

10 Patient Assessment

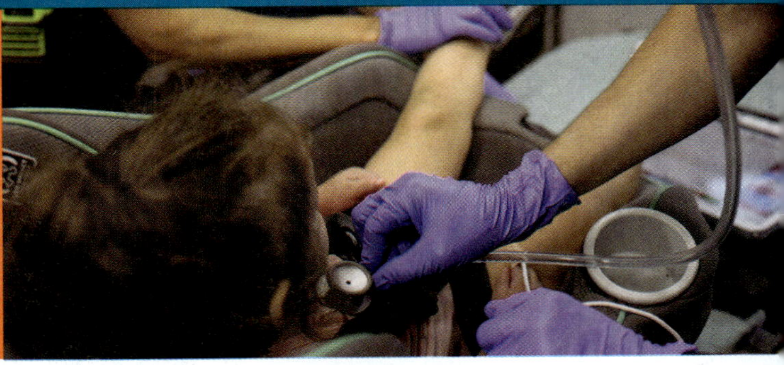

Chapter 10

Patient Assessment

NATIONAL EMS EDUCATION STANDARD COMPETENCIES

Assessment

Applies scene information and patient assessment findings (scene size-up, primary and secondary assessment, patient history, and reassessment) to guide emergency management.

Scene Size-up

- Scene safety/situational awareness (pp 325–326)
- Scene management (pp 326–327)
- Impact of the environment on patient care (pp 326–327)
- Addressing hazards (p 326)
- Violence (p 353)
- Need for additional or specialized resources (p 330)
- Standard precautions (pp 329–330)
- Multiple patient situations (pp 330–331)

Primary Assessment

- Primary assessment for all patient situations (pp 332–347)
- Integration of treatment/procedures needed to preserve life (pp 332–347)

History Taking

- Investigation of the chief complaint (pp 349–350)
- Mechanism of injury/nature of illness (pp 327–328)
- Associated signs and symptoms (pp 349–354)
- Past medical history (pp 349–352)
- Pertinent negatives (p 352)

Secondary Assessment

- Assessment of vital signs (pp 362–375, 382–386)
- Assessment of pain (pp 379–382)
- Techniques of physical examination
  - Respiratory system, including breath sounds (pp 362–366)
  - Cardiovascular system (pp 366–375)
  - Neurologic system (pp 375–379)
  - Musculoskeletal system (pp 379–382)
  - Major anatomic regions (pp 379–382)

Monitoring Devices

- Pulse oximetry (p 383)
- Noninvasive blood pressure (p 384)
- Cardiac monitoring—12-lead electrocardiogram (ECG) acquisition and transmission (Chapter 17, *Cardiovascular Emergencies*)
- Blood glucose determination (p 384)

Reassessment

- How and when to reassess patients (p 388–389)

KNOWLEDGE OBJECTIVES

1. Identify the components of the patient assessment process. (p 323)
2. Explain how the different causes and presentations of emergencies will affect how EMTs perform each step of the patient assessment process. (p 324)
3. Discuss some of the possible environmental, chemical, and biologic hazards that may

be present at an emergency scene, ways to recognize them, and precautions to protect personal safety. (pp 325–327)

4. Discuss the steps EMTs should take to survey a scene for signs of violence and protect themselves and bystanders from real or potential danger. (pp 326–327)
5. Describe how to determine the mechanism of injury (MOI) or nature of illness (NOI) at an emergency and the importance of differentiating trauma patients from medical patients. (pp 327–328)
6. List the minimum standard precautions that should be followed and personal protective equipment (PPE) that should be worn at an emergency scene, including examples of when additional precautions would be appropriate. (pp 329–330)
7. Explain why it is important for EMTs to identify the total number of patients at an emergency scene and how this evaluation relates to determining the need for additional or specialized resources, implementation of the incident command system (ICS), and triage. (pp 330–331)
8. Describe the principal goals of the primary assessment process, including how to identify and treat life threats and determine if immediate transport is required. (pp 332–335, 346–347)
9. Explain the process of forming a general impression of a patient as part of primary assessment and the reasons why this step is critical to patient management. (pp 333–334)
10. Explain the importance of assessing a patient's level of consciousness to determine altered mental status and include examples of different methods used to assess alertness, responsiveness, and orientation. (pp 334–336)
11. Describe the assessment of airway status in patients who are both responsive and unresponsive, including examples of possible signs and causes of airway obstruction in each case as well as the appropriate EMT response. (p 336)
12. Describe the assessment of a patient's breathing status, including the key information EMTs must obtain during this process and the care required for patients who have adequate and inadequate breathing. (pp 336–338)
13. List the signs of respiratory distress and respiratory failure. (p 338)
14. Describe the assessment of a patient's circulatory status, including the different methods for obtaining a pulse and appropriate management depending on the patient's status. (pp 338–340)
15. Explain the variations required to obtain a pulse in infant and child patients compared with adult patients. (pp 338–340)
16. Describe the assessment of a patient's skin color, temperature, and condition, including examples of both normal and abnormal findings and the information this provides related to the patient's status. (pp 340–342)
17. Discuss the process of assessing and methods for controlling external bleeding. (pp 342–343)
18. Explain the steps in the primary assessment of a pediatric patient, including the elements of the pediatric assessment triangle (PAT), hands-on ABCs, transport decision considerations, and privacy issues. (pp 343–346)
19. Explain the significance of the Golden Period. (p 347)
20. List the steps EMTs should follow during the primary assessment of a trauma patient, including examples of abnormal signs and appropriate related actions. (pp 346–347)
21. Explain the process for determining the priority of patient care and transport at an emergency scene and include examples of conditions that necessitate immediate transport. (pp 346–347)
22. List the details that should be documented during the history taking process. (pp 348–349)
23. Discuss the process of determining the chief complaint or chief concern. (pp 349–350)
24. Describe examples of different techniques EMTs may use to obtain information from patients during the history-taking process. (pp 349–352)
25. Discuss different challenges EMTs may face when taking a patient history on sensitive topics and strategies that can be used to facilitate each situation. (pp 353–354)
26. Describe the purpose of a secondary assessment and a physical exam; include how to determine which aspects of the physical exam to use, and the steps. (pp 355–361)
27. Explain the steps in the secondary assessment of a pediatric patient, including what EMTs should look for related to different body areas and the method of injury. (pp 361–362)

28. Explain situations in which patients may receive a focused assessment, including examples by body system of what each focused assessment should include based on a patient's chief complaint. (pp 362–386)
29. List normal blood pressure ranges for adults, children, and infants. (p 374)
30. Explain the GEMS diamond and its role in the assessment and care of the geriatric patient. (p 386)
31. Explain the importance of performing a reassessment of the patient and the steps in this process. (pp 388–389)

SKILLS OBJECTIVES

1. Demonstrate how to use the AVPU scale to test for patient responsiveness. (p 334)
2. Demonstrate how to evaluate a patient's orientation and document their status correctly. (p 335)
3. Demonstrate the techniques for assessing a patient's airway, and correctly obtain information related to respiratory rate and the rhythm, quality, character, and depth of breathing. (pp 336–338)
4. Demonstrate how to assess a radial pulse in a responsive patient and an unresponsive patient. (p 339)
5. Demonstrate how to assess a carotid pulse in an unresponsive patient. (pp 339–340)
6. Demonstrate how to palpate a brachial pulse in a child who is younger than 1 year. (p 339)
7. Demonstrate how to obtain a pulse rate in a patient. (pp 338–340)
8. Demonstrate how to assess capillary refill. (p 342)
9. Demonstrate how to conduct an interview to gather a patient's history. (pp 350–352)
10. Demonstrate how to perform a secondary assessment. (pp 357–360, Skill Drill 10-1)
11. Demonstrate how to measure blood pressure by auscultation. (p 371, Skill Drill 10-2)
12. Demonstrate how to measure blood pressure by palpation. (p 373, Skill Drill 10-3)
13. Demonstrate how to test pupil reaction in response to light in a patient and document their status correctly. (pp 375–377)
14. Demonstrate the assessment of neurovascular status. (pp 377–378, Skill Drill 10-4)
15. Demonstrate the use of a pulse oximetry device to evaluate the effectiveness of oxygenation in the patient. (p 383)
16. Demonstrate the use of electronic devices to assist in determining the patient's blood pressure in the field. (p 384)
17. Demonstrate how to assess a patient's blood glucose level. (p 385, Skill Drill 10-5)

Patient Assessment

Scene Size-Up

Ensure scene safety
Determine mechanism of injury/nature of illness
Take standard precautions
Determine number of patients
Consider additional/specialized resources

↓

Primary Assessment

Form a general impression
Assess level of consciousness
Assess the ABCs (airway, breathing, circulation); identify and treat life threats
Perform primary assessment
Determine priority of patient care and transport

↓

History Taking

Investigate the chief complaint (history of present illness)
Obtain SAMPLE history

↓

Secondary Assessment

Perform a *general* systematic assessment of the patient
Perform a *focused* systematic assessment of the patient

↓

Reassessment

Repeat the primary assessment
Reassess vital signs
Reassess the chief complaint or chief concern
Recheck interventions
Identify and treat changes in the patient's condition
Reassess the patient

- Unstable patients: every 5 minutes
- Stable patients: every 15 minutes

Introduction

One of the most important skills that you can develop as an EMT is the ability to assess your patients. You will assess every patient you meet, and the assessment is the basis for all treatment you will provide as an EMT. This chapter provides the framework and information necessary for you to be able to understand and conduct the patient assessment. The assessment process is divided into five main parts:

1. Scene size-up
2. Primary assessment
3. History taking
4. Secondary assessment
5. Reassessment

Although these steps represent a logical approach to patient assessment, the order in which they are performed may vary depending on the patient's condition and the environment in which you find the patient. For example, the same components of patient assessment used to evaluate a medical patient are used to assess a trauma patient; however, it may be necessary to change the order of some steps after scene size-up based on your findings and the need to prioritize the care of certain conditions. Regardless of the patient's complaint or the environment in which you find yourself, the key to effective patient assessment is to remain organized.

Rarely does one sign or symptom show you the patient's status or underlying problem. Rather, it is the combination of signs and symptoms that will direct the care you provide for your patient. A **symptom** is a subjective condition that the patient feels and tells you about (eg, nausea, abdominal pain). A **sign** is an objective condition that you can observe or measure (eg, vomiting, abdominal distention). Therefore, it is essential to have a basic understanding of the causes and presentations of commonly encountered emergencies, as this information can help you formulate a **field impression**. The field impression is the evident cause of the patient's condition, determined by considering the situation, history, and examination findings. Forming the field impression will help you determine your priorities of care.

For example, consider a person who is experiencing chest pain. Given this information alone, they may be having a heart attack or may have a lung infection, a pulmonary embolism, or a simple strained muscle in the chest. On assessment, the following information is obtained:

- The pain is crushing, radiating down the left arm and up into the jaw.
- The skin is pale (compared to its baseline color) and sweaty.
- The episode began while they were shoveling snow.
- The patient has a history of coronary bypass surgery.
- The patient has been prescribed nitroglycerin.

On the basis of this information, it seems likely the patient is experiencing, and should be treated for, a myocardial infarction.

As an EMT, the treatment you will provide for most patients is based on your assessment, not an exact diagnosis, as many conditions may have similar signs and symptoms.

Words of Wisdom

Although the steps of patient assessment represent a logical approach to the evaluation of a patient, the order in which they are performed may vary based on the patient's condition.

YOU are the EMT

At 1815 hours, you are dispatched with the police to an apartment complex at 3820 121st Street for an unresponsive person. The weather is overcast and rainy, the temperature is 62°F (16.7°C), and the traffic is light. Your response time to the scene is approximately 4 minutes.

1. What are the components of the patient assessment?
2. Will your assessment of the patient differ if the individual is injured versus ill? If so, how?

Patient Assessment

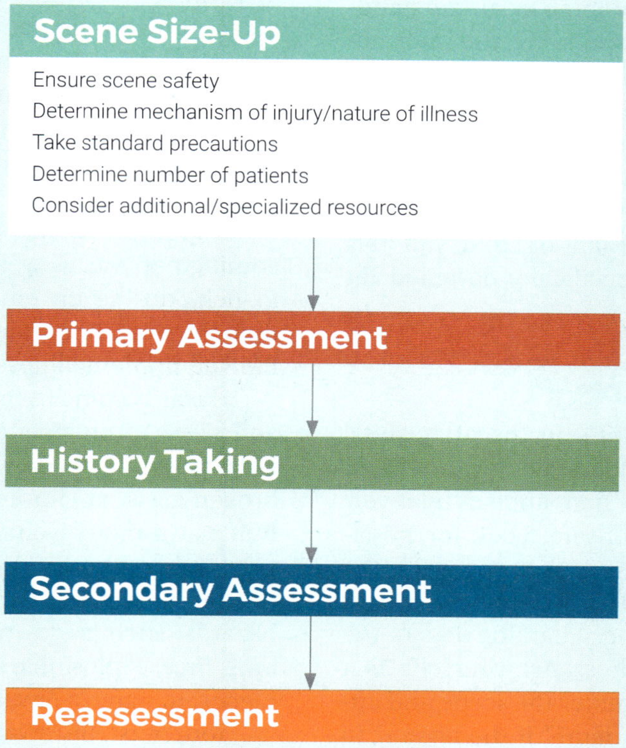

Scene Size-up

Scene size-up refers to your evaluation of the conditions in which you will be treating your patient. Although this will be the focus of your attention when you first arrive on scene, continuous **situational awareness** is necessary throughout the entire call to ensure safety. Situational awareness is paying attention to the conditions and people around you at all times and the potential risks those conditions or people pose. For example, before you know the specific location of the incident, you will need to consider these factors:

- Weather, traffic, and road conditions
- Time of day
- Currently available resources
- Other incidents in the same response district

These considerations will guide your preparations even before receiving a call. For example, during cold weather, ensure you have the proper clothing to stay warm. If you are responding to an incident on the roadway, wear appropriate reflective clothing. Scene size-up is listed at the top of the assessment algorithm because it is the first thing you must consider, and it does not end when you move through the rest of the assessment process.

After you are alerted for an emergency call, the emergency medical dispatcher will provide you with some basic information about the request for your assistance. As you start to build a picture in your mind of what you are responding to, there are additional factors to consider:

- Incident hazards such as fire, hazardous materials, or extrication

- Ingress and egress to the patient's location
- Equipment needed to care for the patient
- Physical threats of violence from people or animals on the scene

Your scene size-up must combine an understanding of conditions prior to responding, the information the dispatcher gave you, and observations of the scene itself to help ensure your own safety and your crew's safety. If the dispatch information includes the patient's age, consider how this information may affect your responsibilities. For example, if you will be caring for an infant or child, you may need to take equipment specifically designed for this population.

Ensure Scene Safety

Issues that you may encounter in the prehospital setting can range from minor difficulties to major dangers. Even scenes that first appear relatively safe and secure can turn unsafe. Look for possible difficulties and dangers as you approach the scene. Signs of danger include, for example, a large crowd, the sound of shouting, a barking dog, or the absence of lights at the address. Ask yourself, "Is it safe for my team and me to enter the scene and approach and manage the patient?" If the answer to this question is, "No, the scene is not yet safe to approach and manage the patient," then take appropriate measures to make it safe or call for additional resources. These resources may include firefighters, utility workers, hazardous materials technicians, or law enforcement personnel. You should listen to your instincts, training, and team when determining if a scene is safe. There are many well-documented cases of EMS clinicians being injured after they entered an unsafe scene despite feeling as though something was wrong.

Use good body mechanics as you exit your ambulance and gather the appropriate equipment to take to the patient. Additionally, remain mindful of special considerations for working at high-risk scenes, such as roadside crashes. See Chapter 2, *Workforce Safety and Wellness*, for further discussion of safe operations.

Working in unfavorable conditions and on unstable surfaces is a large part of prehospital care. Without knowing the infinite number of situations you may become involved in, a good rule to use when faced with a wide variety of possibilities is that any actions you may take to protect yourself (eg, heavy coats, rain gear, life jackets, air conditioned or heated vehicles) should also be considered for the patient. If you are putting on equipment to address environmental hazards and can safely do so, provide the patient with the same or similar equipment. If you move away from the scene to take cover from an environmental hazard, move the patient with you when possible. Taking your time to stay focused on what you are doing will go a long way toward preventing injuries.

If appropriate, help protect bystanders from becoming patients as well. Many bystanders attempt to help during an emergency; always remember that they are not trained to handle complicated EMS equipment, illnesses, or injuries.

Hazards come in many different forms, shapes, and sizes. You may encounter environmental hazards; physical hazards (such as sharp metal and broken glass, or slip-and-fall hazards from leaking fluids at a motor vehicle crash); biohazards (such as blood and body fluids); chemical hazards (such as the release of a hazardous material); electrical hazards (such as downed power lines); water hazards; fires; explosions; and the threat of physical violence, to name a few (**FIGURE 10-1**).

You must be aware of scenes that have the potential for violence due to violent patients, distraught family members, angry bystanders, gangs, or unruly crowds. When you enter a patient's home, scan the patient and immediate area. Do you see any weapons that the patient or others can access?

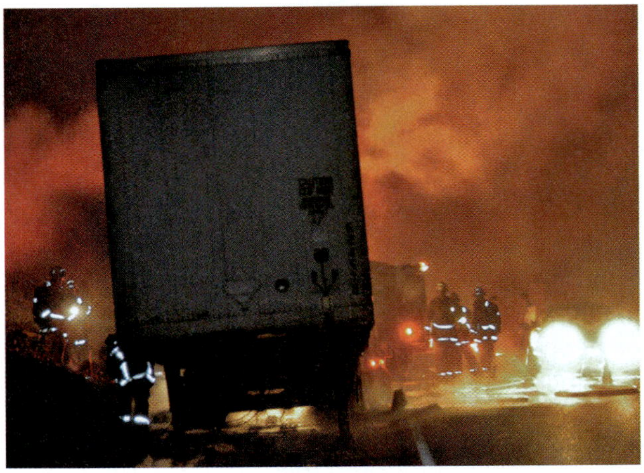

FIGURE 10-1 Evaluate the scene for hazards as soon as you arrive.

Weapons may not be items typically associated with violence, such as a knife or gun; they can be household items such as a screwdriver or hammer, or other readily available objects sitting on the kitchen table or nightstand by the bed. Always be observant for such objects, and if they are not secured, make sure you place yourself between the patient and the potential danger, thus preventing possible access to the object. Immediately request the assistance of law enforcement personnel if the scene presents the potential for violence (**FIGURE 10-2**). Often, law enforcement is dispatched with EMS to help provide safety, redirect traffic, assist with bystanders, and offer medical assistance. If this is not the approach used in your area, you must request law enforcement assistance as soon as you think there may be danger. In some cases, you may need to retreat from the scene or the patient until law enforcement arrives. If you are not yet on the scene but suspect it may be dangerous, stage at a safe location nearby until law enforcement advises that it is safe to proceed to the call. Responding to abandoned buildings and areas of known violence should raise your suspicions for the need for law enforcement.

An emergency scene is a dynamic environment; simply checking the safety of the scene once at the beginning of the call is not enough. As an EMT, you must remain aware of changes in your surroundings that may present safety hazards to you, your EMS team, the patient, or bystanders. Regardless of when the hazards present themselves, it is up to you to either make the scene safe or call for additional resources and move to a safe location.

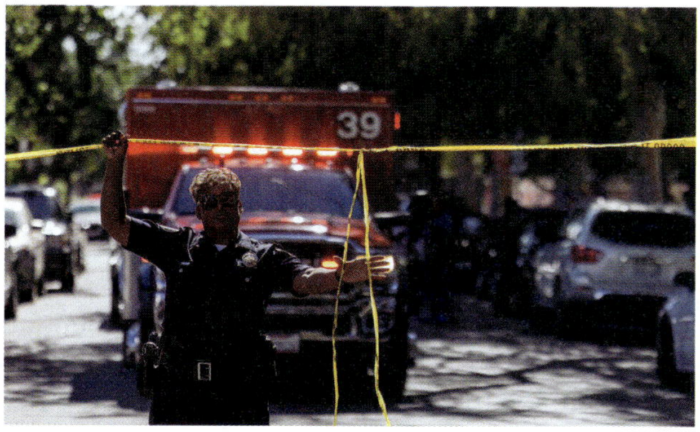

FIGURE 10-2 If the scene is unsafe, request law enforcement support.

Determine Mechanism of Injury/Nature of Illness

Virtually all calls to which you may respond can be categorized as medical conditions, traumatic injuries, or both. Some emergency calls may involve a medical problem that leads to a traumatic injury, such as a patient who becomes weak and dizzy from a low blood glucose level, causing them to stumble, fall, and break their ankle. As an EMT, you will need to be able to identify the general classification and underlying issue or issues of the emergency to which you respond.

Traumatic injuries are the result of physical forces applied to the outside of the body, usually from an object striking the body or a body striking an object. They are generally classified according to the type or amount of force, how long it was applied, and where it was applied to the body. These dynamics constitute the **mechanism of injury (MOI)**. The MOI can be used as a guide to help you focus your assessment.

Certain parts of the body are more easily injured than others. The brain and the spinal cord are fragile and easy to injure. Fortunately, they are protected by the skull, the vertebrae, and several layers of soft tissues. The eyes are also easily injured. Even small forces on the eye may result in serious injury. The bones and certain organs are stronger and can absorb more force without resulting significant injury. A good understanding of anatomy and physiology will help you identify times when the MOI may lead to injury to parts of the body not directly impacted. For example, consider a patient who has fallen off a roof, landing feetfirst. This patient's MOI would direct attention to possible injury to the feet. But significant energy likely transferred to other body areas and may have caused further injury in the patient's legs, pelvis, and even spine.

If the MOI indicates the need for spinal motion restriction, ensure that you or another clinician manually stabilizes the unresponsive patient's cervical spine. Spinal motion restriction is indicated in the context of blunt trauma that presents with any of the following[1]:

- Pain or tenderness on palpation of the neck or spine
- Patient report of pain in neck or back
- Deformity of the spine

- Paralysis or neurologic complaint (numbness, tingling, partial paralysis of the legs or arms)
- Altered mental status
- Intoxication (alcohol or drugs)
- Difficulty communicating or inability to communicate
- Distracting injuries that make assessment of the spine difficult

Spinal motion restriction is also indicated in the presence of a **distracting injury**, which refers to any injury that distracts the patient's attention from other, even severe, injuries. An example is a painful femur or tibia fracture that prevents the patient from noticing back or neck pain.

If it is not possible to both manually stabilize the patient's cervical spine and continue your assessment to identify and correct life threats, do your best to ensure that the patient's spine remains in a stable position while you continue your assessment. You should complete your primary assessment before applying a cervical collar.

Terms commonly associated with MOI include blunt trauma and penetrating trauma. The different types of trauma are further detailed in Chapter 24, *Trauma Overview*.

As an EMT, you will also care for patients experiencing a medical emergency (ie, illnesses or conditions not caused by an outside force). For patients with medical problems, you must evaluate the general type of illness the patient is experiencing, or the **nature of illness (NOI)**. An example would be a patient who tells you that they feel as if they cannot get enough air to breathe. This patient's NOI would be difficulty breathing and, like the MOI, would help direct both your assessment and your care.

There are similarities between the MOI and the NOI. Both require you to search for clues about how the incident occurred or the problem developed. You must make an effort to determine the general type of illness, which is often best described by the patient's **chief complaint**, the most serious sign or symptom the patient is experiencing. However, sometimes what the patient reports as their chief complaint is not the top priority. In this case you will be more focused on the **chief concern**. The chief concern is the condition requiring the most urgent intervention as determined by the clinician's assessment of the patient; it is not always the same as the chief complaint. To quickly determine the NOI, talk with the patient, family, or bystanders about the problem. At the same time, use your senses to check the scene for clues as to the possible problem. You may see open or spilled medication containers, poisonous substances, or unsanitary living conditions. You may smell an unusual or strong odor, such as the odor of fresh paint in a closed room. You may hear a hissing sound, such as a leak from a home oxygen system. Keep these observations of the scene in mind as you begin to assess a medical patient.

Be aware of scenes with multiple patients who are exhibiting similar signs or symptoms. An example would be a couple living together experiencing flulike symptoms, headache, nausea, and vomiting. These symptoms may be indicative of carbon monoxide poisoning, which would also indicate an unsafe scene for you and your partner.

The Importance of the MOI and NOI

Considering the MOI or NOI early can be of value in preparing to care for your patient. For example, when you begin to gather equipment from the unit, what would you take to treat a patient reporting chest pain? How would that equipment differ from the equipment used for a pedestrian struck by a vehicle? The appearance of the scene may also guide your preparation. Other MOIs may include falls, motor vehicle crashes, assaults, burns, and industrial accidents. Examples of NOIs include seizures, heart attacks, syncope, diabetic problems, and poisonings. Family members, bystanders, or even law enforcement personnel may also provide important trauma or medical information to help you assist the patient.

You may be tempted to categorize your patient immediately as a trauma or medical patient. Remember, the fundamentals of a good patient assessment are the same despite the unique aspects of trauma and medical care. If an unconscious patient is found at the bottom of a ladder, did the person fall off the ladder, strike their head and become unconscious, and sustain a ground-level fall? Or did they experience a medical problem that caused them to have a loss of consciousness and then fall off the ladder? Early in the assessment, it can be difficult to identify with absolute certainty whether the problem is of a traumatic or medical origin. Although further assessment is needed to come to a conclusion, considering the MOI or NOI early will help you begin your assessment.

Street Smarts

Although it is always a good idea to start formulating a plan as you respond to the call, it is important to note that there are times when the dispatch information may not match what you find on the scene. EMTs must be able to quickly adapt to that change and reframe their thinking about the call.

Take Standard Precautions

Standard precautions and **personal protective equipment (PPE)** need to be considered and adapted to the prehospital task at hand. PPE includes clothing or specialized equipment that protects the wearer. The type of PPE used depends on the specific job duties required during a patient care interaction. For example, rescue personnel may wear PPE such as helmets, eye protection, boots, gloves, and turnout gear designed to protect them from injury when working to extricate a patient trapped in a damaged motor vehicle. Hazardous materials technicians may don a protective suit designed to prevent contamination by potentially lethal hazardous materials.

Standard precautions are protective measures that have traditionally been recommended by the Centers for Disease Control and Prevention (CDC) for use in dealing with objects, blood, body fluids, and other potential exposure risks of communicable disease. If you have a primary responsibility for patient care, you will need to follow standard precautions when assessing and treating the patient. They are required in every patient encounter. These measures may not provide absolute protection from exposure to infectious diseases or bloodborne pathogens, but they are the most effective way to reduce your risk of exposure. The concept of standard precautions assumes that all blood, body fluids, nonintact skin, and mucous membranes may pose a risk of infection. This includes blood and other potentially infectious materials that are dried, because some diseases can live for days (eg, hepatitis B) or even weeks (eg, hepatitis C) outside the body. During a situation in which there is active community transmission of a virus that can be transmitted by airborne particles or aerosolized particles, this concept of standard precautions must be expanded to recognize the risk associated with non-bloodborne pathogens.

Take standard precautions before actual patient contact, often before you step out of your response vehicle (**FIGURE 10-3**). After you make contact with the patient, it may be too late to think about what precautions should have been considered. The use of standard precautions in EMS, including but not limited to consistent handwashing before and after care, gloves, eye protection, a mask, and a gown, may be dictated by local standards or protocols. At a minimum, gloves and eye protection must be in place before any patient contact. Remember that after contact with a patient, gloves may be contaminated by infectious materials, so avoid handling EMS equipment with the same gloves used during patient contact. Never touch your face or any areas of bare skin with gloves that have been in contact with a patient even if the gloves do not appear to be dirty.

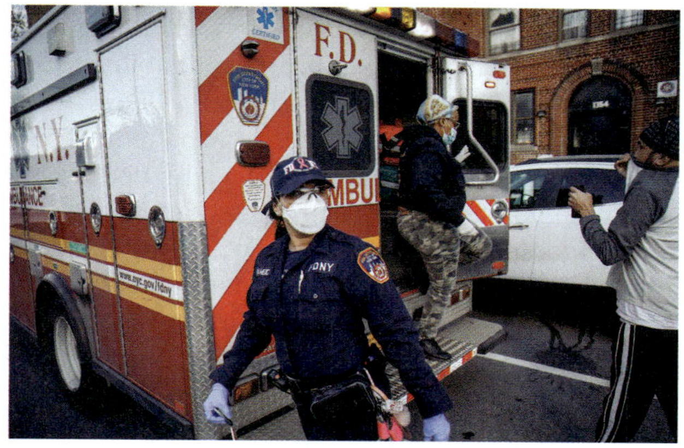

FIGURE 10-3 Taking standard precautions is vital when you are called to a scene in which you may be exposed to infection or blood or other body fluids.

© John Minchillo/AP Photo.

The use of eye protection is recommended for all patient encounters. Patients do not typically give you a warning before they vomit or have a seizure, events that pose a high risk of body fluids splashing into the eye. By wearing eye protection on calls, you will reduce the risk of eye injuries and blood or body fluid exposure. Standard eyeglasses may not offer enough protection because most are not designed with side splash guards. For that reason, eyewear should protect you from potential exposures from many different directions.

A patient displaying signs and symptoms such as coughing, stiff neck with headache, sore throat, or fever with shortness of breath should prompt you to don a mask and ask the patient to wear a mask. A mask will provide protection from some airborne diseases, but its level of protection will depend on the type of mask, a proper fit, and your ability to apply and wear it properly.

After making contact with the patient, if you discover a condition that warrants a higher level of PPE than you are using, do not hesitate to regroup and upgrade your protection. For example, if you discover in your primary assessment that a patient has a productive cough and a history of tuberculosis (TB) and you are not wearing an N95 mask, you and your crew should immediately don appropriate respiratory protection and ask the patient to wear the same type of mask. If you suspect you have been exposed to a communicable disease without the protection of proper PPE, follow your local agency's protocols for postexposure reporting, testing, and prophylaxis.

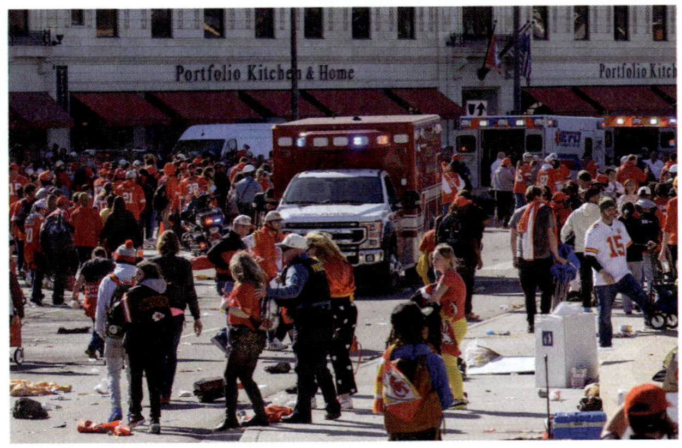

FIGURE 10-4 With multiple patients, use the incident command system, call for additional resources, and then begin triage. A shooting during a celebration for the Kansas City Chiefs in 2024 resulted in the mass-casualty incident shown here.

Words of Wisdom

Standard precautions are the infection prevention practices intended to reduce the risk of transmission of bloodborne and other pathogens from both identified and unrecognized sources of infection. These precautions include hand hygiene; use of PPE such as gloves, eye protection, gowns, and masks when there is a risk of exposure to infectious material; safe injection practices; safe handling of potentially contaminated equipment and surfaces; safe handling of linens; and respiratory hygiene/cough etiquette.[2] The term *standard precautions* has replaced terms for similar concepts, such as *body substance isolation*, and is promoted by both the CDC and World Health Organization (WHO).

Determine Number of Patients

As part of the scene size-up, it is essential that you accurately identify the total number of patients. While you are typically called to care for one patient, this evaluation is critical in determining your need for additional resources, such as firefighters, a specialized rescue group, a hazardous materials team, or additional ambulances. When there are multiple patients, use the incident command system, establish command, identify the number of patients, and then begin triage (**FIGURE 10-4**). Triage and incident command are covered in Chapter 38, *Incident Management.*

Consider Additional/ Specialized Resources

Some situations may require more ambulances, whereas others may have a need for specialized resources. Basic life support units may be all that are needed for some patients; however, advanced life support (ALS) should be requested for patients with severe injuries or complex medical problems, depending on available resources and local protocols. ALS care may be provided by AEMTs or paramedics, depending on how your EMS system is set up. Air medical support or critical care response teams may be another resource for ALS in your area. Follow your local protocols in requesting ALS resources.

In addition to EMS and fire suppression, many resources such as hazardous materials management and technical rescue services, including complex extrication from motor vehicle crashes, wilderness search and rescue, high-angle rope rescue, and water rescue, are typically available through the fire department (**FIGURE 10-5**).

Law enforcement personnel may be needed to assist with traffic or scene control and should be the first to enter crime scenes and hostile environments.

If any situation presents itself as a danger to you, your partner, or your patient, you must retreat to a safe area.

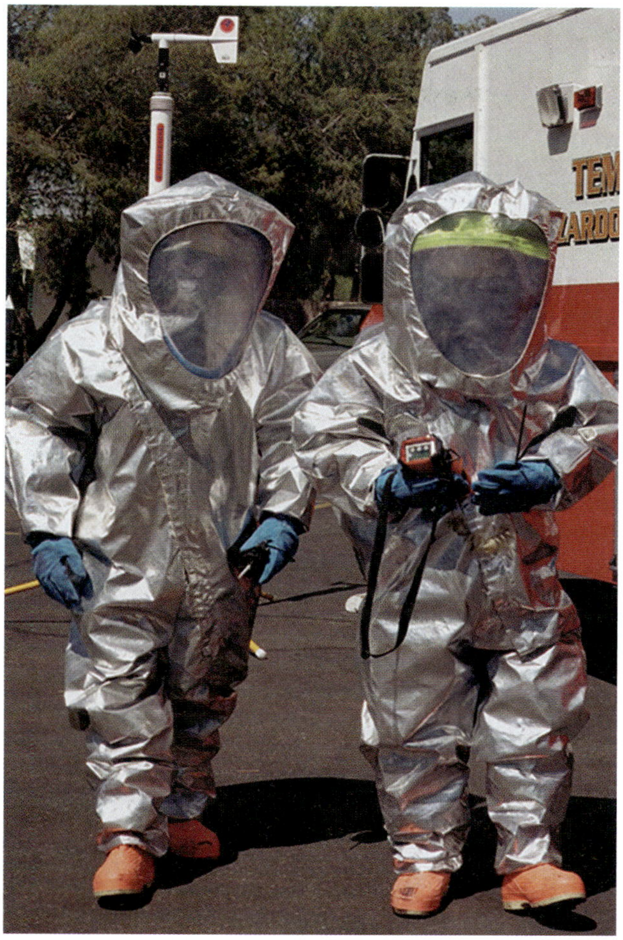

FIGURE 10-5 Scenes involving toxic substances may require specially trained rescuers with extra protective equipment.

Courtesy of Tempe Fire Department.

To determine if you require additional resources, ask yourself the following questions:

- Does the scene pose a threat to myself, my patient, or others?
- How many patients are there?
- Do we have the resources to assess and treat their conditions?

Geriatric Patients: Considerations During Scene Size-up

Geriatric patients are commonly found in their own homes, retirement homes, or skilled nursing facilities, but calls for assistance can come from any location. Many older people live alone. Access to them may be hampered if their condition prevents them from getting to the door to let you in. Police or fire department assistance may be required.

Most older people try to maintain their independence as long as they can. They may or may not have someone who checks on their welfare. You will find some people living in conditions that are not safe or appropriate. Note negative or unsafe environmental conditions. Is the home well maintained and sanitary? Are the utilities working? Look for clues that might explain the patient's medical history or current problem: Is it too hot or too cold? A geriatric patient can have hypothermia or heatstroke in temperatures that are not considered extreme. Is there food available? Is the refrigerator stocked? Is there evidence of physical abuse? Is there evidence of alcohol or illegal drug use? Are there medications on the nightstand in the bedroom or bathroom?

In a nursing home or residential care facility, you will need to locate the patient's room and find a staff member who can explain why you were called. If the patient's mental status is altered, you need to find someone who can confirm the patient's identity and tell you the patient's history and whether the patient's behavior or level of consciousness is normal or altered. The presence of a hospital bed, oxygen tanks, or therapeutic devices can give you a clue to the patient's medical history. The environment may give you the answer to questions when the patient cannot.

The NOI may be difficult to determine in older people who have an altered mental status or dementia. Often it is someone other than the patient who called, so you must ask the family member, caregiver, or bystander for relevant information. Multiple and chronic disease processes may also complicate the determination of the NOI. Complaints from an older person may be vague, such as weakness, dizziness, or fatigue. These symptoms could be indicators of a more serious problem and require more assessment. For example, sudden changes in the ability to talk or walk without assistance could indicate a stroke, or the need to sleep with the upper body propped up by several pillows could suggest early heart failure. Chest pain, shortness of breath, and an altered level of consciousness should always be considered serious.

Knowing how your EMS system is organized will help you determine the additional resources that may be required. The sooner these resources are identified, the sooner they can be requested.

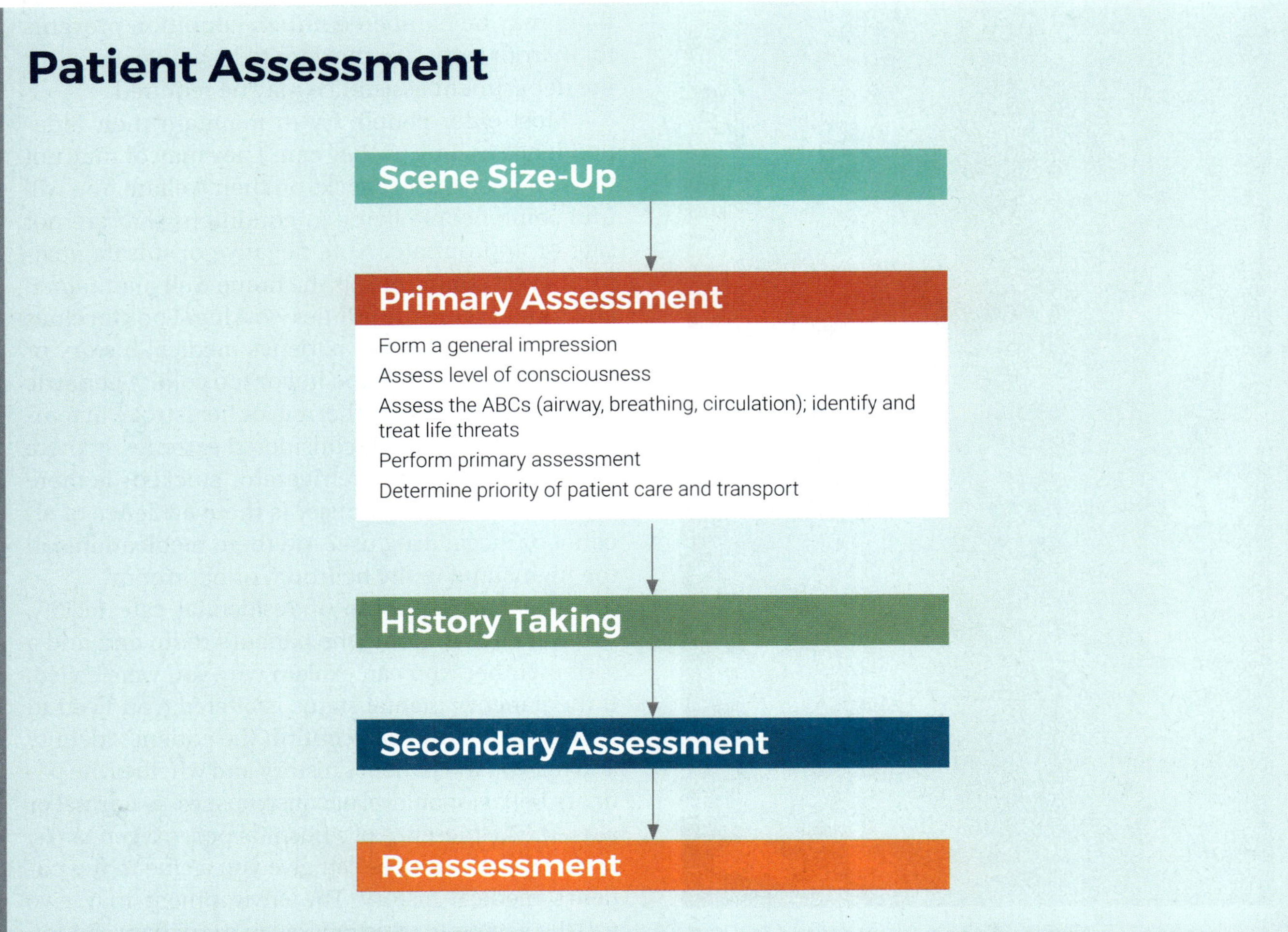

Primary Assessment

During the scene size-up, you evaluated scene hazards and threats, protected yourself and your team, and decided whether you needed additional resources. You also evaluated the dispatch information, the environment in which you are responding, and your initial view of the patient setting to begin to understand what happened and what action you should take. The heart of patient assessment begins when you first greet the patient and begin the **primary assessment**.

The primary assessment has a single, all-important goal: to identify and begin treatment of immediate or imminent life threats. To do this, you must examine the patient and assess the level of consciousness, airway, breathing, and circulation (ABCs). Sometimes this assessment is referred to as XABC, where X stands for eXsanguinating bleeding, because if the patient has obvious life-threatening external bleeding, the bleeding must be stopped first. During the primary assessment, you must identify signs of life threats and immediately work to correct them (**FIGURE 10-6**). From here you will be able to determine the priority of patient care and transport.

Identify and Treat Life Threats

Your role as an EMT is to determine if a life threat is present and, if so, to quickly address it.

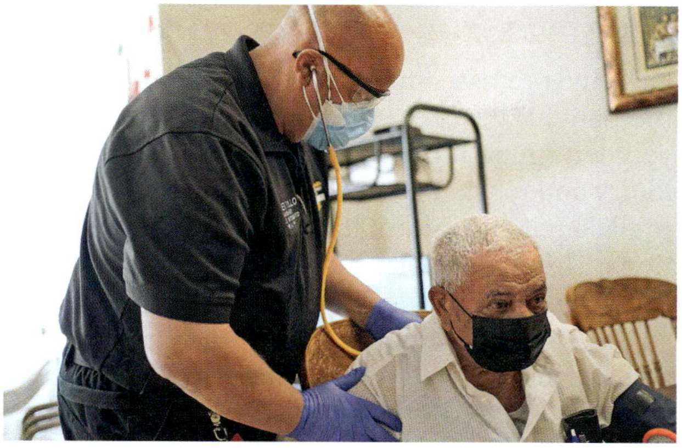

FIGURE 10-6 A survey of the patient's airway, breathing, and circulatory status is used to establish whether the patient has any life-threatening conditions and what you should do.

A life-threatening condition can quickly lead to death; this rapid process may begin with the absence or loss of meaningful communication between you and the patient. In some cases, the patient is unconscious when you arrive. In other cases, a severely sick or injured person becomes less aware of surroundings and stops being able to communicate. Unless an intervention occurs, loss of consciousness may follow. In both situations, the muscles become slack, among them the muscles of the jaw, thus permitting the tongue to lie against the posterior part of the throat, obstructing the airway and preventing air from entering. This causes the patient to stop breathing, stopping the intake of oxygen and the release of carbon dioxide. Without oxygen from the lungs, the heart cannot continue to function and will soon stop beating. Starved of oxygen-rich blood from the heart, brain cells will begin to die within a few minutes, leading to irreversible brain damage.

There are only a few general conditions that cause sudden death: airway obstruction, respiratory failure, respiratory arrest, shock, severe bleeding, cardiac arrest, and an intracranial event such as acute hemorrhage. Often these conditions are manageable or even reversible, but to address them you must be able to recognize them quickly and take immediate steps to correct them. This recognition is the purpose of the general impression and primary assessment.

Form a General Impression

Any time you meet someone new, you form an initial general impression about that person. Forming the **general impression** of a patient is a similar process, but the focus is on rapid identification of potentially life-threatening problems. The general impression is formed to determine the priority of care and is the first part of your primary assessment. Factors such as the person's age, sex, race, level of distress, and overall appearance may lead you to anticipate different problems. A woman of childbearing age who reports abdominal pain, for example, is susceptible to a significantly different spectrum of possible conditions than a middle-aged man with the same complaint because of both physiologic and anatomic differences.

Infants and children pose an additional challenge, as some children can provide helpful medical information and some cannot. While the age at which a child becomes a reliable interviewee varies, taking age into account will help you determine how to go about obtaining information and how strongly to rely on the information offered.

Street Smarts

When performing your initial assessment, you must be aware that assumptions, or bias, can trip you up and lead you down the wrong path. For example, you might assume that a confused patient in a nursing home has dementia when in fact their altered mental status is related to a low blood glucose level. On another call, you might fail to consider pregnancy in a transgender male who was assigned female at birth and is experiencing abdominal pain. Even more commonly, you might assume that a patient known to have alcohol use disorder is unresponsive because they are intoxicated, when in fact they have sustained serious head trauma. These errors are easy to make, which is why having a systematic approach to assessment will help you uncover illnesses or injuries you did not at first suspect.

The initial general impression continues during your introduction (**FIGURE 10-7**). Introduce yourself to the patient by stating something like, "Hi, I'm Sam, an EMT with the ambulance agency. I'm here to help you." After you introduce yourself, ask the patient about the chief complaint. Is the

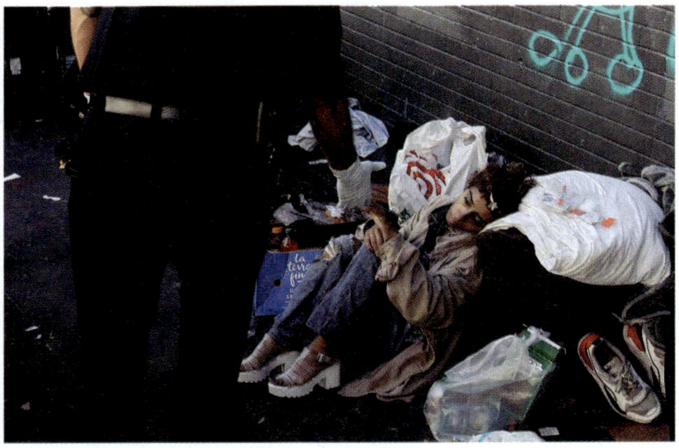

FIGURE 10-7 As you approach the patient, form a general impression of the individual's overall condition.

© Tayfun Coskun/Anadolu Agency/Getty Images.

patient able to respond to your greeting easily and appropriately? The patient's response can give you insight into the level of consciousness, airway patency, respiratory status, and overall circulatory status before you begin your examination. Sometimes life-threatening conditions are obvious even during the general impression. If a life-threatening condition is found, treat it immediately.

Interventions that you may provide as an EMT include administering oxygen or assisting ventilations for a patient who is hypoxic or unable to breathe adequately. Other interventions include performing CPR in cardiac arrest or administering glucose in a patient with diabetes who has altered mental status and a manageable airway. In specific cases, you may also assist with nitroglycerin, aspirin, or inhalers. Pharmacologic interventions require medical direction and are based on local protocol. See Chapter 12, *Principles of Pharmacology and Medication Administration*, for further discussion.

Scan for Signs of Uncontrolled External Bleeding

Uncontrolled external bleeding is a life-threatening emergency that you must recognize during your general impression. A large amount of bleeding that is squirting or gushing, has soaked through clothing, or is pooling under the patient should be considered life threatening, and you should attempt to control it before the assessment continues. Caring for non-life-threatening bleeding can occur following your focused assessment.

Assess Level of Consciousness

Early in your assessment, you will need to evaluate the patient's level of consciousness. This will help you determine if the patient has a life-threatening injury and to what extent the patient will be able to provide reliable information and follow your directions. The patient's level of consciousness can tell you a great deal about neurologic and physiologic status. The brain requires a constant supply of oxygen and glucose to function properly.

The **AVPU scale** tests a patient's **responsiveness**, offering important insight into the patient's level of consciousness. Specifically, the scale is used to assess how well the patient responds to external stimuli, including verbal stimuli (sound) and painful stimuli (such as pinching the trapezius muscle on top of the patient's shoulder). Criteria of the AVPU scale are described as follows:

- **A** **Awake and *a*lert.** The patient's eyes open spontaneously as you approach, and the patient appears to be aware of you and responsive to the environment. The patient is awake, appears to follow commands, and the eyes visually track people and objects.
- **V** **Responsive to *v*erbal stimuli.** The patient is not alert and awake. The patient's eyes do not open spontaneously. However, the patient's eyes do open when you speak them, or the patient is able to respond in some meaningful way when spoken to; for example, by moaning, speaking, or moving. You may need to speak loudly to assess whether the patient is responsive to verbal stimuli.
- **P** **Responsive to *p*ain.** The patient does not respond to your questions but moves or cries out in response to painful stimulus. There are appropriate and inappropriate methods of applying a painful stimulus (**FIGURE 10-8**). Be aware that some methods may not give an accurate result if a spinal cord injury is present.
- **U** ***U*nresponsive.** The patient does not respond spontaneously or to a verbal or painful stimulus. Unresponsive patients usually have no cough or gag reflex and lack the ability to protect their airway. If you are in doubt about whether a patient is truly unresponsive, assume the worst and treat appropriately.

To determine whether a patient who does not respond to verbal stimuli will respond to a

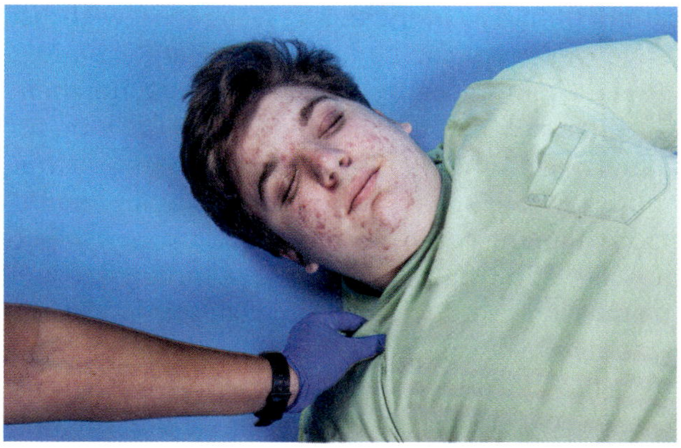

FIGURE 10-8 A patient's responsiveness can be assessed by applying an appropriate painful stimuli, such as gently but firmly squeezing the patient's trapezius muscle on top of the shoulder.

Words of Wisdom

When using the AVPU scale, be sure to note how the patient responded. If the patient is hard of hearing, tap the person's shoulder repeatedly with your fingers. If the patient responds, note that the patient is hard of hearing but responds to being tapped.

painful stimulus, gently but firmly apply pressure or squeeze the patient's tissue. One area where this technique may be applied is the trapezius area (the muscle above the collarbone). Other effective techniques to elicit a central pain response include applying upward pressure along the notch in the ridge of the medial aspect of the orbital rim along the underside of the eyebrow (without applying any pressure to the eyeball) or applying pressure using the flat part of your thumbs to the posterior aspect of the mandible at the temporomandibular joint, gradually increasing the pressure for 10 to 20 seconds.[3] A patient who moans or withdraws is responding to the painful stimulus. Be sure to note the type and location of the stimulus and how the patient responded. Remember the point is to see if the patient responds to or withdraws from the sensation of pain where you have caused it, not to injure the patient. Note that a patient who remains flaccid and does not move or make a sound is considered unresponsive.

For a patient who is alert or responsive or who becomes alert following your stimuli, next evaluate orientation. **Orientation** tests a patient's mental status by checking memory and thinking ability. The most common test evaluates a patient's ability to remember four things:

- **Person.** The patient is able to remember their name.
- **Place.** The patient is able to identify their current location.
- **Time.** The patient is able to tell you the current year, month, and day of the week.
- **Event.** The patient is able to describe what happened (the MOI or NOI).

These questions were not selected at random; it is paramount to assess for all four. They evaluate long-term memory (person and place), intermediate memory (place and time when asking year or month), and short-term memory (time when asking approximate day of the week and event). If the patient knows these facts, the patient is said to be "alert and oriented to person, place, time, and event," or "alert and oriented $\times$ 4."

It is important to determine, if possible, the patient's normal mental status. A number of circumstances, including ongoing illness, history of stroke, traumatic brain injury, developmental delay, Alzheimer disease, and more, may cause a patient to have a baseline of not being fully alert and oriented. Any deviation from alert and oriented to person, place, time, and event, or from a patient's normal baseline is considered an **altered mental status**. If the patient is alert to only person and place, for example, you would say the patient is alert and oriented to person and place but confused to time and event.

In most cases, identifying and correcting life-threatening issues begins with the airway, followed by breathing and circulation (ABC). However, you will find it is possible to assess all of these things quickly and sometimes simultaneously. For example, if a patient greets you and is speaking in full sentences, your assessment is likely to conclude their airway is open, they are breathing, and their heart is pumping blood. However, for some patients, you may need to intervene to address life-threatening injuries. For example, if you find a patient lying in a pool of blood from a leg injury that is vigorously bleeding, you must immediately apply direct pressure to the wound or have your partner do so. Because this is the life-threatening injury you witnessed first, you must take action to fix it, even though you have not yet assessed the airway or breathing. In this case, the ABC sequence becomes XABC. Remember, no part of the primary assessment is more important than the other. While you or your partner are controlling the bleeding, continue assessing the airway, breathing, and circulation.

Assess the Airway

An airway obstruction can result in partial or complete blockage of air movement into and out of the lungs and therefore inadequate **perfusion** of the entire body. As you move through the steps of the primary assessment, stay alert for signs of airway obstruction.

Airway Assessment in Responsive Patients

Patients of any age who are talking or crying have an open airway. However, watching and listening to how patients speak, particularly patients with respiratory problems, may provide important clues about the adequacy of their airway and the status of their breathing. A conscious patient who cannot speak or cry most likely has a severe airway obstruction.

If you identify an airway problem, stop the assessment process and work to clear the patient's airway. This may be as simple as positioning the patient so the air moves in and out, suctioning liquids from the airway, or removing an obvious foreign body from the patient's mouth; it may be as complex as abdominal thrusts or chest compressions to remove a foreign body from the airway. Although airway and breathing problems are not the same, their signs and symptoms often overlap. If your patient has signs of difficulty breathing or is not breathing, immediately take corrective actions using appropriate airway, oxygenation, or ventilation management techniques.

Airway Assessment in Unresponsive Patients

With an unresponsive patient or a patient with a decreased level of consciousness, immediately assess the patency of the airway. If the patient experienced a traumatic injury or the patient is unresponsive and you are unsure of the MOI, use the jaw-thrust maneuver to open the airway. If you cannot obtain a patent airway using the jaw-thrust maneuver or if it can be confirmed that the patient did not experience a significant MOI placing them at risk for spinal trauma, use the head tilt–chin lift maneuver to open and maintain a patent airway. Another cause of airway obstruction in an unconscious patient could be relaxation of the tongue muscles, allowing the tongue to fall to the back of the throat. Address this first by positioning the airway, then by placing an oral or nasal airway. Dentures, blood clots, vomitus, mucus, food, and other foreign objects may also create an obstruction. These obstructions can be cleared with manual techniques and suctioning. Once you have confirmed that the airway is clear, you can continue your assessment. For a detailed discussion of airway interventions, see Chapter 11, *Airway and Ventilation Management*.

Signs of airway obstruction in an unconscious patient include the following:

- Obvious trauma, blood, or other obstruction
- Noisy breathing, such as snoring, bubbling, gurgling, crowing, stridor, or other abnormal sounds (normal breathing is quiet)
- Extremely shallow or absent breathing (airway obstructions may impair breathing)

If any of these conditions exist, the airway is considered inadequate and you should open it using the head tilt–chin lift maneuver, suction as necessary, and use an airway adjunct as necessary. If the patient's airway is not managed quickly and efficiently, the body will not be able to receive the oxygen needed to survive.

Assess Breathing

A patient's breathing status is directly related to the adequacy of the patient's airway. Once you have made sure the patient's airway is open, confirm that the patient's breathing is present and adequate. A patient who is breathing without assistance is said to have **spontaneous respirations**, or spontaneous breathing.

As you assess the patient's breathing, ask yourself the following questions:

- Is the patient breathing?
- What is the patient's breathing rate, rhythm, and quality?
- Is the patient showing signs of hypoxia?

If the patient is not breathing, positive-pressure ventilations should be performed. If the patient is breathing adequately but remains hypoxic, administer oxygen. The goal for oxygenation in most patients is an oxygen saturation of greater than 94%.

If a patient is breathing, assess the rate and depth of breathing to determine if it is adequate for the patient. Remember that air entering the alveoli is the critical issue, not the number of breaths. When there are signs of respiratory failure, or impending respiratory failure, consider providing positive-pressure ventilations with an airway adjunct. Speech is a good indicator of whether a conscious patient is having difficulty breathing. Patients who can speak smoothly without unusual extra pauses are breathing adequately. However, patients who can speak only one word at a time, or must stop every two to three words to catch their breath, a condition known as **two- to three-word dyspnea**, are having significant difficulty breathing. These patients may need oxygen, medication, or assisted ventilation depending on their other assessment findings.

Words of Wisdom

Signs and symptoms of respiratory failure include decreasing consciousness, excessively fast or slow respiratory rate, shallow respirations, diminished breath sounds, decreased oxygen saturation, increased end-tidal carbon dioxide level, and pale, gray, or cyanotic skin color.

When assessing the rhythm of breathing, you will find that most people inhale and exhale over 1 to 2 seconds with a short pause between each breath. This pattern is regular and can be best observed in someone who is sleeping. Breathing that is irregular includes shallow or deep inhalations followed by periods of apnea. Irregular breathing can be observed in someone who is snoring and is often caused by the tongue falling to the back of the throat, obstructing air from entering the trachea. Irregular breathing is also associated with some types of head trauma. **Shallow respirations** can be identified by little movement of the chest wall (reduced tidal volume) or poor chest excursion. Deep respirations cause a significant rise and fall of the chest. Document when the patient's respirations are shallow or deep.

Observe how much effort is required for the patient to breathe when describing the quality of breathing. Breathing should appear effortless and can be described as nonlabored. Deep breathing, breathing that requires effort from the patient, or breathing that requires accessory muscles is described as labored. The presence of **retractions** (indentation above the clavicles and in the spaces between the ribs) or the use of **accessory muscles** of respiration is a sign of labored breathing. Accessory

YOU are the EMT

When you arrive on scene, a police officer directs you to a poorly kept apartment on the second floor. The scene is safe. You find the patient, a young man, lying in a prone position on the floor in the kitchen. He was found by his neighbor, who became concerned when he did not answer the door. You carefully roll the patient to a supine position and begin your assessment. An engine company arrives to provide assistance.

Recording Time: 0 Minutes	
Appearance	Blood draining from the side of the mouth
Level of consciousness	Responsive to pain with moaning and withdrawing
Airway	Bloody secretions and vomitus in the mouth
Breathing	Slow, shallow, and gurgling
Circulation	Radial pulse slow and weak; skin cool and pale (compared to baseline color)

3. Is spinal motion restriction indicated? Why or why not?

4. Which of these assessment findings requires your *most* immediate attention?

muscles include the neck muscles (sternocleidomastoid), the pectoralis major muscles of the chest, and the abdominal muscles. **Nasal flaring** and seesaw breathing in pediatric patients indicate inadequate breathing.[4]

Words of Wisdom

Paradoxical chest motion (or respirations) occurs when the chest, or part of it, moves in a direction opposite to its normal movement. Normally the chest expands (moves outward) when a person inhales, but during paradoxical chest motion, it would instead retract (moves inward). This paradoxical motion can occur in one part of the chest if there are multiple ribs fractured in more than one spot (called flail chest). In this example, only the part of the chest underlying the fractures moves in a paradoxical motion.

Seesaw breathing is a type of paradoxical breathing that occurs when the chest retracts during inspiration while the abdomen expands, then vice versa, creating a seesaw appearance of the chest and abdomen. While this sign can be seen in patients of any age, it is most common in children, especially infants.

Patients who are having marked difficulty breathing will instinctively assume a posture in which it is easier for them to breathe. There are two common postures that indicate the patient is trying to increase air flow. The first position is called the **tripod position**. In this position, a patient is sitting and leaning forward on outstretched arms with the head and chin thrust slightly forward; significant conscious effort is required for breathing. The second position, the **sniffing position**, is most commonly seen in children. The patient sits upright with the head and chin thrust slightly forward, and the patient appears to be sniffing.

Breathing that becomes progressively more difficult requires progressively more effort. When you can see that effort, the patient's breathing is described as **labored breathing**. As breathing becomes more labored, accessory muscles in the chest and neck are used, and the patient may make grunting sounds with each breath. In infants and small children, nasal flaring and supraclavicular and intercostal retractions are commonly associated with labored breathing. Sometimes the patient may be gasping.

Respiratory distress refers to difficulty breathing with an abnormal respiratory rate or effort. It can range from mild to severe and can progress to respiratory failure.

TABLE 10-1 Signs of Respiratory Distress and Failure

Respiratory Distress	Respiratory Failure
Agitation, anxiety, restlessness	Lethargy, difficult to rouse
Stridor, wheezing	Tachypnea with periods of bradypnea or agonal respirations
Accessory muscle use; intercostal retractions, neck muscle use	Inadequate chest rise/poor excursion
Tachypnea	Inadequate respiratory rate or effort
Mild tachycardia	Bradycardia
Nasal flaring, seesaw breathing, head bobbing	Diminished muscle tone

Typically, a person in respiratory distress is dyspneic and has an increase in respiratory effort and rate. Respiratory failure occurs when the blood is inadequately oxygenated or ventilation is inadequate to meet the oxygen demands of the body. Respiratory arrest is the ultimate result of respiratory failure if it is not corrected (**TABLE 10-1**).

Assess Circulation

Assessing circulation helps you to evaluate how well blood is circulating to the major organs, including the brain, lungs, heart, kidneys, and the rest of the body. A variety of problems can impair circulation, including blood loss, shock, and conditions that affect the heart and major blood vessels. Circulation is evaluated by assessing the patient's mental status, pulse, and skin condition. The first step in evaluating any patient is to rapidly scan for, identify, and control severe external bleeding.

Pulse

With each heartbeat, the ventricles contract, forcefully ejecting blood from the heart and propelling it into the arteries. Often referred to as a heartbeat, the **pulse** is the pressure wave that occurs as each heartbeat causes a surge in the blood circulating through the arteries. The pulse is most easily felt at a pulse point where a major artery lies near the surface and can be pressed gently against a bone or solid organ.

Your first consideration when taking a pulse is to determine whether the patient has one. To determine if a pulse is present, you will need to **palpate** (feel) the pulse. Hold together your index and long fingers and place your fingertips over a pulse point. Press gently against the artery until you feel intermittent pulsations. In responsive patients who are older than 1 year, palpate the radial pulse at the wrist (**FIGURE 10-9A**). In unresponsive patients older than 1 year, palpate the carotid pulse in the neck (**FIGURE 10-9B**). When palpating the carotid pulse, place the fingertips of your index and long fingers in the center of the throat on the windpipe and then slide your fingers toward you into the groove between the trachea and the neck muscle. This positions your fingers directly over the carotid artery. Only gentle pressure on one side of the neck should be used. Never press on the carotid arteries on both sides of the neck at the same time. Palpating too hard can occlude the blood flow, especially in a patient who has poor perfusion or is hypotensive.

Sometimes, you may have to slide your fingertips a little to each side and press again until you feel a pulse. When palpating a pulse, do not use your thumb. If you do so, you may mistake the strong pulsing circulation in your thumb for the patient's pulse.

Palpate the brachial pulse, located at the medial area (inside) of the upper arm, in children younger than 1 year (**FIGURE 10-9C**). With the infant lying supine, you can access the brachial pulse by elevating the arm over the infant's head. Because most infants have chubby arms, you need to press your adjacent fingertips firmly along the brachial artery,

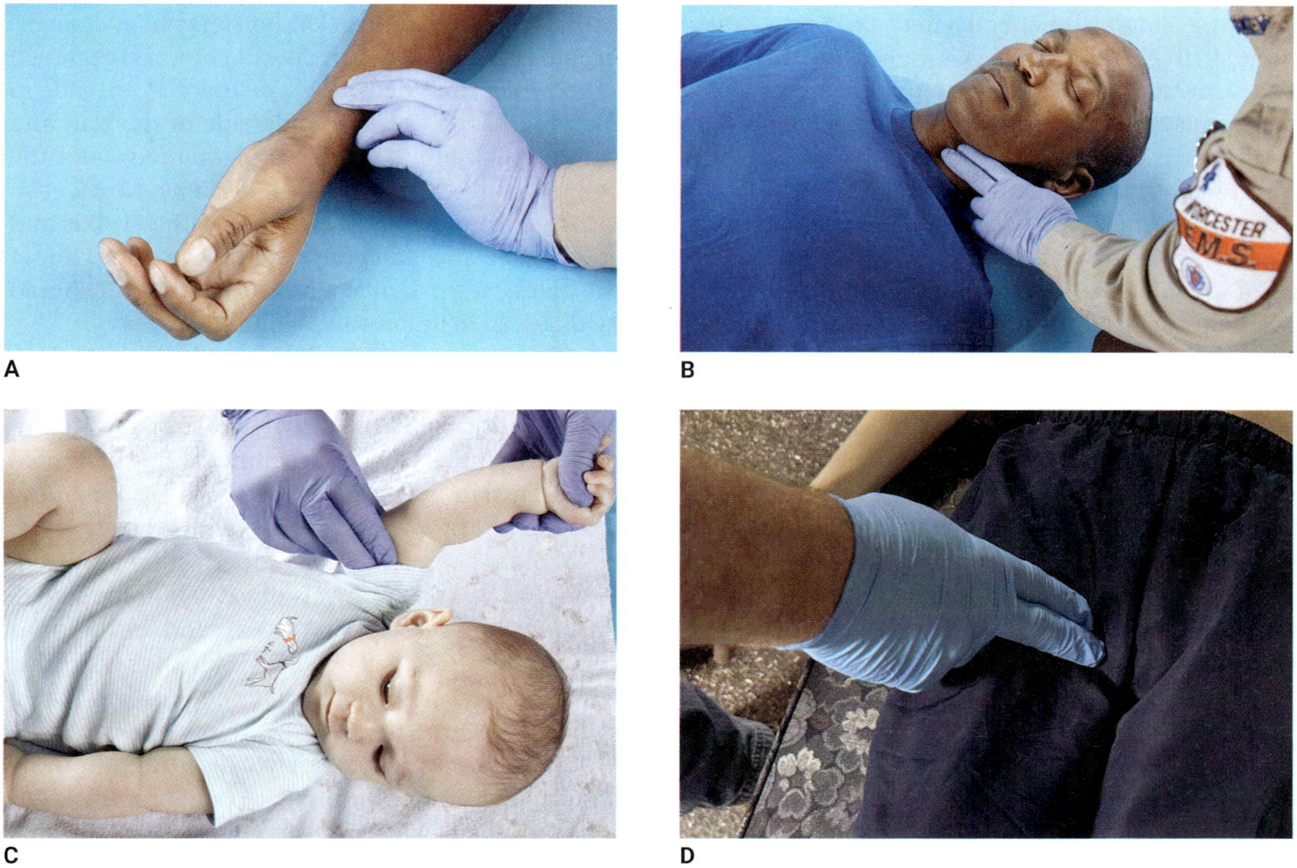

FIGURE 10-9 A. In responsive patients older than 1 year, assess the radial pulse. **B.** In unresponsive patients older than 1 year, assess the carotid pulse. **C.** In infants, assess the brachial pulse. **D.** In children older than 1 year, the femoral pulse may be used instead of the carotid pulse.

A-C: © Jones & Bartlett Learning; **D:** Courtesy of Rhonda Hunt.

which lies parallel to the long axis of the upper arm, to be able to palpate the pulse.

In children older than 1 year, the femoral pulse may be assessed as an alternative to the carotid pulse (**FIGURE 10-9D**).[5] To assess the femoral pulse, place two fingertips firmly in the crease at the groin where the leg meets the lower body between the hip and pubic bones.

If you cannot palpate a carotid pulse in an unresponsive patient, begin CPR. If an automated external defibrillator (AED) is available, have your partner turn it on and follow the voice prompts. An AED is indicated for use on patients who have been assessed to be unresponsive and pulseless. More information about using an AED is available in Chapter 14, *BLS Resuscitation*.

If the patient has a pulse but is not breathing, provide ventilations at a rate of 10 breaths/min for adults and 20 to 30 breaths/min for an infant or a child. Continue to monitor the pulse every 2 minutes to evaluate the effectiveness of your ventilations. If the patient becomes pulseless, start CPR and apply the AED. The apparent absence of a palpable pulse in a responsive patient is not caused by cardiac arrest. Therefore, never begin CPR or use an AED on a responsive patient.

With practice, you will be able to assess whether the pulse is too slow or too fast and whether it is regular or irregular without counting the pulsations. This will help to speed up your assessment of the ABCs and allow you to focus on finding other potentially life-threatening problems. An accurate pulse will be counted later, when you assess the full set of **vital signs**. A pulse rate that is too slow or too fast may change decisions related to transporting your patient. The pulse should be easily felt at the radial, brachial, carotid, or femoral artery and have a regular rhythm. If it is difficult to feel or is irregular, the patient may have problems with the circulatory system that may need further evaluation later in your assessment.

Skin Condition

The skin has many functions. It acts as insulation and protection from infection, helps maintain the water content of the body, and has a role in regulating body temperature by changing the amount of blood circulating through the surface of the skin.

Assessing the skin is one of the most important and most readily accessible ways of evaluating circulation and perfusion, blood oxygen level, and body temperature. Perfusion is assessed by evaluating a patient's skin color, temperature, moisture, and capillary refill. A normally functioning circulatory system perfuses the skin with oxygenated blood, allowing it to maintain an appropriate color, temperature, and moisture level for the environment. Inadequate blood flow to the skin will result in abnormal findings such as pale, cool skin. This may be associated with hypoperfusion to the brain, lungs, heart, and kidneys. The degree of hypoperfusion and how long it lasts will determine if a patient will sustain permanent injuries.

Skin Color

Many blood vessels lie near the surface of the skin. The skin's color is determined by the blood circulating through these vessels and the amount and type of pigment that is present in the skin. In patients with deeply pigmented skin (ie, dark skin), changes in color may be apparent only in certain areas, such as the fingernail beds, the mucous membranes in the mouth, the lips, the underside of the arm and palm (which are usually less pigmented), and the conjunctiva of the lower eyelids. The **conjunctiva** is the delicate membrane that lines the eyelids and covers the exposed surface of the eye. In addition, the palms of the hands and soles of the feet should be assessed in infants and children.

Poor peripheral circulation will cause the skin to appear pale (ie, lighter than its baseline color), ashen, or gray, possibly with a waxy translucent appearance similar to a white candle. Abnormally cold or frozen skin may also appear this way. When the blood is not properly saturated with oxygen, it appears blue. Therefore, in a patient with insufficient air exchange and low levels of oxygen in the blood, the blood and vessels appear blue, and the lips, mucous membranes, nail beds, and skin over the blood vessels appear blue or gray. This condition is called **cyanosis** (**FIGURE 10-10**).

High blood pressure may cause the skin to be abnormally flushed and red. A patient with a significant fever, heatstroke, sunburn, mild thermal burns, or other conditions in which the body is unable to properly dissipate heat will also appear to have red skin.

Changes in skin color may also result from chronic illness. Liver disease or dysfunction may

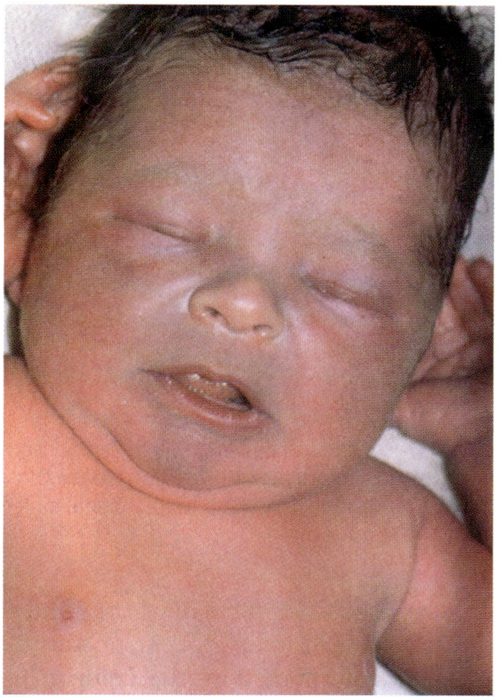

FIGURE 10-10 Cyanosis occurs when the patient has low levels of oxygen in the blood.

Street Smarts

Remember that changes to skin color, whether pallor, cyanosis, flushing, or jaundice, will present differently among patients depending on their baseline skin tone. The EMT must consider what is normal for each patient and may need to look for signs of abnormal perfusion in places such as the oral mucosa, conjunctiva, or nail beds. The observations of friends and family members on scene may also provide valuable insights (eg, "My dad looks really pale.").

cause **jaundice**, resulting in the patient's skin and sclera turning yellow. The **sclera** is the normally white portion of the eye and may show color changes even before skin color change is visible.

Skin Temperature

Normal skin temperature will be warm to the touch; normal body temperature is 98.6°F (37°C). Abnormal skin temperatures are hot, cool, cold, and clammy (moist). When the patient has a significant fever, sunburn, or hyperthermia, the skin feels hot to the touch. The skin will feel cool when the patient is in shock, has mild hypothermia, or has inadequate perfusion. With poor perfusion, the body pulls blood away from the surface of the skin and diverts it to the core of the body. The result is cool, pale, clammy skin; in your primary assessment, this is a good indication of hypoperfusion and shock. The skin will feel cold when the patient is in profound shock, has hypothermia, or has frostbite.

In most cases, it will initially be adequate to assess the patient's skin temperature by feeling the patient's forehead with the back of your gloved hand to see if it is excessively elevated or decreased. A more accurate temperature obtained with a thermometer during the vital signs assessment is often helpful. It is important to obtain a temperature in any patient who you think has an infection or has experienced an environmental emergency and in pediatric patients, because temperature changes can indicate a serious condition.

Fever is a common reason why parents or caregivers call 9-1-1 for children. Simply defined, a fever is an increase in body temperature, usually in response to an infection. Fever is the result of an internal body mechanism in which the body's internal thermostat is reset to adapt to inflammation or infection. Body temperatures of 100.4°F (38°C) or higher are considered abnormal. A fever may have many causes and is rarely life threatening. However, do not underestimate the potential seriousness of a fever that occurs in conjunction with a rash, which is a sign of serious illness, such as meningitis. Common causes of a fever in pediatric patients include infection (eg, pneumonia, meningitis, urinary tract infection), status epilepticus, and cancer.

Note that there are other conditions in which the core body temperature increases. Hyperthermia differs from fever in that it is an increase in body temperature caused by an inability of the body to cool itself. Hyperthermia is typically seen in warm environments, such as a closed vehicle on a hot day, or it can be related to serious adverse drug reactions such as aspirin overdose.

Skin Moisture

Dry skin is normal. Skin that is moist or wet from sweat, or excessively dry and hot, suggests a problem. In the early stages of shock, the skin will become slightly moist. Skin that is only slightly moist but not covered excessively with sweat is described as clammy, damp, or moist. When the skin is bathed in sweat, such as after strenuous exercise or when the patient is in shock, the skin is described as wet or **diaphoretic**.

Because the skin's color, temperature, and moisture are often related signs, you should consider them together. When recording or reporting your assessment of the skin, first describe the color, then the temperature, and last, whether the skin is dry, moist (clammy), or wet. For example, you could say or write, "Skin: pale, cool, and clammy."

Again, these characteristics are important findings in your primary assessment because hypoperfusion can lead to serious consequences if treatment is delayed or ignored.

Words of Wisdom

Remember to assess the following:

- Skin color
- Skin temperature
- Skin moisture

Capillary Refill

Capillary refill is often evaluated in pediatric patients to assess the ability of the circulatory system to perfuse the capillary system in the fingers and toes. When evaluated in an uninjured limb, capillary refill time (CRT) may provide an indication of the pediatric patient's level of perfusion. It should be kept in mind, however, that especially in an adult patient, capillary refill can be affected by the patient's position, age, history as a smoker, history of medical problems such as diabetes, medications the patient is currently taking, and low body temperature related to exposure to a cold environment (**hypothermia**), frozen tissue (**frostbite**), and **vasoconstriction** (narrowing of a blood vessel). Injuries to bones and muscles of the extremities may cause local circulatory compromise, resulting in hypoperfusion of an extremity rather than hypoperfusion of the body in general.

To test capillary refill, place your thumb on the patient's extremity, lifted slightly above the heart, and gently compress (**FIGURE 10-11A**). The blood will be forced from the capillaries in the nail bed. Rapidly release the pressure applied against the tip of the patient's finger. The nail bed will remain blanched (white) for a moment. As the underlying capillaries refill with blood, the nail bed will return to its normal pink color.

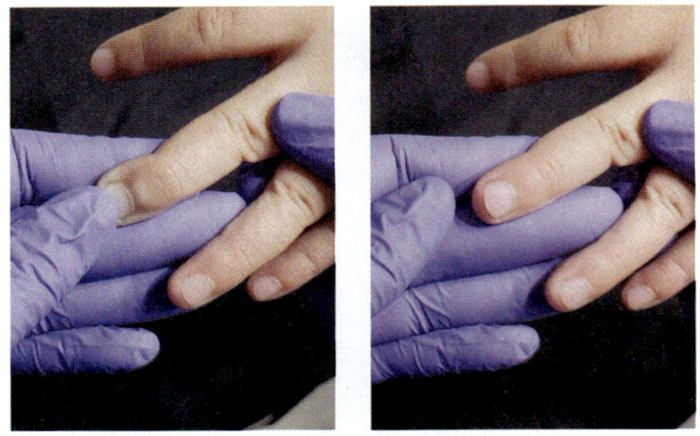

A B

FIGURE 10-11 A. To test capillary refill, gently compress the extremity until it blanches. **B.** Rapidly release the pressure, and count until it returns to its normal pink color.

To assess capillary refill in newborns and young infants, press on the forehead, chin, or sternum.

With adequate perfusion, the color in the infant's or child's nail bed should be restored to its normal pink color within 2 seconds, or about the time it takes to say "capillary refill" at a normal rate of speech (**FIGURE 10-11B**). Report and document the CRT as less than 2 seconds. Suspect poor peripheral circulation when capillary refill takes more than 2 seconds or the nail bed remains blanched. In this case, report and document the CRT as delayed or "CRT > 2." Again, delayed capillary refill is not always considered an accurate indication of poor perfusion, particularly in adult patients.

Words of Wisdom

Children who are in septic shock may have flushed, warm skin and normal capillary refill (<2 seconds), despite their shock state. Other findings such as history that suggests infection, increased temperature, changes in mental status, increased pulse, increased respiratory rate, and low blood pressure are needed to get the full picture in these cases.

Assess and Control External Bleeding

Identify and immediately control major external bleeding. In some cases, blood loss can be very rapid and can quickly result in shock or even death.

Bleeding from an artery is characterized by a spurting flow of blood. Often major blood loss is visible when approaching the patient.

Controlling external bleeding is often very simple. Initially, use direct pressure with your gloved hand; soon thereafter, a sterile bandage over the wound with continued pressure will control bleeding in most cases. Direct pressure stops the bleeding and helps the blood to coagulate, or clot, naturally. Most minor bleeding can be adequately controlled by using direct pressure. When direct pressure is not quickly successful or whenever you encounter obvious arterial hemorrhage of an extremity, apply a tourniquet. More information about applying a tourniquet is found in Chapter 25, *Bleeding*.

Pediatric Patients: Considerations During Primary Assessment

There are several additional challenges you may encounter when caring for a pediatric patient; thus, the primary assessment has some differences. Because young children might not be able to speak, your assessment of their condition must be based largely on what you can see and hear. Family members may be able to provide vital information about an incident or illness. Remember to include parents or caregivers as part of your team. Whenever possible, involve them in decisions and have them help comfort the infant or child during the assessment and any interventions.

As with the adult population, the objective of the primary assessment is to identify and treat immediate or potential threats to life. Infants and small children who have labored breathing for a sustained period, for example, will often become exhausted and eventually lose the strength to breathe. In infants and small children, cardiac arrest is most often caused by respiratory arrest.[5]

Pediatric Assessment Triangle

When you assess an infant or child, use the **pediatric assessment triangle (PAT)** to determine if the patient is sick or not sick. The PAT is a structured assessment tool that allows you to rapidly form a general impression of the child's condition without touching the child. This first-glance assessment or doorway assessment, which can be performed in

YOU are the EMT

Your partner suctioned the airway and begins assisting the patient's ventilations with high-flow oxygen while an EMT from the engine company obtains his vital signs. You ask the police officer to inspect the patient's apartment for anything suspicious. The officer on the engine tells you that the neighbor has no knowledge of the patient's medical history.

Recording Time: 5 Minutes	
Respirations	8 breaths/min and shallow (baseline); ventilations are being assisted
Pulse	42 beats/min; weak and regular
Skin	Cool and pale (compared with baseline)
Blood pressure	76/58 mm Hg
Oxygen saturation (Spo_2)	95% (with assisted ventilation)
Blood glucose level	108 mg/dL

Your primary assessment of the patient reveals no obvious signs of trauma, medical alert tags, or anything else that might explain his condition. The police officer did not find any pill bottles, drug paraphernalia, or anything else suspicious. His driver's license shows that he is 25 years old. You hear on the radio that a paramedic unit is approximately 18 minutes away.

5. Does the patient require further treatment at the scene? If so, what?
6. Should you remain at the scene and wait for the paramedic unit? Why or why not?

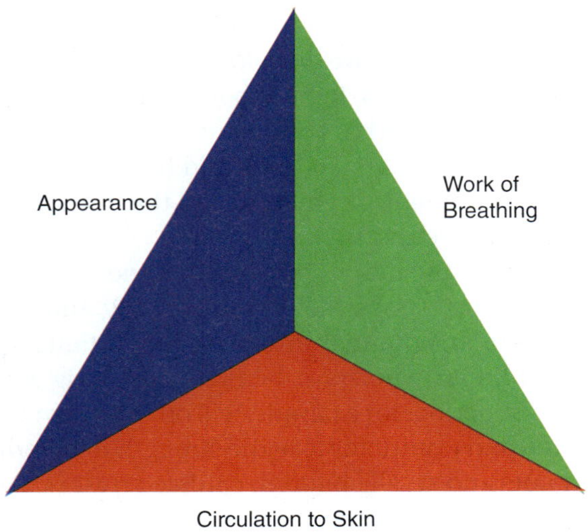

FIGURE 10-12 The three components of the pediatric assessment triangle (PAT) include appearance, work of breathing, and circulation to the skin.

less than 30 seconds, will help you to identify the general category of the patient's physical problem and establish urgency for treatment and/or transport.

The PAT consists of three elements: appearance (muscle tone and mental status), **work of breathing**, and circulation to the skin (**FIGURE 10-12**). The only equipment required for the PAT is your own eyes and ears.

As you evaluate the child's appearance, note the level of consciousness or interactiveness and muscle tone. Much of the information regarding the child's level of consciousness can be obtained by using the PAT. In addition, you can evaluate the child's level of consciousness by using the AVPU scale, modified as necessary for the child's age.

Infants and children with a normal level of consciousness will act appropriately for their age, exhibiting good muscle tone and maintaining good eye contact. An abnormal level of consciousness is characterized by age-inappropriate behavior or level of interactiveness, poor muscle tone, or poor eye contact with the parent or caregiver or with you. Remember, you are unfamiliar to the patient, so the patient may be anxious or frightened by your presence.

The mnemonic TICLS (pronounced "tickles") can also help to determine if the pediatric patient is sick or not sick. TICLS stands for Tone, Interactiveness, Consolability, Look or gaze, and Speech or cry (**TABLE 10-2**).

TABLE 10-2 Characteristics of Appearance: The TICLS Mnemonic

Characteristic	Features to Look For
Tone	Is the child moving or resisting examination vigorously? Does the child have good muscle tone? Or is the child limp, listless, or flaccid?
Interactiveness	How alert is the child? How readily does a person, object, or sound distract the child or draw the child's attention? Will the child reach for, grasp, and play with a toy or examination instrument, like a penlight or tongue blade? Or is the child uninterested in playing or interacting with the parent or caregiver or with the EMT?
Consolability	Can the child be consoled or comforted by the parent or caregiver or by the EMT? Or is the child's crying or agitation unrelieved by gentle reassurance?
Look or gaze	Does the child fix their gaze on a face, or is there a vacant, glassy-eyed stare?
Speech or cry	Is the child's cry strong and spontaneous or weak or high-pitched? Is the content of speech age-appropriate or confused or garbled?

A child's work of breathing increases as the body attempts to compensate for abnormalities in oxygenation and ventilation. Assessment for increased work of breathing in the pediatric patient is described in Chapter 16, *Respiratory Emergencies*.

Similar to adults, an important sign of perfusion is circulation to the skin. When cardiac output falls, the body, through vasoconstriction, shunts blood from areas of lesser need (such as the skin) to areas of greater need (such as the brain, heart, and kidneys). Pallor may result.

Pallor of the skin and mucous membranes may be seen in compensated shock; it may also be a sign

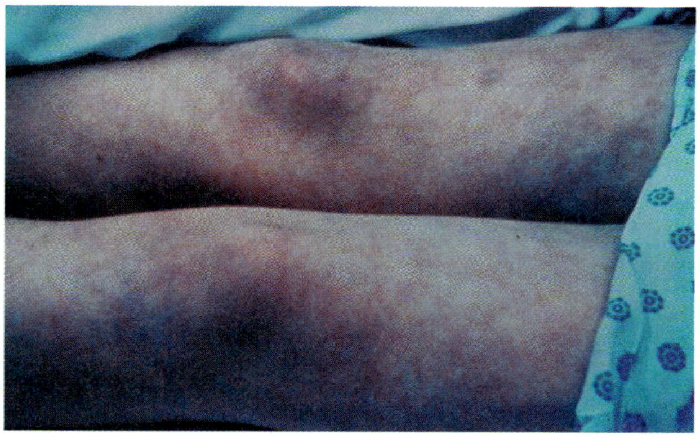

FIGURE 10-13 Mottling of the skin indicates poor perfusion and is the result of constriction of peripheral blood vessels.

Courtesy of Health Resources and Services Administration, Maternal and Child Health Bureau, Emergency Medical Service for Children Program.

of anemia or hypoxia. Mottling is caused by constriction of peripheral blood vessels and is another sign of poor perfusion (**FIGURE 10-13**).

The PAT can be particularly useful in the field when you are confronted with various possible causes of the patient's condition. Based on the PAT findings, you will decide if the child is in stable condition or requires urgent care.

Pediatric Hands-on Primary Assessment

As with adult patients, the primary assessment of the pediatric assessment begins with the ABCs, or the XABC sequence in the presence of life-threatening bleeding.

If the child's airway is open and the patient can keep it open, as is typical in conscious patients, assess respiratory adequacy. If the child is unresponsive or has difficulty keeping the airway clear, you must ensure that the airway is properly positioned and that it is clear of mucus, vomitus, blood, and foreign bodies. To properly assess breathing in infants and small children, expose their chest. Accessory muscle use is easier to see in patients of these ages and can provide valuable clues regarding their effort of breathing. If breathing is inadequate, administer oxygen; when respiratory failure is evident, provide positive-pressure ventilation using a bag-mask device. A detailed discussion of assessing and managing the pediatric patient's airway and breathing, including interventions for opening, clearing, and maintaining the airway, administering oxygen, and performing ventilation, is included in Chapter 11, *Airway and Ventilation Management.*

When you assess circulation, you must determine if the patient has a pulse, is bleeding, or is in shock. Remember, infants and children can tolerate only small amounts of blood loss before circulatory compromise occurs. Assess and control any active bleeding early in your assessment.

A pulse may be difficult to palpate if it is weak, very fast, or very slow. Remember, in infants, palpate the brachial pulse; in children older than 1 year, palpate the carotid or femoral pulse. Note the rate and quality of the pulse just as you do in adults. Strong **central pulses** usually indicate that the child is not hypotensive; however, this does not rule out the possibility of compensated shock. Weak or absent peripheral pulses indicate decreased perfusion. The absence of a central pulse after assessing for 5 to 10 seconds (ie, brachial in infants, carotid or femoral in older children) indicates the need for CPR.

Tachycardia may be an early sign of hypoxia or shock, but it may also reflect less serious conditions such as fever, anxiety, pain, and excitement. Like the respiratory rate and effort, the pulse rate should be interpreted within the context of the overall history, PAT, and the entire primary assessment.

A trend of an increasing or decreasing pulse rate may provide useful information and may suggest worsening hypoxia or shock, or improvement after treatment. When hypoxia or shock becomes critical, bradycardia occurs. As with slowing respirations, bradycardia in a pediatric patient is an ominous sign and often indicates impending cardiopulmonary arrest. When bradycardia develops in an infant or child, the priority intervention is positive-pressure ventilation with high-concentration oxygen. Feel the skin for temperature and moisture at the same time you assess the patient's pulse. Also estimate the CRT as previously described.

Assess the pediatric patient's level of consciousness using the AVPU scale.

Proper exposure of the pediatric patient is necessary to complete the hands-on primary assessment. The PAT requires that the parent or caregiver remove part of the pediatric patient's clothing to allow careful observation of the face, chest wall, and skin. Further exposure may be needed to fully evaluate physiologic functions, anatomic abnormalities, and unsuspected injuries or rashes. Be careful

> **Words of Wisdom**
>
> Remember that infants and children are susceptible to hypothermia because of poor thermoregulation and a larger ratio of body surface area to mass. You must ensure that pediatric patients stay warm, especially when they are ill or injured. Covering the head for newborns is an important measure to maintain body temperature because their head has a large surface area for heat loss.

to avoid heat loss, especially in infants, by covering the patient as soon as possible.

Geriatric Patients: Considerations During Primary Assessment

The general impression is an important aspect of all patient assessment and does not change when caring for a geriatric patient.

Remember that anatomic changes that occur as a person ages predispose geriatric patients to airway problems. Aging and disease can compromise a patient's ability to protect the airway. Gag reflex and normal swallowing mechanisms may be impaired, and changes in level of consciousness, dementia, and weakness or paralysis following a stroke can cause airway obstruction or aspiration. Ensure that the patient's airway is open and is not obstructed by dentures, vomitus, fluids, or blood. Airway and breathing issues should be treated rapidly and monitored constantly. The effects of anatomic changes in the older patient are discussed in Chapter 16, *Respiratory Emergencies*.

Poor perfusion is a serious issue in an older adult. People who normally live with compromised circulation have little in the way of reserves during a circulatory crisis. Physiologic changes may negatively affect circulation. Less responsive nerve stimulation may lower the rate and strength of the heart's contractions, so lower heart rates and weaker and irregular pulses are found in some older patients. Vascular changes and circulatory compromise might make it difficult to feel a radial pulse on an older patient. If choosing an alternative pulse point such as the carotid artery, press gently. Another option is to listen to the apical pulse right over the heart. The pulse may be irregular because of heart rhythm problems. It is important to determine if cardiac abnormalities in an older patient indicate an acute emergency or a chronic condition. Acute emergencies should be managed rapidly.

Patient assessment may be more complicated in an older adult, and multiple problems can exist. Any complaints that suggest compromise of the airway, breathing, or circulation should result in the individual being transported as a priority patient. Older people do not have the reserves that younger adults do, and they can easily decompensate. Older patients may have multiple chronic diseases processes and take multiple medications, both of which can further complicate patient assessment. Even a general complaint of weakness and dizziness can be an indication of something more serious such as a heart problem or pneumonia. Consider early on if ALS treatment and immediate transport is appropriate and available. If possible, try to take the patient to a facility where the patient has been treated before and has an established relationship.

> **Words of Wisdom**
>
> Because of fear related to hospitalization, many older people will delay calling 9-1-1 until their problem is life threatening. Be prepared for a worst-case scenario.

Determine Priority of Patient Care and Transport

The primary assessment will assist you in determining transport priority. If you do not identify any injuries that require treatment or immediate transport when completing your assessment of the ABCs, you may find indications for immediate transport during your secondary assessment. For example, you may identify an internal hemorrhage by the presence of a distended or firm abdomen or bilateral femoral fractures. These types of conditions are indications for immediate transport.

> **Words of Wisdom**
>
> The decision to transport your patient immediately following the primary assessment or to stay on scene and continue the assessment can be considered following the ABCs.

Priority designation is used to determine if a patient needs immediate transport or will tolerate a few more minutes on scene. Patients with any of the following conditions are examples of high-priority patients and should be transported immediately:

- Unresponsive
- Difficulty breathing
- Uncontrolled bleeding
- Altered level of consciousness
- Severe chest pain
- Pale skin or other signs of poor perfusion
- Complicated childbirth
- Severe pain in any area of the body

Recognizing the need to transport serious trauma patients is of such importance that you may hear colleagues refer to the **Golden Period**. This term refers to the time from injury to definitive care, during which treatment of shock and traumatic injuries must occur to maximize the patient's chance of survival (**FIGURE 10-14**). Over time, the body has increasing difficulty in compensating for shock and traumatic injuries. For this reason, you should

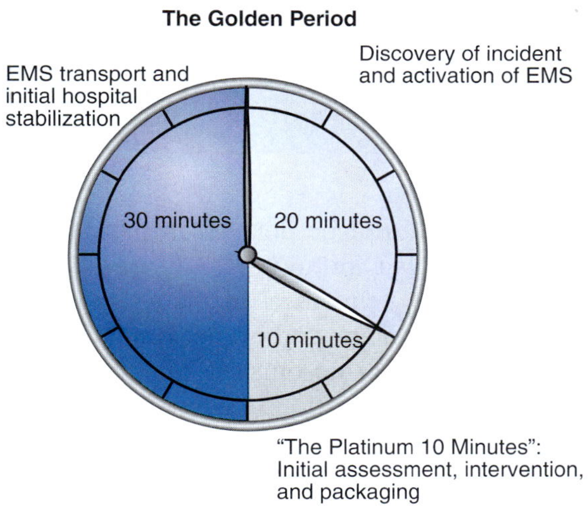

FIGURE 10-14 The Golden Period is the time during which treatment of shock or traumatic injuries is most critical and the potential for survival is best.

Words of Wisdom

The concept of a "Golden Hour" was conceived in the 1960s by R Adams Cowley, MD. The idea was that for a person who has sustained a critical injury, definitive care must be started promptly. Because the Golden *Hour* is not a strict 60-minute time frame and depends on the patient and the injuries, it is better thought of as the Golden *Period*. A related concept, the Platinum 10 Minutes, suggests that transport of a person who has sustained a critical injury should begin within 10 minutes of the injury.

spend only as much time on scene as necessary to treat your patient's life-threatening injuries before beginning transport.

Some patients may benefit from remaining on scene and receiving continuing care. For example, it would be important to apply splinting to a patient who has sustained an isolated injury to a bone, as relief from the pain is more important than immediate transport in an isolated injury. Likewise, an older patient with chest pain may be better served on scene by being administered aspirin and nitroglycerin and waiting for an ALS vehicle than by immediate transport. When indicated, ALS support should be requested if a unit is not already en route to the scene. If ALS is delayed or farther away, coordinating a rendezvous may be a better decision for a high-priority patient. Your decision to stay on scene or transport immediately will be based on your patient's condition, the availability of more advanced help, the distance you must transport the patient, and your local protocols.

Correct identification of high-priority patients is an essential aspect of the primary assessment and helps to improve the outcome in some patients. Although initial treatment is important, remember that immediate transport is one of the keys to the survival of patients who need immediate care that cannot be provided outside the hospital. Transport should be initiated as soon as practical and possible.

Patient Assessment

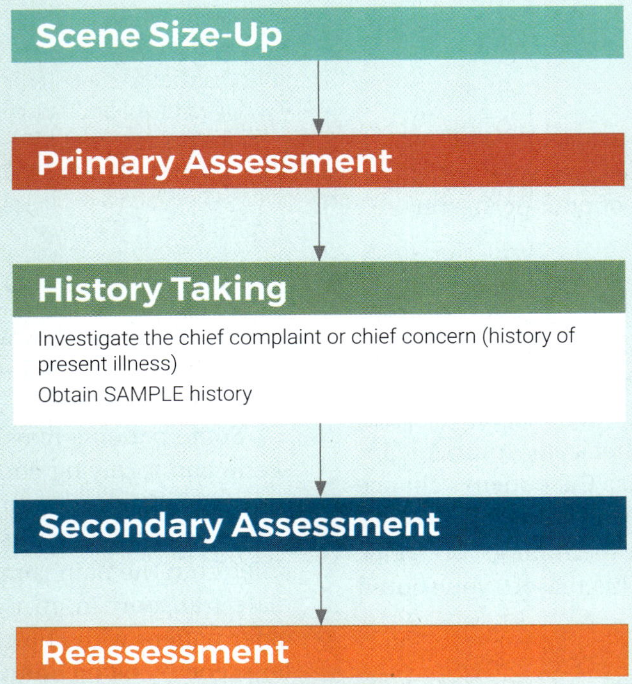

History Taking

Although history taking is listed after the primary assessment, it is an integral part of the assessment. Thus, you may complete the history on scene, in the ambulance, or both. You may work with another responder, allowing one person to ask questions of people in the vicinity while the other initiates patient assessment. It is important to gather as much history as possible on scene from family, friends, and bystanders because this information may not be obtainable once transport is initiated. Also check for medical identification tags or jewelry that may indicate preexisting medical information. If the patient is able to answer questions or a family member is transported in the ambulance with the patient, history taking can be expanded while en route. The history may be essential to determining patient treatment; however, transport should not be delayed in patients who are in an unstable condition.

History taking provides details about the patient's chief complaint and an account of the patient's signs and symptoms. It is important to document all information gathered during this phase of the assessment process. This includes demographic information, past medical history, and current health status of the patient. Be sure to document the following information:

- Date of the incident
- Patient's age
- Patient's sex and gender identity (if it is different than their sex assigned at birth)
- Patient's ethnicity
- Past medical history, including any pertinent information about the patient's condition, such as medical problems, traumatic injuries, and surgical procedures

- Patient's current health status, including diet, medications, drug use, living environment and hazards, physician visits, vaccine history (if relevant), and family history

Investigate the Chief Complaint or Chief Concern (History of Present Illness)

The patient's chief complaint or chief concern is usually the reason EMS was dispatched (**FIGURE 10-15**). After the primary assessment, gather further information about the chief complaint and identify if there are any associated complaints. Use eye contact to encourage the patient to continue speaking, and repeat statements back to the patient to show that you understand the situation. Avoid interrupting, and be empathetic toward the patient's situation.

You must consider the wide range of age groups with which you will interact. Information from infants and children may come from a parent or caregiver. Some older patients may be slow to respond or have multiple complaints. Over time, EMTs develop their own particular method or style to obtain a patient's chief complaint and history. See Chapter 4, *Communications and Documentation.*

You will also gather information about the chief complaint from observable clues and information received from the original dispatch. If the patient is unresponsive, information about the patient, pertinent past medical history, and clues about the immediate incident may be obtained from family members present, a person who may have witnessed the situation, bystanders, medical alert jewelry, or other patient medical history documentation (**FIGURE 10-16**). Observable signs may include things such as the patient not being able to respond using full sentences and appearing to have some respiratory distress. These clues may indicate the patient's chief complaint/concern is "difficulty breathing," or the clues may be part of a bigger problem that has to do with a lengthy history of cardiac problems.

For example, you are called to the home of an older man who fell. This information was provided by the dispatcher, and you can use it to help process all clues that may be presented in what appears to be a simple fall. You find the patient lying at the bottom of the stairs. How many stairs are there, are they carpeted, and is the floor concrete, wood, or tile? Additional observable clues are used to determine a chief complaint or chief concern. The patient states he did fall, which is how the injury occurred, and

Words of Wisdom

Recall the difference between a symptom and a sign: A symptom is a subjective condition that the patient feels and tells you about. A sign is an objective finding that you can detect by observing or examining the patient.

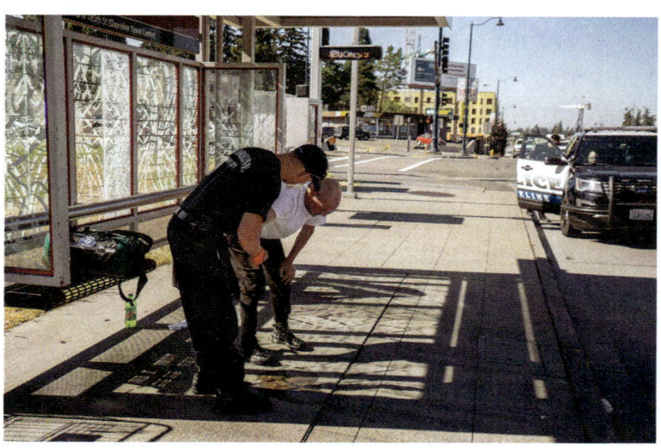

FIGURE 10-15 The patient's initial response to the question, "What's bothering you most today?" is the chief complaint.

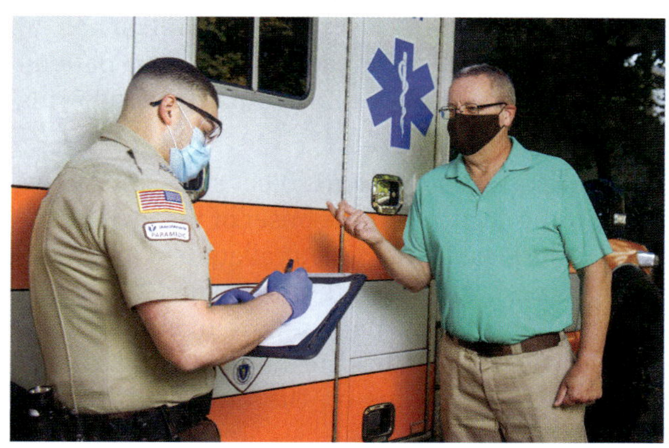

FIGURE 10-16 If the patient is unresponsive, try to obtain a pertinent history or patient information from family or bystanders.

he reports pain in the right arm. However, was the fall the result of tripping on a step, or was it associated with a medical problem such as dizziness, vertigo, or a syncopal episode, any of which may have caused the fall? It is your responsibility to look at the possibilities and ask the appropriate questions to determine the patient's primary complaint.

Street Smarts

In some cases, what the patient tells you is the chief complaint will not be your chief concern. For example, a patient with no prior medical history who has fallen says, "My wrist hurts," but you observe that her speech is slurred and she is not moving her right arm or leg. In this case, your chief concern will be possible stroke even though it is not her chief complaint.

Patient interaction sometimes occurs during the worst possible time in the patient's life. These are emergency situations in which patients are afraid and confused. Some patients assume this could be the end of their lives. Sorting through the clues from the emergency scene itself, from the patient's complaints, and from the patient's signs and symptoms and past medical history will assist you in understanding the cause of your patient's problem and enable you to make appropriate, timely decisions about your patient's care.

Obtain SAMPLE History

As you obtain a patient history, you can use some of the standard techniques for questioning patients. By obtaining a **SAMPLE history**, you will be able to gather important information from the patient. Use the mnemonic SAMPLE to obtain the following information:

- S **Signs and symptoms.** What signs and symptoms occurred at the onset of the incident?
- A **Allergies.** Is the patient allergic to any medication, food, or other substance? What reactions did the patient have to any of them? If the patient has no known allergies, you should note this on the run report as "No known allergies."
- M **Medications.** What medication is the patient prescribed? What dosage is prescribed? How often does the patient take the medication? What prescription, over-the-counter, and herbal medications has the patient taken in the last 12 hours? Are there medications the patient has been prescribed but is not taking? Has the patient taken recreational drugs or ingested alcohol?
- P **Pertinent past medical history.** Does the patient have any history of medical, surgical, or trauma occurrences? Is there important family history that should be known?
- L **Last known.** When and what did the patient last eat or drink? When were they last seen to be well (such as in the setting of a stroke)? When was the patient's last menstrual period (women of childbearing age) or last bowel movement (abdominal pain)?
- E **Events leading up to the injury or illness.** What are the key events that led up to this incident? What occurred between the onset of the incident and your arrival? What was the patient doing when this illness started?

OPQRST

You may find it helpful to use the **OPQRST** mnemonic for gathering additional information about a patient's history of present illness and current symptoms. Although OPQRST can be used most easily for questions about pain, it can be adapted to quantify other symptoms such as dizziness, nausea, or dyspnea (shortness of breath or difficulty breathing).

- O **Onset.** What were you doing when the symptoms began? Did your symptoms begin suddenly or progress slowly? Did you experience any other symptoms with the onset? For example, when the chest pain started, did you feel nauseated?
- P **Provocation/palliation.** Does anything make the symptoms better or worse? How are you most comfortable?
- Q **Quality.** What does the symptom feel like? Is it sharp, dull, crushing, tearing? Does it come in waves? Ask the patient to describe the symptom.
- R **Region/radiation.** Where do you feel the symptom? Does it move anywhere?
- S **Severity.** On a scale of 0 to 10, with 0 being "nothing at all" and 10 being "the worst you can imagine," how would you rate your symptom?
- T **Timing.** How long have you had the symptom? When did it start?

Pediatric Patients: Considerations When Investigating Chief Complaint or Chief Concern

Your approach to the history will depend on the child's age. Historical information for an infant, toddler, or preschool-age child will need to be obtained from the parent or caregiver. When caring for an adolescent, you will usually be able to obtain most of the immediate information from the patient; however, consult the parent or caregiver for a complete history.

Information about sexual activity, the possibility of pregnancy, or the use of illicit drugs or alcohol should be obtained from an adolescent patient in private. Adolescents will be reluctant to provide this information in the presence of their parents or caregivers. When asking sensitive questions, assure the adolescent that this information is important and is needed to provide the most appropriate care.

Question the parent or child about the immediate illness or injury based on the child's chief complaint. Together with an evaluation of the child's medical history, this may provide clues to the underlying illness or injury and other conditions that may exist.

When you interview a parent or caregiver or the older child about the chief complaint, consider inquiring about the following additional information:

- Effects of the illness or injury on the child's behavior
- Patient's typical activity level
- Recent eating, drinking, and urine output
- Change in bowel or bladder habits
- Presence of rashes

Assessment of pain is important. When assessing pain in a child, you must consider their developmental age. The ability to recognize and describe pain improves as a child gets older. For example, crying and agitation in an infant may be the result of a wet diaper or hunger. Meanwhile, a 3-year-old child can say, "My tummy really hurts." In children ages 3 and older, studies by the American Academy of Pediatrics and the Society for Academic Emergency Medicine suggest using a pain scale such as the Wong-Baker scale to assess pain in children and patients with a developmental delay. To use the scale, ask the child to point to the picture that shows how their pain feels and then document the number below the figure they select in your patient report (**FIGURE 10-17**).

If the parent or caregiver is unable to accompany you to the hospital, obtain a name and phone number so hospital staff can call if there are questions. This might be the case when you respond to a day care facility or babysitter's location or when a parent must remain at the scene to care for other children. Most day care facilities require emergency contact information, past medical history, and/or a list of current prescribed medications taken by the child in case of an emergency. Care may be delayed if this information is not discovered early; however, never delay care of a critical patient.

Geriatric Patients: Considerations When Investigating Chief Complaint or Chief Concern

Begin by inquiring about the chief complaint or history of the present illness. Find and account for all medications. If a patient lives alone, look for a list of medications on the refrigerator or a notice by the front door. The Vial of Life is one program that recommends creating a medication history for caregivers or EMS personnel that is to be stored in a vial on the top shelf of the refrigerator door. A similar

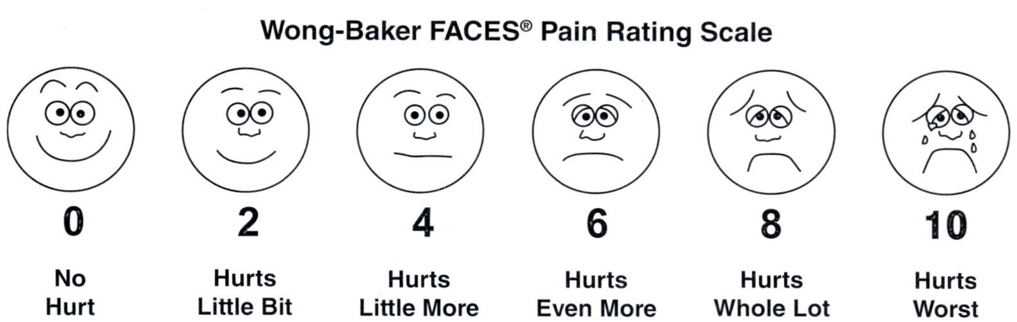

FIGURE 10-17 The Wong-Baker FACES pain rating scale.

program called the File of Life provides a card containing medical information that is stored in a magnetized pouch outside the refrigerator. There may be similar local programs in your area. These programs recommend that the home owner place a decal by the door to alert EMS to the Vial or File of Life.

Communication may be more complicated with an older adult due to changes in hearing and vision, but it is critical that you obtain a thorough patient history. It is best to obtain what information you can directly from the patient, but family or caregivers may need to assist.

The determination should be made early regarding whether an altered level of consciousness or mental status is acute or chronic. Remember that chronic mental status impairment is not a normal process of aging but is caused by a pathologic or disease process. You should never accept confusion as normal. It is important for you to determine your patient's baseline mental status; question family members, if available.

Getting an accurate SAMPLE history can be complicated. The chances are good that the chief complaint is related to a chronic medical problem, and the patient may have experienced it before. Is the patient taking any new medications? Make sure you have a list of the patient's medications, and take the medications with you to the hospital if possible. Patient medications can reveal much information about a patient's history. The hospital will also need to determine if the patient has been taking the medications as instructed. If time and opportunity allow, check the patient's pill sorter if they have one. Has the patient taken every dose this week? Has the patient taken the medications that are scheduled for tomorrow or the next day (**FIGURE 10-18**)?

The last meal is particularly important in a patient with diabetes. A history of last oral intake can indicate that the patient may be dehydrated. Last, what is the event that prompted the call? Again, it is advantageous to provide transport to a facility that "knows" the patient's medical history if the patient's condition and other factors allow.

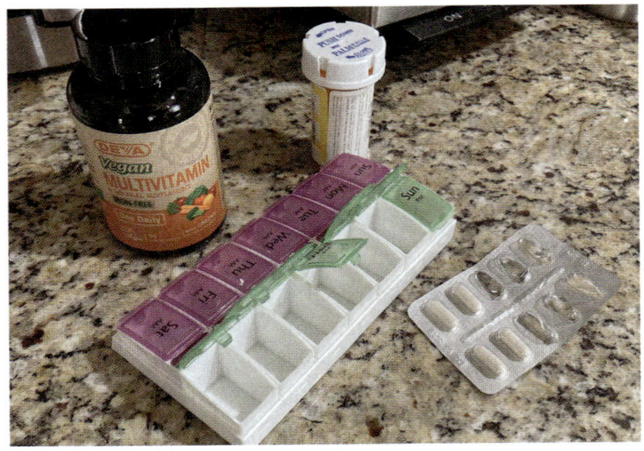

FIGURE 10-18 Many geriatric patients take multiple medications. While obtaining the patient's history, try to determine which medications the patient is taking and whether they have been taken correctly. Observing the patient's pill sorter or medication containers can provide helpful insights.

> **Street Smarts**
>
> Some geriatric patients may appear angry and will be curt in their responses. This may be associated with an underlying illness (eg, dementia), may be a medication side effect, or may relate to the frustration of having lost much of their independence. Be patient and do not take it personally if a geriatric patient seems upset or seems to be yelling at you.

Identify Pertinent Negatives

The process of gathering a patient's past medical history, history of present illness, and signs and symptoms is important, but sometimes just as important are the signs and symptoms that the patient does not have. These important negative findings are referred to as **pertinent negatives**. Often, a patient's complaint would be expected to be associated with other related findings. Examples include chest pain with shortness of breath, palpitations, and sweating or a severe allergic reaction with itching, hives, and trouble breathing. The absence of these findings is relevant, and should be reported and documented. Pertinent negatives are often helpful in identifying a patient's problem and choosing an appropriate treatment.

Critical Thinking and Clinical Decision Making in EMS

Assessment is the logical and ordered process of identifying problems and setting priorities to provide treatment, but it is important that this is not done robotically without understanding. To provide quality patient care in this environment, you must become an expert in gathering facts and other clues; interpreting that data; determining what the problem is; developing a plan; communicating the plan to your team and implementing it; and reassessing to evaluate the effect of your plan. This process of clinical decision making involves critical thinking and must be performed continuously during the dispatch, on-scene, and post-scene phases of a call. Without critical thinking, you will find yourself confused and unable to manage any incident that does not appear exactly the same as described in the textbook. Each of these phases is explained in detail in Chapter 9, *The Team Approach to Health Care*.

Taking History on Sensitive Topics

Alcohol and Drugs

The signs and symptoms a patient may have while under the influence of alcohol or mind-altering drugs may be confusing, hidden, or disguised. Many patients who misuse alcohol and/or drugs may deny having any problems or regularly using them. Families, friends, and coworkers may be unaware that a patient has any drug or alcohol troubles because patients often hide their dependency. The reasons patients deny using alcohol or drugs can vary greatly. It may be out of fear of losing their employment or driver's license, worry about what friends may think about them, and embarrassment or insecurity about their disorder.

The history that you gather from a person with a substance use disorder may be unreliable. The signs and symptoms of alcohol or drug use may be masked by the patient's presentation. Use all your senses when providing patient care. You can assure patients who you suspect are withholding information for fear of penalty that their privacy is protected and their honesty will improve the level of care you can provide.

Work to establish a strong rapport with your patients. Do not judge a patient who may have a chemical dependency, and be professional in your approach. Above all, impress on the patient that information received will be kept in confidence. Then and only then, a patient may open up to you and provide valuable information.

Physical Abuse or Violence

Suspected physical abuse or intimate partner violence must be reported to the appropriate authorities. Follow your state laws and local protocols when dealing with such cases. If you suspect a patient is a victim of physical abuse or intimate partner violence, do not accuse any person of being responsible for the situation. Instead, immediately involve law enforcement (**FIGURE 10-19**).

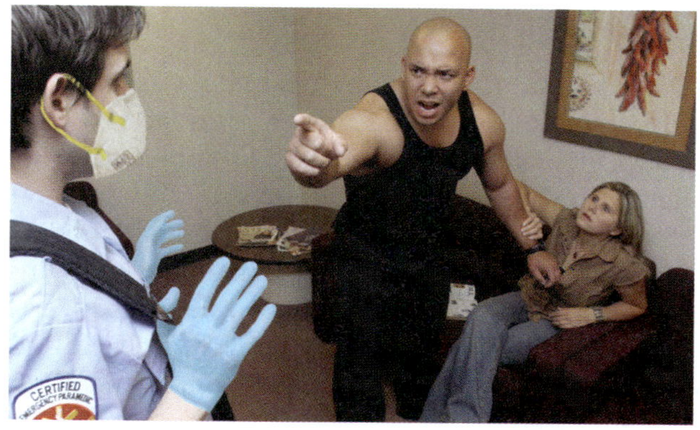

FIGURE 10-19 Do not handle potentially violent calls alone. Summon law enforcement personnel.

Because abuse and physical violence are sensitive situations, look for hidden clues that such a situation exists. When gathering a history, determine if the information provided by the patient and others present at the scene is inconsistent. Do you observe multiple injuries in various stages of healing? Are some bruises red, black, brown, or even green? In some cases, a victim of abuse or violence will not tell you what happened because of fear of further violence when EMS is not present. Victims may not answer your questions because the physical aggressor is still present and is answering questions for the patient. In these cases, separate the people present and interview the patient in a safe place, such as your ambulance. See Chapter 35, *Patients With Special Challenges*, for further discussion of abuse and violence relating to specific patient populations.

When involved with cases of physical abuse, be observant and open-minded, have a high index of suspicion, and be nonjudgmental. Documentation will be very important in cases of abuse and intimate partner violence. Your documentation should be an objective report of the facts. Avoid subjective, judgmental statements, and include any pertinent statements made by the patient or others present using quotation marks. Remember, these prehospital situations could result in legal proceedings. You may be summoned several years later to provide testimony regarding what may have happened, which makes accurate and thorough documentation essential.

Sexual History

Obtaining information about a patient's sexual history may be limited, because a number of factors may influence the details a patient may reveal. Religious beliefs, cultural stereotypes, and society's expectations may have a major role in patients not revealing a very personal side of their life, including practices considered by some people to be bizarre or exotic. In addition, some patients find sharing information regarding their sexual history with others uncomfortable.

As an EMT, you will be involved in the care of female patients reporting pelvic or lower quadrant abdominal pain. You should consider all women of childbearing years who are reporting lower quadrant abdominal pain to be pregnant unless ruled out by history or other information. There are several questions to ask when faced with this prehospital scenario:

- Is there any chance you could be pregnant?
- When was your last menstrual period?
- Are you using any form of birth control?
- *If the patient is bleeding:* How many sanitary pads or tampons have you used?
- Do you have urinary frequency or burning?
- Do you have any unusual vaginal discharge?
- What is the severity of cramping, and are there any foul odors?
- Have you been injured?

When caring for a male patient, you must inquire about urinary symptoms:

- Is there pain associated with urination?
- Do you have any discharge, sores, or an increase in urination?
- Do you have burning or difficulty voiding?
- Have you experienced any trauma?

Street Smarts

As an EMT, you will be caring for patients from all communities and you should work to make your ambulance a safe space. If a patient shares with you a name they prefer or their pronouns, make every effort to use them during your assessment. Ask the patient if they would like you to disclose this information at the hospital or if they would prefer to do so.

YOU are the EMT

As you are packaging the patient and preparing to move him from his building, the paramedic unit is dispatched to another call. There are no other paramedic units in your district. You move the patient from his apartment and load him into the ambulance. With an EMT from the engine company assisting you in the back with the patient, you depart the scene and reassess the patient. The closest appropriate hospital is 25 minutes away.

Recording Time: 12 Minutes	
Level of consciousness	Unconscious and unresponsive
Respirations	6 breaths/min (baseline); ventilations are being assisted at a rate of 10 breaths/min
Pulse	44 beats/min; weak and regular
Skin	Pale and cool; cyanosis noted around mouth
Blood pressure	78/54 mm Hg
Oxygen saturation (Spo_2)	88% (with assisted ventilation)

7. How has your patient's condition changed from the previous assessments?
8. What should you do in response to the patient's change in condition?

Patient Assessment

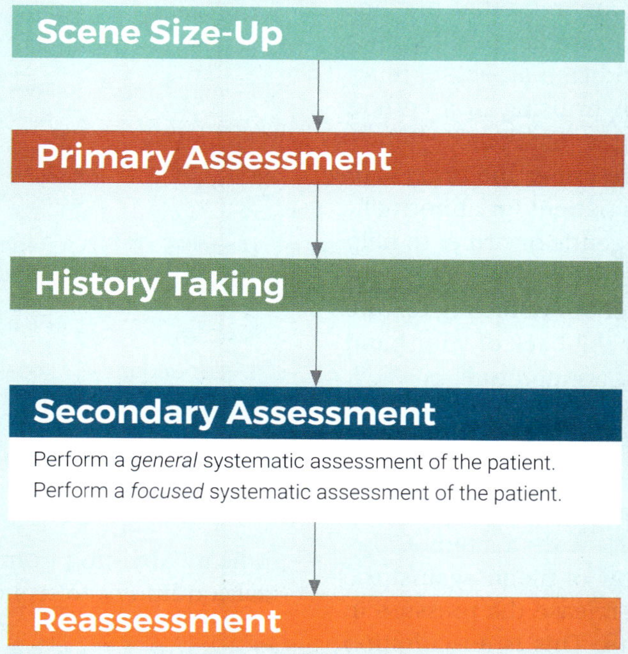

Secondary Assessment

If the patient is in stable condition and has an isolated complaint, you may choose to perform the secondary assessment at the scene. If the secondary assessment is not performed at the scene, it is performed in the back of the ambulance en route to the hospital. However, you may not have time to perform a secondary assessment if you have to continually manage life threats that were identified during the primary assessment.

The purpose of the **secondary assessment** is to perform a systematic physical examination of the patient's condition. The physical examination may be a systematic head-to-toe secondary assessment, as in the case of a multisystem trauma patient, or an assessment that focuses on a certain area or system of the body, as in the case of a medical patient who has abdominal pain or an isolated traumatic injury. Circumstances will determine which aspects of the physical examination will be used.

Words of Wisdom

You will need to expose portions of the patient's body during your secondary assessment. Patients may feel vulnerable during a physical examination. Display compassion during this difficult time. Covering the patient as much as possible and completing the assessment in a private space or the back of the ambulance will help maintain the patient's privacy. Covering the patient and ensuring a warm environment, such as by heating the ambulance, are also important for maintaining the patient's body temperature.

The following techniques are used during a physical examination:

- **Inspection.** Inspection is simply looking at your patient for physical abnormalities. This is done by looking for anything that may indicate a problem. For example, swelling in a lower extremity may indicate an acute injury or a chronic illness, or bruising in a certain area may indicate a history of falls.
- **Palpation.** Palpation describes the process of touching or feeling the patient for abnormalities. Palpation may be gentle or firmer to help you identify where the patient has pain. Your fingertips are best suited for detecting texture and consistency, while the back of your hand is best suited for noting temperature.
- **Auscultation.** Auscultation is the process of listening to sounds the body makes and is often aided by using a stethoscope. For example, when measuring a patient's blood pressure, you listen (**auscultate**) with a stethoscope to the sound of the flow of blood against the brachial artery as you release the pressure in the blood pressure cuff. This is auscultation of blood pressure. Auscultation is also used to assess lung sounds. More information is provided in Chapter 16, *Respiratory Emergencies.*

The mnemonic **DCAP-BTLS** will help remind you what kinds of abnormal findings to look for when inspecting and palpating various body regions (**TABLE 10-3**).

An integral part of your physical examination is to compare findings on one side of the body with the other side when possible. For example, if a patient reports a grating or grinding sensation in one arm, check the other arm before determining that the sensation or noise is caused by fractured bone ends or joints rubbing together (**crepitus**). If one ankle appears swollen, look at the other. If one shoulder feels "out of joint," feel the other one to compare. When listening to breath sounds, listen to both sides of the chest. If possible, find out what conditions are new and which ones the patient has been experiencing for some time. Do not assume that just because a patient has a condition that is causing discomfort, it just happened. As you assess, ask what, if anything, has changed about the condition.

On some occasions, it may even be helpful to note odors during an examination. Odors can indicate anything from infections, to certain medical conditions, to scene safety threats.

TABLE 10-3 The DCAP-BTLS Mnemonic

D—Deformity	Misshapen body part (eg, the arm or leg is no longer straight)
C—Contusions	Bruising; a collection of blood under the skin
A—Abrasions	Loss or damage to the surface of the skin from rubbing or scraping
P—Punctures	A small penetration through the skin into the soft tissue
B—Burns	Redness, blisters, or white areas of skin
T—Tenderness	Pain when an area is palpated
L—Lacerations	A deep cut in the skin
S—Swelling	A raised or enlarged area of soft tissue on the surface of the body

General Systematic (Head-to-Toe) Assessment

The goal of the secondary assessment is to identify hidden injuries or, in the case of a medical patient, to find any additional signs or symptoms that may help confirm the cause of their chief complaint. Any patient who has experienced a significant MOI, has sustained multisystem trauma, is unconscious, or is in critical condition should receive a full head-to-toe examination. An unconscious patient is unable to tell you what is wrong; therefore, this type of examination may give you clues to identify the problem. Because the secondary assessment may provide pertinent clues into the patient's condition, it may be completed prior to obtaining a medical history or vital signs in the multisystem trauma patient.

Street Smarts

Your secondary assessment should be focused on finding and fixing any remaining life threats. You may note contusions or abrasions for eventual treatment; however, life threats, such as a sucking chest wound or unstable pelvis, must be prioritized for treatment.

To perform a secondary assessment of a patient with no suspected spinal injuries, follow the steps in **SKILL DRILL 10-1**:

1. Look at the face for obvious lacerations, bruises, and deformities (**Step 1**).
2. Inspect the area around the eyes and eyelids (**Step 2**).
3. Examine the eyes for redness and for contact lenses. Assess the pupils using a penlight (**Step 3**).
4. Look behind the patient's ears to assess for bruising (Battle sign) (**Step 4**).
5. Use the penlight to look for drainage of spinal fluid or blood in the ears (**Step 5**).
6. Look for bruising and lacerations about the head. Palpate for tenderness, depressions of the skull, and deformities (**Step 6**).
7. Palpate the zygomas for tenderness or instability (**Step 7**).
8. Palpate the maxillae (**Step 8**).
9. Check the nose for blood and drainage (**Step 9**).
10. Palpate the mandible (**Step 10**).
11. Assess the mouth and nose for cyanosis, foreign bodies (including loose teeth or dentures), bleeding, lacerations, and deformities (**Step 11**).

Skill Drill 10-1 Performing the Secondary Assessment[a]

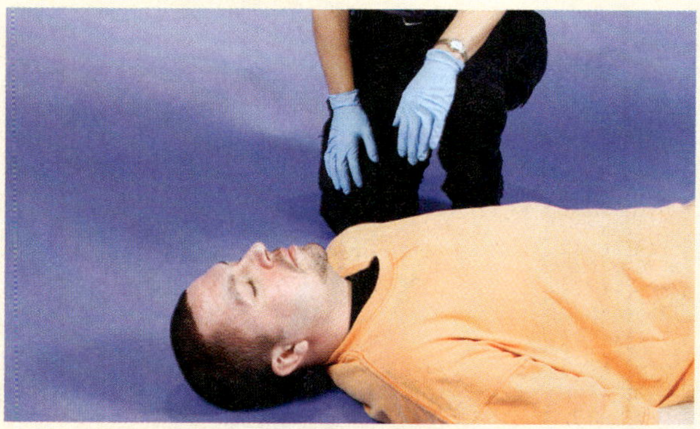

Step 1

Observe the face.

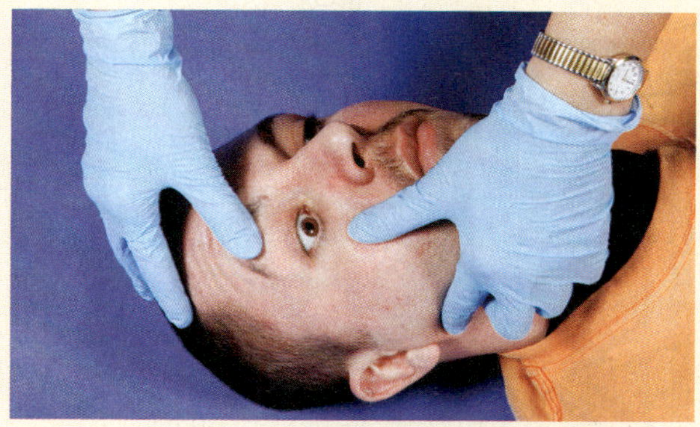

Step 2

Inspect the area around the eyes and eyelids.

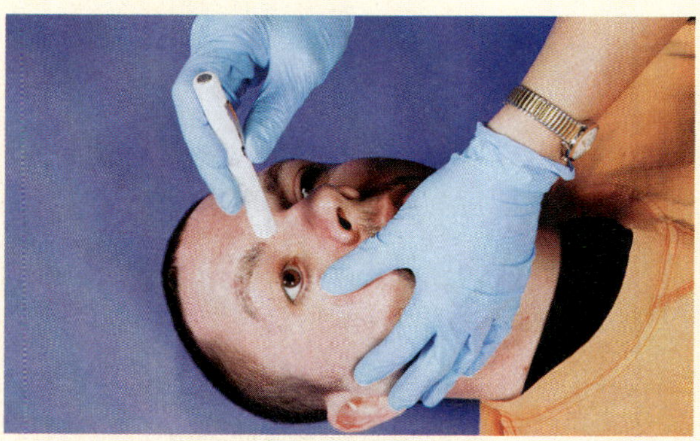

Step 3

Examine the eyes for redness and contact lenses. Check pupil function.

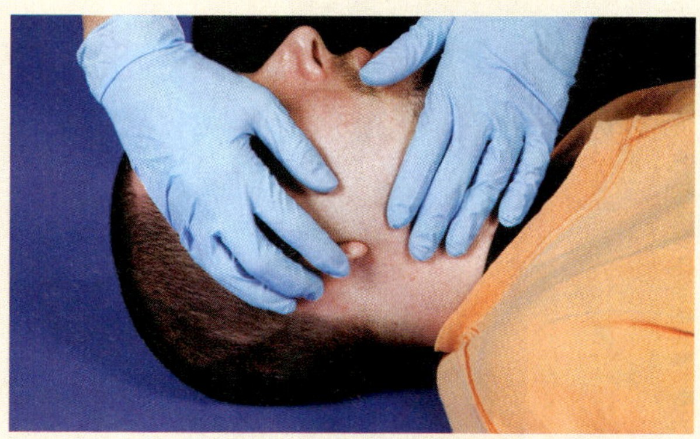

Step 4

Look behind the ears for Battle sign.

(continues)

Skill Drill 10-1 Performing the Secondary Assessment continued

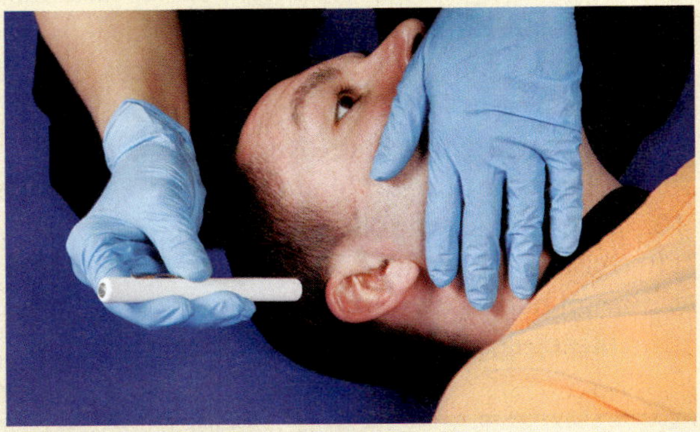

Step 5

Check the ears for drainage or blood.

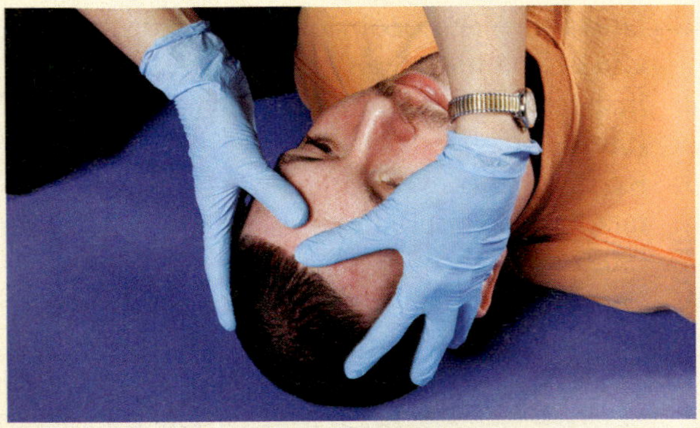

Step 6

Observe and palpate the head.

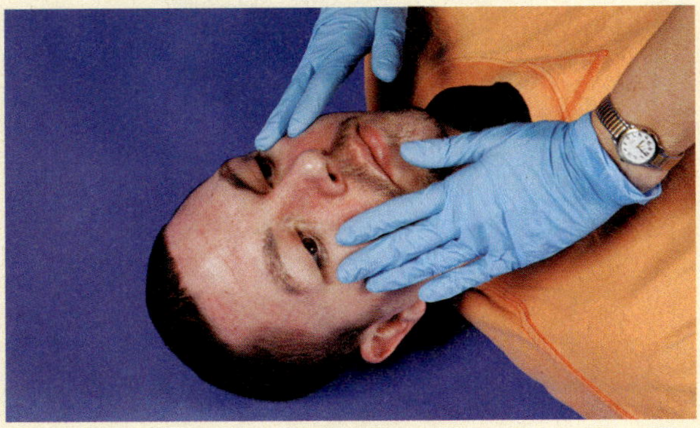

Step 7

Palpate the zygomas.

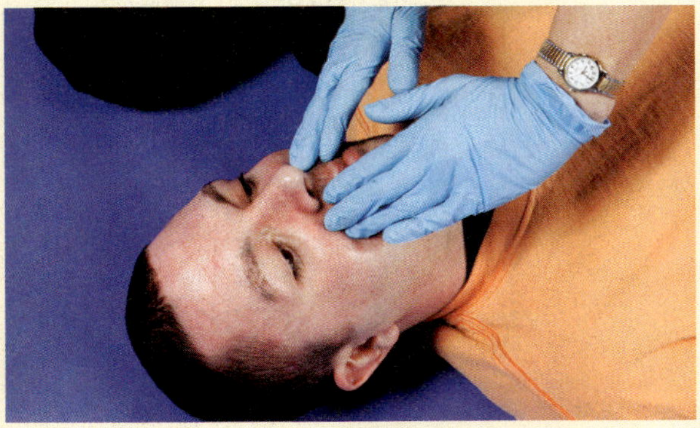

Step 8

Palpate the maxillae.

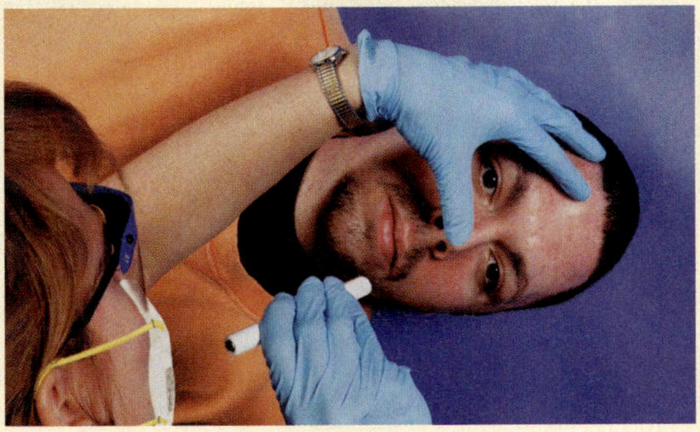

Step 9

Check the nose for blood and drainage.

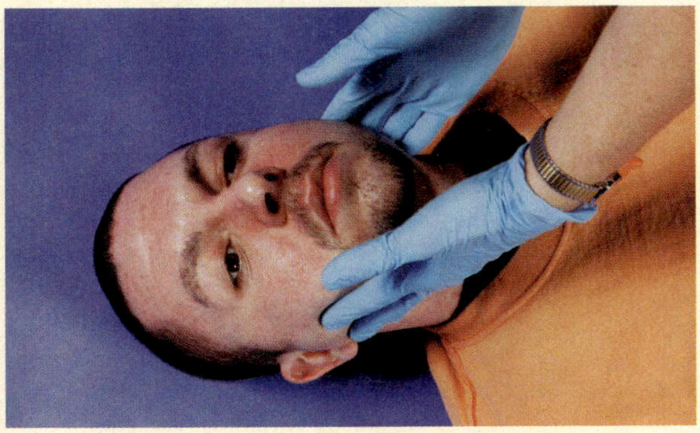

Step 10

Palpate the mandible.

Skill Drill 10-1 Performing the Secondary Assessment *continued*

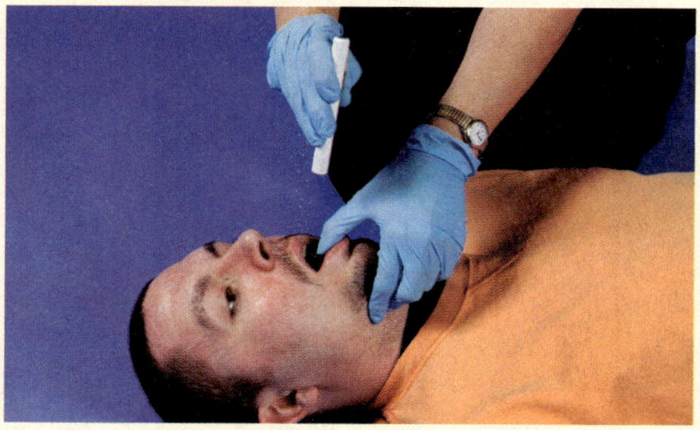

Step 11

Assess the mouth and nose.

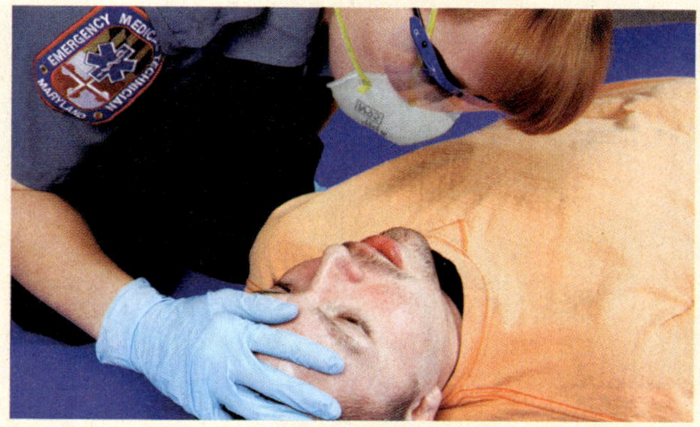

Step 12

Check for unusual breath odors.

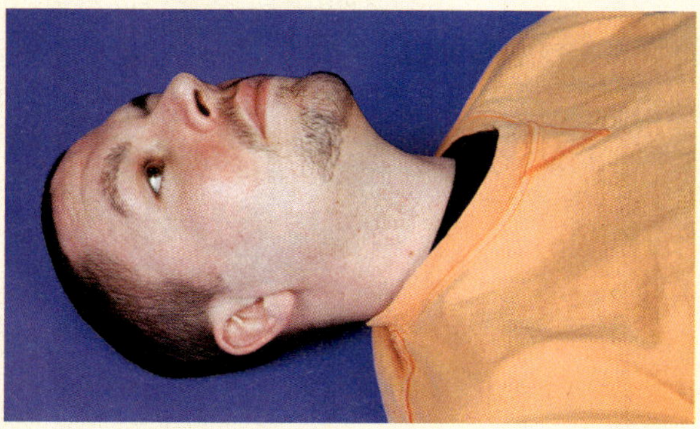

Step 13

Inspect the neck. Observe for jugular venous distention.

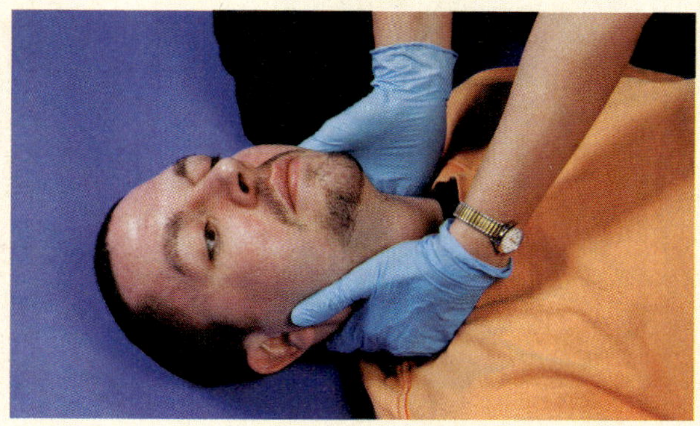

Step 14

Palpate the front and back of the neck.

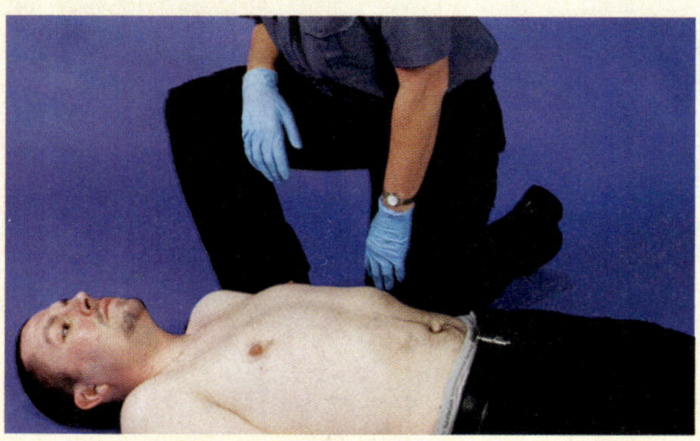

Step 15

Inspect the chest, and observe breathing motion.

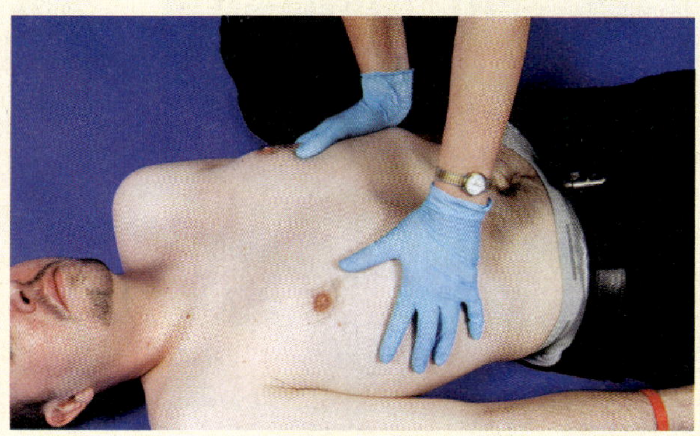

Step 16

Gently palpate over the ribs.

(continues)

Skill Drill 10-1 Performing the Secondary Assessment continued

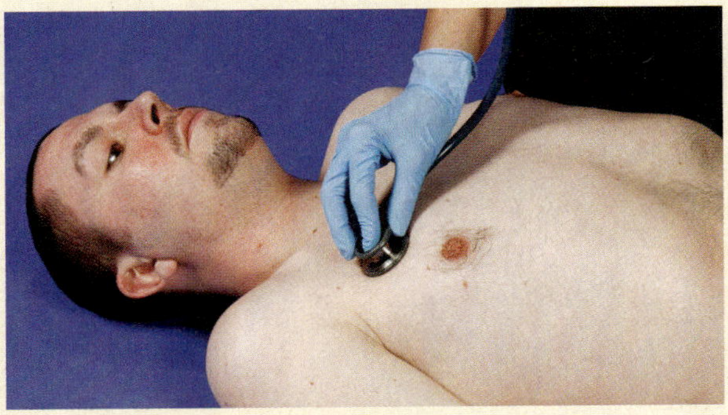

Step 17

Listen to anterior breath sounds (midaxillary, midclavicular).

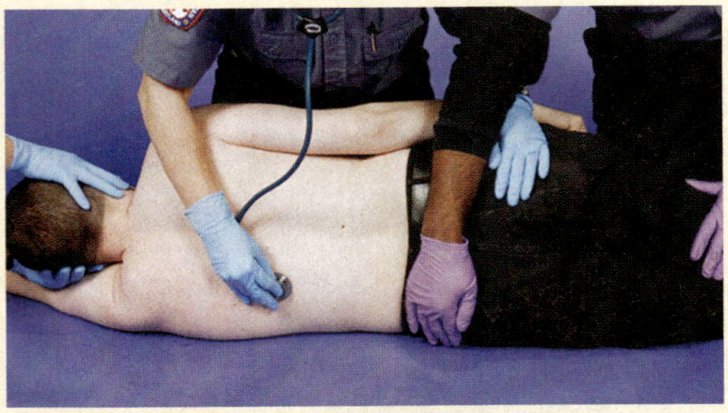

Step 18

Inspect the back. Listen to posterior breath sounds (bases, apices).

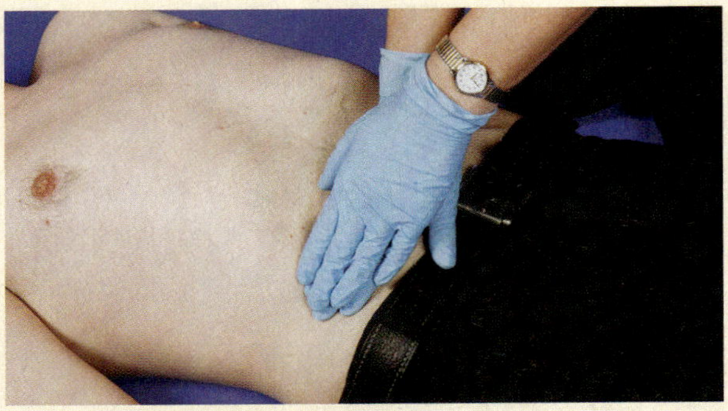

Step 19

Observe and then palpate the abdomen and pelvis.

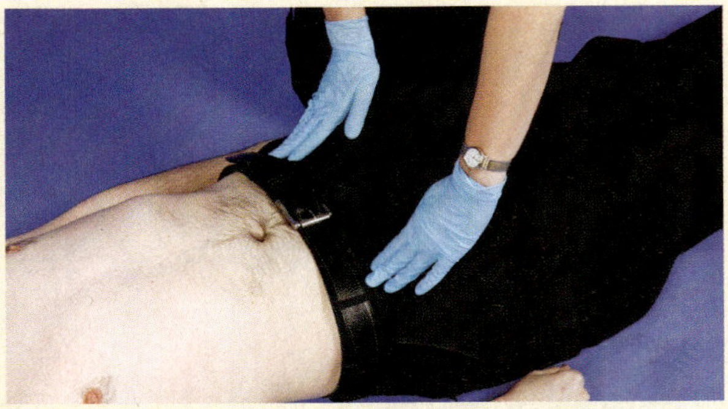

Step 20

Gently press the iliac crests inward and posteriorly.

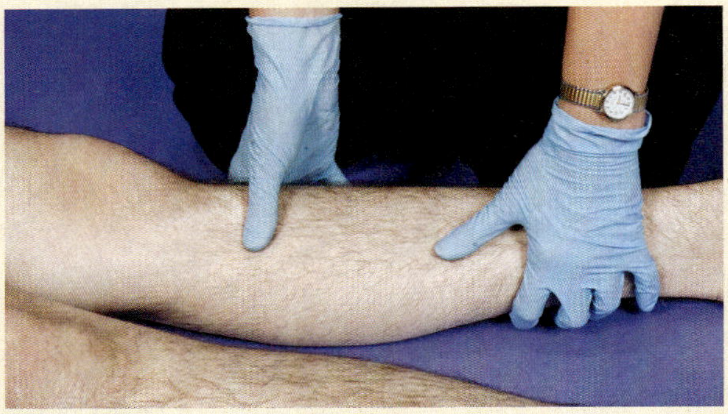

Step 21

Inspect the extremities; assess distal circulation and motor and sensory function.

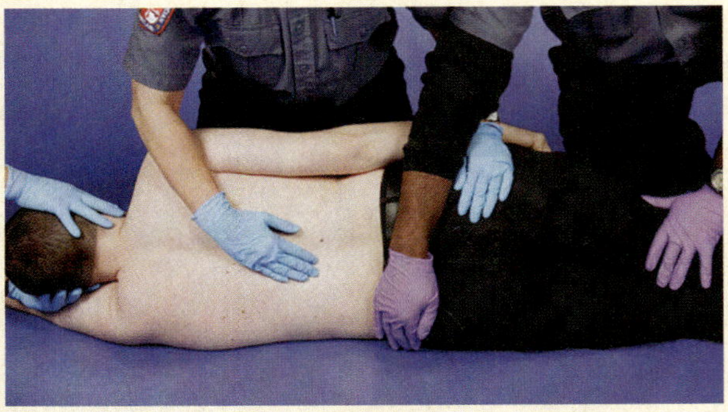

Step 22

Log roll the patient, and inspect the back for tenderness or deformities.

[a]When performing a secondary assessment on a patient who has sustained significant trauma, maintain spinal motion restriction.

12. Check for unusual odors on the patient's breath (**Step 12**).
13. Look at the neck for obvious lacerations, bruises, and deformities. Observe for jugular venous distention. Observe whether the trachea is midline (**Step 13**).
14. Palpate the back of the neck for tenderness, deformity, or spinal step-off (**Step 14**).
15. Look at the chest for obvious signs of injury before you begin palpation. Be sure to watch for movement of the chest with respirations (**Step 15**).
16. Gently palpate over the ribs to elicit tenderness. Avoid pressing over obvious bruises and fractures (**Step 16**).
17. Listen for breath sounds over the midaxillary and midclavicular lines (**Step 17**).
18. Listen also to breath sounds posteriorly at the bases and apices of the lungs (**Step 18**).
19. Look at the abdomen and pelvis for obvious lacerations, bruises, and deformities. Gently palpate the abdomen for tenderness. If the abdomen is unusually tense, describe the abdomen as rigid (**Step 19**).
20. Gently compress the iliac crests of the pelvis inward and posteriorly from the sides to assess for tenderness (**Step 20**).
21. Inspect all four extremities for lacerations, bruises, swelling, deformities, and medical alert anklets or bracelets. Also assess distal pulses and motor and sensory function in all extremities (**Step 22**).
22. Assess the back for tenderness and deformities. Remember, if you suspect a spinal injury, maintain manual stabilization of the neck as you log roll the patient (**Step 23**).

Pediatric Patients: Considerations During the General Systematic Assessment

The secondary assessment in pediatric patients does not differ from that of the assessment in adults. Remember, your patient may not understand why you are conducting this assessment, so an explanation will be important. The patient's family members may be able to help explain some injury findings, such as previous bruising, which is more common in children. Perform a secondary assessment of the entire body in pediatric patients who have the potential for hidden illnesses or injuries, such as unresponsive medical patients or trauma patients with a significant MOI. This type of examination may help to identify problems that were not as obvious during the primary assessment; for example, signs and symptoms of a distended abdomen or possible fractures could become more apparent over time.

Infants, toddlers, and preschool-age children who do not have apparent life-threatening illness or injuries should be assessed starting at the feet and ending at the head; school-age children and adolescents can be assessed using the head-to-toe approach, as with adults. The extent of the physical examination will depend on the situation and may include the following:

- **Head.** The younger the infant or child, the larger the head is in proportion to the rest of the body, increasing the risk for head injury with deceleration (such as in falls or motor vehicle crashes). Look for bruising, swelling, and hematomas. Significant blood loss can occur between the skull and scalp of a small infant. A tense or bulging fontanelle in an upright, noncrying infant suggests elevated intracranial pressure caused by meningitis, encephalitis, or intracranial bleeding. A sunken fontanelle suggests dehydration.
- **Nose.** Young infants are obligate nose breathers, so nasal congestion with mucus can cause respiratory distress. Gentle bulb or catheter suction of the nostrils may bring relief.[6]
- **Ears.** Look for any drainage from the ear canals. Leaking blood suggests a skull fracture. Check for bruises behind the ear or Battle sign, a late sign of skull fracture. The presence of pus may indicate an ear infection or perforation of the eardrum. Bruising or hematomas of the ear may result from abuse, especially if found on both sides.
- **Mouth.** In the trauma patient, look for active bleeding and loose teeth. Note the smell of the breath. Some ingestions are associated with identifiable odors, such as hydrocarbons (eg, gasoline). Acidosis, as in diabetic ketoacidosis, may impart a fruity odor to the breath.
- **Neck.** Examine the area near the trachea for swelling or bruising. Note if the pediatric patient cannot move the neck and has a high

fever. This may indicate that the child has meningitis.

- **Chest.** Examine the chest for penetrating injuries, lacerations, bruises, or rashes. If the patient is injured, feel the clavicles and every rib for tenderness and/or deformity.
- **Back.** Inspect the back for lacerations, penetrating injuries, bruises, or rashes.
- **Abdomen.** Inspect the abdomen for distention. Gently palpate the abdomen and watch closely for guarding or tensing of the abdominal muscles, which may suggest infection, obstruction, or intra-abdominal injury. Note any tenderness or masses. Look for any seat belt abrasions or bruising.
- **Extremities.** Assess for symmetry. Compare both sides for color, warmth, size of joints, swelling, and tenderness. Unless there is obvious deformity of the extremity suggesting a fracture, put each joint through its full range of motion while watching the child's eyes for signs of pain.

Words of Wisdom

Because of the frequency of serious internal injuries in children who show no external signs, it is especially important to investigate and thoroughly document the MOI. Do not let the rush at the scene distract you from determining the MOI, or at least direct another reliable responder to do so. Hospital clinicians need this information.

Some of the guidelines used to assess adult circulatory status (ie, heart rate and blood pressure) have important limitations in children. First, normal heart rates vary with age in children. Second, blood pressure is usually not assessed in patients younger than 3 years; it offers little information about the child's circulatory status and is often difficult to obtain. In these patients, assessment of the skin is a better indication of their circulatory status.

After a physical examination of the whole body has been completed, perform a focused assessment on pediatric patients without life-threatening illnesses or injuries. Focus your physical examination on the area or areas of the body affected by the illness or injury as well as on the chief complaint, MOI or NOI, and the findings of the primary assessment.

Geriatric Patients: Considerations During the General Systematic Assessment

Perform the secondary assessment when appropriate. You may have to remove several layers of clothing. Keep in mind that your older patient may not be comfortable being exposed. Protect the person's modesty. Also remember that older people are often cold due to diminished circulation; consider the need to keep your patient warm during the exam.

Focused Systematic Assessment

A **focused assessment** is generally performed on patients who have sustained nonsignificant MOIs or on responsive medical patients. This type of examination is typically based on the chief complaint. Your assessment may focus on a specific body part that has been affected, such as abrasions to the elbow, or on a particular body system that has been affected, such as the cardiovascular, respiratory, neurologic, musculoskeletal, integumentary, or genitourinary system. For example, if a person has an injury to the arm, that arm will need to be examined for signs of injury and assessed for circulation, movement, and sensation distal to the injury; those same findings should then be compared to the other arm. For a person reporting a headache, carefully and systematically assess the head and the neurologic system. The goal of a focused assessment is to focus your attention on the body part or systems affected by the priority problem or problems. Before the focused assessment, you will obtain the appropriate vital signs that can assist in helping form your general impression.

Respiratory System

When the patient's chief complaint is focused on the respiratory system, you should have identified and managed life threats during the primary assessment. During the secondary assessment, you will perform an examination directed at obtaining clues that will help determine which treatment to perform and protocols to follow.

Expose the patient's chest. Look again for signs of airway obstruction, as well as trauma to the neck and/or chest. Inspect the chest for overall symmetry. Does the right side of the chest look like the left side? Listen carefully to breath sounds, noting abnormalities. Measure the respiratory rate, chest rise and fall (for tidal volume), and effort. Is the patient using accessory muscles to help with breathing, and is there increased work of breathing? For example, sounds of **stridor**, a brassy crowing sound prominent on inspiration, suggest a partially occluded upper airway caused by swelling or a partial upper airway obstruction from a foreign body.

Breathing is normally a rhythmic, spontaneous, automatic process that should occur without interruption, conscious thought, visible effort, marked sounds, or pain. You will assess breathing by *watching* the patient's chest rise and fall and *listening* to **breath sounds** with a stethoscope over each lung. Chest rise and breath sounds should be equal on both sides of the chest.

When assessing breathing, you must obtain the following information:

- Respiratory rate
- Rhythm: regular or irregular
- Quality of breathing
- Breath sounds

Respiratory Rate

The normal respiratory rate varies widely in adults, ranging from approximately 12 to 20 breaths/min. Children breathe at even faster rates. With practice, you will be able to estimate the rate and note whether it is too fast or too slow during the primary survey; however, an exact count is important during the secondary survey.

Respirations are determined by counting the number of breaths the patient takes in 30 seconds and multiplying by two. The result is the number of breaths per minute. For accuracy, count each breath at the same point in its cycle. This is most easily done by counting each peak chest rise. Although you can see peak chest rise, it is easier to place your hand on the patient's chest and feel it. However, be aware that conscious patients will often breathe faster and deeper because they are aware you are counting. To prevent this from happening, check respirations in a conscious, alert patient without making the patient aware of what you are evaluating. This can be easily done by first taking a radial pulse and then, without releasing the wrist or otherwise suggesting a change, counting the chest rise that you see or feel as the patient's forearm rises and falls with the movement of the chest (**FIGURE 10-20**). If the patient coughs, yawns, sighs, or talks during the 30-second period, wait a few seconds and start again.

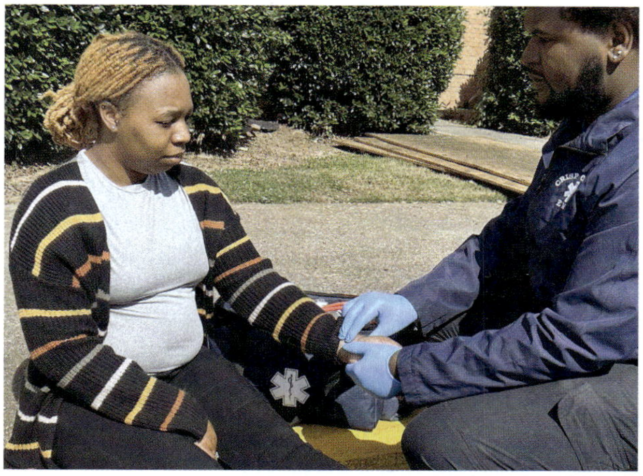

FIGURE 10-20 Assess respirations in a conscious patient by first taking a radial pulse and then, without releasing the patient's wrist, counting the chest rise and fall for 30 seconds.

TABLE 10-4 Normal Ranges for Respirations

Age	Respiratory Rate (breaths/min)
Newborn: 0 to 1 month	30 to 60
Infant: 1 month to 1 year	30 to 53
Toddler: 1 to 3 years	22 to 27
Preschool age: 3 to 6 years	20 to 28
School age: 6 to 12 years	18 to 25
Adults and adolescents (12 years and older)	12 to 20

TABLE 10-4 shows the normal range of respiratory rates of patients who are at rest.

Respiratory Rhythm

While counting the patient's respirations, also note the rhythm. If the time from one peak chest rise to the next is fairly consistent, respirations are considered regular. If the respirations vary or the rate changes frequently, the respirations are considered irregular. When you document the vital signs, be sure to note whether the patient's respirations were regular or irregular.

Quality of Breathing

Normal breathing is almost silent. In a quiet environment, you may hear only the sounds of air movement at the mouth and nose. Breathing accompanied by other sounds may indicate a significant respiratory problem. A snoring sound may indicate an upper airway obstruction and is usually a result of the tongue blocking the airway. When the upper airway has a partial obstruction by a foreign body or swelling, you may hear stridor, a harsh, high-pitched, crowing sound. If you can hear bubbling or gurgling in the upper airway, the patient probably has fluid in those passages, potentially impeding the exchange of gases. Suction the patient's airway to clear the airway and reduce the risk of aspiration of fluid into the lungs. You may hear other sounds, such as wheezes, a whistling sound indicative of a mild lower airway obstruction. The presence of any of these abnormal sounds indicates that an airway or breathing problem exists. Remember that with a complete airway obstruction, the patient will not be able to move any air and will no longer be able to cough or talk. If you hear no sounds, the patient may not be moving any air at all and will require some action to clear the obstruction.

A patient who coughs up thick, yellow or green sputum (matter from the lungs) most likely has a respiratory infection. A patient with a chest injury may cough up blood or frothy white or pink foam-like sputum caused by blood and fluid mixing with air in the lungs. A patient with heart failure may also cough up pink frothy sputum. The presence of either substance, regardless of its cause, indicates that an urgent, potentially critical cardiovascular and respiratory problem exists, possibly requiring oxygenation, ventilation, and other treatments. Without these treatments, the patient's condition may deteriorate rapidly to a point where the patient can no longer breathe.

Quality is also described by the amount of air that the patient is exchanging, as determined by the rate and the tidal volume. **Tidal volume** is a measure of the amount of air that is moved into or out of the lungs during one breath. The quality of the breath determines whether the tidal volume is normal, less than normal, or greater than normal. A normal value is approximately 500 mL in a healthy adult male and 400 mL in a healthy female.[7] You can determine the quality or character of respirations as you are counting the number of respirations. **TABLE 10-5** shows four ways in which the quality or character can be described.

Breath Sounds

When you assess the lungs using a stethoscope you will gain additional important information about the patient's illness or injuries. Stethoscopes have two earpieces that should be placed into the ears so they angle forward toward your nose, following the path of the ear canals. At the other end, most stethoscopes have two sides (**FIGURE 10-21**). The bell is the smaller side and is used to listen to lower-pitched

TABLE 10-5 Characteristics of Respirations

Normal	Breathing is neither shallow nor deep; it appears effortless Equal chest rise and fall No use of accessory muscles
Shallow	Decreased chest or abdominal wall motion
Labored	Increased breathing effort Use of accessory muscles Possible gasping Nasal flaring, supraclavicular and intercostal retractions in infants and children
Noisy	Increase in sound of breathing, including snoring, wheezing, gurgling, crowing, grunting, and stridor

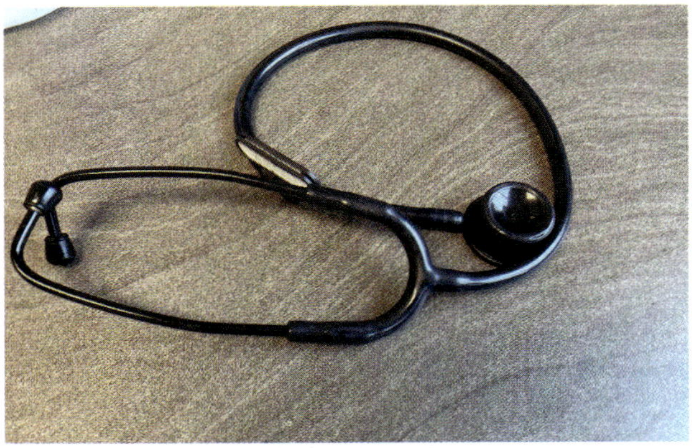

FIGURE 10-21 A stethoscope.

sounds such as heart sounds. The diaphragm is the wider side and is designed to assess breath sounds. To switch between the bell and diaphragm, turn the end of the stethoscope. Tap on the side you wish to listen with to ensure it has clicked into place.

The following describes how and where to listen to assess breathing:

- First, remember that you can almost always hear a patient's breath sounds better from the patient's back; therefore, if the patient's back is accessible, listen (auscultate) there. If you cannot, listen from the front and sides. Move from side to side as you listen so you can compare the breath sounds in each area to the corresponding region on the other lung (**FIGURE 10-22**).
- Auscultate over the upper lungs (apices) at approximately 1 inch (2.5 cm) below the clavicle at the midclavicular line, the midlung fields at

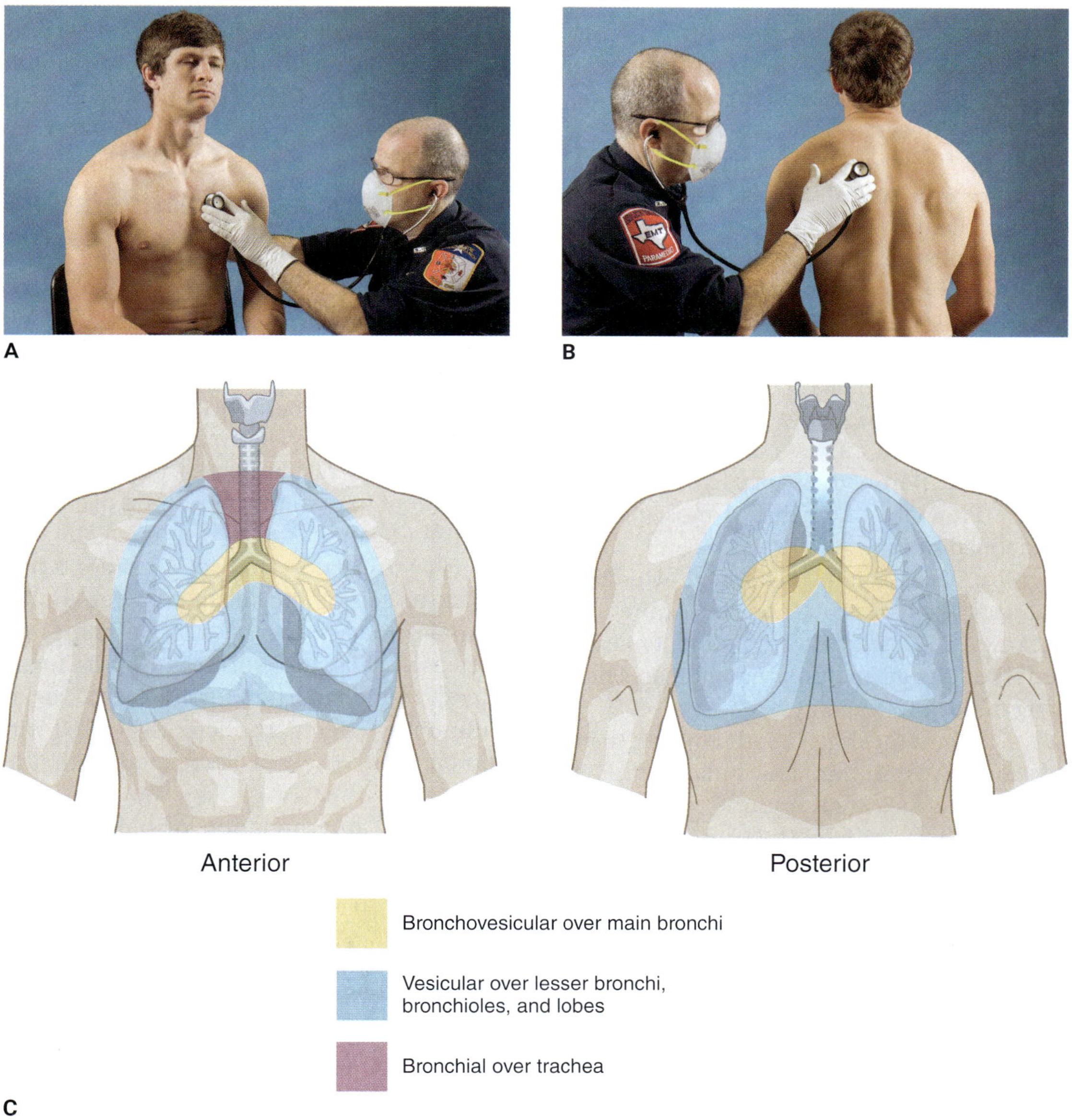

FIGURE 10-22 Locations for auscultating breath sounds: both sides of the chest in multiple lung fields, as shown. **A.** Stethoscope position for auscultating the front of the chest. **B.** Stethoscope position for auscultating the back. **C.** Colors in illustration correspond to areas where sounds are heard.

the third or fourth intercostal space from the patient's posterior, and the lower lungs (bases) at the sixth intercostal space, midaxillary line.

- Lift the clothing or slide the stethoscope under the clothing. If you listen over clothing, you will primarily hear the sound of the stethoscope sliding over the fabric because breath sounds are muted by clothing.
- Place the diaphragm of the stethoscope firmly against the skin to hear breath sounds.

As you listen, you may be able to identify one of the following sounds:

- **Normal breath sounds.** These are clear and relatively quiet during inspiration and expiration. You will hear the air moving into and out of the lungs freely without obstruction.
- **Snoring breath sounds.** These usually indicate a simple, but potentially dangerous, upper airway obstruction, usually caused by the tongue or a foreign body. Snoring is an upper airway sound and does not require a stethoscope to be heard.
- **Stridor.** This is often heard before even listening with a stethoscope and may indicate that the patient has an airway obstruction in the neck or upper part of the chest. Expect to hear a brassy, crowing sound that is most prominent on inspiration.
- **Wheezing**. This is a high-pitched whistling sound that is most prominent on expiration. Wheezing is a lower airway sound typically heard through auscultation that indicates narrowing of the lower airways.
- **Crackles**. Wet, crackling breath sounds (usually found on inspiration) may indicate fluid in the lungs. Crackles are the sound made as the alveoli are popped open; the sound is similar to that of Rice Krispies when milk is added.
- **Rhonchi**. Congested breath sounds may suggest the presence of mucus or fluid in the lungs. Expect to hear low-pitched, noisy sounds that are most prominent on expiration. These lung sounds may be similar to those of blowing bubbles under water. The patient may report a productive cough associated with these sounds.

Note any abnormal breath sounds and document them. The presence of abnormal breath sounds, such as wheezing, may indicate the need for additional treatment based on your protocols.

Pediatric Patients: Considerations During the Respiratory Assessment

Respiratory rates may be difficult to interpret in children because they can be rapid or, in the case of infants, the patient may be crying. Rapid respiratory rates may simply reflect high fever, anxiety, pain, or excitement. Slow rates (ie, lower than normal for age) often signal rapid deterioration requiring intervention. When time and the patient's condition permit, count the respirations for 30 seconds and then double that number. If the patient yawns, sighs, coughs, or talks during the 30-second period, wait a few seconds and begin again. In infants and children younger than 3 years, evaluate respirations by assessing the rise and fall of the abdomen.

Geriatric Patients: Considerations During the Respiratory Assessment

An older patient with a complaint of shortness of breath will want to sit up or assume the tripod position. Accommodate positioning requests when possible. The position in which you found the patient may be maintaining a patent airway. Forcing a patient who is short of breath into a supine position may result in respiratory distress or failure. Allow the patient to maintain a position of comfort unless contraindicated.

The respiratory rate of an older adult should be in the same range as in younger adults, but remember that chest rise may be compromised by increased chest wall stiffness. Be sure to auscultate breath sounds to listen for crackles associated with pulmonary edema, rhonchi associated with pneumonia, and wheezes associated with asthma or anaphylaxis.

Careful interpretation of pulse oximetry data is necessary in older adults because the pulse oximetry device requires adequate perfusion to get an accurate reading. Older adults may have poor circulation, vasoconstriction, hypotension, hypothermia, lack of red blood cells, or carbon monoxide poisoning that could result in an inaccurate reading.

Cardiovascular System

When the patient's chief complaint is associated with chest pain or other discomfort, a physical examination should include looking, listening, and

Special Populations

PEDIATRIC WEIGHT ESTIMATION

Several tools are available to assist the EMT and their ALS partner to assess and care for children in the prehospital setting. Two reference tools commonly used in the field include the Broselow-Luten and the Handtevy systems. One component of both is a **length-based resuscitation tape** (**FIGURE 10-23**). Length-based resuscitation tapes are used to estimate the weight of a critically ill child (typically up to 12 years of age) so that appropriate equipment and medication doses can be quickly determined. The concept is that a child's weight can be adequately determined based on the length of their body.

While both systems are based on average height, weight, and age standards, the Handtevy system focuses more on the child's age in estimating the child's weight. The Handtevy system includes other resources such as cards and an app to aid clinicians with dosing and equipment choices.

Accurate measurement with the length-based tape is crucial. The proper sequence for using the tape is as follows:

1. Place the pediatric patient supine on a flat surface.
2. Lay the tape next to the pediatric patient with the multicolored side facing up.
3. Place the red end of the tape that says "Measure from here" at the top of the pediatric patient's head (red to head).
4. Place one hand with its side down at the top of the pediatric patient's head, covering the red box at the end of the tape, and hold it firmly there.
5. With the other hand, stretch the tape out the full length of the child, stopping at the heel. If the child is longer than the tape, stop here and use the appropriate adult equipment.
6. Note the color or letter block and weight range on the edge of the tape where your hand is. Say the color or letter out loud.
7. Select the appropriate-size equipment by matching the color or letter on the tape to the color or letter on the equipment.

In some cases, ambulance services have an accompanying bag for each color zone that contains the correct airway equipment and vascular access equipment needed to care for a child of that length. Your ALS partner may ask you to measure the child and bring them the corresponding bag for their measured color zone.

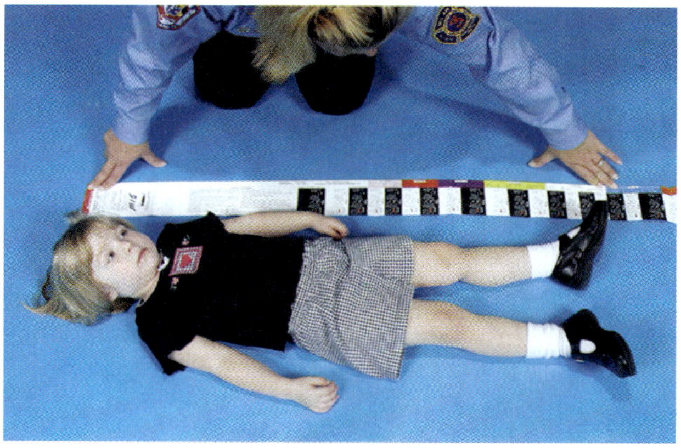

FIGURE 10-23 Length-based resuscitation tape is the best way to estimate the correct size for airway adjuncts in children.

feeling for abnormalities in the patient's thoracic region. Look for trauma to the chest and listen for breath sounds. Scan the chest for evidence of an implanted device such as a pacemaker, automated implanted cardioverter-defibrillator, or ventricular assist device. Also look for a nitroglycerin patch. These findings suggest that the patient has a history of cardiovascular disease. Consider the pulse and respiratory rates and the blood pressure. Pay particular attention to rate, quality, and rhythm. Consider your findings when assessing skin condition, which will allow you to determine how well the cardiovascular and respiratory systems are functioning. Check and compare distal pulses to determine any differences between the right and left sides. If time permits, assess the blood pressure on both arms. A significant difference in values can indicate an aortic aneurysm. Consider auscultation for abnormal heart sounds; however, keep in mind that obtaining these sounds may be difficult in a noisy prehospital setting and is typically assessed by a paramedic. Always remember that a patient's chief complaint may have a medical cause or could be the result of trauma.

Pulse Rate

After you have determined that a pulse is present, next determine its adequacy. This is done by assessing the pulse rate, pulse quality, and pulse rhythm. For an adult, the normal resting pulse rate should be between 60 and 100 beats/min and could be as much as 100 beats/min in older patients. In general,

TABLE 10-6 Normal Ranges for Pulse Rate

Age	Range (beats/min)
Newborn (0 to 1 month)	100 to 205
Infant (1 month to 1 year)	100 to 180
Toddler (1 to 3 years)	98 to 140
Preschool age (3 to 6 years)	97 to 118
School age (6 to 12 years)	75 to 118
Adolescent (12 to 18 years)	60 to 100
Adult (18 years and older)	60 to 100

Data from *Pediatric Advanced Life Support, 2015*, the American Heart Association, Dallas, TX.

in pediatric patients, the younger the patient, the faster the pulse rate. In well-conditioned athletes or in people taking heart medications such as beta blockers, the pulse rate may be considerably lower. Remember, you can always ask patients if they know their normal or resting heart rate. **TABLE 10-6** shows the normal ranges of pulse rates for adults and children.

To obtain the pulse rate in most patients, count the number of pulses felt in a 30-second period and then multiply by two. A pulse that is weak and difficult to palpate, irregular, or extremely slow should be palpated and counted for a full minute. A pulse rate is counted as beats per minute.

In an adult patient, a pulse rate of 100 beats/min or greater is described as **tachycardia**, and a rate of 60 beats/min or less is described as **bradycardia**.

Pulse Quality

Always report the pulse quality whenever reporting or recording the pulse. The pulse is generally palpated at the radial or carotid arteries in adults and at the brachial artery in infants, because it is normally strong and easily palpable at these locations. Therefore, if the pulse feels to be at normal strength, describe it as being strong. Health care practitioners often describe a stronger-than-normal pulse as "bounding" and a pulse that is weak and difficult to feel as "weak" or "thready." With some experience, you will be able to easily make the necessary distinctions.

Special Populations

PEDIATRIC PULSE ASSESSMENT

Assess the child's pulse rate by counting for at least 1 minute, noting its quality and regularity. When you are more rushed due to the critical nature of the child's condition, count the pulse rate for 15 seconds and multiply by 4 to obtain an approximation of the rate.

Words of Wisdom

Counting a very rapid heart rate can be difficult. Try tapping your finger along with each beat to make it easier.

Pulse Rhythm

When you are assessing the pulse, you must also determine whether the rhythm is regular or irregular. Regardless of the rate, the interval between each contraction should be the same, and the pulse should occur at a constant, regular rhythm. Document this rhythm as regular.

The rhythm is considered irregular if the heart periodically has an early or late beat or if a pulse beat is missed. If an irregular pulse is found in a patient with signs and symptoms that suggest a cardiovascular problem, the patient likely needs advanced cardiac assessment and life support. Therefore, depending on your protocols, you should call for ALS backup, arrange for an intercept by paramedics, or initiate prompt transport to definitive care. As with any deviation from expected findings, it is important to determine if this irregular rhythm is new or if it represents either a normal or a chronic condition for the patient.

Blood Pressure

Adequate blood pressure is necessary to maintain proper circulation and perfusion of the vital organs. **Blood pressure** is the pressure of circulating blood against the walls of the arteries. A decrease in the blood pressure may indicate one of the following:

- Loss of blood or its fluid components
- Loss of vascular tone and sufficient arterial constriction to maintain the necessary pressure even without any actual fluid or blood loss
- A cardiac pumping problem

When any of these conditions occurs and results in a drop in circulation, the body's compensatory mechanisms are activated, resulting in an increased heart rate and constriction of the arteries. Normal blood pressure is maintained, and by decreasing the blood flow to the skin and extremities, available blood volume is temporarily redirected to the vital organs so that they remain adequately perfused. However, as shock progresses, eventually the body's defense mechanisms can no longer keep up, and the blood pressure will fall. Decreased blood pressure is a late sign of shock and indicates that the patient is in the critical stage of decompensated shock. Any patient with a markedly low blood pressure has inadequate pressure to maintain proper perfusion of all vital organs and needs to have their blood pressure and perfusion restored to a normal level.

Some people have chronically high blood pressure from progressive narrowing of the arteries that occurs with age, and during an acute episode, their blood pressure may increase to even higher levels. Head injury or any number of other conditions may also cause blood pressure to rise to very high levels. Untreated abnormally high blood pressure may lead to stroke, heart attack, heart failure, and damage to other major organs.

Blood pressure contains two key separate components: systolic pressure and diastolic pressure. **Systolic pressure** is the increased pressure that is caused along the artery with each contraction (systole) of the ventricles and the pulse wave that it produces. **Diastolic pressure** is the residual pressure that remains in the arteries during the relaxing phase of the heart's cycle (diastole), when the left ventricle is at rest. Systolic pressure represents the maximum pressure to which the arteries are subjected, and diastolic pressure represents the minimum amount of pressure that is always present in the arteries.

Blood pressure is measured in millimeters of mercury (mm Hg). Blood pressure is reported as a fraction in the form of systolic pressure over diastolic pressure. Therefore, if the patient's systolic pressure is 120 and the diastolic pressure is 80, you would record it as "BP 120/80 mm Hg." You would report the patient's blood pressure verbally as "120 over 80."

Avoid obtaining a blood pressure reading on an arm if the patient has an intravenous site or other medical device in place, such as an indwelling catheter or dialysis fistula; has had a mastectomy on that side; or has an injury to that arm. You can ask the patient if any of these exist if they are not visible, such as a mastectomy. If a patient has chronic renal failure and is undergoing dialysis, ask if the patient has a fistula or any other reason that you should not take a blood pressure using that arm.

A blood pressure cuff with gauge (sphygmomanometer) contains the following components:

- A wide outer cuff designed to be fastened snugly around the entire arm or leg
- An inflatable wide bladder sewn into a portion of the cuff
- A ball-pump with a one-way valve that allows air to enter and a turn-valve that can be closed or, when opened, will allow air to be released at a controlled speed from the cuff
- A pressure gauge calibrated in millimeters of mercury, which indicates the pressure that exists in the cuff that is being applied against the underlying artery

Most agencies should carry a variety of sizes of blood pressure cuffs to fit a specific arm circumference: infant, child, small adult, adult, large adult, and extra-large adult (**FIGURE 10-24**). You must be sure to select the appropriate-size cuff. A cuff that is too small may result in falsely high readings; a cuff that is too large may result in falsely low readings. The normal size cuff is designed to wrap around the arm 1 to 1.5 times and take up two-thirds the length from the armpit to the crease in the elbow of most adults. Some EMS agencies also carry a

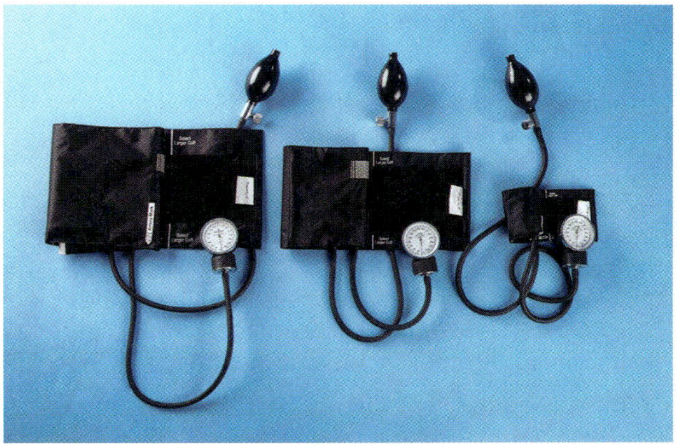

FIGURE 10-24 Three sizes of blood pressure cuffs.

thigh cuff to take the blood pressure of the thigh in patients for whom arm assessment is not possible. Measure blood pressure in all patients older than 3 years.

Auscultation is the most common means of measuring a patient's blood pressure. A blood pressure cuff is applied to a patient's upper arm, allowing for the compression of the brachial artery when inflated. This compression creates turbulence and arterial vibrations that make sounds, known as Korotkoff sounds, that can be heard using a stethoscope. Follow the steps in **SKILL DRILL 10-2** to measure blood pressure by auscultation:

1. Follow standard precautions. Explain the procedure to the patient. Examine for a dialysis fistula, central lines, mastectomy, injury to the arm, or other reason to not use this arm to measure blood pressure. If any are present, use the other arm.
2. With the patient's arm exposed, free of clothing, and extended, and with the palm up, place the appropriate-size cuff so that it lies across the upper arm and is located with its distal edge approximately 1 inch (2.5 cm) above the antecubital space (the crease at the inside of the patient's elbow). Make sure the center of the inflatable bladder, which is usually marked by an arrow on the cuff, lies over the brachial artery. Next, wrap the ends so that the cuff surrounds the upper arm snugly but not tightly. Secure the cuff with the Velcro, making sure to rub your hand over the entire area where the two sides of the Velcro are in contact (**Step 1**).
3. Once the cuff has been properly secured around the upper arm, the arm should be held at about the same level as the heart. With your nondominant hand, palpate the brachial artery (in the antecubital fossa, the anterior aspect of the elbow) to determine where to place the stethoscope (**Step 2**).
4. Place the bell or diaphragm of the stethoscope over the artery and hold it firmly against the artery with the fingers of your nondominant hand.[8] Hold the rubber ball-pump in the palm of your other hand and the turn-valve between your thumb and first finger (**Step 3**).

YOU are the EMT

Following the appropriate interventions, your patient's oxygenation and ventilation status have improved; however, he is still bradycardic, hypotensive, and unresponsive. Because there was no one at the scene to provide information regarding his medical history, you continue to treat him based on his signs and symptoms, perform a reassessment, and call in your radio report to the receiving facility.

Recording Time: 20 Minutes	
Level of consciousness	Unconscious and unresponsive
Respirations	6 breaths/min (baseline); ventilations are being assisted at a rate of 12 breaths per minute.
Pulse	38 beats/min; weak and regular
Skin	Pale and cool; cyanosis has resolved
Blood pressure	84/56 mm Hg
Oxygen saturation (Spo_2)	95% (with assisted ventilation)

You reassess the patient again just before arriving at the emergency department (ED) and note that his condition is unchanged. He is immediately evaluated by the staff physician, who determines that he has overdosed on numerous drugs, including opioids. After further treatment in the ED, he is admitted to the intensive care unit for close observation.

9. What components of the SAMPLE history, if any, can you obtain when your patient is unresponsive? How would you obtain the information?

10. Why is reassessing your interventions so important?

Skill Drill 10-2 Obtaining Blood Pressure by Auscultation

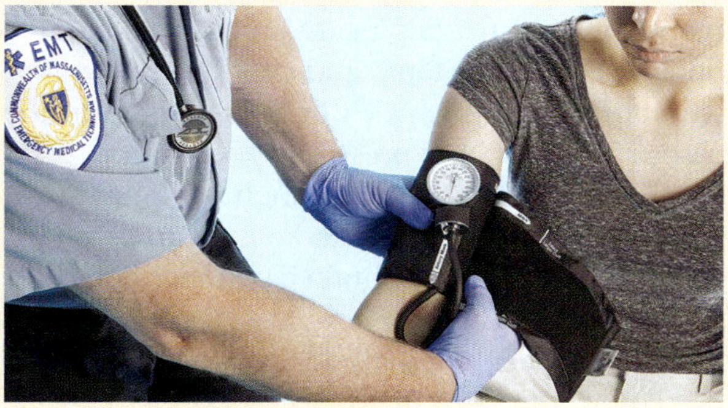

Step 1

Follow standard precautions. Check for a dialysis fistula, central line, previous mastectomy, and injury to the arm. If any are present, use the brachial artery on the other arm. Apply the cuff snugly. The lower border of the cuff should be about 1 inch (2.5 cm) above the antecubital space.

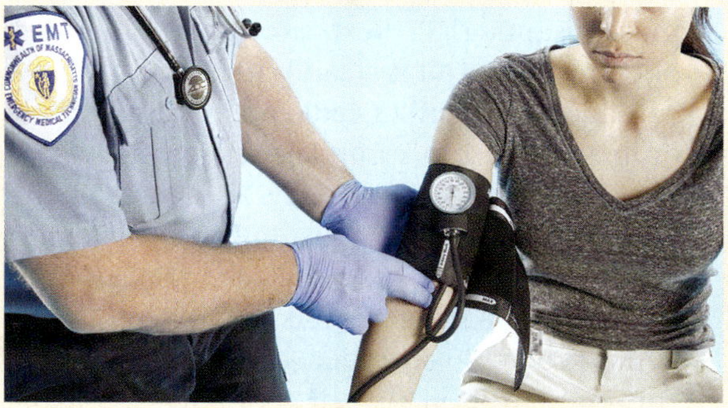

Step 2

Support the exposed arm at the level of the heart. Palpate the brachial artery.

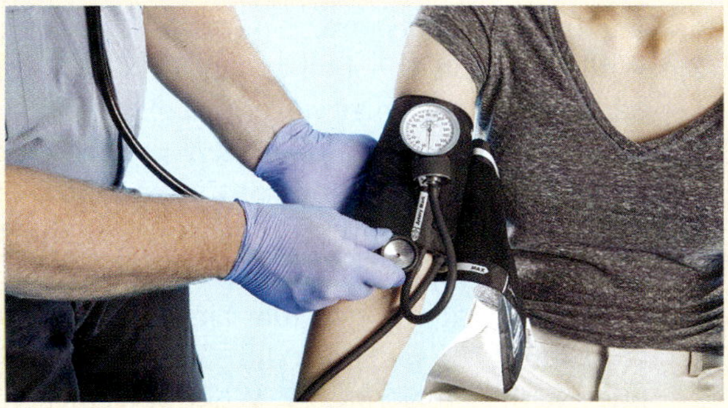

Step 3

Place the stethoscope over the brachial artery, and grasp the ball-pump and turn-valve.

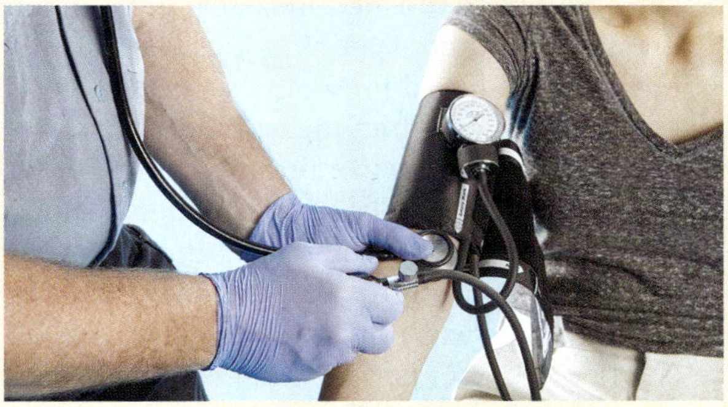

Step 4

Close the valve, and pump to 30 mm Hg above the point at which you stop hearing pulse sounds. Note the systolic and diastolic pressures as you let air escape slowly.

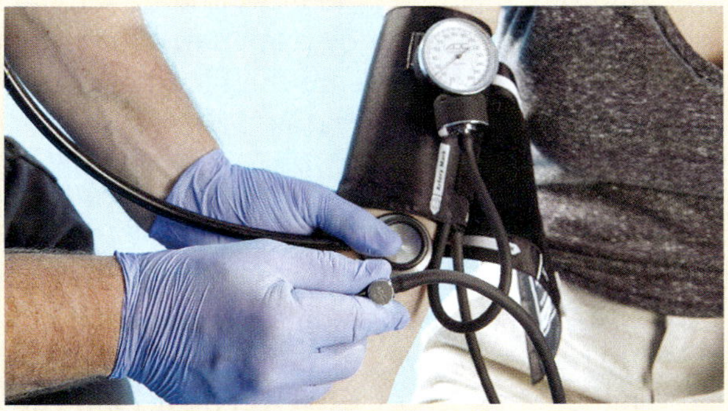

Step 5

Open the valve, and quickly release remaining air

5. Close the valve tightly and pump the ball-pump until you no longer hear pulse sounds. Continue pumping to increase the cuff's pressure to 200 mm Hg (or 30 mm Hg above where the radial pulse disappears[9]). Next, slowly turn the valve, opening it until air is steadily escaping from the cuff and you see the needle of the gauge slowly drop at about 2 to 3 mm Hg per second. Watch the gauge and listen carefully. Note the patient's systolic pressure as the reading on the gauge at which the "taps" or "thumps" of the pulse waves can first be heard clearly. As the pressure in the cuff is progressively reduced, pulse sounds will continue for a time, then suddenly disappear. Note the patient's diastolic pressure as the reading on the gauge at which the sounds stopped (**Step 4**). It is common to see the needle of the sphygmomanometer bounce with the atrial pulsation. Do not mistake these movements as the patient's blood pressure.
6. As soon as the pulse sounds stop, open the valve, and release the remaining air quickly. Once you have finished measuring the blood pressure, document your findings and the time at which the blood pressure was taken. Blood pressure is most often measured by auscultation with the patient in a sitting or semi-Fowler position. Occasionally, when a patient's blood pressure is very low, you will continue to hear pulse sounds from the reading at which they started all the way until the gauge has reached 0. When this occurs, you should record the diastolic pressure as "0" or indicate that it was heard until the gauge read "0" (**Step 5**).[8]

Street Smarts

It is a good idea to ask patients if they know their normal pulse rate or blood pressure. Many people monitor heart rate with a smart watch and can readily provide this information. Very fit people and those taking medicines such as beta blockers may have a normal resting heart rate of less than 60 beats per minute. Likewise, a patient may know that their average blood pressure is very high or runs less than 90 mm Hg systolic. This baseline information helps you gauge whether the values you are finding are normal for your patient.

Obtaining a patient's blood pressure accurately by auscultation may be difficult at times. Noisy environments, patient movement from tremors or seizures, external vibrations from the EMS vehicle, and excessive noises may produce sounds that mimic Korotkoff sounds and provide inaccurate readings. Other variables that may make obtaining an accurate blood pressure reading nearly impossible are uncooperative adults, infants and children, and patients who are hypotensive with poor perfusion. In these cases, measure blood pressure by palpation.

The palpation (feeling) method does not depend on your ability to hear sounds and should be used in these cases to obtain a patient's blood pressure. If possible, it is preferable that you first obtain a baseline auscultated blood pressure.

Follow the steps in **SKILL DRILL 10-3** to measure blood pressure by palpation:

1. Secure the appropriate-size cuff around the patient's upper arm in the manner previously described (**Step 1**).
2. With your nondominant hand, palpate the patient's radial pulse on the same arm as the cuff (**Step 2**). Once you have located it, do not move your fingertips until you have completed taking the blood pressure.
3. While holding the ball-pump in your other hand, close the turn-valve and slowly inflate the cuff until you no longer feel the pulse under your fingertips, then continue to inflate to 200 mm Hg (or 30 mm Hg above where the radial pulse disappears) (**Step 3**).
4. Open the turn-valve so that air slowly escapes (2 to 3 mm Hg/sec) from the cuff, and carefully observe the gauge (**Step 4**). When you can again feel the radial pulse under your fingertips, note the reading on the gauge as the patient's systolic blood pressure. You will not be able to determine the diastolic pressure with this method.
5. Next, open the turn-valve further, and completely deflate the cuff (**Step 5**). Document your findings, including the time, and note that the pressure was taken by palpation. On your patient care report, record the blood pressure as "120/P" and verbalize it as "120 palpated."

Normal Blood Pressure

Blood pressure levels vary with age and sex. **TABLE 10-7** serves as a guideline for normal blood pressure ranges.

A patient has **hypotension** when the blood pressure is lower than the normal range and **hypertension** when the blood pressure is higher than the normal

Skill Drill 10-3 Obtaining Blood Pressure by Palpation

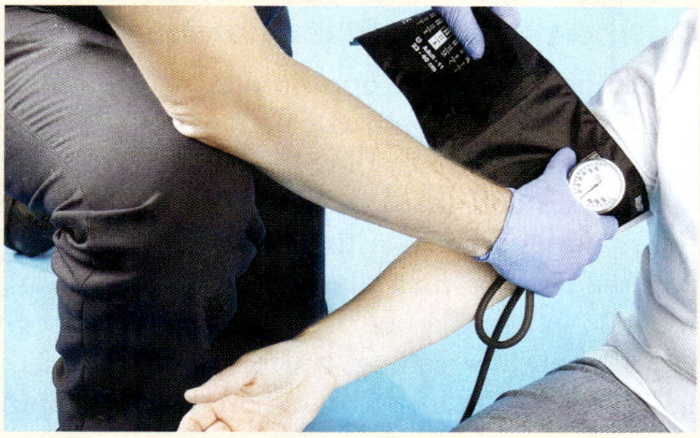

Step 1

Follow standard precautions. Secure the appropriate-size cuff around the patient's upper arm.

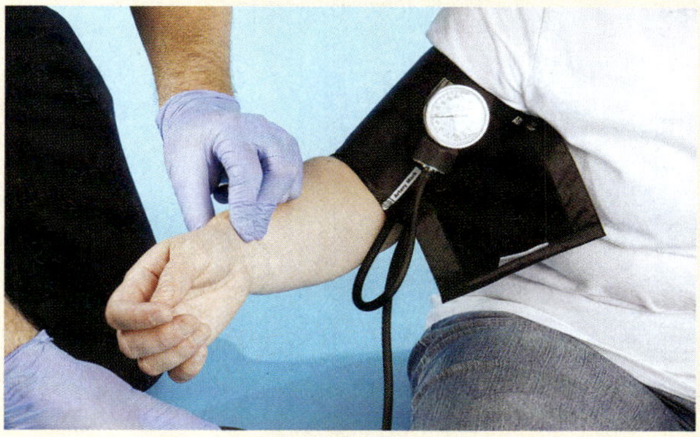

Step 2

With your nondominant hand, palpate the patient's radial pulse on the same arm as the cuff. Once you have located it, do not move your fingertips until you have completed taking the blood pressure.

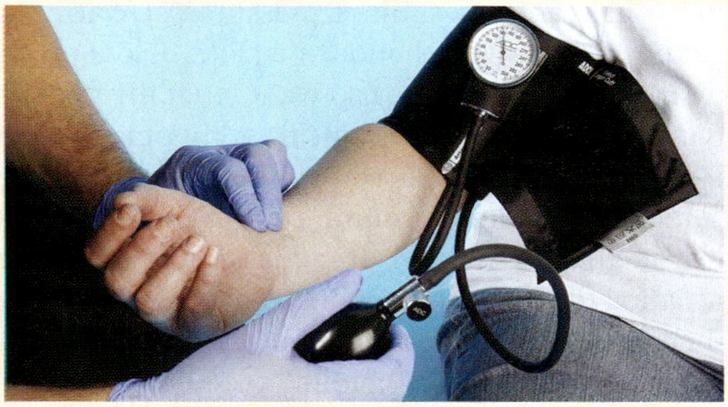

Step 3

While holding the ball-pump in your other hand, close the turn-valve and slowly inflate the cuff until the pulse disappears and then continue to inflate another 30 mm Hg. As the cuff inflates, you will no longer feel the pulse under your fingertips.

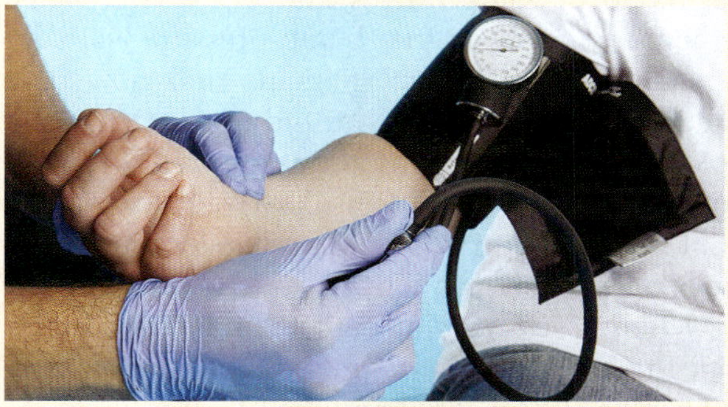

Step 4

Open the turn-valve so that air slowly escapes from the cuff, and carefully observe the gauge. When you can again feel the radial pulse under your fingertips, note the reading on the gauge as the patient's systolic blood pressure.

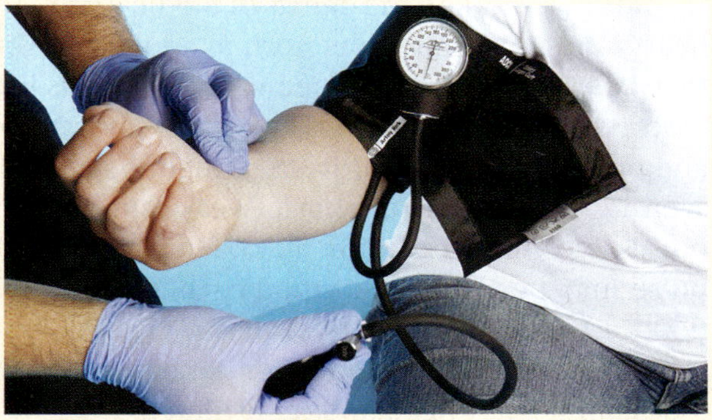

Step 5

Next, open the turn-valve further, and completely deflate the cuff. Document your findings, including the time, and note that the pressure was taken by palpation.

TABLE 10-7 Normal Range for Systolic Blood Pressure

Age	Range (mm Hg)
Newborn (0 to 1 month)	67 to 84
Infant (1 month to 1 year)	72 to 104
Toddler (1 to 3 years)	86 to 106
Preschool age (3 to 6 years)	89 to 112
School age (6 to 12 years)	97 to 115
Adolescent (12 to 18 years)	110 to <120
Adult (18 years and older)	90 to 120

Data adapted from *Pediatric Advanced Life Support, 2015*, the American Heart Association and from the *National Model EMS Clinical Guidelines*, v2.2, 2019, NASEMSO.

range. Typically, you will see children less frequently than adults; therefore, you might not remember the normal ranges for the various age groups. It is a good idea to carry a chart with you that lists normal blood pressure ranges and other vital signs. Remember, however, that blood pressure will vary somewhat with different patients and how they react to the environment around them. Often, the most important information associated with the blood pressure is not the absolute value at any one point but the trend in the pressure over time while you are caring for a patient.

When assessing the patient's general circulation, the blood pressure, pulse, skin temperature, and capillary refill should not be assessed in an injured limb. However, once you have obtained these vital signs from an uninjured limb, you might want to compare the distal skin temperature, quality of the distal pulse, and/or CRT in the injured limb with those found on the uninjured side. This information is useful in evaluating whether the injury may have compromised the circulation in the injured limb.

Words of Wisdom

Automated blood pressure machines often display **mean arterial pressure (MAP)** in addition to systolic and diastolic blood pressures. The MAP is a measure of the average arterial pressure through the systolic and diastolic phases of the cardiac cycle. It is increasingly used as a valuable measurement to determine perfusion in conditions such as sepsis. A MAP of greater than 65 mm Hg is needed to adequately perfuse the vital organs in an adult.

Pediatric Patients: Considerations During the Cardiovascular Assessment

It is important to use appropriate-size equipment when you assess a pediatric patient's vital signs. To obtain an accurate reading of a child's blood pressure, use a cuff that covers two-thirds of the patient's upper arm. As with adults, a blood pressure cuff that is too small may give you a falsely high reading, whereas a cuff that is too large may give you a falsely low reading. The following formula is a useful tool to determine blood pressure in children ages 1 to 10 years (lower limits):

$$70 + (2 \times \text{Child's age in years}) = \text{Lowest expected systolic blood pressure}$$

Remember that your approach to taking vital signs also varies with the age of the pediatric patient. Be gentle, talk to the child, assess respirations and then pulse, and assess blood pressure last. Warm your stethoscope on your hands or a cloth before placing it on the skin. You may also want to let the pediatric patient hold the equipment first; this may help to reduce the child's anxiety. Avoid saying the cuff will "pinch" or "tighten" around the child's arm; instead use language like "hug" or "squeeze" the arm. When inflating the cuff, palpate the radial pulse to estimate the appropriate systolic blood pressure when the pulse disappears and then inflate 30 mm Hg higher before deflating. Avoid excessive inflation in children to avoid causing unnecessary discomfort.[8]

Geriatric Patients: Considerations During the Cardiovascular Assessment

Vital signs may be different in older adults because of the physiologic changes that come with aging, chronic disease, and the effects of medications. The heart rate should be in the normal adult range but may be compromised by medications such as beta blockers. These medications keep the heart rate low and prevent the tachycardia that might be typically seen in dehydration or shock. Weak and irregular pulses are more common in older patients. The pulse may be irregular secondary to atrial fibrillation. Circulatory compromise may make it difficult to feel a radial pulse on an older patient, and other pulse points may need to be considered.

Blood pressure tends to be higher in older people. A geriatric patient who has a blood pressure reading in a normal adult range could be hypotensive. Try to confirm if the patient has missed taking any medications for hypertension.

Capillary refill is not a good assessment tool in older adults because of skin changes and reduced circulation to the skin.

Words of Wisdom

If the pulse is very irregular, it can be difficult to obtain an accurate blood pressure. Deflating the cuff more slowly than normal can be helpful in these situations.

Neurologic System

A neurologic assessment should be performed any time you are confronted with a patient who has changes in mental status, a possible head injury, stupor, dizziness, drowsiness, or syncope. The neurologic assessment starts during your primary assessment and is as simple as talking with the patient, asking questions, and receiving an appropriate reply from the patient during the primary assessment.

Evaluate the level of consciousness and orientation to determine the patient's ability to think and to assess their memory. Use the AVPU scale, if appropriate, to determine the patient's mental status. Is the patient alert and oriented to person, place, time, and events? Is the patient responsive or unresponsive? Does the patient respond to verbal and painful stimuli? If the patient is responsive, evaluate speech for clarity, speed, organization, and logic. What is the patient's activity level? What is the patient's mood and thought content? What do the patient's facial expressions tell you? Is the patient angry, fearful, depressed, anxious, or restless? Does the patient appear uncomfortable? Does the patient make incomprehensible or understandable statements? Is the patient's memory affected? What is the patient's perception or view on what is happening? These are all important considerations when beginning to assess the neurologic system.

Use of the Glasgow Coma Scale (GCS) score can be helpful in providing additional information on patients with changes in mental status. The GCS uses parameters that test a patient's eye opening, best verbal response, and best motor response. The scale provides a numeric score that is associated with the relative severity of a patient's brain dysfunction (**TABLE 10-8**). This information provides baseline data on the patient's overall neurologic status and can be used to help determine if that status is changing for better or worse. A modified GCS is used for children and infants, who respond differently from adults. When you are reporting the GCS score, document or report each section (eg, Eye opening: 3, Verbal response: 4, Motor response: 5 = GCS score of 12) to describe baseline function in each area. Similar to blood pressure, the trending of the patient's GCS is often important. The GCS scale can be difficult to remember and you may need to consult a reference when calculating a patient's GCS. When evaluating patients with neurologic compromise, such as seen with a stroke, there are other assessment tools that can be used. For further discussion of the GCS and other neurologic assessment tools, see Chapter 18, *Neurologic Emergencies*.

Pupils

The pupil is the black center portion of the eye. The pupils are normally round, of approximately equal size, move (react) together, and adjust their size depending on the available light. The diameter and reaction to light of the patient's pupils can reflect the status of the brain's perfusion, oxygenation, and condition. In normal room light, the pupil should appear to be about midsize. With less light, the pupils dilate to allow more light to enter the eye. When a bright light is shined near the eye, the pupils constrict (**FIGURE 10-25A**). When a brighter light is introduced into one eye, both pupils should constrict equally to the appropriate size for the pupil receiving the most light.

In the absence of light, the pupils will become fully dilated (**FIGURE 10-25B**). When light is introduced, each eye sends sensory signals to the brain indicating the level of light it is receiving. Pupil size is regulated by a series of continuous motor commands that the brain automatically sends through the oculomotor nerves to each eye, causing both pupils to constrict to the same appropriate size. Normally, pupil size changes instantly with any change in light level.

Some patients normally have pupils that do not react properly to changes in light as a result of eye surgery or other conditions. A small

TABLE 10-8 Glasgow Coma Scale[a]

Eye Opening		Best Verbal Response		Best Motor Response	
Spontaneous	4	Oriented conversation	5	Obeys commands	6
In response to sound	3	Confused conversation	4	Localizes to pressure	5
In response to pressure	2	Inappropriate words	3	Withdraws from pressure	4
None	1	Incomprehensible sounds	2	Abnormal flexion	3
		None	1	Abnormal extension	2
				None	1

[a]Some systems use a "Not testable (NT)" score for any element that cannot be tested. Eye opening cannot be tested in a patient whose eyes are closed due to a local factor, such as swelling; verbal response cannot be tested in a patient who has a preexisting factor interfering with communication, such as mutism; and motor response cannot be tested in a patient who has preexisting paralysis or some other limiting factor.

Score: 13–15 may indicate mild dysfunction, although 15 is the score a person without neurologic impairment would receive.

Score: 9–12 may indicate moderate dysfunction.

Score: 8 or less is indicative of severe dysfunction.

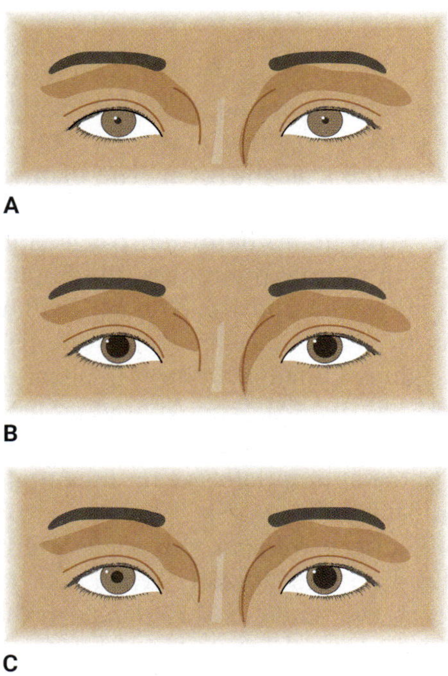

FIGURE 10-25 A. Constricted pupils. **B.** Dilated pupils. **C.** Unequal pupils.

number of patients exhibit normally unequal pupils, a condition called anisocoria (**FIGURE 10-25C**). If the patient or family member cannot confirm the presence of these conditions, you should presume that abnormal pupillary response indicates altered brain function as a result of central nervous system depression or injury. Specifically, evaluate if the pupils react in any of the following ways:

- Become fixed (either dilated or constricted) with no reaction to changes in light
- React sluggishly instead of briskly
- Are unequal in size
- Become unequal in size when a bright light is introduced into or removed from one eye

Some of the causes of depressed brain function include the following:

- Injury of the brain or brainstem
- Trauma or stroke
- Brain tumor
- Inadequate oxygenation or perfusion
- Drugs or toxins (central nervous system depressants)

The mnemonic PERRL is a useful guide in assessing the pupils:

P Pupils
E Equal
R Round
R Regular in size
L React to Light

For patients with normal pupils, you can report "Pupils are Equal and Round, Regular in size, and react properly to Light" or "Pupils = PERRL." Describe any abnormal findings using the longer form, such as "Pupils are equal and round, the left pupil is fixed and dilated, the right pupil is regular in size and reacts to light."

Assessing Neurovascular Status

Now perform a hands-on assessment to determine sensory and motor response. How does the patient move? Check for bilateral muscle strength and weakness. Complete a thorough sensory assessment. Test for sensation, motor function, and position, and compare distal and proximal sensory and motor responses and one side with the other. Remember that a physical examination that deals with a specific chief complaint can be streamlined to assess a specific area of concern.

To assess neurovascular status in a conscious patient, follow the steps in **SKILL DRILL 10-4**:

1. **Pulse.** Palpate the pulse distal to the point of injury. First, palpate the radial pulse in the upper extremity (**Step 1**). Second, in the lower extremity, palpate the posterior tibial and/or dorsalis pedis pulses (**Step 2**).

Skill Drill 10-4 Assessing Neurovascular Status

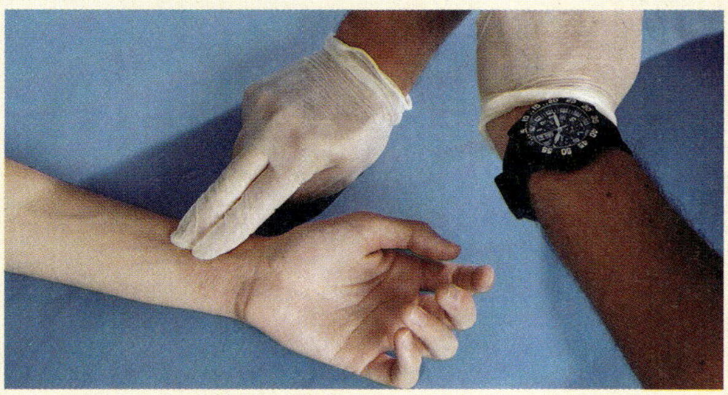

Step 1

Palpate the radial pulse in the upper extremity.

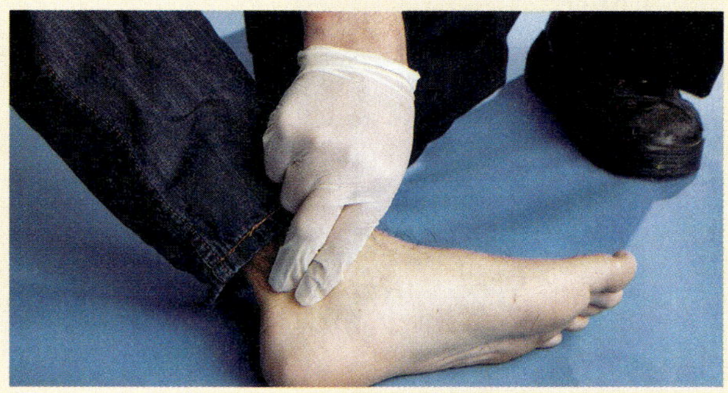

Step 2

Palpate the posterior tibial (shown) and dorsalis pedis pulses in the lower extremity.

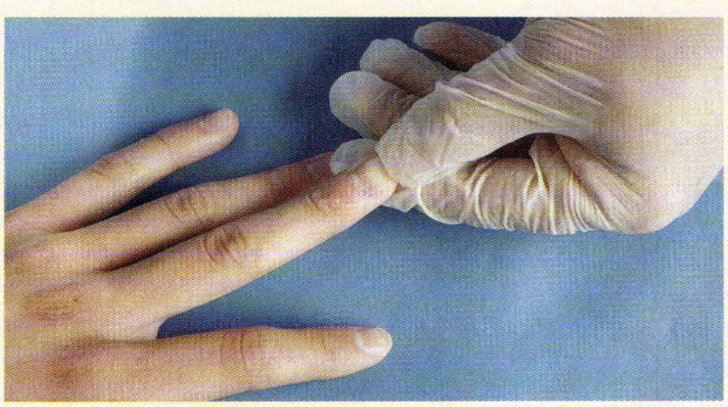

Step 3

Assess capillary refill by blanching a fingernail or toenail.

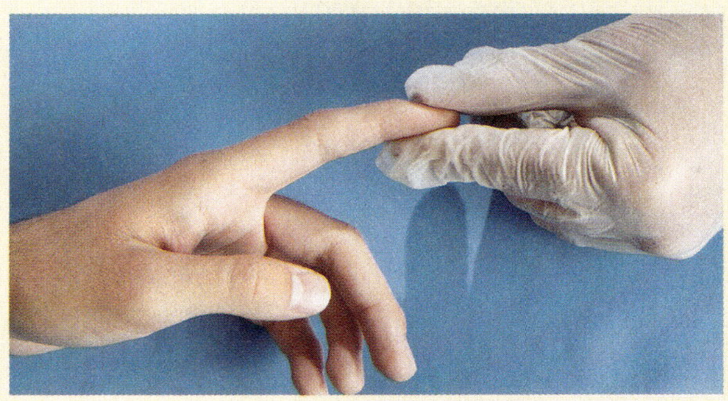

Step 4

Assess sensation on the flesh near the tip of the index finger and thumb, as well as the little finger.

(continues)

Skill Drill 10-4 Assessing Neurovascular Status continued

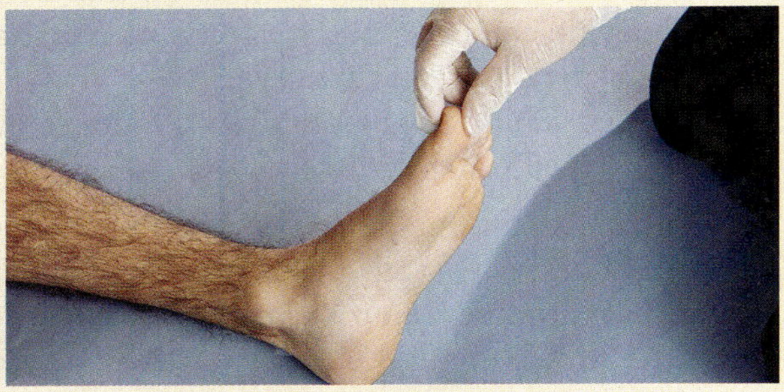

Step 5

On the foot, first check sensation on the flesh near the tip of the big toe.

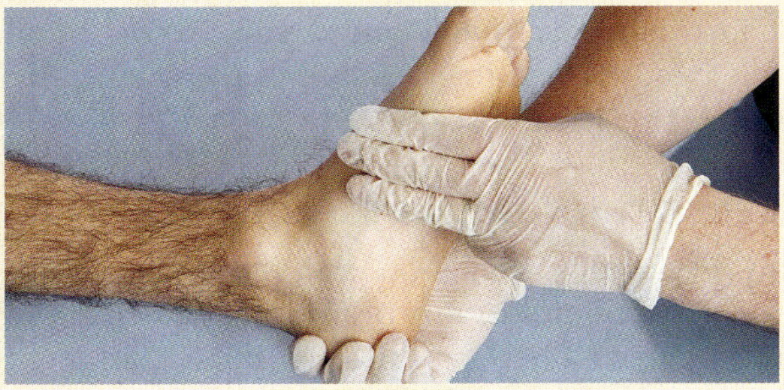

Step 6

Also check sensation on the side of the foot.

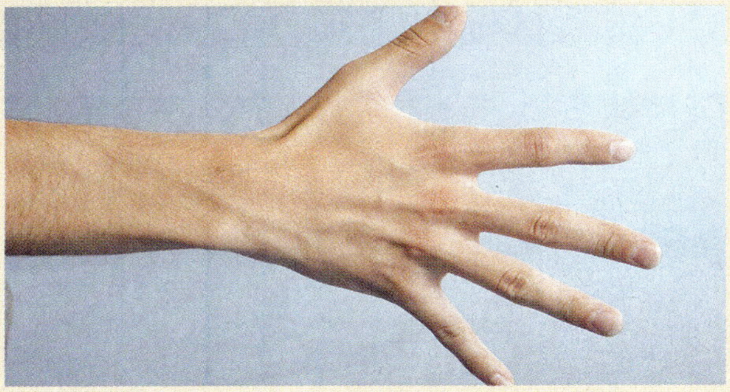

Step 7

For an upper extremity injury, evaluate motor function by asking the patient to open the hand. (Perform motor tests only if the hand or foot is not injured. Stop a test if it causes pain.)

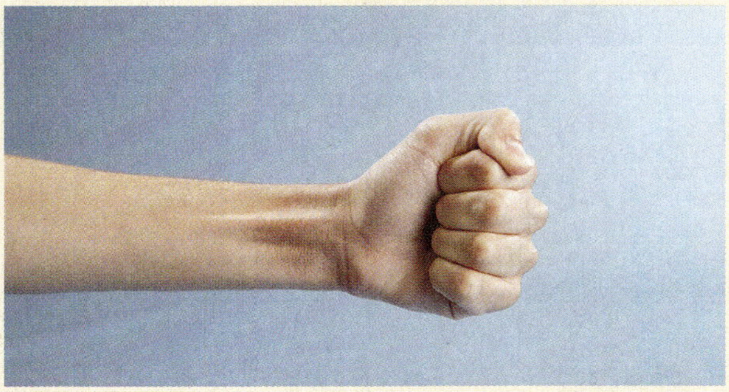

Step 8

Also ask the patient to make a fist.

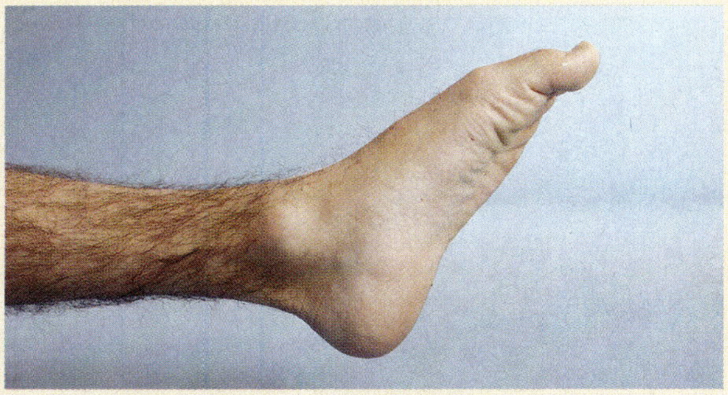

Step 9

For a lower extremity injury, ask the patient to flex the foot and toes (ask the patient to "push down on the gas").

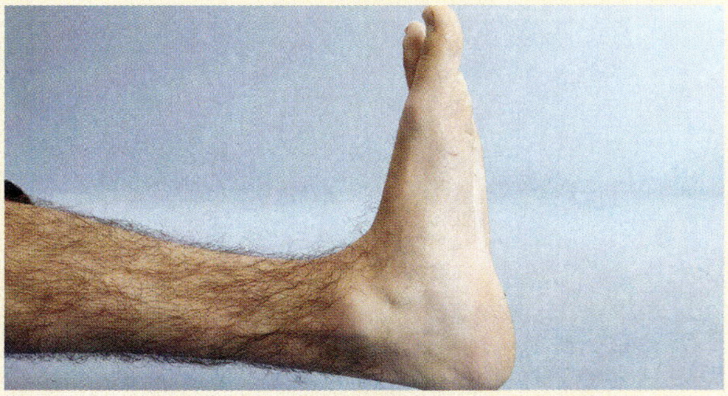

Step 10

Also have the patient extend the foot and ankle and pull the toes and foot toward the nose.

2. **Capillary refill.** Note and record the skin color, identifying any pallor or cyanosis. Then apply firm pressure to the tip of the fingernail or toenail, which will cause the skin to blanch (turn a lighter color). If normal color does not return within 2 seconds after you release the nail, you can assume that circulation is impaired. This test is typically recommended for use in children, although it can also be used in adults (**Step 3**).
3. **Sensation.** In the hand, check the feeling on the flesh near the tip of the index finger and thumb, as well as the little finger (**Step 4**). In the foot, check the sensation on the flesh of the big toe (**Step 5**) and on the side of the foot (**Step 6**). The patient's ability to sense light touch in the fingers or toes distal to the site of a fracture is a good indication that the nerve supply is intact.
4. **Motor function.** Evaluate muscular activity when the injury is proximal to the patient's hand or foot. Ask the patient to open and close a fist for an upper extremity injury and to wiggle the toes and move the foot up and down for a lower extremity injury. Sometimes, an attempt at motion will produce pain at the injury site. If this happens, do not continue this part of the examination. To avoid causing pain, do not perform this test at all if the injury involves the hand or foot itself (**Steps 7 through 10**).

Because many of the steps require patient cooperation, you will not be able to assess sensory and motor functions in an unconscious patient.

Anatomic Regions

Head, Neck, and Cervical Spine

Similar to the head-to-toe assessment, inspect for abnormalities of the head, neck, and cervical spine. Gently palpate the scalp and skull for any pain, deformity, tenderness, crepitus, and bleeding (**FIGURE 10-26**). If the patient is responsive, ask if there is any pain or tenderness. Look at the patient's face. Is it symmetrical? Is there evidence of trauma, such as an **ecchymosis**, which is a buildup of blood beneath the skin caused by an injury that appears as a blue or black discoloration (bruise), or a **hematoma**, which is a mass of blood that has collected within damaged tissue beneath the skin? Does the patient have any facial expressions such as a smile or grimace? Check the patient's eyes, and assess pupillary function, shape, and response. Are the pupils equal in size and reactive to light, or are they constricted, dilated, or unequal? Check the color of the sclera. Assess the patient's cheek bones (zygomas) for possible injury. Check the patient's ears and nose for fluid. Next, before opening the patient's mouth, check the upper (maxillae) and lower (mandible) jaw. Once the patient's jaws have been assessed and it has been determined that movement will not create any additional pain or injury, open the patient's mouth, looking for any broken or missing teeth. If blood and secretions have impaired the airway, this should have been corrected during the primary assessment. Before moving on to the neck, note any unusual odors that may be present in the patient's mouth. This may give an indication of what type of emergency you may be dealing with.

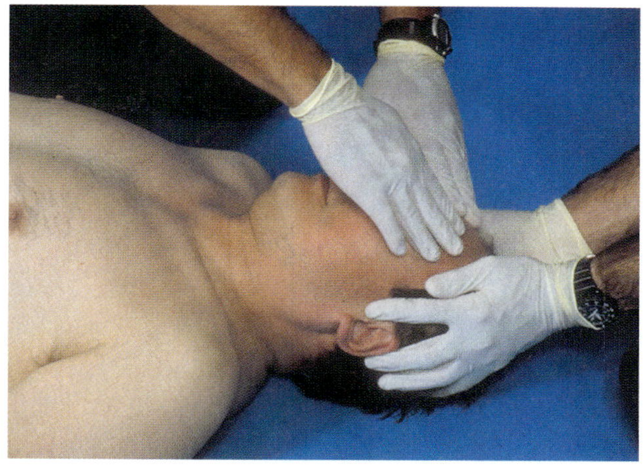

FIGURE 10-26 Gently palpate the head for any pain, deformity, tenderness, crepitus, and bleeding.

Next, check the neck for signs of swelling or bleeding. Palpate the neck for signs of trauma, such as deformities, bumps, swelling, bruising, and bleeding, as well as a crackling sound (crepitus) produced by air bubbles under the skin, known as **subcutaneous emphysema** (**FIGURE 10-27**). Assess if the trachea is midline. Also, in patients in whom spinal injury is not suspected, inspect for pronounced or distended jugular veins with the patient sitting at a 45° angle. This is a normal finding in a person who is lying supine; however, jugular venous distention in a patient who is sitting up suggests a problem

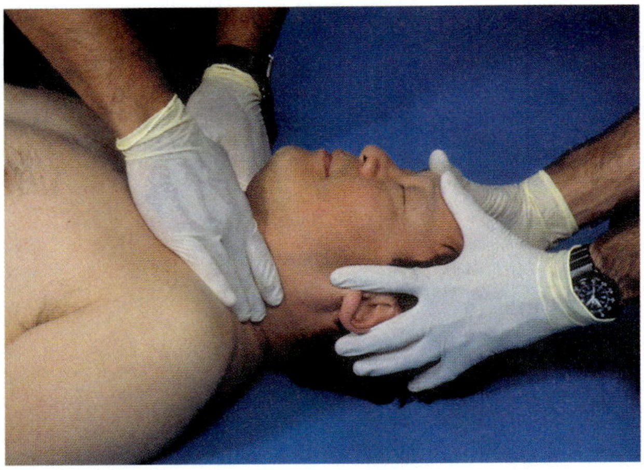

FIGURE 10-27 Gently palpate the neck.

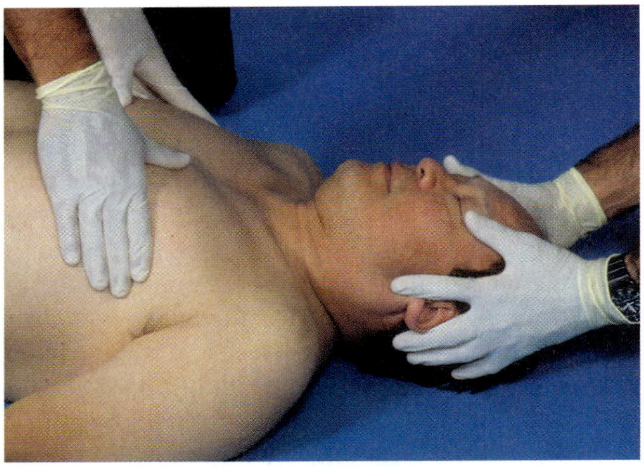

FIGURE 10-28 Inspect, visualize, and palpate over the chest area for injury and signs of trauma.

with blood returning to the heart. Report and record your findings carefully. Palpate the posterior of the neck for tenderness or spinal step-off, which could indicate a spinal column injury.

Chest

When assessing the chest, inspect, visualize, and palpate over the chest area for injury and signs of trauma, including bruising, tenderness, and swelling (**FIGURE 10-28**).

When assessing breathing, watch for both sides of the chest to rise and fall together with normal breathing. Observe for abnormal breathing signs, including retractions or paradoxical chest motion.

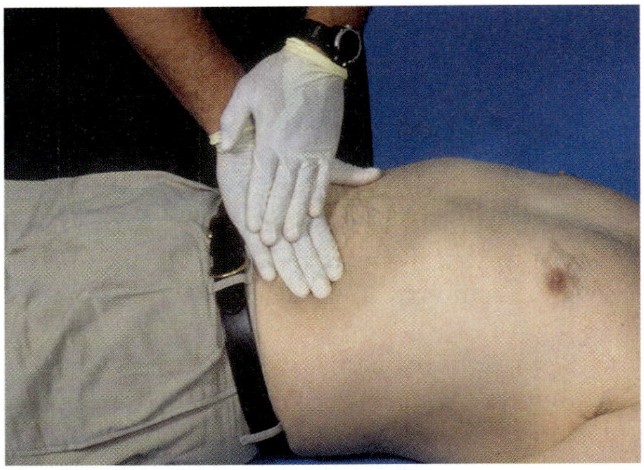

FIGURE 10-29 Palpate the abdomen, evaluating for tenderness and bleeding.

Retractions indicate the patient has some condition, usually medical, that is impairing the flow of air into and out of the lungs. Paradoxical chest motion is associated with a fracture of several ribs (flail), causing a section of the chest to move independently from the rest of the chest wall. Feel for grating of the bones as the patient breathes. Crepitus is often associated with rib fractures. Palpate the chest for subcutaneous emphysema, especially in cases of severe blunt chest trauma, as this could indicate a pneumothorax.

If the patient reports difficulty breathing or has evidence of trauma to the chest, auscultate breath sounds. This helps you to evaluate air movement into and out of the lungs. The goal is to hear and document the presence or absence of breath sounds. If you believe the patient's breathing is abnormal, reassess breathing and, if appropriate, provide appropriate oxygenation and ventilation.

Abdomen

Look for trauma to the abdomen and for distention. Palpate the abdomen for tenderness, rigidity, and patient **guarding** (**FIGURE 10-29**). As you palpate the abdomen, use "firm," "soft," "tender," or "distended" (swollen) to report your findings. If the patient is awake and alert, ask about pain as you perform the examination. The abdomen is divided into four quadrants: left upper quadrant (LUQ), left lower quadrant (LLQ), right upper quadrant (RUQ), and right lower quadrant (RLQ) (**FIGURE 10-30**).

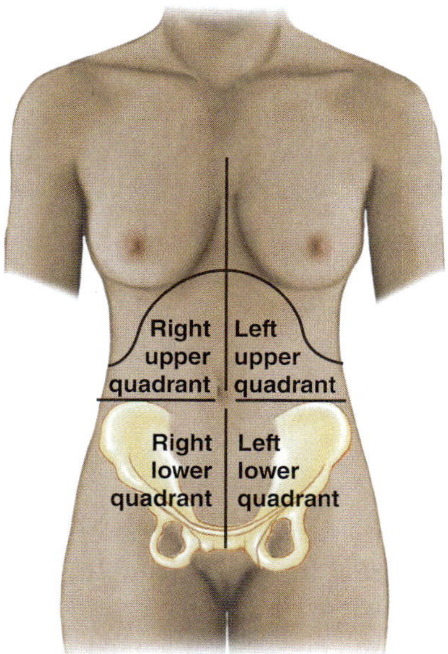

FIGURE 10-30 Quadrants of the abdomen.

Always start the palpation of the abdomen in the quadrant that is farthest from the patient's pain. Do not palpate over obvious soft-tissue injuries, and be careful not to palpate too firmly. Assess for the presence of rebound tenderness, which is pain created when pressure is released. If you note a pulsating mass in the abdomen, do not continue to palpate that area. If there is an abdominal aortic aneurysm, applying further pressure to the area could cause it to rupture, causing massive internal bleeding.

Pelvis

Inspect the pelvis for symmetry and any obvious signs of injury, bleeding, and deformity (**FIGURE 10-31**). If the patient reports no pain, gently press downward and inward on the iliac crests of the pelvic bones. Do not rock the pelvis; this action may result in exacerbation of damage to any unstable bones. If you feel any movement or crepitus or the patient reports pain or tenderness, severe injury may be present. Injuries to the pelvis and surrounding abdomen may bleed profusely without any obvious external signs, so continue to monitor the patient's mental status, skin condition, and vital signs.

Extremities

An assessment of the patient's musculoskeletal system typically is done because of a chief complaint associated with some type of trauma. Do all extremities appear to be properly positioned, and do all extremities appear to be functioning normally? Assess for posture if standing, and look at joints, checking for range of motion. This should be done by asking patients how much they can move the extremity or joint. Never force a painful joint to move. Always compare the right side with the left side, looking for weakness or atrophy, and assess equality of grip strength.

Inspect each extremity for symmetry, cuts, bruises, swelling, obvious injuries, and bleeding (**FIGURE 10-32**). Also palpate along each extremity

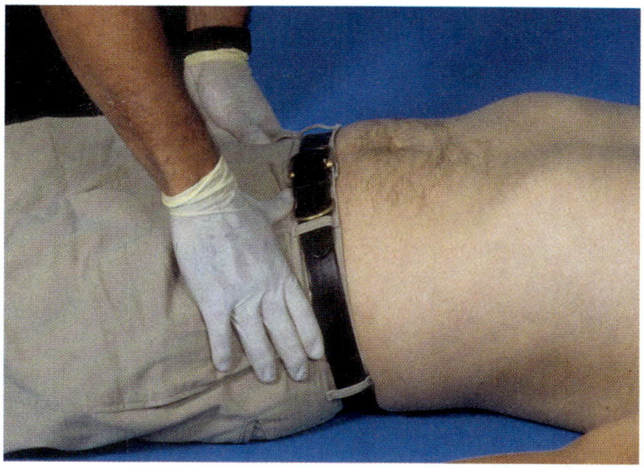

FIGURE 10-31 Inspect the pelvis for any obvious signs of injury, bleeding, and deformity.

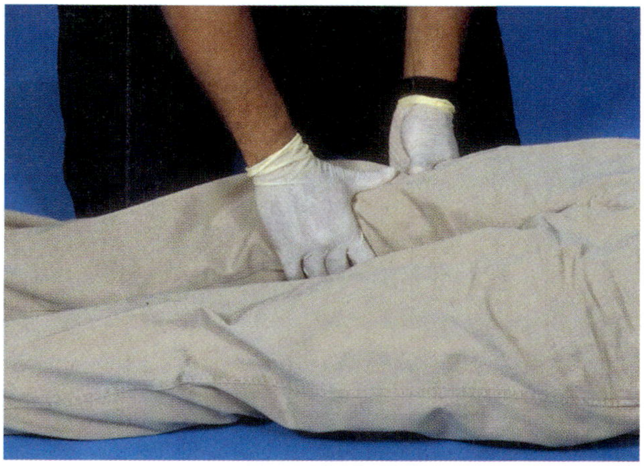

FIGURE 10-32 Inspect each extremity for cuts, bruises, swelling, obvious injuries, and bleeding.

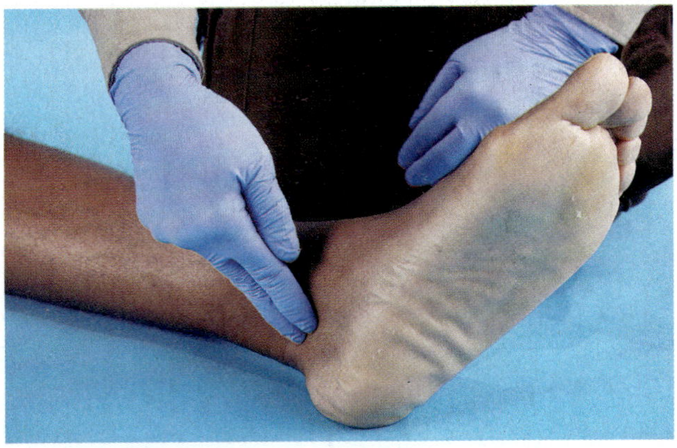

FIGURE 10-33 Palpation of the posterior tibial pulse.

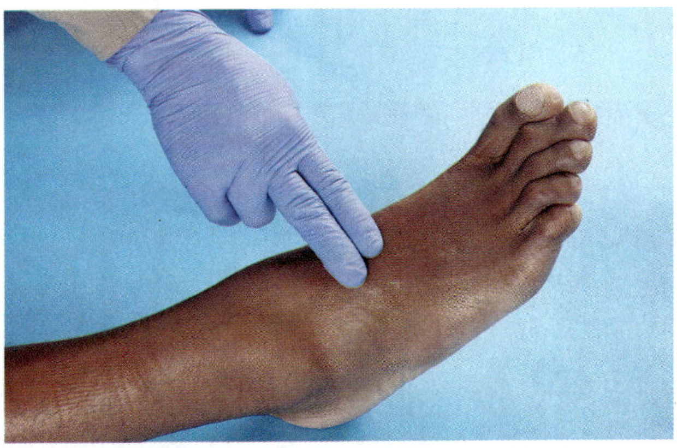

FIGURE 10-34 Palpation of the dorsalis pedis pulse.

for deformities. Ask the patient about any tenderness or pain. As you evaluate the extremities, check for pulses, motor function, and sensory function:

- **Pulse.** Check the distal pulses on the foot (dorsalis pedis or posterior tibial) (**FIGURE 10-33** and **FIGURE 10-34**) and wrist. Assess the pulses in the lower extremities for rate, quality, and rhythm. Is the pulse rate fast, slow, or irregular? Is the pulse weak, thready, or bounding? Also check circulation. Evaluate the skin color and temperature of the hands and feet. Is it normal? How does it compare with the skin color and temperature of the other extremities? Pale or cyanotic skin may indicate poor circulation in that extremity.

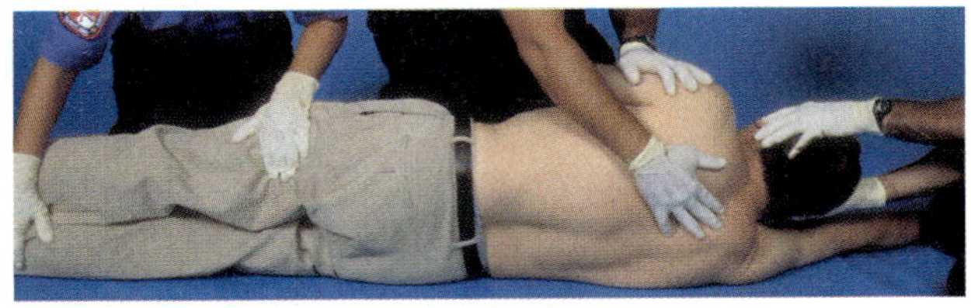

FIGURE 10-35 Feel the back for tenderness, deformity, and open wounds. Carefully palpate the spine from the neck to the pelvis for tenderness and deformity. Look under the clothing for obvious injuries, including bruising and bleeding.

- **Motor function.** Ask the patient to wiggle the fingers and toes. An inability to move a single extremity can be the result of a bone, muscle, or nerve injury. An inability to move several extremities may be a sign of a brain abnormality or spinal cord injury. Verify that you are maintaining spinal motion restriction if indicated.
- **Sensory function.** Evaluate sensory function in the extremity by asking the patient to close the eyes. Gently squeeze or pinch a finger or toe and ask the patient to identify what you are doing. The inability to feel sensation in the extremity may indicate a local nerve injury. The inability to feel sensation in several extremities may be a sign of a spinal cord injury. Ensure that you are maintaining spinal motion restriction.

Posterior Body

Inspect the back for DCAP-BTLS, symmetry, and open wounds (**FIGURE 10-35**). Carefully palpate the spine from the neck to the pelvis for tenderness and deformity.

Assessment of Vital Signs Using the Appropriate Monitoring Device

The use of monitoring equipment in the prehospital setting has continued to expand. EMTs at all levels use a wide variety of devices in the continuous monitoring of patients. It is important to remember that these devices are manufactured and subject to limitations and failures. Such devices should never be used to replace your comprehensive assessment of your patient; think of them as simply adjuncts to the assessment and treatment of your patient. Obtaining and using information from patient monitoring devices includes, but is not limited to, data from pulse oximetry and noninvasive blood pressure monitoring.

Pulse Oximetry

Pulse oximetry is an assessment tool used to evaluate the effectiveness of oxygenation. The pulse oximeter is a photoelectric device that monitors the oxygen saturation of hemoglobin (the iron-containing portion of the red blood cell to which oxygen attaches) in the capillary beds (**FIGURE 10-36**). The parts that make up the pulse oximeter include a monitor and a sensing probe. The sensing probe clips onto a finger or earlobe. The light source must have access to a capillary bed, which may be obstructed by factors such as gel nail polish, but research suggests that removal in the prehospital setting is rarely advised.[10,11] Results appear as a percentage on the display screen. Normally, pulse oximetry values in ambient air will vary depending on the altitude, with most normal oxygen saturation values falling between 94% and 99%. For other considerations when performing pulse oximetry, see Chapter 11, *Airway and Ventilation Management*.

The goal of applying oxygen therapy is to increase oxygen saturation to a normal level. This device is a useful assessment tool to detect hypoxemia in patients with dyspnea or altered consciousness and to determine the effectiveness of oxygen therapy, bronchodilator therapy, and artificial ventilations. However, the pulse oximeter does not take the place of good assessment skills and should not prevent the application of oxygen to any patient who reports difficulty breathing regardless of the pulse oximetry value seen on the monitor.

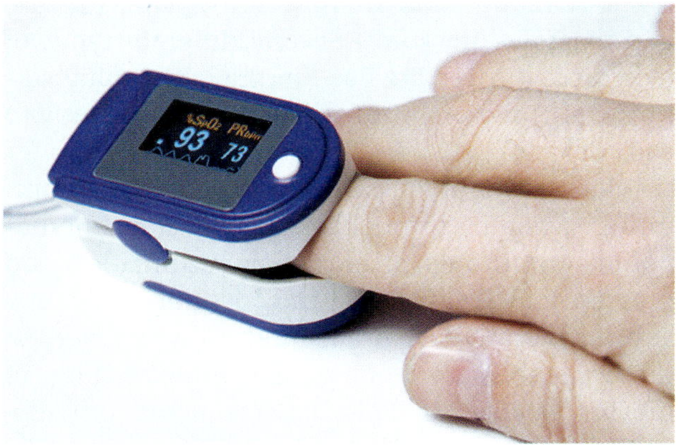

FIGURE 10-36 The pulse oximeter is a device that measures the saturation of oxygen in the blood as a percentage.

Because the device functions properly only with adequate perfusion and numbers of red blood cells, any situation that causes vasoconstriction (such as hypothermia or shock) or loss of red blood cells (such as bleeding or anemia) will result in inaccurate or misleading values. The device also presumes that oxygen is saturating the hemoglobin. Therefore, any chemical that displaces oxygen (such as carbon monoxide) may cause misleading values.

The pulse oximeter is a useful tool as long as you remember that the device is only a tool, not a substitute for a good assessment.

Capnography

Metabolism refers to the chemical reactions that occur in each of the body's cells to maintain life and generate energy. To get an idea about the patient's metabolism and adequacy of ventilation, you can measure exhaled carbon dioxide (CO_2) levels in the air as the patient exhales. Pulse oximetry can measure the amount of oxygen available to the patient's cells for cellular metabolism, but it does not measure how much of that oxygen is being used. **Carbon dioxide** is the by-product of aerobic cellular metabolism and reflects the amount of oxygen being consumed during metabolism. Think of the oxygen as helping to burn the fuel in metabolism, and the carbon dioxide as the exhaust. You can learn a great deal by measuring this "exhaust" from a patient.

When you are working with ALS clinicians, there will be times when they may employ certain techniques to measure the amount of carbon dioxide in exhaled air to help understand the degree to which a patient is adequately perfused and ventilated. For example, **capnography** is a noninvasive method that can quickly and efficiently provide information on a patient's ventilation, circulation, and metabolism. Waveform

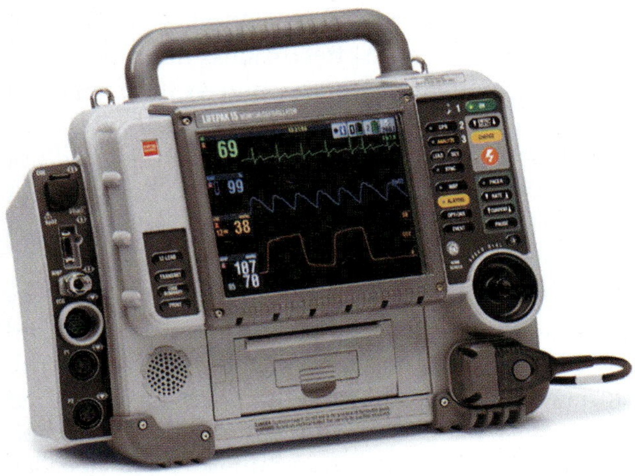

FIGURE 10-37 This device is capable of monitoring multiple functions simultaneously, including continuous capnography (bottom tracing).

The LIFEPAK 15 defibrillator monitor courtesy of Physio-Control. Used with permission of Physio-Control, Inc., and according to the Material Release Form provided by Physio-Control.

capnography shows a graph that indicates how easily, how frequently, and how much carbon dioxide the patient is exhaling (**FIGURE 10-37**). Capnography monitors can be attached to the end of an advanced airway or onto a nasal cannula. Capnography is used to evaluate the effectiveness of breathing treatments and of spontaneous or artificial ventilation and to confirm endotracheal tube placement.

Blood Glucometry

Measuring the blood glucose level of a patient who has altered mental status can prove invaluable. Blood glucometry measures the level of glucose in the patient's bloodstream. If the glucose level is low, this can help you identify the reason a patient is unresponsive. If the level is high in a patient with nausea, vomiting, abdominal pain, and a change in mental status, it may signal dangerous complications of high blood glucose.

Blood glucose level should be assessed in all patients known to have diabetes, all patients who have an altered mental status, and patients with generalized malaise or weakness. In addition, a blood glucose level can be assessed in any patient whom you think has a poor general impression.

To obtain a blood glucose measurement, you will need to use a disposable safety lancet to obtain a drop of blood. Follow the steps in **SKILL DRILL 10-5** to assess blood glucose level:

1. Take standard precautions. Cleanse the site (side of the fingertip) with antiseptic and allow it to dry (**Step 1**).
2. Puncture the site with the disposable safety lancet (**Step 2**).
3. Immediately dispose of the needle in a sharps container (**Step 3**).
4. Obtain a drop of blood on the test strip (you may need to gently squeeze the finger to obtain an adequate sample). Insert the test strip into the glucometer and activate the device per the manufacturer's instructions (**Step 4**).
5. When finished, place a bandage over the puncture site (**Step 5**).

Most newer glucometers take only a few seconds to provide a reading. Glucometers should be calibrated on a regular basis to maintain accuracy. In addition, you should verify that the test strips match the glucometer you are using and that they have not expired.

Noninvasive Blood Pressure Measurement

Auscultation with a sphygmomanometer is the most reliable means of measuring a patient's blood pressure. Electronic measurement is another method of obtaining blood pressure readings on patients. An electronic device measures changes in pressure oscillations that occur during cuff inflation or deflation and are related to systolic, mean, and diastolic pressures. Several different types of electronic devices are used in the prehospital setting; the blood pressure cuff deflates differently in each device.

Standard noninvasive blood pressure monitoring, whether through a manual sphygmomanometer or through an electronic, automatic blood pressure cuff, is easy to use and does not involve any advanced or invasive procedures. However, both of these methods are prone to inaccurate readings in moving vehicles, in noisy environments, or if the cuff is not correctly sized or properly placed on the patient. Electronic automated blood pressure cuffs are further subject to inaccuracy depending on the ability of the sensors to accurately ascertain pressure in the blood vessel. The degree of inaccuracy

Skill Drill 10-5 Assessing Blood Glucose Level

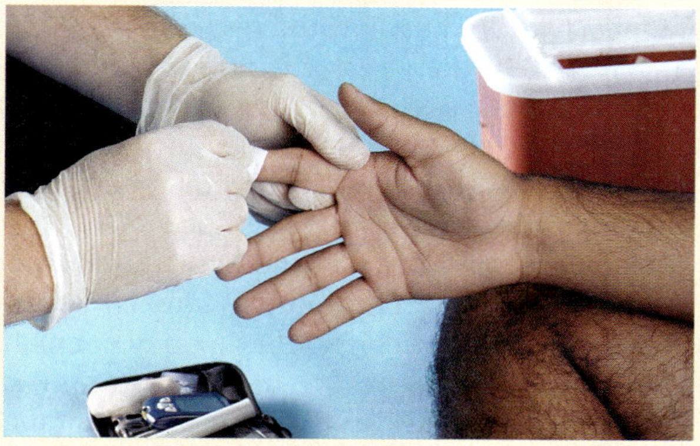

Step 1

Take standard precautions. Cleanse the site (finger) with antiseptic and allow it to dry.

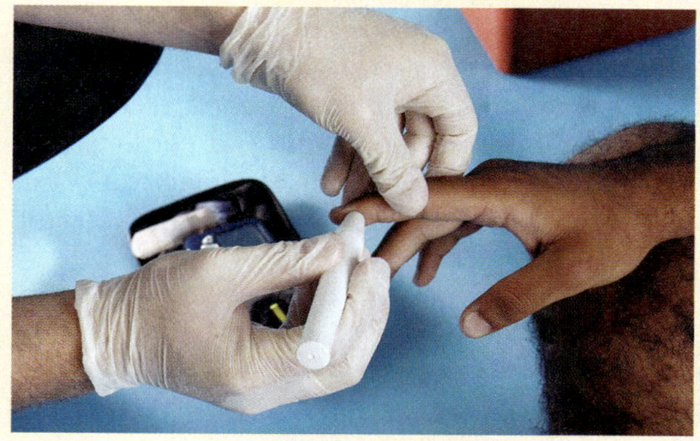

Step 2

Puncture the site with the lancet.

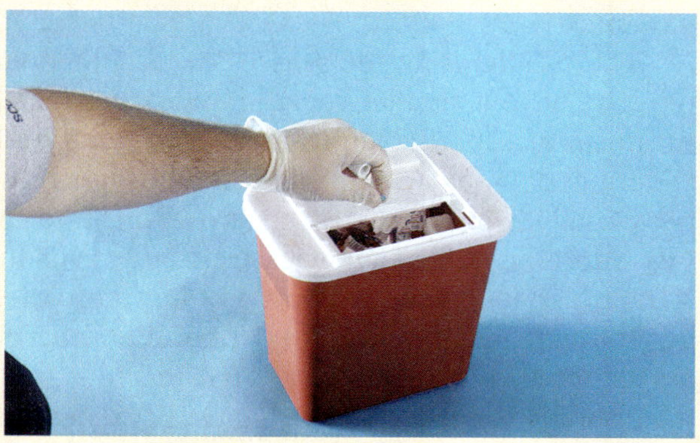

Step 3

Dispose of the needle in a sharps container.

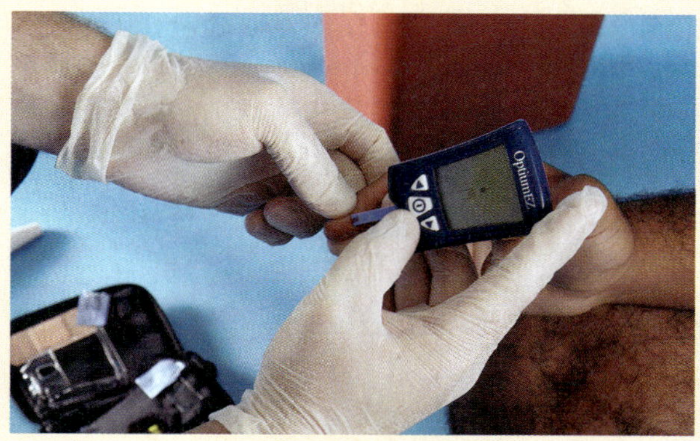

Step 4

Obtain a drop of blood on the test strip. Insert the test strip into the glucometer and activate the device per the manufacturer's instructions.

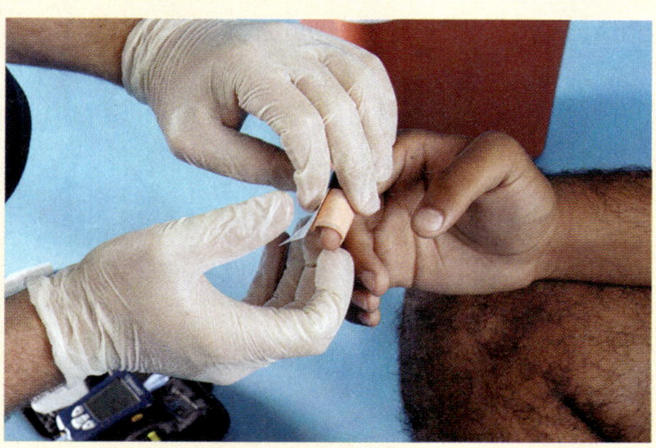

Step 5

Place a bandage over the puncture site.

in these devices can vary substantially from patient to patient depending on several factors. When faced with electronic readings that do not correlate with a patient's clinical presentation, it is best to obtain a manual reading to confirm. As a general rule with each patient, it is good practice to use a manual sphygmomanometer first to obtain a blood pressure reading to confirm that it correlates accurately with the electronic automated cuff prior to relying on the electronic measurement.

Geriatric Patients: Considerations During the Focused Assessment

Assessing an older person can be challenging because of communication issues, hearing and vision deficits, alteration in consciousness, complicated medical histories, and the effects of medications. Previous injury or illnesses that are not associated with the current problem may also alter the assessment findings. These may include medications that mask changes in vital signs that you might expect, such as tachycardia in shock. A previous stroke may have changed a patient's baseline level of consciousness and neurologic status.

The GEMS Diamond

When you are called on to care for older patients, it is important to remember certain key concepts. The GEMS diamond (**TABLE 10-9**) was created to help you remember differences to consider when assessing older patients, as compared with the rest of the population. The GEMS diamond is not intended to be a format for your approach to geriatric patients, nor is it intended to replace the ABCs of care.

The "G" of the GEMS diamond stands for "geriatric patients." When responding to an emergency involving an older patient, you should be familiar with the normal changes of aging and treat older patients with compassion and respect.

The "E" of the GEMS diamond stands for an environmental assessment. Assessment of the environment can help give clues to the patient's condition and the cause of the emergency. Is the temperature in the home appropriate? Is it well kept? Is it secure from intruders? Are hazardous conditions evident? Preventive care is also important for a geriatric patient, who may not realize where risks exist.

The "M" of the GEMS diamond stands for medical assessment. As stated, older patients tend to have a variety of medical problems and may be taking numerous prescriptions, as well as over-the-counter and herbal medications. Obtaining a thorough medical history is important in older patients.

The "S" stands for social assessment. Older people may have a smaller social network because of the death of a spouse, family members, and friends. Older people may also need assistance with activities of daily living (ADLs), such as dressing and eating. Numerous social agencies are readily available to help geriatric patients. Suggest that the patient or their caregiver call the 2-1-1 phone number for assistance and referrals related to caregiving, housing or utility expenses, food programs and benefits, health care expenses, or mental health or substance use concerns.

The GEMS diamond provides an organized way to remember the important issues for older patients. Using this concept will help you make appropriate referrals, and, as a result, you will help older patients maintain their quality of life.

TABLE 10-9 The GEMS Diamond

G Geriatric Patients

- Present atypically
- Deserve respect
- Experience changes with age

E Environmental Assessment

- What is the physical condition of the living space? Is the interior or exterior of the home in need of repair? Is the home secure?
- Are hazardous conditions present (eg, poor wiring, uneven floors, unventilated gas heaters, broken window glass, clutter that prevents adequate egress)?
- Are smoke detectors present and functional?
- Is the home too hot or too cold?
- Is there a fecal or urine odor in the home?
- Are pets well cared for?
- Is food present in the home? Is it adequate and unspoiled?
- Are liquor bottles present (lying empty)?
- Is bedding soiled or dirty?
- If the patient has a disability, are appropriate assistive devices (such as a wheelchair or walker) present and in adequate condition?
- Does the patient have access to a telephone?
- Are medications prescribed, expired, unmarked, or from multiple physicians?
- If living with others, is the patient confined to one part of the home?
- If the patient is residing in a nursing facility, does the care appear to be adequate to meet the patient's needs?

M Medical Assessment

- Older patients tend to have a variety of medical problems, making assessment more complex. Keep this in mind in all cases—that is, both trauma and medical. A trauma patient may have an underlying medical condition related to the traumatic event.
- Obtaining a medical history is very important in older patients, no matter what the primary complaint is.
- Primary assessment
- Reassessment

S Social Assessment

- Assess the activities of daily living (ADLs):
  - Eating
  - Dressing
  - Bathing
  - Toileting
- Are these activities being provided for the patient? If so, by whom?
- Are there delays in obtaining food, medication, or hygiene? The patient may report this, or the environment may be suggestive of this.
- Does the patient have regular visits from family members, live with family members, or live with a spouse?
- If in an institutional setting, is the patient able to feed themself? If not, is food still sitting on the food tray? Has the patient been lying in their own urine or feces for prolonged periods?
- Does the patient have a social network? Does the patient have ways to interact socially with others on a daily basis?

National Association of Emergency Medical Technicians NAEMT. *Geriatric Education for Emergency Medical Services*, Second Edition. Burlington, MA: Jones & Bartlett Learning, 2014.

Patient Assessment

Scene Size-Up

↓

Primary Assessment

↓

History Taking

↓

Secondary Assessment

↓

Reassessment

Repeat the primary assessment
Reassess vital signs
Reassess the chief complaint or chief concern
Recheck interventions
Identify and treat changes in the patient's condition
Reassess the patient

- Unstable patients: every 5 minutes
- Stable patients: every 15 minutes

Reassessment

A **reassessment** is performed at regular intervals during the assessment process. Its purpose is to identify and treat changes in a patient's condition. The role of reassessment cannot be overemphasized, as the patient's condition can change quickly.

Words of Wisdom

Reassessment should take place:

- Every 5 minutes for patients in unstable condition
- Every 15 minutes for patients in stable condition

Repeat the Primary Assessment

The reassessment procedure is to repeat the primary assessment (ABCs) to identify and treat any life-threatening changes in the patient's condition. If you provided any interventions, this is also the time to review that they are working.

Reassess Vital Signs

Reassess and record vital signs. Compare the baseline vital signs obtained during the primary assessment with any and all subsequent vital signs. Look for trends. Have they increased, declined, or stayed the same? If they have changed, how quickly? Reassess the mental status, airway, breathing, and circulation. Monitor skin color and temperature.

Reassess the Chief Complaint or Chief Concern

With all emergency medical services, a reassessment must be completed to determine if the patient care plan is effective. The purpose is to ask and answer the following questions about the patient's chief complaint:

- Is the current treatment improving the patient's condition?
- Has an already identified problem gotten better?
- Has an already identified problem gotten worse?
- What is the nature of any newly identified problems?

Recheck Interventions

In the reassessment process, reevaluate everything that has been done to this point in the patient assessment process. Check all interventions. Most important are the patient's ABCs. In addition, are the bandages, splinting devices, extrication equipment, and patient-securing instruments in place and appropriate for transport?

Identify and Treat Changes in the Patient's Condition

No matter what the patient's condition was prior to your arrival, which interventions were used, or which decisions on treatment and transport priorities were made, a reassessment is necessary to help monitor changes in the patient's condition. If the patient's condition has improved, simply continue whatever treatments you are providing. If the patient's condition deteriorates, prepare to modify treatments as appropriate. Document any changes, whether negative or positive.

Reassess Patient

How and when to perform a reassessment depend on the patient's condition. A patient in unstable condition should be reassessed approximately every 5 minutes, whereas a patient in stable condition should be reassessed approximately every 15 minutes.

Pediatric Patients: Considerations During the Reassessment

When you provide interventions for a pediatric patient, remember that parents and caregivers are often able to assist with administering oxygen or medications via a nebulizer. They can also help you reassess the effectiveness of interventions based on their observations of the child relative to their normal behavior.

Special Challenges in Completing a Patient Assessment

In providing patient care, you will be faced with challenges, many of them new and difficult. Every patient interaction should be viewed as a new experience and handled as an educational opportunity.

Silence

Communicating with patients who say very little, or nothing at all, can be difficult and frustrating. Patience is extremely important in these situations. Patients may be thinking about how to answer you, getting the facts straight, or assessing your crew to determine if they feel comfortable answering you. Using a closed-ended question that requires a simple yes or no answer may work best in certain circumstances. Consider whether the silence is a clue to the patient's chief complaint.

Always look for visual signs that may indicate why a patient is not communicating. This may include nonverbal clues, including facial expressions that may show pain or fear. Is the patient distressed or intimidated by your presence or by the presence of someone else on the scene? Is there a communication problem? Is there a language problem? There are many reasons a patient may be silent during the prehospital encounter. A good EMT will continue to assess the situation and determine a way to communicate with the patient.

Overly Talkative

On the other end of the spectrum is the patient or bystander who is extremely talkative. Some people just talk a lot, and gathering details about their medical condition may be difficult if they talk around your question or you have a difficult time refocusing the patient's conversation. Some possible causes as to why a patient may be overly talkative could include excessive caffeine consumption, nervousness, ingestion of cocaine or methamphetamines, or an underlying psychological issue.

Once you have allowed talkative patients the chance to express themselves, you must keep them focused on the questions presented. Have the patient stick to the facts, and clarify statements for the purpose of making sure the information you are gathering is correct.

Multiple Symptoms

Some patients present with multiple symptoms. Prioritize the patient's complaints as you would in triage; start with the most serious and end with the least serious. Always ask for additional information to determine why EMS was called. Do not limit the patient's complaints; doing so will hinder your ability to gather information.

Keep an open mind, and do not focus on just one complaint or detail to determine a treatment plan. Always remember there may be several possible medical or traumatic causes for a patient's chief complaint.

Intoxication

When you gather a history from an intoxicated patient, be aware that the information may be difficult to get and possibly unreliable. Intoxicated patients may become impatient with you when they are trying to provide you with information. As this impatience increases, so does the anger level. Do not put intoxicated patients in a position where they feel threatened and have no way out. As in other emergency cases, the potential for violence and a physical confrontation is high when a patient is intoxicated.

During the assessment and treatment of a patient who has consumed alcohol, be accepting, diplomatic, objective, and nonjudgmental. Treat the patient with dignity and respect despite the intoxication. Keep in mind that alcohol intoxication may prevent these patients from telling you all the details of their condition. Alcohol dulls a person's senses, including the pain response, compromising a vital source of information.

Crying

A crying patient is a breathing patient. A patient who cries may be sad, in pain, or emotionally overwhelmed. No matter the reason for crying, you need to be calm, patient, reassuring, and confident, and maintain a soft voice.

Your presence may make a crying patient feel more secure. As with all patients, treat a crying patient with respect and dignity.

Confusing Behavior or History

Patients sometimes provide more information to hospital personnel because they were embarrassed or frightened about telling the EMTs or they just forgot to mention it to EMS. Whatever the situation may be, there are medical causes that you must be aware of that can cause a patient to report a confusing history. Conditions such as hypoxia, stroke, diabetes, trauma, medications, and other drugs could alter a patient's explanation of events. It is not uncommon to encounter an older patient who has dementia (eg, Alzheimer disease) or delirium. It is important to verify the normal mental status of each patient. Do not assume that all older patients who demonstrate confusion have one of these conditions.

Confused behavior is not a normal response. After you have properly assessed and treated any life threats, attempt to ask the patient again about the chief complaint or ask someone close to the patient, such as family members or friends, to provide additional details.

Limited Cognitive Abilities

Cognitive disabilities are conditions that impair a person's ability to remember information, process information, make decisions, or communicate in a normal fashion. They can include intellectual disability, autism spectrum disorders, some mental illnesses, and dementia, among other conditions. The level of impairment from cognitive disabilities can range from barely recognizable to severe. You should develop a method of assessing a patient who has limited cognitive abilities. Keep your questions simple, and limit the use of medical terms. Be alert for partial answers, and keep asking questions. In cases of patients with severely limited cognitive function, rely on family, caregivers, and friends to supply answers to your questions.

Cultural Challenges

As an EMT, you are likely to provide care for patients from a variety of backgrounds and cultures. Cross-cultural communication is an important skill for you to develop to provide proper medical care to all patients equally. Just as you may experience physical challenges in providing good field care, you might also need to overcome cultural and literacy barriers to provide proper prehospital services.

For example, you may obtain only a limited patient history if you ask questions using health care terminology. The patient may have limited understanding of medical language and have difficulty answering your questions. Or, you may encounter a female patient who can ride in the ambulance only in the presence of her husband or family member.

Strategies for overcoming cultural challenges include gaining an understanding of the cultures and patient backgrounds you might encounter on emergency calls; gaining the assistance of the patient's friends or family members; and enlisting the help of health care clinicians of the same culture or background. Cultural competence is discussed further in Chapter 2, *Workforce Safety and Wellness*, and Chapter 4, *Communications and Documentation*.

Language Barriers

To overcome language barriers, consider using interpreters, translation resources, and related mobile device apps. The best answer is to find an interpreter, but it is not always that simple. First, determine whether the patient speaks or understands any English by asking the patient or others who may be present. Start by introducing yourself by using your name. Determine whether the patient understands who you are. Patients who can respond by giving you their name have the ability to understand some English. Remember that increasing the volume of your questions will not increase the patient's understanding of what you are asking. Keep questions straightforward and brief. Simple is best in these patient situations. Use of hand gestures may be helpful.

Provide the hospital with advance notice that a non–English-speaking patient will be arriving. This will allow the hospital to make arrangements for an interpreter.

Family and friends on scene may temporarily interpret for you in an emergency, but keep in mind that having a friend or family member translate private health information may pose legal and ethical concerns. Overcoming language barriers is discussed further in Chapter 4, *Communications and Documentation*.

YOU are the EMT SUMMARY

1. What are the components of the patient assessment?

There are five components in the assessment process: scene size-up, primary assessment, history taking, secondary assessment, and reassessment. Each component has an integral role in your overall treatment of the patient. The steps of assessment represent a logical approach to evaluation of a patient, but the order in which they are performed is determined by the patient's condition and the environment in which you are working.

2. Will your assessment of the patient differ if the individual is injured versus ill? If so, how?

The same components of patient assessment used to evaluate a medical patient are used to assess a trauma patient. The differences lie in what you find and how you treat it. For example, during the scene size-up of a trauma patient, you will evaluate the MOI to help focus your assessment of the type and severity of injuries your patient may have; you will also consider the need for spinal motion restriction. In medical patients, the NOI is assessed to help determine what category of medical condition you are dealing with (eg, cardiac, respiratory, endocrine), which will help guide your assessment in the appropriate direction.

Whether you are assessing a medical patient or a trauma patient, the key is to remain organized. Furthermore, you should assess the patient for medical conditions *and* traumatic injuries, especially if you suspect that the patient's injury was preceded by a medical condition.

3. Is spinal motion restriction indicated? Why or why not?

Local protocols for spinal motion restriction vary. If you find that spinal motion restriction is indicated, keep this in mind throughout your assessment

YOU are the EMT SUMMARY continued

process, modifying your assessment as appropriate to ensure that you are not unnecessarily risking additional spinal injury. Remember, however, that any life-threatening injuries *must be addressed immediately*, regardless of your suspicion of a possible spinal injury.

4. Which of these assessment findings requires your *most* immediate attention?

The patient's airway, which contains bloody secretions and vomitus, is in *immediate* jeopardy! Immediately use suction to clear his airway. Suction for up to 10 seconds, and then reassess his airway status. If you hear gurgling, think suction!

After ensuring that his airway is clear of secretions and vomitus, insert a simple airway adjunct while keeping the airway open manually to further help maintain airway patency.

5. Does the patient require further treatment at the scene? If so, what?

At this point, you should continue to support his airway and breathing, monitor his circulatory status (ie, his pulse, which is slow), keep him warm, and be prepared to begin CPR and apply the AED. Apply spinal motion restriction as directed by local protocol and prepare for immediate transport. Remember, there were no witnesses to this event; err on the side of caution and protect the patient's spine.

6. Should you remain at the scene and wait for the paramedic unit? Why or why not?

No, do not remain at the scene! Eighteen minutes is too long to remain at the scene with a patient in unstable condition, not to mention one who still needs to be moved from a second-floor apartment. You should advise the paramedic ambulance of the situation, but do so while you are preparing for immediate transport. The longer you remain at the scene, the greater the chance that the patient's condition will further deteriorate.

If the paramedic ambulance arrives before you depart the scene, it would clearly be prudent to transfer care to them.

Consider an intercept with the paramedic unit at a designated location. Your EMS system protocols should have a plan for coordinating a paramedic intercept when transporting a patient in unstable condition or a patient who requires care that is beyond your level of training. You should be aware of the transport time to the nearest definitive care site and weigh this against the time associated with achieving a paramedic intercept or waiting for ALS to arrive on the scene. Your goal is to reach advanced care in the least amount of time possible.

7. How has your patient's condition changed from the previous assessments?

Your patient's condition has obviously deteriorated. Compared with earlier assessments, which revealed that he was responsive to pain, he is now unconscious and unresponsive. Furthermore, his oxygen saturation is declining despite assisted ventilation with high-flow oxygen, and cyanosis is developing around his mouth (perioral/circumoral cyanosis).

His heart rate and blood pressure, although still unstable, are essentially unchanged compared with previous assessments. However, they must continue to be closely monitored for further deterioration.

The findings of your reassessment (eg, unresponsive, low oxygen saturation level, cyanosis) point to a problem with his oxygenation and ventilation status that may be caused by more than one factor. His head may not be properly positioned, the simple airway adjunct may need to be repositioned, his airway may be filling with blood or vomitus, or he is not being adequately ventilated.

8. What should you do in response to the patient's change in condition?

Deterioration of a patient's condition should immediately prompt you to repeat the primary assessment, which begins by reassessing the ABCs.

Make sure the patient's head is correctly positioned. Look in his mouth for secretions and remove them with suction, if present. If an airway adjunct is used, reevaluate to ensure it is placed correctly. Reassess the mask-to-face seal of the bag-mask device; is it adequate, or is there air leaking? Are you ventilating at the appropriate rate (10 breaths/min in an adult) with the appropriate volume (each breath delivered over 1 second; just enough to cause visible chest rise)?

A rapid, yet careful reassessment of the ABCs will often reveal the cause of the patient's status change, thus allowing you to rapidly correct it.

9. What components of the SAMPLE history, if any, can you obtain when your patient is unresponsive? How would you obtain the information?

In the absence of any family members, caregivers, or bystanders who know the patient, it may not be possible to obtain a complete and accurate SAMPLE history; however, it may be possible to obtain certain

YOU are the EMT SUMMARY continued

components of the SAMPLE history. Obtaining this information relies on your good assessment skills and thinking outside the box.

Signs and symptoms can be established by simply assessing the patient; although signs and symptoms alone will not tell you what the patient's underlying problem is, they will enable you to direct your initial treatment accordingly.

Look for a medical alert bracelet, a medication card carried in the purse or wallet, health information shared on the patient's phone, or medical information posted in the patient's home. Are there any prescription medication bottles present? Is there medical equipment present (eg, home oxygen, nebulizer) that indicates an underlying condition? Although an unresponsive patient cannot speak, you can learn something about the patient's conditions based on the medications found at the scene.

10. Why is reassessing your interventions so important?

The main purpose of reassessing the interventions you have performed on a patient is to determine their effectiveness. If your intervention has been effective, you should see an improvement in the patient's condition. If your intervention has not been effective, the patient's condition will have remained unchanged or will have deteriorated. Intervention reassessment also enables you to determine if you need to make modifications to existing interventions, cease an intervention, or perform another intervention.

For example, if a conscious patient is receiving oxygen via a nonrebreathing mask, and your reassessment reveals that he is now unresponsive, you may need to ensure that the airway is maintained and clear of secretions, and assess to see if the patient is adequately ventilated. Based on these findings, you may need to take measures to maintain the airway and assist with ventilations.

The mere performance of an intervention does not mean that it will cause your patient's condition to improve, nor does it mean that it will prevent your patient's condition from deteriorating. Reassess, reassess, reassess!

Prep Kit

Ready for Review

- The assessment process begins with the scene size-up, which identifies real or potential hazards. The patient should not be approached until any hazards have been dealt with in a way that eliminates or minimizes risk to the EMTs and the patient or patients.
- The primary assessment is performed on all patients. It includes forming an initial general impression of the patient, including the level of consciousness, and identifies any life-threatening conditions to the ABCs. A primary assessment is performed to assist in prioritizing time and mode of transport. Any life threats identified must be treated before moving on to the next step of the assessment.
- The ABCs are assessed to evaluate the patient's general condition.
- History taking includes an investigation of the patient's chief complaint or history of present illness. A SAMPLE history is generally taken during this step of the assessment process. This information may be obtained from the patient, family, friends, bystanders, caregivers, or medical alert devices or documentation.
- By using the SAMPLE mnemonic, you will be able to determine the patient's signs and symptoms, allergies, medications, pertinent past history, last known status, and events leading up to the illness or injury.
- The secondary assessment is a systematic physical examination of the patient. It may involve a systematic head-to-toe physical examination or an assessment that focuses on a certain area or region of the body, often

Prep Kit continued

determined through the chief complaint. Circumstances will dictate which aspects of the physical examination will be used. The secondary assessment is performed on scene or, more often, in the back of the ambulance en route to the hospital. If the patient has serious life threats, you may not have time to perform a secondary assessment.

- The reassessment is performed on all patients. It gives you an opportunity to reevaluate the chief complaint and to reassess interventions to ensure that they are still being delivered correctly. Information from the reassessment may be used to identify and treat changes in the patient's condition.
- A patient in stable condition should be reassessed every 15 minutes, whereas a patient in unstable condition should be reassessed every 5 minutes.
- The assessment process is systematic and dynamic. Each assessment you perform will be slightly different, depending on the needs of the patient. The result will be a process that will enable you to quickly identify and treat the needs of all patients, both medical and trauma related, in a way that meets their unique needs.
- EMTs must understand the special considerations involved in assessing and caring for members of the pediatric and geriatric populations.
  - General rules when caring for pediatric patients of all ages include appearing confident, being calm, remaining honest, and keeping parents or caregivers together with the pediatric patient as much as possible.
  - Because a young child might not be able to speak, your assessment must be based largely on what you can see and hear. Families may be able to provide vital information.
  - Use the pediatric assessment triangle (PAT) to obtain a general impression of the infant or child.
  - The GEMS diamond will help you remember differences to consider when assessing older patients. GEMS stands for Geriatric patients, Environmental assessment, Medical assessment, and Social assessment.

Vital Vocabulary

accessory muscles The secondary muscles of respiration. They include the neck muscles (sternocleidomastoids), the chest pectoralis major muscles, and the abdominal muscles.

altered mental status A change in the way a person thinks and behaves that may signal disease in the central nervous system or elsewhere in the body.

auscultate To listen to sounds within an organ with a stethoscope.

AVPU scale A method of assessing the level of consciousness by determining whether the patient is Awake and alert, responsive to Verbal stimuli or Pain, or Unresponsive; used principally early in the assessment process.

blood pressure The pressure that the blood exerts against the walls of the arteries as it passes through them.

bradycardia A slow heart rate, less than 60 beats/min.

breath sounds An indication of air movement in the lungs, usually assessed with a stethoscope.

capillary refill A test that evaluates distal circulatory system function by squeezing (blanching) blood from an area such as a nail bed and watching the speed of its return after releasing the pressure.

capnography A noninvasive method to quickly and efficiently provide information on a patient's ventilatory status, circulation, and metabolism;

Prep Kit continued

effectively measures the concentration of carbon dioxide in expired air over time.

carbon dioxide A component of air that typically makes up 0.03% of air at sea level; also a waste product exhaled during expiration by the respiratory system.

central pulses Pulses that are closest to the core (central) part of the body where the vital organs are located; include the carotid, femoral, and apical pulses.

chief complaint The reason a patient called for help; also, the patient's response to questions such as "What's wrong?" or "What happened?"

chief concern The condition requiring the most urgent intervention as determined by the clinician's assessment of the patient; it is not always the same as the chief complaint.

cognitive disabilities Conditions that impair a person's ability to remember information, process information, make decisions, or communicate in a normal fashion.

conjunctiva The delicate membrane that lines the eyelids and covers the exposed surface of the eye.

crackles A crackling, rattling breath sound that signals fluid in the air spaces of the lungs.

crepitus A grating or grinding sensation caused by fractured bone ends or joints rubbing together.

cyanosis Skin discoloration that is caused by a reduced level of oxygen in the blood. The blood and vessels appear blue, and the lips, mucous membranes, nail beds, and skin over the blood vessels appear blue or gray.

DCAP-BTLS A mnemonic for assessment in which each area of the body is evaluated for Deformities, Contusions, Abrasions, Punctures/penetrations, Burns, Tenderness, Lacerations, and Swelling.

diaphoretic Characterized by light or profuse sweating.

diastolic pressure The pressure that remains in the arteries during the relaxing phase of the heart's cycle (diastole) when the left ventricle is at rest.

distracting injury Any injury that prevents the patient from noticing other injuries, even severe injuries; for example, a painful femur or tibia fracture that prevents the patient from noticing back pain associated with a spinal fracture.

ecchymosis A buildup of blood beneath the skin caused by an injury that appears as a blue or black discoloration; also called a bruise.

field impression The conclusion about the cause of the patient's condition after considering the situation, history, and examination findings.

focused assessment A type of physical assessment typically performed on patients who have sustained nonsignificant mechanisms of injury or on responsive medical patients. This type of examination is based on the chief complaint and focuses on one body system or part.

frostbite Damage to tissues as the result of exposure to cold; frozen or partially frozen body parts are frostbitten.

general impression The overall initial impression that determines the priority for patient care; based on the patient's surroundings, the mechanism of injury, signs and symptoms, and the chief complaint.

Golden Period The time from injury to definitive care, during which treatment of shock and traumatic injuries should occur because survival potential is best; also called the Golden Hour.

guarding Involuntary muscle contractions (spasm) of the abdominal wall; an effort to protect the inflamed abdomen.

hematoma A mass of blood that has collected within damaged tissue beneath the skin.

history taking A step within the patient assessment process that provides detail about the patient's chief complaint and an account of the patient's signs and symptoms.

Prep Kit continued

hypertension Blood pressure that is higher than the normal range.

hypotension Blood pressure that is lower than the normal range.

hypothermia A condition in which the internal body temperature falls below 95°F (35°C).

jaundice Yellow skin or sclera that is caused by liver disease or dysfunction. In individuals with dark skin, the discoloration may be more evident in the sclera.

labored breathing Breathing that requires greater than normal effort; may be slower or faster than normal and characterized by grunting, stridor, and use of accessory muscles.

length-based resuscitation tape A tape used to estimate an infant's or child's weight on the basis of body length; appropriate drug doses and equipment sizes are listed on the tape.

mean arterial pressure (MAP) The average pressure in the circulatory system during one cardiac cycle.

mechanism of injury (MOI) The forces, or energy transmission, applied to the body that cause injury.

metabolism The biochemical processes that result in production of energy from nutrients within the cells.

nasal flaring Widening of the nostrils, indicating an airway obstruction.

nature of illness (NOI) The general type of illness a patient is experiencing.

OPQRST A mnemonic used in evaluating a patient's pain: Onset, Provocation/palliation, Quality, Region/radiation, Severity, and Timing.

orientation The mental status of a patient as measured by memory of person (name), place (current location), time (current year, month, and approximate date), and event (what happened).

palpate To examine by touch.

paradoxical chest motion Respirations in which the chest moves inward during inhalation and outward during exhalation, opposite of the chest wall's normal motion during breathing.

pediatric assessment triangle (PAT) A structured assessment tool used to rapidly form a general impression of the infant or child without touching them; consists of assessing appearance, work of breathing, and circulation to the skin.

perfusion The flow of blood through body tissues and vessels.

personal protective equipment (PPE) Protective equipment that blocks exposure to a pathogen or a hazardous material.

pertinent negatives Negative findings that warrant no care or intervention.

primary assessment A step within the patient assessment process that identifies and initiates treatment of immediate and potential life threats.

pulse The wave of pressure created as the heart contracts and forces blood out the left ventricle and into the major arteries.

pulse oximetry An assessment tool that measures oxygen saturation of hemoglobin in the capillary beds.

reassessment A step within the patient assessment process performed at regular intervals during the assessment process to identify and treat changes in a patient's condition. A patient in unstable condition should be reassessed every 5 minutes, whereas a patient in stable condition should be reassessed every 15 minutes.

responsiveness The way in which a patient responds to external stimuli, including verbal stimuli (sound), tactile stimuli (touch), and painful stimuli.

retractions Movements in which the skin pulls in around the ribs during inspiration.

rhonchi Coarse, low-pitched breath sounds heard in patients with chronic mucus in the upper airways.

Prep Kit continued

SAMPLE history A brief history of a patient's condition to determine signs and symptoms, allergies, medications, pertinent past history, last known status, and events leading to the injury or illness.

scene size-up A step within the patient assessment process that involves a quick assessment of the scene and the surroundings to provide information about scene safety and the mechanism of injury or nature of illness before you enter and begin patient care.

sclera The tough, fibrous, white portion of the eye that protects the more delicate inner structures.

secondary assessment A step within the patient assessment process in which a systematic physical examination of the patient is performed. The examination may be a systematic exam or an assessment that focuses on a certain area or region of the body, often determined through the chief complaint.

shallow respirations Respirations characterized by little movement of the chest wall (reduced tidal volume) or poor chest excursion.

sign Objective finding that can be seen, heard, felt, smelled, or measured.

situational awareness Knowledge and understanding of one's surroundings and the ability to recognize potential risks to the safety of the patient or EMS team.

sniffing position An upright position in which the patient's head and chin are thrust slightly forward to keep the airway open.

spontaneous respirations Breathing that occurs without assistance.

standard precautions Protective measures that have traditionally been developed by the Centers for Disease Control and Prevention (CDC) for use in dealing with objects, blood, body fluids, and other potential exposure risks of communicable disease.

stridor A harsh, high-pitched, respiratory sound, generally heard during inspiration, that is caused by partial blockage or narrowing of the upper airway; may be audible without a stethoscope.

subcutaneous emphysema A characteristic crackling sensation felt on palpation of the skin, caused by the presence of air in soft tissues.

symptom Subjective finding that the patient feels but that can be identified only by the patient.

systolic pressure The increased pressure in an artery with each contraction of the ventricles (systole).

tachycardia A rapid heart rate, more than 100 beats/min.

tidal volume The amount of air (in milliliters) that is moved into or out of the lungs during one breath.

tripod position An upright position in which the patient leans forward onto two arms stretched forward and thrusts the head and chin forward.

two- to three-word dyspnea A severe breathing problem in which a patient can speak only two to three words at a time without pausing to take a breath.

vasoconstriction Narrowing of a blood vessel.

vital signs The key signs that are used to evaluate the patient's overall condition, including respirations, pulse, blood pressure, level of consciousness, and skin characteristics.

wheezing A high-pitched, whistling breath sound that is most prominent on expiration and that suggests an obstruction or narrowing of the lower airways; occurs in asthma and bronchiolitis.

work of breathing An indicator of oxygenation and ventilation; reflects the patient's attempt to compensate for hypoxia.

Prep Kit continued

References

1. National Association of Emergency Medical Technicians, American College of Surgeons. *PHTLS: Prehospital Trauma Life Support*. 10th ed. Burlington, MA: Jones & Bartlett Learning; 2024.
2. Standard precautions for all patient care. Centers for Disease Control and Prevention website. https://www.cdc.gov/infection-control/hcp/basics/standard-precautions.html. Published April 3, 2024. Accessed October 22, 2024.
3. Nallaluthan V, Tan GY, Murni MF, et al. Pain as a guide in Glasgow Coma Scale status for neurological assessment. *Malays J Med Sci*. 2023;30(5):221–235.
4. Saraya T, Shimoda M, Hirata A, Takizawa H. Paradoxical respiration: "seesaw" motion with massive pulmonary consolidation. *BMJ Case Rep*. 2016;2016:bcr2015213449. doi:10.1136/bcr-2015-213449
5. American Heart Association (AHA). *Pediatric Advanced Life Support Provider Manual*. Dallas, TX: AHA; 2020.
6. Lyng J, Harris M, Mandt M, et al. Prehospital pediatric respiratory distress and airway management training and education: an NAEMSP position statement and resource document. *Prehosp Emerg Care*. 2022;26(sup1):102–110.
7. Hallett S, Toro F, Ashurst JV. Physiology, tidal volume. *StatPearls*. National Library of Medicine website. https://www.ncbi.nlm.nih.gov/books/NBK482502/. Updated May 1, 2023. Accessed October 22, 2024.
8. Pickering TG, Hall JE, Appel LJ, et al. Recommendations for blood pressure measurement in humans and experimental animals: part 1: blood pressure measurement in humans: a statement for professionals from the Subcommittee of Professional and Public Education of the American Heart Association Council on High Blood Pressure Research. *Circulation*. 2005;111(5):697–716.
9. Smith L. New AHA recommendations for blood pressure measurement. *Am Fam Physician*. 2005;72(7):1391–1398
10. Yeganehkhah M, Dadkhahtehrani T, Bagheri A, Kachoie A. Effect of glittered nail polish on pulse oximetry measurements in healthy subjects. *Iran J Nurs Midwifery Res*. 2019;24(1):25–29.
11. Yek JLJ, Abdullah HR, Goh JPS, Chan YW. The effects of gel-based manicure on pulse oximetry. *Singapore Med J*. 2019;60(8):432–435.

Additional Resources

American Heart Association. *2020 American Heart Association Guidelines for Cardiopulmonary Resuscitation and Emergency Cardiovascular Care*. https://professional.heart.org/en/science-news/2020-aha-guidelines-for-cpr-and-ecc. Published October 21, 2020. Accessed October 22, 2024.

Berg KM, Bray JE, Ng KC, et al. 2023 International consensus on cardiopulmonary resuscitation and emergency cardiovascular care science with treatment recommendations: summary from the Basic Life Support; Advanced Life Support; Pediatric Life Support; Neonatal Life Support; Education, Implementation, and Teams; and First Aid Task Forces. *Circulation*. 2023;148(24):e187–e280. doi:10.1161/CIR.0000000000001179

National Association of Emergency Medical Technicians. *PHTLS: Prehospital Trauma Life Support*. 10th ed. Burlington, MA: Jones & Bartlett Learning; 2024.

National Association of State EMS Officials. *National Model EMS Clinical Guidelines: Version 3.0.* https://nasemso.org/wp-content/uploads/National-Model-EMS-Clinical-Guidelines_2022.pdf. Updated March 2022. Accessed October 22, 2024.

National Highway Traffic Safety Administration. *National Emergency Medical Services Education Standards*. EMS.gov website. https://www.ems.gov/assets/EMS_Education-Standards_2021_FNL.pdf. Published January 2021. Accessed October 22, 2024.

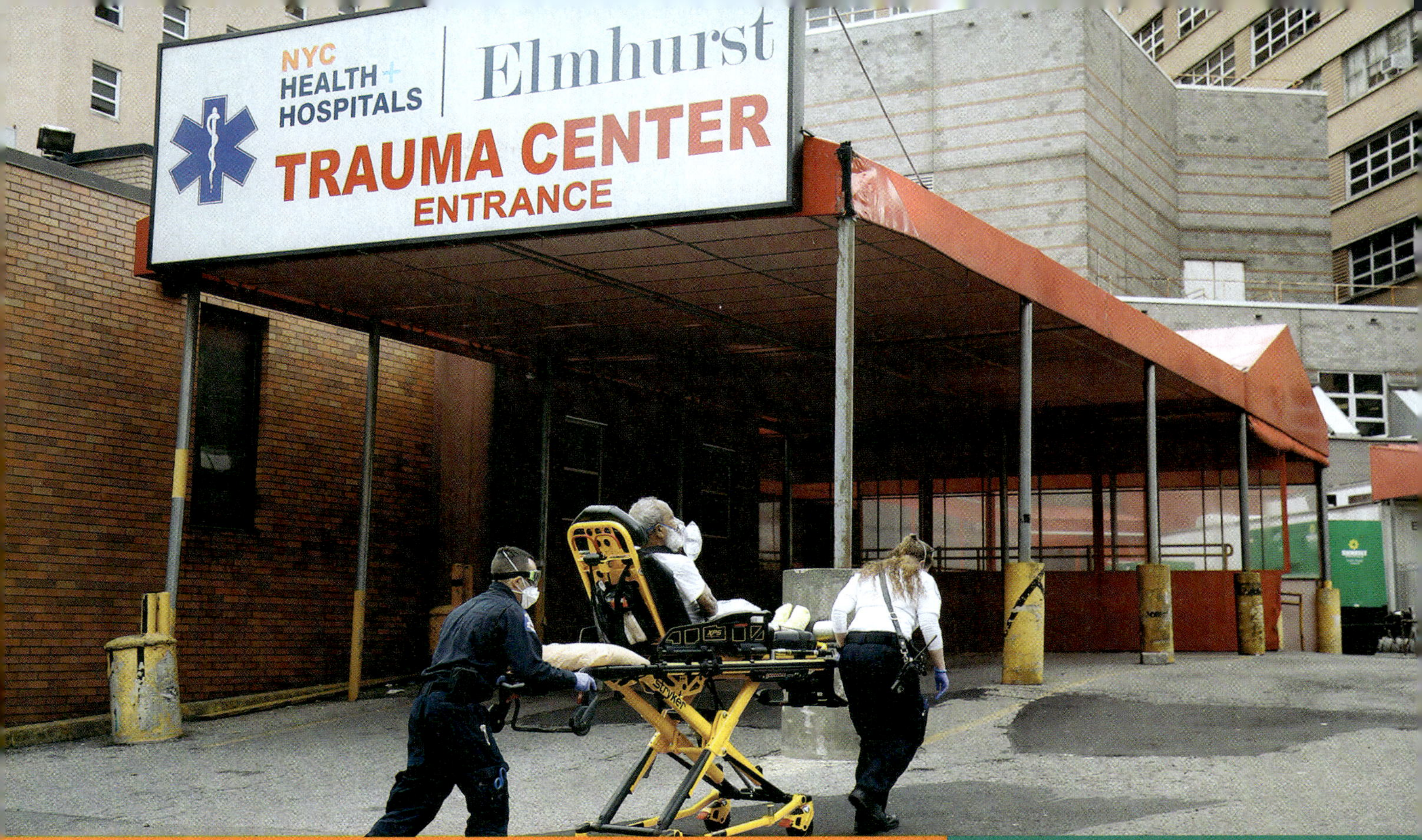

SECTION 3

Airway

11 Airway and Ventilation Management

Chapter 11

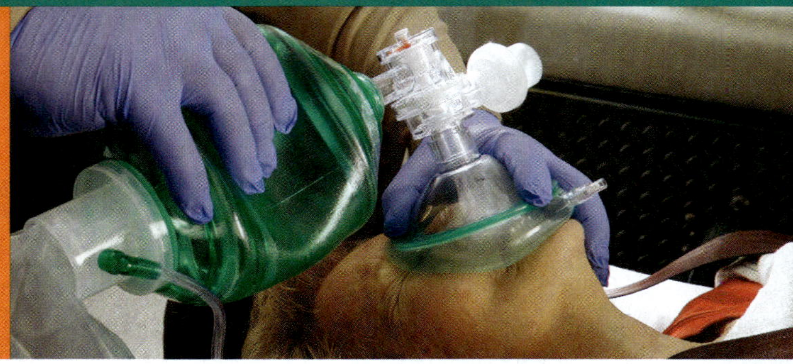

Airway and Ventilation Management

NATIONAL EMS EDUCATION STANDARD COMPETENCIES

Airway Management, Respiration, and Artificial Ventilation

Applies knowledge of anatomy and physiology to patient assessment and management in order to assure a patent airway, adequate mechanical ventilation, and respiration for patients of all ages.

Airway Management

- Airway anatomy (pp 402–407)
- Airway assessment (pp 416–424)
- Techniques of assuring a patent airway (pp 424–431)

Respiration

- Anatomy of the respiratory system (pp 402–407)
- Physiology and pathophysiology of respiration
  - Pulmonary ventilation (pp 408–411)
  - Oxygenation (p 411)
  - Respiration (pp 411–413)
    - External (p 412)
    - Internal (p 412)
    - Cellular (pp 408, 412–413)
- Assessment and management of adequate and inadequate respiration (pp 431–437)
- Supplemental oxygen therapy (pp 437–443)

Ventilation

- Assessment and management of adequate and inadequate ventilation (pp 446–459)
- Effect of ventilation on cardiac output (pp 419–448)

Pathophysiology

Applies knowledge of the pathophysiology of respiration and perfusion to patient assessment and management.

KNOWLEDGE OBJECTIVES

1. Describe the major structures of the respiratory system. (pp 402–407)
2. Discuss the physiology of breathing. (pp 407–411)
3. Give the signs of adequate breathing. (p 416)
4. Give the signs of inadequate breathing. (pp 416–417)
5. Describe the assessment and care of a patient with apnea. (p 418)
6. Explain how to assess for adequate and inadequate respiration, including the use of pulse oximetry. (pp 419–424)
7. Explain how to assess for a patent airway. (p 424)
8. Describe how to perform the head tilt–chin lift maneuver. (p 426)
9. Describe how to perform the jaw-thrust maneuver. (pp 427–428)

10. Explain the importance of and techniques for suctioning. (pp 428–431)
11. Explain how to measure and insert an oropharyngeal airway. (pp 431–434)
12. Describe how to measure and insert a nasopharyngeal airway. (pp 435–436)
13. Explain the use of the recovery position to maintain a clear airway. (pp 436–437)
14. Describe the importance of giving supplemental oxygen to patients who are hypoxic. (p 437)
15. Discuss the basics of how oxygen is stored and the various hazards associated with its use. (pp 437–443)
16. Explain the use of a nonrebreathing mask and the oxygen flow requirements for its use. (p 443)
17. Describe the indications for using a nasal cannula rather than a nonrebreathing face mask. (p 444)
18. Describe the indications for using a humidifier during supplemental oxygen therapy. (p 445)
19. Describe how to perform mouth-to-mouth or mouth-to-mask ventilation. (p 448)
20. Describe the use of a bag-mask device. (pp 448–453)
21. Describe the signs associated with adequate and inadequate artificial ventilation. (pp 446–454)
22. Describe the use of continuous positive airway pressure (CPAP). (pp 454–459)
23. Explain care for patients who have undergone a tracheostomy. (pp 459–461)
24. Explain how to recognize and care for a foreign body airway obstruction. (pp 461–464)
25. Describe the unique management considerations when caring for children who are experiencing an airway emergency. (pp 464–469)
26. Describe the emergency medical technician's (EMT's) role in assisting with intubation. (pp 469–476)
27. Discuss the importance of preoxygenation when performing endotracheal (ET) intubation. (p 469)
28. Describe the signs that indicate a complication with an intubated patient. (p 474)

SKILLS OBJECTIVES

1. Demonstrate how to apply the pulse oximeter. (p 421, Skill Drill 11-1)
2. Demonstrate how to position the unconscious patient. (p 425, Skill Drill 11-2)
3. Demonstrate how to perform the head tilt–chin lift maneuver. (p 426)
4. Demonstrate how to perform the jaw-thrust maneuver. (pp 427–428)
5. Demonstrate how to operate a suction unit. (pp 428–431)
6. Demonstrate how to suction a patient's airway. (pp 430–431, Skill Drill 11-3)
7. Demonstrate the insertion of an oropharyngeal airway with a 90° rotation. (p 433, Skill Drill 11-4)
8. Demonstrate the insertion of an oropharyngeal airway with a 180° rotation. (p 434, Skill Drill 11-5)
9. Demonstrate the insertion of a nasopharyngeal airway. (pp 435–436, Skill Drill 11-6)
10. Demonstrate how to place a patient in the recovery position. (p 436)
11. Demonstrate how to place an oxygen cylinder into service. (p 441, Skill Drill 11-7)
12. Demonstrate the use of a partial rebreathing mask in providing supplemental oxygen therapy to patients. (p 444)
13. Demonstrate the placement of a nasal cannula in providing supplemental oxygen therapy to patients. (p 444)
14. Demonstrate the use of a Venturi mask in providing supplemental oxygen therapy to patients. (p 444)
15. Demonstrate the use of a humidifier in providing supplemental oxygen therapy to patients. (p 445)
16. Demonstrate how to assist a patient with ventilations using the bag-mask device. (p 451, Skill Drill 11-8)
17. Demonstrate the use of an automatic transport ventilator to assist in delivering artificial ventilation to the patient. (pp 453–454)
18. Demonstrate the use of CPAP. (pp 457–458, Skill Drill 11-9)
19. Demonstrate how to provide ventilation to a patient wearing dentures. (p 464)
20. Demonstrate how to provide ventilation to a pediatric patient. (pp 464–469)
21. Demonstrate how to insert an oropharyngeal airway in a pediatric patient. (p 466, Skill Drill 11-10)
22. Demonstrate the insertion of a supraglottic airway. (pp 474–476)

Introduction

The single most important step in caring for patients is to ensure that all life-threatening conditions are rapidly identified and addressed. A primary component of that step is to ensure that patients have an intact airway and can breathe adequately. When the ability to breathe is disrupted, oxygen delivery to the body tissues and cells is compromised. Cells require a constant supply of oxygen to survive. Within seconds of being deprived of oxygen, vital organs such as the heart and brain may not function normally. Therefore, it is imperative that you recognize airway and breathing inadequacies and correct them immediately. Without oxygen, brain tissue will begin to die within 4 to 6 minutes.

Oxygen reaches body tissues and cells through two separate but related processes: breathing and circulation. During inhalation, oxygen moves from the atmosphere into the lungs, crosses the alveolar membrane, and attaches to hemoglobin by a process called **diffusion**. Diffusion is a process in which gas molecules move from an area of higher concentration to an area of lower concentration. Next, red blood cells carry the hemoglobin, with the bound oxygen, through the body, ultimately delivering it to the capillaries to oxygenate the body's cells. At the same time, carbon dioxide, the by-product of normal cellular metabolism, moves from the cells into the blood and is carried back to the lungs where it moves into the alveoli by diffusion. The blood, enriched with oxygen, is sent through the body by the pumping action of the heart. The carbon dioxide then leaves the body during exhalation.

As an EMT, you must be able to identify the anatomic structures of the respiratory system, understand how the system works, and be able to recognize which patients are breathing adequately and which patients are breathing inadequately. This knowledge will enable you to determine how best to treat your patients. You also play a pivotal role by bringing emergency medicine into patients' homes, assisting with advanced patient care skills, and ensuring the effective transfer of patient care to emergency department (ED) staff when you arrive at the hospital.

This chapter reviews the anatomy, physiology, and pathophysiology of the respiratory system. It describes how to assess patients quickly and to carefully determine their airway and ventilation status. The equipment, procedures, and guidelines that you will need to manage a patient's airway and breathing are described in detail. You will learn several ways to open a patient's airway and specific techniques for removing foreign objects or fluids that may be compromising the airway. Because airway management equipment, like any piece of medical equipment, can be dangerous if used improperly, the chapter thoroughly discusses airway adjuncts, oxygen therapy devices, and artificial ventilation methods.

Anatomy of the Respiratory System

The respiratory system consists of all the structures in the body that make up the **airway** and help us breathe, or ventilate (**FIGURE 11-1**). The airway is divided into the upper and the lower airways. Structures that help us breathe include the diaphragm, the intercostal muscles (muscles in between the ribs), and the nerves from the brain and spinal cord that innervate those muscles. In times of increased distress, muscles that are ordinarily not used during normal breathing, called accessory muscles, can be employed. Ventilation is the simple act of moving air into and out of the lungs. The diaphragm and intercostal muscles are responsible for the regular rise and fall of the chest that accompany normal breathing.

Anatomy of the Upper Airway

The upper airway consists of all anatomic airway structures above the level of the vocal cords. These include the nose, mouth, oral cavity, pharynx, and larynx. Its major functions are to warm, filter, and humidify air as it enters the body through the nose and mouth. The pharynx (throat) is a muscular tube that extends from the nose and mouth to the level of the esophagus and trachea. The pharynx is composed of the nasopharynx, oropharynx, and the laryngopharynx (also called the hypopharynx) (**FIGURE 11-2**). The laryngopharynx is the lowest portion of the pharynx. At the base, it splits into two lumens, the larynx (and ultimately, the trachea) anteriorly and the esophagus posteriorly.

Nasopharynx

During inhalation, air typically enters the body through the nose and passes into the **nasopharynx**.

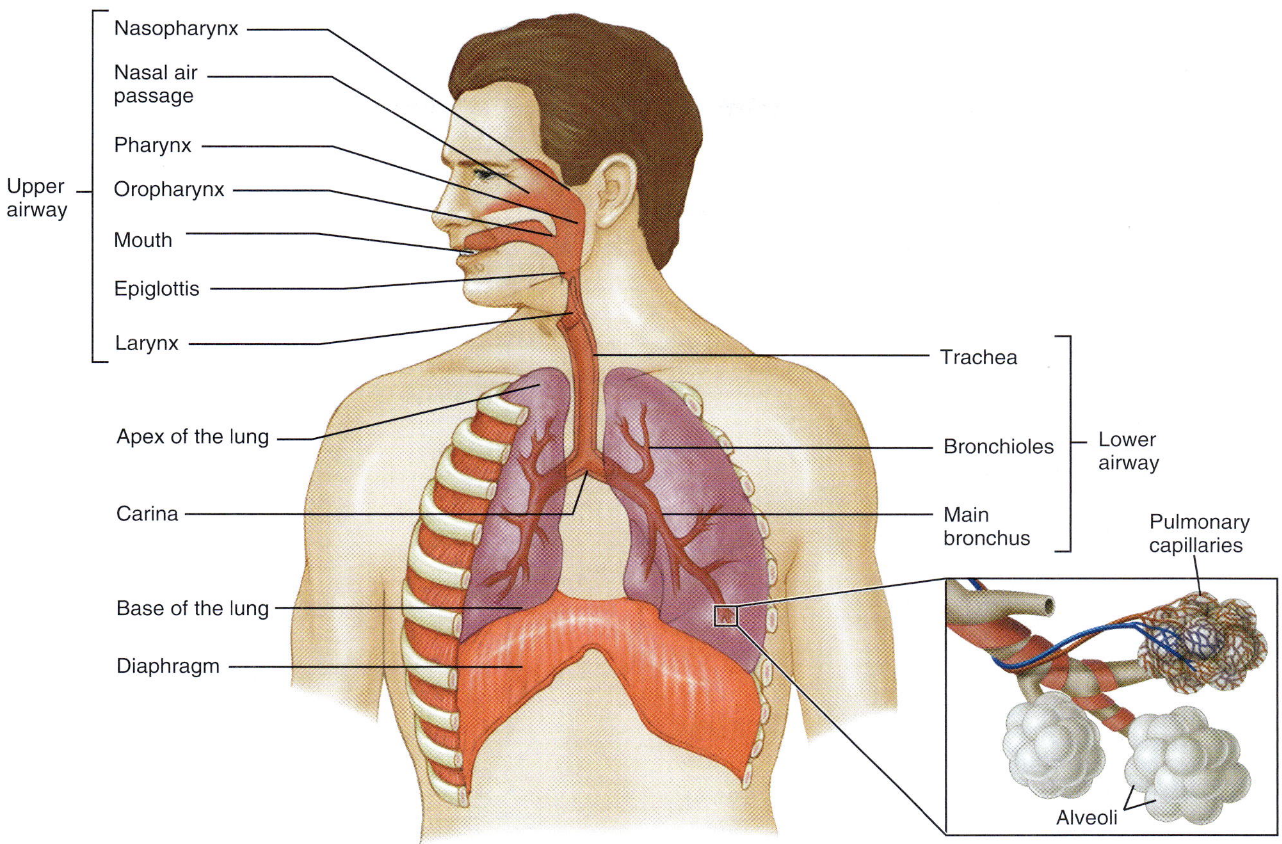

FIGURE 11-1 The upper and lower airways contain the structures in the body that help us breathe.

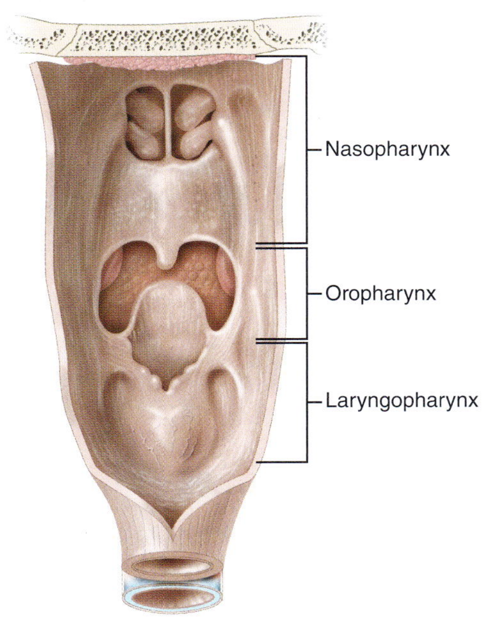

FIGURE 11-2 The pharynx.

The nasopharynx is lined with a specialized mucous membrane that includes cilia (hairlike cells that help move mucus) to keep contaminants such as dust and other small particles out of the respiratory tract. In addition, the mucous membranes warm and humidify air as it enters the body.

Oropharynx

The **oropharynx** forms the posterior portion of the oral cavity, which is bordered superiorly by the hard and soft palates, laterally by the cheeks, and inferiorly by the tongue (**FIGURE 11-3**). Superior to the larynx, the epiglottis helps separate the digestive system from the respiratory system. Its function is to prevent food and liquid from entering the larynx during swallowing. When swallowing occurs, the larynx is elevated and the epiglottis folds over the glottis to prevent **aspiration** of contents into the trachea.

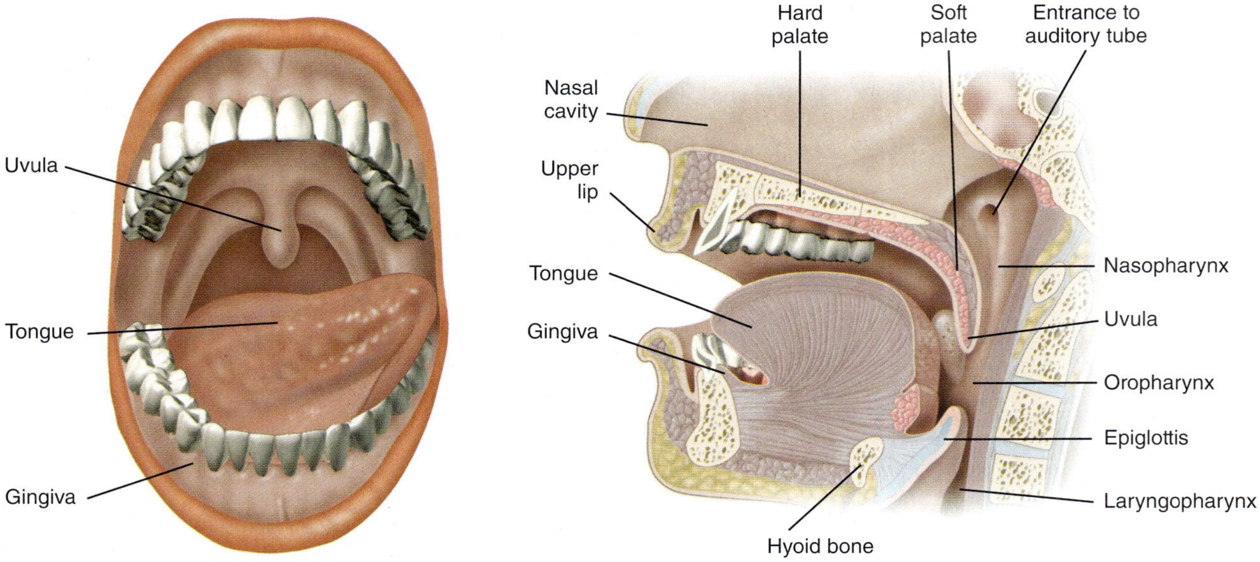

FIGURE 11-3 The oral cavity.

Larynx

The **larynx** is a complex structure formed by many independent cartilaginous structures (**FIGURE 11-4**). Anatomically, this is where the upper airway ends and the lower airway begins.

The thyroid cartilage is a shield-shaped structure formed by two plates that join in a V shape anteriorly to form the laryngeal prominence known as the Adam's apple. The thyroid cartilage is the most prominent anatomic structure on the anterior neck in both sexes and is typically more prominent in males than in females.

The cricoid cartilage, or cricoid ring, lies inferiorly to the thyroid cartilage; it forms the lowest portion of the larynx. The cricoid cartilage is the first ring of the trachea and the only lower airway structure that forms a complete ring. The cricothyroid membrane is the elastic tissue that connects the thyroid cartilage superiorly to the cricoid ring inferiorly.

The **glottis**, also called the glottic opening, is the space between the vocal cords and the narrowest portion of the adult's airway. The **vocal cords** are situated at the lateral borders of the glottis. These white bands of thin smooth muscle tissue are partially separated at rest and serve as the primary center for speech production. In addition, the vocal cords contain defense reflexes that protect the lower airway, causing a spasmodic closure to the lower airway to prevent substances, such as water or vomitus, from entering the trachea.

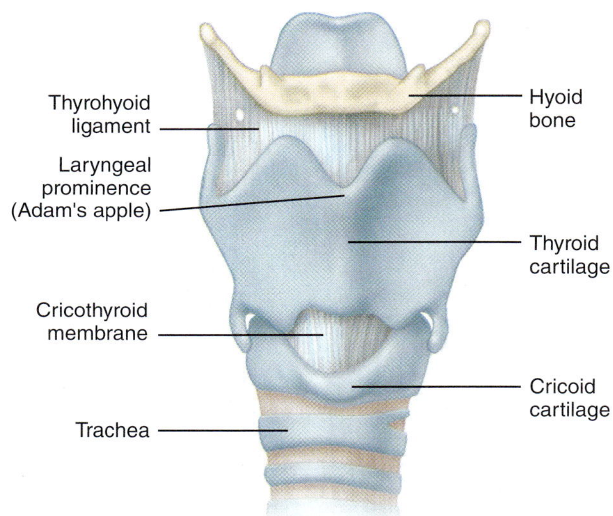

FIGURE 11-4 The larynx.

Anatomy of the Lower Airway

The function of the lower airway is to deliver oxygen to the alveoli. Its external boundaries are the fourth cervical vertebra and the xiphoid process, which is the narrow, cartilaginous, inferiormost part of the sternum. Internally, the lower airway spans the glottis to the pulmonary capillary membrane.

Special Populations

PEDIATRIC AIRWAY MANAGEMENT

Generally, the maneuvers, techniques, and indications for airway management are the same in children as they are in adults. However, several anatomic differences in the child require modification of certain techniques.

Infants who are 4 months or younger are obligate nose breathers, meaning they must breathe through their nose. Obstruction of both nares with mucus or blood can result in airway obstruction. Suctioning the nares may be the only intervention needed to relieve this obstruction.[1]

Infants and small children have a proportionately larger occiput (posterior portion of the cranium), which causes the neck to flex, moving the head forward and the tongue backward, when the child lies supine; this position itself can cause an airway obstruction. Note that while extreme flexion is the more common cause of airway obstruction, extreme extension can also cause obstruction. When positioning the airway of an infant or child, place a folded towel under the child's shoulders to maintain a neutral position of the head (**FIGURE 11-5**).

Compared with adults, children have a proportionately smaller mandible and a proportionately larger tongue (**FIGURE 11-6**). Both factors increase the incidence of airway obstruction in children.

The child's epiglottis is floppier and more omega-shaped than an adult's (**FIGURE 11-7**).

In general, the airway of an infant or child is smaller and narrower at all levels. The larynx lies more superior and anterior than that of an adult. The larynx is also funnel-shaped due to the narrow, underdeveloped cricoid cartilage. In children younger than 8 years, the narrowest portion of the airway is at the cricoid ring. Further narrowing of the child's inherently narrow airway, such as that caused by soft-tissue swelling or foreign body aspiration, can significantly increase airway resistance and cause breathing inadequacy.

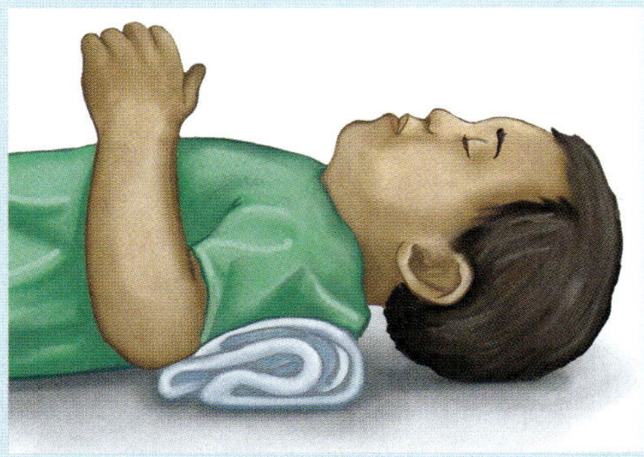

FIGURE 11-5 A folded towel placed under the child's shoulders can help to maintain a neutral head position.

Children do not have well-developed chest musculature, and their ribs and cartilage are softer and more pliable than those of an adult. As a result, the thoracic cavity cannot optimally contribute to lung expansion. Children rely heavily on their diaphragm for breathing, which moves their abdomen in and out. For this reason, infants and small children are commonly referred to as belly breathers.

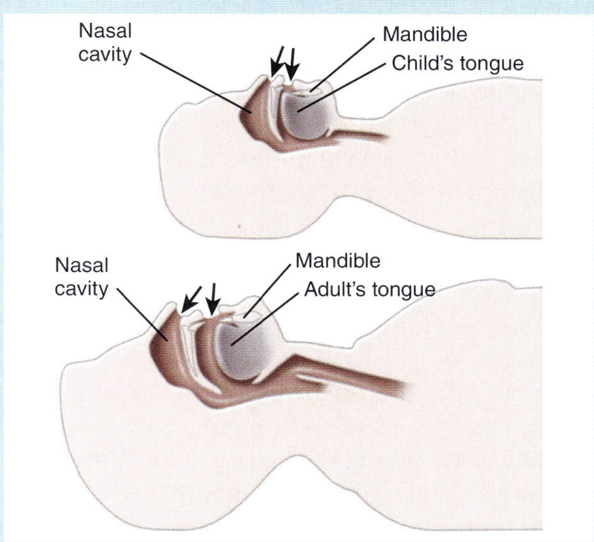

FIGURE 11-6 In children, the mandible is proportionately smaller and the tongue is proportionately larger than in an adult.

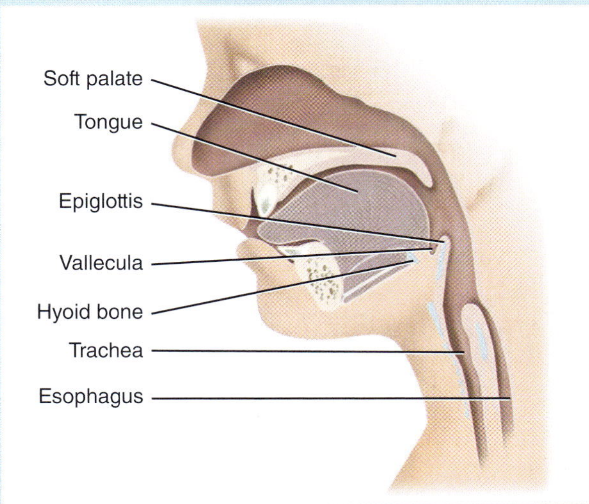

FIGURE 11-7 The child's epiglottis and surrounding structures.

The trachea, or windpipe, is the conduit for air entry into the lungs. This tubular structure is approximately 4 to 5 inches (10 to 12 cm) in length and consists of C-shaped cartilaginous rings. The trachea begins directly below the cricoid cartilage and descends anteriorly down the midline of the neck into the thoracic cavity. Once in the thoracic cavity, the trachea divides at the level of the **carina** into the two main stem bronchi (right and left). The hollow bronchi are supported by cartilage and distribute air into the right and left lungs.

The lungs consist of the entire mass of tissue that includes the smaller bronchi, bronchioles, and alveoli (**FIGURE 11-8**). The pleurae are thin serous membranes that cover the lungs and line the thoracic cavity. The **visceral pleura** covers the outer surface of the lung tissue, and the **parietal pleura** lines the inside of the thoracic cavity. A small amount of fluid is found between these two pleural layers and serves as a lubricant to prevent friction during breathing.

On entering the lungs, each bronchus divides into increasingly smaller bronchi, which in turn subdivide into bronchioles. The **bronchioles** are thin, hollow tubes made of smooth muscle. The tone of these smooth muscles allows the bronchioles to dilate or constrict in response to various stimuli. The smaller bronchioles branch into alveolar ducts that end at the alveolar sacs.

The alveoli, located at the end of the airway, are millions of thin-walled, balloonlike sacs that serve as the functional site for the exchange of oxygen and carbon dioxide. Surrounding each of these sacs is an intricate bed of blood vessels, known as pulmonary capillaries. Oxygen diffuses through the lining of the alveoli into the pulmonary capillaries where, depending on adequate blood volume and pressure, it is carried back to the heart for distribution to the rest of the body. At the same time, carbon dioxide (waste) diffuses from the pulmonary capillaries into the alveoli, where it is exhaled and removed from the body.

The thoracic cage (thorax) surrounds and protects many organs, including the lungs, heart, trachea, great vessels, liver, and spleen. The thoracic cavity, the superior part of the thoracic cage, contains the lungs, one on each side (**FIGURE 11-9**). The boundaries of the thoracic cavity are the rib cage anteriorly, superiorly, and posteriorly and the diaphragm inferiorly. Each individual rib plays a part in the overall protection of the organs contained within the thorax. In between each rib are intercostal muscles that, in conjunction with the diaphragm, facilitate normal breathing. Within the thoracic cavity, you will find the lungs. Between the lungs is a space called the **mediastinum**, which is surrounded by tough connective tissue. This space contains the heart, the great vessels, the esophagus, the trachea,

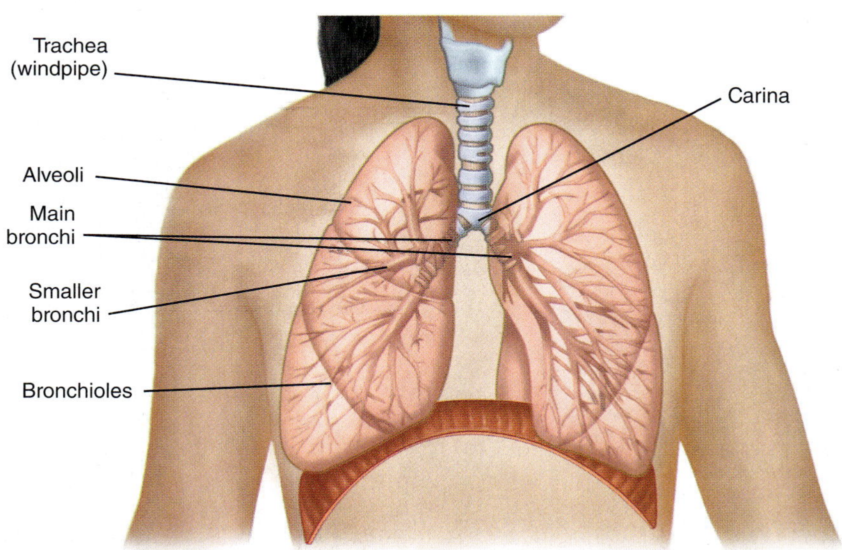

FIGURE 11-8 The trachea and the lungs are lower airway structures.

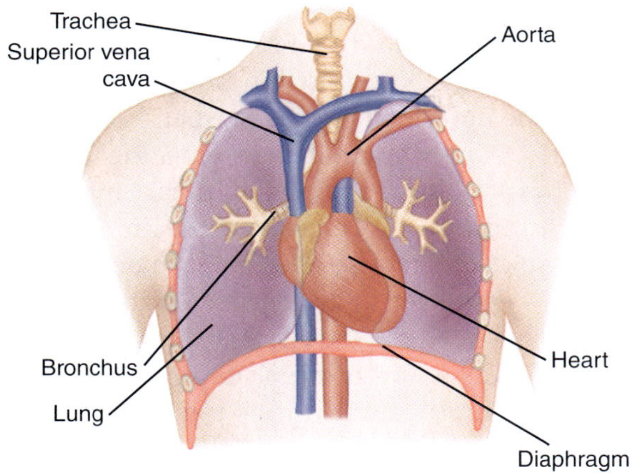

FIGURE 11-9 The thoracic cavity contains important anatomic structures for ventilation, oxygenation, and respiration, including the lungs and bronchi, heart, great vessels (the venae cavae and aorta), and trachea.

the major bronchi, and many nerves. The mediastinum effectively separates the right lung space from the left lung space. In addition to the respiratory and circulatory structures found in the thoracic cavity, important structures of the nervous system are also found: the **phrenic nerves**. The phrenic nerves, which originate from the third, fourth, and fifth cervical nerves, innervate the diaphragm muscle, allowing it to contract. Contraction of the diaphragm occurs in a downward direction and is necessary for adequate breathing to occur.

Physiology of Breathing

The respiratory and cardiovascular systems work together to ensure that a constant supply of oxygen and nutrients is delivered to every cell in the body and that carbon dioxide and waste products are removed from every cell. The following sections will describe the processes of ventilation, oxygenation, and respiration; however, you first need to understand how the processes of breathing and circulation are connected.

As described earlier, air enters the body through the oral and nasal cavities and travels into the lungs. This occurs because a negative pressure is created in the chest when the thoracic cavity enlarges due to contraction of the diaphragm and intercostal muscles. Eventually the air reaches the alveolar sacs, where oxygen diffuses across the alveolar membrane and binds to hemoglobin in the bloodstream. At the same time, carbon dioxide diffuses from the bloodstream into the alveoli. The carbon dioxide is exhaled from the lungs, and the oxygen is transported back to the heart, where it is distributed to the rest of the body.

The heart pumps blood to the tissues of the body through a series of arteries and veins. Arteries carry blood away from the heart and eventually branch into capillaries. In the capillaries, the exchange of nutrients and waste products takes place. Oxygen and nutrients leave the capillaries and enter the cells. At the same time, waste products, such as carbon dioxide, diffuse from the cells back into the capillary blood. From here, the deoxygenated blood travels back to the heart. The deoxygenated blood enters the right side of the heart through the right atrium. The right ventricle pumps the blood to the lungs for oxygenation and removal of carbon dioxide. The oxygenated blood then travels back to the heart and into the left atrium. The left ventricle then pumps the oxygenated blood to the rest of the body. Refer to Chapter 6, *The Human Body*, for an illustration of this process.

It is important to understand that the respiratory and circulatory systems work together to facilitate oxygen delivery to the tissues of the body and removal of waste products from the body (**TABLE 11-1**). When one of these systems is compromised, oxygen delivery is not effective, waste products cannot be removed, and cellular death can result.

Words of Wisdom

Ventilation is the physical act of moving air into and out of the lungs. Although adequate ventilation is required for optimal oxygenation, it cannot be assumed that a patient who is ventilating is also oxygenating. For example, a patient who is trapped in an area that has very low oxygen levels (eg, structural fire, grain silo) may continue to ventilate; however, oxygenation in this case would be impaired. If ventilation is inadequate, oxygenation and respiration will be impaired. Examples of injuries or conditions that can impair ventilation include flail chest; foreign body airway obstruction; injury to the spinal cord that disrupts the phrenic nerves, which innervate the diaphragm; and opioid overdose.

TABLE 11-1 Ventilation, Oxygenation, and Respiration

Function	Definition
Ventilation	The physical act of moving air into and out of the lung.
Oxygenation	The process of loading oxygen molecules onto hemoglobin molecules in the bloodstream.
Respiration	The actual exchange of oxygen and carbon dioxide in the alveoli as well as the tissues of the body. It can be classified by the following three processes: • External respiration: exchange of gases between the lungs and blood. • Internal respiration: exchange of gases between the blood and tissue cells. • **Cellular respiration** (or cellular metabolism): use of oxygen by the cells to carry out their specific activities.

Ventilation

Pulmonary ventilation, the process of moving air into and out of the lungs, is necessary for oxygenation and respiration to occur. Adequate, continuous ventilation is essential for life and therefore is one of the highest priorities in treating any patient. If a patient is not breathing or is breathing inadequately, you must immediately intervene to ensure adequate ventilation.

Inhalation

The active, muscular part of breathing is called **inhalation**. When a person inhales, the diaphragm and intercostal muscles contract, allowing air to enter the body and travel to the lungs. When it contracts, the diaphragm moves down slightly, enlarging the thoracic cage from top to bottom. When the intercostal muscles contract, they lift the ribs up and out. The combined actions of these structures enlarge the thorax in all directions. Take a deep breath to see how your chest expands.

The lungs have no muscle tissue; therefore, they cannot move on their own. They need the help of other structures to be able to expand and contract during inhalation and exhalation. Therefore, the ability of the lungs to function properly is dependent on the movement of the chest and supporting structures. These structures include the thoracic cage (chest), thoracic cavity, diaphragm, intercostal muscles, and accessory muscles of breathing. Accessory muscles are not used during normal breathing but can be employed in times of respiratory distress.

Partial pressure is the term used to describe the amount of gas in air or dissolved in fluid, such as blood. Partial pressure is measured in millimeters of mercury (mm Hg). The partial pressure of oxygen in air (Pao_2) within the alveoli is approximately 104 mm Hg. Carbon dioxide enters the alveoli from the blood and causes a partial pressure of approximately 40 mm Hg.

When the blood from the right side of the heart reaches the lungs to bypass the alveoli, it has very low levels of oxygen (Pao_2) and very high levels of carbon dioxide ($Paco_2$) as compared to the alveoli. After the patient inhales, the Pao_2 in the alveoli is much higher, and the $Paco_2$ is much lower, than in this blood. This pressure imbalance causes oxygen to diffuse from the high levels in the alveoli into the blood at the same time carbon dioxide moves from the blood into the alveoli. The carbon dioxide is then eliminated from the lungs as waste during exhalation. This process occurs in reverse when the arterial blood reaches the tissues. Oxygen diffuses into the tissue fluid and then into the cells, and carbon dioxide diffuses out of the cells and then into the tissue fluid and blood.

The air pressure outside the body, called the atmospheric pressure, is normally higher than the air pressure within the thoracic cavity. During inhalation, the thoracic cage expands and the air pressure within the thoracic cavity decreases, creating a slight vacuum. This pulls air in through the trachea, causing the lungs to fill, a process called negative-pressure ventilation. When the air pressure outside equals the air pressure inside, air stops moving. Gases, such as oxygen, will move from an area of higher pressure to an area of lower pressure until the pressures are equal. At this point, the air stops moving, and inhalation stops.

It may help you to understand this if you think of the thoracic cage as a bell jar in which balloons are suspended. In this example, the balloons are the lungs. The base of the jar is the diaphragm, which

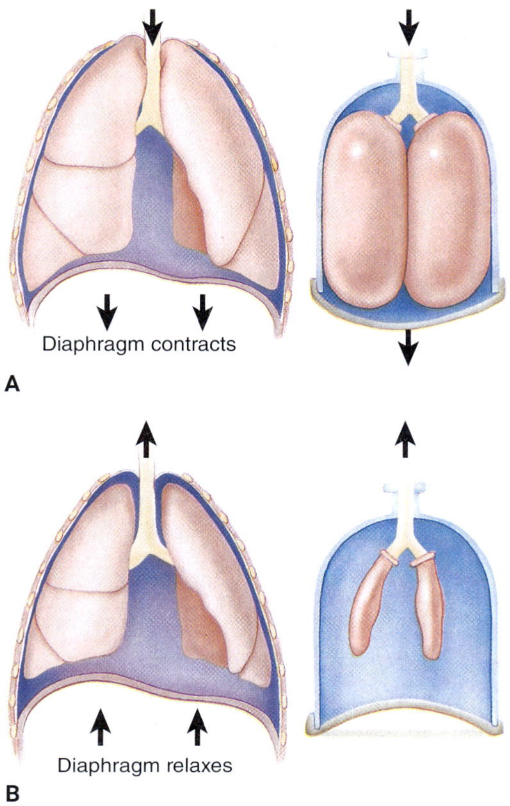

FIGURE 11-10 The mechanism of ventilation can be illustrated by using a bell jar. **A.** Inhalation and chest expansion, anatomic (left) and bell jar (right). **B.** Exhalation and chest contraction, anatomic (left) and bell jar (right).

TABLE 11-2 Ventilation Terminology

Term	Definition
Tidal volume	The amount of air (in milliliters) that is inhaled or exhaled during one breath.
Residual volume	The air that remains in the lungs after maximal expiration.
Alveolar ventilation	The volume of air that reaches the alveoli; calculated by subtracting the amount of dead space air from the tidal volume.
Minute volume	The volume of air moved through the lungs in 1 minute; calculated by multiplying tidal volume and respiratory rate.
Minute alveolar ventilation	The volume of air moved through the lungs in 1 minute minus the dead space; calculated by multiplying tidal volume (minus dead space) and respiratory rate.
Vital capacity	The amount of air that can be forcibly expelled from the lungs after breathing in as deeply as possible.
Dead space	The portion of the tidal volume that does not reach alveoli and thus does not participate in gas exchange.

moves up and down slightly with each breath. The ribs, which are the sides of the jar, maintain the shape of the chest. The only opening into the jar is a small tube at the top, similar to the trachea. During inhalation, the bottom of the jar moves down slightly, causing a decrease in pressure in the jar and creating a slight vacuum. As a result, the balloons fill with air (**FIGURE 11-10**).

The entire process of inspiration is focused on delivering oxygen to the alveoli. However, not all the air you breathe actually reaches the alveoli. **TABLE 11-2** reviews terminology as it relates to the processes of inspiration and expiration. The average tidal volume is the amount of air in milliliters (mL) moved into or out of the respiratory tract (ie, from the nose and mouth to the alveolar sacs) during a single breath. It is approximately 500 mL

YOU are the EMT

You and your partner are dispatched to a residence for a 53-year-old man who passed out. The 9-1-1 caller told the dispatcher that the patient appears to be breathing but will not wake up. The time is 1345 hours, the temperature outside is 77°F (25°C), and the weather is cloudy. A fire squad with two additional EMTs is dispatched simultaneously.

1. Based on the dispatch information, what type of call should you and your partner mentally prepare for? Why?
2. How do tidal volume and respiratory rate influence minute alveolar ventilation?

for a healthy male and 400 mL for a healthy female.[2] Breathing becomes deeper as the tidal volume responds to the increased metabolic demand for oxygen. However, as noted previously, not all inspired air reaches the alveoli for gas exchange. Dead space is described as the portion of inspired air that fails to reach the alveoli and deliver oxygen. These processes of inhalation are discussed further in Chapter 6, *The Human Body*.

Exhalation

Unlike inhalation, **exhalation** does not normally require muscular effort; therefore, it is a passive process. During exhalation, the diaphragm and the intercostal muscles relax. In response, the thorax decreases in size, and the ribs and muscles assume a normal resting position. When the size of the thoracic cavity decreases, air in the lungs is compressed into a smaller space. The air pressure within the thoracic cavity then becomes higher than the outside pressure, and the air is pushed out through the trachea.

Remember that air will reach the lungs only if it travels through the trachea. This is why clearing and maintaining an open airway is so important. Clearing the airway means removing obstructing material, tissue, or fluids from the nose, mouth, and throat. Maintaining an open airway means keeping the airway **patent** so that air can enter and leave the lungs freely (**FIGURE 11-11**).

Air may also pass into the chest cavity through an abnormal opening in the throat or chest wall as a result of trauma, remaining outside the bronchi and never reaching the alveoli. In later chapters, you will learn how to recognize and manage these potentially life-threatening conditions.

Regulation of Ventilation

The body's need for oxygen is dynamic, depending on the metabolic needs at any given time. The respiratory system must be able to accommodate the changes in oxygen demand by altering the rate and depth of ventilation. The regulation of ventilation involves a complex series of receptors and feedback loops that sense gas concentrations in the body fluids and send messages to the respiratory centers in the brainstem to adjust the rate and depth of ventilation accordingly. Failure to meet the body's needs for oxygen may result in **hypoxia**. Hypoxia is an extremely dangerous condition in which the tissues and cells of the body do not get enough oxygen. Hypoxia can be fatal if not promptly recognized and corrected.

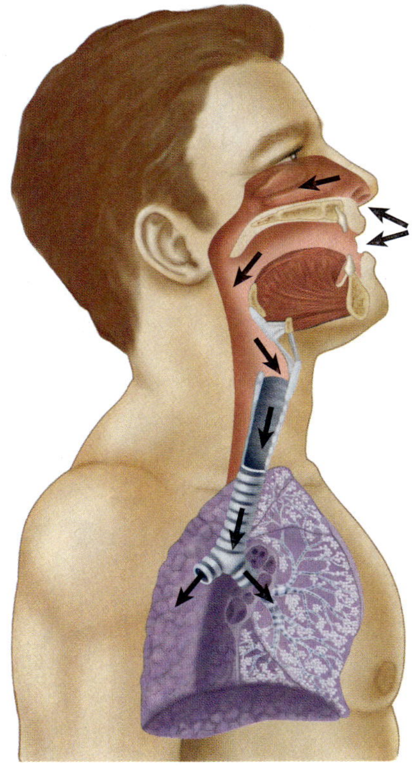

FIGURE 11-11 Air reaches the lungs only if it travels through the trachea. Maintaining the airway means keeping the trachea and the entirety of the airway patent so that air can enter and leave the lungs freely.

For most people, the drive to breathe is based on pH changes (related to carbon dioxide levels) in the blood and cerebrospinal fluid (CSF). When carbon dioxide levels in the blood increase, the pH of the CSF decreases. When this occurs, a message is sent to the respiratory centers in the pons and medulla (located in the brainstem), which stimulates breathing. However, patients with a chronic obstructive pulmonary disease (COPD), such as emphysema or chronic bronchitis, have difficulty eliminating carbon dioxide through exhalation; thus, they may have higher levels of carbon dioxide. This condition potentially alters their respiratory drive. The theory is that the respiratory centers in the brain gradually adjust to accommodate high levels of carbon dioxide. In patients with COPD who have chronically high carbon dioxide levels, the body uses a backup system to control breathing. This theory of secondary control of breathing, called **hypoxic drive**, is based on levels of oxygen dissolved in plasma. This method is different from the primary control of breathing that uses carbon dioxide as the driving force. Hypoxic drive is typically found in end-stage COPD. Providing high concentrations of oxygen over time will increase the amount of oxygen dissolved in plasma. Some believe this could potentially negatively affect the body's drive to breathe in COPD patients who have chronically high levels of carbon dioxide. It is important to remember that high concentrations of oxygen should *never* be withheld from any patient who needs it. Patients with severe respiratory and/or circulatory compromise should receive high concentrations of oxygen regardless of their underlying medical conditions. In these patients, as in all patients, the rate and depth of breathing should be monitored continuously. Carbon dioxide levels should also be monitored, if possible.

Patients who are breathing inadequately will show varying signs and symptoms of hypoxia. The onset and degree of tissue damage caused by hypoxia often depend on the quality of ventilations. Early signs of hypoxia include restlessness, irritability, apprehension, fast heart rate (tachycardia), and anxiety. Late signs of hypoxia include mental status changes, a weak (thready) pulse, slow heart rate or lethal rhythm changes, and cyanosis. Conscious patients will complain of shortness of breath (**dyspnea**) and may not be able to talk in complete sentences. The best time to give a patient oxygen is before signs and symptoms of hypoxia appear.

In children, hypoxia is the leading cause of a slow heart rate (bradycardia). A slow heart rate in children is not typically adequate to provide oxygenated blood to all organs. When a child is found to have a heart rate slower than normal for their age with a low blood pressure, signs of shock, or a sudden change in mental status, administer positive-pressure ventilation with supplemental oxygen.[3]

Street Smarts

If the initial assessment reveals a patient who is very anxious and restless, the EMT should rule out hypoxia as a possible cause before assuming the patient is experiencing a behavioral emergency.

Words of Wisdom

Although the terms hypoxemia and hypoxia are often used interchangeably, they are, in fact, separate processes. Hypoxemia is a low level of oxygen in arterial blood, whereas hypoxia is a low level of oxygen at the cellular level. Uncorrected hypoxemia will lead to hypoxia.

Oxygenation

Oxygenation is the process of loading oxygen molecules onto hemoglobin molecules in the bloodstream. The hemoglobin then transports the oxygen to the cells of the body. Oxygenation requires that the air used for ventilation contain an adequate percentage of oxygen. Ventilation without oxygenation can occur in places where oxygen levels in the breathing air have been depleted, such as in mines, in confined spaces, or inside a burning structure. Ventilation without adequate oxygenation can also occur in climbers who ascend too quickly to an altitude of lower atmospheric pressure. At high altitudes, the percentage of oxygen remains the same, but the lower atmospheric pressure makes it difficult to adequately bring enough oxygen into the body.

Words of Wisdom

Oxygenation can be disrupted through carbon monoxide poisoning. Carbon monoxide has a much greater affinity for hemoglobin than oxygen (250 times more); in other words, carbon monoxide binds to hemoglobin more readily than oxygen. If oxygen cannot bind to hemoglobin, it cannot be transported to the tissues and cells.

Respiration

All living cells perform a specific function and need energy to survive. Cells take energy from nutrients through a series of chemical processes. The name given to these processes is **metabolism**. During metabolism, each cell combines nutrients (such as glucose [sugar]) and oxygen and produces energy (in the form of adenosine triphosphate [ATP]) and waste products, primarily water and carbon dioxide. Each cell in the body requires a continuous supply of oxygen and a regular means of disposing of waste (carbon dioxide). The body provides for these requirements through respiration.

Respiration is the process of exchanging oxygen and carbon dioxide. This exchange occurs by diffusion, a process in which a gas moves from an area of greater concentration to an area of lower concentration. In the body, gases diffuse rapidly across a distance of micrometers.

External Respiration

External respiration (pulmonary respiration) is the process of breathing fresh air into the respiratory system and exchanging oxygen and carbon dioxide between the alveoli and the blood in the pulmonary capillaries (**FIGURE 11-12**).

Fresh air that is inspired into the lungs contains approximately 21% oxygen, 78% nitrogen, and 0.3% carbon dioxide. As this air reaches the alveoli, it encounters a chemical compound that coats them called **surfactant**. Surfactant reduces surface tension within the alveoli and keeps them expanded, making it easier for the gas exchange between oxygen and carbon dioxide to occur. It is important to remember that although adequate ventilation is necessary for external respiration to occur, it does not guarantee that external respiration is being achieved.

Once the oxygen crosses the alveolar membrane, it binds to hemoglobin, an iron-containing molecule that has a great affinity for oxygen molecules. Found in red blood cells, hemoglobin molecules that are low in oxygen concentration are pumped from the right side of the heart through the pulmonary circulation, which ends in the capillaries in the lungs. The capillaries surround alveoli, which contain high concentrations of oxygen (from inspired air). The hemoglobin molecules bind to oxygen as it crosses the alveolar membrane and transport it back to the left side of the heart, where it is pumped out to the rest of the body. Under normal conditions, 96% to 100% of the hemoglobin receptor sites contain oxygen.

Internal Respiration

The exchange of oxygen and carbon dioxide between the systemic circulation and the cells of the body is called **internal respiration**. As blood travels through the body, it supplies oxygen and nutrients to tissues and cells. Oxygen passes from the blood in the capillaries to the cells in the body's tissues. At the same time, carbon dioxide and cell waste pass from the cells into the capillaries. Once in the capillaries, these products are transported in the venous system back to the lung, where the carbon dioxide is exhaled (**FIGURE 11-13**).

Every cell in the body needs a constant supply of oxygen to survive. Whereas some tissues are more resilient than others, eventually, all cells will die if deprived of oxygen (**FIGURE 11-14**). To deliver sufficient oxygen to the tissues of the body, adequate ventilation and perfusion must occur.

In the presence of oxygen, cells convert glucose into energy through a process known as **aerobic metabolism**. Energy is produced through a series of

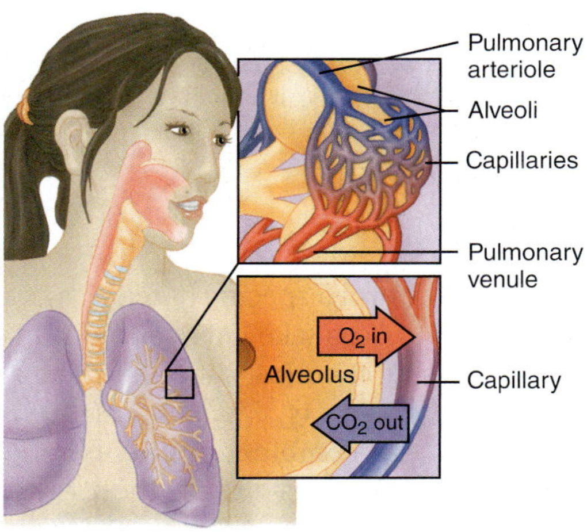

FIGURE 11-12 External respiration.

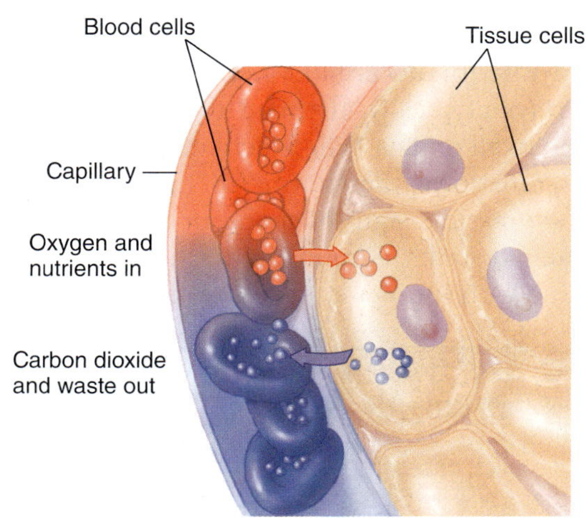

FIGURE 11-13 Internal respiration.

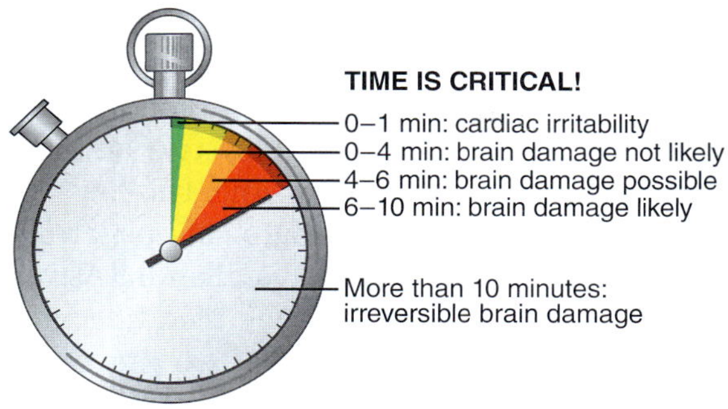

FIGURE 11-14 Cells need a constant supply of oxygen to survive. Some cells may be severely or permanently damaged after 4 to 6 minutes without oxygen.

biochemical reactions. Without adequate oxygen, the cells do not completely convert glucose into energy, and lactic acid and other toxins accumulate in the cell. This process, **anaerobic metabolism**, cannot meet the metabolic demands of the cell. If this process is not corrected, the cells will eventually die. Therefore, adequate perfusion (circulation of blood within an organ or tissue) and ventilation must be present for aerobic metabolism to occur. However, although these elements are necessary for aerobic metabolism, they do not guarantee that aerobic metabolism will occur.

When cells use oxygen to convert glucose to energy, carbon dioxide, the main waste product, accumulates in the cell. Carbon dioxide is then transported through the circulatory system and back to the lungs for elimination from the body through exhalation.

It is important to understand the processes of ventilation, oxygenation, and respiration. The ultimate goal of these mechanisms is to deliver an adequate supply of oxygen to the cells of the body. When one of these processes fails or becomes disrupted, cells die. By recognizing the signs and symptoms of inadequate tissue perfusion and oxygenation, you can immediately intervene and correct a potentially life-threatening condition.

Pathophysiology of Respiration

Multiple conditions inhibit the body's ability to effectively deliver oxygen to the cells. Disruption of ventilation, oxygenation, or respiration will cause immediate effects on the body. As an EMT, you need to recognize these conditions and correct them immediately.

Factors in the Nervous System

Chemical factors are commonly involved in respiratory control issues because of the level of complexity of the human body. A complex series of chemical reactions are constantly taking place. For example, **chemoreceptors** monitor the levels of oxygen and carbon dioxide and the hydrogen ion concentration (indicated by the pH level of the CSF), and then provide feedback to the respiratory centers in the brainstem to modify the rate and depth of breathing based on the body's needs at any given time. Central chemoreceptors in the medulla respond quickly to slight elevations in carbon dioxide level or a decrease in the pH of the CSF. The peripheral chemoreceptors, located in the carotid arteries and the aortic arch, are sensitive to decreased levels of oxygen in arterial blood as well as to low pH levels.

When serum carbon dioxide or hydrogen ion levels increase because of a medical or traumatic condition, chemoreceptors stimulate the medulla to increase the respiratory rate, thus removing more carbon dioxide or acid from the body. One area in the medulla is responsible for initiating inspiration based on the information received from the chemoreceptors. Another area in the medulla is primarily responsible for motor control of the inspiratory and expiratory muscles.

In addition, stimulation from the pons affects the rate and depth of respirations. If one item in this process is disrupted, then the respiratory process will be affected.

Ventilation/Perfusion Ratio and Mismatch

The lungs must place ambient air close enough to circulating blood to permit gas exchange by diffusion. To accomplish this action, air and blood flow must be directed to the same place at the same time. In other words, ventilation (air flow, $\dot{V}$) and perfusion (blood flow, $\dot{Q}$) must be matched. A failure to match ventilation and perfusion (ventilation/perfusion [$\dot{V}/\dot{Q}$] mismatch) lies behind most abnormalities in oxygen and carbon dioxide exchange.

When ventilation is compromised but perfusion continues, blood passes over some alveolar membranes without any oxygen available for gas exchange to take place. This results in a lack of oxygen diffusing across the membrane and into the bloodstream. Carbon dioxide is also not able to diffuse across the membrane from the capillaries into the lungs and is therefore recirculated within the bloodstream. This condition could lead to severe hypoxemia, and eventually hypoxia, if not recognized and treated. It may also result in the accumulation of excess carbon dioxide within the circulating bloodstream that eventually leads to acidosis.

Similar problems can occur when lung tissue lacks adequate blood flow. The lack of blood flow in the affected region of the lung disrupts perfusion across the alveolar capillaries. Although the alveoli are filled with oxygen, disruption in blood flow does not allow for optimal exchange of gases across the membrane. This condition results in less oxygen diffusion into the bloodstream and less carbon dioxide removal. It can also lead to hypoxemia. If this occurs, you need to provide immediate intervention to prevent cellular damage or death.

An example of this type of $\dot{V}/\dot{Q}$ mismatch can be seen with a pulmonary embolism. When a thrombus (blood clot) lodges in a pulmonary artery, blood flow from the right side of the heart to the lungs is partially or completely obstructed, depending on the size and location of the thrombus. Even though the patient continues to ventilate (ie, move air into and out of the lungs), external respiration will be impaired because of decreased blood flow to the lungs.

Factors Affecting Pulmonary Ventilation

Maintaining a patent airway is critical to the delivery of oxygen to the tissues of the body. There are many intrinsic and extrinsic factors that cause airway obstructions.

Intrinsic Factors

Intrinsic (internal) conditions such as infections, allergic reactions, and unresponsiveness (tongue obstruction) can significantly compromise airway patency. Swelling from infections and allergic reactions can be fatal if not aggressively managed with medications and possibly advanced airway techniques.

Some factors affecting pulmonary ventilation are not necessarily directly part of the respiratory system. The central and peripheral nervous systems play key roles in the regulation of breathing. Interruptions to these systems can have a drastic effect on the ability to breathe efficiently. Medications, such as opioids (eg, fentanyl) and sedatives, can depress the central nervous system and lower the respiratory rate and tidal volume. This lower rate and volume will decrease minute volume, alveolar volume, and minute alveolar ventilation. As a result, the amount of oxygen in the blood decreases (hypoxemia) and the amount of carbon dioxide in the bloodstream increases, a condition called **hypercapnia**. Trauma to the head and spinal cord can also interrupt nervous control of ventilation, resulting in decreased respiratory function and even respiratory failure. In addition to medications and trauma, conditions such as muscular dystrophy can affect nervous system control of breathing. This disease causes degeneration of muscle fibers, resulting in a gradual weakening of muscles (such as the diaphragm and intercostal muscles), slowing of motor development, and loss of muscle contractility. Curvature of the spine is also likely in patients with muscular dystrophy and can impair pulmonary function.

Words of Wisdom

It is important for the EMT to recognize the differences between respiratory distress, respiratory failure, and respiratory arrest.

- **Respiratory distress** refers to difficulty breathing and involves an abnormal respiratory rate or effort. It can range from mild to severe and can progress to respiratory failure.
- **Respiratory failure** occurs when oxygen levels are too low to meet the body's needs and ventilation is impaired, leading to high carbon dioxide levels. Respiratory failure is accompanied by serious signs and symptoms and must be corrected quickly.
- **Respiratory arrest** refers to complete cessation of breathing (apnea) or agonal gasps that will lead to cardiac arrest if the EMT does not intervene immediately.

The tongue is the most common airway obstruction in the unresponsive patient. This airway obstruction, while easily corrected, can result in hypoxemia (and ultimately hypoxia) and hinder adequate tissue perfusion. Obstruction of the airway by the tongue is also associated with hypercapnia;

after all, if oxygen cannot get in, carbon dioxide cannot get out. Snoring respirations and the position of the head and/or neck are good indicators that the tongue may be obstructing the airway. Prompt correction of this obstruction is necessary for adequate ventilation and oxygenation.

Patients with allergic reactions not only have a potential airway obstruction from swelling, but may also have a decrease in pulmonary ventilation from bronchoconstriction. As the bronchioles constrict, air is forced through smaller lumens, resulting in decreased ventilation. This condition can also be found in patients with COPD such as chronic bronchitis.

Extrinsic Factors

Extrinsic (external) factors affecting pulmonary ventilation can include trauma or foreign body airway obstruction. Trauma to the airway or chest requires immediate evaluation and intervention. The effect of an injury such as a broken jaw is often overlooked. Patients with a fracture to the mandible, especially unconscious patients, may not be able to maintain an open airway and may require the insertion of an airway adjunct. Blunt or penetrating trauma and burns can disrupt airflow through the trachea and into the lungs, quickly resulting in oxygenation deficiencies. In addition, trauma to the chest wall can result in structural damage to the thorax, leading to inadequate pulmonary ventilation. Swelling, punctures, and bruising can have a tremendous effect on the ability to deliver oxygen to the alveoli and into the bloodstream. Proper airway management and supplemental oxygen are crucial to the patient's outcome in these situations.

Factors Affecting Respiration

External elements in the environment can affect the overall process of respiration. For proper respiration to take place at the cellular level, both oxygenation and perfusion need to function efficiently.

External Factors

Adequate respiration requires adequate ventilation and oxygenation. Here, external factors such as atmospheric pressure and the partial pressure of oxygen in the ambient air play a key role in the overall process of respiration. At high altitudes, the percentage of oxygen remains the same, but the partial pressure decreases because the total atmospheric pressure decreases. The low partial pressure of oxygen can make it difficult (or impossible) to adequately oxygenate tissue, thus interrupting internal respiration. In addition, closed environments, such as mines and trenches, may have decreased levels of ambient oxygen, resulting in poor oxygenation and respiration.

Carbon monoxide, along with other toxic and poisonous gases, displaces oxygen in the environment and makes proper oxygenation and respiration difficult. In particular, carbon monoxide has a much greater affinity for hemoglobin than does oxygen (250 times more) and will occupy all sites on hemoglobin that are normally occupied by oxygen. Loading the hemoglobin with carbon monoxide instead of oxygen prohibits oxygen delivery to the tissues. This results in severe hypoxemia which, if uncorrected, can rapidly lead to death.

Internal Factors

Conditions that reduce the surface area for gas exchange also decrease the body's oxygen supply, leading to inadequate tissue perfusion. Medical conditions such as pneumonia, pulmonary edema, and emphysema may also result in a disturbance of cellular metabolism. These conditions decrease the surface area of the alveoli either by damaging the alveoli or by leading to an accumulation of fluid in the lungs.

Nonfunctional alveoli inhibit the diffusion of oxygen and carbon dioxide, creating a $\dot{V}/\dot{Q}$ mismatch. As a result, blood entering the lungs from the right side of the heart bypasses the alveoli and returns to the left side of the heart in an unoxygenated state, a condition called **intrapulmonary shunting**. The greater the degree of intrapulmonary shunting, the greater the degree of hypoxemia.

Drowning victims and/or patients with pulmonary edema have fluid in the alveoli. This accumulation of fluid inhibits adequate gas exchange across the alveolar membrane and results in decreased oxygenation and respiration. In addition, exposure to certain environmental conditions such as high altitude or occupational hazards such as epoxy resins can result in fluid accumulation over time, or other abnormal conditions, resulting in impaired oxygenation. These conditions can interrupt the process of aerobic metabolism at the cellular level, resulting in anaerobic metabolism and an increase in lactic acid accumulation.

Circulatory Compromise

For respiration to occur, the circulatory system must function efficiently to deliver oxygen to the tissues of the body. When this system becomes compromised, perfusion is inadequate to meet the metabolic demands of the tissues.

Obstruction of blood flow to individual cells and tissue can be related to traumatic injuries. These conditions include a **hemothorax** or a **pneumothorax** (whether a simple or **tension pneumothorax**), open pneumothorax (sucking chest wound), or hemo-pneumothorax. Although not a traumatic injury, a pulmonary embolism can have the same obstructive effects. All of these conditions limit the ability for gas exchange to occur at the tissue level because of their effects on the respiratory and circulatory systems. In addition, conditions such as heart failure and pericardial tamponade inhibit the ability of the heart to effectively pump oxygenated blood to the tissues.

Blood loss and anemia, a deficiency of red blood cells, result in a decreased ability of blood to carry oxygen. Without sufficient circulating red blood cells, there is not enough hemoglobin to carry oxygen to the tissues.

When the body is in a state of shock, oxygen is not delivered to the cells efficiently. Hypovolemic shock is an abnormal decrease in circulating volume that causes inadequate oxygen delivery to the body. In contrast, vasodilatory shock is not determined by the amount of circulating blood, but by the size of the blood vessels. As the diameter of the blood vessels increases, the blood pressure in the circulatory system decreases. As the systemic blood pressure decreases, oxygen is not delivered effectively to the tissues. Both forms of shock result in poor tissue perfusion that leads to anaerobic metabolism. Any patient suspected of being in shock should be treated aggressively to prevent further interruptions in tissue perfusion.

Street Smarts

Just as you need to know *how* to perform a particular airway procedure, you must also know *why* it is performed. Performing the wrong procedure, however skillfully, will not benefit your patient. Without sufficient knowledge of respiratory anatomy, physiology, and pathophysiology, you will not know which intervention is best for your patient. Airway management is not a guessing game. Remember, your patients need your knowledge as much as they need your hands.

Patient Assessment

To ensure your safety during a call that involves a patient with breathing difficulties, wear a mask and protective eyewear that includes eye shields (not glasses) whenever airway management involves suctioning or some other **aerosol-generating procedure (AGP)**. Any airway manipulation that induces the production of aerosols constitutes an AGP, such as cardiopulmonary resuscitation (CPR), manual ventilation, endotracheal (ET) intubation or extubation, open suctioning of airways, and non-invasive ventilation such as continuous positive airway pressure (CPAP) or bilevel positive airway pressure (BPAP).[4] Body fluids can become aerosolized, and exposure to the mucous membranes of your mouth, nose, and eyes can easily occur. If the patient has a highly contagious respiratory disease, a high-efficiency particulate air (HEPA) filter (eg, N95), air-purifying respirator (APR), or powered air-purifying respirator (PAPR) and gown should also be worn (if there is risk such as tuberculosis or COVID-19 spread).

Recognizing Adequate Breathing

Most of the time, you are not aware of your own breathing or the breathing of others around you. Breathing should be a smooth, effortless flow of air moving into and out of the lungs. In general, unless you are directly assessing the patient's airway, *you should not be able to see or hear a patient breathe.* Signs of normal (adequate) breathing are as follows:

- A normal rate (**TABLE 11-3**)
- A regular pattern of inhalation and exhalation
- Clear and equal lung sounds on both sides of the chest (**bilateral**)
- Regular and equal chest rise and fall (chest expansion)
- Adequate depth (tidal volume)

Recognizing Abnormal Breathing

A patient who is awake, alert, and talking to you generally has no *immediate* airway or breathing problems. However, you should always have supplemental oxygen and a **bag-mask device** or pocket

TABLE 11-3 Normal Respiratory Rate Ranges

Age	Respiratory Rate (breaths/min)
Newborn: 0 to 1 month	30 to 60
Infant: 1 month to 1 year	30 to 53
Toddler: 1 to 3 years	22 to 27
Preschool age: 3 to 6 years	20 to 28
School age: 6 to 12 years	18 to 25
Adults and adolescents (12 years and older)	12 to 20

mask close at hand to assist with breathing if necessary. Patients who are breathing normally will have adequate tidal volume (depth) and a rate that is consistent with their age.

If a patient is breathing slower or faster than normal, you should assess the depth of respirations. *Patients with shallow depth of breathing (reduced tidal volume) may require assisted ventilations, even if the respiratory rate is otherwise normal.*

A patient with inadequate breathing may appear to be working hard to breathe, which is called **labored breathing**. It requires effort and, especially among children, may involve the use of accessory muscles, including the neck muscles (sternocleidomastoid), the pectoralis major muscles of the chest, and the abdominal muscles.

Signs of inadequate breathing are as follows:

- Respiratory rate outside of the normal range in the presence of shortness of breath (dyspnea)
- Irregular rhythm, such as a patient taking a series of deep breaths followed by periods of **apnea** (lack of spontaneous breathing)
- Diminished, absent, or noisy auscultated breath sounds
- Use of tripod position, where patient is sitting upright and leaning forward onto arms and hands to facilitate inspiration and expiration (**FIGURE 11-15**).
- Reduced flow of expired air at the nose and mouth
- Unequal or inadequate chest expansion, resulting in reduced tidal volume
- Increased effort of breathing (use of accessory muscles)

Words of Wisdom

The accurate respiratory status of a patient is so important that it should be noted at the beginning of your radio report, after mental status. Any changes during treatment or transport should be immediately reported to the receiving hospital. Respiratory status, along with any changes, should also be clearly documented in your patient care report.

YOU are the EMT

You arrive at the scene and find the patient lying supine in a small bathroom. You quickly move him to a more open area and begin your assessment. He is unresponsive, is making a loud snoring sound, and has slow, irregular breathing. His face is cyanotic. A carotid pulse can be felt, but it is slow, and his radial pulses are bounding.

Recording Time: 0 Minutes	
Appearance	Cyanosis to the face (patient has dark skin and lips appear purple)
Level of consciousness	Unresponsive
Airway	Snoring; no obvious oral secretions
Breathing	Slow and irregular
Circulation	Skin, cyanotic; radial pulse, slow and bounding

3. What are your immediate priorities of care?
4. Anatomically, what causes snoring in an unresponsive patient?

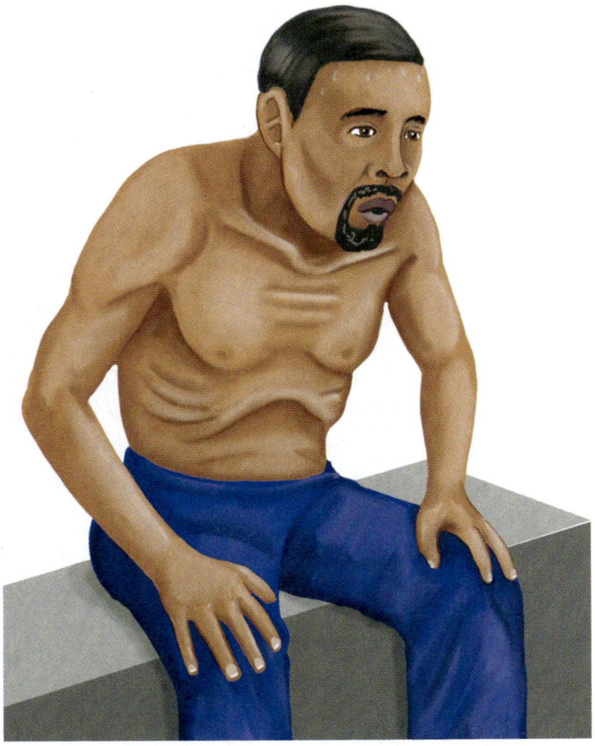

FIGURE 11-15 The use of the tripod position, in which the patient sits or stands with hands on knees or another surface as demonstrated here, is commonly seen in patients with labored breathing to facilitate inhalation and exhalation.

- Shallow depth (reduced tidal volume)
- Skin that is pale, cyanotic, cool, or moist (clammy)
- Skin pulling in around the ribs or above the clavicles during inspiration (**retractions**)

Street Smarts

Becoming short of breath or having the sensation you cannot get enough air to breathe is a scary situation. Work quickly to help patients with difficulty breathing and realize that they are anxious because they are scared.

When you are assessing a patient with potential airway compromise, pay particular attention to the external environment. Conditions such as high altitude and enclosed spaces alter the partial pressure of oxygen in the environment, hindering the process of oxygenation. In addition, poisonous gases, such as carbon monoxide, displace oxygen in the environment and alter overall cellular

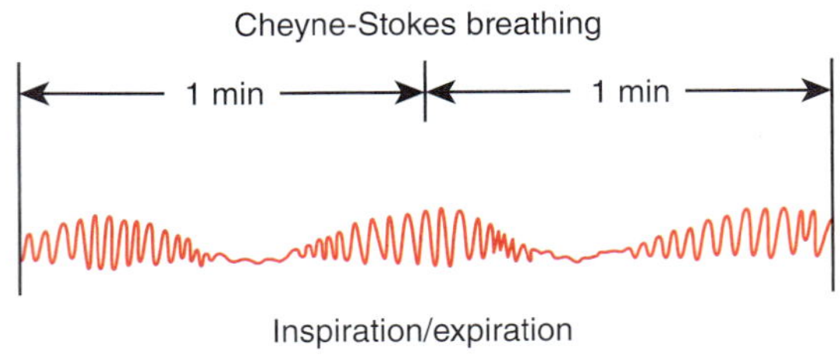

FIGURE 11-16 Cheyne-Stokes breathing is characterized by a crescendo–decrescendo pattern of breathing followed by a period of apnea.

metabolism. Severe hypothermia may result in a slow respiratory rate. The external environment should be considered when deciding on the appropriate treatment.

If the patient is breathing faster than the normal rate for their age without signs of respiratory distress, consider other causes. Nonrespiratory causes of tachypnea include anemia, fever, dehydration, metabolic acidosis (ie, diabetic ketoacidosis and some toxicities), pain, and sepsis.

You should be aware that a patient may appear to be breathing after their heart has stopped. These occasional, gasping breaths are called **agonal gasps**. They occur when the respiratory center in the brain continues to send signals to the respiratory muscles. These gasps do not provide adequate tidal volume because they are infrequent, gasping respiratory efforts. In patients with agonal gasps, you will need to provide artificial ventilations and, most likely, chest compressions.

Some patients may have irregular respiratory breathing patterns that are related to a specific condition. For example, **Cheyne-Stokes respirations** are a respiratory pattern in which the patient breathes with an increasing rate and depth, followed by a decreasing rate and depth (a "crescendo–decrescendo" pattern), followed by periods of **apnea** (**FIGURE 11-16**). This breathing pattern can be seen in patients who have experienced a stroke or serious head injury.

Serious head injuries may cause other changes in the normal respiratory rate and pattern of breathing. These injuries may produce irregular, ineffective respirations that may or may not have an identifiable pattern (**ataxic respirations**).

Patients experiencing a metabolic or toxicologic disorder may display other abnormal respiratory patterns such as Kussmaul respirations. Kussmaul respirations are characterized by deep, rapid respirations commonly seen in diabetic patients with metabolic acidosis.

Whereas rapid breathing is a compensatory mechanism to help patients in respiratory distress, some patients are so ill that their bodies are unable to compensate for their respiratory distress. You need to be vigilant when monitoring patients in respiratory distress because their condition may decline rapidly.

Patients with inadequate breathing have inadequate minute volume and need to be treated immediately. If a patient can speak using only minimal words while at rest, they are attempting to preserve residual volume in the lungs; this is a sign of inadequate ventilation. Likewise, a slow or fast respiratory rate may result in a reduction in tidal volume and decreased ventilation adequacy. Emergency medical care includes airway management, supplemental oxygen, and ventilatory support.

Assessment of Respiration

Even though a patient may be ventilating adequately, the actual exchange of oxygen and carbon dioxide at the tissue level may be compromised. You must assess for signs of adequate and inadequate respiration in all patients.

Environmental factors can dramatically affect respiration and alter cellular metabolism. If there is more than one patient with similar symptoms, consider the presence of poisonous or toxic gases or an infectious cause. If your EMS unit carries a handheld carbon monoxide detector, assess ambient air before entering the location. However, if you enter a space and suspect the quality of the ambient air is not safe, remove yourself and the patient (if possible) from the scene immediately and contact the appropriate resources.

A patient's level of consciousness and skin color and condition are excellent indicators of respiration. During normal respiration, oxygen and carbon dioxide diffuse into and out of tissues. When you are assessing mental status and skin color and condition, it will be apparent if the patient has adequate oxygen levels reaching these areas. A patient with an altered level of consciousness may not have adequate oxygen levels reaching the brain. If adequate oxygen is not reaching the brain, you should expect that the patient is retaining carbon dioxide as well. This lack of oxygen and increase in carbon dioxide can cause rapid changes in the patient's mental status. Therefore, when treating patients with an altered mental status, always consider the possibility that these patients may not be getting adequate oxygen to their brain and that you need to consider the possible underlying causes. Be sure to determine the patient's baseline mental status, considering that the baseline mental status may be abnormal because of a preexisting medical condition (eg, previous stroke, traumatic brain injury). Ask someone familiar with the patient to describe the patient's normal mental status.

Poor skin color can indicate inadequate respiration, just as an altered level of consciousness does. As oxygen fails to reach the skin tissue of the body, either from a lack of perfusion or poor oxygenation, the color of the skin changes to reflect inadequate oxygenation. Pallor is typically associated with poor perfusion caused by illness or shock. As this condition worsens, cyanosis becomes noticeable first peripherally, in the fingertips or palms, and then centrally, in the mucous membranes and around the lips. Eventually, if the poor perfusion or oxygenation is not corrected, anaerobic metabolism will occur. This could cause the skin to become marked with blotches of different colors, commonly referred to as mottling.

Words of Wisdom

When using skin color to assess a patient's condition, keep in mind that pallor, cyanosis, flushing, or jaundice will present differently among patients depending on their baseline skin color. For patients with a dark baseline skin tone, you may need to look for signs of abnormal perfusion in places such as the oral mucosa, conjunctiva, nail beds, or palms.

Several methods can be used to assess proper oxygenation, including the use of **pulse oximetry**. The oxygen saturation (Spo_2) level measures the percentage of hemoglobin molecules that are bound in arterial blood. Because hemoglobin delivers 97% of the oxygen delivered to the body's tissues, oxygen saturation serves as a useful adjunct to assess the amount of oxygen available to the end organs. Oxygen dissolved in plasma (the partial pressure of oxygen [Pao_2]) delivers the other 3% to the body's tissues.

Assessment of oxygen saturation is the standard of care in the management of patients with respiratory or circulatory problems. The pulse oximeter provides a rapid, reliable, noninvasive measurement of a patient's oxygenation status; however, a pulse oximetry reading should not be the sole determinant of a patient's overall respiratory status. This value should be interpreted together with a full clinical assessment of the patient. This device can be used to assess the adequacy of oxygenation during positive-pressure ventilation and to assess the overall effect of interventions on your patient.

Words of Wisdom

The pulse oximeter simply tells you the percentage of hemoglobin that is bound (saturated); *it does not tell you what the hemoglobin is bound to.* Therefore, pulse oximetry must be used in conjunction with a careful physical assessment of the patient. A patient who has been exposed to carbon monoxide or who is anemic may have an Spo_2 reading that is normal or high, but the cells are not receiving the oxygen they need. Do not take an Spo_2 number at face value, especially if the patient is experiencing clinical signs of poor oxygenation.

Under normal conditions, the Spo_2 should be 94% or greater while breathing room air. Although no definitive threshold exists for normal values, an Spo_2 of less than 94% in a nonsmoker may indicate hypoxemia and often requires treatment unless the patient has a chronic condition causing perpetually low oxygen saturation levels. In acute conditions such as stroke, oxygen is indicated when the Spo_2 drops below 94%, with a goal of maintaining an Spo_2 of 94% to 98%. Pulse oximeters can take as long as 60 seconds to reflect changes in a patient's oxygenation status, a situation referred to as Spo_2 "lag." Essentially, a pulse oximeter placed on a patient's finger typically reflects a patient's oxygenation status approximately 1 minute ago. This time delay is important to understand because respiratory insufficiency can develop in a patient well before the pulse oximetry values begin to decline. It is critical to monitor the patient and supplement your assessment with the information from the pulse oximeter.

Words of Wisdom

When caring for patients who live at high altitudes, remember that their normal pulse oximetry reading may be lower than the normal values for individuals living at lower altitudes. When living at high altitude, the body adapts to the decreased pressure of oxygen, resulting in a lower normal Spo_2 reading. Your medical assessment must take this adaptation into account.

Pulse oximetry is considered a routine vital sign and can be used as part of any patient assessment. While there are no contraindications to using pulse oximetry, you must be aware of the limitations associated with this device. To function properly, the pulse oximeter must find a pulsation in the selected tissue. The most commonly used site is a finger. Follow the steps in **SKILL DRILL 11-1** to apply the pulse oximeter:

1. Clean the patient's finger. Place the index or middle finger into the pulse oximeter probe. Turn on the pulse oximeter and note the light-emitting diode (LED) reading of the Spo_2 (**Step 1**).
2. Palpate the radial pulse to ensure that it correlates with the LED display on the pulse oximeter (**Step 2**).

In patients with significant vasoconstriction or very low perfusion (including decompensated shock and cardiac arrest), there may not be enough peripheral perfusion to be detected by the pulse oximeter sensor. In these cases, move the sensor to a more central location (bridge of the nose or earlobe).[5]

Always consult the manufacturer's guidelines for proper placement and troubleshooting of these devices. An inaccurate pulse oximetry reading may be caused by the following:

- Hypovolemia
- Anemia (decreased level of circulating red blood cells and therefore hemoglobin)
- Severe peripheral vasoconstriction (chronic hypoxia, smoking, or hypothermia)
- Time delay in detecting respiratory insufficiency
- Possibly certain types of nail polish, such as gel nail polish, though research has suggested its effect is not clinically significant and may not justify removal in the prehospital setting[6,7]

Skill Drill 11-1 Applying the Pulse Oximeter

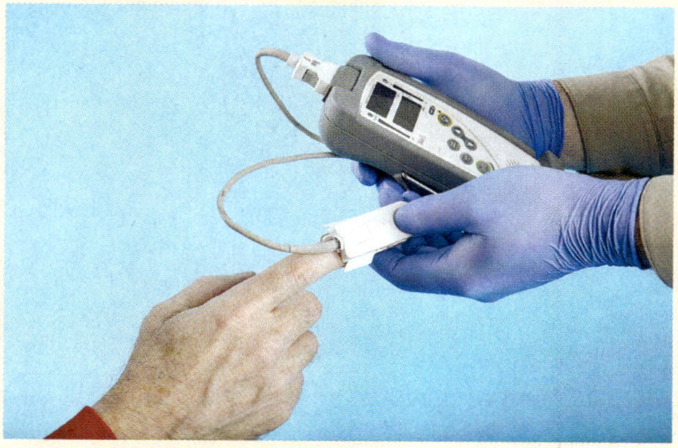

Step 1

Clean the patient's finger and place the index or middle finger into the pulse oximeter probe. Turn on the pulse oximeter and note the LED reading of the Spo_2.

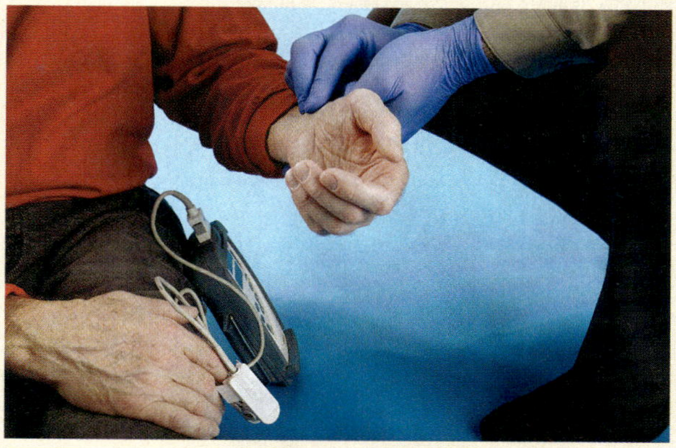

Step 2

Palpate the radial pulse to ensure that it correlates with the LED display on the pulse oximeter.

Special Populations

PULSE OXIMETRY IN NEWBORNS AND INFANTS

Accurate assessment of Spo_2 levels in newborns and infants requires a special flexible probe. The probe is placed on the hand of the newborn and on the palm, foot, or toe of an infant (**FIGURE 11-17**).

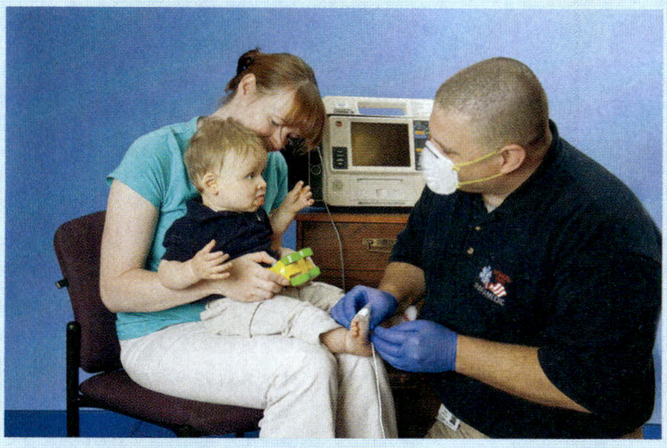

FIGURE 11-17 A pulse oximeter is applied to an infant's palm, foot, or toe.

- Dirty fingers
- Carbon monoxide poisoning

When carbon monoxide is present in the inspired gas, it displaces oxygen from the hemoglobin. Pulse oximetry measures hemoglobin saturation, but it is unable to distinguish between oxygen and carbon monoxide. Therefore, in cases of carbon monoxide poisoning, the Spo_2 reading can be normal in the context of hypoxia.

The pulse oximeter is a valuable adjunct to aid in decision making but is not a replacement for a complete assessment. Many factors may cause the pulse oximeter to give false high or low readings. When you are conducting a complete patient assessment, consider using pulse oximetry readings as one additional measure while obtaining all other comprehensive information you need. Assess the patient for signs and symptoms of adequate oxygenation. If a patient has signs such as cyanosis or pale or clammy skin, or symptoms such as shortness of breath, but a normal Spo_2, treat the patient's condition, not the device. Bear in mind that otherwise healthy patients may maintain a normal Spo_2 for several minutes, even in the face of acute respiratory compromise.

Special Populations

PULSE OXIMETRY IN PATIENTS WITH DARK SKIN

Research suggests that the amount of hemoglobin saturated with oxygen may be lower in Asian, Black, and Hispanic patients than the Spo_2 reading suggests.[8,9] As a result, even in children the EMS clinician may fail to recognize hypoxemia and decide oxygen is not needed.[10] It is vital for the EMT to remember that pulse oximetry is only one tool in the overall assessment of a patient.

Pulse oximetry cannot measure the effectiveness of ventilation or provide information about cellular metabolism. To assess ventilation, you will need to measure exhaled carbon dioxide levels. Carbon dioxide can be described as the "smoke" of metabolism. The body uses oxygen as its fuel and makes carbon dioxide as its by-product. As long as oxygen is delivered to the cells and tissues, carbon dioxide production continues. A helpful analogy is a motor vehicle engine. As long as gasoline continues to burn, exhaust is produced. In the human body, carbon dioxide is the exhaust.

End-tidal carbon dioxide ($ETCO_2$) is the measure of the maximal concentration of carbon dioxide at the end of an exhaled breath. A low carbon dioxide level could indicate several conditions. Patients who are hyperventilating are eliminating carbon dioxide faster than the body is making it; this would cause a low carbon dioxide level. A low carbon dioxide level could also indicate decreased carbon dioxide return to the lungs because of reduced carbon dioxide production at the cellular level secondary to conditions such as shock and cardiac arrest. When cardiac output increases, $ETCO_2$ levels generally increase, a reflection of improved oxygen delivery. By contrast, a carbon dioxide level that is higher than normal may indicate that the patient is retaining carbon dioxide secondary to ventilation inadequacy. An absence of carbon dioxide can indicate that the patient is not breathing at all.

$ETCO_2$ is measured by using capnometry and capnography devices. **Capnometry** refers to a device that provides a digital numeric reading of the $ETCO_2$ level (**FIGURE 11-18**). **Capnography** provides both a numeric reading and a graphic waveform of the $ETCO_2$ levels from breath to breath; specifically, this is called quantitative waveform capnography. The digital display of $ETCO_2$ is expressed in millimeters of mercury (mm Hg). The normal range is 35 to 45 mm Hg.

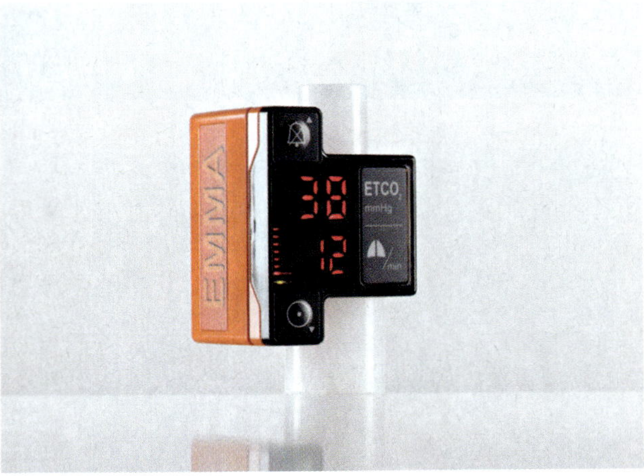

FIGURE 11-18 A capnometer.

Courtesy of Marianne Gausche-Hill, MD, FACEP, FAAP.

$ETCO_2$ monitoring is used as the primary, and most reliable, method to assess proper advanced airway placement. However, it has many clinical applications and is widely used to assess exhaled carbon dioxide in patients with respiratory, cardiac, or neurologic emergencies, as well as patients in shock. $ETCO_2$ monitoring is valuable to determine appropriate bag-mask ventilation as long as there is a tight mask seal and the patient has adequate perfusion.[11] Paramedic or other advanced life support (ALS) clinicians use these devices to determine proper placement of an advanced airway, assess a patient's ventilatory status, and avoid inadvertent hyperventilation of patients with head injuries, which has been linked to poor outcomes. Additionally, quantitative waveform capnography provides data that can be used to determine changes in cardiac output. It also provides the first indication of return of spontaneous circulation (ROSC) after cardiac arrest.

Quantitative waveform capnography can be monitored in spontaneously breathing patients with an adequate airway by applying a special nasal cannula device to the patient and connecting the sampling line to the cardiac monitor (**FIGURE 11-19**). If an advanced airway device is in place (ie, ET tube, supraglottic airway), an inline adapter is placed between the advanced airway device and the ventilation device. The sampling line is then connected to the cardiac monitor (**FIGURE 11-20**).

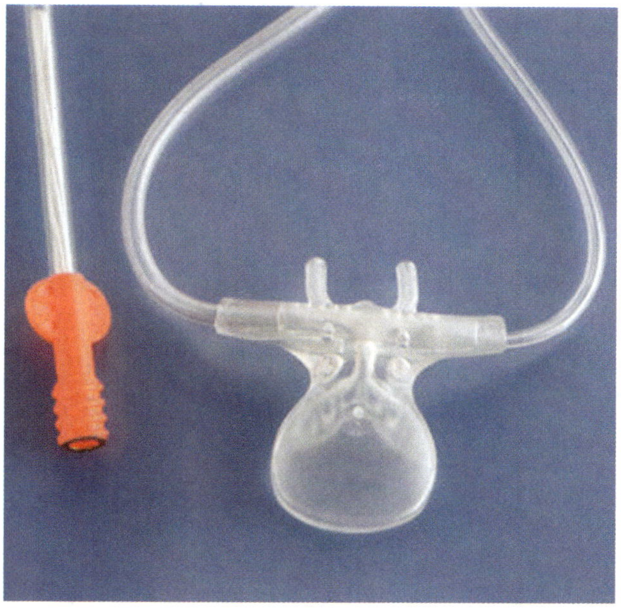

FIGURE 11-19 Nasal cannula device for monitoring end-tidal carbon dioxide in a spontaneously breathing patient.

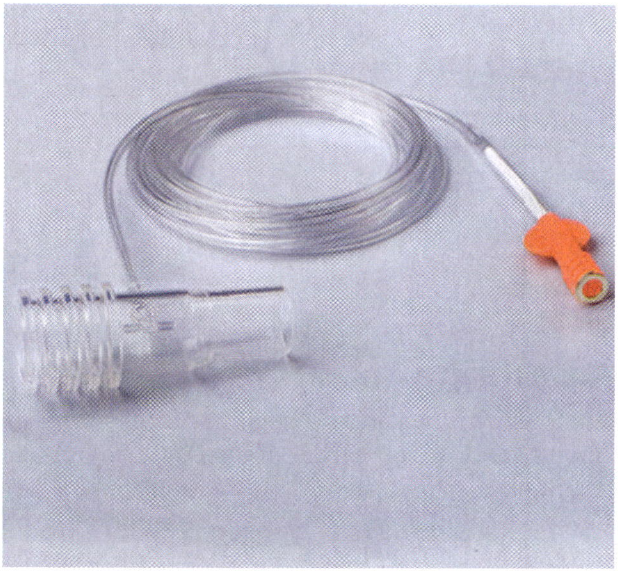

FIGURE 11-20 Inline end-tidal carbon dioxide device for use in the patient with an advanced airway in place.

A normal capnographic waveform has four distinct phases (**FIGURE 11-21**). Phase 1 (**A–B**), also known as the respiratory baseline, is the initial stage of exhalation; the gas sample is dead space gas, free of carbon dioxide (which explains why phase 1 is

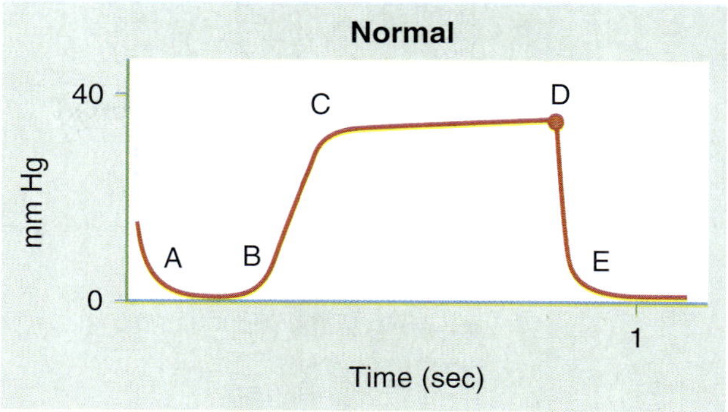

FIGURE 11-21 Normal capnographic waveform with points A through E shown.

flat). Phase 2 (**B–C**) is called the expiratory upslope. At point B, alveolar gas, which contains a high level of carbon dioxide, mixes with dead space gas, resulting in an abrupt rise in exhaled carbon dioxide (which explains why phase 2 abruptly rises from the baseline). The alveolar plateau is represented by phase 3 (**C–D**), and the gas sampled is all alveolar. Point D is the maximal $ETCO_2$ level, the best reflection of the alveolar carbon dioxide level. The height of the waveform at point D correlates with the numeric value of exhaled carbon dioxide that is displayed on the cardiac monitor. Phase 0 (**D–E**), called the inspiratory downstroke, occurs when the patient inhales and fresh gas is breathed into the lungs. During inhalation, carbon dioxide is displaced, causing the waveform to return to the baseline level of carbon dioxide, approximately 0 mm Hg. The duration (width) of each waveform corresponds to the duration of ventilation, and the space between waveforms corresponds to the patient's respiratory rate.

The EMT can recognize abnormalities in carbon dioxide levels by noting the height of the capnographic waveform. Patients who are hypoventilating, such as may be seen in cases of opioid overdose, are retaining too much carbon dioxide; therefore, one would expect a tall capnographic waveform (**FIGURE 11-22**). By contrast, if the patient is hyperventilating and eliminating too much carbon dioxide, or if carbon dioxide return to the lungs is decreased (ie, shock, cardiac arrest), the capnographic waveform would be correspondingly smaller (**FIGURE 11-23**). The absence of a capnographic waveform indicates that

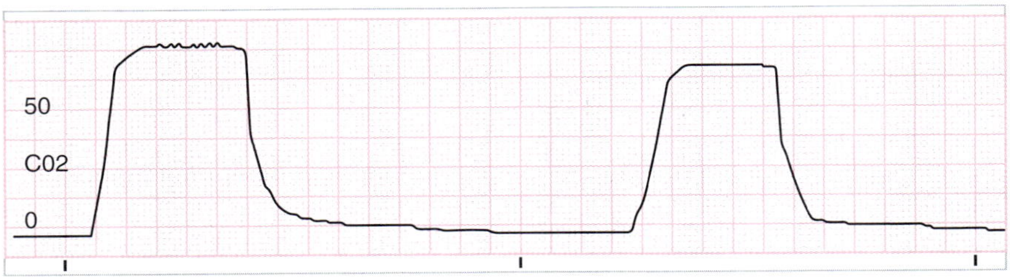

FIGURE 11-22 Capnographic waveform caused by hypoventilation.

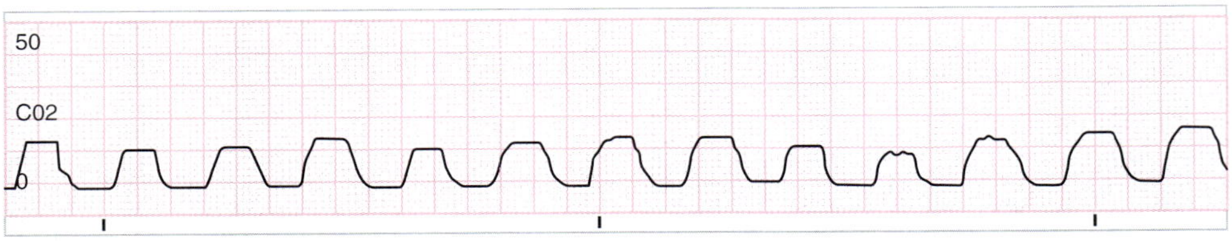

FIGURE 11-23 Capnographic waveform caused by hyperventilation, or reduced carbon dioxide return to the lungs.

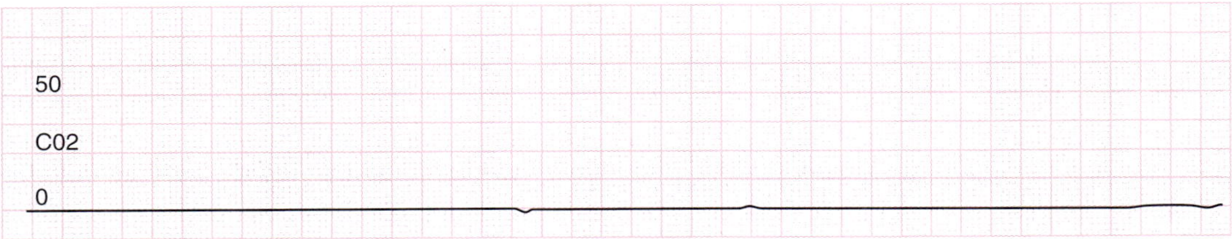

FIGURE 11-24 The absence of a capnographic waveform in the intubated patient indicates that the endotracheal tube is in the esophagus, not the trachea.

the sensor is not detecting any carbon dioxide. In a patient with an advanced airway device, such as an ET tube, this indicates that the ET tube is in the esophagus, which contains almost no carbon dioxide (**FIGURE 11-24**).

Street Smarts

Effective airway management is accomplished by a team, not an individual. Never leave a partner to struggle, attempting to establish a patent airway and adequate ventilation alone! When practicing airway skills (which should be frequently), practice as a team. Plan how you will manage the next airway problem before you receive the call. Remember, practice like you play.

Opening the Airway

Emergency medical care begins with ensuring an open airway. If you cannot immediately open and maintain a patent airway, you cannot ensure adequate oxygenation, ventilation, respiration, and ultimately, perfusion. Regardless of the patient's condition, the airway must remain patent at all times.

When you respond to a call and find an unconscious patient, you need to quickly assess for a pulse and breathing; this should be done simultaneously and within a few seconds. If the patient has a pulse, you need to determine whether breathing is adequate. Remember that airway and breathing are two separate components that are closely related to each other. However, you must understand that an adequate airway does not always equate to adequate breathing.

Airway and breathing assessment should occur in an unresponsive patient when they are in a supine position. However, if your patient is in a situation that delays placement in a supine position (eg, entrapped in a vehicle), the patient's airway must be opened and assessed in the position in which you find the patient. Patients found in the prone position (lying facedown) must be repositioned to allow for assessment of airway and breathing and to begin CPR, should it become necessary.

Currently, health care workers are taught to begin CPR with high-quality compressions if cardiac arrest is suspected. The patient should be log rolled as a unit so the head, neck, and spine all move together without twisting. Although care should be taken to avoid injury, remember that airway management almost always takes priority and should not be delayed when caring for patients with life-threatening conditions. Unconscious patients, especially when there are no witnesses who can rule out trauma, should be moved as a unit because of the potential for spinal injury. To position the unconscious patient to open the airway, follow the steps in **SKILL DRILL 11-2**:

1. Kneel beside the patient. Make sure you kneel far enough away so that the patient, when rolled toward you, does not come to rest in your lap. Place your hands behind the patient's head and neck to support the cervical spine as your partner straightens the patient's legs (**Step 1**).

Skill Drill 11-2 Positioning the Unconscious Patient

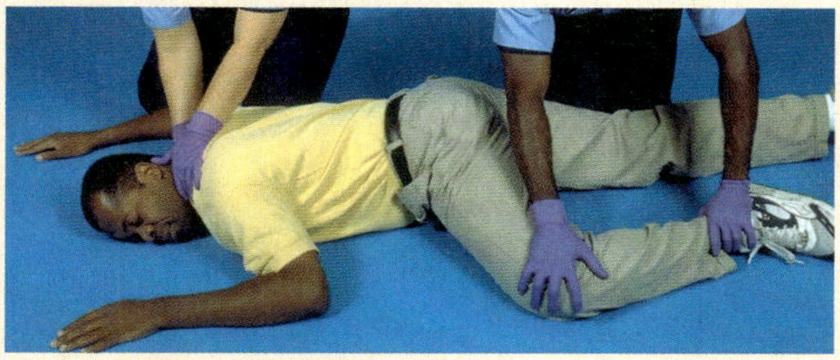

Step 1

Support the head while your partner straightens the patient's legs.

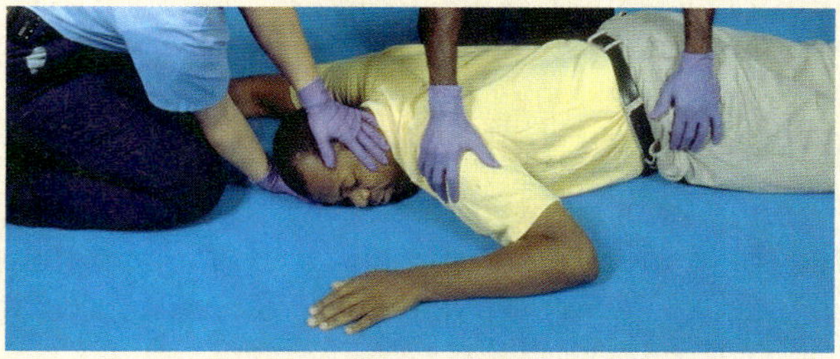

Step 2

Have your partner place a hand on the patient's far shoulder and hip.

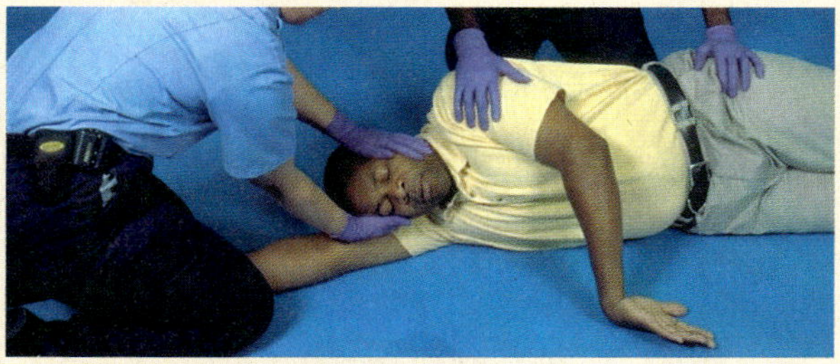

Step 3

Roll the patient as a unit with the EMT at the patient's head calling the count to begin the move.

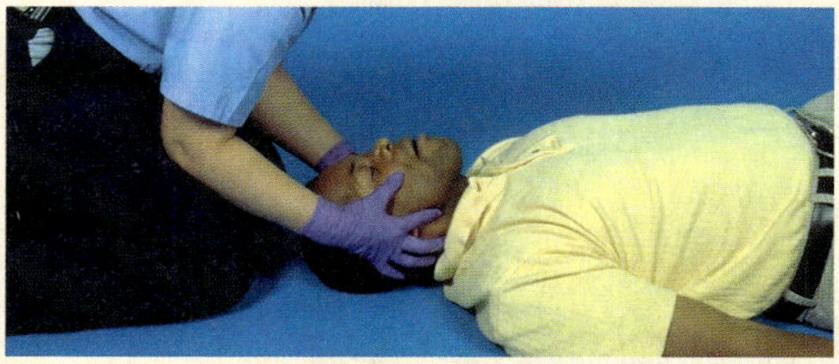

Step 4

Open and assess the patient's airway and breathing status.

2. Have your partner place their hands on the patient's far shoulder and hip (**Step 2**).
3. As you call the count to control movement, have your partner turn the patient toward you by pulling on the far shoulder and hip. Control the head and neck so that they move as a unit with the rest of the torso. In this way, the head and neck stay in the same vertical plane as the back. This single motion will minimize aggravation of any potential spine injury. Place the patient's arms at their side (**Step 3**).
4. Once the patient is positioned, maintain an open airway and check for breathing (**Step 4**).

In an unconscious patient, the most common airway obstruction is the patient's tongue, which falls back into the throat when the muscles of the throat and tongue relax (**FIGURE 11-25**). Dentures (false teeth), blood, vomitus, mucus, food, and other foreign objects may also compromise the airway. Therefore, always be prepared to help clear and maintain a patent airway with the use of suction and placement of an airway adjunct, such as an oropharyngeal or nasopharyngeal airway.

Head Tilt–Chin Lift Maneuver

Opening the airway to relieve an obstruction can often be done quickly and easily by simply tilting the patient's head back and lifting the chin in what is known as the **head tilt–chin lift maneuver**. For patients who have not sustained or are not suspected of having sustained spinal trauma, this simple maneuver is sometimes all that is needed for the patient to resume breathing.

To perform the head tilt–chin lift maneuver, follow these steps:

1. With the patient in a supine position, position yourself beside the patient's head.
2. Place the heel of one hand on the patient's forehead and apply firm backward pressure with your palm to tilt the patient's head back. This extension of the neck will move the tongue forward, away from the back of the throat, and clear the airway if the tongue is blocking it.
3. Place the fingertips of your other hand under the lower jaw near the bony part of the chin. Do not compress the soft tissue under the chin, as this may block the airway.
4. Lift the chin upward, bringing the entire lower jaw with it, helping to tilt the head back. Do not use your thumb to lift the chin. Lift so that the teeth are nearly brought together, but avoid closing the mouth completely. Continue to hold the forehead to maintain the backward tilt of the head (**FIGURE 11-26**).

Words of Wisdom

Causes of airway obstruction include the following:

- Relaxation of the tongue in an unresponsive patient
- Foreign objects (food, small toys, dentures)
- Blood clots, broken teeth, or damaged oral tissue following trauma
- Airway tissue swelling (infection, allergic reaction)
- Aspirated vomitus (stomach contents)

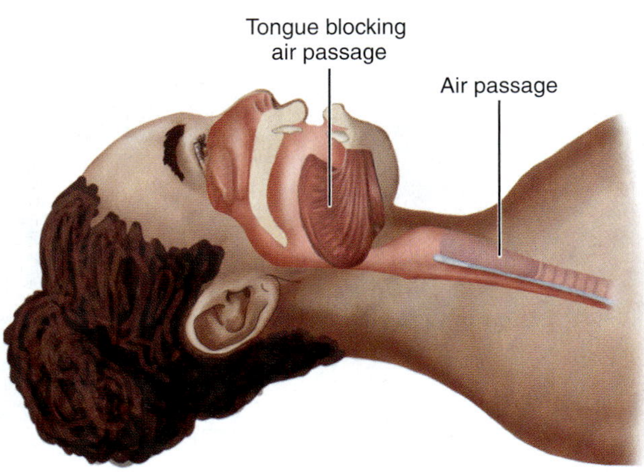

FIGURE 11-25 The most common airway obstruction is the patient's own tongue, which falls back into the throat when the muscles of the throat and tongue relax.

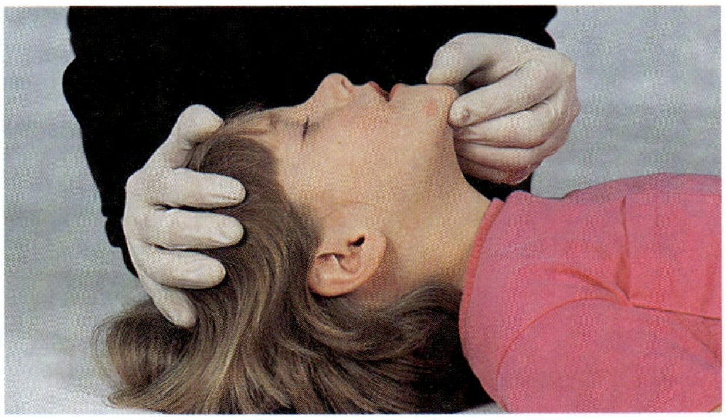

FIGURE 11-26 The head tilt–chin lift maneuver is a simple technique for opening the airway in a patient without a suspected cervical spine injury.

Jaw-Thrust Maneuver

The head tilt–chin lift maneuver will open the airway in most patients. However, if you suspect a cervical spine injury, use the jaw-thrust maneuver. The **jaw-thrust maneuver** is a technique to open the airway by placing the fingers behind the angle of the jaw and lifting the jaw upward. You can easily seal a mask around the mouth while doing the jaw-thrust maneuver. In fact, the jaw-thrust maneuver can be used in *any* patient, not just those with a suspected spinal injury. Refer to Chapter 28, *Head and Spine Injuries*, for a more detailed discussion of these types of injuries.

Perform the jaw-thrust maneuver using the following steps (**FIGURE 11-27**):

1. Kneel above the patient's head. Place your fingers behind the angles of the lower jaw, and move the jaw upward. Use your thumbs to help position the lower jaw to allow breathing through the mouth and nose.
2. The completed maneuver should open the airway with the mouth slightly open and the jaw jutting forward.

Patients who have a pulse may start to breathe on their own once the airway has been opened. Assess whether breathing has returned by quickly looking at the chest and observing for obvious movement (**FIGURE 11-28**).

Special Populations

AIRWAY MANAGEMENT IN PATIENTS WITH RHEUMATOID ARTHRITIS OR DOWN SYNDROME

Patients with a history of rheumatoid arthritis or Down syndrome are predisposed to instability of the cervical spine, specifically at the first and second cervical vertebrae. The head tilt–chin lift maneuver should be avoided on these patients. Excessive force or hyperextension of the neck can injure the cervical spine, which can potentially lead to paralysis. It is often better to open the airway of these patients using a jaw-thrust maneuver.

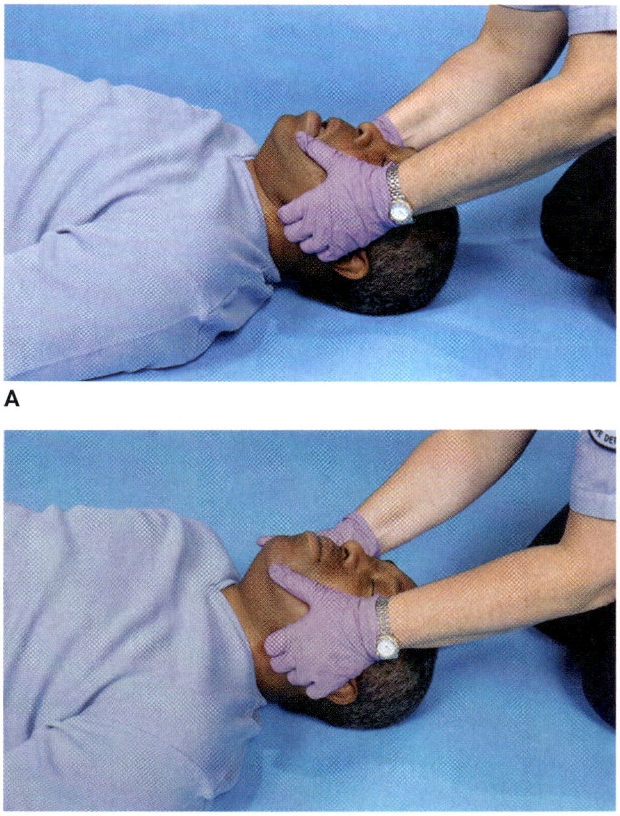

A

B

FIGURE 11-27 Performing the jaw-thrust maneuver. **A.** Kneeling above the patient's head, place your fingers behind the angles of the lower jaw, and move the jaw upward. Use your thumbs to help position the lower jaw. **B.** The completed maneuver should look like this.

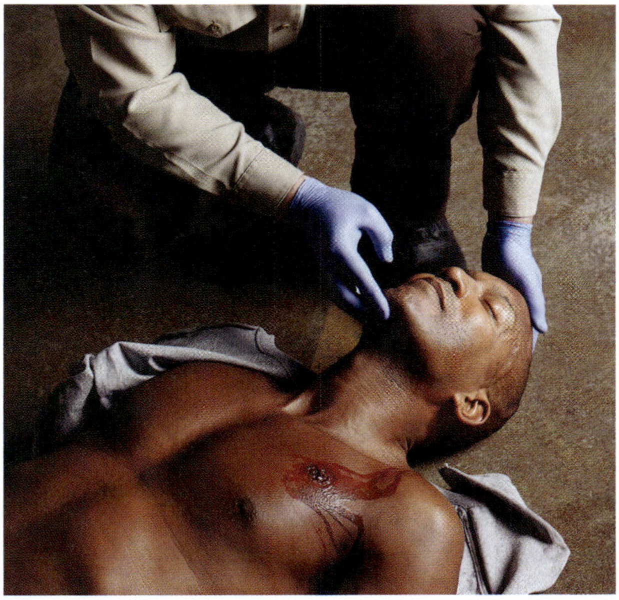

FIGURE 11-28 Looking at the chest and observing for obvious movement can be used to assess whether breathing has spontaneously returned.

With complete airway obstruction, there will be no movement of air. However, you may see the chest and abdomen rise and fall considerably with the patient's frantic attempts to breathe. This is why the presence of chest wall movement alone does not indicate if adequate breathing is present. Regular chest wall movement indicates a respiratory effort is present. Observing chest and abdominal movement is often difficult with a fully clothed patient. You may see little, if any, chest movement, even with normal breathing. This is particularly true in some patients with chronic lung disease if you discover that there is no movement of air.

Opening the Mouth

Even though you may have opened the airway with a head tilt–chin lift or jaw-thrust maneuver, the patient's mouth may still be closed. To open the mouth, place the tips of your index finger and thumb on the patient's teeth. Then, open the mouth by pushing your thumb on the lower teeth and index finger on the upper teeth. This pushing motion will cause the index finger and thumb to cross over each other, which is why this is called the cross-finger technique.

Suctioning

You must keep the airway clear so that you can ventilate the patient properly. If the airway is not clear, you will force the fluids and secretions into the lungs, resulting in aspiration. If aspiration occurs, mortality increases significantly. Therefore, suctioning is your next priority. If you have any doubt about the situation, remember this rule: If you hear gurgling, the patient needs suctioning!

Suctioning Equipment

Portable, hand-operated, and fixed (mounted) suctioning equipment is essential for resuscitation (**FIGURE 11-29**).

A portable suctioning unit must generate enough vacuum pressure to allow you to suction the mouth and nose effectively. Hand-operated suctioning units with disposable chambers are reliable, effective, and relatively inexpensive. A fixed suctioning unit should generate a vacuum of more than 300 mm Hg when the tubing is clamped.

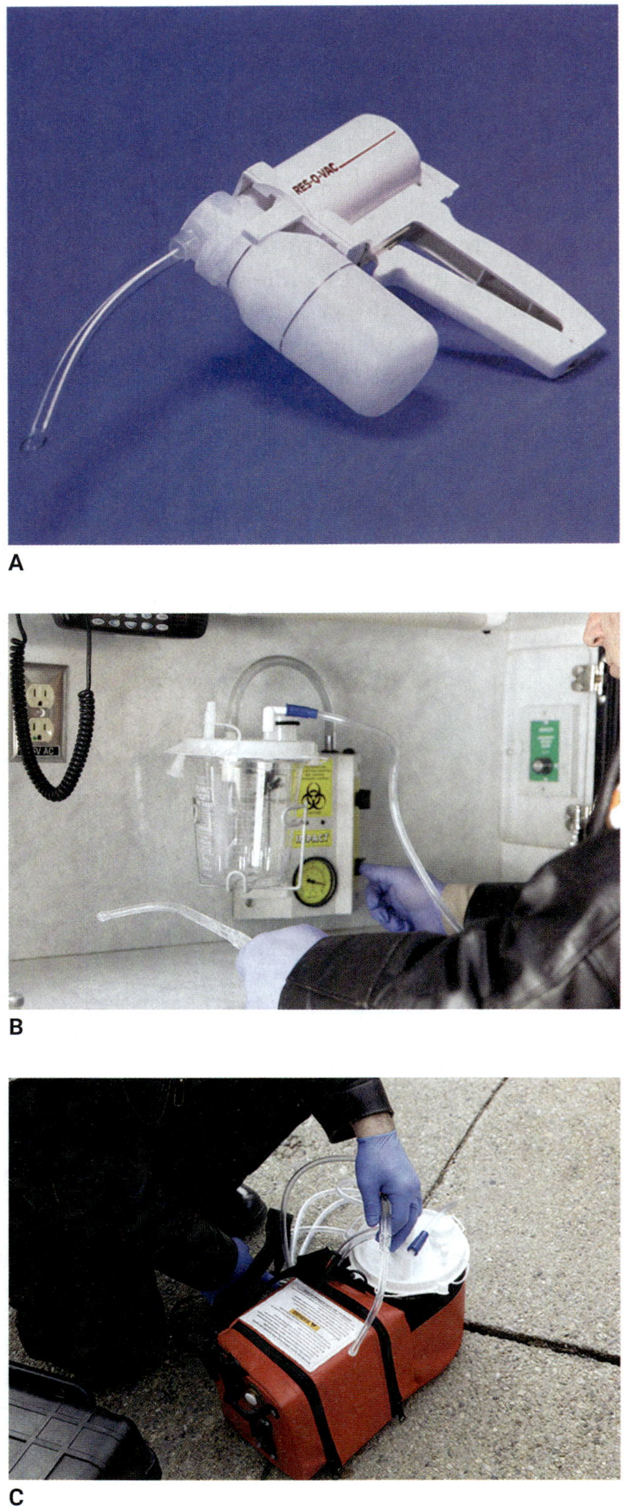

FIGURE 11-29 Suctioning equipment is essential for resuscitation. **A.** Hand-operated unit. **B.** Fixed unit. **C.** Portable unit.

A portable or fixed suctioning unit should be fitted with the following:

- Wide-bore, thick-walled, nonkinking tubing
- Plastic, rigid pharyngeal suction tips, called **tonsil tips** (Yankauer tips or DuCanto catheter)
- Nonrigid plastic catheters, called French or whistle-tip catheters
- A nonbreakable, disposable collection bottle
- Water for rinsing the tips

A **suction catheter** is a hollow, cylindrical device that is used to remove fluids from the patient's airway. The Yankauer tonsil-tip catheter, while rigid and noncollapsible, has a small bore at the end and is therefore more useful for removing thin secretions. Another type of suction catheter, the DuCanto catheter, is designed for routine and emergency airway management. It has a larger distal bore capable of removing copious thick secretions, large debris, or clotted blood (**FIGURE 11-30**).

Tips with a curved contour allow for easy, rapid placement in the oropharynx. Nonrigid plastic catheters, sometimes called French or whistle-tip catheters, are used to suction the nose and thin secretions in the back of the mouth and in situations in which you cannot use a rigid catheter, such as for a patient with a **stoma** (**FIGURE 11-31**). A stoma is an opening through the skin that goes into an organ or other structure.

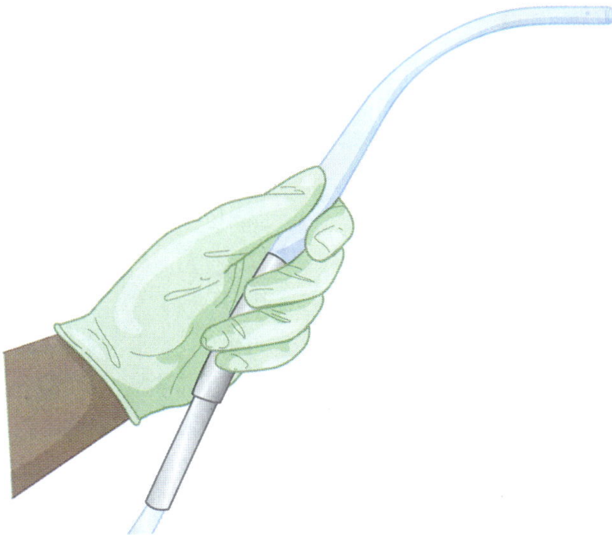

FIGURE 11-30 A large-bore suction catheter used for routine and emergency airway management.

For example, a rigid catheter could break off a patient's tooth, whereas a flexible catheter may be inserted along the cheeks without injury. Before you insert any catheter, make sure to measure for the proper size. Use the same technique you would use when measuring for an oropharyngeal airway. Be careful not to touch the back of the airway with a suction catheter. This can stimulate the gag reflex, causing vomiting, and increase the possibility of aspiration. Aggressive suctioning can also stimulate the vagus nerve and cause bradycardia, especially in infants and small children.

Words of Wisdom

Any time there are fluids in the airway, the risk of aspiration increases. Aspiration significantly increases mortality.

Techniques of Suctioning

Inspect your suctioning equipment regularly to make sure it is in proper working condition. Turn on the suction, clamp the tubing, and make sure the unit generates a vacuum of more than 300 mm Hg. Check that a battery-charged unit has charged batteries. Ensure that your suctioning equipment is placed at the patient's head and is easily accessible.

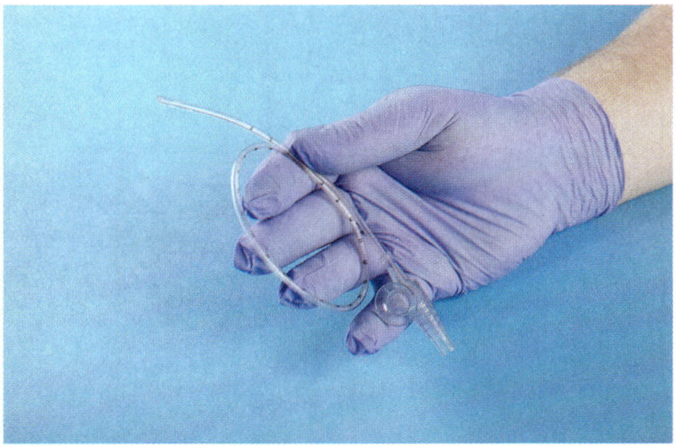

FIGURE 11-31 French, or whistle-tip, catheters are used in situations in which rigid catheters cannot be used, such as for a patient who has a stoma, for patients whose teeth are clenched, or if suctioning the nose is necessary.

Generally suction must create a vacuum force of 80 to 120 mm Hg to clear secretions. When suctioning infants and children, the suction should be regulated to have adequate force to clear secretions while minimizing trauma to the tissues.[3]

Because mortality increases significantly if a patient aspirates, it is important to suction the airway until it is clear of liquids or other debris. Ventilating a patient whose airway is full of blood, vomitus, or other secretions virtually guarantees aspiration. Repeat suctioning as needed to keep the airway clear, ensuring that the patient remains adequately ventilated and oxygenated. Consider limiting each suctioning attempt to 10 seconds. Between suction attempts, rinse the catheter and tubing with water to prevent clogging of the tube with dried vomitus or other secretions.

Use extreme caution when suctioning a conscious or semiconscious patient. Put the tip of the suction catheter in only as far as you can visualize. Be aware that suctioning may induce vomiting.

To properly suction a patient, follow the steps in **SKILL DRILL 11-3**:

1. Turn on the assembled suction unit. To test the suction, clamp the tubing, and make sure the unit generates a vacuum of more than 300 mm Hg (**Step 1**).
2. Measure the catheter to the correct depth by measuring the catheter from the corner of the patient's mouth to the earlobe or angle of the jaw (**Step 2**).
3. Before applying suction, turn the patient's head to the side (unless you suspect cervical spine injury) or log roll the patient onto the side if needed. Open the patient's mouth using the cross-finger technique or tongue-jaw lift, and insert the tip of the catheter to the depth measured. Do not suction while inserting the catheter (**Step 3**).
4. Insert the catheter to the premeasured depth and apply suction in a circular motion as you withdraw the catheter (**Step 4**).

Skill Drill 11-3 Suctioning a Patient's Airway

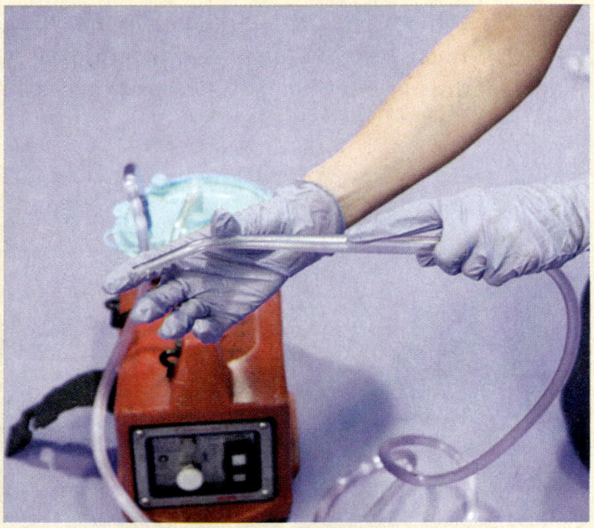

Step 1

Make sure the suctioning unit is properly assembled and turn it on. Clamp the tubing, and make sure the unit generates a vacuum of more than 300 mm Hg.

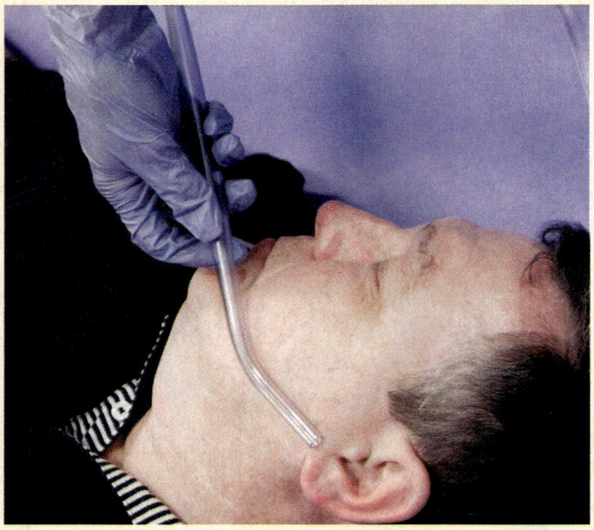

Step 2

Measure the catheter from the corner of the mouth to the earlobe or angle of the jaw.

Skill Drill 11-3 Suctioning a Patient's Airway continued

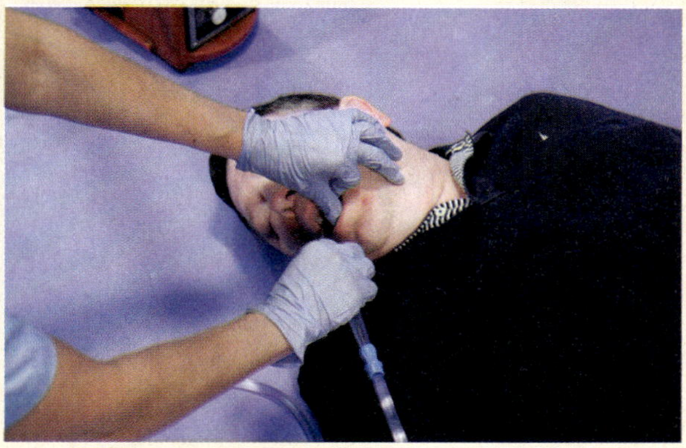

Step 3

Turn the patient's head to the side (unless you suspect cervical spine injury) or log roll the patient onto the side if needed, open the mouth using the cross-finger technique or tongue-jaw lift, and insert the catheter to the predetermined depth without suctioning.

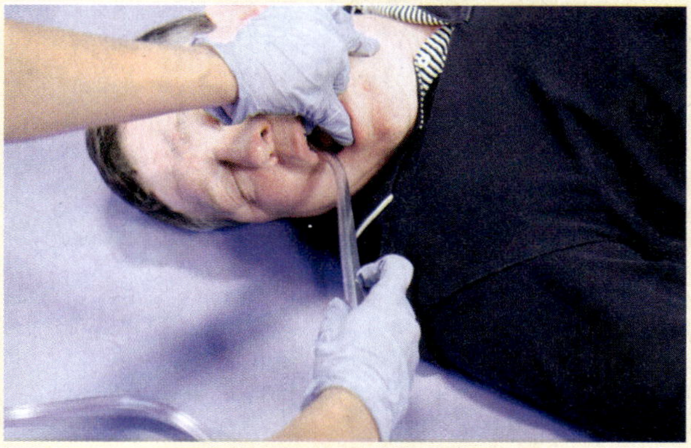

Step 4

Apply suction in a circular motion as you withdraw the catheter.

At times, a patient may have secretions or vomitus that cannot be suctioned quickly and easily, and some suction units cannot effectively remove solid objects such as teeth, foreign bodies, and food. In these cases, you should remove the catheter from the patient's mouth, log roll the patient to the side, and then clear the mouth carefully with your gloved finger. Only attempt to remove an object if it is visible during examination of the open mouth; blind sweeps of the back of the oropharynx may push an object farther down in the airway, making the obstruction worse. A patient who requires assisted ventilations may also produce secretions as quickly as you can suction them from the airway. In this situation, alternate suctioning with ventilations, ensuring that the airway remains as clear of secretions as possible. Do not continuously ventilate a patient if vomitus or other debris are present in the airway.

Clean and decontaminate your suctioning equipment after each use according to the manufacturer's guidelines. Place all disposable components (eg, catheter, suction tubing) in a biohazard bag.

Basic Airway Adjuncts

The primary function of an airway adjunct is to prevent obstruction of the upper airway by the tongue and allow the passage of air and oxygen to the lungs.

Oropharyngeal Airways

An **oropharyngeal airway** has two principal purposes. The first is to lift the tongue away from the posterior pharynx, thus creating a path for airflow. The second is to make it easier to suction the oropharynx if necessary. Suctioning is possible through an opening down the center or along either side of the oropharyngeal airway (**FIGURE 11-32**).

Indications for the oropharyngeal airway include the following:

- Unresponsive patients without a gag reflex (breathing or apneic)
- Any apneic patient being ventilated with a bag-mask device

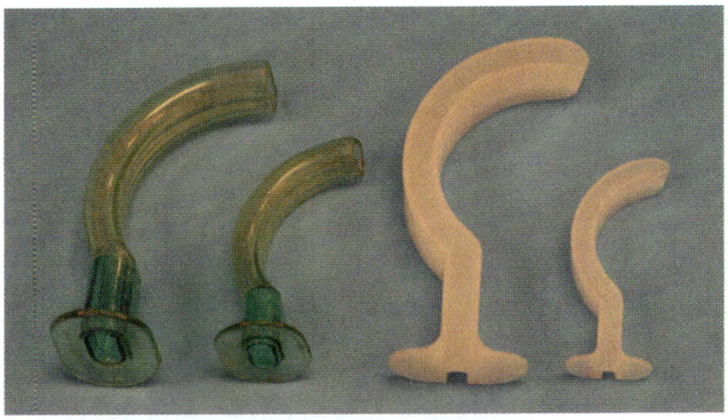

FIGURE 11-32 An oropharyngeal airway is used for unconscious patients who have no gag reflex. It lifts the tongue away from the posterior pharynx, thus creating a path for airflow, and makes suctioning the airway easier.

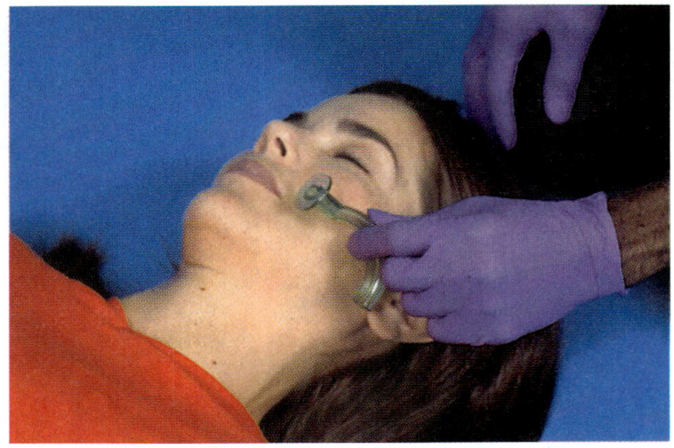

FIGURE 11-33 To select the proper size of oropharyngeal airway, measure from the patient's earlobe or angle of the jaw to the corner of the mouth.

Contraindications for the oropharyngeal airway include the following:

- Conscious patients
- Any patient (conscious or unconscious) who has an intact gag reflex

The **gag reflex** is a protective reflex mechanism that prevents food and other particles from entering the airway. If you try to insert an oropharyngeal airway in a patient with an intact gag reflex, the result may be vomiting or a spasm of the vocal cords (laryngospasm). If the patient gags while you are attempting to insert an oropharyngeal airway, immediately remove the adjunct and prepare to log roll the patient and suction the oropharynx, should vomiting occur. An oropharyngeal airway is also a safe, effective way to help maintain the airway of a patient with a possible spinal injury. The use of an oropharyngeal airway may make manual airway maneuvers such as the head tilt–chin lift and the jaw thrust easier to maintain; however, manual maneuvers are often still needed to ensure that the airway remains open.

You must clearly understand when and how this device is used. If the oropharyngeal airway is too large, it could push the tongue back into the pharynx, blocking the airway. Conversely, an oropharyngeal airway that is too small could block the airway directly, just like any foreign body obstruction. The process of selecting the proper size is shown in **FIGURE 11-33**. The following steps should be used when inserting an oropharyngeal airway (**SKILL DRILL 11-4**):

1. Holding the oropharyngeal airway in one hand, use a tongue depressor or bite stick to depress the tongue, ensuring the tongue remains forward (**Step 1**).
2. Insert the oropharyngeal airway sideways from the corner of the mouth, until the flange reaches the teeth (**Step 2**).
3. Rotate the oropharyngeal airway 90°, removing the depressor or bite stick as you exert gentle backward pressure on the oropharyngeal airway until it rests securely in place against the lips and teeth (**Step 3**).

In some cases, a patient may become responsive and regain the gag reflex after you have inserted an oropharyngeal airway. If this occurs, gently remove the airway by pulling it out, following the normal curvature of the mouth and throat. Be prepared for the patient to vomit. Have suction available, and

Special Populations

OROPHARYNGEAL AIRWAY INSERTION IN CHILDREN

In children, the only acceptable method of inserting an oropharyngeal airway is to use a tongue blade to hold the tongue down while inserting the airway. Because the airways of children are undeveloped, rotating an oropharyngeal airway in the posterior pharynx may cause damage.

Skill Drill 11-4 Inserting an Oropharyngeal Airway With a 90° Rotation

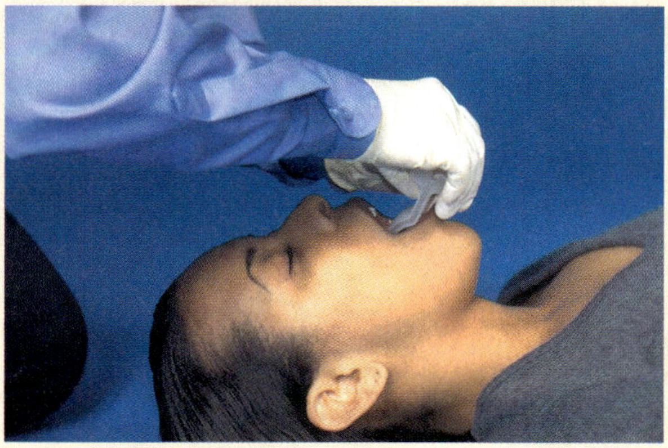

Step 1

Depress the tongue so that it remains forward.

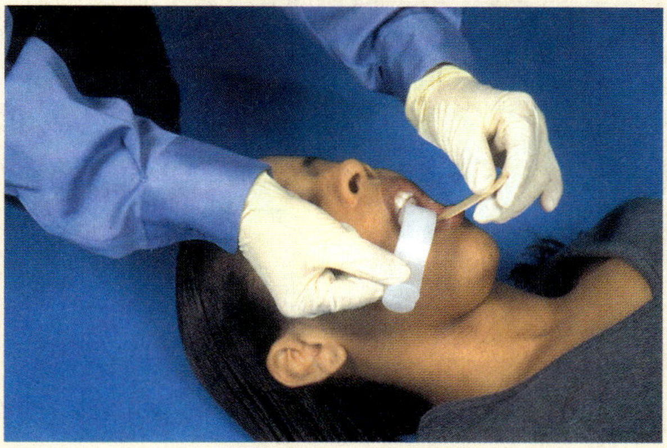

Step 2

Insert the oropharyngeal airway sideways from the corner of the mouth, until the flange reaches the teeth.

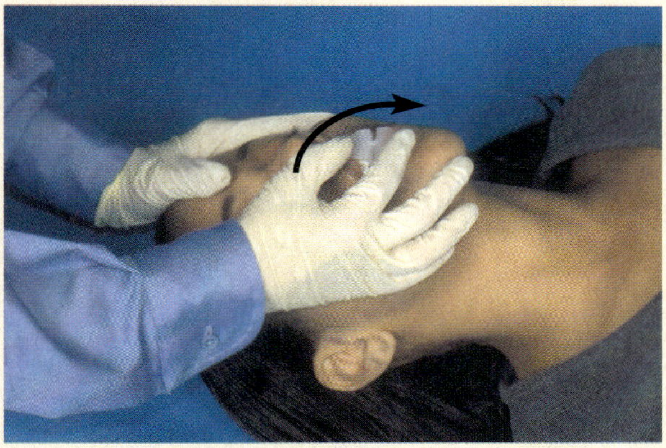

Step 3

Rotate the oropharyngeal airway 90°. Remove the bite stick as you exert gentle backward pressure on the oropharyngeal airway until it rests securely in place against the lips and teeth.

log roll the patient onto the side and allow any fluids to drain out.

An alternative approach to oropharyngeal insertion uses a 180° rotation rather than the 90° rotation described in Skill Drill 11-4. Note, however, that EMS agencies are moving away from this approach because it poses a risk of injury to the hard and soft palates. Insertion with a 180° rotation involves the following steps (**SKILL DRILL 11-5**):

1. Holding the oropharyngeal airway in one hand, open the patient's mouth with the other hand by using the cross-finger technique. Hold the airway upside down and insert it with the tip facing the roof of the mouth (**Step 1**).
2. Rotate the airway 180°. When inserted properly, the airway will rest in the mouth with the curvature of the airway following the contour of the anatomy. The flange should rest against the lips or teeth, with the other end opening into the pharynx (**Step 2**).

Take care to avoid injuring the hard palate (roof of the mouth) as you insert the airway. Roughness

Skill Drill 11-5 Inserting an Oropharyngeal Airway With a 180° Rotation

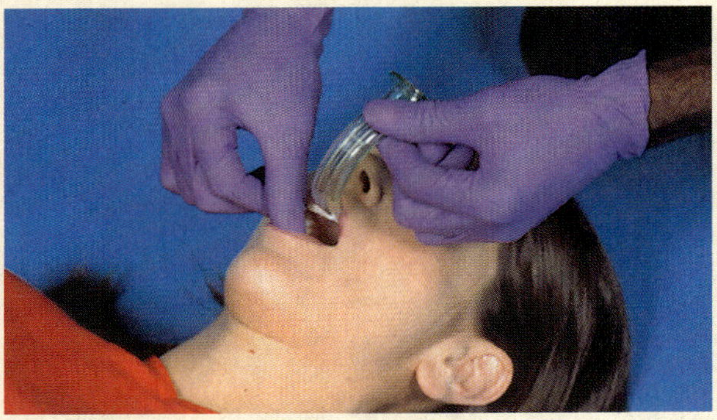

Step 1

Open the patient's mouth with the cross-finger technique. Hold the airway upside down and insert it with the tip facing the roof of the mouth.

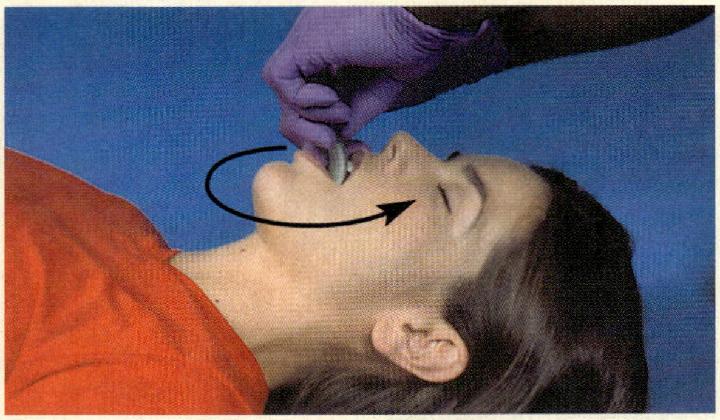

Step 2

Rotate the airway 180°. Insert the airway until the flange rests on the patient's lips and teeth. In this position, the airway will hold the tongue forward.

can cause bleeding that may aggravate airway problems or even cause vomiting.

Nasopharyngeal Airways

A **nasopharyngeal airway** is usually used with an unresponsive patient or a patient with an altered level of consciousness who has an intact gag reflex and is not able to maintain the airway spontaneously (**FIGURE 11-34**).

Special Populations

AIRWAY MANAGEMENT IN OLDER ADULTS

When you are managing the airway of an older patient, be aware of the presence of dentures or other dental appliances. If dentures are tight-fitting and allow for effective airway management, leave them in place. However, if the dentures are loose, remove them to avoid potential airway obstruction.

Patients with an altered mental status or who have just had a seizure may also benefit from a nasopharyngeal airway. If a patient has sustained severe trauma to the head or face, use of a nasopharyngeal airway should be avoided. If the nasopharyngeal airway is accidentally pushed through a hole caused by a fracture of the base of the skull, it may enter the cranial vault. Although this is rare, it is possible.

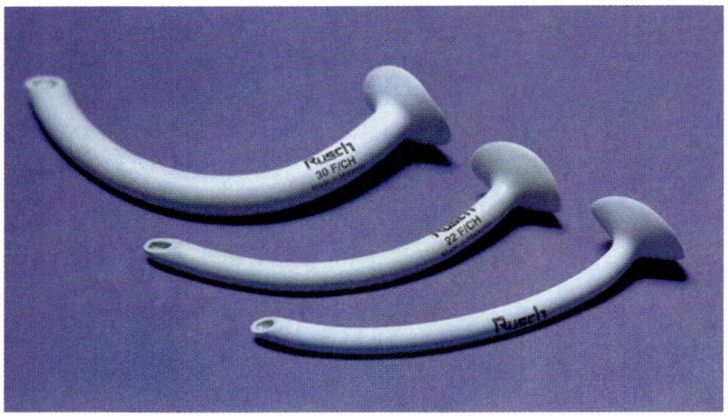

FIGURE 11-34 A nasopharyngeal airway is better tolerated than an oropharyngeal airway by patients who have an intact gag reflex.

This type of airway is usually better tolerated than an oropharyngeal airway by patients who have an intact gag reflex. It is not as likely to cause vomiting. Coat the airway well with a water-soluble lubricant before inserting it. Be aware that slight bleeding may occur even when the airway is inserted properly. However, never force the airway into place.

Indications for the nasopharyngeal airway include the following:

- Semiconscious or unconscious patients with an intact gag reflex
- Patients who otherwise will not tolerate an oropharyngeal airway

Contraindications for the nasopharyngeal airway include the following:

- Severe head injury with blood draining from the nose
- Nasal bone fracture

Follow these steps to ensure correct placement of the nasopharyngeal airway (**SKILL DRILL 11-6**):

1. Before inserting the airway, be sure you have selected the proper size. Measure from the tip of the patient's nose to the earlobe. Coat the tip with a water-soluble lubricant (**Step 1**).
2. In almost all patients, one nostril is larger than the other, typically the right nare. The airway should be placed in the larger nostril, with the curvature of the device following the curve of the floor of the nose. If using the right nare, the bevel should face the septum (**Step 2**). If using the left nare, insert the airway with the tip of the airway pointing upward, which will allow the bevel to face the septum.
3. Advance the airway gently (**Step 3**). If using the left nare, insert the nasopharyngeal airway until resistance is met. Then rotate the nasopharyngeal airway 180° into position. This rotation is not required if using the right nare.
4. When completely inserted, the flange rests against the nostril. The other end of the airway opens into the posterior pharynx and depresses the soft palate away from the tongue (**Step 4**). If the patient becomes intolerant of

Skill Drill 11-6 Inserting a Nasopharyngeal Airway

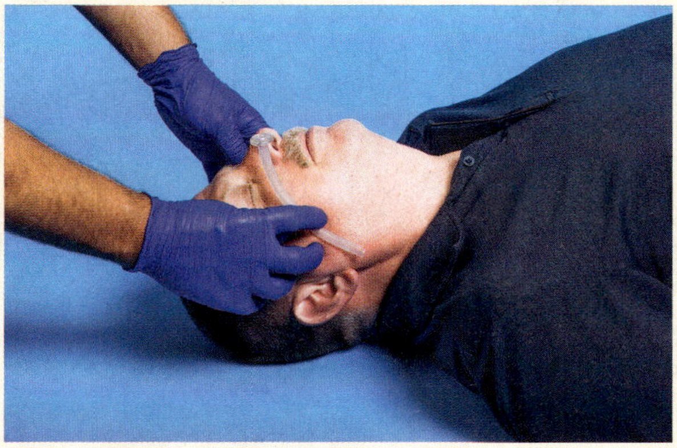

Step 1

Size the airway by measuring from the tip of the nose to the patient's earlobe. Coat the tip with a water-soluble lubricant.

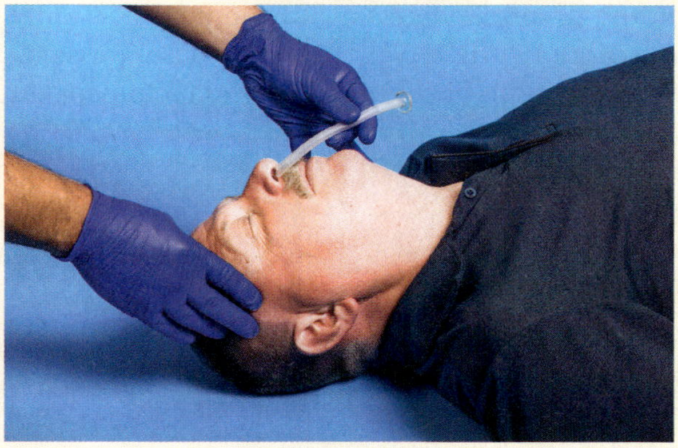

Step 2

Insert the lubricated airway into the larger nostril with the curvature following the floor of the nose. If using the right nare, the bevel should face the septum. If using the left nare, insert the airway with the tip of the airway pointing upward, which will allow the bevel to face the septum.

(continues)

Skill Drill 11-6 Inserting a Nasopharyngeal Airway continued

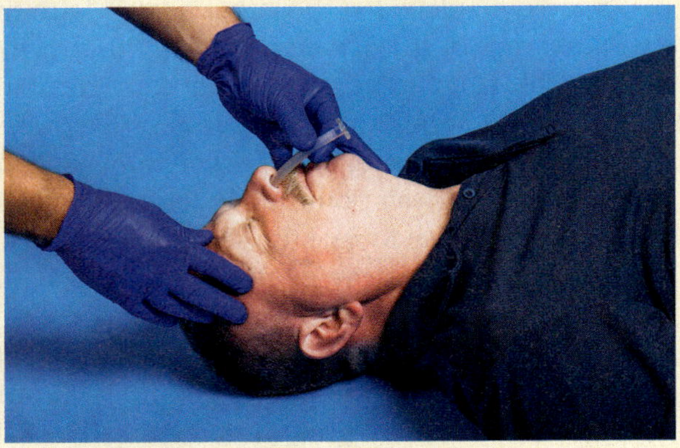

Step 3

Gently advance the airway. If using the left nare, insert the nasopharyngeal airway until resistance is met. Then rotate the nasopharyngeal airway 180° into position. This rotation is not required if using the right nostril.

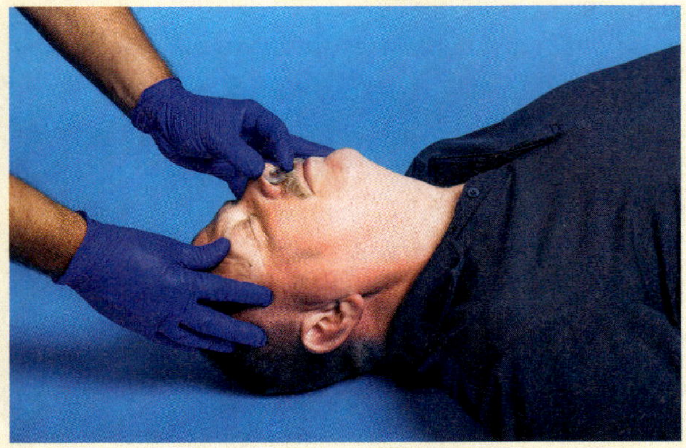

Step 4

Continue until the flange rests against the nostril. If you feel any resistance or obstruction, remove the airway and insert it into the other nostril.

the nasopharyngeal airway, remove it. Gently withdraw the airway from the nasal passage. Precautions like those used when removing an oropharyngeal airway should be followed.

Words of Wisdom

The patient's airway should be reassessed after insertion of any airway device, including oropharyngeal and nasopharyngeal airways. Reassessment ensures that the device has not inadvertently been misplaced or obstructed the airway and that the airway is now patent.

Maintaining the Airway

The **recovery position** is used to help maintain a clear airway in an unconscious patient who is not injured and is breathing on their own with a normal respiratory rate and adequate tidal volume (depth of breathing) (**FIGURE 11-35**).

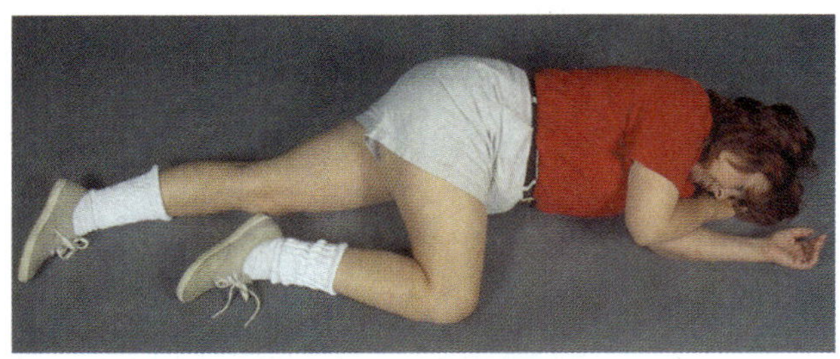

FIGURE 11-35 In the recovery position, the patient is rolled onto the left or right side.

Take the following steps to put the patient in the recovery position:

1. Roll the patient onto either side so that the head, shoulders, and torso move at the same time without twisting.
2. Extend the patient's lower arm and place the upper hand under the cheek.

For patients who have resumed spontaneous breathing after being resuscitated, the recovery position will prevent the aspiration of vomitus. However, this position is not appropriate for patients with suspected spinal, hip, or pelvic injuries or for patients who are unconscious and require ventilatory assistance. Reposition such patients to provide adequate access to the airway while maintaining appropriate spinal stabilization.

Supplemental Oxygen

Supplemental oxygen is indicated for patients who are hypoxemic (Spo_2 level <94%) because there is not enough oxygen in the blood to adequately supply the tissues and cells of the body. Deliver supplemental oxygen in a concentration sufficient to maintain an Spo_2 level between 94% and 98%. Some tissues and organs, such as the heart, central nervous system, lungs, kidneys, and liver, need a constant supply of oxygen to function normally. *Never withhold oxygen from any patient who might benefit from it, especially if you must assist ventilations.* When ventilating any patient in cardiac or respiratory arrest, use high-concentration supplemental oxygen.

Supplemental Oxygen Equipment

In addition to knowing when and how to give supplemental oxygen, you must understand how oxygen is stored and the various hazards associated with its use.

Oxygen Cylinders

The oxygen that you will give to patients is usually supplied as a compressed gas in green, seamless, steel or aluminum cylinders. Some cylinders may be silver or chrome with a green area around the valve stem on top. Newer cylinders are often made of lightweight aluminum or spun steel; older cylinders are much heavier.

Check to make sure the cylinder is labeled for *medical oxygen.* Look for letters and numbers stamped into the metal on the collar of the cylinder (**FIGURE 11-36**). The month and year stamps are particularly important because they indicate when the cylinder was last tested. Generally, aluminum cylinders are tested every 5 years; composite cylinders are tested every 3 years.

Oxygen cylinders are available in several sizes. The two sizes that you will most often use are the D (or jumbo D) and M cylinders (**FIGURE 11-37**). The D (or jumbo D) cylinder can be carried from your unit to the patient. The M cylinder remains on board your unit as a main supply tank. Other sizes that you may see are A, E, G, H, and K (**TABLE 11-4**). Another naming system for identifying the size of the oxygen cylinder has been introduced. Per this naming convention, cylinders are labeled with M (for medical), followed by a number.

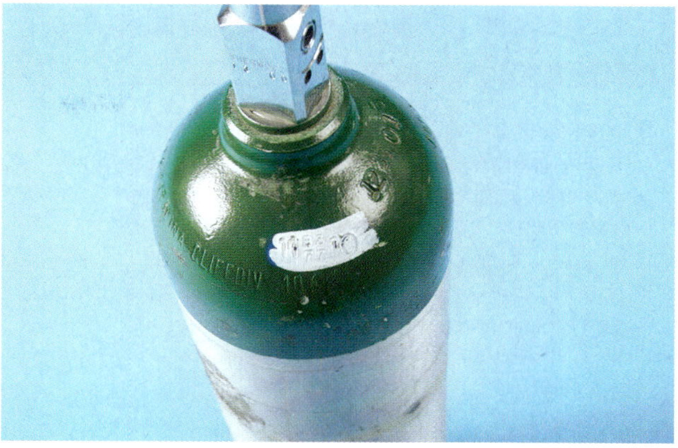

FIGURE 11-36 Oxygen tanks for medical use have a series of letters and numbers stamped into the metal on the collar of the cylinder.

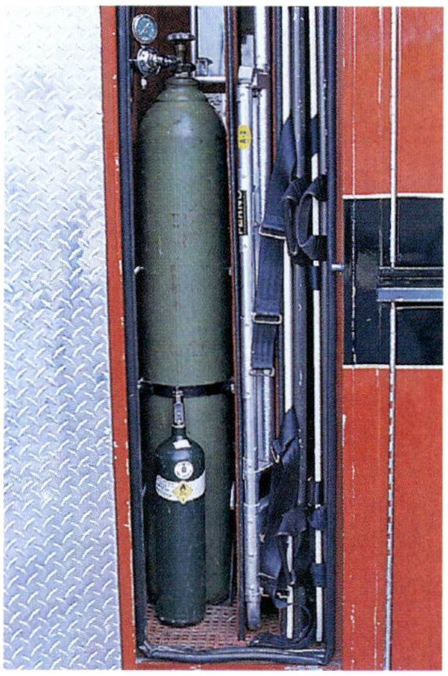

FIGURE 11-37 The cylinders that are most commonly found on an ambulance are the D (or jumbo D) and M size cylinders. D, jumbo D, and E sizes are typically portable tank systems while the M, G, H, A, and K sizes are mounted inside the ambulance.

Words of Wisdom

Some patients require oxygen continuously. Many of these patients have liquid oxygen at home. Liquid oxygen containers hold a large volume of oxygen and do not need to be filled as often, depending on the flow rate. Liquid oxygen tanks generally need to be kept upright and have special requirements for filling, large-volume storage, and cylinder transfer.

The length of time you can use an oxygen cylinder depends on the pressure in the cylinder and the oxygen flow rate. A method of calculating cylinder duration is shown in **TABLE 11-5**.

TABLE 11-4 Oxygen Cylinder Sizes Carried on the Ambulance

Size	Volume, Liters
D	350
Jumbo D	500
E	625
M (MM)	3,000
G	5,300
H, A (M4), K	6,900

Words of Wisdom

If you are preparing to transfer a patient who is on oxygen a long distance, it is important to calculate cylinder duration before leaving the hospital to ensure there will be sufficient oxygen for the entire trip. Electronic oxygen tank duration calculators are available online.

Safety Considerations

Handle compressed gas cylinders carefully because their contents are under pressure. Cylinders are fitted with pressure regulators to make sure patients receive the right amount and type of gas. Make sure the correct pressure regulator is firmly attached before you transport the cylinders. A puncture or hole in the tank can cause the cylinder to become a deadly missile. Do not handle a cylinder by the neck assembly alone. Secure cylinders with mounting brackets when they are stored on the ambulance. Oxygen cylinders that are in use during transport should be positioned and secured to prevent the tank from falling, damaging the valve-gauge assembly, or becoming a dangerous projectile during a collision.

Pin-Indexing System

The compressed gas industry has established a **pin-indexing system** for portable cylinders to prevent an oxygen regulator from being connected to a carbon dioxide cylinder, a carbon dioxide regulator

TABLE 11-5 Oxygen Cylinders: Duration of Flow

Formula

$$\frac{(\text{Gauge pressure in psi} - \text{Safe residual pressure}) \times \text{Cylinder constant}}{\text{Flow rate in L/min}} \times \text{Duration of flow in minutes}$$

Safe residual pressure = 200 psi

Cylinder constant for a given cylinder size:
A = 3.14 G = 2.41 D = 0.16 H = 3.14 E = 0.28 K = 3.14 M = 1.56

Determine the life of an M cylinder that has a pressure of 2,000 psi and a flow rate of 10 L/min.

$$\frac{(2{,}000 - 200) \times 1.56}{10} = \frac{2{,}808}{10} = 281 \text{ min, or 4 h 41 min}$$

psi = pounds per square inch.

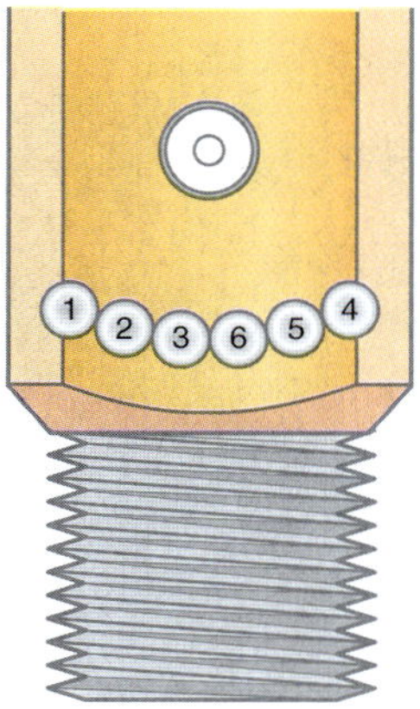

FIGURE 11-38 The locations of the pin-indexing safety system holes in a cylinder valve face. Each cylinder of a specific gas has a given pattern and a given number of pins.

from being connected to an oxygen cylinder, and so on. In preparing to administer oxygen, always check to be sure that the pinholes on the cylinder *exactly* match the corresponding pins on the regulator.

The pin-indexing system features a series of pins on a yoke that must be matched with the holes on the valve stem of the gas cylinder. The arrangement of the pins and holes varies for different gases according to accepted national standards (**FIGURE 11-38**). Other gases that are supplied in portable cylinders, such as acetylene, carbon dioxide, and nitrogen, use regulators and flowmeters that are similar to those used with oxygen. Each cylinder of a specific gas type has a given pattern and a given number of pins. These safety measures make it impossible for you to attach a cylinder of a different type of gas to an oxygen regulator. The oxygen regulator will not fit.

The outlet valves on portable oxygen cylinders are designed to accept yoke-type pressure-reducing gauges, which conform to the pin-indexing system (**FIGURE 11-39**).

The safety system for the large cylinders is known as the **American Standard Safety System**. In this system, oxygen cylinders are equipped with threaded gas outlet valves. The inside and outside thread sizes of these outlets vary depending on the gas in the cylinder. The cylinder will not accept a regulator valve unless it is properly threaded to fit that regulator. The purpose of these safety devices is the same as in the pin-indexing system: to prevent the accidental attachment of a regulator to the wrong cylinder.

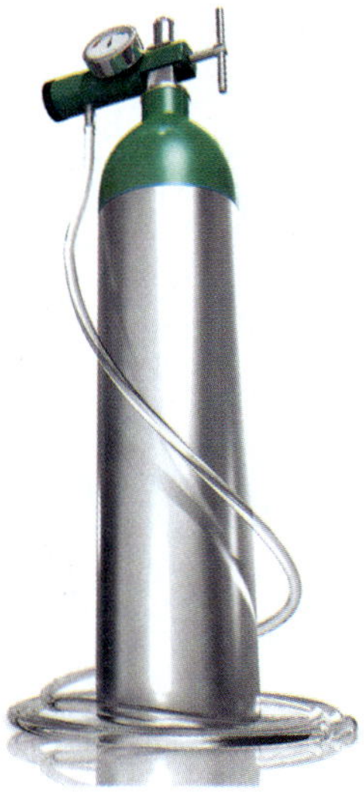

FIGURE 11-39 A yoke-type pressure-reducing gauge is used with a portable oxygen cylinder.

Pressure Regulators

The pressure of the gas in a full oxygen cylinder is approximately 2,000 pounds per square inch (psi).[12] This is far too much pressure for safe patient administration. Pressure regulators reduce the pressure to a more useful range, usually 40 to 70 psi. Most pressure regulators currently in use reduce the pressure in a single stage, although multistage regulators exist. A two-stage regulator will reduce the pressure first to 700 psi and then to 40 to 70 psi.

After the pressure is reduced to a workable level, the final attachment for delivering the gas to the patient is usually one of the following:

- A quick-connect female fitting that will accept a quick-connect male plug from a pressure hose or ventilator/resuscitator
- A flowmeter that will permit the regulated release of gas measured in liters per minute

Flowmeters

Flowmeters are usually permanently attached to pressure regulators on emergency medical equipment. The two types of flowmeters that are used are pressure-compensated flowmeters and Bourdon-gauge flowmeters.

A pressure-compensated flowmeter incorporates a float ball within the tapered calibrated tube. The flow of gas is controlled by a needle valve

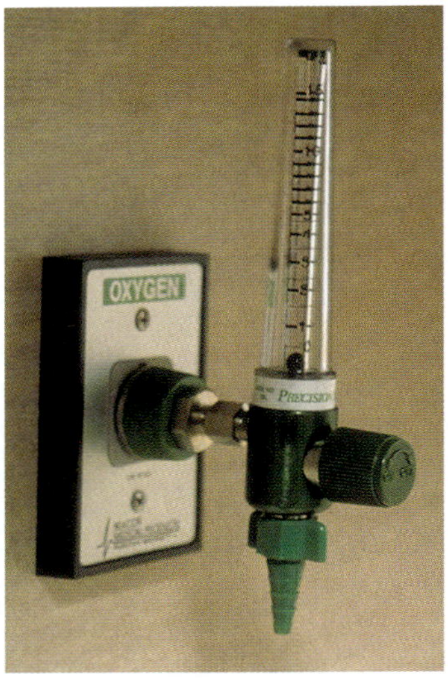

FIGURE 11-40 A pressure-compensated flowmeter contains a float ball that rises or falls according to the gas flow within the tube. It must be maintained in an upright position for an accurate reading.

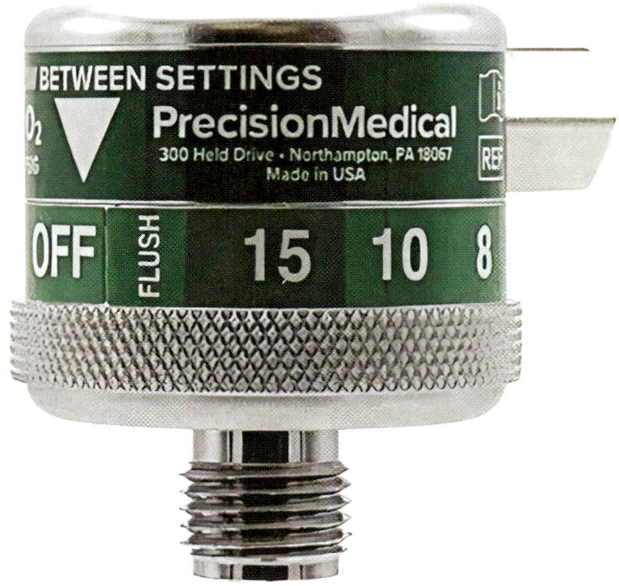

FIGURE 11-41 The Bourdon-gauge flowmeter is not affected by gravity and can be used in any position.

located downstream from the float ball. This type of flowmeter is affected by gravity and must always be maintained in an upright position for an accurate flow reading (**FIGURE 11-40**). For this reason, pressure-compensated flowmeters are rarely used on portable oxygen cylinders that are taken to the patient's side.

The Bourdon-gauge flowmeter is not affected by gravity and can be used in any position (**FIGURE 11-41**). It is a pressure gauge that is calibrated to record flow rate. This type of flowmeter, however, is now generally considered outdated. Newer flowmeters incorporate a fixable setting with either a dial or a knob that sets the flow. With these regulators, a Bourdon gauge is not necessary.

Procedures for Operating and Administering Oxygen

To place an oxygen cylinder into service and administer medical oxygen to a patient, follow the steps in **SKILL DRILL 11-7**:

1. Inspect the cylinder and its markings. If the cylinder was commercially filled, it will have a plastic seal around the valve stem covering the opening in the stem. Remove the seal and inspect the opening to make sure it is free of dirt and other debris. The valve stem should not be sealed or covered with adhesive tape or any petroleum-based substances. These can contaminate the oxygen and can contribute to combustion when mixed with pressurized oxygen.
2. "Crack" the cylinder by slowly opening and then reclosing the valve to help make sure dirt particles and other possible contaminants do not enter the oxygen flow. Never face the tank toward yourself or others when cracking the cylinder. Open the tank by attaching a tank key (wrench) to the valve and rotating the valve counterclockwise. You should be able to clearly hear the rush of oxygen coming from the tank. Close the tank by rotating the valve clockwise (**Step 1**).
3. Attach the regulator/flowmeter to the valve stem after clearing the opening. On one side of the valve stem, you will find three holes. The larger one, on top, is a true opening through which the oxygen flows. The two smaller holes below it do not extend to the inside of the tank. They provide stability to the regulator. Following the design of the pin-indexing system, these two holes are very precisely located in positions that are unique to the oxygen cylinders.
4. Above the pins on the inside of the collar is the actual port through which oxygen flows from

Skill Drill 11-7 Placing an Oxygen Cylinder Into Service

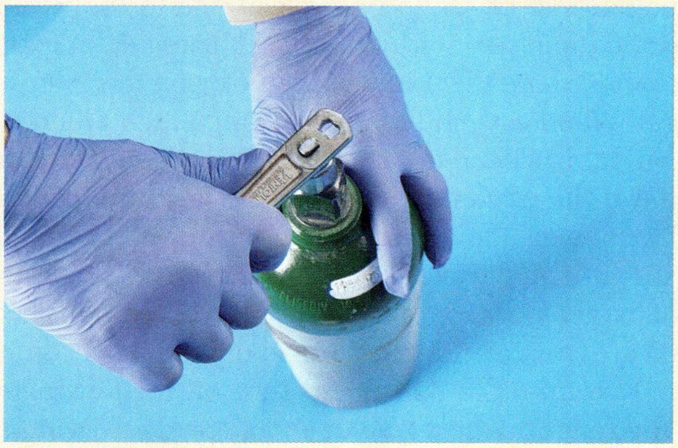

Step 1

Using an oxygen wrench, turn the valve counterclockwise to slowly "crack" the cylinder. Gently retighten the valve to stop the oxygen flow to allow the regulator to be attached.

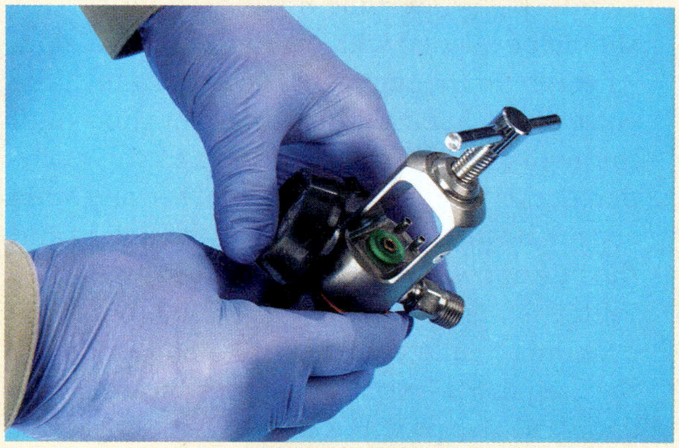

Step 2

Attach the regulator/flowmeter to the valve stem using the two pin-indexing holes and make sure the washer/gasket is in place over the larger hole.

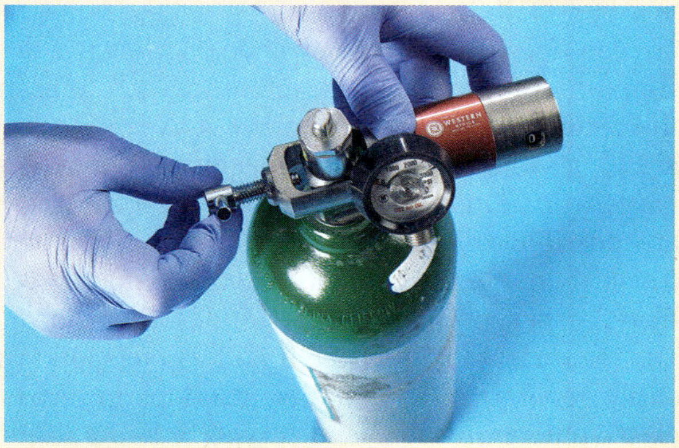

Step 3

Align the regulator so that the pins fit snugly into the correct holes on the valve stem, and hand tighten the regulator.

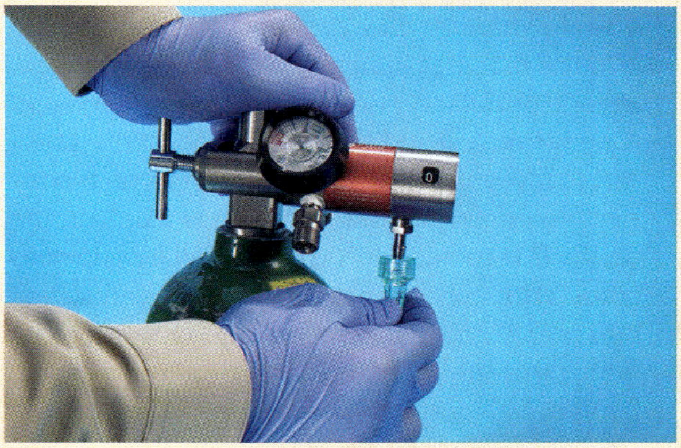

Step 4

Attach the oxygen connective tubing to the flowmeter. Use the wrench to fully open the tank.

the cylinder to the regulator. A metal-bound elastomeric sealing washer (also called a gasket) is placed around the oxygen port to optimize the airtight seal between the collar of the regulator and the valve stem (**Step 2**). In the past, crush gaskets made of plastic and nylon were used, but they are no longer recommended. If used, crush gaskets can be used only once and then they must be replaced.

5. Place the regulator collar over the cylinder valve, with the oxygen port and pin-indexing pins on the side of the valve stem that has the

three holes. Open the screw bolt just enough to allow the collar to fit freely over the valve stem. Move the regulator so that the oxygen port and the pins fit into the correct holes on the valve stem. The screw bolt on the opposite side should be aligned with the dimple depression. As you hold the regulator securely against the valve stem, hand tighten the screw bolt until the regulator is firmly attached to the cylinder. At this point, you should not see any open spaces between the sides of the valve stem and the interior walls of the collar (**Step 3**).

6. With the regulator firmly attached, open the cylinder completely, check for air leaking from the regulator–oxygen cylinder connection, and read the pressure level on the regulator gauge. Most portable cylinders have a maximum pressure of approximately 2,000 psi. Most EMS systems consider a cylinder with less than 500 to 1,000 psi to be too low to keep in service. Learn your department's policies regarding safe/minimal residual pressure in the tank and follow them.
7. The flowmeter will have a second gauge or a selector dial that indicates the oxygen flow rate. Several popular types of devices are widely used. Attach the selected oxygen device to the flowmeter by connecting the universal oxygen connecting tubing to the "Christmas tree" nipple on the flowmeter. Most oxygen-delivery devices come with this tubing permanently attached; however, some oxygen masks do not. You must attach this tubing to the oxygen-delivery device if it is not already attached (**Step 4**).

Safety Tips

Slowly open the oxygen tank after attaching the regulator and check for leaks. Remember that although oxygen itself is not combustible, it supports combustion, and any ignition source may cause fire or an explosion in an oxygen-rich environment, especially if oxygen is being released too quickly from the cylinder at the time or if the seal between the regulator and oxygen cylinder is not secure.

Open the flowmeter to the desired flow rate. Flow rates will vary based on the oxygen-delivery device being used. Remember that you must be completely familiar with the equipment before attempting to use it on a patient. Once the oxygen is flowing at the desired rate, apply the oxygen device to the patient and make any necessary adjustments. Monitor the patient's response to the oxygen and to the oxygen device, and periodically recheck the regulator gauge to make sure there is sufficient oxygen in the cylinder. When oxygen therapy is complete or when the patient has been transferred to the hospital, first remove the oxygen delivery device from the patient. Disconnect the tubing from the flowmeter nipple and turn off the cylinder. In a few seconds, the sound of oxygen flowing from the nipple will cease. This indicates that all the pressurized oxygen has been removed from the flowmeter. Turn off the flowmeter. The gauge on the regulator should read zero with the tank valve closed. This reading confirms that there is no pressure left above the valve stem. If there is *any* pressure reading on the regulator gauge, it is not safe to remove the regulator from the valve stem.

Hazards of Supplemental Oxygen

Combustion

Oxygen does not burn or explode. However, it does support combustion. The more oxygen present, the faster the combustion process. A small spark, even a glowing cigarette, can become a flame in an oxygen-rich atmosphere. Therefore, you must keep any possible source of fire away from the area while oxygen is in use. Make sure the area is adequately ventilated, especially in industrial settings where hazardous materials may be present and where sparks are easily generated. Be extremely cautious in any enclosed environment in which oxygen is being administered, as an oxygen-rich environment increases the chance of fire if a spark or flame is introduced. A bystander who is smoking or sparks generated during vehicle extrication are possible sources of ignition. Never leave an oxygen cylinder standing unattended. The cylinder can be knocked over, which could injure the patient or damage the equipment.

Oxygen Toxicity

The administration of oxygen to patients is a common practice. Although many patients in the prehospital environment require high concentrations of oxygen, some patients do not require oxygen at all. Excessive supplemental oxygen can have a detrimental effect on patients with certain illnesses (ie, COPD, stroke, and myocardial infarction) When initially ventilating newborns, it is recommended to use room air.

Research has shown that although the administration of oxygen benefits many patients and is rarely problematic, high concentrations of oxygen are potentially harmful for a select population.[13] **Oxygen toxicity** refers to damage to cellular tissue due to excessive oxygen levels in the blood. Years ago, high concentrations of oxygen were thought to benefit all patients in the prehospital environment. However, current evidence suggests that increased cellular oxygen levels contribute to the production of oxygen free radicals. These free radicals may lead to tissue damage and cellular death in some patients.

Current guidelines recognize there may be negative effects of oxygen toxicity and recommend that oxygen be administered to patients experiencing signs of a myocardial infarction when they have signs of heart failure, are short of breath, or have a room air Spo_2 less than 90%.[14] In addition, patients experiencing signs of shock should be placed on oxygen. Understand that hypoxemia is immediately life threatening, whereas oxygen toxicity is not; when in doubt, or if unable to measure oxygen saturation reliably, supplemental oxygen should be administered.

Pulse oximetry is not always available to the EMT. When pulse oximetry is available and oxygen is indicated, tailor oxygen therapy to the patient's needs, and administer the minimum amount of oxygen necessary to maintain Spo_2 between 94% and 98%. Exceptions to these minimums include patients who have been exposed to carbon monoxide, patients with potential anemia, or patients with shock.

Oxygen-Delivery Equipment

In general, the oxygen delivery equipment used in the field is limited to nonrebreathing masks, bag-mask devices, and nasal cannulas, depending on local protocol (**TABLE 11-6**). Other devices you may encounter during transports between medical facilities, such as partial rebreathing masks, are also described in this section. Note that while the bag-mask device is used to deliver oxygen, it provides positive-pressure ventilation for patients who do not have adequate spontaneous breathing; thus, it is discussed in the next section, Assisted and Artificial Ventilation.

TABLE 11-6 Oxygen-Delivery Devices

Device	Flow Rate	Oxygen Delivered
Nonrebreathing mask with reservoir	10 to 15 L/min	Up to 95%
Nasal cannula	1 to 6 L/min	24% to 44%
Bag-mask device with reservoir	15 L/min	Up to 95%

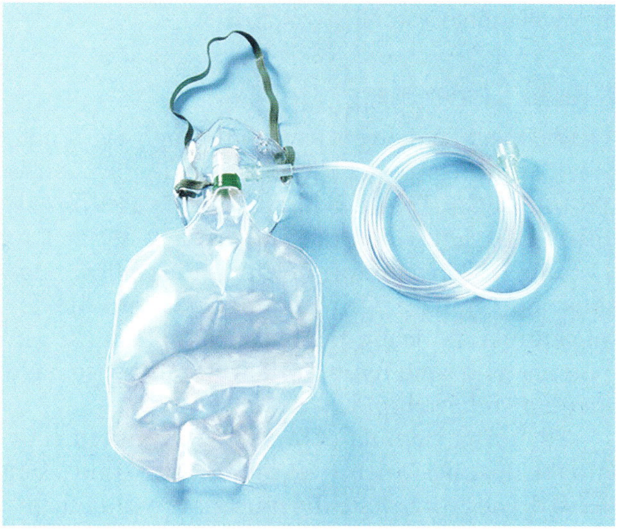

FIGURE 11-42 The nonrebreathing mask contains flapper valve ports at the cheek areas of the mask to prevent the patient from rebreathing exhaled gases.

Nonrebreathing Masks

The **nonrebreathing mask** is used to administer high concentrations of oxygen to significantly hypoxemic patients who otherwise have adequate tidal volume. With a good mask-to-face seal and a flow rate of 15 L/min, the nonrebreathing mask can provide up to 95% inspired oxygen.[3]

The nonrebreathing mask is a combination mask and reservoir bag system. Oxygen fills a reservoir bag that is attached to the mask by a one-way valve. The system is called a nonrebreathing mask because the exhaled gas escapes through flapper valve ports at the cheek areas of the mask (**FIGURE 11-42**). These valves prevent the patient from rebreathing exhaled gases, namely carbon dioxide.

When using this system, you must be sure that the reservoir bag is full before the mask is placed on the patient. Adjust the flow rate so that the bag does not fully collapse when the patient inhales, to about two-thirds of the bag volume, or 10 to 15 L/min. Make sure the bag stays inflated. Should the bag collapse when the patient inhales, increase the flow rate of oxygen. In addition, if oxygen therapy is discontinued, remove the mask from the patient's face. Leaving the mask in place while oxygen is not flowing allows the patient to rebreathe exhaled carbon dioxide. Use a pediatric nonrebreathing mask, which has a smaller reservoir bag, with infants and children, as they will inhale a smaller volume.

Nasal Cannulas

A **nasal cannula** delivers oxygen through two small, tubelike prongs that fit into the patient's nostrils (**FIGURE 11-43**). This device can provide 24% to 44% inspired oxygen when the flowmeter is set at 1 to 6 L/min. For the comfort of your patient, flow rates above 6 L/min are not recommended with the nasal cannula. Typically, the nasal cannula is used in patients with mild hypoxemia who otherwise have adequate tidal volume.

The nasal cannula delivers dry oxygen directly into the nostrils, which, over prolonged periods, can cause dryness or irritate the mucous membrane lining of the nose. Therefore, when you anticipate a long transport time, consider the use of humidification.

The nasal cannula does have some limitations. For example, a patient who breathes through the mouth or who has a nasal obstruction will likely get little or no benefit from a nasal cannula. Use a nonrebreathing mask if the patient is significantly hypoxemic, coaching the patient if necessary. If the patient will not tolerate a nonrebreathing mask, you will have to use a nasal cannula, which some patients find more comfortable. Another option is to allow the patient to hold the nonrebreathing mask to their face as they feel comfortable. As always, a good assessment of your patient will guide your decision.

Partial Rebreathing Masks

The partial rebreathing mask is similar to a nonrebreathing mask except that there is no one-way valve between the mask and the reservoir. Consequently, patients rebreathe a small amount of their exhaled air. The oxygen enriches the air mixture and delivers a gas mix of approximately 80% to 90% oxygen. You can easily convert a nonrebreathing mask to a partial rebreathing mask by removing the one-way valve between the mask and the reservoir bag.

Venturi Masks

A Venturi mask has several attachments that enable you to vary the percentage of oxygen delivered to the patient while a constant flow is maintained from the regulator (**FIGURE 11-44**). This is accomplished by the Venturi principle, which causes air to be drawn into the flow of oxygen as it passes a hole in the line. The Venturi mask is a medium-flow device that delivers 24% to 40% oxygen, depending on the manufacturer.

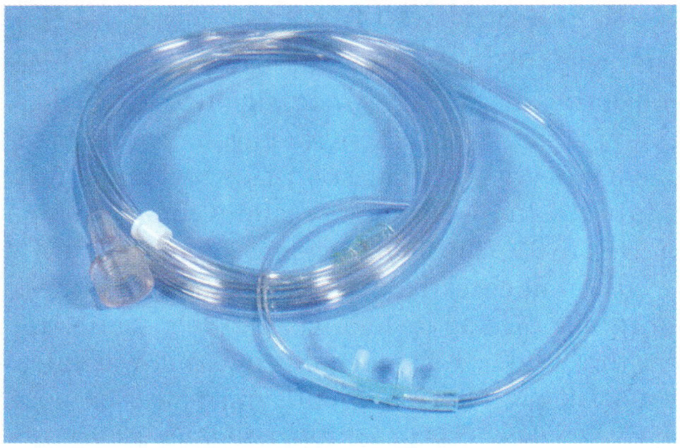

FIGURE 11-43 The nasal cannula delivers oxygen directly through the nostrils.

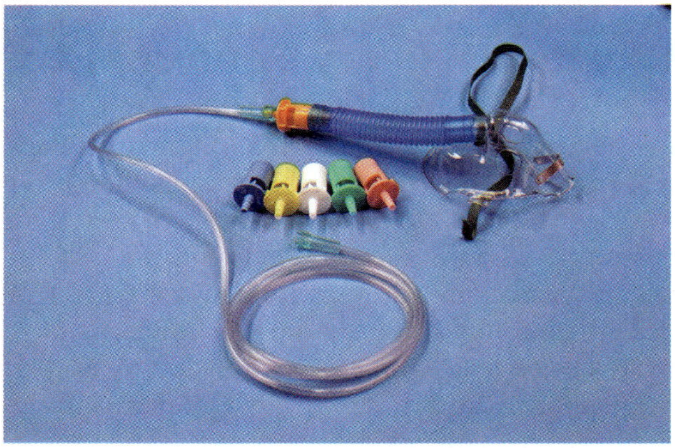

FIGURE 11-44 The Venturi mask.

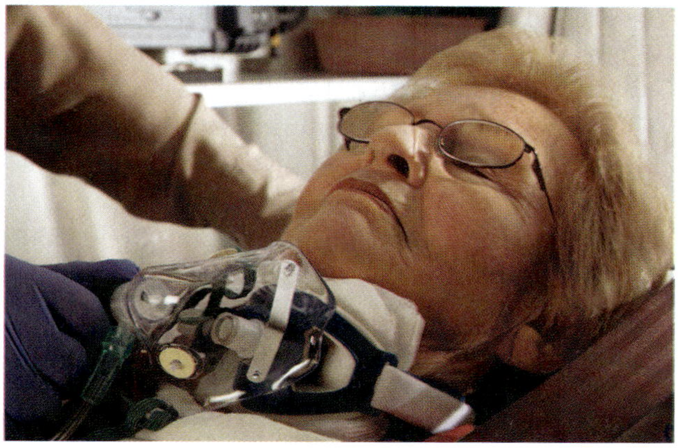

FIGURE 11-45 For a patient with a tracheostomy, if you do not have a tracheostomy mask, use a face mask instead.

The main advantage of the Venturi mask is the use of its fine adjustment capabilities in the long-term management of physiologically stable patients. However, in the emergency setting, such fine adjustments are not necessary. When you need to adjust the oxygen concentration in an emergency, it is typically done by adjusting the flow rate or changing the delivery device. You are far more likely to encounter a Venturi mask when doing an interfacility transfer.

Tracheostomy Masks

Patients with tracheostomies do not breathe through their mouth or nose. A face mask or nasal cannula therefore cannot be used to treat them. Masks designed specifically for these patients cover the tracheostomy hole and have a strap that goes around the neck. These masks are usually available in intensive care units, where many patients have tracheostomies, and may not be available in an emergency setting. If you do not have a tracheostomy mask, you can improvise by placing a face mask over the stoma. Even though the mask is shaped to fit the face, you can usually get an adequate fit over the patient's neck by adjusting the strap (**FIGURE 11-45**).

Humidification

Some EMS systems provide humidified oxygen to patients during extended transport or for certain conditions such as croup (**FIGURE 11-46**). However, humidified oxygen is usually indicated only for long-term oxygen therapy and in patients who have thick secretions. Dry oxygen is not considered harmful and generally does not cause patient discomfort when used for short periods, especially at flow rates of 4 L/min or less. An oxygen humidifier consists of a small single-patient-use bottle of sterile water through which the oxygen leaving the cylinder becomes moisturized before it reaches the patient. Because the humidifier must be kept in an upright position, however, it is practical only for the fixed oxygen unit in the ambulance. Humidification may be associated with an increased generation of aerosolized droplets of fluid that may increase the degree to which the patient can transmit disease to other people in the same ambulance compartment. This fact is particularly relevant when a patient has a disease that can be transmitted through respiratory droplets.

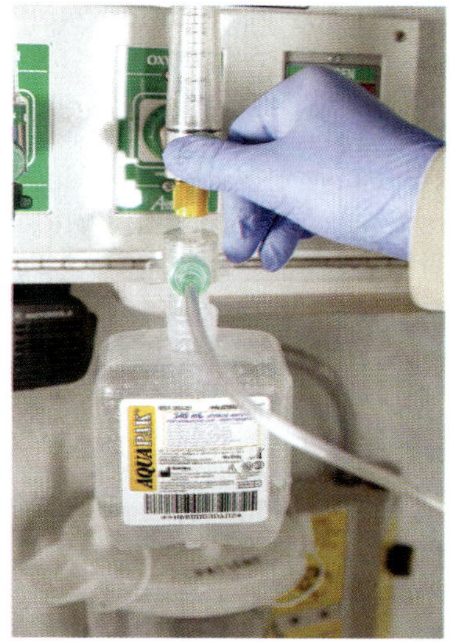

FIGURE 11-46 Giving humidified oxygen is preferred with long transport times, although it increases the aerosolization of droplets and may increase the risk of disease transmission to others in the same ambulance compartment as the patient.

Assisted and Artificial Ventilation

A patient who is not breathing needs artificial ventilation and 100% supplemental oxygen. Assisted ventilation and artificial ventilation are critical skills for any EMS clinician, regardless of certification level. Too often emphasis is placed on advanced airway techniques, making the basic airway maneuvers seem ineffective. This cannot be further from the truth. Basic airway and ventilation techniques are extremely effective when administered appropriately. Mastery of these techniques at the EMT level, and continued mastery at the AEMT and paramedic levels, is imperative.

Patients who are breathing inadequately may be unable to speak in complete sentences. An irregular breathing pattern may also require artificial ventilation to assist patients in maintaining adequate minute volume. Keep in mind that fast, shallow breathing can be just as dangerous as very slow breathing. Fast, shallow breathing moves air primarily in the larger airway passages (dead air space) and does not allow for adequate exchange of air and carbon dioxide in the alveoli. Patients with inadequate breathing require assisted ventilations with some form of positive-pressure ventilation. Remember to follow standard precautions as needed when managing the patient's airway.

Assisting Ventilation in Respiratory Distress/Failure

When a patient is in severe respiratory distress or respiratory failure and not breathing adequately, you must intervene quickly to prevent further deterioration of the patient. Two treatment options are available in these situations: assisted ventilation (invasive) and CPAP, or noninvasive ventilation. CPAP is discussed later in this chapter; the focus of this section will be on assisted ventilation.

The purpose of assisted ventilations is to improve the overall oxygenation and ventilatory status of the patient. Patients who require assisted ventilations are no longer able to maintain adequate oxygen levels for the body and need assistance to prevent further hypoxia.

You need to be familiar with the signs and symptoms associated with inadequate ventilation. Signs of altered mental status and shallow breathing (reduced tidal volume) are indications for assisted ventilation. In addition, excessive accessory muscle use and fatigue from labored breathing are signs of potential respiratory failure. Patients exhibiting these signs need immediate treatment.

Follow these steps to assist a spontaneously breathing patient's ventilations using a bag-mask device:

1. Explain the procedure to the patient.
2. Place the mask over the patient's nose and mouth.
3. Squeeze the bag each time the patient breathes, maintaining the same rate as the patient.
4. After the initial 5 to 10 breaths, slowly adjust the rate and deliver an appropriate tidal volume.
5. Adjust the rate and tidal volume to maintain an adequate minute volume.
6. Use pulse oximetry and capnography (if available) to quantify effective oxygenation and ventilation.

Artificial Ventilation

Patients who are in respiratory arrest need immediate treatment. Without it, they will die. However, the act of breathing for a patient, or artificial ventilation, is not a skill you should take lightly. Once you determine that a patient is not breathing, begin artificial ventilation immediately. The methods that you may use to provide artificial ventilation include the mouth-to-mask technique (used only in off-duty situations when a bag-mask device is not available) and the one- or two-person bag-mask device technique.

Normal Ventilation Versus Positive-Pressure Ventilation

It is important to understand that although artificial ventilations are necessary to sustain life, they are not the same as normal breathing. As discussed earlier, the act of air moving into and out of the lungs is based on pressure changes within the thoracic cavity. During normal ventilation, the diaphragm contracts and negative pressure is generated in the chest cavity. This essentially sucks air into the chest from the trachea to equalize the pressure in the chest with the atmospheric pressure. The same vacuum that sucks air into the chest also pulls blood back to the right side of the heart. However, positive-pressure ventilation generated by a device, such as a bag-mask device, forces air into the chest cavity from the external environment, rather than using pressure changes. This difference between normal ventilation and positive-pressure ventilation can create some challenges (**TABLE 11-7**).

The physical act of the chest wall expanding and retracting during breathing helps the circulatory system return blood to the heart. During normal ventilation, the chest wall movement works similarly to a pump. The pressure changes in the thoracic cavity help draw venous blood back to the

TABLE 11-7 Normal Ventilation Versus Positive-Pressure Ventilation

	Normal Ventilation	Positive-Pressure Ventilation
Air movement	Air is sucked into the lungs due to the negative intrathoracic pressure created when the diaphragm contracts.	Air is forced into the lungs through a means of mechanical ventilation.
Blood movement	Normal breathing allows blood to naturally be pulled back to the heart.	Intrathoracic pressure is increased as air is driven into the lungs, which can reduce blood return to the heart and therefore reduce the amount of blood pumped by the heart.
Airway wall pressure	Not affected during normal breathing.	More volume is required to have the same effects as normal breathing. As a result, the walls are pushed out of their normal anatomic shape.
Esophageal opening pressure	Not affected during normal breathing.	Air may be forced into the stomach, especially with aggressive ventilation, causing gastric distention that could result in vomiting and aspiration. The esophagus opens at approximately 20 cm H_2O. Higher pressure levels cause gastric distention.
Overventilation	Overventilation is not typical of normal breathing.	Too much volume and/or a fast ventilation rate results in increased intrathoracic pressure, gastric distention, and decrease in cardiac output, resulting in hypotension.

heart. However, when positive-pressure ventilation is initiated, more air is needed to achieve the same oxygenation and ventilatory effects of normal breathing. This increase in airway wall pressure causes the walls of the chest cavity to push out of their normal anatomic shape. As a result, there is an increase in the overall intrathoracic pressure. This pressure increase affects the return of venous blood to the heart. Considering that the left side of the heart receives only what the right side gives it,

YOU are the EMT

Following the appropriate corrective action, the patient's airway is now patent. As your partner continues to manage the airway and assist the patient's ventilations, you assess baseline vital signs. The patient's wife, who called 9-1-1, tells you that her husband has a history of hypertension but does not take his medication as he should. He was taking a nap, and when she checked on him, she found him in his present condition.

Recording Time: 4 Minutes	
Respirations	6 breaths/min and irregular (baseline); 10 breaths/min (assisted)
Pulse	40 beats/min, weak
Skin	Cool and dry; facial cyanosis resolving
Blood pressure	178/102 mm Hg
Oxygen saturation (Spo_2)	93% (with assisted ventilation and high-flow oxygen)

5. What are some indications of effective positive-pressure ventilation?

6. What effect, if any, does positive-pressure ventilation have on cardiac output?

reduced venous return would result in reduced cardiac output. Therefore, it is imperative that you regulate the rate and volume of artificial ventilations to help prevent this drop in cardiac output.

Words of Wisdom

It is important to know the correct ventilation rates for apneic patients with a pulse:

- Adult: One breath every 6 seconds (10 breaths/min)
- Child or infant: One breath every 2 to 3 seconds (20 to 30 breaths/min)

Mouth-to-Mouth and Mouth-to-Mask Ventilation

As you learned in your CPR course, mouth-to-mouth ventilations should be done with a **barrier device**, such as a face shield. Barrier devices provide some protection, but not from diseases transmitted by airborne pathogens or aerosolized droplets such as SARS-CoV-2 or tuberculosis (**FIGURE 11-47**). *Mouth-to-mouth ventilations with or without a barrier device should be provided only in extreme situations.* To help prevent possible disease transmission, performing mouth-to-mask ventilations with a pocket mask containing a one-way valve with an adequate filter is a safer option. This method is used only when the EMT is off duty in a situation where no bag-mask device is available.

The Bag-Mask Device

With an oxygen flow rate of 15 L/min and an adequate mask-to-face seal, a bag-mask device with an oxygen reservoir can deliver up to 95% oxygen (**FIGURE 11-48**). Most commercially available bag-mask devices include reservoirs that permit the delivery of oxygen concentrations up to 95%; however, the device can deliver only as much volume as you can squeeze out of the bag by hand. The bag-mask device provides less tidal volume than mouth-to-mask ventilation; however, it delivers a higher concentration of oxygen. The bag-mask device is the most common method used to ventilate patients in the field. Although an experienced EMT will be able to supply adequate tidal volume with a bag-mask device, as a new EMT you should develop proficiency at ventilating airway-training manikins before using a bag-mask device on a patient. If you

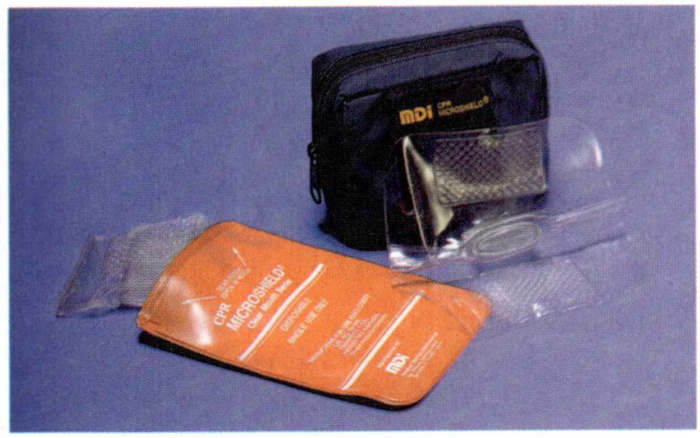

A

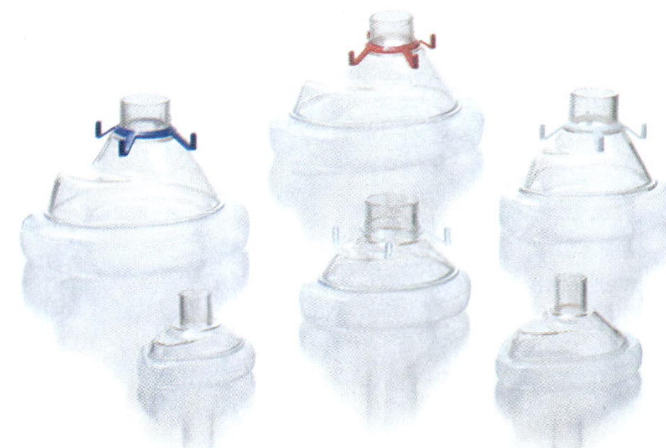

B

FIGURE 11-47 A barrier device **(A)** or pocket mask with a one-way valve **(B)** provides some protection from certain diseases but inadequate protection from aerosolized droplets.

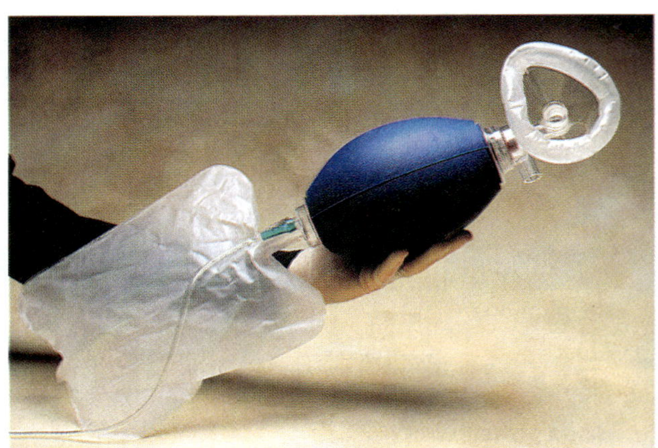

FIGURE 11-48 A bag-mask device with an oxygen reservoir can deliver up to 95% oxygen if a good seal between the mouth and mask is achieved and if supplemental oxygen is used.

have difficulty adequately ventilating a patient with a bag-mask device, reposition the airway, adjust the mask seal, or ask another EMT to assist.

A bag-mask device should be used when you need to deliver high concentrations of oxygen to patients who are not ventilating adequately. The device is also used for patients in respiratory arrest, cardiopulmonary arrest, and respiratory failure. It may be used with or without oxygen. However, in most cases, to ensure the highest concentration of delivered oxygen, you must attach supplemental oxygen and a reservoir. Use an oropharyngeal or nasopharyngeal airway adjunct in conjunction with the bag-mask device.

Bag-Mask Device Components

All adult bag-mask devices should have the following components:

- A disposable self-inflating bag
- No pop-off valve, or if one is present, the capability of disabling the pop-off valve
- An outlet valve that is a true valve for nonrebreathing
- An inline viral filter
- An oxygen reservoir that allows for delivery of high-concentration oxygen
- A one-way, no-jam inlet valve system that provides an oxygen inlet flow at a maximum of 15 L/min with standard 15/22-mm fittings for face mask and ET tube (or other advanced airway adjunct) connection
- A transparent face mask
- Ability to perform under extreme environmental conditions, including extreme heat or cold

The total volume in the bag of an adult bag-mask device is usually 1,200 to 1,600 mL. The pediatric bag volume is 500 to 700 mL, and the infant bag volume is 150 to 240 mL.

The volume of air delivered to the patient is based on one key observation: chest rise and fall. Essentially, this is the only means of assessing tidal volume in the field. In most situations, you will be using the bag-mask device attached to high-flow oxygen (15 L/min). When using the bag-mask device with high-flow oxygen on an adult patient, you should squeeze the bag enough to cause a noticeable rise of the patient's chest: a volume of about 600 mL (approximately 6 to 8 mL/kg of ideal body weight) over 1 second.

By delivering just enough tidal volume to see the chest rise, and not ventilating at a rate that is too fast, the risks of gastric distention (and associated complications of vomiting and aspiration) and cardiac compromise are reduced.

It is not practical for you to accurately measure tidal volume in milliliters per kilogram for each patient ventilated in the field. The key is to watch for good chest rise and fall.

Words of Wisdom

While adequate ventilation can be achieved using a bag-mask device, ventilation can be enhanced by adding a positive end-expiratory pressure (PEEP) valve to the bag-mask device (**FIGURE 11-49**).[11] Unlike continuous positive airway pressure (CPAP), which maintains a small amount of pressure throughout the respiratory cycle, PEEP maintains that extra pressure only at the end of exhalation. When PEEP is added, it decreases the work of breathing and improves oxygenation by preventing collapse of alveoli between each breath, improving the alveoli's availability to participate in gas exchange. It may be especially helpful in patients suspected to have pneumonia, pulmonary edema, or drowning. Just as in CPAP, PEEP can reduce the venous return to the heart, which can potentially decrease the preload and subsequently the blood pressure. This risk is small when a small amount of PEEP is added; however, PEEP should not be used when the patient's systolic blood pressure is less than 90 mm Hg. It is important to recognize that, just like ventilation, PEEP will not be delivered unless there is a good mask seal. You can best achieve this by using a two-person bag-mask technique when possible.

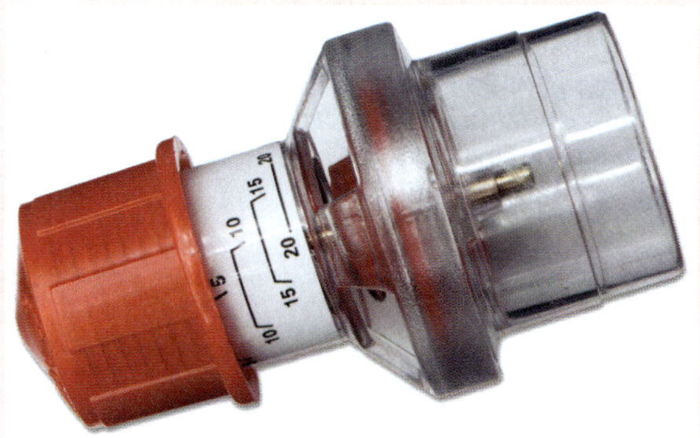

FIGURE 11-49 Positive end-expiratory pressure valve.

Bag-Mask Device Technique

Whenever possible, you and your partner should work together to provide bag-mask ventilation. One EMT can maintain a good mask seal by securing the mask to the patient's face with two hands while the other EMT squeezes the bag using a few fingers of one hand in a controlled manner. Ventilation using a bag-mask device is a challenging skill: it may be very difficult for one EMT to maintain a proper seal between the mask and the face with one hand while squeezing the bag well enough to deliver an adequate volume to the patient. This skill can be difficult to maintain if you do not have many opportunities to practice. Effective one-person bag-mask ventilation requires considerable practice and experience. Also, performance of this skill depends on having enough personnel to carry out other actions that need to be done at the same time, such as chest compressions, putting the stretcher in place, or helping to lift the patient onto the stretcher.

Follow these steps to use the one-person adult bag-mask device technique (**SKILL DRILL 11-8**):

1. Select the proper size mask and assemble your equipment. Kneel above the patient's head. Maintain the patient's neck in an extended position (with the head elevated up to 30° when possible) unless you suspect a cervical spine injury (**Step 1**). In that case, stabilize the patient's head and neck and use the jaw-thrust maneuver. Have your partner hold the head, or, if you are alone, use your knees to stabilize the head.
2. Open the patient's mouth, and suction as needed. Insert an oropharyngeal or nasopharyngeal airway to maintain airway patency (**Step 2**).
3. Place the mask on the patient's face (**Step 3**). Make sure the top is over the bridge of the nose and the bottom is in the groove between the lower lip and the chin. If the mask has a large, round cuff around the ventilation port, center the port over the patient's mouth. Adjust the amount of air in the mask to obtain a better fit and seal to the face if necessary.
4. Create a seal by using the EC-clamp method to hold the mask to the patient's face: Form a *C* by holding your index finger over the lower part of the mask and your thumb over the upper part of the mask. Then form an *E* by using your remaining fingers to pull the lower jaw into the mask. This EC technique will maintain an effective face-to-mask seal.
5. Bring the lower jaw up to the mask with the last three fingers of your hand. This will help to maintain an open airway. Make sure you do not grab the fleshy part of the neck; doing so will push the tongue against the roof of the mouth and block the airway.

YOU are the EMT

The fire squad arrives to assist you and your partner. The closest appropriate hospital is located 9 miles away. You assess the patient's blood glucose level and reassess his vital signs. The patient is then secured to the stretcher and loaded into the ambulance. Your assessment thus far has not revealed any obvious causes of his condition.

Recording Time: 8 Minutes	
Level of consciousness	Unresponsive
Respirations	6 breaths/min and irregular (baseline); 10 breaths/min (assisted)
Pulse	44 beats/min, bounding
Skin	Baseline color, warm and dry
Blood pressure	170/100 mm Hg
Oxygen saturation (Spo_2)	95% (with assisted ventilation and high-flow oxygen)
Blood glucose	132 mg/dL

7. How does an adult's heart rate typically respond to hypoxemia initially? Why?

Skill Drill 11-8 Performing One-Rescuer Bag-Mask Ventilations

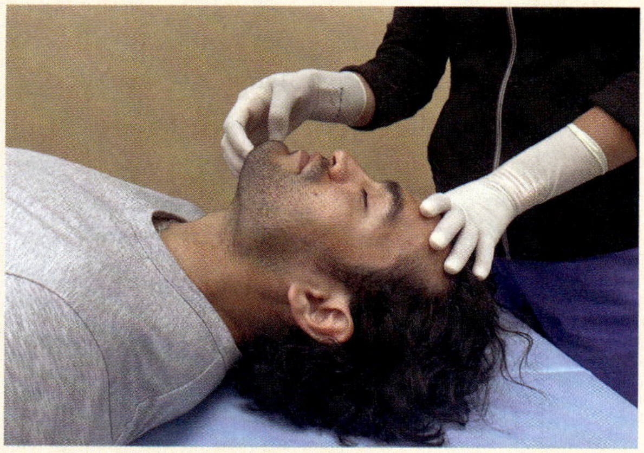

Step 1

Assemble your equipment and position yourself above the patient's head. Open the airway using the head tilt–chin lift or jaw-thrust maneuver.

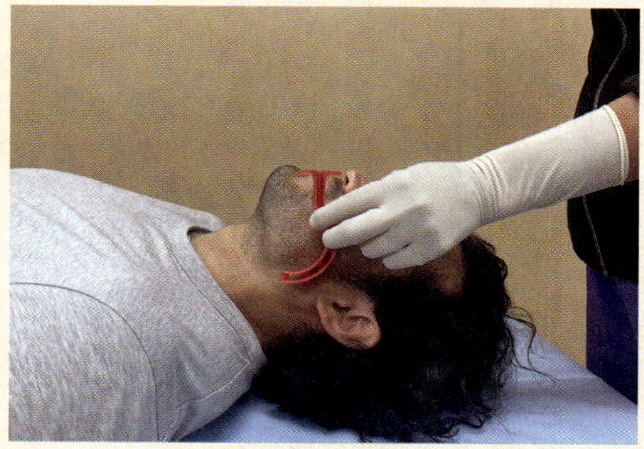

Step 2

Open the patient's mouth and suction as necessary to clear secretions. Insert an oropharyngeal or nasopharyngeal airway.

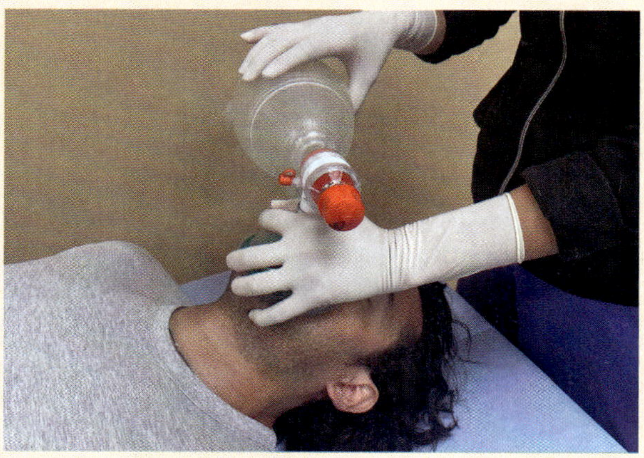

Step 3

Select the appropriate mask and position it properly on the patient's face. Following the EC-clamp method, make a seal by holding your index finger over the lower part of the mask and your thumb over the upper part of the mask. Then use your remaining fingers to pull the lower jaw into the mask. Bring the lower jaw up to the mask with the last three fingers of your hand. Avoid the fleshy soft tissue of the neck.

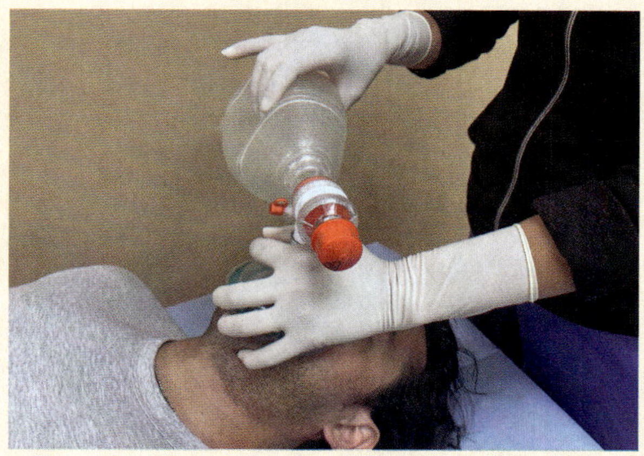

Step 4

Squeeze the bag with your other hand until you see adequate chest rise. For adults, squeeze once every 6 seconds. For infants and children, squeeze once every 2 to 3 seconds. In patients undergoing CPR and with an advanced airway in place, use a rate of 1 breath every 6 seconds (10 breaths/min) for adults and a rate of 1 breath every 2 to 3 seconds (20 to 30 breaths/min) for infants and children until puberty.

6. Squeeze the bag with your other hand until you see adequate chest rise (**Step 4**). Perform this in a rhythmic manner once every 6 seconds for an adult and once every 2 to 3 seconds for infants and children. According to the American Heart Association, you can deliver 2 breaths after every 30 compressions for adults in cardiac arrest, *or* you can perform continuous chest compressions with 1 breath every 6 seconds (10 breaths/min) before an advanced airway device (eg, ET tube, King airway, i-gel) has been inserted. Once an advanced airway device has been inserted, use a ventilation rate of 1 breath every 6 seconds (10 breaths/min), without pausing chest compressions.[3]

If two EMTs are available to manage the airway and ventilate the patient, have one EMT use both hands to hold the mask in position, using an EC clamp on both sides of the mask and drawing the lower jaw up to the mask. This helps to seal the mask to the face and maintain an open airway. The second EMT squeezes the bag with *a few fingers* of one hand until the chest rises adequately in the same manner as the one-person technique (**FIGURE 11-50**).

If you are unable to obtain a mask seal using the EC technique, consider one of the following methods:

- To perform the one-handed EO grip, encircle the neck of the mask with the first two digits of one hand while the other fingers lift the chin.
- To perform an alternate two-handed technique, position yourself at the patient's head and then firmly press down on the sides of the mask with the thenar eminence (the mound formed on the palm at the base of the thumb) of each hand while lifting each side of the jaw with the remaining fingers on each hand.

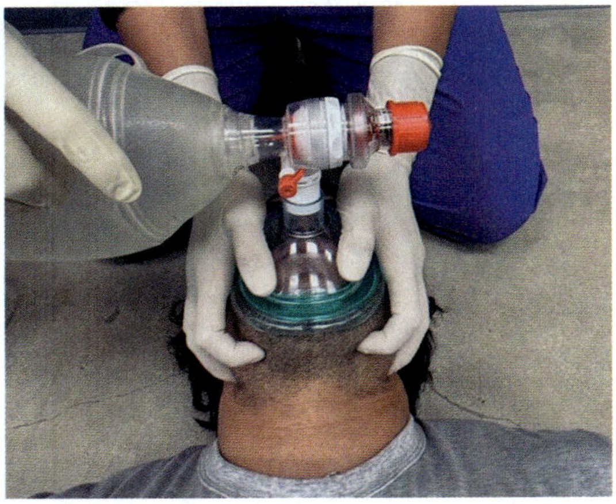

FIGURE 11-50 With two-person bag-mask ventilation, you hold the mask in place while your partner squeezes the bag with *a few fingers* of one hand until the patient's chest rises adequately.

When using the device to assist ventilations of a patient who is breathing too slowly (hypoventilation) with reduced tidal volume, squeeze the bag as the patient tries to breathe in. Then, for the next 5 to 10 breaths, slowly adjust the rate and delivered tidal volume until clinical improvement (ie, increased Spo_2 level, decreased $ETCO_2$ level, improvement in skin condition) is observed.

Words of Wisdom

In certain situations, you will need to perform ventilations with a bag-mask device before supplemental oxygen is available. If you are unable initially to attach your bag-mask device to an oxygen source, do not withhold ventilations. Provide ventilations using the standard technique and attach the bag-mask device to an oxygen source as soon as it is available.

To assist ventilations of a patient who is breathing too fast (hyperventilation) with reduced tidal volume, you must first explain the procedure to the patient if the patient is coherent. Initially assist ventilations at the rate at which the patient has been breathing, squeezing the bag each time the patient inhales. Then, for the next 5 to 10 breaths, slowly adjust the rate and the delivered tidal volume until clinical improvement is observed.

As you are assisting ventilations with a bag-mask device, you should evaluate the effectiveness of your delivered ventilations. You will know that artificial ventilations are not adequate if the patient's chest does not rise and fall with each ventilation, the rate at which you are ventilating is too slow or too fast, the heart rate does not return to normal, or oxygen saturation does not improve. If too much air is escaping from under the mask, reposition the mask for a better seal. If the patient's chest does not rise and fall, you may need to reposition the head or use an airway adjunct. If the patient's chest still does not rise and fall after you have made these corrections, check for an airway obstruction. If an obstruction is not present, attempt ventilations using an alternative method, such as the mouth-to-mask technique.

The bag-mask device may also be used in conjunction with an ET tube or with other advanced airway devices. Advanced airway techniques are beneficial when a good seal is difficult to maintain, the patient has a cervical spine injury, or the patient's condition warrants. These techniques are discussed later in the text.

Safety Tips

A viral filter should be placed between the mask, or advanced airway device, and the bag. While this was specifically emphasized during the COVID-19 pandemic,[15] EMS systems should have *always* been using an inline filter to minimize exposure to any potentially contagious respiratory diseases. If a contagious respiratory disease is suspected or confirmed, use a HEPA filter.

Gastric Distention

When using a bag-mask device or any other ventilation device, be alert for **gastric distention**, inflation of the stomach with air. Although gastric distention most commonly affects children, it also affects adults. Gastric distention is most likely to occur when you ventilate the patient too forcefully or too rapidly with a bag-mask device or pocket mask. It may also occur when the airway is obstructed because of a foreign body or improper head position. For this reason, give slow, gentle breaths during artificial ventilation over 1 second (enough to see the chest rise) in any patient. As compliance decreases, you will notice it becoming increasingly difficult to squeeze the bag-mask device to get air into the lungs. Slight gastric distention is not of concern; however, severe inflation of the stomach is dangerous because it may cause vomiting and increase the risk of aspiration during CPR. Gastric distention can also significantly reduce available lung volume by elevating the diaphragm, especially in infants and children.

To prevent or alleviate distention, do the following: (1) ensure that the patient's airway is appropriately positioned, (2) ventilate the patient at the appropriate rate, and (3) ventilate the patient with the appropriate volume.

If the patient's stomach appears to be distending, recheck and reposition the head, and ventilate for 1 second, just until you observe the chest begin to rise. Avoid rapid, forceful breaths. If the patient vomits, roll them onto a side and suction before resuming ventilation.

ALS Assist

Prior to and during placement of an ET tube (a procedure performed by ALS clinicians), consider applying a nasal cannula and setting the flow rate at 15 L/min. This initiates the processes of preoxygenation and denitrogenation. **Denitrogenation** attempts to replace alveolar nitrogen with oxygen; the goal is to increase oxygen reserve in the lungs, thus minimizing the risk of oxygen desaturation during periods of forced apnea that will occur during the intubation attempt.

Words of Wisdom

Indications that positive-pressure ventilation is adequate:

- Visible and equal chest rise and fall with ventilation
- Ventilations delivered at the appropriate rate
  - 10 breaths/min for adults (in apneic patients with a pulse)
  - 20 to 30 breaths/min for infants and children (in apneic patients with a pulse)
  - In patients with ongoing CPR with an advanced airway in place, 1 breath every 6 seconds
- Heart rate returns to normal range
- Patient's color improves
- Oxygen saturation increases
- $ETCO_2$ values are improving

Automatic Transport Ventilator/Resuscitator

The **automatic transport ventilator (ATV)** is a ventilation device attached to a control box that allows the variables of ventilation (ie, rate and tidal volume) to be set (**FIGURE 11-51**). An EMT must be properly trained and credentialed by the medical director to use these devices. Furthermore, the ATV is almost always used in conjunction with an advanced airway device, usually an ET tube. Although some ATVs may not offer the same controls as a hospital ventilator, some are very advanced and are similar to a hospital ventilator but with a simpler interface; these devices free you to perform other tasks, such as maintaining a mask seal or ensuring continued patency of the airway. You can even perform non–airway-related tasks if the patient has an advanced airway in place and is being ventilated with the ATV. As recommended for all ventilators, always have a bag-mask device or a backup ventilator ready in case of mechanical malfunction.

Most models have adjustments for respiratory rate and tidal volume; more sophisticated models allow you to regulate the percentage of oxygen delivered to the patient and may offer a pressure cycle. In most cases, the respiratory rate is set at the midpoint or average for the patient's age. Tidal volume is usually estimated using the formula of 6 to 8 mL/kg of ideal body weight because ATVs are oxygen-powered and provide oxygen-enriched breathing gas. The tidal volume can be adjusted based on the patient's chest rise and physiologic response.

The ATV is generally oxygen-powered, although some models may require an external power source. Even though the ATV requires oxygen to run, in some cases it will consume as little as 5 L/min. In other cases, the consumed oxygen is the amount used by the patient only, considered a "zero drive" oxygen consumption. In comparison, a typical bag-mask device uses 15 to 25 L/min.

Compliance is the ability of the alveoli to expand when air is drawn in during inhalation. Poor lung compliance is the inability of the alveoli to fully expand during inhalation. When ventilating a patient, you would recognize this by noting an increase in resistance when you attempt to ventilate.

Whereas ATVs potentially leave you free to perform other tasks, constant reassessment of the patient is necessary. Damage to the tissue of the respiratory organs caused by the increased pressure in the chest, known as barotrauma, can occur in patients being ventilated. Keep in mind the potentially negative effects of positive-pressure ventilation on cardiac output, as discussed earlier in the chapter.

Continuous Positive Airway Pressure

Continuous positive airway pressure (CPAP) is a noninvasive means of providing ventilatory support for patients experiencing respiratory distress. Many people with diagnosed obstructive sleep apnea wear a CPAP unit at night to maintain their airway while they sleep (**FIGURE 11-52**). CPAP in the prehospital environment has proven to be an excellent adjunct in the treatment of respiratory failure associated with COPD, acute pulmonary edema, and acute bronchospasm (such as in asthma). In asthma and COPD, it is used in conjunction with bronchodilator medications (eg, albuterol).[16] Many of these patients would have otherwise been managed with advanced airway techniques, such as ET intubation.[17,18] Early intervention with CPAP is an alternative means of providing ventilatory support to patients; it helps to decrease overall morbidity and mortality, and it can prevent the need to

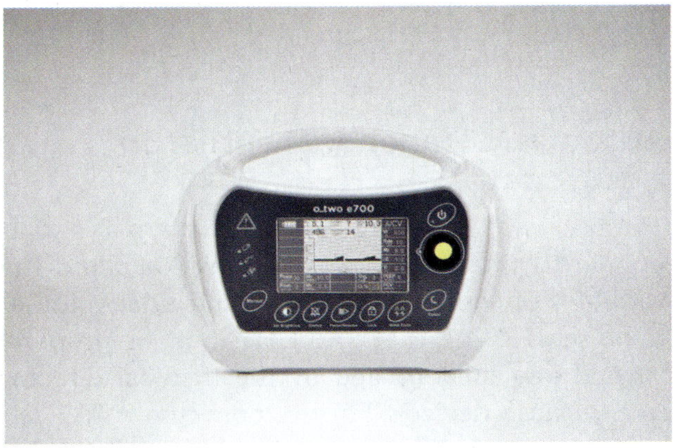

FIGURE 11-51 Automatic transport ventilator.

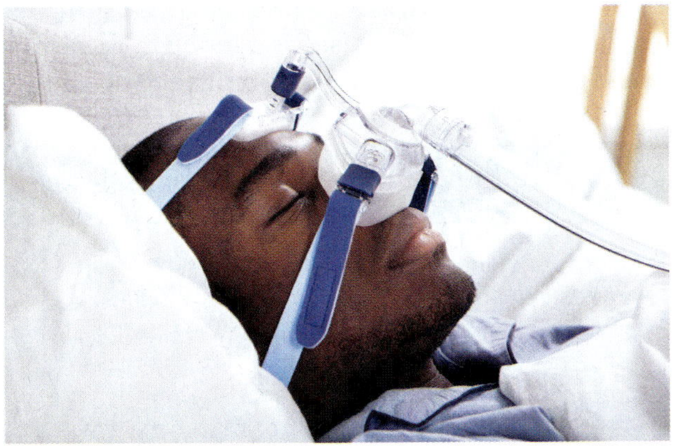

FIGURE 11-52 Many people with diagnosed obstructive sleep apnea wear a continuous positive airway pressure unit at night to maintain their airway while they sleep.

intubate the patient. Because of the simplicity of the device and its great benefit to the patient, CPAP is widely used at the EMT level. Follow your local protocols regarding the use of CPAP in your agency or department.

Safety Tips

CPAP systems without viral filters may increase the risk of aerosolization of secretions, which may increase the risk of these patients transmitting certain diseases, such as COVID-19 or tuberculosis, to people around them when they sleep.

Mechanism

CPAP works through the following mechanisms:

- Decreases the work of breathing
- Increases pressure in the lungs
- Opens collapsed alveoli and prevents further alveolar collapse (atelectasis), a process called alveolar recruitment
- Pushes more oxygen across the alveolar membrane
- Forces interstitial fluid back into the pulmonary circulation

The desired effect of CPAP is to improve pulmonary compliance and make spontaneous ventilation easier for the patient. The therapy is delivered through a mask that is held to the face with a strapping system. A good seal with minimal leakage between the face and mask is essential.

Many CPAP systems use oxygen as the driving force to deliver the positive-pressure ventilation to the patient. Frequently check the oxygen regulator when administering CPAP; depending on the flow and the patient's respiratory rate, some CPAP units can empty a D cylinder in under 15 minutes, depending on the oxygen flow rate.[19]

The CPAP device is fitted with a valve that determines the amount of pressure that is maintained throughout the respiratory cycle. During exhalation, this pressure helps to keep the alveoli open. The CPAP unit's pressure setting typically ranges between 5 and 20 cm H_2O. The CPAP protocol in most EMS agencies ranges from 5 to 10 cm H_2O.[20] As the patient breathes against this pressure, positive pressure is redirected to the lower airway, thereby recruiting more alveoli. Therefore, patients benefit the most from CPAP during exhalation rather than inhalation. The effect of CPAP is similar to hanging your head out the window while driving on the highway. In order to exhale, you must first overcome the high inspiratory flow created by the fast-moving air. Although this may appear to require a great deal of effort on the part of a patient who is already in distress, many patients improve dramatically when CPAP is applied.

YOU are the EMT

Transport to the hospital is initiated. One of the EMTs from the fire squad accompanies you in the back of the ambulance. En route, you note that the patient's abdomen has become somewhat distended, although bag-mask ventilation is still adequate. After reassessing the patient, you call in your report to the ED.

Recording Time: 12 Minutes	
Level of consciousness	Unresponsive
Respirations	6 breaths/min and irregular (baseline); 10 breaths/min (assisted)
Pulse	50 beats/min, bounding
Skin	Baseline color, warm, and dry
Blood pressure	172/98 mm Hg
Oxygen saturation (Spo_2)	97% (with assisted ventilation and high-flow oxygen)

8. Would you expect a hypoventilating patient's $ETCO_2$ level to be low, normal, or high? Why?
9. How can gastric distention interfere with bag-mask ventilation?

Because CPAP increases pressure inside the chest, it reduces the amount of blood flow returning to the heart. As the pressure in the thoracic cavity increases, venous blood returning to the heart meets the resistance of the increased pressure in the chest. The result is a decrease in the preload of the heart and a drop in cardiac output. This is not common with lower levels of CPAP; however, caution should be used when considering CPAP in patients with low blood pressure. Continually monitor blood pressure in patients receiving CPAP treatment.

Indications

CPAP is indicated for patients experiencing respiratory distress in which their own compensatory mechanisms are not enough to keep up with their oxygen demand (ie, respiratory failure). Whereas most patients improve after the application of CPAP, it is important to remember that CPAP is merely treating the symptoms and not the underlying pathology.

The following are general indications for using CPAP:

- Patient is alert and able to follow commands.
- Patient is displaying obvious signs of moderate to severe respiratory distress (eg, accessory muscle use, tripod position, retractions) from an underlying pathology, such as pulmonary edema, obstructive pulmonary disease (ie, COPD), or bronchospasm.
- Respiratory distress occurs after a submersion incident.
- Patient is breathing so rapidly that it affects overall minute volume.
- Pulse oximetry reading is less than 90%.

Although these guidelines should be considered when assessing the need for CPAP, it is important that you follow your local guidelines and protocols.

Contraindications

The following are general contraindications for CPAP use:

- Patient is in respiratory arrest or has agonal respirations.
- Patient is hypoventilating (slow respiratory rate and/or reduced tidal volume).
- Patient cannot speak.
- Patient is unresponsive or otherwise unable to follow verbal commands.
- Patient cannot protect their own airway.
- Patient has hypotension (systolic blood pressure less than 90 mm Hg).
- Signs and symptoms of a pneumothorax or chest trauma are present.
- Patient has a tracheostomy.
- Active gastrointestinal bleeding, nausea, or vomiting is present.
- Patient has experienced facial trauma.
- Patient is in cardiogenic shock.
- Patient cannot sit upright.
- CPAP system mask and strap cannot be properly fit.
  - Excessive facial hair, lack of teeth, or dysmorphic facial features can impede your ability to ensure a properly fitting mask.
  - Various mask sizes are available for smaller patients.
- Patient cannot tolerate the mask.

In addition to these contraindications, always reassess the patient for signs of deterioration and/or respiratory failure. CPAP is an excellent tool to improve ventilation; however, not all patients will improve with this therapy. Once signs of respiratory failure worsen or the patient is no longer able to follow commands, remove CPAP from the patient, and initiate positive-pressure ventilation with a bag-mask device attached to high-flow oxygen.

Application

Most CPAP devices used in the prehospital setting are disposable and connect directly to an oxygen source; less commonly you may encounter a CPAP unit that is powered by a mechanical ventilator. This discussion focuses on disposable devices, which are far more common in EMS. The CPAP device contains a mask, a circuit with corrugated tubing, a viral/bacterial filter, and a connected pressure valve. The continuous flow of oxygen creates resistance throughout the respiratory cycle. This resistance creates a back pressure into the airways that pushes open the smaller airway structures, such as bronchioles and alveoli, as the patient exhales. In many systems the amount of pressure can be determined by adjusting the pressure valve. A pressure of 7 to 10 cm H_2O is generally an acceptable therapeutic range for a patient on CPAP. Always consult the operations manual of any CPAP device for proper assembly instructions.

Because disposable CPAP units are powered by a continuous flow of oxygen, it is important to have a full cylinder of oxygen when using CPAP and to continuously monitor the amount of available oxygen in the cylinder. Some newer CPAP devices allow the clinician to adjust the percentage of oxygen delivered to the patient, called the fraction of inspired oxygen (FIO_2), from between 30% to as high as 95%. Older devices are set to deliver a fixed FIO_2 of 30% to 35%.

Most CPAP devices permit the EMT to attach a nebulizer to administer bronchodilator medications. This capability is useful when treating patients who have asthma or COPD and are wheezing at the time the CPAP is being delivered.

As noted earlier, CPAP therapy can deplete a full D cylinder of oxygen in a very short time, depending on the FIO_2 setting. Therefore, proper planning for oxygen consumption is necessary when considering applying CPAP.

Follow the steps in **SKILL DRILL 11-9** to use CPAP:

1. Take standard precautions. Assess the patient for indications and contraindications of CPAP. Confirm the patient's blood pressure, explain the procedure to the patient, and prepare the device for assembly (**Step 1**).
2. Connect the face mask to the corrugated circuit tubing (**Step 2**).
3. Connect the tubing to the oxygen tank and ensure that oxygen is flowing from the device (**Step 3**).
4. Place the patient in a high Fowler position to facilitate breathing, and coach the patient through the initial application of the mask. Instruct the patient to place the mask over the mouth and nose, creating the most airtight seal possible (**Step 4**). Allowing the patient to hold the mask to their face initially may help reduce some of the stress and anxiety associated with the application of CPAP; however, some patients may resist application of the mask while in severe respiratory distress.
5. After the mask is placed on the face and the patient adjusts to it, use the strapping mechanism to secure it to the patient's head. Ensure the seal between the mask and face remains

Skill Drill 11-9 Using CPAP

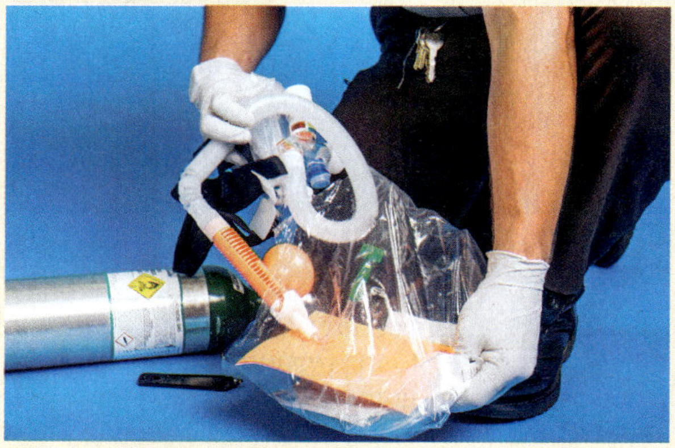

Step 1

Take standard precautions. Assess the patient for indications and contraindications of CPAP. Confirm the patient's blood pressure, explain the procedure to the patient, and prepare the device for assembly.

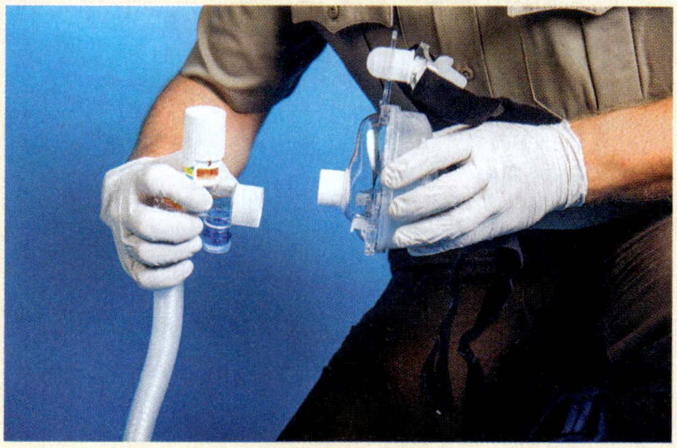

Step 2

Connect the face mask to the corrugated circuit tubing.

(continues)

Skill Drill 11-9 Using CPAP continued

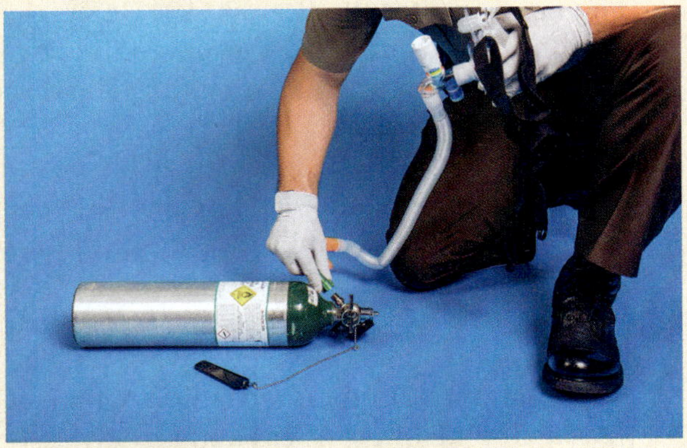

Step 3

Connect the tubing to the oxygen tank and ensure that oxygen is flowing from the device.

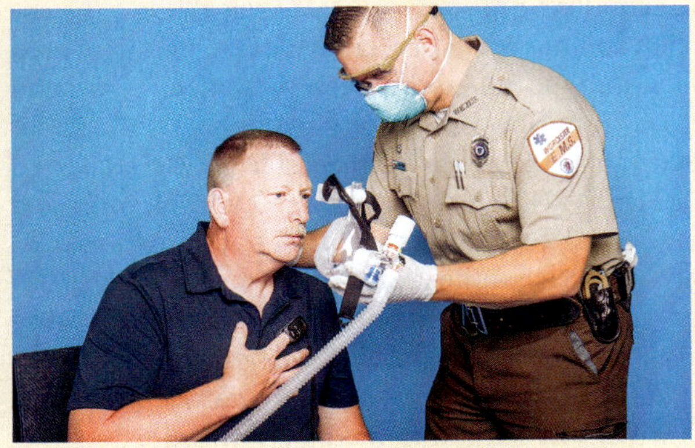

Step 4

Place the patient in a high Fowler position to facilitate breathing, and coach the patient through the initial application of the mask. Instruct the patient to place the mask over the mouth and nose, creating the most airtight seal possible.

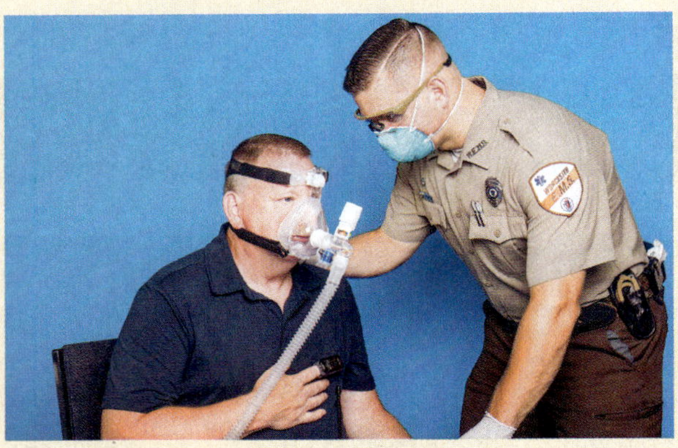

Step 5

After the mask is placed on the face and the patient adjusts to it, use the strapping mechanism to secure it to the patient's head. Ensure the seal between the mask and face remains intact.

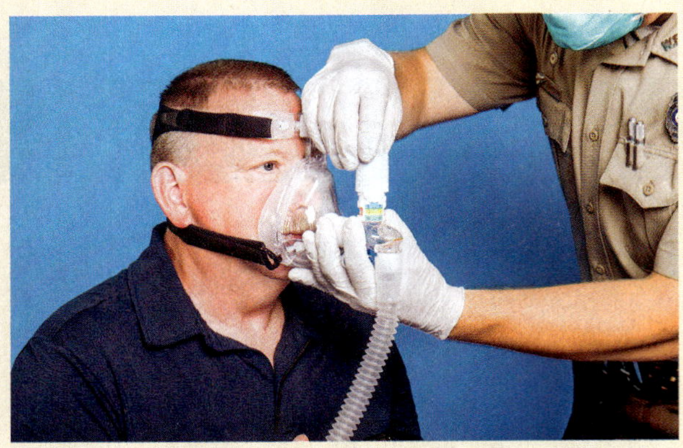

Step 6

Adjust the pressure control valve and the F_{IO_2} according to the manufacturer's recommendations to maintain adequate oxygenation and ventilation. With CPAP in place, the patient's oxygenation saturation level should improve, the work of breathing should decrease, and the ability to speak should improve. Constantly reassess the patient for signs of clinical deterioration and/or complications (eg, pneumothorax, hypotension).

intact (**Step 5**). Consult the manufacturer's guidelines for specific strapping instructions.

6. Adjust the pressure control valve and the FIO_2 according to the manufacturer's recommendations to maintain adequate oxygenation and ventilation. With CPAP in place, the patient's oxygenation saturation level should improve, the work of breathing should decrease, and the ability to speak should improve. Constantly reassess the patient for signs of clinical deterioration and/or complications (eg, pneumothorax, hypotension) (**Step 6**).

Complications

The application and administration of CPAP is a relatively easy process. However, some patients may find CPAP claustrophobic and will resist the application. As patients become more hypoxic, the application of a mask to their face is sometimes perceived as suffocation, rather than helping them breathe. In any event, it is important to explain the application to patients and coach them through the process. Do not force the mask on patients. This will create a higher level of anxiety and increase their oxygen demand. Coach patients through the application of CPAP, allowing them to adjust to the situation. Coaching patients is not always an easy task; it takes practice and a willingness to work closely with your patient during a difficult time.

Due to the high volume of pressure generated by CPAP, there is the possibility of causing a pneumothorax. Although the medical literature suggests that this is highly unlikely, you should be aware of this risk and continually assess your patients for signs and symptoms of a pneumothorax.

Due to the tight fit of the mask, aspiration can occur if the patient vomits. Monitor the patient continuously.

In addition to pneumothorax, high pressure in the chest can lower a patient's blood pressure. As the intrathoracic pressure increases, venous blood returning to the heart meets resistance from the increased pressure in the chest. This can result in hypotension. Although this is not common with lower levels of CPAP, continuous monitoring of blood pressure is necessary.

CPAP has consistently shown positive results with patients experiencing moderate and severe respiratory distress; however, there are still cases in which patients deteriorate. It is important that you reassess the patient for signs of deterioration. If the patient is no longer able to follow verbal commands and/or goes into respiratory failure/arrest, you must act quickly to remove CPAP and begin positive-pressure ventilation using a bag-mask device attached to high-flow oxygen.

Stomas and Tracheostomy Tubes

A **tracheostomy** is a surgical procedure that creates a stoma, or opening, through the patient's anterior neck. The stoma connects the trachea directly to the skin (**FIGURE 11-53**). This provides a pathway directly into the trachea where a **tracheostomy tube** may be placed to maintain a patent airway (**FIGURE 11-54**).

Tracheostomy tubes are generally placed in patients who have had a laryngectomy (surgical removal of the larynx) or who require long-term mechanical ventilation, require frequent tracheal suctioning, or have recurrent pulmonary infections due to the inability to adequately control oral and airway secretions. The tracheostomy may be permanent or temporary, depending on the condition that required its placement. Because these tubes

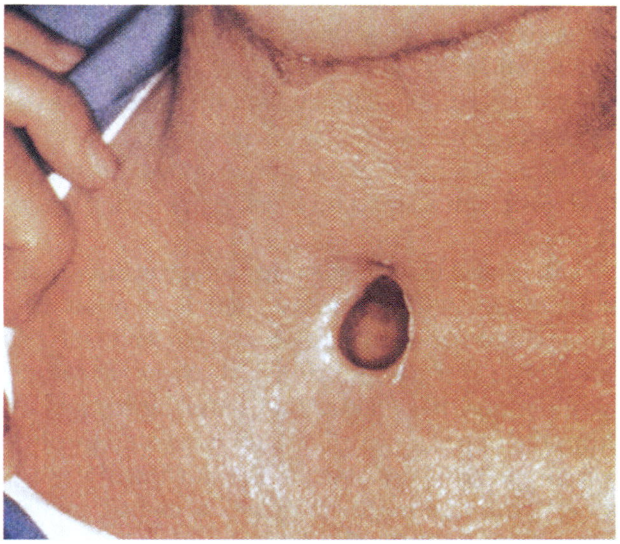

FIGURE 11-53 A tracheal stoma is typically located in the midline of the neck. The midline opening is the only one that can be used to ventilate the patient.

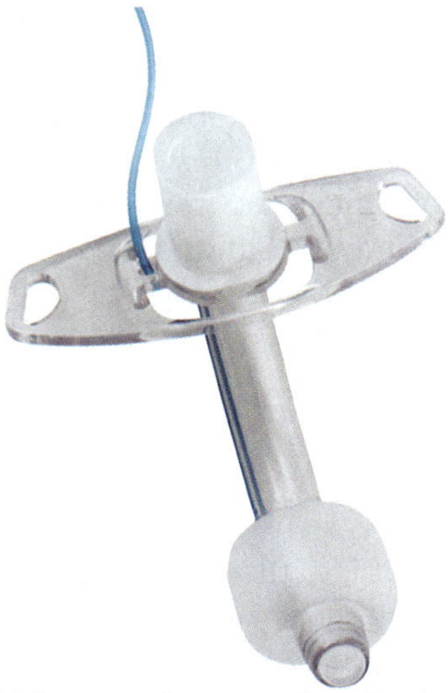

FIGURE 11-54 Some patients require a tracheostomy tube to breathe.

Portex® Blue Line® Ultra Tracheostomy courtesy of Smiths Medical.

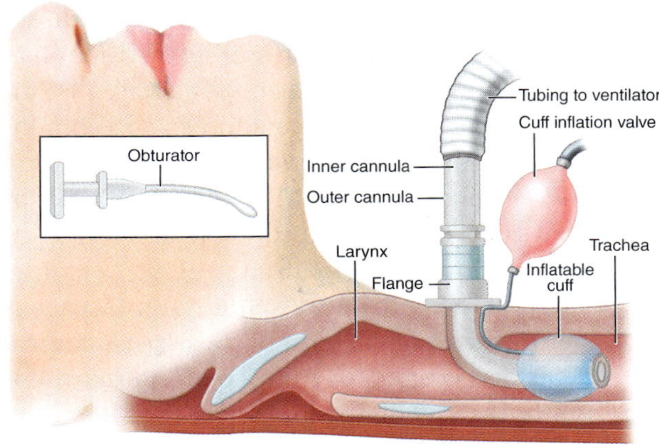

FIGURE 11-55 A tracheostomy is a surgical procedure in which an opening is placed in the trachea below the cricoid ring. A tracheostomy tube can be inserted into the opening (stoma) to maintain it. The tube can also be attached to a mechanical ventilator or bag-mask device to assist with ventilations.

are foreign to the respiratory tract, the body reacts by building up secretions in and around the tube. At times the secretions are thick and dry because the humidifying effects of the upper airway are lost. Therefore, they are susceptible to obstruction by mucus plugs or foreign bodies. Routine care that is provided by caregivers includes keeping the inner cannula of the tracheostomy tube clean and dry and suctioning any secretions.

Some patients who have a tracheostomy tube in place may be dependent on a mechanical ventilator. Almost all patients with a tracheostomy tube can still be ventilated manually with a bag-mask device, either attached to the tracheostomy tube itself, with a small mask over the stoma, or over the mouth and nose with a standard mask if the upper airway is intact.

The standard tracheostomy tube has three main components (**FIGURE 11-55**). There is an outer cannula with a flange that helps support and stabilize the device as it passes through the neck. The outer cannula may have a cuff that seals the trachea off from the upper airway. This cuff is inflated through a pilot balloon and valve on the outside of the device. Within the outer cannula is a slightly smaller inner cannula through which the patient is ventilated. The inner cannula has a 15-mm adaptor that allows for a bag-mask device or mechanical ventilator circuit to be attached. Most, but not all, inner cannulas are capable of being removed for cleaning or in case a mucus plug has developed. The final component of a tracheostomy tube setup is a rigid obturator. This blunt-tipped (rounded) device is curved and long enough to reach the distal end of the outer cannula. It is used when reinserting the flexible inner cannula. It may also be used to occlude the tracheostomy tube when ventilations are being provided by mask over the nose and mouth during an emergency. Some patients use a valve attached to the end of the tracheostomy to help them speak. This valve needs to be removed to suction or ventilate through the tracheostomy (**FIGURE 11-56**).

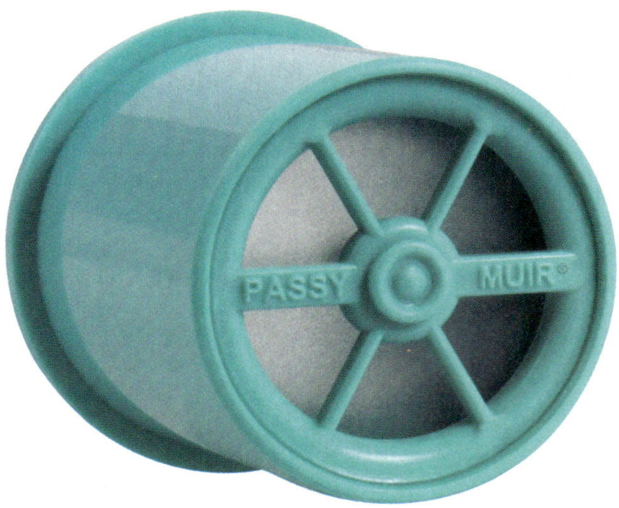

FIGURE 11-56 Speaking valve.

Image courtesy of Passy-Muir, Inc. Irvine, CA.

Words of Wisdom

The tracheostomy opening provides a direct pathway into the respiratory tract. Emergency tracheostomy care is an AGP. The EMT should wear eye protection and a face mask. If the patient is suspected of having a communicable respiratory disease, additional PPE such as an N95 mask, an APR, or a PAPR and gown are needed.

An obstructed tracheostomy tube is an emergency that requires immediate intervention. This type of emergency can be stressful. A useful mnemonic in these situations is DOPE:

- **D** Displaced, dislodged, or damaged tube
- **O** Obstructed tube (secretions, blood, mucus, vomitus)
- **P** Pneumothorax
- **E** Equipment failure (kinked tubing, ventilator malfunction, empty oxygen supply)

The DOPE mnemonic facilitates troubleshooting a problem with the tracheostomy so that it can be rapidly corrected. Failure to clear an obstructed tracheostomy tube could lead to cardiopulmonary arrest.

There may be bleeding or air leaking around the tube. This is more likely to happen with new tracheostomies. The tube can become loose or dislodged. Occasionally, the opening around the tube may become infected. Your care of the patient with a tracheostomy tube includes maintaining airway patency, placing the patient in a position of comfort, administering supplemental oxygen as needed, and providing transport to the hospital.

Some patients with tracheostomy tubes and special health care needs may have muscle contractions that will not allow you to place them in the typical semi-Fowler position; in these cases, suction the tracheostomy tube with the patient in a position of comfort. If trauma is involved, protect the cervical spine.

If suctioning of the tracheostomy tube is necessary, first attempt to use the patient's suction device. It is probably already sized correctly and readily available. If the size of the suction catheter is unknown, estimate the size by doubling the inner diameter of the tracheostomy tube. To determine the length of the suction tubing, ask a family member or measure the length of a spare tracheostomy tube. If the length of the patient's tracheostomy tube cannot be determined, insert the suction catheter no more than 1 to 2 inches (3 to 6 cm) deep. The suction unit should be set to 100 mm Hg. You may need to instill 2 to 3 mL of sterile saline before suctioning thick tracheal secretions. Do not suction for more than 10 seconds, and do not force the suction catheter into the cannula. Oxygenate before and after the procedure. Call for ALS backup.

Words of Wisdom

If a tracheostomy tube becomes plugged, ask the caregiver to remove the tube and reinsert a new one. Their spare tracheostomy tube should slide into the existing stoma once lubricated. Caregivers should be trained to do this and should have spare tracheostomy tubes in a "go bag" with the patient. They may need your encouragement to do so but it can be lifesaving. You can assist them by placing a folded towel under the patient's shoulders to make the tracheostomy more accessible. A completely obstructed tracheostomy tube results in hypoxia and leads to cardiac arrest if not corrected quickly. When you are providing an ALS assist, the paramedic may ask you for a small ET tube if there is no spare tracheostomy tube available to reinsert in the stoma.

Foreign Body Airway Obstruction

A foreign body that *completely* blocks the airway in a patient is a true emergency that will result in death if not treated immediately. In an adult, sudden foreign body airway obstruction usually occurs during a meal. In a child, it occurs while eating, playing with small toys, or crawling around the house. An otherwise healthy child who has sudden difficulty breathing should be assumed to have a foreign body airway obstruction.

The most common airway obstruction in an unconscious patient is the tongue, which relaxes and falls back against the posterior pharynx. There are other causes of airway obstruction that do not involve foreign bodies in the airway. These include swelling from infection, acute allergic reaction, and trauma (tissue damage from injury). With airway obstruction from medical conditions such as infection and acute allergic reactions, repeated attempts to clear the airway as if there were a foreign body will be unsuccessful and potentially dangerous. These patients require specific emergency medical care for their condition. In the case of anaphylaxis, epinephrine should be administered urgently. In other medical conditions, rapid transport to the hospital is critical.

Recognition

Early recognition of airway obstruction is crucial in providing effective emergency medical care. Obstruction from a foreign body can result in a **mild airway obstruction** or a **severe airway obstruction**.

Patients with a mild airway obstruction are still able to exchange air but will have varying degrees of respiratory distress. Great care must be taken to prevent a mild airway obstruction from becoming a severe airway obstruction. The patient will usually have noisy breathing and may be coughing. Assess the patient and determine whether the patient has **good air exchange** or **poor air exchange**.

With good air exchange, the patient can cough forcefully, although you may hear **wheezing** (the production of whistling sounds during breathing) between coughs. Wheezing is usually indicative of a mild lower airway obstruction. If the patient can breathe effectively, cough forcefully, or talk, you should not interfere with the patient's efforts to expel the foreign object on their own. Continue to monitor the patient closely and encourage the patient to continue coughing. Abdominal thrusts are not indicated for a patient with a mild airway obstruction and good air exchange. Attempts to remove the object manually could force the object farther down into the airway and cause a severe airway obstruction. Continually reassess the patient's condition and be prepared to provide treatment if the air exchange becomes poor or a mild obstruction becomes a severe obstruction.

With poor air exchange, the patient has a weak, ineffective (not forceful) cough and severe difficulty breathing, **stridor** (a high-pitched noise heard on inspiration), and cyanosis. Stridor is an indication of an upper airway obstruction. You must quickly recognize this situation and provide immediate care.

For patients with mild airway obstruction with poor air exchange, treat immediately as if there is a severe airway obstruction.

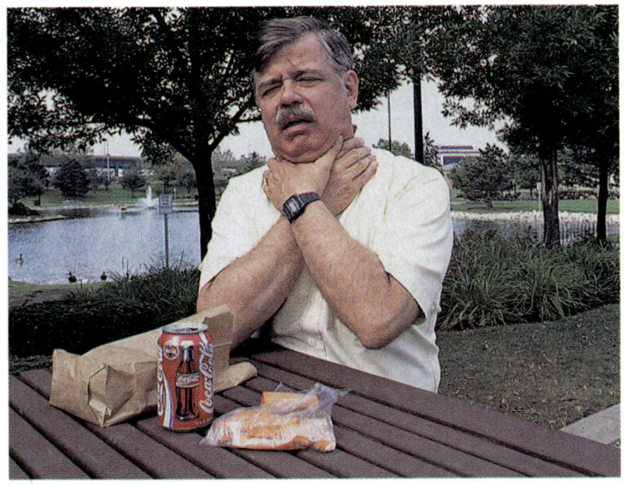

FIGURE 11-57 The universal sign of choking is a person who grasps the throat and has difficulty breathing.

Patients with a severe airway obstruction cannot breathe, talk, or cough. One sure sign of a severe obstruction is the sudden inability to speak or cough during or immediately after eating. The person may clutch or grasp the throat (universal distress signal), start to become cyanotic, and have extreme difficulty breathing (**FIGURE 11-57**). There is little or no air movement. Ask the conscious patient, "Are you choking?" If the patient nods "yes," provide immediate treatment. If the obstruction is not cleared quickly, the amount of oxygen in the patient's blood will decrease dramatically. If not treated, the patient will become unconscious and die.

Some patients with a severe airway obstruction will be unconscious when you arrive and perform your initial assessment. You may not know that an airway obstruction is the cause of their condition. There are many other causes of unconsciousness and respiratory failure, including stroke, heart failure, trauma, seizures, and drug overdose. A complete and thorough patient assessment by you, therefore, is essential to providing appropriate emergency medical care.

If the patient is found unresponsive, does not appear to be breathing, and does not have a pulse, begin CPR with high-quality chest compressions. When you open the airway and attempt two ventilations following chest compressions, it will be obvious to you if the airway is blocked (**FIGURE 11-58**). The compressions may have been enough to clear the airway; however, if you are unable to ventilate the patient after several attempts (no chest rise and fall) or you feel resistance while ventilating, consider the possibility of an airway obstruction. Resistance to ventilation can also be due to poor lung compliance. As discussed, compliance is the ability of the alveoli to expand when air is drawn in during inhalation; poor lung compliance is the inability of the alveoli to fully expand during inhalation.

Emergency Medical Care for Foreign Body Airway Obstruction

Perform the head tilt–chin lift maneuver to clear an obstruction that has been caused by the tongue and throat muscles relaxing back into the airway in any person who is found unconscious. This should be performed on unresponsive patients with adequate or inadequate breathing who are not suspected of having spinal trauma. If spinal trauma is suspected, open the airway with the jaw-thrust maneuver. Large pieces of vomited food, mucus, loose dentures, or blood clots in the mouth should be swept forward and out of the mouth with your gloved index finger. Use suction to clear the airway of thinner secretions.

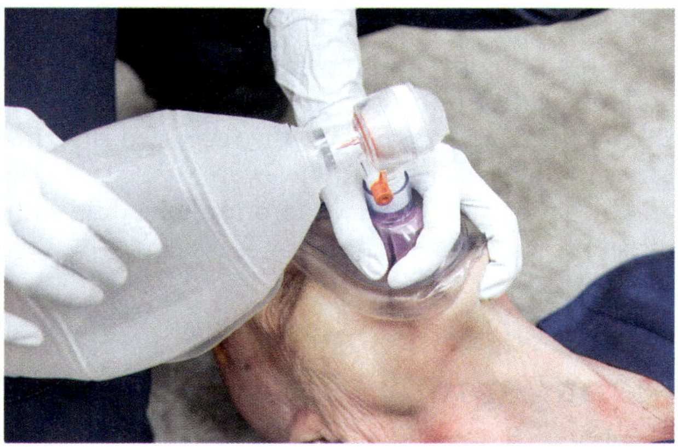

FIGURE 11-58 When you open the airway and attempt ventilations, it will be obvious to you if the airway is blocked.

Alternating between five back slaps and five abdominal thrusts is the most effective method of dislodging and forcing an object out of the airway of a conscious adult or child (age 1 year and older). Residual air, which is always present in the lungs, is compressed upward and used to expel the object. Use back slaps and abdominal thrusts until the object dislodges or the patient becomes unconscious. If a conscious infant is choking, alternate between five backslaps and five chest thrusts (**TABLE 11-8**).

For the unresponsive patient with a severe foreign body airway obstruction, reassess to confirm apnea and inability to ventilate. Begin chest compressions just as you would for CPR. At the completion of the 30 compressions, perform a tongue-jaw lift by grasping the jaw with your thumb and index finger. Place your thumb onto the tip of the patient's lower teeth and tongue while placing your index finger under the bony portion of the chin. Be careful not to compress the soft tissues under the chin. Pull the jaw/mouth open and look at the back of the oropharynx for any foreign objects. If an object is observed, carefully remove it with a gloved index finger or suction. Attempt to remove an object only if it is visible during examination of the open mouth; blind sweeps of the back of the oropharynx may push an object farther down in the airway, making the obstruction worse. If the object is removed, attempt to

TABLE 11-8 Steps to Relieve Foreign Body Airway Obstruction in a Conscious Patient

Adults and Teenagers	Children (1 Year to Puberty)	Infants (Younger than 1 Year)
1. Ask, "Can you speak?"	**1.** Ask, "Can you speak?"	**1.** Conscious infant is not making any sound or breathing and suspected to have choked.
2. Perform five back slaps followed by five abdominal thrusts (chest thrusts if the patient is pregnant or has obesity).	**2.** Perform five back slaps followed by five abdominal thrusts.	**2.** Perform up to five back slaps, followed by up to five chest thrusts.
3. Repeat step 2 until the obstruction is relieved or the patient loses consciousness.	**3.** Repeat step 2 until the obstruction is relieved or the patient loses consciousness.	**3.** Repeat step 2 until the obstruction is relieved or the infant loses consciousness.

Data from *Basic Life Support Provider Manual*. American Heart Association; 2020.

ventilate. If no object was seen during the tongue-jaw lift, continue chest compressions.

If you are unable to clear a severe airway obstruction with your initial attempts, begin rapid transport and continue your efforts to relieve the obstruction with back slaps and abdominal thrusts (conscious patients) or chest compressions (unconscious patients) on the way to the hospital.

Remember to treat patients with a mild airway obstruction with poor air exchange as if they have a severe airway obstruction.

Patients with a mild airway obstruction and good air exchange should be monitored closely for deterioration of their condition. If the patient is unable to clear the obstruction and remains conscious, support (or let the patient control) the airway position that is most efficient and comfortable. Provide supplemental oxygen, and transport to the hospital.

Words of Wisdom

If spinal trauma is suspected, open the airway using the jaw-thrust maneuver.

Dental Appliances

Many dental appliances can cause an airway obstruction. If a dental appliance, such as a crown or bridge, dentures, or even a piece or section of braces, has become loose, manually remove it before providing ventilations. Simple manual removal may relieve the obstruction and allow the patient to breathe on their own.

Providing bag-mask or mouth-to-mask ventilation is usually much easier when dentures can be left in place. Leaving the dentures in place provides more structure to the face and will generally assist you in being able to provide a good face-to-mask seal, thus delivering adequate tidal volume. However, loose dentures make it difficult to perform artificial ventilation by any method and can easily obstruct the airway. Therefore, dentures and dental appliances that do not stay in place should be removed. Dentures and appliances may become loose or be completely out of place following trauma or as you are providing care. Periodically reassess the patient's airway to make sure these devices are firmly in place. If dentures become dislodged, place them in a container and transport with the patient, if possible.

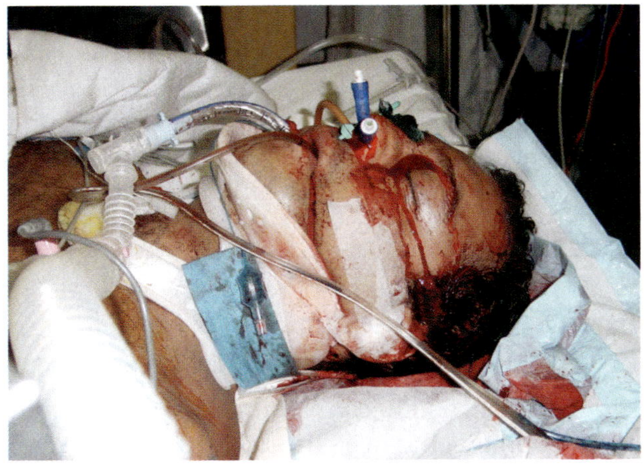

FIGURE 11-59 Airway problems can be especially challenging in patients with serious facial injuries.

Courtesy of Dr. Ken Harrison, Careflight/NSW Institute of Trauma & Injury Management.

Facial Bleeding

Airway problems can be especially challenging in patients with serious facial injuries (**FIGURE 11-59**). Because the blood supply to the face is so rich, injuries to the face can result in severe tissue swelling and bleeding into the airway. Control bleeding with direct pressure and suction as necessary.

Pediatric Airway Management

Respiratory failure is the leading cause of cardiopulmonary arrest in the pediatric population.[21] Failure to recognize and treat declining respiratory status will result in death. During respiratory distress, the child is working harder to breathe but still has the compensatory mechanisms needed to facilitate oxygen intake and carbon dioxide removal. Respiratory failure occurs when the patient has exhausted all compensatory mechanisms and waste products begin to collect. If respiratory failure is not treated, a total shutdown of the respiratory system (ie, respiratory arrest) will occur.

In the early stages of respiratory distress, you may note changes in the child's behavior, such as anxiety, restlessness, or combativeness. As the body attempts to maximize the amount of air going into the lungs, the work of breathing increases. Signs and symptoms of increased work of breathing include nasal flaring; abnormal breath sounds; grunting; retractions; seesaw breathing; use of accessory muscles of the neck, chest, or abdomen; and the tripod position.

As the pediatric patient progresses to possible respiratory failure, efforts to breathe decrease; inhalation becomes less effective, and the respiratory rate may slow. The body has used up its available energy stores and cannot continue to support the extra work of breathing under these conditions. At this point, without care, cyanosis may develop (a late sign). Be aware that not all pediatric patients develop cyanosis. You should be just as concerned about a child with pallor as one with cyanosis.

Changes in behavior will also occur until the patient demonstrates an altered level of consciousness. The child may experience periods of apnea. As the lack of oxygen becomes more serious, the heart muscle itself becomes hypoxic and slows down. This leads to bradycardia, which is almost always an ominous sign in children. If the heart rate is fast, you need to investigate the cause. However, if the heart rate is slow (less than 60 beats/min) despite bag-mask ventilation with high-flow oxygen, especially with signs of poor perfusion (eg, pallor, cyanosis, decreased level of consciousness), you must begin CPR immediately. Without aggressive airway management, bradycardia may quickly progress to cardiopulmonary arrest.

Of course, respiratory failure does not always indicate airway obstruction. It may indicate trauma, nervous system problems, dehydration (often caused by vomiting and diarrhea), or metabolic disturbances. For example, a pediatric patient who ingested an opioid may have inadequate, slow breathing, or a child might have a pH imbalance, as can happen with certain diseases. Regardless of the cause, your first step is always to ensure adequate oxygenation and ventilation.

A pediatric patient can progress from respiratory distress to respiratory failure very quickly. Therefore, continuous monitoring and reassessment are imperative. It is concerning if after oxygen is administered, oxygen saturation remains low.

A child or infant in respiratory distress needs supplemental oxygen and careful, continuous monitoring. To minimize anxiety, agitation, or crying, which may increase the effort or work of breathing, use whichever method seems least upsetting (ie, face mask, blow-by, or nasal cannula). If necessary, distract the child with games, a toy, or conversation. Allow the pediatric patient to remain in a comfortable position. A small child may be most comfortable sitting on the parent's or caregiver's lap. Ventilate the infant or child with a bag-mask device and 100% oxygen if signs of respiratory failure become apparent.

Give nothing by mouth if the patient has severe respiratory distress in case the patient's condition deteriorates suddenly. If the patient's condition progresses to respiratory failure, begin assisted ventilation immediately, and continue to provide supplemental oxygen.

Airway Adjuncts

In children with inadequate ventilation, an airway adjunct, such as an oropharyngeal or nasopharyngeal airway, may be needed to maintain an open airway while assisting their ventilations with a bag-mask device. Placing the adjuncts correctly starts with choosing the appropriate-size equipment. Many EMS agencies use pediatric resuscitation systems that include tools such as a color-coded, **length-based resuscitation tape** (eg, Broselow tape) or the Handtevy method to help EMS clinicians select the appropriate equipment for infants and children. It is essential to be properly trained to use these systems effectively. See Chapter 10, *Patient Assessment*, for a description of these methods.

Oropharyngeal Airway

An oropharyngeal airway should be used for pediatric patients who are unconscious and in respiratory failure. This adjunct should not be used in either conscious pediatric patients or those who have a gag reflex. In addition, this adjunct should not be used in children who may have ingested a caustic or petroleum-based product because it may induce vomiting.

SKILL DRILL 11-10 shows the steps for inserting an oropharyngeal airway in a child:

1. Determine the appropriate-size airway by placing the airway next to the face with the flange at the level of the central incisors and the bite block segment parallel to the hard palate. The tip of the airway should reach the angle of the jaw (**Step 1**). Or, use your department's resuscitation system to determine the appropriate-size airway.
2. Position the pediatric patient's airway. If the emergency is medical, use the head tilt–chin lift maneuver. Avoid hyperextension; you may

Skill Drill 11-10 Inserting an Oropharyngeal Airway in a Pediatric Patient

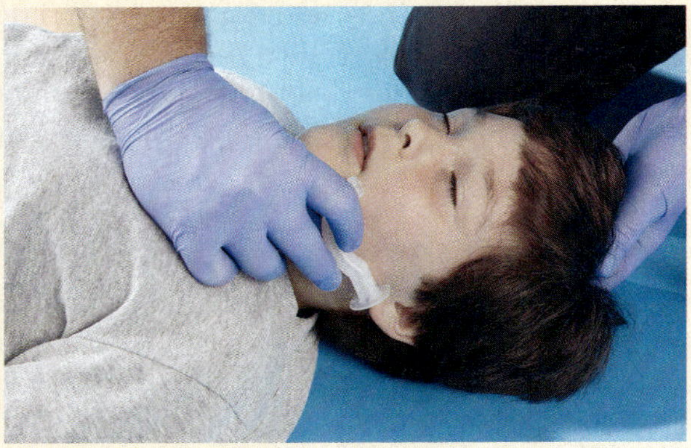

Step 1

Determine the appropriate-size airway. Confirm the correct size visually, by placing it next to the pediatric patient's face.

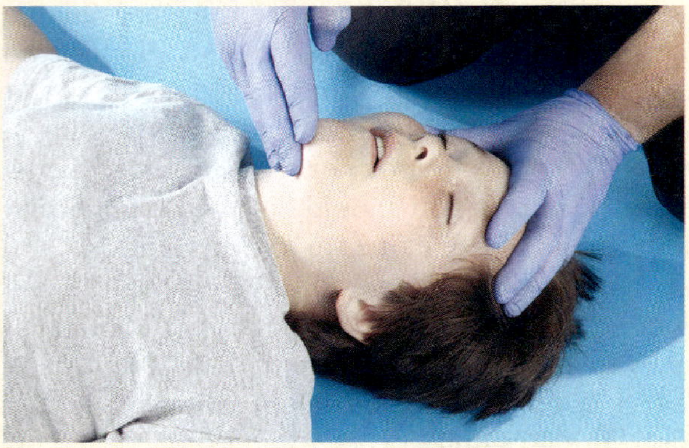

Step 2

Position the pediatric patient's airway using the appropriate method.

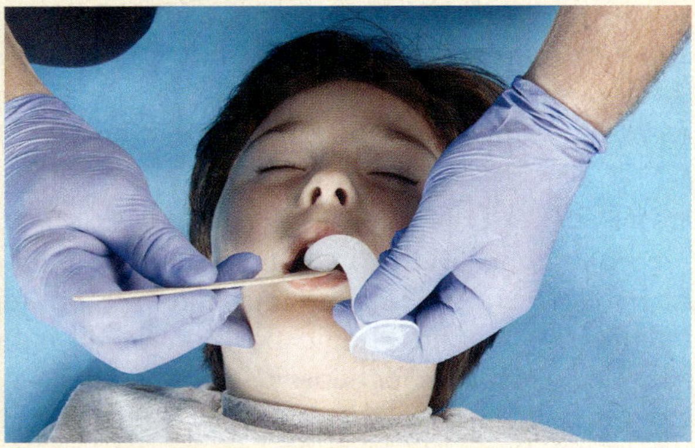

Step 3

Open the mouth by depressing the tongue with the tongue blade. Insert the airway until the flange rests against the lips. Reassess the airway.

place a towel under the child's shoulders. If the patient has a traumatic injury, use the jaw-thrust maneuver and provide manual in-line stabilization (**Step 2**).

3. Open the mouth by applying pressure on the chin with your thumb.
4. Insert the airway by depressing the tongue with a tongue blade applied to the base of the tongue and inserting the airway directly over the tongue blade (**Step 3**). Insert the airway until the flange rests against the lips.
5. Reassess the airway after insertion. Take care to avoid injuring the hard palate as you insert the airway. Rough insertion can cause bleeding, which can aggravate airway problems and may even cause vomiting. Note also that if the oropharyngeal airway is too large, it can push the tongue back into the pharynx, obstructing the airway. If the oropharyngeal airway is too small, it may become an airway obstruction itself.

Nasopharyngeal Airway

A nasopharyngeal airway is usually well tolerated and is not as likely as the oropharyngeal airway to cause vomiting. The nasopharyngeal airway can be used for children who are responsive or unresponsive. In pediatric patients, the nasopharyngeal airway is typically used in association with possible respiratory failure or after a seizure. It is rarely used in infants younger than 1 year.

A nasopharyngeal airway should not be used in pediatric patients with nasal obstruction, fracture of the nasal bone, facial fractures, or head trauma with fluid draining from the nose. In children with moderate to severe head trauma, the nasopharyngeal airway could increase intracranial pressure. The steps to insert the nasopharyngeal airway in a child are the same as for the adult (see Skill Drill 11-6).

As with the oropharyngeal airway, there can be problems with the nasopharyngeal airway. An airway with a small diameter may easily become obstructed by mucus, blood, vomitus, or the soft tissues of the pharynx. If the airway is too long, it may stimulate the vagus nerve and slow the heart rate or enter the esophagus, causing gastric distention. Inserting the airway in responsive patients may cause a spasm of the larynx and result in vomiting. Nasopharyngeal airways should not be used when pediatric patients have facial trauma because the device may tear soft tissues and cause bleeding into the airway.

Oxygen Delivery Devices

When treating infants and children who require more than the usual 21% oxygen found in room air, you have several options:

- Blow-by technique at 6 L/min provides more than 21% oxygen concentration.
- Simple face mask at 6 to 10 L/min provides 35% to 60% oxygen concentration.
- Nasal cannula at 1 to 6 L/min provides 24% to 44% oxygen concentration.
- Nonrebreathing mask at 10 to 15 L/min provides up to 95% oxygen concentration (unassisted ventilations).
- Bag-mask device (with oxygen reservoir) at 10 to 15 L/min provides up to 95% oxygen concentration (assisted ventilations), depending on tidal volume and pressure.

Pediatric patients need enough air to be delivered for adequate gas exchange in the lungs. Therefore, use of a nonrebreathing mask, a nasal cannula, or a simple face mask is indicated only for pediatric patients who have adequate tidal volume. The tidal volume is the amount of air that moves in or out of the respiratory tract in one breath. Children with a decreased level of consciousness who are breathing slower or faster for their age with inadequate tidal volume should receive assisted ventilation with a bag-mask device.

Blow-by oxygenation is a noncontact method of oxygen administration that is not as effective as a face mask or nasal cannula for delivering oxygen. In the blow-by technique, an oxygen tube or mask is held near the infant or child's nose and mouth. It is often used after childbirth to deliver a small amount of oxygen to the newborn. On rare occasions when other adjuncts cannot be used, the child will not tolerate any other oxygen administration device, or the child is feeding, this technique may be necessary, but only for infants or young children. Although the blow-by technique does not provide a reliable or high concentration of oxygen, it is better than no oxygen. Take the following steps to administer blow-by oxygen:

1. Connect a simple pediatric face mask to 10 L/min oxygen flow.
2. Hold the mask approximately 1 to 2 inches (2 to 5 cm) below the child's nose and mouth.[22]

Words of Wisdom

It is important to use the appropriate-size equipment to assess Spo_2 and $ETCO_2$ values, administer oxygen, or perform bag-mask ventilation on infants and children. Using adult equipment on an infant or small child can result in inaccurate assessment results and improper or inadequate oxygenation or ventilation.

Nasal Cannula

Some pediatric patients prefer the nasal cannula, whereas others find it uncomfortable. Take the following steps to apply a nasal cannula:

1. Choose the appropriate-size pediatric nasal cannula. The prongs should not fill the nares entirely (**FIGURE 11-60**). If the nares blanch, select a smaller cannula.
2. Connect the tubing to an oxygen source set at 1 to 6 L/min.

Nonrebreathing Mask

A properly applied nonrebreathing mask delivers up to 95% oxygen and allows the patient to

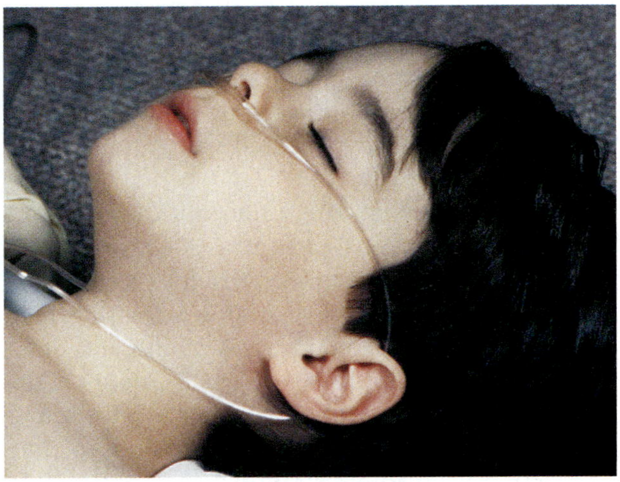

FIGURE 11-60 The prongs of a pediatric nasal cannula should not fill the nares entirely.

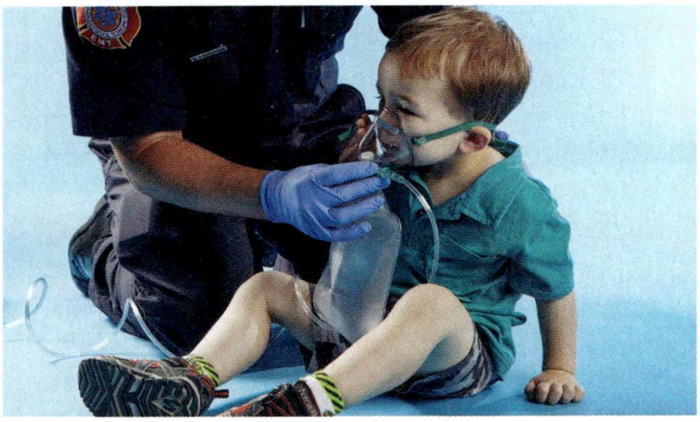

FIGURE 11-61 A pediatric nonrebreathing mask delivers up to 95% oxygen and allows the patient to exhale carbon dioxide without rebreathing it.

exhale all carbon dioxide without rebreathing it (**FIGURE 11-61**). Use the following steps to apply a nonrebreathing mask:

1. Select the appropriate-size pediatric nonrebreathing mask. The mask should extend from the bridge of the nose to the cleft of the chin.
2. Connect the tubing to an oxygen source set at 10 to 15 L/min.
3. Adjust oxygen flow as needed to match the pediatric patient's respiratory rate and depth. The reservoir bag should neither deflate completely nor fill to bulging during the respiratory cycle.

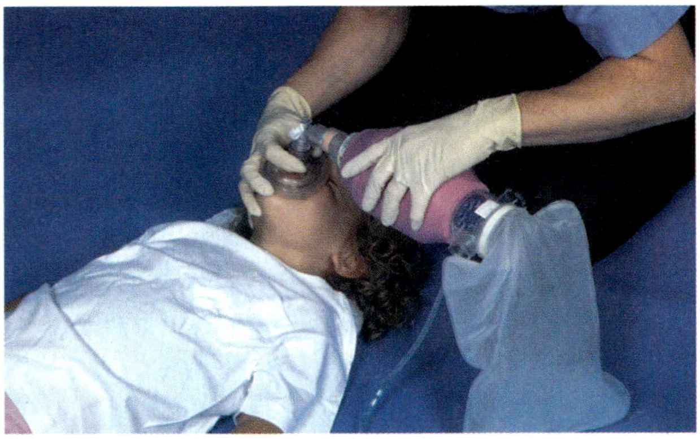

FIGURE 11-62 Proper mask size for bag-mask ventilation is critical. The mask should extend from the bridge of the nose to the cleft of the chin, avoiding compression of the eyes.

Bag-Mask Device

Ventilation with a bag-mask device is indicated for pediatric patients who are apneic or who have signs of respiratory failure, such as a decreased level of consciousness and fast or slow breathing with inadequate tidal volume.

Ventilate an infant or child using a bag-mask device in the following way:

1. Ensure that you have the appropriate-size equipment. The proper-size mask will extend from the bridge of the nose to the cleft of the chin, avoiding compression of the eyes (**FIGURE 11-62**). The mask is transparent, so you can observe for cyanosis and vomiting. In addition, mask volume should be small to decrease dead space and avoid rebreathing; however, the bag should contain at least 450 mL of air. Use an infant bag, not a neonatal bag, for infants younger than 1 year; use a pediatric bag for children older than 1 year. Older children and adolescents may need an adult bag. Make sure there is no pop-off valve on the bag; if the bag has a pop-off valve, make sure you can hold it shut as necessary to achieve chest rise. Proper mask size for bag-mask ventilation is critical.
2. Maintain a good seal with the mask on the face (**FIGURE 11-63**). With infants and toddlers, support the jaw with only your third fingertip. Be careful not to compress the area under the chin because you may push the tongue into the back of the mouth and block the airway.

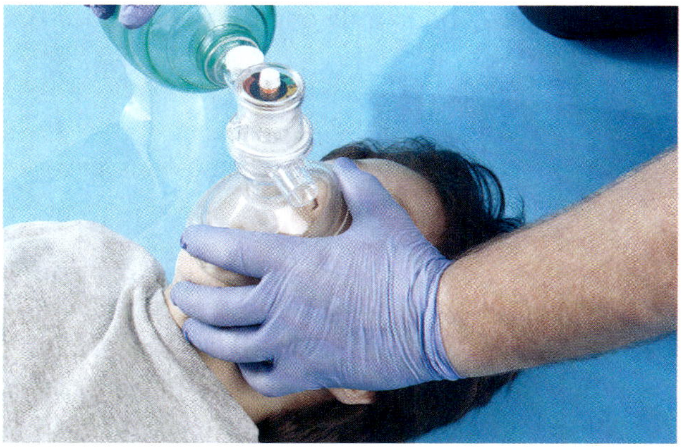

FIGURE 11-63 Hold the mask on the pediatric patient's face with a one-handed head tilt–chin life maneuver (EC-clamp method). Ensure a good mask-to-face seal while maintaining the airway.

3. Ventilate at the appropriate rate and volume using a slow, gentle squeeze, not a sharp, quick one. Stop squeezing and begin to release the bag as soon as the chest wall begins to rise. To keep from ventilating too rapidly, use the phrase "Squeeze, release, release." Say "Squeeze" as you squeeze the bag; when you see the chest start to rise, release pressure on the bag and slowly say "Release, release."

Words of Wisdom

One-person bag-mask device ventilation can be difficult, especially without regular practice. Errors in technique, such as providing too much volume with each breath, squeezing the bag too forcefully, or ventilating at a rate that is too fast, can result in gastric distention or overinflation of the lung, which may decrease cardiac output or result in a pneumothorax. An inadequate mask seal or improper head position can lead to hypoventilation or hypoxia.

Two-Person Bag-Mask Ventilation on a Pediatric Patient

As with adult patients, this procedure requires two EMTs: one to hold the mask to the pediatric patient's face and maintain the pediatric patient's head position, the other to ventilate the patient. This technique is usually more effective in maintaining a tight seal, as it provides an open airway due to proper body position.

Special Populations

AIR SWALLOWING IN THE PEDIATRIC PATIENT

One of the problems associated with abdominal injuries in children is the presence of air in the stomach. Pediatric patients, especially those who have had a traumatic injury, tend to swallow air when they cry. Air in the stomach can cause distention and increase the risk of vomiting. Air can also accumulate in the stomach with artificial ventilation, pushing upward on the diaphragm and making it harder to ventilate adequately.

Assisting With ALS Airway Procedures

Many EMTs work as a team with a paramedic partner. When a critical patient needs an advanced airway intervention, the paramedic will perform the skill, but the EMT partner will play an essential role in helping set up for the procedure, performing BLS airway and ventilation maneuvers, and helping to monitor the patient.

Assisting With Intubation

Endotracheal (ET) intubation is the insertion of a tube into the trachea to maintain and protect the airway. The ET tube can be inserted through the mouth or through the nose. In either case, the ET tube passes directly between the vocal cords and then into the trachea. You may also be asked to assist with the placement of other advanced airway devices.

Patient Preparation

The first step in preparing a patient for ET intubation is oxygenation. Good oxygenation often includes bag-mask ventilation (including the use of an oropharyngeal or nasopharyngeal airway) and ensuring a proper seal, ventilation rate, volume of ventilation, and time for patient exhalation. Oxygen enters the bloodstream through the process of diffusion. The more oxygen that is available in the alveoli, the longer the patient can maintain adequate gas exchange in the lungs while the intubation procedure is being performed. This critical phase of the intubation procedure is called **preoxygenation**.

During the preoxygenation phase, apply a nasal cannula to the patient and set the flow rate at 15 to

25 L/min. Leave the nasal cannula in place during the intubation attempt, during which bag-mask ventilation is not being performed. This technique, called **apneic oxygenation**, allows for continuous oxygen delivery down the airways during all phases of the intubation procedure.

Preoxygenation is a critical step in advanced airway management. Always follow your local protocols regarding the sequence of this procedure.

Equipment Setup

Equipment sets vary depending on local protocols, clinician preference, and whether **direct laryngoscopy** or **video laryngoscopy** will be used. Direct laryngoscopy is direct visualization of the vocal cords with a laryngoscope, whereas video laryngoscopy is visualization of the vocal cords using a video camera and monitor. These differences emphasize why it is important for team members to train and practice together. Typically, intubation equipment sets include the following:

- Personal protective equipment, including face mask and eye shield
- Suction unit with rigid, tonsil-tip (Yankauer or DuCanto) and nonrigid, whistle-tip (French) catheters
- Laryngoscope handle and blade (sized for the patient)
- Magill forceps
- ET tube (sized for the patient)
- Stylet or tube introducer (elastic bougie)
- Water-soluble lubricant
- 10-mL syringe
- Confirmation device, specifically a waveform $ETCO_2$ monitor (capnography)
- Commercial ET tube securing device
- Alternate airway management devices, such as a supraglottic airway and/or cricothyrotomy kit

Words of Wisdom

When assembling the intubation equipment, ensure that the ET tube is properly shaped (straight with a slight curve at the distal end, like a hockey stick). Attach a 10-mL syringe to the pilot balloon and ensure that the distal cuff holds air and does not leak. Avoid contaminating the tube. Check the laryngoscope (direct or video) to ensure that it is functioning properly.

YOU are the EMT

The patient's condition remains unchanged during transport. Shortly before arriving at the hospital, you reassess his vital signs. You also note that the patient exhibits abnormal extension in response to painful stimuli.

Recording Time: 19 Minutes	
Level of consciousness	Unresponsive
Respirations	4 breaths/min and irregular (baseline); 10 breaths/min (assisted)
Pulse	46 beats/min, bounding
Skin	Baseline color, warm, and dry
Blood pressure	174/100 mm Hg
Oxygen saturation (Spo_2)	98% (with assisted ventilation and high-flow oxygen)

After transferring patient care to the ED staff, the attending physician intubates the patient, further stabilizes him, and sends him to get a computed tomography (CT) scan of the brain. On returning to your station, you follow up and learn that the patient had an intracerebral hemorrhage.

10. What types of abnormal respiratory patterns can be observed in patients with an intracerebral hemorrhage?

11. With the knowledge of the patient's diagnosis, is there anything different that you could have done regarding airway management of this patient?

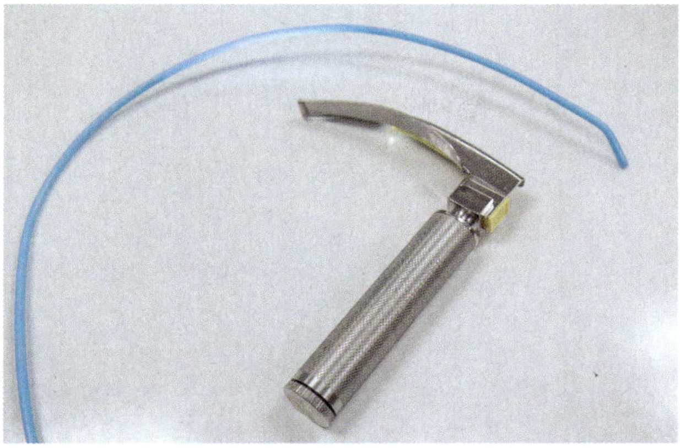

FIGURE 11-64 An elastic bougie is shown next to a laryngoscope.

The **elastic bougie**, also called an ET tube introducer or bougie, is a flexible device that is 0.2 inch (5 mm or 15 Fr) in diameter and approximately 2 feet (70 cm) long. A 30° bend is found at the distal tip (**FIGURE 11-64**). Although reusable versions are available, most are disposable and are available in both adult and pediatric sizes. The bougie is used to facilitate intubation when the vocal cords cannot be completely visualized, such as an epiglottis-only view. It can make intubation possible in some difficult situations. The bougie is rigid enough that it can be easily directed through the glottic opening, yet flexible enough that it does not damage the tracheal wall. Many ALS clinicians routinely use a bougie when intubating patients, even if they have an unobstructed view of the vocal cords.

The bougie is inserted through the glottic opening under laryngoscopy. The angle at its distal tip facilitates entry into the glottic opening and enables the clinician to "feel" the cartilaginous rings of the tracheal wall (**FIGURE 11-65**). After the bougie is placed deeply into the trachea, it serves as a guide for the ET tube, which is simply slid over the bougie and into the trachea.

Performing the Procedure

While specific details of ET intubation may vary depending on available equipment, difficulties encountered, and clinician preference, you can remember the six typical steps by using the BE MAGIC mnemonic:

B Perform *Bag-mask* preoxygenation.
E *Evaluate* for airway difficulties.

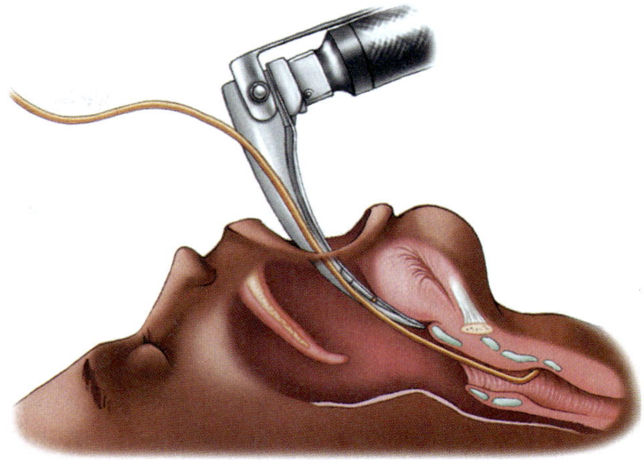

FIGURE 11-65 The angle of the distal tip of the bougie facilitates entry into the glottic opening and enables the intubator to feel the tracheal rings.

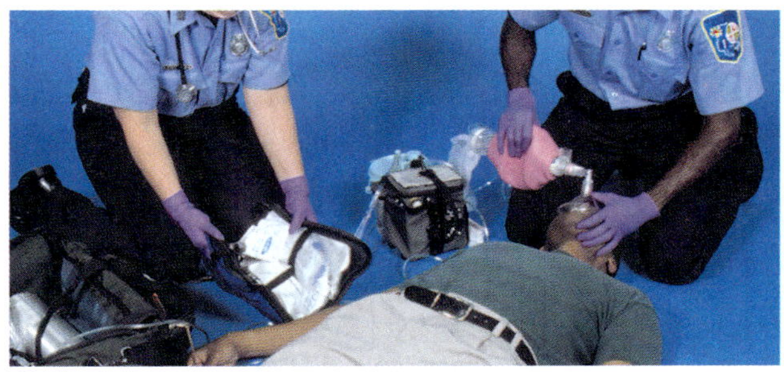

FIGURE 11-66 One EMT or the paramedic may prepare the intubation equipment while another EMT continues to ventilate and preoxygenate the patient.

M *Manipulate* the patient.
A *Attempt* first-pass intubation.
GI Use a supra*Glottic* airway if unable to intubate.
C *Confirm* successful intubation/*Correct* any issues.

Bag-Mask Device Preoxygenation

As discussed previously, it is crucial that you adequately preoxygenate the patient before the intubation procedure, especially critical patients (**FIGURE 11-66**). Do not hyperventilate the patient during the preoxygenation phase, because this may cause gastric distention and increase the risk of aspiration. Hyperventilation may also cause hypotension by reducing venous blood return to the heart. Focus on maintaining a good seal, achieving chest rise and fall, and delivering breaths at a rate appropriate for the patient's age (1 breath every 6 seconds for an adult, and 1 breath every 2 to 3 seconds for an infant or child).

Evaluate for Airway Difficulties

While you preoxygenate the patient, an ALS clinician should evaluate the patient to identify any factors that will present difficulties during the procedure; for example, trauma or anatomic deformities to the airway. It is crucial that difficulties be identified before the procedure begins. You may assist with this process, as well as the preparation of any equipment that will be needed to address the problem or problems.

ALS Assist

It may be difficult for the ALS clinician to visualize the vocal cords in bariatric and pediatric patients or patients with suspected cervical spine injuries. The EMT plays a crucial role in assisting with the intubation procedure, whether there are anticipated difficulties or not. If the patient has a cervical collar in place because of a suspected neck injury, remove the anterior part of the collar, which will facilitate better opening of the mouth, and maintain manual cervical spine stabilization while the ALS clinician attempts intubation. Good communication and coordination between team members is critical during these advanced procedures.

Manipulate the Patient

Before the procedure can begin, position the patient so that the ALS clinician can visualize the vocal cords. The ideal position is achieved when the patient's ear canal is on the same horizontal plane as the sternal notch, known as the sniffing position. The sniffing position can be achieved with the EMT placing a hand under the back of the patient's head and lifting until the ears and sternal notch are on the same horizontal plane, being careful to avoid flexing or extending the head. Alternatively, padding can be placed behind the shoulders and occiput to achieve this position (**FIGURE 11-67**).[23]

Attempt Intubation

When the ALS clinician is ready to begin the intubation attempt, remove the oropharyngeal airway and disconnect the mask from the bag in preparation for connecting the bag to the ET tube. Always keep the mask and airway within reach in case the first attempt is unsuccessful and you need to resume bag-mask ventilation. Likewise, keep suction equipment at hand in case you need to suction the patient's airway. The ALS clinician will begin by inserting the laryngoscope blade into the patient's mouth and will use it to move structures in the airway, such as the tongue and epiglottis, to gain a view of the vocal cords, through which the ET tube will pass (**FIGURE 11-68**).

The ALS clinician may ask you for assistance in manipulating the patient's larynx (external laryngeal manipulation) or otherwise positioning the patient

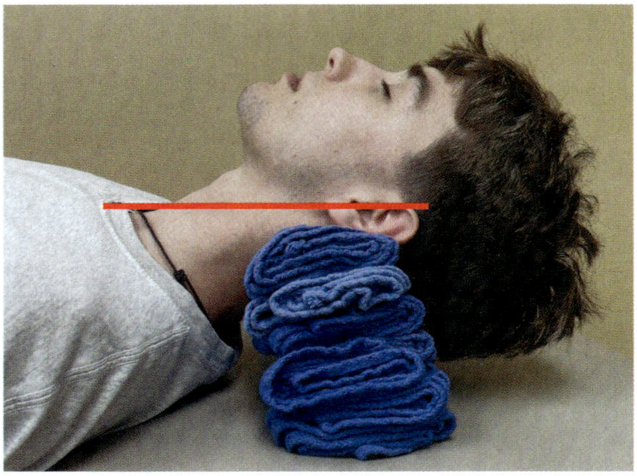

FIGURE 11-67 The sniffing position: Position the patient so that the ear canal is on the same horizontal plane as the sternal notch.

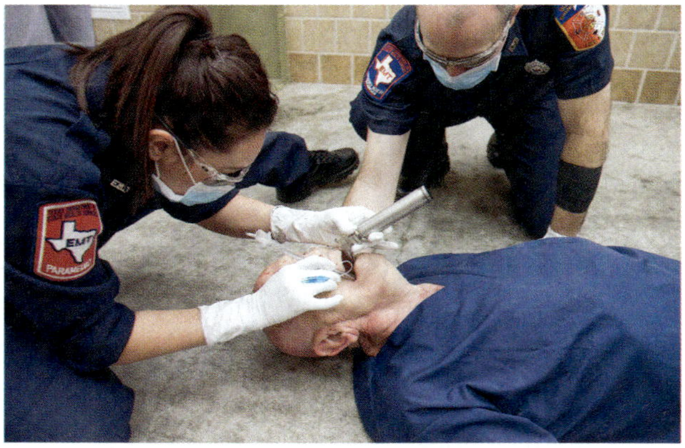

FIGURE 11-68 The ALS clinician will use the laryngoscope blade to visualize the target of the vocal cords, through which the endotracheal tube will pass.

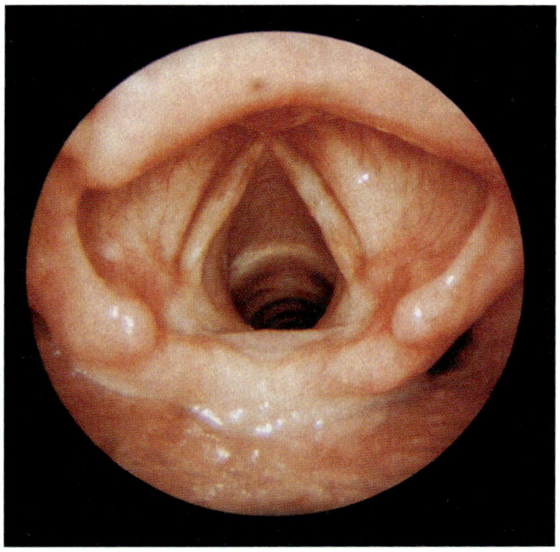

FIGURE 11-69 The cuff of the ET tube must pass through the vocal cords.

for a better view of the vocal cords (**FIGURE 11-69**). You may also be asked to hand the ET tube, elastic bougie, suction catheter, or other equipment to the ALS clinician.

ALS Assist

Quantitative waveform capnography, discussed earlier in this chapter, is the *most* reliable method of confirming proper ET tube placement. If the ET tube is correctly placed in the trachea, a consistent waveform and numeric value will be displayed. In the absence of a waveform and digital reading, the ET tube must be assumed to be in the esophagus.

Confirm Intubation and Correct Issues

Following the intubation procedure, you must work with your team to confirm intubation success. Attach the $ETCO_2$ waveform detector in line between the ET tube and the bag. You may also either ventilate the patient while another clinician checks for positive breath sounds and the absence of gastric sounds or listen while another team member ventilates (**FIGURE 11-70**). In a successfully intubated patient, the $ETCO_2$ waveform will be consistent, bilateral breath sounds will be present, and gastric (or epigastric) sounds will be absent. Either absence of breath sounds or presence of gastric sounds suggests the ET tube was improperly inserted into the esophagus; however, $ETCO_2$ monitoring is the most

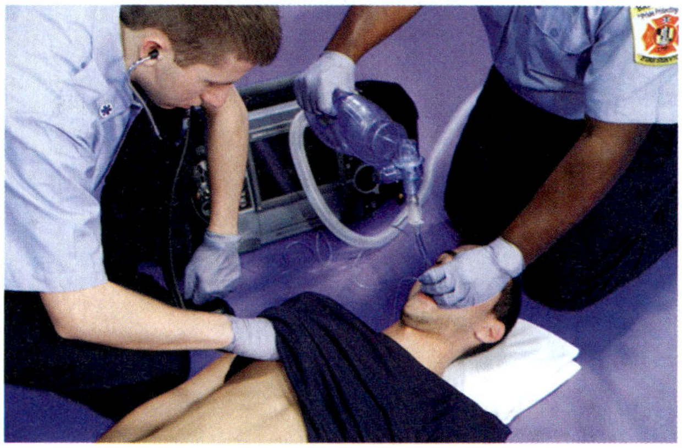

FIGURE 11-70 Ventilate while listening for breath sounds to confirm successful placement of the ET tube.

reliable confirmation source. If the intubation is confirmed as successful, then you may assist in securing the ET tube (**FIGURE 11-71**). If the intubation cannot be confirmed, or if the ET tube appears to be properly placed but airway or breathing issues remain, then you may assist other team members in correcting these issues.

ALS Assist

The paramedic may indicate they will use the suction-assisted laryngoscopy and airway decontamination (SALAD) technique if the airway is filled with vomit, blood, or other debris. If a DuCanto suction catheter is available, it will be used for continuous suction during this procedure. As an EMT, familiarity with the SALAD technique may allow you to assist the paramedic, such as by having a flexible catheter ready so that once the paramedic has placed the ET tube in the trachea, the suction connection tubing can be switched to the flexible catheter, allowing the paramedic to suction the trachea.

Words of Wisdom

Until the ET tube is secured, its position is unstable. A commercial device is the preferred method for the ALS clinician to secure the tube. The team must reassess to be sure the ET tube is not dislodged by movement at this point in the procedure or at any time during patient care.

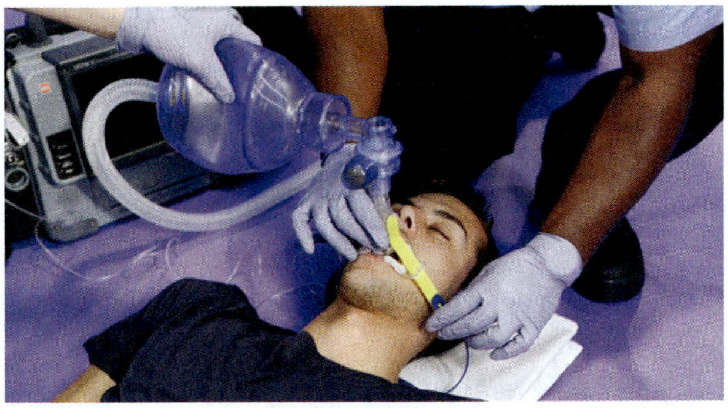

FIGURE 11-71 Ensure the ET tube does not move while it is being secured or at any point during patient care.

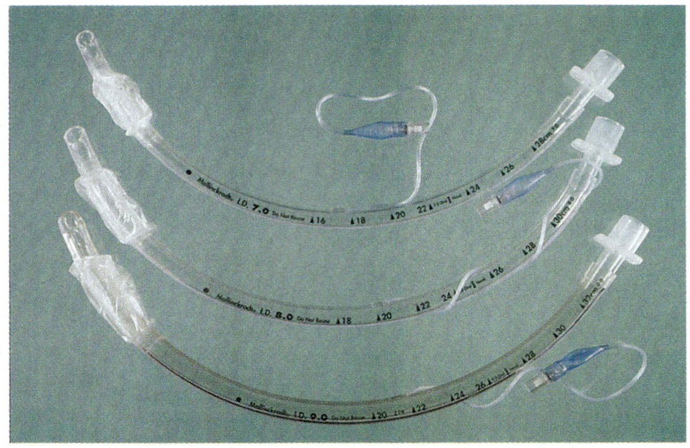

FIGURE 11-72 Centimeter markings on the ET tube are used to ensure insertion to the appropriate depth.

Continuing Care

Once an intubation attempt has been confirmed as successful, the job of airway management is not over for the EMS team. You must continue to observe all of the patient's monitor readings, as well as monitoring for signs of potential complications, including the following:

- **Absence of an $ETCO_2$ level.** Alert team members if the $ETCO_2$ waveform suddenly disappears. This indicates that the ET tube has shifted out of the proper position. Remember, quantitative waveform capnography is the most reliable indicator that the tube is correctly positioned in the trachea.
- **Decreasing SpO_2 level.** Alert team members if the SpO_2 level begins to drop, especially below 94%. This is a sign the ET tube may have shifted out of the proper position. It could also indicate an underlying oxygenation issue.
- **Increasing resistance when ventilating.** The person assigned the task of ventilation should monitor for increasing resistance when the bag is squeezed for ventilation. When increasing resistance is felt, it could indicate a critical airway or breathing problem that must be addressed, such as the advanced airway device has been mistakenly placed into the esophagus rather than into the trachea, referred to as **esophageal intubation**. When the ET tube is placed in the esophagus, ventilation results in air being pumped into the stomach, which increases the size of the patient's stomach and leads to gastric distention. When this happens, oxygen does not enter the lungs.
- **Other physical signs of poor ventilation and perfusion.** Physical signs include pallor and cyanosis.
- **Improper positioning or dislodgement of the ET tube.** Each time the patient is moved, it is important to reassess the placement of the ET tube. Verify proper ET tube position by ensuring breath sounds are present, gastric sounds are absent, an $ETCO_2$ waveform is visible during ventilation, SpO_2 values are stable or rising, and the ET tube is secured at the proper depth marking (**FIGURE 11-72**).

Safety Tips

When caring for a patient with a potentially highly contagious respiratory disease, emergency care clinicians must consider not only the device most appropriate for the patient's emergency condition, but also the safety of using those devices for rescuers. There is a difference in the distance that aerosols are dispersed from various devices. Therefore, some simple modifications may be made for some patients. For example, it may be safer to use a nonrebreathing mask rather than a nasal cannula in these patients.

Assisting With Supraglottic Airway Placement

Should intubation attempts fail, or if the ALS clinician elects not to attempt intubation, it may be your responsibility to assist with placement of a supraglottic airway device. Unlike an ET tube, which is placed into the trachea, a supraglottic airway comes to rest above the glottis and does not enter the trachea, hence the term supraglottic (*supra* = above) airway. While several supraglottic airway devices are available on the market, they all fundamentally work the same by providing a seal around the glottis, which facilitates airflow into the trachea.

The King LT airway is a single-lumen airway that is blindly inserted into the esophagus. The device consists of a curved tube with ventilation ports located between two inflatable cuffs. Both cuffs are inflated simultaneously using a single valve. When the device is properly placed in the esophagus, the distal cuff seals the esophagus, and the proximal cuff seals the oropharynx (**FIGURE 11-73**). Openings located between these two cuffs provide for ventilation of the lungs until proper positioning is confirmed. The King LT airway is an alternative to bag-mask ventilation or ET intubation.

Two types of King LT airways are available: the King LT-D (see Figure 11-73) and the King LTS-D. The King LTS-D is the more commonly used device; it is available in seven sizes, which are based on the patient's height. Each size has a different color of proximal connector and requires different cuff inflation pressures.

The King LT-D and the King LTS-D share most of the same features. Both have a proximal pharyngeal cuff and a distal cuff, as well as several ventilation outlets at the distal part of the tube. The distal end of the King LT-D is closed, whereas the distal end of the King LTS-D is open (**FIGURE 11-74**). This opening permits insertion of a suction catheter through a gastric access lumen on the proximal end of the King LTS-D to perform gastric decompression.

The i-gel supraglottic airway is also a blindly inserted supraglottic airway device. It was designed to create a noninflatable, anatomic seal of

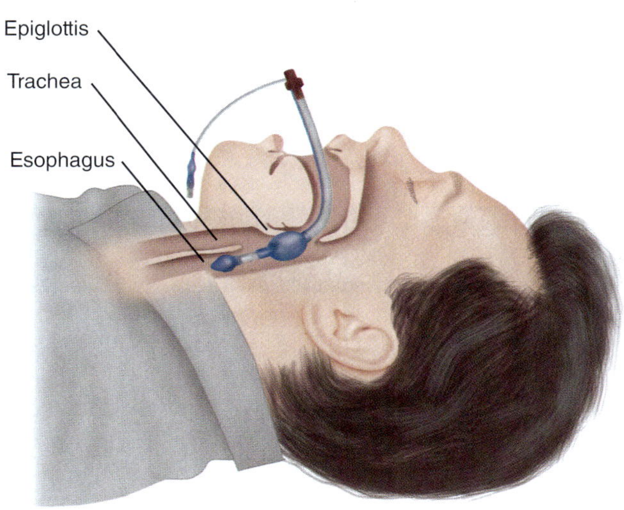

FIGURE 11-73 The King LT airway is a single-lumen airway that is blindly inserted into the esophagus. When properly placed, the distal cuff seals the esophagus and the proximal cuff seals the oropharynx.

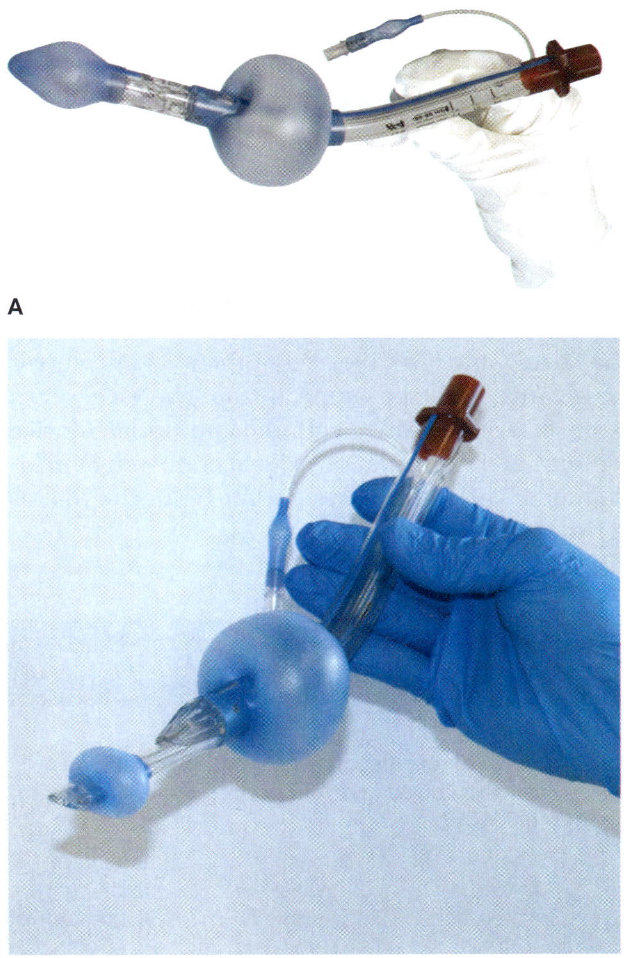

A

B

FIGURE 11-74 A. The distal end of the King LT-D is closed. **B.** The distal end of the King LTS-D is open.

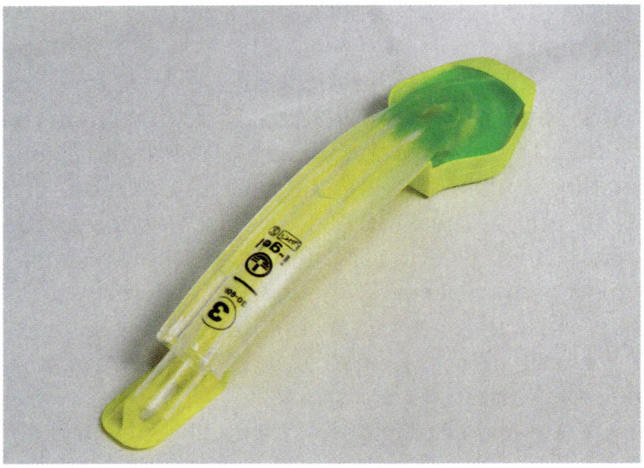

FIGURE 11-75 The i-gel airway device.

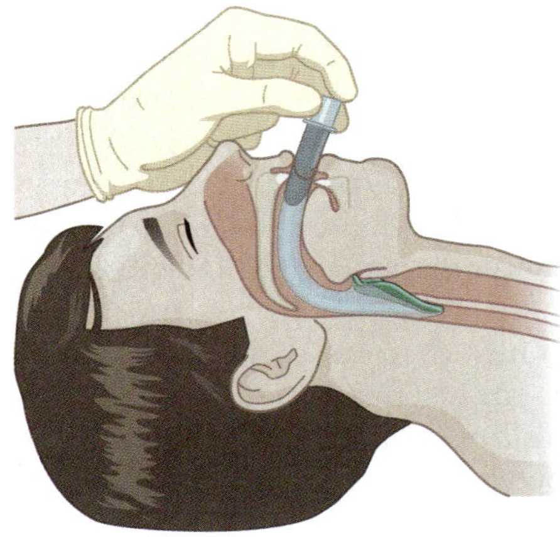

FIGURE 11-76 Correct position of the i-gel in the airway.

the pharyngeal, laryngeal, and perilaryngeal structures, while avoiding the compression trauma that may occur from devices with an inflatable cuff (**FIGURE 11-75**). The i-gel is a commonly used supraglottic airway device and is a reasonable alternative to intubation.

The i-gel features an integral bite block, a gastric access channel that allows for placement of a gastric tube for gastric decompression, a supplemental oxygen inlet port, and a support strap to secure the airway in position. A color-coded, proximal hook ring indicates the size of the i-gel and serves as an anchor for the support strap. There are seven sizes of i-gel available, with the appropriate device determined by the patient's ideal body weight in kilograms. The size and weight range for the i-gel is printed directly on the device.

The tip of the i-gel is designed to fit into the proximal esophagus, while the sides form a seal around the hypopharynx. This position facilitates air entry into the trachea (**FIGURE 11-76**).

ALS Assist

As with the bag-mask device, supraglottic airway devices rely on a good seal to function properly. Supraglottic airways are advanced airways and must be confirmed by clinical assessment and continuous waveform capnography. These devices should be secured according to the manufacturer's instructions and the patient monitored continuously for signs that the tube is no longer in the proper location.

YOU are the EMT SUMMARY

1. Based on the dispatch information, what type of call should you and your partner mentally prepare for? Why?

When you are dispatched for an unresponsive patient and the presence of normal breathing cannot be confirmed, you should mentally prepare for a cardiac arrest. All you know from the dispatch information is that the patient "appears" to be breathing. Agonal gasps, which are ineffective, irregular breaths, are commonly observed shortly after a patient experiences sudden cardiac arrest. If not evaluated carefully when the dispatcher is gathering information, these gasps could be mistaken for a patient who is breathing. This is why it is critical for the dispatcher to ask if the patient is breathing *normally*, rather than simply asking if the patient is breathing.

2. How do tidal volume and respiratory rate influence minute alveolar ventilation?

Minute alveolar ventilation is the volume of air that actively participates in pulmonary gas exchange each minute. Tidal volume is the volume of air

YOU are the EMT SUMMARY continued

(in mL) that is breathed into and out of the respiratory tract with each breath, and minute volume is the amount of air breathed into and out of the respiratory tract each minute. It is important to understand that not all the patient's tidal volume physically enters the lungs. Approximately 30% remains in the upper airway and larger bronchi; this area is called anatomic dead space. For example, if a patient has a tidal volume of 450 mL, only about 315 mL would physically enter the lungs and participate in pulmonary gas exchange; the remaining 135 mL would stay in the anatomic dead space. Minute alveolar ventilation is influenced by tidal volume and respiratory rate. If tidal volume is reduced, the respiratory rate would need to increase to maintain minute alveolar ventilation. Conversely, if the respiratory rate is decreased, the tidal volume would need to increase accordingly. This interplay is why it is so important to assess rate, depth, and regularity of breathing when determining if it is adequate or not. The patient can have a "normal" respiratory rate; however, if tidal volume is reduced (shallow breathing), minute alveolar ventilation will be reduced as well.

3. What are your immediate priorities of care?

The most obvious immediate life threats are a partially obstructed airway, as evidenced by the patient's snoring, and ineffective breathing (slow and irregular). Obtaining and maintaining a patent airway and ensuring adequate ventilation are paramount in any patient. Manually open the patient's airway using either the head tilt–chin lift or jaw-thrust maneuver; if you suspect a spinal injury, avoid the head tilt–chin lift maneuver. After opening the airway, inspect the oropharynx for secretions and use suction as needed to remove them. Insert a properly sized nasopharyngeal airway; if a gag reflex is absent, consider inserting an oropharyngeal airway.

Slow, irregular breathing will not provide adequate minute alveolar ventilation and should be treated with positive-pressure ventilation. Attach a bag-mask device to high-flow oxygen and assist the patient's breathing; augment the patient's own breaths with more tidal volume and provide additional breaths to ensure a rate of 10 breaths/min. Do not ventilate the patient aggressively; provide just enough volume to cause visible chest rise.

4. Anatomically, what causes snoring in an unresponsive patient?

In the unresponsive patient, the tongue is the most common cause of airway obstruction. Snoring occurs any time the tongue and posterior pharynx contact one another. In a supine patient, the tongue falls back against the posterior pharynx; in a prone patient, the posterior pharynx relaxes forward and contacts the tongue. Manual techniques, such as the head tilt–chin lift and jaw-thrust maneuvers, essentially create a space between the tongue and the posterior pharynx, allowing for unobstructed air movement. Simple adjuncts, such as the nasopharyngeal and oropharyngeal airway accomplish the same goal but replace the need for manual airway positioning.

5. What are some indications of effective positive-pressure ventilation?

Signs of effective positive-pressure ventilation include, but are not limited to, bilateral chest rise with each ventilation; the presence of auscultated breath sounds during ventilation; a ventilation rate that is appropriate for the patient's age (10 breaths/min in adults; 20 to 30 breaths/min in children); improved skin condition, such as resolving cyanosis; increasing Spo_2 level; and decreasing $ETCO_2$ level.

6. What effect, if any, does positive-pressure ventilation have on cardiac output?

During normal, unassisted breathing, air is pulled into the lungs through a process called negative-pressure ventilation. Mechanically, this occurs because of diaphragmatic contraction and descension, which decreases intrathoracic pressure and creates a vacuum effect. The same negative pressure that pulls air into the lungs facilitates venous blood return to the right side of the heart. By contrast, positive-pressure ventilation is the process of pushing air into the lungs (eg, bag-mask ventilation). As air is pushed into the lungs, intrathoracic pressure increases rather than decreases, as it does with negative-pressure ventilation. The effects of positive-pressure ventilation on cardiac output depend on how conservatively or aggressively the patient is being ventilated. If the ventilation rate and volume are *tightly regulated* (ie, ventilating just enough to produce visible chest rise and not ventilating too rapidly), then the effects on cardiac output are minimal. However, with aggressive positive-pressure ventilation, intrathoracic pressure can become dangerously high secondary to hyperinflation of the lungs. As a result, inward pressure is placed on the heart, which can restrict its ability to relax (diastole). If the heart cannot relax, it cannot adequately refill with blood. With less blood refilling the right side of the heart, less blood is delivered to the left side of the heart. As a result, cardiac output decreases. This effect will be more evident in patients whose blood pressure is low.

YOU are the EMT SUMMARY continued

7. How does an adult's heart rate typically respond to hypoxemia initially? Why?

When a systemic oxygen deficit in arterial blood (hypoxemia) occurs, the adult's heart rate typically responds with tachycardia initially. This is a sympathetic nervous system response to hypoxemia in which catecholamines are released into the bloodstream to move blood (and oxygen) around faster in the circulatory system. As oxygen levels are restored, the tachycardia should begin to resolve, unless there are other underlying problems that can also cause tachycardia (ie, hypovolemia). It is important to understand, however, that if the hypoxemia is not corrected, the heart rate will begin to slow; this is a sign of impending cardiac arrest. Children also respond to hypoxemia with tachycardia initially; however, their heart rate falls more quickly than that of an adult. For these reasons, it is critical to monitor the heart rate in any patient with hypoxemia.

8. Would you expect a hypoventilating patient's $ETCO_2$ to be low, normal, or high? Why?

Carbon dioxide is the by-product of aerobic metabolism (ie, metabolism in the presence of oxygen). $ETCO_2$ monitoring is used to assess cellular perfusion by indicating how much carbon dioxide is being produced at the cellular level and how much carbon dioxide is being eliminated from the body. $ETCO_2$ monitoring works by sampling air at the end of exhalation and translating the value into a digital reading and waveform (quantitative waveform capnography). If cellular perfusion is normal, and the respiratory system is functioning normally, you would expect to see a normal (35 to 45 mm Hg) $ETCO_2$ value. However, if the patient is hypoventilating (ie, reduced tidal volume [shallow breathing], slow respiratory rate), then the respiratory tract will not effectively remove the carbon dioxide produced by the body; as a result, a high (> 45 mm Hg) $ETCO_2$ value would be observed. A low (< 35 mm Hg) $ETCO_2$ value may be observed in several situations. If the respiratory system is eliminating carbon dioxide faster than the body produces it (ie, hyperventilation), $ETCO_2$ readings would be low. Poor cellular perfusion, such as shock and cardiac arrest, would also be expected to cause low $ETCO_2$ readings. If oxygen delivery to the cells is inadequate, the body will make less carbon dioxide and, therefore, return less carbon dioxide to the lungs because of anaerobic metabolism. $ETCO_2$ is an important tool to use when assessing a patient's respiratory adequacy, or the adequacy of cellular perfusion.

9. How can gastric distention interfere with bag-mask ventilation?

Esophageal opening pressure is approximately 20 cm H_2O, which is why the esophagus is closed during normal breathing; inspiratory force during normal negative-pressure ventilation is much lower than 20 cm H_2O. Positive-pressure ventilation with a bag-mask device, however, can generate pressures higher than 20 cm H_2O, especially when the bag is squeezed too quickly and forcefully. As the stomach becomes distended with air, it pushes superiorly into the diaphragm. Because of upward pressure on the diaphragm, the lungs cannot descend far enough; this situation can impair bag-mask ventilation. A hallmark sign that this is occurring is decreased compliance (increased resistance) when ventilating. If gastric distention is severe, it can make ventilating the patient nearly impossible; it also markedly increases the risks of vomiting and aspiration. When ventilating a patient with a bag-mask device, tightly regulated ventilation rates and volumes are crucial. Provide just enough volume to cause chest rise; the patient should appear to be taking a normal breath, not a deep one. Ventilate the adult patient at a rate of one breath every 6 seconds (10 breaths/min).

10. What types of abnormal respiratory patterns can be observed in patients with an intracerebral hemorrhage?

Several abnormal respiratory patterns can be observed in patients with an intracerebral hemorrhage, and they are caused by injury to (or pressure on) the brainstem because of increased intracranial pressure. Cheyne-Stokes respirations are a respiratory pattern in which the patient breathes with an increased rate and depth, followed by a decreasing rate and depth (crescendo–decrescendo), followed by periods of apnea. Another abnormal respiratory pattern that may be observed is called central neurogenic hyperventilation, which is characterized by deep, rapid respirations. The patient may also exhibit ataxic respirations, which are irregular (slow or fast), ineffective respirations that have no identifiable pattern. Your patient's slow irregular breaths are characteristic of ataxic respirations.

11. With the knowledge of the patient's diagnosis, is there anything different that you could have done regarding airway management of this patient?

Your job is to recognize life-threatening conditions, provide emergency care, and transport the patient to the hospital. There will be times in your career

YOU are the EMT SUMMARY continued

in which the underlying cause of the patient's problem will either not be apparent or not be possible to determine without further testing at the hospital. In these cases, treat the patient's signs and symptoms and transport without delay. In this instance, the patient was found unresponsive, his airway was compromised, he was breathing inadequately, and he was clearly hypoxic. A patient's airway must remain patent and breathing must remain adequate, regardless of the underlying problem (whether identified or not). Even if you knew that the patient had an intracerebral hemorrhage, your treatment of his airway and breathing status would not have changed.

Prep Kit

Ready for Review

- The upper airway includes the nose, mouth, jaw, oral cavity, pharynx, and larynx. Its function is to warm, filter, and humidify air as it enters the nose and mouth.
- The lower airway includes the trachea and lungs; its function is to exchange oxygen and carbon dioxide.
- Aerosol-generating procedures (AGPs) require enhanced PPE.
- Adequate breathing is characterized by a normal rate for the person's age, a regular pattern of inhalation and exhalation, adequate depth, bilaterally clear and equal lung sounds, and regular and equal chest rise and fall.
- Inadequate breathing for an adult or pediatric patient features a respiratory rate that is slower or faster for their age, shallow depth (reduced tidal volume), an irregular pattern of inhalation and exhalation, and breath sounds that are diminished, absent, or noisy.
- Patients who are breathing inadequately show signs of hypoxia, a dangerous condition in which the body's tissues and cells do not have enough oxygen.
- Patients with inadequate breathing need to be treated immediately. Emergency medical care includes airway management, supplemental oxygen, and ventilatory support.
- Basic techniques for opening the airway include the head tilt–chin lift maneuver or, if trauma is suspected, the jaw-thrust maneuver.
- One basic airway adjunct is the oropharyngeal, or oral, airway, which keeps the tongue from blocking the airway in unconscious patients with no gag reflex. If the oropharyngeal airway is not the proper size or is inserted incorrectly, it can cause an obstruction.
- Another basic airway adjunct is the nasopharyngeal, or nasal, airway, which is typically used with patients who have a gag reflex and is better tolerated than the oropharyngeal airway.
- Suctioning is the next priority after opening the airway. Rigid tonsil-tip catheters are the best catheters to use when suctioning the pharynx; soft plastic catheters are used to suction the nose and liquid secretions in the back of the mouth.
- The recovery position is used to help maintain the airway in patients without traumatic injuries who are unconscious and breathing adequately.
- You must provide immediate artificial ventilations with supplemental oxygen to patients who are not breathing on their own. Patients with inadequate breathing may also require artificial ventilations to maintain effective tidal volume.
- Excessive supplemental oxygen can have a detrimental effect on patients with certain illnesses when administered for a prolonged time. Patients who require oxygen include

Prep Kit continued

(1) patients with signs of dyspnea, (2) patients with signs of shock, and (3) patients experiencing signs of a myocardial infarction with an Spo_2 level lower than 94%. Use pulse oximetry, when available, to tailor oxygen administration to the patient's needs, but do not rely on it exclusively.

- Handle compressed gas cylinders carefully; their contents are under pressure. Always make sure the correct pressure regulator is firmly attached before transporting a cylinder. The pin-indexing safety system features a series of pins on a yoke that must be matched with the holes on the valve stem of the gas cylinder. Pressure regulators reduce the pressure of gas in an oxygen cylinder to between 40 and 70 psi. Pressure-compensated flowmeters and Bourdon-gauge flowmeters permit the regulated release of gas measured in liters per minute.
- When oxygen therapy is complete, disconnect the tubing from the flowmeter nipple and turn off the cylinder valve, then turn off the flowmeter. As long as there is a pressure reading on the regulator gauge, it is not safe to remove the regulator from the valve stem. Keep any possible source of fire away from the area while oxygen is in use.
- Nasal cannulas and nonrebreathing masks are used most often to deliver oxygen in the field. The nonrebreathing mask is the delivery device of choice for providing supplemental oxygen to patients who are breathing adequately but are suspected of having or are showing signs of hypoxia. With a flow rate set at 15 L/min and the reservoir bag preinflated, the nonrebreathing mask can provide more than 90% inspired oxygen. If the patient will not tolerate a nonrebreathing mask, apply a nasal cannula.
- The methods of providing artificial ventilation include mouth-to-mask ventilation, two-person bag-mask ventilation, and one-person bag-mask ventilation. A bag-mask device with an oxygen reservoir and supplemental oxygen can deliver up to 95% oxygen.
- CPAP is a noninvasive method of providing ventilatory support for patients in respiratory distress or experiencing sleep apnea.
- When you are providing artificial ventilation, remember that ventilating too forcefully can cause gastric distention. Slow, gentle breaths during artificial ventilation can help to prevent gastric distention. Patients who have a tracheal stoma or a tracheostomy tube need to be ventilated through the tube or the stoma.
- Foreign body airway obstruction usually occurs during a meal in an adult or while a child is eating, playing with small objects, or crawling about the house. The earlier you recognize an airway obstruction, the better. You must learn to recognize the difference between airway obstruction caused by a foreign object and that caused by a medical condition.
- Foreign body airway obstructions are classified as being mild or severe. Patients with a mild airway obstruction are able to move adequate amounts of air and should be left alone. Patients with a severe airway obstruction cannot move any air at all and require immediate treatment. Perform back slaps and abdominal thrusts on conscious adults and children older than 1 year; infants require back slaps and chest thrusts. If the patient becomes unconscious, open the airway and look in the mouth (do not perform blind finger sweeps), attempt to ventilate the patient, and perform chest compressions if ventilations are unsuccessful.
- Check for loose dental appliances in a patient before assisting ventilations. Loose appliances should be removed to prevent them from obstructing the airway. Tight-fitting appliances should be left in place.
- In children, the tongue is large relative to other structures, so it poses a higher risk of airway obstruction than in an adult. The airway in a child has a smaller diameter than the

Prep Kit continued

airway in an adult and is therefore more easily obstructed.

- The three keys to successful use of the bag-mask device in a child are (1) have the appropriate equipment in the right size; (2) maintain a good face-to-mask seal; and (3) ventilate at the appropriate rate and volume.
- As an EMT, you may be asked to assist the paramedic in establishing an advanced airway. You must have a fundamental understanding of the equipment and methods involved in procedures such as intubating a patient and placing a supraglottic airway device.

Vital Vocabulary

aerobic metabolism Metabolism that can proceed only in the presence of oxygen.

aerosol-generating procedure Any airway manipulation, such as CPR, that induces the production of aerosols that may present a risk for airborne transmission of pathogens.

agonal gasps The reflexive, slow, and inadequate breathing that some patients in cardiac arrest exhibit as the brainstem becomes hypoxic.

airway The upper airway tract or the passage above the larynx, which includes the nose, mouth, and throat.

alveolar ventilation The volume of air that reaches the alveoli. It is determined by subtracting the amount of dead space air from the tidal volume.

American Standard Safety System A safety system for large oxygen cylinders, designed to prevent the accidental attachment of a regulator to a cylinder containing the wrong type of gas.

anaerobic metabolism The metabolism that takes place in the absence of oxygen; the main by-product is lactic acid.

apnea Absence of spontaneous breathing.

apneic oxygenation A technique in which oxygen via nasal cannula set at 15 to 25 L/min is left in place during an intubation attempt, allowing for continuous oxygen delivery into the airways during all phases of the intubation procedure.

aspiration In the context of the airway, the introduction of vomitus or other foreign material into the lungs.

ataxic respirations Irregular, ineffective respirations that may or may not have an identifiable pattern.

automatic transport ventilator (ATV) A ventilation device attached to a control box that allows the variables of ventilation to be set. It frees the EMT to perform other tasks while the patient is being ventilated.

bag-mask device A device with a one-way valve and a face mask attached to a ventilation bag; when attached to a reservoir and connected to oxygen, it delivers up to 95% supplemental oxygen.

barrier device A protective item, such as a pocket mask with a valve, that limits exposure to a patient's body fluids.

bilateral A body part or condition that appears on both sides of the midline.

bronchioles Subdivisions of the smaller bronchi in the lungs; made of smooth muscle and dilate or constrict in response to various stimuli.

capnography A noninvasive method to quickly and efficiently provide information on a patient's ventilatory status, circulation, and metabolism. It effectively measures the concentration of carbon dioxide in expired air over time.

capnometry The use of a capnometer, a device that measures the amount of expired carbon dioxide.

carina Point at which the trachea bifurcates (divides) into the left and right main stem bronchi.

Prep Kit continued

cellular respiration Use of oxygen by the cells to carry out their specific activities; also called cellular metabolism.

chemoreceptors Receptors that monitor the levels of oxygen, carbon dioxide, and pH of the cerebrospinal fluid and then provide feedback to the respiratory centers to modify the rate and depth of breathing based on the body's needs at any given time.

Cheyne-Stokes respirations A cyclical pattern of abnormal breathing that increases and then decreases in rate and depth, followed by a period of apnea.

compliance The ability of the alveoli to expand when air is drawn in during inhalation.

continuous positive airway pressure (CPAP) A method of noninvasive ventilation used primarily in the treatment of critically ill patients with respiratory distress; can prevent the need for endotracheal intubation.

dead space Any portion of the airway that contains air but cannot participate in gas exchange, such as the trachea and bronchi.

denitrogenation The process of replacing nitrogen in the lungs with oxygen to maintain a normal oxygen saturation level during advanced airway management.

diffusion Movement of a gas from an area of higher concentration to an area of lower concentration.

direct laryngoscopy Visualization of the airway with a laryngoscope.

dyspnea Shortness of breath.

elastic bougie A flexible device that is inserted between the glottis under direct laryngoscopy; the endotracheal tube is threaded over the device, facilitating its entry into the trachea.

endotracheal (ET) intubation Insertion of an ET tube directly through the larynx between the vocal cords and into the trachea to maintain and protect an airway.

end-tidal carbon dioxide ($ETCO_2$) The amount of carbon dioxide present at the end of an exhaled breath.

esophageal intubation Improper placement of an advanced airway device into the esophagus rather than into the trachea.

exhalation The passive part of the breathing process in which the diaphragm and the intercostal muscles relax, forcing air out of the lungs.

external respiration The exchange of gases between the lungs and the blood cells in the pulmonary capillaries; also called pulmonary respiration.

gag reflex A normal reflex mechanism that causes retching; activated by touching the soft palate or the back of the throat.

gastric distention A condition in which air fills the stomach, often as a result of high volume and pressure during artificial ventilation.

glottis The space in between the vocal cords that is the narrowest portion of the adult's airway; also called the glottic opening.

good air exchange A term used to distinguish the degree of distress in a patient with a mild airway obstruction. With good air exchange, the patient is still conscious and able to cough forcefully, although wheezing may be heard.

head tilt–chin lift maneuver A combination of two movements to open the airway by tilting the forehead back and lifting the chin; not used for trauma patients.

hemothorax A collection of blood in the pleural cavity.

hypercapnia Increased carbon dioxide level in the bloodstream.

hypoxia Deficient oxygen concentration in the tissues.

hypoxic drive A "backup system" to control respiration; senses drops in the oxygen level in the blood.

Prep Kit continued

inhalation The active, muscular part of breathing that draws air into the airway and lungs.

internal respiration The exchange of gases between the blood and the tissue cells.

intrapulmonary shunting Bypassing of oxygen-poor blood past nonfunctional alveoli to the left side of the heart.

jaw-thrust maneuver Technique to open the airway by placing the fingers behind the angle of the jaw and bringing the jaw forward; used for patients who may have a cervical spine injury.

labored breathing The use of muscles of the chest, back, and abdomen to assist in expanding the chest; occurs when air movement is impaired.

larynx A complex structure formed by many independent cartilaginous structures that all work together; where the upper airway ends and the lower airway begins; also called the voice box.

length-based resuscitation tape A tape used to estimate an infant's or child's weight on the basis of body length; appropriate drug doses and equipment sizes are listed on the tape.

mediastinum Space within the chest that contains the heart, major blood vessels, vagus nerve, trachea, major bronchi, and esophagus; located between the two lungs.

metabolism The biochemical processes that result in production of energy from nutrients within the cells.

mild airway obstruction Occurs when a foreign body partially obstructs the patient's airway. The patient is able to move adequate amounts of air, but also experiences some degree of respiratory distress.

minute alveolar ventilation The volume of air moved through the lungs in 1 minute minus the dead space; calculated by multiplying tidal volume (minus dead space) and respiratory rate.

minute volume The volume of air that moves into and out of the lungs per minute; calculated by multiplying the tidal volume and respiratory rate; also called minute ventilation.

nasal cannula An oxygen-delivery device in which oxygen flows through two small, tubelike prongs that fit into the patient's nostrils; delivers 24% to 44% supplemental oxygen, depending on the flow rate.

nasopharyngeal airway Airway adjunct inserted into the nostril of an unresponsive patient or a patient with an altered level of consciousness who is unable to maintain airway patency independently; also referred to as a nasal airway.

nasopharynx The part of the pharynx that lies above the level of the roof of the mouth, or palate.

nonrebreathing mask A combination mask and reservoir bag system that is the preferred way to give oxygen in the prehospital setting; delivers up to 90% inspired oxygen and prevents inhaling the exhaled gases (carbon dioxide).

oropharyngeal airway Airway adjunct inserted into the mouth of an unresponsive patient to keep the tongue from blocking the upper airway and to facilitate suctioning the airway, if necessary; also referred to as an oral airway.

oropharynx A tubular structure that forms the posterior portion of the oral cavity, which is bordered superiorly by the hard and soft palates, laterally by the cheeks, and inferiorly by the tongue.

oxygenation The process of delivering oxygen to the blood by diffusion from the alveoli following inhalation into the lungs.

oxygen toxicity A condition of excessive oxygen consumption resulting in cellular and tissue damage.

parietal pleura Thin membrane that lines the chest cavity.

partial pressure The term used to describe the amount of gas in air or dissolved in fluid, such as blood.

patent Open, clear of obstruction.

phrenic nerves The two nerves that innervate the diaphragm; necessary for adequate breathing to occur.

Prep Kit continued

pin-indexing system A system established for portable cylinders to ensure that a regulator is not connected to a cylinder containing the wrong type of gas.

pneumothorax An accumulation of air or gas in the pleural cavity.

poor air exchange A term used to describe the degree of distress in a patient with a mild airway obstruction. With poor air exchange, the patient often has a weak, ineffective cough, increased difficulty breathing, or possible cyanosis and may produce a high-pitched noise during inhalation (stridor).

preoxygenation The process of providing oxygen, often in combination with ventilation, prior to intubation in order to raise the oxygen levels of body tissues; a critical step in advanced airway management. This extends the time during which an advanced airway can be placed in an apneic patient, because the more oxygen that is available in the alveoli, the longer the patient can maintain adequate gas exchange in the lungs during the procedure.

pulse oximetry An assessment tool that measures oxygen saturation of hemoglobin in the capillary beds.

recovery position A side-lying position used to maintain a clear airway in unconscious patients without injuries who are breathing adequately.

residual volume The air that remains in the lungs after maximal expiration.

respiration The process of exchanging oxygen and carbon dioxide.

respiratory arrest Complete cessation of breathing (apnea) or agonal gasps that will lead to cardiac arrest if intervention does not occur immediately.

respiratory distress A condition marked by difficulty breathing and an abnormal respiratory rate or effort; can range from mild to severe and can progress to respiratory failure.

respiratory failure A condition in which oxygen levels are too low to meet the body's needs and ventilation is impaired, leading to high carbon dioxide levels; accompanied by serious signs and symptoms and must be corrected quickly.

retractions Movements in which the skin pulls in around the ribs during inspiration.

severe airway obstruction Occurs when a foreign body completely obstructs the patient's airway. The patient cannot breathe, talk, or cough.

stoma An opening through the skin and into an organ or other structure.

stridor A harsh, high-pitched respiratory sound, generally heard during inspiration, that is caused by partial blockage or narrowing of the upper airway; may be audible without a stethoscope.

suction catheter A hollow, cylindrical device used to remove fluid from the patient's airway.

surfactant A liquid protein substance that coats the alveoli in the lungs, decreases alveolar surface tension, and keeps the alveoli expanded; a low level in a premature infant contributes to respiratory distress syndrome.

tension pneumothorax An accumulation of air or gas in the pleural cavity that progressively increases pressure in the chest and that interferes with cardiac function, with potentially fatal results.

tidal volume The amount of air (in mL) that is moved into or out of the lungs during one breath.

tonsil tips Large, semi-rigid suction tips recommended for suctioning the pharynx.

tracheostomy A surgical procedure to create an opening (stoma) into the trachea; a stoma in the neck connects the trachea directly to the skin.

tracheostomy tube A plastic tube placed within the tracheostomy site (stoma).

ventilation The exchange of air between the lungs and the environment; occurs spontaneously by the patient or with assistance from another person, such as an EMT.

Prep Kit continued

video laryngoscopy Visualization of the vocal cords, and thereby placement of the endotracheal tube, that is facilitated by use of a video camera and monitor.

visceral pleura Thin membrane that covers the lungs.

vital capacity The amount of air that can be forcibly expelled from the lungs after breathing in as deeply as possible.

vocal cords Thin white bands of tough muscular tissue that are lateral borders of the glottis and serve as the primary center for speech production.

wheezing A high-pitched, whistling breath sound that is most prominent on expiration, and which suggests an obstruction or narrowing of the lower airways; occurs in asthma and bronchiolitis.

References

1. Lyng J, Harris M, Mandt M, et al. Prehospital pediatric respiratory distress and airway management training and education: an NAEMSP position statement and resource document. *Prehosp Emerg Care*. 2022;26(sup1):102–110.
2. Hallett S, Toro F, Ashurst JV. Physiology, tidal volume. *StatPearls*. National Library of Medicine website. https://www.ncbi.nlm.nih.gov/books/NBK482502/. Updated May 1, 2023. Accessed August 6, 2024.
3. American Heart Association (AHA). *Pediatric Advanced Life Support Provider Manual*. Dallas, TX: AHA; 2020.
4. Clinical safety: occupationally acquired infections and healthcare workers. Centers for Disease Control and Prevention website. https://www.cdc.gov/infection-control/hcp/safety/index.html. Published April 3, 2024. Accessed August 6, 2024.
5. Hamber EA, Bailey PL, James SW, et al. Delays in the detection of hypoxemia due to site of pulse oximetry probe placement. *J Clin Anesth*. 1999;11(2):113–118.
6. Yeganehkhah M, Dadkhahtehrani T, Bagheri A, Kachoie A. Effect of glittered nail polish on pulse oximetry measurements in healthy subjects. *Iran J Nurs Midwifery Res*. 2019;24(1):25–29.
7. Yek JLJ, Abdullah HR, Goh JPS, Chan YW. The effects of gel-based manicure on pulse oximetry. *Singapore Med J*. 2019;60(8):432–435.
8. Al-Halawani R, Charlton PH, Qassem M, Kyriacou PA. A review of the effect of skin pigmentation on pulse oximeter accuracy. *Physiol Meas*. 2023;44(5):05TR01. doi:10.1088/1361-6579/acd51a
9. Gottlieb ER, Ziegler J, Morley K, Rush B, Celi LA. Assessment of racial and ethnic differences in oxygen supplementation among patients in the intensive care unit. *JAMA Intern Med*. 2022;182(8):849–858.
10. Andrist E, Nuppnau M, Barbaro RP, Valley TS, Sjoding MW. Association of race with pulse oximetry accuracy in hospitalized children. *JAMA Netw Open*. 2022;5(3):e224584. doi:10.1001/jamanetworkopen.2022.4584
11. Lyng JW, Guyette FX, Levy M, Bosson N. Prehospital manual ventilation: an NAEMSP position statement and resource document. *Prehosp Emerg Care*. 2022;26(sup1):23–31.
12. Cylinder/tank specifications chart. Tri-Med website. http://www.tri-medinc.com/page12.htm#cyl-spec. Accessed August 6, 2024.
13. Weekley MS, Bland LE. Oxygen administration. *StatPearls*. National Library of Medicine website. https://www.ncbi.nlm.nih.gov/books/NBK551617/. Updated July 18, 2023. Accessed August 6, 2024.
14. Rao SV, O'Donoghue ML, Ruel M, et al. 2025 ACC/AHA/ACEP/NAEMSP/SCAI guideline for the management of patients with acute coronary syndromes: a report of the American College of Cardiology/American Heart Association Joint Committee on Clinical Practice Guidelines. *Circulation*. 2025. doi:10.1161/CIR.0000000000001309
15. Whittle JS, Pavlov I, Sacchetti AD, Atwood C, Rosenberg MS. Respiratory support for adult patients with COVID-19. *ACEP Open*. 2020;1(2):95–101.
16. McCoy AM, Morris D, Tanaka K, Wright A, Guyette FX, Martin-Gill C. Prehospital noninvasive ventilation: an NAEMSP position statement and resource document. *Prehosp Emerg Care*. 2022;26(sup1):80–87.
17. Taylor DM, Bernard SA, Masci K, et al. Prehospital noninvasive ventilation: a viable treatment option in the urban setting. *Prehosp Emerg Care*. 2008;12(1):42–45. Erratum in: *Prehosp Emerg Care*. 2009;13(1):151.
18. Warner GS. Evaluation of the effect of prehospital application of continuous positive airway pressure therapy in acute respiratory distress. *Prehosp Disaster Med*. 2010;25(1):87–91.
19. Daily JC, Wang HE. Noninvasive positive pressure ventilation: resource document for the National Association of EMS Physicians position statement. *Prehosp Emerg Care*. 2011;15(3):432–438.
20. Schwerin DL, Kuhl EA, Goldstein S. EMS prehospital CPAP devices. *StatPearls*. National Library of Medicine website. https://www.ncbi.nlm.nih.gov/books/NBK470429/. Updated June 22, 2024. Accessed August 6, 2024.

Prep Kit continued

21. Muhanuzi B, Sawe HR, Kilindimo SS, Mfinanga JA, Weber EJ. Respiratory compromise in children presenting to an urban emergency department of a tertiary hospital in Tanzania: a descriptive cohort study. *BMC Emerg Med*. 2019;19(1):21.
22. Davies P, Cheng D, Fox A, Lee L. The efficacy of noncontact oxygen delivery methods [published correction appears in *Pediatrics*. 2006 Sep;118(3):1325]. *Pediatrics*. 2002;110(5):964–967.
23. Weingart S. EMCrit 226: airway update—bougie and positioning. EMCrit website. https://emcrit.org/emcrit/bougie-and-positioning/. Published June 13, 2018. Accessed August 6, 2024.

Additional Resources

American Heart Association. *Highlights of the 2020 American Heart Association Guidelines Update for CPR and ECC*. https://cpr.heart.org/-/media/cpr-files/cpr-guidelines-files/highlights/hghlghts_2020_ecc_guidelines_english.pdf. Accessed April 22, 2024.

Berg KM, Bray JE, Ng KC, et al. 2023 International consensus on cardiopulmonary resuscitation and emergency cardiovascular care science with treatment recommendations: summary from the Basic Life Support; Advanced Life Support; Pediatric Life Support; Neonatal Life Support; Education, Implementation, and Teams; and First Aid Task Forces. *Circulation*. 2023;148(24):e187–e280. doi:10.1161/CIR.0000000000001179

National Association of State EMS Officials. *National Model EMS Clinical Guidelines*. Version 3.0. https://nasemso.org/wp-content/uploads/National-Model-EMS-Clinical-Guidelines_2022.pdf. Updated March 2022. Accessed March 27, 2024.

Rafay K. Oxygen tank duration calculator. Omni Calculator website. https://www.omnicalculator.com/other/oxygen-tank-duration. Updated July 18, 2024. Accessed December 6, 2024.

Wyckoff MH, Greif R, Morley PT, et al. 2022 International consensus on cardiopulmonary resuscitation and emergency cardiovascular care science with treatment recommendations: summary from the Basic Life Support; Advanced Life Support; Pediatric Life Support; Neonatal Life Support; Education, Implementation, and Teams; and First Aid Task Forces. *Circulation*. 2022;146(25):e483–e557. doi:10.1161/CIR.0000000000001095

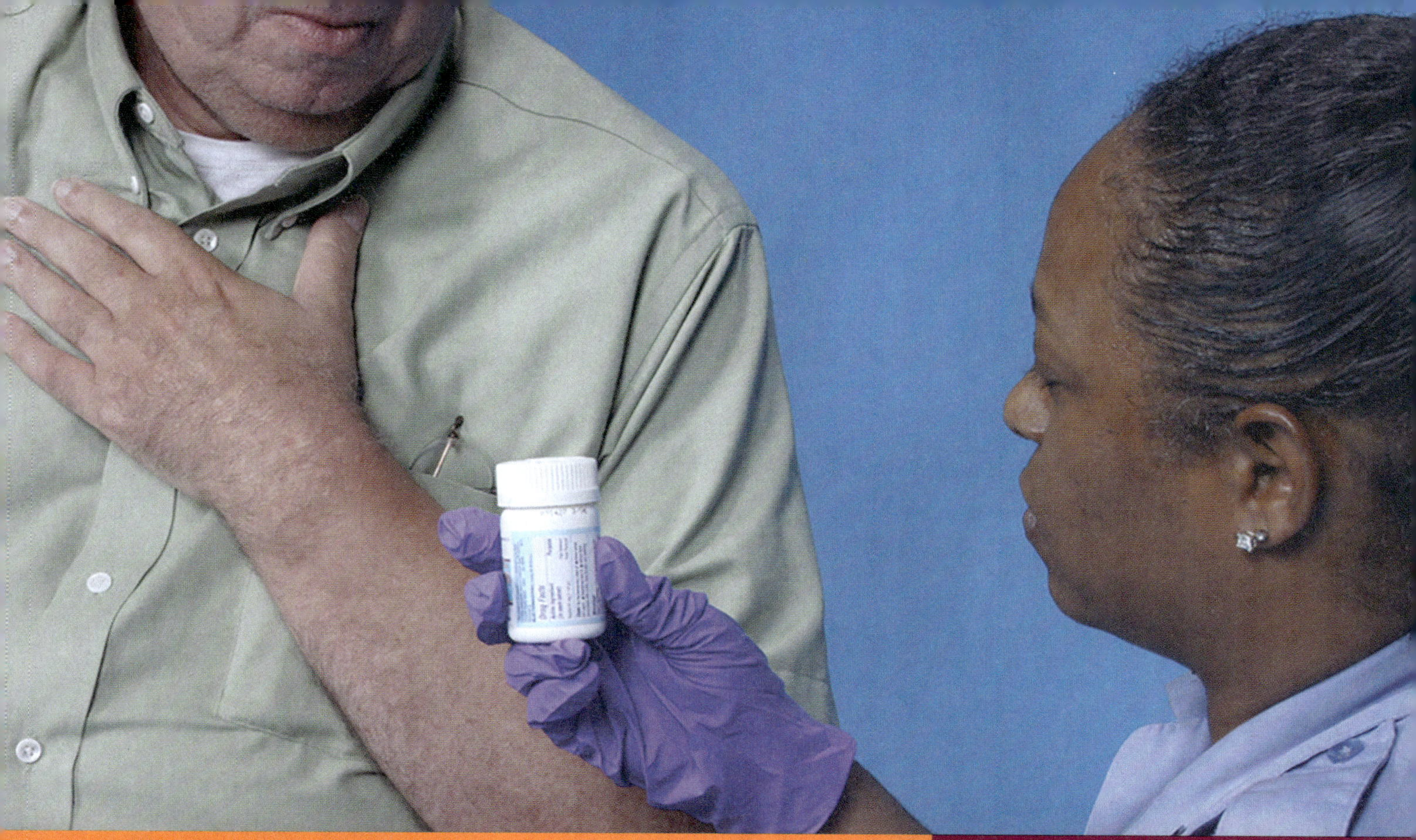

SECTION 4

Pharmacology

12 Principles of Pharmacology and Medication Administration

Chapter 12

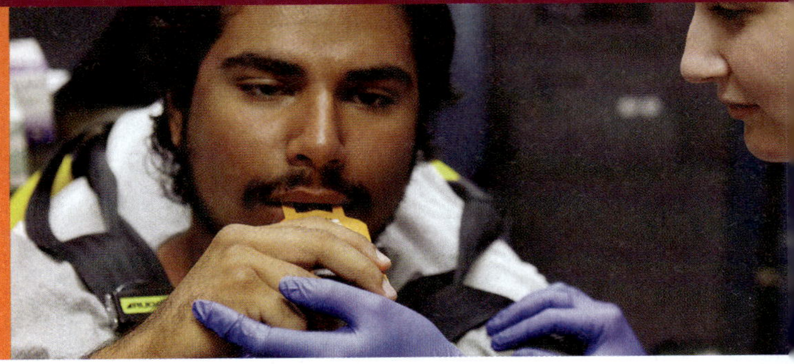

Principles of Pharmacology and Medication Administration

NATIONAL EMS EDUCATION STANDARD COMPETENCIES

Pharmacology

Applies knowledge of the medications the emergency medical technician (EMT) may administer to a patient during an emergency and chronic or maintenance medications the patient may be taking.

Principles of Pharmacology

- Medication safety (pp 490–492, 498–501)
- Medication legislation (pp 491, 498–501)
- Naming (p 492)
- Classifications (p 490)
- Storage and security (pp 492–495)
- Medication interactions (pp 491–492)
- Adverse drug reactions (pp 491–492)
- Metabolism and excretion (pp 493–495)
- Mechanism of action (pp 491, 493–495)
- Medication response relationships (pp 490–495)

Medication Administration

- Use a medication cross-check procedure (p 500)
- Use an auto-injector (pp 514–515)
- Use a unit-dose, premeasured intranasal device (pp 415–416)
- Withdraw medication from a multidose vial with a syringe (p 511)
- Administer medications to a patient (pp 498–501)
- Provide pain management, including ethical and safety considerations (pp 502–505)
- Routes of administration (pp 492–495)

Acute Medications (pp 501–520)

- Names
- Effects
- Indications
- Contraindications
- Side effects
- Routes of administration
- Dosages
- Actions
- Complications
- Interactions

Chronic or Maintenance Medications (pp 501–520)

- Class names
- Class indications
- Class complications
- Class side effects
- Polypharmacy

KNOWLEDGE OBJECTIVES

1. Define the terms pharmacodynamics, therapeutic effects, indications, adverse effects, pharmacokinetics, onset of action, peak, duration, elimination, unintended effects, and untoward effects. (pp 490–492)
2. Explain medication contraindications; include an example. (p 491)
3. Explain the differences between a generic medication name and a trade medication name; provide an example of each. (p 492)
4. Differentiate enteral and parenteral routes of medication administration. (p 493)
5. Describe rectal, oral, intravenous, intraosseous, subcutaneous, intramuscular, intranasal, inhalation, sublingual, and transdermal routes of medication administration; include the rates of absorption. (pp 492–495)
6. Explain the solid, liquid, and gas forms of medication and the routes of administration; provide examples of each. (pp 495–497)
7. List the "rights" of medication administration; include how each one relates to emergency medical services (EMS). (pp 498–500)
8. Explain the difference between direct orders (online) and standing orders (off-line) and the role of medical oversight. (p 501)
9. Discuss the medication administration circumstances involving peer-assisted medication, patient-assisted medication, and EMT-administered medication. (pp 501–506)
10. Know the generic and trade names, actions, indications, contraindications, routes of administration, adverse effects, interactions, and doses of medications that may be administered by an EMT in an emergency as dictated by state protocols and local medical direction. (pp 501–506)
11. Describe the medication administration considerations related to special populations, including pediatric, geriatric, and pregnant patients. (pp 501, 516, 518)
12. Describe the circumstances in which EMTs may administer vaccines. (pp 512, 515)
13. State the steps to follow when administering medications to a patient using an auto-injector. (p 514)
14. Explain why determining what prescription and over-the-counter medications a patient is taking is a critical aspect of patient assessment during an emergency. (pp 520–524)
15. State the steps to take if a medication error occurs. (p 524)

SKILLS OBJECTIVES

1. Apply the rights of medication administration. (pp 498–500)
2. Perform the medication cross-check procedure prior to administering a medication. (pp 500–501)
3. Demonstrate how to administer oral medication to a patient. (pp 506–507)
4. Demonstrate how to administer oral glucose to a patient with hypoglycemia. (p 506)
5. Demonstrate how to administer aspirin to a patient with chest pain. (p 507)
6. Demonstrate how to assist a patient with the sublingual administration of a medication. (pp 507–509)
7. Demonstrate how to withdraw a medication or vaccine from a vial. (p 511; Skill Drill 12-1)
8. Demonstrate how to administer an IM medication in the deltoid muscle. (p 513; Skill Drill 12-2)
9. Demonstrate how to administer a medication by auto-injector. (p 514)
10. Demonstrate how to administer an intranasal medication. (pp 515–516)

Introduction

Medications are an important intervention available to you as an EMT. You must understand the medications within your scope of practice, just as paramedics and nurses must understand the medications they administer. Used appropriately, a medication may alleviate pain or improve a patient's condition. Failure to administer medications safely and competently can lead to serious consequences for the patient, including death. Therefore, it is essential that you have the knowledge and skills to administer or assist in administration of these medications.

This chapter describes the various forms of medications, the different ways in which they can be administered, and how they work. It then takes a close look at each of the forms of medications you may be asked to administer or help patients to self-administer. It will also explain when it is dangerous to administer these medications.

How Medications Work

Pharmacology is the science of drugs, including their ingredients, preparation, uses, and actions on the body. Although the terms *drugs* and *medications* are often used interchangeably, the term *drugs* may make some people think of illegal substances. For this reason, it is best to use the word *medications* whenever the intent may be unclear, especially when interviewing patients and families or providing patient care. In general terms, a **medication** is a substance that is used to treat or prevent disease or relieve pain.

Words of Wisdom

It is important for you to become familiar with the "street" names of commonly used and misused drugs. Most users will not tell you they took methylenedioxymethamphetamine; most likely you will hear terms such as ecstasy, XTC, Molly, rolling, or popping. Research these street names using a reliable source, such as the National Institutes of Health (NIH) or the Centers for Disease Control and Prevention (CDC). Popular street drugs evolve and are modified over time. Local, regional, or national EMS publications and continuing education events will help you obtain the most current information about street drugs that you are likely to encounter in your service area.

Pharmacodynamics is the process by which a medication works on the body. Different types of receptors are located throughout the body. Receptors are sites on cells where medications or chemicals produced in the body can bind and produce an effect. When medications are given, they bind to these sites and either stimulate the receptors to produce an effect or block the receptors to prevent other chemicals or medications from binding. Thus, a medication can either increase or decrease a normal function of the body. A medication that causes stimulation of receptors is called an **agonist**. A medication that binds to a receptor and blocks other medications or chemicals from attaching is called an **antagonist**, or blocker.

There are various other ways that medications affect the body. Certain medications may add electrolytes such as potassium to the body. Other medications target the cell walls of invasive organisms. For example, an **antibiotic** targets bacteria, and an **antifungal** medication targets fungi. Finally, medications might change the concentration of substances in certain body compartments, prompting the movement of water molecules and chemicals from one area of the body to another.

The **dose** is the amount of the medication that is given. It often depends on the patient's weight or age. The dose also depends on the desired action of the medication. The **action** is the intended **therapeutic effect** that a medication is expected to have on the body. The therapeutic effect is also referred to as the desired or intended effect. These factors, among others, can help to explain why one dose of medication works quickly and efficiently on one patient and the same dose has little effect on another patient. Doses may need to be decreased for older adults because they cannot process medications as efficiently as younger people.

ALS Assist

Doses of medications are usually decreased for infants and children because they have smaller bodies, and in some cases, process the drugs differently. Scales in homes, day care centers, schools, and medical offices can be used to obtain an accurate patient weight on scene during EMS responses for infants and children. These devices can offer the most accurate means to calculate weight-based medications to assist your ALS partner. Because scales are not always available, length-based approximation of patient weight is also an important skill. See Chapter 10, *Patient Assessment*, for a description of pediatric weight estimation.

When administering a medication or treating an overdose, you should also consider how the body absorbs, distributes, changes, or eliminates a particular substance. These actions refer to the **pharmacokinetics** of a medication, or actions of the body on the medication (or chemical).

Pharmacokinetic properties for a medication include the following:

- **Onset of action**. Time from medication administration until clinical effects occur.
- **Duration**. Length of time that the clinical effects persist.
- **Elimination**. How medications or chemicals are removed from the body.
- **Peak**. The point or period when the maximum clinical effect is achieved. For EMS clinicians, these times become particularly important when treating pain with opioid medications or managing an opioid overdose with naloxone (Narcan).

Many medications are transformed by the liver and/or eliminated by the kidneys. Patients with liver or kidney disease will have altered pharmacokinetics of many medications compared to healthy individuals. EMTs should understand both the pharmacodynamics and the pharmacokinetics of a medication when assessing a patient's response to a medication, monitoring for adverse effects, or considering the administration of repeat doses of a medication. These two sets of factors will determine how quickly a medication will begin to work, when its effects will peak, how long it will last, and when additional doses would be safe to administer. The route of administration will often have a significant effect on both the pharmacodynamics and the pharmacokinetics of a particular medication or substance. Shock states, altered vital signs, and medication interactions can profoundly alter both the pharmacodynamics and the pharmacokinetics of medications administered by prehospital clinicians.

Indications are the reasons or conditions for which a particular medication is given. For example, nitroglycerin relaxes the walls of all blood vessels, both veins and arteries. This increases the blood flow and the supply of oxygen to the heart muscle. In this way, nitroglycerin may relieve the discomfort that can occur with the cardiac condition called angina. Therefore, nitroglycerin may be indicated for chest pain associated with angina.

There are times when you should not give a medication, even if it usually is indicated for that person's condition. Such situations are called **contraindications**. A medication is contraindicated when it would harm the patient or have no positive effect on the patient's condition. For example, aspirin is an important treatment for patients experiencing a heart attack (acute myocardial infarction), yet it would be contraindicated in a patient reporting acute gastrointestinal bleeding. Some contraindications are absolute, meaning the medication should never be given if the contraindication is present. For example, severe hypotension is an absolute contraindication for nitroglycerin. Some contraindications are relative, meaning the benefits of administering the drug may outweigh the risks. For example, glaucoma (a condition of increased pressure within the eye) is a relative contraindication for many drugs. Consider a patient with anaphylaxis and a history of glaucoma. Glaucoma is a relative contraindication to the use of epinephrine; however, it would likely be more dangerous to withhold epinephrine from this patient than to administer it.

Adverse effects are any actions of a medication other than the desired ones. Adverse effects can occur even when medications are administered correctly. There are two types of adverse effects: unintended effects and untoward effects. **Unintended effects** are undesirable but pose little risk to the patient, such as a slight headache after

YOU are the EMT

You and your partner are dispatched to a residence at 4864 Prospect Avenue for a geriatric patient with "diabetic problems." The time is 0600 hours, the weather is clear, the traffic is light, and your response time to the scene is approximately 5 minutes.

1. What is pharmacology?
2. Why is knowledge of pharmacology important to patient care?

taking nitroglycerin. **Untoward effects** can be harmful to the patient, such as hypotension after taking nitroglycerin.

Consider diphenhydramine (Benadryl). People take this medication for allergic reactions (indication). The medication is supposed to block the effects of histamine (intended effect). Its adverse effects include dry mouth and drowsiness (unintended effect) and it can increase the pressure of the vitreous fluid within the eye (untoward effect). Asthma is a relative contraindication for diphenhydramine because it can worsen lower airway constriction.

Medication Names

Medications usually have two names. The **generic name** (such as ibuprofen) is a simple, clear, nonproprietary name. The generic name is not capitalized. Sometimes a medication is called by its generic name more often than by any of its trade names. For example, you may hear "nitroglycerin" used more often than the trade names NitroMist and Nitrostat. All medications that are licensed for use in the United States are listed by their generic names in the *United States Pharmacopoeia and National Formulary (USP-NF)*. The generic name is approved by the US Food and Drug Administration (FDA) for new drugs. The FDA regulates drug safety and effectiveness in the United States. The Federal Food, Drug, and Cosmetic Act of 1938 gives the FDA authority to enforce drug safety standards.

A **trade name** is the brand name that a manufacturer gives to a medication, such as Tylenol (acetaminophen). As a proper noun, a trade name begins with a capital letter. Trade names are used in every aspect of our daily lives, not just in medications.

Words of Wisdom

Many medication labels use tall man lettering to avoid confusion of medications with similarly spelled names. Capitalized letters are used to highlight the portion of a medication's name that is different from an otherwise similar medication name to help distinguish their names. Examples include DOBUTamine and DOPamine, and diphenhydrAMINE and dimenhyDRINATE.

Well-known examples include Jell-O, Band-Aid, Kleenex, and Coke. A medication may have many different trade names, depending on how many companies manufacture it. Advil, Nuprin, and Motrin all are trade names for the generic medication ibuprofen. A trade name is sometimes designated by use of a raised registered symbol (eg, Advil®).

Medications may be **prescription medications** or **over-the-counter (OTC) medications**. Prescription medications are distributed to patients only by pharmacists according to a physician's order. OTC medications may be purchased without a prescription. Over time, as the effects of a prescription medication are studied and the safety profile is better understood, its status may be changed to allow OTC sales. Examples include Nasacort, Nexium, and Flonase.

You may be called to care for patients who have taken recreational drugs such as heroin or cocaine. Other patients may take herbal remedies, enhancement drugs, vitamin supplements, or alternative medicines. Keep in mind that a patient may have taken more than one of these substances and may additionally be taking prescription or OTC medications. Thus, you may need to consider the actions of more than a single agent or the complex interactions of multiple agents. Your assessment must take into account any and all substances in the patient's system.

Street Smarts

Because many herbal medications, supplements, and OTC medications can interact with prescription medicines, the EMT should document a list of all substances the patient has taken, including prescription and OTC medications, herbal supplements, and recreational substances, so the physician has a full picture of the patient's medication use.

Routes of Administration

Medications can enter the body through a variety of routes. To simplify this topic, the routes of medication administration are divided into two categories: enteral and parenteral. **Enteral medications** enter the body through the digestive system. Typically, the form of the medication will be a pill or a liquid, such as cough medicine. Medications administered via this route tend to absorb slowly. Most emergency medications are not administered orally because the delayed absorption would limit their efficacy when time is crucial. Aspirin and certain **antipyretics** (fever-reducing medications) are common exceptions and may be administered orally by EMS clinicians in many systems.

Parenteral medications enter the body by a route other than the digestive tract, the skin, or the mucous membranes. Parenteral medications are often in a liquid form and are generally administered using syringes and needles. Because these medications enter directly into the bloodstream, they are absorbed much more quickly and offer a more predictable and measurable response.

Certain medications may be administered by both enteral and parenteral routes. Examples include benzodiazepine medications, such as midazolam (Versed) and lorazepam (Ativan), as well as naloxone (Narcan), which is used to reverse opioid overdoses.

Regardless of a medication's route of administration, the end goal is to get the medication into the bloodstream. **Absorption** is the process by which medications travel through body tissues until they reach the bloodstream. Often, the rate at which a medication is absorbed into the bloodstream depends on its route of administration (**TABLE 12-1**). Common routes of medication administration are described as follows:

- **Per rectum (PR)**. Per rectum literally means through the rectum. This route of delivery is most commonly used with children because of easier administration and more reliable absorption. (Children may regurgitate or refuse to take some or all of a medication.) For similar reasons, many medications that are used for nausea and vomiting come in a rectal suppository form. Some medications to control seizures are administered PR when it is impossible to administer them intravenously. The PR route also is used to give some medications when the patient cannot swallow, is actively seizing, or is unconscious. If there is a large amount of stool present, or if the patient has a bowel movement shortly after administration, rectal drug absorption can be slowed.
- **Oral**. Many medications are taken by mouth, or **per os (PO)**, and enter the bloodstream through the digestive system. This process often takes as long as 1 hour but may be surprisingly rapid, depending on the substance or form of preparation. One of the advantages of using this route is that it is noninvasive. Patients are often much happier to take a pill than to have a needle stuck in them. It is also often less expensive to use enteral medications than to use parenteral forms. The main disadvantage of this administration route is the unpredictability of medication absorption. If the patient has vomiting or diarrhea, the amount of medication that is absorbed will be altered. Some medication preparations, referred to as orally disintegrating tablets (ODTs), are put directly onto the tongue, where they dissolve. This is an alternative administration form for patients who may have difficulty swallowing. Some forms of medications are adversely affected by stomach acids, so dissolving them directly on the tongue avoids breakdown by gastric acids. An example of this type of medication is ondansetron (Zofran), which is used to treat nausea and vomiting.

TABLE 12-1 Routes of Administration and Rates of Absorption

Route	Rate
Enteral	
Sublingual (SL)	Rapid
Per rectum (PR)	Rapid
By mouth (PO)	Slow
Parenteral	
Intravenous (IV)	Immediate
Endotracheal (ET)	Unpredictable
Intraosseous (IO)	Immediate
Inhalation	Rapid
Intranasal (IN)	Rapid
Intramuscular (IM)	Moderate
Subcutaneous	Slow
Transdermal	Slow

- **Intravenous (IV) injection**. Intravenous means *into the vein*. Medications that need to enter the bloodstream immediately may be injected directly into a vein. This is the fastest way to deliver a chemical substance, but the IV route cannot be used for all chemicals. For example, aspirin, albuterol, and oxygen cannot be given by the IV route.

ALS Assist

EMTs are generally not permitted to perform IV access. Nonetheless, EMTs may need to assist advanced EMTs (AEMTs) and paramedics with setting up equipment or positioning the patient. It is often necessary for a second person to help hold a patient's hand or arm in a particular position while the vein is located or cannulated by the IV catheter, then secured in place. Planning, effective communication, and standard infection control precautions are essential because these situations present a high risk of accidental needlestick injuries or bloodborne pathogen exposure.

- **Intraosseous (IO) injection**. Intraosseous means into the bone. Medications that are given by this route reach the bloodstream through the bone marrow. Giving a medication by the IO route, into the marrow, requires drilling a needle through the outer layer of the bone. Because this is painful, the IO route is used by ALS clinicians most often in patients who are unconscious as a result of cardiac arrest or extreme shock. Often, the IO route is used for children who have fewer available (or difficult to access) IV sites. In general, any medication that can be given by the IV route can be given by the IO route. This route may be more desirable in critical patients in whom IV access will take longer.
- **Subcutaneous injection**. Subcutaneous means under the skin. A subcutaneous injection is given into the fatty tissue between the skin and the muscle. Because there is less blood here than in the muscles, medications that are given by this route are generally absorbed more slowly, and their effects last longer. A subcutaneous injection is a useful way to give medications that cannot be taken by mouth, as long as they do not irritate or damage the tissue. Daily insulin injections for patients with diabetes are given by the subcutaneous route. Some forms of epinephrine can be given by the subcutaneous route.
- **Intramuscular (IM) injection**. Intramuscular means into the muscle. Usually, medications that are administered by IM injection are absorbed quickly because muscles have many blood vessels. However, not all medications can be administered by the IM route. Possible problems with IM injections are damage to muscle tissue and uneven, unreliable absorption, especially in people with decreased tissue perfusion or who are in shock.

  You will typically use the IM route of medication administration with an auto-injector. These devices deliver a predetermined amount of medication into the patient when pressed firmly into the thigh. Examples of this delivery method would be the EpiPen auto-injector, which is used for anaphylactic reactions, and the DuoDote auto-injector and Antidote Treatment-Nerve Agent Auto-Injector (ATNAA), which are used for nerve agent exposure. During public health emergencies, EMTs also administer vaccines intramuscularly. When giving IM vaccines to adults and older children, administer the injections in the deltoid muscle of the upper arm. (For discussion of the EpiPen and DuoDote/ATNAA, see Chapter 21, *Allergy and Anaphylaxis*, and Chapter 39, *Terrorism Response and Disaster Management*, respectively.)
- **Inhalation**. Some medications are inhaled into the lungs so that they can be absorbed into the bloodstream more quickly. Others are inhaled because they work in the lungs. Generally, inhalation helps minimize the effects of the medication in other body tissues. Such medications come in the form of aerosols, fine powders, and sprays.
- **Endotracheal**. On rare occasions when an ALS clinician is unable to establish IV or IO access, they may administer some medications down the endotracheal tube during cardiac arrest. This route delivers the medication directly into the lungs and is generally considered to have unpredictable absorption; therefore, the doses are much higher than the IV or IO

routes. Administering medications by the endotracheal route requires a momentary pause in chest compressions while the drug is administered to prevent the drug from immediately spraying back up out of the tube.[1]

- **Sublingual (SL)**. Sublingual means under the tongue. Medications given by the SL route, such as nitroglycerin tablets, enter through the oral mucosa under the tongue and are absorbed into the bloodstream within minutes. This route is faster than the oral route, and it protects medications from chemicals in the digestive system, such as acids that can weaken or inactivate them. Sublingual absorption may be delayed if the patient has an unusually dry mouth in situations such as profound dehydration or shock.
- **Transdermal (transcutaneous)**. Transdermal means through the skin. Some medications can be absorbed transdermally, such as the nicotine in patches used by people who are trying to quit smoking. On occasion, a medication that also comes in another form is administered transdermally to achieve a longer-lasting effect. Example are adhesive patches containing nitroglycerin or fentanyl.

Words of Wisdom

Transdermal patches may contain massive quantities of medication that may be released rapidly if the patches are chewed or taken orally through accident or misuse. Children, often toddlers, may face a life-threatening overdose emergency if they chew adult medication patches such as nitroglycerin or fentanyl (Sublimaze) or apply one or more of them to their skin.[2,3] Even adults can overdose if old medication patches are left on the skin when a new one is applied or if a patch is applied to skin with cuts or abrasions. Consult a Poison Control Center or online medical direction in these situations. Consult local protocols or guidelines regarding the removal of transdermal patches during resuscitation or overdose situations.

- **Intranasal (IN)**. In the intranasal route of medication administration, a liquid medication is pushed through a specialized device called a **mucosal atomizer device (MAD)** (**FIGURE 12-1**). The liquid medication is aerosolized and is administered into a nostril. The mucous membranes lining the sinuses and passageways within the head and neck are very vascular; therefore, absorption is rather quick with this route.

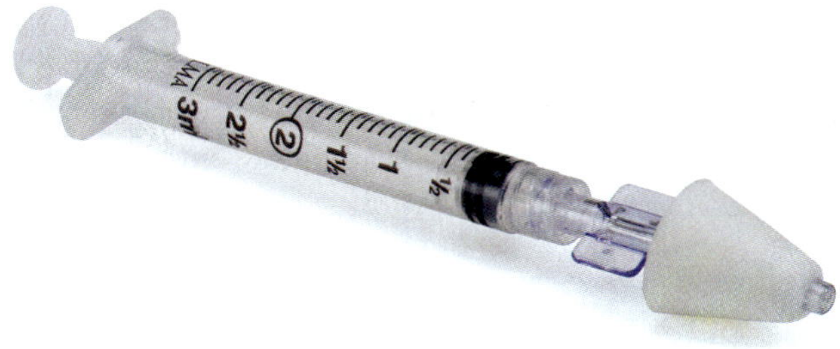

FIGURE 12-1 Mucosal atomizer device can be used for drugs approved for intranasal use.

TABLE 12-2 lists the words that are used for routes of medication delivery, along with their general rates of absorption.

Safety Tips

Make absolutely certain you take standard precautions when administering any medication, particularly topical drugs. If the medication can be absorbed into the patient's skin, it can be absorbed into yours as well.

Medication Forms

The form of a medication usually dictates the route of administration. For example, a tablet or a spray cannot be given through a needle. The manufacturer chooses the form to ensure the proper route of administration, the timing of its release into the bloodstream, and its effects on the target organs or body systems. As an EMT, you should be familiar with the following seven medication forms.

Tablets and Capsules

Most medications that are given by mouth to adult patients are in tablet or capsule form. Capsules are gelatin shells filled with powdered or liquid medication. If the capsule contains liquid, the shell is sealed and usually soft. If the capsule contains powder, the shell can usually be pulled apart. Tablets often contain other materials that are mixed with the medication.

Some tablets are designed to dissolve quickly in small amounts of liquid so that they can be given sublingually (under the tongue) and absorbed rapidly. An example is the sublingual nitroglycerin tablet used to treat chest pain in patients with cardiac conditions. Orally dissolving tablets are another rapidly acting tablet form. These medications are especially useful in emergency situations

TABLE 12-2 Routes of Administration: Words and Their Meanings

This Word...	From These Latin/Greek Words...	Means
Endotracheal	*endo* (within) and *tracheia* (windpipe)	within the windpipe
Inhalation	*inhalatio* (drawing air into the lungs)	inhaling or breathing in
Intramuscular (IM)	*intra* (into) and *muscularis* (of the muscles)	into muscle
Intraosseous (IO)	*intra* (into) and *osse* (bone)	into bone
Intravenous (IV)	*intra* (into) and *venosus* (of the veins)	into vein
Per os (PO)	*per* (by) and *os* (mouth)	by mouth
Per rectum (PR)	*per* (by) and *rectum* (rectum)	by rectum
Subcutaneous	*sub* (under) and *cutis* (skin)	under the skin
Sublingual (SL)	*sub* (under) and *lingua* (relating to the tongue)	under the tongue
Transdermal	*trans* (through) and *derma* (skin)	through the skin
Intranasal	*intra* (into) and *nasal* (nose)	into the nose

YOU are the EMT

You arrive at the scene and find the patient, a 68-year-old woman, sitting in a recliner in her living room. Her son, who called 9-1-1, tells you that she is not "acting right." He also tells you that she has taken her medications today but is not sure when she last ate. You assess the patient as your partner opens the jump kit and prepares to begin treatment.

Recording Time: 0 Minutes	
Appearance	Confused; diaphoretic; pale for baseline
Level of consciousness	Conscious but confused
Airway	Open; clear of secretions or foreign bodies
Breathing	Increased rate; shallow depth
Circulation	Radial pulses rapid and weak; skin pale for baseline and diaphoretic

As your partner gives the patient high-concentration oxygen via nonrebreathing mask, her son tells you that she has diabetes, heart disease, and depression. Her medication list includes eight different prescription medications, including glimepiride (Amaryl) for her diabetes, nitroglycerin (Nitrostat) for her heart disease, and sertraline (Zoloft) for her depression. You assess her blood glucose level, which reads 36 mg/dL. The patient is disoriented to place and time but able to speak and follow simple commands.

3. Other than oxygen, what other medication does this patient require, and why?

4. Why is it significant to know the patient took her medications on an empty stomach?

because medications that must be swallowed and then digested require more time to have an effect. For example, an oral pain medication is less useful than an IV pain medication when pain relief is needed immediately.

Solutions and Suspensions

A **solution** is a liquid mixture of one or more substances that cannot be separated by filtering or allowing the mixture to stand. Solutions can be given by almost any route. When given by mouth, solutions may be absorbed from the stomach rather quickly because the medication is already dissolved.

Specifically prepared solutions labeled for injection only can be given as an IV, IM, or subcutaneous injection. If a patient has an anaphylactic reaction, you may help the patient to self-administer a solution of epinephrine using an auto-injector (EpiPen).

Many substances do not dissolve well in liquids. Some of these can be ground into fine particles and evenly distributed throughout a liquid by shaking or stirring. This type of mixture is called a **suspension**. An example is acetaminophen (Tylenol) suspension, given to infants and children for fever control or pain relief.

Suspensions separate if they stand or are filtered. It is important that you shake or swirl a suspension before administering it to ensure that the patient receives the right amount of medication.

Suspensions usually are administered by mouth but sometimes are given rectally. Occasionally, suspensions are applied directly to the skin to treat skin problems. You may have used calamine lotion in this way. Injectable suspensions are given via IM or subcutaneous injection only. Certain hormone shots or vaccinations are given this way because of the suspended particles. They cannot be given by IV injection because the suspended particles do not remain dissolved.

Metered-Dose Inhalers

If liquids or solids are broken into small enough droplets or particles, they can be inhaled. A **metered-dose inhaler (MDI)** is a miniature spray canister used to direct such substances through the mouth and into the lungs (**FIGURE 12-2**) and is often used by a patient with a respiratory illness such as asthma or emphysema. An MDI delivers the same amount of medication each time it is used. Because an inhaled medication usually is suspended in a propellant, the MDI must be shaken vigorously before the medication is administered. When possible, a spacer should be added between the patient and the MDI. The spacer helps to assure that more medication reaches the lungs. Many patients who use MDI medications also self-administer medications with a nebulizer. Use of MDIs and nebulizers will be discussed later in this chapter.

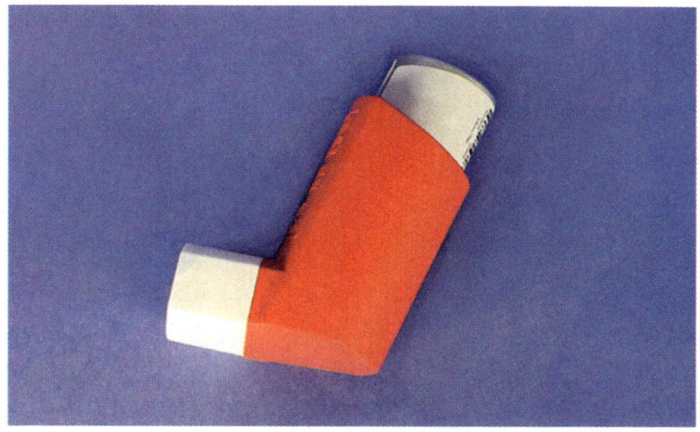

FIGURE 12-2 Some medications are inhaled into the lungs with a metered-dose inhaler so that they can be absorbed into the bloodstream near the site of desired action more quickly.

Topical Medications

Lotions, creams, and ointments are **topical medications**; that is, they are applied to the surface of the skin and affect only that area. Lotions contain the most water, and ointments contain the least. Lotions (such as calamine lotion) are absorbed the most rapidly, and ointments (such as triple antibiotic ointment [Neosporin]) the most slowly. Hydrocortisone cream, to diminish skin itching, is an example of a medical cream that can also be given in ointment form.

Transdermal Medications

Transdermal medications are designed to be absorbed through the skin, or transdermally. Medications such as nitroglycerin ointment usually have properties or delivery systems that help to dilate the blood vessels in the skin and, thus, speed absorption into the bloodstream. In contrast to most topical medicines, which work directly on the application site, transdermal medications are usually

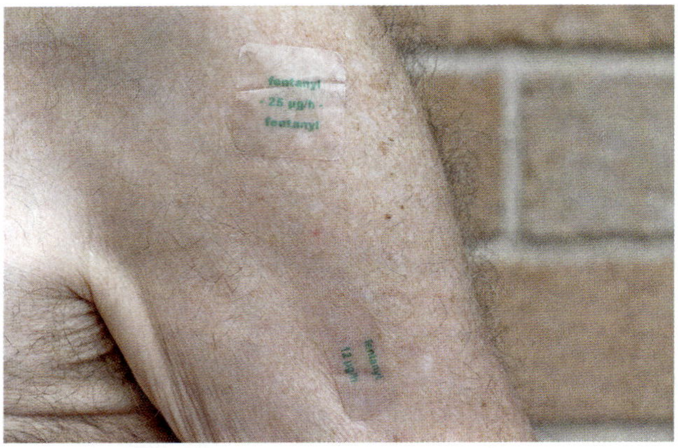

FIGURE 12-3 Some medications are transdermal, or administered through the skin, such as the fentanyl patch shown.

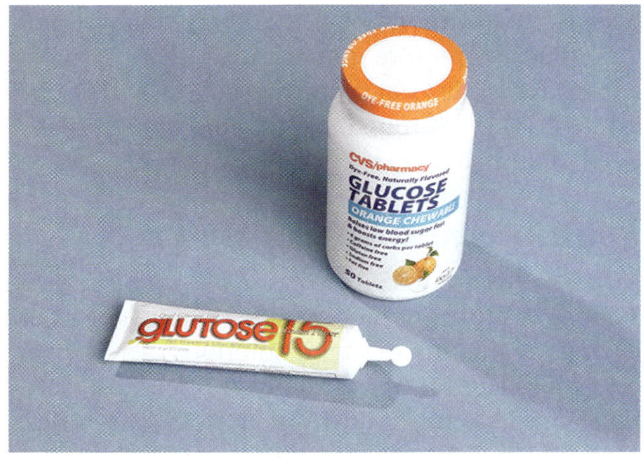

FIGURE 12-4 Oral glucose, used in diabetic emergencies, is available in gel and tablet forms.

intended for systemic (whole-body) effects. A note of caution: If you touch such a medication with your bare skin while administering it, you will absorb it just as readily as the patient will. This can be very dangerous. For example, if you absorb nitroglycerin paste, your blood pressure may drop and cause you to faint while driving the ambulance to the hospital.

One delivery system for transdermal medications is the adhesive patch. Patches attach to the skin and allow even absorption of a medication for many hours (**FIGURE 12-3**). Prescription and OTC medications come in this form. Common examples are nitroglycerin, nicotine, some pain medications, and some hormones.

Gels

A **gel** is a semiliquid substance that is administered orally in capsule form or through plastic tubes. Gels usually have the consistency of pastes or creams but are transparent (clear) or translucent (allowing some light to pass through). "Gelatinous" means thick and sticky, like gelatin. Depending on your local medical directives, as an EMT, you may give oral glucose in gel form to a patient with diabetes (**FIGURE 12-4**).

Gases for Inhalation

Gaseous medications are neither solid nor liquid. The medication most commonly used in gaseous form is oxygen. You might not think of oxygen as a medication; however, in its concentrated form, it is a potent medication that has systemic effects. You will deliver this gas through a nonrebreathing mask, nasal cannula, or bag-mask device. Current guidelines and potential risks of oxygen administration are discussed in Chapter 11, *Airway and Ventilation Management*.

Words of Wisdom

When you document the use of oxygen, include the liter flow rate, the time oxygen was delivered (usually recorded in military time), and the type of device used. For example, "0915—Nonrebreathing mask at 15 L/min. Patient states shortness of breath has improved." *Always* remember to document the patient's response to oxygen administration.

General Steps in Administering Medication

As an EMT, you may only administer medications for which you have an order from medical direction. Medical oversight may be provided online or off-line based on local protocol. You must be familiar with the general steps of administering any medication to a patient, including the "rights" of medication administration:

- Right patient
- Right medication and indication

- Right dose
- Right route
- Right time
- Right documentation

Medication errors, which will be discussed later in this chapter, are disturbingly common and almost always result from failure to follow these rights. After the medication has been administered, you will need to reassess the patient to see if it worked. You should look for adverse effects and then be prepared to document your findings and your actions.

When administering or assisting with the administration of patient medications, you must have an order from medical oversight to do so. If this order is given to you directly through online medical direction, it is important that you repeat the order back to the physician. This is referred to as the echo technique, and it is done to ensure that you heard the order correctly.

The following example illustrates the correct way to acknowledge orders for medications. EMT Johnson is talking on the radio to medical direction and has already given the physician all of the patient assessment information and vital signs. EMT Johnson now asks, "Do you have any orders?" Dr. Ortez says, "Yes, please assist the patient with one nitroglycerin tablet. Make sure the tablet is administered sublingually. Reassess the patient's pain and blood pressure and contact me for further orders if needed." EMT Johnson should reply, "Dr. Ortez, I copy one nitroglycerin tablet sublingual, reassess the patient's pain and blood pressure, and contact you again if needed." Dr. Ortez says, "That is correct. ABC Hospital clear."

If at any point while you are receiving an order for a medication you are confused or unclear about what to do, you should tell medical direction. It is essential that you understand what the physician wants you to do. With all of the noise on a hectic scene, or in the back of an ambulance, it is important to err on the side of caution. If you are not sure what to do, say so and ask for the order to be clarified. If you believe a medication order may be harmful to the patient, it is your responsibility to address your concerns with the ordering physician.

The other way to receive orders to administer or assist with medications is through indirect or off-line medical oversight. Protocols are documents that contain standing orders for the administration of certain medications in specific circumstances. For example, your system may use a protocol that describes how the medical director wants you to deal with a patient who is having respiratory difficulties. Part of this protocol may direct you to use a nonrebreathing mask to deliver oxygen at 15 L/min. You may do this without calling online medical direction if the patient meets the criteria of the protocol.

The "rights" of medication administration are as follows:

- **Right patient.** Make sure the medication is the patient's own and does not belong to a friend or relative, or possibly another patient on scene. You should never give a patient a medication that was prescribed for someone else.
- **Right medication and indication.** Verify the proper medication and prescription, if applicable. Once received, confirm the medication order and determine that the patient is still a candidate for the medication. Make sure the patient does not have any contraindications for the medication. It is always a good idea to have your partner confirm the medication before you administer it. Carefully read the label. If it is the patient's own prescription, the bottle may show the trade name or the generic name. If you have any questions, contact online medical direction.
- **Right dose.** Verify the form and dose of the medication. Once you have confirmed the order and verified that the medication is the correct one to give, you must make sure the form of the medication and the dose are correct. This is where it is important to pay close attention to detail. If you are ordered to give 324 mg of aspirin, you will need to read the bottle to determine how many milligrams are in each tablet. If aspirin is available in 81-mg tablets, how many will you need to give the patient? Again, it is always a good idea to have your partner confirm the dosage before administering it.
- **Right route.** Verify the route of the medication. You must make sure the route matches the order you received. For example, suppose you are told to give the patient a sublingual nitroglycerin tablet. The patient's nitroglycerin tablet bottle is empty, but he has another bottle of nitroglycerin capsules. These are to be swallowed four times per day. The medication is the same, even the dose may be the same,

but the route of delivery is different from the order given. You may not substitute the capsules for the tablets without specific orders from medical direction.

- **Right time.** The concept of right time has different meanings depending on the setting. In health care facilities, medications are typically administered on a particular schedule, based on specific times or intervals. In EMS, an initial dose of a medication is typically given immediately (or "stat"). Subsequent repeat doses may require a specific time interval, depending on the medication, dose, and route.

  The concept of right time also includes checking the expiration date and condition of the medication. The last step before administering a medication is to make sure the expiration date has not passed. Prescription and OTC medications have an expiration date. Check the label. If no date can be found, you should examine the medication with suspicion. If you find discoloration, cloudiness, or particles in a liquid medication, you should not use it. If a patient with asthma gives you an MDI and the expiration date on it is smudged, you should not use it.
- **Right documentation.** Remember this EMS expression: "The work is not done until the paperwork is done." Once the medication has been given, you must document your actions and the patient's response. This includes the time you gave the medication and the name, dose, and route of administration. Did the patient's condition improve, worsen, or not change? Were there any adverse effects? A second EMS expression says, "If you did not write it down, it did not happen." Should your performance ever be questioned, accurate documentation is your best defense.

Street Smarts

Many patients who have a history of cardiovascular problems may be prescribed nitroglycerin to take "just in case" they have chest pain. By the time it is needed during an emergency, the medication may have expired and not be as effective. Be sure to note the expiration date and communicate this situation to medical direction.

After the medication is administered, you will need to reassess the patient to see if it has worked. Does the patient still have the same complaint as before you administered the medication? Has it changed? Is the patient experiencing any adverse effects? You should reassess the vital signs, especially heart rate and blood pressure, at least every 5 minutes if the patient's condition changes. If the medication is being administered to help reduce pain, you should ask the patient to rate the pain both before and after medication administration. A 0 to 10 scale or the visual pain scale is often used to help patients quantify their pain level. In addition, if the physician orders you to repeat the medication, it is important to do so at the right time. For example, if you are advised by medical direction to repeat administration of nitroglycerin in 10 minutes if the patient's pain is unresolved, you should not wait 15 minutes.

Medication Administration Cross-Check Procedure

Merely reviewing the rights of medication administration in your head is often not a sufficient safeguard to prevent a medication error. Using a verbal cross-check procedure that verifies you are giving the right drug to the right patient at the right dose has been found to reduce medication errors. This procedure, initially developed by Sedgwick County EMS in Kansas, should be stated aloud for each medication administration. It uses closed-loop communication and provides a time-out to reflect on whether the proper drug administration is being performed.

To perform the procedure, the person who is prepared to give the medicine alerts their partner that an important communication is happening by saying, "Medication check." The partner then replies, "Ready." Then the EMT who will give the medicine says, "I am going to give [medication name, dose, and route] for [indication]." If the partner thinks this information is correct, they respond, "Contraindications?" This is a chance to reflect on whether the patient has allergies or other reasons the medicine should not be given. If there are none, the EMT reports, "None." The partner then asks, "Volume?" and the EMT presents the medication container and the syringe, tablets, or device with the appropriate dose measured. If the partner agrees it is correct, they state, "I agree with administration."

This procedure can be done with another EMT, an EMR, or even aloud, alone in the back of the ambulance. The mere act of pausing and consciously verifying these steps aloud may help you catch an error before it is too late.

Medication Administration and the EMT

There are several medications that may be carried on the EMS unit, including oxygen, oral glucose, aspirin, naloxone, medicines to treat wheezing (eg, albuterol, ipratropium), and epinephrine. When used wisely, each can be a powerful tool. Keep in mind, however, that you may give these medications only according to standing orders in a protocol (off-line medical direction) or a direct order (online medical direction). Along with the several different medications that can be given by EMTs, there are several different routes of administration that will be used to deliver these medications to the patient.

Before specific medications are discussed, the circumstances surrounding the administration of the medications need to be discussed. Over the years, EMTs have been allowed increasing responsibility to work with medications, but this growth has come with some degree of confusion and worry. Many departments throughout the United States have strict controls on when an EMT is allowed to administer a medication. The circumstances are as follows:

- **Peer-assisted medication**
- **Patient-assisted medication**
- **EMT-administered medication**

In peer-assisted medication administration, you are administering medication to yourself or your partner. At times it may be necessary for an EMS crew to receive medications because they were exposed to a toxic nerve agent, such as during a terrorism incident. In this case, you would first treat yourself and then your partner. Typically, nerve agent antidotes are administered via an auto-injector. (See Chapter 39, *Terrorism Response and Disaster Management*, for more information on nerve agent antidotes.)

In patient-assisted medication administration, you are assisting the patient with the administration of their own medication, such as an EpiPen, an MDI bronchodilator, or nitroglycerin. Perhaps the patient cannot find their medication. Maybe the patient is so upset that they cannot open the pill bottle or hold the MDI steady. In this circumstance, the patient is trying to administer the medication, but you need to offer some help so the task can be completed.

The last circumstance is EMT-administered medications. Here you are directly administering the medication to the patient. It can certainly be difficult to find the exact point where assisting a patient ends and actually administering a medication begins. The patient may be severely ill, too confused, or unable to understand the need for the medication. Common medications that you will administer in this circumstance are oxygen, oral glucose, epinephrine, nitroglycerin, bronchodilators (albuterol, ipratropium), naloxone, and aspirin.

It is important for you to understand that the medication itself does not necessarily dictate whether you will be assisting or directly administering. Medical oversight, state guidelines, and local protocols will be the determining factors that define the role of the EMT. The EpiPen is an example of a medication that is both patient-assisted and EMT-administered. Refer to your local standards to obtain a listing of how and when EMTs can administer medications.

Special Populations

MEDICATIONS AND THE PREGNANT PATIENT

Pregnant patients are limited in the medications they can take because of the risk to the fetus.

Medications Used by EMTs

The following is a discussion of medications that may be administered by EMTs. Again, your state, department, and medical director will ultimately define what medications are carried on your ambulance. **TABLE 12-3** provides an overview of these medications and their actions, indications, contraindications, routes of administration, adverse effects, interactions, and doses.

The 2019 National EMS Scope of Practice Model recognizes that some regions of the country may need EMTs to be involved in the administration of medications beyond oxygen, oral glucose, aspirin

TABLE 12-3 EMT Medication Overview

Generic/ Trade	Action	Indications	Contraindications	Routes	Adverse Effects	Interactions	Dose[a]	Administration Concerns
Medications EMTs Administer or May Assist in Administering								
Aspirin (Bayer)	Anti-inflammatory agent and anti-fever agent; prevents platelets from clumping, thereby decreasing formation of new clots	Relief of mild pain, headache, muscle aches, fever; chest pain of cardiac origin	Hypersensitivity; recent bleeding; suspected stroke prior to CT scanning; fevers in children	PO	Nausea, vomiting, stomach pain, bleeding, allergic reactions	Caution should be used in patients who are taking anticoagulants	160 to 325 mg; 160- to 325-mg chewable tablets for chest pain	Do not administer for pain caused by trauma; patients with chest pain must be able to chew tablets
Albuterol (Proventil, Ventolin)[b], ipratropium (Atrovent)	Albuterol stimulates the sympathetic nervous system, causing bronchodilation. Ipratropium blocks an action of the parasympathetic nervous system to relax bronchial smooth muscles, causing bronchodilation	Asthma/ difficulty breathing with wheezing	Hypersensitivity; tachycardia (relative); chest pain of cardiac origin	Inhalation	Hypertension, tachycardia, anxiety, restlessness	Increases effects of other nervous system stimulants	Adult nebulizer: 2.5 mg albuterol alone or with ipratropium 0.5 mg (as Combivent or DuoNeb) in 2.5 mL 0.9% normal saline MDI: 1 to 2 inhalations; wait 5 minutes before repeating dose Pediatric albuterol: <44 pounds (20 kg), 2.5 mg/ dose diluted in 2 mL of 0.9% NS; MDI 4 puffs with spacer Pediatric ipratropium: 250 to 500 mcg by MDI or nebulizer every 20 min	Patient must inhale all medication in one breath; coach patient to hold breath for 5 seconds after inhalation

Epinephrine (EpiPen)	Stimulates nervous system, causing bronchodilation	Anaphylactic reaction	Chest pain of cardiac origin; hypothermia; hypertension	IM	Hypertension, tachycardia, anxiety, restlessness	Increases effects of other nervous system stimulants	Adult: 0.3 mg Pediatric: <55 pounds (25 kg), 0.15 mg IM in lateral thigh; >55 pounds (25 kg), 0.3 mg IM in lateral thigh	Medication will last approximately 5 minutes; can repeat dose every 5 to 15 minutes; ensure ALS is en route for continuing treatment
Naloxone (Narcan, EVZIO auto-injector)	Reverses respiratory depression secondary to opioid overdose	Opioid poisoning	Hypersensitivity	IM, IN	Nausea, vomiting	Additional doses may be required for severe opioid overdoses	Adult: 2 mg IN or IM auto-injector Pediatric: 0.1 mg/kg IM, max dose 2 mg; 0.1 mg/kg NAS, max dose 4 mg; naloxone nasal spray in a single-use bottle contains 4 mg/0.1 mL (Refer to medical oversight guidance for dosing, as naloxone is supplied in a variety of concentrations. Naloxone autoinjectors contain 0.4 mg/0.4 mL or 2 mg/0.4 mL)	Patients may wake up combative
Nitroglycerin (Nitrostat, NitroMist)	Dilates blood vessels	Chest pain of cardiac origin	Hypotension; use of sildenafil (Viagra) or another treatment for erectile dysfunction within the previous 24 hours; head injury	SL tablet or spray	Headache, burning under tongue, hypotension, nausea	Increases dilating effects of other blood vessel–dilating medications	0.3 to 0.4 mg SL; 0.4 mg spray SL	Ensure ALS is en route

(continues)

TABLE 12-3 EMT Medication Overview (*continued*)

Generic/Trade	Action	Indications	Contraindications	Routes	Adverse Effects	Interactions	Dose[a]	Administration Concerns
Oral glucose (Glutose)	When absorbed, provides glucose for cell use	Low blood glucose (hypoglycemia)	Decreased level of consciousness; nausea; vomiting	PO	Nausea, vomiting	None	½ to 1 tube	Patient must be awake, have control of airway, and be able to follow commands
Oxygen (no trade name)	Reverses hypoxia; provides oxygen to be absorbed by lungs	Hypoxia or suspected hypoxia. *Routine use of supplemental oxygen without underlying hypoxia is no longer indicated for many conditions.*	Use in suspected stroke and STEMI restricted to the presence of dyspnea OR unable to obtain Spo_2 OR suspected myocardial infarction with Spo_2 <90% OR suspected stroke with Spo_2 <94% Do not use near open flames, as oxygen will support combustion	Inhalation	In patient with normal Spo_2, may decrease oxygenation to the heart in myocardial infarction and to the brain in stroke	Can support combustion	Adult: use oxygen delivery devices to administer 28% to 100% oxygen Pediatric: 1 to 6 L/min nasal cannula (up to 4 L/min if <2 years); 10 to 15 L/min NRB mask	No open flames nearby; do not withhold oxygen from patients in respiratory distress
Common Over-the-Counter Medications								
Acetaminophen (Tylenol)	Analgesic and fever reducer	Relief of mild pain or fever, headache, muscle aches	Hypersensitivity	PO	Allergic reaction	Take caution to avoid potential overdosing; many OTC medications contain acetaminophen	Adult: 500 to 1,000 mg every 4 hours as needed Pediatric: <12 years, 15 mg/kg every 6 h, max single dose 1,000 mg; >12 years, same as adult	Weight of child is more important than age

Diphenhydramine (Benadryl)	Antihistamine (blocks histamine)	Mild allergic reactions	Asthma; glaucoma; pregnancy; hypertension; infants	PO	Sleepiness (although can stimulate children), dry mouth and throat	Do not take with alcohol or MAO inhibitors (a type of psychiatric medication)	Adult: 25 to 50 mg Pediatric: 1 mg/kg PO, max dose 25 mg	Can use in severe allergic reaction; however, epinephrine is administered first
Ibuprofen (Advil, Motrin, Nuprin)	NSAID that reduces inflammation and fever; analgesic	Mild pain or fever, headache, muscle aches	Hypersensitivity	PO	Nausea, vomiting, stomach pain, bleeding, allergic reactions	Do not take with aspirin	Adult: 200 to 400 mg every 4 to 6 hours Pediatric: 10 mg/kg every 4 to 6 hours, max dose 400 mg	Do not take for pain caused by trauma; weight of child is more important than age

[a]Pediatric dosing must always be approved by medical oversight, either in standing orders or by online medical direction.
[b]Albuterol and ipratropium are often packaged together in the same inhaler or prefilled medication dose for inhalation under the trade name Combivent or DuoNeb.

Abbreviations: ALS, advanced life support; CT, computed tomography; IM, intramuscular; IN, intranasal; MDI, metered-dose inhaler; MAO, monoamine oxidase; NRB, nonrebreathing; NSAID, nonsteroidal anti-inflammatory drug; OTC, over the counter; PO, per os (taken by mouth); SL, sublingual; Spo_2, oxygen saturation; STEMI, ST-elevated myocardial infarction for chest pain of ischemic origin, oral OTC analgesics for pain or fever, inhaled beta agonists, naloxone, auto-injectors for chemical/hazardous materials exposures, epinephrine, and nitroglycerin for chest pain (must be the patient's medication). The exact list of medications that you will be allowed to manage is ultimately controlled by the state in which you practice and medical director of your agency. In public health emergencies, EMTs may also be asked to assist with vaccination efforts.

Oral Medications

There are several medications that you may be asked to administer or to assist with administration. Oral glucose, aspirin, and several OTC medications can be administered by this route. As discussed, the advantages of this route are its ease of access and comfort level for the patient. One of the disadvantages of administering medications orally is that the digestive tract can be easily affected by food, stress, and illness. The speed of movement of food through the tract dramatically changes the speed of absorption. As with all medications, you need to start with the rights of administration. Follow these steps to perform oral medication administration:

1. Take standard precautions.
2. Obtain medical direction per local protocol.
3. Confirm the medication is not expired and the other rights of medication administration.
4. If possible, place the patient in a semi-Fowler or high-Fowler position.
5. Confirm that the patient has a patent airway and is able to swallow and follow instructions, then instruct the patient to swallow or chew the medication and follow with small sips of water if needed (**FIGURE 12-5**).
6. Monitor the patient's condition and document.

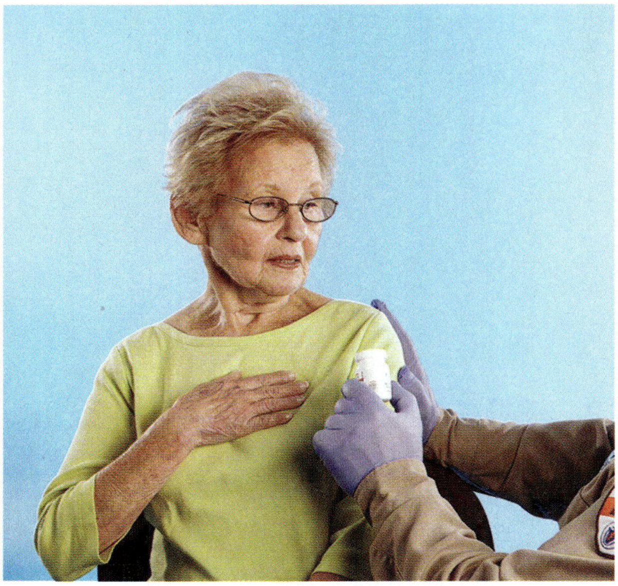

FIGURE 12-5 Instruct the patient to chew (eg, baby aspirin) or swallow the medication.

Oral Glucose

Glucose is a sugar that our cells use as fuel. Although some cells can use other sugars, brain cells must have glucose. If the level of glucose in the blood gets too low, a person can experience a loss of consciousness, have seizures, and ultimately die.

The medical term for an extremely low blood glucose level is **hypoglycemia**. Hypoglycemia can be caused by an excess of insulin, which is taken to control blood glucose levels. Patients with diabetes who use insulin regularly usually understand the effects of this medication on the body. The **oral glucose** that is carried in the EMS unit, as well as glucose tablets, can counteract the effects of hypoglycemia in the same way as a caloric beverage such as juice or a non-diet soda, but faster. This is because common table sugar (sucrose) and fruit sugars (fructose) are complex sugars and must be broken down before they can be absorbed. Glucose is a simple sugar that is readily absorbed by the bloodstream.

As an EMT, you can give glucose only by mouth. Hospital personnel and advanced clinicians (AEMTs and paramedics) can also give a form of glucose (dextrose) intravenously. Glucose is available as a gel designed to be spread on the mucous membranes between the cheek and gum; however, absorption through this route is not as quick as with injection. Because the patient may be conscious one moment and unconscious the next, you must be very careful when administering oral glucose. Never administer oral medications to an unconscious patient or to a patient who is unable to swallow or protect the airway. See Chapter 20, *Endocrine and Hematologic Emergencies*, for more information on the administration of oral glucose.

Safety Tips

Never attempt to give anything by mouth to a patient with a decreased level of consciousness (LOC). Remember, an altered LOC may be an indication for a medication such as oral glucose; however, a decreased LOC can be a contraindication for oral medications, due to the potential for airway compromise.

Aspirin

Aspirin (acetylsalicylic acid or ASA) is an antipyretic (reduces fever), analgesic (reduces pain), and anti-inflammatory (reduces inflammation) medication that also inhibits platelet aggregation (clumping). This last property makes it one of the most used medications today. Research has shown that clumping of platelets to form clots in the coronary arteries under certain conditions is one of the direct causes of heart attack. Patients at high risk for coronary artery disease are often prescribed one or two low-dose (often called baby or children's) aspirins per day. During a potential heart attack, aspirin may be lifesaving.

Contraindications for aspirin include documented hypersensitivity to aspirin (absolute), preexisting liver damage (absolute), bleeding disorders (relative), and asthma (relative). Because of the association of aspirin with Reye syndrome (a rare but serious condition that causes swelling in the brain and liver), it should not be given to children younger than 16 years.

Sublingual Medications

The sublingual route of administration has many advantages. Assuming the patient is awake, alert, and able to follow commands, it is easy to instruct the patient to place a pill under the tongue. The membranes that line the mouth and the undersurface of the tongue receive large amounts of blood flow; as a result, when taken sublingually, a medication is absorbed faster but has a shorter duration of action than when it is taken orally. Be aware, however, that any medication placed in the mouth requires constant evaluation of the airway. You must also be alert to any signs of choking on the pill. If the patient is uncooperative or unconscious, this route of medication administration should not be used.

Nitroglycerin

Many patients with cardiac conditions carry some form of fast-acting nitroglycerin to relieve the pain of angina. **Nitroglycerin** has been used medically since the 1800s. Nitroglycerin is typically the only medication that you will help to administer sublingually (**FIGURE 12-6**).

YOU are the EMT

After administering 15 g of oral glucose to the patient, you reassess her and note that her condition has improved. She is conscious and alert and asks you what happened. As you explain what happened to her, your partner takes her vital signs.

Recording Time: 5 Minutes	
Respirations	22 breaths/min; regular and adequate
Pulse	112 beats/min; strong and regular
Skin	Baseline color; slightly moist
Blood pressure	122/72 mm Hg
Oxygen saturation (Spo_2)	98% (on oxygen)
Blood glucose	70 mg/dL

5. What are the "rights" of medication administration, and why are they important?

6. What medications are typically carried on an ambulance staffed by EMTs?

7. As an EMT, what medications can you assist the patient to self-administer?

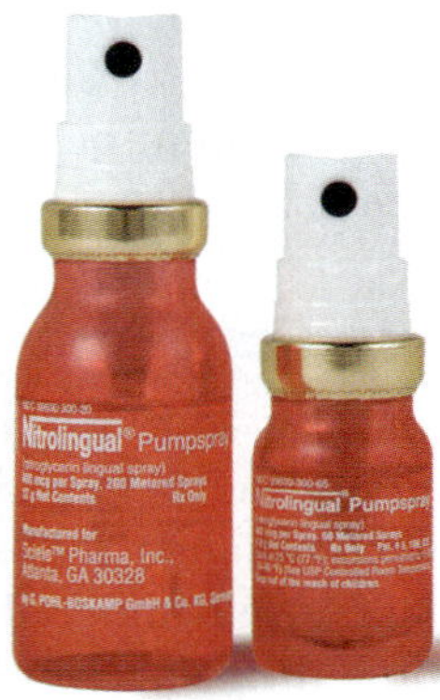

A

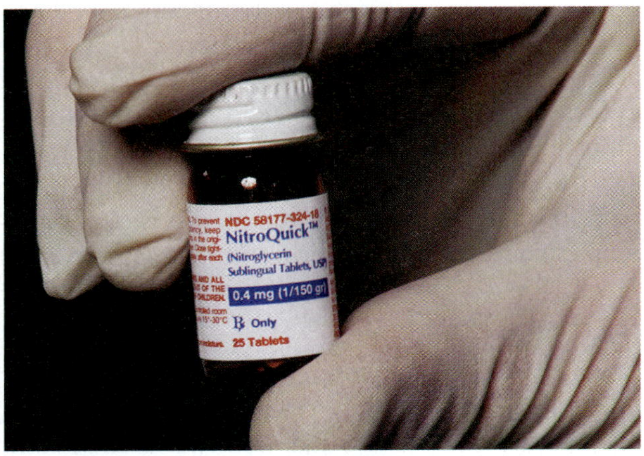

B

FIGURE 12-6 Nitroglycerin, which is prescribed for chest pain, can be given sublingually as a spray (**A**) or tablet (**B**).

If you have ever run for a prolonged period, you probably remember your muscles developed a painful, heavy, burning sensation. This is because the demand for oxygen by the muscles exceeded the supply. When a similar pain develops in heart muscle, it is called angina pectoris. The cause is the same: insufficient oxygen. In this case the pain is due to a blockage or narrowing in the blood vessels that supply the heart. Occasionally, the cause is a spasm in these blood vessels. Unlike a runner with sore legs, the heart muscle cannot stop and rest until the pain goes away.

The purpose of nitroglycerin is to increase blood flow by relieving the spasms or causing the arteries to dilate. It does this by relaxing the muscular walls of the coronary arteries and veins. Nitroglycerin also relaxes veins throughout the body, so less blood is returned to the heart and the heart does not have to work as hard each time it contracts. However, in some patients nitroglycerin also decreases blood pressure. Because of this, it is important that you always take the patient's blood pressure before administering nitroglycerin. If the systolic blood pressure is less than 100 mm Hg, the nitroglycerin may have the harmful effect of lowering the blood flow to the heart's own blood vessels. Even a patient who has adequate blood pressure should sit or lie down with the head elevated before taking this medication. A patient who is standing may faint when blood flow to the brain is reduced as the nitroglycerin starts to work. If a significant decrease in the patient's blood pressure (15 to 20 mm Hg) occurs and the patient suddenly feels dizzy or sick, have the patient lie down.

During a heart attack (myocardial infarction [MI]), a narrowing or blockage in a coronary artery blocks the blood flow to a section of the heart muscle (myocardium). If the blockage is not cleared in time, the section of the heart muscle beyond the clot will die. If nitroglycerin no longer brings relief to a person in whom it has previously worked, the person may be experiencing an MI instead of an angina attack. Therefore, it is important to know how much nitroglycerin a patient has needed in the past to relieve chest pain and how much has been taken during the current emergency, including the use of nitroglycerin patches. Always report this information to medical direction. Remember, you cannot administer this medication without direct online medical direction or standing orders.

There are important interactions to consider when administering nitroglycerin. Erectile dysfunction medications, such as sildenafil (Viagra), tadalafil (Cialis), and vardenafil (Levitra), can have potentially fatal interactions with nitroglycerin. When taken together, nitroglycerin and these drugs can cause a dramatic drop in blood pressure. Always ask a patient who has been prescribed nitroglycerin if they have used any medication for the treatment of erectile dysfunction within the previous 24 hours. If so, do not administer the nitroglycerin, and report this to medical direction. Keep in mind that drugs for erectile dysfunction may be used by both men and women; do not assume women have not taken erectile dysfunction drugs.

Nitroglycerin has the following effects:

- Relaxes the muscular walls of coronary arteries and veins, improving blood flow to the heart muscle

- Dilates veins, resulting in less blood returning to the heart and decreasing the preload
- Relaxes arteries throughout the body, decreasing afterload
- Decreases blood pressure in some patients[4]
- Often causes a mild headache and/or burning under the tongue after administration

By decreasing the preload and afterload, nitroglycerin reduces the heart's workload, thereby lowering its oxygen demand.

Administering Nitroglycerin by Tablet

Nitroglycerin is usually taken sublingually. The patient places a tiny tablet under the tongue, where it dissolves. The tablet should create a slight tingling or burning sensation under the tongue. Exposure to light, heat, or air may degrade the strength of the medication. If the nitroglycerin does not produce the typical burning sensation, it may have lost potency because of aging or improper storage. If you notice any signs of improper storage, be sure to include that information in the patient's medical history. In addition, be sure to check the expiration date on the bottle.

Sublingual nitroglycerin tablets should be stored in their original glass container with the cap screwed on tightly. Nothing else should be placed in the container, as it can rob nitroglycerin of its power.

Street Smarts

Do not pour nitroglycerin tablets directly from the bottle into the patient's mouth; doing so may cause you to inadvertently administer multiple tablets. Patients who have an unusually dry mouth might benefit from the metered-dose spray form of nitroglycerin, as the tablets may not dissolve fully in a timely manner.

Administering Nitroglycerin by Metered-Dose Spray

Some patients who take nitroglycerin use a metered-dose spray, which deposits medication on or under the tongue. Each spray is equivalent to one tablet. To ensure direct, proper dosing on the bottom of the tongue, hold the canister upright when administering, and do not use a spacer with the metered-dose canister when giving nitroglycerin by this method. Do not shake the canister before spraying it.

Whether using the tablets or the metered-dose spray, you should wait 5 minutes for a response before repeating the dose. Closely monitor the patient's vital signs, particularly the blood pressure. Give repeated doses per medical direction and/or local protocol. Remember, always wear gloves when handling nitroglycerin tablets or spray, because this medication can be absorbed by your skin.

Next, you must reconfirm that the medication is still indicated for the patient. For example, suppose you have received and verified the order to give one sublingual nitroglycerin tablet to a patient with a cardiac condition. While you are getting the order, however, the patient begins to sweat more and becomes less responsive. Reassessment of the blood pressure reveals a pressure of 80/60 mm Hg. Using your knowledge of nitroglycerin, you recognize the contraindication and decide not to give the medication. Instead, you notify medical direction of the changes in the patient's condition and seek new orders.

Knowing and understanding the local protocols under which you will be working are absolutely essential, as is a thorough knowledge of the medications within your scope of practice. Refer to Table 12-3 for a review of all medications and the important information needed for their administration. See Chapter 17, *Cardiovascular Emergencies*, for more information on how to administer nitroglycerin.

Words of Wisdom

Remember these general steps in administering medication:

1. Obtain an order from medical direction.
2. Verify the rights of medication administration.
3. Complete a cross-check procedure.
4. Reassess the vital signs, especially heart rate and blood pressure, at least every 5 minutes or as the patient's condition changes.
5. Document your actions and the patient's response.

Intramuscular Medications

The intramuscular (IM) route of administration provides quick and easy access to the circulatory system without the need for placing a needle within a vein. Blood flow to the muscles is relatively stable, even during circumstances of severe illness or injury. This advantage makes the IM route an efficient means to deliver some medications. A disadvantage for this route is the use of a needle and the subsequent pain it can cause. Patients may be reluctant for you to use the needle for fear of pain or injury. With proper technique, you can administer medications via the IM route and limit the amount of pain delivered to the patient.

Administering an IM Injection

Drawing Medication From a Vial

When drawing medication from a vial, you must avoid introducing pathogens that may cause an infection from the time you begin to prepare your supplies and the environment, until you are completely finished. When withdrawing medication, changing the needles, or administering the injection, you must clean your hands, put on clean gloves, clean the vial top with antiseptic, and avoid touching any part of the needle or the tip of the syringe to any unsterile surface. If you accidently contaminate the needle or tip of the syringe prior to administering the drug, you will need to discard the contaminated equipment in the appropriate sharps container and start again.

Follow these steps to draw medication from the vial.[5] First, prepare your supplies and the environment:

1. Gather your supplies: medicine vial, syringe with tapered or blunt-tip needle (used only for withdrawing medication), antiseptic wipe (alcohol or chlorhexidine-alcohol), and sharps container.
2. Clean your hands.

Next, carefully check your medicine:

1. Check the label. Make sure you have the right medicine. Also check the date on the vial; do not use expired medicine.
2. You may have a multidose vial, or you may have a vial with powder that you mix with liquid. If it must be mixed, read the medication's instructions or ask another clinician for instructions.
3. If you will use the medicine more than once, write the date on the vial so you remember when you opened it.
4. Look at the medicine in the vial. Check for a change in color, small pieces floating in the liquid, cloudiness, or any other changes from its original or expected appearance.

Prepare your medicine vial:

1. Take the cap off the vial.
2. Wipe the rubber top clean with an alcohol pad.

Follow these steps to fill the syringe with medicine:

1. Hold the syringe in your hand like a pencil, with the needle pointed up.
2. Pull back the plunger to the line on your syringe for the volume needed to administer your dose. This fills the syringe with air.
3. Insert the needle into the rubber top. Do not touch or bend the needle.
4. Push the air into the vial. This keeps a vacuum from forming. If you put in too little air, you will find it hard to draw out the medicine. If you put in too much air, the medicine may be forced out of the syringe.
5. Turn the vial upside down and hold it up in the air. Keep the needle tip in the medicine.
6. Pull back the plunger to the line on your syringe for your dose. For example, if you need 1 milliliter (mL) of medicine, pull the plunger to the line marked 1 mL on the syringe.

To remove air bubbles from the syringe:

1. Keep the syringe tip in the medicine.
2. Tap the syringe with your finger to move air bubbles to the top. Then push gently on the plunger to push the air bubbles back into the vial.
3. If the syringe contains a lot of bubbles, push the plunger to return all of the medicine to the vial. Draw medicine out again slowly and tap air bubbles out. Double-check that you still have the right amount of medicine drawn up.
4. Remove the syringe from the vial and keep the needle clean.
5. Put the cover back on the needle using a one-handed technique. Remove the needle used to draw up the medicine and discard it in a sharps container. Replace the needle used to draw up the medication with a needle of the appropriate size (gauge) and length for the injection. This may vary based on patient size and/or injection site being used.
6. Before administering, confirm medication volume and dose with a partner using the medication administration cross-check procedure discussed earlier.

The steps for drawing medication from a vial are summarized in **SKILL DRILL 12-1**.

Skill Drill 12-1 Drawing Medication From a Vial

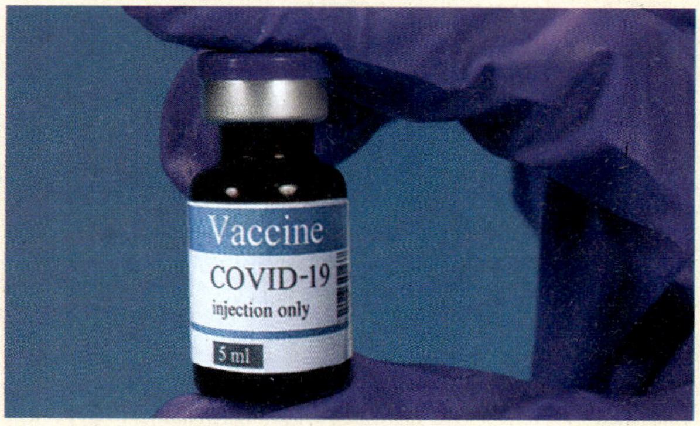

Step 1

Check the label. Make sure you have the right medicine and it is not expired. Look at the medicine in the vial and make sure there are no small pieces floating in the liquid, cloudiness, or any other changes from its expected appearance. Prepare the vial by taking off the cap and wiping the rubber top clean with an alcohol pad.

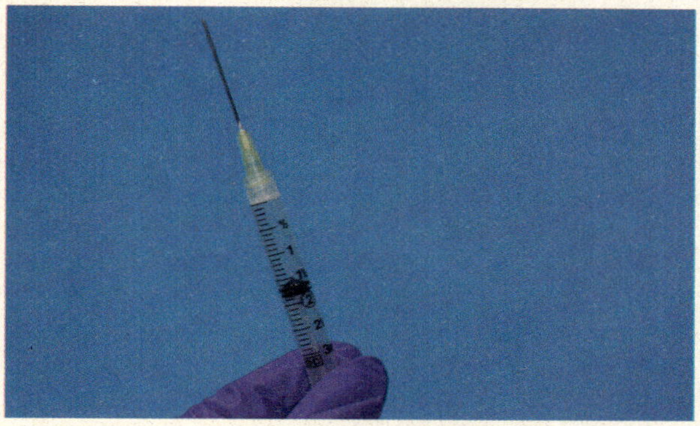

Step 2

Determine the amount of medication that you will need, and draw that amount of air into the syringe. Allow a little extra room to expel some air while removing air bubbles.

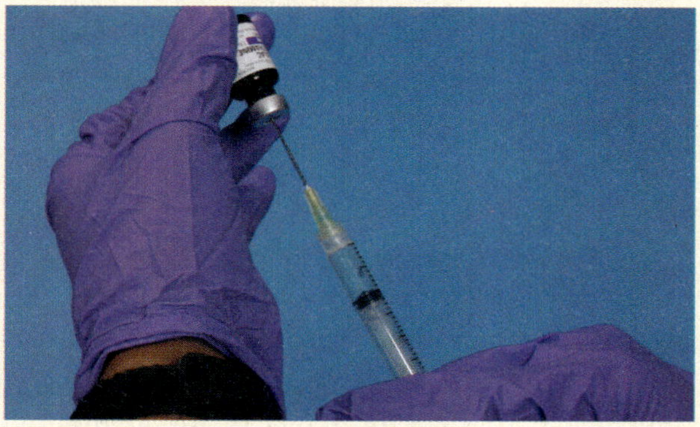

Step 3

Insert the needle into the rubber top, push the air into the vial, and turn the vial upside down with the needle tip in the medicine. Pull back the plunger to the correct line on the syringe. After drawing the medicine into the syringe, remove air bubbles by keeping the syringe tip in the medicine, tapping the syringe with your finger to move air bubbles to the top, and gently pushing the plunger until the air bubbles return to the vial.

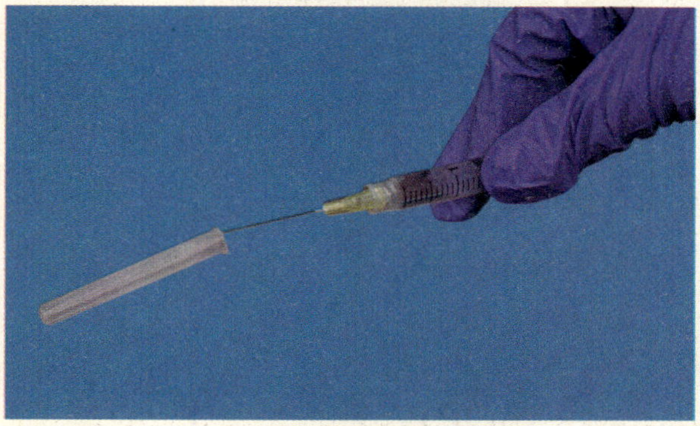

Step 4

Put the cover back on the needle using a one-handed technique. Remove the needle used to draw up the medicine and discard it in a sharps container.

Safety Tips

A tapered needle has a sharp end that easily punctures the skin. Some agencies also carry blunt-tipped needles to withdraw medication from a vial. These blunt needles reduce the risk of puncturing your hand when withdrawing the medication. Blunt needles cannot be used to administer the medication to the patient; however, even a tapered needle, if used to draw up the medication, must be changed. When preparing the injection, the tapered needle is changed out prior to patient administration because medication residue on the tip of the needle may be painful.

Words of Wisdom

The CDC recommends that medications packaged as single dose be used for only one patient and that, when possible, multidose vials also be used for a single patient only.[6] Some vaccines, which as an EMT you may be involved in administering during a community disease outbreak, come in multidose vials. If you must administer a vaccine from a multidose vial, the stopper must be cleaned with antiseptic each time and a new syringe and needle must be used for each dose. If the entire vial is not used, note the date/time the vial was opened. It is important to note, however, that some vaccines may not be reused after a prolonged time due to their stringent storage requirements.

Locating the Deltoid Muscle for IM Injections

Find the acromion process, which is the bony structure that sticks out from your shoulder, just above the deltoid muscle. The deltoid injection site is approximately two to three fingerbreadths (about 2 inches [5 cm]) below the acromion process, and sitting just above the level of the armpit, in the central part of the upper arm.

Administering an Injection Into the Deltoid Muscle

1. Locate the deltoid injection site, and use a needle long enough to reach the deep muscle. For vaccinations in adults, this is usually a 22- to 25-gauge needle, which is 1 inch (25 mm) long

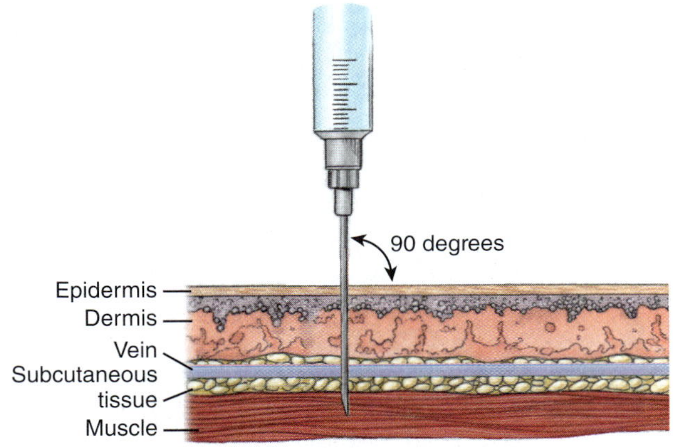

FIGURE 12-7 An intramuscular injection delivers medication below the dermis and subcutaneous layer and into muscle.

2. Use your thumb and index finger to stretch the skin around the injection site.
3. Insert the needle with a deep thrust at a 90° angle to the skin (straight up and down) (**FIGURE 12-7**). Push down on the plunger of the syringe slowly, then withdraw the needle once all the contents have been administered.
4. Apply pressure with a gauze pad and place a Band-Aid on the area if there is any bleeding.

The steps for administering medication by the IM route are summarized in **SKILL DRILL 12-2**.

Epinephrine

Epinephrine is the main hormone that controls the body's fight-or-flight response and is the primary medication that you will administer intramuscularly. Epinephrine is a sympathomimetic medication, which mimics the effect of the sympathetic nervous system. The body releases epinephrine when there is sudden stress, such as during exercise or when the patient is suddenly scared. Because epinephrine is secreted by the adrenal glands, it is also known as adrenaline. Epinephrine has different effects on different body tissues and is used as a medication in several forms. Generally, epinephrine will constrict blood vessels, increase the heart rate and blood pressure, and dilate passages in the lungs. It can ease breathing problems caused by the bronchial spasms common in asthma and allergic reactions. In a person who is close to anaphylactic shock as a result of an allergic reaction, epinephrine

Skill Drill 12-2 Administering Medication via the Intramuscular Route

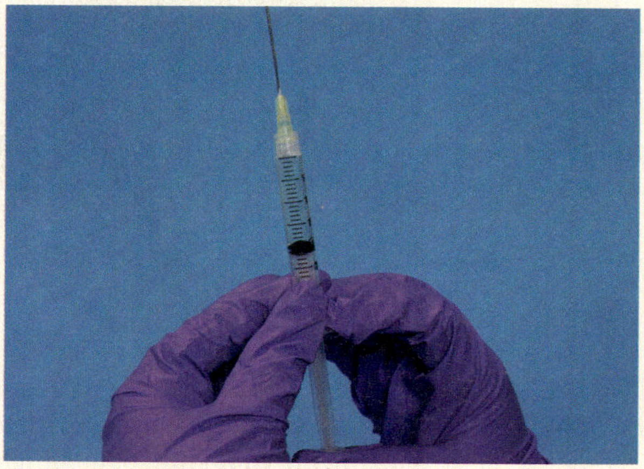

Step 1

Take standard precautions. Confirm the rights of medication administration, and ensure the medicine is not cloudy or discolored and has not expired. Assemble and check equipment needed: alcohol preps and the correct size of syringe and needle. Draw up the correct dose of medication and dispel air while maintaining sterility.

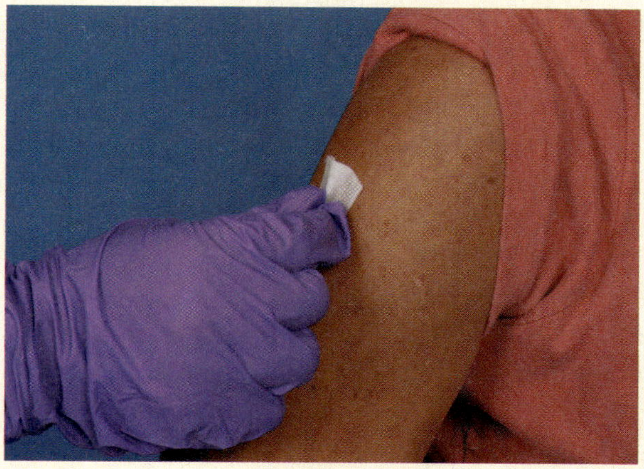

Step 2

Locate the deltoid injection site. Cleanse the area for administration using aseptic technique.

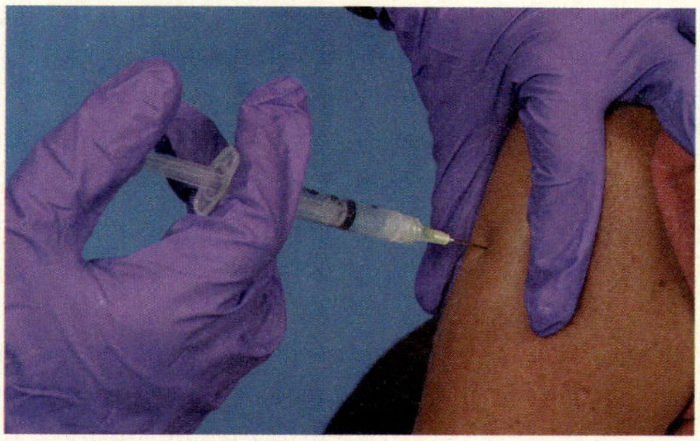

Step 3

Stretch the skin over the cleansed area, advise the patient they will feel a stick, and insert the needle at a 90° angle. Push down on the plunger of the syringe slowly, then withdraw the needle once all the contents have been administered.

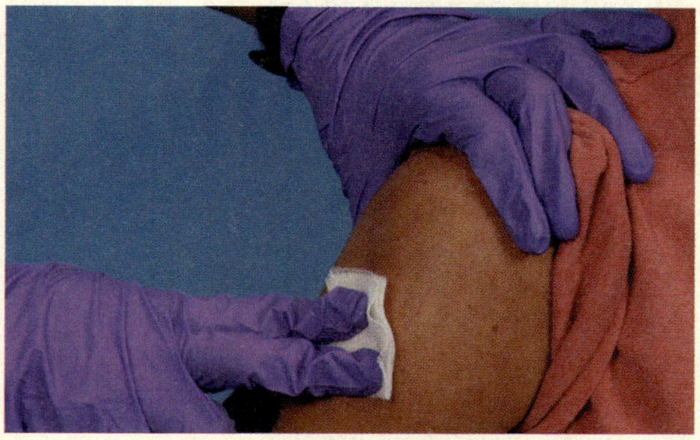

Step 4

Immediately dispose of the needle and syringe in the sharps container. Apply pressure with a gauze pad and place a Band-Aid on the area if there is any bleeding.

may also help to maintain the patient's blood pressure. However, epinephrine is not indicated for patients who do not show signs of airway obstruction or wheezing due to an allergic reaction. In addition, this medication should not be given to patients with hypertension or hypothermia, or if you believe the patient may be experiencing an MI.

Epinephrine has the following characteristics:

- Secreted naturally by the adrenal glands
- Dilates passages in the lungs
- Constricts blood vessels, causing increased blood pressure
- Increases heart rate

Refer to Chapter 6, *The Human Body*, for more information on epinephrine.

Administering Epinephrine by Injection

Most states and EMS agencies now authorize the use of epinephrine by EMTs for the treatment of life-threatening anaphylaxis. In certain patients, insect venom or other allergens cause the body to overrelease histamine, which lowers blood pressure by relaxing the small blood vessels and allowing them to leak. The over-release of histamine may also cause wheezing from bronchial spasms and swelling of the airway tissues (edema), which make it difficult for the patient to breathe. Epinephrine acts as a specific antidote to reverse the effects of histamines, countering both of their harmful effects. It constricts the blood vessels, allowing blood pressure to rise and reducing the swelling. In the lungs, it has the opposite effect: It dilates the air passages, so the flow of air is less restricted.

Epinephrine may be dispensed from an auto-injector, which automatically delivers a preset amount of the medication, usually 0.3 mg of epinephrine (**FIGURE 12-8**). This is the method that you will most likely use. Some states may authorize EMTs to draw epinephrine from a vial if an auto-injector is not available.

Some areas may allow epinephrine to be administered by IM injection using a vial of 1 mg/mL concentration with a needle and syringe. Older references or medication labels might refer to epinephrine concentration using "1:1,000" or "1:10,000." This practice has been phased out and replaced by the "mg/mL" concentration language for epinephrine and other medications that previously used that same concentration language.[7]

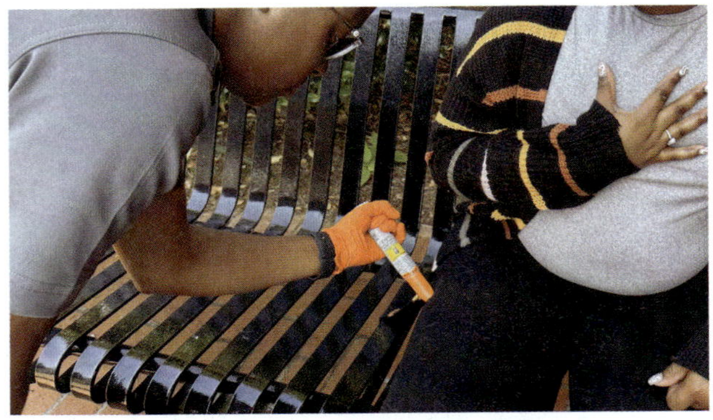

FIGURE 12-8 An EpiPen auto-injector may be used to administer a preset dose of epinephrine.

Courtesy of Rhonda Hunt.

Familiarize yourself with the procedures for using the auto-injector on your unit. The general procedure for devices such as the EpiPen are as follows:

1. Grasp the unit with the tip pointing downward.
2. Do *not* place your thumb over either end of the unit.
3. With the other hand, pull off the activation cap.
4. Hold the tip near the outer part of the patient's thigh.
5. Press the device firmly into the outer thigh so that the unit is perpendicular (at a 90° angle) to the thigh. Do not allow the unit to bounce.
6. Hold firmly in the thigh for several seconds.
7. Immediately place the unit in an appropriate sharps container after administration.

Some auto-injectors, such as the Auvi-Q, include verbal instructions for administration, and an epinephrine nasal spray called Neffy is available. Administration of epinephrine is discussed further in Chapter 21, *Allergy and Anaphylaxis*.

Epinephrine causes a burning sensation where it is injected, and the patient's heart rate will increase after the injection, so be prepared for these

Words of Wisdom

It is important to count to 10 once the EpiPen is activated against the patient's thigh. If pressure on the thigh is released too soon, it is possible that the entire dose of epinephrine will not be administered.

adverse effects. Some services do not permit EMTs to carry epinephrine but do allow them to assist patients in administering their own epinephrine in life-threatening anaphylactic reactions.

Naloxone (IM Route)

The FDA has approved an auto-injector device that delivers an IM or subcutaneous injection of naloxone (Narcan) to reverse the effects of an opioid overdose. This medication can be administered by family members or caregivers to help reverse dangerous adverse effects of opioid overdose, such as life-threatening respiratory depression. One version of auto-injectable naloxone, called EVZIO, provides verbal instructions for administration similar to those provided by automated external defibrillators.

Administering Naloxone by Injection

There are several important considerations for EMTs related to auto-injectable naloxone:

- Follow your local protocol. Consider requesting assistance from ALS personnel, if available, for any suspected opioid overdose. Ensure that another rescuer is ventilating and oxygenating the patient or performing CPR, if needed, while you prepare the medication.
- Find out if naloxone has been administered by a bystander prior to your arrival.
- Be aware that the effects of naloxone may not last as long as those of opioids. Repeat doses of naloxone may be needed.
- Administration of naloxone to opioid-dependent patients can cause severe withdrawal symptoms, including seizures and, rarely, cardiac arrest.
- You must consider your safety, as patients may become violent following naloxone administration. Make sure you are wearing proper personal protective equipment, including eye protection, mask, and gloves.

Most prefilled naloxone IM preparations are administered in increments of 2 mg, then gradually increase based on the patient response, or lack thereof, to achieve the desired effect of restoring respirations while avoiding withdrawal symptoms and associated complications. Refer to medical oversight instructions for naloxone administration in infants and children.

Vaccines

EMTs in various states may be permitted to administer vaccines either through state scope of practice or public health order, such as those issued during the coronavirus disease 2019 (COVID-19) pandemic. Training and supervision requirements vary by jurisdiction. The CDC distributes Vaccine Information Statements (VISs) that outline risks and benefits to vaccine recipients. Prior to administering any vaccine, you should understand the indications, contraindications, potential adverse reactions, and emergency treatment steps in the event of a life-threatening adverse or anaphylactic reaction.

Vaccines typically arrive in either a sterile vial for injection or a prefilled syringe. It is common for vaccines to require refrigeration and special handling until immediately before administration. Adults and most children older than 3 years receive injectable vaccines as an IM injection into the deltoid muscle near the shoulder. Different sites should be used if multiple vaccine injections are needed. Other vaccines may require oral or nasal administration rather than injection. Certain vaccines are combination preparations designed to protect against several organisms from a single dose.

Intranasal Medications

Naloxone (Intranasal Route)

Not all EMS departments will use naloxone IM auto-injectors, due to their expense. The most common technique for naloxone administration is via the intranasal route. Other common routes of administration include intravenous and intramuscular. All of the same considerations described for administering injectable naloxone apply when administering naloxone in any another form.

Administering Naloxone Intranasally

For patients who you suspect have experienced an opioid overdose and who have respiratory depression or arrest with a palpable pulse, provide bag-mask ventilation immediately. Continue this ventilation as naloxone is prepared and administered until the patient's breathing status returns to normal.

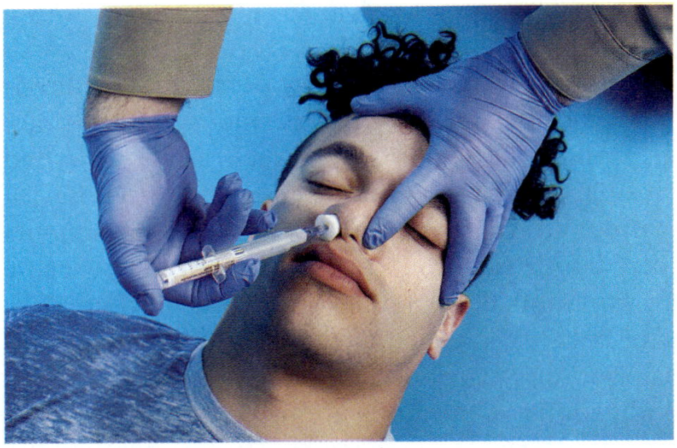

FIGURE 12-9 Some EMTs may administer naloxone intranasally to treat an opioid overdose.

Follow these steps to administer a medication intranasally:

1. Obtain medical direction per local protocol.
2. Confirm correct medication and expiration date.
3. Attempt to determine if the patient is allergic to any medications.
4. Prepare the medication and attach the atomizer. *Never* use a needle.
5. Tip the patient's head back and place the atomizer in one nostril, pointing upward (**FIGURE 12-9**).
6. Administer according to manufacturer and medical direction instructions. In some cases, one-half of the dose is sprayed into each nostril, and in other cases, the entire dose is given in one nostril and the dose is repeated if there is no response to the first dose.
7. Reassess the patient and document appropriately.

Words of Wisdom

When documenting a medication, include the name of the medication, dose and route, and vital signs before and after administration. For example:

1030 hours—vital signs: pulse, 88 beats/min; respirations, 18 breaths/min; blood pressure, 128/68 mm Hg; nitroglycerin, 0.4 mg SL.

1035 hours—vital signs: pulse, 80 beats/min; respirations, 18 breaths/min; blood pressure, 124/60 mm Hg. Patient states the pain remains at 6/10.

Special Populations

MEDICATIONS AND THE GERIATRIC PATIENT

Geriatric patients often take many medications. They might also save medications left over from previous medical conditions. Make every effort to identify which medications are current and the conditions they are being used to treat. Ask family members to help distinguish current from outdated medications, or look at the expiration dates on the medication labels. If possible, bring the medications with you to the emergency department (ED).

Geriatric patients can become confused about their medication regimen. Uncertainty about whether they missed a dose may cause a patient to repeat the medication, possibly leading to an overdose. If you think an overdose has occurred, contact medical direction.

Remember, medications can interact with each other, creating potentially harmful conditions. Even though a medication may be indicated for a special condition, it might be contraindicated in the presence of another medication. For example, if the patient is taking the heart medication metoprolol (Lopressor, Toprol) and has an acute episode of shortness of breath, some asthma treatments might be made less effective by the heart medication.

Kidney and liver functions decline with advanced age. These two organs are primarily responsible for the breakdown and elimination of medications and other potentially harmful substances from the body. As organ function declines, the risk of toxicity increases. It becomes increasingly difficult to effectively and safely prescribe and administer medications, especially as numerous medications interact with each other in patients.

Although medications help people to recover from acute conditions and adjust to chronic diseases, they can pose serious problems for geriatric patients. You should distinguish current from previous medications, suspect accidental or intentional overdoses, and be prepared for potentially lethal medication interactions. Document all findings and inform medical direction.

Inhalation Medications

Oxygen

Oxygen is, by far, the most commonly administered medication in the prehospital setting. All cells need **oxygen** to function properly. The heart and brain, especially, cannot function for long if oxygen levels

ALS Assist

Nonpharmacologic pain control measures such as extremity elevation, positioning, splinting, and ice packs can assist when analgesic medications are not available. Consider using these techniques until analgesic medications can be administered. These adjuncts may be especially helpful in children. They can still be used when AEMTs or paramedics are simultaneously administering analgesic medications.

decrease, which is why oxygen is an onboard medication for EMS units. If a patient is not breathing, has a low oxygen saturation level, or is dyspneic, you should administer supplemental oxygen. In general, you will be giving oxygen via either a nonrebreathing mask at 10 to 15 L/min or via nasal cannula at 2 to 6 L/min based on the patient's condition. However, if the patient is not breathing adequately, you must also provide artificial ventilations, so you will need to use a bag-mask device. Oxygen is usually delivered at 15 L/min with this technique.

Outside a hospital, the nonrebreathing mask is the preferred method of giving oxygen to patients who are experiencing significant respiratory difficulties or shock. With a good mask-to-face seal, this mask can provide up to 95% inspired oxygen. With a nasal cannula, oxygen flows through two small, tubelike prongs that fit into the patient's nostrils.

Words of Wisdom

Oxygen is not helpful, and prolonged use of supplemental oxygen may actually be harmful, in patients who are having a heart attack when breathing is normal and the oxygen saturation is 90% or greater, or in patients experiencing a stroke when the oxygen saturation is 94% or greater.[8] Nonetheless, the evidence is very strong that even brief periods of hypoxemia in these patients can be very dangerous. Patients who need supplemental oxygen should receive it promptly. Administer oxygen in any of the following situations:

- There is no means available to measure oxygen saturation.
- The patient becomes dyspneic.
- The oxygen saturation level drops below 90% for suspected heart attack or below 94% for suspected stroke.

This device can provide up to 44% inspired oxygen if the flowmeter is set at 6 L/min.

Remember that, although oxygen itself does not burn, it is a catalyst for combustion. If there is extra oxygen in the air, objects will burn more easily. Ensure there are no open flames, lit cigarettes, or sparks in the area in which you are administering oxygen.

MDIs and Nebulizers

MDIs and small-volume nebulizers (SVNs) are used to administer liquid medications that have been turned into a fine mist by a flow of air or oxygen (**FIGURE 12-10**). Respiratory illness can be spread through SVNs. When the medication is atomized, it is breathed into the lungs and delivered to the alveoli. Blood flow to the alveoli is very high and absorption rates are close to those found with IV medications. This route is fast and relatively easy to access. MDIs are commonly used because of their convenience and portability. The major disadvantage of an MDI is that the patient needs to be cooperative and control their breathing. If the patient is unconscious, an MDI cannot be used, although you could use a nebulizer. Nebulizers are often used for more severe problems.

Sometimes, a respiratory condition such as asthma is not severe enough to require the use of epinephrine. In such cases, patients may use one of the chemical "cousins" of epinephrine, such as albuterol, that are more narrowly focused on the lungs. These medications are delivered using an MDI or SVN.

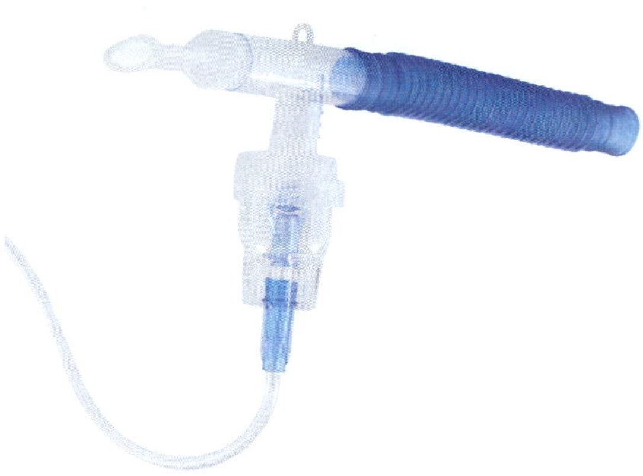

FIGURE 12-10 Metered-dose inhalers and small-volume nebulizers (shown here) convert liquid medications into a fine mist.

Special Populations

UNIQUE CONSIDERATIONS FOR THE PEDIATRIC PATIENT

Children are not small adults, especially when it comes to the administration of medications. The approach to children differs from that for adults. First, doses of medications are different. Most of the assisted medications will be smaller doses. Children often do not have the coordination needed to use an MDI. It will be more effective if a spacer device is added to the inhaler to ensure the child receives the full benefit of the medicine. A little more time and effort may be required to explain each procedure. It is also in your best interest to tell the child the truth. You do not have much time to bond with the child, so establishing trust quickly is important.

Asthma, also known as reactive airway disease, can be a life-threatening condition. Therefore, some patients use rescue inhaler MDIs to relieve bronchial spasms quickly. A few of the more common OTC MDIs include Primatene Mist, Bronitin Mist, and Bronkaid Mist. Each of these MDIs contains epinephrine and can cause significant adverse effects, such as tachycardia, hypertension, and restlessness. Therefore, as mentioned earlier, most patients with asthma use certain chemical cousins of epinephrine that produce fewer adverse effects and act more specifically on the bronchi of the lungs. Common prescription MDIs include albuterol (ProAir, Proventil, and Ventolin), ipratropium bromide (Atrovent), and levalbuterol (Xopenex). Often albuterol and ipratropium are combined in one preparation (eg, Combivent, DuoNeb).

Another type of MDI used by respiratory patients is the maintenance, or controller, inhaler. These MDIs are slow acting and are meant to be used regularly to be effective. Maintenance inhalers are *not* useful for a patient experiencing acute respiratory distress and in need of immediate relief. Common maintenance inhalers include fluticasone propionate (Flovent Diskus), budesonide (Pulmicort), mometasone furoate (Asmanex Twisthaler), beclomethasone dipropionate (Qvar), and ciclesonide (Alvesco).

There are dozens of different MDIs on the market, and often patients may be prescribed several of them at once. The only medications that will

YOU are the EMT

The patient is placed onto the stretcher and loaded into the ambulance. She remains conscious and alert. Her son tells you that he has to retrieve some items from her house and will follow the ambulance in his car. Shortly before departing the scene, you reassess the patient's vital signs.

Recording Time: 13 Minutes	
Level of consciousness	Conscious and alert
Respirations	18 breaths/min; regular and adequate
Pulse	84 beats/min; strong and regular
Skin	Baseline color, warm, and slightly moist
Blood pressure	128/74 mm Hg
Spo_2	99% (on oxygen)
Blood glucose	94 mg/dL

The patient tells you that she thinks she may have accidentally taken too much of her Amaryl. You reassess her blood glucose level and note that it is 94 mg/dL.

8. You are unfamiliar with the medication Amaryl. What should you do?

9. If you were unable to obtain a blood glucose reading on this patient, would you still administer oral glucose? Why or why not?

be effective during an acute attack of shortness of breath will be the fast-acting rescue inhalers, such as albuterol (Proventil, Ventolin) and levalbuterol (Xopenex). Whether you are assisting the patient with an MDI or an SVN medication, be sure you have the right medication for a patient with acute respiratory distress.

Using an MDI

Proper use of an MDI requires some degree of coordination, something that may be difficult to achieve when a person is having trouble breathing. Patients must aim properly and spray just as they start to inhale. If administered improperly, most of the medication ends up on the roof of the patient's mouth. An adapter, called a spacer, fits over the inhaler like a sleeve and should be used whenever possible to avoid misdirecting the spray (**FIGURE 12-11**). The patient sprays the prescribed dose into the chamber and then breathes in and out of the mouthpiece until the mist is completely inhaled. Spacer devices are especially useful with young children who have difficulty using an MDI.

You can activate the spray by pressing the canister into the adapter just as the patient starts to inhale. If relief is not achieved, wait 3 to 5 minutes and repeat this sequence according to the patient's prescription. Above all, it is important to ensure that the patient inhales all of the medication in a single sprayed dose.

MDIs contain both the medication and a propellant, a chemical used to help push the medication out of the inhaler. It is possible for the medication

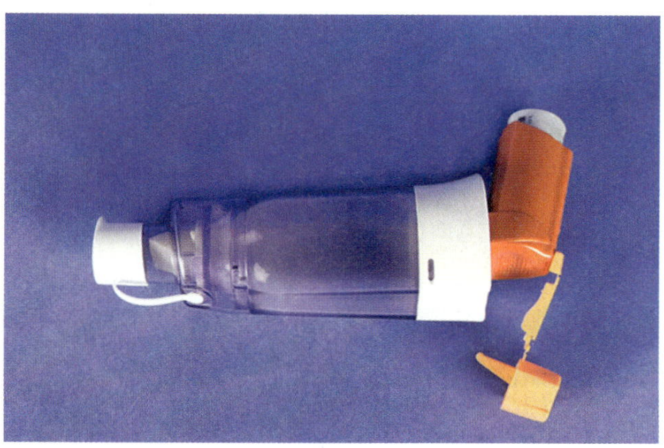

FIGURE 12-11 Some inhalers have spacer devices to better direct the medication spray.

to be depleted in the MDI, even though it continues to spray. It may be difficult to determine whether a patient's MDI is still providing needed medicine. Some albuterol MDIs have a dose counter that will indicate if there is still medication in the inhaler.

Using an SVN

SVNs are much easier to use than MDIs; however, they take longer to deliver the medication and require an external air or oxygen source. An SVN can be more effective than an MDI in moderate to severe respiratory distress. An SVN can also be used while a patient is on continuous positive airway pressure and during bag-mask ventilation. An SVN can easily be adapted to a nonrebreathing mask for patients unable to hold an SVN. This can be especially helpful with children.

Assisting a patient with an SVN involves placing the medication into the nebulizer and then running a flow of oxygen through the device, which will atomize the liquid and allow the patient to breathe in the medication (**FIGURE 12-12**). You will typically use an oxygen tank to deliver an SVN treatment; however, many patients with respiratory conditions have a portable SVN machine at home that can be used. Consult your local protocol to determine if use of an SVN is within the EMT scope of practice for your agency.

Follow these steps to administer a medication via SVN:

1. Obtain medical direction per local protocol.
2. Confirm the rights of medication administration.
3. Confirm that the patient is *not* allergic to the medication.
4. Add the appropriate medication and dose to the nebulizer reservoir and assemble according to the manufacturer's instructions.
5. Perform the medication cross-check.
6. Connect to the nebulizer machine (often in the patient's home) or oxygen tank at 6 to 8 L/min (or the oxygen flow recommended by the manufacturer).
7. Place the nebulizer in the patient's mouth and instruct the patient to breathe until the medication is gone (usually about 5 minutes).
8. Reassess the patient and document appropriately.

Note: Some nebulizers come preconnected to an oxygen mask for easier administration for

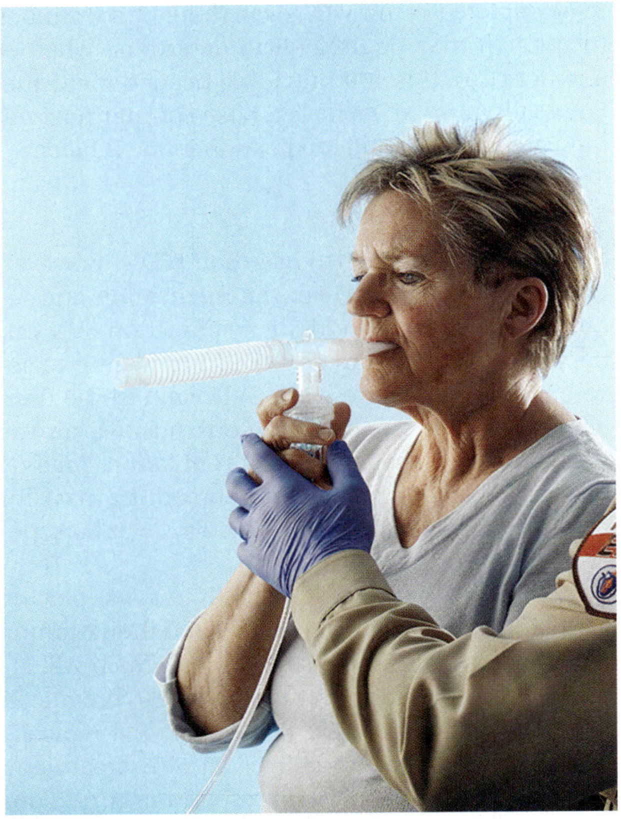

FIGURE 12-12 With a small-volume nebulizer, liquid medication is atomized by the flow of oxygen. The patient then breathes in the medication through a mouthpiece or a mask.

patients who are unable to hold the nebulizer. See Chapter 16, *Respiratory Emergencies*, for more information on steps for using MDIs and SVNs.

Patient Medications

Part of your patient assessment includes finding out what medications your patient is currently taking. This information may provide vital clues to your patient's condition that may help guide your treatment or be extremely useful to the ED physician. Often, knowing what medications a patient takes may be the only way you can determine what chronic or underlying conditions your patient may have, such as when a patient is unable to relate their medical history to you. The patient may be unresponsive, confused, or uncooperative; may not know certain details about their medical history; or may be unable to communicate. Discovering what the patient takes and transporting the medications or a list of medications with you to the ED can be crucial in assessing your patient's needs.

Special Populations

POLYPHARMACY

Polypharmacy refers to the use of multiple medications by one person. It is not uncommon today to encounter patients, especially older patients, who take many medications on a regular basis. Often, the prescription regimens can be complex and confusing. The medications may be prescribed by multiple physicians. The person may also be taking nonprescription and herbal medicines. Add to this the possibility of failing memory and confusion, and the potential for overdosing, underdosing, and harmful interactions increases exponentially.

In addition to prescription medications, patients often take nonprescription OTC medications, herbal medications, or other supplements. Many times, they do not consider these substances to be medications and will not report them to you unless you ask about them specifically. Yet, they may be as potent as prescription medications and can have interactions and effects on a patient's health and condition that are just as important. Be sure to ask specifically about these substances.

Implications for EMS Clinicians

EMS clinicians must not underestimate the importance of obtaining a thorough medication history during patient encounters. Medications are frequently not taken as prescribed. There may be huge gaps between a patient's medication list (or reported history) and what the patient is actually receiving.

Street Smarts

When possible, EMS clinicians should verbally verify which medications are actually being taken, even when presented with a printed medication list.

A patient may take medications correctly yet still have many opportunities for medication toxicity, adverse medication reactions, or body changes that alter the pharmacodynamics and pharmacokinetics in that individual. Acute illness, dehydration, liver or kidney dysfunction, and a vast array of other variables can alter how a medication affects the body, even if a patient has been stable on that medication for many years. EMS clinicians should consider a patient's medication in the context of the particular clinical encounter, assessing for clues that the two might be related.

Patient medications may significantly alter the clinical presentation of many acute medical conditions or injuries. Beta adrenergic blocking agents, such as metoprolol (Lopressor) and atenolol (Tenormin), along with calcium channel blocking agents such as amlodipine (Norvasc) and diltiazem (Cardizem), can prevent the patient's heart rate from increasing in sepsis, trauma, hemorrhage, and other conditions that normally would present with tachycardia. Patients who take these medications may demonstrate normal or low heart rate, even when perfusion is impaired and shock is worsening.

Antiplatelet and anticoagulant medications will also complicate EMS assessment and treatment of many patients. **Antiplatelet** medications, such as aspirin and clopidogrel (Plavix), decrease the ability of blood platelets to aggregate (stick together). **Anticoagulant** medications, such as warfarin (Coumadin), apixaban (Eliquis), and rivaroxaban (Xarelto), interfere with other blood clotting mechanisms in the body. Both groups of medications are prescribed to patients who are susceptible to dysfunctional blood clotting conditions, including acute coronary syndrome, ischemic cerebrovascular accident (stroke), peripheral or pulmonary blood clots, and similar conditions. Patients taking medications from either of these groups are predisposed to bleeding. This bleeding risk becomes more significant when the patient sustains trauma, has an otherwise manageable hemorrhage such as a nosebleed, or a hemorrhage develops that cannot be easily controlled, such as a gastrointestinal bleed. In each instance, hemorrhage control can become quite difficult. EMS clinicians should strongly suspect intracranial hemorrhage in patients who present with altered mental status or other neurologic symptoms. When a complicated hemorrhage is present, EMS clinicians should consider transport to a health care facility with the capabilities to manage these situations. Some of these medications have approved antidotes, whereas others require aggressive supportive countermeasures to manage the hemorrhage. **TABLE 12-4** lists common antiplatelet and anticoagulant medications that EMS clinicians may encounter.

Several of the most commonly prescribed drugs for adults in the United States are used to treat cardiovascular disease, high cholesterol, and diabetes. **TABLE 12-5** lists medications frequently prescribed in the United States and their uses. There are also excellent mobile apps that can help you quickly look up unfamiliar medications.

Patients are naturally reluctant to tell you about any illegal drugs or medications they may have

TABLE 12-4 Common Antiplatelet and Anticoagulant Medications

Antiplatelet Medications	Anticoagulant Medications
aspirin	apixaban (Eliquis)
clopidogrel (Plavix)	dabigatran (Pradaxa)
dipyridamole (Aggrenox, Persantine)	edoxaban (Savaysa)
prasugrel (Effient)	enoxaparin (Lovenox); injectable medication given to patients in their homes
ticagrelor (Brilinta)	rivaroxaban (Xarelto)
vorapaxar (Zontivity)	warfarin (Coumadin)

Courtesy of Andrew Bartkus.

TABLE 12-5 Commonly Prescribed Medications in the United States

Generic Name (Trade Name)	Use
adalimumab (Humira)	Treats rheumatoid arthritis, Crohn disease, and ulcerative colitis
alprazolam (Xanax)	Treats anxiety disorders
amlodipine (Norvasc)	Treats high blood pressure or cardiac conditions
amoxicillin (Moxatag)	Treats infection caused by bacteria
aripiprazole (Abilify)	Treats psychosis, depression
atenolol (Tenormin)	Beta blocker; treats hypertension
atorvastatin (Lipitor)	Treats high cholesterol
azithromycin (Zithromax)	Treats infection caused by bacteria
buprenorphine and naloxone (Suboxone)	Prescribed to prevent opioid withdrawal
bupropion (Wellbutrin; Zyban)	Treats depression; also used for smoking cessation
celecoxib (Celebrex)	Treats pain
citalopram hydrobromide (Celexa)	Treats depression
cyclobenzaprine (Amrix, Fexmid)	Treats pain from muscle spasms
dextroamphetamine (Adderall)	Treats attention-deficit/hyperactivity disorder
donepezil HCl (Aricept)	Treats dementia
dulaglutide (Trulicity)	Treats type 2 diabetes
duloxetine (Cymbalta)	Treats depression and anxiety disorders
empagliflozin (Jardiance)	Treats type 2 diabetes
escitalopram (Lexapro)	Treats depression and anxiety
esomeprazole (Nexium)	Treats gastric reflux, heartburn
etanercept (Enbrel)	Treats rheumatoid arthritis
furosemide (Lasix)	Diuretic; treats hypertension, heart failure
gabapentin (Neurontin)	Treats seizures and nerve pain
hydrochlorothiazide (Microzide)	Diuretic treats hypertension, heart failure
hydrocodone (Vicodin)	Opioid analgesic; pain reliever
insulin glargine (Lantus)	Medicine used to treat diabetes that is administered subcutaneously
levetiracetam (Keppra)	Treats seizures
levothyroxine (Synthroid)	Treats hypothyroidism
lisinopril (Zestril)	Angiotensin-converting enzyme (ACE) inhibitor; treats hypertension

Generic Name (Trade Name)	Use
loratadine (Claritin)	Antihistamine
losartan (Cozaar)	Angiotensin receptor blocker; treats hypertension
metformin (Glucophage)	Lowers blood glucose level in type 2 diabetes
metoprolol (Lopressor)	Beta blocker, treats hypertension, heart failure
montelukast (Singulair)	Treats asthma
olanzapine (Zyprexa)	Treats schizophrenia and bipolar disorder
omeprazole (Prilosec)	Treats gastric reflux, heartburn
oxycodone (Oxycontin; also known as Percocet when combined with acetaminophen)	Treats pain (analgesic)
pantoprazole (Protonix)	Reduces stomach acid
pembrolizumab (Keytruda)	Treats various cancer types
phenytoin (Dilantin)	Treats seizures
prednisone	Anti-inflammatory agent that treats asthma, skin infections, autoimmune diseases
risankizumab (Skyrizi)	Treats plaque psoriasis, psoriatic arthritis, and Crohn disease
rosuvastatin (Crestor)	Treats high cholesterol
salmeterol (Advair)	Inhaled glucocorticoid and long-acting beta-2 agonist; prevents asthma attacks, chronic obstructive pulmonary disease
semaglutide (Ozempic, Rybelsus)	Treats type 2 diabetes; off-label use for weight loss
semaglutide (Wegovy)	Assists in weight loss
sitagliptin (Januvia)	Treats type 2 diabetes
sertraline HCl (Zoloft)	Treats depression
sildenafil (Viagra)	Treats erectile dysfunction
simvastatin (Zocor)	Treats high cholesterol
tamsulosin (Flomax)	Treat urinary disorders related to an enlarged prostate
triamcinolone acetonide (Nasacort)	Treats inflammatory conditions
ustekinumab (Stelara)	Treats psoriasis and psoriatic arthritis
valsartan (Diovan)	Treats high blood pressure and congestive heart failure
varenicline (Chantix)	Used for smoking cessation
zolpidem (Ambien)	Treats insomnia

taken. It is important to ask, and you can assure them that your only interest in asking is to be able to treat them appropriately.

Medication Errors

As discussed earlier, medication errors are common. A **medication error** is inappropriate use of a medication that could lead to patient harm. For example, this could include incorrect communication of a dose or administration of an incorrect dose. An estimated 1.3 million people in the United States are harmed each year due to medication errors in hospitals, extended care facilities, and outpatient clinics.[9] EMS professionals are not immune to committing medication errors. Medication errors are preventable, so you must be extremely vigilant any time medications are administered to a patient.

Errors can stem from different causes. Administration of a medication that is outside one's scope of practice is a rules-based error. Choosing the wrong medication to administer is a knowledge-based error. Using incorrect equipment or an incorrect procedure for administering a medication is an example of a skills-based error.

If the circumstances of the errors are understood, it may be possible to minimize them. Ensure that the environment does not contribute to errors: lighting is sufficient, equipment is organized, and distractions are limited as much as possible. Consider using a cheat sheet or application to help yourself remember all crucial steps to medication administration. Finally, before administering a medication, stop to ask yourself, "Why am I doing this?" Pausing for a moment allows you to sharpen your focus and ensure that what you are doing is correct.

If a medication error does take place, take the following steps. First, rapidly provide any appropriate patient care that is required. Second, notify medical direction as quickly as possible. Third, follow your local protocols and document the incident thoroughly, accurately, and honestly. Additionally, talk with your partner, supervisor, or medical director. This is an opportunity for you to learn how to prevent such errors in the future. These discussions can also help identify areas for your agency to target during quality improvement.

YOU are the EMT

The patient's condition remains stable during transport. You transport in nonemergency mode, reassess her vital signs, and then call in your radio report to the hospital, where you expect to arrive in approximately 8 minutes.

Recording Time: 19 Minutes	
Level of consciousness	Conscious and alert
Respirations	18 breaths/min; regular and adequate
Pulse	74 beats/min; strong and regular
Skin	Baseline color, warm, and dry
Blood pressure	126/72 mm Hg
Spo_2	98% (on oxygen)
Blood glucose	94 mg/dL

You arrive at the hospital and give your verbal report to the charge nurse. The patient's son arrives shortly thereafter and presents the nurse with a plastic bag containing seven medications, including those that you have already noted. After further assessment, treatment, and observation in the ED, the patient is discharged home with modification of her medication regimen and instructions to follow up closely with her primary care clinician.

10. What does the term "polypharmacy" mean, and why is it important?

YOU are the EMT SUMMARY

1. What is pharmacology?

Pharmacology is the study of medications, including their therapeutic uses and actions on the body. Several terms are used when discussing pharmacology. The *dose* is the amount of medication that is given to the patient. The *action* is the therapeutic effect that the medication is expected to have on the body. *Indications* are the reasons or conditions for which a particular medication is given. *Contraindications* are the reasons or conditions for which a particular medication should not be given because it may cause further harm. *Adverse effects* are any actions of a medication other than the desired effects.

2. Why is knowledge of pharmacology important to patient care?

Giving a medication to a patient without understanding how it will affect the person is dangerous. Prior to administering *any* medication, including oxygen, you must understand what effect or effects it will have on the patient. In addition, you must perform a careful and accurate assessment to determine if medication therapy is even indicated.

The patient may have a condition for which a particular drug is indicated; however, various factors that are unique to the patient (eg, known allergy to the drug, unstable vital signs) may otherwise contraindicate its use. Even medications that are normally taken by the patient may be contraindicated at the current time. For example, the nitroglycerin a patient takes for angina should not be administered if the patient's blood pressure is too low. The only way you will be able to determine whether a particular medication should be given is through a careful assessment.

It is easy enough to memorize the indications, contraindications, doses, and adverse effects of the drugs that you may administer as an EMT, but if you do not know how the drug will affect the patient's body, you should not be giving it. *Once you give it, you cannot take it back!*

3. Other than oxygen, what other medication does this patient require, and why?

This patient is a candidate for oral glucose. A normal blood glucose level is 80 to 120 mg/dL. This patient's glucose level is 36 mg/dL, which is critically low (hypoglycemia) and would explain the patient's present mental status.

Oral glucose is available as a gel or as tablets. If authorized by medical direction, you should administer oral glucose to any patient with a decreased LOC, an ability to protect their own airway, and a history of diabetes. The only contraindications to oral glucose are an inability to swallow and decreased LOC, because of the risk of aspiration.

4. Why is it significant to know the patient took her medications on an empty stomach?

If a patient with diabetes takes their medication but does not eat, either before or right after taking the medication, there is a significant risk of symptomatic hypoglycemia developing. If the blood glucose level becomes too low, a person can experience a loss of consciousness, experience seizures, and, ultimately, die.

5. What are the "rights" of medication administration, and why are they important?

Prior to assisting a patient with a prescribed medication or prior to administering a drug from your ambulance, you should review the rights of medication administration, a concept used to promote safe and accurate medication administration, and verify the drugs and dose with your partner using a cross-check procedure, if possible. Most medication errors result from failure to follow the rights.

- **Right patient.** If you are assisting the patient with their own medication, look at the medication label to ensure that it reads the same name as your patient.
- **Right medication and indication.** Check the medication label to make sure it is the right medication for the patient's condition.
- **Right dose.** Check the medication label and take note of the dose. The dosing information should be on the medication container. If it is not, contact medical direction or follow your local protocols.
- **Right route.** A medication given by the wrong route, even if it is the correct medication, may be ineffective or may even cause harm to the patient.
- **Right time.** Medications that can be repeated must be given at the correct time intervals. After administering the medication, document the time. After the proper time has passed, follow your local protocols or contact medical direction again if the drug needs to be readministered.
- **Right documentation.** After administering any medication to any patient, you must document the drug, dose, route, time or times of

YOU are the EMT SUMMARY continued

administration, and reassessment findings after the medication has been given. Proper documentation will ensure that the receiving facility is aware of the medications the patient received in the field and the effects they may have had.

6. What medications are typically carried on an ambulance staffed by EMTs?

There are five medications typically carried on an ambulance that is staffed by EMTs: oxygen, aspirin, oral glucose, naloxone, and epinephrine. Depending on local protocol, other medications may be carried on the ambulance, including nitroglycerin, and MDI or nebulized medications such as albuterol.

It is important to note that just because these medications are carried on the ambulance, you cannot administer them at will. They may be given only on the direct order of a physician (online medical direction) or according to standing orders in your local protocol (off-line medical oversight).

7. As an EMT, what medications can you assist the patient to self-administer?

You may be asked to help patients self-administer certain prescription medications, including epinephrine auto-injectors (EpiPens), MDI medications (albuterol [Proventil, Ventolin]), or nitroglycerin (Nitrostat).

First, perform a careful assessment of your patient to determine if medication therapy is indicated. Just because the patient is prescribed a particular medication does not mean that it is indicated. For example, nitroglycerin (a vasodilator drug) is contraindicated if the patient's systolic blood pressure is less than 100 mm Hg. By dilating the patient's blood vessels, nitroglycerin may cause a dangerous drop in blood pressure.

8. You are unfamiliar with the medication Amaryl. What should you do?

The simplest and most obvious way of determining the purpose of a medication is to ask the patient. She is conscious and will likely be able to answer your question. If the patient is unsure what it is used for, you should refer to an EMT field guide, drug reference text, or mobile app, or contact medical direction. In this case, glimepiride (Amaryl) is an oral medication commonly used by patients with type 2 diabetes mellitus to help lower their blood glucose level.

As an EMT, you will often encounter patients who take numerous medications. Just because it is not one that you carry on the ambulance or are authorized to assist the patient in taking does not mean you should not determine its purpose. Much information about a patient's medical history can be obtained by looking at the medications they are taking, especially when the patient is not able to speak and there is no one else who can provide the patient's medical history.

9. If you were unable to obtain a blood glucose reading on this patient, would you still administer oral glucose? Why or why not?

Patients with hypoglycemia can experience a rapid loss of consciousness, experience seizures, and even die. Withholding glucose from a patient who needs it is far more dangerous than administering it to a patient who does not. Be sure to follow local protocol regarding administration of any medication.

10. What does the term "polypharmacy" mean, and why is it important?

Polypharmacy refers to the use of multiple medications by the same patient. It is not uncommon to encounter patients, especially older patients, who are taking multiple prescribed medications, OTC medications, and herbal remedies on a regular basis; this often makes a patient's medication regimen complex and confusing.

The potential for inadvertent underdosing and overdosing and harmful drug interactions increases in patients who take multiple medications. Furthermore, the primary problem may be the result of one or more of the medications the patient is taking. Often older patients see several medical clinicians for different problems, each of which may prescribe medications without knowing what other medications the patient is taking. In some cases, the prescribed medications may either interfere with other medications or may dangerously increase adverse effects in combination.

You should carry a field guide or similar reference that lists common prescription and nonprescription medications. In cases where the patient is unable to communicate with you and a reliable source (eg, family member, caregiver) is not available to answer your questions, the patient's medications can give you important clues as to their medical history.

Prep Kit

Ready for Review

- Pharmacology is the science of drugs, including their ingredients, preparation, uses, and actions on the body.
- Medications may be administered through the following routes: injection (intravenous, intramuscular, subcutaneous, or intraosseous), intranasal, oral, sublingual, endotracheal, transdermal, inhalational, and rectal.
- These routes of administration often determine the speed with which the medication takes effect.
- Medications come in seven forms: tablets and capsules, solutions and suspensions, MDIs, topical medications, transdermal medications, gels, and gases.
- The administration of any medication requires approval by medical oversight, through direct orders given online or standing orders that are part of the local protocols.
- The sequence of administering medications begins with receipt of an order from medical direction. Next, verify the rights of medication administration (right patient, right medication and indication, right dose, right route, right time, and right documentation). Once the medication has been administered, reassess vital signs and document the patient's history, assessment, treatment, and response findings.
- Five medications are typically carried on an EMT ambulance: oxygen, aspirin, oral glucose, naloxone, and epinephrine. Depending on local protocol, some EMS units may carry other medications, such as nitroglycerin, and MDI medications.
- There are several medications that you may assist the patient to self-administer, including epinephrine auto-injectors (EpiPens), MDI medications (eg, albuterol [Proventil, Ventolin]), and nitroglycerin (Nitrostat). Remember, medication assistance permissions may differ depending on local protocol.
- Knowing what medications a patient takes may be the only way you can determine what chronic or underlying conditions your patient may have.
- You must be extremely vigilant when administering medications. If a medication error occurs, provide any appropriate patient care required, notify medical direction as soon as possible, and document the incident.
- EMTs may be permitted to administer vaccines, as was the case in many states during the COVID-19 pandemic. This expanded scope of practice often requires additional training.

Vital Vocabulary

absorption The process by which medications travel through body tissues until they reach the bloodstream.

action The therapeutic effect of a medication on the body.

adverse effects Any unwanted clinical results of a medication.

agonist A medication that causes stimulation of receptors.

antagonist A medication that binds to a receptor and blocks other medications.

antibiotic A medication used to treat infections caused by a bacterium.

anticoagulant A medication that impairs the ability of blood to clot.

antifungal A medication used to treat infections caused by a fungus.

antiplatelet A medication that prevents blood platelets from clumping or sticking together.

antipyretics Medications that treat or reduce a fever.

Prep Kit continued

aspirin (acetylsalicylic acid or ASA) A medication that is an antipyretic (reduces fever), analgesic (reduces pain), anti-inflammatory (reduces inflammation), and potent inhibitor of platelet aggregation (clumping).

contraindications Conditions that make a particular medication or treatment inappropriate because it would not help, or may actually harm, a patient.

dose The amount of medication given on the basis of the patient's size and age.

duration The amount of time that clinical effects of a medication last.

elimination The process of removing a medication or chemical from within the body.

EMT-administered medication Administration of a medication by the EMT directly to the patient.

endotracheal Through the tracheal tube; a rarely used medication administration method.

enteral medications Medications that enter the body through the digestive system.

epinephrine A medication that increases heart rate and blood pressure but also eases breathing problems by decreasing muscle tone of the bronchial tree.

gel A semiliquid substance that is administered orally in capsule form or through plastic tubes.

generic name The original chemical name of a medication (in contrast with one of its proprietary or trade names); the name is not capitalized.

hypoglycemia An abnormally low blood glucose level.

indications The therapeutic uses for a specific medication.

inhalation The active, muscular part of breathing that draws air into the airway and lungs; a medication delivery route.

intramuscular (IM) injection An injection into a muscle; a medication delivery route.

intranasal (IN) A delivery route in which a medication is pushed through a specialized atomizer device called a mucosal atomizer device (MAD) into the naris.

intraosseous (IO) injection An injection into the bone; a medication delivery route.

intravenous (IV) injection An injection directly into a vein; a medication delivery route.

medication A substance that is used to treat or prevent disease or relieve pain.

medication error Inappropriate use of a medication that could lead to patient harm.

metered-dose inhaler (MDI) A miniature spray canister used to direct medications through the mouth and into the lungs.

mucosal atomizer device (MAD) A device that is used to change a liquid medication into a spray and push it into a nostril.

nitroglycerin A medication that increases cardiac perfusion by causing blood vessels to dilate; EMTs may be allowed to assist the patient to self-administer this medication.

onset of action The amount of time from the administration of a medication to the onset of clinical effects.

oral By mouth; a medication delivery route.

oral glucose A simple sugar that is readily absorbed by the bloodstream; it is carried on the EMS unit.

over-the-counter (OTC) medications Medications that may be purchased directly by a patient without a prescription.

oxygen A gas that all cells need for metabolism; the heart and brain, especially, cannot function without oxygen.

parenteral medications Medications that enter the body by a route other than the digestive tract, skin, or mucous membranes.

patient-assisted medication When the EMT assists the patient with the administration of their own medication.

Prep Kit continued

peer **peak** The point or period when the maximum clinical effect of a drug is achieved.

peer-assisted medication When the EMT administers medication to self or to a partner.

per os (PO) Through the mouth; a medication delivery route; same as oral.

per rectum (PR) Through the rectum; a medication delivery route.

pharmacodynamics The process by which a medication works on the body.

pharmacokinetics The processes that the body performs on a medication, including how it is absorbed, distributed, possibly changed, and eliminated.

pharmacology The study of the properties and effects of medications.

polypharmacy The use of multiple medications on a regular basis.

prescription medications Medications that are distributed to patients only by pharmacists according to a physician's order.

solution A liquid mixture that cannot be separated by filtering or allowing the mixture to stand.

subcutaneous injection Injection into the fatty tissue between the skin and muscle; a medication delivery route.

sublingual (SL) Under the tongue; a medication delivery route.

suspension A mixture of ground particles that are distributed evenly throughout a liquid but do not dissolve.

therapeutic effect The desired or intended effect a medication is expected to have on the body.

topical medications Lotions, creams, and ointments that are applied to the surface of the skin and affect only that area; a medication delivery route.

trade name The brand name that a manufacturer gives a medication; the name is capitalized.

transdermal (transcutaneous) Through the skin; a medication delivery route.

unintended effects Actions that are undesirable but pose little risk to the patient.

untoward effects Actions that can be harmful to the patient.

References

1. Meloni S, Mastenbjörk M. *Advanced Cardiovascular Life Support: Provider Manual*. Medical Creations; 2021.
2. Accidental exposure to fentanyl patches continue to be deadly to children. US Food and Drug Administration website. https://www.fda.gov/consumers/consumer-updates/accidental-exposures-fentanyl-patches-continue-be-deadly-children. Updated September 4, 2024. Accessed November 4, 2024.
3. Using skin patch medicines safely. Poison Control website. https://www.poison.org/articles/using-skin-patch-medicines-safely. Accessed November 4, 2024.
4. Popp LM, Lowell LM, Ashburn NP, Stopyra JP. Adverse events after prehospital nitroglycerin administration in a nationwide registry analysis. *Am J Emerg Med*. 2021;50:196–201.
5. Drawing medicine out of a vial. MedlinePlus Medical Encyclopedia website. https://medlineplus.gov/ency/patientinstructions/000530.htm#:~:text=Turn%20the%20vial%20upside%20down,1%20cc%20on%20the%20syringe. Reviewed February 8, 2024. Accessed November 4, 2024.
6. One needle, one syringe, only one time. Centers for Disease Control and Prevention website. https://stacks.cdc.gov/view/cdc/31799. Published June 26, 2014. Accessed November 4, 2024.
7. Cocchio C. Medication safety win: no more epinephrine ratio expressions. Pharmacy Times website. https://www.pharmacytimes.com/contributor/craig-cocchio-pharmd/2016/01/medication-safety-win-no-more-epinephrine-ratio-expressions. Published January 20, 2016. Accessed November 4, 2024.
8. American Heart Association (AHA). *2020 Handbook of Emergency Cardiovascular Care*. AHA; 2020.
9. Naseralallah L, Stewart D, Price M, Paudyal V. Prevalence, contributing factors, and interventions to reduce medication errors in outpatient and ambulatory settings: a systematic review. *Int J Clin Pharm*. 2023;45(6):1359–1377.

Prep Kit continued

Additional Resources

Guy JS. *Pharmacology for the Prehospital Professional*. 2nd ed. Burlington, MA: Jones & Bartlett Learning; 2020.

Misasi P, Keebler JR. Medication safety in emergency medical services: approaching an evidence-based method of verification to reduce errors. *Ther Adv Drug Safety*. 2019;10:2042098678821916. doi:10.1177/2042098618821916.

National Association of State EMS Officials. *National EMS Scope of Practice Model 2019*. Washington, DC: National Highway Traffic Safety Administration; February 2019. Report No. DOT HS 812-666. https://www.ems.gov/pdf/National_EMS_Scope_of_Practice_Model_2019.pdf. Accessed November 4, 2024.

Neiman AB, Ruppar T, Ho M, et al. CDC grand rounds: improving medication adherence for chronic disease management—innovations and opportunities. *Morb Mortal Wkly Rep*. 2017;66(45):1248–1251.

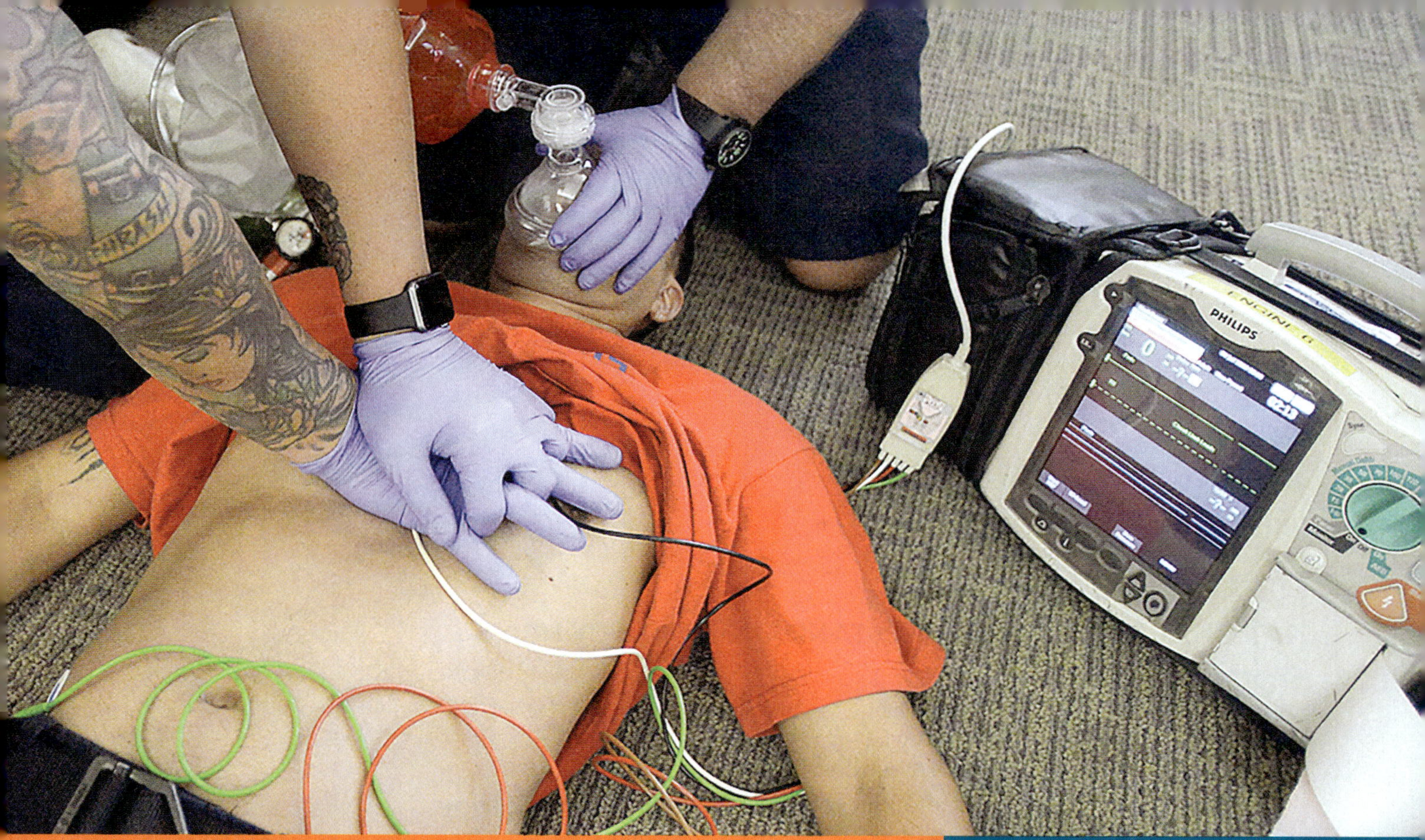

Shock and Resuscitation

SECTION

5

13 Shock

14 BLS Resuscitation

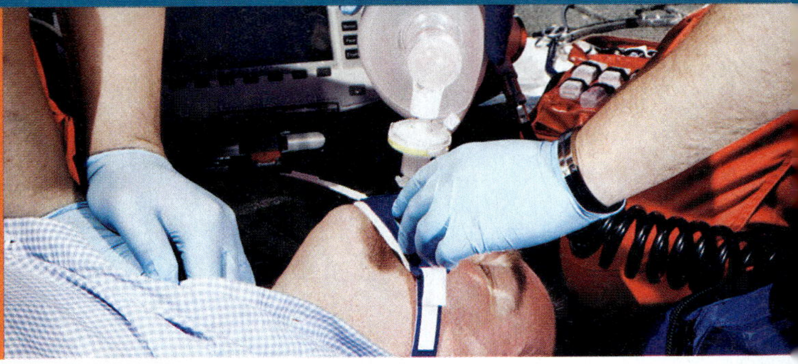

Chapter 13

Shock

NATIONAL EMS EDUCATION STANDARD COMPETENCIES

Shock and Resuscitation

Applies knowledge of the causes, pathophysiology, and management of shock, respiratory failure or arrest, cardiac failure or arrest, termination of resuscitation efforts, and postresuscitation management.

Shock

- Essential components in normal perfusion (pp 533–536)
- Physiologic response (pp 533–536)
- Types of shock (pp 536–543)
- Treatment of shock (pp 546–554)

Pathophysiology

Applies fundamental knowledge of the pathophysiology of respiration and perfusion to patient assessment and treatment.

KNOWLEDGE OBJECTIVES

1. Describe the pathophysiology of shock (hypoperfusion). (pp 533–536)
2. Identify the causes of shock. (p 536)
3. Differentiate among the various types of shock. (pp 536–543)
4. Describe the signs and symptoms of shock, including compensated and decompensated. (p 543)
5. Discuss key components of patient assessment for shock. (pp 544–546)
6. Describe the steps to follow in the emergency care of the patient with various types of shock. (pp 546–551)
7. Discuss the special treatment considerations for pediatric and geriatric patients experiencing shock. (pp 551–554)

SKILLS OBJECTIVES

1. Demonstrate how to assess and treat shock. (pp 544–554)

Introduction

In this chapter, **shock** is defined as inadequate cellular perfusion. Cells require oxygen, water, and glucose to carry out cellular processes to produce energy in the form of adenosine triphosphate. When the cells do not receive these requirements via the bloodstream, they cannot create energy and are categorized as hypoperfused. If cells are hypoperfused, tissues and organs are also hypoperfused. In the early stages of shock, the body will attempt to compensate by maintaining **homeostasis** (a balance of all systems of the body); however, as shock progresses from tissues and organs to organ systems and the whole body, blood circulation slows and eventually ceases. This state of inadequate oxygen and nutrient delivery to the cells of the body causes organs and then organ systems to fail. If not treated promptly, shock can be fatal.

Shock can occur because of several medical or traumatic events, such as a heart attack, severe allergic reaction, infection, bleeding, or spinal injury. As an emergency medical technician (EMT), you will respond to these types of emergencies to provide care and transport for these patients. Therefore, you must be constantly alert to the signs and symptoms of shock and be able to provide the necessary treatment.

This chapter begins with a close look at perfusion. It then examines the physiologic causes of shock, describes each of its major forms, and discusses the emergency treatment of shock. See Chapter 14, *BLS Resuscitation*, for resuscitation techniques.

Pathophysiology

Perfusion

Perfusion is the circulation of blood to the tissues in adequate amounts to meet the cells' needs. It includes delivery of oxygen and removal of toxic waste products. The circulatory system is a complex arrangement of connected tubes, including the arteries, arterioles, capillaries, venules, and veins, in which blood circulates throughout to the body. There are two circuits in the body: the systemic circulation between the heart and the body and the pulmonary circulation between the heart and the lungs. The systemic circulation carries oxygen-rich blood from the left ventricle through the body and back to the right atrium. In the systemic circulation, as blood passes through the tissues and organs, it delivers oxygen and nutrients. Adequate perfusion is also important for the removal of waste products such as carbon dioxide, a by-product of energy production. The circulatory system carries these waste products for excretion or exhalation.

Organs, tissues, and cells must have adequate oxygenation to survive. Each time you take a breath, the alveoli, which are microscopic, thin-walled air sacs, receive a supply of oxygen-rich air. Oxygen diffuses through the walls of the alveoli into the bloodstream and attaches to hemoglobin, a protein that makes up red blood cells. The red blood cells then circulate the oxygen to the tissues where it can be offloaded.

Oxygen and carbon dioxide pass rapidly across the thin walls of the alveoli by the process of diffusion. Diffusion is a passive process in which molecules move from an area of higher concentration to an area of lower concentration. When the air reaches your alveoli, there is more oxygen in the air than in the bloodstream. Therefore, the oxygen molecules slip between the thin layers of the alveoli into the blood. Carbon dioxide does the same thing in the other direction. When blood is returned to the lungs from the tissues, there is more carbon dioxide in the blood than in the alveoli; thus, it diffuses into the alveoli, where it is exhaled.

Whereas most oxygen is carried to the tissues while attached to hemoglobin, carbon dioxide can

YOU are the EMT

At 2022 hours, your alert tones sound: "Medic 4, respond to the Westlake Urgent Care at 1111 University Avenue for a 39-year-old woman in shock." You and your partner proceed to the clinic, which is approximately 9 minutes from your station. It is cloudy outside, the temperature is 66°F (18.9°C), and the traffic is light.

1. What additional information should you attempt to gather about the patient while en route to the clinic?
2. What is shock and how does it relate to perfusion?

be transported in the blood back to the lungs in three ways: dissolved in the plasma, combined with water in the form of bicarbonate, or attached to hemoglobin. Carbon dioxide waste products released from cells can combine with water in the bloodstream to form bicarbonate. Bicarbonate concentrations become higher as more carbon dioxide is produced and blood moves back toward the lungs. Once it reaches the lungs, the bicarbonate breaks down again into carbon dioxide and water and the carbon dioxide is exhaled. In cases of poor perfusion (shock), the transportation of carbon dioxide out of the tissues becomes impaired, resulting in a dangerous buildup of waste products, which may damage cells and tissues.

To protect vital organs from hypoperfusion, the body attempts to compensate by directing blood flow away from organs that are more tolerant of shock (such as the skin and intestines) to organs that cannot tolerate shock (such as the heart, brain, and lungs). If these tissues do not have adequate perfusion restored, they can die, resulting in permanent damage to the tissues and organ.

Recall that the cardiovascular system consists of three parts: a pump (the heart), a set of pipes (the blood vessels or arteries that act as the container), and the contents of the container (the blood) (**FIGURE 13-1**). These three parts can be referred to as the perfusion triangle (**FIGURE 13-2**). When a patient is in shock, one or more of the three parts is not working properly. For further review of the cardiovascular system, see Chapter 6, *The Human Body*.

Blood is the vehicle for carrying oxygen and nutrients through the vessels to the capillary beds and

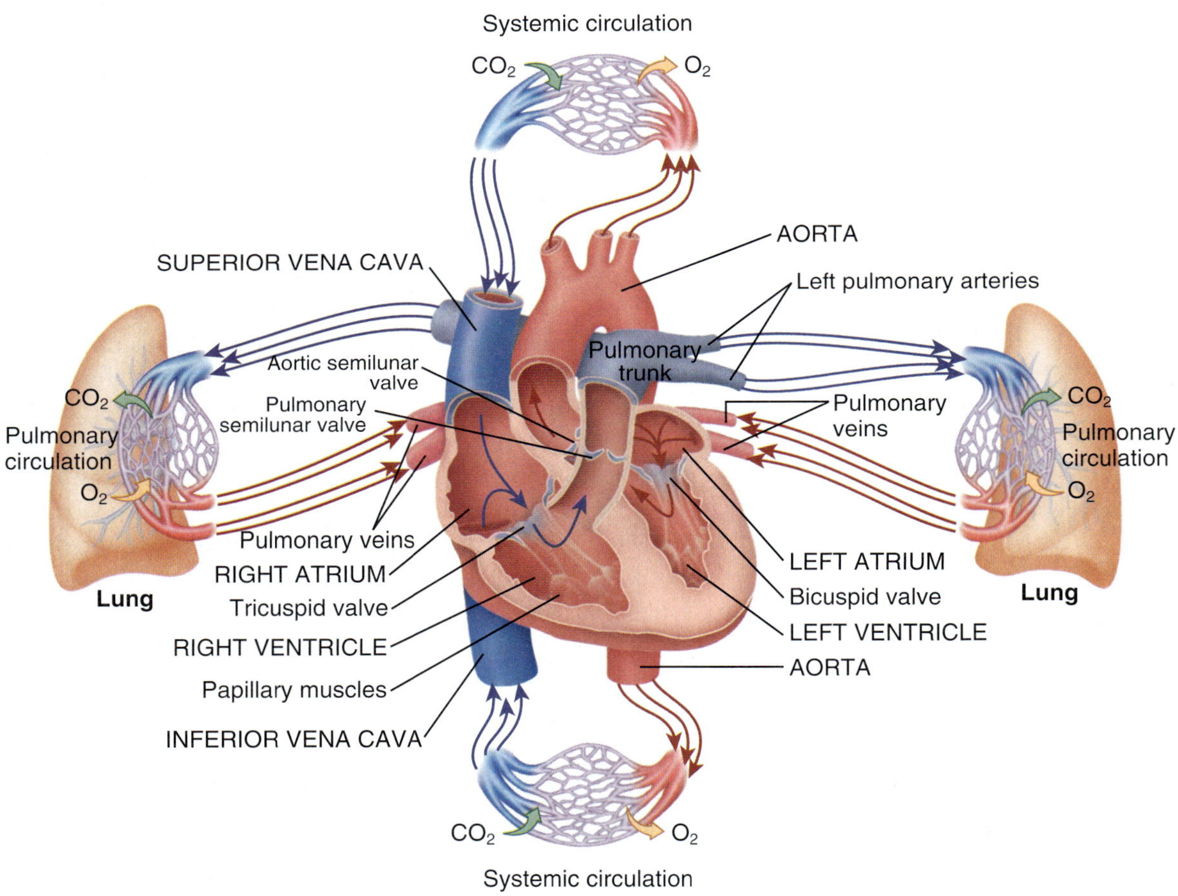

FIGURE 13-1 The cardiovascular system consists of three parts: the pump (heart), the container (vessels), and the contents (blood). The blood carries oxygen and nutrients through the vessels to the capillary beds, where they diffuse into the tissue; in exchange, waste products diffuse into the bloodstream.

Abbreviations: CO_2, carbon dioxide; O_2, oxygen

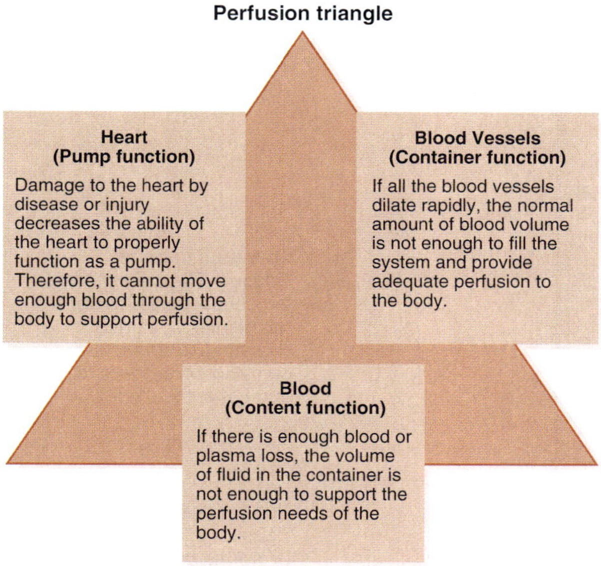

FIGURE 13-2 The heart, the blood vessels, and the blood represent the three parts of perfusion (the perfusion triangle).

tissue, where they are exchanged for waste products. For this process to happen, the vessels (container) must be intact. Blood is composed of red blood cells, white blood cells, platelets, and a liquid called plasma. Red blood cells are responsible for transporting oxygen to the cells and transporting carbon dioxide away from the cells to the lungs, where it is exhaled and removed from the body. Each component of blood has an important role in overall health: white blood cells help the body fight infection, platelets assist in forming blood clots, and plasma contains electrolytes and fluid, which are important for cells to function.

These components are all vital to maintain homeostasis. If, at any time, tissue is hypoperfused, the body will attempt to compensate by regulating the blood pressure, or the amount of blood delivered to any given part of the body, thereby preventing shock.

Words of Wisdom

When shock patients do not have adequate perfusion, the cells switch from aerobic metabolism (with oxygen) to anaerobic metabolism (without oxygen). Anaerobic metabolism creates lactic acidosis and greatly reduces the body's ability to create adenosine triphosphate to provide energy for cellular functions.

As shock progresses, patients are unable to maintain their blood pressure. Remember, blood pressure is the pressure of blood within the vessels at any moment in time. The *systolic* pressure is the peak arterial pressure, or pressure generated when the heart contracts; the *diastolic* pressure is the pressure maintained within the arteries while the heart is at rest, or between beats. **Pulse pressure** is the difference between the systolic and diastolic pressures (Systolic – Diastolic = Pulse pressure). It signifies the amount of force the heart generates with each contraction.

Blood flow through the capillary beds is regulated by the capillary sphincters, circular muscular walls that constrict and dilate. These **sphincters** are under the control of the **autonomic nervous system**, which regulates involuntary functions such as sweating and digestion. Capillary sphincters also respond to other stimuli such as heat, cold, the need for oxygen, and the need for waste removal. This regulation is important because not all organs require the same amount of blood. Whereas your brain requires a constant amount of blood, your digestive tract requires more blood while digesting food and less when you are not eating.

Thus, regulation of blood flow is determined by cellular need and is accomplished by vessel constriction or dilation and capillary sphincter constriction or dilation. This team effort of the heart, blood, and vessels helps ensure blood gets to the tissues when it is needed.

Perfusion requires more than just having a working cardiovascular system, however. It also requires adequate oxygen exchange in the lungs, adequate nutrients in the form of glucose, and adequate waste removal, primarily through the lungs. Carbon dioxide is one of the primary waste products of cellular work (metabolism) in the body and is removed from the body by the lungs. This is the reason adequate ventilation and oxygenation are among the EMT's primary concerns. The body has neural and endocrine or hormonal mechanisms in place to help support the respiratory and cardiovascular systems when the need for perfusion of vital organs is increased. These mechanisms include the autonomic nervous system and hormones, which are triggered when the body senses that the pressure in the system is falling. The sympathetic side of the autonomic nervous system, which is responsible for the fight-or-flight response, assumes more control of the body's functions during a state of shock. This response by the autonomic nervous system causes the release of the hormones epinephrine and norepinephrine. These hormones stimulate receptor sites (known as alpha and beta sites) of the heart, lungs, and blood vessels, causing changes in certain body functions. When the beta-1 sites are triggered, the heart rate increases and there is a greater force of contraction. When beta-2 sites are triggered, the bronchioles in the lungs dilate and allow in more oxygenated air. Triggering the alpha sites causes the blood vessels to selectively distribute blood to essential organs such as the heart, brain, and lungs while simultaneously decreasing blood flow to nonessential areas such as the skin and gastrointestinal tract by constricting blood vessels in those organs. Together, these actions help maintain pressure in the system and, as a result, sustain perfusion to the vital organs. The response of the autonomic nervous system and these hormones comes within seconds. It is this response that causes the signs and symptoms of shock in a patient.

Other compensatory responses occur more slowly. Eventually, hormones are released that cause reabsorption of fluid into the bloodstream when it passes through the kidneys in an attempt to increase the circulating blood volume.

Causes of Shock

In all cases of shock, the damage occurs because of insufficient perfusion of organs and tissues. As soon as perfusion becomes impaired, cells and tissues start to die. Organs and systems begin to fail due to the damaged and dying tissue. If the conditions causing shock are not promptly stopped and reversed, death will follow.

> **Words of Wisdom**
>
> Shock is a complex physiologic process that gives subtle signs of its presence before it becomes severe. These early signs relate closely to the body's attempts to compensate for shock. It is important for you to know the underlying processes of shock thoroughly. If you understand what causes shock, and how the body attempts to compensate, you will be able to recognize it in many patients before it progresses.

Understanding the basic physiologic causes of shock will better prepare you to treat it (**FIGURE 13-3** and **TABLE 13-1**).

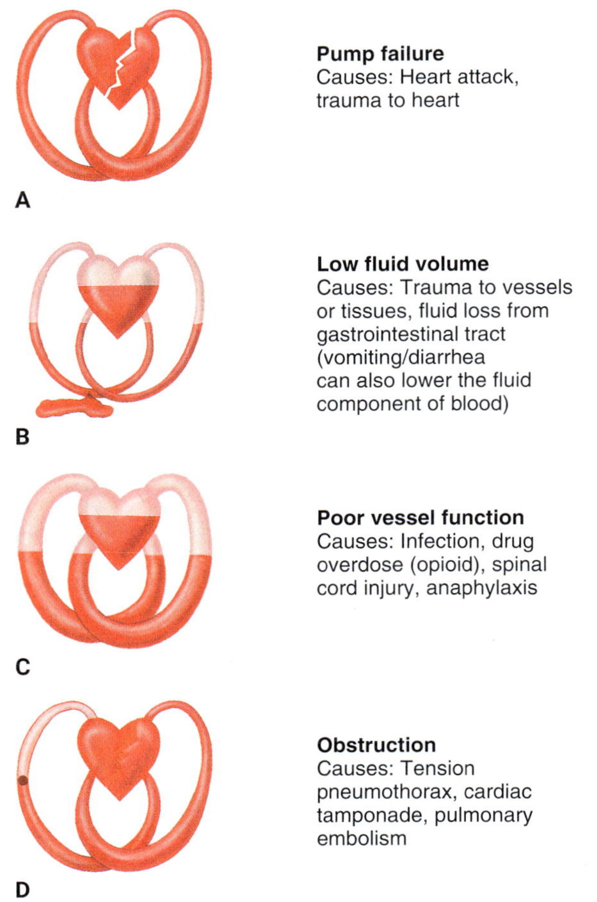

FIGURE 13-3 There are four basic causes of shock and impaired tissue perfusion. **A.** Pump failure occurs when the heart is damaged by disease or injury. **B.** Low fluid volume is often a result of bleeding. **C.** The blood vessels can dilate excessively so that the blood within them is inadequate to fill the system. **D.** An obstruction prevents blood from effectively reaching or leaving the heart.

Types of Shock

Cardiogenic Shock

Cardiogenic shock is caused by inadequate function of the heart, or pump failure. Circulation of blood throughout the vascular system requires the constant pumping action of the heart muscle. Many diseases or injuries can cause destruction or inflammation of heart muscle. Within certain limits, the heart can adapt. If too much muscular damage occurs, however, as sometimes happens after a heart attack, the heart no longer functions well.

The muscular contraction of the heart moves blood through the vessels at distinct pressures. For blood to circulate efficiently throughout the entire

TABLE 13-1 Causes of Shock

Cause	Type of Shock
Pump failure	Cardiogenic shock
Poor blood vessel function	Distributive shock • Septic shock • Neurogenic shock • Anaphylactic shock
Low fluid volume	Hypovolemic shock • Hemorrhagic shock • Nonhemorrhagic shock
Obstructed blood flow	Obstructive shock • Tension pneumothorax • Cardiac tamponade • Pulmonary embolism

system, the amount of pressure must be adequate and there must be a sufficient number of heartbeats.

Cardiogenic shock develops when the heart cannot maintain enough output (cardiac output) to meet the demands of the body. Cardiac output is the volume of blood that the heart can pump per minute and depends on several factors. First, the heart must have adequate strength, which is largely determined by the ability of the heart muscle to contract. This ability to contract is referred to as **myocardial contractility**. Second, the heart must receive adequate blood to pump. As the volume of blood coming to the heart increases, the pressure in the heart builds up. This pressure is known as **preload**. As preload increases, the volume of blood within the ventricles increases, which causes the heart muscle to stretch. When the muscle is stretched, myocardial contractility increases, leading to greater force of contraction and increased cardiac output. Last, the resistance to flow in the peripheral circulation must be appropriate. The force, or resistance against which the heart pumps, is known as **afterload**. In general, as afterload increases, cardiac output decreases. Increased afterload may also cause the heart to overwork while trying to maintain adequate cardiac output. Chronically high afterload is often the reason heart failure develops in patients with hypertension. Cardiogenic shock may result from low cardiac output due to high afterload, low preload, poor contractility, or any combination of the three.

When severe heart failure occurs, a major effect is the backup of blood into the pulmonary vessels.

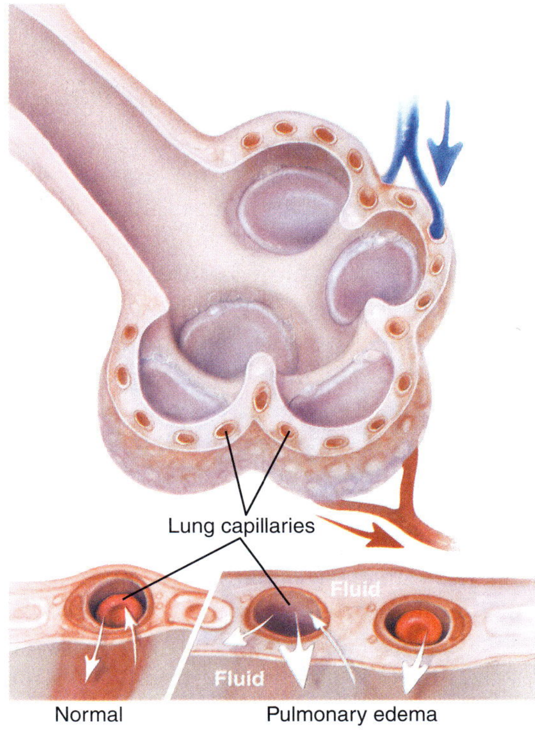

FIGURE 13-4 Pulmonary edema develops as a result of fluid buildup within the pulmonary tissue. This edema causes swelling and leads to impaired oxygenation.

The resulting buildup forces fluid out of the capillary beds that surround the alveoli and may lead to pulmonary edema. **Edema** is the presence of abnormally large amounts of fluid between cells in body tissues, causing swelling of the affected area (**FIGURE 13-4**). Red blood cells cannot easily leave the capillaries; however, as blood backs up, the fluid in the vessels is forced out and accumulates in the alveoli. Oxygen cannot diffuse across the fluid-filled alveoli, causing hypoxemia. This results in tachypnea (rapid respirations), decreased oxygen saturation (Spo_2), and crackles (a rattling sound that may be heard during breathing, typically on inhalation). When pulmonary edema occurs during cardiogenic shock, treatment is more complicated and tissue hypoxia occurs more rapidly.

Obstructive Shock

Obstructive shock is caused by an obstruction that blocks blood from returning to the heart, filling the ventricles, or leaving the heart. This condition decreases the cardiac output, preventing an adequate volume of blood from being pumped to the body.

Three of the most common examples of obstructive shock are cardiac tamponade, tension pneumothorax, and pulmonary embolism.

A collection of fluid between the pericardial sac and the myocardium is called a **pericardial effusion**. If the effusion becomes large enough, it can prevent the ventricles from filling with blood, a condition called **cardiac tamponade** or pericardial tamponade. This life-threatening condition may also be caused by blunt or penetrating trauma that causes hemorrhage around the heart. Large pericardial effusions leading to cardiac tamponade can also be seen in patients with cancer and autoimmune diseases. Cardiac tamponade occurs when blood or fluid leaks into the space between the tough fibrous membrane known as the pericardium and the outer walls of the heart, an area called the pericardial sac. As more blood or fluid accumulates in this confined space, the outer walls of the heart become compressed. Because the pericardium has a limited ability to stretch, the accumulated blood or fluid in the pericardial space eventually exerts back-pressure on the outer walls of the heart, compressing the walls of the heart and preventing the heart from completely refilling with blood. Continued pressure within the pericardial sac obstructs the flow of blood into the heart, resulting in decreased outflow from the heart (**FIGURE 13-5**). Signs and symptoms of cardiac tamponade are referred to as the Beck triad: the presence of jugular venous distention, muffled heart sounds, and a narrowing pulse pressure, where the systolic and diastolic blood pressures start to merge (systolic pressure decreases and the diastolic pressure increases). Of these findings, jugular venous distention may be the most notable. If a patient has a low blood pressure, the jugular veins should not be distended. If hypotension and distended jugular veins are noted, consider obstructive shock.

Tension pneumothorax is another obstructive condition (**FIGURE 13-6**). A tension pneumothorax is caused by damage to the lung tissue. This damage allows air normally held within the lung to escape into the chest cavity. The lung eventually collapses, causing a pneumothorax. If a pneumothorax is allowed to progress, air will accumulate within the chest cavity and apply pressure to the heart and greater vessels. When the trapped air begins to shift the chest organs toward the uninjured side, a pneumothorax becomes known as a tension pneumothorax, which is a serious, life-threatening condition. As pressure from one side of the chest begins to push the mediastinum toward the other

YOU are the EMT

You arrive at the clinic and are escorted to the patient by a clinic technician. You find the patient lying supine on an examination table. She is conscious, but restless, and staff confirms her skin is notably pale and diaphoretic compared to its baseline tone. She is covered by a blanket and is receiving oxygen via a nasal cannula at 4 L/min. Several attempts at establishing intravenous (IV) access were unsuccessful. Your assessment of the patient reveals the following:

Recording Time: 0 Minutes	
Appearance	Restless, pale, and diaphoretic
Level of consciousness	Conscious and restless
Airway	Open and patent
Breathing	Increased rate
Circulation	Radial pulses weak and rapid; skin cool, pale, and diaphoretic

The clinic physician tells you that the patient presented approximately 15 minutes ago, reporting abdominal pain and rectal bleeding, which apparently started about 24 hours ago. The patient has a history of irritable bowel syndrome, takes lubiprostone (Amitiza) and dicyclomine hydrochloride (Bentyl), and is allergic to codeine.

3. Based on your assessment, what changes, if any, in the patient's current treatment are required?

4. How do the patient's signs and symptoms correlate with the body's response to inadequate perfusion?

side, the superior and inferior venae cavae lose their ability to stay fully expanded. This compression of these large vessels leads to reduced blood return to the right side of the heart and blood pressure drops. As the patient has more difficulty breathing, the heart also has more difficulty pumping. You may notice difficulty when attempting to ventilate the patient with a bag-mask device. The affected side will have absent lung sounds, and the patient may become cyanotic. Tracheal deviation is a late sign of tension pneumothorax and is difficult to see. As with cardiac tamponade, distended jugular veins may be noted.

A pulmonary embolism can also lead to obstructive shock. A **pulmonary embolism** is a blood clot that occurs in the pulmonary arteries and blocks the flow of blood through the lungs. When a massive pulmonary embolism occurs, it can

Words of Wisdom

Understanding the main differences among the types of shock is as simple as considering the terms themselves.

- **Cardiogenic shock.** Consider the parts of the word *cardiogenic*. *Cardio* suggests the heart, and *genic* means produced by.
- **Obstructive shock.** Think of obstructive shock as an *obstruction* blocking blood flow into or out of the ventricles.
- **Distributive shock.** Think of distributive shock as a problem *distributed* throughout the body.
- **Hypovolemic shock.** Consider the parts of the word *hypovolemic*. *Hypo* means less than normal, and *volemic* suggests volume—specifically, the volume of fluid in the circulatory system. Hemorrhagic shock is a form of hypovolemic shock caused by bleeding. Hypovolemic shock can also be caused by factors such as vomiting and diarrhea. Remember, hemorrhagic shock is always hypovolemic; however, hypovolemic shock is not always hemorrhagic.

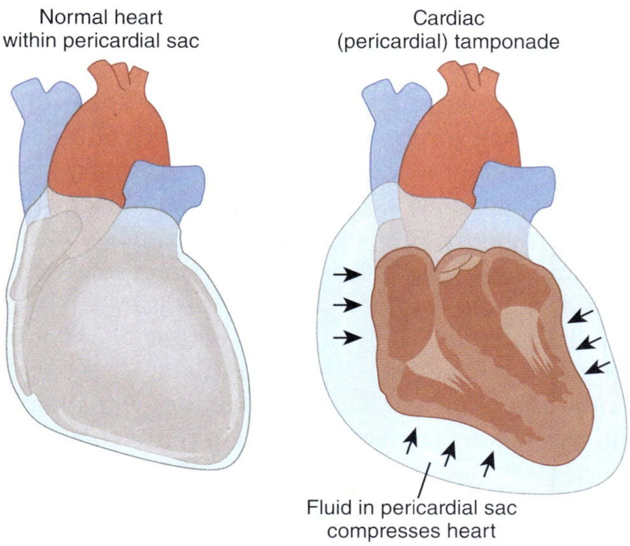

FIGURE 13-5 Impaired ventricular filling from a pericardial effusion causes cardiac tamponade.

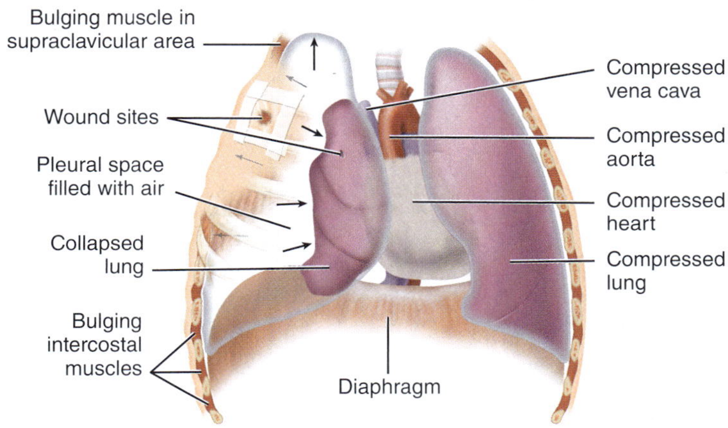

FIGURE 13-6 A tension pneumothorax is an accumulation of air in the pleural space, which eventually compresses the heart and great vessels.

prevent blood from being pumped from the right side of the heart to the left, resulting in complete backup of blood in the right ventricle and catastrophic obstructive shock.

Distributive Shock

Distributive shock results when there is widespread dilation of the small arterioles, small venules, or both. As a result, the circulating blood volume pools in the expanded vascular beds and tissue perfusion decreases when less blood returns to the heart to pump. The three most common types of distributive shock are septic shock, neurogenic shock, and anaphylactic shock.

Septic Shock

Septic shock occurs as a result of severe infections or after other major trauma. Infectious pathogens that cause septic shock are usually bacterial. Toxins (poisons) are generated by the bacteria and released into the blood. When sepsis and subsequent septic shock occurs, the body has an extreme inflammatory response as it attempts to fight off infections with white blood cells and other elements of the immune system. Because infections are typically in the tissue, the immune system makes the blood vessels larger and more permeable, or leaky, so the white blood cells can move into the tissue and fight the pathogens.

Septic shock is a complex problem. First, there is an insufficient volume of fluid in the container (hypovolemia), because much of the plasma has leaked out of the vessels. Second, the fluid that has leaked out often collects in the alveoli, interfering with respiration. Third, the vasodilation leads to a larger-than-normal vascular volume. This increase in space combined with smaller-than-normal volume of intravascular fluid leads to decreased preload and, subsequently, shock, which coupled with small blood clots in the capillaries can cause organ failure and death (**FIGURE 13-7**).

Neurogenic Shock

Damage to the spinal cord, particularly at the upper cervical levels, may cause loss of control to the musculature and vessels below the injury site. **Neurogenic shock** is usually the result of high spinal cord injury. Although very rare, there are medical causes as well. These include brain infection, tumors, inflammatory diseases, pressure on the spinal cord, and some toxins. In neurogenic shock, the muscles in the walls of the blood vessels are cut off from the nerve impulses of the sympathetic nervous system that cause them to contract. Therefore, all vessels below the level of the spinal injury dilate widely, increasing the size and capacity of the vascular system (**FIGURE 13-8**) and causing blood

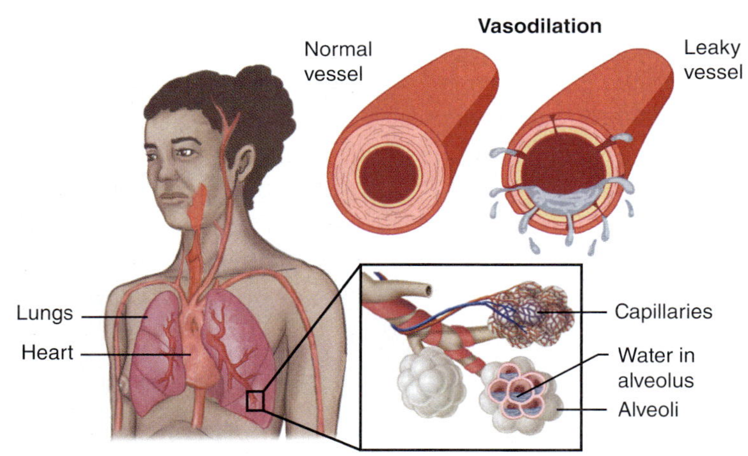

FIGURE 13-7 In septic shock, plasma leaks from the blood vessels, resulting in hypovolemia. This fluid often collects in the alveoli, interfering with respiration. Vasodilation leads to a larger-than-normal vascular volume. The decreased blood volume in the vessels paired with the increased vessel diameter results in dangerously low blood pressure and, potentially, a state of shock.

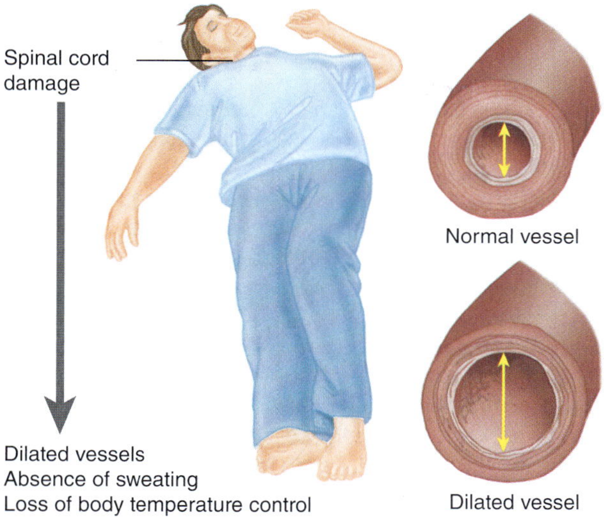

FIGURE 13-8 Damage to the spinal cord can cause significant injury to the part of the nervous system that controls the size and muscle tone of blood vessels. If the muscles in the blood vessels are cut off from their impulses to contract, the vessels dilate widely, increasing the size and capacity of the vascular system. The blood in the body can no longer fill the enlarged vessels, and shock ensues.

to pool. The available blood in the body can no longer fill the enlarged vascular system. Even if there is no blood or fluid loss, perfusion of organs and tissues becomes inadequate and shock occurs. In this condition, a change in the size of the vascular system has caused shock. Characteristic signs of this type of shock are the absence of sweating below the level of injury, normal and low heart rate in the presence of hypotension, and normal, warm skin. This is the only type of shock that presents without the characteristic pale (compared with baseline), cool skin, because the peripheral vasoconstriction cannot be triggered through the autonomic nervous system.

With neurogenic shock, many other functions that are under the control of the same part of the nervous system are also lost. The most important of them, in an acute injury setting, is the ability to control body temperature. Body temperature in a patient in neurogenic shock can rapidly fall to match that of the environment. In many situations, significant hypothermia occurs, severely complicating the situation. **Hypothermia** is a condition in which the internal body temperature falls below 95°F (35°C), usually after prolonged exposure to cool or freezing temperatures. Maintenance of body temperature is always an important element of treatment for a patient in shock. Cover the patient with blankets, or, if possible, wrap the patient in a warmed blanket.

Anaphylactic Shock

Anaphylaxis, or **anaphylactic shock**, occurs when individuals react quickly to a substance to which they have been sensitized. **Sensitization** means becoming sensitive to a substance that did not initially cause a reaction. Do not be misled by a patient who reports no history of allergic reaction to a substance on first or second exposure. Each subsequent exposure after sensitization tends to produce a more severe reaction.

Instances that cause severe allergic reactions commonly fall into the following four categories of exposure:

- Injections (tetanus antitoxin, penicillin, stings/bites)
- Ingestion (fish, shellfish, nuts, eggs, medication)
- Inhalation (dust, pollen, mold)
- Absorption, primarily through the skin (poison ivy, latex, personal care products)

Anaphylactic reactions can develop within minutes after contact with the substance to which the patient is allergic. The signs of such allergic reactions are distinct and not seen with other forms of shock. **TABLE 13-2** lists the signs of anaphylactic shock (the number of signs vary). Note that **cyanosis** (blue discoloration of the skin) is a late sign of anaphylactic shock. Cyanosis can be difficult to detect in persons with dark skin. Look at the fingernail beds and inside the inner lower eyelid.

In anaphylactic shock, there is widespread vascular dilation, increased permeability, and bronchoconstriction. The combination of poor oxygenation and poor perfusion in anaphylactic shock may rapidly prove fatal.

For more information on allergic reactions and anaphylaxis, see Chapter 21, *Allergy and Anaphylaxis*.

Words of Wisdom

Biphasic anaphylaxis is a condition in which the initial symptoms of an allergic exposure resolve but then recur within 48 hours, despite no reexposure to the allergen. The incidence of biphasic anaphylaxis is unclear; however, it may occur in up to 20% of anaphylaxis cases.[1]

TABLE 13-2 Signs and Symptoms of Anaphylactic Shock

System	Signs and Symptoms
Skin	• Flushed (red or dark compared with baseline), itchy, or burning, especially over the face and upper part of the chest • Urticaria (hives), which may spread over large areas of the body • Edema, especially of the face, tongue, and lips • Pallor (lighter, gray, or ashen skin compared with baseline), which in patients with dark skin may be easier to detect by examining capillary refill and the mucous membranes inside the inner lower eyelid • Cyanosis (a blue cast to the skin resulting from poor oxygenation of circulating blood) about the lips, which in persons with dark skin may be observed by examining mucous membranes inside the inner lower eyelid and capillary refill
Circulatory system	• Dilated peripheral blood vessels • Increased vessel permeability • Drop in blood pressure • Weak, barely palpable pulse
Respiratory system	• Sneezing or itching in the nasal passages • Stridor • Upper airway obstruction • Tightness in the chest, with a persistent dry cough • Wheezing and dyspnea (difficulty breathing) • Secretions of fluid and mucus into the bronchial passages, alveoli, and lung tissue, causing coughing • Constriction of the bronchi; difficulty drawing air into the lungs • Forced expiration, requiring exertion and accompanied by wheezing • Cessation of breathing
Other	• Abdominal cramping • Nausea • Vomiting • Altered mental status • Dizziness • Fainting and coma

Words of Wisdom

Sometimes a patient has a sudden reaction of the nervous system that produces temporary, generalized vasodilation, resulting in fainting, or **syncope**. The non-life-threatening events that cause syncope include receiving bad news, experiencing fear, standing still in one position for a prolonged time, or encountering an unpleasant sight, such as blood. In these cases, syncope occurs when blood pools in the dilated vessels, reducing the blood supply to the brain; as a result, the brain temporarily ceases to function normally, and the patient faints. When this happens, the fainting episode is temporary and the patient rouses before, or soon after, they are placed in the supine position. The person may initially appear to be in shock, with pale skin and a rapid heart rate, but their vital signs and appearance quickly return to normal.

There are many causes of syncope, and it is important to realize that some are serious. All patients who have a syncopal or near-syncopal event should have a thorough assessment, often by an advanced life support (ALS) crew. Syncope that is potentially life threatening may be caused by events such as an irregular heartbeat or an aortic or brain **aneurysm**.

Hypovolemic Shock

Hypovolemic shock is the result of an inadequate amount of fluid in the circulatory system. There are hemorrhagic and nonhemorrhagic causes of hypovolemic shock. For example, injuries involving bleeding may result in hemorrhagic shock, whereas vomiting and diarrhea may result in nonhemorrhagic hypovolemic shock.

Hypovolemic shock also occurs with severe thermal burns. In this case, intravascular plasma (the colorless part of the blood) loss is caused when fluid leaks from the capillaries into the surrounding tissue. Likewise, crushing injuries may result in the loss of blood and plasma from damaged vessels into injured tissues. These injuries can be thought of as excessive swelling.

Dehydration, the loss of water or fluid from body tissues, can cause shock. Fluid loss may be a result of severe vomiting and/or diarrhea. Patients who are very young or old are particularly susceptible to fluid loss and therefore at risk for the development of shock through dehydration. People who exercise in hot weather and are not acclimated to it may experience dehydration if they do not drink enough fluids. In these circumstances, the common factor is an insufficient volume of fluid within the vascular system to provide adequate circulation to the organs of the body.

ALS Assist

The use of whole blood transfusion for prehospital resuscitation of hemorrhagic shock is becoming more common. If your EMS agency uses whole blood, you will learn how to assist your paramedic partner in maintaining the strict requirements for storing the blood at a controlled temperature and preparing and administering it to patients experiencing hemorrhagic shock. Note that after use, the blood bags must not be discarded. The paramedic will turn the empty bag over to the receiving facility for additional testing after documenting the appropriate identifying numbers from the bag.

The Progression of Shock

The signs and symptoms of shock can become apparent as a patient progresses through them (**TABLE 13-3**). The early stage of shock, while the body can still compensate for blood loss, is called **compensated shock**. The late stage, when blood pressure is falling and the mental status is declining, is called **decompensated shock**. When shock progresses too far, it becomes irreversible (**irreversible shock**); however, there is no way to know when a patient has reached that point. It is therefore important to recognize and treat shock early, before the patient has developed irreversible shock.

TABLE 13-3 Progression of Shock

Progression	Signs and Symptoms
Compensated shock	• Agitation • Anxiety • Restlessness • Feeling of impending doom • Weak, rapid (thready) pulse • Clammy (pale, cool, moist) skin • Pallor, with cyanosis about the lips • Shallow, rapid breathing • Nausea or vomiting • Capillary refill of longer than 2 seconds in infants and children • Marked thirst • Narrowing pulse pressure
Decompensated shock	• Falling blood pressure (systolic blood pressure of 90 mm Hg or lower in an adult) • Declining mental status, altered level of consciousness • Labored or irregular breathing • Ashen, mottled, or cyanotic skin • Thready or absent peripheral pulses • Dull eyes, dilated pupils • Poor urinary output

Words of Wisdom

You should suspect shock when an adult's systolic blood pressure is less than their heart rate.

Remember that blood pressure may be the last measurable factor to change in shock. As we have seen, the body has several automatic mechanisms to compensate for initial blood loss and to help maintain blood pressure. Thus, by the time you detect a decrease in blood pressure, shock is well developed. This is particularly true in infants and children, who can maintain their blood pressure until they have sustained blood loss equivalent to more than one-half their blood volume. By the time blood pressure drops in infants and children who are in shock, they are close to death.

You should expect shock in many emergency medical situations. For example, you would expect shock to accompany massive external or internal bleeding. You should also expect shock if a patient has any one of the following conditions:

- Multiple severe fractures
- Abdominal or chest injury
- Spinal injury
- Severe infection

- Significant burns
- Major heart attack
- Anaphylaxis

Words of Wisdom

Frequently obtaining and recording vital signs, and observing perfusion indicators such as skin condition and mental status, will give you a window into the progression of shock. Monitoring vital signs every 5 minutes may reveal a pattern that will alert you to the presence of evolving shock. If suspected, expedite transport and begin treatments for shock immediately.

Patient Assessment for Shock

Scene Size-up

As you approach the scene, be alert to potential hazards to your safety. If this is a trauma scene or bleeding is suspected, put on gloves and eye protection, at a minimum.

Street Smarts

Put several pairs of gloves in your pocket for easy access in case your gloves tear or there are multiple patients with bleeding.

In incidents involving violence, such as assaults or gunshot wounds, make sure police are on scene. At times, you may need to stage several blocks away until law enforcement personnel have secured the area.

When you first see the patient, observe the scene and patient for clues to determine the nature of the illness or the mechanism of injury. This could help you anticipate the potential for development of shock.

Primary Assessment

The primary assessment for a patient with suspected shock should include a rapid exam to look for evidence of severe or exsanguinating hemorrhage, determine level of consciousness, identify and manage life-threatening concerns as they are found, and determine priority of the patient and transport. A patient with massive hemorrhage may require a tourniquet or wound packing *before* the airway is opened. In the case of obvious life-threatening external bleeding, the usual ABC (Assessment, Breathing, Circulation) sequence becomes XABC, where X represents eXsanguinating bleeding.[2] Once bleeding is controlled, the ABCs can be assessed and treated. If cardiac arrest is suspected, the order becomes CAB because circulation (via chest compressions) is the first priority.

When treating a patient in shock, provide high-concentration oxygen to assist in perfusion of damaged tissues. If the patient has bled out, saturating the red blood cells they have left will help prevent hypoxia. If the patient has signs of hypoperfusion, treat aggressively and provide rapid transport to the hospital. Request ALS as necessary to assist with more aggressive shock management. Do not delay transport of the seriously injured trauma patient to complete non-lifesaving treatments in the field, such as splinting extremity fractures; instead, complete these types of treatments en route to the hospital.

When you first visually inspect your patient, quickly form an initial general impression. This will help you develop an early sense of urgency for care of a patient who appears sick.

Once you are close to the patient, determine the need for manual spinal stabilization, and assess the patient's level of consciousness using the AVPU (Awake and alert, responsive to Verbal stimuli, responsive to Pain, Unresponsive) scale. A patient who has an altered level of consciousness may need emergency airway management. If the patient is awake and alert, determine a chief complaint.

Next, quickly assess the airway to ensure it is patent. Be alert to abnormal airway sounds such as gurgling (indicating the need to suction the airway) or stridor (indicating partial airway obstruction). Consider an adjunct such as an oropharyngeal or nasopharyngeal airway for a patient with an altered level of consciousness.

Quickly assess breathing in the patient. Observe the patient for signs of accessory muscle use such as movement in the neck muscles, intercostal retractions, or abnormal use of the abdominal muscles. An increased respiratory rate is often an early sign of impending shock and can be overlooked even by experienced providers. Administer high-concentration oxygen or, if needed, assist respirations with a bag-mask device to achieve an Spo_2 of 94% to 98%.

Assessing the patient's circulatory status can reveal important clues regarding the presence of shock. Check for the presence of a distal pulse. If you cannot obtain a distal pulse, assess for a central pulse. Make a rapid determination if the pulse is fast, slow, weak, strong, or altogether absent. A rapid pulse is found in both compensated and uncompensated shock. The pulse will weaken and become thready as the patient moves into uncompensated shock. In shock, the skin may be cool, clammy, or ashen. If the patient has no pulse and is not breathing, immediately begin cardiopulmonary resuscitation (CPR). Assess for and identify any life-threatening bleeding in trauma patients; if serious bleeding is discovered, treat it immediately. You must also quickly assess skin temperature, condition, and color, and check for capillary refill time.

Words of Wisdom

If the shock patient's mental status is starting to deteriorate, the brain is no longer receiving adequate blood flow and the patient is progressing from compensated to decompensated shock.

Once you have assessed perfusion, determine whether the patient should be treated as high priority, whether ALS is needed, and the transport destination.

History Taking

After the life threats have been managed during the primary assessment, determine the chief complaint. Obtain a medical history and be alert for injury-specific signs and symptoms as well as any pertinent negatives such as loss of sensation. Quickly obtain a SAMPLE history (Signs and symptoms, Allergies, Medications, Pertinent past medical history, Last oral intake, Events leading up to the illness or injury) from the patient. Anticoagulants can increase bleeding and worsen shock. Blood pressure medicines such as beta blockers can prevent the heart rate from rising to compensate for shock.

Secondary Assessment

The secondary assessment is a more detailed, comprehensive examination of the patient that is used to uncover injuries that may have been missed during the primary assessment. The secondary assessment begins by repeating the primary assessment followed by a focused assessment. In some instances, such as a critically injured patient or short transport time, you may not have time to conduct a secondary assessment.

YOU are the EMT

You continue with the treatment initiated by the clinic; however, you remove the nasal cannula and apply high-concentration oxygen via a nonrebreathing mask. Your partner obtains the patient's vital signs and reports them to you and the clinic physician.

Recording Time:	4 Minutes
Respirations	24 breaths/min; shallow
Pulse	120 beats/min; weak
Skin	Pale, cool, and diaphoretic
Blood pressure	108/58 mm Hg
Oxygen saturation (Spo_2)	94% (on oxygen)

You bring the stretcher into the room and prepare the patient for immediate transport. The patient remains conscious and alert, but is becoming increasingly restless and reports feeling dizzy.

5. Is the patient in compensated or decompensated shock? How can you tell?

If your patient is a trauma patient with a significant mechanism of injury or multiple injuries, if the patient gives you a poor initial general impression, or if you found problems in the primary assessment, perform a secondary assessment of the entire body. If your patient has a medical problem but is not responsive or if problems were noted in the primary assessment, perform a secondary assessment of the entire body. These assessments should be performed quickly but thoroughly to ensure that you do not miss any significant or life-threatening problems or delay needed care.

If your patient has a simple mechanism of injury, such as a lacerated wrist, focus your examination on the specific area affected. Whether your examination is of the entire body or of a specific area, if a life-threatening problem is found, treat it immediately.

When time permits and the patient's condition is stable, perform a thorough examination of the patient, which includes a complete neurologic assessment.

Obtain a complete set of baseline vital signs. If the patient's condition is unstable or could become unstable, reassess vital signs every 5 minutes. If the patient is in stable condition, reassess vital signs every 10 to 15 minutes. Baseline vital signs will help you trend changes in your patient.

In addition to hands-on assessment, use monitoring devices to quantify the patient's oxygenation and circulatory status. Use a noninvasive technique to monitor blood pressure and a pulse oximeter to evaluate the effectiveness of oxygenation. It is recommended that you assess the patient's blood pressure with a sphygmomanometer (blood pressure cuff) and stethoscope (manually), before using a noninvasive blood pressure monitor, to establish a baseline blood pressure and to determine the accuracy of the noninvasive blood pressure monitor.

Reassessment

Reassess the patient's vital signs, interventions, chief complaint, and mental status. You must determine what interventions are needed for your patient based on the assessment findings. Focus on supporting the cardiovascular system. Treat for shock early and aggressively by providing oxygen, if needed, to achieve an Spo_2 of 94% to 98%, and keeping the patient warm.

Emergency Medical Care for Shock

You must begin immediate treatment for shock as soon as you realize that the condition may exist. As with any type of patient care, you should begin by following standard precautions. Control all obvious external bleeding. Apply direct pressure with dry, sterile dressings over the bleeding sites, and secure with bandages. If direct pressure is not rapidly successful in the control of bleeding from an extremity, apply a tourniquet proximal to the bleeding site (**FIGURE 13-9**). Make sure the patient has an open airway. Maintain manual in-line stabilization if necessary, and check breathing and pulse. The use of tourniquets is further described in Chapter 25, *Bleeding*.

Comfort, calm, and reassure the patient, while maintaining the patient in the supine position unless they have severe respiratory distress. Never allow patients to eat or drink prior to being evaluated by a physician.

Apply spinal motion restriction if there is a concern about neck or back injuries. Do not delay transport to apply individual splints in the field when shock is present. If time allows, splint individual extremity fractures during transport. Splinting minimizes pain, bleeding, and discomfort, all of which can aggravate shock. It also prevents the broken bone ends from further damaging adjacent soft tissue.

Remember that inadequate ventilation may be a major factor in the development of shock. Provide

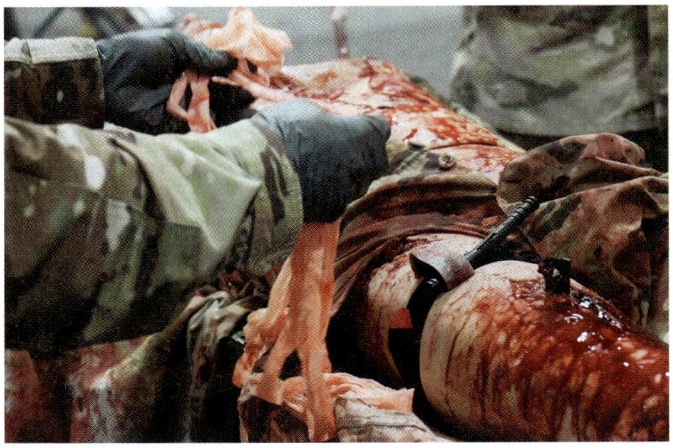

FIGURE 13-9 If direct pressure does not quickly control bleeding from an extremity, a tourniquet should be applied proximal to the bleeding site.

oxygen, assist with ventilations, and use airway adjuncts as needed, and continue to monitor the patient's breathing. To prevent the loss of body heat, place blankets under and over the patient. Do not use external heat sources, such as hot water bottles or heating pads. They may harm a patient in shock by causing vasodilation and decreasing blood pressure even more.

Transport the patient and treat additional injuries en route. Consider ALS rendezvous if possible, and consider aeromedical transport if transport times by ground are extended.

Accurately record the patient's vital signs approximately every 5 minutes throughout treatment and transport. It is essential to transport trauma patients to the ED as rapidly as possible for definitive treatment. The critically important period for the early resuscitation and treatment of severely injured trauma patients is often referred to as the Golden Period. This concept underscores the importance of rapid evaluation, stabilization, and transport. The goal of EMS is to limit on-scene time (time on scene until transport to hospital is started) to 10 minutes or less. Remember to speak calmly and reassuringly to a conscious patient throughout assessment, care, and transport.

TABLE 13-4 lists the general supportive measures for the major types of shock. Not every measure is used for every type of shock.

Words of Wisdom

Know these six critical interventions for shock:

1. Patients experiencing anaphylaxis need epinephrine immediately.
2. Control external bleeding.
3. Place the patient supine unless this position compromises breathing.
4. Provide high-concentration oxygen to achieve an Spo_2 of 94% to 98%.
5. Prevent heat loss.
6. Provide rapid transport to the appropriate facility.

Treating Cardiogenic Shock

The patient who is in shock as a result of a heart attack or heart failure simply cannot generate the necessary contraction to pump blood throughout the circulatory system. An acute myocardial infarction is the most common cause of cardiogenic shock, and these patients may complain of chest pain.

These patients may have taken nitroglycerin before your arrival and may want to take more. Hypotensive patients in cardiogenic shock should

Words of Wisdom

Keep in mind that chronic lung disease will aggravate cardiogenic shock. If the patient has chronic obstructive pulmonary disease and heart disease, oxygenation of the blood passing through the lungs is impaired. Because fluid is collecting in the lungs, this patient is often able to breathe better in a sitting or semi-sitting position and may tell you so.

TABLE 13-4 Types of Shock

Type of Shock	Examples of Potential Causes	Signs and Symptoms	Treatment
Cardiogenic	Inadequate heart function Disease of muscle tissue Impaired electrical system Disease or injury	Chest pain Irregular pulse Weak pulse Low blood pressure Cyanosis (lips, under nails) Cool, clammy skin Anxiety Delayed capillary refill Rapid breathing Crackles Pulmonary edema	Position comfortably. Administer oxygen to target 94% to 98% Spo_2. Assist ventilations. Transport promptly. Provide ALS assist and/or rapid transport.

(continues)

TABLE 13-4 Types of Shock *(continued)*

Type of Shock	Examples of Potential Causes	Signs and Symptoms	Treatment

Obstructive	Mechanical obstruction of the cardiac muscle causing a decrease in cardiac output
	• Tension pneumothorax
	• Cardiac tamponade
	• Pulmonary embolism
		Dependent on cause:
		• Dyspnea
		• Rapid, weak pulse
		• Low blood pressure
		• Rapid, shallow breaths
		• Decreased lung compliance
		• Unilateral, decreased, or absent breath sounds
		• Jugular venous distention
		• Subcutaneous emphysema
		• Cyanosis
		• Tracheal deviation toward unaffected side
		• Beck triad (cardiac tamponade):
		  • Jugular venous distention
		  • Narrowing pulse pressure
		  • Muffled heart tones
			Dependent on cause:
			• Administer oxygen to target 94% to 98% Spo_2.
			• Provide ALS assist and/or rapid transport.

Septic	Severe infection	Warm skin or fever (early) Low blood pressure Pale, gray, mottled skin (late) Tachycardia	Administer oxygen to target 94% to 98% Spo_2. Assist ventilations. Keep patient warm. Provide ALS assist and/or rapid transport.
Neurogenic	Damaged cervical spine, which causes widespread blood vessel dilation	Bradycardia (slow pulse) or normal heart rate Low blood pressure Baseline skin color, temperature below the level of the injury Signs of neck injury	Secure airway. Maintain spinal motion restriction. Assist ventilations. Administer oxygen to target 94% to 98% Spo_2. Preserve body heat. Provide ALS assist and/or rapid transport
Anaphylactic	Extreme life-threatening allergic reaction	Can develop within seconds Mild itching or rash (hives) Burning or flushed skin Wheezing Vascular dilation Generalized edema Coma Rapid death	Administer epinephrine. Manage the airway. Assist ventilations. Administer oxygen to target 94% to 98% Spo_2. Determine cause. Provide ALS assist and/or rapid transport
Hypovolemic	Loss of blood or fluid	Rapid, weak pulse Low blood pressure Change in mental status Cyanosis (lips, under nails) Cool, clammy skin Increased respiratory rate	Secure airway. Assist ventilations. Administer oxygen to target 94% to 98% Spo_2. Control external bleeding. Keep warm. Provide ALS assist and/or rapid transport

Abbreviations: ALS, advanced life support; Spo_2, oxygen saturation not receive nitroglycerin.[3,4] In addition to low blood pressure, other signs include a weak, irregular pulse; cyanosis about the lips and underneath the fingernails; anxiety; and nausea.

Treatment of cardiogenic shock should begin by placing the patient in the position in which breathing is easiest as you administer high-concentration oxygen. Be ready to assist ventilations as necessary, and have suction nearby in case the patient vomits. Provide prompt transport to the emergency department (ED). If an ALS crew is not already on the scene, consider a rendezvous en route to the hospital if available. Frequently check for a pulse in an unresponsive patient to identify early whether CPR and an automated external defibrillator (AED) are needed.

Words of Wisdom

Acute pulmonary edema may occur without hypotension. In fact, often the blood pressure is very high. In these cases, treatments such as continuous positive airway pressure (CPAP) and ALS administration of nitroglycerin can help the patient. However, when pulmonary edema occurs in cardiogenic shock and the patient is hypotensive, both CPAP and nitroglycerin are contraindicated. Acute pulmonary edema is discussed further in Chapter 16, *Respiratory Emergencies*.

Street Smarts

Provide calm reassurance to a patient who has had a suspected heart attack.

Treating Obstructive Shock

As discussed previously, two of the most common examples of obstructive shock are cardiac tamponade and tension pneumothorax.

Increasing cardiac output should be the priority in treating cardiac tamponade. The preload must be increased because increasing pressure in the pericardium is squeezing the heart. Apply high-concentration oxygen. The only definitive treatment for cardiac tamponade is surgery. Pericardiocentesis involves penetrating the pericardium with a needle to withdraw the accumulated blood from the pericardial sac. This procedure is an advanced skill, and it is rarely performed in the field.

To treat a tension pneumothorax, administer high-concentration oxygen via nonrebreathing mask early to prevent hypoxia. Usually, the only action that can prevent eventual death from a tension pneumothorax is decompression of the injured side of the chest, relieving the pressure in the chest and allowing the heart to expand fully again. Chest decompression is an ALS skill. Ask for ALS assistance early in the call if available; however, do not delay transport waiting for the arrival of ALS.

YOU are the EMT

The patient is placed onto the stretcher and loaded into the ambulance. You quickly gather the patient records from the clinic physician and begin transport to a hospital that is only 10 minutes away. En route, you continue with your treatment and reassess the patient's condition.

Recording Time: 11 Minutes	
Level of consciousness	Responsive to pain only
Respirations	30 breaths/min; shallower
Pulse	130 beats/min; absent radial pulses (carotid pulse present)
Skin	Pale, cool, and diaphoretic
Blood pressure	84/44 mm Hg
Oxygen saturation (Spo_2)	89% (on oxygen)

6. How has your patient's condition changed?
7. Are adjustments in your current interventions required? If so, what?

ALS Assist

It is important to notify your ALS partner immediately if you are ventilating a patient with a bag-mask device and note gastric distention or experience increased difficulty ventilating the patient (ie, poor bag compliance). These findings may indicate the presence of airway obstruction, displaced airway adjunct, or tension pneumothorax.

Treating Distributive Shock

Treating Septic Shock

The proper treatment of septic shock requires complex hospital management, including expeditious administration of antibiotics. If you suspect that a patient has septic shock, use appropriate standard precautions and transport as promptly as possible, administering high-concentration oxygen during transport. Ventilatory support may be necessary to maintain adequate tidal volume. Use blankets to conserve body heat. Sepsis has become an increasingly common illness. Some hospitals have instituted specialized sepsis teams, which, when notified, will meet the patient in the ED. Sepsis teams have protocols that decrease the amount of time spent in identification of the infectious agent and initiation of the appropriate treatment, thereby decreasing the mortality from septic shock. EMS agencies may have sepsis protocols in which EMTs alert the hospital to the potential for sepsis when giving their radio report. Be familiar with your local protocols for sepsis alerts and notifications. Remember to protect yourself from the infection affecting the patient. Some infections causing sepsis are respiratory and can be transmitted through breathing. Wear proper protective equipment and clean your ambulance thoroughly after the call.

Treating Neurogenic Shock

Shock that accompanies spinal cord injury is best treated by a combination of all known supportive measures. Emergency treatment must be directed toward obtaining and maintaining a proper airway, providing spinal motion restriction, assisting inadequate breathing as needed, conserving body heat, and ensuring the most effective circulation possible.

A patient in neurogenic shock is usually not losing blood; however, the capacity of the blood vessels has become significantly larger than the available volume of the blood inside the vessels. Supplemental oxygen will boost the concentration of oxygen in the blood. If respirations are weak or inadequate, assist ventilations. Because the injury may have disabled the body's normal temperature controls, keep the patient as warm as possible with blankets. Transport the patient promptly to a facility capable of managing spinal injuries.

Treating Anaphylactic Shock

The most effective emergency treatment of a severe, acute allergic reaction is to administer epinephrine by way of intramuscular injection. A patient who is aware of having a specific sensitivity may carry a kit containing epinephrine. If the patient is unable to inject the medication, you may have to do so if you are allowed by local protocol. Many EMT-staffed ambulances carry prefilled epinephrine injectors on the ambulance to administer during anaphylaxis. In some cases, EMTs with appropriate authorization and training by the medical director draw up and administer intramuscular epinephrine from a vial or ampule.[5] If the patient's signs and symptoms recur or the patient's condition deteriorates, consult medical control for authorization to administer a repeat injection, if available. For more information on the emergency care for allergic reactions, see Chapter 21, *Allergy and Anaphylaxis*.

A patient with anaphylaxis requires immediate transport to the ED after administration of the epinephrine. Additional emergency care includes high-concentration oxygen. Assist ventilations with a bag-mask device if necessary. If possible, attempt to determine what agent caused the reaction (eg, drug, insect bite or sting, food item) and how it was received (ie, by mouth, inhalation, absorption, or injection). The severity of allergic reactions can vary greatly, with symptoms ranging from mild itching to profound coma and rapid death. Keep in mind that a mild reaction may worsen suddenly or over time. Because of the potential for airway compromise, consider requesting ALS backup, if available.

Treating Hypovolemic Shock

The emergency treatment of hypovolemic or hemorrhagic shock includes the control of all obvious external bleeding. The best initial method to control external bleeding is direct pressure. To prevent continued bleeding, you must apply sufficient pressure to control obvious external bleeding. If severe extremity bleeding is not controlled with direct pressure, apply a tourniquet. Ensure that you use great care to handle the patient gently and keep the patient warm. Bleeding control, including application of a tourniquet and wound packing, is discussed in detail in Chapter 25, *Bleeding*.

Although you cannot control internal bleeding in the field, it is important to recognize its existence and provide general support and rapid transport. Secure and maintain an airway, and provide respiratory support, including supplemental oxygen and, if needed, assisted ventilations. Start oxygen as soon as you suspect shock and continue it during transport; with too little circulating blood, additional oxygen may be lifesaving. Watch to ensure that the patient does not aspirate blood or vomitus, and transport the patient as rapidly as possible to the ED.

Treating Shock in Infants and Children

Circulation Emergencies and Management

Compared to adults, children have more effective compensatory mechanisms (initially) when cardiovascular compromise occurs. Cardiac output is influenced by stroke volume and heart rate. While stroke volume is relatively fixed, particularly in infants and young children, heart rate can be increased to help maintain cardiac output.[6] Once this mechanism begins to fail, peripheral vasoconstriction occurs, enabling a sufficient volume of blood to return to the heart. This combination of increased heart rate and vasoconstriction can help stabilize blood pressure initially until the child has lost a significant amount of blood. Once these compensatory mechanisms are overwhelmed, the blood pressure drops quickly and decompensated shock may occur.

In pediatric patients, the most common causes of shock include the following:

- **Hypovolemic**
  - Traumatic injury with blood loss (especially abdominal)
  - Dehydration from diarrhea and vomiting
  - Large burns
  - Inadequate fluid intake

Words of Wisdom

Children have less circulating blood than adults do. Remember that a relatively small amount of blood loss may represent a serious threat of shock, regardless of what the blood pressure indicates.

YOU are the EMT

You ask your partner to call ahead to the hospital because you are busy caring for the patient and cannot free up your hands. The noninvasive automatic vital signs machine records another set of vital signs. With an estimated time of arrival at the hospital of 5 minutes, you reassess the patient.

Recording Time: 16 Minutes	
Level of consciousness	Responsive to pain only
Respirations	30 breaths/min and shallow (baseline); ventilations are being assisted
Pulse	128 beats/min; absent radial pulses (carotid pulse present)
Skin	Pale, cool, and diaphoretic
Blood pressure	80/40 mm Hg
Oxygen saturation (Spo_2)	96% (with assisted ventilation; on oxygen)

You arrive at the hospital and give your report to the charge nurse. IV access is rapidly obtained, the attending physician quickly assesses the patient, and additional treatment is given.

8. What part of the patient's perfusion triangle has failed?

9. How does shock caused by volume failure differ from shock caused by container failure?

- **Distributive**
  - Severe infection
  - Neurologic injury, such as severe head trauma
  - A severe allergic reaction to an allergen (anaphylaxis), such as an insect bite or food allergy
- **Cardiogenic**
  - Congenital heart disease
  - Infection of the heart muscle
  - Diseases that weaken the heart muscle
- **Obstructive**
  - A collapsed lung (tension pneumothorax)
  - Blood or fluid around the heart (cardiac tamponade or pericarditis)

Begin treating shock by assessing the ABCs, intervening immediately as required; do not wait until you have performed the complete assessment to take action. If there is an obvious life-threatening external hemorrhage, the order becomes XABC, because bleeding control is the priority. If cardiac arrest is suspected, the order becomes CAB because chest compressions are essential.

When you assess circulation, pay particular attention to the following:

- **Pulse.** Assess the rate, quality, and location of the pulse. A weak, thready pulse is a sign that there is a problem. Absence of a peripheral pulse (radial or pedal) is an indicator of poor perfusion. The appropriate rate depends on age; however, suspect shock or another serious medical condition in infants and children younger than 2 years who have a heart rate of 180 beats/min or greater and in children older than 2 years who have a heart rate of 160 beats/min or greater.[6]
- **Skin signs.** Assess the temperature and moisture of the hands and feet. How does the temperature of the extremities compare with that of the skin on the trunk of the body? Is the skin dry and warm, or cold and clammy? Are the mucous membranes in the mouth dry?
- **Capillary refill time.** Squeeze a finger or toe for several seconds until the skin blanches, and then release it. Does the fingertip return to its normal color within 2 seconds, or does it take longer (delayed capillary refill)?
- **Color.** Assess the patient's skin color. Is the pediatric patient pale, ashen, or cyanotic? This sign can be more difficult to assess in children with dark skin pigmentation. Reliance on other signs is necessary.
- **Changes.** Changes in pulse rate, color, skin signs, and capillary refill time are all important clues in recognizing shock.

Blood pressure is the most difficult vital sign to measure in pediatric patients. The cuff must be the proper size: two-thirds the length of the upper arm. Also, normal blood pressure values are age specific. In general, the following rule can be used to recognize hypotension in children 1 to 10 years of age:

$$\text{Blood pressure should be} \geq 70 \text{ mm Hg} + (2 \times \text{Child's age in years})$$

For example, a 4-year-old is considered hypotensive if their blood pressure is less than 78 mm Hg: 70 mm Hg + (2 × 4 years). Remember that blood pressure may be normal with compensated shock. Low blood pressure is a sign of decompensated shock. All shock in infants and children requires care from an ALS team and rapid transport.

Part of your assessment should also include talking with the parents or caregivers to determine when the signs and symptoms first appeared and whether any of the following has occurred:

- Decrease in urine output (with infants, are there fewer wet diapers than normal?)
- Absence of tears, even when the child is crying
- A sunken or depressed fontanelle (infant patient)
- Changes in level of consciousness and behavior

Limit your management to these simple interventions. Do not waste time performing field procedures. Control life-threatening bleeding if present, ensure that the airway is open, prepare for artificial ventilation, and give supplemental oxygen by mask. Continue to monitor the airway and breathing. Place the child in a position of comfort in an appropriate restraint system. Keep the child warm with blankets and by turning up the heat in the patient compartment. Provide immediate transport to the nearest appropriate facility and continue monitoring vital signs en route. Call for ALS intercept as needed. Allow a parent or caregiver to accompany the child whenever possible.

Dehydration Emergencies and Management

Dehydration occurs when fluid losses are greater than fluid intake. The most common cause of dehydration in pediatric patients is vomiting and diarrhea. If left untreated, dehydration can lead to shock and eventually death. Infants and children are at greater risk than adults for dehydration because their fluid reserves are smaller than those in adults. Life-threatening dehydration can overcome an infant in a matter of hours.

Dehydration can be mild, moderate, or severe. The severity of the dehydration can be gauged by looking at several clues (**TABLE 13-5**). For example, an infant with mild dehydration may have dry lips and gums, decreased saliva, and fewer wet diapers throughout the day. As the dehydration grows more severe, the lips and gums may become very dry, the eyes may look sunken, and the infant may be sleepy and/or irritable, refusing bottles. The skin may be loose and have no elasticity, a condition called poor skin turgor (**FIGURE 13-10**). Also, infants may have sunken fontanelles.

Young children can compensate for fluid losses by decreasing blood flow to the extremities and directing blood flow to vital organs such as the brain and heart. Children who are moderately to severely dehydrated may have mottled, cool, clammy skin and delayed capillary response time. Respirations will usually be increased. Be aware that blood pressure may remain within a normal range while the pediatric patient is in shock, because the compensatory mechanisms are still in place.

Emergency medical care should include assessing the ABCs and obtaining baseline vital signs. However, if the dehydration is severe, ALS backup may be necessary so that IV access can be obtained and rehydration can begin. All pediatric patients with signs and symptoms of moderate to severe dehydration should be transported to the ED for further evaluation and treatment.

ALS Assist

If local protocol allows EMTs to set up IV lines, this can be extremely helpful for ALS providers. To reduce the risk of infection or air embolism, be sure you are properly trained and credentialed to perform this task.

TABLE 13-5 Vital Signs and Symptoms of Dehydration

	Mild Dehydration	Moderate Dehydration	Severe Dehydration
Pulse	Normal	Increased	Marked tachycardia Weak or absent peripheral pulses
Level of activity	Normal or slowed	Slowed	Variable, weak to unresponsive
Urine output	Decreased	Decreased	No output
Skin	Normal	Cool, mottled; poor turgor	Cool, clammy; poor turgor; delayed capillary refill time
Mouth	Decreased saliva	Dry mucous membranes	Dry mucous membranes
Eyes	Normal	No tears	Sunken eyes
Anterior fontanelle (<18 months)	Normal to sunken	Sunken	Very sunken
Level of consciousness	Normal	Altered	Markedly altered
Blood pressure	Normal	Normal	Hypotension

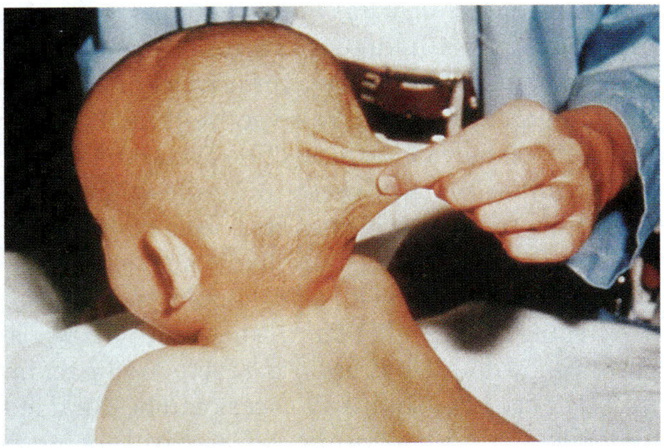

FIGURE 13-10 An infant with dehydration may exhibit "tenting" or poor skin turgor.

Courtesy of Ronald Dieckmann, MD.

Treating Shock in Older Patients

Use caution when caring for older patients who are experiencing shock. As a result of the aging process, older patients generally have less ability to compensate for shock than younger patients. For example, the immune system is not as effective in older adults, which increases the likelihood of septic shock developing. Moreover, older patients frequently have existing illnesses that impair their compensatory mechanisms or complicate assessment for shock. Such conditions include the following:

- Chronic obstructive pulmonary disease, which can interfere with normal oxygenation and ventilation
- Heart failure, which impairs the heart's ability to increase contractility to maintain cardiac output and makes it more likely the patient will decompensate quickly
- Dementia, which makes assessment of the patient's mental status difficult

In each of these situations, an understanding of the patient's baseline vital signs and mental status will help you determine if the patient's condition is deteriorating.

In addition, many older patients take numerous medications that could either mask or mimic signs of shock. Anticoagulants such as dabigatran (Pradaxa) and warfarin (Coumadin) inhibit blood clotting, making it more difficult to control bleeding. Drugs used to lower blood pressure, such as metoprolol (Toprol), prevent the heart rate from increasing in response to shock.

Keep in mind the following signs of the normal aging process when treating geriatric patients:

- The central nervous system often has a delayed response; thus, tachypnea and vasoconstriction may be slower to respond to shock.
- The cardiovascular system has a variety of changes that result in a decrease in the efficiency of the system. On assessment, be alert for higher resting heart rates and irregular pulse rates.
- The respiratory system undergoes significant changes as the elasticity of the lungs and their size and strength decrease. On assessment, be alert for higher respiratory rates, lower tidal volume, and a decreased gag reflex. In addition, remember that cervical arthritis may be present and that dentures may cause an airway obstruction.
- The skin becomes thinner, drier, less elastic, and more fragile, thus providing less protection and thermal regulation (cold and hot).
- The renal system decreases in function and may not respond well to unusual demands such as illness or dehydration.
- The gastrointestinal system sustains changes in gastric motility that may lead to slower gastric emptying.

The principles of treating a geriatric patient in shock are, in some cases, slightly different than they are for any other shock patient:

1. Provide in-line spinal motion restriction if indicated. Geriatric patients with conditions such as arthritis may need additional padding for comfort and support. If spinal motion restriction is not indicated, place the patient who is in shock supine unless they experience difficulty breathing in this position.
2. Control life-threatening hemorrhage immediately with direct pressure or tourniquet application when appropriate.
3. Suction as necessary and provide high-concentration oxygen via a nonrebreathing mask to achieve an Spo_2 of 94% to 98%.
4. Maintain body temperature.
5. Provide rapid transport.

YOU are the EMT SUMMARY

1. What additional information should you attempt to gather about the patient while en route to the clinic?

The description of "a woman in shock" tells you very little. The patient could have a severe injury with internal bleeding, could be experiencing a severe allergic reaction, or may have simply fainted. When you are dispatched to *any* call with minimal information provided, attempt to gather additional information while you are en route. In many cases, the dispatcher will provide additional patient information without you asking for it as it becomes available. In other cases, you will need to ask the dispatcher to try to make contact with the caller to obtain a patient update. Many EMS systems use an emergency medical dispatcher (EMD); if this is the case, the EMD should be able to provide you with more detailed information, as well as give prearrival instructions to the caller.

2. What is shock and how does it relate to perfusion?

Shock is a state of inadequate perfusion (hypoperfusion) and is the result of failure of one or more components of the perfusion triangle or the respiratory system. Perfusion is the delivery of blood and oxygen and other essential nutrients to the body's cells to keep them alive. While delivering these essential items to the body's cells, waste products such as carbon dioxide are removed from the cell and eliminated from the body. Adequate perfusion is maintained by the perfusion triangle, which consists of three essential components: a functioning pump (the heart), adequate volume (the blood and water), and an intact container (the blood vessels). The respiratory system is also a critical component for adequate perfusion; if oxygen cannot get into the lungs, the heart cannot pump it through the blood vessels and to the cells.

The type of shock that a patient is experiencing describes the component of the perfusion triangle that has failed. Regardless of the type of shock, the result is the same: inadequate perfusion of the body's tissues and cells, which will lead to death if untreated.

3. Based on your assessment, what changes, if any, in the patient's current treatment are required?

The patient clearly has signs of shock (ie, restlessness; tachypnea; tachycardia; weak radial pulses; and cool, pale, diaphoretic skin), and the treatment that has been provided thus far is essentially appropriate. She is being kept warm, and she is receiving oxygen. However, patients with signs of hemorrhagic shock need *high-concentration* oxygen. She is presently receiving oxygen via a nasal cannula; this should be changed to a nonrebreathing mask with the flow rate set at 15 L/min. Based on this patient's presentation, which includes abdominal pain and rectal bleeding, you should suspect blood loss (bleeding into the intestines) as the cause of shock. Blood carries oxygen; if the blood volume decreases, so does the ability of oxygen to get to the cells. Providing a high concentration of oxygen will oxygenate the red blood cells that remain in the circulatory system. In addition to receiving high-concentration oxygen, the patient needs IV access and volume replacement to help circulate the oxygenated blood. The physician has been unable to obtain IV access, and since IV therapy is beyond the EMT's scope of practice, you must prepare the patient for immediate transport. If your transport time to the hospital will be prolonged, you should consider an intercept with ALS, because ALS is trained to establish IV access.

4. How do the patient's signs and symptoms correlate with the body's response to inadequate perfusion?

During shock, the body mounts a physiologic response aimed at maintaining adequate perfusion, most of which is the result of increased activity of the sympathetic nervous system releasing greater quantities of epinephrine (adrenaline) and norepinephrine. Restlessness, perhaps one of the earliest signs of shock, is caused by a decrease in oxygen to the brain. As a result, the number of signals the brain sends to the respiratory muscles increases, which causes an increase in the patient's respiratory rate (tachypnea). Increased levels of epinephrine cause an increase in heart rate and cardiac contractility, and as a result, blood is pumped faster and with greater force throughout the body to compensate for decreased perfusion. Increased levels of norepinephrine cause the blood vessels to constrict (vasoconstriction), thus maintaining the patient's blood pressure. Early in shock, blood is shunted away from areas of lesser need (ie, the skin and muscles) to areas of greater need (ie, heart, lungs, liver, kidneys) by vasoconstriction. This causes the skin to turn pale (pallor) and become cool to the touch. When the sympathetic nervous system activity increases, sweat gland activity increases as well, resulting in diaphoresis (profuse sweating).

YOU are the EMT SUMMARY continued

5. Is the patient in compensated or decompensated shock? How can you tell?

Signs of compensated shock include restlessness, anxiety, or agitation; tachycardia; rapid, weak (thready) peripheral pulses; tachypnea; and marked thirst. In compensated shock, however, the patient's systolic blood pressure is maintained, usually above 90 mm Hg in adults. Your patient's current blood pressure is 108/58 mm Hg. These signs and symptoms indicate that the patient is in compensated shock. Signs of decompensated shock include systolic blood pressure of 90 mm Hg or lower in an adult; absent peripheral pulses; dilated pupils; ashen, mottled, or cyanotic skin; and a decreasing level of consciousness. It is important to note that the patient's blood pressure is often a very late factor to change in shock. By the time a low blood pressure (hypotension) is detected, shock is well developed. In decompensated shock, the body's compensatory mechanisms are no longer able to maintain adequate perfusion. Survival is less likely, even with rapid transport and aggressive treatment at the hospital.

6. How has your patient's condition changed?

Your patient's condition has changed for the worse. Her level of consciousness has decreased (responsive to pain only), her respirations have increased in rate and decreased in depth (reduced tidal volume), her heart rate has increased and her radial pulses are no longer palpable, her blood pressure is below 90 mm Hg (84/44 mm Hg), and her oxygen saturation has fallen, despite the administration of high-concentration oxygen. Based on these reassessment findings, your patient is now in decompensated shock with inadequate breathing. As previously discussed, decompensated shock occurs when the body's compensatory mechanisms begin to fail and are no longer able to maintain adequate perfusion. At the clinic, the patient had signs of shock but was still conscious and alert, although restless, and her systolic blood pressure was maintained. Patients can decompensate within a matter of minutes; this fact underscores the criticality of frequent reassessments.

7. Are adjustments in your current interventions required? If so, what?

In terms of shock treatment, you are doing everything you can. The patient is being kept warm with a blanket and is receiving high-concentration oxygen. An intercept with an ALS unit is not practical because you are too close to the hospital. However, the patient's breathing is no longer adequate (30 breaths/min and shallow) and requires assistance. Because of her decreased level of consciousness, you should insert a nasopharyngeal airway, as she is responsive to pain and likely has an intact gag reflex. Begin assisting her ventilations with a bag-mask device attached to high-concentration oxygen at the appropriate rate and depth. Monitor her closely for signs of improvement or further deterioration. Many EMS systems carry noninvasive blood pressure monitoring devices that automatically measure the patient's blood pressure and other vital signs. If you have this capability, set the device to reassess the patient's vital signs *at least* every 5 minutes or as deemed appropriate by the patient's condition. You are the only EMT in the back with the patient; managing her airway and assisting her ventilations clearly has priority over obtaining a manual blood pressure measurement.

8. What part of the patient's perfusion triangle has failed?

There are three components to the perfusion triangle, each of which must function well at all times to maintain adequate perfusion: the heart (pump), the blood vessels (container), and the blood (content or volume). Recalling the patient's chief complaint—abdominal pain and rectal bleeding—the patient is in shock secondary to blood loss (hemorrhagic shock). Therefore, the content function of the perfusion triangle has failed. If there is enough blood or plasma loss, internally or externally, the volume of fluid that remains in the container (blood vessels) will not be able to carry sufficient oxygen to the cells to adequately perfuse them.

9. How does shock caused by content (volume) failure differ from shock caused by container failure?

Shock caused by content failure refers to insufficient oxygen delivery to the cells because of inadequate volume and is called hypovolemic shock. Hypovolemia is a generic term that simply means low volume; it could be blood, plasma, water, or a combination. Common causes of hypovolemic shock include blunt or penetrating trauma, burns, and dehydration. Shock that is caused by blood loss specifically is called hemorrhagic shock. The signs of hypovolemic shock include tachycardia; pale, cool, clammy skin; tachypnea; restlessness, agitation, or anxiety; and as a late sign, hypotension. Shock caused by container failure refers to inadequate perfusion

YOU are the EMT SUMMARY continued

because of excessive dilation of the blood vessels, resulting in a decrease in pressure within the circulatory system. Although the volume of blood has not changed, the container that it circulates within has increased; therefore, the normal volume of blood is insufficient to fill the system and provide adequate perfusion. Common causes of shock caused by container failure include anaphylaxis, overdose with drugs that suppress the nervous system (ie, narcotics), and spinal cord injury. The classic signs of hypovolemic shock—specifically, tachycardia, pallor, and diaphoresis—will be absent. Instead, the patient's skin is usually warm and dry, and the heart rate is normal or low.

Prep Kit

Ready to Review

- Perfusion requires an intact cardiovascular system and a functioning respiratory system.
- Remember, most types of shock (hypoperfusion) are caused by dysfunction in one or more parts of the perfusion triangle:
  - The pump (the heart)
  - The pipes, or container (blood vessels)
  - The content, or volume (blood)
- Shock (hypoperfusion) is a condition in which the cardiovascular system fails to provide sufficient circulation to maintain normal cellular functions. Shock can lead to organ failure and death.
- Blood is the vehicle for carrying oxygen and nutrients through the vessels to the capillary beds and tissue cells, where these supplies are exchanged for waste products.
- Blood contains red blood cells, white blood cells, platelets, and a liquid called plasma.
- The *systolic* pressure is the peak arterial pressure, or pressure generated every time the heart contracts; the *diastolic* pressure is the pressure maintained within the arteries while the heart rests between heartbeats.
- The various types of shock are cardiogenic, obstructive, septic, neurogenic, anaphylactic, and hypovolemic.
- Signs of compensated shock include anxiety or agitation; tachycardia; pale, cool, moist skin; increased respiratory rate; nausea and vomiting; and increased thirst. If there is any question on your part, treat for shock. Early recognition and rapid treatment are important.
- Signs of decompensated shock include labored or irregular respirations, ashen gray or cyanotic skin color, weak or absent distal pulses, dilated pupils, and profound hypotension (systolic blood pressure of 90 mm Hg or lower in an adult).
- Remember, by the time a decrease in blood pressure is detected, shock is usually in an advanced stage.
- Anticipate shock in patients who have the following conditions:
  - Severe infection
  - Significant blunt force trauma or penetrating trauma
  - Massive external bleeding or index of suspicion for major internal bleeding
  - Spinal cord injury
  - Chest or abdominal injury
  - Major heart attack
  - Anaphylaxis
- While children may compensate for shock longer than adults, and older adults often have less effective compensatory mechanisms, treating these patient in shock is often very similar to treating any other shock patient. The EMT should be familiar with age-appropriate vital signs and the impact of

Prep Kit continued

other illness or medications on assessment and treatment.

- Treat all patients suspected to be in shock from any cause as follows and in this order:
  - Control life-threatening hemorrhage immediately with direct pressure or tourniquet application when appropriate.
  - Open and maintain the airway.
  - Provide high-concentration oxygen, and as needed, provide bag-mask assisted ventilations.
  - Maintain normal body temperature with blankets.
  - Provide calm reassurance.
  - Provide prompt transport to the appropriate hospital.

Vital Vocabulary

afterload The force or resistance against which the heart pumps.

anaphylactic shock Severe shock caused by an allergic reaction.

anaphylaxis An extreme, life-threatening, systemic allergic reaction that may include shock and respiratory failure.

aneurysm A swelling or enlargement of a part of an artery, resulting from weakening of the arterial wall.

autonomic nervous system The part of the nervous system that regulates involuntary activities of the body, such as heart rate, blood pressure, and digestion of food.

cardiac tamponade Compression of the heart as the result of buildup of blood or other fluid in the pericardial sac, leading to decreased cardiac output.

cardiogenic shock A state in which not enough oxygen is delivered to the tissues of the body, caused by low output of blood from the heart. It can be a severe complication of a large acute myocardial infarction, as well as other conditions.

compensated shock The early stage of shock, in which the body can still compensate for blood loss.

cyanosis A blue skin discoloration that is caused by a reduced level of oxygen in the blood. Although pallor, or a decrease in blood flow, can be difficult to detect in people with dark skin, it may be observed by examining mucous membranes inside the inner lower eyelid and capillary refill. On general observation, the patient may appear ashen or gray.

decompensated shock The late stage of shock when blood pressure is falling.

dehydration Loss of water from the tissues of the body.

distributive shock A condition that occurs when there is widespread dilation of the small arterioles, small venules, or both.

edema The presence of abnormally large amounts of fluid between cells in body tissues, causing swelling of the affected area.

homeostasis A balance of all systems of the body.

hypothermia A condition in which the internal body temperature falls below 95°F (35°C).

hypovolemic shock A condition in which low blood volume, due to massive internal or external bleeding or extensive loss of body water, results in inadequate perfusion.

irreversible shock A condition defined by the inability to successfully achieve resuscitation regardless of the methods employed.

myocardial contractility The ability of the heart muscle to contract.

neurogenic shock Circulatory failure caused by paralysis of the nerves that control the size of the blood vessels, leading to widespread dilation; seen in patients with spinal cord injuries.

obstructive shock Shock that occurs when there is a block to blood flow in the heart or great

Prep Kit continued

vessels, causing an insufficient blood supply to the body's tissues.

perfusion The flow of blood through body tissues and vessels.

pericardial effusion A collection of fluid between the pericardial sac and the myocardium.

preload The precontraction pressure in the heart as the volume of blood builds up.

pulmonary embolism A blood clot that breaks off from a large vein and travels to the blood vessels of the lung, causing obstruction of blood flow.

pulse pressure The difference between the systolic and diastolic pressures.

sensitization Developing a sensitivity to a substance that initially caused no allergic reaction.

septic shock Shock caused by severe infection, usually a bacterial infection.

shock A condition in which the circulatory system fails to provide sufficient circulation to maintain normal cellular functions; also called hypoperfusion.

sphincters Muscles that encircle and, by contracting, constrict a duct, tube, or opening.

syncope A fainting spell or transient loss of consciousness.

References

1. Dribin TE, Sampson HA, Camargo CA Jr, et al. Persistent, refractory, and biphasic anaphylaxis: a multidisciplinary Delphi study. *J Allergy Clin Immunol.* 2020;146(5):1089–1096.
2. Berry C, Gallagher JM, Goodloe JM, Dorlac WC, Dodd J, Fischer, PE. Prehospital hemorrhage control and treatment by clinicians: a joint position statement. *Prehosp Emerg Care.* 2023;27(5):544–551.
3. Teirney P, Ahmed B, Nichol A. Shock: causes, initial assessment and investigations. *Anaesth Intens Care Med.* 2017;18(3):118–121.
4. American Heart Association (AHA). *2020 Handbook of Emergency Cardiovascular Care*. AHA; 2020.
5. National Association of State EMS Officials. *National EMS Scope of Practice Model 2019: Including Change Notices 1.0 and 2.0.* Washington, DC: National Highway Traffic Safety Administration; August 2021. Report No. DOT HS 813-151.
6. American Heart Association (AHA). *Pediatric Advanced Life Support Provider Manual*. Dallas, TX: AHA; 2020.

Additional Resources

Guyette FX, Fowler RL, Kitch BB, Beck EH. Hypotension and shock. In: Cone DCB, Delbridge JH, Myers TR, Brent J, eds. *Emergency Medical Services: Clinical Practice and Systems Oversight*. 3rd ed. vol. 1. Hoboken, NJ: Wiley-Blackwell; 2021:71–82.

National Association of Emergency Medical Technicians. *PHTLS: Prehospital Trauma Life Support*. 10th ed. Burlington, MA: Jones & Bartlett Learning; 2023.

National Association of State EMS Officials. *National Model EMS Clinical Guidelines: Version 3.0.* https://nasemso.org/wp-content/uploads/National-Model-EMS-Clinical-Guidelines_2022.pdf. Updated March 2022. Accessed October 4, 2024.

National Highway Traffic Safety Administration. *National Emergency Medical Services Education Standards*. https://www.ems.gov/assets/EMS_Education-Standards_2021_FNL.pdf. EMS.gov website. Published January 2021. Accessed October 4, 2024.

Wang EN, Chan C, Anand S, et al. Considerations in the management of shock in the pediatric trauma patient. *Ped Emerg Med Rep.* 2006:11(11):129–144.

Chapter 14

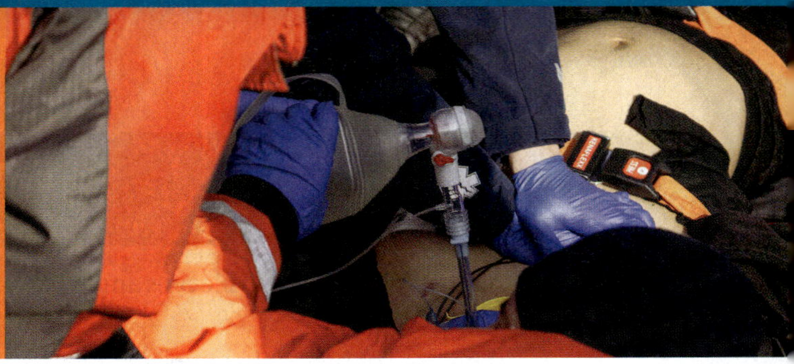

BLS Resuscitation

NATIONAL EMS EDUCATION STANDARD COMPETENCIES

Shock and Resuscitation

Applies knowledge of the causes, pathophysiology, and management of shock, respiratory failure or arrest, cardiac failure or arrest, termination of resuscitative efforts, and postresuscitation management.

Resuscitation From Cardiac Arrest

- Ethical issues in resuscitation (pp 595–596, 604–605)
- CPR physiology (pp 566–572)
- Resuscitation system components (pp 564–566)
- Special arrest and peri-arrest situations (pp 603–604)
- Postresuscitation support (pp 581–583)
- Termination of resuscitation (pp 595–596)

KNOWLEDGE OBJECTIVES

1. Explain the elements of basic life support (BLS), how it differs from advanced life support (ALS), and why BLS must be applied rapidly. (p 562)
2. Explain the goals of cardiopulmonary resuscitation (CPR) and when it should be performed on a patient. (pp 562–564)
3. Explain the components of CPR, the six links in the American Heart Association (AHA) chain of survival, and how each one relates to maximizing the survival of a patient. (pp 564–566)
4. Describe the proper way to position an adult patient to receive BLS care. (p 566)
5. Describe the purpose of external chest compressions. (p 566)
6. Describe the two techniques EMTs may use to open an adult patient's airway and the circumstances that would determine when each technique would be used. (pp 569–570)
7. Describe the recovery position and circumstances that would warrant its use, as well as situations in which it would be contraindicated. (pp 570–571)
8. Describe the process of providing artificial ventilations to an adult patient, ways to avoid gastric distention, and modifications required for a patient with a stoma. (pp 571–572)
9. Explain the steps in providing single-rescuer adult CPR. (pp 572–573)
10. Explain the steps in providing two-rescuer adult CPR, including the method for switching positions during the process. (pp 572–576)
11. Explain the general purpose and function of automated external defibrillators (AEDs). (pp 576–577)
12. Describe how to use an AED. (pp 577–579)
13. Describe the components of patient care following AED shocks. (pp 581–582)
14. Discuss the importance of coordinating with ALS personnel. (p 582)
15. Describe AED maintenance procedures. (p 583)
16. Explain the role of medical direction in the use of AEDs. (p 583)
17. Describe the different mechanical devices that are available to assist emergency care

clinicians in delivering improved circulatory efforts during CPR. (pp 583–586)

18. Describe the different possible causes of cardiopulmonary arrest in children. (pp 587–588)
19. Explain the steps of pediatric BLS procedures and how they differ from BLS procedures used in an adult patient. (pp 586–594)
20. Describe the ethical issues related to patient resuscitation, including examples of when not to start CPR on a patient. (pp 594–595)
21. Explain the various factors involved in the decision to stop CPR after it has been started on a patient. (pp 595–596)
22. Explain common causes of foreign body airway obstruction in both children and adults and how to distinguish mild or partial airway obstruction from complete airway obstruction. (pp 596–597, 599–600)
23. Describe the different methods for removing a foreign body airway obstruction in an infant, child, and adult, including the procedure for a patient with an obstruction who becomes unresponsive. (pp 597–599, 600–603)
24. Discuss how to provide grief support for a patient's family members and loved ones after resuscitation has ended. (pp 604–605)
25. Discuss the importance of frequent CPR training for EMTs, as well as public education programs that teach compression-only CPR. (p 605)

SKILLS OBJECTIVES

1. Demonstrate how to position an unresponsive adult for CPR. (p 566)
2. Demonstrate how to check for a pulse at the carotid artery in an unresponsive child or adult. (p 566)
3. Demonstrate how to perform external chest compressions on an adult. (pp 566–568, Skill Drill 14-1)
4. Demonstrate how to perform a head tilt–chin lift maneuver on an adult. (p 569)
5. Demonstrate how to perform a jaw-thrust maneuver on an adult. (p 570)
6. Demonstrate how to place a patient in the recovery position. (p 570)
7. Demonstrate how to perform rescue breathing in an adult. (pp 571–572)
8. Demonstrate how to perform one-rescuer adult CPR. (pp 572–573, Skill Drill 14-2)
9. Demonstrate how to perform two-rescuer adult CPR. (pp 572–575, Skill Drill 14-3)
10. Demonstrate the use of an AED. (pp 577–579, Skill Drill 14-4)
11. Demonstrate the use of mechanical devices that assist emergency responders in delivering improved circulatory efforts during CPR. (pp 585–586)
12. Demonstrate how to check for a pulse at the brachial artery in an unresponsive infant. (p 588)
13. Demonstrate how to perform external chest compressions on an infant. (p 589, Skill Drill 14-5)
14. Demonstrate how to perform CPR on a child who is between 1 year of age and the onset of puberty. (pp 590–591, Skill Drill 14-6)
15. Demonstrate how to perform a head tilt–chin lift maneuver on a pediatric patient. (p 593)
16. Demonstrate how to perform a jaw-thrust maneuver on a pediatric patient. (p 593)
17. Demonstrate how to perform rescue breathing on a child. (pp 593–594)
18. Demonstrate how to perform rescue breathing on an infant. (pp 593–594)
19. Demonstrate how to remove a foreign body airway obstruction in a responsive adult patient using back slaps and abdominal thrusts. (pp 597–598)
20. Demonstrate how to remove a foreign body airway obstruction in a responsive pregnant or obese patient using back slaps and chest thrusts. (p 598)
21. Demonstrate how to remove a foreign body airway obstruction in a responsive child older than 1 year using back slaps and abdominal thrusts. (pp 599–601)
22. Demonstrate how to remove a foreign body airway obstruction in an unresponsive child. (pp 601–602, Skill Drill 14-7)
23. Demonstrate how to remove a foreign body airway obstruction in an infant. (pp 601–603)

Introduction

The principles of basic life support (BLS) were introduced in 1960. Since then, the specific techniques for the management of cardiac arrest and the delivery of emergency and cardiac care have been reviewed and revised regularly. The goal is to produce the best recommendations possible given the available scientific evidence and to maximize the chance of successful resuscitation. The updated guidelines are published in peer-reviewed journals: *Circulation* in the United States and *Resuscitation* in Europe. Reviews are conducted and published by the International Liaison Committee on Resuscitation (ILCOR) based on availability of new relevant information. The most recent revision (2023) occurred as a result of a rigorous and systematic review of the newest scientific evidence relating to treatment for patients in cardiac arrest.[1]

This chapter begins with definitions and general discussions of BLS and **cardiopulmonary resuscitation (CPR)**. It then reviews methods for opening and maintaining a patent (open) airway, providing artificial ventilation to a person who is not adequately breathing, providing artificial circulation to a person with no pulse, and removing a foreign body airway obstruction. Each of these topics is followed by a review of the changes in technique that are necessary to treat infants and children. Chapter 2, *Workforce Safety and Wellness*, discusses the methods of preventing the transmission of infectious diseases during CPR. Chapter 6, *The Human Body*, discusses the anatomy and physiology of the respiratory and cardiovascular systems. Chapter 9, *The Team Approach to Health Care*, discusses how to work as an effective team in the health care setting. During any emergency, working as a team is critical to giving the patient the best chance for a successful outcome.

Words of Wisdom

In normal situations, the risk of acquiring an infectious disease while performing CPR is very low. During situations posing a high risk of infection, EMS personnel should consider wearing enhanced personal protective equipment (PPE), such as goggles, an N95 mask, gloves, and gown. This level of protection can make the physical exertion of CPR more difficult.

Principles of BLS

Basic life support (BLS) is noninvasive emergency lifesaving care that is used to treat medical conditions, including airway obstruction, respiratory arrest, and cardiac arrest. BLS follows a specific sequence for adults and for infants and children. This care focuses on the ABCs: Airway (obstruction), Breathing (respiratory arrest), and Circulation (cardiac arrest or severe bleeding). If the EMT immediately recognizes cardiac arrest after the initial assessment, then a CAB sequence (Compressions, Airway, Breathing) is used for resuscitation because chest compressions are essential and must be started as quickly as possible (**FIGURE 14-1**). If the patient presents with life-threatening external bleeding, then an XABC sequence (eXsanguination, Airway, Breathing, Circulation) is used. Ideally, only seconds should pass between the time you recognize that a patient needs BLS and the start of treatment. Remember, brain cells die every second they are deprived of oxygen. Permanent brain damage is possible after as little as 4 to 6 minutes without oxygen (**FIGURE 14-2**).

The basic principles of BLS resuscitation are the same for infants, children, and adults, but CPR techniques differ slightly for each group. For the purposes of BLS, anyone younger than 1 year is considered an infant. A child is between 1 year of age and the onset of puberty (approximately 12 to 14 years of age), as signified by breast development in girls and underarm, chest, and facial hair in boys. For purposes of BLS, a patient is an adult from the onset of puberty and older.

BLS differs from **advanced life support (ALS)**, which involves additional lifesaving procedures such as administration of intravenous (IV) fluids and medications, and the use of advanced airway devices. However, BLS care is the foundation for ALS care. Without early, effective BLS, there is no ALS.

The Goal of CPR

The goal of CPR is to reestablish circulation and artificial ventilation in a patient who is not breathing and has no pulse; however, defibrillation and advanced interventions (ie, medication therapy) are often necessary to achieve **return of spontaneous circulation (ROSC)**. The steps for CPR include the following:

1. Restore circulation by performing 30 chest compressions at a depth of at least 2 inches

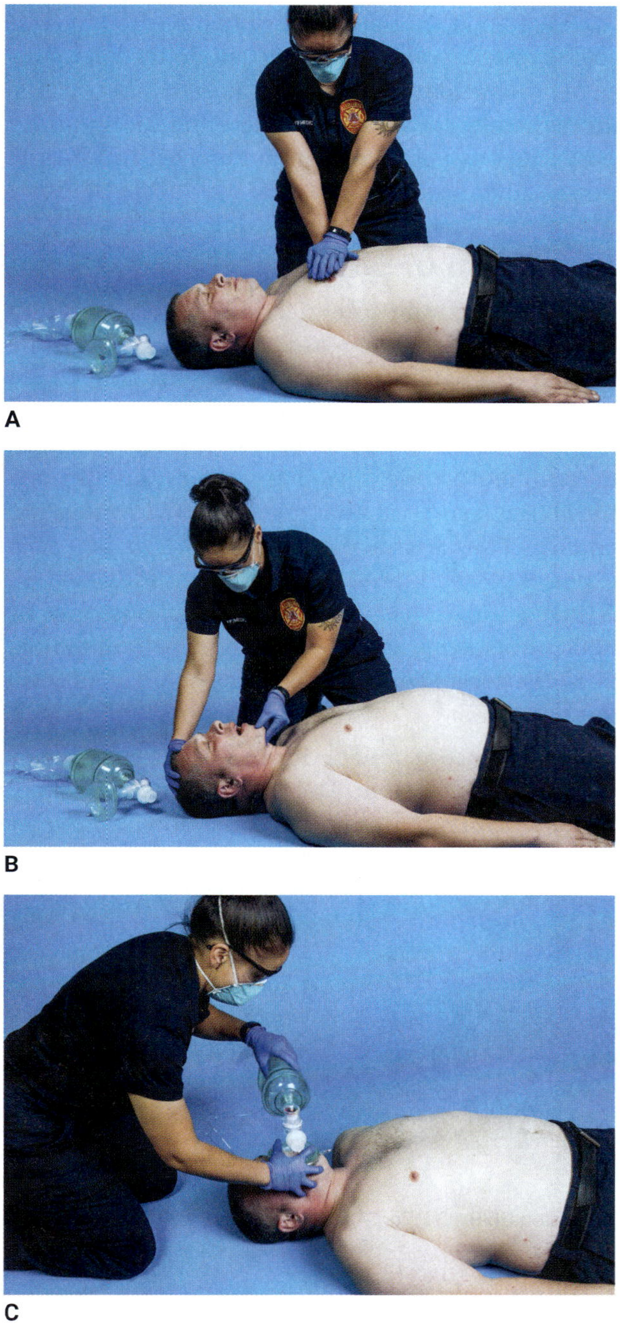

FIGURE 14-1 Use the CAB sequence for resuscitation of an unresponsive patient who appears to be in cardiac arrest: Chest compression (*C*, shown in part **A**), Airway (*A*, shown in part **B**), Breathing (*B*, shown in part **C**).

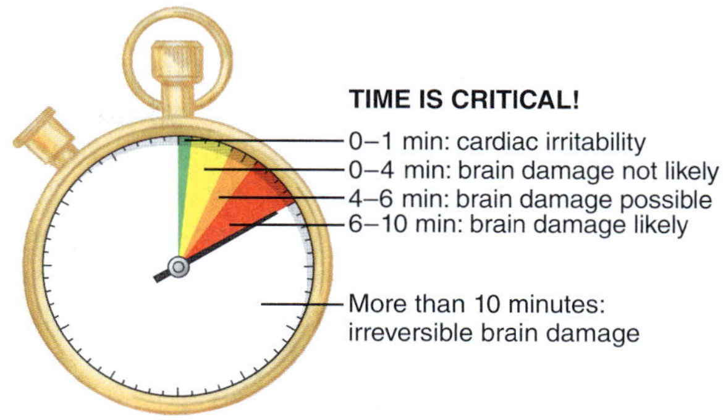

FIGURE 14-2 Time is critical for patients who are not adequately breathing. If the brain is deprived of oxygen for 4 to 6 minutes, brain damage is possible.

(5 cm) but not greater than 2.4 inches (6 cm) to circulate blood to the vital organs of the body. After each compression, the chest must completely recoil to allow the heart to refill. The rate of compressions should be at least 100 compressions per minute but no more than 120 per minute. Interruptions between compressions should be no longer than 10 seconds for any reason.

2. Open the airway with the jaw-thrust or head tilt–chin lift maneuver to restore breathing by providing rescue breaths (via bag-mask device). Administer two breaths, each more than 1 second, while visualizing for chest rise. Repeat this sequence.

Recognizing the Need for CPR

Because of the urgent need to start CPR in a pulseless patient who is not breathing, you must complete a primary assessment as soon as possible and begin CPR, starting with chest compressions. After determining that the scene is safe to enter and taking standard precautions, the first step is to determine unresponsiveness. Tap the patient on the shoulder and shout, "Are you okay?" (**FIGURE 14-3**). Clearly, a patient who is responsive does not need CPR. If the patient is not responsive, assess for absent or inadequate breathing (breathing only slowly or occasionally, known as **agonal breathing**), and at the same

Words of Wisdom

Patients in cardiac arrest will sometimes take a few slow breaths. This breathing, called agonal breathing, occurs as a natural reflex as the brainstem loses oxygen. It will be clear to you that the patient's breathing is not adequate to support life.

time check for the adult patient's carotid pulse for no more than 10 seconds. If you do not note a definite pulse, assume the person is in cardiac arrest.

If a patient has inadequate breathing or breathing is absent, you may be able to restore breathing simply by opening the airway. However, if the patient has no pulse, then you must combine artificial ventilation with artificial circulation (chest compressions). If breathing stops before the heart stops, then the patient may have enough oxygen in the lungs for the heart to continue beating for several minutes. When cardiac arrest occurs first, the heart and brain stop receiving oxygen immediately.

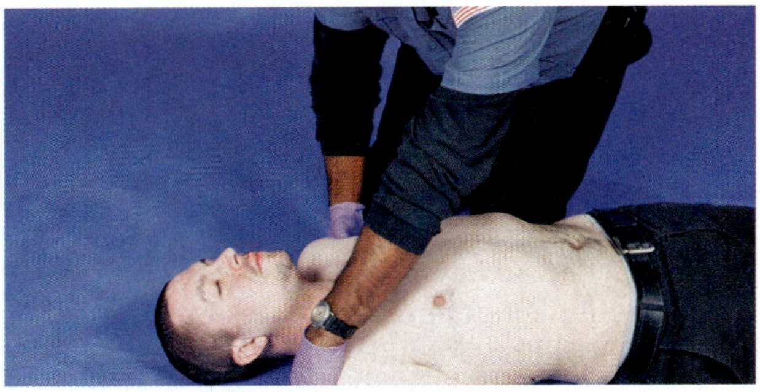

FIGURE 14-3 Assess an unresponsive patient by first attempting to rouse the person by tapping on the shoulder.

Keep in mind that some patients who are conscious when you arrive, will suddenly lose consciousness and go into cardiac arrest. If this occurs, immediately check for adequate breathing and a pulse, just as you would if you arrived to find the person unconscious.

The Chain of Survival

According to the American Heart Association (AHA), 70% of sudden cardiac arrests occur in the home.[2] Few patients who experience cardiac arrest in the prehospital environment survive unless a rapid sequence of events take place. The AHA has determined an ideal sequence of events, termed the chain of survival, that together can improve the chance of successful resuscitation of a patient who experiences sudden cardiac arrest (**FIGURE 14-4**). A successful resuscitation is defined not only by ROSC, but also by the survival of the patient to hospital discharge. The six links in the chain of survival are as follows:

1. **Recognition and activation of the emergency response system.** The first step in the chain of survival requires public education and awareness. Lay people must learn to recognize the early warning signs of a cardiac emergency;

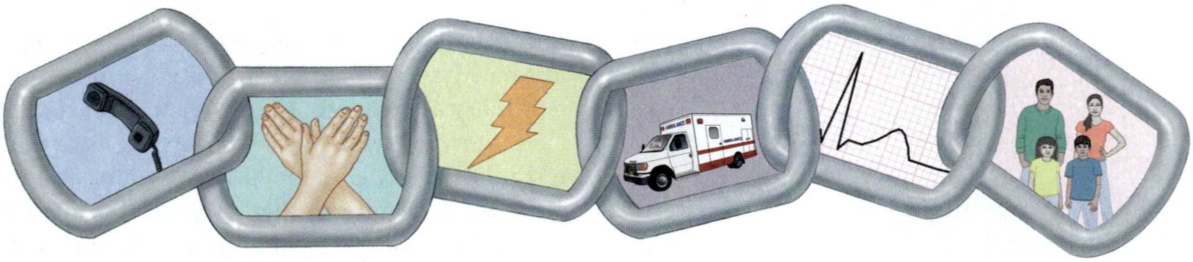

FIGURE 14-4 The six links of the chain of survival.

Data from the American Heart Association.

YOU are the EMT

At 1445 hours, you and your partner respond to a local supermarket at 400 Main St. where a 54-year-old man reportedly collapsed in the parking lot. While you are en route to the scene, dispatch advises you that bystander CPR is in progress. Your response time is less than 5 minutes.

1. What should you immediately do on receiving this update from dispatch?
2. What should be your initial actions on arriving at this scene?

immediately activate EMS by calling 9-1-1; and begin chest compressions. These steps ensure that emergency responders are dispatched to the scene quickly, thus allowing the other links of the chain to be more effective. In modern EMS systems, the 9-1-1 dispatcher can provide prearrival instructions and direct the caller to provide high-quality CPR.

2. **Immediate, high-quality CPR with emphasis on compressions.** The initiation of immediate, effective CPR by a bystander is essential for resuscitation of a person in cardiac arrest. Immediate, high-quality CPR markedly increases the patient's chance of survival, whereas a delay in CPR leads to poor patient outcomes. The lay public as well as emergency responders should all be trained in CPR. In addition, emergency telecommunicators (also known as call takers, dispatchers, and 9-1-1 operators) should be trained to quickly recognize and provide instructions and coaching for bystanders to provide CPR, even if they have never been trained.

   Unfortunately, many bystanders are hesitant to perform CPR on a stranger for fear of contracting a disease from mouth-to-mouth breathing, or out of fear of liability. A perception that bystander CPR involves mouth-to-mouth breathing persists. EMS has a role in educating laypeople in performing compressions-only (hands-only) CPR.

   For chest compressions to be most effective, they must be given hard and fast. Compressions should be between 2 and 2.4 inches in depth (5 to 6 cm) and given at a rate of 100 to 120 per minute. The chest should completely recoil between each compression to maximize blood return to the heart. The rescuer should never lean on the chest between compressions. For EMTs, high-quality CPR includes basic airway management (ie, oral airway insertion, bag-mask ventilation with high-concentration oxygen).

3. **Rapid defibrillation.** Coupled with early, high-quality CPR, defibrillation offers the best opportunity to achieve a successful patient outcome. Automated external defibrillators (AEDs) have become readily available in many schools, fitness clubs, airports, sports arenas, government buildings, and other mass gathering places. The simple design of the AED makes it easy for emergency medical clinicians and laypeople to use with little training. Manual interpretation of the heart rhythm and defibrillation can be used by advanced-level clinicians, including some advanced EMTs, paramedics, and others.

4. **Advanced EMS.** This link in the chain describes care provided by ALS clinicians including paramedics, nurses, physicians, and other advanced health care practitioners. In addition to high-quality CPR and defibrillation, such care includes advanced airway management (ie, endotracheal [ET] intubation or use of supraglottic airways), manual defibrillation, vascular access, administration of medications, and other interventions. This fourth link emphasizes that high-quality CPR and defibrillation must be established before advanced care can begin either in or out of the hospital.

5. **Post–cardiac arrest care.** If the resuscitation is successful and the patient regains a pulse, further cardiopulmonary and neurologic support may be provided. Maintain ventilation at 10 breaths/min, oxygen saturation between 92% and 98%, and systolic blood pressure above 90 mm Hg. Additional support includes an advanced airway if one is needed, medication therapy to support blood pressure, a 12-lead electrocardiogram (ECG), in-hospital targeted temperature management (ie, therapeutic hypothermia), an electroencephalogram to detect brain activity; other advanced circulatory support interventions, and admission to the intensive care unit for critical care management.

Street Smarts

If a bystander has initiated CPR before your arrival, thank the individual for helping as you assess the patient's pulse and assume control of CPR. You may say, "Thank you, we appreciate your help and will take over now." Even if the CPR they provided was not optimal, be careful not to criticize the person. Doing so may discourage them from providing help in the future, and if the patient does not survive, they may blame themselves for not saving the person.

6. **Recovery and survivorship.** Physical and emotional recovery can take a year or longer for people who are successfully resuscitated. After cardiac arrest, survivors can have physical, cognitive, and emotional challenges and may need ongoing therapies and interventions.

If any one of the links in the chain is not maintained, the patient is more likely to die. For example, fewer patients survive cardiac arrest if CPR is not administered within the first few minutes, if the CPR is not high quality, or if defibrillation is not quickly available. The patient's best chance of survival occurs when all links in the chain are maintained.

Street Smarts

Cardiac arrest calls are highly emotional. Planning your initial actions and roles en route to the call can avoid confusion and help ensure that the priorities of high-quality CPR and early defibrillation are achieved quickly.

Performing CPR

Positioning the Patient

For CPR to be effective, the patient must be lying supine on a firm, flat surface, with enough clear space around the patient for two rescuers to perform CPR and use the AED. If the patient is lying on the side or facedown (prone), then you will need to move them to a supine position. If the patient is found in a bed or on a couch, then move them to the floor. Be mindful that you cannot rule out a spinal injury in an unresponsive patient; therefore, protect the patient's neck and move them as a unit as best you can without twisting. However, do not delay initiating high-quality CPR.

Checking for Adequate Breathing and a Pulse

After you have determined that the patient is unresponsive, quickly check for adequate breathing and a pulse. These assessments can occur simultaneously and should take no longer than 10 seconds in total.

Visualize the chest for signs of adequate breathing while palpating for a carotid pulse. Feel for the carotid artery by locating the larynx at the front of the neck and then sliding two fingers toward one side (the side closest to you). The pulse is felt in the groove between the larynx and sternocleidomastoid muscle, with the pads of the index and middle fingers held side by side (**FIGURE 14-5**). Light pressure is sufficient to palpate the pulse.

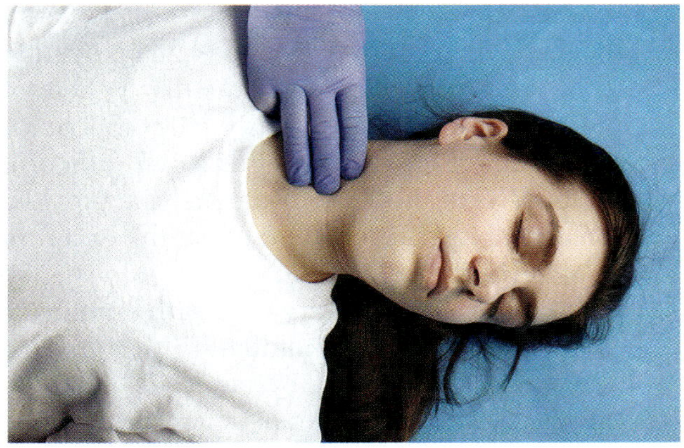

FIGURE 14-5 Feel for the carotid artery by locating the larynx, then slide your index and middle fingers toward one side. You can feel the pulse in the groove between the larynx and sternocleidomastoid muscle.

Performing External Chest Compressions

If the patient is not adequately breathing and does not have a pulse, then begin CPR, starting with chest compressions. It is critical to perform compressions properly. Chest compressions are administered by applying rhythmic pressure and relaxation to the lower half of the sternum. The heart is located slightly to the left of the middle of the chest between the sternum and the spine (**FIGURE 14-6**). Compressions squeeze the heart, thereby acting as a pump to circulate blood. Allow the chest to completely recoil between compressions, which enhances blood return to the heart. Do not lean on the chest between compressions. When artificial ventilation is provided, the blood that is circulated through the lungs during chest compressions is likely to receive adequate oxygen to maintain tissue perfusion. However, even when external chest compressions are performed properly, they circulate only one-third of the blood that is normally pumped by the heart.

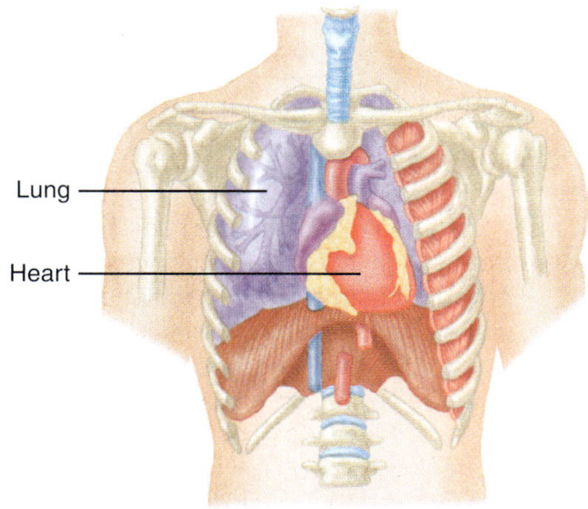

FIGURE 14-6 The heart lies slightly to the left of the middle of the chest between the sternum and spine.

Proper Hand Position and Compression Technique

With the adult patient, correct hand position is established by placing the heel of one hand on the sternum in the center of the chest over the lower half of the sternum. Follow the steps in **SKILL DRILL 14-1**:

1. Take standard precautions.
2. Place the heel of one hand on the center of the chest over the lower half of the sternum (**Step 1**).
3. Place the heel of your other hand over the first hand (**Step 2**).
4. With your arms straight, lock your elbows and position your shoulders directly over your hands, so that the thrust of each compression is straight down on the sternum. Your technique may be improved or made more

Skill Drill 14-1 Performing Adult Chest Compressions

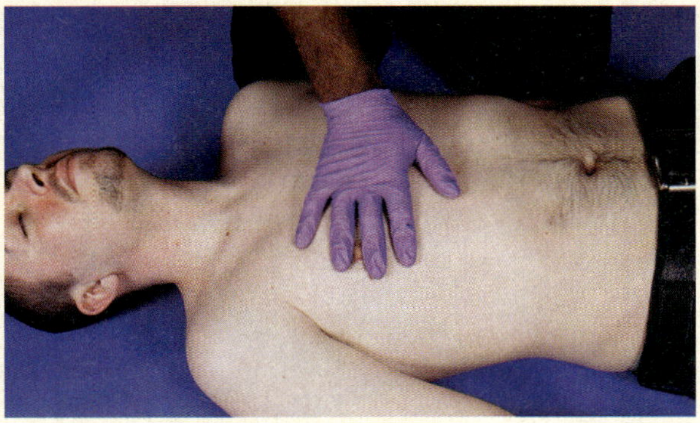

Step 1

Take standard precautions. Place the heel of one hand on the center of the chest (lower half of the sternum).

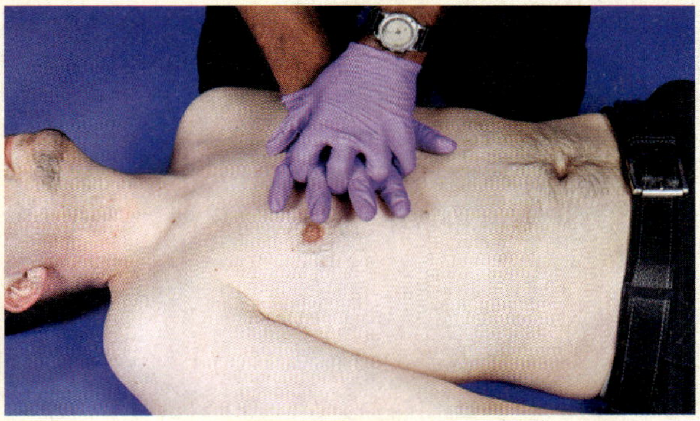

Step 2

Place the heel of your other hand over the first hand.

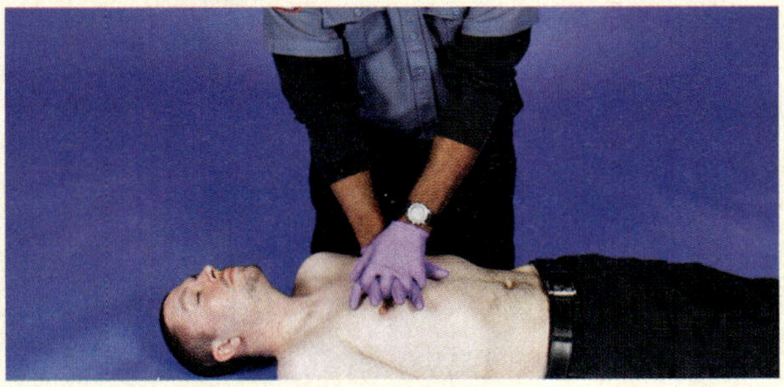

Step 3

With your arms straight, lock your elbows and position your shoulders directly over your hands. Depress the sternum at a rate of 100 to 120 compressions per minute, and to a depth of 2 inches (5 cm) using a downward movement. Allow the chest to return to its normal position; do not lean on the chest between compressions. Compression and relaxation should be of equal duration.

comfortable if you interlock the fingers of your lower hand with the fingers of your upper hand; either way, keep your fingers off the patient's ribs.

5. Depress the sternum to a depth of 2 inches (5 cm), using direct downward movement and then rising gently upward (**Step 3**). This motion allows pressure to be delivered vertically from your shoulders. Downward pressure produces a compression that must be followed immediately by an equal period of relaxation. The ratio of time devoted to compression versus relaxation should be 1:1. It is important that you allow the chest to return to its normal position; do not lean on the patient's chest between compressions. Compression and relaxation should be of equal duration.

Complications from chest compressions are rare but can include fractured ribs, a lacerated liver, and a fractured sternum, among other injuries.[3] Although these injuries cannot be entirely avoided, you can minimize the chance that they will occur if you use good technique and proper hand placement. Risk of injury to the patient should not delay your initiation of CPR or performance of high-quality CPR.

Your motions must be smooth, rhythmic, and uninterrupted (**FIGURE 14-7A**). Short, jabbing compressions are not effective in producing artificial blood flow. Do not remove the heel of your hand from the patient's chest during relaxation, but make sure that you completely release pressure on the sternum so that it can return to its normal resting position between compressions (**FIGURE 14-7B**).

Words of Wisdom

For most people, the focus of CPR is on the downstroke of compressions, "pressing hard (2 inches) and fast (100 to 120 per minute)." However, a common mistake is not releasing all pressure from the chest between compressions. Chest recoil is crucial to effective circulation. The pressure in the chest must be allowed to drop for blood to return from the body through the superior and inferior venae cavae into the heart. Further, the heart must be allowed to expand fully for the chambers to refill with blood to pump out in the next compression. Similarly, expansion allows the coronary arteries, which supply oxygen to the heart muscle, to refill during diastole. An easy way to keep in mind the importance of the "down and up" cycle of CPR is to think that the compression pushes blood out to the brain and recoil pulls blood back to the heart. Therefore, each compression–recoil cycle gives blood to the brain, then heart, then brain, then heart, and so on.

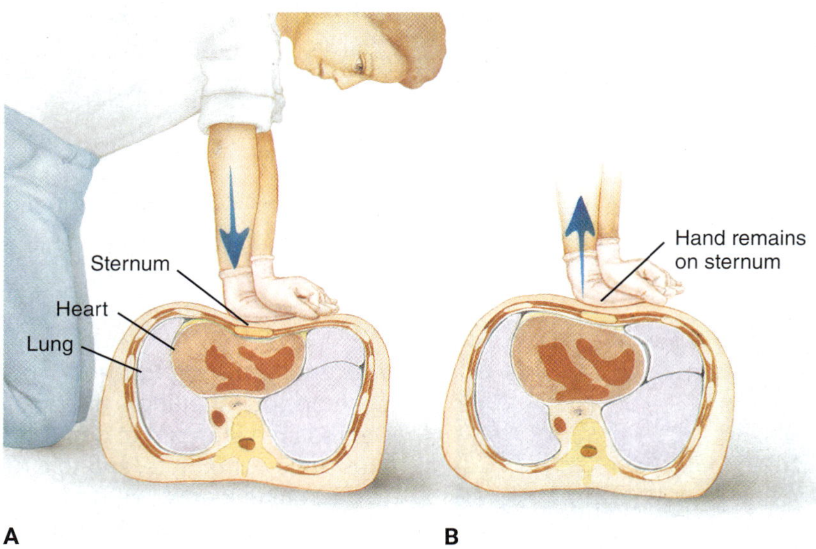

FIGURE 14-7 A. Compression and relaxation should be rhythmic and of equal duration (a 1:1 ratio). **B.** Pressure on the sternum must be released so that the sternum can return to its normal resting position between compressions.

Words of Wisdom

When performing chest compressions on an adult, it is difficult to achieve a precise depth of 2 inches (5 cm) without the use of a monitoring device that provides immediate feedback (**FIGURE 14-8**). Research continues to support the use of compression feedback devices to improve CPR and continues to determine their role in cardiac arrest survivability.[4]

It is more dangerous to compress the chest too lightly than it is to compress too forcefully. Compressing hard can lead to fatigue, and as you become tired, your compressions will become shallower. Therefore, it is critical to push hard and push fast and switch compressors (the person providing chest compressions) every 2 minutes, even if the compressor does not feel tired.

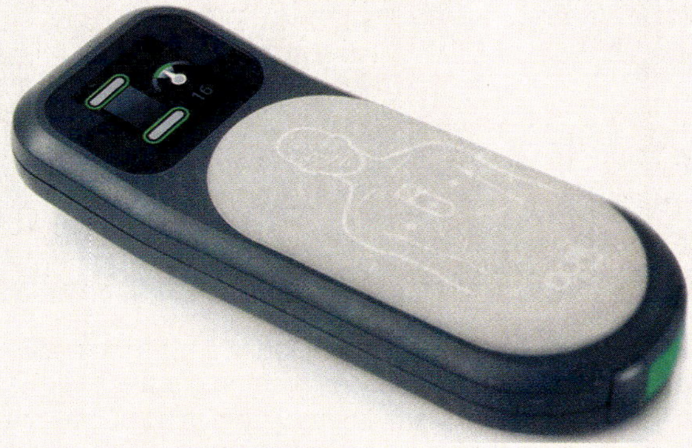

FIGURE 14-8 CPR feedback devices help ensure a consistent rate and depth of compressions.

Words of Wisdom

Chest compressions create blood flow to the heart through filling of the coronary arteries. Every time compressions are stopped, blood flow (and thus, perfusion) to the heart (and brain) drops to zero. It takes 5 to 10 compressions to reestablish effective blood flow to the heart after chest compressions are resumed. Avoid frequent or prolonged interruptions greater than 10 seconds in chest compressions, which lead to poor patient outcomes.

Opening the Airway in Adults

Without an open airway, rescue breathing will not be effective. The two techniques for opening the airway in adults are the head tilt–chin lift maneuver and the jaw-thrust maneuver. These manual maneuvers are designed to bring the tongue forward and off the throat. Once the airway has been opened, it will need to be maintained in that position unless the patient regains consciousness.

Head Tilt–Chin Lift Maneuver

The **head tilt–chin lift maneuver** is effective for opening the airway in most patients when there is no indication of a spinal injury (**FIGURE 14-9**). See Chapter 11, *Airway and Ventilation Management*, for further review of opening the airway.

In patients who have not sustained trauma, this simple maneuver is sometimes all that is required for the patient to resume breathing. If the

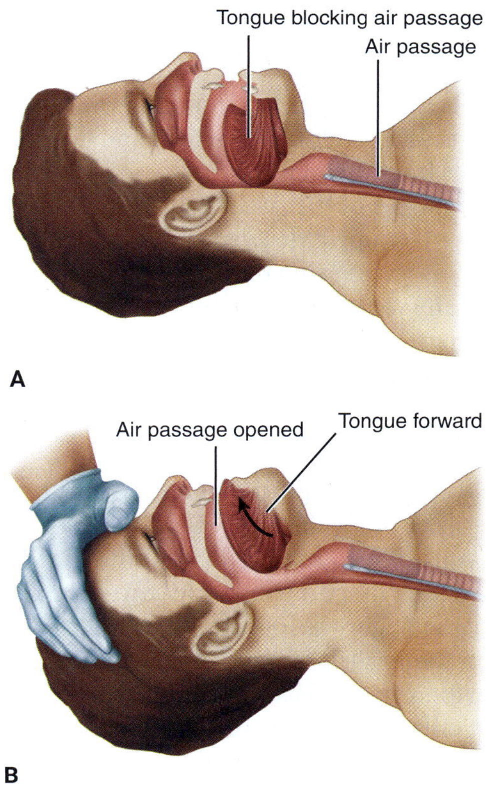

FIGURE 14-9 A. Relaxation of the tongue back into the throat causes airway obstruction. **B.** The head tilt–chin lift maneuver combines two movements of opening the airway; head tilt is shown here.

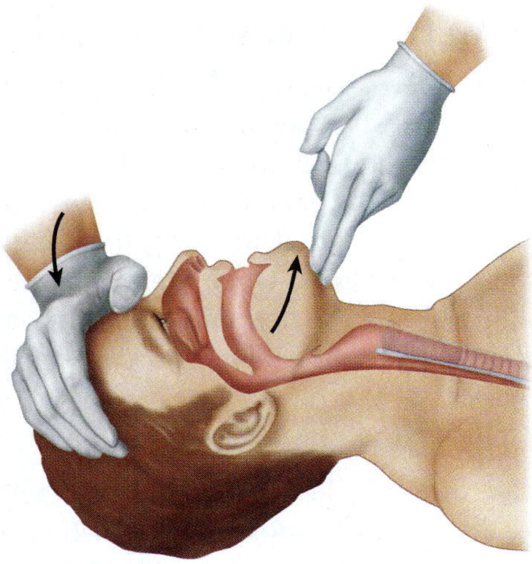

FIGURE 14-10 To perform the head tilt–chin lift maneuver, place one hand on the patient's forehead and apply firm backward pressure with your palm to tilt the head back. Next, place the tips of the index and middle fingers of your other hand under the lower jaw near the bony part of the chin. Lift the chin upward, bringing the entire lower jaw with it, helping to tilt the head back.

patient has any foreign material or vomitus in the mouth, then quickly remove it. Remove any liquid materials from the mouth with a suction device; locate the angles of the patient's lower jaw and then move the jaw upward. Keep the head in a neutral position as you move your hooked index finger to remove any visible solid material. **FIGURE 14-10** reviews how to perform the head tilt–chin lift maneuver in an adult.

Jaw-Thrust Maneuver

If spinal injury is suspected, then use the **jaw-thrust maneuver**. Do not tilt the patient's head back, because you want to minimize movement of the patient's neck. To perform a jaw-thrust maneuver, place your fingers behind the jaw and lift upward to open the mouth. If the patient's mouth remains closed, then you can use your thumbs to pull down the patient's lower lip to allow breathing. If the jaw thrust fails to open the airway, then the head tilt–chin lift should be used to open the airway. An open airway is the primary goal when caring for trauma patients, and you must ensure an open airway to improve survival. **FIGURE 14-11** reviews how to perform the jaw-thrust maneuver.

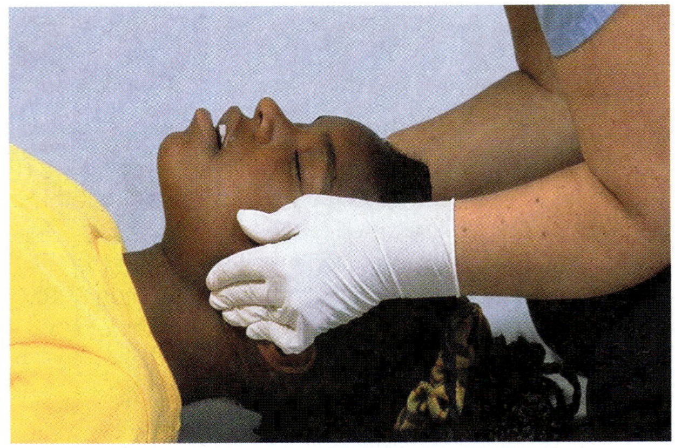

FIGURE 14-11 To perform the jaw-thrust maneuver, maintain the head in neutral alignment and place your fingers behind the angles of the lower jaw, and move the jaw upward.

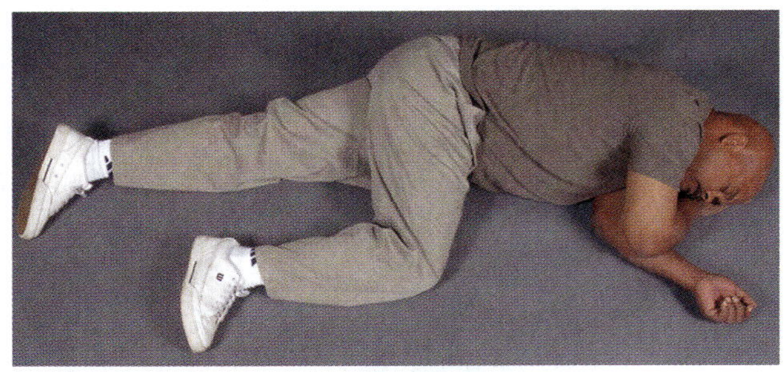

FIGURE 14-12 The recovery position is used to maintain an open airway in an adequately breathing patient with a decreased level of consciousness who has no spinal injury. It allows vomitus, blood, and any other secretions to drain from the mouth.

Recovery Position

If the patient is breathing adequately on their own and has no signs of injury to the spine, hip, or pelvis, then place the patient in the **recovery position**. This position helps to maintain a clear airway in a patient with a decreased level of consciousness who has not sustained traumatic injuries and is breathing adequately on their own (**FIGURE 14-12**). It also allows vomitus to drain from the mouth. Roll the patient onto the side so that the head, shoulders, and torso move as a unit, without twisting. Then place the top hand under the patient's cheek. Avoid placing a patient who has a suspected head or spinal injury in the recovery position because in this position, the spine is not aligned, spinal stabilization is not possible, and further spinal injury could result.

Providing Artificial Ventilations

A lack of oxygen (hypoxia), combined with too much carbon dioxide in the blood (hypercapnia), is lethal. To correct this condition, you must provide slow, deliberate ventilations that last 1 second. This gentle, slow method of ventilating the patient prevents air from being forced into the stomach (discussed later in this chapter).

Ventilations can be given by one or two EMS clinicians. Use a bag-mask device when you administer ventilations in the prehospital environment. Use devices that supply supplemental oxygen when possible. Devices with an oxygen reservoir will provide higher percentages of oxygen to the patient. Regardless of whether you ventilate the patient with or without supplemental oxygen, you should observe the chest for visible rise to assess the effectiveness of your ventilations.

The specific steps of CPR are discussed later in this chapter. Adult BLS procedures are summarized in **TABLE 14-1**. Pediatric BLS procedures are summarized in Table 14-2 later in this chapter. Resuscitation of a newborn is discussed in Chapter 34, *Obstetrics and Neonatal Care*.

Words of Wisdom

Ventilation is the physical act of moving air into and out of the lungs. Ventilation is required for adequate respiration. Examples of conditions that hinder ventilation include trauma such as flail chest, foreign body airway obstruction, and an injury to the spinal cord that disrupts the phrenic nerve that innervates the diaphragm.

Avoiding Hyperventilation and Gastric Distention

Hyperventilation (ventilating too fast or with too much force) may cause increased intrathoracic pressure (pressure inside the chest cavity) by putting pressure on the venae cavae, thus reducing the amount of blood that returns to the heart. This increased intrathoracic pressure decreases the effectiveness of chest compressions and results in the heart and brain receiving decreased amounts of oxygen.

Artificial ventilation may result in the stomach becoming filled with air, a condition called **gastric distention**. Gastric distention is likely to occur if you hyperventilate the patient. If you ventilate too forcefully, or if the patient's airway is not opened adequately, then the excess gas under pressure opens

YOU are the EMT

You arrive at the scene and find two bystanders performing CPR on the patient, who appears to be in his mid 50s. You perform a primary assessment as your partner retrieves the AED.

Recording Time: 0 Minutes	
Appearance	Motionless; cyanosis of the face
Level of consciousness	Unresponsive
Airway	Open; clear of secretions or foreign bodies
Breathing	Absent
Circulation	No carotid pulse; skin cool and pale compared with baseline; no gross bleeding

Your partner takes over ventilations while the bystanders, whose chest compressions are good, continue performing chest compressions, alternating every 2 minutes. One of the bystanders tells you that the patient was about to get into his vehicle when he suddenly grabbed his chest, slumped against the vehicle, and eased himself to the ground. By the time the bystander reached him, he was unresponsive with gasping breaths. The bystander further tells you that he immediately called 9-1-1 and then began CPR.

3. What links in the chain of survival have been maintained at this point?
4. Why is it so critical to minimize interruptions in CPR?

TABLE 14-1 Review of Adult BLS Procedures

Procedure	Notes
Circulation	
Pulse check	Carotid artery
Compression area	Two hands on the lower half of the sternum
Compression depth	2 in. (5 cm)
Compression rate	100 to 120/min
Compression-to-ventilation ratio (until advanced airway is inserted)	30:2
Severe foreign body obstruction	Responsive: back slaps and abdominal thrusts, or chest thrusts if patient is pregnant or has obesity Unresponsive: CPR No need to assess pulse Check mouth for foreign body before delivering breaths and remove if visible
Airway	
Airway positioning	Head tilt–chin lift; jaw-thrust maneuver if spinal injury is suspected
Breathing	
Ventilations	1 breath every 6 seconds (a rate of 10 breaths/min); visible chest rise
Ventilations with advanced airway placed	1 breath every 6 seconds (a rate of 10 breaths/min)

up the collapsible tube (the esophagus) and allows air to enter the stomach. Therefore, it is important for you to give slow, gentle breaths. Such breaths are also more effective in ventilating the lungs. Excessive inflation of the stomach is dangerous because it can cause the patient to vomit during CPR, blocking the airway. It can also reduce lung volume by elevating the diaphragm.

If massive gastric distention occurs, first check for adequate ventilation; if it interferes with adequate ventilation, contact medical direction. Check the airway again and reposition the patient, watch for rise and fall of the chest, and avoid giving forceful breaths. Have a suction unit available in case the patient vomits. Remember, mortality increases significantly if aspiration occurs. If an ALS clinician is available, then this person can insert an orogastric or nasogastric tube to decompress the stomach.

One-Rescuer Adult CPR

When you provide CPR alone, you must provide a continuous cycle of 30 chest compressions followed by two artificial ventilations (a ratio of 30:2). To perform one-rescuer adult CPR, follow the steps in **SKILL DRILL 14-2**:

1. Take standard precautions. Establish unresponsiveness and call for additional help (**Step 1**).
2. Position the patient properly (supine) on a flat surface.
3. Quickly visualize the chest for signs of breathing while simultaneously palpating for a carotid pulse. Take no more than 10 seconds in total to do this (**Step 2**).
4. If pulse and breathing are absent, then perform CPR until an AED is available. Place your hands in the proper position for delivering external chest compressions, as described previously (**Step 3**). Give 30 chest compressions at a rate of 100 to 120 per minute for an adult. Each set of 30 compressions should take about 17 seconds.
5. Open the airway according to your suspicion of spinal injury (**Step 4**).
6. Give two ventilations of 1 second each, and observe for visible chest rise (**Step 5**).
7. Continue cycles of 30 chest compressions and two ventilations until additional personnel arrive or the patient starts to move.

Two-Rescuer Adult CPR

You and your team should be able to perform one-rescuer and two-rescuer CPR with ease. Two-rescuer CPR is always preferable because it is less tiring and it facilitates effective chest compressions. In fact, a team approach to CPR and AED use is far superior to the one-rescuer approach. Once one-rescuer CPR is in progress, additional rescuers

Skill Drill 14-2 Performing One-Rescuer Adult CPR

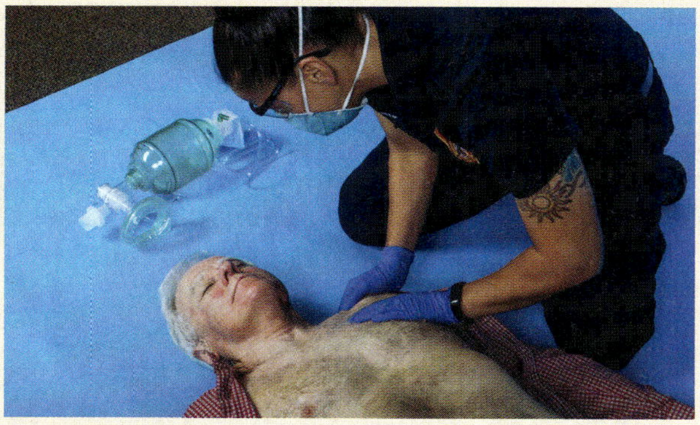

Step 1

Take standard precautions. Establish unresponsiveness and call for help. Use your mobile phone if needed.

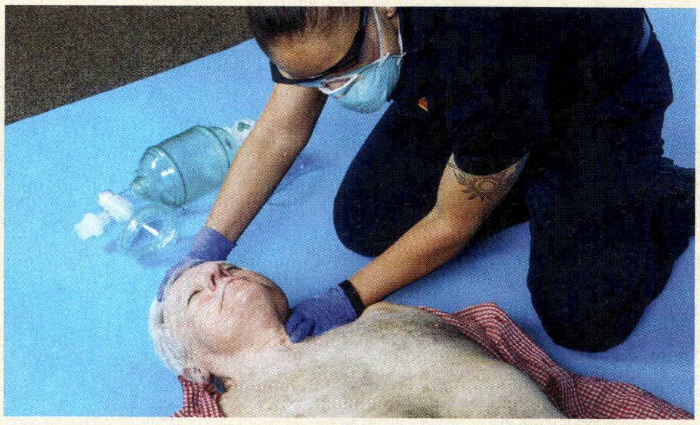

Step 2

Check for breathing and a carotid pulse for no more than 10 seconds.

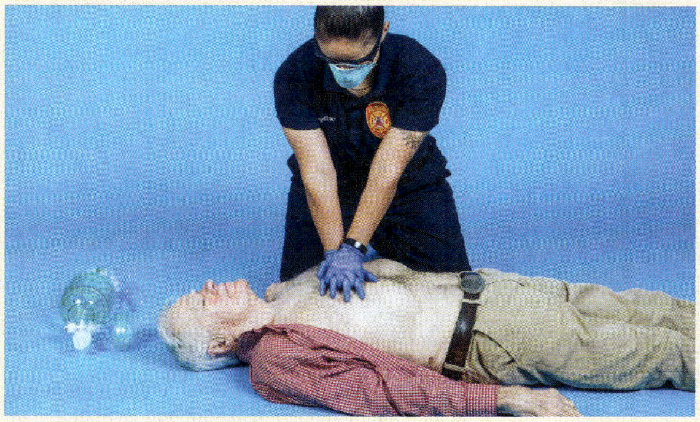

Step 3

If breathing and pulse are absent, then perform CPR until an AED is available. Give 30 chest compressions at a rate of 100 to 120 per minute.

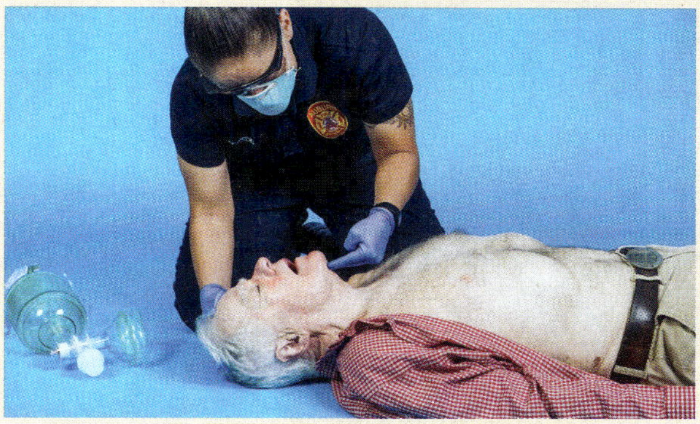

Step 4

Open the airway according to your suspicion of spinal injury.

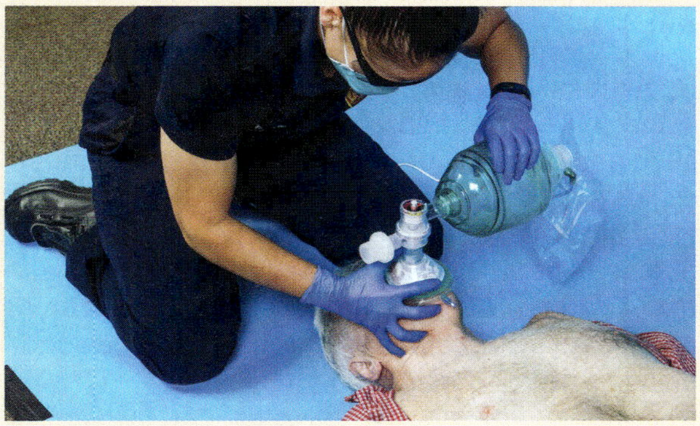

Step 5

Give two ventilations of 1 second each and observe for visible chest rise. Continue cycles of 30 chest compressions and two ventilations until additional personnel arrive or the patient starts to move.

can be added to the procedure easily. Before assisting with CPR, a second rescuer should incorporate the use of airway adjuncts, including a bag-mask device and suction, and insert an oropharyngeal (oral) airway. If CPR is in progress, then the second rescuer should enter the procedure after the AED and then cycle of 30 compressions and two ventilations. To perform two-rescuer adult CPR, follow the steps in **SKILL DRILL 14-3**:

1. Take standard precautions. Establish unresponsiveness while your partner moves to the

Skill Drill 14-3 Performing Two-Rescuer Adult CPR

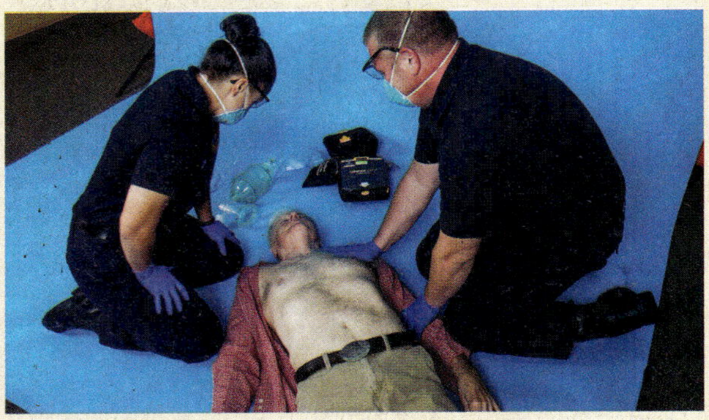

Step 1

Take standard precautions. Establish unresponsiveness and take positions.

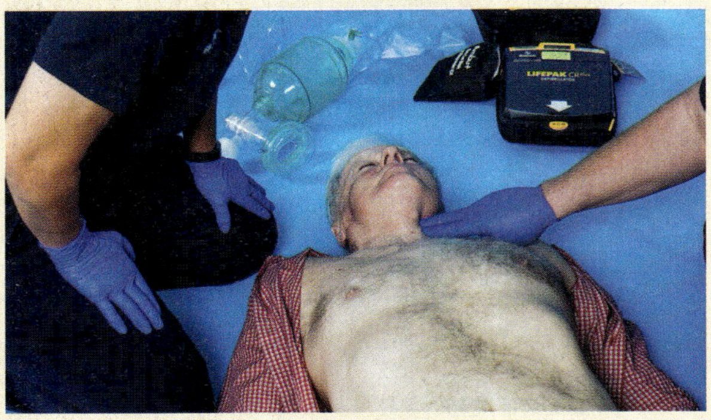

Step 2

Check for breathing and a carotid pulse.

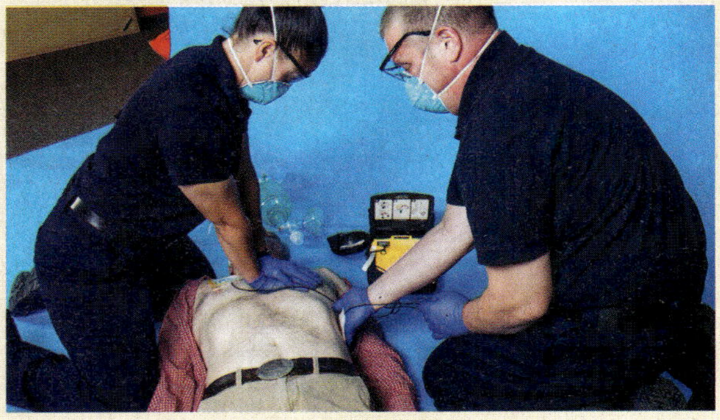

Step 3

Begin CPR, starting with chest compressions. Give 30 chest compressions at a rate of 100 to 120 per minute. If the AED is available, then apply it and follow the voice prompts.

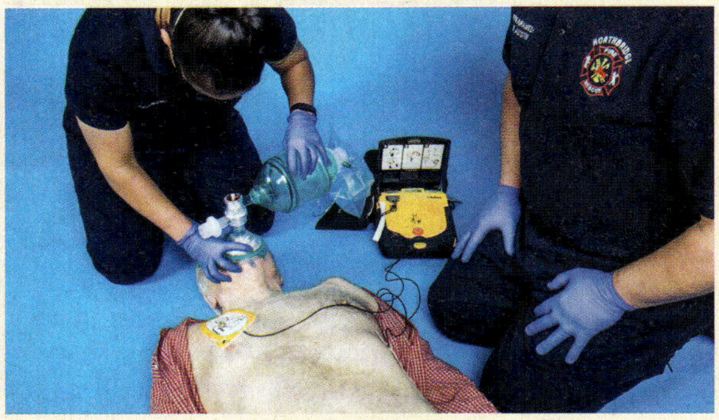

Step 4

Open the airway according to your suspicion of spinal injury. Give two ventilations of 1 second each and observe for visible chest rise. Continue cycles of 30 chest compressions and two ventilations (switch roles every five cycles [2 minutes]) until ALS clinicians take over or the patient starts to move. Reanalyze the patient's cardiac rhythm with the AED every 2 minutes and deliver a shock if indicated.

patient's side to be ready to deliver chest compressions (**Step 1**).
2. If the patient is unresponsive, then simultaneously check for breathing and palpate for a carotid pulse; take no more than 10 seconds to do this (**Step 2**).
3. If the patient is not breathing adequately and has no pulse, then begin CPR, starting with chest compressions. Give 30 chest compressions at a rate of 100 to 120 per minute. If an AED is available, then apply it and follow its voice prompts. Do not interrupt chest compressions to apply the AED pads (**Step 3**).
4. Open the airway according to your suspicion of spinal injury (**Step 4**).
5. Give two ventilations of 1 second each and observe for visible chest rise (**Step 5**).
6. Perform five cycles of 30 compressions and two ventilations (this should take approximately 2 minutes). After 2 minutes of CPR, the compressor and the ventilator should switch positions. The switch time should take no longer than 5 seconds. Reanalyze the patient's cardiac rhythm with the AED every 2 minutes and deliver a shock if indicated.
7. Continue cycles of 30 chest compressions and two ventilations until ALS clinicians take over or the patient starts to move.

Words of Wisdom

When CPR is in progress on a patient who has an advanced airway device in place (ie, ET tube or supraglottic airway), stopping compressions to provide a breath is not necessary. Compressions should be continuous at a rate of 100 to 120 per minute and ventilations should occur at a rate of one breath every 6 seconds (10 breaths/min). Do not pause between compressions to deliver breaths.

Switching Positions

It is critical to switch rescuers during CPR to maintain high-quality compressions. After five cycles of CPR (approximately 2 minutes), the rescuer providing compressions to the patient (the compressor) will begin to tire, and compression quality will decrease. Therefore, compressors should switch positions every 2 minutes. If there are only two rescuers on scene, then the two rescuers will alternate positions. If additional rescuers are available, the compressor should rotate every 2 minutes. During switches, every effort should be made to minimize the time that no compressions are being administered. It should take less than 10 seconds to switch compressors.

The switch between the two rescuers can be easily accomplished. Rescuer one (the first compressor) should finish the cycle of 30 compressions

Words of Wisdom

Even if the EMT providing compressions does not feel tired after 2 minutes, the compressions being provided are probably less effective. Rotate compressors every 2 minutes, even if you do not feel tired.

Words of Wisdom

Many EMS systems have implemented a pit crew approach to the management of cardiac arrest. The term originated in motor racing, in which teams of technicians rapidly assess and repair vehicles in a matter of seconds. Following this model, each resuscitation team member is assigned a specific role before beginning care of the cardiac arrest patient. The following provides an example:

- EMT 1 will be the team leader.
- EMT 2 and EMT 3 will perform CPR.
- EMT 4 will operate the AED.

This model clarifies each team member's role and responsibilities and minimizes confusion on the scene. Depending on the size and level of response, the "pit crew" may be more than four people and may involve different roles, including ALS skills.

If there are only two EMTs on scene initially, as is the situation in many cases, then a plan should be developed to integrate additional rescuers into the resuscitation effort as they arrive. This preplanned approach allows rescuers to accomplish multiple steps and assessments simultaneously, rather than in the slower, sequential manner used by individual rescuers. Therefore, the pit crew model minimizes the time to first compression. The success of this team approach depends on preplanning, practice, and thorough familiarity with the cardiac arrest algorithm. See Chapter 9, *The Team Approach to Health Care*, for more information.

while the second rescuer moves to the opposite side of the chest and moves into position to begin compressions. Rescuer one should deliver two rescue breaths and then rescuer two should take over compressions by administering 30 chest compressions. Rescuer one will then deliver two ventilations and the CPR cycles will continue as needed until the next 2-minute mark (five cycles) is reached, at which time the process will be repeated.

Automated External Defibrillation

Most prehospital cardiac arrests occur as the result of a sudden disturbance (dysrhythmia) in the cardiac rhythm. The normal heart rhythm is known as normal sinus rhythm. Heart rhythms in cardiac arrest include "shockable" rhythms that may be successfully defibrillated, including ventricular fibrillation (VF) or pulseless ventricular tachycardia (VT). VF is the disorganized quivering of the ventricles, resulting in no blood flow and a state of cardiac arrest. VT is a rapid contraction of the ventricles that does not allow for normal filling of the heart. Defibrillation may interrupt VF or pulseless VT, allowing the heart to resume normal sinus rhythm. The likelihood of survival decreases rapidly as long as VF or pulseless VT persists.

There are also "nonshockable" rhythms that do not respond to defibrillation, including asystole (flatline) and pulseless electrical activity (PEA), where there is no electrical activity in the heart at all. Asystole indicates that no electrical activity remains and therefore defibrillation will not help. PEA refers to a state of cardiac arrest that exists despite an organized electrical complex; defibrillation could possibly make this situation worse. In both cases, high-quality, minimally interrupted CPR should be initiated as soon as possible, beginning with chest compressions.

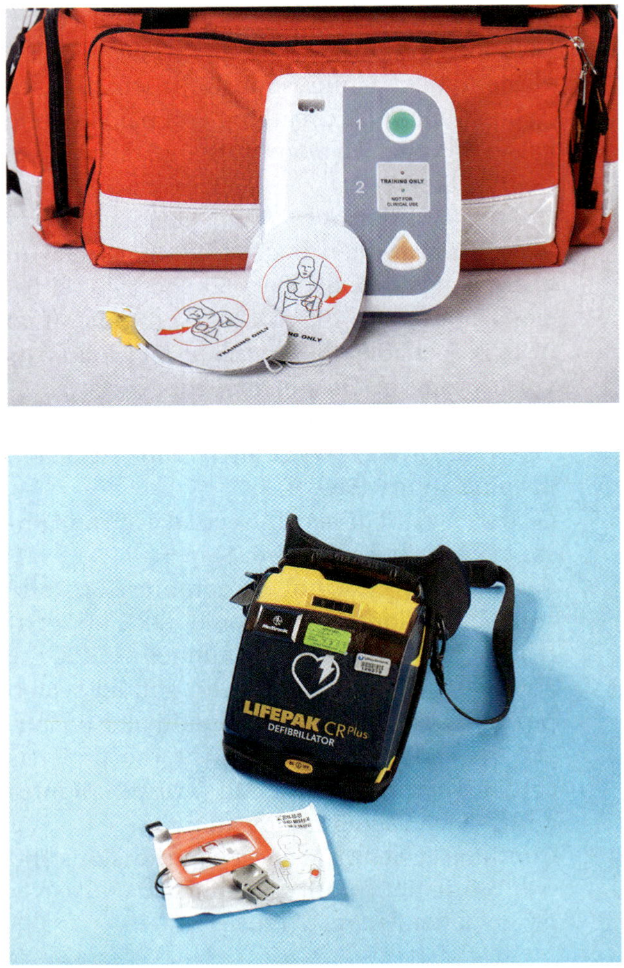

FIGURE 14-13 Automated external defibrillators vary in their design, features, and operation. Two types of defibrillators are shown here.

Top: © Photographee.eu/Shutterstock; **Bottom:** © Jones & Bartlett Learning.

Overview of AEDs

AED machines come in different models with different features (**FIGURE 14-13**). All of them require a certain degree of operator interaction, beginning with turning on the machine and applying the pads. For most models, the operator also has to push a button to deliver an electrical shock. Many AEDs use a computer voice synthesizer to advise the operator which steps to take on the basis of the AED's analysis. Some have a button that tells the computer to analyze the heart's electrical rhythm; other models start doing this as soon as they are turned on. Even though most defibrillators are semiautomated, the term AED is still used to describe all of these machines.

Words of Wisdom

In the late 1970s and early 1980s, scientists developed a small computer that could analyze electrical signals from the heart. This development, along with improved battery technology, made the automated portable defibrillator possible.

AEDs deliver electrical energy from one pad to the other (and then back to the first pad) to electrically stun the heart and allow it to resume normal function. The amount of electricity delivered by the machine varies among the manufacturers, but each one has shown that the energy delivered is adequate to defibrillate the heart. The factors involved in the defibrillation include voltage, current, and impedance. Most AEDs are set up to adjust the voltage based on the impedance (or resistance of the body to the flow of electricity) to deliver the proper amount of current, which is what causes the cells to defibrillate.

The computer inside the AED is programmed to recognize rhythms that require defibrillation to be corrected, most commonly VF. AEDs are extremely accurate. It would be rare for an AED to recommend a shock when a shock is not required, and an AED rarely fails to recommend one when it would be helpful. Therefore, if the AED recommends a shock, you can trust that it is indicated.

An AED has several advantages. First, the machine is fast, and it delivers the most important treatment for a patient in VF: an electrical shock. It can be delivered within 1 minute of your arrival at the patient's side. Second, AEDs are easy to operate. ALS clinicians do not have to be on the scene to provide this lifesaving care.

Words of Wisdom

If you witness a patient's cardiac arrest and an AED is available, use the AED immediately and then begin CPR. However, if you did not witness the patient's cardiac arrest or if an AED is unavailable, then perform CPR and apply the AED as soon as it is available. If two or more rescuers are present, one rescuer should begin CPR while the other prepares to defibrillate using the AED.

AED Use

If you are in a tiered system and the patient is in cardiac arrest, call for ALS assistance. If you suspect that the patient may be in cardiac arrest, discuss who will perform which resuscitation responsibilities prior to arrival on the scene. Preparation tasks should be done concurrently, so that time to defibrillation is minimized. For example, one clinician begins compressions while another prepares for ventilation and another prepares the AED. Working as a well-organized team will improve the chances for a successful resuscitation.

If you witness a patient's cardiac arrest, begin CPR, starting with chest compressions, and turn on the AED as soon as it is available. As soon as the AED is turned on and the pads are attached, follow the instructions to analyze and deliver shocks to the patient. Minimize the time when you are not performing chest compressions; research has shown the best survival rates for patients in whom compressions were interrupted for the least amount of time. At each defibrillation, the person performing compressions should switch places with the person providing ventilations so that neither person becomes overtired. Immediately after each defibrillation, resume CPR with compressions first. The steps for using the AED are listed here and shown in **SKILL DRILL 14-4**:

1. If bystander CPR is in progress, assess the effectiveness of chest compressions by palpating for a carotid or femoral pulse. If compressions are effective, you should be able to feel a pulse. If you do, leave your fingers in that position and stop compressions (**Step 1**). If you lose the pulse when compressions stop, immediately resume compressions. It is important to limit the amount of time compressions are interrupted. If the patient is responsive, do not apply the AED.
2. If the patient is unresponsive and CPR has not been started yet, begin providing chest compressions and rescue breaths at a ratio of 30 compressions to two breaths and a rate of 100 to 120 compressions per minute, continuing until an AED arrives and is ready for use. It is important to start chest compressions and use the AED as soon as possible.
3. Turn on the AED. Remove clothing from the patient's chest area. Apply the pads to the chest: one just to the right of the breastbone (sternum) just below the collarbone (clavicle), the other on the left lower chest area with the top of the pad 2 to 3 inches (5 to 7.5 cm) below the armpit (**Step 2**). Do not place the pads on top of breast tissue in women. If necessary, move the breast out of the way with the back of your hand and place the pad underneath. It may be helpful to shave the hairy chest of a

Skill Drill 14-4 Using an AED

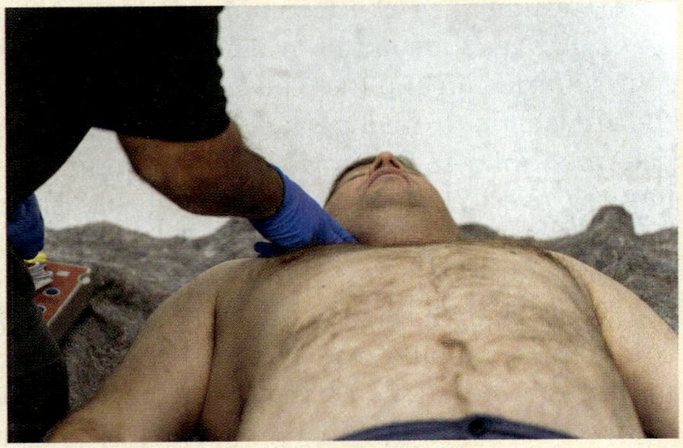

Step 1

Take standard precautions. Determine scene safety. Question bystanders. Determine responsiveness. Assess compression effectiveness if CPR is already in progress. If the patient is unresponsive and CPR has not been started yet, begin providing chest compressions and rescue breaths at a ratio of 30 compressions to two breaths and a rate of 100 to 120 compressions per minute, continuing until an AED arrives and is ready for use.

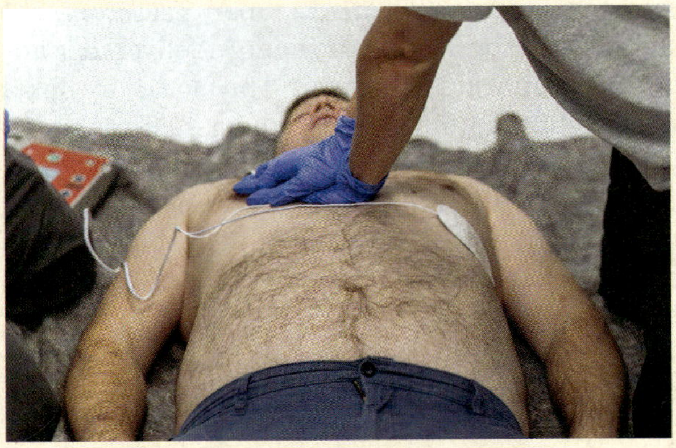

Step 2

Turn on the AED. Apply the AED pads to the chest and attach the pads to the AED.

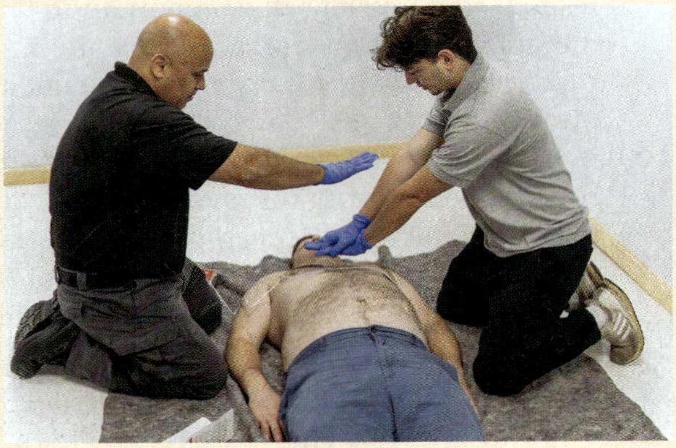

Step 3

Push the Analyze button, if there is one, and wait for the AED to determine whether a shockable rhythm is present. Stop CPR when the AED instructs you to so it can analyze the rhythm.

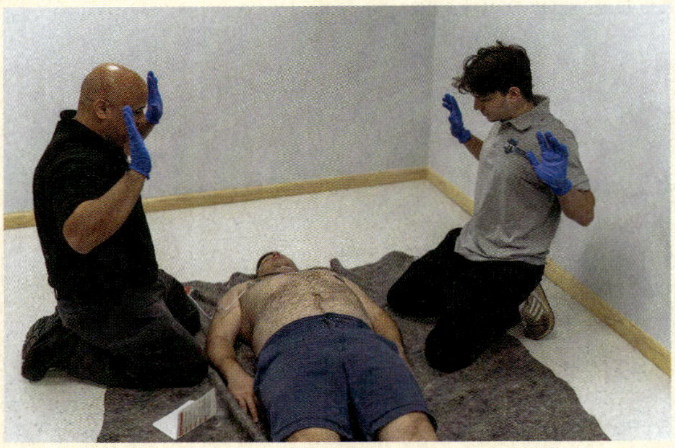

Step 4

If a shock is advised, state aloud, "Clear the patient," and ensure that no one is touching the patient. Reconfirm that no one is touching the patient and push the Shock button. Continue CPR for five cycles (2 minutes) after the shock is delivered *without stopping* to check for a pulse after the shock has been delivered! If no shock is advised, immediately return to chest compressions and ventilations.

Skill Drill 14-4 Using an AED continued

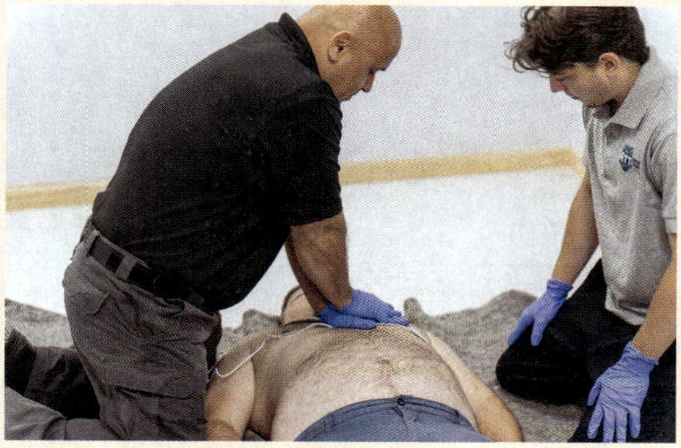

Step 5

After five cycles (or 2 minutes), pause CPR and allow the AED to analyze the rhythm. If a shock is advised, clear the patient, push the Shock button, and immediately resume CPR compressions. If no shock is advised, immediately resume CPR compressions and be sure to switch rescuers. Repeat the cycle of five cycles (2 minutes) of CPR, one shock (if indicated), and 2 minutes of CPR. Transport, and contact medical control as needed.

patient before pad placement to increase conductivity. Ensure that the pads are attached to the patient cables (and that they are attached to the AED in some models). Plug in the pads' connectors to the AED.

4. Push the Analyze button, if there is one, and wait for the AED to determine whether a shockable rhythm is present. Stop CPR when the AED instructs you to (**Step 3**). If a shock is advised, consider performing chest compressions while the AED is charging.
5. If a shock is advised, state aloud, "Clear the patient," and ensure that no one is touching the patient. Reconfirm that no one is touching the patient and push the Shock button (**Step 4**). Immediately resume CPR.
6. If a shock is not advised, perform five cycles (approximately 2 minutes) of CPR, beginning with chest compressions, and then reanalyze the cardiac rhythm. If at any time the AED advises to check the patient, quickly assess for a carotid or femoral pulse. This should not take longer than 10 seconds. If you feel a pulse, the patient has experienced ROSC. ROSC is defined as the return of a pulse and effective blood flow to the body in a patient who previously was in cardiac arrest. Continue to monitor the patient.
7. After any shock is delivered, immediately resume CPR, beginning with chest compressions. Remember to change to a different person for chest compressions each time CPR is paused to prevent rescuer fatigue.
8. After five cycles (approximately 2 minutes) of CPR, reanalyze the patient's cardiac rhythm (**Step 5**). Do not interrupt chest compressions for more than 10 seconds.
9. Gather additional information about the arrest event.
10. Repeat the cycle of 2 minutes of CPR, one shock (if indicated), and 2 minutes of CPR.
11. Transport, and contact medical control as needed.

A summary of how to manage cardiac arrest in adults is shown in **FIGURE 14-14**.

Special AED Situations

It is important to ensure the safety of yourself, others at the scene, and the patient. As such, keep the following factors in mind when using an AED.

Pacemakers and Implanted Defibrillators

You may encounter a patient who has an automated implanted cardioverter-defibrillator (AICD) or pacemaker that delivers shocks directly to the heart if necessary. These devices are used in patients who are at a high risk for certain cardiac dysrhythmias and cardiac arrest. It is easy to recognize AICDs

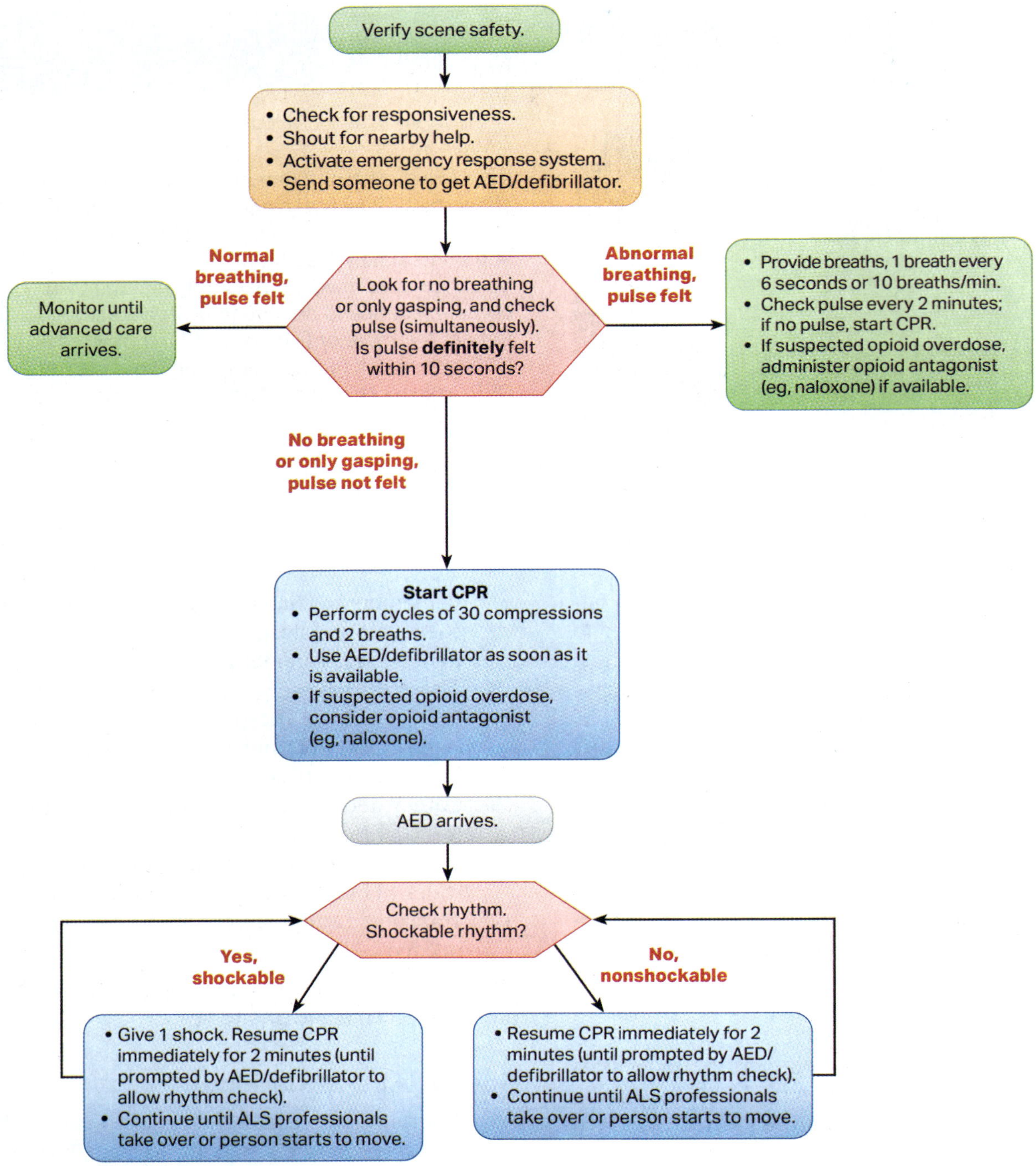

*If signs of puberty, treat as adult.

FIGURE 14-14 Adult basic life support algorithm for health care clinicians.

Abbreviations: AED, indicates automated external defibrillator; ALS, advanced life support; CPR, cardiopulmonary resuscitation or pacemakers because they create a hard lump beneath the skin, usually on the upper left side of the chest (just below the clavicle). If the AED pads are placed directly over the device, then the effectiveness of the shock delivered by the AED may be reduced, and the shock could potentially damage the implanted device. Therefore, if you identify an AICD or pacemaker, then you should place the AED pad at least 1 inch (2.5 cm) away from the device.

Occasionally, the implanted device will deliver shocks to the patient. If you observe the patient's muscles twitching as if they were just shocked, then continue CPR and wait 30 to 60 seconds before delivering a shock from the AED.

Wet Patients

Do not defibrillate a patient who is in pooled water. Although there is some danger to you if you are also in the water, there is another problem. Electricity follows the path of least resistance; instead of traveling between the pads and through the patient's heart, it will flow into the water. Therefore, the heart will not receive enough electricity to convert the heart rhythm. You can defibrillate a wet patient but try first to dry the patient's chest.

If the patient is submerged in water, then pull the patient out of the water and quickly dry the skin before attaching the AED pads. Do not delay CPR to dry the patient thoroughly; instead, quickly wipe off as much moisture as possible from the chest. If the patient is lying in a small puddle of water or in the snow, the AED can be used, but again, the patient's chest should be quickly dried as much as possible.

Safety Tip

As the operator of the AED, you are responsible for making sure the electricity does not injure anyone, including yourself. Remote defibrillation using pads allows you to distance yourself safely from the patient. As long as you place the pads in the correct position and make sure no one is touching the patient, you should be safe. Also, because metal conducts electricity, do not defibrillate someone who is touching metal that others are touching.

Transdermal Medication Patches

You may encounter a patient who is receiving medication, such as nitroglycerin, through a transdermal medication patch. The medication is absorbed through the skin. The patch could reduce the flow of the electrical current from the AED to the heart and may burn the skin. If the medication patch interferes with AED pad placement, then remove the patch with your gloved hands and wipe the skin to remove any residue prior to attaching the AED pad.

Words of Wisdom

Some areas have begun using new technologies to improve access to AEDs. For example, the PulsePoint app allows first responders to locate a nearby AED if it is registered with their system.[5] Some rural/frontier areas are testing the use of drones to deliver AEDs before EMS arrival.[6] Be familiar with the technology-enhanced resuscitation options in your community.

Patient Care Following AED Use

Care of a patient after the AED delivers a shock depends on your location and EMS system; therefore, you should follow your local protocols. After the AED protocol is completed, one of the following outcomes is likely:

- Pulse is regained (ROSC).
- No pulse is present, and the AED indicates that no shock is advised.
- No pulse is present, and the AED indicates that a shock is advised.

Patients who do not regain a pulse on the scene of the cardiac arrest usually do not survive. What you do with these patients, again, depends on your EMS system. Whether you should transport the patient or wait for ALS to arrive should be in the local protocols established by medical control. If paramedics or another ALS service is responding to the scene, the best option usually is to stay where you are and continue the sequence of shocks and CPR. The best chance for patient survival occurs when the patient is resuscitated where found, unless the location is unsafe. Administering CPR while patients are being moved or transported is usually not very effective. If moving the patient is necessary with CPR in progress, consider the use of a mechanical chest compression device (discussed in the following section) if one is available and you are trained to use it.

If an ALS service is not responding to the scene and your local protocols agree, you should begin transport when one of the following occurs:

- The patient regains a pulse.
- Six to nine shocks have been delivered (or as directed by local protocol).
- The AED gives three consecutive messages (separated by 2 minutes of CPR) that no shock is advised on a pulseless patient (or as directed by local protocol).

If you transport a patient while performing CPR, you need a plan for managing the patient in the ambulance. Performing compressions in a moving vehicle is dangerous to the clinician and should be avoided if possible. A mechanical chest compression device enables chest compressions without placing the clinician at risk.

Ideally, you will have two EMTs in the patient compartment while a third EMT drives. You may deliver additional shocks at the scene or en route with the approval of medical control. Keep in mind that AEDs cannot analyze the rhythm as effectively while the vehicle is in motion, and it is less safe to defibrillate in a moving ambulance. Therefore, you should consider coming to a complete stop if more shocks are needed. Be sure to memorize the protocol of your EMS system.

Cardiac Arrest During Transport

If you are traveling to the hospital with an unconscious patient, check for breathing at least every 30 seconds. If breathing is not present, check for a pulse. If a pulse is not present, take the following steps:

1. Stop the vehicle.
2. If the AED is not immediately ready, perform CPR, beginning with chest compressions, until the AED is ready.
3. Call for help in the form of ALS or any other available resources as appropriate based on circumstances and local protocol.
4. Analyze the rhythm.
5. Deliver one shock, if indicated, and immediately resume CPR.
6. Continue resuscitation according to your local protocol.

If you are en route with a conscious adult patient who is experiencing chest pain and becomes unconscious, take the following steps:

1. Check for breathing and, if there is none, a pulse.
2. Stop the vehicle.
3. If the AED is readily available, apply it and assess for the need to shock. If it is not immediately ready, perform CPR, beginning with chest compressions, until the AED is ready.
4. Analyze the rhythm.
5. Deliver one shock, if indicated, and immediately resume CPR.
6. Begin compressions, and continue resuscitation according to your local protocol, including transporting the patient.

Coordination With ALS Personnel

The time to defibrillation is critical to survival after cardiac arrest. As an EMT equipped with an AED, you have the one tool that a dying patient in VF needs most. Furthermore, it is impossible to hurt someone in cardiac arrest with an AED. Therefore, if you have an AED available, do not wait for the paramedics to arrive to administer a shock to a patient in VF. Waiting might seem like a good idea, but it is throwing away the patient's best chance for survival.

If the patient is unresponsive and does not have a pulse, apply the AED, turn it on, and push the Analyze button (if there is one) as quickly as you can. Notify the ALS personnel as soon as possible after you recognize a cardiac arrest, but do not delay defibrillation. After the paramedics arrive at the scene, inform them of your actions to that point and then interact with them according to your local protocols.

Management of ROSC

If you are able to restore a heartbeat during CPR or through the use of an AED (ie, ROSC), what is done next can be critical to the patient's survival. Monitor for spontaneous respirations; if there are none, ventilate with oxygen via bag-mask device at 10 breaths/min, and maintain an oxygen saturation between 92% and 98%.[7] Assess the patient's blood pressure, and see if the person can follow simple commands such as "Squeeze my fingers." If ALS is not on scene or en route, leave the AED pads on and immediately begin transport to the closest appropriate hospital, depending on local protocol.

AED Maintenance

You must become familiar with the maintenance procedures required for the brand of AED your system uses. Read the operator's manual. If your defibrillator does not work on the scene, someone will want to know what went wrong. That person may be your system's administrator, your medical director, the local newspaper reporter, or the family's attorney. You will be asked to show proof that you maintained the defibrillator properly and attended any mandatory in-service sessions.

The main legal risk in using the AED is failing to deliver a shock when one was needed. The three most common errors in using certain AEDs are failure of the machine to shock fine VF; applying the AED to a patient who is moving, squirming, or being transported; and turning off the AED before analysis or shock is complete. Operator errors include failing to apply the AED to a patient in cardiac arrest, not pushing the Analyze or Shock buttons when the machine advises you to do so, or pushing the Power button instead of pushing the Shock button when a shock is advised. Like any other manufactured item, the AED can fail, although this is rare. Ideally, you will encounter any such failure while doing routine maintenance, not while caring for a patient in cardiac arrest.

Another risk is failure to deliver a shock due to a battery that did not work, usually because it was not properly maintained. Check your equipment, including your AED, daily at the beginning of each shift and maintain the battery as often as the manufacturer recommends. Ask the manufacturer for a checklist of items that should be checked daily, weekly, or less often (**FIGURE 14-15**).

If the AED fails while you are caring for a patient, you must report the problem to the manufacturer and the US Food and Drug Administration. Be sure to follow the appropriate EMS procedures for notifying these organizations.

Words of Wisdom

An error can also occur when the AED is applied to a responsive patient with a rapid heart rate. Most AEDs identify a regular rhythm faster than 150 or 180 beats/min as VT, which should be shocked if the patient is pulseless. However, shocking VT in a patient with a pulse may result in the patient losing the pulse and going into cardiac arrest. To avoid this problem, you should apply the AED only to unresponsive *pulseless* patients.

Medical Direction and Incident Review Relating to AED Use

Defibrillation of the heart is a medical procedure. Although AEDs have made the process of delivering electricity much simpler, there is still a benefit in having a physician's involvement. The medical director of your service should approve the written protocol that you will follow in caring for patients in cardiac arrest.

There should be a review of each incident in which the AED is used. After returning from the hospital or the scene, discuss with the rest of the team what happened. This discussion will help all members of the team learn from the incident. Review such events by following your departmental procedure and the device's recordings, if applicable.

Most departments conduct some type of review of cardiac arrest responses. This review may include your service's medical director or quality improvement officer. It should include a focus on the time from the first contact with the patient to the time CPR was initiated and the first shock is delivered. Additionally, when the monitor can record it, the review should include the quality of CPR (to include timing of pauses). Few systems will achieve the ultimate goal: shocking 100% of patients within 1 minute of initial patient contact. However, all systems can continuously work on improving patient care. Continuing education with skill competency review should be required for all EMS clinicians.

Additional Devices and Techniques to Assist Circulation

The effectiveness of CPR depends on the amount of blood circulated throughout the body as a result of chest compressions. Even under ideal conditions, however, manual chest compressions cannot equate to normal cardiac output. In addition,

AUTOMATED EXTERNAL DEFIBRILLATOR
Inspection Checklist

Serial # ______________ **Date** ______________ **Time** ______________

Model # ______________ **Inspected by** ______________

Item	Pass	Fail
Exterior/Cables		
Nothing stored on top of unit		
Carry case intact and clean		
Exterior/LCD/cables connectors clean and undamaged		
Cables securely attached to unit		
Batteries		
All chargers plugged in and operational (if applicable)		
All batteries fully charged (battery in unit, spare battery)		
Valid expiration date on both batteries		
Supplies		
Two sets of electrodes in sealed packages with valid expiration dates		
Razor		
Hand towel		
Alcohol wipes		
Memory/voice recording device—module, card, microcassette		
Manual override—module, key (if applicable)		
Printer paper (if applicable)		
Operation		
Unit self-test per manufacturer's recommendation/instructions		
Display (if applicable)		
Visual indicators		
Verbal prompts		
Printer (if applicable)		
Attach AED to simulator/tester		
Recognizes shockable rhythm		
Charges to correct energy level within manufacturer's specifications		
Delivers charge		
Recognizes nonshockable rhythm		
Manual override system in working order (if applicable)		

Signature:

FIGURE 14-15 A sample checklist for the automated external defibrillator (AED).

Special Populations

PATIENTS WITH VENTRICULAR ASSIST DEVICES

On occasion, you may encounter a patient who has a ventricular assist device (VAD), usually a left ventricular assist device (LVAD). The LVAD is a mechanical pump that is implanted in the chest and helps pump blood from the left ventricle to the aorta. A tube from the device passes through the skin and is attached to an external power source that the patient wears on their belt or an over-the-shoulder harness. The LVAD is commonly implanted in patients with severe heart failure or in those who are awaiting a heart transplant.

If the LVAD is working, then you will hear a humming sound when listening to the chest with a stethoscope because blood flows continuously through the LVAD. The more assistance the LVAD is providing to the heart, the weaker the patient's pulse will be. In some patients with an LVAD, you may not feel a pulse at all, even though they are responsive and alert. If the patient is unresponsive with no breathing, poor skin color, and poor or no capillary refill, and the hum of the device is heard, CPR is indicated. If the hum of the device is not heard, check to ensure that all cables are connected and that the power supply is working (batteries have a charge or the device is plugged into an outlet). When transporting a patient who has an LVAD, be sure to bring all LVAD equipment with you and ensure that the receiving facility is capable of caring for the patient's specific needs.

You should know the location of patients with an LVAD in your service area. If possible, visit with the patient prior to any emergency to determine the patient's specific device and to obtain instructions. Family members are usually knowledgeable about the device; use them as a source of information.

LVAD coordinators are usually available for consultation 24 hours per day. These medical professionals can help troubleshoot problems with the LVAD. Follow your local protocols or contact medical direction regarding the treatment of a patient with an LVAD. VADs are discussed further in Chapter 17, *Cardiovascular Emergencies*.

factors such as rescuer fatigue or inaccurate depth or rate of compressions can further impede the resuscitation process. Before you consider the use of mechanical devices to assist circulation, ensure that your manual chest compressions are of consistently high quality. If you decide to use a CPR assist device, the device should be applied quickly with minimal interruptions to CPR. Knowledge about, and frequent training with, the CPR assist device you may use is crucial for best patient outcome.

Mechanical Piston Device

A **mechanical piston device** depresses the sternum via a compressed gas-powered or electric-powered plunger mounted on a backboard (**FIGURE 14-16**). The patient is positioned supine on the backboard, with the piston positioned on top of the patient with the plunger centered over the patient's thorax in the same manner as with manual chest compressions. The device is then secured to the backboard.

The mechanical piston device, when applied correctly, provides consistent depth and rate of compressions. This frees the rescuer to complete other tasks and eliminates rescuer fatigue that results from continuous delivery of manual chest compressions.

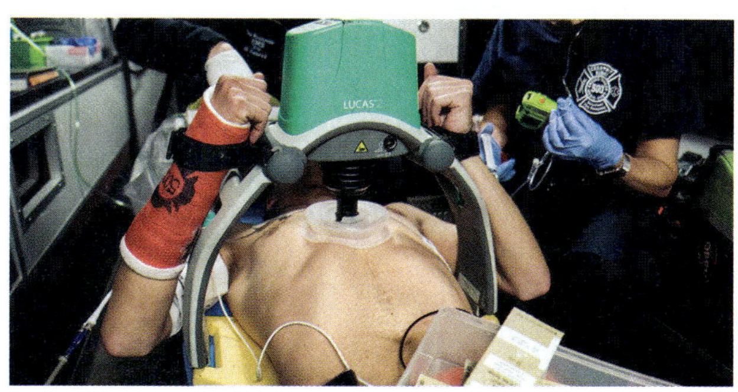

FIGURE 14-16 A mechanical piston device in use.

Load-Distributing Band CPR or Vest CPR

The **load-distributing band (LDB)** is a circumferential chest compression device composed of a constricting band and backboard (**FIGURE 14-17**). The

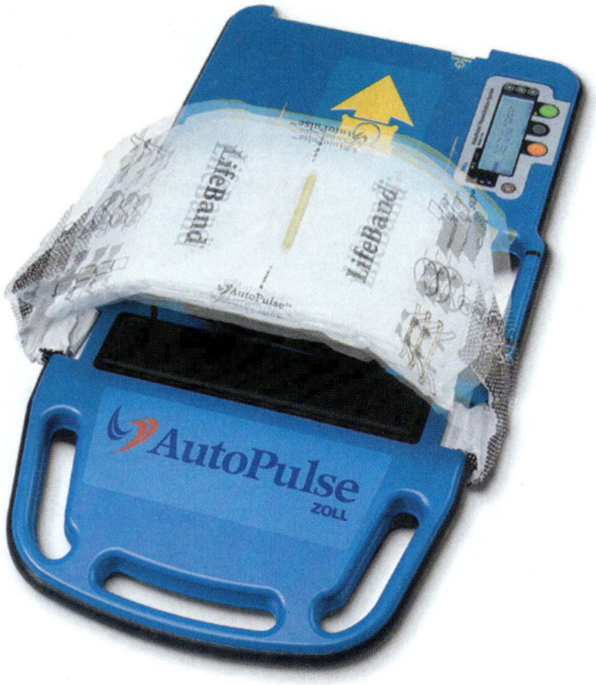

FIGURE 14-17 A load-distributing band.

Provided with permission by ZOLL Medical.

device is either electrically or pneumatically driven to compress the heart by putting inward pressure on the thorax.

The use of mechanical CPR devices may be reasonable in specific settings where the delivery of high-quality manual compressions may be challenging or dangerous for the clinician. Mechanical CPR devices can be programmed to deliver continuous compressions or compressions at a 30:2 ratio. The EMT should ventilate at the same rate or ratio as for traditional CPR, depending on which mode the agency protocols dictate.

EMTs must strictly limit interruptions in CPR during changeover from manual CPR to the mechanical device. If your EMS system uses a mechanical CPR device, then it is critical to practice frequently to ensure that you can apply it smoothly. Remember to minimize interruptions to chest compressions while the device is being applied.

Infant and Child CPR

In most cases, cardiac arrest in infants and children follows respiratory arrest, which triggers hypoxia and **ischemia** (decreased oxygen supply) of

YOU are the EMT

With CPR ongoing, you open the AED pads and prepare to apply them to the patient's chest. A second EMT unit arrives on the scene to assist with care. You note that the patient has a medication patch on the right upper part of his chest. You also see a bulge with a scar over it on the left upper part of his chest. You apply the AED pads, analyze the patient's cardiac rhythm, and receive a "shock advised" message. After delivering the shock, your partner and another EMT resume CPR.

Recording Time: 4 Minutes	
Level of consciousness	Unresponsive
Respirations	Absent (baseline); two breaths are being given after every 30 chest compressions; chest rise is visible with each breath
Pulse	Absent (baseline); femoral pulse is palpable with chest compressions
Skin	Ashen
Blood pressure	Not measurable
Oxygen saturation (Spo_2)	Not measurable

5. Should you remove the medication patch or leave it in place? Explain your decision.
6. What does the bulge and scar over the patient's left chest indicate? How will this affect the way you treat the patient?

the heart. Children consume oxygen two to three times more rapidly than adults, so you must first focus on opening the airway and providing artificial ventilation. Often, this will be enough to allow the child to resume spontaneous breathing and, thus, prevent cardiac arrest. Therefore, airway and breathing are the focus of pediatric BLS (**TABLE 14-2**).

Respiratory issues leading to cardiopulmonary arrest in children can have a number of different causes. These causes include the following:

- Traumatic injury
- Infections of the respiratory tract or another organ system such as croup or epiglottitis
- Foreign body in the airway
- Submersion (drowning)

TABLE 14-2 Review of Pediatric BLS Procedures

Procedure	Infants (between age 1 month and 1 year[a])	Children (age 1 year to onset of puberty[b])
Circulation		
Pulse check	Brachial artery	Carotid or femoral artery
Compression area	In the center of the chest, just below the nipple line on the lower half of the sternum	On the lower half of the sternum
Compression width	Two-thumb-encircling-hands technique or heel of one hand	Heel of one or both hands
Compression depth	At least one-third anterior-posterior diameter (about 1.5 in. [4 cm])	At least one-third anterior-posterior diameter (approximately 2 in. [5 cm])
Compression rate	100 to 120/min	100 to 120/min
Compression-to-ventilation ratio (until advanced airway is inserted)	30:2 (one rescuer); 15:2 (two rescuers)[c]	30:2 (one rescuer); 15:2 (two rescuers)[c]
Foreign body obstruction	Responsive: Back slaps and chest thrusts Unresponsive: CPR	Responsive: Abdominal thrusts Unresponsive: CPR
Airway		
	Head tilt–chin lift; jaw-thrust maneuver if spinal injury is suspected	Head tilt–chin lift; jaw-thrust maneuver if spinal injury is suspected
Breathing		
Ventilations	1 breath every 2 to 3 seconds (20 to 30 breaths/min); visible chest rise	1 breath every 2 to 3 seconds (20 to 30 breaths/min); visible chest rise
Ventilations with advanced airway placed	1 breath every 2 to 3 seconds (a rate of 20 to 30 breaths/min)	1 breath every 2 to 3 seconds (a rate of 20 to 30 breaths/min)

[a] The AHA defines neonatal patients as birth to age 1 month, and infants as age 1 month to 1 year. Neonatal resuscitation is covered in Chapter 34, *Obstetrics and Neonatal Care*.
[b] Onset of puberty is at approximately 12 to 14 years of age, as defined by secondary characteristics (eg, breast development in girls and armpit hair in boys).
[c] Pause compressions to deliver ventilations.

- Electrocution
- Poisoning or drug overdose
- Sudden infant death syndrome

Determining Responsiveness

Never shake a child to determine whether the child is responsive, especially if the possibility of a neck or back injury exists. Instead, gently tap the child on the shoulder, and say loudly, "Are you okay?" (**FIGURE 14-18**). With an infant, gently tap the soles of the feet. If a child is responsive but struggling to breathe, allow the child to remain in whatever position is most comfortable.

If you find an unresponsive, apneic, and pulseless child while you are alone and off duty, and you did not witness the child's collapse, perform CPR beginning with chest compressions for approximately five cycles (approximately 2 minutes), and then stop to call 9-1-1 and retrieve an AED. Remember that cardiopulmonary arrest in children is most often the result of respiratory failure, not a primary cardiac event. Therefore, children will require immediate restoration of oxygenation, ventilation, and circulation, which can be accomplished by immediately performing five cycles (approximately 2 minutes) of CPR before activating the EMS system.

Although uncommon, you may encounter a child whose cardiac arrest was caused by a primary cardiac event rather than a respiratory problem. If an otherwise healthy child without an apparent respiratory condition suddenly collapses and you witness it, first confirm that the child is in cardiac arrest. If you are alone without a mobile phone, then leave the child to call 9-1-1 and get an AED before beginning CPR. If you are not alone, then send someone to call 9-1-1 and get an AED while you begin CPR. The sudden collapse of an otherwise healthy child does not indicate a respiratory problem; instead, it suggests a primary cardiac event that may respond to defibrillation. Therefore, it is critical to get the AED to the child's side as soon as possible.

Words of Wisdom

Be familiar with the laws and policies that apply in your service area regarding your duty to act. If you choose to intervene while off duty, then you must continue to provide competent care until an equal or higher medical authority assumes care of the patient. See Chapter 3, *Medical, Legal, and Ethical Issues*, for more information.

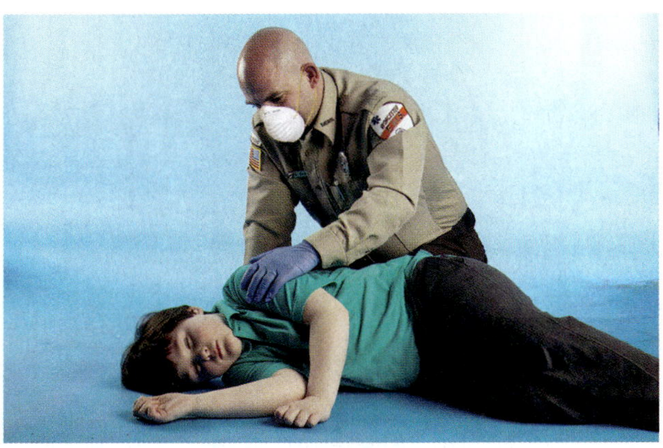

FIGURE 14-18 Never shake a child to determine responsiveness. Rather, gently tap on the shoulder (child) or tap the soles of the feet (infant), and speak loudly.

Checking for Breathing and Pulse

After you establish responsiveness, you need to assess adequacy of breathing and circulation. As with an adult, this assessment in a child can occur simultaneously and should take no longer than 10 seconds. Visualize the chest for signs of adequate breathing and palpate for a pulse in a large central artery. As with an adult, agonal gasps should be treated as "no breathing." In infants, palpate the brachial artery, which is located on the inner side of the arm, midway between the elbow and shoulder. Place your thumb on the outer surface of the arm between the elbow and shoulder. Then place the tips of your index and middle fingers on the inside of the biceps, and press lightly toward the bone. CPR will be required if the infant or child is not breathing or is not breathing normally (agonal gasps), and a pulse is absent or less than 60 beats/min.

As with an adult, an infant or child must be lying on a hard, flat surface for effective chest compressions. If you need to carry an infant while providing CPR, then your forearm and hand can serve as the flat surface. Use your palm to support the infant's head. In this way, the infant's shoulders are elevated, and the head is slightly tilted back in a position that will keep the airway open. Ensure that the infant's head is not higher than the rest of the body.

The technique for chest compressions in infants and children differs from that in adults because of several anatomic differences, including the position of the heart, the size of the chest, and the fragile organs of a child. The liver (immediately under the right side of the diaphragm) is relatively large and fragile, especially in infants. The spleen, on the left, is smaller and more fragile in children than in adults. These organs are easily injured if you are not careful in performing chest compressions, so be sure that your hand position is correct before you begin. The chest of an infant is smaller and more pliable than that of an older child or adult; therefore, you should use only the thumbs to compress the chest. Use the two-thumb-encircling-hands technique to deliver chest compressions just below the nipple line on the lower half of the sternum, making sure to avoid the xiphoid process (**FIGURE 14-19**). Alternatively, you may use the heel of one hand to provide chest compressions to the infant.

Follow the steps in **SKILL DRILL 14-5** to perform infant chest compressions:

1. Take standard precautions. Place the infant on a firm surface. You can also use a pad or wedge under the shoulders and upper body to keep the head from tilting forward (**Step 1**).

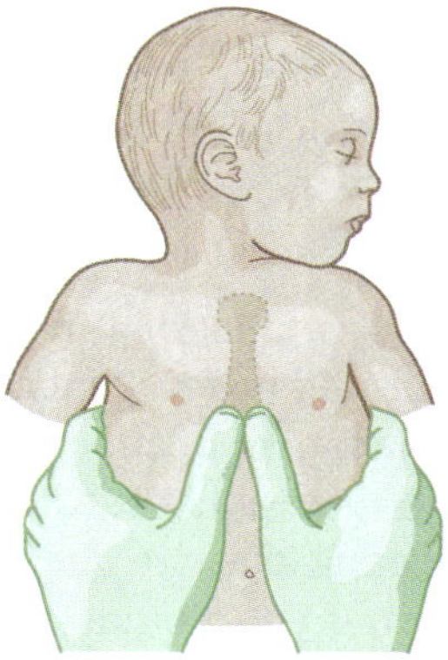

FIGURE 14-19 Hand positions for infant CPR.

Skill Drill 14-5 Performing Infant Chest Compressions

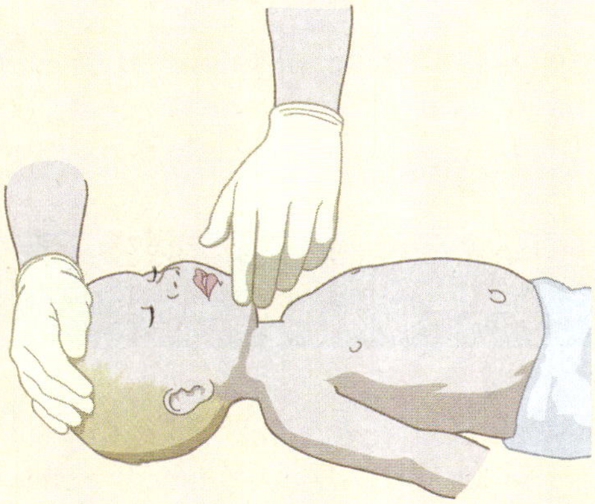

Step 1

Take standard precautions. Position the infant on a firm surface while maintaining the airway.

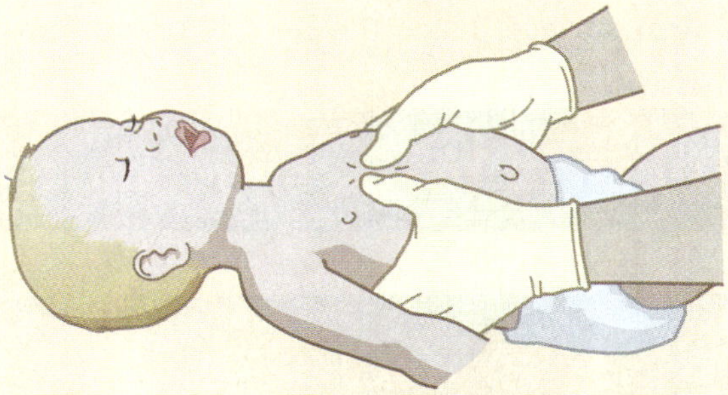

Step 2

Place your thumbs in the middle of the sternum and compress the chest at least one-third its depth at a rate of 100 to 120 per minute. Allow the sternum to return to its normal position between compressions. Infant compressions may also be performed using the heel of one hand.

2. Imagine a line drawn between the nipples. Place your thumbs in the middle of the sternum, just below the nipple line.
3. Compress the sternum at least one-third the anterior-posterior diameter of the chest (approximately 1.5 inches [4 cm] in most infants). Compress the chest at a rate of 100 to 120 per minute (**Step 2**).
4. After each compression, allow the sternum to return to its normal position. Allow equal time for compression and relaxation of the chest. Do not remove your thumbs from the sternum, and avoid jerky movements.

Coordinate compressions and ventilations in a 30:2 ratio if you are working alone, and in a 15:2 ratio if you are working with a trained bystander or another health care clinician. Ensure the infant's chest fully recoils in between compressions and that the chest visibly rises with each ventilation. If your hands do not encircle the infant's chest, you may perform chest compressions by placing the heel of one hand on the sternum. If the chest does not rise, or rises only a little, then use a head tilt–chin lift to open the airway. Use the AED as soon as it is available. Reassess the infant for signs of spontaneous breathing or a pulse after five cycles (approximately 2 minutes) of CPR.

SKILL DRILL 14-6 shows the steps for performing CPR in children between 1 year of age and the onset of puberty:

1. Take standard precautions. Place the child on a firm surface. Place the heel of one or two hands in the center of the chest, on the lower half of the sternum. Avoid compression over the lower tip of the sternum, which is called the xiphoid process (**Step 1**).
2. Compress the chest at least one-third the anterior-posterior diameter of the chest (approximately 2 inches [5 cm] in most children) at a rate of 100 to 120 per minute. With pauses for ventilation, the actual number of compressions delivered will be about 80 per minute. In between compressions, allow the chest to fully recoil; do not lean on the chest. Compression and relaxation time should be the same duration. Use smooth movements. Hold your fingers off the child's ribs, and keep the heel of your hand or hands on the sternum.
3. Coordinate compressions and ventilations in a 30:2 ratio for one rescuer and 15:2 for two rescuers, making sure the chest rises with each ventilation. At the end of each cycle, pause for two ventilations (**Step 2**).
4. After five cycles (approximately 2 minutes) reassess for a pulse.
5. If the child regains a pulse of greater than 60 beats/min and resumes effective breathing, place the child in a position that allows for frequent reassessment of the airway and vital signs during transport (**Step 3**).

Switching rescuer positions is the same for children as it is for adults, every five cycles (2 minutes) of CPR. Remember, if the child is past the onset of

Skill Drill 14-6 Performing CPR on a Child

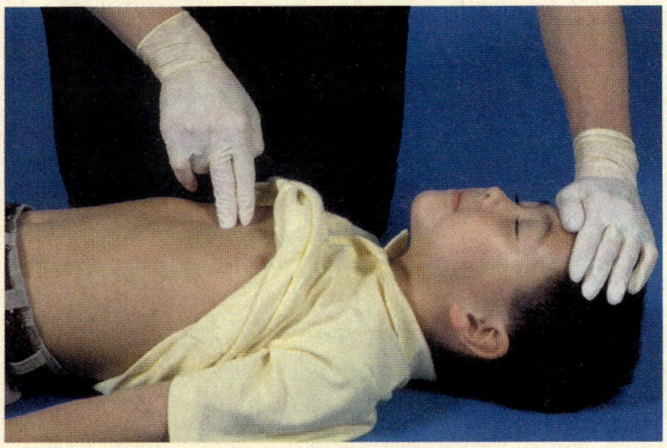

Step 1

Take standard precautions. Place the child on a firm surface. Identify the location for hand placement, as shown here. Place the heel of one or two hands in the center of the chest, on the lower half of the sternum, avoiding the xiphoid process. Use the AED as soon as it is available.

Skill Drill 14-6 Performing CPR on a Child continued

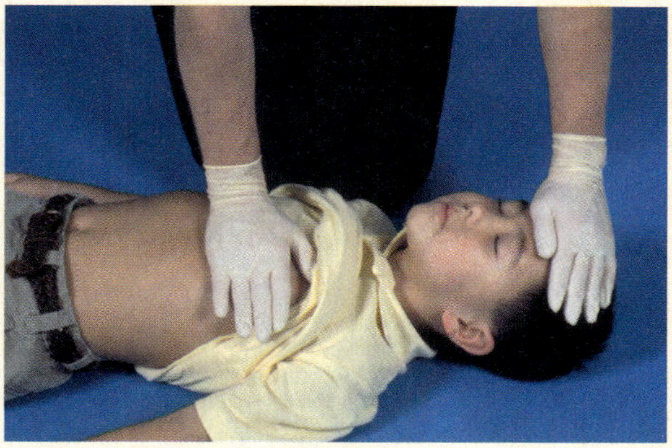

Step 2

Compress the chest at least one-third the anterior-posterior diameter of the chest at a rate of 100 to 120 times/min. Coordinate compressions with ventilations in a 30:2 (one rescuer) or 15:2 (two rescuers) ratio, pausing for two ventilations. Reassess for a pulse after 2 minutes.

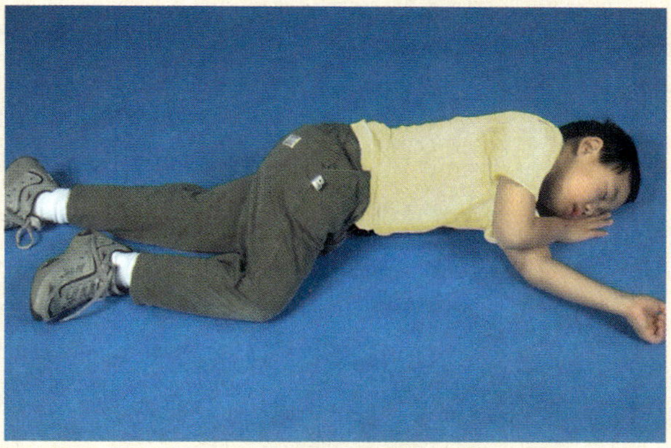

Step 3

If the child regains a pulse of greater than 60 beats/min and resumes effective breathing, then place the child in a position that allows for frequent reassessment of the airway and vital signs during transport.

puberty, use the adult CPR sequence, including the use of the AED.

A summary of how to manage cardiac arrest in children is shown in **FIGURE 14-20**. The algorithm for neonatal resuscitation is shown in Chapter 34, *Obstetrics and Neonatal Care*.

Opening the Airway in Children

Infants and toddlers often put toys and other objects, as well as food, in their mouths; therefore, foreign body obstruction of the upper airway is common. You must make sure that the upper airway is open when managing pediatric respiratory emergencies or cardiopulmonary arrest. If the child is unresponsive and lying in a supine position, then the airway may become obstructed when the tongue and throat muscles relax and the tongue falls backward.

If the child is unresponsive but breathing adequately, then place them in the recovery position to maintain an open airway and allow drainage of saliva, vomitus, or other secretions from the mouth. Do not use this position if you suspect injury to the spine, hips, or pelvis unless you can secure the child to a backboard that can be tilted to the side. If the child is responsive and breathing, but in a labored fashion, then provide supplemental oxygen and prompt transport to the closest appropriate hospital.

Opening the airway in an infant or child is done by using the same techniques as used for an adult. However, because a child's neck is so flexible, the techniques should be slightly modified. The jaw-thrust maneuver is the best method to use if you suspect a spinal injury in a child. If a second rescuer is present, they should immobilize the child's cervical spine. If spinal injury is not suspected, then use the head tilt–chin lift maneuver but modified so that, as you tilt the head back, you are moving it only into the neutral position or a slightly extended position (**FIGURE 14-21**).

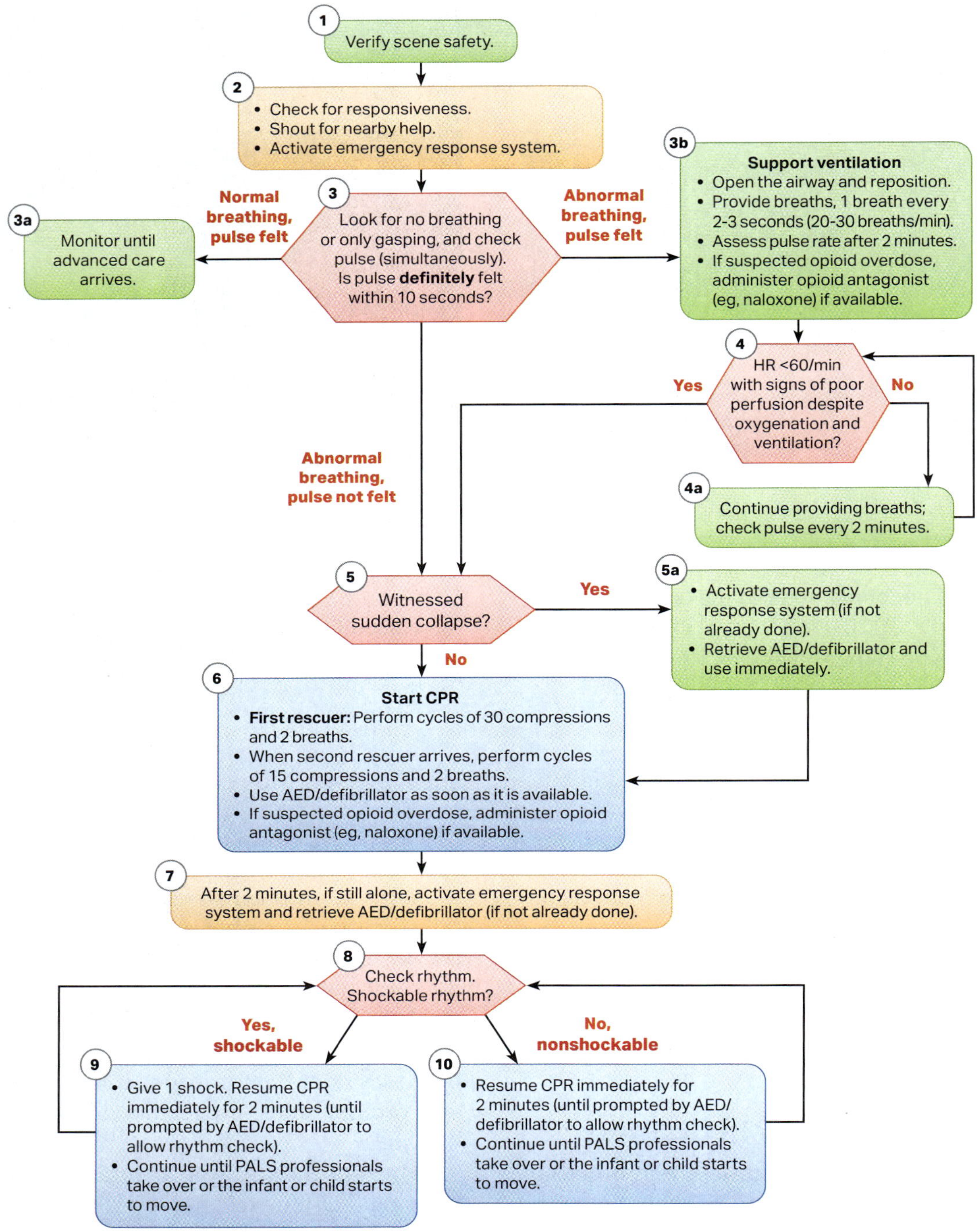

FIGURE 14-20 Pediatric basic life support algorithm for a single rescuer.

Abbreviations: AED, automated external defibrillator; CPR, cardiopulmonary resuscitation; HR, heart rate; PALS, Pediatric Advanced Life Support

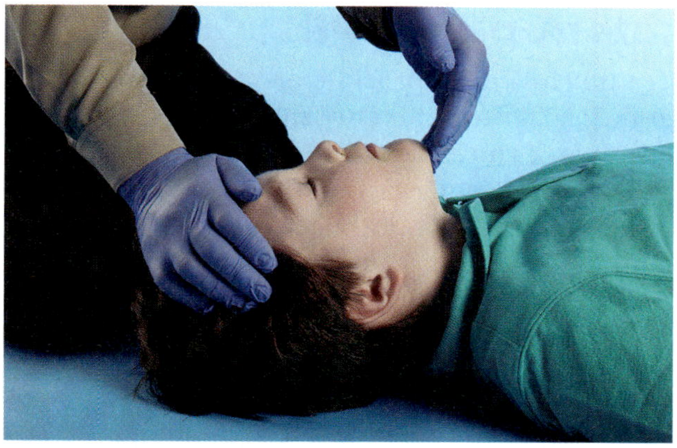

FIGURE 14-21 Use the head tilt–chin lift maneuver to open the airway in a child who has not sustained a traumatic injury. Do not overextend the neck.

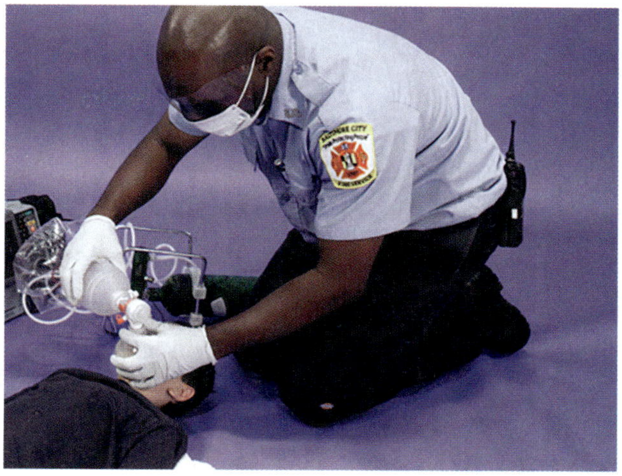

FIGURE 14-22 Open the child's airway and provide rescue breathing.

Head Tilt–Chin Lift Maneuver

Perform the head tilt–chin lift maneuver in a child in the following manner:

1. Place one hand on the child's forehead, and tilt the head back gently, with the neck slightly extended.
2. Place two or three fingers (not the thumb) of your other hand under the child's chin, and lift the jaw upward and outward. Do not close the mouth or push under the chin; either move may obstruct rather than open the airway.
3. Remove any visible foreign body or vomitus.

Jaw-Thrust Maneuver

Perform the jaw-thrust maneuver in a child in the following manner:

1. Place two or three fingers under each side of the angle of the lower jaw; lift the jaw upward and outward.
2. If the jaw thrust alone does not open the airway and cervical spine injury is not a consideration, then tilt the head slightly. If cervical spine injury is suspected, then use a second rescuer to immobilize the cervical spine.

Remember that the head of an infant or young child is disproportionately large in comparison with the chest and shoulders. As a result, when a child is lying flat on their back, especially on a backboard, the head will bend forward (hyperflexion) onto the upper chest. This position can partially or completely obstruct the upper airway. To avoid this possibility, place padding under the child's upper back and shoulders (torso).

Providing Rescue Breathing to Children

If the child is not breathing but has a pulse, then open the airway and deliver one breath every 2 to 3 seconds (20 to 30 breaths/min) (**FIGURE 14-22**). If the child is not breathing and does not have a pulse, then deliver two rescue breaths after every 30 chest compressions (15 chest compressions if two rescuers are present). Each ventilation should last approximately 1 second and should produce visible chest rise. Use the proper-size mask and bag and ensure an adequate mask-to-face seal.

If an infant or small child is breathing, then provide prompt transport. Again, a child who is in respiratory distress should be allowed to stay in whatever position is most comfortable. Children who are unresponsive but breathing with difficulty should be kept in a position that allows you to manage the airway and provide ventilatory support, if needed.

> **Words of Wisdom**
>
> An injured child with a serious airway or breathing problem is likely to need full-time attention from at least two EMS clinicians. Therefore, it is important for you to call for any additional resources you need as soon as possible, perhaps even before you arrive at the scene. In such cases, you will need a driver and often ALS for optimum patient care.

Using an AED in Infants and Children

EMS calls relating to chest pain or cardiac arrest in infants and children are uncommon. Chest pain is usually the result of respiratory failure and not a primary cardiac event. Cardiac emergencies are usually associated with a noncardiac condition or with a child who has a preexisting heart condition, which is usually congenital (present since birth). In pediatric situations, it is vital to see family members or caregivers as a valuable source of information.

The AHA has determined that AEDs are safe to use in infants and children. If ALS is on the scene and it will not delay the shock administration, manual defibrillation is preferred to an AED. When ALS is not on the scene, if the patient is 8 years old or younger, pediatric-size pads and a dose-attenuating system (energy reducer) are preferred when using the AED. If these items are unavailable, use adult-size AED pads. Apply the AED to infants or children as soon as it becomes available. If you use adult-size AED pads on an infant or small child, do not cut the pads to adjust the size. Instead, use the anterior–posterior (front and back, over the heart) placement, following the manufacturer's recommendation.

Some clinicians may be hesitant to use "adult" levels of energy with the AED to defibrillate an infant or child, but it is important to keep in mind that the damage caused by a child remaining in cardiac arrest will always be far worse than any damage caused by "adult" levels of energy to defibrillate.

Remember, if the child is past the onset of puberty, follow the adult CPR sequence, including the use of adult-size AED pads.

Interrupting CPR

Try not to interrupt CPR for more than 10 seconds, except when it is absolutely necessary. For example, if you have to move a patient up or down stairs, you should continue CPR until you arrive at the head or foot of the stairs, interrupt CPR at a mutually agreed-on signal, and move quickly to the next level where you can resume CPR. Do not move the patient until all transport arrangements are made so that interruptions to CPR can be kept to a minimum. See Chapter 8, *Lifting and Moving Patients*, to review patient lifting and moving techniques.

Chest compression fraction is the total percentage of time during a high-quality CPR resuscitation attempt in which chest compressions are being performed. Make every effort to maintain a chest compression fraction greater than 80% (the higher the better). The more frequent the interruptions in chest compressions, the lower the compression fraction will be. Low compression fractions lead to worse patient outcomes. Most modern cardiac monitors will provide information about chest compression fraction that you can review after a cardiac arrest. If possible, routinely review this information after every arrest so that you can learn ways to improve the chest compression fraction and improve on other key performance indicators.

Determining Not to Start CPR

As an EMT, it is your responsibility to start CPR on virtually all patients you encounter who are in cardiac arrest. There are only three general exceptions to this rule.

First, do not start CPR if the scene is unsafe. The concept of ensuring scene safety applies in cardiac arrest situations, just as it does on any other call.

Second, do not start CPR if the patient has obvious signs of death. Obvious signs of death include absence of a pulse and breathing, along with any one of the following findings:

- Rigor mortis, or stiffening of the body after death
- Dependent lividity (livor mortis), a discoloration of the skin caused by pooling of blood
- Putrefaction (decomposition of the body tissues)

- Evidence of nonsurvivable injury, such as decapitation, dismemberment, or being burned beyond recognition.

Rigor mortis and dependent lividity develop after a patient has been dead for a long period.

Third, do not start CPR if the patient and the patient's physician have previously agreed on a do not attempt resuscitation (DNAR) order or no-CPR order. DNAR orders give you permission not to attempt resuscitation. This may apply only to situations in which the patient is known to be in the terminal stage of an incurable disease. In this situation, CPR would only prolong the patient's death. However, end-of-life issues can be complicated. Advance directives, such as living wills and physician orders for life-sustaining treatment (POLST) may express the patient's wishes; however, these documents may not be readily producible by the patient's family or caregiver. In such cases, the safest course is to begin CPR under the rule of implied consent and then contact medical direction for further guidance. However, if a valid DNAR document, living will, or POLST is produced, resuscitative efforts may be withheld. Learn your local protocols and the standards in your EMS system for treating terminally ill patients. Some EMS systems have electronic notes on patients who are preregistered with the system. These notes usually specify the amount and extent of treatment that is desired. Other states have specific DNAR and POLST forms that allow EMS clinicians to withhold care when the patient, family, and physician have agreed in advance that such a course is most appropriate. It is essential that you understand your local protocols and are aware of the specific restrictions these advance directives imply.

In virtually all other cases, begin CPR on anyone who is in cardiac arrest. Factors such as air temperature and the basic health of the tissues and organs can affect the patient's ability to survive. Most legal advisers recommend that, when in doubt, always give too much care rather than too little care. Therefore, always start CPR if any doubt exists.

Obvious signs of death and documentation relating to end-of-life decisions are described further in Chapter 3, *Medical, Legal, and Ethical Issues.*

Stopping CPR

As an EMT, you are generally not responsible for making the decision to stop CPR. After you begin CPR in the field, you must continue until one of the following events occurs (the STOP mnemonic):

- **S** The patient Starts breathing and has a pulse.
- **T** The patient's care is Transferred to another clinician of equal or higher-level training.

YOU are the EMT

After 2 minutes of CPR, you reanalyze the patient's cardiac rhythm and receive a "no shock advised" message. Your partner and the other EMT immediately resume CPR. During CPR, your partner ventilates the patient with a bag-mask device and high-concentration oxygen. As your partner attempts to insert an oral airway, the patient starts to gag. You quickly reassess the patient.

Recording Time: 7 Minutes	
Level of consciousness	Unresponsive
Respirations	Occasional agonal gasps; 4 breaths/min
Pulse	100 beats/min; strong carotid pulse; absent radial pulses
Skin	Skin color is improving
Blood pressure	70/40 mm Hg
Oxygen saturation (Spo_2)	82% (on oxygen)

7. How should you continue to treat this patient?
8. Because the patient is no longer in cardiac arrest, should you remove the AED pads? Why or why not?

- **O** You are Out of strength or too tired to continue CPR.
- **P** A Physician who is present or providing online medical direction assumes responsibility for the patient and directs you to discontinue CPR.

Out of strength means that you are no longer physically able to perform CPR. It does not mean merely weary. If fatigue can be managed by changing the person performing compressions every 2 minutes, per the usual CPR process, then CPR should be continued. In short, always continue CPR until the patient's care is transferred to a physician or higher medical authority in the field. In some cases, your medical director or a designated medical oversight clinician may order you to stop CPR on the basis of the patient's condition. ALS clinicians under Termination of Resuscitation (TOR) protocols may cease resuscitation efforts without online medical direction under specific situations.

Every EMS system should have clear standing orders or protocols that provide guidelines for starting and stopping CPR. Your medical director and your system's legal adviser should agree on these protocols, which should be closely administered and reviewed by your medical director.

Words of Wisdom

The BLS criteria for TOR differ from the ALS criteria. In addition to contacting medical direction, BLS criteria include the following three rules[8,9]:

- Unwitnessed by EMS
- No AED or shock delivered
- No ROSC

ALS criteria include the three BLS rules plus the following additional two rules:

- Unwitnessed by bystander
- No bystander CPR

Words of Wisdom

Patients who do not achieve ROSC may be potential organ donors in select situations (ie, short transport times, rapid access to an organ recovery program). Follow your local protocols regarding the care of potential organ donors.

Documentation and Communication

If you choose not to start CPR on a patient in cardiac arrest, then always comply with your local protocols and provide detailed documentation. In particular, record the physical examination signs that led to your decision and reference the protocol that states these signs are a reason not to start CPR. If special circumstances physically prevent you from making resuscitation attempts (eg, if the patient is entrapped in a vehicle), then document the scene conditions thoroughly. These decisions occasionally raise questions that can be put to rest immediately with reference to a well-written report. See Chapter 4, *Communications and Documentation*, for more information.

Foreign Body Airway Obstruction in Adults

Occasionally, a large foreign body will be aspirated and block the upper airway. An airway obstruction may be caused by various factors, including relaxation of the throat muscles in an unresponsive patient, vomited or regurgitated stomach contents, blood, damaged tissue after an injury, dentures, or foreign bodies such as food or small objects.

Large objects that are visible but cannot be removed from the airway with suction, such as loose dentures, large pieces of food, or blood clots, should be swept forward and out with your gloved index finger. Suctioning can then be used as needed to keep the airway clear of thinner secretions such as blood, vomitus, and mucus.

Recognizing Foreign Body Airway Obstruction

An airway obstruction by a foreign body in an adult usually occurs during a meal. In children, it usually occurs during mealtime or at play. If the foreign body is not removed quickly, then the lungs will not be oxygenated, and unconsciousness and death will follow. Management is based on the severity of the airway obstruction.

Mild Airway Obstruction

Patients with a mild (partial) airway obstruction are able to exchange adequate amounts of air, but still have signs of respiratory distress. Breathing may be noisy; however, the patient usually has a strong, effective cough. Encourage the patient to continue coughing. Your main concern is to prevent a mild airway obstruction from becoming a severe (complete) airway obstruction. Abdominal thrusts are *not* indicated for patients with a mild airway obstruction.

For the patient with a mild airway obstruction, first encourage the patient to cough or to continue coughing if they are already doing so. Do not interfere with the patient's own attempts to expel the foreign body. Instead, give supplemental oxygen if needed and provide prompt transport to the emergency department (ED). Closely monitor the patient and observe for signs of a severe airway obstruction (weak or absent cough, decreasing level of consciousness, cyanosis).

Severe Airway Obstruction in Responsive Patients

A sudden, severe airway obstruction is usually easy to recognize in someone who is eating or has just finished eating. The person is suddenly unable to speak or cough, grasps the throat, becomes cyanotic, and makes exaggerated efforts to breathe. Either air is not moving into and out of the airway, or the air movement is so slight that it is not detectable. At first, the patient will be responsive and able to clearly indicate the problem. Ask the patient, "Are you choking?" The patient will usually answer by nodding yes. Alternatively, the person may use the universal sign to indicate airway blockage (**FIGURE 14-23**).

If there is a minimal amount of air movement, you may hear a high-pitched sound on inspiration called **stridor**. This occurs when the object is not fully blocking the airway, but the small amount of air entering the lungs is not enough to sustain life and the patient will eventually become unconscious if the obstruction is not relieved.

Severe Airway Obstruction in Unresponsive Patients

When you discover an unresponsive patient, your first step is to determine whether the person is breathing and has a pulse. The unconsciousness may be caused by airway obstruction, cardiac arrest, or a number of other conditions. If the patient has a pulse, but is not breathing, then you must make sure that the airway is open and unobstructed.

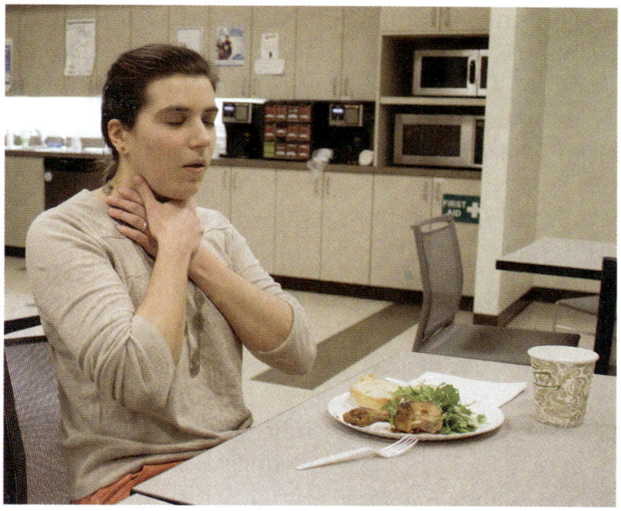

FIGURE 14-23 Placing the hands at the throat is the universal sign to indicate choking.

You should suspect an airway obstruction if the standard maneuvers to open the airway and ventilate the lungs are ineffective. If you feel resistance when attempting to ventilate, the patient probably has some type of obstruction.

Removing a Foreign Body Airway Obstruction in an Adult

The manual maneuvers recommended for removing severe airway obstructions in responsive adults and children older than 1 year are back slaps and the **abdominal thrust maneuver** (also called the Heimlich maneuver). Back slaps are performed by leaning the person forward and striking them between the shoulder blades with the heel of the open hand. If five back slaps do not dislodge the object, they are followed by five abdominal thrusts. This technique creates an artificial cough by causing a sudden increase in intrathoracic pressure when thrusts are applied to the subdiaphragmatic region; it is a very effective method for removing a foreign body obstruction from the airway. If the patient with a severe airway obstruction is unresponsive, then perform chest compressions.

Responsive Patients

Abdominal Thrust Maneuver

The goal of the abdominal-thrust maneuver is to compress the lungs upward and force residual air from the lungs to flow upward and expel the object.

In responsive patients with a severe airway obstruction, repeat the cycle of back slaps and abdominal thrusts until the foreign body is expelled or the patient becomes unresponsive. Each thrust should be deliberate, with the intent of relieving the obstruction.

To perform abdominal thrusts on a responsive adult (**FIGURE 14-24**), use the following technique:

1. Standing behind the patient, first lean the patient forward and deliver five back slaps with the heel of one hand between the shoulder blades. If the object is not dislodged, wrap your arms around their abdomen. Place one of your legs between the patient's legs. This will allow you to easily slide the patient to the ground if they become unresponsive.
2. Make a fist with one hand; grasp the fist with the other hand. Place the thumb side of the fist against the patient's abdomen just above the umbilicus and well below the xiphoid process.
3. Press your fist into the patient's abdomen with a quick inward and upward thrust.
4. Continue this cycle of five back slaps and five abdominal thrusts until the object is expelled from the airway or the patient becomes unresponsive.

Chest Thrusts

You can perform the abdominal thrust maneuver safely on all adults and children. However, for women in advanced stages of pregnancy and patients who have obesity, use chest thrusts instead.

To perform chest thrusts on the responsive adult, use the following technique (**FIGURE 14-25**):

1. Standing behind the patient, first deliver five back slaps. If the object is not dislodged, place your arms directly under the patient's armpits and wrap your arms around the patient's chest.
2. Make a fist with one hand; grasp the fist with the other hand. Place the thumb side of the fist against the patient's sternum, avoiding the xiphoid process and the edges of the rib cage.

Words of Wisdom

If a responsive choking patient is found lying on the floor, then administer abdominal thrusts by placing one leg between the patient's legs, placing your hands just above the umbilicus, and giving rapid thrusts inward and upward under the rib cage, using the heel of your hand with your other hand on top of it.

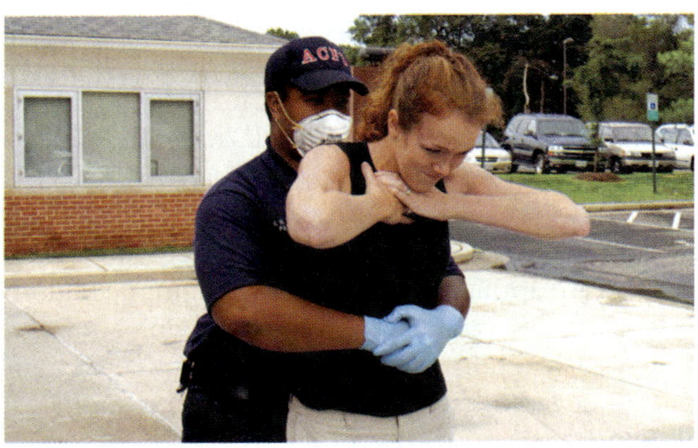

FIGURE 14-24 The abdominal thrust maneuver in a responsive adult. Stand behind the patient and wrap your arms around the patient's abdomen. Place the thumb side of one fist against the patient's abdomen while holding your fist with your other hand. Press your fists into the patient's abdomen, using inward and upward thrusts.

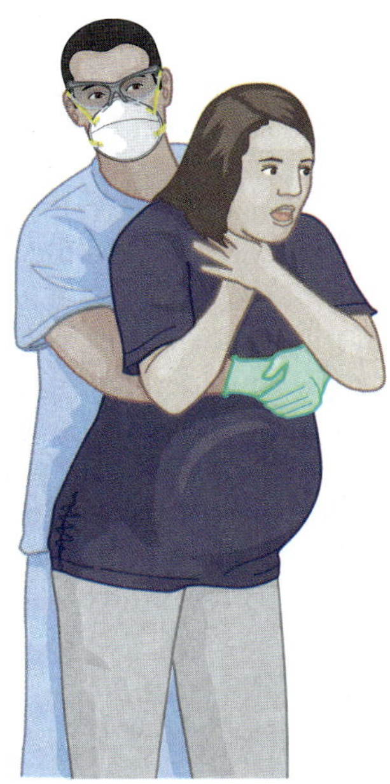

FIGURE 14-25 Removal of a foreign body obstruction in a responsive adult using chest thrusts. Stand behind the patient and wrap your arms around the patient's chest. Place the thumb side of one fist against the chest while holding your fist with your other hand. Press your fists into the patient's chest with backward thrusts.

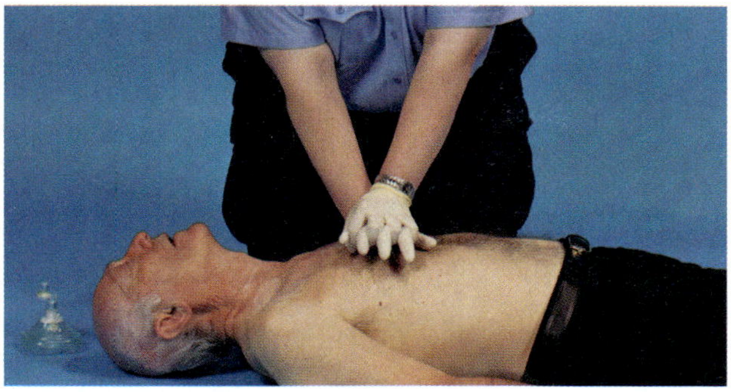

FIGURE 14-26 An unresponsive patient with an airway obstruction requires CPR.

3. Press your fist into the patient's chest with backward thrusts, continuing this cycle of five back slaps and five chest thrusts until the object is expelled or the patient becomes unresponsive.
4. If the patient becomes unresponsive, then begin CPR, starting with chest compressions (**FIGURE 14-26**).

Responsive Patients Who Become Unresponsive

A patient with an airway obstruction may become unresponsive while you are attempting to remove the obstruction. In this case, begin CPR, starting with chest compressions. Use the following steps to manage the patient's airway obstruction:

1. Carefully support the patient to the ground and immediately call for help (or send someone to call for help).
2. Perform 30 chest compressions, using the same landmark as you would for CPR (center of the chest, on the lower half of the sternum). Do not check for a pulse before performing chest compressions.
3. Open the airway and look in the mouth. If you see an object that can easily be removed, then remove it with your fingers and attempt to ventilate. If you do not see an object, then resume chest compressions.
4. Repeat steps 2 and 3 until the obstruction is relieved or ALS clinicians take over.

If you are able to remove an object from the mouth, then attempt to ventilate. If ventilation produces chest rise, then continue to ventilate and check for a pulse. If a pulse is present but the patient is not breathing, then continue rescue breathing and monitor the pulse. If a pulse is absent, then continue CPR (compressions and ventilations) and apply the AED as soon as it is available.

Unresponsive Patients

When a patient is found unresponsive, you may not know what caused the problem. Begin CPR by determining unresponsiveness and checking for breathing and a pulse simultaneously. If a pulse is present but breathing is absent, then open the airway and attempt to ventilate. If the first ventilation does not produce visible chest rise, then reposition the airway and reattempt to ventilate. If both ventilation attempts do not produce visible chest rise, then perform 30 chest compressions, and then open the airway and look in the mouth. If an object is visible and can easily be removed, then remove it with your fingers and attempt to ventilate. Never perform blind finger sweeps on any patient; doing so may push the obstruction farther into the airway. If an object is not visible or cannot easily be removed, then resume chest compressions. Continue the sequence of chest compressions, opening the airway, and looking inside the mouth until the airway is clear or ALS clinicians arrive.

Foreign Body Airway Obstruction in Infants and Children

As mentioned previously, airway obstruction is a common problem in infants and children, usually caused by a foreign body (such as food or a toy) or by an infection, resulting in swelling and narrowing of the airway. Try to identify the cause of the obstruction as soon as possible. In patients who have signs and symptoms of an airway infection, do not waste time trying to dislodge a foreign body. Administer supplemental oxygen if needed and immediately transport the child to the ED.

A previously healthy child who is eating or playing with small toys or an infant who is crawling about the house and who suddenly has difficulty breathing has probably aspirated a foreign body. As in adults, foreign bodies may cause a mild or a severe airway obstruction.

With a mild airway obstruction, the child can cough forcefully, although they may wheeze

Words of Wisdom

If you arrive at the scene and find that the infant or child is not breathing or has cyanosis, then immediate management (including rescue breathing and supplemental oxygen) is essential. Consider requesting additional assistance, if available. If air enters freely with your initial breaths and the chest rises, then the airway is clear. If air does not enter freely, then check the airway for obstruction. Reposition the patient to open the airway, and attempt to give another breath. If air still does not enter freely, then you must take steps to relieve the obstruction.

between coughs. As long as the patient can breathe, cough, or talk, do not interfere with their attempts to expel the foreign body. As with an adult, encourage the child to continue coughing. Administer supplemental oxygen if needed (and tolerated) and provide transport to the ED.

You should intervene only if signs of a severe airway obstruction develop, such as a weak, ineffective cough; cyanosis; stridor; absent air movement; or a decreasing level of consciousness.

Removing a Foreign Body Airway Obstruction in Children

Responsive Patients

If you determine a child older than 1 year has an airway obstruction, then stand or kneel behind the child and provide back slaps and abdominal thrusts in the same manner as an adult, but use less force, until the object is expelled or the child becomes unresponsive. If the child becomes unresponsive, then follow the same steps as for the unresponsive adult.

To clear an airway obstruction in a responsive child who is in a standing or sitting position, follow these steps (**FIGURE 14-27**):

1. Kneel on one knee behind the child. Support the child's chest with one hand as you give five back slaps with the heel of one hand between the shoulder blades. If the object is not dislodged, circle both of your arms around the child's body. Prepare to give abdominal thrusts by placing your fist just above the patient's umbilicus and well below the xiphoid process. Place your other hand over that fist.
2. Give the child abdominal thrusts in an upward direction. Avoid applying force to the lower rib cage or sternum.

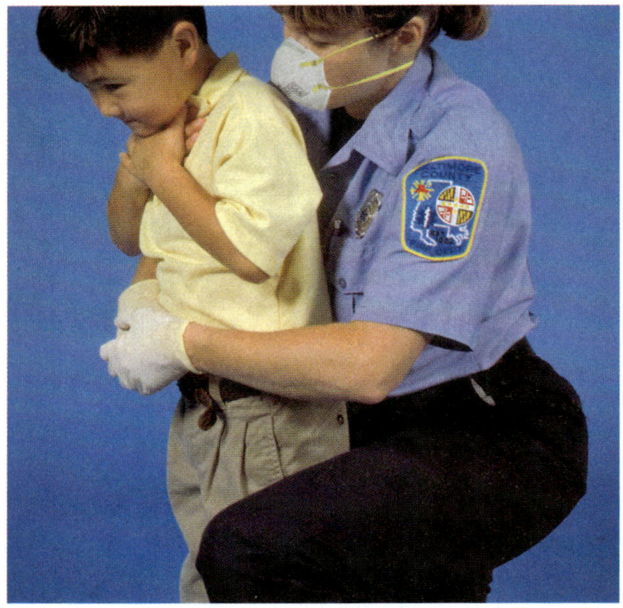

FIGURE 14-27 To perform the abdominal thrust maneuver on a child, kneel behind the child on one knee, wrap your arms around the child's body, and place your fist just above the umbilicus and well below the lower tip of the sternum.

3. Repeat this cycle of five back slaps and five abdominal thrusts until the child expels the foreign body or becomes unresponsive.
4. If the child becomes unresponsive, position the child on a hard surface and immediately call for help (or send someone to call for help).
5. Perform 30 chest compressions (15 compressions if two rescuers are present), using the same landmark as you would for CPR. Do not check for a pulse before performing chest compressions.
6. Open the airway and look inside the mouth. If you see an object that can easily be removed, then remove it with your fingers and attempt to ventilate. If you do not see an object, then resume chest compressions.
7. Repeat steps 5 and 6 until the obstruction is relieved or ALS clinicians take over.

Words of Wisdom

It is possible that you will see a bystander or law enforcement officer use a suction-type device on patients older than 1 year to attempt to remove a foreign body airway obstruction. Currently, the AHA does not find sufficient evidence to recommend the use of suction-based airway clearance devices.[1]

If you manage to clear the airway obstruction in an unresponsive child who continues to have no spontaneous breathing or circulation, then perform CPR (compressions and ventilations) and apply the AED as soon as it is available.

Unresponsive Patients

Care for a child older than 1 year who has an airway obstruction and becomes unresponsive is the same as care provided for an adult. **SKILL DRILL 14-7** demonstrates the steps for removing a foreign body airway obstruction in an unresponsive child:

1. Take standard precautions. Carefully place the child in a supine position on a firm, flat surface (**Step 1**).
2. Perform 30 chest compressions (15 compressions if two rescuers are present), using the same landmark as you would for CPR (lower half of the sternum). Do not check for a pulse before performing chest compressions (**Step 2**).
3. Open the airway and look in the mouth (**Step 3**).
4. If you see an object that can easily be removed, then remove it with your fingers and attempt to ventilate (**Step 4**).
5. If you do not see an object, then resume chest compressions.
6. Repeat the sequence of chest compressions, opening the airway, and looking inside the mouth until the obstruction is relieved or ALS clinicians take over (**Step 5**).

Removing a Foreign Body Airway Obstruction in Infants

Responsive Patients

Do not use abdominal thrusts on a responsive infant with an airway obstruction because of the risk of injury to the immature organs of the abdomen. Instead, perform back slaps and chest thrusts to try to clear a severe airway obstruction in a responsive infant, as follows:

1. Hold the infant facedown, with the body resting on your forearm. Support the infant's jaw and face with your hand and keep the head lower than the rest of the body.
2. Deliver five back slaps between the shoulder blades, using the heel of your hand (**FIGURE 14-28A**).
3. Place your free hand behind the infant's head and back and turn the infant faceup on your other forearm and thigh, sandwiching the infant's body between your two hands and arms. The infant's head should remain below the level of the body.
4. Give five quick chest thrusts in the same location as chest compressions (**FIGURE 14-28B**). Use the heel of one hand, using two thumbs placed on the lower half of the sternum. For larger infants, or if you have small hands, you can perform this step by placing the infant in your lap and turning the infant's whole

YOU are the EMT

You and your partner secure the patient to the cot, load him into the ambulance, and begin transport to a hospital located 5 miles away with one of the other EMTs to assist you. En route, you reassess the patient and then call your radio report to the receiving hospital.

Recording Time: 12 Minutes	
Level of consciousness	Unresponsive
Respirations	8 breaths/min; shallow depth
Pulse	94 beats/min; strong carotid pulse, weak radial pulses
Skin	Circulation assessed as adequate by examination of mucous membranes inside the inner lower eyelid and capillary refill with skin cool and dry
Blood pressure	86/66 mm Hg
Oxygen saturation (Spo_2)	95% (on oxygen)

9. Is ALS care likely to benefit your patient at this point?

10. What further treatment, if any, is indicated for this patient?

Skill Drill 14-7 Removing a Foreign Body Airway Obstruction in an Unresponsive Child

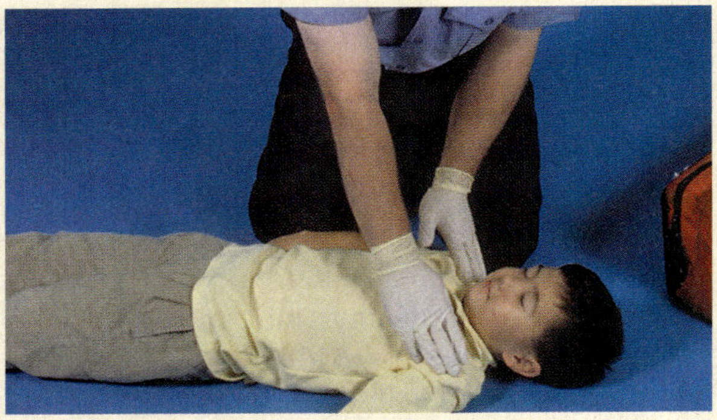

Step 1

Take standard precautions. Position the child on a firm, flat surface.

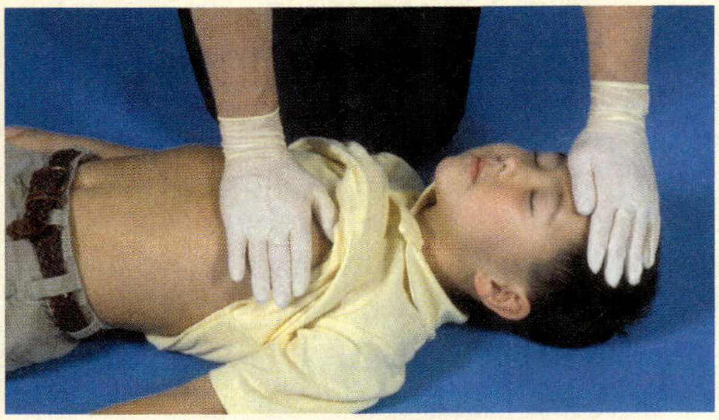

Step 2

Perform chest compressions using the same landmark as you would for CPR.

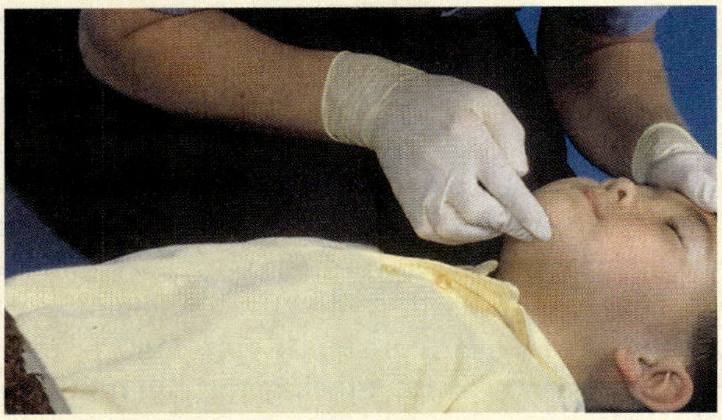

Step 3

Open the airway and look inside the mouth.

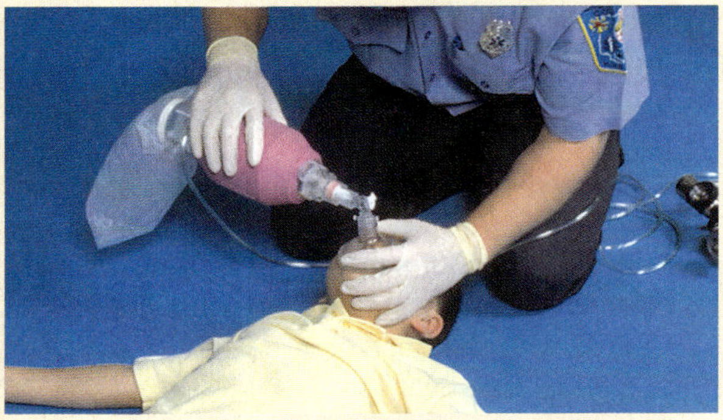

Step 4

If an object is visible and can easily be removed, then remove it with your fingers and attempt rescue breathing.

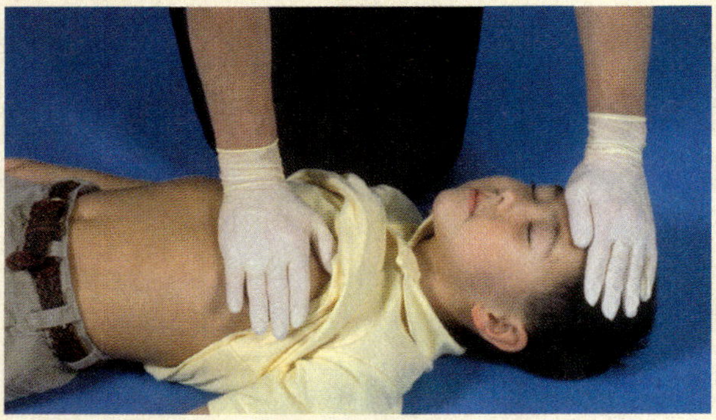

Step 5

If you do not see an object in the mouth, then resume chest compressions. Continue the sequence of chest compressions, opening the airway, and looking inside the mouth until the obstruction is relieved or ALS clinicians take over.

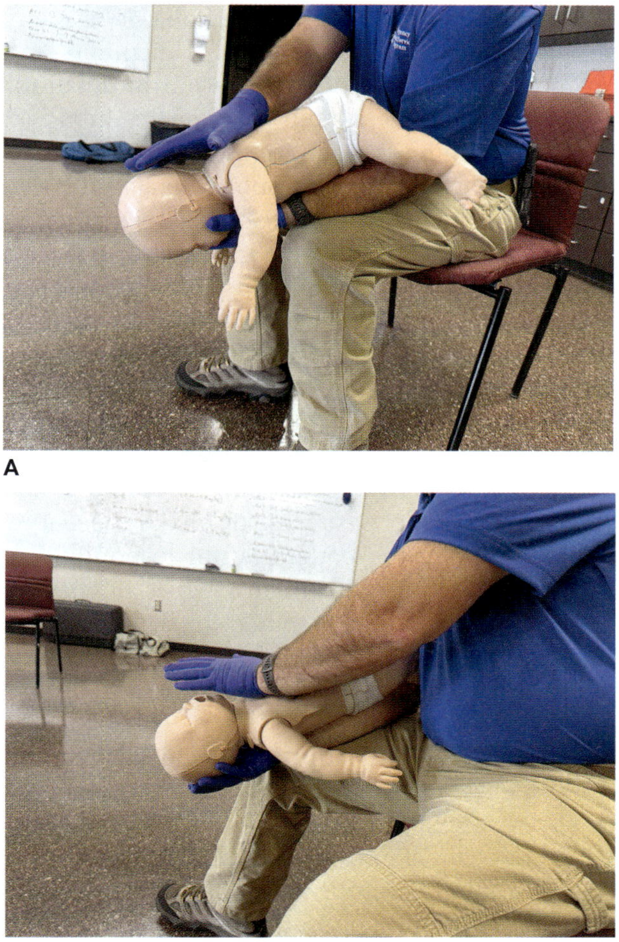

A

B

FIGURE 14-28 A. Delivering back slaps to the infant. **B.** Providing chest thrusts to the infant.

Courtesy of Rhonda Hunt.

body as a unit between back slaps and chest thrusts.

5. Check the airway. If you can see the foreign body, then remove it. If not, then repeat the cycle as often as necessary.
6. If the infant becomes unresponsive, then begin CPR and follow the same sequence as for a child and adult.

Unresponsive Patients

If the infant becomes unresponsive during your attempts to relieve an airway obstruction, then perform CPR starting with chest compressions. Do not check for a pulse before starting compressions. Open the airway and look in the mouth. If you see an object that can easily be removed, then remove it with your finger and attempt to ventilate; if you do not see an object, then resume chest compressions. Continue the sequence of chest compressions, opening the airway, and looking inside the mouth until the obstruction is relieved or ALS clinicians take over.

Special Resuscitation Circumstances

Opioid Overdose

An opioid, when taken in excess, depresses the central nervous system and causes respiratory arrest followed by cardiac arrest. Examples of opioids include heroin and oxycodone. If you suspect opioid poisoning in a patient who is in cardiac arrest, you may consider administering naloxone after beginning effective CPR and using the AED.[7] Opioids are discussed further in Chapter 22, *Toxicology*.

Cardiac Arrest in Pregnancy

If you encounter a pregnant patient who is in cardiac arrest, then your priorities are to provide high-quality CPR and relieve pressure from the aorta and inferior vena cava. When the patient lies supine, the pregnant uterus can compress the aorta and vena cava (aortocaval compression). Compression of the vena cava causes a significant decrease in blood return to the heart and, secondarily, in the forward flow of blood to the vital organs.

A pregnant patient who is not in cardiac arrest should be positioned on the left side to relieve pressure on the great vessels. However, if the patient is in cardiac arrest, then this approach is impractical, because the individual must remain in a supine position to maximize the effectiveness of compressions. Therefore, if the top of the patient's uterus (fundus) can be felt at or above the level of the umbilicus, perform manual displacement of the uterus to the patient's left to relieve aortocaval compression while CPR is being performed. This step will improve the effectiveness of compressions (**FIGURE 14-29**).

Lazarus Syndrome

In rare cases, patients who have been pronounced dead are found to have regained a pulse, and in a few instances, this occurred even after transport to a morgue or funeral home. In some of these situations, insufficient assessment in the health care setting was deemed to be the cause. In other cases,

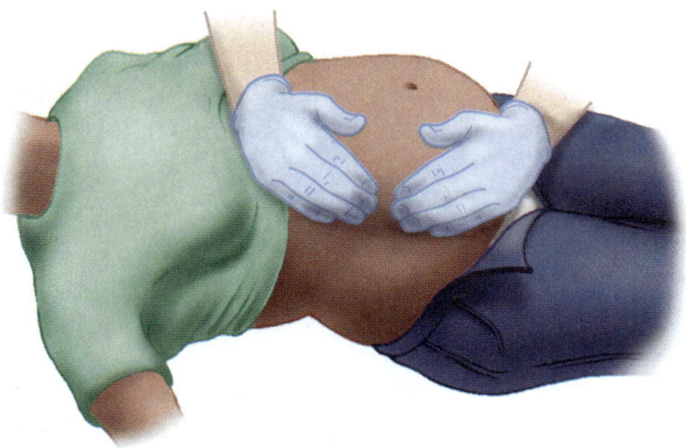

FIGURE 14-29 Manual left displacement of the uterus. The two-handed technique is shown. Alternatively, one hand can be used.

a phenomenon known as Lazarus syndrome, or autoresuscitation, has been implicated. Autoresuscitation refers to the spontaneous return of cardiac activity after the patient has been presumed or pronounced dead.

In general, one or two cases of Lazarus syndrome have been documented each year since the 1980s, and it has been found to occur for virtually all causes of cardiac arrest.[8] The exact causes of Lazarus syndrome are unknown.

While encountering this phenomenon is rare, it underscores the importance of thorough assessment and continuous monitoring during resuscitation efforts. To mitigate the risk of Lazarus syndrome, EMTs should consider monitoring the patient for at least 10 minutes after the cessation of resuscitation efforts.[10] Additionally, clear documentation of resuscitation attempts, including the duration and interventions performed, is essential.

Grief Support for Family Members and Loved Ones

Whenever you assist a patient, remember that the patient's loved ones will also be affected by the emergency. Serious illness, injury, and pediatric patients create an especially high level of anxiety for family members. A health emergency is often hard for family members to understand. In some cases, family members may experience a psychological crisis that turns into a medical crisis, and may become patients themselves.

Whereas a cardiac arrest may be one of many similar calls in your career, family members and loved ones will remember this event in detail for the rest of their lives. Your reaction to them will form a lasting impression. Conversely, a mismanaged death notification or poor interaction could leave the family feeling disrespected or ignored. A compassionate and sensitive approach will leave a positive impression of you and your agency. Most important, appropriate and supportive care at the onset of grief may positively affect the family's grieving process.

Families do not typically expect EMS clinicians to stop resuscitation and leave their loved one on scene. When death appears imminent and resuscitative efforts are unsuccessful, make the family members aware the patient is not responding to treatment. Discuss with them what is happening so they may be better prepared for the inevitable. Keep the family informed throughout the resuscitation process because it may also help them feel more in control.

Sequential notification starts during resuscitative efforts; family members should be updated as the resuscitation progresses, if possible. Designate one clinician to communicate the patient's status to family members, so that information is streamlined from one source rather than from multiple clinicians. Be concise and clear. For example, say, "Your husband is not breathing and his heart has stopped. We are attempting to restart his heart with the AED." After resuscitation efforts have stopped, it is appropriate to tell them, "As you know, when we arrived, your husband wasn't breathing and did not have a pulse. He has not responded to any of our treatments. I'm sorry, but he has died." Avoid euphemisms such as "passed away" or "passed on," because these expressions

Street Smarts

Allowing family members to watch the resuscitation may be beneficial to their emotional healing. Have a clinician sit or stand with the person and explain the process. If it does not interfere with resuscitation attempts and the family member wishes, they may be allowed to hold the loved one's hand or tell the person goodbye before termination of resuscitation efforts.

may be confusing or misinterpreted. Law enforcement personnel may be involved in the official death declaration and will likely be responsible for what happens next, such as determining whether the medical examiner should be notified. See Chapter 4, *Communications and Documentation*, for a detailed discussion of death notification.

Another consideration is to ensure that children are not ignored. They may not understand death. Preschool-age children may be less affected, whereas older children understand death but do not expect it to happen to someone they know. Younger children tend to blame themselves. Teenagers may be highly affected but may mask their feelings.

Last, consider your own feelings in this stressful situation and make sure you seek assistance if needed. See Chapter 2, *Workforce Safety and Wellness*, for a discussion of the emotional aspects of emergency care and stress management.

Education and Training for the EMT

You may go weeks or months without performing CPR on a human, depending on how busy your EMS system is. Like any skill, CPR skills can deteriorate over time. You must practice them often using manikin-based training; ideally, you will practice more frequently than the standard retraining that occurs every 2 years.

During training, the use of manikins that provide feedback about the quality of CPR is encouraged, if your system's budget allows. CPR devices that provide corrective feedback are preferred over devices that only provide voice prompts (ie, a metronome).

CPR self-instruction through video and/or computer-based modules with hands-on practice may be a reasonable alternative to instructor-led courses, because it may facilitate frequent retraining.

Education and Training for the Public

As an EMT, you are a patient advocate. Not only are you responsible for providing the best possible care for your patient, but you must also do your part to facilitate the training of laypeople in the critical skills of CPR and AED operation. Training in CPR and AED usage should not be limited to health care clinicians. Not enough laypeople are trained to perform these lifesaving skills.

As discussed previously, many laypeople assume CPR requires both mouth-to-mouth rescue breathing and chest compressions. As long as this misconception remains, fewer people will be willing to help during an emergency, which means that fewer lives will be saved. If you are asked to train members of your community how to perform compression-only CPR, then you should consider it your professional responsibility and be willing to assist.

It is likely that some citizens in your service area are at increased risk for cardiac arrest. Your agency should make an effort to identify these potential patients and educate their families to recognize cardiac arrest and to train them to perform compression-only CPR.

YOU are the EMT SUMMARY

1. What should you immediately do on receiving this update from dispatch?

After you are informed that CPR is in progress, you should immediately request additional assistance if it has not already been dispatched. Effective treatment of a patient in cardiac arrest requires adequate personnel at the scene and during transport. As an EMT, you must be familiar with the resources that are available to you and know when it is appropriate to request them. If your system protocols permit, bystanders who are performing high-quality chest compressions can assist until other help arrives so the compressors can alternate every 2 minutes.

Regardless of the resources available to you, request them as soon as possible—in this case, as soon as you are advised that CPR is in progress. One EMT cannot effectively treat a patient in cardiac arrest during transport; you would have to perform

YOU are the EMT SUMMARY continued

continuous CPR while your partner drives the ambulance (or vice versa), which could result in rescuer fatigue and decreased effectiveness of chest compressions.

2. What should be your initial actions on arriving at this scene?

After ensuring your own safety, approach this patient as you would any other patient, by performing a primary assessment. Although the dispatcher has advised you that bystander CPR is in progress, you must still assess the patient to confirm he is indeed apneic and pulseless and requires CPR.

Your primary assessment should take only a few seconds, just long enough to confirm the patient is in cardiac arrest. If he is in cardiac arrest, then begin CPR immediately, apply the AED as soon as it is available, and analyze the patient's cardiac rhythm. To avoid interrupting CPR, you should apply the AED as chest compressions are being performed (do not stop compressions to do this).

If the AED advises you to shock, then deliver the shock as soon as your partner eliminates any contact with the patient and immediately resume CPR, starting with chest compressions. If the AED does not advise you to shock, then immediately resume CPR, starting with chest compressions. During CPR, ask the two bystanders if they witnessed the event and determine whether they know anything about the patient (ie, past medical history, events leading up to the cardiac arrest).

Regardless of how a call is dispatched and whether or not you are assuming patient care from bystanders or other health care clinicians, it is important for you to always perform a primary assessment of the patient.

3. What links in the chain of survival have been maintained at this point?

The following links in the chain of survival have been established or maintained:

- *Recognition and activation of the emergency response system*, because the bystanders quickly recognized the patient was experiencing a cardiac emergency and immediately called 9-1-1.
- *Immediate, high-quality CPR*, because the bystanders began CPR directly after calling 9-1-1.

The following links in the chain of survival have not been maintained:

- *Rapid defibrillation*, because it has not yet occurred. Of all the links in the chain of survival, early defibrillation has the most profound effect on patient survival. With early access and early CPR, defibrillation may successfully terminate lethal cardiac dysrhythmias in a significant number of patients. For each minute that defibrillation is delayed, the patient's chance for survival decreases by 7% to 10%.
- *Advanced EMS*, because advanced care, such as IV access and medication administration, has not been started.
- *Post–cardiac arrest care*, because ROSC has not been established and the patient has not arrived at the hospital.
- *Recovery and survivorship*, because it takes place after all the links have been maintained.

4. Why is it so critical to minimize interruptions in CPR?

Even when CPR is performed correctly (that is, at a rate of 100 to 120 compressions per minute at a depth of 2 inches [5 cm] in the adult, with full chest recoil), chest compressions deliver only about one-third of a person's normal cardiac output. When CPR is performed properly and with minimal interruption, it is often enough to keep the patient's vital organs viable until defibrillation and more advanced care can be provided at the scene or at the ED. Of course, this assumes that defibrillation and advanced care are provided within a short period.

Within a few seconds of stopping chest compressions, the pressure generated in the arteries drops to near zero; therefore, frequent or prolonged interruptions in chest compressions will not even provide the minimum perfusion needed to keep the vital organs viable. This has been clearly linked to low survival rates from cardiac arrest. Remember to maintain a chest compression fraction of 80% or greater.

As soon as cardiac arrest has been confirmed, it is crucial to begin CPR immediately and apply the AED as soon as it is available. Even when the AED pads are being applied, your partner should continue chest compressions.

5. Should you remove the medication patch or leave it in place? Explain your decision.

The patch is located on the patient's right upper chest, which is where you will place one of the AED pads. Because of its location, the patch could interfere with the electrical current to the heart and may cause burns to the patient's skin. To prevent this complication, remove the patch, wipe any residue

YOU are the EMT SUMMARY continued

from the skin, and then apply the AED pads. Remember to take standard precautions!

6. What does the bulge and scar over the patient's left chest indicate? How will this affect the way you treat the patient?

A hard lump or bulge on the patient's chest, usually with a corresponding scar, indicates an AICD, or pacemaker. These devices are used in patients who are at high risk for certain cardiac dysrhythmias and cardiac arrest. The AICD will deliver shocks directly to the heart if it detects a lethal cardiac dysrhythmia. Implanted pacemakers are used to increase the patient's heart rate if it falls below a given value. Sometimes the implanted device may have both capabilities.

If the AED pads are placed directly over the device, then shocks delivered by the AED may be less effective. In addition, AED or manual defibrillator shocks given by ALS clinicians may damage the device. Therefore, if you identify an AICD or pacemaker, place the AED pad at least 1 inch (2.5 cm) away from the device. Because most of these devices are implanted in the upper left chest, this should not be an issue. The pads are placed to the right of the upper sternum and to the lower left chest, just below the nipple, so they should be well beyond 1 inch (2.5 cm) from the device. Follow your local protocols regarding patients with AICDs or implanted pacemakers.

7. How should you continue to treat this patient?

You have restored a pulse in your patient; however, his breathing is not adequate. Agonal gasps are ineffective and do not produce adequate minute volume.

Some patients may have an intact gag reflex, despite being unresponsive; in these cases, an oropharyngeal airway is contraindicated. Insert a nasopharyngeal (nasal) airway and continue to provide rescue breathing. Deliver one breath every 6 seconds (10 breaths/min); each breath should be delivered over 1 second (just enough to produce visible chest rise). Closely and carefully monitor the patient's pulse and be prepared to resume CPR if necessary.

Assume the patient has a full stomach and have a suction unit ready in case he regurgitates. Remember that mortality increases significantly if aspiration occurs. It is also important to avoid hyperventilating the patient.

8. Because the patient is no longer in cardiac arrest, should you remove the AED pads? Why or why not?

Although the patient is not in cardiac arrest, he is still at high risk for recurrence of cardiac arrest. Therefore, do not remove the AED pads; simply turn the AED off, continue rescue breathing, and prepare the patient for prompt transport.

9. Is ALS care likely to benefit your patient at this point?

ALS care may benefit this patient. For example, it may help to support blood pressure with fluids and medications, ensure maintenance of a clear airway with an advanced airway device, or evaluate cardiac function with a 12-lead ECG.

10. What further treatment, if any, is indicated for this patient?

Unresponsive patients are at increased risk for regurgitation, which could lead to aspiration and increased mortality. Vigilantly monitor the patient's airway status and be prepared to turn his head to the side if he regurgitates. Maintain his airway with manual positioning and a basic airway adjunct—in this case, a nasal airway.

Although the patient is breathing, his breaths are slow and shallow. Slow, shallow (reduced tidal volume) respirations will not produce adequate minute volume; therefore, you need to continue to assist the patient's ventilations with a bag-mask device, but do not hyperventilate him. Deliver each breath over 1 second while observing for visible chest rise. Start at 10 breaths per minute (1 every 6 seconds) and then monitor his oxygen saturation level and heart rate to help you determine if your assisted ventilations are adequate.

Further treatment of your patient should consist of careful monitoring because he remains at high risk for recurrence of cardiac arrest. In patients who are responsive and alert, the presence of a pulse is obvious; however, when a patient is unresponsive, you must frequently reassess for a pulse.

As mentioned earlier, do not remove the AED pads. Turn the AED off, but be prepared to stop the ambulance if cardiac arrest redevelops to safely defibrillate the patient.

The patient's blood pressure (86/66 mm Hg) is still low. Follow your local protocols regarding positioning of the patient to improve his blood pressure.

Prep Kit

Ready for Review

- BLS is noninvasive emergency lifesaving care that is used to treat medical conditions, including airway obstruction, respiratory arrest, and cardiac arrest.
- BLS care focuses on the ABCs: Airway (obstruction), Breathing (respiratory arrest), and Circulation (cardiac arrest or severe bleeding). If the patient is in cardiac arrest, a CAB sequence (Compressions, Airway, Breathing) should be used.
- CPR is used to establish artificial ventilation and circulation in a patient who is not breathing and has no pulse.
- The goal of CPR is to help restore spontaneous breathing and circulation; however, advanced procedures such as medications and defibrillation are often necessary for this to occur.
- ALS involves advanced lifesaving procedures, such as cardiac monitoring, administration of IV fluids and medications, and use of advanced airway adjuncts.
- The six links in the chain of survival are (1) recognition and activation of the emergency response system; (2) immediate, high-quality CPR; (3) rapid defibrillation; (4) advanced EMS; (5) post–cardiac arrest care; and (6) recovery and survivorship.
- The AED should be applied as soon as it is available to any patient experiencing cardiac arrest.
- When using an AED on a child between ages 1 and 8 years, use pediatric-size pads and a dose-attenuating system (energy reducer). If these items are unavailable, then use adult-size AED pads. If a manual defibrillator is unavailable, then use an AED equipped with pediatric-size pads and a dose attenuator. If neither option is available, then use adult-size AED pads.
- As an EMT, it is your responsibility to start CPR in virtually all patients who are in cardiac arrest. The three general exceptions to the rule are as follows: (1) you should not start CPR if the scene is unsafe, (2) you should not start CPR if the patient has obvious signs of death, and (3) you should not start CPR if the patient and their physician have a previously agreed-on DNAR or no-CPR order.
- As an EMT, you are generally not responsible for making the decision to stop CPR. After you begin CPR in the field, you must continue until one of the following events occurs (the STOP mnemonic):
  - S, the patient *Starts* breathing and has a pulse.
  - T, the patient's care is *Transferred* to another clinician of equal or higher-level training.
  - O, you are *Out* of strength or too tired to continue.
  - P, a *Physician* who is present or providing online medical direction assumes responsibility for the patient and gives direction to discontinue CPR.
- If a patient is not responsive, is not breathing, and does not have a pulse, perform automated external defibrillation. If the patient is 8 years old or younger, pediatric-size pads and a dose-attenuating system (energy reducer) are preferred. If these items are unavailable, use adult-size AED pads.
- The AED requires the operator to apply the pads, power on the unit, follow the AED prompts, and press the Shock button as indicated. The computer inside the AED recognizes rhythms that require shocking and will not mislead you.
- Do not touch the patient while the AED is analyzing the heart rhythm or delivering shocks.
- Effective CPR and early defibrillation with an AED are critical interventions for the survival of a patient in cardiac arrest. Begin CPR starting with high-quality, minimally interrupted chest compressions, and apply the AED as soon as it is available.
- If an ALS service is responding to the scene, stay where you are and continue CPR and defibrillation as needed. If ALS is not responding, begin transport if the patient regains a pulse. If the arrest was not witnessed and there were no shocks advised, the resuscitation efforts may be terminated. Follow your local protocols regarding when it is appropriate to transport the patient.

Prep Kit continued

- If an unconscious patient becomes pulseless during transport, stop the vehicle, reanalyze the rhythm, and defibrillate again or begin CPR, as appropriate.
- An airway obstruction may have various causes, including relaxation of the throat muscles in an unresponsive patient, vomited or regurgitated stomach contents, blood, damaged tissue after an injury, dentures, or foreign bodies such as food or small objects.
- The manual maneuvers recommended for removing severe airway obstructions in the responsive adult and child are back slaps and the abdominal thrust maneuver. Use back slaps and chest thrusts to treat a responsive infant with a severe airway obstruction.
- If the adult, child, or infant with a severe airway obstruction is unresponsive, then perform CPR, starting with chest compressions.
- As an EMT, you will encounter situations in which grief support for family and loved ones will be part of your role. After resuscitation has stopped, turn your attention to the family and loved ones, and provide clear communication and emotional support.

Vital Vocabulary

abdominal thrust maneuver The preferred method, in conjunction with back slaps, to dislodge a severe airway obstruction in adults and children; also called the Heimlich maneuver.

advanced life support (ALS) Advanced lifesaving procedures, including those in the advanced EMS link of the Chain of Survival.

agonal breathing The reflexive, slow, and inadequate breathing that some patients in cardiac arrest exhibit as the brainstem becomes hypoxic.

basic life support (BLS) Noninvasive emergency lifesaving care that is used to treat medical conditions, including airway obstruction, respiratory arrest, and cardiac arrest.

cardiopulmonary resuscitation (CPR) The combination of chest compressions and rescue breathing used to establish adequate ventilation and circulation in a patient who is not breathing and has no pulse.

chest compression fraction The total percentage of time during a resuscitation attempt in which active chest compressions are being performed.

gastric distention A condition in which air fills the stomach, often as a result of high volume and pressure during artificial ventilation.

head tilt–chin lift maneuver A combination of two movements to open the airway by tilting the forehead back and lifting the chin; not used for trauma patients.

hyperventilation Rapid or deep breathing that lowers the blood carbon dioxide level below normal; may lead to increased intrathoracic pressure, decreased venous return, and hypotension when associated with bag-mask device use.

ischemia A lack of oxygen that deprives tissues of necessary nutrients, resulting from partial or complete blockage of blood flow; potentially reversible because permanent injury has not yet occurred.

jaw-thrust maneuver Technique to open the airway by placing the fingers behind the angle of the jaw and bringing the jaw forward; used for patients who may have a cervical spine injury.

load-distributing band (LDB) A circumferential chest compression device composed of a constricting band and backboard that is either electrically or pneumatically driven to compress the heart by putting inward pressure on the thorax.

mechanical piston device A device that depresses the sternum via a compressed gas-powered or electric-powered plunger mounted on a backboard.

recovery position A side-lying position used to maintain a clear airway in unresponsive patients who are breathing adequately and do not have suspected injuries to the spine, hips, or pelvis.

return of spontaneous circulation (ROSC) The return of a pulse and effective blood flow to the

Prep Kit continued

body in a patient who previously was in cardiac arrest.

stridor A harsh, high-pitched respiratory sound, generally heard during inspiration, that is caused by partial blockage or narrowing of the upper airway; may be audible without a stethoscope.

ventilation The exchange of air between the lungs and the environment, spontaneously by the patient or with assistance from another person, such as an EMT.

References

1. Berg KM, Bray JE, Ng KC, et al. 2023 International Consensus on Cardiopulmonary Resuscitation and Emergency Cardiovascular Care Science With Treatment Recommendations: summary from the Basic Life Support; Advanced Life Support; Pediatric Life Support; Neonatal Life Support; Education, Implementation, and Teams; and First Aid Task Forces. *Circulation*. 2023;148(24):e187–e280. doi:10.1161/CIR.0000000000001179
2. Hands-only CPR fact sheet: American Heart Association website. https://cpr.heart.org/-/media/CPR-Files/Resources/Bystander-CPR/2202-updates/DS19398_ECC_CPRWeek_Fact_Flyer_01kk.pdf. Published 2022. Accessed October 23, 2024.
3. Victor C, Poriswanish N. Injuries associated with prehospital CPR provided by professionals and non-professionals in Bangkok EMS. *Int J Paramed*. 2024;5:74–81.
4. Gugelmin-Almeida D, Tobase L, Polastri TF, Peres HHC, Timerman S. Do automated real-time feedback devices improve CPR quality? A systematic review of literature. *Resusc Plus*. 2021 Mar 27;6:100108. doi:10.1016/j.resplu.2021.100108
5. PulsePoint AED website [homepage]. https://aedregistry.pulsepoint.org/index.php. Accessed October 23, 2024.
6. Akman C, Ergun Suzer N, Karcioglu O. Can drones be a solution for defibrillation and blood transfusions? A review on the impact of new technologies in emergency healthcare. *Front Disas Emerg Med*. 2024;2. doi.org/10.3389/femer.2024.1297539
7. American Heart Association (AHA). *2020 Handbook of Emergency Cardiovascular Care*. AHA; 2020.
8. Panchal AR, Bartos JA, Cabañas JG, et al. Part 3: Adult basic and advanced life support: 2020 American Heart Association guidelines for cardiopulmonary resuscitation and emergency cardiovascular care. *Circulation*. 2020;142(16_suppl_2):S366–S468.
9. National Association of EMS Physicians. Termination of resuscitation in nontraumatic cardiopulmonary arrest. *Prehosp Emerg Care*. 2011;15(4):542.
10. Rzeźniczek P, Gaczkowska AD, Kluzik A, Cybulski M, Bartkowska-Śniatkowska A, Grześkowiak M. Lazarus Phenomenon or the Return from the Afterlife-What We Know about Auto Resuscitation. *J Clin Med*. 2023;12(14):4704.

Additional Resources

Cheskes S, Verbeek PR, Drennan IR, et al. Defibrillation strategies for refractory ventricular fibrillation. *N Engl J Med*. 2022;387(21):1947–1956.

Crowley C, Salciccioli J, Wang W, et al. The association between mechanical CPR and outcomes from in-hospital cardiac arrest: an observational cohort study. *Resuscitation*. Published online February 10, 2024. doi:10.1016/j.resuscitation.2024.11014

Gordon L, Pasquier M, Brugger H, Paal P. Autoresuscitation (Lazarus phenomenon) after termination of cardiopulmonary resuscitation: a scoping review. *Scand J Trauma Resusc Emerg Med*. 2020;28(1):14.

Meyers M. *ROSC after death: the Lazarus syndrome*. EMS1.com website. https://www.ems1.com/medical-treatment/articles/rosc-after-death-the-lazarus-syndrome-WfDfxqI9As8diGUq/. Published August 31, 2020. Accessed October 23, 2024.

Nwanne T, Jarvis J, Barton D, Donnelly JP, Wang HE. Advanced airway management success rates in a national cohort of emergency medical services agencies. *Resuscitation*. 2020;146:43–49.

Toronto CE, LaRocco SA. Family perception of and experience with family presence during cardiopulmonary resuscitation: an integrative review. *J Clin Nurs*. 2019;28(1–2):32–46.

Wyckoff MH, Greif R, Morley PT, et al. 2022 International consensus on cardiopulmonary resuscitation and emergency cardiovascular care science with treatment recommendations: summary from the Basic Life Support; Advanced Life Support; Pediatric Life Support; Neonatal Life Support; Education, Implementation, and Teams; and First Aid Task Forces. *Circulation*. 2022;146(25):e483–e557. doi:10.1161/CIR.0000000000001095

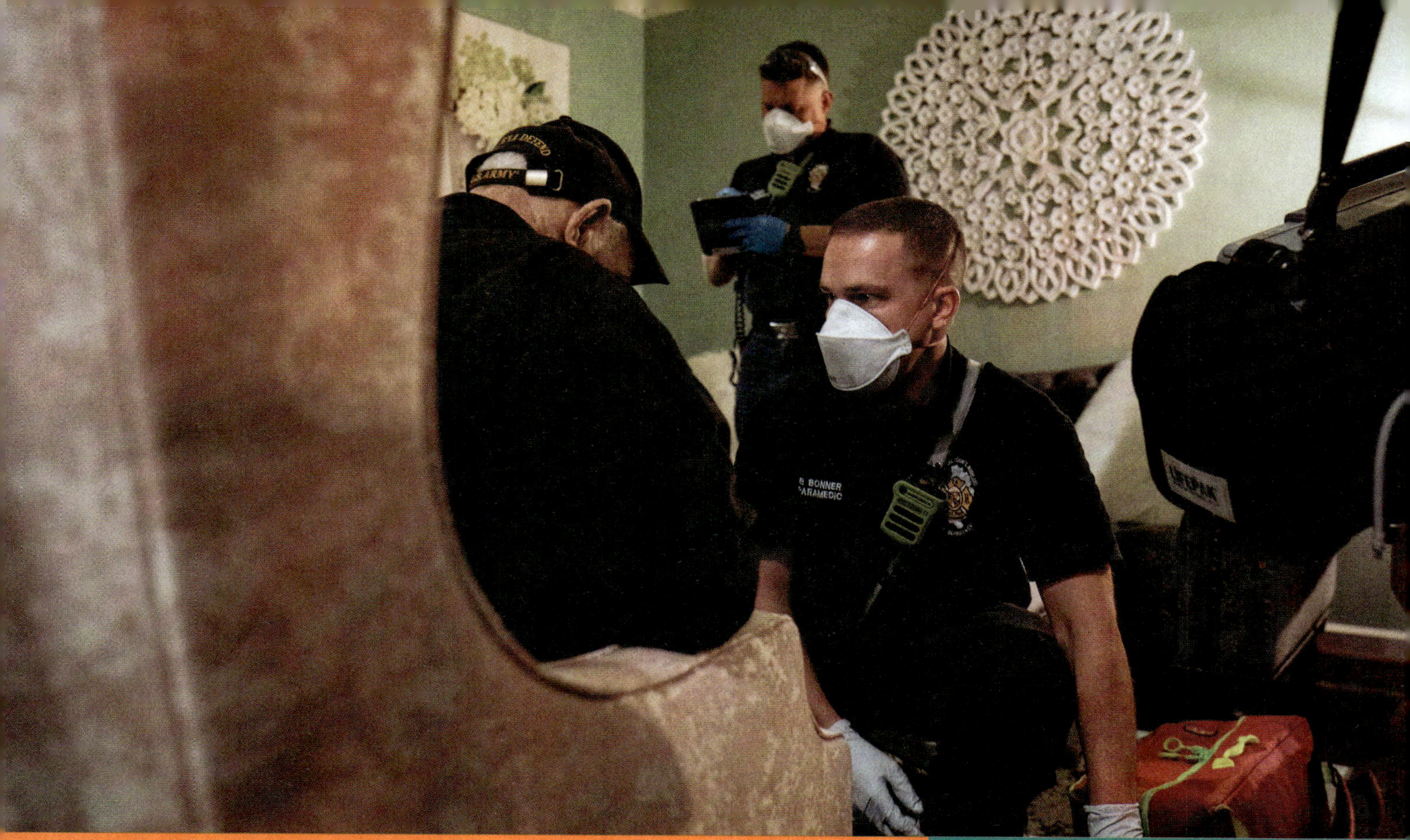

SECTION

6

Medical

15 Medical Overview

16 Respiratory Emergencies

17 Cardiovascular Emergencies

18 Neurologic Emergencies

19 Gastrointestinal and Urologic Emergencies

20 Endocrine and Hematologic Emergencies

21 Allergy and Anaphylaxis

22 Toxicology

23 Behavioral Health Emergencies

Chapter 15

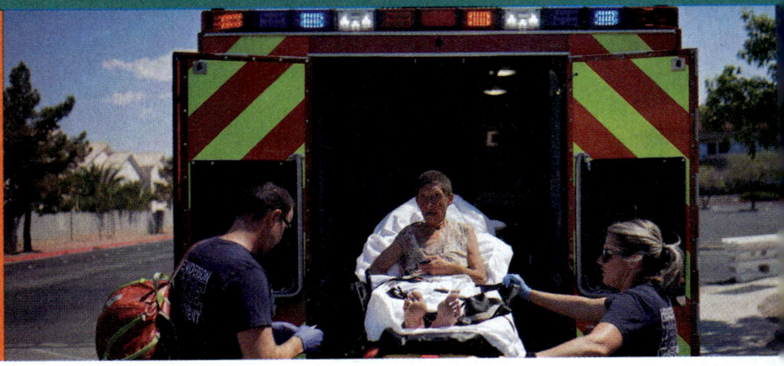

Medical Overview

NATIONAL EMS EDUCATION STANDARD COMPETENCIES

Medicine

Applies knowledge to provide basic emergency care and transportation based on assessment findings for an acutely ill patient.

Medical Overview

- Pathophysiology, assessment, and management of medical complaints to include:
  - Transport mode (pp 620–623)
  - Destination decisions (p 622)

Infectious Diseases

- Assessment and management of a patient who may have an infectious disease (pp 623–632)
- How to decontaminate the ambulance and equipment after treating a patient (Chapter 36, *Transport Operations*)
- Sepsis and septic shock (Chapter 13, *Shock*)

KNOWLEDGE OBJECTIVES

1. Differentiate between medical emergencies and trauma emergencies, remembering that some patients may have both. (p 613)
2. Name the various categories of common medical emergencies and provide examples. (pp 613–614)
3. Describe the evaluation of the nature of illness (NOI). (p 614)
4. Discuss the assessment of a patient with a medical emergency. (pp 615–620)
5. Explain the importance of transport time and destination selection for a medical patient. (pp 620–623)
6. Define infectious disease and communicable disease. (p 623)
7. Discuss diseases of special concern and their routes of transmission, including influenza, herpes simplex, human immunodeficiency virus (HIV)/acquired immunodeficiency syndrome (AIDS), hepatitis, meningitis, tuberculosis, pertussis, methicillin-resistant *Staphylococcus aureus* (MRSA), coronavirus disease 2019 (COVID-19), and Ebola. (pp 624–632)

SKILLS OBJECTIVES

There are no skills objectives for this chapter.

Introduction

Patients who need EMS assistance generally have experienced either a medical emergency or trauma emergency; in some cases, both have occurred. **Trauma emergencies** involve injuries resulting from physical forces applied to the body. **Medical emergencies** involve illnesses or conditions caused by disease. Although it is important for you to be able to distinguish between medical and trauma patients, it is equally important for you to remember that patients may have a combination of medical and trauma conditions affecting their health. For example, a person who experiences a heart attack while driving may be involved in a crash, or a patient with diabetes whose blood glucose level is too low may fall and be injured. This chapter introduces medical emergencies seen in adults, children, and older adults. Chapter 24, *Trauma Overview*, discusses the effects and management of trauma emergencies relating to these same patient populations.

Types of Medical Emergencies

There are many types of medical emergencies (**TABLE 15-1**). In general, they are defined by the body system affected or the cause or nature of the resulting problem.

Respiratory emergencies occur when patients have trouble breathing or when the amount of oxygen supplied to the tissues is inadequate. Diseases that can lead to respiratory emergencies in adults include asthma, emphysema, and chronic bronchitis. Children can experience asthma but are also susceptible to illnesses such as croup and pertussis (whooping cough); emphysema does not develop in children. Patients of all ages are susceptible to contracting viral conditions such as coronavirus disease 2019 (COVID-19), caused by severe acute respiratory syndrome coronavirus 2 (SARS-CoV-2). Viruses tend to affect different age groups differently, and newer viruses, such as the SARS-CoV-2 virus, are somewhat unpredictable in how they present and spread.

Cardiovascular emergencies are caused by conditions affecting the circulatory system. The most common examples that require EMS intervention in adult and geriatric patients include heart attacks (myocardial infarction) and heart failure.

TABLE 15-1 Common Medical Emergencies

Type of Medical Emergency	Related Conditions
Respiratory	Asthma, emphysema, chronic bronchitis, croup, epiglottitis, COVID-19, pertussis, respiratory syncytial virus
Cardiovascular	Heart attack (myocardial infarction), heart failure, congenital defects, hypertensive emergencies, aneurysm
Neurologic	Seizure, stroke, syncope, dementia
Gastrointestinal	Appendicitis, diverticulitis, pancreatitis, GI hemorrhage
Urologic	Kidney stones, urinary tract infection, dialysis complications
Endocrine	Diabetes mellitus
Hematologic	Sickle cell disease, blood clotting disorders
Immunologic	Anaphylactic reaction (severe allergy to bee stings, food, or other substances), sepsis
Toxicologic	Substance misuse, overdose, or withdrawal; food, plant, or chemical poisoning
Behavioral	Alzheimer disease, schizophrenia, depression, suicide, anxiety
Gynecologic	Vaginal bleeding, sexually transmitted infection, pelvic inflammatory disease, ectopic pregnancy

Abbreviation: COVID-19, coronavirus disease 2019; GI, gastrointestinal

Cardiovascular emergencies seen in children are commonly associated with congenital conditions or structural alterations in the heart present at birth, such as tetralogy of Fallot.

Although diseases affecting the heart and lungs represent a high percentage of EMS calls, any body system can experience illness. Neurologic emergencies involve the brain and may be caused by a seizure, stroke, or fainting (syncope). Many gastrointestinal conditions can result in a call to EMS for help. A well-known gastrointestinal condition seen in adults and children is appendicitis, although there are many others, including diverticulitis and pancreatitis. A urologic emergency can involve kidney stones or a urinary tract infection. The most common endocrine emergencies are caused by complications of diabetes mellitus, which can be seen in patients of all age groups. Hematologic (blood) emergencies may be the result of sickle cell disease or various types of blood clotting disorders such as hemophilia. Hematologic disorders are commonly present at birth and thus can affect all age groups. Immunologic emergencies involve the body's response to foreign substances. One type of immunologic emergency is an allergic reaction, in which the body overreacts to a foreign substance. Allergic reactions can range from fairly minor to life threatening. When a patient's immune system is overwhelmed by an infection, sepsis may develop.

Toxicologic emergencies, including poisoning and substance use, result in other types of medical emergencies with various presentations. Geriatric patients commonly take many medications, which can result in adverse effects from drug interactions. Children may mistake pills for candy and unintentionally overdose on medications. Some patients become addicted to a substance and may overdose on the substance, resulting in a medical emergency.

Some medical emergencies are caused by psychological or behavioral problems. Behavioral emergencies may be especially difficult to manage because patients often do not present with typical signs and symptoms. If a patient with a behavioral emergency attempts suicide, trauma and toxicologic emergencies may be involved.

The chapters in this section discuss each of these medical emergencies in greater detail.

Patient Assessment

Assessment of a medical patient is similar to the assessment of a trauma patient, but with a different focus. Whereas trauma assessments focus on the mechanism of injury or physical injuries, some of which can be detected on a physical examination, medical patient assessment focuses on the **nature of illness (NOI)**, symptoms, and the patient's chief complaint. When you are assessing a patient, establish an accurate and complete medical history. Information received from dispatch can help you anticipate what you might find when you arrive on scene, but it is conceivable that what appears to be a traumatic emergency may in fact be a medical emergency, or vice versa. Use the dispatch information to guide your initial response, but do not get locked into a preconceived idea of the patient's condition strictly from what the dispatcher tells you. During assessment, be aware of several challenges. It is possible that a patient has sustained an injury that distracts you from an underlying medical condition. For example, a patient may have a medical condition that resulted in a motor vehicle crash, or the patient may have sustained a large laceration and you fail to recognize that the patient has had a hypoglycemic (low blood sugar) event that caused them to fall and sustain the injury. Tunnel vision occurs when you become focused on one aspect of the patient's condition and exclude all others, which may cause you to miss an important injury or illness.

Patients may sometimes be uncooperative or even hostile toward those who respond to care for them. Patients may be fearful, angry, and confused and may take out their frustrations on you. In some cases, patients with an altered mental status secondary to a metabolic condition or behavioral emergency may not realize what they are doing or saying. It is important that you maintain a professional, calm, and nonjudgmental demeanor at all times.

You are obligated as a medical professional to refrain from labeling patients and displaying personal biases. Never assume that you know what the problem is, even when you are treating patients who frequently call for EMS. This attitude could result in missing a serious condition. For example, an intoxicated patient may call 9-1-1 regularly and then call at another time after a fall resulting in a serious head injury. The head injury may be overlooked if you assume the call is a response only to intoxication. Labeling a patient is dangerous, demeaning, and detrimental to both you and the patient. Personal biases should never affect your care for a patient. We all have biases. Health care clinicians need to acknowledge their biases and work to ensure these biases do not influence patient assessment and treatment. Biased assessment and treatments may have negative consequences. Any biases you may have need to be resolved before you respond to calls.

The major components of patient assessment as they relate to a medical emergency are discussed next. These components include the following:

- Scene size-up
- Primary assessment
- History taking
- Secondary assessment
- Reassessment

The general patient assessment process is detailed in Chapter 10, *Patient Assessment*.

Scene Size-up

You must complete a scene size-up. The most important aspect of this step is to make sure the scene is safe. Hazards may not be as obvious with medical emergencies as with trauma situations, but they still exist and must be considered. Therefore, remain conscious of the safety of you, your crew, and your patient before you enter a scene and throughout the call. The evaluation of scene safety should not occur only at the beginning of the call.

It is also important that you take standard precautions when you respond to an emergency, including wearing the appropriate personal protective equipment (PPE) for the situation. As soon as possible after your arrival, determine the number of patients who need assistance. In most medical cases, there will be only one patient, but anticipate the possibility of more patients, and be prepared. Finally, consider whether you need additional help. If you anticipate needing air transport, an advanced life support (ALS) unit, or police assistance, call for them immediately if you have not already done so, so that they will arrive as soon as possible.

Determine the NOI. What are the patient's signs and symptoms? Evaluation of the NOI for a medical patient will provide you with an **index of suspicion** for different types of serious or life-threatening underlying illnesses. The index of suspicion is your awareness and concern for potentially serious underlying and unseen injuries or illnesses. If there is a concern the patient may have injured their neck secondary to the medical emergency, provide initial stabilization of the spine by holding it in line.

Words of Wisdom

On entering the residence, your general impression will tell you if the patient is "sick or not sick." This determination will guide the speed and detail of your on-scene assessment.

Primary Assessment

As you approach a medical patient, you should develop a general impression of their condition. Perform a rapid examination of the patient to identify life threats. Visual clues include apparent unconsciousness, obvious severe bleeding, or extreme difficulty breathing.

Quickly determine the patient's level of consciousness using the AVPU (Awake and alert, responsive to Verbal stimuli, responsive to Pain, Unresponsive) scale. If the patient is alert on your approach, you can infer several things about their condition, such as the existence of a pulse and breathing, but you must always complete a full primary assessment. If the patient is unconscious as you approach, see if you can get a response to verbal stimuli by speaking to the patient. If the patient does not respond to your verbal stimulation, check whether the patient is responsive to painful

YOU are the EMT

Your unit is dispatched to 125 Green Hills Drive for a 36-year-old with a fever, diarrhea, and vomiting. The time is 1325 hours, there is a fine mist falling, the temperature is 72°F (22.2°C), and the traffic is moderate. You and your partner respond; the scene is located approximately 10 minutes away.

1. What observations should you make when you arrive at the scene before making physical contact with the patient?

stimuli, such as by pinching the trapezius muscle. If there is no response to verbal or painful stimuli, consider the patient unresponsive and quickly continue the assessment. Begin by ensuring the patient is breathing and has a pulse. See Chapter 10, *Patient Assessment*, for further discussion of the AVPU assessment.

Words of Wisdom

Do not let a relatively normal impression lull you into complacency. The conditions of many dangerously ill medical patients may not appear serious at first, and the patient may deteriorate rapidly.

In conscious patients, ensure the airway is open and they are breathing adequately. Check the respiratory rate, depth, and quality. Consider applying oxygen at this time if there is any indication that breathing has been affected. For unconscious patients, open the airway using the proper technique for their condition, and take several seconds to evaluate their breathing. Apply oxygen to patients in shock, with difficulty breathing, and when low oxygen saturation (Spo_2) measurements are obtained (ie, <94%). Consider having your partner administer oxygen as you continue your assessment. Unconscious patients may need airway adjuncts and ventilatory assistance with a bag-mask device.

Quickly assess the circulation in a conscious patient by checking the radial pulse and observing the patient's skin color, temperature, and condition (**FIGURE 15-1**). Because pale skin can be difficult to detect in patients with dark skin, check for pale mucous membranes inside the inner lower eyelid or inner lips, or check for slow capillary refill. On general observation, the patient may appear ashen or gray. For unconscious patients, assess the circulation at the carotid artery because generally this is the site of the strongest pulse, and it is relatively easy to palpate on a supine person. Also, quickly glance around the patient to identify any life threats such as severe bleeding or injury to the chest that affects the breathing. If any life threats are found, address them immediately.

YOU are the EMT

You arrive at the residence and knock on the patient's door. The spouse greets you and shares their significant other has been feeling ill, which has caused them to worry. You note that the spouse refers to the patient as "they" while leading you to the bedroom. You find the patient in a semisitting position in the bed. The patient is conscious and alert, is covered with several blankets, and is shivering. The patient tells you they began feeling ill the day before but then started running a fever last night. Other than diarrhea and vomiting, there are no other symptoms. The patient reports taking 400 mg of ibuprofen approximately 20 minutes ago and having a temperature of 100.6°F (38.1°C) just before you arrived. The patient has diabetes and their spouse is worried because they have not been able to keep anything down, including their diabetes pills.

Your primary assessment reveals the following information:

Recording Time: 0 Minutes	
Appearance	Flushed skin (patient's spouse states their cheeks appear darker than usual)
Level of consciousness	Conscious and alert
Airway	Open; clear of secretions and foreign bodies
Breathing	Adequate rate and depth; no accessory muscle use
Circulation	Radial pulses, rapid and strong; skin, flushed and warm to the touch

2. On the basis of your general impression and primary assessment findings, does this patient require immediate transport?

3. How should you proceed with your care of the patient?

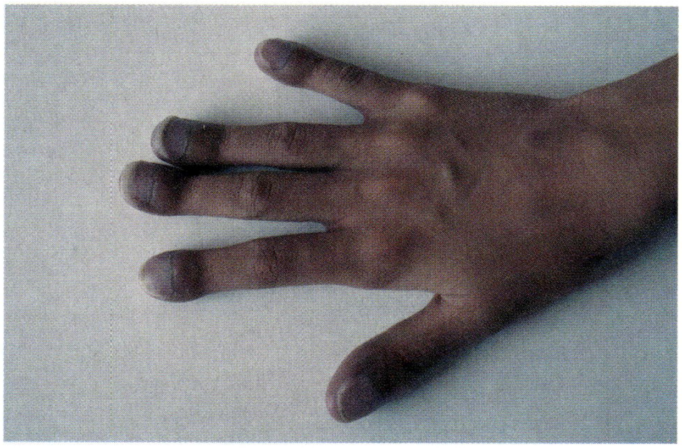

FIGURE 15-1 Skin color can provide an early and fast indication of several disease processes. Cyanosis presents as purple skin in individuals with a baseline dark skin color, such as the person shown here, or as blue skin in patients with a lighter skin color. This photo also shows nail clubbing, which is associated with chronic hypoxemia seen in various lung and heart diseases.

Once you have completed the primary assessment, you should have enough information to make a preliminary transport decision. The following patients should be considered in serious condition and in need of rapid transport: patients who are unconscious or who have an altered mental status, patients with airway or breathing problems, and patients with obvious circulation problems such as severe bleeding or signs of shock. Patients identified as needing rapid transport still require additional assessment and care.

If the patient does not initially meet the criteria for rapid transport, continue your assessment on scene and prepare for transport after you have completed the assessment and treatment. If you find that your patient's condition deteriorates during the primary assessment, prepare the patient for immediate transport and complete the assessment en route to the emergency department (ED).

Words of Wisdom

Once the primary assessment has been completed, a preliminary transport decision should be made. This decision includes determining if ALS or air transport should be called, as well as appropriate hospital destination.

History Taking

With a medical patient, history taking may be the only way to determine what the problem is or what may be causing the problem. It is imperative to gather a thorough history from the patient and/or any family, friends, or bystanders who may have pertinent information. Family members may be the only people aware that a patient sustained a head injury the previous week or that a patient has a history of drug use disorder. Bystanders may have seen clues prior to the 9-1-1 call that will lead you and the hospital staff to identify the cause of a patient's condition.

Investigate the NOI by inquiring about the chief complaint. Identifying signs and symptoms associated with the chief complaint will often help you determine the nature of the condition. Ask about the history of the present illness and ask follow-up questions such as, "Has anything like this ever happened before?" If the patient answers yes, then ask, "What was done at that time?" and "How does this episode compare with previous episodes?"

When assessing a child with a medical emergency, the parents are commonly the best source of information. Ask parents about the onset of symptoms and if the child has any diagnosed medical conditions. Be sure to inquire about immunizations. For newborns, events that occurred during pregnancy may be relevant. Remember that feeling sick can be scary for small children, as can being surrounded by unfamiliar people. Allow parents to hold the child, or at least remain close, and approach gently (**FIGURE 15-2**). Children in their teenage years may respond better without their parents present.

Street Smarts

When assessing a medical patient outside of the home, be conscious of the person's privacy. Onlookers may be tempted to record the event, such as with a smartphone.

If a patient is unconscious, survey the scene for evidence of traumatic events, medication containers, or medical devices the patient may have been using. Try to obtain as much of the patient's medical history as possible from family members, friends,

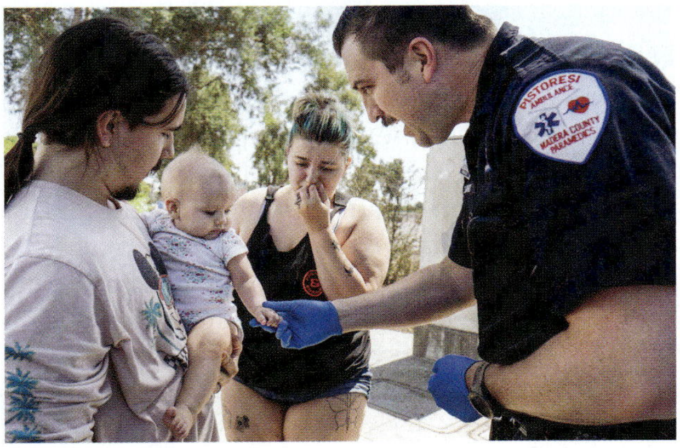

FIGURE 15-2 When assessing a small child, allow parents to comfort the child and provide insights into the current situation.

© Melina Mara/The Washington Post/Getty Images.

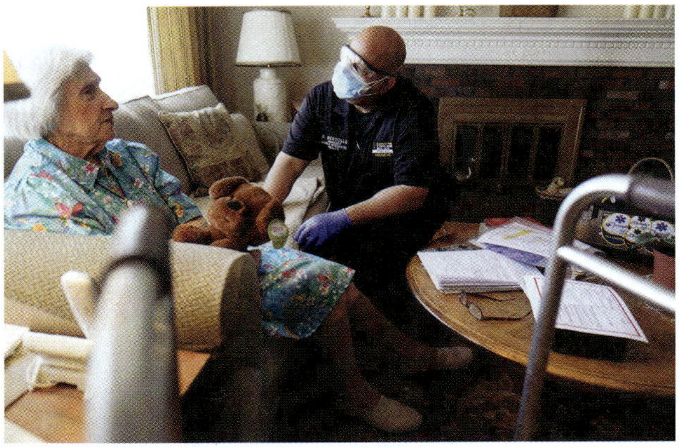

FIGURE 15-3 History taking is an important part of the patient assessment process.

© Seth Wenig/AP Photo.

and bystanders or from the scene itself. Family members or friends may know the patient's allergies, medications, or medical conditions. Look for medical alert bracelets or necklaces, which may offer information about the patient's medical history. Ask whether the patient reported any symptoms before they lost consciousness. If possible, have a family member accompany you to the hospital to answer questions there as well.

As you continue to gather information, remember to obtain a SAMPLE (Signs and symptoms, Allergies, Medications, Pertinent past medical history, Last oral intake, Events leading up to the illness or injury) history and to ask questions about the patient's chief complaint using the OPQRST (Onset, Provocation/palliation, Quality, Region/radiation, Severity, Timing) mnemonic. Ask patients to identify all of the symptoms they are experiencing. Make sure you record any allergies, medical conditions, and medications they take (**FIGURE 15-3**). Ask about prescriptions, over-the-counter medications, and herbal medications.

Sometimes older patients will report taking numerous medications, both prescription and over the counter. In those situations, it is best to take the medications with you to the hospital, and list them in your report. Ask patients about their medical history to help determine the current problem and identify any other conditions that might cause complications. To obtain a complete history, ask about specific conditions such as heart problems, breathing problems, and blood sugar (glucose) problems. Determine if the patient is taking any medications for these conditions and whether they are compliant with the drug regimen. The purpose of these questions is to obtain the most complete medical history possible. In addition, look around the scene for clues, such as prescription pill bottles or home medical equipment, that may help you piece together the patient's medical history and better understand the circumstances surrounding the current medical emergency. The scene may also give clues about alcohol, drug use, and the patient's overall ability to care for themselves.

Secondary Assessment

When the patient is critically ill or the transport time is short, you may not have time to conduct a secondary assessment. In other cases, the secondary assessment may occur on scene or en route to the ED.

Conscious medical patients seldom need a secondary assessment of the entire body or a head-to-toe examination, but all conscious patients should undergo a limited or detailed physical examination based on their chief complaint. For example, you should check for pulse, motion, and sensation in all of the patient's extremities and check the patient's pupillary reaction if you suspect a neurologic problem. Likewise, patients with chest pain should have an assessment focusing on the thorax and the organs in the thorax. Unconscious patients are unable to tell you what is wrong, so you should always perform a secondary assessment of the entire body or a head-to-toe examination. A full body assessment should help you obtain clues to assess the problem, but this assessment should be performed quickly so it does not delay transport to the hospital.

Words of Wisdom

Just as medical alert jewelry can provide insights into a patient's condition, so too can a patient's cell phone. Most phones have a feature on the home screen where medical information can be viewed without the need to unlock the phone.

If the patient's condition warrants the secondary assessment, begin by carefully examining the head, scalp, and face. Look for evidence of possible trauma, and monitor the patient for any signs of pain with palpation throughout the assessment. Examine the head and face for symmetry, making sure to check the pupils for equality and reactivity to light. Look at the conjunctiva of the eyes for moisture and the ears and nose for any drainage. Look for nasal flaring, and examine the mouth for foreign bodies (including loose teeth or dentures) and pink, moist mucosa. Note any unusual odors on the patient's breath. For example, an acetone smell on the breath may indicate high blood glucose level in a patient with diabetes or severe dehydration in a child who has experienced vomiting and diarrhea.

Examine the neck closely for any evidence of accessory muscle use with respirations. Check for jugular venous distention and tracheal deviation, which can be indicators of respiratory or cardiac problems. While you are examining the neck, make sure to move any clothing so that you can check for a tracheostomy or stoma.

Next, assess the chest and abdomen. At the chest, listen to breath sounds and ensure that the patient is breathing adequately with equal chest rise and fall on each side. Carefully inspect and palpate the chest and abdomen to identify any areas of tenderness or swelling. Look for medication patches on the chest or abdomen and any implanted medical devices (which may be suggested by surgical scars), which usually can be palpated just under the skin. Check for rigidity and distention in the abdomen, and look for scars on the chest or abdomen that might indicate previous surgeries, including scars from laparoscopic surgery that may be difficult to notice. Finally, check the pelvis and genital area, asking about pain and looking for signs of incontinence or bleeding.

Palpate the legs and arms for swelling and other abnormalities, making sure to check for distal motion, sensation, and circulation in all four extremities. Note any scars or track marks along the veins, which are indicators of intravenous (IV) drug use. Fistulas or shunts in the arm may indicate a patient with kidney failure who is on dialysis. Look for medical alert jewelry at the wrists as well. Finally, examine the patient's back to note any irregularities, pain, or scars. At this point, your full assessment of the patient should be complete, and treatment of non-life-threatening conditions should be instituted. Treatment will depend on each condition and your local protocols.

Words of Wisdom

Although the use of an automatic blood pressure cuff is convenient, you should always attempt to obtain at least one manual blood pressure reading to be sure it correlates with the automatic reading.

Obtaining an accurate set of vital signs is critical. Often your partner can begin this process while you are asking about the medical history. Assess the pulse for rate, quality, and regularity at the most appropriate site, either at the radial artery if the patient is conscious, or at the carotid artery if the patient is unconscious. Assess respirations as you assess the pulse to prevent the patient from modifying their respirations in response to your observation. Identify the rate, quality, and regularity of the respirations and any difficulties that may be apparent. Finally, obtain an initial blood pressure reading, measuring both systolic and diastolic pressures.

Consider using the automatic blood pressure cuff for future assessments at regular intervals. Depending on your local protocol, other important information to consider obtaining includes a blood glucose level and a pulse oximetry reading.

Reassessment

After completing the assessment and treatment, begin reassessment and continue it throughout transport. During the reassessment, repeat the primary assessment and reassess the chief complaint. Look for any changes in the level of consciousness, reassess the ABCs (Airway, Breathing, and Circulation), and reexamine the transport decision. Consider the need for ALS backup or transport to a closer hospital. Obtain another full set of vital signs every 5 minutes for unstable patients or every 15 minutes for stable patients. Reassessment also includes repeating your physical examination to identify and treat changes in the patient's condition.

Finally, the reassessment includes reviewing all treatments that have been performed. Reassess oxygen delivery, any bandages or splints applied, and any other treatment that has been performed. If medications were administered, watch the patient for the desired effect, known side effects, or other adverse effects. Remember that some medications may need to be repeated depending on the transport time.

Document any changes that have developed as a result of the treatments and, if needed, adjust any of the treatments accordingly. Reassessment is an important step in patient assessment; it allows you to modify care as needed and ensures you have the most current information on the patient's condition when you arrive at the hospital.

Management, Transport, and Destination

Most medical emergencies require a level of treatment beyond that available in the prehospital setting. Also, the treatments depend on an accurate diagnosis of the exact medical condition, which may require advanced testing that is available only in a hospital. The primary prehospital treatments for medical emergencies address the symptoms more than the actual disease process.

Medication administration by EMTs should be guided by the national EMS scope of practice, state regulations, and medical oversight. In general, EMTs may administer the patient's own nitroglycerin to them when they have chest pain that suggests myocardial infarction.

Administration of medications that are stored in the ambulance is also limited for EMTs. During a medical emergency, some protocols include administering the following medications:

- Aspirin for patients having chest pain
- Epinephrine (auto-injector) for anaphylaxis
- Oral glucose to a patient with diabetes and a low blood glucose level
- Inhaled albuterol or ipratropium to a patient experiencing respiratory difficulty

YOU are the EMT

Your partner obtains the patient's vital signs. He also obtains a blood glucose level of 242 mg/dL and notes that the patient seems to be showing some signs of dehydration, such as dry mucous membranes. Palpation of the patient's abdomen shows it to be soft and nontender. The patient agrees to transport and requests transport to a hospital where they have been treated before, which is located 25 miles away. There is another hospital located only 10 miles away.

Recording Time:	5 Minutes
Respiration	18 breaths/min; regular and adequate
Pulse	110 beats/min; strong and regular
Skin	Flushed and dry; warm to the touch
Blood pressure	124/70 mm Hg
Oxygen saturation (Spo_2)	99%

4. Is it appropriate to transport the patient to the hospital they requested, or should you transport them to the closer facility?

- Intranasal naloxone for suspected opioid overdose
- Nonprescription analgesics such as ibuprofen (eg, Motrin, Advil) or acetaminophen (eg, Tylenol) for fever or mild pain

Never administer any medication without authorization from medical oversight, and always follow your state and local protocols.

You may also use an automated external defibrillator (AED) on a patient who is pulseless and apneic. Familiarize yourself with the equipment and medications carried on your ambulance, and use them appropriately under a medical director's instruction. The AED is discussed in more detail in Chapter 17, *Cardiovascular Emergencies*.

Scene Time

In many cases, the time on scene may be longer for medical patients than for trauma patients. If the patient is not in critical condition, gather as much information as possible from the scene so that you can transmit that information to the physician at the ED. Briefly check the patient's living conditions: heating, air conditioning, cleanliness of environment, adequate food, and so on. When assessing children, watch for signs of abuse or neglect by the parent or caretaker. Critical patients include those with altered mental status, airway or breathing difficulties, or any sign of circulatory compromise. In some circumstances, a patient who is very old or very young may be considered critical even if the patient appears to be relatively stable. Patients in critical condition or with a time-critical diagnosis such as heart attack or stroke often need expeditious transport. The time on scene should be limited to 10 minutes or less for these patients.

Type of Transport

Serious consideration should be given to how best to transport a medical patient. If a life-threatening condition exists, transport may be meaningfully accelerated by the use of lights and siren, but if the patient is not critical, or if using lights and siren would not substantially decrease transport times, consider nonemergency transport. Many patients experiencing a medical emergency can be transported without the use of lights and siren. This is a much safer method of transport and will often result in arrival only a few minutes later than an emergency transport using lights and siren.

Differentiating a high-priority transport from a low-priority transport is a skill developed with experience, but it is a skill that can be learned. A general rule for determining the priority of transport is to consider the results of the patient's primary assessment. Patients with an altered mental status, especially if it is still present at the completion of your assessment and treatment, should be considered a high-priority transport. Patients with circulatory compromise, including signs and symptoms of shock, should also be considered a high-priority transport. Most patients with circulatory problems cannot be stabilized in the prehospital setting and need to undergo treatment at a hospital quickly but safely. Patients with difficulty breathing often require high-priority transport. However, if the patient has responded well to your initial treatment, such as oxygen and albuterol administration, lights and siren may not be necessary. As a rule, if you choose to use lights and siren, you should be able to specifically describe in your report why such emergency transport was medically necessary and why the improved arrival time justified the increased risk to which you exposed the patient and public at large (**FIGURE 15-4**).

Modes of transport ultimately come in one of two categories: ground (**FIGURE 15-5**) or air (**FIGURE 15-6**). Ground transportation EMS units are generally staffed by EMTs and paramedics. Air transportation EMS units or critical care transport

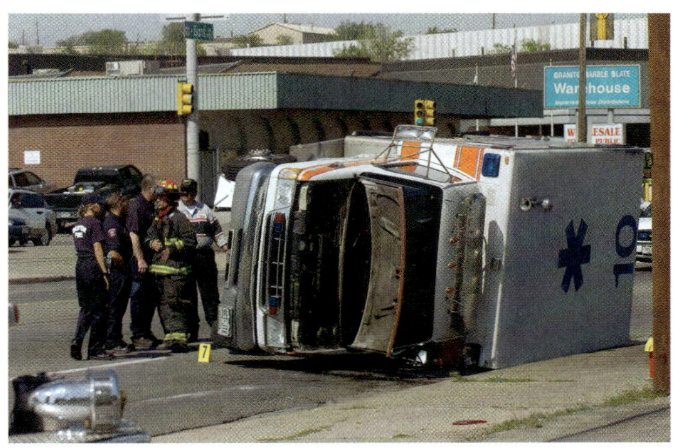

FIGURE 15-4 Ambulance crash. Additional risk may be posed to the population on the roads by use of lights and siren.

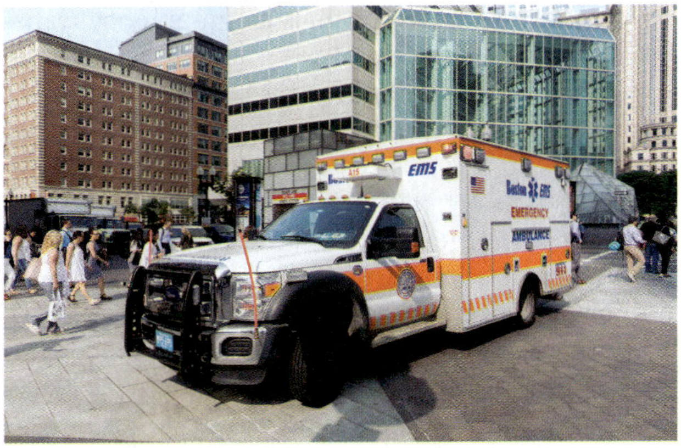

FIGURE 15-5 Ground transport.

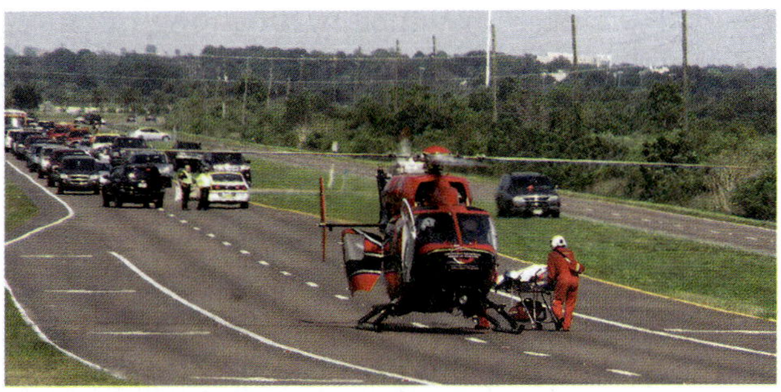

FIGURE 15-6 Air transport.

units are generally staffed by critical care transport professionals such as critical care nurses and paramedics. Although it is not as common to summon an air ambulance for a medical patient, it is sometimes advisable. In rural areas with long ground transport times, patients who have possibly experienced a heart attack, stroke, or complication of pregnancy could benefit from air transport. Children with certain medical conditions may also benefit from air transport. When you are considering ALS support for a patient, compare the total time for a ground ALS unit to respond and transport to the time required for an ALS helicopter to respond and transport; also consider the urgent resources needed by the patient. Follow local protocols and medical direction.

Street Smarts

Transporting a patient using lights and siren or transporting via helicopter can cause additional anxiety for the patient. Reassure the patient that the mode of transport is most appropriate for their needs.

Destination Selection

It is generally appropriate to select the closest ED as your destination. However, there are times when the closest hospital is not necessarily the most appropriate choice. Patients with chest pain as a result of a heart attack may need a facility that is capable of performing cardiac catheterization, which may not necessarily be available at the closest hospital. If the patient is in cardiac arrest or experiences cardiac arrest during transport, immediately reroute to the closest hospital with emergency facilities. Stroke patients can also benefit from specialized hospital selection. Some hospitals have designated stroke teams and interventional neurology capabilities. Taking a possible stroke patient to a hospital without these resources may result in a delay in definitive treatment and may lead to a worse outcome for the patient. Pediatric patients, especially those born with a congenital condition, may require transport to a pediatric center. Most EDs can treat children, but not all can treat children with special medical needs.

An increasing number of hospitals have geriatric-accredited EDs, as defined by the American College of Emergency Physicians. These hospitals improve care for the older adult by meeting benchmarks related to staffing, geriatric protocols, patient outcomes, and equipment and physical resources.[1] Their criteria incorporate the 4Ms framework[2]:

- What **M**atters. Understand the current and future needs/desires of each patient, and align care accordingly.
- **M**edication. Determine whether medication is necessary and prioritize options that do not interfere with "what matters" to the patient.
- **M**entation. Use a standard guideline to assess for delirium or dementia.
- **M**obility. Assess for fall risk and follow guidelines to improve mobility.

An older adult may benefit from transport to a geriatric-accredited ED; however, a patient who has experienced heart attack, stroke, or trauma should be transported to an ED accredited to treat these conditions when possible.

Selecting the transport type and destination constitutes an intervention and involves shared decision making with the patient and possibly caregivers. When the most appropriate hospital is not the patient's choice and the person has decision-making capacity, it is your job to explain why you are recommending an alternative. Consult with medical direction if the patient continues to refuse transport to the most appropriate hospital.

Infectious Diseases

An **infectious disease** is a medical condition caused by the growth and spread of small, harmful organisms, such as bacteria or viruses, within the body (**TABLE 15-2**). A **communicable disease** is a disease that can be spread from one person or species to another. Most of these diseases are not spread as easily as is commonly believed. In addition, there are many immunizations, protective techniques, and devices that clinicians can use to minimize their risk of infection. When clinicians use these protective measures, their risk of contracting a serious infectious disease is substantially decreased. When a pathogen that was not previously known to be contractible by humans begins causing illness, it is unknown how easily it may spread from person to person. During these events, greater protective measures, on multiple levels, may be implemented to ensure protection of the health care workforce. The worldwide response to COVID-19 illustrates the many ways that public health stakeholders, including governments of all levels, schools, and the full breadth of the medical community, must work together to address such disease outbreaks.

As an EMT, you will be called on to treat and transport patients with a variety of infectious or communicable diseases. In Chapter 2, *Workforce Safety and Wellness*, the routes of transmission and standard precautions that responders need to take to reduce risk and increase prevention and awareness are described. The assessment and treatment of a patient who may have a communicable or infectious disease also are covered. Chapter 36, *Transport Operations*, discusses decontamination techniques after transport.

General Assessment Principles

The assessment of a patient suspected of having an infectious disease should be approached much like the assessment of any other medical patient. With most patients who have a potentially infectious disease in the prehospital setting, the next step after scene size-up and primary assessment is to gather patient history using OPQRST to elaborate on the patient's chief complaint. Typical chief complaints include fever, nausea, rash, pleuritic chest pain, difficulty breathing, vomiting, and diarrhea. Obtain a SAMPLE history and a set of baseline vital signs, paying particular attention to medications the patient is currently taking and the events leading up to the current problem. Also ask whether the patient has recently traveled or has come in contact with someone who has traveled, especially out of the country. Always show respect for the feelings of the patient, family members, and others at the scene.

TABLE 15-2 Causes of Infectious Disease

Organism	Description	Example
Bacteria	Grow and reproduce outside the human cell in the appropriate temperature and with the appropriate nutrients	*Salmonella*
Viruses	Smaller than bacteria; multiply only inside a host and die when exposed to the environment	Influenza
Fungi	Similar to bacteria in that they require the appropriate nutrients and organic material to grow	Mold
Protozoa (parasites)	Single-celled microscopic organisms, some of which cause disease	Amoebas
Helminths (parasites)	Invertebrates with long, flexible, rounded, or flattened bodies	Worms

Having contracted an illness can be frightening, especially if the illness is unknown.

General Management Principles

The general management of the patient with a suspected infectious disease first focuses on any life-threatening conditions that were identified in the primary assessment (airway management, oxygen and ventilatory assistance, and circulatory support). Remember to be empathetic. Because most patients who have an infectious disease involving the respiratory system will have a fever or mild to significant breathing problems, place the patient in a position of comfort on the stretcher and keep them warm. Remember to use appropriate PPE based on the nature of the call. Always follow your agency's exposure control plan regarding cleaning equipment, properly discarding any disposable supplies, and washing linens. Infectious diseases causing prolonged vomiting and diarrhea can cause life-threatening dehydration and shock. Infants, young children, and older adults are especially vulnerable and their condition may deteriorate quickly.

Epidemic and Pandemic Considerations

An **epidemic** occurs when new cases of a disease in a human population substantially exceed the number expected based on recent experience. A **pandemic** is an outbreak that occurs on a global scale. A flu pandemic occurs when a new influenza virus emerges for which people have little or no immunity. The disease can spread easily from person to person, cause serious illness, and be found in multiple countries in a short time. Because it is a new virus, there would be no specific vaccine immediately available. Local and global response to such an event can involve quarantine and isolation to limit the spread of the virus.

Common or Serious Communicable Diseases

Influenza

Influenza, commonly known as flu, is primarily an animal respiratory disease that has mutated to infect humans. It can affect all people, but those with chronic medical conditions, compromised immune systems, the very young, and the very old are particularly susceptible to complications of the disease. All strains of influenza are transmitted by direct contact with nasal secretions and aerosolized droplets from coughing and sneezing by infected people.

Words of Wisdom

The H1N1 virus provides an example of how viral mutations can affect the human population. Previous forms of H1N1 found in pigs (swine) mutated and in 2009 began infecting humans. The resulting disease, commonly referred to as the swine flu, quickly resulted in a global pandemic. In 2009 and 2010, swine flu is thought to have caused nearly 300,000 deaths worldwide.[3] The pandemic ended in 2010, but H1N1 still circulates as a seasonal virus and is included in yearly flu vaccines.

Mutations from another type of influenza are posing concern for public health officials today. The H5N1 virus, more commonly called avian influenza (or bird flu), was first detected in wild birds in 1959 and at the time spread only among birds. However, the virus has since mutated, with reported outbreaks in domestic poultry and cattle since 2020. By 2024, more than 60 human cases had been reported in the United States. The cases were associated with exposure to infected animals, mostly on poultry or dairy farms. In early 2025, the first US human death from avian influenza was reported in Louisiana.[4] Currently, there is no evidence that the H5N1 virus can be spread from person to person; however, if mutations were to allow human-to-human transmission, a pandemic could result.[5]

Many potentially serious diseases can be spread by the respiratory route; therefore, you need to wear PPE, such as gloves, eye protection, and a high-efficiency particulate air (HEPA) respirator or an N95 mask, at a minimum. Viruses can live for several days on surfaces, so frequent handwashing is also important. Maintain your vaccinations and stay up to date on the latest Centers for Disease Control and Prevention (CDC) recommendations. Place a surgical mask or N95 mask on patients with suspected or confirmed respiratory disease. Wear a HEPA respirator or an N95 mask during any aerosol-generating procedures such as suctioning of airway secretions, performing cardiopulmonary resuscitation, or assisting with endotracheal intubation. A HEPA respirator has a pleated air filter that removes at least 99.97% of airborne particles that are 0.3 micron in size.

An annual influenza immunization is important, especially for EMS personnel, to protect both clinicians and patients. The influenza virus is constantly changing. Experts adjust vaccines from year to year to provide protection against the strains most likely to affect the population. Vaccination effectively decreases transmission rates and limits (but does not eliminate) the disease incidence. Complications of the vaccine are far less common and severe than complications of the flu. Depending on many factors (eg, characteristics of the circulating viruses, distribution/efficacy of the year's vaccine), the seasonal flu can contribute to more than 50,000 deaths in a given year in the United States.[6]

Words of Wisdom

In the 1990s, false claims associated the measles, mumps, rubella (MMR) vaccine with autism, contributing to widespread distrust in all vaccines by some people. Research has definitively disproven the theory that immunizations cause autism.[7,8] Unfortunately vaccination distrust has persisted, and outbreaks of the highly contagious measles virus have recently occurred in United States, causing several deaths.

Herpes Simplex

Herpes simplex is a common virus strain carried by humans. Eighty percent of people carrying the virus are asymptomatic, but symptomatic infections cause eruptions of tiny fluid-filled blisters called *vesicles* that often appear on the lips or genitals. Herpes simplex can cause more serious illnesses such as pneumonia and meningitis in very young, very old, and immunocompromised patients. The primary mode of infection is through close personal contact, so standard precautions are generally sufficient to prevent spread to or from health care workers.

Words of Wisdom

Herpes zoster, or shingles, is a painful rash that occurs in approximately 1 million people each year in the United States.[9] It is caused by reactivation of the varicella-zoster virus that causes chickenpox. The virus lies dormant on nerve fibers after a person recovers from their initial illness and reactivates later in life, often when a person is older or has a weakened immune system. The shingles rash appears as blisters that follow a nerve route. Direct contact with fluid from the blisters or inhaling particles from the vesicular fluid can lead to chickenpox in people who have never had it. Use PPE when caring for a patient who is suspected to have shingles. Cover any lesions that have not dried and scabbed over.

HIV Infection

Exposure to the human immunodeficiency virus (HIV) is a risk that EMTs face on a regular basis. It is this prospect that led to the development of standard precautions. There is no vaccine to protect against HIV infection, and despite great progress in drug treatments, infection may still result in acquired immunodeficiency syndrome (AIDS). However, with treatment, patients can expect a near-normal life span. In fact, recent advances in medicine have led to some patients having no detectable circulating virus in their bloodstream. HIV attacks the body's immune system, making it difficult for the natural defenses to fight disease. If the AIDS develops as a result of HIV infection, minor illnesses can become fatal to the patient.

Fortunately, HIV is not easily transmitted in your work setting. For example, it is far less contagious than hepatitis B, which is why immunization for hepatitis B is important. HIV infection is a potential hazard only when the virus comes in contact with mucous membranes or is directly transmitted into the bloodstream. Transmission can occur via sexual contact or exposure to blood or body fluids, meaning your risk of infection is limited to exposure to an infected patient's blood and body fluids. Exposure can take place in the following ways:

- The patient's blood is splashed or sprayed into your eyes, nose, or mouth or into an open sore or cut, however tiny; even a microscopic opening in the skin is an invitation for infection with a virus.
- You have blood from the infected patient on your hands and then touch your own eyes, nose, mouth, or an open sore or cut.
- A needle used to inject the patient breaks your skin. Although the risk to you from a single injection, even with a hollow-bore needle, is small, this is by far the most dangerous form of exposure.

- Broken glass at a motor vehicle crash or other incident penetrates your glove (and skin), which may have already been covered with blood from an infected patient.

As with several other bloodborne illnesses, many patients who are infected with HIV do not show any symptoms. This is why health care workers should wear gloves any time they are likely to come into contact with secretions or blood from any patient and take other precautions to prevent the spread of disease.

If you have any reason to think that a patient's blood or secretions may have entered your system, especially through contact with a patient's blood, seek medical advice as soon as possible and notify your infectious disease officer. If you know that the patient is infected with HIV, your physician may suggest immediate treatment to try to prevent you from becoming infected. However, if the patient is an unlikely candidate for HIV infection, your physician may recommend that you and the patient be tested before you undergo therapy. As scientists learn more about HIV infection, testing and treatment recommendations change. It is important that you immediately see your physician (or your program's designated physician) any time you have a significant exposure to a communicable or infectious disease. Know the policy for your system, and take time now to consider what you would do in the event of exposure.

Words of Wisdom

A patient may report to you that they are taking pre-exposure prophylaxis (PrEP). PrEP is a prevention strategy in which a person who is at increased risk of HIV exposure takes antiretroviral medication(s) to reduce the likelihood of infection. PrEP has been found to reduce the risk of contracting HIV from sexual intercourse by 99% and the risk from injection drug use by 74%.[10]

Hepatitis

The term *hepatitis* refers to an inflammation (and often infection) of the liver. Hepatitis can be caused by a number of different viruses and toxins. Early signs of viral hepatitis include loss of appetite, vomiting, fever, fatigue, sore throat, cough, and muscle and joint pain. Several weeks later, jaundice (yellow coloration of the eyes and skin) and right upper quadrant abdominal pain develop (**FIGURE 15-7**). The severity of toxin-induced hepatitis depends on the amount of agent absorbed and the duration of exposure. Toxin-induced hepatitis is not contagious. There is no definitive way in the prehospital environment to tell which patients with hepatitis have a contagious form of the disease and which do not.

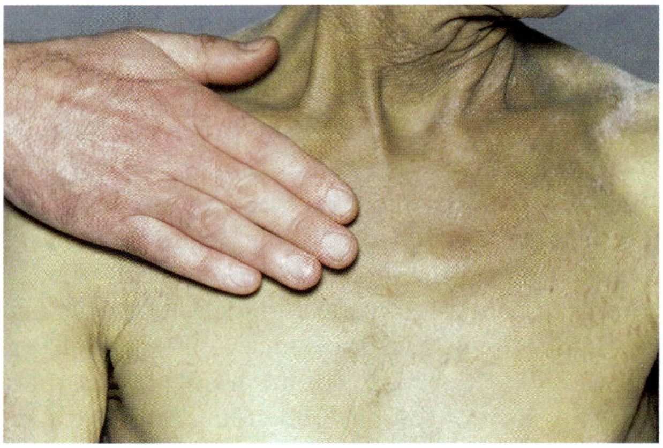

FIGURE 15-7 Jaundice is a sign of a hepatitis infection. Other causes of jaundice may include alcohol-related liver disease, blocked bile ducts, pancreatic cancer, and certain medications such as acetaminophen, penicillin, birth control pills, and steroids.

TABLE 15-3 shows the characteristics of different types of hepatitis, from which you can assess your risk of exposure. Hepatitis A can be transmitted only from a patient who has an acute infection, whereas hepatitis B and hepatitis C can be transmitted from long-term carriers who have no signs of illness. A carrier is a person (or animal) in whom an infectious organism has taken up permanent residence and may or may not cause any active disease. Carriers may never know that they harbor the organism; however, they can infect other people.

Hepatitis A is transmitted orally through oral or fecal contamination. This means that, generally, you must eat or drink something that is contaminated with the virus. Contamination is the presence of an infectious organism on or in an object. The organisms that cause hepatitis B and C are transmitted through vehicles other than food or water. For example, these organisms may enter the body through a transfusion or needlestick with

TABLE 15-3 Characteristics of Hepatitis

Type	Route of Infection	Incubation Period	Chronic Infection	Vaccine and Treatment	Comments
Viral Hepatitis					
Hepatitis A (infectious)	Fecal–oral, infected food or drink	2–6 wk	Chronic condition does not exist.	Vaccine is available; no specific treatment is available; body will clear the infection on its own.	Mild illness; rarely results in death; mortality is highest in older adults; after acute infection, the patient has lifelong immunity.
Hepatitis B	Blood, sexual contact, saliva, breast milk, at birth from mother	4–12 wk	Chronic infection affects up to 2% to 6% of patients and up to 90% of newborns who have the disease.	Vaccine is available; treatment is aimed at reducing risk of serious liver disease and liver cancer.	Some patients are asymptomatic and without signs of liver disease, but they may infect others; injecting drugs is the highest risk factor; most deaths relate to liver failure or liver cancer.
Hepatitis C	Blood, sexual contact	2–10 wk	Chronic infection affects more than 50% of patients.	No vaccine is available; treatment is costly but effective for many strains of hepatitis C.	Approximately 40% of patients with chronic hepatitis C do not know they are infected; chronic infection increases the risk of cancer of the liver.
Hepatitis D	Blood, sexual contact	4–12 wk	Chronic infection is common.	No vaccine is available; however, vaccination against hepatitis B also protects against hepatitis D; no treatment is available.	Occurs only in patients with active hepatitis B infection; illness is often more severe than in those with hepatitis B alone.
Toxin-Induced Hepatitis					
Medications, drugs, and alcohol	Inhalation, skin or mucous membrane exposure, oral ingestion, or intravenous administration	Within hours to days following exposure	Some chemicals may initiate an inflammatory response that continues to cause liver damage long after the chemical is out of the body.	No vaccine is available; treatment is to stop exposure; in patients with an overdose of acetaminophen, certain drugs may minimize liver injury if given early enough.	This type of hepatitis is not contagious; patients with toxin-induced hepatitis may have liver damage and jaundice; not every exposure to a toxin will cause liver damage.

Data from: Numbers and rates of deaths with hepatitis A virus infection listed as a cause of death among residents, by demographic characteristics—United States, 2016–2020. Centers for Disease Control and Prevention website. https://www.cdc.gov/hepatitis/statistics/2020surveillance/hepatitis-a/table-1.4.htm. Reviewed August 17, 2022. Accessed December 3, 2024; Hepatitis B basic information. US Department of Health and Human Services website. https://www.hhs.gov/hepatitis/learn-about-viral-hepatitis/hepatitis-b-basics/index.html. Reviewed March 31, 2023. Accessed December 3, 2024; Hepatitis C basic information. US Department of Health and Human Services website. https://www.hhs.gov/hepatitis/learn-about-viral-hepatitis/hepatitis-c-basics/index.html. Reviewed November 30, 2022. Accessed December 3, 2024; Hepatitis D basics. Centers for Disease Control and Prevention website. https://www.cdc.gov/hepatitis-d/about/index.html. Published April 24, 2024. Accessed December 3, 2024.

infected blood, which puts health care workers at high risk for contracting hepatitis B, the more contagious and virulent form. **Virulence** is the strength or ability of a pathogen to produce disease. Hepatitis B is far more contagious than HIV. For this reason, vaccination with the hepatitis B vaccine is highly recommended for EMTs. Unfortunately, not everyone who is vaccinated develops immediate immunity to the virus. Sometimes, but not always, an additional dose will provide immunity. You should be tested after vaccination to determine your immune status.

If you are stuck with a needle or injured in some other way while caring for a patient who might have hepatitis, see your physician immediately.

Words of Wisdom

Track marks (scars or increased pigmentation along a person's veins) may indicate a person's use of illicit injection drugs. Injection drug use, particularly the reuse and sharing of needles, increases a person's risk for hepatitis B, hepatitis C, and HIV infection.

Meningitis

Meningitis is an inflammation of the meningeal coverings of the brain and spinal cord. Patients with meningitis will have signs and symptoms such as fever, headache, stiff neck, and altered mental status. It is an uncommon but frightening infectious disease. Meningitis can be caused by viruses or bacteria, most of which are not contagious.

Meningococcal meningitis, one form of meningitis, however, is highly contagious. Meningococcal meningitis is an inflammation of the meningeal coverings of the brain and spinal cord. The bacteria that cause meningococcal meningitis can be spread by the exchange of respiratory secretions through coughing and sneezing. The effects are lethal in some cases. Victims who survive can be left with brain damage, hearing loss, or learning disabilities. Patients may present with flulike symptoms, but high fever, severe headache, photophobia (light sensitivity), and a stiff neck in adults are symptoms that are highly suggestive of meningitis. Patients sometimes have an altered level of consciousness. When the disease is advanced, patients may have small, flat, purple-red blotches on the skin that do not blanch when pressure is applied, known as

YOU are the EMT

You place the patient onto the stretcher, load them into the ambulance, and begin transport to the hospital. You decide to reassess the patient's vital signs every 15 minutes. En route, their vital signs and overall condition are reassessed and remain stable. The patient continues to have nausea and has one episode of vomiting that results in a small amount of yellow liquid. Before vomiting, the patient reported some abdominal discomfort that they rated at about 2 out of 10, but the reported discomfort decreased to 0 after vomiting.

Recording Time: 12 Minutes	
Level of consciousness	Conscious and alert
Respiration	20 breaths/min; regular and adequate
Pulse	104 beats/min; strong and regular
Skin	Flushed, warm, and dry
Blood pressure	122/68 mm Hg
Oxygen saturation (Spo_2)	98%

5. Should you reassess the patient's vital signs at shorter intervals? Why or why not?
6. Based on the patient's chief complaint, what additional information can you obtain by using the OPQRST mnemonic?

petechiae. Use respiratory protection, provide rapid transport, and provide early notification to the ED so they can make specific preparations for accepting a highly contagious patient.

Only laboratory tests can sort out the different forms of meningitis; therefore, you should take standard precautions with any patient who is suspected of having meningitis. Wearing gloves and a mask, and having the patient wear a mask, will go a long way to prevent the patient's secretions from getting into your nose and mouth. Again, the risk of infection is small, even if the organism is transmitted.

Despite the lower risk of transmission, because the disease can cause death or severe disability, several vaccines are available for most types of meningococcus. The CDC recommends that children 11 to 12 years of age receive the MenACWY vaccine, with a booster at age 16 years. If the MenB vaccine is also recommended, it should be given near the time of highest risk, such as prior to college entry. Doctors may advise that children or adults with other risk factors be vaccinated with one or more of these vaccines.[11] Meningitis can be treated following exposure with antibiotics.

After treating a patient with meningitis, contact your designated infection control officer. Many states consider meningococcal infection reportable and will notify you that meningitis was diagnosed in one of your patients. Prophylactic treatment may be recommended for you.

Tuberculosis

Most patients who are infected with *Mycobacterium tuberculosis* (the tubercle bacillus) feel well most of the time. If the disease involves the brain or kidneys, the patient is only slightly contagious. In the United States, however, **tuberculosis** is a chronic disease that usually strikes the lungs. Patients have tuberculosis disease when they exhibit signs and symptoms and can spread the disease. People who have latent tuberculosis infection have no signs or symptoms and cannot spread the disease. Latent tuberculosis is diagnosed using a skin test, a blood test, and, if either of these is positive, a chest radiograph. If latent tuberculosis infection is not treated, it can develop into tuberculosis disease. After the initial infection, the tubercle bacillus is rendered dormant by the patient's immune system. However, even after decades of lying dormant, this germ can reactivate. Tuberculosis is difficult to treat, especially because an increasing number of tuberculosis strains have grown resistant to most antibiotics. The risk of developing tuberculosis disease is high in patients who have diabetes, untreated HIV infection, or immunosuppression from disease or medication; are younger than 5 years; or have had inadequately treated tuberculosis infection.[12]

When tuberculosis disease develops in patients and their lungs are affected, they typically report a cough of more than 3 weeks' duration that produces mucus (sometimes bloody) and chest pain. They often report other general signs and symptoms such as fever, weight loss, night sweats, fatigue, and decreased appetite.

Although tuberculosis is often hard to distinguish from other diseases, patients who have tuberculosis disease almost invariably have a cough, some with blood-tinged mucus. Therefore, for your safety, you should immediately use respiratory precautions if tuberculosis is suspected. The droplets produced by coughing are not the real problem. The real problem is the droplet nuclei, which are the remnants of the droplets after the excess water has evaporated. These particles are tiny enough to be invisible and can remain suspended in the air for a long time. In fact, as long as these particles are shielded from ultraviolet light, they can remain alive for decades. Particles that are the size of droplet nuclei are not stopped by routine surgical masks. Inhaled, they are carried directly to the alveoli of the lungs, where the bacteria may begin to grow. N95 or HEPA masks are required to stop droplet nuclei (**FIGURE 15-8**).

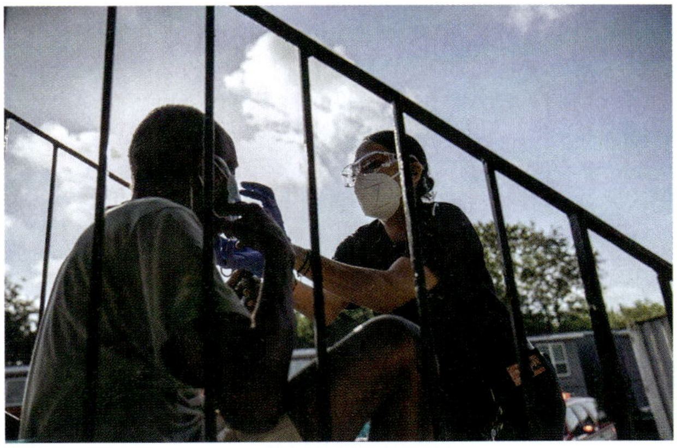

FIGURE 15-8 Wear an N95 mask when treating a patient whom you suspect has tuberculosis, just as you would a patient who you suspect has COVID-19.

According to the World Health Organization, approximately one-fourth of the world's population has been infected with tuberculosis.[13] The vaccine for tuberculosis, called BCG, is rarely used in the United States. Under normal circumstances, however, the mechanism of transmission used by *M tuberculosis* is not very efficient. Infected air is easily diluted with uninfected air. *M tuberculosis* typically causes no illness in a new host. Tuberculosis is most contagious in crowded environments with poor ventilation, where the disease spreads more easily.

Special Populations

PATIENTS AT INCREASED RISK OF INFECTION

The aging process may alter the body's natural defense mechanisms against invading microorganisms. As a person ages, their physical defenses weaken or are eliminated. The skin's thinning and loss of supportive collagen, along with a reduction in the number of blood vessels, allow bacteria or viruses to enter the body with less resistance. The respiratory system cannot trap and eliminate bacteria and viruses in the airways as efficiently as it once did. Additionally, the gastrointestinal system allows easier entry for bacteria or viruses through the intestines. As the body ages, physical barriers to entry weaken, the immune system deteriorates, and invading organisms are not as easily identified. Infectious agents can take hold in older people much more easily because of reduced defenses.

When transporting an older patient, protect the patient from the environment because extremes in heat or cold can further reduce the body's defenses. If the patient has a cold or the flu, protect yourself by wearing an N95 mask and placing a surgical or oxygen mask on the patient, if doing so is indicated.

People who are immunosuppressed from chronic illnesses, cancer treatment, or organ transplants may also lack the ability to fight certain infections. Ensure that these patients are not exposed to any additional conditions that could lead to an infection.

Young children do not have fully developed immune systems. This younger population may be at increased risk of becoming ill after exposure to a disease. Also consider that when transporting a sick child, you are at risk of contracting an illness from them. When obtaining a history on a child, be sure to ask if they are up to date on their immunizations.[14]

If you are exposed to a patient who is found to have pulmonary tuberculosis, you will be given a tuberculin skin test. This simple skin test determines whether you have been infected with *M tuberculosis*. A positive result means that exposure has occurred; it does not mean that you have active tuberculosis. It takes at least 6 weeks for the bacteria to show up in the laboratory test. The purpose of having the test near the time of an exposure (ie, sooner than 6 weeks) is to establish that you were negative prior to the exposure; if you test negative, you will be tested again after 6 weeks to ensure you are still negative. If at that time you test positive, you will know the likely cause, or at least the timing, of your infection. If your initial test result is positive, you will know that you were exposed to tuberculosis at an earlier time, in which case you will probably never identify the source. Most transmissions occur silently, so it is necessary that you have tuberculin skin tests regularly. If the infection is found before you become ill, preventive therapy is almost 100% effective. Usually, a daily dose of the medication isoniazid will prevent the development of active infection.

Pertussis

Pertussis, also called whooping cough, is an airborne disease caused by bacteria that mostly affects children younger than 6 years. Signs and symptoms in the first week or two are similar to the common cold and are followed by fever, excess mucus, and bursts of prolonged coughing followed by a long inspiration that often produces a "whoop" sound in children. During the coughing attacks, children and infants may become cyanotic and appear very ill. They may vomit when it concludes. Complications such as pneumonia (especially in infants), dehydration, and seizures (related to hypoxia) may occur. While pertussis can develop in adults, their disease is not often as severe; however, they can transmit the disease to others.

Cases of pertussis are on the rise due to a decrease in the number of children who are vaccinated to protect against infection and the waning effectiveness of the vaccine over time.[15] The best way to prevent infection from pertussis is to be vaccinated with a diphtheria, tetanus, and pertussis (DTaP) vaccine. Clinicians who have previously had this vaccine should make sure they are up to date with a booster. For added protection, place a mask on the patient and on yourself.

Methicillin-Resistant *Staphylococcus aureus*

Each year in the United States, approximately 20,000 people die from bloodstream infection with *S aureus*.[16] Resistance to the antibiotics that treat *S aureus* infection, such as methicillin, significantly increases a person's risk of mortality. Approximately 2% of individuals are asymptomatic but carry **methicillin-resistant *Staphylococcus aureus* (MRSA)**, although serious MRSA infections will not develop in most of these individuals.[17]

In health care settings, MRSA is believed to be transmitted from patient to patient via the unwashed hands of health care clinicians. MRSA is also spread in the broader community; for example, children with no health care exposure can present with MRSA. The bacterium can be transmitted through broken skin from surfaces or objects such as towels that were contaminated with it hours or days before.[18] Factors that increase the risk for the development of MRSA include antibiotic therapy, prolonged hospital stays, a stay in an intensive care or burn unit, and exposure to an infected patient.

The incubation period for MRSA appears to be between 5 and 45 days. The communicable period varies, as patients who have active infection may carry MRSA for months. MRSA results in soft-tissue infections. Its signs and symptoms may involve localized skin abscesses, and sepsis may be found in older patients with the infection.

Global Health Issues

Coronavirus Disease 2019

Coronaviruses are typically responsible for minor respiratory illnesses such as the common cold, which in most people is not a lethal illness. Past outbreaks of novel (new) strains of coronavirus, such as SARS in 2002–2003 and the Middle East respiratory syndrome (MERS) in 2012, introduced the world to more lethal types of these viruses.

The virus responsible for the COVID-19 pandemic (SARS-CoV-2) spreads rapidly between people and is susceptible to mutation. The global response beginning in 2019 was to mandate social distancing and immunizations. Since the initial outbreak in 2019, much of the world population has been immunized or exposed, with authorized immunizations becoming available in 2021 and new vaccines developed since then to address variations in the virus.[19] Natural immunities to the virus have also begun to develop. While COVID-19 is still present and contagious, more has been learned about the virus, and mandates for social distancing and immunizations have relaxed.

Although the mortality rate has decreased substantially since the disease's initial appearance, there have been more than 1.2 million deaths related to COVID-19 in the United States.[20] Currently, most deaths caused by COVID-19 are seen in people who are already ill with other chronic medical conditions and in geriatric patients.[21] As with all viral diseases, the virus responsible for COVID-19 has and will continue to mutate. The WHO and the CDC continue to monitor COVID-19, as well as other coronavirus-related diseases, and make recommendations for public safety.

Ebola

In 2014, an outbreak of the Ebola virus in West Africa caused international concern. Several infected people with the virus traveled to other countries, including the United States, where two nurses caring for these patients were infected.[22] These cases motivated EMS and health care facilities to prepare for further outbreaks. Ebola is one of a number of viral hemorrhagic fevers most frequently seen in several African countries. The incubation period is approximately 6 to 12 days after exposure; however, symptoms may not begin to appear for as long as 21 days after infection. Symptoms include watery diarrhea, vomiting, fever, body aches, and bleeding. The fatality rate can be as high as 70% if effective supportive treatment in an intensive care unit is not initiated promptly.

If you suspect your patient may have this condition, enhanced PPE is needed. Don an N95 mask, face shield, foot covers, surgical hood, a second pair of gloves, and gown. When viral hemorrhagic fever is known or suspected, follow the specific instructions for donning and doffing PPE, as outlined by local protocols and by the CDC, which provides detailed guidance for EMS clinicians.[23] Immediately notify the receiving facility that your patient may have or may have been exposed to the Ebola virus.

Travel Medicine

Every day, thousands of people travel to various countries. Although humans share many common germs, some are confined to certain areas of the world. As an EMS clinician, you must be aware of this when assessing a patient who recently traveled outside the United States.

Patients who acquire an illness from another country can present with a variety of symptoms depending on the illness. They may have a fever, cough, vomiting, bloody diarrhea, body aches, and rashes. In many cases, the patient experiences mild symptoms and does not require EMS. However, some patients become extremely ill, requiring urgent evaluation and treatment. When you encounter an ill patient with a recent travel history, place a mask on the patient and gather as much information as possible. Important questions to ask the patient include:

- Where did you recently travel?
- Did you receive any vaccinations before your trip?
- Were you exposed to any infectious diseases?
- Is there anyone else in your travel party who is sick?
- What types of food did you eat?
- What was your source of drinking water?

If you suspect the patient has a communicable illness, follow appropriate PPE precautions and notify the receiving facility. Although treatment for many travel-related illnesses is primarily supportive in the prehospital environment, always be prepared to treat life-threatening conditions should the patient become unstable.

Words of Wisdom

The ability of your EMS system to support you in the event of exposure to a communicable disease depends on your understanding of how an exposure to potentially infectious materials can occur and your immediate reporting of the exposure. Make notes right away to ensure that you remember all pertinent information, and report the possible exposure immediately after the response, following your service's guidelines. Wash your hands frequently and keep your equipment clean.

Conclusion

Although trauma patients often present with dramatic signs and symptoms, the assessment and treatment you provide for them are fairly straightforward. The assessment and treatment of medical patients, in comparison, can be challenging and interesting because of the highly variable nature of medical conditions. The condition of a medical patient may not be as apparent as that of a trauma patient, and, therefore, treatment may not be as straightforward. Additionally, patients may have

YOU are the EMT

With an estimated time of arrival at the hospital of 5 minutes, you reassess the patient and call in your radio report. The hospital acknowledges your report and is awaiting your arrival. The patient reports feeling better but being very thirsty. The patient is delivered to the hospital without incident, and you give your verbal report to a staff nurse, who assumes care. The receiving nurse reassesses the patient's temperature and notes a reading of 99.8°F (37.7°C). After cleaning the ambulance, you return to service.

Recording Time: 21 Minutes	
Level of consciousness	Conscious and alert
Respiration	18 breaths/min; regular and adequate
Pulse	102 beats/min; strong and regular
Skin	Warm, dry; flushed
Blood pressure	120/72 mm Hg
Oxygen saturation (Spo_2)	98%

7. Do the patient's vital signs differ from your initial readings? If so, why might there be a difference?

multiple disease processes, which may complicate your assessment. Children who present with a medical emergency may not have any history of a medical condition. This may be their first medical problem. You must remember that delays of any kind in an attempt to diagnose a condition can be harmful to the patient and thus are not recommended. Your best approach is to keep calm, use your patient assessment skills, treat the patient's symptoms, report to medical control, and transport the patient safely to the ED. Finally, keep in mind that patients sometimes have more than one problem, so you must be prepared to handle any combination of conditions, including conditions of medical patients who have been involved in traumatic situations.

YOU are the EMT SUMMARY

1. What observations should you make when you arrive at the scene before making physical contact with the patient?

When arriving at any scene, your first priority is to assess for any actual or potential hazards that could pose a safety risk to you or your partners. Remember to take standard precautions before making contact with the patient! Additional precautions or protective equipment may be added based on the dispatch information or findings at the scene. Next, assess the environment in which the patient is found. As you approach the patient, form a general impression that will help you rapidly recognize life-threatening conditions even before making physical contact with the patient. Apparent unconsciousness, obvious external bleeding, and severe difficulty breathing are only a few of the visual clues that you may recognize during the initial general impression. After visually assessing the scene, the patient's environment, and the patient, proceed with the primary assessment.

2. On the basis of your general impression and primary assessment findings, does this patient require immediate transport?

Your patient is clearly sick; they have a fever and report weakness. However, they are conscious and alert and do not have any airway, breathing, or circulation problems. Their heart rate and respiratory rate are both increased; however, their pulse is strong and palpable at the radial artery, and their breathing is producing adequate tidal volume. Tachypnea and tachycardia are common physiologic responses to fever. At the present time, there are no signs indicating the need for immediate transport, although the history of diabetes is an added reason for having the patient evaluated at the hospital.

3. How should you proceed with your care of the patient?

You have already determined the patient's chief complaint and have begun initial treatment. Because their condition is stable, immediate transport is not indicated; therefore, proceed by inquiring about the history of the present illness, taking vital signs, obtaining a SAMPLE history, and performing a secondary assessment. The secondary assessment of a medical patient should primarily focus on the chief complaint and presenting signs and symptoms. A baseline set of vital signs, including pulse oximetry and a blood glucose level, may be obtained by your partner while you are assessing the patient. The baseline vital signs can then be compared with future readings (trending) to determine if the patient's condition is unchanged, has improved, or has worsened.

4. Is it appropriate to transport the patient to the hospital they requested, or should you transport them to the closer facility?

Generally, patients should be transported to the hospital of their choice when at all possible, especially if they have been there previously. Ultimately, however, the destination facility should be dictated by the patient's condition as well as local protocols and medical direction. Your patient is in stable condition; that is, they currently have no airway, breathing, or circulation problems. Therefore, it is not unreasonable to comply with their request and transport them to the hospital of their choice. However, you should inform the patient that if their condition worsens, it may be necessary to divert to a closer facility. If the patient's spouse will be following you in a personal vehicle, ask for their mobile phone number, if they have one, so you can contact them should diversion to a closer facility become necessary. Documenting the reason for your transport destination choice can influence payment from insurers.

5. Should you reassess the patient's vital signs at shorter intervals? Why or why not?

On the basis of your patient's stable condition, reassessing the vital signs every 15 minutes is appropriate at this time. If the condition worsens, you can

YOU are the EMT SUMMARY continued

always record the vital signs at shorter intervals. Vital signs are only one component of reassessment. You should also monitor the patient's level of consciousness and other parameters (eg, skin condition and temperature, breathing status, pulse regularity and strength) en route. In many cases, these parameters change when a patient's condition is deteriorating even before the vital signs change.

6. Based on the patient's chief complaint, what additional information can you obtain by using the OPQRST mnemonic?

Not every component of the OPQRST mnemonic will apply to every patient; however, there are some components that will. Your patient's chief complaint was fever, diarrhea, and vomiting with weakness. Details leading up to the event, including an acute onset of fever versus fever that developed slowly, are important to note; this can aid the ED physician in making a diagnosis. The presence of provoking or palliating factors can also be established. In a patient with a fever, ask if any antipyretics (fever-reducing medications), such as ibuprofen or acetaminophen, were taken and if they seemed to help. Ask if there is a particular position that improves or worsens symptoms. In this case, the patient had taken ibuprofen, but there is no information on what the fever was prior to taking it, so its effectiveness is not as easy to determine. Although the patient did not report pain initially, you can ask if there is discomfort during vomiting or diarrhea episodes and what that feels like (quality). Radiating or referred pain would be less likely in this patient by history but may be discovered during palpation of the abdomen in the secondary exam. If the patient does have any pain or discomfort, ask the patient to assign it a number initially (severity) and then ask again at regular intervals. In this case, the patient did report some discomfort, rated as 2 out of 10, before they vomited, and the pain disappeared after the vomiting. When establishing the time of onset, you are asking for a specific time that the symptoms began (eg, yesterday around 1500 hours). If the patient is unable to give a specific time, they may be able to give a duration (eg, 8 hours) that they have been feeling ill.

7. Do the patient's vital signs differ from your initial readings? If so, why might there be a difference?

The patient's blood pressure has remained consistent throughout your encounter. This is important as the patient is showing some signs of dehydration (thirst, dry mucous membranes). If there had been a large amount of vomiting, the blood pressure may have decreased and the pulse rate would have likely increased.

Fever can cause shivering, which causes the patient to expend a lot of energy and can make them feel weak. Fever also increases a person's metabolic rate, resulting in the production of more heat energy. Physiologically, the body responds to an increased metabolic rate by increasing its vital functions; namely, respirations and heart rate. Additionally, the heart rate and respirations may increase with vomiting episodes. As the temperature decreases after administration of an antipyretic, the heart rate and respiratory rate may decrease.

When a person is actively "running a fever," the skin is typically flushed, abnormally warm or hot, and dry. As the fever begins to subside, sweating usually occurs, which is the body's way of removing heat through evaporation. However, if as in this case, a person is dehydrated, perspiration cannot increase to cool the body. Note that "flushed" does not always mean "red" or "pink" skin. In a patient with dark baseline skin tone, such as this patient, the increased flow of blood to the skin may be difficult to detect. By suspecting that the patient's face was uncharacteristically dark and confirming with the spouse, you were able to obtain a helpful assessment finding.

<table>
<tr><th colspan="6">EMS Patient Care Report (PCR)</th></tr>
<tr><td>Date: 7-29-25</td><td>Incident No.: 011109</td><td colspan="2">Nature of Call: Sick person</td><td colspan="2">Location: 125 Green Hills Dr</td></tr>
<tr><td>Dispatched: 1325</td><td>En Route: 1325</td><td>At Scene: 1335</td><td>Transport: 1348</td><td>At Hospital: 1402</td><td>In Service: 1413</td></tr>
<tr><th colspan="6">Patient Information</th></tr>
<tr><td colspan="3">Age: 36
Sex: M
Weight (in kg [lb]): 79 kg (175 lb)</td><td colspan="3">Allergies: No known allergies
Medications: Ibuprofen, metformin (oral diabetic medication)
Past Medical History: Type 2 diabetes
Chief Complaint: Fever, diarrhea, and vomiting with weakness</td></tr>
</table>

YOU are the EMT SUMMARY continued

Vital Signs				
Time: 1340	**BP:** 124/70	**Pulse:** 110	**Respirations:** 18	**Spo_2:** 99%
Time: 1347	**BP:** 122/68	**Pulse:** 104	**Respirations:** 20	**Spo_2:** 98%
Time: 1356	**BP:** 120/72	**Pulse:** 102	**Respirations:** 18	**Spo_2:** 98%
EMS Treatment (circle all that apply)				
Oxygen @ ___ L/min via: NC NRM BVM		**Assisted Ventilation**	**Airway Adjunct**	**CPR**
Defibrillation	**Bleeding Control**	**Bandaging**	**Splinting**	**Other:** Position of comfort

Narrative

9-1-1 dispatch for a 36-year-old with fever with diarrhea and vomiting. Patient states they are biologically male.

Chief Complaint: Fever, diarrhea, vomiting, feeling weak

History: Patient stated that they began feeling bad the day before and began running a fever last night. Patient also reported diarrhea and vomiting all night and now feels a bit weak, but denied any other symptoms. Approximately 20 minutes prior to EMS arrival, patient took 400 mg of ibuprofen. Spouse took patient's temperature just prior to EMS arrival and noted a reading of 100.6°F (38.1°C).

Assessment: On arrival at the scene, found the patient in a semisitting position in bed. Patient was conscious and alert, airway was patent, and breathing was adequate. Obtained vital signs and performed additional assessment. Patient's skin was noted to be flushed, warm to touch, and dry. Breath sounds were clear to auscultation bilaterally and patient denied a cough. Abdomen was soft and nontender on palpation. Patient further denied any significant past medical history other than diabetes, for which patient takes an oral diabetic medication. Patient stated no allergies to medications. A blood glucose reading of 242 mg/dL was obtained.

Treatment (Rx): None administered.

Transport: Patient took two steps with assistance from crew to the stretcher. Began transport to the hospital of patient's choice with the patient in position of comfort. En route, continued to monitor patient's condition and vital signs as indicated. Patient remained conscious and alert with little change in vital signs. Patient stated feeling better but being very thirsty. They had one episode of vomiting, which consisted of a small amount of clear yellow liquid. Remainder of transport was uneventful. Delivered patient to ED without incident and gave verbal report to staff nurse, Jimenez. On arrival, receiving nurse reassessed patient's temperature; a reading of 99.8°F (37.7°C) was noted. Medic 14 returned to service at 1413.

End of report

Prep Kit

Ready for Review

- Trauma emergencies are injuries that are the result of physical forces applied to the body. Medical emergencies require EMS attention because of illnesses or conditions not caused by an outside force.
- The assessment of a medical patient is similar to the assessment of a trauma patient but with a different focus. Whereas a trauma assessment focuses on physical injuries, some of which may be detectable by physical examination,

Prep Kit continued

medical patient assessment is usually more focused on symptoms and depends more on establishing an accurate medical history.

- Many seriously ill medical patients may not appear to be in critical condition at first glance.
- For conscious medical patients, obtaining a thorough patient history can be one of the most beneficial aspects of the patient assessment. Try to determine the NOI by asking questions about the patient's chief complaint.
- Conscious medical patients seldom need a secondary assessment of the entire body, but all should get a detailed physical examination based on their chief complaint. However, you should always perform a secondary assessment of the entire body on unconscious patients; this head-to-toe assessment may give you clues to help identify the problem. Your secondary assessment of an unconscious or unstable patient should never delay transport.
- Most medical emergencies require a level of treatment beyond what is available in the prehospital setting. Also, the treatments depend on an accurate diagnosis of the exact medical condition; therefore, advanced testing in the hospital may be required.
- If the patient is not in critical condition, you should gather as much important information as possible from the scene so that you can transmit that information to the physician at the ED.
- Many medical emergency patients do not have immediately life-threatening conditions. If a life-threatening condition exists, transport might be meaningfully expedited by the use of lights and siren, but if that is not the case, careful consideration should be given to nonemergency transport.
- Modes of transport ultimately come in one of two categories: ground or air.
- Many medical patients will benefit from being transported to a specific hospital capable of handling their particular condition.
- Because it is often impossible to tell which patients have infectious diseases, you should avoid direct contact with the blood and body fluids of all patients.
- If you think you may have been exposed to an infectious disease, see your physician (or your employer's designated physician) immediately.
- Diseases of special concern include influenza, HIV infection, hepatitis, meningitis, pertussis, tuberculosis, COVID-19, and Ebola.
- Infection control should be an important part of your daily routine. Be sure to follow the proper steps when dealing with potential exposure situations.
- Patients who recently traveled outside of the United States should be screened for possible infectious illnesses. If you suspect the patient has a travel-related illness, place a mask on them, follow appropriate PPE, and gather as much information as possible.

Vital Vocabulary

communicable disease A disease that can be spread from one person or species to another.

epidemic A disease outbreak in which new cases of a disease in a human population substantially exceed the number expected based on recent experience.

herpes simplex A common virus that is asymptomatic in 80% of people carrying it, but characterized by small blisters on the lips or genitals in symptomatic infections.

index of suspicion Awareness that unseen life-threatening injuries or illness may exist.

infectious disease A medical condition caused by the growth and spread of small, harmful organisms within the body.

influenza A disease caused by a virus that has crossed the animal–human barrier and infected

Prep Kit continued

humans and that kills thousands of people every year.

medical emergencies Emergencies that are caused by disease (illnesses or conditions) rather than a physical force acting on the body (ie, trauma).

meningitis An inflammation of the meningeal coverings of the brain and spinal cord; usually caused by a virus or a bacterium.

meningococcal meningitis An inflammation of the meningeal coverings of the brain and spinal cord; can be highly contagious.

methicillin-resistant *Staphylococcus aureus* (MRSA) A disease caused by a bacterium that can cause infections in different parts of the body and is often resistant to commonly used antibiotics. It is transmitted by different routes, including the respiratory route, and can be found on the skin, in surgical wounds, or in the bloodstream, lungs, or urinary tract.

nature of illness (NOI) The general type of illness a patient is experiencing.

pandemic A disease outbreak that occurs on a global scale.

pertussis A highly contagious bacterial disease that causes episodes of uncontrolled coughing followed by prolonged inspiration often accompanied by a "whoop" sound; also called whooping cough.

petechiae Small, flat, purple-red blotches on the skin that do not blanch when pressure is applied; may be seen in individuals with meningococcal infection.

trauma emergencies Emergencies that are the result of physical forces applied to the body; injuries.

tuberculosis A chronic bacterial disease, caused by *Mycobacterium tuberculosis*, that usually affects the lungs but can also affect other organs such as the brain and kidneys; it is spread by cough and can lie dormant in a person's lungs for decades and then reactivate.

virulence The strength or ability of a pathogen to produce disease.

References

1. Geriatric emergency department criteria. American College of Emergency Physicians website. https://www.acep.org/siteassets/sites/geda/media/documnets/geda-criteria.pdf. Updated April 2024. Accessed December 3, 2024.
2. Age-friendly health systems: guide to recognition for geriatric emergency department accredited sites. Institute for Healthcare Improvement website. https://forms.ihi.org/hubfs/Guide%20to%20Recognition%20for%20GEDA%20Sites_FINAL.pdf. Published July 2024. Accessed December 3, 2024.
3. Learning from pandemic flu. Centers for Disease Control and Prevention. https://www.cdc.gov/museum/pdf/cdcm-pha-stem-learning-from-pandemic-flu-lesson.pdf. Accessed December 3, 2024.
4. Bird flu is raising red flags among health officials. Johns Hopkins website. https://publichealth.jhu.edu/2025/bird-flu-is-raising-red-flags-among-health-officials. Published January 14, 2025. Accessed February 18, 2025.
5. How CDC is monitoring influenza data among people to better understand the current avian influenza A (H5N1) situation. Centers for Disease Control and Prevention website. https://www.cdc.gov/bird-flu/index.html. Published February 8, 2025. Accessed February 18, 2025.
6. Influenza. Centers for Disease Control and Prevention website. https://www.cdc.gov/nchs/fastats/flu.htm. Reviewed September 4, 2024. Accessed December 3, 2024.
7. Taylor LE, Swerdfeger AL, Esclick GD. Vaccines are not associated with autism: an evidence-based meta-analysis of case-control and cohort studies. *Vaccine*. 2014;32:3623–3629.
8. Maglione MA, Das L, Raaen L, et al. Safety of vaccines used for routine immunization of US children: a systematic review. *Pediatrics*. 2014;134(2):325–337.
9. About shingles (herpes zoster). Centers for Disease Control and Prevention website. https://www.cdc.gov/shingles/about/index.html. Published May 10, 2024. Accessed December 3, 2024.
10. Let's stop HIV together: PrEP. Centers for Disease Control and Prevention website. https://www.cdc.gov/stophivtogether/hiv-prevention/prep.html. Reviewed February 7, 2024. Accessed December 3, 2024.
11. Meningococcal vaccine recommendations. Centers for Disease Control and Prevention website.

Prep Kit continued

https://www.cdc.gov/meningococcal/hcp/vaccine-recommendations/index.html. Published October 24, 2024. Accessed December 3, 2024.

12. TB 101 for healthcare workers. Centers for Disease Control and Prevention website. https://www.cdc.gov/tb/webcourses/TB101/page5108.html. Accessed December 3, 2024.
13. Tuberculosis. World Health Organization website. https://www.who.int/health-topics/tuberculosis. Published November 7, 2023. Accessed December 3, 2024.
14. National Center for Immunization and Respiratory Diseases. Children and adolescent immunization schedule by age. Centers for Disease Control and Prevention website. https://www.cdc.gov/vaccines/schedules/hcp/imz/child-adolescent.html. Reviewed November 16, 2023. Accessed December 3, 2024.
15. About whooping cough outbreaks. Centers for Disease Control and Prevention website. https://www.cdc.gov/pertussis/outbreaks/index.html. Published August 23, 2024. Accessed December 3, 2024.
16. Kourtis AP, Hatfield K, Baggs J, et al. Vital signs: epidemiology and recent trends in methicillin-resistant and in methicillin-susceptible *Staphylococcus aureus* bloodstream infections—United States. *MMWR Morb Mortal Wkly Rep*. 2019;68(9):214–219.
17. Clinical overview of methicillin-resistant *Staphylococcus aureus* (MRSA) in healthcare settings. Centers for Disease Prevention and Control website. https://www.cdc.gov/mrsa/hcp/clinical-overview/index.html. Published April 12, 2024. Accessed December 3, 2024.
18. Preventing methicillin-resistant *Staphylococcuss aureus* (MRSA). Centers for Disease Control and Prevention website. https://www.cdc.gov/mrsa/prevention/index.html#cdc_prevention_exposure-exposure. Published July 8, 2024. Accessed December 3, 2024.
19. Doshi RH, Nsasiirwe S, Dahlke M, et al. COVID-19 vaccination coverage: World Health Organization African Region, 2021–2023. *MMWR Morb Mortal Wkly Rep*. 2024;73(14):307–311.
20. Provisional COVID-19 mortality surveillance. Centers for Disease Control and Prevention website. https://www.cdc.gov/nchs/nvss/vsrr/covid19/index.htm. Reviewed November 27, 2024. Accessed December 3, 2024.
21. Choi WY. Mortality rate of patients with COVID-19 based on underlying health conditions. *Disaster Med Public Health Prep*. 2021 May 3:1–6.
22. Ebola outbreak. Centers for Disease Control and Prevention website. https://www.cdc.gov/ebola/outbreaks/index.html. Published May 6, 2024. Accessed December 3, 2024.
23. Viral hemorrhagic fevers (VHFs): interim guidance for emergency services. Centers for Disease Control and Prevention website. https://www.cdc.gov/viral-hemorrhagic-fevers/hcp/emergency-guidance/index.html. Published May 15, 2024. Accessed December 3, 2024.

Additional Resources

National Association of State EMS Officials. *National Model EMS Clinical Guidelines: Version 3.0*. https://nasemso.org/wp-content/uploads/National-Model-EMS-Clinical-Guidelines_2022.pdf. Updated March 2022. Accessed December 3, 2024.

National Highway Traffic Safety Administration. *National Emergency Medical Services Education Standards*. https://www.ems.gov/assets/EMS_Education-Standards_2021_FNL.pdf. EMS.gov website. Published January 2021. Accessed December 3, 2024.

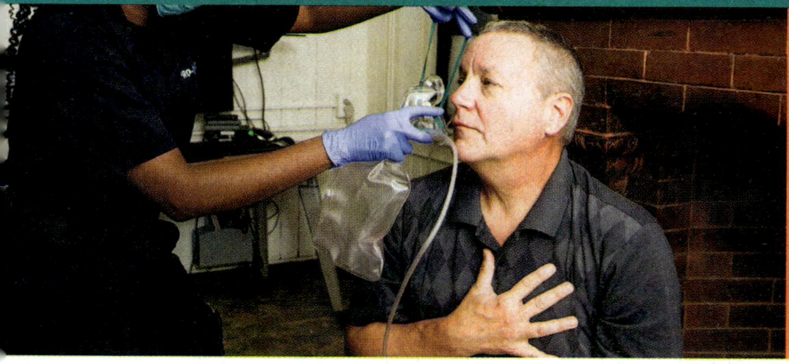

Chapter 16

Respiratory Emergencies

EMS EDUCATION STANDARD COMPETENCIES

Medicine

Applies knowledge to provide basic emergency care and transportation based on assessment findings for an acutely ill patient.

Respiratory

- Respiratory distress/failure/arrest (Chapter 11, *Airway and Ventilation Management*)
- Upper airway obstruction (pp 676–677)
- Lower airway disease:
  - Asthma (pp 671–675)
  - Bronchiolitis (pp 665–666)
  - Pneumonia (p 666)
  - Chronic obstructive pulmonary disease (COPD) (pp 670–671)
- Spontaneous pneumothorax (pp 675–676)
- Other respiratory disorders to be determined locally

KNOWLEDGE OBJECTIVES

1. List the structures and functions of the upper and lower airways, lungs, and accessory structures of the respiratory system. (pp 641–643)
2. Describe the differences in the anatomy and physiology of the pediatric airway compared to the adult patient and implications for emergency medical technicians (EMTs). (pp 641–643)
3. Discuss the physiologic changes associated with the aging process and the age-related assessment and treatment modifications that result. (pp 643, 647)
4. Explain the special patient assessment and care considerations that are required for geriatric patients who are experiencing respiratory distress. (pp 643, 647)
5. Explain the physiology of respiration; include the signs of normal breathing. (pp 643–644)
6. Discuss the pathophysiology of respiration, including examples of the common signs and symptoms a patient with inadequate breathing may present with in an emergency situation. (pp 644–649)
7. Describe different respiratory conditions that cause dyspnea, including their causes, assessment findings and symptoms, complications, and specific prehospital management and transport decisions. (pp 647–648, 664–679)
8. List the characteristics of infectious diseases that are frequently associated with dyspnea. (pp 648–649)
9. Describe the assessment of a patient who is in respiratory distress and the relationship of the assessment findings to patient management and transport decisions. (pp 649–653)
10. Explain the special patient assessment and care considerations that are required for pediatric patients who are experiencing respiratory distress. (pp 650–651, 664–675)

11. Describe the differences in the pathophysiology of respiration in the pediatric patient compared to the adult patient and implications for EMTs. (pp 650–651)
12. List different types of abnormal breath sounds, their signs and symptoms, and the disease process associated with each one. (pp 652–654)
13. Describe the primary emergency medical care of a person who is in respiratory distress. (pp 657–664)
14. State the generic name, medication forms, dose, administration, indications, actions, and contraindications for medications that are administered via metered-dose inhalers (MDIs) and small-volume nebulizers. (pp 657–664)
15. Discuss some pandemic considerations related to the spread of the influenza type A virus and coronavirus and strategies EMTs should employ to protect themselves from infection during a possible crisis situation. (pp 667–668)
16. Describe the assessment findings and emergency care for a patient who has experienced a spontaneous pneumothorax. (pp 675–676)
17. Describe the causes and risk factors of aspiration and steps the EMT can take to prevent aspiration from occurring in their patients. (p 677)

SKILLS OBJECTIVES

1. Demonstrate the process of history taking to obtain more information related to a patient's chief complaint based on a case scenario. (pp 654–655)
2. Demonstrate how to use the OPQRST assessment to obtain more specific information about a patient's breathing problem. (p 655)
3. Demonstrate how to use the PASTE assessment to obtain more specific information about a patient's breathing problem. (p 655)
4. Demonstrate how to assist a patient with the administration of a metered-dose inhaler. (p 662, Skill Drill 16-1)
5. Demonstrate how to assist a patient with the administration of a small-volume nebulizer. (p 663, Skill Drill 16-2)
6. Demonstrate how to administer a nasal midturbinate specimen test for coronavirus disease 2019 (COVID-19) infection. (pp 667–668)

Introduction

As an EMT, you will often encounter the patient complaint of **dyspnea**, when a patient reports shortness of breath or has difficulty breathing. It is a symptom of many different conditions, from the common cold or asthma, to heart failure or pulmonary embolism. You may not be able to determine what is causing dyspnea in a particular patient; this can be difficult even for physicians. Also, several different problems may be contributing to a patient's dyspnea at the same time, including some that are life threatening. However, even without making a definitive diagnosis, you will often be able to improve the patient's symptoms or save the patient's life.

This chapter begins with a basic review of respiratory anatomy and physiology. The chapter then looks at common medical problems that can impair normal respiratory functioning and cause dyspnea. Next, it explains specific strategies you can use to assess a patient who has difficulty breathing, using the patient assessment template and organized approach. You will learn the signs and symptoms of each condition and cover topics such as foreign body and anatomic airway obstruction, lung infections, and chronic airway disease. You should keep all of these medical possibilities in mind as you obtain the patient's history and perform a physical assessment; these processes will be described in detail in this chapter. The information you collect will help you to decide on the proper treatment, which can differ according to the probable cause of the dyspnea. For a more thorough review of the anatomy and physiology of the respiratory system, see Chapter 11, *Airway and Ventilation Management*. For a more detailed discussion of assessing a patient with breathing difficulty, see Chapter 10, *Patient Assessment*.

Remember, the sensation of not getting enough air can be terrifying, regardless of its cause. As an

EMT, you should be prepared to fully treat your patient, addressing not just the symptom and the underlying problem, but also the anxiety it produces.

Anatomy of the Respiratory System

The respiratory system consists of the structures of the body that contribute to the breathing process (**FIGURE 16-1**). These structures include the diaphragm, the muscles of the chest wall, the accessory muscles of breathing, and the nerves from the brain and spinal cord to those muscles.

The upper airway consists of all anatomic airway structures above the level of the vocal cords. These include the nose, mouth, jaw, oral cavity, pharynx, and larynx. Air enters the upper airway through the nose and mouth, and it is here that the air is filtered, warmed, and humidified. The upper airway ends at the larynx, which is protected by the epiglottis. This leaf-shaped valve folds over the larynx during swallowing and diverts food and fluid into the esophagus. During normal breathing, the epiglottis returns to an upright position, allowing air to flow freely between the vocal cords into and out of the trachea. Air moves through the trachea into and out of the lungs.

The principal function of the lungs is **respiration**, which is the exchange of oxygen and carbon dioxide. To reach the lower airways, air travels through the trachea into each lung, first passing through the left and right main stem bronchi (larger airways), then on to the bronchioles (smaller airways), and finally into the alveoli. The alveoli are microscopic, thin-walled air sacs where the actual exchange of oxygen and carbon dioxide occurs.

The Pediatric Respiratory System

To manage the pediatric airway effectively, you must understand the anatomic differences between the adult and pediatric airway. To start with, the pediatric airway is smaller in diameter and shorter in length, the lungs are smaller, and the heart is higher in a child's chest. The glottic opening (vocal cords) is higher and positioned more anteriorly (toward the front), and in infants and young children, the neck appears to be nonexistent. As the child develops, the neck gets proportionally longer as the vocal cords and epiglottis achieve their anatomically correct adult position.

The anatomy of a pediatric airway and other important structures differs from that of an adult in the following ways (**FIGURE 16-2**):

- A larger, rounder occiput, or back of the head, which requires more careful positioning of the airway

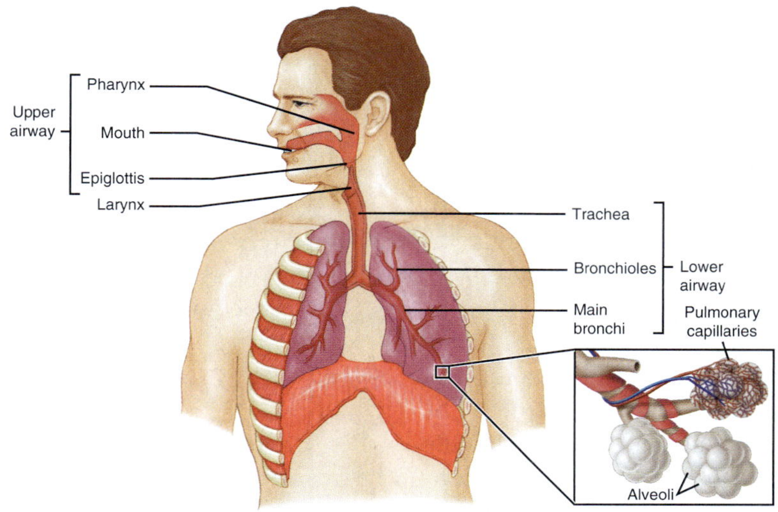

FIGURE 16-1 The upper airway includes the nose, mouth, jaw, oral cavity, pharynx, and larynx. The lower airway includes the trachea, bronchi, bronchioles, and alveoli surrounded by the pulmonary capillaries.

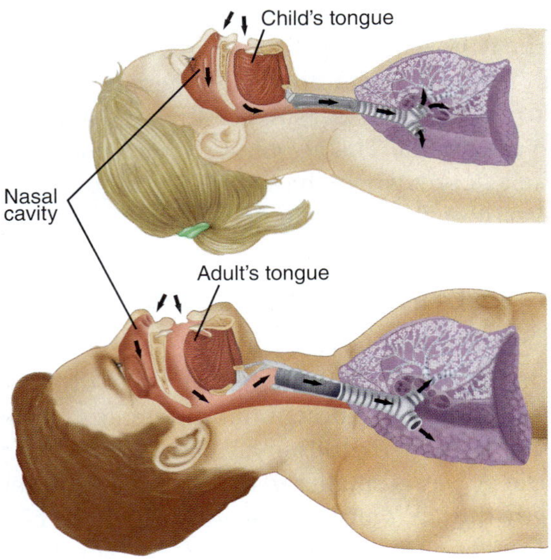

FIGURE 16-2 The anatomy of a child's airway differs from that of an adult in several ways. The back of the head is larger in a child. The tongue is proportionately larger and is located more anterior in the mouth. The trachea is smaller in diameter and more flexible. The airway itself is lower and narrower (funnel-shaped).

- A proportionately larger tongue relative to the size of the mouth and a more anterior location in the mouth. The child's tongue is also larger relative to the small mandible and can easily block the airway.
- Less-developed rings of cartilage in the trachea that may easily collapse if the neck is flexed or hyperextended
- A narrowing funnel-shaped (wide to narrow) upper airway compared to that of a cylinder-shaped (same width) lower airway

These differences will influence the treatment decisions that you make about pediatric patients, including whether intervention is needed and, if so, what procedure to use.

Because of the smaller diameter of the trachea in infants, which is about the same diameter as a drinking straw, their airway is easily obstructed by secretions, blood, or swelling. Infants are obligate nose breathers, which may require diligent suctioning or reassessment and management to maintain a clear airway.

An infant needs to breathe faster than an older child (**TABLE 16-1**). Children's lungs grow and develop increased abilities to handle the exchange

TABLE 16-1 Pediatric Respiratory Rates

Age	Respiratory Rate (breaths/min)
Newborn: 0 to 1 month	30 to 60
Infant: 1 month to 1 year	30 to 53
Toddler: 1 to 3 years	22 to 27
Preschool age: 3 to 6 years	20 to 28
School age: 6 to 12 years	18 to 25
Adolescent: 12 to 18 years	12 to 20

Data From: *Pediatric Advanced Life Support, 2015*, the American Heart Association.

of oxygen as they age. A respiratory rate of 30 to 60 breaths/min is normal for the newborn, whereas the adolescent is expected to have rates closer to the adult range (12 to 20 breaths/min). Children have not only a higher metabolic rate, but also a higher oxygen demand, which in infants is roughly twice that of an adult.[1] This is partly related to the actual size of the lung tissues and the volume that can be exchanged. Smaller lungs mean that the oxygen reserves are smaller. This higher oxygen demand, combined with a smaller oxygen reserve, increases the risk of hypoxia because of apnea or ineffective **ventilation** efforts.

Words of Wisdom

Reference materials such as pediatric protocols, field guides, or mobile device apps can help you with the assessment and care of a child. Refer to these resources during your care, and document your specific observations and treatment decisions. This information-intensive approach to pediatric care helps ensure good care and thorough documentation and can reduce any anxiety you may feel about assessing children.

Breathing also requires the use of the chest muscles and diaphragm. Because intercostal muscles are not well developed in infants and young children, movement of the diaphragm, their major muscle of respiration, dictates the amount of air that they inspire. Young children also experience muscle fatigue much more quickly than older children. This can lead to respiratory failure if a child has to physically fight to breathe for long periods. Any pressure on the abdomen of a young child can block the movement of the diaphragm and cause respiratory compromise. Gastric distention can also interfere with movement of the diaphragm and lead to hypoventilation. Use caution when applying straps to a spinal motion restriction device because this may hinder full symmetric chest wall expansion and thus limit tidal volume.

Safety Tips

In a pediatric patient, the lung tissues are susceptible to a simple or tension pneumothorax if excessive ventilatory pressures occur during assisted ventilations with a bag-mask device. To prevent hypoxia and to avoid damaging the lung tissues, use the appropriate-size mask and reservoir bag to avoid administering an excessively large tidal volume. Only use enough force to make the chest rise slightly. Focus your attention on the rise and fall of the chest wall, versus just simply squeezing the reservoir bag. Although it is rarely indicated, if it is evident that there is inadequate ventilation and oxygenation and the child has some rapid spontaneous respirations, ventilate with the patient's underlying respiratory rate, and be careful not to ventilate against the patient's efforts.[2] If the child's ineffective spontaneous respirations are too slow, assist ventilation by delivering a breath once every 2 to 3 seconds.

Breath sounds in children are easier to hear because of their thinner chest walls, but because less air is exchanged with each breath, detection of poor air movement or complete absence of breath sounds may be more difficult.

The Geriatric Respiratory System

Age-related changes in the respiratory system can predispose an older adult to respiratory illness. Even a minor lung infection can become a life-threatening event. One of the conditions contributing to breathing problems is the weakening of the airway musculature that can cause decreased breathing capacity. This decreased muscle mass means that older patients have less help from muscles in the chest wall when they have trouble breathing.

As one gets older, the alveoli in lung tissue can become enlarged and the elasticity decreases, making it harder to expel used air (air trapping). This change in lung tissue quality is comparable to a balloon that has been expanded and then deflated; the balloon loses some of its ability to contract to its original state. The lack of elasticity results in a decreased ability to bring in oxygen and push out carbon dioxide.

The body's chemoreceptors, which monitor the changes in oxygen and carbon dioxide levels in the blood, become less sensitive with age. As a result, the body may respond more slowly to hypoxia, a dangerous condition in which the body tissues and cells do not have enough oxygen.

In addition, loss of mechanisms that protect the upper airway include decreased cough and gag reflexes. There is also a decrease in the cilia that line the bronchial tree. These changes lessen an older person's ability to cough and clear secretions, thereby increasing the risk of infection.

Physiology of Respiration

The two ventilatory processes that facilitate respiration are inspiration, the act of breathing in (inhaling), and expiration, the act of breathing out (exhaling). During respiration, oxygen is provided

YOU are the EMT

It is 0430 hours when the alert tones sound: "Medic 81, respond to 109 East Lawler for a 72-year-old woman with shortness of breath." You recognize the address as one to which you have responded on numerous occasions. The woman lives alone; has emphysema, hypertension, and gout; and routinely refuses EMS transport. You and your partner proceed to the scene. The weather is clear, and the temperature is 65°F (18.3°C).

1. What is emphysema? What is the typical cause?

2. Why is it especially significant that *this* patient called 9-1-1?

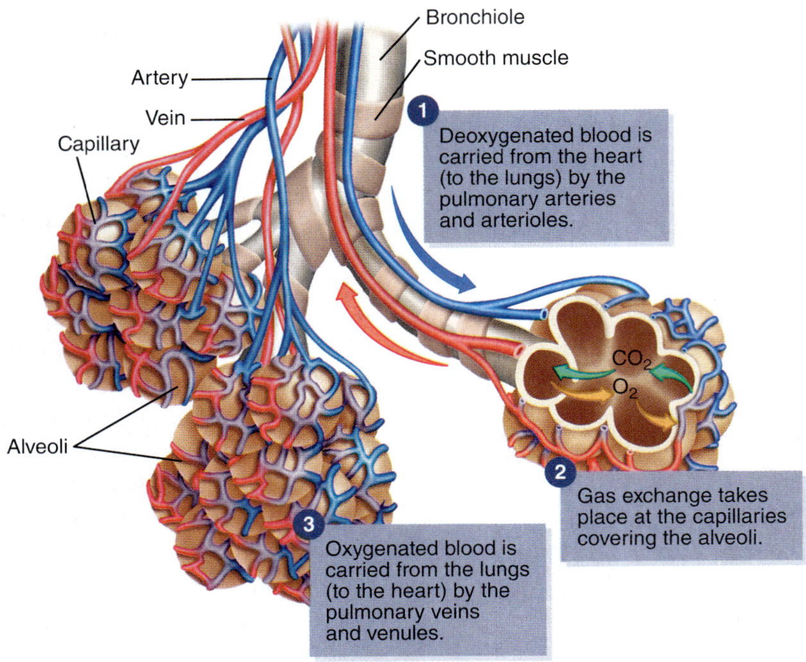

FIGURE 16-3 An enlarged view of a single alveolus (air sac) showing where the exchange of oxygen and carbon dioxide between air in the sac and blood in the pulmonary capillaries takes place.

to the blood, and carbon dioxide is removed from it. In healthy lungs, this exchange of gases takes place rapidly at the level of the alveoli (**FIGURE 16-3**). The alveoli lie against the pulmonary capillary vessels, and as oxygen enters the alveoli from inhalation, it passes freely through tiny passages in the alveolar wall into these capillaries through the process of diffusion. The oxygen binds to the hemoglobin in the red blood cells and is carried to the heart, which then pumps the oxygen-rich blood around the body, where it is released to the tissues that need oxygen. Carbon dioxide produced by the body's cells returns to the lungs in the blood that circulates through and around the alveolar air spaces. The carbon dioxide diffuses back into the alveoli and travels back up the bronchial tree and out through the upper airways during exhalation (**FIGURE 16-4**). Again, carbon dioxide is exchanged for oxygen, which travels in the opposite direction (during inhalation).

Throughout the whole process of respiration, the brainstem constantly senses the level of carbon dioxide in the arterial blood. The level of carbon dioxide bathing the brainstem stimulates a healthy person to breathe. If the level of carbon dioxide drops too low, the person automatically breathes at a slower rate and less deeply. As a result, less carbon dioxide is expired, allowing carbon dioxide levels in the blood to return to normal. Although considered a waste gas, some level of carbon dioxide in the blood is necessary: In addition to stimulating breathing, it helps balance the pH level. If the level of carbon dioxide in the arterial blood rises above normal, the person breathes more rapidly and more deeply. When more fresh air is brought into the alveoli, more carbon dioxide diffuses out of the bloodstream, thereby lowering the level of carbon dioxide in the blood.

Pathophysiology

The pathophysiology of respiration refers to conditions under which body processes are not working as they should and, as a result, interfere with normal respiration. Abnormal or pathologic conditions in the anatomy of the airway, disease processes, and traumatic conditions can prevent the proper exchange of oxygen and carbon dioxide. In addition, the pulmonary blood vessels themselves may have abnormalities that interfere with blood flow and thus with the transfer of gases.

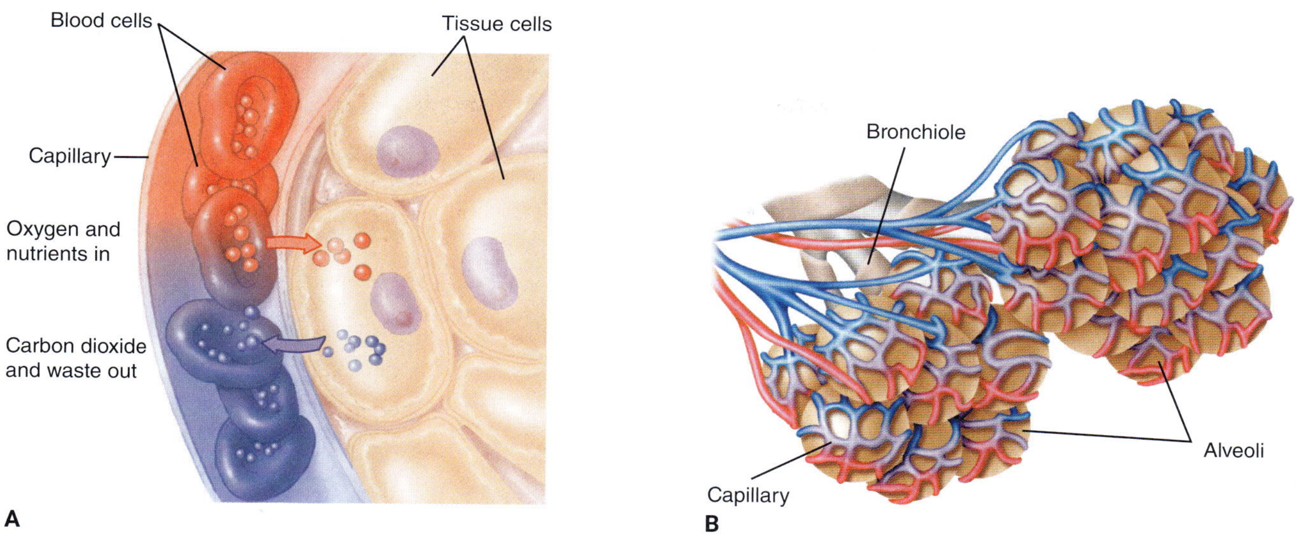

FIGURE 16-4 The exchange of oxygen and carbon dioxide in the tissues. **A.** Oxygen passes from the blood through capillaries to tissue cells. Carbon dioxide passes from tissue cells through capillaries to the blood. **B.** In the lungs, oxygen is picked up by the blood, and carbon dioxide is given off.

TABLE 16-2 Signs of Normal Breathing

- A normal rate (adults and children ≥12 years: 12 to 20 breaths/min; child <12 years: 18 to 28 breaths/min; newborn/infant: 30 to 60 breaths/min)
- A regular pattern of inhalation and exhalation
- Clear and equal breath sounds on both sides of the chest
- Regular and equal chest rise (chest expansion) and fall
- Adequate depth (tidal volume)
- Unlabored; without adventitious (abnormal) breath sounds (wheezing, stridor)

Regardless of the reason for difficulty breathing, you must be able to immediately recognize the signs and symptoms of inadequate breathing and know what to do about it. **TABLE 16-2** gives the signs of normal (adequate) breathing, which is measured by rate, rhythm, and quality. **TABLE 16-3** lists the clues that will help you determine if your patient is having difficulty breathing. **TABLE 16-4** provides key signs and symptoms to help you recognize and differentiate among various respiratory-related complaints.

Carbon Dioxide Retention and Hypoxic Drive

You will sometimes encounter patients who have an elevated level of carbon dioxide in their arterial

TABLE 16-3 Signs and Symptoms of Inadequate Breathing

- The patient reports difficulty breathing or shortness of breath.
- The patient has an altered mental status associated with shallow or slow breathing.
- The adult patient appears anxious or restless; the pediatric patient appears sleepy or listless.
- The respiratory rate is too fast or too slow (see Table 16-2).
- The breathing rhythm is irregular.
- The skin is pale, cool, clammy, or cyanotic.
- Adventitious breath sounds are heard, including wheezing, gurgling, snoring, crowing, or stridor (harsh, high-pitched, barking sounds).
- Decreased or noisy breath sounds are heard on one or both sides of the chest.
- The patient cannot speak more than a few words between breaths. Ask the patient, "How are you doing?" A patient who cannot speak at all most likely has a respiratory emergency.
- You observe accessory muscle use, retractions, or labored breathing.
- The patient has unequal or inadequate chest expansion.
- The patient is coughing excessively.
- The patient is sitting up, leaning forward with palms flat on the bed or the arms of the chair. This is called the tripod position because the patient's back and both arms are working together to support the upper body.
- The patient has pursed lips (pursed-lip breathing) or nasal flaring.

TABLE 16-4 Signs and Symptoms Seen in Various Respiratory Conditions

Condition	Signs and Symptoms
Asthma	• Wheezing on inspiration/expiration • Dyspnea • Thick mucus
Anaphylaxis	• Flushed skin or hives (urticaria) • Generalized edema • Decreased blood pressure (hypotension) • Laryngeal edema with dyspnea • Wheezing or stridor • Dyspnea
Bronchiolitis	• Dyspnea • Wheezing • Coughing • Fever • Dehydration • Tachypnea (increased breathing rate) • Tachycardia • Excessive mucus
Bronchitis	• Chronic cough (with sputum production) • Wheezing • Cyanosis • Tachypnea
Coronavirus disease 2019 (COVID-19)	• Cough • Fever • Dyspnea • Chest pain • Inability to smell
Croup	• Fever • Barking cough • Stridor • Mostly seen in pediatric patients • Dyspnea
Diphtheria	• Difficulty breathing and swallowing • Sore throat • Thick, gray buildup in throat or nose • Fever
Emphysema	• Barrel chest • Pursed-lip breathing • Dyspnea on exertion • Cyanosis • Wheezing/decreased breath sounds • Mostly seen in older patients
Epiglottitis	• Dyspnea • High fever • Stridor • Drooling • Difficulty swallowing • Severe sore throat • Tripod or sniffing position
Heart failure	• Dependent (lower extremity) edema • Crackles (pulmonary edema) • **Orthopnea** • **Paroxysmal nocturnal dyspnea**
Influenza type A (flu)	• Cough • Fever • Sore throat • Fatigue
Pertussis (whooping cough)	• Coughing spells • "Whooping" sound • Fever
Pneumonia	• Dyspnea • Chills, fever • Cough • Green, red, or rust-colored sputum • Localized wheezing or crackles
Pulmonary embolus	• Dyspnea • Occasionally will have sharp chest pain • Sudden onset • Tachycardia • Clear breath sounds initially
Respiratory syncytial virus	• Cough • Wheezing • Fever • Dehydration • Copious secretions
Spontaneous pneumothorax	• Sudden chest pain with dyspnea • Decreased breath sounds (affected side) • Subcutaneous emphysema
Tension pneumothorax	• Severe shortness of breath • Diminished or absent breath sounds on one side • Decreased/altered level of consciousness • Neck vein distention • Tracheal deviation (late sign) • Hypotension; signs of shock
Tuberculosis	• Cough • Fever • Fatigue • Productive/bloody sputum

blood. The level can increase for many reasons. The exhalation process may be impaired by various types of lung disease. The body may also produce too much carbon dioxide, either temporarily or chronically, depending on the disease or abnormality. If, for a period of years, arterial carbon dioxide levels rise to an abnormally high level and remain there, the respiratory centers in the brain, which sense the carbon dioxide level and control breathing, may work less efficiently.

The failure of these centers to respond normally to a rise in arterial levels of carbon dioxide is due to chronic **carbon dioxide retention**. Normally, the brain senses the levels of carbon dioxide (based on the pH) in the blood and cerebrospinal fluid. When carbon dioxide levels become elevated, the respiratory centers in the brain adjust the rate and depth of ventilation accordingly. However, patients with chronic lung diseases such as chronic bronchitis or emphysema have difficulty eliminating carbon dioxide through exhalation; thus, they may always have higher levels of carbon dioxide. This condition potentially alters their drive for breathing. The theory is that the brain gradually accommodates high levels of carbon dioxide and then uses a backup system to control breathing based on low levels of oxygen, rather than high levels of carbon dioxide. This condition is called **hypoxic drive**.

Hypoxic drive is frequently found in end-stage chronic obstructive pulmonary disease (COPD). Some experts advocate withholding high concentrations of oxygen, for extended periods, from patients with chronic lung diseases for fear that the increased oxygen level in the blood could depress, or completely stop, the patient's respiratory drive. Use caution when providing high concentrations of oxygen on a long-term basis to patients with chronic lung disease, but *never* withhold oxygen therapy from a patient who needs it. Closely monitor patients who are experiencing respiratory distress and be prepared to assist with ventilations if needed.

Special Populations

AGING-RELATED CHANGES IN THE RESPIRATORY SYSTEM

As a result of the normal aging process, geriatric patients may have greater difficulties with the exchange of carbon dioxide and oxygen. In respiratory emergencies, begin oxygen therapy early in the assessment and treatment process.

Words of Wisdom

It is important for you to properly ventilate a patient; both underventilation and overventilation can cause harmful alterations in the level of carbon dioxide in the blood. Avoid hyperventilation when performing bag-mask ventilation. Hyperventilation can increase the risk of vomiting and cause serious alterations in pH, increased intrathoracic pressure, impaired venous return, and hypotension.

Causes of Dyspnea

Many medical problems may cause dyspnea. Be aware that if the patient's problem is severe and the brain is deprived of oxygen, the patient may not be alert enough to report shortness of breath. Altered mental status may be a sign that the brain is dysfunctional because of severe **hypoxia**, a condition in which the body's cells and tissues do not get enough oxygen.

In addition to the conditions discussed in Table 16-4, patients often have abnormal breathing and/or hypoxia related to trauma or other medical conditions such as the following:

- Pleural effusion
- Obstruction of the airway
- Hyperventilation syndrome
- Acidosis
- Environmental/industrial exposure
- Carbon monoxide or other toxic exposures
- Drug overdose

As you treat patients with disorders of the lungs, be aware that one or more of the following situations most likely exists:

- Gas exchange between the alveoli and pulmonary circulation is obstructed by fluid in the lung, infection, or collapsed alveoli (**atelectasis**).
- The alveoli are damaged and cannot transport gases properly across their own walls.
- The air passages are obstructed by muscle spasm, mucus, or weakened airway walls.
- Blood flow to the lungs is obstructed by blood clots.
- The pleural space is filled with air or excess fluid, so the lungs cannot properly expand.

All of these conditions prevent the proper exchange of oxygen and carbon dioxide. In addition, the pulmonary blood vessels themselves may have abnormalities that interfere with blood flow and thus with the transfer of gases.

Besides shortness of breath, a patient with dyspnea may report the sensation of chest tightness and air hunger. Air hunger is when a person reports the feeling of "not getting enough air" and has a strong need to breathe. Chest tightness is described as an uncomfortable feeling in the chest, and it is commonly reported by patients with asthma.

Dyspnea is also a common complaint in patients with cardiopulmonary diseases. In some cases, it may be caused by physical exertion that has been made difficult because the patient's heart is damaged. Left-side heart failure (often called congestive heart failure) is a troublesome cause of breathlessness because the heart is not pumping efficiently and, therefore, the body does not have adequate oxygen. Another condition commonly associated with left-side heart failure is pulmonary edema, in which the alveoli are filled with fluid.

Words of Wisdom

When the left side of the heart fails, blood backs up into the lungs, causing congestion of fluid that interferes with normal gas exchange; thus, left-side heart failure is often called congestive heart failure. Left-side heart failure can be mild, causing the patient to have shortness of breath only on exertion. If you auscultate the patient's lungs, you may hear only faint crackles in the lung bases. If left-side heart failure is not treated, or progresses, the patient's dyspnea may increase, even at rest. At this point, the condition may interfere with the person's ability to perform normal life tasks. In these cases, crackles may be auscultated farther up the lung fields on both sides. Over time, left-side heart failure usually causes right-side heart failure, because the right ventricle must work harder to eject blood into the lungs due to the congestion in them. Right-side heart failure results in a backup of fluid in the body's veins and can lead to symptoms such as jugular venous distention and swelling in dependent areas of the body, such as the feet. The life-threatening emergency called pulmonary edema occurs when an abrupt drop in the function of the left ventricle results in a flood of fluid into the lungs that causes sudden severe dyspnea, hypoxia, and panic.

Severe pain can cause a patient to experience rapid, shallow breathing without the presence of a primary pulmonary problem. In some patients, breathing deeply causes pain because it causes expansion of the chest wall.

When you assess your patient for complaints of dyspnea, ask about chest pain; conversely, when you are evaluating your patient for chest pain, ask about dyspnea. It is sometimes difficult to distinguish a cardiac problem from a respiratory problem.

Upper or Lower Airway Infection

Infectious diseases causing dyspnea may affect all parts of the airway. Some cause mild discomfort; others require aggressive respiratory support. Infections that impair airflow through the airways are problems of respiration. Inadequate oxygen delivery to the tissues is a problem of **oxygenation**. Infections may cause dyspnea by obstructing airflow in the larger airways due to production of mucus and secretions (colds, diphtheria) or by causing swelling of soft tissues located in the larger, upper airways (epiglottitis, croup). Infections may also impair the exchange of gases between the alveoli and the capillaries (pneumonia).

In patients with infectious diseases, you will be in close contact, so be diligent about your use of appropriate personal protective equipment (PPE). Immunizations, protective techniques, and handwashing can dramatically minimize your risk of contracting an infectious disease. Follow your local protocols, and stay up to date on the latest Centers for Disease Control and Prevention (CDC) recommendations. At a minimum, gloves, eye protection,

Words of Wisdom

Placing a surgical mask on a patient with a respiratory infection helps stop the transmission of the pathogen, but it can also increase the patient's difficulty breathing and produce anxiety. In these cases, if oxygen by nasal cannula is indicated, apply the surgical mask over the nasal cannula, or if higher concentrations of oxygen are needed, apply a nonrebreathing oxygen mask over the surgical mask. Oxygen molecules will diffuse effectively through the surgical mask, while larger viral particles can be stopped.[3,4]

and a surgical mask or a high-efficiency air particulate (N95) respirator should be mandatory. Place a surgical mask on patients with suspected or confirmed respiratory disease. Remember to completely disinfect your unit prior to returning to service. See Chapter 2, *Workforce Safety and Wellness*, for more information on protecting yourself from infection.

Infectious diseases that may be associated with complaints of dyspnea include croup, epiglottitis, respiratory syncytial virus, bronchiolitis, pneumonia, pertussis, influenza type A, COVID-19, and tuberculosis. These specific conditions are discussed later in the chapter.

Patient Assessment

Your assessment of patients in respiratory distress should be a calm and systematic process. These patients are usually anxious, and they may be some of the most ill and challenging patients you will encounter.

Scene Size-up

As always, first consider standard precautions and use of PPE. The patient may have a respiratory infection that could be passed to you through sputum and/or airborne droplets. Follow local protocols.

Next, consider whether the respiratory emergency may have been caused by a toxic substance that was inhaled, absorbed, or ingested.

Once you have determined the scene is safe, determine how many patients there are and whether you need additional or specialized resources. If there are multiple people with dyspnea, consider the possibility of an airborne hazardous material release.

If the nature of illness (NOI) is in question, ask why 9-1-1 was activated. By questioning the patient, family, and/or bystanders, you should be able to determine the NOI.

Words of Wisdom

If there are several patients presenting with the same complaints, there is a good chance the scene is not safe and there is something in the air causing the illness. Do not place yourself in danger. Remember that not all scene safety concerns are visible.

Primary Assessment

Perform a rapid examination to identify immediate life threats, which includes problems with the ABCs: Airway, Breathing, and Circulation (discussed next). If any major problem is identified,

YOU are the EMT

After arriving at the scene and entering the patient's house, you smell cigarette smoke. There are numerous full ashtrays in the living room. The patient is sitting on the edge of her couch; she is wearing a nasal cannula attached to a home oxygen concentrator, is smoking a cigarette, and is experiencing obvious breathing difficulty. She tells you, in two-word sentences, that her shortness of breath has worsened. You perform a primary assessment as your partner prepares to begin treatment.

Recording Time: 0 Minutes	
Appearance	Obvious breathing difficulty; breathing through pursed lips
Level of consciousness	Conscious and alert
Airway	Open; no secretions or foreign bodies
Breathing	Rapid and labored
Circulation	Radial pulse: rapid and weak; skin: baseline color, warm, and dry

3. What should be your *most* immediate action?
4. How does emphysema differ from chronic bronchitis?

treat it immediately. If you find life-threatening issues, provide rapid transport.

Note your general impression of the patient. What is the patient's age and position? A patient in significant respiratory distress will want to sit up. In a serious scenario, you will arrive to see the patient in the tripod position.

Does the patient appear calm? Is the patient anxious and restless, or listless and tired? How severe is the patient's breathing complaint? This initial impression will help you decide whether the patient's condition is stable or unstable.

Use the AVPU (Awake and alert, responsive to Verbal stimuli, responsive to Pain, Unresponsive) scale to check for responsiveness. If the patient is alert or responding to verbal stimuli, you know that the brain is still receiving oxygen. Ask the patient about the chief complaint. If the patient is responsive only to painful stimuli or unresponsive, the brain may not be oxygenating well and the potential for an airway or breathing problem is more likely. If there is no gag or cough reflex, you need to immediately assess the patient's airway status. Within seconds you will be able to determine if there are any immediate threats to life.

Assessing ABCs in Respiratory Patients

Assess the airway; air must flow into and out of the chest easily for the airway to be considered patent. If there is any question about airway patency, immediately open the airway using the head tilt–chin lift maneuver in nontrauma patients and the jaw-thrust maneuver in patients with suspected spinal trauma and then insert an oral airway (for patients without a gag reflex) or nasal airway (for patients who have a gag reflex).

If the airway is patent, next evaluate whether the patient's breathing is adequate. What are the rate, rhythm, and quality of the breaths? Is the rate within normal limits for the patient's age? Is the patient using accessory muscles to assist the respiratory effort, and can you see retractions? Is there abdominal breathing? What is the depth of breathing, and is the tidal volume adequate? Is there adequate rise and fall of the chest? What are the color, temperature, and moisture conditions of the patient's skin? Although cyanosis resulting from low oxygen in the blood can be difficult to detect in individuals with dark skin, it may be observed by examining the palms or the mucous membranes of the lips, which may appear pale, ashen, or gray.

Is the patient's breathing labored? If the patient can speak only one or two words at a time before gasping for a breath, ventilations are considered labored. If the respiratory effort is inadequate, you must provide the necessary intervention. Place patients who are in respiratory distress in a position that best facilitates breathing (generally sitting upright in a full or semi-Fowler position) and administer oxygen at 15 L/min via nonrebreathing mask. If the patient's breathing has inadequate depth or the rate is too slow, assist ventilations with a bag-mask device.

Ask yourself the following questions:

1. Is air going in and out?
2. Does the chest rise and fall with each breath?
3. Is the rate appropriate for the patient's age?

If the answer to any of these questions is "no," something is wrong. After you open the patient's airway, continue to monitor the airway for fluid, secretions, and other problems as you move on to assess the adequacy of your patient's breathing. Refer to Chapter 11, *Airway and Ventilation Management*, for a review of airway management and ventilation techniques.

Special Populations

SPECIAL CONSIDERATIONS IN PEDIATRIC RESPIRATORY EMERGENCIES

Respiratory problems are the leading cause of cardiopulmonary arrest in the pediatric population. Failure to recognize and treat declining respiratory status will result in death. A pediatric patient in respiratory distress is using compensatory mechanisms and has the ability to exchange oxygen and carbon dioxide. During respiratory distress, the child is working harder to breathe and will eventually go into respiratory failure if left untreated. Respiratory failure occurs when the patient has exhausted all compensatory mechanisms and waste products begin to collect. If this is not treated, a total shutdown of the respiratory system will occur; this condition is called respiratory arrest.

In the early stages of respiratory distress, you may note changes in the child's behavior, such as anxiety, restlessness, or combativeness. As the body attempts to maximize the amount of air going into the lungs, the **work of breathing** increases. Increased work of breathing often manifests as follows:

- **Abnormal airway noise.** Grunting or wheezing
- **Accessory muscle use.** Contractions of the muscles above the clavicles (supraclavicular)
- **Retractions.** Drawing in of the muscles between the ribs (intercostal retractions) or of the sternum (substernal retractions) during inspiration (**FIGURE 16-5**)
- **Head bobbing.** The head lifting and tilting back during inspiration, then moving forward during expiration
- **Nasal flaring.** The nostrils (the external openings of the nose) widening; usually seen during inspiration
- **Tachypnea**. Increased respiratory rate
- **Tripod position**. An upright position used by older children to maximize the effectiveness of the airway (**FIGURE 16-6**)

As the pediatric patient progresses to possible respiratory failure, efforts to breathe decrease; the chest rises less with inspiration and the respiratory rate may slow. The body has used up its available energy stores and cannot continue to support the extra work of breathing under these conditions. At this point, without care, cyanosis may develop (a late sign). Be aware that not all pediatric patients experience cyanosis. You should be just as concerned by the appearance of pallor.

Changes in behavior will also occur until the patient demonstrates an altered level of consciousness. The child may experience periods of apnea (absence of breathing). As the lack of oxygen becomes more serious, the heart muscle itself becomes hypoxic and slows down. This leads to bradycardia, which is almost always an ominous sign in children. If the heart rate is fast, you need to investigate the cause. However, if the heart rate is slow (less than 60 beats/min) or absent, despite bag-mask ventilation with high-concentration oxygen, especially in an unconscious infant or child, you must begin CPR immediately. Without aggressive airway management, bradycardia may quickly progress to cardiopulmonary arrest.

Respiratory distress or failure does not always originate from an airway or respiratory problem; it may also be caused by trauma, nervous system problems, dehydration (often caused by vomiting and diarrhea), or metabolic disturbances. For example, a pediatric patient who ingested an opioid may have inadequate, slow breathing, or a child might have a pH imbalance related to a very high blood glucose level. Regardless of the cause, your first step is always to ensure adequate oxygenation and ventilation.

Remember, because respiratory status can deteriorate quickly, you must reassess the child frequently.

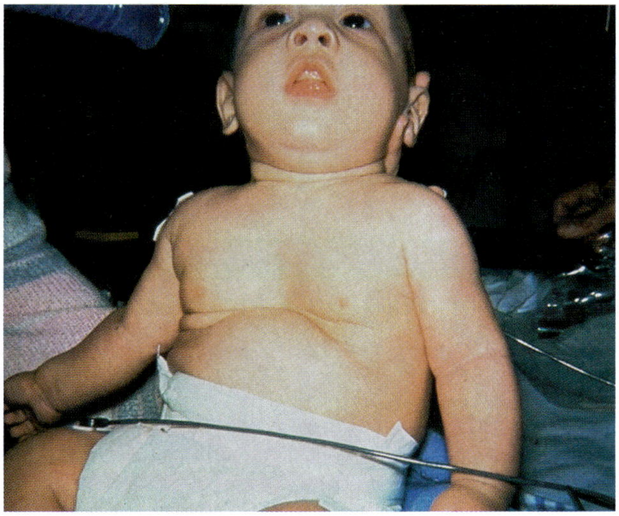

FIGURE 16-5 Retractions of the intercostal muscles or sternum indicate increased work of breathing.

Courtesy of Health Resources and Services Administration, Maternal and Child Health Bureau, Emergency Medical Service for Children Program.

The next step in assessing breathing in a patient with a respiratory emergency is to assess breath sounds. Techniques for this assessment are described at the end of this section.

After assessing breath sounds, assess circulation: the pulse rate, quality, and rhythm. If the pulse rate is too fast or too slow, the patient may not be getting enough oxygen. Determine the quality of the pulse. Is it strong, bounding, or weak? Also determine whether the rhythm is regular or irregular. Irregular beats could indicate a cardiac problem.

Assessing a patient's circulation includes an evaluation for the presence of shock and bleeding. Respiratory distress in a patient could be caused by an insufficient number of red blood cells to transport the oxygen. Assess the patient's perfusion by evaluating skin color, temperature, and condition.

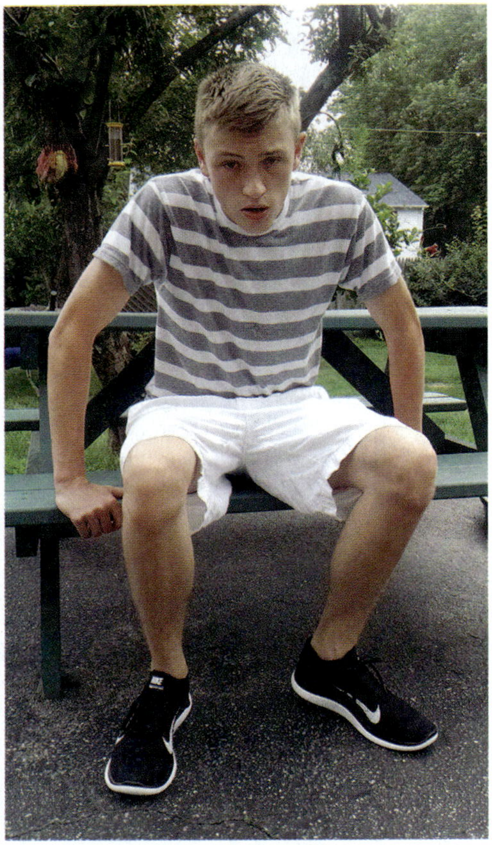

FIGURE 16-6 A patient in the tripod position will sit leaning forward on outstretched arms with the head and chin thrust slightly forward.

Assess capillary refill in infants and children. Normal capillary refill is less than 2 seconds; abnormal capillary refill is greater than 2 seconds. Capillary refill is not considered a reliable assessment tool in the adult patient.

An insufficient concentration of oxygen in the blood can produce a life-threatening situation as rapidly as vascular causes of shock, even if the volume of blood, the volume of the vessels, and the action of the heart are all normal. Without oxygen, the organs in the body cannot survive, and their cells promptly start to deteriorate.

If the patient's condition is unstable and there is a possible life threat, address the life threat and proceed with rapid transport. This means you will keep your scene time short, providing only lifesaving interventions. Perform a secondary assessment en route to the hospital. If the patient's condition is stable and there are no life threats, you may decide to perform a thorough secondary assessment on scene, after obtaining the patient history.

Assessing Breath Sounds

Obtaining breath sounds, or lung sounds, is an important step when you assess a patient who is experiencing respiratory distress. Place the diaphragm of the stethoscope firmly over the skin of the chest. Trying to listen over clothing or chest hair may give you inaccurate information. If possible, patients who are

YOU are the EMT

Your partner obtains the patient's vital signs as you continue your assessment. You notice she is breathing through pursed lips and has a prolonged exhalation phase, and cyanosis is present in her fingernail beds. You auscultate her breath sounds and hear scattered wheezing in all lung fields. When you talk to her, you note she is now confused, is slow to answer your questions, and appears fatigued.

Recording Time: 3 Minutes	
Respirations	28 breaths/min, labored; prolonged exhalation phase
Pulse	110 beats/min; weak
Skin	Cyanotic, cool, clammy
Blood pressure	116/54 mm Hg
Oxygen saturation (Spo_2)	88% (on 4 L/min oxygen by nasal cannula)

5. Why do patients with emphysema breathe through pursed lips?
6. What does a prolonged exhalation phase indicate in patients with obstructive lung disease?
7. What treatment is indicated for the patient at this point?

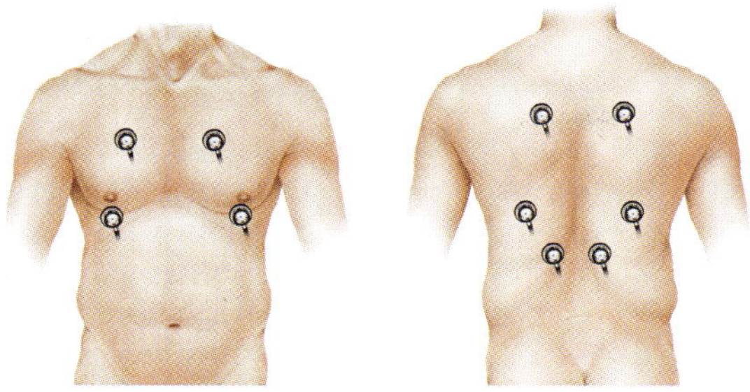

FIGURE 16-7 Locations of the stethoscope bell for auscultation of breath sounds.

lying down should be brought to a sitting position, which is a better position for assessing breath sounds.

You need to determine whether your patient's breath sounds are normal (**vesicular breath sounds**, **bronchial breath sounds**) or decreased, absent, or abnormal (**adventitious breath sounds**). With your stethoscope, check breath sounds on the right and left sides of the chest, alternating from side to side so you can compare each side (**FIGURE 16-7**). When listening on the patient's back, place the stethoscope between and below the scapulae, not over them, or you will have an inaccurate assessment.

Make sure you listen for a full respiratory cycle at each location on the chest so you can detect the adventitious sounds that may be heard at the end of the inspiratory or expiratory phase. When you assess for fluid collection, pay special attention to the lower lung fields. Start from the bottom up and determine at which level you start hearing clear breath sounds.

You want to hear clear flow of air in both lungs. Not hearing the flow of air is considered an absent lung sound. The lack of air movement in the lung is a significant finding. Listen carefully and do not confuse absent breath sounds with clear breath sounds. See **TABLE 16-5** for examples of breath sounds and the diseases that may be associated with them.

Street Smarts

When auscultating lung sounds, clinicians commonly ask patients to breathe in and out. Do not place patients in further respiratory distress by asking them to breathe too quickly or too slowly just so you can hear lung sounds.

TABLE 16-5 Signs, Symptoms, and Adventitious Breath Sounds Associated With Specific Respiratory Diseases

Breath Sounds	Condition
Wheezing: High- or low-pitched sound heard usually during expiration; indicates a partial lower airway obstruction	Asthma COPD Pulmonary edema (rarely) Pneumonia Bronchitis Anaphylaxis Foreign body aspiration Bronchiolitis
Rhonchi: Low-pitched rattling sounds caused by secretions or mucus in the larger airway	COPD Pneumonia Bronchitis
Crackles: A crackling or bubbling sound typically heard on inspiration; indicates inflammation or infection	Left-side heart failure/pulmonary edema Pneumonia
Stridor: High-pitched inspiratory sound; indicates a partial upper airway obstruction	Croup Epiglottitis Foreign body airway obstruction
Grunting: An *uh* sound heard during exhalation; reflects pediatric patient's attempt to keep alveoli open by increasing pressure in chest cavity; indicates inadequate oxygenation	Respiratory distress syndrome
Decreased or absent breath sounds	Asthma COPD Pneumonia Pneumothorax Atelectasis Foreign body aspiration or obstruction Impending respiratory failure Respiratory arrest (if absent)

Abbreviation: COPD, chronic obstructive pulmonary disease

Words of Wisdom

Adventitious breath sounds are sounds heard by auscultation of abnormal lungs. These sounds can include wheezing, crackles, rhonchi, gurgling, snoring, crowing, and stridor. The ability to hear and distinguish different kinds of breath sounds can give you important clues as to what is wrong with your patient. The only way to develop your ability to identify breath sounds is through practice. Ask your instructor if you can accompany a physician, nurse, or respiratory therapist in the hospital to help you develop this skill.

Street Smarts

Although it is easy to assume that patients with a history of a respiratory illness (such as asthma) are having an exacerbation of their condition when they present with dyspnea, it may lead to misdiagnosis and delayed or incorrect treatment. It is critical to keep an open mind and consider all the signs and symptoms in addition to the history before deciding on a treatment plan. A person with asthma may have an anaphylactic reaction, or a patient with COPD may have an acute onset of pulmonary edema caused by left-side heart failure. It is important to get as much information as possible and consider all possibilities before developing a treatment plan.

History Taking

The next step of your assessment will provide more information specific to the patient's chief complaint (history of present illness) through history taking. The information you obtain during history taking will be subjective (what the patient expresses, or symptoms) and objective (what you observe, or signs). Both sets of information are important in building a general assessment. Rule out any findings that warrant no care or intervention. Report pertinent negatives to health care clinicians or emergency department (ED) staff members. Recall that a pertinent negative is any sign or symptom that commonly accompanies a particular condition, but is absent. Examples of pertinent negatives would be a patient in respiratory distress who denies chest pain, or a patient with rapid deep breathing who denies shortness of breath.

Find out what the patient has done for the breathing problem. Does the patient have home oxygen? Does the patient use a prescribed inhaler or a small-volume nebulizer? If so, when was it used last? How many doses have been taken? Does the patient use more than one inhaler or treatment? Be sure to record the name of each device and when it was used.

Chronic Respiratory Conditions

Different respiratory complaints offer different clues and different challenges. Patients with chronic conditions may have long periods in which they are able to live relatively normal lives but then sometimes experience acute worsening of their conditions. That is when you are called, and it is important for you to be able to determine your patient's baseline status—in other words, the patient's normal condition (and what is different this time that made the patient call you). Ask the patient, "What is different today?" Your knowledge of the signs and symptoms of specific respiratory conditions, discussed later in this chapter, will enable you to recognize the patient's needs.

Questioning a Patient With Difficulty Breathing

With patients in respiratory distress, many of the SAMPLE (Signs and symptoms, Allergies, Medications, Pertinent past medical history, Last oral intake, Events leading up to the illness or injury) questions can be answered by the family or bystanders if they are present. Limit the number of questions directed to the patient by asking only pertinent ones; a patient who is in respiratory distress does not need to use any additional air to answer questions.

Ask the following questions about a patient in respiratory distress:

- What is the patient's general state of health?
- Has the patient had any childhood or adult diseases?
- Have there been any recent surgical procedures or hospitalizations?
- Have there been any traumatic injuries?

To help determine the cause of your patient's problem, be a detective. Look for medications, medical alert bracelets, environmental conditions, and other clues to what may be causing the problem. Each part of the SAMPLE history may give you clues, so be thorough. For example, you forget to ask about allergies, only to find out later that your patient has a severe allergy to cat dander and that their 8-year-old child had been playing with a cat shortly before the onset of her problem. You would have missed important and possibly lifesaving information.

The OPQRST assessment, generally used for determining the specifics of pain, can also be modified to obtain more specific information about the breathing problem. Begin by asking the patient to describe the problem. Pay close attention to OPQRST and include the following open-ended questions:

- When and how did the breathing problem begin, suddenly or gradually? (Onset)
- What makes the breathing difficulty better or worse? (Provocation or palliation)
- How does the breathing feel? (Quality)
- Does the discomfort move? (Radiation/region)
- How much of a problem is the patient having? (Severity)
- Is the problem continuous or intermittent? If it is intermittent, how frequently does it occur and how long does it last? (Timing)

An additional assessment for a complaint of shortness of breath or difficulty breathing uses the mnemonic PASTE:

P **Progression.** Similar to the O in OPQRST, you want to know if the problem started suddenly or has worsened over time.

A **Associated chest pain.** Dyspnea can be a significant symptom of a cardiac problem.

S **Sputum.** Has the patient been coughing up sputum? Yellow-, green-, or rust-colored sputum could indicate a respiratory infection; pink frothy sputum is indicative of fluid in the lungs; and a problem such as a pulmonary embolus may not result in any sputum at all.

T **Talking tiredness.** This is an indicator of how much distress the patient is having. Ask the patient to repeat a sentence and see how many words they can speak without needing to take a breath. The assessment results would be reported as the patient "speaks in full sentences" or, perhaps, "speaks in two- to three-word sentences."

E **Exercise tolerance.** Ask the patient a question about what they were able to do before this problem started, such as walk across the room, and then ask if the patient could do it now. If the answer is "no," then it is another indicator that your patient is in distress. Exercise tolerance will decrease as the breathing problem and hypoxia increase.

Secondary Assessment

During the secondary assessment, further investigate the specific chief complaint (eg, dyspnea) by performing a physical examination and taking vital signs.

In respiratory emergencies, as in all other emergencies, do not proceed to history taking and the secondary assessment until all life threats have been identified and treated during the primary assessment. If you are busy treating airway or breathing problems, you may not have the opportunity to proceed to a physical examination prior to arriving at the ED. Never compromise the assessment and treatment of airway and breathing problems to conduct a physical examination.

Sometimes it is not possible to quickly and definitively determine what is causing your patient's respiratory distress. If your patient is a 20-year-old at a picnic in whom difficulty breathing and hives rapidly develop after being stung by a bee, you have a clear-cut diagnostic picture. Conversely, if your patient is an older person in a nursing home who is receiving 12 medications and has a cough and increasing shortness of breath that developed during the past week, this is more perplexing. Keep an open mind, gather as complete a history as possible, and perform a secondary assessment.

Conduct an in-depth assessment when a patient reports shortness of breath. In addition to the signs of air hunger present in all patients with respiratory distress, such as the tripod position, rapid breathing, and use of accessory muscles, restriction of the small lower airways in patients with asthma often causes wheezing. Patients may have a prolonged expiratory phase of breathing as they attempt to exhale trapped air from the lungs. In severe cases, you may actually not hear wheezing because of insufficient airflow. Remember that the brain needs a constant, adequate supply of oxygen to function normally. As your patient tires from the effort of breathing and oxygen levels drop, the respiratory and heart rates may drop, and you will notice an altered level of consciousness. This may manifest itself as confusion, lack of coordination, bizarre behavior, or even combativeness. Your patient may seem to relax or fall asleep. These findings indicate respiratory failure. A change in affect or level of consciousness is one of the early warning signs of respiratory inadequacy, and you must act immediately.

When you perform a secondary assessment on the respiratory system, look for overall symmetry of the chest, adequate rise and fall of the chest, and evidence of retractions or accessory muscle use. Is the patient's breathing labored or unlabored? Assess breath sounds, and perform additional physical assessment if warranted.

A secondary assessment of the cardiovascular system, especially when there is associated chest pain, should include checking and comparing distal pulses, reassessing the skin condition, and being alert for bradycardia and tachycardia.

Feel for the skin temperature, and look for color changes in the extremities and in the core of the body. Cyanosis is an ominous sign that requires immediate, aggressive intervention.

Blood pressure should be auscultated when possible to obtain the systolic and diastolic numbers. If you are in an environment where you cannot hear well enough to auscultate the blood pressure, then palpation of the blood pressure is an alternative.

It is important to assess the neurologic system because the level of consciousness can change. Check the patient's mental status, and determine if the patient's activity can be described as anxious or restless. If so, that would be an indicator of hypoxia. Does the patient have clear thought processes? Disorientation may be another indicator of hypoxia.

Use monitoring devices if you have them available, including, but not limited to, a pulse oximeter. Pulse oximetry is an effective diagnostic tool when used in conjunction with experience, good assessment skills, and clinical judgment. Pulse oximeters measure the percentage of hemoglobin that is saturated by oxygen. In patients with normal levels of hemoglobin, pulse oximetry can be an important tool in evaluating oxygenation. To use pulse oximetry properly, it is important for you to be able to evaluate the quality of the reading and correlate it with the patient's condition. For example, it is doubtful a patient with left-side heart failure in severe respiratory distress will have a pulse oximetry reading of 98% or that a pulse oximetry reading of 80% is reliable in a conscious, alert, active patient with healthy skin color.

Words of Wisdom

Be aware of conditions that can skew pulse oximetry results. Bright light, darkly pigmented skin, and in some cases, dark-colored nail polish can cause errors in the readings. Remember that pulse oximetry measures the percentage of hemoglobin that is saturated, but it does not tell you how much hemoglobin the patient has; nor does it tell you whether it is oxygen that has bound to the hemoglobin (the typical and desired condition) or carbon monoxide.

Waveform capnography, sometimes referred to as the "ventilation vital sign," is an excellent tool and should be used when available on patients who have dyspnea. Use a special nasal cannula to measure the end-tidal carbon dioxide level in patients who are breathing spontaneously, and connect the capnographic monitor between the bag and mask or between the ventilator device and any airway device when monitoring patients who need assisted ventilation. The normal capnography reading is 35 to 45 mm Hg. Monitoring this value helps determine whether the patient is ventilating adequately and whether any treatments you provide are improving their condition.

Waveform capnography can provide even more information. Instead of the normal box-shaped waveform (**FIGURE 16-8A**), a patient whose airways are narrowed, such as in asthma or COPD, may have a waveform that looks like a shark fin with a slow rising upstroke during inhalation (**FIGURE 16-8B**). When a patient has a large pulmonary embolism, the carbon dioxide in the alveoli of the affected lung tissue has no blood flow to diffuse into; thus, there will be a decreased amount of carbon dioxide in the patient's exhaled breath, resulting in a flattened end-tidal carbon dioxide waveform (**FIGURE 16-8C**). See Chapter 11, *Airway and Ventilation Management*, for further discussion of waveform capnography.

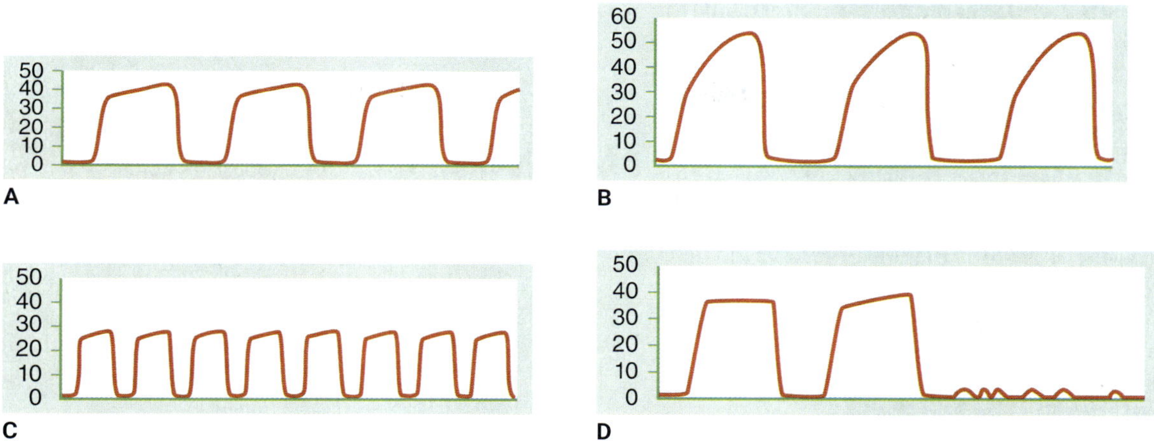

FIGURE 16-8 A. Normal capnographic waveform. **B.** Shark-fin waveform, suggestive of a narrowed airway. **C.** Flattened waveform, suggestive of hyperventilation (decreased carbon dioxide level). **D.** Waveform that suddenly drops, suggestive of cardiac arrest or displaced advanced airway.

If you get a good reading consistent with your patient's condition, the pulse oximeter can help you determine the severity of the respiratory component of the patient's problem. In addition, if the reading goes steadily up or down, it can give you an indication of improvement or deterioration of the patient's oxygenation status, sometimes even prior to changes in the patient's appearance or vital signs.

Reassessment

Once assessment and treatment have been completed, you need to reassess the patient and closely watch patients with shortness of breath. Repeat the primary assessment and maintain an open airway. Monitor the patient's breathing and reassess circulation.

Determine if there have been changes in the patient's condition. Confirm the adequacy of interventions and patient status. Is the current treatment improving the patient's condition? Has an already identified problem improved? Has an already identified problem gotten worse? What is the nature of any newly identified problems?

If the changes you find are improvements, simply continue the treatments; however, if your patient's condition deteriorates, prepare to modify treatments. Be prepared to assist ventilations with a bag-mask device. Monitor the skin color and temperature. Reassess and record vital signs at least every 5 minutes for a patient in unstable condition and/or after the patient uses an inhaler. If the patient's condition is stable and no life threat exists, vital signs should be obtained at least every 15 minutes.

General Care for Respiratory Emergencies

Interventions for respiratory problems may occur during the primary assessment, when life threats are identified in the secondary assessment, or following reassessment of the patient. They may include the following:

- Using airway management techniques such as an oropharyngeal (oral) airway, a nasopharyngeal (nasal) airway, suctioning, or airway positioning
- Providing oxygen via a nonrebreathing mask at 15 L/min
- Providing positive-pressure ventilations using a bag-mask device
- Providing noninvasive ventilatory support with continuous positive airway pressure (CPAP)
- Positioning the patient in a high Fowler position or a position of choice to facilitate breathing
- Administering intramuscular epinephrine if anaphylaxis is suspected

- Assisting with respiratory medications found in a patient-prescribed metered-dose inhaler or administering a bronchodilator with a small-volume nebulizer

Before discussing the specific respiratory conditions you may encounter, this chapter will review two interventions that are required at many different types of respiratory emergency: oxygen administration and use of a metered-dose inhaler or small-volume nebulizer.

Administering Oxygen

You will usually administer oxygen to patients in respiratory distress. If a patient reports breathing difficulty, administer supplemental oxygen immediately. Supplemental oxygen should be administered to maintain an oxygen saturation of 94% to 98%. Depending on the level of distress, some patients may benefit from CPAP (discussed later in the chapter). In addition, patients may require ventilatory support with a bag-mask device, particularly if their mental status is declining, if they are in moderate to severe respiratory distress, or if their depth of breathing is inadequate.

Take great care in monitoring the patient's breathing as you provide oxygen. Reevaluate the breathing and the patient's response to oxygen repeatedly, at least every 5 minutes, until you reach the ED. In a person with a chronically high carbon dioxide level (eg, certain patients with COPD), this is important, because the supplemental oxygen may cause a rapid rise in the arterial oxygen level, which may depress the patient's hypoxic drive, particularly if there is a prolonged transport time.

In patients who have long-standing COPD and probable carbon dioxide retention, administer low-flow oxygen (2 L/min) to start, with adjustments to 3 L/min, then 4 L/min with a goal of reaching an oxygen saturation range of 88% to 92% and improved patient symptoms.[5,6] Pulse oximetry will help you understand the degree of oxygen deprivation and adjust oxygen therapy accordingly. In these patients, the target for oxygen saturation is 90% or higher.[7] When in doubt, err on the side of more oxygen, and monitor the patient closely. It is important to note that regardless of the initial oxygen flow rate, for the small-volume nebulizer to adequately disperse medication, the manufacturer's guidelines for oxygen flow rate (often 6 to 8 L/min) should be followed.

Words of Wisdom

When caring for patients with a chronic respiratory condition, ask them or their caregiver what their normal oxygen saturation level is; they often know. This can be an essential piece of information to guide your care.

Remember, do *not* withhold oxygen for fear of depressing or stopping breathing in a patient with COPD who needs oxygen. If the respiratory rate is slow and the patient becomes unconscious, assist breathing with a bag-mask device with high-concentration oxygen.

A child or infant in respiratory distress needs supplemental oxygen. Anxiety, agitation, or crying may increase the effort or work of breathing, so use whichever method seems least upsetting: mask, blow-by, or nasal cannula. You may need to get creative by distracting the child with games, a toy, or conversation. Assist ventilation with a bag-mask device and 100% oxygen for infants and children who are in possible respiratory failure.

Always provide emotional support to the patient who is anxious. Always speak with assurance and assume a concerned, professional approach to reassure the patient, who is probably very frightened.

Using Metered-Dose Inhalers and Small-Volume Nebulizers

Patients who call for help because of difficulty breathing are likely to have had the same problem before. They probably have prescribed medications to use that are delivered by an inhaler or small-volume nebulizer. If so, you may be able to help them use these devices, depending on local protocols. Some of the most common medications used for shortness of breath are inhaled beta agonists, which dilate breathing passages. Some medications may be administered via a **metered-dose inhaler (MDI)**, which is a miniature spray canister used to direct such substances through the mouth and into the lungs. MDIs are used to administer medications such as albuterol (Proventil, Ventolin), albuterol/ipratropium (Combivent), levalbuterol (Xopenex), and terbutaline (Brethine).

The **small-volume nebulizer** works by providing a means for a fine mist of aerosolized medicine to get deep into the patient's lungs and start to work quickly. The patient inhales the mist through a mouthpiece or a mask. When the medicine is breathed in correctly, it goes directly into the lungs. Medications typically administered by small-volume nebulizer include, but are not limited to, albuterol, ipratropium, and levalbuterol.

Words of Wisdom

Some states allow EMTs to administer medication by inhalers or small-volume nebulizers or to assist patients in the administration of their own inhalers. With this increased scope of practice comes the responsibility to know the names, doses, indications, contraindications, side effects, and precautions of the numerous medications given by this route. Patients sometimes do not know the difference between their rescue inhalers (immediately effective medication, such as albuterol) and their maintenance inhalers (such as corticosteroids, which have no immediate effect). It is essential, then, that *you* know the difference! For further discussion, see Chapter 12, *Principles of Pharmacology and Medication Administration*.

Medical Oversight

Consult medical direction (online), or follow standing orders (off-line). Remember to report what the medication is, when the patient last self-administered a treatment, how much medication was used at that time, and what the label states regarding dosage. If medical control or standing orders permit, you may administer a medication or assist the patient to self-administer their own medication. When using the patient's medication, be certain that the inhaler belongs to the patient, it contains the correct medication, the expiration date has not passed, and the correct dose is being administered. There may be times when the prescribed dose is not explicitly listed on the inhaler. In this situation, ask the patient how many inhalations of the medication they take. Administer repeated doses of the medication if the maximum dose has not been exceeded and the patient is still experiencing shortness of breath.

Unlike an MDI, a small-volume nebulizer must be assembled prior to use. An oxygen tank, or air compressor, is also required to administer the aerosolized medication. The patient may have a tank available, or you will need to use your own tank.

Indications and Contraindications

Before helping a patient to self-administer any MDI or small-volume nebulizer medication, make sure the medication is indicated; that is, make sure the patient has signs and symptoms of shortness of breath. The most common use for an MDI is asthma, and a small-volume nebulizer is used in asthma, bronchiolitis, COPD, and anaphylaxis. Check that there are no contraindications for its use, such as the following:

- The patient is unable to help coordinate inhalation with depression of the trigger on an MDI or is too confused to effectively administer medication through a small-volume nebulizer. These devices will be only minimally effective when patients are in respiratory failure and have only minimal air movement.
- The MDI or small-volume nebulizer is not prescribed for this patient.
- You did not obtain permission from medical control and/or it is not permissible by local protocol.
- The patient has already taken the maximum prescribed dose before your arrival.
- The medication is expired.
- There are other contraindications specific to the medication.

Actions

Most respiratory inhalation medications relax the muscles that surround the air passages in the lungs, leading to enlargement (dilation) of the lower airways and easier movement of air. See **TABLE 16-6** for a list of respiratory inhalation medications. Note that some medications are used only for chronic (day-to-day) treatment, with the goal of preventing signs and symptoms; these drugs do not help reduce dyspnea in an acute worsening of signs and symptoms. The medications used for acute symptoms are designed to give the patient rapid relief from symptoms if the

TABLE 16-6 Respiratory Medications

Medication			Indications			Use: Acute Versus Chronic Disease	
Generic Drug Name	**Trade Names**	**Action**	**Asthma**	**Bronchitis**	**COPD**	**Acute**	**Chronic**
Albuterol	Proventil, Ventolin, ProAir	Dilates bronchioles	Yes	Yes	Yes	Yes	No
Beclomethasone	Beclovent, Beconase, Qvar, Vanceril	Anti-inflammatory, reduces swelling	Yes	No	No	No	Yes
Cromolyn	Intal	Decreases release of histamines	Yes	No	No	No	Yes
Fluticasone	Flovent Diskus	Anti-inflammatory, reduces swelling	Yes	No	No	No	Yes
Fluticasone and salmeterol (combination drug)	Advair Diskus	Decreases secretions	Yes	No	No	No	Yes
Ipratropium bromide	Atrovent	Dilates bronchioles	Yes	Yes	Yes	Yes	No
Levalbuterol	Xopenex	Dilates bronchioles	Yes	Yes	Yes	Yes	No
Montelukast	Singulair, oral tablet	Anti-inflammatory, reduces swelling	Yes	No	Yes	No	Yes
Salmeterol	Serevent Diskus	Dilates bronchioles	Yes	Yes	Yes	No	Yes

YOU are the EMT

After initiating the appropriate treatment, you place the patient onto the stretcher, load her into the ambulance, and begin transport to the hospital. You reassess her and note that her condition has acutely deteriorated.

You insert a nasopharyngeal airway and begin assisting her ventilations with a bag-mask device and high-flow oxygen.

Recording Time: 9 Minutes	
Level of consciousness	Responsive only to pain
Respirations	8 breaths/min; shallow
Pulse	124 beats/min; weak
Skin	Cool and dry; cyanosis of the nail beds and around the lips
Blood pressure	108/50 mm Hg
Oxygen saturation (Spo_2)	82% (on oxygen)

8. Why is cyanosis a later sign of hypoxemia in patients with emphysema?

9. Why does tachycardia develop in patients with hypoxemia?

condition is reversible. Medications used for chronic symptoms are administered for preventive measures or as maintenance doses. The medications for long-term use will provide little relief of acute symptoms.

Side Effects

Common side effects of inhalers used for acute shortness of breath include increased pulse rate, nervousness, and muscle tremors. Often, a patient will begin coughing *after* administration of an inhaler as the airways are opened and secretions start to loosen and clear.

If the patient has a prescribed MDI or small-volume nebulizer, read the label carefully to make sure the medication is to be used for shortness of breath and has been prescribed by a physician. When in doubt, consult medical control.

Dose and Route

Medication from an inhaler is delivered through the respiratory tract to the lung. The dose is one puff for an MDI or continuation of the small-volume nebulizer until all the medication has been administered or the patient's signs and symptoms are resolved.

Administration of an MDI

To help a patient self-administer medication from an inhaler, follow the steps in **SKILL DRILL 16-1**:

1. Take standard precautions.
2. Obtain an order from medical control or local protocol.
3. Check that you have the right medication, right patient, right dose, and right route, and that the medication is not expired.
4. Make sure the patient is alert enough to use the inhaler.
5. Check whether the patient has already taken any doses.
6. Make sure the inhaler is at room temperature or warmer (**Step 1**).
7. Shake the inhaler vigorously several times. Attach the spacer (if available) to the MDI (**FIGURE 16-9**).
8. Stop administering supplemental oxygen, and remove any mask from the patient's face.
9. Ask the patient to exhale deeply and, before inhaling, to put their lips around the opening of the inhaler (**Step 2**).

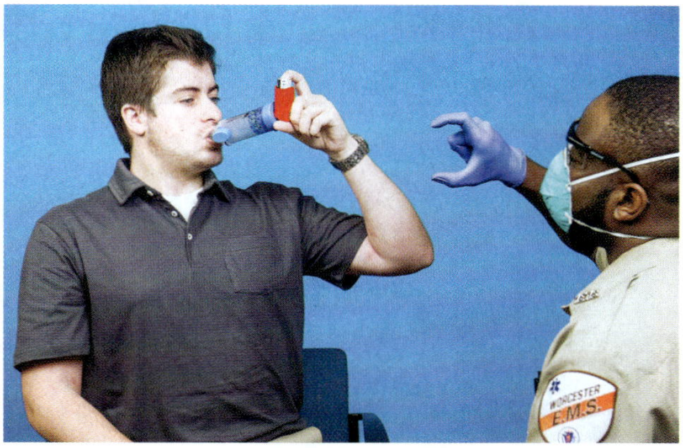

FIGURE 16-9 Some inhalers have spacer devices to better control the medication delivery to the patient.

10. Have the patient begin to inhale deeply just before depressing the inhaler and to continue inhaling for 3 to 5 seconds.
11. Instruct the patient to hold their breath for as long as is comfortable to help the body absorb the medication (**Step 3**).
12. If a spacer is used, the patient may need to take several breaths from the mouthpiece, without depressing the inhaler again, to get the full initial dose of the medication.
13. Continue to administer supplemental oxygen (replace the oxygen mask).
14. Allow the patient to breathe a few times, then repeat a second dose per direction from medical control or local protocol (**Step 4**).

Administration of a Small-Volume Nebulizer

To help a patient self-administer medication from a small-volume nebulizer, follow the steps in **SKILL DRILL 16-2**:

1. Take standard precautions.
2. Obtain an order from medical control or local protocol.
3. Check that you have the right medication, right patient, right dose, and right route, and that the medication is not expired. Ensure there are no issues with contamination, discoloration, or clarity of the medication (**Step 1**).
4. Make sure the patient is alert enough to use the device.
5. Check whether the patient has already taken any treatments.

Skill Drill 16-1 Assisting a Patient With a Metered-Dose Inhaler

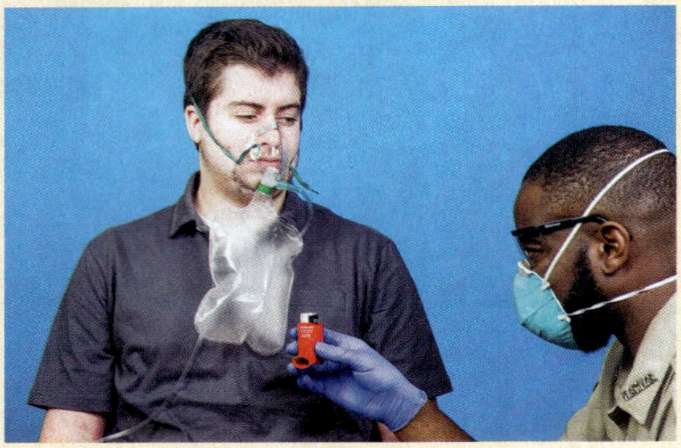

Step 1

Check that you have the correct medication for the correct patient. Check the expiration date. Ensure the inhaler is at room temperature or warmer.

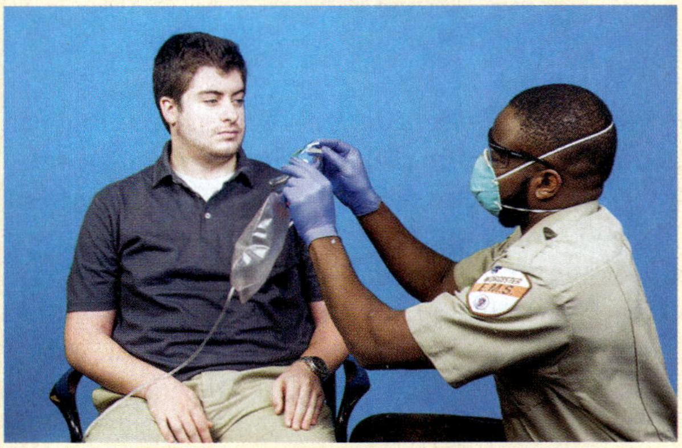

Step 2

Remove the oxygen mask. Hand the inhaler to the patient. Instruct the patient to exhale deeply and to then place their lips around the mouthpiece before inhaling.

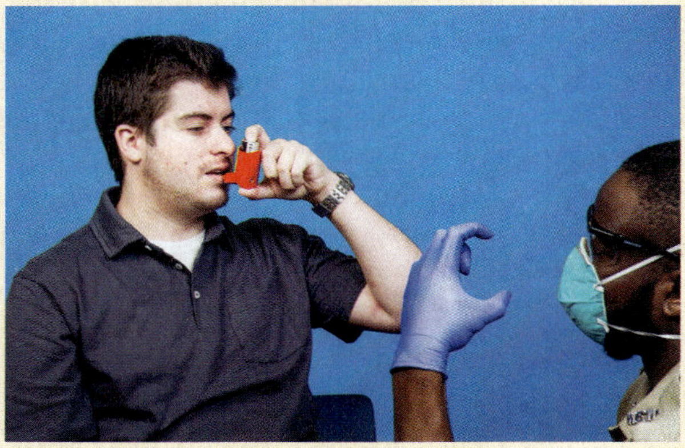

Step 3

Instruct the patient to press the inhaler and inhale one puff. Instruct about breath holding.

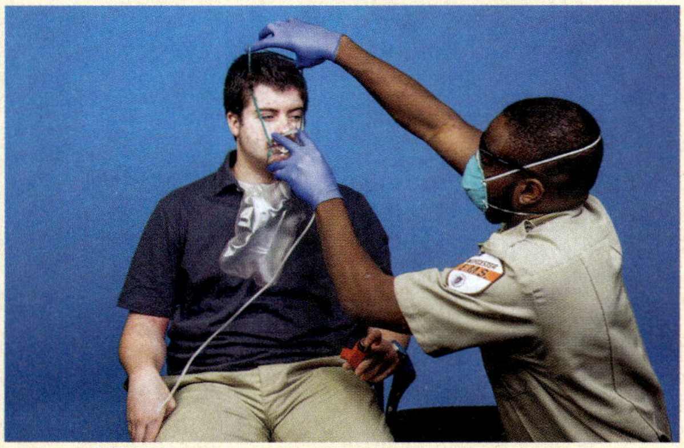

Step 4

Reapply oxygen. After a few breaths, have the patient repeat the dose if the medical order or protocol allows.

6. If assisting to assemble the device, maintain aseptic technique.
7. Open the medication container on the nebulizer and pour the medication (generally the whole volume of the medication) into the container. In some cases, sterile saline may be added (about 3 mL) to achieve the optimal volume of fluid for the nebulized application (**Step 2**).
8. Attach the medication container to the nebulizer mouthpiece and to the oxygen tubing. Attach the oxygen tubing to the oxygen tank.

Skill Drill 16-2 Assisting a Patient With a Small-Volume Nebulizer

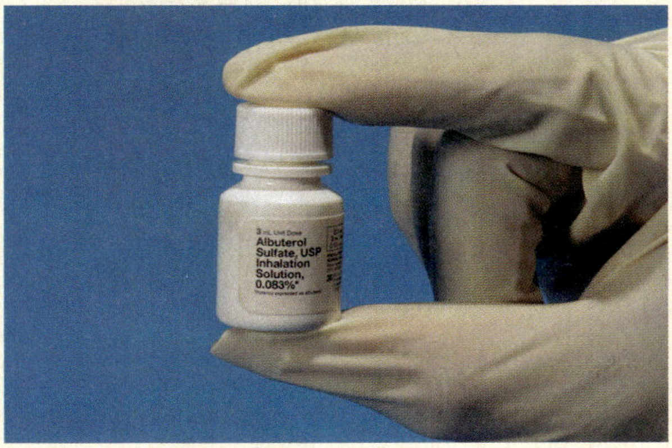

Step 1

Check that you have the correct medication for the patient. Check the expiration date. Confirm you have the correct patient and the correct dose.

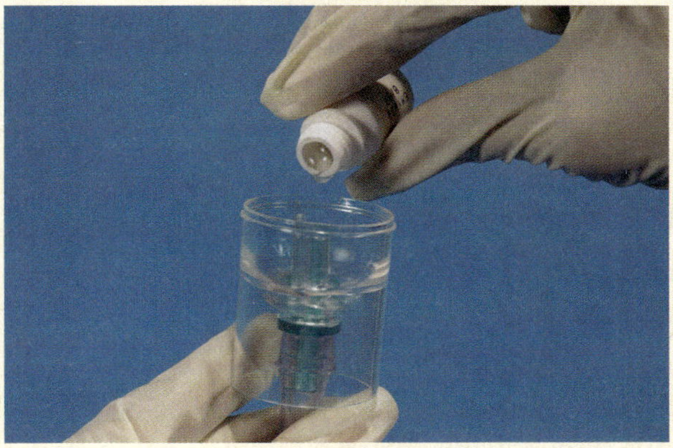

Step 2

Pour the medication into the container on the nebulizer. In some cases, sterile saline may be added (about 3 mL) to achieve the optimal volume of fluid for the nebulized application.

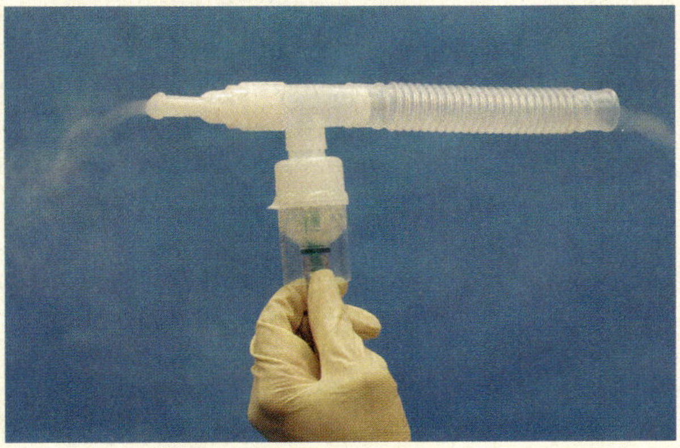

Step 3

Attach the medication container to the nebulizer, mouthpiece, and tubing. Attach the oxygen tubing to the oxygen tank. Set the flowmeter at 6 L/min.

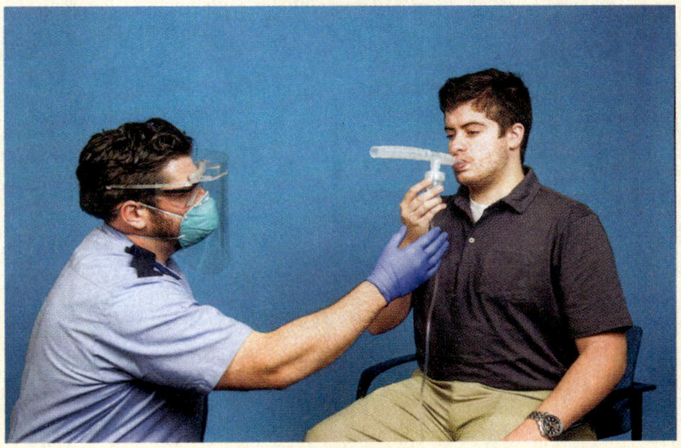

Step 4

Instruct the patient to put their lips around the mouthpiece, inhale the mist, and hold it for 3 to 5 seconds before exhaling.

9. Adjust oxygen flow to 6 L/min to establish a misting effect (**Step 3**).
10. Stop administering supplemental oxygen, and remove the nonrebreathing mask from the patient's face.
11. Ask the patient to put their lips around the mouthpiece of the device, inhale the mist, and hold it for 3 to 5 seconds before exhaling (**Step 4**).
12. When the mist dissipates and the container is empty or the patient is no longer experiencing

shortness of breath, discontinue use of the device.
13. Place the nonrebreathing mask back on the patient if the patient continues to report shortness of breath.
14. Reassess vital signs, and document your actions and the patient's response.
15. Consult with medical control and/or follow local policy if repeated doses are necessary.

Recognition and Management of Specific Conditions

Respiratory Infections

Dyspnea associated with acute infections is common. In patients with pneumonia, acute bronchitis, bronchiolitis, or epiglottitis, it can become extremely serious. The acute congestion and stuffiness of a common cold hardly ever require emergency care. Indeed, most people with colds treat themselves with over-the-counter medications. However, people with a common cold who have underlying problems such as asthma or heart failure may experience a worsening of their condition as a result of the additional stress of the infection. In addition, medications for colds may have stressful side effects, such as agitation, increased heart rate, and increased blood pressure. Some people with influenza or other, more serious respiratory viral infections such as COVID-19 may initially mistake their symptoms for those occurring secondary to a common cold. Severe pneumonia with significant respiratory deterioration can rapidly develop in these patients.

General management for patients with upper airway infections and dyspnea typically involves administering humidified oxygen (if available) and providing prompt transport to the hospital. Management of specific conditions is discussed in the following sections.

Croup

Croup (laryngotracheobronchitis) is inflammation of the larynx and trachea and is usually caused by an infection, typically viral infection (**FIGURE 16-10**).[8] This disease is often secondary to an acute viral infection of the upper respiratory tract and is typically seen in children between ages 6 months and 3 years. It is easily passed between children. Peak seasonal outbreaks of this disease occur in the late fall and during the winter.

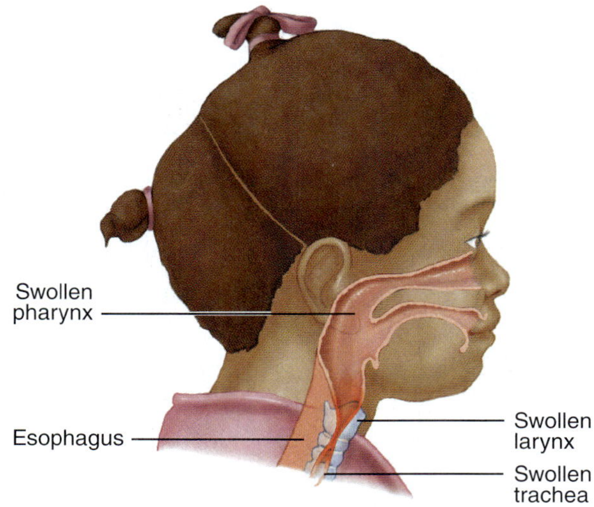

FIGURE 16-10 Croup results in swelling of the whole airway: pharynx, larynx, and trachea.

The disease starts with a cold, cough, and a low-grade fever that develops over a few days. The hallmark signs of croup are stridor and a seal-bark cough, which signal a narrowing of the air passage of the trachea that may progress to significant obstruction.

Croup is rarely seen in adults because their breathing passages are larger and can accommodate the inflammation and mucus production without producing symptoms. The airways of adults are wider, and the supporting tissue is firmer than that in children.

Note that bronchodilators are not indicated for croup and can worsen a patient's symptoms. Advanced life support (ALS) assist or transport is needed to administer medicines that are needed to treat croup.

Epiglottitis

Epiglottitis is a life-threatening inflammatory disease of the epiglottis, the small flap of tissue at the back of the throat that protects the larynx and trachea during swallowing. Bacterial infection is the most common cause (**FIGURE 16-11**). The overall incidence of epiglottitis is low. In the past, it was most often seen in infants and children, but it is now more prevalent in adults.[9] The development of a childhood vaccine against *Haemophilus influenzae*

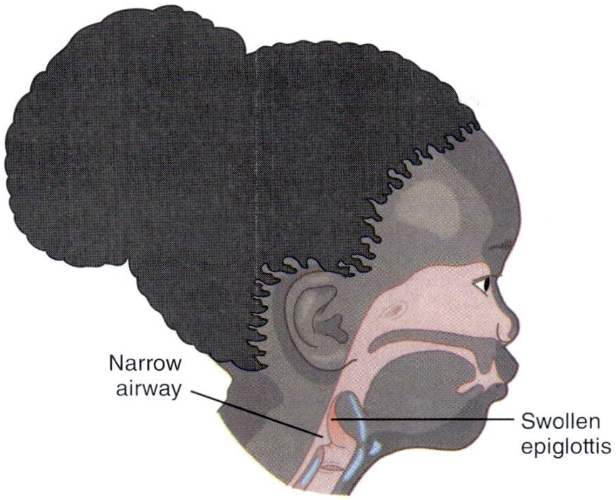

FIGURE 16-11 Acute epiglottitis is caused by a bacterial infection that results in severe swelling of the epiglottis, which could obstruct the airway.

type B has dramatically decreased the incidence of this disease in children.

In preschool and school-age children especially, the epiglottis can swell to two to three times its normal size. This puts the airway at risk of complete obstruction. The condition usually develops in otherwise healthy children, and symptoms are sudden in onset. Patients with this infection look ill, report a very sore throat, and have a high fever. They will often be found in the tripod position and drooling. Stridor is a late sign in the development of airway obstruction.

Treat patients with suspected epiglottitis gently and in the case of children, try not to do anything that will cause them to cry. Keep these patients in a position of comfort, and give them high-flow oxygen. Do not force a patient with epiglottitis to lie supine, as doing so may cause upper airway obstruction that could result in death. Do not attempt to suction the airway or place an oropharyngeal airway in a patient with suspected epiglottitis. These maneuvers may cause a spasm and complete airway obstruction.

Deterioration can occur quickly in adults with acute epiglottitis. You should be concerned if your adult patient presents with stridor or any other sign of airway obstruction without an obvious mechanical cause. Focus on maintaining a patent (adequate) airway, and provide prompt transport to the ED.

Respiratory Syncytial Virus

Respiratory syncytial virus (RSV) is a common cause of illness in young children. It causes an infection in the upper airway, lungs, and breathing passages and can lead to other serious illnesses such as bronchiolitis and pneumonia, as well as serious heart and lung problems in premature infants and in children who have depressed immune systems.

RSV is highly contagious and can be spread through droplets when the patient coughs or sneezes. The virus can also survive on surfaces, including hands and clothing. Therefore, the infection tends to spread rapidly through schools and child care centers.

When you assess a child with suspected RSV, look for signs of dehydration. Infants with RSV often refuse liquids. The thick mucus found in RSV infection can obstruct an infant's airway, as they are obligate nose breathers. Using a bulb syringe or suction catheter to suction the nose and/or mouth can reduce their respiratory distress. Treat airway and breathing problems as appropriate. The recently released vaccines to prevent RSV are expected to decrease the incidence of infection and hospitalization, especially in infants if the community achieves widespread immunization.

Bronchiolitis

Bronchiolitis is a respiratory illness that often occurs due to RSV infection and results in severe inflammation of the bronchioles. Bronchioles, the tiny airways that lead from the larger airways (bronchi) to the alveoli in the lungs, become inflamed, swell, and fill with mucus. This condition occurs most frequently in newborns and toddlers, especially boys, whose airways can easily become blocked. Infections are common during the winter and spring. Signs and symptoms include dyspnea, nasal congestion, coughing, fever, and wheezing. Look for signs of dehydration; infants with RSV often refuse liquids. If the RSV has progressed to bronchiolitis, shortness of breath and fever may be present.

The treatment for a child suffering from bronchiolitis is mainly supportive. Although many of these patients do well, there is still a risk for significant respiratory compromise. You should provide appropriate oxygen therapy to maintain an oxygen saturation level of 94% to 98% and allow the patient to remain in a position of comfort. Suction thick mucus from the nostrils if present. Reassess frequently for signs of worsening respiratory distress. Drugs such as albuterol are often not helpful to improve wheezing, and ipratropium should not be administered.[7] Be prepared to provide airway management and positive-pressure ventilation should the patient experience respiratory failure. Young children who require hospitalization for bronchiolitis are at increased risk for experiencing childhood asthma.

Pneumonia

According to the World Health Organization, pneumonia is a significant cause of morbidity worldwide and is the leading cause of death from infection in the United States for individuals older than 65 years. **Pneumonia** is a general term that refers to an infection of the lungs. The infection collects in the surrounding normal lung tissues, impairing the lung's ability to exchange oxygen and carbon dioxide.

Pneumonia is often a secondary infection, meaning it begins after an upper respiratory tract infection such as a cold or sore throat. It can be caused by a virus or bacterium, or by a chemical injury after an accidental ingestion or a direct lung injury from a submersion incident. Interventions such as intubation and tracheostomy can increase the risk of pneumonia developing. Pneumonia commonly affects people who are younger than 5 years or older than 65 years; have heart, lung, or liver disease; or are immunocompromised.[10]

Symptoms of pneumonia vary, depending on the age of the person and the cause of the illness; however, the following are common:

- Productive cough (with green, yellow, or bloody mucus)
- Fever
- Dyspnea
- Tachypnea
- Chest pain described as sharp or stabbing
- Loss of appetite

Children often present with unusually rapid or labored breathing or breathing characterized by grunting or wheezing sounds. Assess the work of breathing by observing for signs of accessory muscle use. The patient may also exhibit unilateral diminished breath sounds or crackles over the infected lung segments.

In severe cases where oxygen exchange at the alveoli is markedly impaired, the lips and fingernails may be blue or gray. If the pneumonia is in the lower part of the lungs near the abdomen, there may be fever, abdominal pain, and vomiting rather than dyspnea.

Bacterial pneumonia results in severe symptoms more quickly, including high fevers, which put the child at risk for febrile seizures. A viral pneumonia presents more gradually and is less severe.

Other signs and symptoms include dry skin, decreased skin turgor, exertional dyspnea, a productive cough, chest discomfort or pain that varies with inspiration and expiration, nasal flaring, tachypnea, headache, nausea and vomiting, musculoskeletal pain, weight loss, and confusion. The patient may be febrile, tachycardic, or even hypotensive. Assessment of the lungs may reveal diminished breath sounds or wheezing, crackles, or rhonchi. If possible, assess temperature to determine the presence of fever. Pulse oximetry readings, if available, may be low.

Regardless of the cause, treatment includes airway support and providing supplemental oxygen. Use oxygen with appropriate adjuncts, and provide supportive measures if needed. Evaluate patient treatment through reassessment, and prepare for possible deterioration in the patient's condition.

Pneumonia is particularly serious in infants because they have an increased oxygen demand and less respiratory reserve than older children or adults. For a pediatric patient with suspected pneumonia, your primary treatment will be supportive. Monitor the patient's airway and breathing status and administer supplemental oxygen if required. If the child is wheezing, administer a bronchodilator if permitted in your EMS system. A diagnosis of pneumonia must be confirmed in the hospital setting with a chest radiograph, followed by the administration of antibiotics as the primary treatment.

Maintain a high index of suspicion for pneumonia in individuals 65 years or older and those who are chronically and terminally ill. The process of aging causes some degree of immune suppression and increases the risk of contracting infections such as pneumonia. Increased mucus production, pulmonary secretions, and the inflammatory effects of infection all interfere with the ability of the alveoli to oxygenate the blood. While earlier recognition of pneumonia in these patients is important, your management remains the same.

Pertussis

Pertussis (whooping cough) is an airborne bacterial infection that primarily affects children younger than 6 years with the highest incidence in infants.[11] It is highly contagious and is passed through droplet infection.

A patient with pertussis will be feverish and exhibit a "whoop" sound on inspiration after a coughing attack. Symptoms are generally similar to colds, but coughing spells can last for more than 1 minute, during which the child may turn red or purple. This may frighten the parents or caregivers into calling 9-1-1.

Some infants and younger children with pertussis should be treated in a hospital because they are at greater risk for complications such as pneumonia, which occurs mostly in children younger than 1 year. In infants younger than 6 months, pertussis can be life threatening.

Children with pertussis may vomit or not want to eat or drink. Watch for signs of dehydration. You may have to suction thick secretions to clear the airway. Give oxygen by the most appropriate means.

Pertussis can also occur in adults either because they were not vaccinated as children or, more commonly, because the vaccine did not confer lifelong immunity. When it does occur, it can cause a severe upper respiratory infection, which can lead to pneumonia in geriatric patients or people with compromised immune systems. The infection can cause coughing spells that last for weeks and can be so severe that patients find it hard to breathe, eat, or sleep. In the worst cases of infection, particularly in geriatric patients, coughing can lead to cracked ribs. For patients who are already weak from other chronic conditions, such as asthma or COPD, pertussis can lead to hospitalization. According to the CDC, in 2024 more than six times the cases of the disease were reported compared to the prior year.[12] Pertussis has become a serious issue, and physicians are becoming more aggressive about immunizing adults with the pertussis vaccine as vaccine effectiveness fades over time.

Influenza Type A

Influenza type A is an animal respiratory disease that has mutated to infect humans. In 2009, the H1N1 strain of influenza type A became **pandemic** (an outbreak that occurred on a global scale). Influenza type A strains prevalent in 2024 are related to this H1N1 strain.[13] Infection with influenza may make chronic medical conditions worse. All strains of influenza type A are transmitted by direct contact with nasal secretions and aerosolized droplets from coughing and sneezing by infected people. Influenza type A viruses cause fever, cough, sore throat, muscle aches, headache, and fatigue and may lead to pneumonia or dehydration. Serious illness is more likely to occur in older adults, those who have chronic illnesses such as asthma or COPD, pregnant people, and children younger than 5 years (especially those younger than 2 years). Annual influenza vaccines are known to reduce the risk of contracting or becoming seriously ill from the flu, or spreading it to vulnerable friends or family members.

COVID-19

Coronavirus disease 2019 (COVID-19) is a respiratory disease caused by the virus SARS-CoV-2. The virus is a coronavirus, similar to the one that causes the common cold. It is believed to have initially been native to bats and transferred to humans by contact in China, in the fall of 2019. Because the virus is extremely contagious, it spread rapidly across the entire world, creating a severe pandemic. The virus preferentially affects older adults, patients living in close quarters with one another, and those with weakened immune systems, but it has also sickened and even killed many people who were otherwise young and healthy.[13]

COVID-19 is transmitted by aerosol droplets, through airborne particles generated by sneezing or coughing, and by direct contact. The virus may survive on surfaces for several days, although the risk of transmission by contact is low.[14] Equipment and surfaces in contact with a patient suspected to be infected with COVID-19 should be disinfected. Incubation after exposure is 2 to 12 days. Signs and symptoms include fever, cough, dyspnea, congestion, chest pain during inspiration, sore throat, vomiting, diarrhea, fatigue, muscle aches, and loss of taste or smell.[15] Respiratory deterioration in these patients can be dramatic and rapid. COVID-19 vaccines are known to reduce the incidence of the disease and of serious illness related to it.

> **Words of Wisdom**
>
> In 2021, the National EMS Scope of Practice Model expanded the EMT role to include specimen collection via nasal swab. This expanded role greatly enhanced public health efforts to detect and slow the spread of COVID-19 infections.
>
> The collection process varies widely based on the test manufacturer's guidelines. The EMT must be familiar with the testing instructions. In most cases, the tests require an anterior sample, obtained by swabbing just inside each nostril. However, some tests indicate a midturbinate swab, which requires the swab to be advanced just until resistance is encountered in each nostril (**FIGURE 16-12**).[16] Regardless of the test being used, the EMT should take appropriate infection control precautions, including gloves, mask, and eye protection.

Tuberculosis

Tuberculosis (TB) is a bacterial infection caused by *Mycobacterium tuberculosis*. TB spreads by cough and is dangerous because many strains are resistant to antibiotics. It most commonly affects the lungs but can rarely be found in almost any organ of the body, particularly the kidneys, spine, and lining of the brain and spinal cord (meninges). In some cases, TB remains latent for years without causing symptoms or being infectious to other people. However, when the person is in a state of weakened immunity, TB disease can activate. The patient may not even be aware of having the disease.

Patients with TB disease involving the lungs will report fever, coughing, fatigue, night sweats, and weight loss. If the lung infection becomes severe, the patient will experience shortness of breath, coughing, productive sputum, bloody sputum, and chest pain.

TB has a higher prevalence among people who live in close contact, such as prison inmates, nursing home residents, and people in homeless shelters. TB is also found in people who abuse intravenous drugs or alcohol and people whose immune systems are compromised by an infection such as human immunodeficiency virus (HIV). Anyone who comes into close contact with people who have active TB or is in contact with people from countries that have a high prevalence of TB is at risk for contracting the disease. As an EMT, you are also at risk.

If you suspect your patient may have active TB, you need to wear (at a minimum) your gloves, eye protection, and an N95 respirator. These respirators are fit-tested to the individual to ensure no contaminated air can pass through. Also place a surgical mask or oxygen mask (if indicated) on the patient.

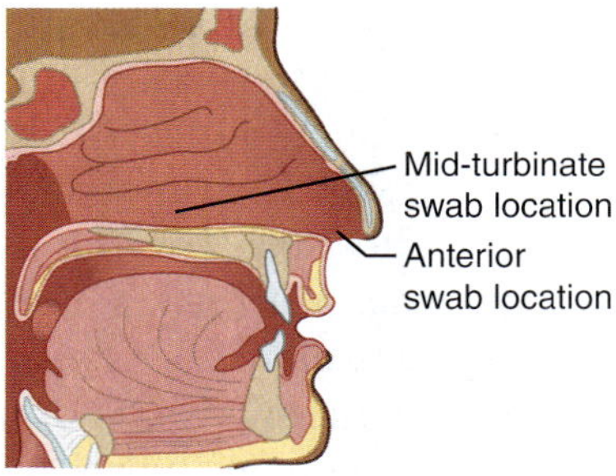

FIGURE 16-12 COVID-19 swab sample locations.

Acute Pulmonary Edema

Sometimes, the heart muscle is so damaged after a heart attack or other illness that it cannot contract forcefully enough to circulate blood properly. In these cases, the left side of the heart cannot eject blood delivered from the lung as fast as the right side delivers it. As a result, fluid builds up within the alveoli and in the lung tissue between the alveoli and the pulmonary capillaries. This accumulation of fluid is referred to as **pulmonary edema**, and it is usually a result of left-side heart failure. By physically separating the alveoli from the pulmonary capillary vessels, the edema interferes with the exchange of carbon dioxide and oxygen (**FIGURE 16-13**). High blood pressure and low cardiac output often trigger this acute (flash) pulmonary edema. These patients are among the most

> **Words of Wisdom**
>
> Not all patients with pulmonary edema have heart disease. Poisonings from inhaling large amounts of smoke or toxic chemical fumes can produce pulmonary edema, as can traumatic injuries of the chest and exposure to high altitudes. In these cases, fluid collects in the alveoli and lung tissue in response to damage to the tissues of the lung or the bronchi.

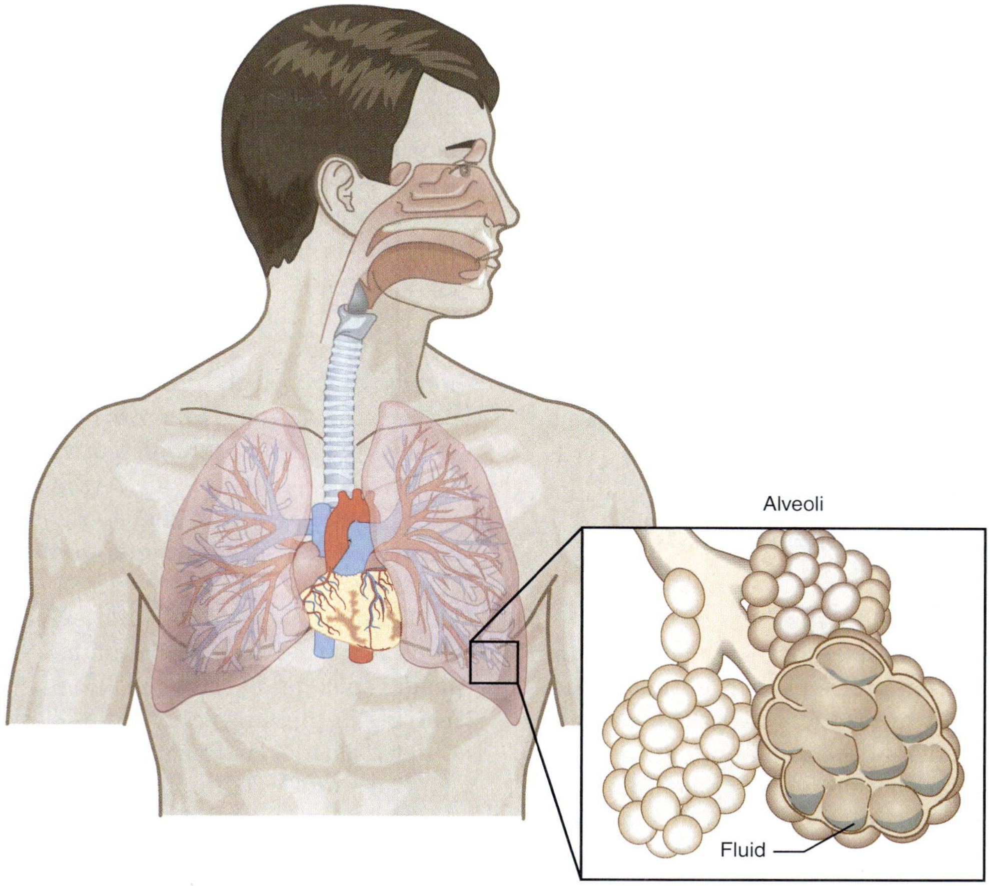

FIGURE 16-13 In pulmonary edema, fluid fills the alveoli and separates the capillaries from the alveolar wall, interfering with the exchange of oxygen and carbon dioxide.

sick, frightened, and worrisome patients you will encounter. They are literally drowning in their own fluid. The patient experiences dyspnea with rapid, labored breathing. In the most severe cases, you will see frothy pink sputum at the nose and mouth.

Dyspnea caused by acute pulmonary edema may be associated with cardiac disease or direct lung damage. In either case, administer high-concentration oxygen, and, if necessary, carefully suction any secretions from the airway. The best position for a conscious patient who has acute pulmonary edema is the position in which it is easiest to breathe. Usually, this is sitting up. An unconscious patient with acute pulmonary edema may require full ventilatory support, including placement of an airway adjunct, positive-pressure ventilation with a bag-mask device, oxygen, and suctioning.

Continuous positive airway pressure (CPAP) is a noninvasive means of providing ventilatory support for patients experiencing respiratory distress associated with obstructive pulmonary disease (such as emphysema) and acute pulmonary edema. CPAP increases pressure in the lungs, opens collapsed alveoli, pushes more oxygen across the alveolar membrane, and forces interstitial fluid back into the pulmonary circulation. CPAP systems use oxygen to deliver the positive ventilatory pressure to the patient. Many patients show dramatic improvement with the use of CPAP. CPAP can be used for patients who have moderate to severe respiratory distress from an underlying disease, such as pulmonary edema or obstructive pulmonary disease (including emphysema), are alert and able to follow commands, have tachypnea, or have a pulse oximetry reading of less than 90%. One potential contraindication to the use of CPAP is low blood pressure. Because of the increased pressure inside the chest, blood flow returning to the heart is diminished, further decreasing blood pressure. CPAP is also not used in patients in respiratory arrest or who have signs and symptoms of a pneumothorax or chest trauma, a tracheostomy, a decreased level of consciousness, inability to follow commands, or active gastrointestinal bleeding.

If you are authorized to apply CPAP for acute pulmonary edema according to your local protocols, do so. Call for ALS or provide prompt transport to the nearest appropriate ED. Continue to reassess patients using CPAP for signs of deterioration and/or respiratory failure. See Chapter 11, *Airway and Ventilation Management*, for a complete discussion on using CPAP.

Chronic Obstructive Pulmonary Disease

Chronic obstructive pulmonary disease (COPD), is a lung disease characterized by chronic obstruction of lung airflow that interferes with normal breathing and is not fully reversible.[17] In the United States, COPD has been diagnosed in more than 16 million people, and millions more people have COPD and do not know it. According to the CDC, it is one of the top 10 leading causes of death in the United States.[18] COPD is an umbrella term used to describe several lung diseases, including emphysema and **chronic bronchitis**, an ongoing irritation of the trachea and bronchi.

COPD may be a result of direct lung and airway damage from repeated infections or inhalation of toxic gases and particles, but most often it results from cigarette smoking. Although it is well known that cigarettes are a direct cause of lung cancer, their role in the development of COPD is far more significant and less publicized.

Tobacco smoke is a bronchial irritant and can create chronic bronchitis. With bronchitis, excess mucus is constantly produced, obstructing small airways and alveoli. Protective cells and lung mechanisms that remove foreign particles are destroyed, further weakening the airways. Chronic oxygenation problems can also lead to right-side heart failure, which leads to fluid retention, such as edema in the legs.

Pneumonia develops easily when the air passages are persistently obstructed. Ultimately, repeated episodes of irritation and pneumonia cause scarring in the lungs and some dilation of the obstructed alveoli, leading to COPD (**FIGURE 16-14**).

The most common form of COPD is **emphysema**. Emphysema is a loss of the elastic material in the lungs that occurs when the alveolar air spaces are chronically stretched due to inflamed airways and obstruction of airflow out of the lungs.

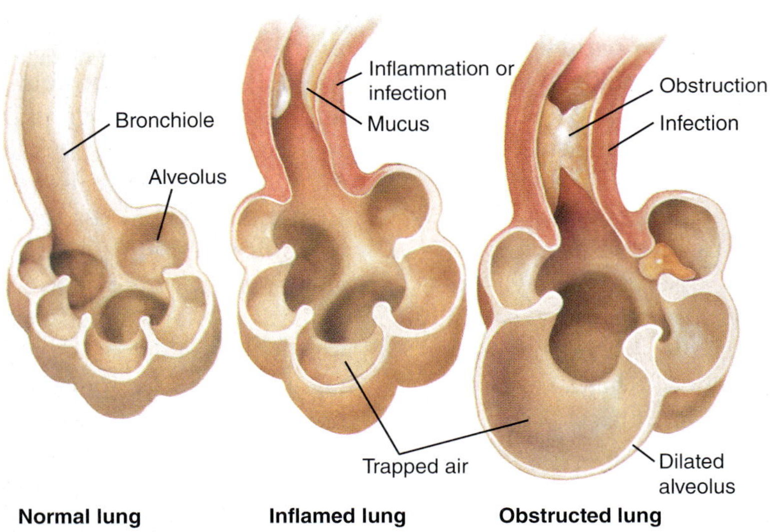

FIGURE 16-14 Repeated episodes of irritation and inflammation in the alveoli result in the obstruction, scarring, and some dilation of the alveolar sac characteristic of COPD.

Smoking can also directly destroy the elasticity of the lung tissue. Normally, the lungs act like spongy balloons that are inflated; once they are inflated, they will naturally recoil because of their elastic nature, expelling gas rapidly. However, when they are constantly obstructed or when the elasticity is diminished, air is no longer expelled rapidly, and the walls of the alveoli eventually fall apart, leaving large holes in the lung that resemble large air pockets or cavities.

Most patients with COPD have elements of both chronic bronchitis and emphysema. Some patients will have more elements of one condition than the other; few patients will have only emphysema or bronchitis. Therefore, most patients with COPD will chronically produce sputum, have a chronic cough, and have difficulty expelling air from their lungs, with long expiration phases and wheezing. Patients may present with adventitious breath sounds such as crackles, rhonchi, and wheezes, or may have severely diminished breath sounds due to poor air movement.

Patients with COPD may have an altered level of consciousness or may be unresponsive from hypoxia or carbon dioxide retention. Patients with COPD often find breathing difficult when lying down. Assist with the patient's prescribed inhaler if there is one. Often, a patient with COPD will overuse an inhaler, so watch for side effects. If approved by medical direction, the use of CPAP may be helpful for these patients. Promptly transport patients with COPD to the ED, allowing them to sit upright if this is most comfortable.

Asthma and Anaphylaxis

Asthma and anaphylaxis are the result of an allergic reaction to an inhaled, ingested, or injected substance. The substance itself (**allergen**) is not the cause of the allergic reaction; rather, it is an

Words of Wisdom

Be aware that the signs and symptoms of sudden deterioration of COPD and pulmonary edema significantly overlap. Many patients suffer from both diseases, and it is often difficult to determine which disease is causing the patient's shortness of breath. Lung sounds are one way to help you tell the difference. Patients with pulmonary edema caused most often by heart failure will often have wet lung sounds (crackles), and patients with COPD will often have dry lung sounds (wheezes). However, do not assume *all* patients with COPD have wheezes and *all* heart failure patients have crackles. **TABLE 16-7** compares COPD and heart failure.

To help illustrate the distinction between heart failure and COPD, suppose you are called to assist an 80-year-old man who has experienced shortness of breath for 45 minutes. Physical examination reveals that his pulse and respiratory rate are elevated, and you observe pedal edema (swollen legs and feet) and jugular venous distention. His lung sound check reveals wheezing. He has a history of hypertension, heart failure, and myocardial infarction; however, he has no history of smoking, asthma, or COPD. What is your initial general impression?

This patient's elevated blood pressure, pedal edema, jugular venous distention, and history of heart failure should lead you in the direction of pulmonary edema related to heart failure. Unlike a typical patient with COPD, he has no history of smoking and takes diuretics and medication for hypertension. In this case, the alveoli are so full of fluid that bubbles (the condition that gives the sound of crackles) cannot form. The bronchi also become constricted, which produces wheezing. The wheezing this patient is experiencing is called cardiac asthma, which is not a form of asthma, but rather a type of coughing or wheezing that occurs with left-side heart failure. The treatment for this type of wheezing requires different medications than those used for asthma or COPD.

Patients with COPD wheeze because of bronchial constriction and present with shortness of breath. Their breathing gets progressively worse, and they have the most trouble breathing on exertion. Patients with COPD have chronic coughing and thick sputum. They are usually long-term smokers with a thin, barrel-chest appearance. Their medications would include home oxygen, bronchodilators, and corticosteroids.

Patients with COPD often have a slower onset of symptoms because their disease is worsened by infection and other stressors. Patients with heart failure experience a fluid overload in the lung, which may develop quickly from a failing pump.

As you try to discern between COPD and heart failure, keep an open mind so that you do not miss important differences. The best advice is to treat the patient, not the lung sounds.

TABLE 16-7 Comparison of COPD and Heart Failure

	COPD	Heart Failure
Description	• A slow process of dilation and disruption of the airways and alveoli caused by chronic bronchial obstruction • Usually in long-term smokers	• A disease of the heart characterized by shortness of breath, edema, and weakness
Pathophysiology	Emphysema: • Destruction of the airways distal to the bronchioles • Destruction of the pulmonary capillary bed • Decreased ability to oxygenate the blood • Lower cardiac output and hyperventilation • Development of muscle wasting and weight loss Chronic bronchitis: • Excessive mucus production with airway obstruction • Pulmonary capillary bed undamaged • Compensation by decreasing ventilation and increasing cardiac output • Poorly ventilated lungs, leading to hypoxemia • Increased carbon dioxide retention	• Damaged left ventricle and failure of heart as a pump • Attempt by heart to compensate with increased rate • Enlarged left ventricle • Backup of fluid into the lungs and, if the right heart fails, the body, as the heart fails to pump adequately
Signs/symptoms	• Use of accessory muscles Emphysema: • Thin appearance with barrel chest • "Puffing" (pursed-lip) style of breathing • Tripod position Chronic bronchitis: • May be obese • Difficulty with expiration	• Abdominal distention • Dependent edema (sacral or pedal) • Tachycardia • Increased respiratory rate • Anxiety • Inability to lie flat • Dyspnea that awakens them at night • Ashen or cyanotic
Level of consciousness	Normal or altered	Confusion
Neck veins	• Flat • Distended when heart failure also present	Distended
Skin color	• In emphysema, flushed • In chronic bronchitis, often cyanotic	Cyanotic or pale
Lung condition	• In emphysema, dry • In chronic bronchitis, wet when heart failure also present	Wet
Breathing	• Shortness of breath (mostly on exertion) • Breathing worsens over time (progressive) • May have pursed-lip breathing	• Shortness of breath all the time • Sudden onset of shortness of breath
Breath sounds	Rhonchi, wheezing	Crackles, wheezing
Circulation	No dependent edema	Dependent edema
Cough	• In emphysema, little or none • In chronic bronchitis, frequent or chronic cough	Coughing may be present; increases when supine

	COPD	Heart Failure
Sputum	• In emphysema, no mucus • In chronic bronchitis, excessive, thick mucus	Pink, frothy sputum
Medications	Home oxygen, bronchodilators, and steroids help open the airways	Diuretics and antihypertensives help promote cardiac function and reduce fluid loads on the heart

exaggerated response of the body's immune system to the substance that causes it. In some cases, however, there is no identifiable allergen that triggers the body's immune system.

Asthma Emergencies

Asthma is an acute spasm of the bronchioles accompanied by excessive mucus production and swelling of the mucous lining of the respiratory passages (**FIGURE 16-15**). According to the Asthma and Allergy Foundation of America, nearly 26 million people in the United States have asthma, and it is a leading chronic disease in children, affecting approximately 4.8 million children.[19] Asthma affects people of all ages, but the highest prevalence rate is seen in children ages 5 to 17 years. It is rare in children younger than 1 year.

Common causes (triggers) for an asthma episode include upper respiratory infection, exercise, exposure to cold air or smoke, allergens, and emotional stress.

People with asthma will wheeze as they attempt to exhale through partially obstructed lower air passages; you may be able to hear loud wheezing without a stethoscope. In other cases, the airways are completely blocked and no air movement is heard. Between attacks, patients may breathe normally. In severe cases, cyanosis and/or respiratory arrest may quickly develop.

Asthma patients in respiratory distress will typically assume a position of comfort, such as the tripod position, to allow for maximum respiratory effort. In severe cases, the actual work of exhaling is tiring, and cyanosis and/or respiratory arrest may quickly develop. Cyanosis is the result of poor oxygenation of the blood as it passes through the capillaries around the alveoli. It can be seen first in the lips and mucous membranes.

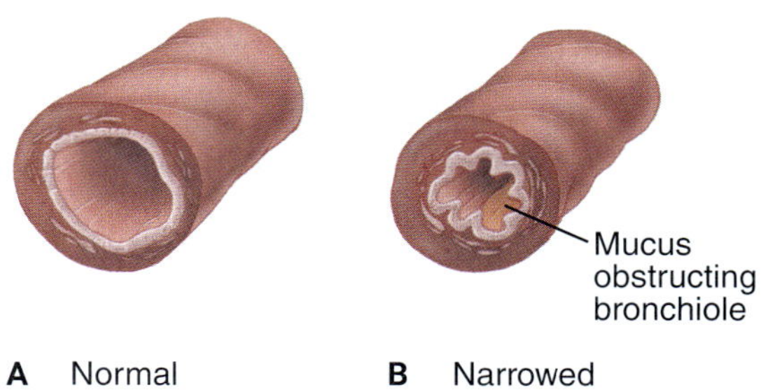

FIGURE 16-15 Asthma is an inflammation of the lungs associated with excessive mucus production and swelling of the bronchioles. **A.** Cross section of a normal bronchiole. **B.** The bronchiole in spasm; a mucus plug has formed and partially obstructed the bronchiole.

Words of Wisdom

Many lung problems are incorrectly labeled "asthma"; therefore, you must critically assess the patient. Asthma is often a recurring pathologic condition. Confirm whether the patient is able to breathe normally at other times. If possible, ask family members to describe the patient's asthma. When wheezing is the only problem identified, be aware that some forms of heart failure, foreign body aspiration, toxic fumes inhalation, or allergic reactions may cause wheezing.

Keep in mind that a cough is not always a symptom of a cold; it could signal pneumonia or asthma. Even if you do not hear much wheezing, the presence of a cough can indicate that some degree of reactive airway disease or an acute asthma attack may be taking place.

Because the effort to breathe during an asthma attack is very tiring, the patient may be exhausted by the time you arrive. An exhausted pediatric

Special Populations

ASTHMA AND THE PEDIATRIC PATIENT

When treating pediatric patients experiencing an asthma attack, allow the child to assume a position of comfort in the parent's or caregiver's lap if possible. Avoid overexciting the child because doing so may worsen the condition. Administer supplemental oxygen via a route that is tolerated by the child. Many small children will not tolerate (or may refuse to wear) a face mask. Rather than fighting with the child, provide blow-by oxygen by holding the oxygen mask in front of the child's face or ask the parent or caregiver to hold the mask (**FIGURE 16-16**). Allow the parent or caregiver to assist the team by gathering any medications, calming the patient, or holding blow-by oxygen or a nonrebreathing mask.

When you assess a pediatric patient, look for retractions of the skin above the sternum and between the ribs. Retractions are typically easier to see in children than in adults. Cyanosis is a late finding in children.

Many children with asthma will have prescribed handheld MDIs or small-volume nebulizers. Use these inhalers or nebulizers just as you would with an adult. Pediatric patients and some geriatric patients are more likely to use spacers to assist in inhaler use. Treat as in adult asthma. A bronchodilator such as albuterol alone or with ipratropium via an MDI with a spacer-mask device or by nebulizer may be administered based on local agency protocols. Often the parents or caregivers have attempted multiple dosages of albuterol. In this case, administer an additional dose while ALS clinicians are dispatched to meet you en route for additional medication administration and advanced care.

patient may have stopped feeling anxious or even struggling to breathe. It may look as if this patient is recovering; however, the patient is at a critical stage and is likely to stop breathing. Aggressive airway management, oxygen administration, and prompt transport are essential in this situation. Consider calling for ALS backup, if available, rapidly. Follow local protocol.

As you assess the patient's vital signs, note that the pulse rate will be normal or elevated, the blood pressure may be slightly elevated, and the respiratory rate will be increased. Ask questions about how and when the symptoms began.

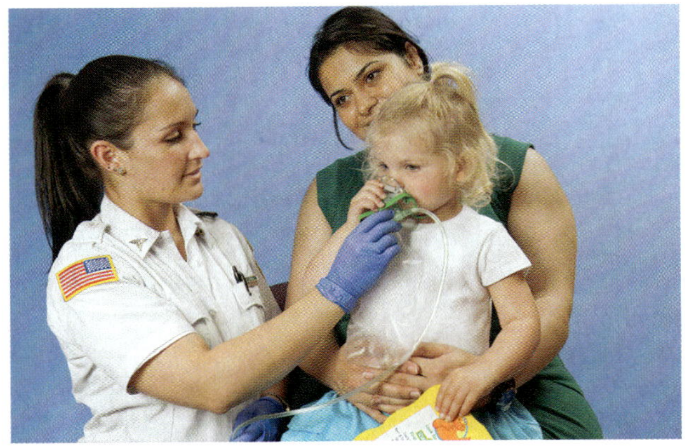

FIGURE 16-16 Because children may refuse to wear an oxygen mask, you may have to hold the mask in front of the child's face or ask the parents or caregivers for help holding the mask for their child.

Special Populations

ASTHMA AND THE GERIATRIC PATIENT

Asthma, like any chronic disease, can become life threatening in older people, especially in patients who have problems with airway control. The condition is made worse by anxiety and dehydration, which is typical in older people. Geriatric patients with asthma tend to have both inspiratory and expiratory wheezes.

If the patient has medication, such as an inhaler for an asthma attack, you may help with its administration, as directed by local protocol. If your agency has protocols to administer an inhaled bronchodilator that is carried on the ambulance, administer it using a small-volume nebulizer. Even patients who use their inhaler may continue to get worse. Reassess breathing frequently and be prepared to assist ventilations with a bag-mask device in severe cases. If you must assist ventilations in a patient who is having an asthma attack, use slow, gentle breaths.

Street Smarts

Most patients with asthma are familiar with their symptoms. Listen carefully to what a patient with asthma tells you; they often know exactly what they need.

Remember, the problem in asthma is getting the air out of the lungs, not into them. Resist the temptation to squeeze the bag hard and fast.

A prolonged asthma attack that is unrelieved by bronchodilators may progress into a condition known as **status asthmaticus**. The patient is likely to be frightened, frantically trying to breathe, and using all of their accessory muscles. Status asthmaticus is a true emergency. Give oxygen and promptly transport to the ED while continuing care.

Anaphylactic Reactions

Anaphylaxis, or anaphylactic shock, is a severe allergic reaction characterized by airway swelling and dilation of blood vessels all over the body, which may significantly lower blood pressure. Anaphylaxis may be associated with widespread hives (urticaria), itching, signs of shock, and signs and symptoms similar to asthma. The airway may swell so much that breathing problems can progress to total airway obstruction in a matter of minutes. Most anaphylactic reactions occur within 30 minutes of exposure to the allergen, which can be anything from food (eg, peanuts), to an insect sting, to a medication (eg, penicillin). For some patients, the episode of anaphylaxis may be their first; therefore, they may not know what caused the reaction. Other patients may be aware of substances they are sensitive to but unaware that an exposure has occurred, such as eating food that was not supposed to contain nuts.

An anaphylactic reaction is a life-threatening emergency. The first steps should be to administer epinephrine (adrenalin) and remove the offending agent. For example, if the patient has a stinger from a bee sting still in place, you may need to remove the stinger. Remember to scrape the stinger off because you can inject more venom into the patient if you pinch or squeeze the stinger.

Patients may have their own prescribed automatic epinephrine injector (EpiPen) or nasal spray (Neffy). Because epinephrine has immediate action, it can rapidly reverse the effects of anaphylaxis. If the patient continues to have signs of anaphylaxis after the first dose, it may be repeated at the same dose in 5 to 15 minutes according to protocol. If wheezing persists after epinephrine administration, protocols may permit administration of a nebulized bronchodilator. Recall that the bronchodilator may reverse wheezing but not airway swelling and hypotension, so epinephrine administration is always the priority. Use of an EpiPen is discussed further in Chapter 21, *Allergy and Anaphylaxis*.

Allow patients who are awake to assume a position that does not compromise breathing. Use an appropriate oxygen device for supplemental oxygen administration, if indicated. Be prepared to assist breathing as needed. Rapid transport and the early administration of epinephrine should be a priority.

Words of Wisdom

Some patients experience mild allergic reactions that do not develop into anaphylaxis. In these cases, there may be itching and hives that develop slowly, but none of the life-threatening signs and symptoms such as airway obstruction, wheezing, or hypotension seen in anaphylaxis. In the patient with a simple allergic reaction, medical direction will not order epinephrine, but rather may simply advise the patient to take an antihistamine such as diphenhydramine to provide relief from their discomfort.

Spontaneous Pneumothorax

Pneumothorax is a partial or complete accumulation of air in the pleural space. Pneumothorax is most often caused by trauma, but it can also be caused by some medical conditions. In these cases, the condition is called a spontaneous pneumothorax.

Normally, the negative pressure in the pleural space creates a vacuum that keeps the lung inflated. When the surface of the lung is disrupted, however, air escapes into the pleural cavity and results in a loss of negative vacuum pressure. The natural elasticity of the lung tissue causes the lung to collapse. The accumulation of air in the pleural space may be mild or severe (**FIGURE 16-17**).

Spontaneous pneumothorax may occur in patients with asthma, emphysema, or certain chronic lung infections (eg, TB), or in young people born with weak areas of the lung. Tall, thin young men are also more susceptible to experiencing spontaneous pneumothorax.

Patients with spontaneous pneumothorax may have severe respiratory distress, or they may have no distress at all and report only **pleuritic chest pain**, a sharp, stabbing pain on one side that is

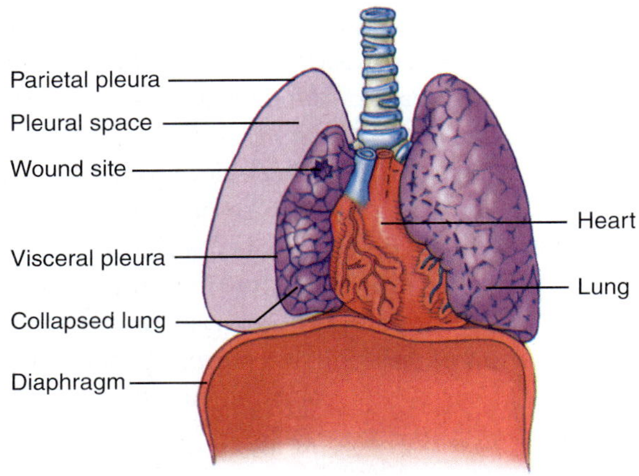

FIGURE 16-17 A pneumothorax occurs when air leaks into the pleural space from an opening in the chest wall or the surface of the lung. The lung collapses as air fills the pleural space and the two pleural surfaces are no longer in contact.

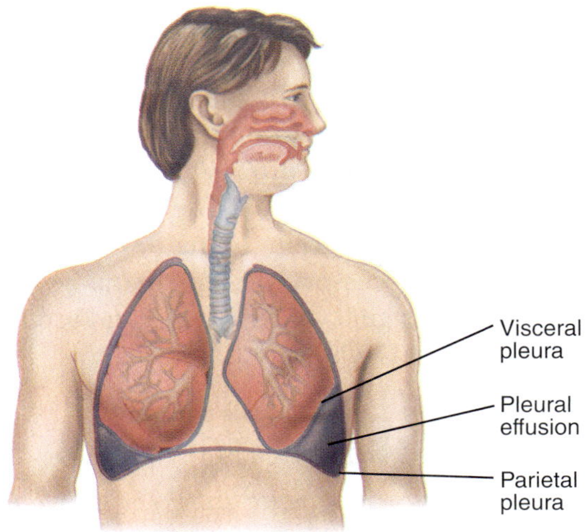

FIGURE 16-18 With a pleural effusion, fluid may accumulate in large volumes on one or both sides, compressing the lungs and causing dyspnea.

worse during inspiration and expiration or with certain movement of the chest wall. By listening to the chest with a stethoscope, you can sometimes detect that breath sounds are absent or decreased on the affected side. However, altered breath sounds are very difficult to detect in a patient with severe emphysema. A spontaneous pneumothorax has the potential to evolve into a life-threatening tension pneumothorax. Continually reassess for anxiety, increased dyspnea, hypotension, absent or severely decreased breath sounds on one side, the presence of jugular venous distention, and cyanosis.

Provide supplemental oxygen and prompt transport to the hospital. Like most dyspneic patients, those with spontaneous pneumothorax are usually more comfortable sitting up. Monitor the patient carefully, watching for any sudden deterioration in the respiratory status. Be ready to support the airway, assist breathing, and provide CPR if it becomes necessary.

Pleural Effusion

A **pleural effusion** is a collection of fluid outside the lung on one or both sides of the chest. It compresses the lung or lungs and causes dyspnea (**FIGURE 16-18**). This fluid may collect in large volumes in response to any form of irritation such as infection, heart failure, or lung cancer. Although it can build up gradually, over days or even weeks, patients often report that their dyspnea came on suddenly.

When you auscultate the chest of a patient with dyspnea resulting from pleural effusion, you will hear decreased breath sounds over the region of the chest where fluid surrounds the lung. These patients frequently feel better if they are sitting upright.

Treatment of pleural effusion consists of removal of fluid collected outside the lung, which must be done by a physician in a hospital setting. However, you should provide oxygen and other routine support measures to these patients.

Obstruction of the Airway

As an EMT, you must always be aware of the possibility that a patient with dyspnea may have a mechanical obstruction of the airway and be prepared to treat it quickly. If the patient is a small child or someone who was eating just before dyspnea developed, you start by assuming that the problem is an inhaled or aspirated foreign body. If the patient is old enough to talk but cannot make any noise, upper airway obstruction is the likely cause. A patient's airway may also be compromised by other causes, such as obstruction of a tracheostomy tube.

There is no condition more immediately life threatening than a complete airway obstruction. The obstructing body must be removed before any other actions will be effective. Chapter 11, *Airway and Ventilation Management*, discusses conditions that may result in an obstructed airway. Chapter 14, *BLS Resuscitation*, describes methods of clearing an airway obstruction, including in an infant and small child.

Words of Wisdom

Aspiration occurs when foreign material such as fluid or food enters the lungs. It typically occurs in adults or children who have conditions that make swallowing difficult, cause reflux of stomach contents into the esophagus, or alter their mental status. Congenital problems, such as cleft palate, increase the risk of aspiration in infants and young children. Ingestion of toxins, such as oils (eg, mineral oil, castor oil) and hydrocarbons (eg, gasoline, kerosene), may also result in aspiration. Larger objects can cause a complete airway obstruction; however, in most cases the aspirated substance moves through the trachea into the lungs.

Complications of aspiration may include pneumonia or other infections, damage to the lung tissue, sepsis, and respiratory failure, which may lead to death. Signs and symptoms of aspiration may have a slow or rapid onset, depending on the substance that passes through the vocal cords. Aspiration may cause pain when swallowing, chest discomfort, dyspnea, or fever and may cause the person to cough or choke constantly while eating. Assessment of breath sounds may reveal crackles, rhonchi, expiratory wheezes, or diminished breath sounds if pneumonia has developed.

Prevention of aspiration is an important goal for the EMT. The risk of this complication can be minimized by positioning patients who have altered mental status in the left lateral recumbent position or positioning an alert patient who has had a stroke with the head elevated at least 30°. When performing bag-mask ventilation, the risk of aspiration is minimized by delivering breaths at the proper rate or depth. If the patient vomits, the mouth should be suctioned promptly.

Pulmonary Embolism

An **embolus** is anything in the circulatory system that moves from its point of origin to a distant site and lodges there, obstructing subsequent blood flow in that area. Beyond the point of obstruction, circulation can be significantly decreased or completely blocked, which can result in a life-threatening condition. Emboli can be blood clots in an artery or vein that break off and travel through the bloodstream, or foreign bodies that enter the circulation, such as a bubble of air.

A **pulmonary embolism** is a condition that occurs when a blood clot formed in a vein (ie, an embolus), usually in the legs or pelvis, breaks off and circulates through the venous system until it reaches the lung. The embolus can also come from the right atrium in a patient with atrial fibrillation. The clot moves through the right side of the heart and into the pulmonary artery, typically becoming lodged in a smaller artery of the lung and significantly decreasing or blocking blood flow (**FIGURE 16-19**). Even though the lung itself can continue the process of inhalation and exhalation, no exchange of oxygen or carbon dioxide takes place in the areas of blocked blood flow because there is no effective circulation. In this circumstance, oxygen levels in the bloodstream may drop enough to cause cyanosis. The severity of cyanosis and dyspnea is directly related to the size of the embolism and the amount of blood flow affected.

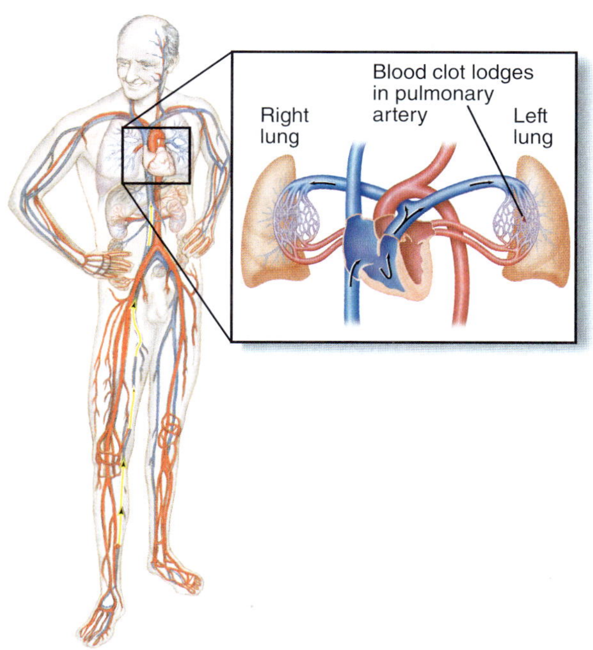

FIGURE 16-19 A pulmonary embolism occurs when a blood clot from a vein breaks off, circulates through the venous system, and moves through the right side of the heart into the pulmonary artery. Here, it can become lodged and significantly obstruct blood flow.

Pulmonary emboli may occur as a result of damage to the lining of vessels, a tendency for blood to clot unusually fast, or, most often, slow blood flow in a lower extremity. Slow blood flow in the legs is usually caused by long-term bed rest, which can lead to the collapse of veins. Pregnancy, active cancer, and recent surgery in the legs or pelvis are other risk factors.

Although they are fairly common, pulmonary emboli are difficult to diagnose. According to the CDC, over 100,000 deaths related to pulmonary embolism occur each year in the United States.[20] Symptoms and signs of pulmonary emboli include the following:

- Dyspnea (often sudden onset)
- Tachycardia
- Tachypnea
- Varying degrees of hypoxia
- Cyanosis (uncommon)
- Pleuritic chest pain
- Hemoptysis (coughing up blood) (rare)

With a large enough embolus, complete, sudden obstruction of the output of blood flow from the right side of the heart can result in cardiac arrest and sudden death.

Because a considerable amount of lung tissue may not be functioning, supplemental oxygen is mandatory in a patient with a pulmonary embolism. Place the patient in a comfortable position, usually sitting, and assist breathing as necessary. Hemoptysis, if present, is usually not severe, but any blood that has been coughed up should be cleared from the airway. The patient may have an unusually rapid and possibly irregular heartbeat. Transport the patient to the ED promptly.

Hyperventilation

Hyperventilation is defined as rapid breathing to the point that the level of arterial carbon dioxide falls below normal. It may be an indicator of a life-threatening illness. For example, a patient with diabetes who has a high blood glucose level, a patient who has taken an overdose of aspirin, or a patient with a severe infection is likely to hyperventilate. In these cases, rapid, deep breathing is the body's attempt to stay alive. The body is trying to compensate for **acidosis**, the buildup of excess acid in the blood or body tissues that results from the primary illness. Because carbon dioxide, mixed with water in the bloodstream, can add to the blood's acidity, lowering the level of carbon dioxide helps to compensate for the other acids.

Similarly, in an otherwise healthy person, blood acidity can be diminished by hyperventilation because the person is blowing off too much carbon dioxide. The result is a relative lack of acids. The resulting condition, **alkalosis**, is the buildup of excess base (lack of acids) in the body fluids.

Alkalosis is the cause of many of the symptoms associated with **hyperventilation syndrome**, including anxiety, dizziness, numbness, tingling of the hands and feet, and painful spasms of the hands and/or feet (carpopedal spasms). Patients often feel as if they cannot catch their breath despite the rapid breathing. Although hyperventilation can be a response to illness and a buildup of acids, hyperventilation syndrome is not caused by these conditions. Instead, this syndrome occurs in the absence of other physical problems. It commonly occurs when a person is experiencing psychological stress. The respiratory rate of an individual who is experiencing hyperventilation syndrome may be as high as 40 shallow breaths/min or as low as 20 deep breaths/min.

When you respond to a patient who is hyperventilating, complete a primary assessment and gather a history of the event. Is the patient having chest pain? Is there a history of cardiac problems or diabetes? You must always assume a serious underlying problem even if you suspect that the underlying

Words of Wisdom

Do *not* have the patient breathe into a paper bag, even though it was once thought to be the technique for managing hyperventilation syndrome. In theory, breathing into a paper bag causes the patient to rebreathe exhaled carbon dioxide, allowing the level of carbon dioxide in the blood to return to normal. In fact, if the patient is hyperventilating because of a serious medical problem, this maneuver could make things worse. A patient with underlying pulmonary disease who breathes into a bag may become severely hypoxic. Treatment should instead consist of reassuring the patient in a calm, professional manner; supplying supplemental oxygen; and providing prompt transport to the ED.

problem is stress. The decision whether hyperventilation is being caused by a life-threatening illness or a panic attack should not be made outside the hospital. After assessing for life-threatening causes of the rapid or deep breathing, you can verbally instruct the patient to slow their breathing; however, if that does not work, give supplemental oxygen and provide transport to the hospital where physicians will determine the cause of the hyperventilation.

Environmental/Industrial Exposure

Many exposures that cause inhalation injury and dyspnea occur at industrial sites. Pesticides, cleaning solutions, chemicals, chlorine, and other gases can be accidentally released and inhaled by employees. Sometimes chemicals such as ammonia and chlorine bleach are mixed and create a hazardous by-product.

In many cases, industrial sites have their own medical, fire, and/or hazardous materials teams that are familiar with all of the chemicals used at their site and know what to do in case of an exposure. They will begin immediate decontamination, if it is needed, and medical care. In these cases, the patient needs to be decontaminated by trained responders before you take responsibility.

Once the patient is decontaminated, gather information from the first responders about the substance and the cause of dyspnea. Assess the patient, paying special attention to breath sounds. Inhalation injuries can cause aspiration pneumonia that can result in eventual pulmonary edema. The inhaled substance can also cause lung damage. Blood coming from the airway is an ominous sign.

Treat with oxygen, adjuncts, and suction on the basis of the presentation, level of consciousness, and level of distress observed in your patient. If the patient is wheezing, medical direction may order treatment with a bronchodilator. Chapter 38, *Incident Management*, discusses hazardous materials in more detail.

Carbon Monoxide Poisoning

Toxic gases can also affect people outside the industrial setting. One common type of exposure is **carbon monoxide**, a colorless, odorless, tasteless, and highly poisonous gas known as "the silent killer." Carbon monoxide is the leading cause of nondrug accidental poisoning deaths in the United States.[21] People who survive carbon monoxide poisoning can have permanent brain damage.

Carbon monoxide is produced by fuel-burning household appliances such as gas-fueled water heaters, space heaters, grills, and generators. The onset of cold weather commonly leads to an increase in carbon monoxide poisonings as people turn on heaters for the first time. The combined effects of incomplete combustion and a poorly ventilated building can cause a buildup of carbon monoxide. Another common source of carbon monoxide poisoning is motor vehicle exhaust. By running the engine inside a closed garage and inhaling the fumes, whether accidentally or in a suicide attempt, the person may become poisoned.

Carbon monoxide has a much stronger bond with hemoglobin than does oxygen; therefore, oxygen is not being delivered to the tissues of the body.

People who are exposed to carbon monoxide may think they have the flu. They initially complain of headache, dizziness, fatigue, and nausea and vomiting. They may report dyspnea on exertion and chest pain and display nervous system symptoms such as impaired judgment, confusion, or coma. The worst exposures may result in rapid onset of syncope or seizure. This can lead to cellular death and organ failure if uncorrected.

When you assess the scene, do not put yourself at risk of exposure (**FIGURE 16-20**). Consider toxic gas exposure if more than one patient in the same environment is experiencing the same signs and symptoms. The symptoms of patients will start to improve as soon as they are removed from the toxic environment. High-concentration oxygen by nonrebreathing mask is the best treatment for conscious patients. Patients who are unconscious or have an altered level of consciousness may need full airway control with insertion of an airway adjunct and ventilation using a bag-mask device. In the worst cases, patients may be treated with hyperbaric or pressurized oxygen therapy.

Cystic Fibrosis

Cystic fibrosis (CF) is a genetic disorder that affects the lungs and digestive system. CF disrupts the normal function of cells that make up the sweat glands in the skin and that also line the lungs and

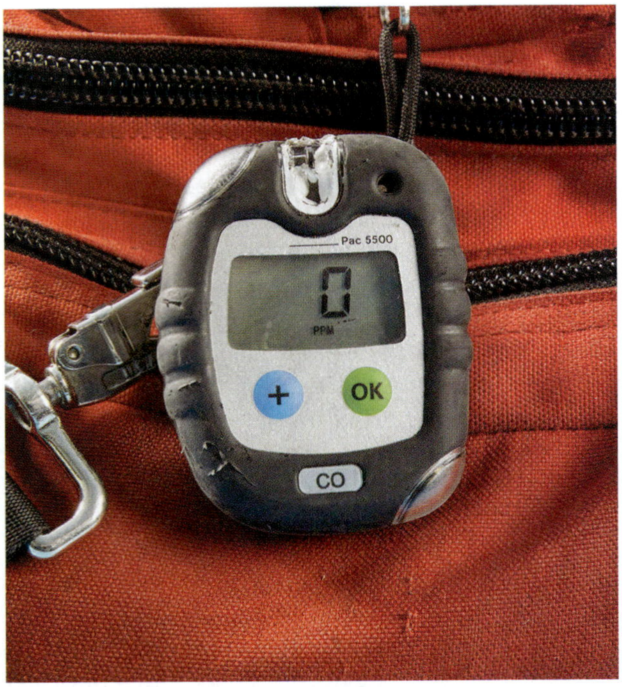

FIGURE 16-20 A portable carbon monoxide alarm can be attached to your medical bag to alert you to its presence at potential toxic scenes.

the digestive and reproductive systems. The disease predisposes the child to repeated lung infections.

The disease process in CF disrupts the essential balance of salt and water necessary to maintain a normal coating of fluid and mucus inside the lungs and other organs. The end result is that the mucus becomes thick, sticky, and hard to move. The mucus holds germs, causing the lungs to become infected.

Special Populations

RESPIRATORY ASSESSMENT IN THE GERIATRIC PATIENT

Most geriatric patients take medications, sometimes many, to treat various ailments that are part of the aging process. Some of these medications will blunt the body's normal reactions to stress and the mechanisms the body uses to compensate for respiratory compromise and hypoxia. For example, beta blockers, used for a variety of conditions, prevent heart rate from increasing to compensate for a decrease in blood pressure. Keep this in mind when you evaluate vital signs in geriatric patients.

YOU are the EMT

With an estimated time of arrival at the hospital of 8 minutes, you ask your partner to radio in the patient report. The patient's level of consciousness has not changed; however, the cyanosis around her mouth and in her nail beds has resolved and her oxygen saturation has improved. You complete your reassessment and continue treatment.

Recording Time: 15 Minutes	
Level of consciousness	Responsive to pain only
Respirations	10 breaths/min assisted
Pulse	118 beats/min; weak
Skin	Cool and dry; cyanosis has resolved
Blood pressure	112/70 mm Hg
Oxygen saturation (Spo_2)	90% (with bag-mask device and oxygen)

You deliver the patient to the ED staff and give your verbal report to the nurse. Because of the patient's decreased level of consciousness and the need for ongoing ventilation assistance, the physician elects to intubate her. She is diagnosed with acute exacerbation of her emphysema and is admitted to the intensive care unit.

10. How can positive-pressure ventilation cause a decrease in a patient's blood pressure?

11. What does *exacerbation* mean?

12. Should oxygen ever be withheld from a patient with COPD?

In CF, the child's symptoms range from sinus congestion to wheezing and asthmalike complaints. A chronic cough that produces thick, heavy, discolored mucus may develop in the child. As lung function decreases, so does the ability to breathe effectively. The child often has dyspnea; this generally results in the parents or caregivers calling EMS. Treat the child with suction and oxygen using age-appropriate adjuncts.

CF may cause death in childhood because of chronic pneumonia secondary to the thick, pathologic mucus in the airway. It also causes malabsorption of nutrients in the intestines. New treatments mean patients who have CF are living longer, often into their sixties.[22] Adults with CF are predisposed to other medical conditions, including arthritis, osteoporosis, diabetes, and liver problems.

YOU are the EMT SUMMARY

1. What is emphysema? What is the typical cause?

Emphysema, a form of COPD, is a disease of the respiratory system in which chronic inflammation develops in the airways, and destruction of alveoli and small airways leads to a loss of lung elasticity. As a result, the expiratory phase of respiration becomes difficult and gas exchange in the lungs becomes impaired. Although emphysema is an irreversible condition, its symptoms can be reduced and the disease progression slowed with lifestyle changes (eg, quitting smoking) and certain medications.

The single most common cause of emphysema is heavy, long-term cigarette smoking. Other causes include frequent pulmonary infections and long-term exposure to toxic agents, such as from working in an industrial setting for a long period.

2. Why is it especially significant that *this* patient called 9-1-1?

Patients with chronic diseases call 9-1-1 when something is different or has gotten worse. The patient could be experiencing an acute flare-up of her emphysema, a secondary respiratory illness to which she is predisposed (such as pneumonia), or complete respiratory failure. Just because she has refused EMS transport in the past does not mean that she will this time; she has a known respiratory illness, which you should assume has gotten worse, and she should be treated no differently from any other patient with a respiratory emergency.

3. What should be your *most* immediate action?

Oxygen and lit cigarettes, or any other source of fire, do not go together! Ask the patient to immediately extinguish her cigarette and then continue your assessment. Although oxygen is not flammable or explosive, it does support the process of combustion. A small spark or lit cigarette can become a flame in an oxygen-rich atmosphere. Oxygen will cause a fire to burn more vigorously, as well as hotter. The patient could literally light her face on fire; you and your partner could be injured as well.

4. How does emphysema differ from chronic bronchitis?

Emphysema is a disease in which small airways and the inner walls of alveoli are progressively destroyed, resulting in a loss of lung elasticity. Chronic bronchitis is caused by persistent inflammation in larger airways. With chronic bronchitis, excess mucus is constantly produced, which obstructs the bronchioles and alveoli. As a result, pulmonary gas exchange is less efficient. Many patients with chronic bronchitis have a chronic productive cough. In some patients, however, the cough reflex is weakened; this causes sputum to settle in the lungs and become infected, resulting in pneumonia. Emphysema and chronic bronchitis are both forms of COPD, and both are usually caused by heavy, long-term cigarette smoking.

5. Why do patients with emphysema breathe through pursed lips?

With emphysema, the force of exhalation increases intrathoracic pressure and causes premature closure of the small airways, causing air to be trapped in the alveoli. The harder the patient tries to push air out, the more air gets trapped in the alveoli. Chronic air trapping in the lungs explains why many patients with long-term emphysema have a characteristic barrel-shape appearance to their chest. Over time, patients with emphysema learn that if they push air out slowly at a higher residual airway pressure, they can exhale more air than if they try to push it out faster because their airways will remain open for longer. One of the ways they do this is by breathing through pursed lips during exhalation. Pursed-lip breathing allows the patient to push air out slowly under controlled pressure.

YOU are the EMT SUMMARY continued

6. What does a prolonged exhalation phase indicate in patients with obstructive lung disease?

A prolonged exhalation phase indicates that the patient is experiencing difficulty exhaling air from the lungs, which, as a result, causes chronic air trapping in the lungs. The inhalation-to-exhalation ratio in healthy people during normal breathing is typically 1:2. In other words, it takes about twice as long to exhale as it does to inhale. Depending on the severity of their disease process, patients with obstructive lung disease may have an inhalation to exhalation ratio of 1:4, 1:5, or longer. Because the patient's bronchioles significantly narrow during exhalation, wheezing (a whistling sound) is often heard during the exhalation phase while auscultating the lungs.

7. What treatment is indicated for the patient at this point?

Compared with the patient's condition during your initial assessment, it has deteriorated. She is now confused and slow to answer your questions, which indicates decreased oxygen delivery to the brain. Her oxygen saturation level of 88% indicates significant hypoxemia, and the fatigue indicates that she is less able to compensate for her condition. She clearly needs a higher concentration of oxygen than what her nasal cannula is supplying. Apply a nonrebreathing mask, set the flow rate at 12 to 15 L/min, and reassess her condition. CPAP might be helpful, but remember that altered mental status is a contraindication to its use for patients with COPD. If oxygenation does not improve, assisted ventilation with a bag-mask device may be necessary. If you must assist the patient's breathing, however, ensure that you allow *complete* exhalation between positive-pressure breaths. Remember, patients with emphysema have a lot of air trapped in the alveoli.

8. Why is cyanosis a later sign of hypoxemia in patients with emphysema?

Patients with emphysema maintain chronically low blood oxygen levels and chronically elevated carbon dioxide levels. Unlike in otherwise healthy people, cyanosis often does not develop in patients with emphysema until significantly more hemoglobin is desaturated (not carrying oxygen). The absence of cyanosis does not rule out hypoxemia in any patient, especially a patient with alveoli who needs a longer period of time to move air out of the lungs.

9. Why does tachycardia develop in patients with hypoxemia?

Whenever the body's demand for oxygen increases and its supply decreases (eg, hypoxemia), the nervous system increases the production of epinephrine from the adrenal glands. Epinephrine is a hormone that causes tachycardia (rapid heart rate) and an increase in the strength of cardiac contraction. Tachycardia is a critical physiologic compensatory mechanism that circulates oxygenated blood faster, thus helping to maintain adequate perfusion of the body's vital organs. However, if the underlying cause of the patient's hypoxemia is not corrected, the nervous system, which also requires oxygen, will no longer be able to compensate and the patient's heart rate will begin to fall.

10. How can positive-pressure ventilation cause a decrease in a patient's blood pressure?

Recall that negative-pressure ventilation, the process that occurs with normal breathing, involves contraction of the diaphragm and intercostal muscles and a decrease in intrathoracic pressure; as a result, air is pulled into the lungs. The decreased intrathoracic pressure also increases blood return to the heart by allowing the venae cavae to enlarge. Positive-pressure ventilation involves pushing air into the lungs, as occurs with artificial ventilation. It is critical to perform positive-pressure ventilation correctly. Deliver each breath over a period of 1 second, just enough to produce visible chest rise, at a rate that is appropriate for the patient (10 breaths/min for adults; 20 to 30 breaths/min for infants and children). If positive-pressure ventilation is delivered too fast or with too much force (hyperventilation), the resultant increase in intrathoracic pressure may impair blood return to the right atrium. The reduced blood return to the right side of the heart reduces the amount it can supply to the left side of the heart. If blood supply to the left side of the heart is reduced, less blood is pumped from the left ventricle per contraction (stroke volume). As a result, the patient's blood pressure (and perfusion status) will deteriorate.

11. What does *exacerbation* mean?

Exacerbation means to intensify or worsen in severity. In acute exacerbation of COPD, sometimes no other condition exists that would clearly explain the patient's sudden deterioration (ie, heart failure, pneumonia). Patients with COPD often experience acute exacerbation of their disease secondary to a change in environmental conditions, such as

YOU are the EMT SUMMARY continued

weather, humidity, or sudden activation of central heating or cooling in the home. Like diseases such as asthma, COPD can also be exacerbated by certain triggers, such as cat dander, dust, and seasonal allergens. In some cases, acute exacerbation is idiopathic (of unknown cause). As the patient's disease progresses, they will eventually reach a point at which the lungs simply cannot support oxygenation and ventilation (end-stage COPD). In end-stage COPD, it can be difficult to determine whether the patient is experiencing an exacerbation that can be treated effectively or if they have reached the end of the disease process. This will not affect your treatment, however, which involves airway management and ensuring adequate oxygenation and ventilation.

12. Should oxygen ever be withheld from a patient with COPD?

Although the brain uses the carbon dioxide level in the blood in regulating respiratory rate, some patients with COPD have a chronically high carbon dioxide level because of the difficulty removing it during exhalation. In those patients, the oxygen level in the blood becomes the stimulus for the respiratory process (hypoxic drive). Some patients who depend on hypoxic drive may decrease their respiratory effort if given increased oxygen. If a patient is hypoxic, however, it is essential that increased oxygen be given. If the respiratory rate and depth start to decrease, the problem can be managed by providing bag-mask ventilation.

Prep Kit

Ready for Review

- Children are not only smaller than adults and more vulnerable, they are also anatomically, physiologically, and psychologically different from adults in important ways.
  - The tongue is large relative to other structures in the pediatric patient, so it poses a higher risk of airway obstruction than in an adult.
  - An infant breathes faster than an older child.
  - Breathing requires the use of chest muscles and the diaphragm.
  - The airway in a child has a smaller diameter than the airway in an adult and is therefore more easily obstructed.
- Dyspnea is a common complaint that may be caused by numerous medical problems, including infections of the upper or lower airways, acute pulmonary edema, COPD, spontaneous pneumothorax, asthma, allergic reactions, pleural effusion, mechanical obstruction of the airway, pulmonary embolism, and hyperventilation.
- Each of these lung disorders has the capability to interfere with the exchange of oxygen and carbon dioxide that takes place during respiration. This interference may take the form of damage to the alveoli, separation of the alveoli from the pulmonary vessels by fluid or infection, obstruction of the air passages, or air or excess fluid in the pleural space.
- Patients with chronic lung diseases often have high levels of blood carbon dioxide; in some cases, giving them too much oxygen may depress or stop respirations (hypoxic drive). However, never withhold oxygen from patients with dyspnea.
- Breathing difficulty and/or hypoxia often develop in patients with the following medical conditions: respiratory infection, acute pulmonary edema, COPD, asthma, anaphylaxis, spontaneous pneumothorax, and pleural effusion.
- Infectious diseases associated with dyspnea include epiglottitis, bronchitis, TB, pneumonia, and pertussis.

Prep Kit continued

- Breath sounds (lung sounds) are some of the most important vital signs you should assess when treating a patient in respiratory distress.
- Signs and symptoms of breathing difficulty include adventitious breath sounds (wheezing, stridor, crackles, and rhonchi); nasal flaring; pursed-lip breathing; cyanosis; inability to talk; use of accessory muscles to breathe; and sitting in the tripod position, which allows the diaphragm the most room to function.
- Interventions for respiratory problems may include the following:
  - Oxygen via a nonrebreathing mask at 15 L/min, or positive-pressure ventilations using a bag-mask device
  - Airway management techniques such as use of an oropharyngeal (oral) airway, a nasopharyngeal (nasal) airway, suctioning, or airway positioning
  - Providing noninvasive ventilatory support with CPAP
  - Positioning the patient in a high Fowler position or a position of comfort to facilitate breathing
  - Assistance with respiratory medications found in a prescribed MDI or a small-volume nebulizer (Consult medical control to assist with its use or follow standing orders if the orders allow for this.)
- A patient who is breathing rapidly may not be getting enough oxygen as a result of respiratory distress from a variety of problems, including pneumonia or a pulmonary embolism; trying to blow off more carbon dioxide to compensate for acidosis caused by a poison, a severe infection, or a high blood glucose level; or having a stress reaction.
- In every case, prompt recognition of the problem, administration of oxygen, and prompt transport are essential.

Vital Vocabulary

acidosis The buildup of excess acid in the blood or body tissues that can result from a primary illness.

adventitious breath sounds Abnormal breath sounds such as wheezing, stridor, rhonchi, and crackles.

alkalosis The buildup of excess base (lack of acids) in the body fluids.

allergen A substance that causes an allergic reaction.

anaphylaxis An extreme, life-threatening, systemic allergic reaction that may include shock and respiratory failure.

aspiration A respiratory emergency that occurs when foreign material such as fluid or food enters the lungs and prevents effective breathing.

asthma An acute spasm of the smaller air passages, called bronchioles, associated with excessive mucus production and with swelling of the mucous lining of the respiratory passages.

atelectasis Collapse of the alveolar air spaces of the lungs.

bronchial breath sounds Normal breath sounds made by air moving through the bronchi.

bronchiolitis Inflammation of the bronchioles that usually occurs in children younger than 2 years and is often caused by the respiratory syncytial virus.

bronchitis An acute or chronic inflammation of the lung that may damage lung tissue; usually associated with cough and production of sputum and, depending on its cause, sometimes fever.

carbon dioxide retention A condition characterized by a chronically high blood level of carbon dioxide in which the respiratory center no longer responds to high blood levels of carbon dioxide.

carbon monoxide An odorless, colorless, tasteless, and highly poisonous gas that results from incomplete oxidation of carbon in combustion.

Prep Kit continued

chronic bronchitis Irritation of the major lung passageways from long-term exposure to infectious disease or irritants such as smoke.

chronic obstructive pulmonary disease (COPD) A lung disease characterized by chronic obstruction of lung airflow that interferes with normal breathing and is not fully reversible.

continuous positive airway pressure (CPAP) A method of ventilation used primarily in the treatment of critically ill patients with respiratory distress; can prevent the need for endotracheal intubation.

coronavirus disease 2019 (COVID-19) A respiratory disease caused by the virus SARS-CoV-2. The virus is a coronavirus, similar to the one that causes the common cold.

crackles Crackling, rattling breath sounds that signal fluid in the air spaces of the lungs.

croup A viral inflammatory disease of the upper respiratory system that may cause a partial airway obstruction and is characterized by a barking cough; usually seen in children.

diphtheria An infectious disease in which a pseudomembrane forms, lining the pharynx; this lining can severely obstruct the passage of air into the larynx.

dyspnea Shortness of breath.

embolus A blood clot or other substance in the circulatory system that travels to a blood vessel where it causes a blockage of blood flow.

emphysema A disease of the lungs in which there is extreme dilation and eventual destruction of the pulmonary alveoli with poor exchange of oxygen and carbon dioxide; it is one form of chronic obstructive pulmonary disease.

epiglottitis A bacterial infection in which the epiglottis becomes inflamed and enlarged and may cause an upper airway obstruction.

grunting A sign of increased work of breathing, heard as an *uh* sound during exhalation; reflects a pediatric patient's attempt to keep the alveoli open.

hyperventilation Rapid, usually deep, breathing that lowers the blood carbon dioxide level below normal.

hyperventilation syndrome This syndrome occurs in the absence of physical problems. The respiratory rate of a person who is experiencing hyperventilation syndrome may be as high as 40 shallow breaths/min or as low as only 20 very deep breaths/min. This syndrome is often associated with panic attacks.

hypoxia A dangerous condition in which the body tissues and cells do not have enough oxygen.

hypoxic drive A condition in which chronically low levels of oxygen in the blood stimulate the respiratory drive; seen in patients with chronic lung diseases.

influenza type A Virus that has crossed the animal/human barrier and has infected humans, recently reaching a pandemic level with the H1N1 strain.

metered-dose inhaler (MDI) A miniature spray canister used to direct medications through the mouth and into the lungs.

orthopnea Severe dyspnea experienced when lying down and relieved by sitting up.

oxygenation The process of delivering oxygen to the blood by diffusion from the alveoli following inhalation into the lungs.

pandemic An outbreak that occurs on a global scale.

paroxysmal nocturnal dyspnea Severe shortness of breath, especially at night after several hours of reclining; the person is forced to sit up to breathe.

pertussis (whooping cough) An airborne bacterial infection that affects mostly children younger than 6 years. Patients will be feverish and exhibit a "whoop" sound on inspiration after a coughing attack; highly contagious through droplet infection.

pleural effusion A collection of fluid between the lung and chest wall that may compress the lung.

Prep Kit continued

pleuritic chest pain Sharp, stabbing pain in the chest that is worsened by a deep breath or other chest wall movement; often caused by inflammation or irritation of the pleura.

pneumonia An infectious disease of the lung that damages lung tissue.

pneumothorax An accumulation of air or gas in the pleural cavity.

pulmonary edema A buildup of fluid in the lungs, often as a result of heart failure.

pulmonary embolism A condition in which a blood clot (embolus) breaks off from a large vein and travels to the blood vessels of the lung, causing obstruction of blood flow.

respiration The process of exchanging oxygen and carbon dioxide.

respiratory syncytial virus (RSV) A virus that causes an infection of the lungs and breathing passages; can lead to other serious illnesses that affect the lungs or heart, such as bronchiolitis and pneumonia. RSV is highly contagious and spread through droplets.

rhonchi Coarse, low-pitched breath sounds heard in patients with chronic mucus in the upper airways.

small-volume nebulizer A respiratory device that holds liquid medicine that is turned into a fine mist. The patient inhales the medication into the airways and lungs as a treatment for conditions such as asthma.

status asthmaticus An emergency that occurs when standard treatments fail to relieve asthma symptoms, resulting in acute respiratory failure.

stridor A harsh, high-pitched respiratory sound, generally heard during inspiration, that is caused by partial blockage or narrowing of the upper airway; may be audible without a stethoscope.

tachypnea Rapid respiratory rate.

tripod position An upright position in which the patient leans forward onto outstretched arms with the head and chin thrust slightly forward.

tuberculosis (TB) A contagious disease that attacks the lungs and that can remain dormant in a person's lungs for decades, then reactivate; many strains are resistant to antibiotics. TB is spread by cough.

ventilation Exchange of air between the lungs and the environment, spontaneously by the patient or with assistance from another person, such as an EMT.

vesicular breath sounds Normal breath sounds made by air moving into and out of the alveoli.

wheezing A high-pitched, whistling breath sound that is most prominent on expiration, and which suggests an obstruction or narrowing of the lower airways; occurs in asthma and bronchiolitis.

work of breathing An indicator of oxygenation and ventilation; reflects the child's attempt to compensate for hypoxia.

References

1. Alexander P. Respiratory physiology for intensivists. In: Ungerleider RM, Meliones JN, McMillan KN, Cooper DS, Jacobs JP, eds. *Critical Heart Disease in Infants and Children*. 3rd ed. Elsevier; 2019:134–149.
2. American Heart Association (AHA). *Pediatric Advanced Life Support Provider Manual*. Dallas, TX: AHA; 2020.
3. Interim guidance for healthcare providers caring for pediatric patients. American Heart Association website. https://cpr.heart.org/-/media/cpr-files/resources/covid-19-resources-for-cpr-training/interim-guidance-pediatric-patients-march-27-2020.pdf. Updated March 23, 2020. Accessed December 19, 2024.
4. Binks AC, Parkinson SM, Sabbouh V. Oxygen: under or over a surgical facemask for COVID-19 patients? *Anaesthesia*. 2020;75(12):1691–1692.
5. Kopsaftis Z, Carson-Chahhoud KV, Austin MA, Wood-Baker R. Oxygen therapy in the pre-hospital setting for acute exacerbations of chronic obstructive pulmonary disease. *Cochrane Database Syst Rev*. 2020;1(1):CD005534. doi:10.1002/14651858.CD005534.pub3
6. Berg KM, Bray JE, Djärv T, et al. Executive Summary: 2025 International Liaison Committee on Resuscitation Consensus on Science With Treatment Recommendations. *Circulation*. 2025;152(16_suppl_1):S2–S22.

Prep Kit continued

7. National Association of State EMS Officials. *National Model EMS Clinical Guidelines: Version 3.0.* https://nasemso.org/wp-content/uploads/National-Model-EMS-Clinical-Guidelines_2022.pdf. Updated March 2022. Accessed December 19, 2024.
8. Croup in children. Johns Hopkins Medicine website. https://www.hopkinsmedicine.org/health/conditions-and-diseases/croup#:~:text=A%20virus%20is%20the%20most,Parainfluenza%20virus. Accessed February 25, 2025.
9. Sutton AE, Guerra AM, Waseem M. Epiglottitis. *StatPearls*. National Library of Medicine website. https://www.ncbi.nlm.nih.gov/books/NBK430960/. Updated October 5, 2024. Accessed December 19, 2024.
10. Risk factors for pneumonia. Centers for Disease Control and Prevention website. https://www.cdc.gov/pneumonia/risk-factors/index.html#cdc_risk_factors_who-people-at-increased-risk. Published October 17, 2023. Accessed December 19, 2024.
11. Pertussis cases by year (1922–2022). Centers for Disease Control and Prevention website. https://www.cdc.gov/pertussis/php/surveillance/pertussis-cases-by-year.html. Published July 23, 2024. Accessed December 19, 2024.
12. Pertussis surveillance and trends. Centers for Disease Control and Prevention website. https://www.cdc.gov/pertussis/php/surveillance/index.html. Published January 13, 2025. Accessed February 25, 2025.
13. Types of influenza viruses. Centers for Disease Control and Prevention website. https://www.cdc.gov/flu/about/viruses-types.html. Published September 18, 2024. Accessed December 19, 2024.
14. Infection prevention and control. COVID protocols v2.0 website. https://covidprotocols.org/en/chapters/infection-prevention-and-control/. Accessed December 19, 2024.
15. Symptoms of COVID-19. Centers for Disease Control and Prevention website. https://www.cdc.gov/covid/signs-symptoms/index.html. Published June 25, 2024. Accessed December 19, 2024.
16. COVID-19 test basics. US Food and Drug Administration website. https://www.fda.gov/consumers/consumer-updates/covid-19-test-basics. Updated September 7, 2023. Accessed December 19, 2024.
17. Chronic obstructive pulmonary disease (COPD). World Health Organization website. https://www.who.int/news-room/fact-sheets/detail/chronic-obstructive-pulmonary-disease-(copd). Published November 6, 2024. Accessed December 19, 2024.
18. COPD. Centers for Disease Control and Prevention website. https://www.cdc.gov/cdi/indicator-definitions/chronic-obstructive-pulmonary-disease.html. Published June 3, 2024. Accessed December 19, 2024.
19. Asthma facts. Asthma and Allergy Foundation of America website. https://aafa.org/asthma/asthma-facts/. Updated September 2024. Accessed December 19, 2024.
20. Data and statistics on venous thromboembolism. Centers for Disease Control and Prevention website. https://www.cdc.gov/blood-clots/data-research/facts-stats/index.html. Published May 15, 2024. Accessed December 19, 2024.
21. Shin M, Bronstein AC, Glidden E, et al. Morbidity and mortality of unintentional carbon monoxide poisoning: United States 2005 to 2018. *Ann Emerg Med*. 2023;81(3):309–317.
22. Understanding changes in life expectancy. Cystic Fibrosis Foundation website. https://www.cff.org/managing-cf/understanding-changes-life-expectancy. Accessed February 25, 2025.

Additional Resources

Cramer N, Jabbour N, Tavarez MM, Taylor RS. Foreign body aspiration. *StatPearls*. National Library of Medicine website. https://www.ncbi.nlm.nih.gov/books/NBK531480/. Updated July 31, 2023. Accessed December 19, 2024.

Diphtheria symptoms and complications. Centers for Disease Control and Prevention website. http://www.cdc.gov/diphtheria/about/symptoms.html. Published February 12, 2024. Accessed December 19, 2024.

Diphtheria vaccination. Centers for Disease Control and Prevention website. https://www.cdc.gov/diphtheria/vaccines/. Published June 26, 2024. Accessed December 19, 2024.

King KC, Goldstein S. Congestive heart failure and pulmonary edema. *StatPearls*. National Library of Medicine website. https://www.ncbi.nlm.nih.gov/books/NBK554557/. Updated September 19, 2022. Accessed December 19, 2024.

Kukla P, McIntyre WF, Koracevic G, et al. Relation of atrial fibrillation and right-sided cardiac thrombus to outcomes in patients with acute pulmonary embolism. *Am J Cardiol*. 2015;115(6):825–830.

National Center for Immunization and Respiratory Diseases, Division of Viral Diseases. Respiratory syncytial virus infection (RSV): symptoms and care. Centers for Disease Control and Prevention website. http://www.cdc.gov/rsv/about/symptoms.html. Reviewed September 6, 2023. Accessed December 19, 2024.

Pneumonia in children. World Health Organization website. https://www.who.int/news-room/fact-sheets/detail/pneumonia. Updated November 11, 2022. Accessed December 19, 2024.

Chapter 17

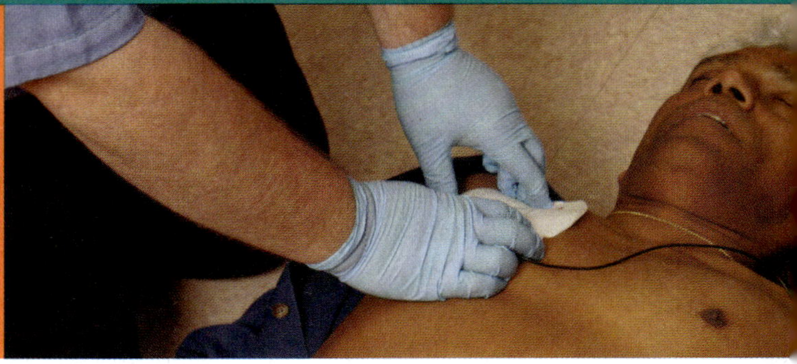

Cardiovascular Emergencies

NATIONAL EMS EDUCATION STANDARD COMPETENCIES

Pathophysiology

Applies knowledge of the pathophysiology of respiration and perfusion to patient assessment and management.

Medicine

Applies knowledge to provide basic emergency care and transportation based on assessment findings for an acutely ill patient.

Cardiovascular

- Acute coronary syndrome (pp 699–702)
- Hypertensive emergencies (pp 705–706)
- Aortic aneurysm/dissection (pp 705–706)
- Thromboembolism (pp 698–699)
- Heart failure (pp 702–705)

Assessment

Applies scene information and patient assessment findings (scene size-up, primary and secondary assessment, patient history, and reassessment) to guide emergency management.

Monitoring Devices

- Cardiac monitoring: 12-lead electrocardiogram acquisition and transmission (pp. 714–718)

KNOWLEDGE OBJECTIVES

1. Discuss the basic anatomy and physiology of the cardiovascular system. (pp 689–698)
2. Describe the anatomy, physiology, pathophysiology, assessment, and management of thromboembolism. (pp 698–699)
3. Describe the anatomy, physiology, pathophysiology, assessment, and management of angina pectoris. (pp 699–700)
4. Describe the anatomy, physiology, pathophysiology, assessment, and management of myocardial infarction. (pp 700–702)
5. Describe the anatomy, signs and symptoms, and management of hypertensive emergencies. (pp 705–706)
6. Describe the anatomy, physiology, pathophysiology, assessment, and management of aortic aneurysm/dissection. (p 705)
7. Explain the assessment for patients with cardiovascular problems. (pp 706–711)
8. Explain the relationship between airway management and the patient with cardiac compromise. (p 707)
9. Give the indications and contraindications for the use of aspirin and nitroglycerin. (pp 711–714)

10. Recognize that many patients will have had cardiac surgery and may have implanted pacemakers or defibrillators. (pp 718–722)
11. Define cardiac arrest. (p 722)
12. Explain the importance of prompt compressions and defibrillation for patients who experience sudden cardiac arrest outside a hospital. (p 723)

SKILLS OBJECTIVES

1. Perform the steps of assessment of a patient with chest pain or discomfort. (pp 706–711)
2. Demonstrate how to provide emergency medical care for a patient with chest pain or discomfort. (pp 711–714)
3. Demonstrate how to administer nitroglycerin. (p 713, Skill Drill 17-1)
4. Demonstrate how to attach a cardiac monitor to obtain an electrocardiogram. (pp 716–717, Skill Drill 17-2)

Introduction

Heart disease is the leading cause of death in the United States among both men and women, including individuals of most racial and ethnic groups.[1] In 2022, an estimated 702,880 people died from heart disease, which is approximately 1 in every 5 deaths. Fortunately, since about 1950, advances in technology have resulted in better medical care and thus improved survivability of cardiovascular disease; further, reductions in risk factors such as smoking, high blood pressure, and high cholesterol have led to declines in heart disease morbidity and mortality.[1,2]

It is important for EMS clinicians to understand that many deaths caused by cardiovascular disease occur because of problems that may have been avoided by people living more healthful lifestyles and by access to improved medical technology. The number of deaths can be reduced with better public awareness, early access to medical care, increased numbers of laypeople trained in cardiopulmonary resuscitation (CPR), increased use of evolving technology in dispatch and cardiac arrest response, public access to defibrillation devices, the recognition of the need for advanced life support (ALS) services, and use of cardiac specialty centers when they are available.

This chapter begins with a brief description of the heart and how it works. It then discusses the relationship between chest pain or discomfort and ischemic heart disease, hypertension, and aortic aneurisms. It explains how to recognize and treat acute myocardial infarction (classic heart attack) and its complications: sudden death, cardiogenic shock, and heart failure. The use of nitroglycerin and aspirin are described. See Chapter 14, *BLS Resuscitation*, for a focused discussion of automated external defibrillators (AEDs).

Anatomy and Physiology

The heart is a relatively simple organ with a simple job. It pumps blood to supply oxygen-enriched red blood cells to the tissues of the body. The heart is divided down the middle into two sides (left and right) by a wall called the septum. Each side of the heart has an **atrium**, or upper chamber, to receive incoming blood, and a **ventricle**, or lower chamber, to pump outgoing blood (**FIGURE 17-1**). Blood leaves each of the four chambers of the heart through a one-way valve. These valves keep the blood moving through the circulatory system in the proper direction. The **aorta**, the body's main artery, receives the blood ejected from the left ventricle and delivers it to all the other arteries so they can carry blood to the tissues of the body.

The right side of the heart receives oxygen-poor (deoxygenated) blood from the veins of the body (**FIGURE 17-2A**). Blood from the superior and inferior venae cavae enters the right atrium and passes through the tricuspid valve into the right ventricle. After contraction of the right ventricle, blood flows through the pulmonic valve and into the pulmonary artery, then travels through the pulmonary circulation in the lungs, where it is reoxygenated. As the blood reaches the lungs, it receives fresh oxygen from the alveoli and carbon dioxide waste is removed from the blood and moved into the alveoli. The blood then returns to the heart through the pulmonary veins. The left side of the heart receives oxygen-rich (oxygenated) blood from the lungs through the pulmonary veins (**FIGURE 17-2B**). Blood enters the left atrium and then passes through

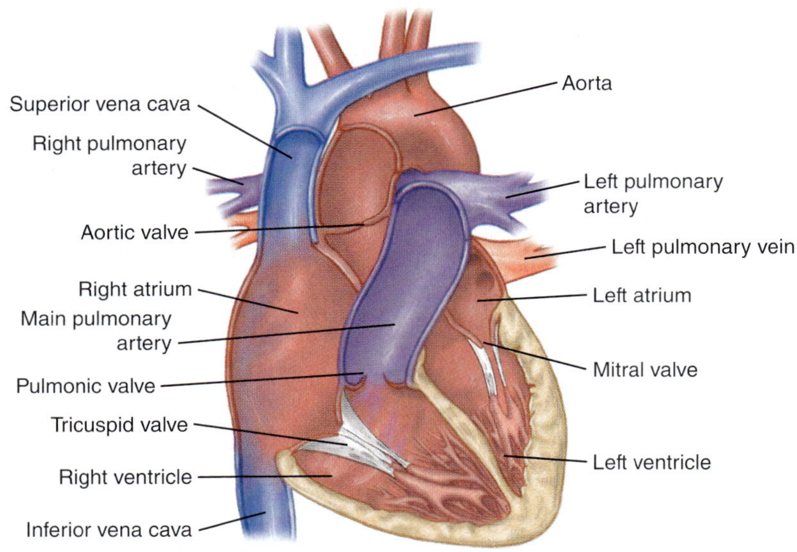

FIGURE 17-1 The heart is a four-chambered muscle that pumps blood to all parts of the body.

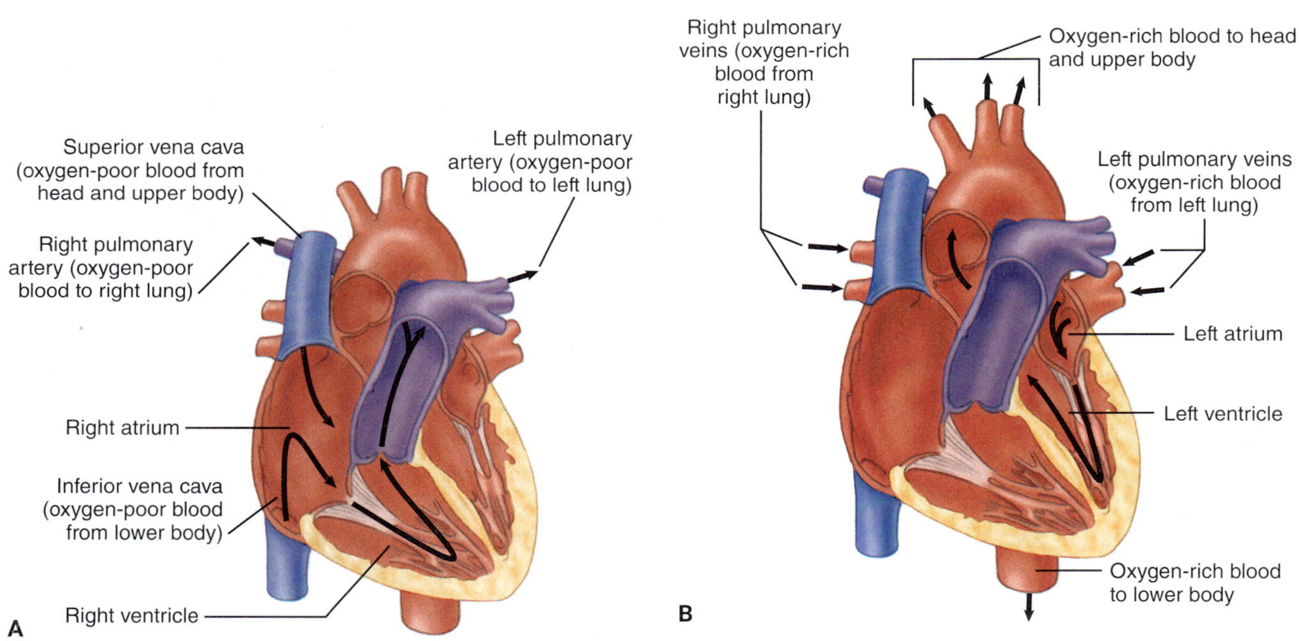

FIGURE 17-2 A. The right side of the heart receives oxygen-poor blood from the venous circulation. **B.** The left side of the heart receives oxygen-rich blood from the lungs through the pulmonary veins.

the mitral (bicuspid) valve, into the left ventricle, through the aortic valve, and into the aorta. The left ventricle is more muscular than the right ventricle because it must pump blood against more pressure into the aorta to supply all the other arteries of the body.

The heart contains more than muscle tissue. The heart's electrical conduction system controls heart rate and enables the atria and ventricles to work together (**FIGURE 17-3**). Normal electrical impulses begin in the sinus node, which is in the upper part of the right atrium and is also known as

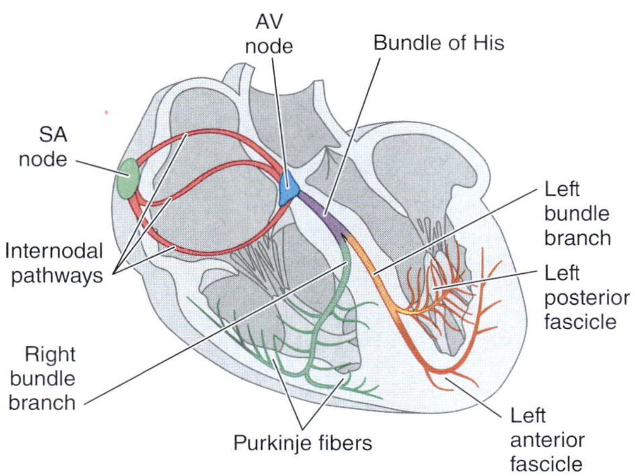

FIGURE 17-3 The electrical conduction system of the heart controls most aspects of heart rate and enables the four chambers to work together.

Abbreviations: AV = atrioventricular; SA = sinoatrial.

the sinoatrial (SA) node. The impulses travel across both atria, stimulating them to contract. Between the atria and the ventricles, the impulses cross a bridge of special electrical tissue called the atrioventricular (AV) node. Here, the signal is slowed for about one- to two-tenths of a second to allow blood time to pass from the atria to the ventricles. The impulses then exit the AV node and spread throughout both ventricles via the bundle of His, the right and left bundle branches, and the Purkinje fibers, ultimately causing the muscle cells of the ventricles to contract.

Cardiac muscle cells have a special characteristic called **automaticity** that is not found in any other type of muscle cells. Automaticity allows a cardiac muscle cell to contract spontaneously without a stimulus from a nerve source. Normal impulses in the heart start at the SA node. As long as impulses come from the SA node, the other myocardial cells will contract when the impulse reaches them. However, if no impulse arrives, the other myocardial cells are capable of creating their own impulses and stimulating a contraction of the heart, although at a generally slower rate.

The stimulus that originates in the SA node is controlled by impulses from the brain, which arrive by way of the **autonomic nervous system**. The autonomic nervous system is the part of the brain that controls the functions of the body that do not require conscious thought, such as the heartbeat, respirations, dilation and constriction of blood vessels, and digestion of food. The autonomic nervous system has two parts, the **sympathetic nervous system** and the **parasympathetic nervous system**. The sympathetic nervous system is also known as the fight-or-flight system and makes adjustments to the body to compensate for increased physical activity. The sympathetic nervous system speeds up the heart rate, increases respiratory rate and depth, dilates blood vessels in the muscles, and constricts blood vessels in the digestive system. The parasympathetic nervous system directly opposes the sympathetic nervous system. It slows the heart and respiratory rates, constricts blood vessels in the muscles, and dilates blood vessels in the digestive system. Normally, these two systems balance each other, but in times of stress, the sympathetic nervous system gains primary control, whereas in times of relaxation, the parasympathetic system takes control.

Circulation

To perform the function of pumping blood, the **myocardium**, or heart muscle, must have a continuous supply of oxygen and nutrients. During periods

YOU are the EMT

You and your partner are returning to your station after completing a call when you are dispatched to 1152 Blanco Road for a 60-year-old woman with chest pain. Dispatch advises you that the patient's son, who called 9-1-1, stated that she has a history of heart problems. You proceed to the scene, which is approximately 5 minutes away. The time is 0942 hours, traffic is light, the weather is clear, and the temperature is 80°F (27°C).

1. What is the function of the heart?
2. What does the heart require to function effectively?
3. What should you include in your primary assessment of a patient with cardiac problems?

of physical exertion or stress, the myocardium requires more oxygen. The heart must increase cardiac output to meet the increased metabolic requirements of the body. Cardiac output is increased by increasing the heart rate or **stroke volume**. In the normal heart, this increased oxygen demand of the myocardium itself is accomplished by increasing the amount of blood flowing (and therefore the amount of oxygen being delivered) to the myocardium by **dilation**, or widening, of the coronary arteries. The **coronary arteries** are the blood vessels that supply blood to the heart muscle (**FIGURE 17-4**). They begin at the first part of the aorta, just above the **aortic valve**. The right coronary artery supplies blood to the right atrium and right ventricle and, in most people, the bottom part, or inferior wall, of the left ventricle. The left coronary artery divides into two major branches just a short distance from the aorta: the left anterior descending artery and the circumflex artery. The left anterior descending artery supplies a large portion of blood to the left ventricle.

Two major arteries branching from the upper aorta supply blood to the head and arms (**FIGURE 17-5**). The right and left carotid arteries supply the head and brain with blood. The right

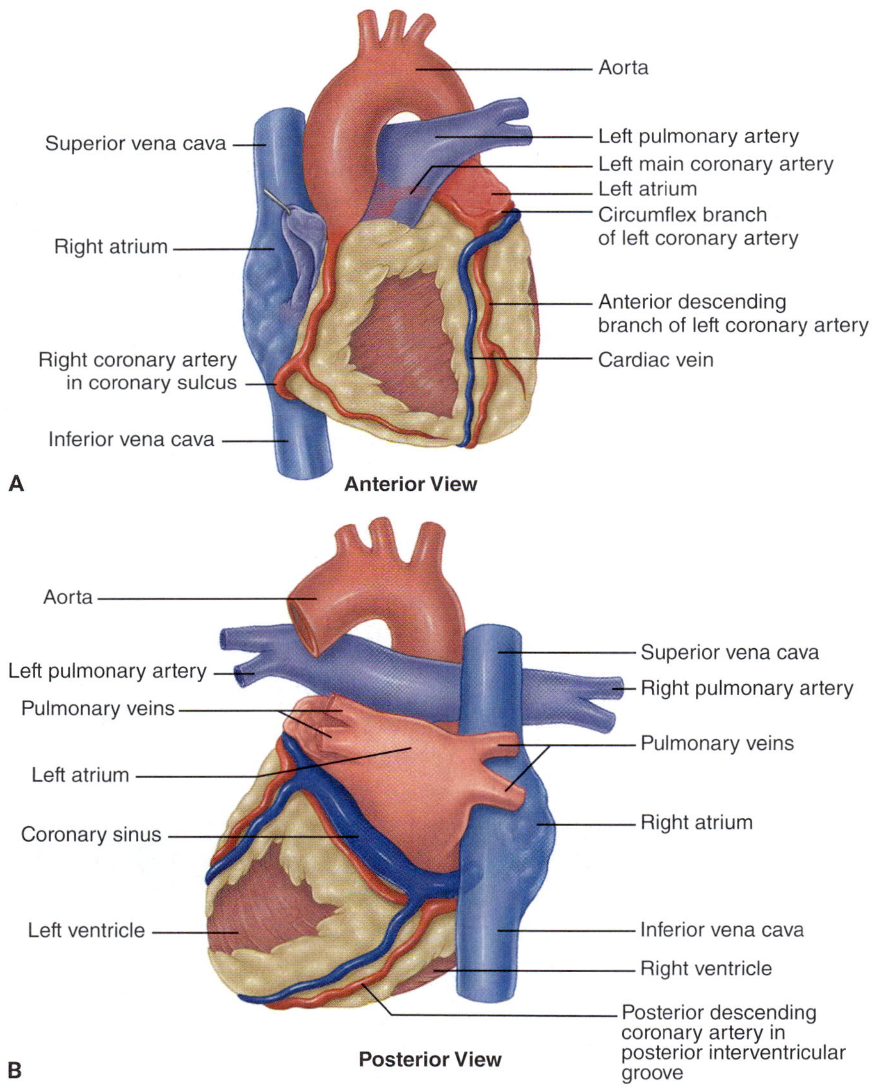

FIGURE 17-4 Blood flow to the heart. **A.** Coronary arteries (anterior view). **B.** Coronary arteries (posterior view).

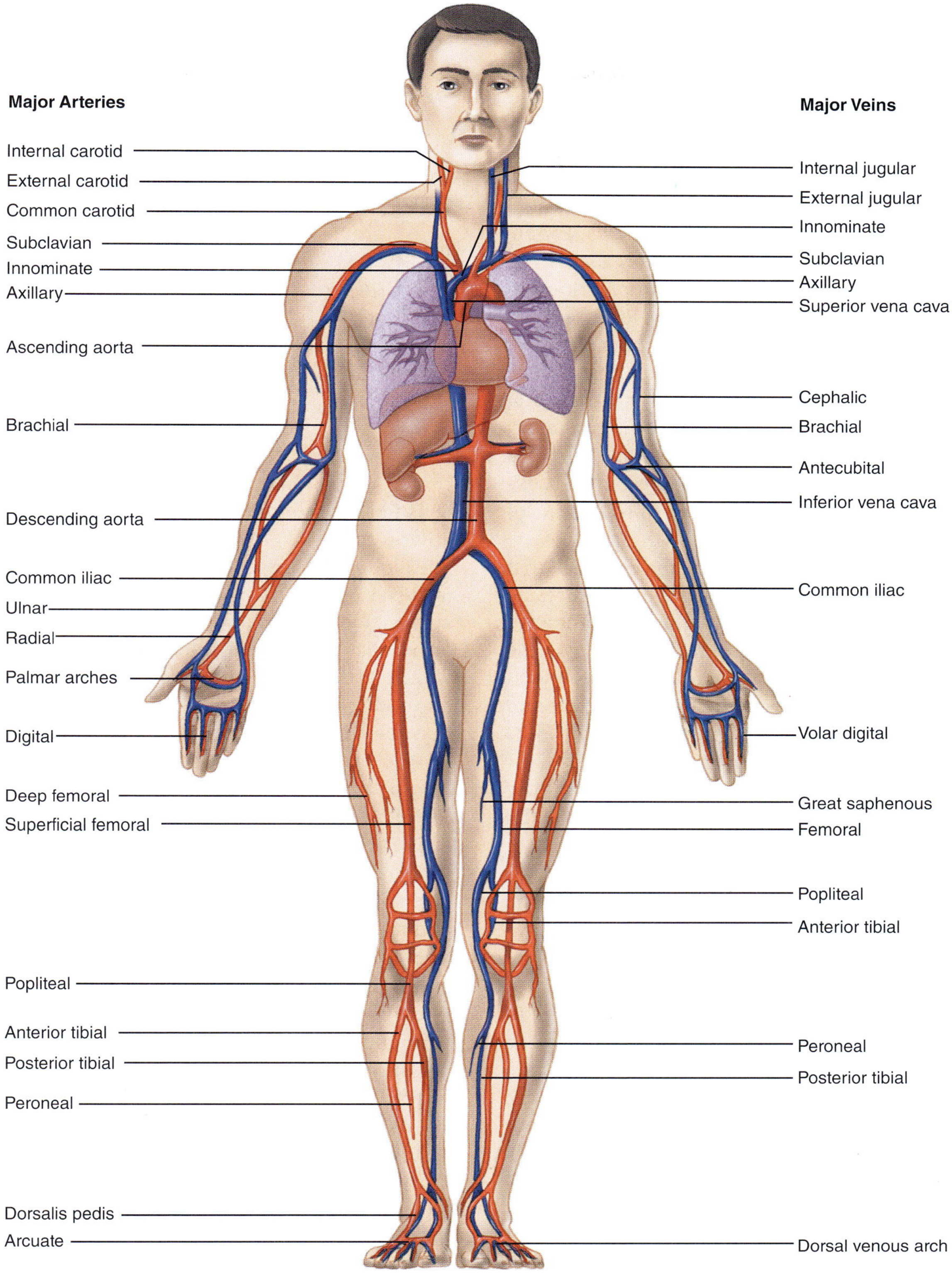

FIGURE 17-5 The major arteries of the body carry oxygen-rich blood to all parts of the body. The major veins of the body carry deoxygenated blood back to the heart.

and left subclavian arteries (under the clavicles) supply blood to the upper extremities. As the subclavian artery enters each arm, it becomes the brachial artery, the major vessel that supplies blood to each arm. Just below the elbow, the brachial artery divides into two major branches: the radial and ulnar arteries, supplying blood to the lower arms and hands.

At the level of the umbilicus, the descending aorta divides into two main branches called the right and left iliac arteries, which supply blood to the groin, pelvis, and legs. As the iliac arteries enter the legs through the groin, they become the right and left femoral arteries. At the level of the knee, the femoral artery divides into the **anterior** (front) and **posterior** (back) tibial arteries and the peroneal artery, supplying blood to the lower legs and feet.

After blood travels through the arteries, it enters smaller and smaller vessels called arterioles and eventually enters the capillaries. Capillaries are tiny blood vessels approximately one cell thick that connect arterioles to venules. Capillaries, which are found in all parts of the body, allow the exchange of nutrients and waste at the cellular level. As the blood passes through the capillaries, it gives up oxygen to the tissues and picks up carbon dioxide and other waste products to be removed from the body.

Venules are the smallest branches of veins. After traveling through the capillaries, oxygen-poor blood enters the system of veins, starting with the venules, on its way back to the heart. The veins become larger and larger and eventually form the two large venae cavae: the superior vena cava and the inferior vena cava. The **superior** (upper) vena cava carries blood from the head and arms back to the right atrium. The **inferior** (lower) vena cava carries blood from the abdomen, pelvis, and legs back to the right atrium. The superior and inferior venae cavae join at the right atrium of the heart, where blood is then returned to the pulmonary circulation for oxygenation.

Blood consists of fluid and several components (**FIGURE 17-6**). Red blood cells are the most numerous and give the blood its color: bright red when oxygenated and darker red when low on oxygen. Red blood cells carry oxygen to the body's tissues and help remove carbon dioxide. Larger white blood cells help to fight infection. Platelets, which help the blood to clot, are much smaller than either red or white blood cells. Plasma is the fluid in which the cells float. It is a mixture of water, salts, nutrients, and proteins.

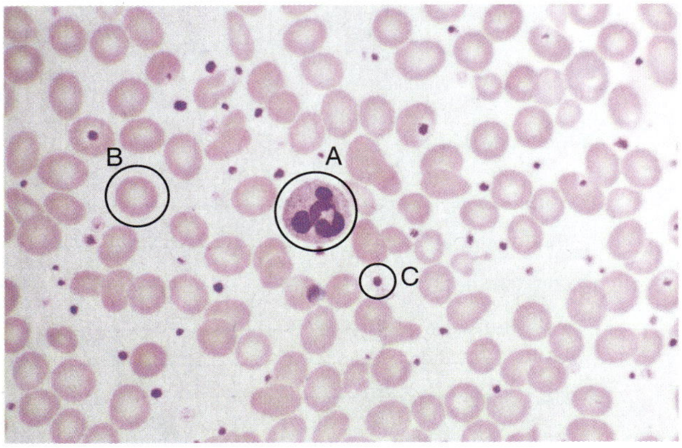

FIGURE 17-6 Blood consists of fluid and several components, including white blood cells (**A**), red blood cells (**B**), and platelets (**C**).

Blood pressure is the force of circulating blood against the walls of the arteries. Systolic blood pressure is the maximum pressure generated in the arms and legs during the contraction of the left ventricle, during the time period known as systole. As the left ventricle relaxes in the stage known as diastole, the arterial pressure falls. When the left ventricle relaxes, the aortic valve closes and blood flow between the left ventricle and the aorta stops. The diastolic blood pressure is the pressure exerted against the walls of the arteries while the left ventricle is at rest. Remember that the top number in a blood pressure reading is the systolic pressure, and the bottom number is the diastolic, or resting, pressure. The cardiac cycle consists of one systolic and one diastolic time period. The mean arterial pressure (MAP) measures the average blood pressure and is displayed when a noninvasive blood pressure is measured. The MAP is a good measure of perfusion.

As the blood passes through an artery during systole, a wave of blood generates a pulse. Pulses felt in the extremities, such as the radial and the posterior tibial, are called peripheral pulses, whereas pulses near the trunk of the body, such as the femoral and carotid pulses, are known as central pulses.

The rate of cardiac contractions can be increased or decreased by the autonomic nervous system. The heart also has the capability to increase or decrease the volume of blood it pumps with each

Words of Wisdom

EMTs should be skilled at finding multiple pulse points and should compare proximal and distal pulses bilaterally, when applicable, to determine any differences in quality or strength that could indicate the patient's condition is progressing to decompensated shock or that blood supply in an artery is interrupted by a clot or an aneurysm.

Common places to feel for a pulse include the following (**FIGURE 17-7**):

- The carotid pulse can be felt in the neck by placing two fingertips in the center of the throat on the trachea, and then sliding them toward you into the groove between the trachea and the neck muscle. Do not assess both carotid pulses at the same time, as this could greatly reduce blood flow to the brain.
- The femoral pulse can be felt in the groin at the crease dividing the lower abdomen from the leg.
- The brachial pulse can be felt on the anterior aspect of the elbow at the level of the crease. This is the pulse that you listen for when you obtain a blood pressure measurement. Pulsations also can be palpated on the medial side of the arm midway between the elbow and armpit.
- The radial pulse can be felt on the thumb side of the wrist, about one fingerbreadth above the wrist crease.
- The posterior tibial pulse can be felt on the inside of the ankle, just behind the medial malleolus. The medial malleolus is the bony bump at the bottom end of the tibia.
- The dorsalis pedis pulse can be felt at the top of the foot. To find the pulse, have the patient lift their great toe until you see the extensor tendon, then gently slide your fingers up the foot just lateral to the tendon toward the ankle until a pulsation is felt. Once you feel something that might be a pulse, use your fingertips to confirm that finding.

Practice feeling for these pulses on yourself and on friends and family members.

contraction based on the autonomic nervous system response. To obtain an accurate measure of the efficiency of the heart, the volume of blood pumped and the heart rate are used to calculate the cardiac output. The **cardiac output** is calculated by multiplying the heart rate by the volume of blood ejected with each contraction, or the stroke volume. This is the volume of blood that passes through the heart in 1 minute and is the best measure of the output of the heart. In the field, we have no way of directly measuring the volume of blood being pumped; therefore, we must rely on the heart rate and the strength of the pulse to estimate the cardiac output.

The constant flow of oxygenated blood to the tissues is known as **perfusion**. Good perfusion requires three primary components. The first is a well-functioning heart, or pump. The heart must beat at an appropriate rate and with adequate force because a rate that is too slow or too fast, or contractions that are not strong enough, can reduce the volume of blood circulated and, thus, reduce the cardiac output. When the heart beats too rapidly, there is not enough time between contractions for the heart to refill completely, and when the heart beats too slowly, the volume of blood circulated per minute decreases due to the slow pulse rate. The second component of good perfusion is an adequate volume of fluid, or blood. If there is blood loss through hemorrhage, the reduced volume will limit the amount of tissue that can be perfused. Third, the blood must be carried in a proper-size

Words of Wisdom

Cardiac output is an important predictor of the patient's condition. In the prehospital setting, your ability to estimate it and interpret its implications will depend on your understanding of the underlying principles.

$$\text{Cardiac output} = \text{Heart rate} \times \text{Stroke volume}$$

Cardiac output is the amount of blood pumped out of the left ventricle in 1 minute.

Heart rate is the number of times the heart contracts in 1 minute.

Stroke volume is the volume of blood pumped out by the left ventricle in one contraction.

Stroke volume is affected by preload, afterload, and contractility. Preload is related to the amount of blood returning to the right ventricle and therefore, ultimately, to the left ventricle. Afterload is the pressure that the left ventricle pumps against, and it is associated with systemic vascular resistance, which is a function of the constriction of the systemic blood vessels. As the blood vessels constrict, it becomes harder for the ventricle to push the blood into them. Contractility refers to how forcefully the myocardium contracts.

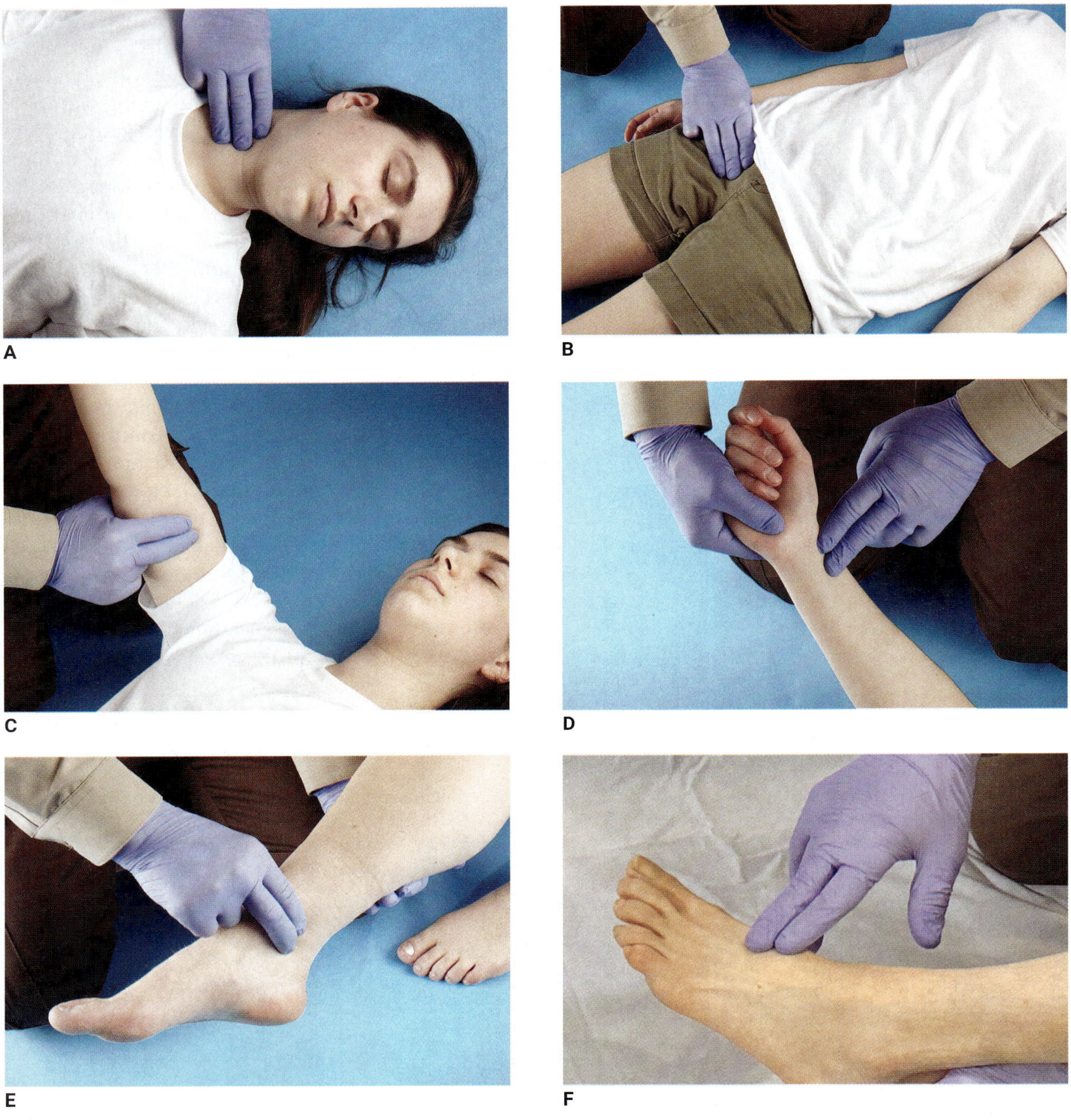

FIGURE 17-7 Common pulse points. **A.** The carotid pulse is felt in the neck. **B.** The femoral pulse is felt in the groin area. **C.** The brachial pulse is felt on the inside of the upper arm. **D.** The radial pulse is felt on the thumb side of the wrist. **E.** The posterior tibial pulse is felt on the inside of the ankle. **F.** The dorsalis pedis pulse is felt on the top of the foot.

container. This means that the blood vessels must be appropriately constricted to match the volume of blood available so that circulation can occur without problems. If the blood vessels dilate, thereby increasing the size of the container, and the volume of fluid remains the same, there will not be enough blood to fill the blood vessels and perfusion will be reduced. If there is a problem with the functioning of the heart, the functioning of the blood vessels, or the volume of blood, perfusion will fall, which will lead to cellular death and, eventually, death of the patient.

The Geriatric Circulatory System

Various changes occur in the cardiovascular system as a person ages, with the net effect of a decrease in the efficiency of the system. Specifically, the heart tends to hypertrophy (enlarge) with age, usually in response to the chronically increased afterload imposed by stiffening blood vessels. However, bigger is not better for the heart. Over time, cardiac output may decline, mostly as a result of a decreasing stroke volume, but the heart rate also has less ability to quickly respond to changes in preload.

Cardiac output is a measure of the workload of the heart. A younger person's body normally compensates for an increased demand on the cardiovascular system by increasing the heart rate, increasing the contraction of the heart, and constricting the blood vessels to nonvital organs. However, with aging, a person's ability to speed up contractions, increase contraction strength, and constrict or narrow blood vessels (vasoconstriction) is often decreased because of stiffer vessels. As stroke volume is reduced, cardiac output decreases. The heart may lose its ability to increase cardiac output to meet the needs of the body. Older patients may also be taking beta blockers for hypertension that reduces their ability to increase their heart rate.

With aging, the blood vessels themselves become stiff, which results in a higher systolic blood pressure. When this happens, the left ventricle, which pushes blood out into the body, becomes thicker and eventually loses elasticity, resulting in decreased filling of the left ventricle, which in turn causes decreased cardiac output.

Other anatomic changes include stiffening and degeneration of the heart valves, which may impede normal blood flow in and out of the heart. Aging also alters the heart's electrical conduction system. The sinoatrial node is the normal pacemaker of the heart, but by age 75 years, the number of the cells in the sinoatrial node will decrease by 90%. This event, combined with fibrosis and fatty deposits attaching to the electrical pathway, makes it likely that the patient will have some kind of heart rhythm disturbance, or dysrhythmia. This can cause a heart rate that is too fast, too slow, or too erratic to provide effective blood flow to the body.

Another condition that affects many older people is orthostatic hypotension (postural hypotension), which is a decrease in blood pressure caused by a change in position. When a person moves from a sitting to a standing position, gravity pulls blood down, away from the brain. This causes heart rate and contractility to increase. In younger people, the body's ability to compensate keeps them from passing out. Because older people become less sensitive to rapid changes in blood pressure, you may see a drop in the systolic blood pressure of 20 mm Hg when an older patient moves from a sitting position to a standing position. This may lead to syncope (fainting) that can result in injury. The body, therefore, is less able to adapt to rapid postural changes.

Patients with diabetes can experience reduced circulation to the hands and feet, which makes peripheral pulses harder to detect. It also puts the hands and feet at particular risk for infection and ulceration.

Other conditions to which older adults are susceptible, including atherosclerosis and aneurysm, are discussed later in this chapter.

The Pediatric Circulatory System

The pulse ranges for younger children are higher than those of adults. From birth to 3 months, a typical range is 85 to 205 beats/min; from 3 months to 2 years, it is 100 to 190 beats/min; and from 2 to 10 years, it is 60 to 140 beats/min. By age 10 years, the pulse rate is similar to an adult's: 60 to 100 beats/min. It is important to know the normal pulse ranges when evaluating children. An infant's heart can beat extremely fast if the body needs to compensate for injury or illness. This increased rate is the body's primary method to compensate for decreased perfusion. A slow heart rate in a young child is commonly a critical finding and may need to be managed with CPR if a trial of positive-pressure ventilation with a bag-mask device does not increase the rate. A common cause of a slow heart rate (bradycardia) in children in hypoxia.

Children are able to compensate for decreased perfusion by constricting the vessels in the skin. Constriction of the blood vessels can be so profound that blood flow to the extremities can be diminished. Signs of vasoconstriction include pallor (early sign), weak distal (eg, radial or pedal) pulses in the extremities, delayed capillary refill time, and cool hands or feet.

Pathophysiology

Chest pain or discomfort that is related to the heart usually stems from a condition called **ischemia**, which is decreased blood flow, in this case, to the myocardium. A partial or complete blockage of blood flow through the coronary arteries can cause a portion of the myocardium to be deprived of enough oxygen and nutrients. The tissue soon begins to starve and, if blood flow is not restored, eventually dies. Ischemic heart disease, then, is disease involving a decrease in blood flow to one or more portions of the heart muscle.

Atherosclerosis

Most often, the low blood flow to heart tissue is caused by coronary artery atherosclerosis. **Atherosclerosis** is a disorder in which calcium and a fatty material called cholesterol build up and form a plaque inside the walls of blood vessels, obstructing flow and interfering with their ability to dilate or contract (**FIGURE 17-8**). Eventually, atherosclerosis can even cause complete **occlusion**, or blockage, of a coronary artery. Atherosclerosis usually involves other arteries of the body as well.

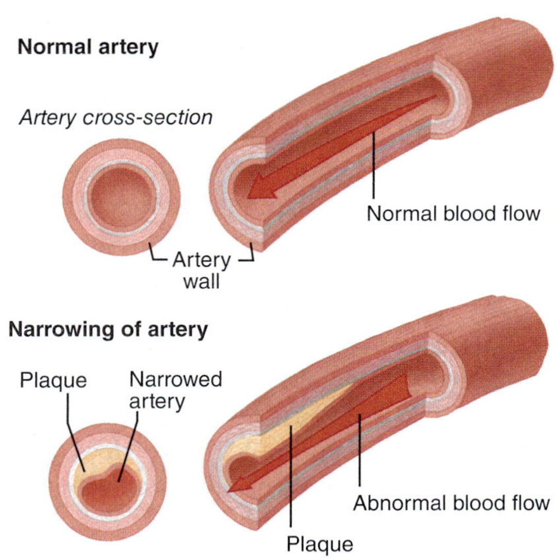

FIGURE 17-8 In atherosclerosis, calcium and cholesterol build up inside the walls of the coronary blood vessels, causing an obstruction in blood flow to the heart.

The problem begins when the first trace of cholesterol is deposited on the inside of an artery. This may happen as early as the teenage years. As a person ages, more of this fatty material is deposited; the **lumen**, or the inside diameter of the artery, narrows. As the cholesterol deposits grow, calcium deposits can form as well. The inner wall of the artery, which is normally smooth and elastic, becomes rough and brittle with these atherosclerotic plaques. Damage to the coronary arteries may become so extensive that they cannot accommodate increased blood flow during times of maximum stress.

A brittle plaque will sometimes develop a crack, exposing the inside of the atherosclerotic wall. Acting like a torn blood vessel, the ragged edge of the crack activates the blood-clotting system, just as when an injury has caused bleeding. In this situation, however, the resulting blood clot will partially or completely block the lumen of the artery. If it does not occlude the artery at that location, the blood clot may break loose and begin floating in the blood, becoming what is known as a thromboembolism. A **thromboembolism** is a blood clot that is floating through blood vessels until it reaches an area too narrow for it to pass, causing it to stop and block the blood flow at that point. Tissues downstream from the blood clot will experience a lack of oxygen (hypoxia). If blood flow is restored in a short time, the hypoxic tissues will recover. However, if too much time goes by before blood flow returns, the hypoxic tissues will die. If a blockage occurs in a coronary artery, the condition results in an **acute myocardial infarction (AMI)**, a heart attack (**FIGURE 17-9**). **Infarction** means the death of tissue. The same sequence may also cause the death of cells in other organs, such as the brain. The death of heart muscle decreases the heart's ability to pump and can also cause it to completely stop pumping (**cardiac arrest**).

In the United States, coronary artery disease is the number one cause of death for men and women. The incidence of heart disease is highest among individuals 45 years and older, but it can strike even in a person's teens.[2] You must be alert to the possibility that, although less likely, a 26-year-old with chest pain could be having an AMI, especially if the individual has increased risk factors. The major controllable risk factors are cigarette smoking, high blood

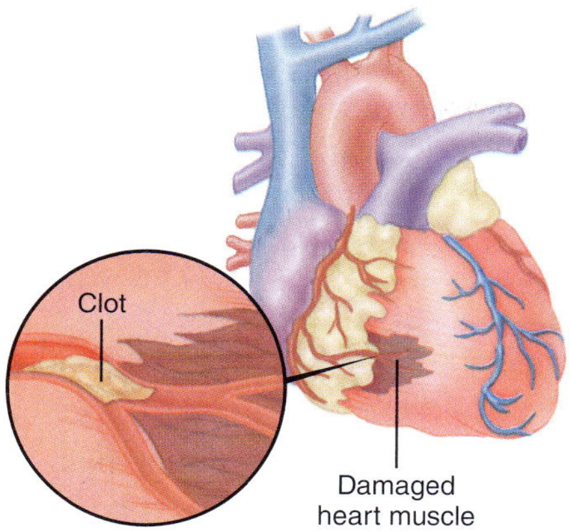

FIGURE 17-9 An acute myocardial infarction (heart attack) occurs when a blood clot prevents blood flow to an area of the heart muscle. If left untreated, death of myocardium can result.

pressure, elevated cholesterol level, elevated blood glucose level (diabetes), lack of exercise, and obesity. The major risk factors that cannot be controlled are older age, family history of atherosclerotic coronary artery disease, race, ethnicity, and male sex. Other factors that play a role in heart disease are stress, excessive alcohol use, and poor diet.

Acute Coronary Syndrome

Many patients who call for EMS assistance because of chest pain have **acute coronary syndrome (ACS)**, which is a term used to describe a range of symptoms and conditions caused by myocardial ischemia. As discussed earlier, myocardial ischemia is a decrease in blood flow to the heart, which leads to chest pain through reduced supply of oxygen and nutrients to the tissues of the heart. This can be a temporary situation known as angina pectoris, or a more serious condition, an AMI. Because the signs and symptoms of these two conditions are very similar, they are treated the same under the designation of ACS. To understand them better, we will examine each one separately.

Angina Pectoris

Chest pain does not always mean that a person is having an AMI. When, for a brief time, heart tissues are not getting enough oxygen, the pain is called **angina pectoris**, or angina. Although angina can result from a spasm of an artery, it is most often a symptom of atherosclerotic coronary artery disease. Angina occurs when the heart's need for oxygen exceeds its supply, usually during periods of physical or emotional stress when the heart is working hard. When the increased oxygen demand goes away (eg, the person stops exercising), the pain typically goes away.

Anginal pain is commonly described as crushing, squeezing, or "like somebody standing on my chest." It is usually felt in the midportion of the chest, under the sternum. However, it can radiate to the jaw, the arms (frequently the left arm), the midportion of the back, or the epigastrium (the upper-middle region of the abdomen). The pain, which is typically triggered by physical exertion or emotional stress, usually gets more intense, typically lasting only a few minutes.[3] It may be associated with shortness of breath, nausea, or sweating. It usually disappears promptly with rest and the administration of nitroglycerin, both of which decrease the need for or increase the supply of oxygen to the heart. Although angina pectoris is frightening, it does not mean that heart cells are dying, nor does it usually lead to death or permanent heart damage. It is, however, a warning that you and the patient should take seriously. With angina, the electrical system can be compromised because the oxygen supply to the heart is diminished, and the person is at risk for problems with cardiac rhythm.

Angina can be further differentiated into stable and unstable angina. Unstable angina is characterized by pain or discomfort in the chest of coronary origin that occurs in the absence of a significant increase in myocardial oxygen demand. If untreated, it is associated with a very high risk of spontaneous AMI. Stable angina is characterized by pain in the chest of coronary origin that occurs in response to exercise or some activity that increases the demand on the heart muscle beyond the heart's capacity to increase its own blood flow. Stable angina is often predictable; pain typically resolves by stopping physical exertion or taking nitroglycerin. EMS often becomes involved when stable angina becomes unstable, such as when a patient whose pain is normally relieved by sitting down and taking one nitroglycerin tablet has taken three tablets with no relief. Keep in mind that it can be difficult, even for physicians in hospitals, to distinguish between the pain of angina and the pain of an AMI. Patients experiencing chest pain or discomfort, therefore, should always be treated initially as if they are having an AMI.

> **Words of Wisdom**
>
> According to the American Heart Association (AHA), "Chest pain means more than pain in the chest."[3] Symptoms that can be considered equivalent to chest pain include pressure, tightness, or discomfort in the chest, shoulders, arms, neck, back, upper abdomen, and jaw, as well as dyspnea and fatigue. These symptoms are as important as chest pain when considering the possibility of ACS.

Acute Myocardial Infarction

The pain of an AMI signals the actual death of cells in the area of the heart muscle where blood flow is obstructed. Once dead, the cells cannot be revived. Instead, they will eventually turn to scar tissue and become a burden to the beating heart. Therefore, fast action is critical in treating an AMI. The sooner the arterial blockage can be cleared, the fewer the cells that may die. About 30 minutes after blood flow is cut off, some heart muscle cells begin to die. After approximately 2 hours, as many as one-half of the cells in the area can be dead; in most cases, after 4 to 6 hours, more than 90% will be dead. In many cases, however, opening the coronary artery with clot-busting (thrombolytic) medications or angioplasty (mechanical clearing of the artery) can prevent permanent damage to the heart muscle if done within the first few hours after the onset of symptoms. Therefore, immediate prehospital treatment and transport to the emergency department (ED) are essential.

An AMI is more likely to occur in the larger, thick-walled left ventricle, which needs more blood and oxygen than the right ventricle.

Signs and Symptoms of AMI

A patient with an AMI may show any of the following signs and symptoms:

- Sudden onset of weakness, nausea, and sweating without an obvious cause
- Chest pain, discomfort, or pressure that is often crushing or squeezing and that does not change with each breath
- Pain, discomfort, or pressure in the lower jaw, arms, back, abdomen, or neck
- Irregular heartbeat and **syncope** (fainting)
- Shortness of breath, or dyspnea
- Nausea/vomiting
- Pink, frothy sputum (indicating possible pulmonary edema)
- Sudden death

The Pain of AMI

The pain of an AMI differs from the pain of angina in three ways:

- It may or may not be caused by exertion but can occur at any time, sometimes when a person is sitting quietly or even sleeping.
- It does not resolve in a few minutes; rather, it can last between 30 minutes and several hours.
- It may or may not be relieved by rest or nitroglycerin.

Not all patients who are having an AMI experience pain or recognize it when it occurs. Approximately one-third of patients never seek medical attention. This can be attributed, in part, to the fact that people are afraid of dying and do not want to face the possibility that their symptoms may be serious (cardiac denial). While chest pain is the most common finding in acute myocardial infarction, some patients, particularly people older than 75 years, women, and people with diabetes, may not experience any pain during an AMI but may have other signs or symptoms associated with ischemia. Complaints of stabbing or sharp pain or discomfort in the throat or abdomen may be seen more often in these groups, as well as other findings such as nausea, vomiting, light-headedness, confusion, and dizziness or syncope.[3] Others may feel only mild discomfort and call it indigestion. AMI without the classic chest pain is often referred to as a silent myocardial infarction.

EMTs should be mindful that heart disease is the number one killer of women in the United States, and although chest pain is the most common symptom, it is important to recognize that palpitations, jaw and neck pain, back pain, nausea, fatigue, and dyspnea are more common in women than in men. Therefore, EMTs should consider AMI, especially in women 65 years and older, even when the classic symptom of chest pain is not present.

When you are called to a scene where the chief complaint is chest pain, complete a thorough assessment, no matter what the patient says. Patients with cardiac risk factors should also be carefully assessed if they have any of the associated symptoms, even if no chest pain is present. Any complaint of chest discomfort is a serious matter. The best thing you can do is assume the worst.

Street Smarts

Patients who are Black or Hispanic and patients who are covered by Medicaid or are uninsured are less likely to be treated appropriately when presenting with chest pain.[3] The EMT should complete the same thorough assessment for all patients presenting with chest pain.

Street Smarts

If a patient has signs of ACS, be sure the AED is close by. That way, if it is needed, the delay to the first shock will be minimized.

Physical Findings of AMI and Cardiac Compromise

The physical findings of AMI vary, depending on the extent and severity of heart muscle damage. The following are common:

- **General appearance.** The patient often appears frightened. There may be nausea, vomiting, and a cold sweat. The skin is often pale or ashen gray because of poor cardiac output and the loss of perfusion, or blood flow through the tissue. Occasionally, the skin, nailbeds, or mucous membranes will have a blue tint, called cyanosis; this is the result of poor oxygenation of the circulating blood.
- **Pulse.** Generally, the pulse rate increases as a normal response to pain, stress, fear, or actual injury to the myocardium. Because dysrhythmias are common in an AMI, you may feel an irregularity or even a slowing of the pulse. The pulse may also be dependent on the area of the heart that has been affected by the AMI. Damage to the inferior area of the heart often presents with bradycardia.
- **Blood pressure.** Blood pressure may decrease as a result of diminished cardiac output and diminished capability of the left ventricle to pump. However, most patients with an AMI will have a normal or possibly even elevated blood pressure.
- **Respiration.** The respiratory rate is usually normal unless the patient has heart failure. In that case, respirations may become rapid and labored with a higher likelihood of cyanosis and possibly frothy sputum. A complaint of difficulty breathing is common with cardiac compromise, so even if the rate seems normal, look at the work of breathing, and treat the patient as if respiratory compromise were present.
- **Mental status.** Patients with AMIs often experience fear or anxiety and sometimes experience an almost overwhelming feeling of impending doom. If a patient tells you, "I feel like I'm going to die," pay attention. Older patients may exhibit signs of confusion during AMI.

Words of Wisdom

Documenting exactly how a patient describes chest discomfort, in the patient's own words, is a valuable source of information for hospital staff. Remember OPQRST (Onset, Provocation/Palliation, Quality, Radiation, Severity, Time of onset).

Consequences of AMI

An AMI can have three serious consequences:

- Sudden death
- Cardiogenic shock
- Heart failure

Sudden Death

Sudden death is usually the result of cardiac arrest, in which the heart fails to generate effective blood flow. Although you cannot feel a pulse in someone experiencing cardiac arrest, the heart may still be twitching, though erratically. The heart is using up energy without pumping any blood. Such an abnormality of heart rhythm is a ventricular **dysrhythmia**, known as ventricular fibrillation.

A variety of other lethal and nonlethal dysrhythmias may follow an AMI, usually within the first hour. In most cases, premature ventricular contractions, or extra beats in the damaged ventricle, occur. Premature ventricular contractions by themselves may be harmless and are common among healthy people, as well as sick people. Other dysrhythmias include the following:

- **Tachycardia**. Rapid beating of the heart, 100 beats/min or more.
- **Bradycardia**. Unusually slow beating of the heart, 60 beats/min or less.
- **Ventricular tachycardia (VT)**. Rapid heart rhythm, usually at a rate of 150 to 200 beats/min. The electrical activity starts in the ventricle instead of the atrium. This rhythm usually does not allow adequate time between beats for the left ventricle to fill with blood. Therefore, the heart pumps less volume and the patient's blood pressure may fall. The patient may also feel weak or light-headed, or may even become unresponsive or the pulse may be lost altogether. In some cases, existing chest pain may worsen or chest pain that was not there before onset of the dysrhythmia may develop. Most cases of VT will be sustained but may deteriorate into ventricular fibrillation.
- **Ventricular fibrillation (VF)**. Disorganized, ineffective quivering of the ventricles. No blood is pumped through the body, and the patient becomes unconscious within seconds. The only way to convert this dysrhythmia is to defibrillate the heart. To **defibrillate** means to shock the heart with a specialized electric current in an attempt to stop the chaotic, disorganized contraction of the myocardial cells and allow them to start again in a synchronized manner to restore a normal rhythmic beat. Defibrillation is most likely to be lifesaving if delivered within the first few minutes of sudden death. The importance of prompt defibrillation cannot be overstated, with studies showing the highest rates of out-of-hospital cardiac arrest survival in patients who received defibrillation by lay responders using an AED before EMS could arrive on scene.[4] If a defibrillator is not immediately available, CPR must be initiated until the defibrillator arrives.

If uncorrected, unstable VT or VF will eventually lead to **asystole**, the absence of all heart electrical activity. Without CPR, asystole may occur within minutes. Asystole usually reflects a long period of ischemia, and almost all patients you find in asystole will die.

Cardiogenic Shock

Heart failure involving impairment of the left ventricle can result in the backup of blood into the pulmonary vessels. This backup in turn forces fluid out of the capillary beds that surround the alveoli and causes fluid accumulation in the lungs, a condition known as pulmonary edema. Pulmonary edema, which causes severe dyspnea, crackles, and hypoxia, can greatly compromise the delivery of oxygen to the body's tissues. When the reduced cardiac output caused by impairment of the left ventricle is very severe, blood pressure can drop and tissue ischemia can occur rapidly throughout the body (**TABLE 17-1**).

The discussion of shock in this chapter is limited to cardiac problems; however, many other medical problems and injuries may cause shock. See Chapter 13, *Shock*, for a more detailed discussion.

When a person is experiencing shock, the body tissues do not get enough oxygen, causing body organs to malfunction. In **cardiogenic shock**, often caused by an AMI, the problem is that the heart lacks enough power to force the proper volume of blood through the circulatory system. Cardiogenic shock is more commonly found after an AMI that affects the anterior wall of the left ventricle of the heart because this ventricle provides circulation to most of the body. Cardiogenic shock can develop immediately or sometime after an AMI. The various signs and symptoms of cardiogenic shock are produced by the improper functioning of the body's organs. The challenge for you is to recognize shock in its early stages, when treatment is much more likely to be successful.

Heart Failure

Heart failure occurs when the ventricular myocardium is so profoundly damaged that it can no longer keep up with the return flow of blood from the atria. **Heart failure** can occur at any time after a myocardial infarction when heart muscle is damaged or

TABLE 17-1 Cardiogenic Shock and Heart Failure Facts

Cardiogenic Shock	Heart Failure and Pulmonary Edema
Signs and Symptoms • Patient becomes anxious or restless as the brain becomes relatively starved for oxygen. • Patient reports shortness of breath associated with other signs of shock. • Skin becomes pale, cool, and clammy as blood is shunted to vital organs. • Heart rate increases to compensate for shock, often >120 beats/min. • As the shock progresses, the pulses may become irregular and weak. • Later, the systolic blood pressure falls to <90 mm Hg, a late finding that indicates decompensated shock. • Do not assume that shock is not present just because the blood pressure is normal (compensated shock). • MAP decreases	***Signs and Symptoms*** • Patient may have a history of heart failure. • Shortness of breath is the primary symptom. • Chest pain may or may not be present. • Patient may have distended neck veins that do not collapse even when sitting. • The patient may have swollen ankles from dependent edema (backup of fluid). • The patient generally will have high blood pressure, a rapid heart rate, and rapid respirations as compensation for the shortness of breath caused by fluid accumulation in the alveoli. • The patient will usually be using accessory breathing muscles of the neck and ribs, reflecting the additional hard work of breathing. • Skin is usually pale or cyanotic and sweaty. • The fluid surrounding small airways may produce crackles, best heard on either side of the patient's chest, about midway down the back. In pulmonary edema, crackles can be heard even at the top of the lung.
Treatment of Cardiogenic Shock Treat the patient with signs and symptoms of cardiogenic shock urgently. Call for ALS backup. **1.** Some patients will be more comfortable in a semi-Fowler position (head and knees slightly elevated); however, patients with low blood pressure may not tolerate a semi-upright position and may be more comfortable in a supine position. **2.** Administer oxygen at a rate to keep the oxygen saturation between 94% and 98%. **3.** Assist ventilations as necessary; if a PEEP valve is available to use with the bag-mask device, do so. **4.** Cover the patient with sheets or blankets as necessary to preserve body heat. Cover the top of the patient's head in very cold weather, as this is where much heat is lost. **5.** Provide prompt transport to the ED.	***Treatment of Pulmonary Edema*** Treat a patient with heart failure and pulmonary edema urgently. Call for ALS backup. **1.** Take the vital signs, and give oxygen by CPAP to help move some of the fluid out of the lungs and improve oxygenation. If CPAP is not available or not tolerated by the patient, you may give oxygen by mask or cannula to keep the oxygen saturation between 94% and 98%. **2.** Allow the patient to remain sitting in an upright position with the legs down. **3.** Be reassuring; many patients with heart failure are quite anxious because they feel as if they cannot breathe. **4.** Gather the patient's medications and take them along with you to the hospital. **5.** Nitroglycerin may be of value in reducing pulmonary edema if the patient's systolic blood pressure is more than 100 mm Hg. If medical direction or standing orders advise you to do so, administer nitroglycerin sublingually.

Abbreviations: ALS, advanced life support; CPAP, continuous positive airway pressure; ED, emergency department; PEEP, positive end-expiratory pressure.

dies, in the setting of heart valve damage, or as a consequence of long-standing high blood pressure. Any condition that weakens the pumping strength of the heart may cause heart failure, and this often happens after an AMI. Patient risk factors for heart failure include hypertension, AMI, and a history of coronary artery disease and/or atrial fibrillation, a condition in which the atria no longer contract, but instead quiver.

Just as the pumping function of the left ventricle can be damaged by coronary artery disease, it can also be damaged by diseased heart valves or chronic hypertension. In any of these cases, when the muscle can no longer contract effectively, the heart tries other ways to maintain an adequate cardiac output. Two specific changes in heart function occur: The heart rate increases, and the left ventricle enlarges to increase the amount of blood pumped each minute.

When these adaptations can no longer make up for the decreased heart function, heart failure eventually develops. With left-side heart failure, the lungs become congested with fluid because the left side of the heart fails to pump the blood effectively, which is why this condition is often referred to as *congestive* heart failure. Blood tends to back up in the pulmonary veins, increasing the pressure in the capillaries of the lungs. When the pressure in the capillaries rapidly exceeds a certain level, fluid (mostly water) passes through the walls of the capillary vessels and into the alveoli. This condition is called pulmonary edema. It may occur suddenly, as in an AMI, or slowly over months, as in chronic left-side heart failure.

With right-side heart failure, blood backs up in the venae cavae and fluid collects in the body, often resulting in edema in the lower extremities (swelling in the feet and legs) or distention of the veins in the neck. The collection of fluid in the part of the body that is closest to the ground is called **dependent edema**. The swelling causes relatively few symptoms other than discomfort. However, chronic dependent edema may indicate underlying heart disease even in the absence of pain or other symptoms. Because the right side of the heart supplies the preload for the left side of the heart, right-side heart failure can result in an inadequate supply of blood to the left ventricle, resulting in a drop in the systemic blood pressure. It is important to realize that some patients may present with signs of both left- and right-side heart failure because left-side failure often leads to right-side failure.

Signs and symptoms of heart failure include difficulty breathing with exertion because the heart cannot keep up with the body's need for oxygen. Patients may also report a sudden attack of respiratory distress that wakes them at night when they are in a reclining position. This is caused by fluid accumulation in the lungs. Patients also report coughing, feeling suffocated, cold sweats, and tachycardia. In your primary assessment, you might find the patient has cool, diaphoretic, cyanotic skin, and you

YOU are the EMT

You arrive at the scene and are escorted by the patient's son to her bedroom. She is sitting up in bed with her fist clutched against her chest. She is conscious and alert, but is notably anxious. Her skin is pale and diaphoretic. Your partner opens the jump kit as you assess the patient.

Recording Time: 0 Minutes	
Appearance	Anxious, pale (compared with baseline skin color), and diaphoretic
Level of consciousness	Conscious and alert
Airway	Open; clear of secretions and foreign bodies
Breathing	Increased respiratory rate; adequate depth
Circulation	Radial pulse rapid and irregular; skin pale and diaphoretic

After confirming that she has not taken any medication and that she is not allergic to any medications, you give the patient four 81-mg aspirin tablets to chew and swallow according to your protocols. As you continue your assessment and further inquire about her medical history, your partner applies the pulse oximeter, which shows that the patient's oxygen saturation is 89%. Based on this, he applies oxygen via nasal cannula at 4 L/min and prepares to take her vital signs. She tells you that she had a heart attack 3 years ago, has high blood pressure, and takes enalapril (Vasotec), nitroglycerin, and one aspirin per day.

4. Why is aspirin given to patients with an acute cardiac event?

5. What type of medication is nitroglycerin? How may it help relieve chest pain, pressure, or discomfort?

6. When is nitroglycerin indicated for a patient? What is the typical dose?

will hear adventitious breath sounds such as crackles or wheezing. The patient's pulse will be tachycardic. The patient may have hypertension early, followed by deterioration to hypotension as a late finding. Sometimes, in patients with an acute onset of heart failure, acute, severe pulmonary edema will develop, in which the patient has pink, frothy sputum and severe dyspnea.

Once heart failure develops, it can be treated but not cured. Regular use of medications may alleviate the symptoms. However, patients with heart failure often become ill again and are occasionally hospitalized. Approximately one-half will die within 5 years of the onset of symptoms.[5]

Hypertensive Emergencies

Hypertension is defined as any systolic blood pressure consistently at or greater than 130 mm Hg or a diastolic blood pressure greater than 80 mm Hg. Another cardiac-related condition is a hypertensive emergency. A **hypertensive emergency** is defined as a systolic pressure greater than 180 mm Hg and/or diastolic pressure higher than 120 mm Hg in the presence of impending or progressive organ damage. Because patients do not feel their blood pressure rising, the signs and symptoms of hypertensive emergency are related to the effects of the hypertension. Some patients with chronic hypertension may not experience signs or symptoms until their systolic pressure is significantly higher than this value. One of the most common signs is a sudden severe headache. If described as "the worst headache I have ever felt," this may also be a sign of cerebral hemorrhage. Other signs and symptoms include strong bounding pulse, ringing in the ears, nausea and vomiting, dizziness, warm skin (dry or moist), nosebleed, altered mental status, and even the sudden development of pulmonary edema. Untreated hypertensive emergencies can lead to heart failure, a stroke, or a dissecting aortic aneurysm.

Words of Wisdom

The definitions and treatment for hypertensive emergencies during pregnancy and immediately after birth vary from those discussed here. See Chapter 34, *Obstetrics and Neonatal Care*, for a discussion of conditions related to pregnancy and hypertension.

If you suspect your patient is experiencing a hypertensive emergency, attempt to make the individual comfortable and monitor the blood pressure regularly. Position the patient with the head elevated, and transport rapidly to the ED. Depending on the distance and time involved in transport, you should consider ALS assistance for the patient. Paramedics may be able to administer medications to lower the blood pressure to a safer level. If ALS personnel can be on the scene quickly, contact them early and allow them to transport the patient from the scene. If the transport distance is long, consider asking for an ALS unit to meet you along the way and take over patient care and transport from that point. Remember that getting the patient with a hypertensive emergency to the hospital as quickly and safely as possible is the best prehospital treatment you can provide.

An **aortic aneurysm** is an abnormal, blood-filled dilation of the wall of the aorta. The aorta dilates at the weakened area, which makes it susceptible to tear and rupture. A **dissecting aneurysm** occurs when the inner layers of the aorta become separated, allowing blood (at high pressures) to flow between the layers. Uncontrolled hypertension is the primary cause of dissecting aortic aneurysms. This separation of layers weakens the wall of the aorta significantly, making it more likely to be ruptured under conditions of continued high blood pressure. If the aorta ruptures, the amount of internal blood loss will be so large that the patient will die almost immediately. The signs and symptoms of a dissecting aortic aneurysm include very sudden chest pain located in the anterior part of the chest or in the back between the shoulder blades. It may be difficult to differentiate the chest pain of a dissecting aortic aneurysm from that of an AMI, but several distinctive features may help. The pain from an AMI is often preceded by other symptoms, such as nausea, indigestion, weakness, and sweating, and tends to come on gradually, getting more severe with time and often described as "pressure" rather than "stabbing." By contrast, the pain of a dissecting aortic aneurysm usually comes on full force from one minute to the next (**TABLE 17-2**). A patient with a dissecting aortic aneurysm also may exhibit a difference in blood pressure between arms or diminished pulses in the lower extremities. Aortic aneurysms are often difficult to diagnose in the prehospital setting, but you must consider them a possibility in any patient

TABLE 17-2 AMI Versus Dissecting Aortic Aneurysm

	AMI	Dissecting Aneurysm
Onset of pain	Gradual, with additional symptoms	Abrupt, without additional symptoms
Quality of pain	Tightness or pressure	Sharp or tearing
Severity of pain	Increases with time	Maximal from onset
Timing of pain	May wax and wane	Does not abate once it has started
Region/radiation	Substernal; back is rarely involved	Back possibly involved, between the shoulder blades
Clinical signs	Peripheral pulses equal	Blood pressure discrepancy between arms or decrease in a femoral or carotid pulse; may present with syncope, stroke, heart failure, or AMI.

with chest and abdominal pain and significant hypertension. Transport the patient without delay.

Patient Assessment

While en route to the scene, consider the standard precautions that will be needed. The precautions can be as simple as gloves for a patient with chest pain or full precautions for a patient in cardiac arrest. Remember, the patient's condition can change rapidly between the time you are dispatched and your arrival.

Scene Size-up

Do not let your guard down on medical calls. Always ensure that the scene is safe for all. As you approach the scene, look for and address any hazards. Determine the necessary standard precautions and whether you will need additional resources.

Identification of the nature of illness is important to start your patient assessment in the right direction. Use the information you get from the dispatcher, clues at the scene, and comments of bystanders or family members to begin to develop an idea about the type of problem your patient might be experiencing. For patients with cardiac problems, the clues often include a report of chest pain, difficulty breathing, syncope, or sudden loss of consciousness. Once you establish a preliminary nature of illness, you will be able to guide your assessment to find the important information much more effectively. Just remember not to become fixated on a specific condition at this early point in the assessment; sometimes the situation turns out to be very different from how it initially appeared.

Primary Assessment

As you approach the patient, form a general impression of their condition to recognize and address life threats. You will likely begin by determining whether the patient is responsive. Perform a primary assessment of the patient. If the patient is unresponsive and pulseless, begin CPR, starting with chest compressions, and call for an AED. Generally, an AED should be applied immediately if the patient is pulseless, not breathing (apneic), and unresponsive, or if you suspect ACS and the patient's vital signs are not normal. Consider calling for ALS backup if possible. See Chapter 14, *BLS Resuscitation*, for a detailed review of CPR and AED use.

Once you have formed a general impression, the next step in the primary assessment of a conscious patient is to assess airway and breathing. Unless the patient is unresponsive, the airway will most likely be patent. Responsive patients should be able to maintain their own airway. Some episodes of cardiac compromise may produce dizziness or even fainting spells (syncope). If dizziness or fainting from a standing position or height has occurred, consider the possibility of a spinal injury from a fall. Assess and treat the patient as appropriate.

Assess the patient's breathing to determine if it is adequate. If the rate is too fast or too slow, the depth of respiration seems to be too shallow, or if the patient is struggling to breathe, respirations are inadequate. Listen for abnormal breath sounds at this time because these can also be important indicators of respiratory distress. Some patients feel shortness of breath even though there are no obvious signs of respiratory distress. Pulse oximetry is a valuable tool in treatment of cardiac disease and should be applied at this time. If the patient is having any difficulty breathing or if oxygen saturation is less than 90%, administer oxygen at 4 L/min via a nasal cannula.[6] If the saturation does not improve quickly, increase the oxygen concentration. If you cannot get a pulse oximetry reading and the patient has signs and symptoms of dyspnea or shock, apply a nonrebreathing mask at 15 L/min. In general, the goal is to maintain the oxygen saturation level between 94% and 98%.[6] If the patient is not breathing or has inadequate breathing, ensure adequate ventilations with a bag-mask device and 100% oxygen.

Patients experiencing pulmonary edema may require positive-pressure ventilation with CPAP or, if respiratory failure or arrest develops, ventilation with a bag-mask device. CPAP is the most effective way to assist a person with left-side heart failure to breathe effectively and prevent the need to use an invasive airway management technique. Be aware of the indications and contraindications of CPAP and be competent in utilizing this equipment.

After assessing airway and breathing, assess the patient's circulation. Determine the rate and quality of the patient's pulse. Is the pulse rhythm regular or irregular? Is the pulse too fast or too slow? If you find abnormalities in the pulse, you should be more suspicious. Assess the patient's skin condition, color, moisture, and temperature, as well as the capillary refill time. Pallor and cyanosis can be difficult to detect in people with dark skin; these signs may be observed by examining mucous membranes inside the inner lower eyelid, lips, and nail beds and capillary refill. On general observation, the patient may appear ashen or gray. Changes in perfusion may indicate more serious cardiac compromise. Consider treatment for cardiogenic shock early to reduce the workload of the heart. Place the patient in a comfortable position, usually sitting up and well supported. Provide reassurance that appropriate treatment is being given for the condition to reduce the patient's anxiety.

Make a preliminary transport decision based on whether you were able to stabilize life threats during the primary assessment. If the decision is immediate transport, the remainder of the assessment can be initiated en route. If you can acquire and transmit a 12-lead electrocardiogram (ECG), do so after the primary assessment has been completed and medications such as aspirin and nitroglycerin have been administered. The ECG can provide information that helps determine the appropriate patient destination. In general, most patients with chest pain should be transported immediately after these initial actions are complete.

Whether to transport using the lights and siren is determined for each specific patient and may be partially based on the estimated transport time, road conditions, traffic, and local protocols. As a general rule, however, patients with cardiac problems should be transported in the most gentle, stress-relieving manner possible. You may save a little time using lights and siren, but you can do a lot to calm your patient and reduce the release of heart-damaging adrenaline through your reassurance and by creating a ride to the hospital that is as pleasant as possible. Try to help the patient avoid exerting physical effort, such as walking. By default, these patients should not walk to the stretcher or to the ambulance but instead should be carried or wheeled gently.

Your decision as to where to transport the patient will depend on your local protocol. Patients are generally transported to the closest appropriate facility. If your service is served by only one hospital, the transport decision is easy. In larger urban areas, there may be several hospitals within the service areas. Some medical directors have written protocols calling for patients with suspected cardiac emergencies to be transported to cardiac specialty centers with certain capabilities. Other protocols call for the patient to be transported to the nearest facility for stabilization before transporting to a specialty hospital. In most cases, cardiac arrest patients are transported to the closest hospital. Be sure you know your local protocol.

Special Populations

CIRCULATORY ASSESSMENT IN OLDER ADULTS

Remember when assessing the pulse of older patients that it is not uncommon for a geriatric person to have an irregular pulse that is normal for them.

Words of Wisdom

Hospitals certified by the AHA and the Joint Commission as Comprehensive Heart Attack Centers strive to meet specific criteria known to optimize the care for patients who are having an AMI.[7] The Level I Comprehensive Heart Attack Center is the highest tier and provides cardiac surgical services and primary percutaneous coronary intervention around the clock.

History Taking

Once you have stabilized life threats, determine and investigate the chief complaint and discover more about the history of the present illness. For a conscious medical patient, begin with obtaining a brief past medical history, identifying associated signs and symptoms, and identifying pertinent negatives. Friends, caregivers, or family members who are present may also have helpful information.

Remember that not all patients experiencing an AMI have the same signs and symptoms. A chief complaint of chest pain or discomfort, shortness of breath, or dizziness should be taken seriously. Many patients who suspect that something is wrong experience restlessness, appear anxious, and perhaps have a sense of impending doom. Act professionally; be calm. Speak to the patient in a normal voice that is neither too loud nor too soft. Let the patient know that trained responders, including you, are present to provide care and transport to the hospital. Remember, some patients may act less concerned, whereas others may be demanding. Most patients, however, are frightened. Your professional attitude may be the single most important factor in winning the patient's cooperation and helping the patient through this event. Patients often have a good idea about what is happening, so do not lie or offer false reassurance. If asked, "Am I having a heart attack?" you can say, "I don't know for sure, but in case you are, we're taking care of you. We're going to help you now by taking you to the hospital. You're in good hands."

Begin by asking questions about the current situation. Determine whether the patient is experiencing chest pain or discomfort and whether there are any other signs and symptoms. Determine whether the patient is having respiratory difficulty, because this is common among patients with chest pain. If the patient is experiencing dyspnea, find out whether it is related to exertion or whether it is related to the patient's position. Often, patients with chest pain experience worse difficulty breathing when they are lying down. Also determine whether the dyspnea is continuous or if it changes, especially with deep breathing. Note whether the patient has a cough and whether the cough produces sputum. Ask about other signs and symptoms that are commonly found, such as nausea and vomiting, fatigue, headache, and palpitations (a feeling of the heart skipping a beat or racing). Also ask about any trauma the patient might have experienced during the past few days. Be sure to record your findings, including those that are negative (known as pertinent negatives).

Words of Wisdom

When assessment reveals an unusual heart rate, try to determine whether this finding is appropriate for the patient and situation or a cause for concern. Athletes may have a slower (bradycardic; <60 beats/min) heart rate as a result of normal physiologic changes related to physical conditioning. Older patients may have slower heart rates controlled by medications to regulate high blood pressure (hypertension). Tachycardia (>100 beats/min) is a normal physiologic response to exercise to ensure adequate tissue perfusion and is normal in small children. Pain, fear, and excitement may also cause a person to be tachycardic.

If the patient is responsive, obtain the SAMPLE history, and ask the following questions specific to a cardiovascular emergency:

- Have you ever had a heart attack?
- Have you been told that you have heart problems?
    - Have you ever been diagnosed with angina, heart failure, or heart valve disease?
    - Have you ever had high blood pressure?
    - Have you ever been diagnosed with an aneurysm?
    - Do you have any respiratory diseases such as emphysema or chronic bronchitis?
    - Do you have diabetes or have you ever had any problems with your blood sugar?
    - Have you ever had kidney disease?

- Do you have any risk factors for coronary artery disease, such as smoking, high blood pressure, or high cholesterol?
  - Is there a family history of heart disease?
  - Do you currently take any medications?

The SAMPLE history provides basic information on the patient's overall medical history. You will want to determine as many signs and symptoms as you can. For example, you may determine that the patient has chest pain at rest or absence of chest pain with respirations or movement. The more signs and symptoms a patient has, the easier it is to identify a particular problem. In addition, ask whether the patient has had the same pain before. If so, ask "Do you take any medications for the pain?" and "Do you have any of the medication with you?" If the patient has had an AMI or angina before, ask whether the pain is similar.

Make sure to ask about allergies and confirm prior to administering any medication. If the patient is taking medications, determine whether they are prescribed, over the counter, and/or recreational drugs. Even when a patient may not be able to articulate an exact medical condition, knowing the patient's medications may give you important clues. For example, a patient may say he has "heart problems." You see that he is taking furosemide (Lasix), atorvastatin (Lipitor), and metoprolol (Toprol). Furosemide is a diuretic, atorvastatin lowers cholesterol, and metoprolol lowers blood pressure. These medications are often prescribed together for patients with heart failure and may alert you to carefully evaluate the lungs for the presence of crackles, which indicate fluid in the lungs and a need to increase the amount of oxygen being delivered or consider CPAP. When you ask about medical conditions, be sure to ask whether the patient takes medications for any other condition. If the patient reports taking prescription medications, ask what condition they are taken to treat. Asking about the last oral intake may seem unnecessary, but this information can be important; it is always better to have too much information than too little. Similarly, remember to ask about any home remedies the patient might have used, because this information may also prove helpful.

Be sure to include the OPQRST questions when you are obtaining the symptoms as part of the SAMPLE history. Using OPQRST helps you to understand the details of specific complaints, such as chest pain (**TABLE 17-3**).

Secondary Assessment

Circumstances will determine which aspects of the physical examination will be performed. The secondary assessment of a conscious patient with chest pain or discomfort would likely focus on the patient's cardiac and respiratory systems.

The physical examination of a patient with chest pain begins with the cardiovascular system. Evaluate the patient's circulation by assessing

YOU are the EMT

The patient took two of her prescribed nitroglycerin tablets before her son called 9-1-1; however, she is still experiencing chest pain, which she rates as a 7 on a scale of 0 to 10. Your partner takes her vital signs as you perform a more focused examination, inquire about her past medical history, and prepare for further treatment.

Recording Time: 2 Minutes	
Respirations	20 breaths/min; adequate depth
Pulse	118 beats/min; strong and irregular
Skin	Pale compared with baseline, cool, and diaphoretic
Blood pressure	150/90 mm Hg
Oxygen saturation (Spo_2)	98% (on 4 L/min oxygen)

7. What is significant about the patient's vital signs?
8. Should you give her additional nitroglycerin? Why or why not?

TABLE 17-3 OPQRST Mnemonic for Assessing Pain

Onset	When did the problem begin, and what does the patient think may have caused it?
Provocation/palliation	Ask what makes the pain or discomfort better or worse. Is it positional? Does a deep breath or palpation of the chest make it worse? Did you take anything for it (including anything nonprescribed)?
Quality	Ask the patient to describe the pain. Let the patient use their own words to describe what is happening. If the patient is unable to describe the pain, try to avoid supplying only one option. Do not ask, "Does it feel like an elephant is sitting on your chest?" Instead, say, "Tell me what the pain feels like." If the patient cannot answer an open-ended question, then provide a list of alternatives: "There are lots of different kinds of pain. Is your pain more like heaviness, pressure, burning, tearing, dull ache, stabbing, or needlelike?"
Region/radiation	Ask where the pain is located and whether the pain has spread to another part of the body.
Severity	Ask the patient to rate the pain on a simple scale. Often, a scale ranging from 0 to 10 is used; a 10 represents the worst pain imaginable. Do not use the patient's answer to determine whether the pain has a serious cause. Instead, use it to check whether the pain is getting better or worse. After a few minutes of oxygen or administration of nitroglycerin, ask the patient to rate the pain again.
Timing	Find out how long the pain lasts when it is present and whether it has been intermittent or continuous.

pulses at various locations, and assessing skin color, temperature, and condition. Is the skin cool or moist? How do the mucous membranes look? Are they pink, ashen, or cyanotic? Are the pulses of equal strength bilaterally? Does the patient have any edema in the extremities, especially the lower extremities? All of these physical findings can help identify poor circulation, which may be caused by a failure of the cardiovascular system.

In addition to the cardiovascular system, examine the respiratory system for signs of inadequate ventilation. These two systems are closely related, and cardiovascular issues can cause problems with the respiratory system. Are the lung sounds clear? Wet-sounding lungs indicate fluid is being moved into the lungs from the circulatory system, possibly because of a problem with the heart. Are the breath sounds equal? Are the neck veins distended? Is the trachea deviated, or is it midline? The answers to these questions can help determine whether a problem exists with the lungs or with the heart. Although the physical examination is not usually as important as the history in a patient with a possible cardiac problem, it may produce important clues to the patient's condition. Note the presence of any devices such as a pacemaker or automatic implanted defibrillator on the patient's chest; either one suggests a significant past heart problem.

Measure and record the patient's vital signs, including pulse, respirations, and blood pressure. You must obtain readings for systolic and diastolic blood pressures. Measure blood pressure on both arms if time allows. Use pulse oximetry to measure the oxygen saturation of the blood and use the pulse rate reading only to confirm your manually obtained pulse rate. Pulse oximetry may not give an accurate measurement if the patient has poor circulation, has been exposed to a toxin such as carbon monoxide or cyanide, or is in cardiac arrest, but it should be used and the readings noted for all patients with possible cardiac problems.

Be sure to engage in continuous blood pressure monitoring if you have access to it, ensuring that you obtain an accurate manual blood pressure first. Obtain repeat vital signs at appropriate intervals and use the settings on the automatic blood pressure monitoring machine to remind you when it is time to recheck and record the vital signs. Note the time that each set of vital signs is obtained.

Reassessment

Repeat the primary assessment by checking to see whether the patient's chief complaint and condition have improved or are deteriorating. Vital signs should be reassessed at least every 5 minutes or any time significant changes in the patient's condition occur. It is essential to closely monitor the patient with a suspected AMI because sudden cardiac arrest is always a risk. If cardiac arrest occurs, you must be ready to begin automated defibrillation or chest compressions immediately. If an AED is immediately available, use it; if not, perform CPR until the AED is available. Reassess your interventions to see whether they are helping and whether the patient's condition is improving. Reassessment will also determine whether further interventions are indicated or contraindicated.

Street Smarts

In some cases, patients who experience sudden cardiac arrest will have what appears to be brief seizure activity as they lose consciousness. This is related to the sudden loss of oxygenation to the brain. An experienced EMT recognizes this situation, checks for a pulse, and if there is none begins chest compressions until the AED can be used.

Transport the patient. Early, prompt transport to the ED or cardiac specialty center is critical so that treatments such as clot-busting medications or angioplasty can be initiated. To be most effective, these treatments must be started as soon as possible after the onset of the attack. If the patient does not have prescribed nitroglycerin and you do not have permission from medical direction to administer nitroglycerin, complete your patient assessment, prepare to transport as soon as possible, and consider ALS intercept.

Alert the ED staff about the status of your patient's condition and your estimated time of arrival. Follow the instructions of medical direction. Describe the patient's condition to the ED staff on arrival.

It is important to document your assessment and treatment of the patient. All interventions should be initiated according to protocol. If the intervention required an order from medical direction document the intervention and/or medication requested and that prior approval was granted. It must be clear in your documentation that the patient was reassessed appropriately following any intervention. The patient's response to the intervention and the time of each intervention must also be recorded.

Emergency Medical Care for Chest Pain or Discomfort

Your treatment of the patient begins with proper positioning. As mentioned before, some patients will not tolerate being positioned supine, so they should be allowed to sit up (leaning back on the stretcher). Also loosen tight clothing, trying to make the patient as comfortable as possible.

If it is indicated, you should be giving the patient oxygen by this time, but continually reassess the oxygen saturation and the patient's respiratory status. For patients with mild dyspnea, a nasal cannula may be all that is needed, whereas patients with more serious respiratory difficulty may require a nonrebreathing mask. If signs of pulmonary edema are present, CPAP may be indicated. Remember to begin oxygen administration if the oxygen saturation is less than 90% and titrate it to obtain an oxygen saturation between 94% and 98%, unless ongoing difficulty breathing suggests that respiratory distress is present despite a high pulse oximetry reading. A patient who is unconscious or in obvious respiratory distress may need assistance with breathing. Use a bag-mask device. Be aware that ALS may be valuable to support the use of positive end-expiratory pressure, CPAP, bilevel positive airway pressure, and transport ventilators.

Depending on local protocol, prepare to administer low-dose chewable aspirin and nitroglycerin. Aspirin (acetylsalicylic acid) prevents new clots from forming or existing clots from getting bigger. Aspirin is a lifesaving medication for those with a partially occluded coronary vessel. Low-dose aspirin comes in 81-mg chewable tablets. The recommended dose is 162 mg (two tablets) to 324 mg (four tablets). Be sure you have verified that the patient is not allergic to aspirin before you give it and that the vital signs are appropriate. Also, ask if the patient has any history of gastrointestinal bleeding such as stomach ulcers, and, if so, contact medical direction before giving the patient aspirin.

Nitroglycerin may help to relieve the pain of angina or myocardial infarction. As indicated for acute chest pain, it comes either as a small white tablet, placed sublingually (under the tongue), or as a spray, also administered sublingually. In either form, the effect is the same. Nitroglycerin relaxes the muscle of systemic blood vessel walls, slightly dilates coronary arteries, and decreases the workload of the heart, thus decreasing the oxygen demand of the cardiac muscle. Because nitroglycerin dilates blood vessels in other parts of the body, it can cause a decrease in blood pressure and a severe headache. Other side effects include changes in the patient's pulse rate, including tachycardia or bradycardia. Therefore, you should obtain the patient's blood pressure before administering each dose and again within 5 minutes after each dose. If the systolic blood pressure is less than 100 mm Hg, do not give nitroglycerin.[6] Also do not give this drug if the patient's heart rate is less than 50 beats/min or greater than 100 beats/min,[8] a head injury is present, the patient has used erectile dysfunction drugs within the previous 24 to 48 hours, or the maximum prescribed dose of nitroglycerin has already been given (usually three doses). Drugs used for erectile dysfunction include sildenafil (Viagra), tadalafil (Cialis), avanafil (Stendra), and vardenafil (Levitra, Staxyn).

Administering Nitroglycerin

Check the condition of the medication and its expiration date, and do not administer contaminated or expired medications. Always make sure the medication is prescribed for your patient or from your ambulance stock. Occasionally, patients will try to take medications prescribed for their spouse or a friend if they think it will help them. Be sure to wear gloves when handling nitroglycerin tablets or spray because it is easily absorbed through the skin. If you handle tablets with bare fingers or get the spray on your fingers, it may be absorbed into your body, causing you to experience a painful headache. If the patient is hypotensive or in cardiac arrest and has a nitroglycerin patch on when you arrive, be sure to carefully remove it before using the AED.

After you obtain permission from medical direction, administer the nitroglycerin if required. Nitroglycerin works in most patients within 5 minutes. Most patients who have been prescribed nitroglycerin carry a supply with them. Nitrostat is one of the trade names for nitroglycerin. The most frequent dose for sublingual tablets is 0.4 mg, although 0.3 mg is sometimes prescribed for patients who experience side effects at the higher dose. Sublingual spray is supplied as a dose of 0.4 mg per spray. Patients are instructed to take one dose of nitroglycerin under the tongue whenever they have an episode of angina that does not immediately go away with rest. If the pain is still present after 5 minutes, patients are typically instructed by their physicians to take a second dose. If the second dose does not work, most patients are told to take a third dose and then call for EMS. If the patient has not taken all three doses, you can administer the medication, if you are allowed to do so by local protocol.

Be aware that nitroglycerin will lose its potency over time, especially if exposed to light and/or heat. Patients who take it only rarely may keep a bottle in their pocket for months. It may lose its potency even before its expiration date. When the nitroglycerin tablet loses its potency, patients may not feel the fizzing sensation when the tablet is placed under their tongue, and they may not experience the normal burning sensation and headache that often accompany nitroglycerin administration. Note that the fizzing occurs only with a potent tablet, not with the spray form.

To safely assist the patient with nitroglycerin, follow the steps listed in **SKILL DRILL 17-1**:

1. Obtain an order from medical direction, either online or through off-line protocol.
2. Take the patient's blood pressure. Administer nitroglycerin only if the systolic blood pressure is greater than 100 mm Hg (**Step 1**).
3. Check that you have the right medication, the right patient, the right dose, and the right delivery route. Check the expiration date. Make sure the patient has no contraindications, such as having taken medication for erectile dysfunction in the past 24 hours.
4. Ask the patient about the last dose taken and its effects. Make sure the patient understands the route of administration. Be prepared to have the patient lie down to prevent fainting if the nitroglycerin substantially lowers the patient's blood pressure (the patient gets dizzy or feels faint) (**Step 2**).
5. Ask the patient to lift the tongue. Place the tablet or spray the dose under the tongue (while wearing gloves). Have the patient lower the tongue and keep the mouth closed with the tablet or spray under the tongue until it is dissolved and absorbed. Caution the patient against chewing or swallowing the tablet (**Step 3**).

Skill Drill 17-1 Administering Nitroglycerin

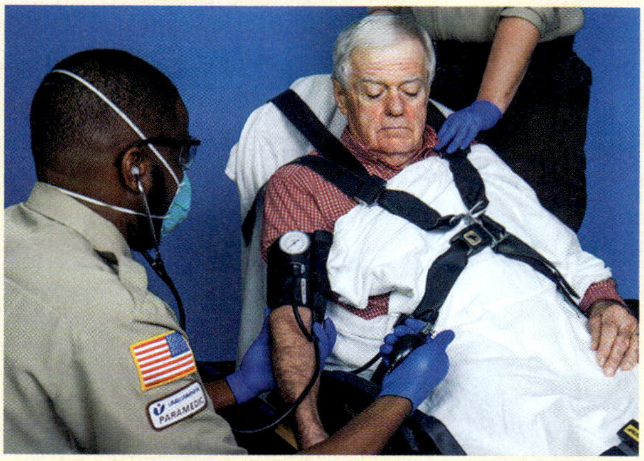

Step 1

Obtain an order from medical direction. Take the patient's blood pressure. Administer nitroglycerin only if the systolic blood pressure is greater than 100 mm Hg.

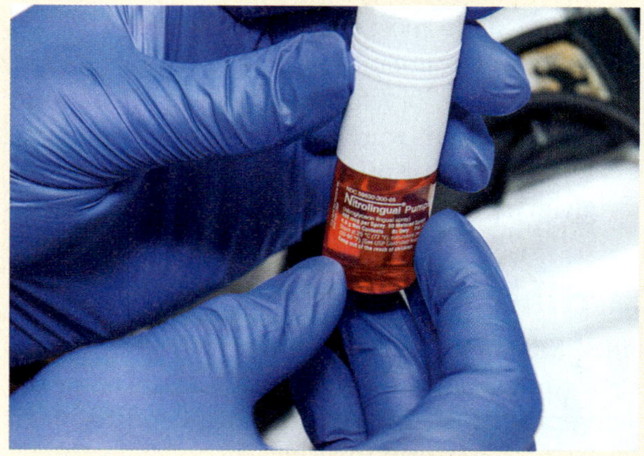

Step 2

Check the medication and expiration date. Ask the patient about the last dose taken and its effects. Make sure that the patient understands the route of administration. Prepare to have the patient lie down to prevent fainting.

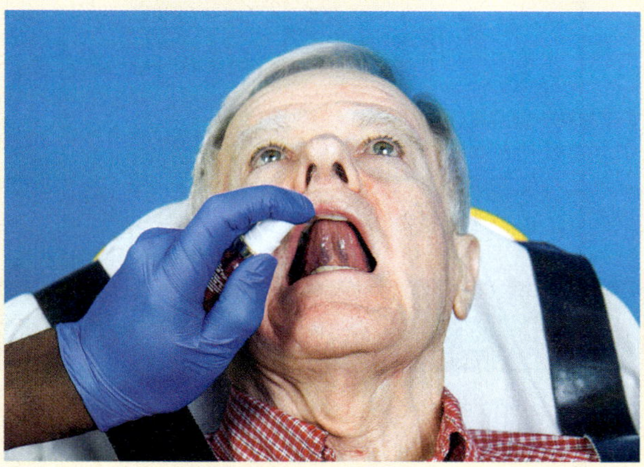

Step 3

Ask the patient to lift the tongue. Place the tablet or spray the dose under the tongue (while wearing gloves), or have the patient do so. Have the patient keep the mouth closed with the tablet or spray under the tongue until it is dissolved and absorbed. Caution the patient against chewing or swallowing the tablet.

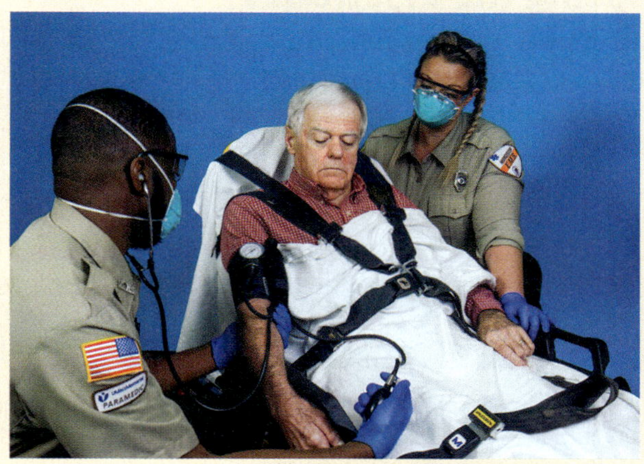

Step 4

Recheck the blood pressure within 5 minutes. Record each medication and the time of administration. Reevaluate the chest pain and blood pressure, and repeat treatment if necessary.

6. Recheck the blood pressure within 5 minutes. Record the name and dose of medication given and the time of administration. Reevaluate the chest pain and note the response to the medication. If the chest pain persists and the patient still has a systolic blood pressure greater than 100 mm Hg, repeat the dose every 5 minutes as authorized by medical direction. In general, a maximum of three doses of nitroglycerin is given for any one episode of chest pain (**Step 4**).

Cardiac Monitoring

Some EMS systems allow EMTs to place electrodes, attach the leads, and obtain and transmit an ECG tracing prior to or during transport. If your service allows you to perform this skill, the following information will guide you. The goal is to obtain the ECG within 10 minutes of your first contact with the patient. Be sure to familiarize yourself with the operation of the monitor that your service uses, including how to obtain and transmit ECG tracings before using it on a call.

Placing the Electrodes

For an ECG to be reliable and useful, the electrodes must be placed in consistent positions on each patient. **FIGURE 17-10** shows placement of limb lead electrodes, which are used to obtain a rhythm strip. **FIGURE 17-11** shows placement of limb lead electrodes and 12-lead ECG electrodes, both of which are used when obtaining a 12-lead ECG. To maintain consistency in monitoring and obtaining a useful ECG, there are specific predetermined locations for each electrode. Electrodes used in the prehospital setting are generally adhesive and have a gel center to aid in skin contact. Whichever type is used, certain basic principles should be followed to achieve the best skin contact and minimize **artifact**

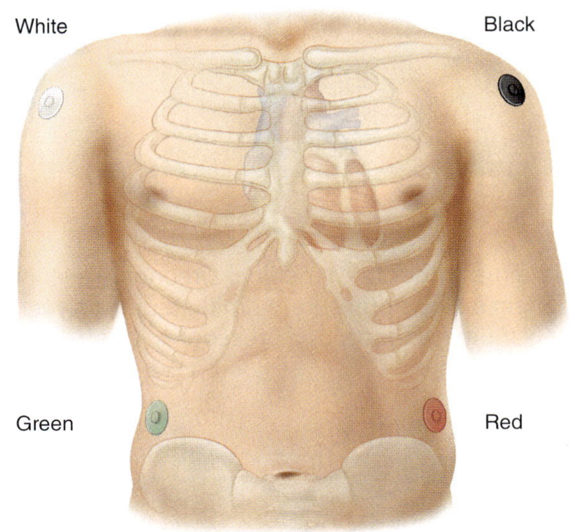

FIGURE 17-10 Limb electrode placement for cardiac monitoring.

YOU are the EMT

After completing the remainder of your assessment and initial treatment, you place the patient onto the stretcher, load her into the ambulance, and proceed to a hospital located 20 miles away. You ask your partner to notify the hospital to alert the staff as you reassess the patient.

Recording Time: 10 Minutes	
Level of consciousness	Conscious and alert; still anxious
Respirations	18 breaths/min; adequate depth
Pulse	84 beats/min; strong and irregular
Skin	Pale compared with baseline and cool; less diaphoretic
Blood pressure	136/84 mm Hg
Oxygen saturation (Spo_2)	96% (on oxygen)

9. Why is early notification of the receiving facility so important for patients with an acute coronary event?

10. Should you apply the AED to determine if this patient is experiencing a cardiac dysrhythmia? Why or why not?

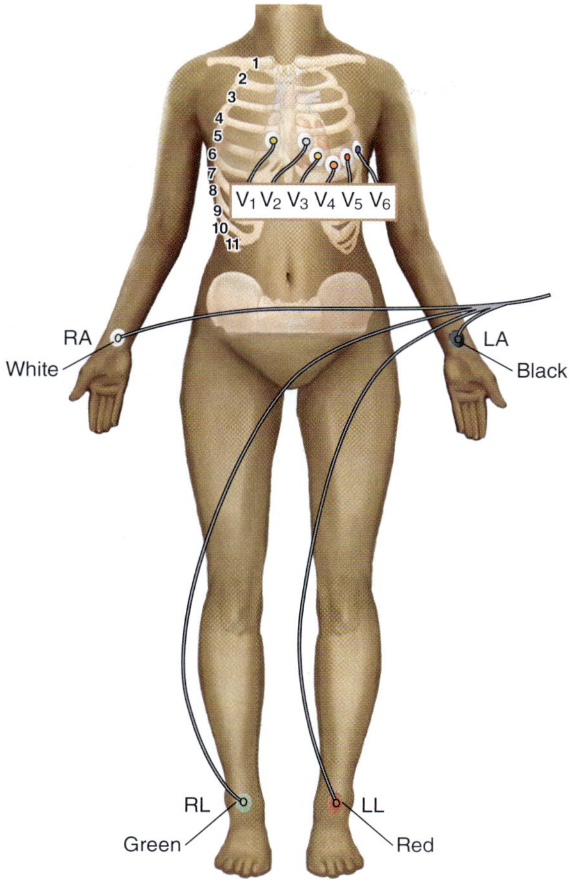

Lead	Location	View
V_1	4th intercostal space, right sternal border	Ventricular septum
V_2	4th intercostal space, left sternal border	Ventricular septum
V_3	Between V_2 and V_4	Anterior wall of left ventricle
V_4	5th intercostal space, midclavicular line	Anterior wall of left ventricle
V_5	Lateral to V_4 at the anterior axillary line	Lateral wall of left ventricle
V_6	Lateral to V_5 at the midaxillary line	Lateral wall of left ventricle

FIGURE 17-11 Twelve-lead ECG electrode placement.

in the signal. Artifact refers to an ECG tracing with waves that are the result of interference, such as patient movement, rather than the heart's electrical activity. Guiding principles are as follows:

- To maintain the correct lead placement, it may occasionally be necessary to shave body hair from the electrode site. Do not be fooled by a hairy chest. It may initially appear that you have good skin contact, but the electrode will rise off the skin and stick to the hair. If you must shave the site, be very careful to avoid nicking the skin. If one is available, it is best to use an electric razor to remove hair, because single-blade manual razors irritate the skin and can easily cut a patient.

ALS Assist

Recent research suggests an improved survival benefit to patients receiving double-sequential external defibrillation (DSED), also called vector change defibrillation. DSED is a technique in which a paramedic applies a second set of defibrillation pads attached to a second cardiac monitor. A paramedic delivers a defibrillation shock first from one cardiac monitor and then the other monitor in rapid succession. The pad placement is referred to as anterior–posterior because one pad is placed medially to the pad on the chest and the second is placed posteriorly on the back. The strategy is meant to provide the shock in a different direction than the first. It is not about the amount of electricity delivered, but rather the direction in which the heart receives the electricity. DSED can be performed only with cardiac monitors and is not to be performed with AEDs.

- To remove oils and dead tissues from the surface of the skin, rub the electrode site briskly with an alcohol swab before application. Wait for the alcohol to dry before applying electrodes or dry it with a quick wipe of a 4 × 4–inch (10 × 10–cm) gauze pad. This step may have to be repeated if the patient is very sweaty, as many cardiac patients are.
- Attach the electrodes to the ECG cables before placement. Confirm that the appropriate electrode now attached to the cable is placed at the correct location on the patient's chest or limbs (each cable is marked and color coded as to the correct location for placement).

Performing Cardiac Monitoring

Once all electrodes are in place, switch on the monitor, and print a sample rhythm strip. If the strip shows any interference (artifact), verify that the electrodes are firmly applied to the skin and the monitor cable is plugged in correctly. Artifact caused by patient movement, including deep breathing or muscle tremor, may appear as a wavy baseline or small up-and-down squiggles on the baseline. Artifact will prevent the ECG from being usable. Make sure the patient is resting comfortably in the position of comfort (ideally supine with the head elevated about 30°) and not moving while obtaining the rhythm strip. Also make sure the patient's arms are relaxed by their sides and feet are uncrossed.

SKILL DRILL 17-2 shows the steps for performing cardiac monitoring:

1. Take standard precautions (**Step 1**).
2. Explain the procedure to the patient. Prepare the skin for electrode placement (**Step 2**).
3. Attach the electrodes to the leads before placing them on the patient (**Step 3**).
4. Position the limb electrodes on the patient's limbs if you will be acquiring a 12-lead ECG. These electrodes may be placed on the torso only if performing continuous monitoring and a 12-lead ECG will not be required. The RA electrode goes on the right arm distal to the shoulder or on the wrist (avoid placing electrodes

Skill Drill 17-2 Performing Cardiac Monitoring

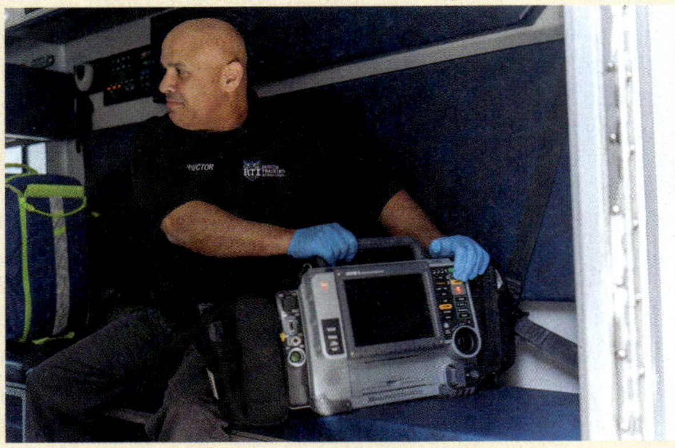

Step 1

Take standard precautions.

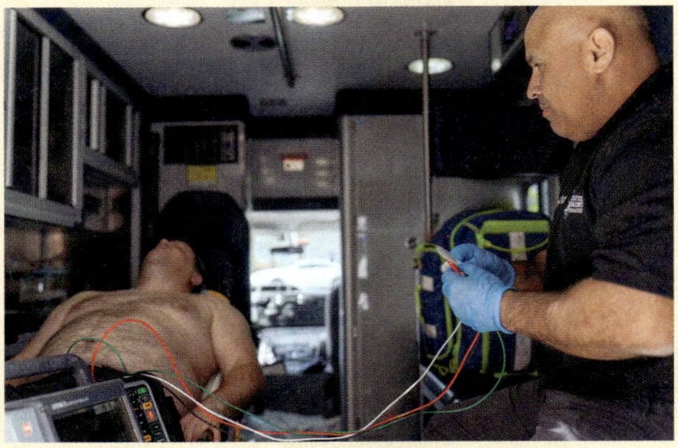

Step 2

Explain the procedure to the patient. Prepare the skin for electrode placement.

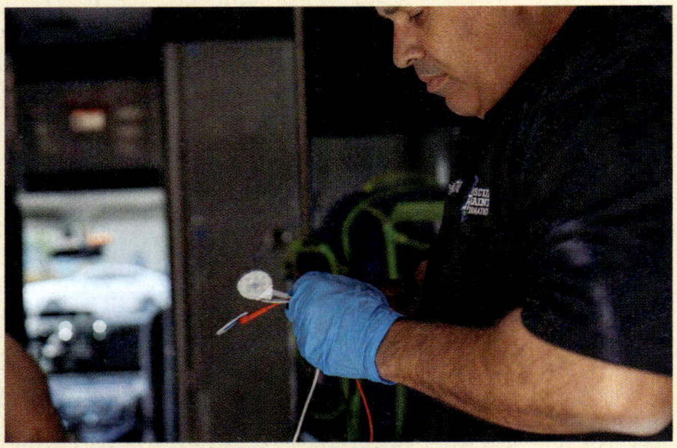

Step 3

Attach the electrodes to the leads before placing them on the patient.

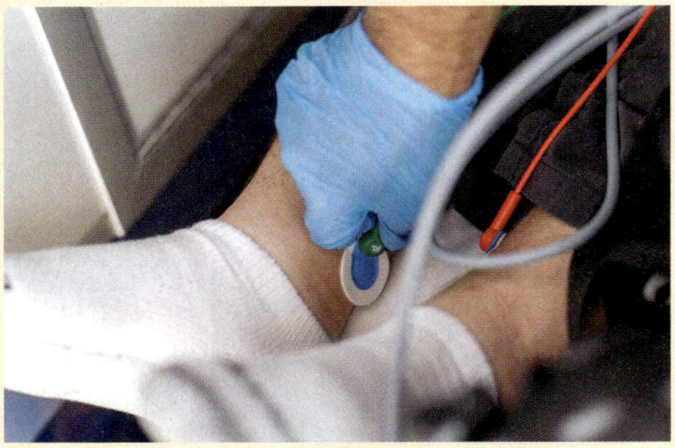

Step 4

Position the limb electrodes on the patient. Place the leads on the torso if performing continuous monitoring, and on the limbs if you will be acquiring a 12-lead ECG.

Skill Drill 17-2 Performing Cardiac Monitoring continued

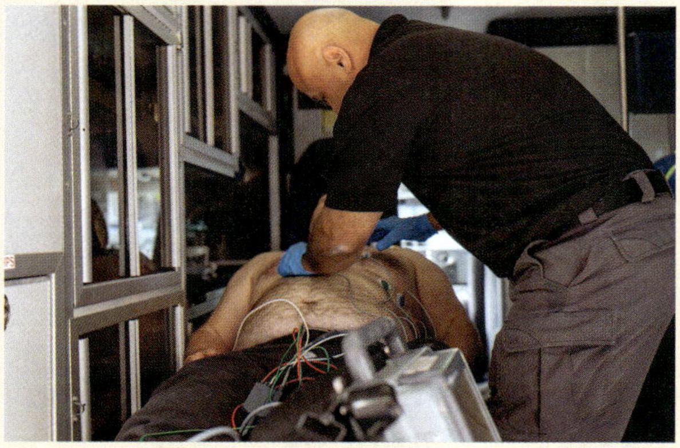

Step 5

If you plan to obtain a 12-lead ECG tracing, place the chest (V) leads on the chest.

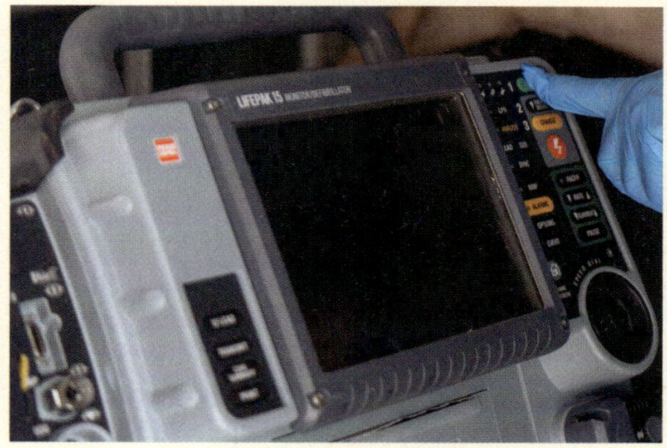

Step 6

Turn on the monitor.

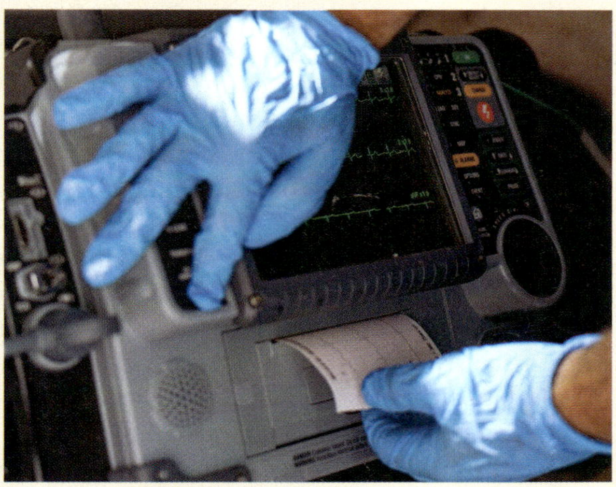

Step 7

Record tracings.

All images courtesy of Aura Prep/Rescue Training International.

directly over a bone). The LA electrode goes on the left arm at the same location as you placed the RA electrode on the right arm. The LL electrode is placed on the left leg on the thigh or ankle, although if you do not plan to obtain a 12-lead ECG tracing, this electrode may be placed on the lower left side of the abdomen (slightly lower than an AED pad would be placed). Place the RL electrode at the same location on the right side of the body as the LL electrode on the left. Each electrode should be approximately an equal distance from the heart (or the bottom of the sternum) (**Step 4**).

5. If you plan to obtain a 12-lead ECG tracing, place the chest leads on the chest as shown. The V_1 electrode is placed on the right side of the sternum between the fourth and fifth ribs. To find this location, place your finger on the angle of Louis (where the manubrium meets the body of the sternum) and slide it to the right. Your finger should now be on the second rib. You can move it down to the third and then fourth rib and place the electrode below this location, between the fourth and fifth ribs. The V_2 electrode is placed on the left side of the sternum directly across from V_1. The V_4 electrode

is placed next, between the fifth and sixth ribs in a straight line down from the middle of the clavicle. The V_3 electrode is then placed halfway between V_2 and V_4 in between the fifth and sixth ribs (not on top of a rib). The V_6 electrode is placed next and is located horizontally even with V_4 in a straight line down from the middle of the armpit. Finally, the V_5 electrode is placed halfway between V_4 and V_6 (**Step 5**).
6. Turn on the monitor (**Step 6**).
7. Record tracings. As soon as a rhythm is visible on the screen, press the print button on the monitor and print a strip while counting slowly to six or seven. Then press the print button again to stop the printout. If the time is not printed correctly on the strip, write it on the edge of the strip. If you are obtaining a 12-lead ECG tracing, ask the patient to hold their breath or to take very shallow breaths. Press the 12-lead button and wait for the machine to acquire, analyze, and print or transmit the 12-lead ECG tracing. Gently tear off the tracing when the printer automatically stops (**Step 7**).
8. Transmit the tracing to the facility where you are transporting the patient. This may be performed electronically on the monitor, or it might require you to scan (or take a photo of) the printout and send it as you would a fax, text, or email attachment. Whichever method your service uses, make sure you are familiar with it and have practiced it.
9. Add the ECG into your electronic patient care report (if this feature is not done automatically).

Reviewing the ECG Tracing

After obtaining an ECG tracing, it is important to make sure you have a high-quality printout. You should be able to see the QRS complexes (the largest, usually narrow, deflections on the ECG) clearly without interference from artifact. Each QRS complex represents one contraction of the ventricles, so the closer together they are, the faster the heartbeat.

You may also see a small, rounded wave before the QRS called a P wave, which represents the contraction of the atria. After each QRS complex, you should see a T wave that represents the repolarization (or recharging) of the ventricles. The horizontal line between all of the waves is called the baseline and segments of the baseline are often identified by the waves they connect. For example, the ST segment connects the end of the QRS complex and the beginning of the T wave.

> **ALS Assist**
>
> Identification of cardiac rhythms and interpretation of 12-lead ECGs are paramedic-level skills. As an EMT, you will typically assist with the application of the electrodes or acquire the 12-lead ECG so your paramedic partner can interpret it. Correct lead placement is essential to ensure the tracing accurately displays the heart's electrical activity.

Heart Surgeries and Cardiac Assistive Devices

During the past 40 years, hundreds of thousands of open-heart surgeries have been performed to bypass damaged segments of coronary arteries in the heart. In a coronary artery bypass graft, a blood vessel from the chest or leg is sewn directly from the aorta to a coronary artery beyond the point of the obstruction. Another procedure is percutaneous transluminal coronary angioplasty, which aims to dilate, rather than bypass, the coronary artery. In this procedure, which is usually called angioplasty or balloon angioplasty, a tiny balloon is attached to the end of a long, thin tube. The tube is introduced through the skin into a large artery, usually in the groin or wrist, and then threaded using imaging into the narrowed coronary artery. Once the balloon is in position inside the coronary artery, it is inflated. The balloon is then deflated, and the tube is removed from the body. Sometimes, a metal mesh cylinder called a stent is placed inside the artery instead of or after the balloon. The stent is usually coated in medicine to prevent new clots from forming. It is left in place permanently to help keep the artery from narrowing again.

A patient who has had an AMI or angina in the past will possibly have had one of these procedures. Patients who have had a bypass graft may have a long surgical scar on their chest from the operation. Newer minimally invasive cardiac surgical procedures may produce only one or two smaller scars lateral to the sternum. Patients who have undergone angioplasty or coronary artery stent placement usually will not have a scar. Chest pain in a patient who has undergone any of these procedures should be treated in the same manner as chest pain in patients who have not had any heart surgery.

Perform all the described tasks, and transport the patient promptly to the ED. If CPR is required, perform it in the usual way, regardless of the scar on the patient's chest. Likewise, if indicated, an AED should be used.

In the United States, many people with heart disease have cardiac pacemakers to maintain a regular cardiac rhythm and rate. Pacemakers are inserted when the electrical control system of the heart no longer functions properly. These battery-powered devices deliver an electrical impulse through wires that are in direct contact with the myocardium. The generating unit is generally placed under a heavy muscle or a fold of skin. It typically resembles a small silver dollar under the skin in the left upper portion of the chest (**FIGURE 17-12**).

Normally, you do not need to be concerned about problems with pacemakers. Thanks to modern technology, an implanted unit will not require replacement for years. Wires are well protected and rarely broken. Every patient with a pacemaker should be aware of the precautions, if any, that must be taken to maintain its proper functioning.

If a pacemaker does not function properly, as when the battery wears out, the patient may experience syncope, dizziness, or weakness because of an excessively slow heart rate. The pulse ordinarily will be less than 60 beats/min because the heart is beating without the stimulus of the pacemaker and without the regulation of its own electrical system, which may be damaged. In these circumstances, the heart tends to assume a fixed slow rate that is not fast enough to allow the patient to function normally. A patient with a malfunctioning pacemaker should be promptly transported to the ED; repair of the problem may require surgery. When an AED is used, the patches should not be placed directly over the pacemaker.

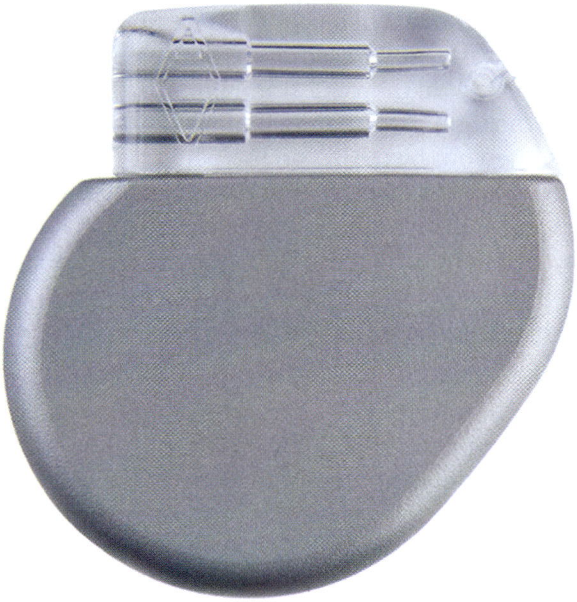

FIGURE 17-12 A pacemaker, which is typically inserted under the skin in the left upper portion of the chest, delivers an electrical impulse to regulate the heartbeat.

Words of Wisdom

The AHA recommends that individuals with a pacemaker or automatic implantable cardiac defibrillator avoid any device or power source that may interfere with the function of their implanted device.[9] Examples may include batteries, metal detectors, jumper cables, welders, and even headphones. Cell phones and earbuds should be kept at least 6 inches (15 cm) away from an implanted defibrillator. Patients should understand the risks relating to their medical equipment. As an EMT, be mindful that electromagnetic waves can disrupt the function of these devices.

Automatic Implantable Cardiac Defibrillators

More and more patients who survive cardiac arrest resulting from VF have a small automatic implantable cardiac defibrillator (**FIGURE 17-13**). It is nearly impossible to tell the difference between an implanted defibrillator and a pacemaker from their appearance, and many devices can function as both, depending on the patient's need. Some patients who are at particularly high risk for a cardiac arrest have them as well. These devices are attached directly to the heart and can prolong the lives of certain patients. They continuously monitor the heart rhythm, delivering shocks as needed.

Regardless of whether a patient having an AMI has an automatic implantable cardiac defibrillator, the individual should be treated like all other patients having an AMI. Treatment should include typical assessment and monitoring; if the patient is in cardiac arrest, it should include performing CPR and using an AED.

It is also likely that you will care for someone who has had their implanted defibrillator deliver a shock to them. This patient likely experienced VF

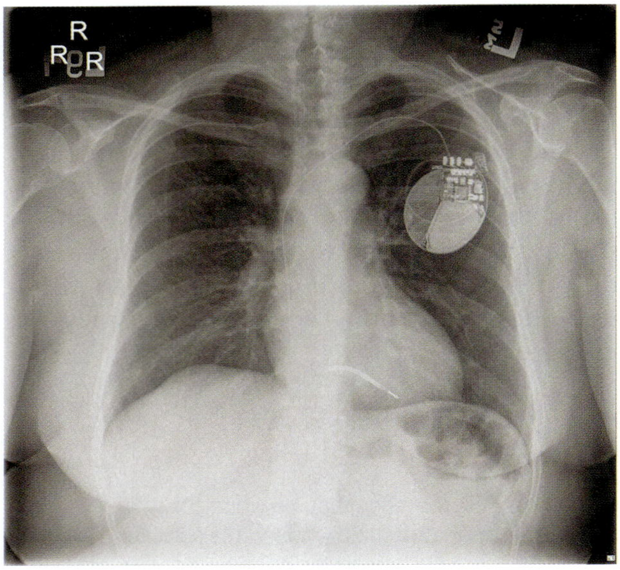

FIGURE 17-13 An automatic implantable cardiac defibrillator is attached directly to the heart and continuously monitors heart rhythm, delivering shocks as needed. The electricity from the defibrillator is so low that it has no effect on rescuers.

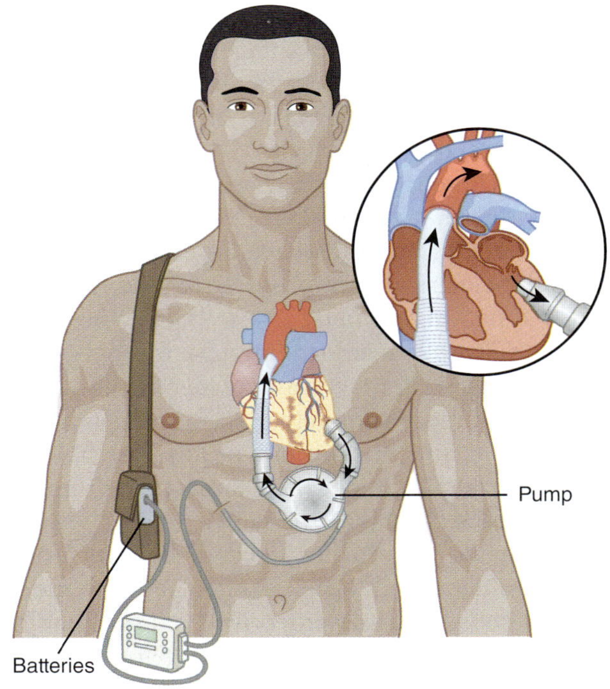

FIGURE 17-14 Left ventricular assist device.

or VT and the defibrillator delivered an electrical charge to restore a normal heart rhythm. These patients should be transported to the hospital to have the event investigated and ensure it does not occur again. You should be highly alert that VT or VF could occur again and the defibrillator will shock the patient again. If you are touching the patient when a shock is delivered, you may feel a slight tingle; however, it will not harm you.

External Defibrillator Vest

A temporary alternative to the implantable cardiac defibrillator is the external defibrillator vest. This device is a vest with built-in monitoring electrodes and defibrillation pads, which is worn by the patient under the clothing. The vest is attached to a monitor worn on a belt or hung from a shoulder strap. The monitor provides alerts and voice prompts when it recognizes a dangerous rhythm and before a shock is delivered. It takes 25 to 60 seconds from detection of the rhythm problem to delivery of the shock. Unlike the implantable defibrillator, this device uses high-energy shocks similar to an AED, so you should avoid contact with the patient if the device warns that it is about to deliver a shock. An audible warning alerting rescuers to stay clear will state, "Bystanders, do not interfere," before the shock is delivered. Blue gel under the large defibrillation pads indicates that the device has already delivered at least one shock.

If the patient is in cardiac arrest, the vest should remain in place while CPR is being performed unless it interferes with compressions. If it is necessary to remove the vest, simply remove the battery from the monitor and then remove the vest. You can then use your own AED on the patient. Any patient who is wearing a device that has already delivered a shock should be transported to the hospital for further evaluation.

Ventricular Assist Devices

Ventricular assist devices (VADs) are used to enhance the pumping function of one or both ventricles in patients with severe heart failure or in patients who need a temporary boost due to a myocardial infarction (**FIGURE 17-14**). Left ventricular assist devices (LVADs) are the most common type of VAD encountered in the field. There are several types of LVADs; the most common ones have an internal pump unit and an external battery pack. These pumps are almost all continuous, so many of these patients will not have any palpable pulses.

Obtaining an automated blood pressure measurement is possible only about 50% of the time in these patients, so you may need to assess blood pressure manually. When an automated blood pressure is present, look at the mean arterial pressure; a value greater than 60 mm Hg indicates that adequate tissue perfusion is likely. When the pulse is not detected, you must rely on assessment findings such as level of consciousness, skin color, and capillary refill to determine if circulation is adequate. End-tidal carbon dioxide monitoring is also a helpful adjunct to determine perfusion. A value of 35 to 40 mm Hg can help confirm that the patient's ventilation and perfusion are adequate, and lower values may indicate poor perfusion. If the pulse oximetry value is normal, consider it accurate; however, it is often difficult or impossible to obtain on these patients if their VAD has continuous flow.

If you are treating a patient who has a VAD and has lost consciousness, listen for a hum that indicates the pump is working. If it is not present, check that all connections on the device are secure and that the power (either a battery pack or an AC source) is connected.

Patients who have VADs often have a complex medical history. Be sure to consider causes other than the VAD when vital signs are not normal. Because the pulse check is not reliable, cardiac arrest in a patient who has a VAD is detected by assessing level of consciousness, absence of breathing, and skin color or capillary refill. If cardiac arrest is suspected, begin chest compressions (**FIGURE 17-15**).

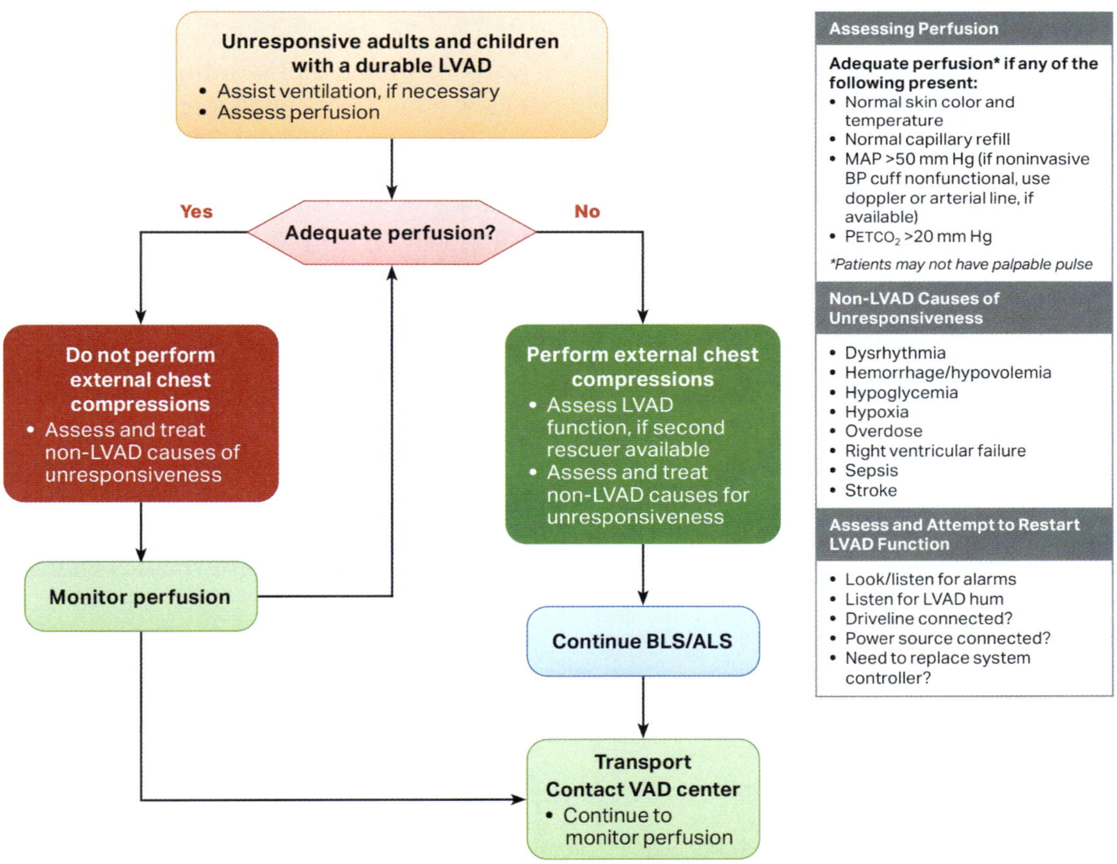

FIGURE 17-15 Response algorithm for a patient with a left ventricular assist device (LVAD).

Abbreviations: ALS, indicates advanced life support; BLS, basic life support; BP, blood pressure; ET, endotracheal; LVAD, left ventricular assist device; MAP, mean arterial pressure; PETCO2, partial pressure of end-tidal carbon dioxide; VAD, ventricular assist device

Almost all patients who have a VAD also have an automatic implantable cardiac defibrillator that will deliver a shock if the patient's rhythm is VF or VT.

A patient with an LVAD (or their family members) may be able to tell you about the unit. Unless it malfunctions, you should not need to deal with it. If you are unsure of what to do, contact medical direction for assistance. Also, LVADs provide a number to call for assistance and 24-hour emergency assistance is available. Transport all LVAD supplies and battery packs to the hospital with the patient. If the patient's condition and distance permit, it is preferred to transport the patient to a hospital with a VAD program.

ALS Assist

Other methods of circulatory assistance that the EMT may encounter in the prehospital setting include the Impella device and extracorporeal membrane oxygenation (ECMO). The Impella is a temporary catheter-based heart pump used when a patient has cardiogenic shock. These devices may be inserted to maintain the patient's perfusion until they can be transported to a higher level of care. ECMO uses a machine to circulate blood around the body and oxygenate it using an artificial lung. When ECMO is used in the prehospital setting, it is often referred to as ECPR (extracorporeal cardiopulmonary resuscitation). This intervention may be used when traditional CPR and defibrillation have failed to restore circulation. Specialized training is needed to care for patients who have undergone either Impella insertion or ECMO. Your role as an EMT will largely be related to helping move the patient or drive the ambulance.

Cardiac Arrest

Cardiac arrest is the complete cessation of cardiac activity. It is indicated in the field by the absence of a carotid pulse. Until the advent of CPR and external defibrillation in the 1960s, cardiac arrest was almost always a terminal event. With good initial CPR, early defibrillation, and access to advanced care, it is now possible for some patients to survive a cardiac arrest without neurologic damage.

When you arrive to find a patient who appears to be in cardiac arrest, you should automatically follow your CPR training. Start with high-quality chest compressions and apply an AED as soon as it is available. Defibrillate immediately if indicated. Chapter 14, *BLS Resuscitation*, covers CPR and AED use in detail.

YOU are the EMT

The patient is still conscious and alert and appears less anxious. She tells you that her chest pain has decreased in severity and is now a 3 on a 0 to 10 scale. After reassessing her, you contact the receiving facility and give the staff a patient update.

Recording Time: 17 Minutes	
Level of consciousness	Conscious and alert; less anxious
Respirations	16 breaths/min; adequate depth
Pulse	80 beats/min; strong and irregular
Skin	Baseline color, cool, and dry
Blood pressure	128/78 mm Hg
Oxygen saturation (Spo_2)	98% (on oxygen)

You deliver the patient to the ED, where the cardiac team greets you and assumes care of the patient. The physician obtains a 12-lead ECG and determines that she is experiencing an AMI. Within 15 minutes, she is taken to the cardiac catheterization laboratory, where two coronary stents are successfully placed.

11. What is the difference between angina pectoris and an AMI?

12. As an EMT, how can you distinguish angina pectoris from an AMI?

Words of Wisdom

Few patients who experience sudden cardiac arrest outside a hospital survive unless a rapid sequence of events takes place. The chain of survival is a way of describing the ideal sequence of events that can take place when such an arrest occurs. The six links in the chain of survival are as follows:

1. Recognition of early warning signs and immediate activation of EMS
2. Immediate CPR with emphasis on high-quality chest compressions
3. Rapid defibrillation
4. Advanced EMS
5. Postarrest care
6. Recovery and survivorship

If any one of the links in the chain is absent, the patient is less likely to be resuscitated. If all links in the chain are strong, the patient has the best possible chance of survival. The link that is the most common determinant for survival is the third link: rapid defibrillation. This link and those for immediate high-quality CPR and basic and advanced EMS are where EMTs are most involved. See Chapter 14, *BLS Resuscitation*, for further discussion of the chain of survival.

YOU are the EMT SUMMARY

1. What is the function of the heart?

The heart receives deoxygenated blood from the body, sends it to the lungs to be reoxygenated, and then pumps oxygenated blood throughout the body. The heart must pump effectively to ensure that the body's tissues and cells receive an uninterrupted supply of oxygen and that metabolic waste (eg, carbon dioxide) is removed from the tissues and cells and returned, through the heart, for elimination from the body by the respiratory system.

2. What does the heart require to function effectively?

Like any other critical organ or muscle, the heart requires a constant supply of oxygen, which it receives from the coronary arteries. It also relies on electricity to stimulate the contraction of the muscular layer of the heart (myocardium). Adequate blood volume is also required for effective cardiac function. As blood returns to the heart, it enters the chambers, stretches their walls, and causes them to contract with greater force. If blood volume is low, the heart will stretch less, and its contractile force will decrease.

3. What should you include in your primary assessment of a patient with cardiac problems?

Your primary assessment of a patient with cardiac problems should be no different from your primary assessment of any other patient: to find and immediately correct problems with airway, breathing, and circulation. Look for signs of impaired cardiac function, such as an irregular heartbeat, a fast or slow heart rate, a weak (thready) pulse, and poor skin condition (eg, pallor, diaphoresis).

4. Why is aspirin given to patients with an acute cardiac event?

Aspirin has clearly been shown to reduce mortality from AMI. Unless the patient is allergic to aspirin, it should be given as soon as possible if an acute cardiac event is suspected. An AMI occurs when an atherosclerotic plaque ruptures and occludes a coronary artery. When this occurs, platelets rush to the area and aggregate (clump together), which further occludes the coronary artery. Aspirin makes the platelets less "sticky," which makes them less likely to aggregate. Although aspirin will not dissolve the existing clot that is occluding the coronary artery, it may help prevent it from getting larger by reducing the amount of platelet aggregation.

5. What type of medication is nitroglycerin? How may it help relieve chest pain, pressure, or discomfort?

Nitroglycerin is a vasodilator. It relaxes the smooth muscle that regulates the diameter of the blood vessels, causing them to dilate (open). Nitroglycerin is used by patients with coronary artery disease who are experiencing chest pain, pressure, or discomfort. It dilates the coronary arteries and increases blood flow to the heart. As a result, the myocardial oxygen supply and demand are rebalanced, and the pain subsides or resolves completely. In some cases, however, nitroglycerin does not relieve the patient's

YOU are the EMT SUMMARY continued

chest pain. In a patient with a cardiac history, this should make you more suspicious that the individual is experiencing an AMI.

6. When is nitroglycerin indicated for a patient? What is the typical dose?

Nitroglycerin is indicated for patients with coronary artery disease who experience chest pain, pressure, or discomfort. Many patients with coronary artery disease have been prescribed nitroglycerin, which they self-administer. If the patient has not taken any of their prescribed nitroglycerin, you may administer it after ensuring that the patient's systolic blood pressure is at least 100 mm Hg and that approval from medical direction has been obtained. The most common dose for nitroglycerin found on an ambulance is 0.4 mg per tablet or spray. Patients may have 0.3-mg tablets or rarely other strengths prescribed by their physicians. Because nitroglycerin is a vasodilator, it can cause hypotension. Therefore, it is important to reassess the patient's blood pressure within a few minutes after administering nitroglycerin to ensure that it is at least 100 mm Hg. Nitroglycerin is contraindicated in patients with a systolic blood pressure of less than 100 mm Hg and in patients who have taken drugs for erectile dysfunction within the past 24 to 36 hours. Drugs for erectile dysfunction are also vasodilators; if given together with nitroglycerin, significant hypotension may occur.

7. What is significant about the patient's vital signs?

Skin that is pale compared with its baseline color, cool, and clammy (diaphoretic) is not exclusive to a cardiac problem. However, in the context of the patient's chief complaint and history of heart problems, it is highly suggestive that her chest pain is of cardiac origin. An irregular heartbeat indicates a disturbance in the cardiac electrical conduction system (dysrhythmia). Again, in the context of her chief complaint and cardiac history, this should further increase your index of suspicion that she is experiencing a cardiac event. An irregular heartbeat in a patient with a cardiac problem could indicate an impending life-threatening dysrhythmia. The patient's rapid heart rate (tachycardia) and relatively elevated blood pressure (150/90 mm Hg) are also clinically significant; they indicate that her heart is working harder than normal. As the heart rate and blood pressure increase, the heart consumes and requires more oxygen. If the heart is already deprived of oxygen, the patient's condition could worsen.

8. Should you give her additional nitroglycerin? Why or why not?

Despite taking two of her prescribed nitroglycerin doses before your arrival, the patient is still experiencing significant chest pain (7 on a scale of 0 to 10). Because her systolic blood pressure is well above 100 mm Hg, you should contact medical direction and request permission to assist her with one more nitroglycerin dose. Remember to reassess her blood pressure within a few minutes after administering the medication.

9. Why is early notification of the receiving facility so important for patients with an acute coronary event?

The longer it takes to reestablish blood flow distal to an occluded artery, the greater the amount of cardiac muscle damage (hence the phrase, "time is muscle"). Early reperfusion, with fibrinolytic medications (clot busters) or cardiac catheterization and stent placement, has clearly been shown to minimize the amount of cardiac damage and improve the patient's outcome. The earlier you notify the receiving facility that you are transporting a patient with a possible AMI, the more time the staff will have to allocate the resources needed to facilitate rapid cardiac reperfusion. The physician determines the reperfusion strategy. Your job is to recognize that the patient may be experiencing an AMI, provide immediate lifesaving care, promptly notify the appropriate receiving facility, and transport without delay.

10. Should you apply the AED to determine if this patient is experiencing a cardiac dysrhythmia? Why or why not?

No. Currently, your patient is breathing and has a pulse. Even if you did use the AED, it would not analyze her cardiac rhythm. An AED will not analyze the cardiac rhythm if it detects patient movement. You should have the AED readily available in case she experiences cardiac arrest, but its application is not indicated at this point.

11. What is the difference between angina pectoris and an AMI?

Angina pectoris occurs when the heart's demand for oxygen temporarily exceeds its available supply (ischemia), resulting in chest pain or discomfort. Angina is typically triggered by exertion, which increases myocardial oxygen consumption and demand. When the patient ceases exertion, oxygen

YOU are the EMT SUMMARY continued

supply and demand are rebalanced and the pain resolves, usually within a few minutes. In more severe cases, a combination of rest and nitroglycerin are required for resolution of the patient's chest pain or discomfort.

An AMI occurs when a portion of the heart muscle is completely deprived of oxygen because of complete occlusion of one or more coronary arteries. Unlike angina, the chest pain, pressure, or discomfort associated with an AMI typically does not resolve with rest or nitroglycerin and persists for greater than a few minutes. The patient experiencing an AMI needs prompt treatment in the hospital, which is aimed at removing the clot in the coronary artery and reestablishing distal blood flow.

12. As an EMT, how can you distinguish angina pectoris from an AMI?

The signs and symptoms of angina and an AMI are essentially the same and usually cannot be distinguished without advanced diagnostic procedures. In both conditions, the chest pain or discomfort may be described as a feeling of pressure or heaviness. The patient requires physician evaluation, blood analysis, and other tests to diagnose an AMI. You should assume that any patient with nontraumatic chest pain or discomfort is experiencing an AMI until ruled out by a physician.

Prep Kit

Ready for Review

- The heart is divided down the middle into two sides, right and left, each with an upper chamber called the atrium and a lower chamber called the ventricle.
- The heart valve that keeps blood moving through the circulatory system in the proper direction is the aortic valve, which lies between the left ventricle and the aorta, the body's main artery.
- The heart's electrical system controls the heart rate and helps the atria and ventricles work together to pump the blood.
- During periods of exertion or stress, the myocardium requires more oxygen. The oxygen is supplied by dilation of the coronary arteries, which increases blood flow.
- Common places to feel for a pulse include the carotid, femoral, brachial, radial, posterior tibial, and dorsalis pedis arteries.
- Low blood flow to the heart is usually caused by coronary artery atherosclerosis, a disease in which cholesterol plaques build up inside blood vessels, eventually occluding them.
- Occasionally a brittle plaque in an artery will crack, causing a blood clot to form. Heart tissue downstream will experience a lack of oxygen and, within 30 minutes, will begin to die. This condition is called an AMI, or heart attack.
- Heart tissues that are not getting enough oxygen but are not yet dying can cause pain called angina. The pain of an AMI is different from the pain of angina in that it can come at any time, not just with exertion; it lasts up to several hours, rather than just a few moments; and it is not relieved by rest or nitroglycerin.
- In addition to crushing chest pain, signs of AMI include sudden onset of weakness, nausea, and sweating; sudden dysrhythmia; pulmonary edema; and even sudden death.
- AMIs can cause sudden death, usually the result of cardiac arrest caused by abnormal heart rhythms called dysrhythmias. These include tachycardia, bradycardia, VT, and, most commonly, VF.
- A second consequence of an AMI is cardiogenic shock. Symptoms include restlessness; anxiety;

Prep Kit continued

pale, clammy skin; pulse rate higher than normal; and blood pressure lower than normal. Patients with these symptoms should receive oxygen, assisted ventilations as needed, and immediate transport.

- A third consequence of an AMI is heart failure, in which damaged heart muscle can no longer contract effectively enough to pump blood through the system. The lungs become congested with fluid, breathing becomes difficult, the heart rate increases, and the left ventricle enlarges.
- Signs of heart failure include swollen ankles from dependent edema, rapid heart rate and respirations, crackles, and, sometimes, pink sputum and dyspnea if acute pulmonary edema is present.
- Treat a patient with heart failure as you would a patient with chest pain. Monitor the patient's vital signs. Apply CPAP if it is available and you are authorized to use it. Give the patient oxygen via a nonrebreathing mask if they will not tolerate CPAP or it is not available. Allow the patient to remain sitting up.
- When treating patients with chest pain or discomfort, obtain a SAMPLE history, following the OPQRST mnemonic to assess the pain; measure and record vital signs; ensure the patient is in a comfortable position (usually semireclining or half sitting up); administer aspirin, prescribed nitroglycerin, and oxygen; and transport the patient, reporting to medical direction as you do.
- The chain of survival, which is the sequence of events that must happen for a patient with cardiac arrest to have the best chance of survival and recovery, includes recognition of early warning signs and immediate activation of EMS, immediate high-quality CPR, rapid defibrillation, advanced EMS, postarrest care, and recovery and survivorship.

Vital Vocabulary

acute coronary syndrome (ACS) A group of symptoms caused by myocardial ischemia; includes angina and myocardial infarction.

acute myocardial infarction (AMI) A heart attack; death of heart muscle following obstruction of blood flow to it. "Acute" in this context means "new" or "happening right now."

angina pectoris Transient (short-lived) chest discomfort caused by partial or temporary blockage of blood flow to the heart muscle; also called angina.

anterior The front surface of the body; the side facing you in the standard anatomic position.

aorta The main artery, which receives blood from the left ventricle and delivers it to all the other arteries that carry blood to the tissues of the body.

aortic aneurysm A weakness in the wall of the aorta that makes it susceptible to rupture.

aortic valve The one-way valve that lies between the left ventricle and the aorta and keeps blood from flowing back into the left ventricle after the left ventricle ejects its blood into the aorta; one of four heart valves.

artifact A tracing on an ECG that is the result of interference, such as patient movement, rather than the heart's electrical activity.

asystole The complete absence of all heart electrical activity.

atherosclerosis A disorder in which cholesterol and calcium build up inside the walls of blood vessels, eventually leading to partial or complete blockage of blood flow.

atrium One of the two upper chambers of the heart.

automaticity The ability of cardiac muscle cells to contract without stimulation from the nervous system.

Prep Kit continued

autonomic nervous system The part of the nervous system that controls the involuntary activities of the body such as the heart rate, blood pressure, and digestion of food.

bradycardia A slow heart rate, less than 60 beats/min.

cardiac arrest An event in which the heart fails to generate effective and detectable blood flow; pulses are not palpable in cardiac arrest, even if muscular and electrical activity continues in the heart.

cardiac output A measure of the volume of blood circulated by the heart in 1 minute, calculated by multiplying the stroke volume by the heart rate.

cardiogenic shock A state in which not enough oxygen is delivered to the tissues of the body, caused by low output of blood from the heart. It can be a severe complication of a large acute myocardial infarction, as well as other conditions.

coronary arteries The blood vessels that carry blood and nutrients to the heart muscle.

defibrillate To shock a fibrillating (chaotically shaking) heart with specialized electric current in an attempt to restore a normal, rhythmic beat.

dependent edema Swelling in the part of the body closest to the ground, caused by collection of fluid in the tissues; a possible sign of heart failure.

dilation Widening of a tubular structure such as a coronary artery.

dissecting aneurysm A condition in which the inner layers of an artery, such as the aorta, become separated, allowing blood (at high pressures) to flow between the layers.

dysrhythmia An irregular or abnormal heart rhythm.

heart failure A disorder in which the heart loses part of its ability to effectively pump blood, usually as a result of damage to the heart muscle and usually resulting in a backup of fluid into the lungs if the left ventricle is involved.

hypertensive emergency An emergency situation created by excessively high blood pressure, which can lead to serious complications such as stroke or aneurysm.

infarction Death of a body tissue, usually caused by interruption of its blood supply.

inferior Below a body part or nearer to the feet.

ischemia A lack of oxygen that deprives tissues of necessary nutrients, resulting from partial or complete blockage of blood flow; potentially reversible because permanent injury has not yet occurred.

lumen The inside diameter of an artery or other hollow structure.

myocardium The heart muscle.

occlusion A blockage, usually of a tubular structure such as a blood vessel.

parasympathetic nervous system The part of the autonomic nervous system that controls vegetative functions such as digestion of food and relaxation.

perfusion The circulation of oxygenated blood within an organ or tissue in adequate amounts to meet the cells' current needs.

posterior The back surface of the body; the side away from you in the standard anatomic position.

stroke volume The volume of blood ejected with each ventricular contraction.

superior Above a body part or nearer to the head.

sympathetic nervous system The part of the autonomic nervous system that controls active functions such as responding to fear (also known as the fight-or-flight system).

syncope A fainting spell or transient loss of consciousness.

tachycardia A rapid heart rate, more than 100 beats/min.

thromboembolism A blood clot that has formed within a blood vessel and is floating within the bloodstream.

Prep Kit continued

ventricle One of the two lower chambers of the heart.

ventricular fibrillation (VF) Disorganized, ineffective quivering of the ventricles, resulting in no blood flow and a state of cardiac arrest.

ventricular tachycardia (VT) A rapid heart rhythm in which the electrical impulse begins in the ventricle (instead of the atria), which may result in inadequate blood flow and eventually deteriorate into cardiac arrest.

References

1. Heart disease facts. Centers for Disease Control and Prevention website. https://www.cdc.gov/heart-disease/data-research/facts-stats/. Published October 24, 2024. Accessed February 21, 2025.
2. National Center of Health Statistics. Health, United States. Heart disease prevalence. Centers for Disease Control and Prevention website. https://www.cdc.gov/nchs/hus/topics/heart-disease-prevalence.htm. Reviewed August 5, 2024. Accessed December 19, 2024.
3. Gulati M, Levy PD, Mukherjee D, et al. 2021 AHA/ACC/ASE/CHEST/SAEM/SCCT/SCMR guideline for the evaluation and diagnosis of chest pain: a report of the American College of Cardiology/American Heart Association Joint Committee on Clinical Practice Guidelines. *Circulation*. 2021;144(22):e368–e454. doi:10.1161/CIR.0000000000001029
4. Bμkgaard JS, Viereck S, Møller TP, Ersbøll AK, Lippert F, Folke F. The effects of public access defibrillation on survival after out-of-hospital cardiac arrest: a systematic review of observational studies. *Circulation*. 2017;136(10):954–965.
5. Terry K. What's behind major rise in heart failure deaths? WebMD website. https://www.webmd.com/heart-disease/heart-failure/news/20240503/heart-failure-mortality-rate-continues-to-rise. Published May 3, 2023. Accessed December 19, 2024.
6. National Association of State EMS Officials. *National Model EMS Clinical Guidelines: Version 3.0.* https://nasemso.org/wp-content/uploads/National-Model-EMS-Clinical-Guidelines_2022.pdf. Updated March 2022. Accessed December 19, 2024.
7. New heart attack care certification available for hospitals and health systems. American Heart Association website. https://newsroom.heart.org/news/new-heart-attack-care-certification-available-for-hospitals-and-health-systems. Published August 17, 2022. Accessed December 19, 2024.
8. 2020 American Heart Association Guidelines for Cardiopulmonary Resuscitation and Emergency Cardiovascular Care. American Heart Association website. https://professional.heart.org/en/science-news/2020-aha-guidelines-for-cpr-and-ecc. Published October 21, 2020. Accessed December 19, 2024.
9. Devices that may interfere with ICDs and pacemakers. American Heart Association website. https://www.heart.org/en/health-topics/arrhythmia/prevention--treatment-of-arrhythmia/devices-that-may-interfere-with-icds-and-pacemakers. Reviewed October 29, 2024. Accessed December 19, 2024.

Additional Resources

American Heart Association (AHA). *Pediatric Advanced Life Support Provider Manual*. Dallas, TX: AHA; 2020.

Berg KM, Bray JE, Ng KC, et al. 2023 International consensus on cardiopulmonary resuscitation and emergency cardiovascular care science with treatment recommendations: summary from the Basic Life Support; Advanced Life Support; Pediatric Life Support; Neonatal Life Support; Education, Implementation, and Teams; and First Aid Task Forces. *Circulation*. 2023;148(24):e187–e280. doi:10.1161/CIR.0000000000001179

Martin SS, Aday AW, Almarzooq ZI, et al. 2024 heart disease and stroke statistics: a report of US and global data from the American Heart Association [published correction appears in *Circulation*. 2024 May 7;149(19):e1164]. *Circulation*. 2024;149(8):e347–e913. doi:10.1161/CIR.0000000000001209

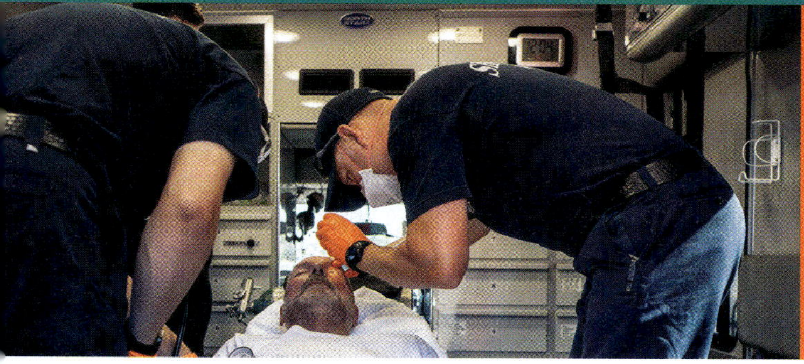

Chapter 18

Neurologic Emergencies

NATIONAL EMS EDUCATION STANDARD COMPETENCIES

Medicine

Applies fundamental knowledge to provide basic emergency care and transportation based on assessment findings for an acutely ill patient.

Neurology

- Decreased level of responsiveness (pp 743–745)
- Seizure (pp 738–743, 757–758)
- Stroke (pp 734–738, 756–757)
- Dementia vs delirium (Chapter 23, *Behavioral Health Emergencies*)
- Alzheimer disease (Chapter 23, *Behavioral Health Emergencies*)
- Headache (pp 732–733, 755–756)
- Brief resolved unexplained event (BRUE) (Chapter 35, *Patients With Special Challenges*)

KNOWLEDGE OBJECTIVES

1. Describe the anatomy, physiology, and functions of the brain and spinal cord. (pp 730–731)
2. Discuss the different types of headaches, the possible causes of each, and how to distinguish a harmless headache from a potentially life-threatening condition. (pp 732–733)
3. Explain the various ways blood flow to the brain may be interrupted and cause a cerebrovascular accident. (pp 734–736)
4. Discuss the causes, similarities, and differences of an ischemic stroke, hemorrhagic stroke, and transient ischemic attack. (pp 734–736)
5. List the general signs and symptoms of stroke and how those symptoms manifest if the left hemisphere of the brain is affected and if the right hemisphere of the brain is affected. (p 737)
6. List three conditions with symptoms that mimic stroke and the assessment techniques emergency medical technicians (EMTs) may use to identify them. (p 738)
7. Define a general seizure, focal-onset seizure, and status epilepticus; include how they differ from each other and their effects on patients. (pp 738–740)
8. Describe how the different stages of a seizure are characterized. (pp 738–740)
9. Discuss the importance for EMTs to recognize when a seizure is occurring or whether one has already occurred in a patient. (pp 741–742)
10. Explain the postictal state and the specific patient care interventions that may be necessary. (p 742)
11. Discuss the clinical significance of syncope. (pp 742–743)
12. Define altered mental status; include possible causes and the patient assessment considerations that apply to each. (pp 743–745, 757)
13. Discuss scene safety considerations when responding to a patient with a neurologic emergency. (pp 745–746)

14. Explain the special considerations required for pediatric patients who exhibit altered mental status. (p 745)
15. Explain the primary assessment of a patient who is experiencing a neurologic emergency and the necessary interventions that may be required to address all life threats. (pp 746–748)
16. Describe the process of history taking for a patient who is experiencing a neurologic emergency and how this process varies depending on the nature of the patient's illness. (pp 748–749)
17. Explain the secondary assessment of a patient who is experiencing a neurologic emergency. (p 749)
18. Explain how to use stroke assessment tools to rapidly identify a stroke patient; include two commonly used tools. (pp 749–752)
19. Explain the concept of a stroke alert and the important time frame for the most successful treatment outcome for a patient who is suspected of having a stroke. (p 749)
20. List the key information EMTs must obtain and document for a stroke patient during assessment and reassessment. (pp 752–755)
21. Explain the care, treatment, and transport of patients who are experiencing headaches, stroke, seizure, and altered mental status. (pp 755–757)
22. Explain the special considerations required for geriatric patients who are experiencing a neurologic emergency. (p 756)

SKILLS OBJECTIVE

1. Demonstrate how to use a stroke assessment tool such as the Cincinnati Prehospital Stroke Scale or the BE-FAST mnemonic to test a patient for aphasia, facial weakness, and motor weakness. (pp 749–755)

Introduction

Stroke is the fifth leading cause of death and a leading cause of disability in the United States, according to the American Stroke Association.[1] Although stroke is common in geriatric patients, it may happen to anyone. Contributing factors for stroke include family history and race and ethnicity: people of African American, Hispanic, and Asian descent have an increased risk of stroke. Fortunately, treatments are available for stroke, and many hospitals are certified stroke centers. Stroke centers vary in capabilities, as discussed later in this chapter. Some patients can avoid the devastating consequences of an acute stroke if they reach a hospital in time for treatment. Seizures and altered mental status may occur in patients with brain disorders. Seizures may occur as a result of a recent or a prior head injury, a brain tumor, a metabolic disease, fever, or a genetic disposition. Your ability to recognize when a seizure has occurred or is occurring is a critical step because you can then provide the appropriate treatment.

Altered mental status is common in patients with a wide variety of medical conditions. However, avoid making assumptions about the cause of a patient's altered mental status. Many causes are possible, some obvious, some not: intoxication, head injury, hypoxia, stroke, metabolic disturbances, and many more. Treatment also varies based on what causes the altered mental status. Caring for patients with altered mental status can be challenging because they may not be able to answer questions or follow instructions, and their behavior may be unpredictable or combative. This chapter will help you better understand, communicate with, and care for patients experiencing neurologic emergencies. Remember, your professionalism is paramount in these situations.

This chapter describes the structure and function of the brain and reviews the most common causes of brain disorders, including stroke, transient ischemic attacks (TIAs), seizures, headaches, and altered mental status. The signs and symptoms of each condition are explained as well as how to approach and assess a patient with a neurologic emergency and why prompt transport to an appropriate medical facility is so important.

Anatomy and Physiology

The brain is the body's computer. It controls breathing, speech, and all other body functions. All thoughts, memories, needs, and desires reside in the brain. Different parts of the brain perform different functions. For example, some parts of the brain receive input from the senses, including sight, hearing, taste, smell, and touch; some control the muscles and movement; and some control the formation of speech. The brain also regulates emotion, which can play a role in many different patient encounters.

The brain is divided into three major parts: the brainstem, the cerebellum, and the cerebrum, which is the largest part (**FIGURE 18-1**). The brainstem controls the most basic functions of the body, such as breathing, blood pressure, swallowing, and pupil constriction. Located just behind the brainstem is the cerebellum, which controls muscle and body coordination. The cerebellum is responsible for coordinating complex tasks that involve many muscles, such as standing on one foot without falling, walking, writing, picking up a coin, and playing the piano.

The cerebrum, located above the cerebellum, is divided down the middle into the right and left cerebral hemispheres. Each hemisphere controls activities on the opposite side of the body. The front part of the cerebrum controls emotion and thought, and the middle part controls sensation and movement. The back part of the cerebrum processes sight. In most people, speech is controlled on the left side of the brain, near the middle of the cerebrum.

Messages sent to and from the brain travel through nerves. Twelve pairs of cranial nerves run directly from the brain to various parts of the body, especially in the head, such as the eyes, ears, nose, and face. The remaining nerves join in the spinal cord and exit the brain through a large opening in the base of the skull called the foramen magnum (**FIGURE 18-2**). At each vertebra in the neck and back, two nerves, called spinal nerves, branch out from the spinal cord, one on each side, and carry signals to and from the body.

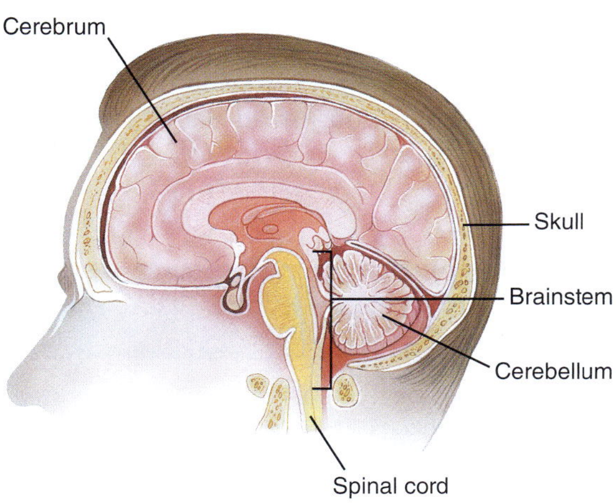

FIGURE 18-1 The brain is well protected within the skull. The brain's major parts are the cerebrum, the cerebellum, and the brainstem.

Special Populations

AGING-RELATED CHANGES IN THE NERVOUS SYSTEM

Aging produces changes in the nervous system that are reflected in the neurologic examination. Changes in thinking speed, memory, and postural stability are the most common normal findings in older people. Studies have documented age-associated declines in mental function, especially slower central processing of sensory stimuli and language, and longer retrieval times for short- and long-term memory.

The brain decreases in mass as a person ages. This increases the amount of space in the cranium, thus increasing the chance for brain injuries. In addition, there is a loss of white matter, the nerve fibers that contain myelin, in older people. These nerve fibers are responsible for transmission of impulses, so the motor and sensory neural networks slow with age. This affects the control of the rate and depth of breathing, heart rate, blood pressure, hunger, thirst, and body temperature. However, the functional significance of these changes is not clear. The human brain has an enormous reserve capacity, and having a smaller, lighter brain does not necessarily interfere with the mental capabilities of all older people.

A growing body of research has identified modifiable risk factors that can delay or prevent dementia or stroke related to aging. It suggests that to reduce risk, individuals should not smoke and should try to maintain weekly aerobic physical activity, a healthy body weight, social engagement, low stress levels, a healthy diet, 7 to 8 hours of sleep per night, and normal blood pressure, blood glucose, and blood cholesterol levels.[2]

Pathophysiology

Many different disorders may cause brain dysfunction or other neurologic symptoms and may affect the patient's level of consciousness, speech, and

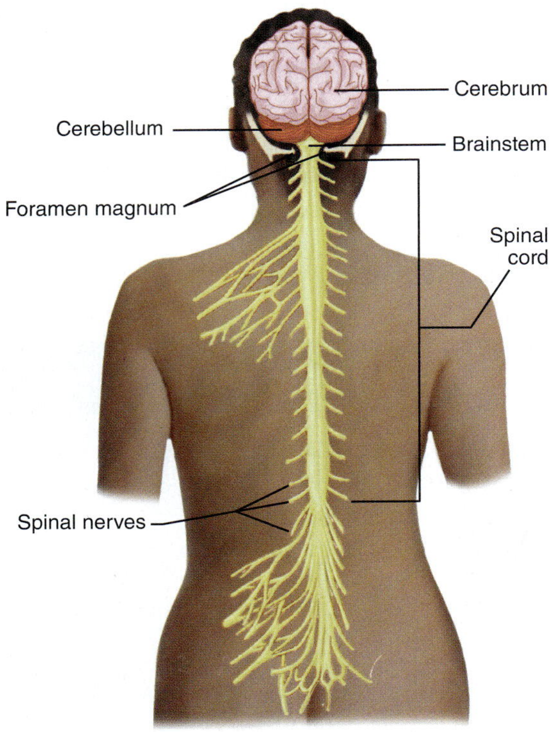

FIGURE 18-2 The spinal cord is the continuation of the brainstem. It exits the skull at the foramen magnum and extends down to the level of the second lumbar vertebra.

voluntary muscle control. The brain is most sensitive to changes in oxygen, glucose, and temperature levels. A significant change in any one of these three levels will result in a neurologic change. In general, if the problem is caused primarily by disorders in the heart and lungs, the entire brain will be affected. For example, when blood flow is stopped (cardiac arrest), the patient will go into a **coma**, a state of profound unconsciousness, and permanent brain damage can result within minutes. However, if the primary problem is in the brain, such as a poor blood supply to one side of the brain, the patient may have signs and symptoms affecting only one side of the body. A low oxygen level in the bloodstream will affect the entire brain, often causing anxiety, restlessness, and confusion. Low blood glucose levels (hypoglycemia) can cause a wide spectrum of symptoms ranging from mild confusion to symptoms that mimic stroke.

Headache

One of the most common complaints of pain you will hear from your patients is headache. Because a headache is subjective, it is often treated as a symptom of another condition; however, a headache may be considered a neurologic condition on its own. Every year, millions of people experience a headache, but only a small percentage of these are caused by a serious medical condition. The brain and skull do not actually sense pain because neither contain pain receptors. The pain associated with a headache is felt from the surrounding areas of the face, scalp, meninges (membranes that cover the brain and spinal cord), larger blood vessels, and muscles of the head, neck, and face.

Tension headaches, migraines, and sinus headaches are the most common types of headaches. These types of headaches are not considered life threatening, although they may be debilitating for the patient. Tension headaches are caused by muscle contractions in the head and neck and are attributed to stress. Patients usually describe the pain as squeezing, dull, or an ache. This type of

YOU are the EMT

At 1823 hours, your unit is dispatched to 106 Scottie Drive. The dispatcher states that a 58-year-old woman is reported to be experiencing a seizure. Bystanders report the patient is unresponsive, with shaking of her extremities and torso. You respond to the scene, which is located approximately 4 miles from your station. The weather is cloudy, the traffic is moderate, and the temperature is 87°F (30.6°C). While en route, you and your partner discuss the different types of seizures.

1. On the basis of the dispatch information, what type of seizure is the patient most likely experiencing?
2. What are some common causes of seizures in this patient's age group?

headache typically does not have any associated symptoms and usually does not require medical attention.

Migraine headaches are thought to be caused by changes in blood vessel size in the base of the brain. Both adults and children can experience migraine headaches. Women are three times as likely as men to experience migraines. Frequently, the patient will have a history of migraines and will tell you that this episode is similar to one in the past. Pain from a migraine headache is usually described as pounding, throbbing, or pulsating. Migraines are often associated with nausea and vomiting and may be preceded by visual warning signs such as flashing lights or partial vision loss. These headaches can last for several hours to days.

Sinus headaches are caused by pressure that is the result of fluid accumulation in the sinus cavities. Patients may also have coldlike signs and symptoms of nasal congestion, cough, and fever if they have a sinus infection. Patients may report increased pain when they bend over or when their heads are moved forward. This type of headache is usually self-limiting, and prehospital emergency care is not required.

Although most headaches are not life threatening, some patients with a chief complaint of headache will require medical attention. Hemorrhagic stroke (bleeding in the brain), brain tumor, and meningitis are serious neurologic conditions that may include headache as a symptom. Be concerned if the patient reports a sudden-onset, severe headache or a sudden-onset headache that has associated symptoms. An incident with multiple patients reporting a headache may indicate carbon monoxide poisoning. Headaches accompanied by a high blood pressure, fever, stiff neck, seizures, or altered mental status or following a head trauma are potentially life threatening and require a complete assessment and transport to the hospital.

A patient who is having a hypertensive crisis may also present with a chief complaint of headache. According to the American Heart Association, a hypertensive crisis occurs when the blood pressure is higher than 180/120 mm Hg with signs and symptoms such as headache, weakness, vision changes, confusion, headache, dizziness, vomiting, chest pain, or shortness of breath.[3]

A hemorrhagic stroke will often present with a complaint of headache that is described as "the worst headache of my life." If a patient describes a headache this way, you should have a high index of suspicion and transport expeditiously to the hospital. The blood from a ruptured blood vessel irritates the tissues of the brain and can cause increased intracranial pressure (ICP), resulting in severe headache pain. This type of pain may initially be localized and then become more diffuse as the irritation in the meninges spreads. You should suspect a hemorrhagic stroke in patients with a severe headache, seizures, and altered mental status. Signs of increased ICP include headache, vomiting, altered mental status, and seizures. Increasing ICP may also be caused by a tumor or by head trauma that may have occurred hours or days before this event. During your patient assessment, ask if the patient has experienced any recent head trauma.

Bacterial meningitis, an inflammation of the meninges caused by a bacterial infection, is a central nervous system infection in which the patient may complain of a headache, stiff neck, fever, and sensitivity to light. This is a serious condition requiring prompt medical attention and is highly contagious. Take standard precautions, and provide supportive care of the ABCs (Airway, Breathing, and Circulation). Provide a quiet, darkened environment when possible, and avoid using lights and siren.

Words of Wisdom

A patient who has a headache associated with any of the following red flags should be evaluated for a potentially life-threatening condition:

- Sudden onset of symptoms
- Headache described by the patient as "the worst headache of my life"
- Explosive/thunderclap pain
- Altered mental status
- Age older than 50 years
- Depressed immune system (known to be at higher risk for infection)
- Neurologic deficits
- Neck stiffness/pain
- Fever
- Changes in vision
- One-sided paralysis or weakness
- Blood pressure higher than 180/120 mm Hg

Stroke

A **cerebrovascular accident (CVA)**, or **stroke**, is an interruption of blood flow to an area within the brain that results in the loss of brain function. In the context of a total lack of oxygen, brain cells stop functioning and begin to die within minutes. Medical science currently has little to offer in the way of treatment once brain cells are dead. However, when oxygen levels are decreased, but not absent, brain cells may be damaged more slowly. It may take several hours or more for brain cells to die in this situation. When brain cells die or are injured, severe disability may result. For example, if cells that are responsible for controlling the left arm are starved for oxygen, the patient will not be able to move that arm. The brain cells will develop **ischemia**, a reduction in blood supply that results in inadequate oxygen being supplied to the brain cells. This causes those cells to stop functioning properly. If normal blood flow is restored to that area of the brain in time, the cells will not die and the patient may regain full use and control of the arm.

Unfortunately, many patients experiencing a stroke deny or ignore their symptoms and delay seeking medical attention. The delay in seeking care can result in devastating consequences, because "time is brain."

Words of Wisdom

Stroke patients who receive treatment within the first few hours of the onset of stroke symptoms have a much greater chance of surviving and avoiding long-term brain damage. Patients with ischemic strokes, the most common type of stroke, may be candidates for treatment with medications to lyse, or dissolve, the clot that is causing the stroke, or with treatment to remove the clot by inserting a tiny catheter into an artery and guiding it to the site of the clot using fluoroscopic imaging that allows a real-time view of the blood vessels. These treatments must be completed soon after a stroke to have the best chance of reversing the symptoms. Note the time of symptom onset, and transport to a stroke center depending on local protocol. Sometimes the gap from last known well time to initiation of effective treatment can be 24 hours or longer, but sooner is better in terms of restoring long-term function.

Types of Stroke

The two main types of stroke are ischemic and hemorrhagic. An ischemic stroke occurs when blood flow through the cerebral arteries is blocked. In hemorrhagic stroke, a blood vessel ruptures and

YOU are the EMT

You arrive at the scene, where you are greeted by the patient's sister. She tells you they were having a conversation when the patient suddenly grabbed both sides of her head and then began "shaking all over." The patient is lying on the floor in her living room with a pillow under her head. She is conscious but confused and reports a severe headache. You perform an assessment as your partner opens the jump bag.

Recording Time: 0 Minutes	
Appearance	Skin is dry and slightly pale (compared with baseline skin color)
Level of consciousness	Conscious, but confused
Airway	Open; clear of secretions and foreign bodies
Breathing	Rapid rate; adequate depth
Circulation	Radial pulse rapid and bounding

Your partner prepares to take the patient's vital signs. The patient's sister tells you her sister has never had a seizure before. The patient is wearing a medical alert bracelet, which identifies her medical history of high blood pressure, heart disease, and type 2 diabetes.

3. What additional questions should you ask the patient's sister?
4. What prehospital assessments can you perform to determine the possible cause of the patient's seizure?
5. What treatment is indicated at this point?

the accumulated blood causes increased pressure in the brain.

Ischemic Stroke

According to the American Stroke Association, **ischemic stroke** is the most common type of stroke, accounting for 87% of all strokes.[4] When blood flow to a specific part of the brain is stopped by a blockage inside a blood vessel, the result is an ischemic stroke. Patients who experience an ischemic stroke may have dramatic symptoms, including loss of movement on the side of the body opposite the side where the occlusion has occurred.

This blockage may be due to **thrombosis**, where a clot forms at the site of a damaged blood vessel (referred to as a thrombus) and obstructs blood flow, or an **embolism**, where the blood clot forms in a remote area, such as a diseased heart, and then travels to the site (referred to as an embolus) and obstructs blood flow. Patients with atrial fibrillation (a heart rhythm where the atria shake rather than squeeze) are susceptible to ischemic strokes caused by an embolus and often take blood thinners (anticoagulants) to reduce the risk of these events.

As with coronary artery disease, atherosclerosis in the blood vessels is often the cause of ischemic stroke. **Atherosclerosis** is a disorder in which calcium and cholesterol build up, forming plaque inside the walls of the blood vessels. This plaque may obstruct blood flow and interfere with the vessels' ability to dilate. Eventually, atherosclerosis may cause complete occlusion of an artery (**FIGURE 18-3**). In other cases, an atherosclerotic plaque in the carotid artery in the neck ruptures. A blood clot forms over the crack in the plaque. Sometimes, it grows large enough to completely block all blood flow through that artery. The parts of the brain supplied by the artery are deprived of oxygen and stop functioning.

Even if the blockage in the carotid artery is not complete, smaller pieces of the blood clot may embolize (break off and be carried by the normal flow of blood) deep into the brain, where they may become lodged in a smaller branch of a blood vessel. This cerebral embolism then blocks blood flow (**FIGURE 18-4**). Depending on the location of the lodged blood clot, the patient's symptoms can vary widely, from nothing at all to complete paralysis or loss of function to the areas or functions of the body controlled by that portion of the brain.

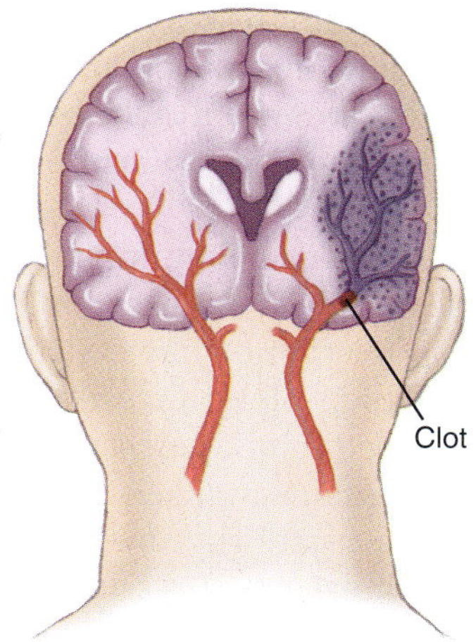

FIGURE 18-3 Atherosclerosis can damage the wall of a cerebral artery, producing narrowing and/or a blood clot. When a vessel is narrowed or completely blocked, blood flow to part of the brain may be blocked, causing brain cells to die because of the lack of adequate oxygenation.

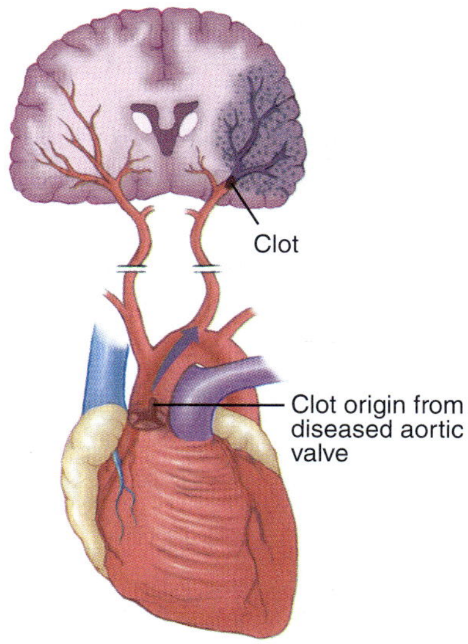

FIGURE 18-4 An embolus, a blood clot formed elsewhere in the body, such as on a diseased heart valve, can travel through the body's vascular system, lodge in a cerebral artery, and cause a stroke.

Hemorrhagic Stroke

Hemorrhagic stroke occurs as a result of bleeding inside the brain. According to the American Stroke Association, hemorrhagic strokes account for 13% of all strokes.[5] In hemorrhagic stroke, a blood vessel ruptures, and the accumulated blood then forms a blood clot, which compresses the brain tissue next to it. The compression prevents oxygenated blood from getting into the area, and the brain cells begin to die. Cerebral hemorrhages are often massive and rapidly fatal.

Hemorrhagic stroke commonly occurs in people experiencing stress or exertion. The people at highest risk for hemorrhagic stroke are those with extremely high blood pressure or long-term untreated elevated blood pressure. Many years of high blood pressure weaken the blood vessels in the brain. If a vessel ruptures, the bleeding in the brain will increase the pressure inside the cranium. Proper treatment of high blood pressure can help prevent this long-term damage to the blood vessels, decreasing the risk of this devastating complication.

Some people are born with a weakness in the walls of an artery. An **aneurysm**, a swelling or enlargement of the wall of an artery resulting from a defect or weakening of the arterial wall, may then develop (**FIGURE 18-5**). The most notable symptom of a ruptured cerebral aneurysm is often a sudden-onset, severe headache, typically described by the patient as the worst headache they have ever had. A headache will result if the bleeding irritates or puts pressure on the nerves surrounding the brain, such as those in the meninges. The brain tissue itself does not contain pain-sensing fibers, so it is possible for a patient to have a hemorrhagic stroke with no headache and only the neurologic deficits. For this reason, it may be difficult for the EMT to determine if the stroke is hemorrhagic or ischemic. Treat all potential strokes as an emergency.

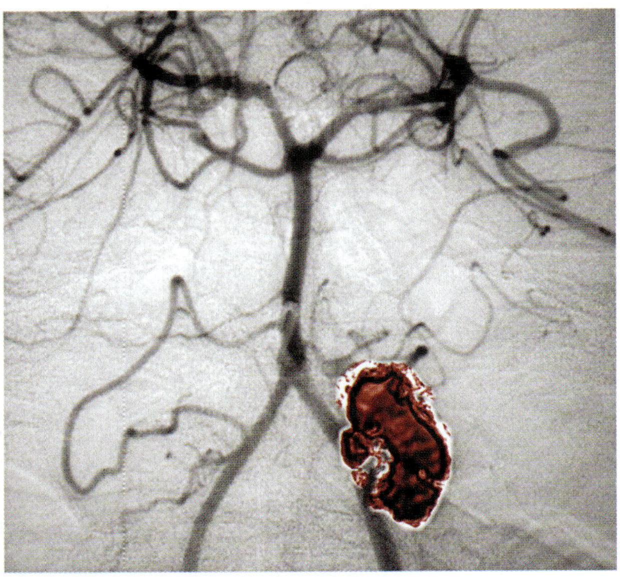

FIGURE 18-5 An angiogram showing a cerebral aneurysm. (Color has been added for illustrative purposes.)

A hemorrhagic stroke in an otherwise healthy young person is often caused by a weakness in a blood vessel called a *berry aneurysm*. This type of aneurysm resembles a tiny balloon (or berry on a stem) that juts out from the artery. When the aneurysm is overstretched and ruptures, blood spurts into an area between two of the coverings of the brain called the subarachnoid space. These types of hemorrhagic strokes are called subarachnoid hemorrhages. If the patient reaches the hospital quickly, surgical repair of the aneurysm may be possible. However, like other brain bleeding and cerebral hemorrhage, this condition is often fatal.

Transient Ischemic Attack

In a patient with coronary artery disease, blood flow to the heart muscle may be obstructed, causing chest pain (angina), which is considered a warning sign of a potential myocardial infarction. Similarly, when blood flow to the brain is obstructed due to atherosclerosis or a small blood clot, the patient may exhibit signs of a stroke. When these stroke-like symptoms resolve on their own (usually within 5 minutes but in less than 24 hours), the event may be caused by a **transient ischemic attack (TIA)**. Some people call these *mini strokes*. As with angina, no actual death of tissue (infarction) occurs if a TIA is confirmed. However, because symptoms of a TIA can last up to 24 hours, you will not be able to differentiate between a stroke and a TIA in the prehospital setting. Even if the symptoms last only a few minutes, the patient needs to be evaluated in the hospital and have specialized testing to determine if any tissue damage has occurred.[6]

Although most patients with TIAs do well, every TIA is an emergency. It may be a warning sign that a more significant stroke may occur in the future. Approximately one in five patients who have a TIA will experience a stroke within 90 days of the TIA.[6] For this reason, all patients with a TIA should be evaluated by a physician to determine whether preventive action should be undertaken.

Signs and Symptoms of Stroke

The general signs and symptoms of stroke depend on the type of stroke and location of the disrupted blood flow. They include the following:

- Facial drooping
- Sudden weakness or numbness in the face, arm, leg, or one side of the body
- Decreased or absent movement and sensation on one side of the body
- Lack of muscle coordination (ataxia) or loss of balance
- Sudden vision loss in one eye; blurred or double vision or abnormal eye movements
- Difficulty swallowing (a primary reason for good airway management in a patient with a stroke)
- Decreased level of responsiveness
- Hearing loss
- Aphasia; difficulty expressing thoughts or inability to use the right words (expressive aphasia) or difficulty understanding spoken words (receptive aphasia)
- Slurred speech (**dysarthria**)
- Sudden and severe headache
- Confusion
- Dizziness
- Weakness
- Combativeness
- Nausea and vomiting
- Restlessness
- Tongue deviation
- Coma

Left Hemisphere

If the left cerebral hemisphere has been affected by a stroke, the patient may exhibit a speech disorder called **aphasia**, the inability to produce or understand speech. Speech problems can vary widely. Some patients will have trouble understanding speech, which is known as receptive aphasia, but will be able to speak clearly. These patients may misinterpret information, have trouble understanding written information, and respond inappropriately. Expressive aphasia occurs when patients understand the question but cannot produce the right sounds or words or leave out words when providing an answer. You can detect this problem by asking the patient a question such as "What day is today?" The patient may respond with an inappropriate answer such as "Green." The speech is clear, but it does not make sense. Some patients have both receptive and expressive aphasia. Strokes that affect the left side of the brain can also cause paralysis of the right side of the body.

Right Hemisphere

If the right cerebral hemisphere of the brain is not getting enough blood, the patient will have trouble moving the muscles on the left side of the body. Usually, the patient will understand language and be able to speak, but the words may be slurred and hard to understand.

Interestingly, patients with right-hemisphere strokes may be completely oblivious to their problems. If you ask these patients to lift their left arm and they cannot, they will lift their right arm instead. Patients will seem to have forgotten that their left arm even exists. This symptom is called neglect. Patients with conditions affecting the back part of the cerebrum may neglect certain parts of their vision. Generally, this is hard to detect in the field because patients compensate without conscious effort. Nevertheless, be aware of the possibility. Sit or stand on the patient's unaffected side because they may be unable to see things on the affected side.

Neglect and lack of pain cause many patients who have had strokes to delay seeking help. A patient may be unaware of a problem until someone points it out.

Bleeding in the Brain

Patients with bleeding in the brain (cerebral hemorrhage) may have very high blood pressure. High blood pressure can either cause the bleeding or be a compensatory response to the bleeding. Blood pressure increases as the body attempts to force more oxygen to the area of the brain where the damage is occurring. Remember, the brain is located inside a box (skull) with only a few openings. When bleeding occurs inside the brain, the pressure inside the skull increases. The body must increase the blood pressure to get blood to the brain's tissues, increasing the pressure even further. A trend of increasing blood pressure is an important sign. Blood pressure may then taper off and return to normal. Significant drops in blood pressure may also occur as the patient's condition worsens. Therefore, it is important to monitor the blood pressure for changes in these patients. The patient who has had a hemorrhagic stroke is more likely to deteriorate quickly than those who have had an ischemic stroke. Their level of consciousness may decline quickly, they are more likely to vomit, and they may experience arrythmias and pulmonary edema if there is a subarachnoid hemorrhage.

Conditions That May Mimic Stroke

The following conditions may appear to be a stroke:

- Hypoglycemia
- A postictal state
- Subdural or epidural bleeding

Because oxygen and glucose are needed for brain metabolism, a patient with hypoglycemia may present in a manner similar to a patient who is experiencing a stroke. Good patient assessment includes finding out whether the patient's medical history includes diabetes. Always check the blood glucose level in patients with altered mental status.

Postictal state refers to the period following a seizure that is characterized by labored respirations and some degree of altered mental status. A patient in a postictal state may resemble a patient experiencing a stroke. However, in most cases, a patient who has had a seizure will recover rapidly, typically within 5 to 30 minutes.

Subdural and epidural bleeding refers to a collection of blood near the skull that presses on the brain. It usually occurs as a result of trauma. The dura is the leathery covering of the brain that lies next to the skull. A fracture near the temples may cause an artery to bleed on top of the dura, resulting in pressure on the brain (**FIGURE 18-6A**). The onset of epidural bleeding is usually very rapid after injury. When the veins just below the dura bleed, this is referred to as subdural bleeding (**FIGURE 18-6B**). Subdural bleeding is slower than epidural bleeding, sometimes occurring over a period of several days. See Chapter 28, *Head and Spine Injuries*, for further discussion.

Words of Wisdom

With epidural hemorrhage after a head injury, the patient may have normal mental status for a period (usually minutes to hours), only to deteriorate markedly. This period between injury and deterioration is called a *lucid interval.* See Chapter 28, *Head and Spine Injuries*, for further discussion.

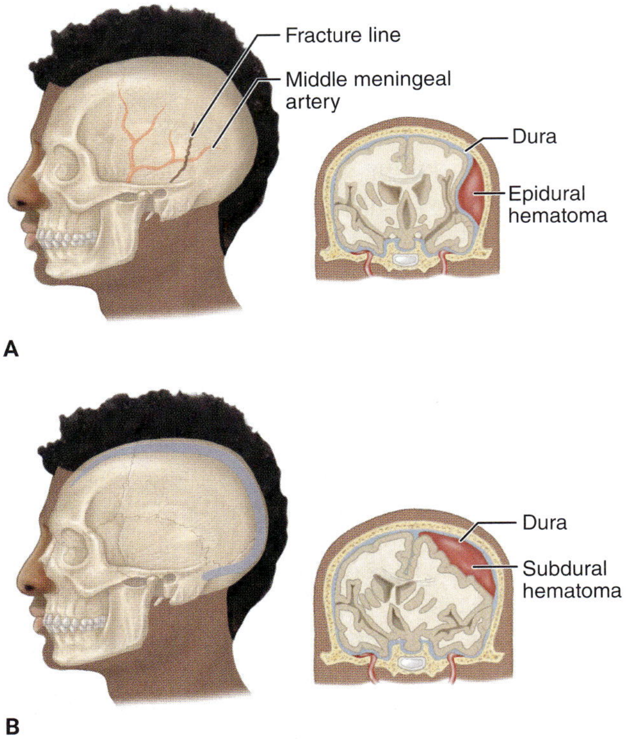

FIGURE 18-6 Trauma to the head may result in intracranial bleeding. **A.** Bleeding outside the dura and under the skull is called epidural bleeding. **B.** Bleeding beneath the dura but outside the brain is called subdural bleeding.

With subdural and epidural bleeding, the onset of strokelike signs and symptoms may be subtle. The patient or family may not even remember the original injury that is causing the bleeding.

Seizures

EMS calls frequently involve seizures. A **seizure** is a neurologic episode caused by a surge of electrical activity in the brain. It can take the form of a convulsion, characterized by generalized, uncoordinated muscle activity, and/or possibly a temporary alteration in consciousness. Nearly 3.5 million people in the United States have **epilepsy**, which is a common cause of seizures.[7] Seizures are classified as either generalized or focal, and their underlying cause can be either known (such as secondary to a brain tumor or a metabolic disorder) or unknown (idiopathic).

A **generalized seizure** results from abnormal electrical discharges from large areas of the brain, involving both hemispheres. It is typically characterized by unconsciousness and a generalized severe twitching of the body's muscles that lasts several minutes or longer (identified as "motor"). In generalized motor seizures (sometimes classified as tonic-clonic), almost all of the muscles in the body are contracting at the same time, causing twitching or jerking motions. In other cases, the seizure may simply be characterized by a brief lapse of consciousness in which the patient seems to stare and not to respond to anyone. This type of seizure does not involve any changes in motor activity and is called a generalized-onset absence seizure.

A **focal seizure** begins in one part of the brain. Focal-onset seizures are classified as either aware or impaired-awareness, and either type can be motor or nonmotor (absence).

In a focal-onset aware seizure, no change occurs in the patient's level of consciousness. Patients may report numbness, weakness, or dizziness. The senses may also be involved; the patient may report visual changes and unusual smells or tastes. A focal-onset aware (motor) seizure may also cause twitching of the muscles and the extremities that may spread slowly from one part of the body to another, but it is not characterized by the dramatic severe twitching and muscle movements seen in a generalized seizure. The patient may also experience brief paralysis.

In a focal-onset, impaired-awareness seizure, the patient has an altered mental status and does not interact normally with the environment. This type of seizure results from abnormal discharges from the temporal lobe of the brain. Other signs may include lip smacking, eye blinking, and isolated convulsions or jerking of the body or one part of the body such as an arm. The patient may experience unpleasant smells and visual hallucinations, exhibit uncontrollable fear, or exhibit repetitive physical behavior such as constant sitting and standing. In impaired-awareness seizures, the patient usually does not remember events occurring during the seizure.

Some focal-onset seizures remain on only one side of the body. Others begin on one side and gradually progress to the entire body. In focal-onset aware seizures, the patient may have no loss of consciousness but still experience body shaking or muscle tremors. Most people with lifelong or chronic seizures tolerate these events reasonably well without complications, but in some patients, seizures may signal life-threatening conditions.

Often, a patient who has epilepsy may experience a warning sign prior to the event. This is referred to as an **aura**. An aura can include visual changes (flashing lights or blind spots in the field of vision) or hallucinations (seeing, hearing, or smelling things that are not actually present). People with a history of seizures recognize their auras and usually take steps to minimize injury, such as sitting or lying down. However, be aware that auras do not occur prior to every seizure, and not all patients with a seizure disorder experience an aura. The experience of an aura is more often associated with focal seizures.

A generalized motor seizure may be characterized by sudden loss of consciousness followed by chaotic muscle movement and tone. The patient may experience a tonic phase, usually lasting only seconds, in which there is a period of extreme muscular rigidity. This period is usually followed immediately by a clonic phase, lasting much longer, of constant muscle contraction and possibly trembling, tongue biting, or **incontinence** (loss of bowel or bladder control). During a generalized seizure, the patient typically may exhibit bilateral movement characterized by a cycle of muscle rigidity and relaxation. Throughout a generalized seizure, the patient exhibits tachycardia, hyperventilation, sweating, and intense salivation; however, other responses are also possible.

Generalized motor seizures typically last less than 5 minutes and are followed by a postictal state (typically 5 to 30 minutes), in which a patient is unresponsive at first and gradually regains consciousness. The postictal state is over when the patient completely returns to a normal level of consciousness. In most cases, the patient will gradually begin to recover and awaken but appear dazed, confused, and fatigued. In contrast, a generalized nonmotor or absence seizure may last for just seconds, after which the patient fully recovers with only a brief lapse of memory of the event.

Status epilepticus refers to abnormally prolonged seizures that can lead to long-term consequences, including brain damage if not interrupted. A continuous seizure lasting more than 5 minutes or repeated convulsive seizures continuing every few minutes without the person regaining consciousness must be treated as quickly as possible to prevent brain injury. If the seizure lasts longer than 30 minutes, permanent damage may occur.[8]

Recurring or prolonged seizures should be considered immediately life-threatening situations in which patients need emergency medical care. Protect the patient from self-harm, and call for advanced life support (ALS) backup. These patients need medication and possibly advanced airway management to stop the seizure.

Causes of Seizures

Some seizure disorders, such as epilepsy, are congenital. Other types of seizures may be caused by high fevers, structural problems in the brain, or metabolic or chemical problems in the body (**TABLE 18-1**). In addition, a percentage of the population will experience a seizure for which the cause cannot be determined (idiopathic). Epileptic seizures can usually be controlled with medications. Medications patients may take at home to prevent seizures include the following:

- Levetiracetam (Keppra)
- Phenytoin (Dilantin)
- Oxcarbazepine (Trileptal, Oxtellar XR)
- Ethosuximide (Zarontin)
- Lamotrigine (Lamictal)
- Carbamazepine (Tegretol)
- Valproic acid (Depakote)
- Topiramate (Topamax)
- Phenobarbital (Luminal, Solfoton)
- Clonazepam (Klonopin)

Family or caregivers may also have rescue medications to treat the patient if their daily medications fail to prevent a seizure. Rescue medications may include rectal diazepam and intranasal midazolam or diazepam. Remind them to administer these medications if they are available. After they have been administered, monitor the patient's breathing carefully, as these medications have the potential to depress respirations.

Patients with epilepsy will often have seizures if they stop taking their medications or if they do not take the prescribed dose on a regular basis. Other factors that increase the likelihood a patient who has epilepsy will have a seizure include illness, infection, or exposure to alcohol or other toxins.

Seizures may also be caused by abnormalities in the brain, such as a benign or cancerous tumor, an infection (brain abscess, meningitis), or scar tissue from some type of injury within the skull. These seizures are said to have a structural cause. Seizures from a metabolic cause may result from abnormal levels of certain blood chemicals (eg, extremely low sodium level), **hypoglycemia** (low blood glucose level), **hyperglycemia** (high blood glucose level), poisons, drug overdoses, or sudden withdrawal from routine heavy alcohol or sedative drug use, or even from prescribed medications. Phenytoin, a drug that is used to control seizures, may itself cause seizures if the person takes too much.

Seizures may also result from sudden high fevers, primarily in children. This type of seizure, called a **febrile seizure**, is frightening for parents but is generally well tolerated by the child. Always transport a child who has had a febrile seizure to the hospital, as the seizure may be a sign of a serious medical condition. If a child is younger than 6 months or older than 6 years and has a seizure with a fever, it signals a cause other than a simple febrile seizure, such as a brain infection (eg, meningitis, encephalitis) that requires urgent transport to an appropriate facility.[9] All children who experience a brief resolved unexplained event (BRUE) should be transported for evaluation. BRUEs include seizures and syncope.

TABLE 18-1 Common Causes of Seizures

Type	Cause
Epileptic	Congenital origin
Structural	Tumor (benign or cancerous) Infection (brain abscess) Scar tissue from injury (within the skull) Head trauma Stroke
Metabolic	Hypoxia Abnormal blood chemical values Hypoglycemia Poisoning Drug overdose Sudden withdrawal from alcohol or medications
Febrile	Sudden high fever (primarily in children)

Special Populations

SEIZURES IN CHILDREN

Seizures in children may manifest in a wide variety of ways, depending on the age of the child. Seizures in infants can be subtle, consisting of only an abnormal gaze, sucking motions, or "bicycling" motions.
In older children, seizures are more obvious and typically consist of repetitive muscle contractions and unresponsiveness.

The Importance of Recognizing Seizures

Regardless of the type or the cause of a seizure, it is important for you to recognize when a seizure is occurring or whether one has already occurred. You must also determine whether this episode differs from any previous ones. For example, if the previous seizure occurred on only one side of the body and this seizure occurs over the entire body, an additional or new problem may be involved. In addition to recognizing that seizure activity has occurred and/or that something different may now be occurring, you must recognize the postictal state and the complications of seizures.

Most seizures involve vigorous muscle twitching. This excessive demand consumes oxygen that is needed for the vital functions of the body. As a result, there is a buildup of acids in the bloodstream, and the patient may turn cyanotic from the lack of oxygen. Often, the seizures themselves prevent the patient from breathing normally, making the problem worse. In a patient with diabetes, the blood glucose level may decrease because of the excessive muscular contraction of a seizure. If possible, closely monitor the blood glucose level after a patient with diabetes has a seizure.

Recognizing seizure activity also means examining other problems associated with the seizure. For example, the patient may have fallen during the seizure episode and been injured; head injury is the most serious possibility. Some patients may experience bowel or bladder incontinence during a generalized seizure. Therefore, one clue that unresponsive or confused patients may have had a seizure is to find that they were incontinent. Although incontinence can occur with other medical conditions, sudden incontinence is likely a sign of a seizure. The patient will likely be embarrassed on regaining consciousness by this temporary loss of control. Minimize the patient's discomfort by covering the patient and assuring them that incontinence is part of the loss of control that accompanies a seizure.

YOU are the EMT

Your partner reports the patient's vital signs. The patient tells you she is nauseated and her headache, which is still severe, is located on both sides of her head. She further tells you the last thing she remembers was the sudden, severe headache. When she woke up, she was lying on the floor with a pillow under her head. She appears to be having difficulty moving her left side. Her sister tells you she caught the patient before she struck the ground.

Recording Time: 4 Minutes	
Respirations	14 breaths/min; adequate depth
Pulse	100 beats/min; strong and regular
Skin	Baseline skin color
Blood pressure	200/112 mm Hg
Oxygen saturation (Spo_2)	96% (on ambient air)

The patient's blood glucose level is assessed and noted to be 97 mg/dL. Her sister hands you the patient's medication list, which includes benazepril (Lotensin), hydrochlorothiazide, and metformin. The patient says she is noncompliant with her medication regimen.

6. What is your field impression of this patient? Why?
7. On the basis of your field impression, you should monitor the patient for which additional signs and symptoms?

Words of Wisdom

The physician's examination of a patient who has had a seizure will be aided greatly by information you provide about the seizure pattern and changes in that pattern. Record all pertinent information about the seizure in terms of duration, areas of body movement, and possible triggering factors. This requires effective interviewing of available witnesses, family members, and/or caregivers.

The Postictal State

Once a seizure has stopped, the patient's muscles relax, becoming almost flaccid or floppy, and the breathing becomes labored (fast and deep) to compensate for the buildup of acids in the bloodstream. By breathing faster and more deeply, the body can balance the acidity in the bloodstream. With normal circulation and liver function, the acids clear away within minutes, and the patient will begin to breathe more normally. The longer and more intense the seizures, the longer it will take for this imbalance to correct itself. Likewise, longer and more severe seizures will result in longer postictal unresponsiveness and confusion. Once the patient regains a normal level of consciousness, the postictal state is over.

Words of Wisdom

Interventions during the postictal state are important. Patients may be unable to maintain an open airway because of their relaxed and exhausted state; therefore, patient positioning, clearing the airway of secretions, and preventing aspiration are critical steps for achieving the best patient outcomes.

In some situations, the postictal state may be characterized by **hemiparesis**, or weakness and numbness on one side of the body, resembling a stroke. However, unlike a stroke, hypoxic hemiparesis soon resolves. Most commonly, the postictal state is characterized by lethargy and confusion to the point that the patient may be combative. Be prepared for these circumstances in your approach to scene control and in your treatment of the patient's symptoms. If the patient's condition does not improve, consider other possible underlying conditions such as hypoglycemia or infection.

Another seizure complication that results in the inability to move the arm on one or both sides is dislocation of one or both shoulders. In contrast to hemiparesis, this is a very painful injury.

Special Populations

STATUS EPILEPTICUS IN OLDER ADULTS

Status epilepticus is harmful at any age, but because of physical changes caused by the normal aging process, geriatric patients are at greater risk of hypoxia, hypotension, and/or cardiac dysrhythmias.

Syncope

Syncope (fainting) presents with a sudden, temporary, complete loss of consciousness accompanied by loss of muscle tone, followed by a rapid and spontaneous recovery.[10] In some cases, syncope results from a brief episode of postural hypotension that occurs when a person (often an older adult) stands up too quickly, causing their blood pressure to drop. This medical emergency may be complicated by injuries sustained if the person subsequently falls.

Although syncope resolves quickly, it can signal a serious underlying problem, such as the rupture of a brain aneurysm, hemorrhagic stroke, hypotension, internal bleeding, or heart rhythm or structural abnormality. When an adult older than 60 years has a syncopal episode, their risk of hospitalization and death is higher than in younger adults; however, patients of all ages may experience syncope. Other factors that may point to a serious underlying cause for the syncope include the following:

- Absence of other signs and symptoms prior to the syncopal episode
- Syncope that occurred during exertion
- History of structural heart disease or heart failure
- Cerebrovascular disease
- Abnormal vital signs that do not resolve
- Trauma or obvious bleeding
- Abnormal electrocardiogram

Seizures are often mistaken for syncope. Fainting often occurs while the patient is standing, whereas seizures may occur in any position.

Fainting is not associated with a postictal state. Syncope in any patient warrants a thorough history, physical exam, and transport for further evaluation.

Altered Mental Status

Aside from stroke and seizures, the most common type of neurologic emergency you will encounter is a patient with altered mental status. Simply put, **altered mental status** means the patient is not thinking clearly or is incapable of being awakened. In some cases, the patient will be unconscious; other times, the patient may be alert but confused. The range of problems is wide and the causes are many, including hypoglycemia, hypoxemia, intoxication, delirium, drug overdose, unrecognized head injury, brain infection, body temperature abnormalities, brain tumors, and poisonings.

Causes of Altered Mental Status

Hypoglycemia

The clinical picture of patients with altered mental status caused by hypoglycemia is complex. Because oxygen and glucose are needed for brain function, hypoglycemia commonly results in confusion and diminishing level of consciousness, mimicking conditions in the brain associated with stroke. In rare cases, the patient may have hemiparesis similar to that seen with a stroke. The principal difference is that a patient who has experienced a stroke may be alert and attempting to communicate normally, whereas a patient with hypoglycemia almost always has an altered or decreased level of consciousness (**FIGURE 18-7**).

Patients with hypoglycemia commonly, but not always, take medications that lower their blood glucose level. Thus, if the patient appears to have signs and symptoms of stroke and altered mental status, report your findings to medical direction and treat the patient accordingly. Remember, patients with a decreased level of consciousness should not be given anything by mouth.

Patients with hypoglycemia may also experience seizures, and you may arrive at the scene to find a patient in a postictal state: confused and disoriented or unresponsive. The mental status of a patient who has had a typical seizure is likely to improve soon after the seizure stops. In a patient with hypoglycemia, however, mental status is not likely to improve, even after several minutes. Consider the possibility of hypoglycemia in a patient who has had a seizure, especially if the patient has a history of diabetes.

Likewise, consider hypoglycemia in a patient who has altered mental status after an injury such as a motor vehicle crash, particularly if they have a history of diabetes, even when there is the possibility of an accompanying head injury. As with any other patient, look for medical identification jewelry or medications that might confirm your suspicions.

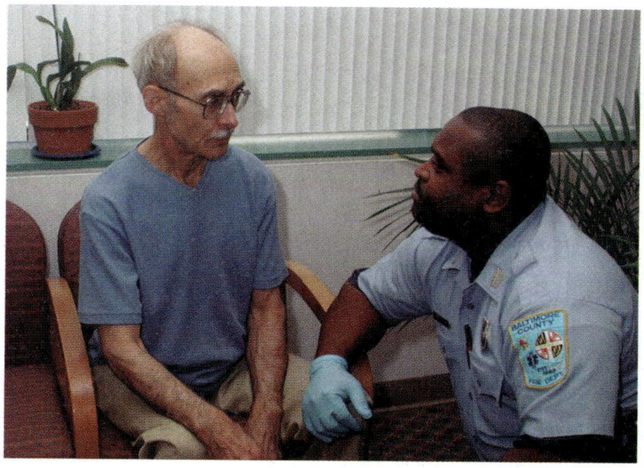

FIGURE 18-7 During your assessment of a patient with an altered or decreased level of consciousness, consider the possibility of hypoglycemia.

Words of Wisdom

Always remember that altered mental status is a symptom, not a disease.

Words of Wisdom

A helpful mnemonic to use when reviewing the possible causes of altered mental status is AEIOU TIPS:

A Alcohol
E Epilepsy, endocrine, electrolytes
I Insulin
O Opioids and other drugs
U Uremia (kidney failure)
T Trauma, temperature
I Infection
P Poisoning, psychogenic causes
S Shock, stroke, seizure, syncope, space-occupying lesion, subarachnoid hemorrhage

Delirium

Delirium is a sudden alteration in cognition and attention during which a person is less able to direct, focus, sustain, or shift attention and awareness. It is a symptom, not a disease. Delirium presents as a new complaint, rather than a long-standing alteration in behavior. It is a temporary state that often has a physical or mental cause (eg, infection, changes in medications, hypoxia) and may be reversed with proper treatment.

Signs and symptoms include confusion and disorientation, disorganized thoughts, inattention, memory loss, striking changes in personality and affect, hallucinations, delusions, or a decreased level of consciousness.[11] The patient may experience a rapid alteration between mental states such as lethargy and agitation. Symptoms of delirium may mimic drug/alcohol intoxication or severe psychological disorders such as schizophrenia.

Special Populations

DELIRIUM IN OLDER ADULTS

In older adults, delirium can be the result of medical conditions such as a urinary tract infection, bowel obstruction, dehydration, fever, cardiovascular disease, hypoglycemia, hyperglycemia, malnutrition, and vitamin deficiencies. Assess the patient for the following specific conditions that can be managed at the prehospital level:

- Hypoxia
- Hypovolemia
- Hypoglycemia
- Hypothermia

Any of these four conditions, if unrecognized or untreated, can be fatal. With these conditions, delirium has a rapid onset and is usually curable if identified early. The onset may be described in terms of minutes, hours, or days. Critical prehospital interventions may include supplemental oxygen, treatment of shock, administration of glucose, and rewarming measures.

During the physical examination, you may see changes in circulation, breath sounds, motor function, and pupillary response. Hypotension can be an indication of hypovolemia. Dilated pupils may suggest brain damage from hypoxia; earlier hypoxia can lead to pupil constriction. Wheezing, crackles, and rhonchi are the result of disease processes that impair breathing and oxygenation.

Treatment will depend on the results of your assessment but should include airway, ventilatory, and circulatory support appropriate to the patient's condition if tolerated by the patient. ALS personnel will attempt venous access to introduce fluids that will help correct hypovolemia. Never assume that altered mental status in an older person is just a normal part of aging.

Dementia

Dementia is a progressive decline in cognitive function that impairs memory function and leads to behavior change. Key characteristics of dementia are a slow decline in attention, memory, ability to learn, language skills, or ability to make decisions. These changes interfere with the person's ability to function independently. Although medication can slow the progression of the signs and symptoms associated with it, dementia is usually irreversible.

Alzheimer disease is the most common type of dementia in older adults.[12] Other forms include Parkinson disease dementia and dementia with Lewy bodies.[13] Other causes of dementia that are reversible in some cases, can occur in younger adults and include diseases of the blood vessels (eg, stroke, hypertension), infections such as Lyme disease and bacterial meningitis, traumatic brain injury, exposure to toxins (eg, alcohol, lead), and problems with metabolism.

The patient who has dementia may also develop delirium related to an illness or injury. This condition will be more difficult to assess. It is important to ask the caregivers if the patient's behavior represents a sudden change from their normal level of functioning.

Street Smarts

When in a home caring for a patient who has Alzheimer disease, it is important to be empathetic to their caregiver. Many people caring for individuals with dementia report stress associated with coordinating care, navigating the health system, obtaining assistance so they can take a break, and affording the resources required to manage health care needs. You can suggest they contact the free Alzheimer's Association helpline (800-272-3900). This service is available around the clock and provides information about resources, crisis assistance, and emotional support for these caregivers.[14]

Other Causes of Altered Mental Status

Other causes of altered mental status include unrecognized head injury and severe alcohol intoxication. Considering other possibilities is important because a patient with altered mental status may be combative and may refuse treatment and transport. Be prepared for difficult patient encounters and follow local protocols for dealing with these situations.

In most cases, a patient who appears intoxicated is just that; however, you must consider other causes as well. A person with chronic alcoholism may have decreased liver function, impaired blood clotting, and immune system abnormalities, causing a predisposition to intracranial bleeding, brain and bloodstream infections, and hypoglycemia.

Psychological disorders and medication complications are also possible causes of altered mental status. A person who appears to have a psychological disorder may also have an underlying medical condition.

Infections, particularly those involving the brain or bloodstream, are another possible cause of altered mental status. Infections in the brain and bloodstream are life threatening and require immediate medical attention. Patients may not demonstrate the typical signs of infection, such as fever, particularly if they are very young or very old or have an impaired immune system. Altered mental status may also be caused by a drug overdose or poisoning.

Patient Assessment

Scene Size-up

The dispatcher may obtain a lot of information about your patient or very little. In some calls, the description of the patient's signs and symptoms will give you a fairly good idea of what the problem may be (the patient has slurred speech or one-sided paralysis). In other calls, the description may be vague (the patient has a headache). Dispatchers are frequently given information regarding a seizure by the caller. Even if the caller has never seen a seizure before, based on the caller's description of the convulsions, the dispatcher will be able to convey this information to the responding crew.

Patients with altered mental status may exhibit a wide range of signs and symptoms and behaviors. The most significant difference between a patient with altered mental status and other emergencies is that a patient with altered mental status cannot reliably tell you what is wrong, and there may be more than one cause. Make an early determination whether the call is medical or trauma related because this will help determine the approach of care for the patient.

Special Populations

ALTERED MENTAL STATUS IN CHILDREN

Children can have altered mental status caused by strokes, seizures, high or low blood glucose levels, infection (eg, meningitis), poisoning, or tumors. Hemorrhagic strokes in children are usually caused by congenital defects in blood vessels, such as berry aneurysms. Ischemic strokes can be caused by disorders such as sickle cell anemia. Children who have sickle cell anemia are at particularly high risk for ischemic stroke. Treat stroke and altered mental status in children the same way you would in adults.

Remember that in children, seizures can result from a rapid increase in body temperature. They are not associated with a specific body temperature and can occur even with a fever as low as 100.4°F (38°C).[15] Also remember that although febrile seizures are generally well tolerated by children, you must provide transport to the hospital to assess for the underlying cause of the seizure. The possibility of a second seizure makes transport mandatory for an evaluation of life-threatening conditions and so that if other problems develop, the child is in the hospital and can receive immediate definitive care.

Do not be distracted by the seriousness of the situation or by frightened family members who want you to rush. Look first for threats to your safety, and take standard precautions.

Consider the need for spinal motion restriction based on dispatch information and your assessment of the scene as you approach the patient. Many calls involving a neurologic emergency would benefit from ALS assistance if it is available. Call for additional resources early.

Look for clues to help you determine the nature of the illness. Special considerations for a patient with a suspected neurologic emergency include an evaluation of the patient's environment, assessing for any signs of potential trauma (mechanism of injury); indications of a medical condition, such as diabetic supplies or medical alert tags; and evidence of a seizure. Answers to the following questions may help you determine the nature of the illness: Did anyone witness what happened? When was the last time the patient appeared normal? Is the patient's bed or furniture in disarray? Most patients with a neurologic emergency display a change in their level of consciousness and their ability to interact with their environment and others.

Primary Assessment

Your first priority is to look for and treat any life-threatening conditions. Perform a rapid exam. Patients become unresponsive or have an altered level of consciousness, especially from a neurologic cause, for many reasons. Use a sound approach to assessing whether the patient is bleeding and the patient's airway, breathing, and circulation to have significant effect on how well these systems respond to your care and treatment.

As you approach the patient, gather information from the scene (is this medical or trauma related?) and note the patient's body position and level of consciousness. This initial impression will help you determine the severity of the situation and help set the pace of your call. A patient lying on the ground in an unnatural position is more likely to have a potentially life-threatening condition than one sitting up in bed. On a call that indicates that a seizure is taking place, you should be able to tell whether the patient is still experiencing a seizure. Unless your arrival time is 1 minute or less, most seizures will be over by the time you arrive. If the seizure is still occurring, the potentially life-threatening condition of status epilepticus may be present. A patient in a postical state may be unresponsive or starting to regain awareness of the surroundings. When you treat any patient with altered mental status, first determine the patient's level of consciousness. To assess the patient's level of consciousness, use the AVPU scale (Awake and alert, responsive to Verbal stimuli, responsive to Pain, Unresponsive).

As with any other situation, focus on the patient's airway and breathing on arrival. Stroke affects how the body functions in many ways. Patients may have difficulty swallowing and are at risk for choking on their own saliva. This risk is especially high if the patient has had a hemorrhagic stroke because vomiting and a rapid decline in alertness are

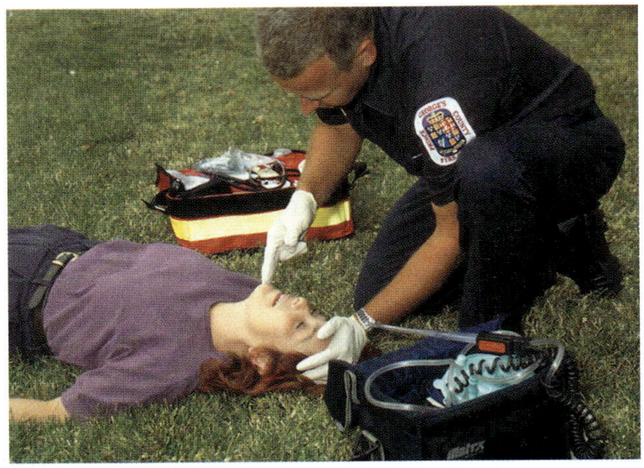

FIGURE 18-8 Securing and maintaining the airway in a patient who is unconscious is extremely important. Have suction readily available in case the patient vomits.

more likely. Evaluate the airway of an unresponsive patient to make sure it is patent and will remain so (**FIGURE 18-8**). If the patient requires assistance maintaining their airway, consider an oropharyngeal or nasopharyngeal airway. The nasopharyngeal airway is often a good choice in a postictal patient, who may gag on an oropharyngeal airway as they become more alert. Be prepared to provide suction, and position the patient to prevent aspiration. If you determine that the patient cannot protect their airway, place the patient in the recovery position to help prevent secretions from entering the airway.

A patient who has had or is experiencing a seizure may have been eating or chewing gum at the time of the seizure, so check for foreign body obstruction. Bystanders may have tried to put objects in the patient's mouth to keep the person from "swallowing their tongue," even though this practice is not advised.[16] Note that it is impossible for a person to literally swallow their tongue, but it is possible for the tongue to fall back and obstruct the entrance to the trachea; the usual airway management techniques, such as the head tilt–chin lift maneuver, will resolve or prevent this threat.

Assess the patient's breathing. Some causes of altered mental status, such as opioid overdose, can also cause alterations in the patient's breathing and ability to manage their own airway. Alternatively, hypoxia can be the cause of an altered mental state, as in the case of unconsciousness from airway obstruction. Seizures cause patients to use oxygen quickly, resulting in hypoxia. Again, in the immediate postictal state following a seizure, you should anticipate rapid, deep respirations and an accompanying fast heart rate resulting from the stress of the severe convulsions. However, the respirations and the heart rate should begin to slow to normal rates after several minutes.

If the adult patient's breathing is absent or inadequate, it is important to ventilate the patient at the appropriate rate with the proper volume. Deliver each breath over a period of about 1 second (with just enough volume to produce visible chest rise) at a rate of 10 breaths/min. Do not hyperventilate the patient; doing so may have several negative consequences. Hyperventilation overinflates the lungs, which can impair blood return to the right atrium and cause a decrease in blood pressure and cardiac output. Hyperventilation also increases the risks of regurgitation and aspiration. In addition to the risks already discussed, hyperventilation may cause severe injury in patients with intracerebral bleeding and increased ICP; it causes cerebral vasoconstriction, which shunts blood (and oxygen) away from the brain. This decrease in cerebral perfusion may cause further injury to the brain.

Circulation should be confirmed as normal or treated as necessary. Your assessment of the patient's circulation should begin with checking the pulse if the patient is unresponsive. If no pulse is found, immediately begin cardiopulmonary resuscitation (CPR), and attach an automated external defibrillator (AED). If a pulse is present, determine whether the pulse is fast or slow, weak or strong. Oxygen administration if the patient's oxygen saturation level is low helps limit the effects of hypoperfusion of the brain. Evaluate the patient quickly for external bleeding. A patient experiencing a stroke is unlikely to have sustained trauma; it is more likely in a patient who has had a seizure. Consider this possibility and assess appropriately.

Establish your priorities of care based on your assessment of the patient's level of consciousness and the ABCs. How the patient presents will guide you as to whether you stay at the scene for further

Street Smarts

When caring for patients with neurologic issues such as stroke or seizures, good interpersonal skills are crucial. Good communication, including active listening with everyone involved, makes potentially difficult calls easier. Compassion and empathy are important in caring for these patients. The patient and family may regard the emotional support you provide as more valuable than the physical skills you perform. Your ability to reassure and make the patient comfortable during assessment and transport is always beneficial.

YOU are the EMT

An engine crew arrives shortly before you load the patient onto the stretcher. Shortly after loading her into the ambulance, you reassess her and note that her condition has deteriorated. One of the engine crew EMTs accompanies you in the back of the ambulance, and you proceed to the hospital.

Recording Time: 10 Minutes	
Level of consciousness	Unconscious and unresponsive
Respirations	6 breaths/min; snoring, irregular, and shallow
Pulse	60 beats/min; bounding
Skin	Nail beds and mucous membranes appear cyanotic
Blood pressure	198/110 mm Hg
Oxygen saturation (Spo_2)	78% (on ambient air)

8. What should be your most immediate action?
9. What additional treatment does this patient require?

assessment or proceed to immediate transport. If you suspect the patient is experiencing a stroke, provide rapid transport to an appropriate facility. Prompt treatment is a critical action to minimize the disability caused by an ischemic stroke.

History Taking

If the patient is unresponsive, you will need to gather any history of the present illness from family or bystanders. If no one is around, quickly look for explanations for the altered mental status (eg, signs of trauma, medical alert tags, track marks resulting from intravenous drug injections, environmental clues such as empty alcohol or medication containers).

To determine the chief complaint in a responsive patient, begin by asking the patient what happened. Look for signs and symptoms that may indicate a cause for the patient's altered mental status, such as a stroke (eg, hemiparalysis or one-sided weakness), or any evidence of a seizure (eg, incontinence, bitten tongue). Evaluate the patient's speech. Is the patient making sense? Is the patient's speech slurred?

If you know that the patient has had a seizure and is now in a postictal state, you will not be able to obtain a history from the patient. Look for any obvious trauma or explanations as to why the patient may have had a seizure. Check whether the patient is wearing medical jewelry or has medical information on their cell phone.

If the patient is responsive and breathing, obtain a SAMPLE history. Also speak with family or friends who may be able to explain the events leading up to the altered mental status, remembering that time is crucial in a neurologic emergency. Make a special effort to determine the exact time that the patient last appeared to be healthy, often referred to as the "last known well" time. In the case of a patient experiencing a stroke, this information will help physicians decide whether it is safe to begin certain treatments that must be given within the first hours after the onset of stroke symptoms. You may be the only person with the opportunity to speak with bystanders to obtain this critical information. Many times, you will be able to find out only that the patient was healthy when they went to sleep the night before. In those cases, the time the patient was last seen to be healthy was at bedtime, not when the patient awoke with symptoms. Collect or list all medications the patient has taken. When possible, determine allergies and the patient's last oral intake.

Although a patient who has had a stroke may appear to be unconscious and unable to speak, the patient may still be able to hear and understand what is taking place. Therefore, avoid making unnecessary or inappropriate remarks. Communicate with the patient by looking for indications that the patient may understand you, such as a glance, gaze, motion or pressure of the hand, effort to speak, or head nod. Reassure your patient that you understand that communication between the two of you may be difficult at this point but that you will provide continuous information as to what you and the other team members are doing. Establish effective communication to help you calm the patient and lessen the fear that accompanies an inability to communicate (**FIGURE 18-9**). Keep in mind that the patient has just experienced a potentially life-threatening event and that anxiety, frustration, and embarrassment may inhibit communication with you.

With patients who have had a seizure, your SAMPLE (Signs and symptoms, Allergies, Medications, Pertinent past medical history, Last oral intake, Events leading up to the illness or injury) history should reveal if the patient has a history of

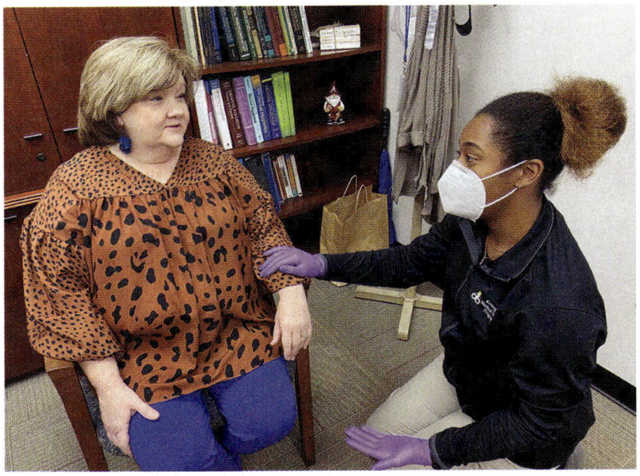

FIGURE 18-9 Make a special effort to establish communication with a patient who may have had a stroke, seizure, or other neurologic emergency that impairs the patient's ability to communicate. Look for indications that the patient understands you, such as a glance, gaze, squeeze of the hand, efforts to speak, or nodding of the head.

Courtesy of Rhonda Hunt.

seizures. If so, it is important to find out how the patient's seizures typically occur and whether this episode differs in some way from previous episodes. Also, ask what medications the patient has been taking, and note medications used to treat a seizure disorder. You might find that the patient ran out of medication or stopped taking the medication for a time. A patient who has a history of seizures *and* diabetes may use up all the glucose in the body to fuel the seizure.

If a patient with no history of seizures suddenly has a seizure, a serious condition should be suspected, such as a brain tumor, intracranial bleeding, or serious infection. This part of the patient assessment process is the time to determine whether the patient takes medications that lower blood glucose, such as insulin or oral hypoglycemic agents. In other situations, you may want to inquire about illicit drug use or exposure to poisons.

Words of Wisdom

When assessing a patient who might have had a stroke, it is important to pinpoint when the symptoms first started. Outcomes are best when treatment is initiated as soon after onset of symptoms as possible. In select cases, there may be a possibility of some recovery of neurologic function, with treatment initiated as long as 24 hours after onset of symptoms. During transport, notify the receiving hospital of when the patient's symptoms first began. If possible, get the phone number of the person who witnessed when the patient was last known well, as the hospital personnel may wish to speak to them. When appropriate, this information will allow hospitals to activate stroke alerts and be ready to immediately start treating these patients as soon as they enter the emergency department (ED). Follow your local protocols.

Secondary Assessment

Your assessment of the patient should continue with a secondary assessment of the entire body, paying particular attention to the system involved. If you suspect your patient is experiencing a stroke, then you should direct particular attention to the neurologic assessment. As always, your secondary assessment should include a complete set of vital signs using the monitoring devices you have available.

Patients with significant intracranial bleeding (hemorrhagic stroke) may have a great deal of pressure in the skull that is compressing the brain, thus slowing the pulse and causing respirations to be erratic. Blood pressure is usually high to compensate for poor perfusion in the brain. Unequal pupil size and reactivity indicate significant bleeding and pressure on the brain. If the patient has altered mental status (regardless of the cause), check the blood glucose level if your local protocol allows. Most commonly, this is done using a portable blood glucose monitor (glucometer), similar to the one your patient may use at home. The portable blood glucose monitor measures the glucose level in whole blood, using capillary or venous samples. Chapter 10, *Patient Assessment*, discusses the use of a glucometer in more detail.

Evaluating vital signs is impossible during most active seizures, and this should not be your priority. In most cases, the vital signs of a patient in a postictal state will be within normal limits. Obtain pulse rate, rhythm, and quality; respiratory rate, rhythm, and quality; blood pressure; skin color, temperature, and condition; oxygen saturation; and pupil size and reactivity. Administer oxygen if the patient's oxygen saturation is 94% or less.[17]

It is recommended that the first blood pressure reading be obtained manually, with a sphygmomanometer (blood pressure cuff) and a stethoscope. You may also use automated noninvasive methods to monitor blood pressure if they are available and you are approved to use them.

Stroke Assessment

A stroke assessment tool should be part of your secondary assessment in patients with a neurologic disorder. It is advisable to use stroke scales to rapidly identify stroke in the field.[18,19] If the patient does not have a normal response to these evaluations, you should strongly suspect a stroke. Rapid transport to a designated stroke center is indicated.

In the prehospital setting, the most commonly used stroke screening tools is the Cincinnati Prehospital Stroke Scale (**TABLE 18-2**) and the Los Angeles Prehospital Stroke Screen (**TABLE 18-3**).

While the Cincinnati Prehospital Stroke Scale and Los Angeles Prehospital Stroke Screen offer fair reliability in detecting anterior circulation ischemic strokes, which are the most common, they are less

TABLE 18-2 Cincinnati Prehospital Stroke Scale

Test	Normal Response	Abnormal Response
Facial droop (**FIGURE 18-10**) (Ask patient to show teeth or smile.)	Both sides of face move equally well.	One side of face does not move as well as the other (droops).
Arm drift (**FIGURE 18-11**) (Ask patient to close eyes and hold both arms out with palms up.)	Both arms move the same, or neither arm moves. (The latter response requires a retest because it may indicate the patient did not understand the instructions.)	One arm does not move, or one arm drifts down and turns toward the body (pronation) compared with the other side.
Speech (Ask patient to say, "You can't teach an old dog new tricks.")	Patient uses correct words with no slurring.	Patient slurs words, uses inappropriate words, or is unable to speak.

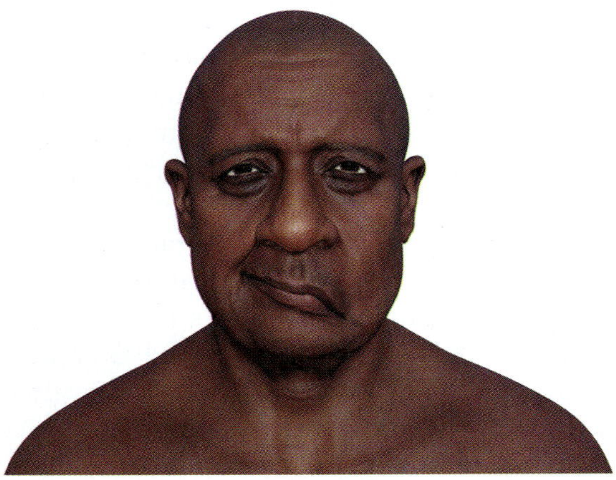

FIGURE 18-10 Facial drooping characteristic of a stroke.

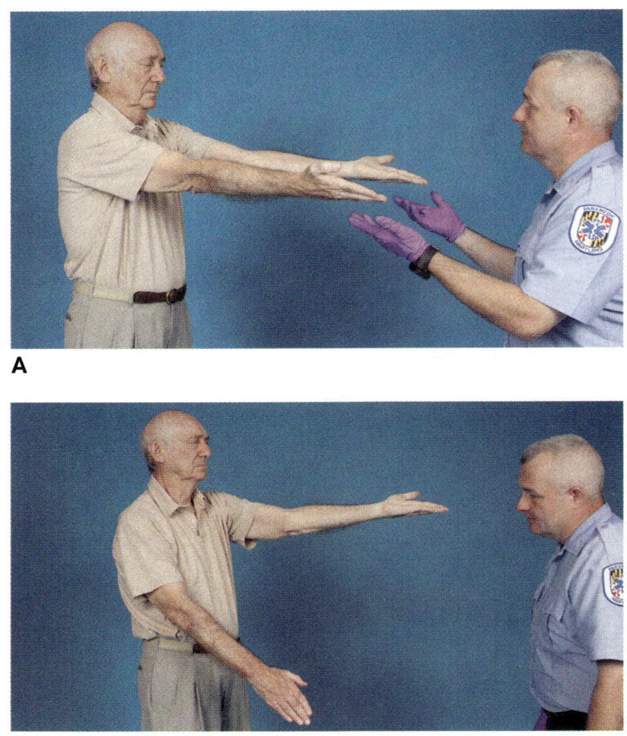

FIGURE 18-11 A. A person who has not had a stroke will be able to hold both arms in front of their body even with their eyes closed. **B.** A person who has had a stroke might not be able to maintain this position. One arm will drift down and turn toward the body.

Words of Wisdom

In the hospital, the most commonly used instrument for evaluating a possible stroke is the NIH Stroke Scale. This 11-step numerical grading system takes approximately 10 minutes to conduct and provides the hospital with very specific information about the patient's condition. In addition, the NIH evaluation can be repeated throughout the patient's hospital stay to compare numerical values related to any changes in condition. This scale is rarely used in the prehospital setting due to its complexity; however, some components of this evaluation can be assessed by asking the patient to identify common objects in the room and to read a short, written passage.

likely to identify posterior circulation strokes.[20,21] A different tool, the BE-FAST stroke scale, evaluates balance and eyes in addition to the face, arms, and speech elements (**TABLE 18-4**). The addition of

TABLE 18-3 Los Angeles Prehospital Stroke Screen

Criterion	Yes	Unknown	No
Interpretation: If all criteria 1–6 are marked yes, the probability of a stroke is 97%.			
1. Age older than 45 years	☐	☐	☐
2. History of seizures or epilepsy absent	☐	☐	☐
3. Symptoms <24 hours	☐	☐	☐
4. At baseline, patient is not wheelchair-bound or bedridden	☐	☐	☐
5. Blood glucose between 60 and 400 mg/dL	☐	☐	☐
6. Obvious asymmetry (right versus left) in any of the following three exam categories (must be unilateral):	☐	☐	☐
	Equal	**Right Weak**	**Left Weak**
Facial smile/grimace	☐	☐ Droop	☐ Droop
Grip	☐	☐ Weak grip ☐ No grip	☐ Weak grip ☐ No grip
Arm strength	☐	☐ Drifts down ☐ Falls rapidly	☐ Drifts down ☐ Falls rapidly

TABLE 18-4 BE-FAST Stroke Assessment

Balance	Did the patient experience a sudden loss of balance or inability to walk?
Eyes	Is there a change in vision? Loss of vision, double vision, or absence of side or top vision?
Facial droop (Ask patient to show teeth or smile.)	Does one side of the patient's face droop when smiling?
Arm drift (Ask patient to close eyes and hold both arms out with palms up.)	Does the patient demonstrate weakness or the inability to move one of the arms?
Speech	Is the patient slurring words or using words that do not make sense?
Time	When did the symptoms first appear? Do not delay transport to an appropriate stroke facility.

these findings has been shown to increase the detection of posterior circulation strokes.

To test speech, ask the patient to repeat a simple sentence such as "You can't teach an old dog new tricks." If the patient does this correctly, you know the patient understands and can produce speech. If the patient cannot repeat the phrase, the problem may be with either understanding speech or producing it.

To test facial movement, ask the patient to smile, showing their teeth (or gums if the patient does not have teeth). Watch whether both sides of the face around the mouth move equally. If only one side is moving well, you know something is wrong with the control of the muscles on the other side.

To test arm movement, ask the patient to hold both arms in front of their body, palms up toward the sky, with eyes closed and without moving. During the next 10 seconds, watch the patient's hands. If you see one side drift down toward the ground, you know that side is affected. If both arms stay up and do not move, you know both sides of the brain are functioning. If both arms fall to the ground, you have not really identified any problems. Perhaps the patient did not understand your instructions. Perform the arm test again, but this time move the patient's arms into position yourself.

Recently, it has been determined that large vessel occlusion (LVO) strokes, which are a subtype of ischemic stroke, can be identified by EMS with fair reliability using specific stroke scales. These strokes, caused by an occlusion of a large blood vessel in the brain, respond well to fibrinolytics or mechanical thrombectomy but require rapid identification and transport to the appropriate level of stroke center to provide the best results (**TABLE 18-5**). Three scales used to detect LVO are the Rapid Arterial oCclusion Evaluation (RACE) scale (**TABLE 18-6**), the Los Angeles Motor Scale (LAMS), and the Vision, Aphasia, Neglect (VAN) scale. A 2021 study of more than 13,500 prehospital patients compared these assessment tools to the Cincinnati Prehospital Stroke Scale with a score of 2 or higher and showed a similar ability to detect LVO.[22]

The LAMS, which is based on the Los Angeles Prehospital Stroke Screen, was developed to identify LVO strokes faster and more accurately to guide EMS to the best transport destination for the patient. The LAMS gives points for facial droop (absent = 0, present = 1), arm drift (absent = 0, slow drift = 1, rapid fall = 2), and grip strength (normal = 0, weak grip = 1, no grip = 2). A score of 4 or more is a strong indication of an LVO stroke and indicates consideration of transport to a comprehensive stroke center, if available.

Become familiar with whatever assessment method and cut-off scores are used by your EMS system.

You should calculate the Glasgow Coma Scale (GCS) score (**TABLE 18-7**) for all patients with altered mental status (ie, stroke, TIA, seizure of unknown cause).

Reassessment

The reassessment should focus on reassessing the ABCs, vital signs, and interventions provided so far. Patients who are experiencing a stroke may lose their airway, or their breathing may stop without warning. Multiple interventions may be necessary. The effectiveness of airway adjuncts, positive-pressure ventilations, and other treatments can be

TABLE 18-5 Stroke Center Levels and Capabilities

Stroke Center Level	Capabilities
Acute Stroke Ready	Has stroke team and computed tomography available 24 hours per day Can administer thrombolytic drug for stroke
Primary Stroke Center	All of the above and: • Has advanced brain imaging 7 days per week • Can diagnose stroke causes and manage complications • Has dedicated stroke unit
Thrombectomy-Capable Stroke Center	All of the above and can perform thrombectomy
Comprehensive Stroke Center	All of the above and: • Admits hemorrhagic stroke • Treats ruptured aneurysms • Has dedicated neurologic intensive care unit

TABLE 18-6 Rapid Arterial oCclusion Evaluation (RACE) Scale

Item	Instruction	Criteria	Score
Facial palsy	Ask patient to show their teeth.	Absent (symmetrical) Mild (slightly asymmetrical) Moderate to severe (completely asymmetrical)	0 1 2
Arm motor function	Extend patient's arm 90° if patient is sitting, or 45° if supine.	Normal to mild function (holds limb up for >10 sec) Moderate dysfunction (holds limb up <10 sec) Severe dysfunction (unable to raise arm, flaccid)	0 1 2
Leg motor function	Ask supine patient to lift leg 30° and hold it.	Normal to mild dysfunction (holds limb up for >5 sec) Moderate (holds limb up <5 sec) Severe (unable to lift leg)	0 1 2
Head and gaze deviation	Observe patient's eyes and head for deviation to one side.	Absent (eye moves to both sides and no head deviation observed) Present (deviation of eyes and head to one side observed)	0 1
Aphasia (if right hemiparesis)	Give two verbal orders: **1.** "Close your eyes." **2.** "Make a fist."	Performs both tasks correctly Performs one task correctly Performs neither task	0 1 2
Agnosia (if left hemiparesis)	Ask the patient: **1.** "Whose arm is this?" (while showing them their impaired arm) **2.** "Can you move your arm?"	Recognizes their arm and impairment Does not recognize their arm or impairment Does not recognize arm nor impairment	0 1 2
Score Total (Any score above 0 prompts a stroke alert.)			

Adapted from Pérez de la Ossa N, Carrera D, Gorchs M, et al. Design and validation of a prehospital stroke scale to predict large arterial occlusion. *Stroke*. 2014;45(1):87–91.

TABLE 18-7 Glasgow Coma Scale[a]

Eye Opening		Best Verbal Response		Best Motor Response	
Spontaneous	4	Oriented conversation	5	Obeys commands	6
In response to sound	3	Confused conversation	4	Localizes to pressure	5
In response to pressure	2	Inappropriate words	3	Withdraws from pressure	4
None	1	Incomprehensible sounds	2	Abnormal flexion (**FIGURE 18-12**)	3
		None	1	Abnormal extension	2
				None	1

[a]Some systems use a "Not testable (NT)" score for any element that cannot be tested. Eye opening cannot be tested in a patient whose eyes are closed due to a local factor, such as swelling; verbal response cannot be tested in a patient who has a preexisting factor interfering with communication, such as mutism; and motor response cannot be tested in a patient who has preexisting paralysis or other limiting factor.

Score: 13–15 may indicate mild dysfunction, although 15 is the score a person without neurologic disabilities would receive.

Score: 9–12 may indicate moderate dysfunction.

Score: 8 or less indicatives severe dysfunction.

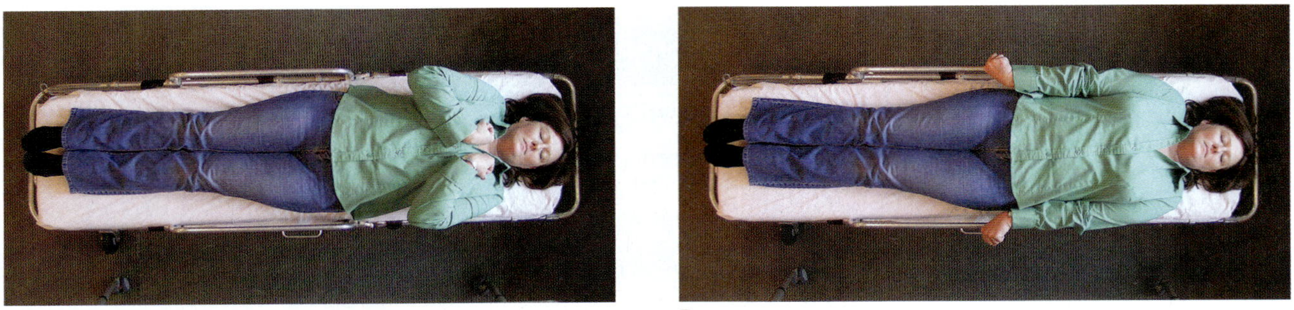

A B

FIGURE 18-12 Decorticate (**A**) or decerebrate posturing (**B**) is a reflexive body position that suggests altered mental status.

Courtesy of Chuck Sowerbrower, MED, NREMT-P.

Words of Wisdom

The following is key information to document for a patient who may have had a stroke:

- Time of onset of the signs and symptoms
- Score on the GCS
- Results of a stroke assessment tool
- Changes noted on reassessment

Establishing the time of onset is critical information because it helps determine whether the patient is a candidate for treatment with blood clot–dissolving drugs or clot-retrieval therapy. If the person who last saw the person well cannot come to the hospital, ask for their phone number to give to hospital personnel.

determined only with immediate and continuous observation after providing the intervention. If an intervention is not working, try something else.

You have already established baseline vital signs during your assessment, as well as a GCS score. Now is the time to compare that baseline information with updated information. Any changes may indicate if treatments are effective. Watch carefully for changes in pulse, blood pressure, respirations, and GCS scores. If time permits during transport and you have the capability to perform it, acquire and transmit a 12-lead electrocardiogram to the receiving facility.[9]

Notify the receiving facility of your patient's chief complaint and your assessment findings. Your

YOU are the EMT

You continue treatment en route to the hospital. You reassess the patient and note that her condition has deteriorated further. Her pupils are unequal, and she exhibits decorticate posturing (flexion posturing to painful stimulus). You call in your report to the receiving facility, with an estimated time of arrival of 6 minutes.

Recording Time: 17 Minutes	
Level of consciousness	Unconscious and unresponsive
Respirations	10 breaths/min via bag-mask device
Pulse	64 beats/min; bounding
Skin	Nail beds and mucous membranes appear cyanotic
Blood pressure	194/104 mm Hg
Oxygen saturation (Spo_2)	98% (on oxygen via bag-mask device)

You arrive at the hospital and transfer patient care to the ED staff. After further treatment in the ED, a CT scan of the patient's brain was performed and revealed massive intracerebral hemorrhage. Despite aggressive treatment in the intensive care unit, the patient died the next day.

10. What do unequal pupils indicate?

11. On the basis of your last assessment, what is the patient's GCS score?

local protocol will tell you if the designated stroke centers in your call area want you to call in a stroke alert for patients you have assessed and suspect to be experiencing a stroke. This will alert the stroke team members at the hospital and give them time to assemble their resources to be ready to treat the patient without delay. Report the time the patient last appeared to be well, the findings of your neurologic examination, and the time you anticipate arriving at the hospital.

A key piece of information to document is the time of onset of the patient's signs and symptoms. If the diagnosis is an ischemic stroke, time of onset of the signs and symptoms is critical information in determining whether the patient is a candidate for clot-retrieval or for blood clot–dissolving drugs. It is also important to document your findings from your stroke scale and the GCS score, along with any changes you found in your reassessment. Document airway management and interventions performed, including the position in which the patient was placed.

For patients who have had a seizure, give a description of the seizure activity, if known. Include bystanders' comments if they witnessed the seizure. Document the onset and duration of the seizure. Did the patient mention noticing an aura? Record any evidence of trauma and interventions performed. Document whether this is the patient's first seizure or whether the patient has a history of seizures. If the patient has a history of seizure activity, determine how often the seizures occur and if there is any history of status epilepticus. Document your interventions, and record the time the intervention was performed, the patient's response to the intervention, and the findings of continued reassessments.

Emergency Medical Care

A patient experiencing stroke, seizure, hypoglycemia, or hypoxia typically shows relatively easily identifiable signs or symptoms, and treatment options are readily available. With other neurologic emergencies, the cause of the patient's symptoms will not always be obvious, and more time and diagnostic testing may be needed at the hospital to determine the cause. This may make it difficult for you to provide definitive treatment in the field. Most of your interventions will be based on your assessment findings. For example, if the blood glucose level is low, you may give oral glucose according to your local protocol; if a patient is unresponsive, you may need to position the person in the recovery position to protect the airway. Remember, never give anything orally to a patient with altered mental status or to a patient who is unable to swallow normally, as doing so may result in aspiration. Your best treatment in these situations is to perform a thorough assessment and maintain the ABCs.

> **Special Populations**
>
> **CHILDREN WITH A HISTORY OF SEIZURES**
>
> Parents or caregivers of infants or children with a history of seizures may have given the child an intranasal dose of midazolam or diazepam or a rectal dose of diazepam (Diastat) to stop the seizure prior to your arrival. Monitor breathing and level of consciousness carefully in these patients. Transport the child to the appropriate facility.

In all cases, show patience and tolerance because many of these patients are likely to be confused, and occasionally frightened, after a seizure. Many patients who experience seizures are frustrated with their condition and may refuse transport. Kindness and professional behavior are required to help convince the patient that transport is necessary for definitive care.

> **Words of Wisdom**
>
> Use the same process as with all other patients in determining whether an adequate airway is present and whether the patient is able to sufficiently maintain that airway on their own. Do not assume that a patient who has had a seizure needs an airway adjunct. Conversely, do not assume that a patient who has had a seizure has an intact airway. Conduct a thorough assessment, and then decide.

Headache

As discussed earlier, most headaches are harmless and do not require emergency medical care. However, be concerned if the patient complains of a sudden-onset, severe headache or a sudden headache that has associated symptoms. Headaches with fever, seizures, or altered mental status, or following head trauma, are potentially life threatening. Complete a thorough patient assessment, and transport the patient to the hospital.

Treatment of a migraine headache is supportive; however, always assess the patient for other signs and symptoms that might indicate a more serious condition. Applying high-flow oxygen, if tolerated, may help ease the patient's condition in the case of a cluster headache, which may be mistaken for a migraine headache.[23] When possible, provide a darkened and quiet environment because patients with migraines are sensitive to light and sound. Do not use lights and siren during transport.

Stroke

Caring for a patient experiencing a stroke in the field is based on supporting the ABCs and providing rapid transport to a stroke center. Depending on the location of the stroke in the brain and the signs and symptoms, the patient may require manual airway positioning. Patients may have difficulty swallowing and controlling their own secretions; therefore, be prepared to use suction as needed. Provide oxygen to maintain an oxygen saturation of 94% to 98%, and monitor the patient's oxygen saturation with a pulse oximeter. Routine use of oxygen therapy in a stroke patient is not recommended if the patient clearly demonstrates no evidence of respiratory distress and has no signs of hypoxia. If there is any doubt, however, err on the side of providing oxygen therapy, as the adverse consequences of hypoxemia, even for brief periods, are far greater than the potential consequences of excess oxygenation for brief periods. If the patient's extremities are paralyzed, they will require protection from injury because the patient may not be able to feel the extremities or move them out of harm's way as you prepare and move the patient for transport. Continuously talk to the patient and describe what is going on. Many patients who are experiencing or who have had a stroke understand what is going on, even though they may not be able to communicate with you. The patient may not be able to speak or may use inappropriate words. Regardless, the patient will be scared. Reassure the patient and provide emotional support throughout the call.

Fibrinolytic therapy (blood clot–dissolving drugs) and endovascular therapy to mechanically remove the blood clot may reverse stroke symptoms and even stop the stroke if implemented quickly enough from the onset of symptoms; this window is 3 to 4.5 hours (for selected patients) in the case of drug therapy or 6 hours for mechanical methods.[17,24] In some very specific situations at centers with advanced capabilities, the window during which mechanical removal of the clot may offer

Special Populations

AGING-RELATED CHANGES IN THE BRAIN

The brain gradually deteriorates and shrinks as a part of the normal aging process. These processes increase the risk of brain injury from minor forces because the brain can more readily impact the inside of the skull as a result of the increased space and because the veins that connect the brain to the dura are stretched. A reduced brain mass may also reduce the patient's mental status and capacity. A smaller brain can impair memory function. A geriatric patient with lapses in short-term memory may often ask the same or similar questions repeatedly.

When you are called to care for a geriatric patient with altered mental status, consider the possibility of a stroke or TIA. At the scene of a motor vehicle crash involving an older driver, consider a stroke or TIA as a possible cause in the crash. Be alert for altered mental status and unusual pupil responses (eg, constricted pupils in dim light, unequal pupils).

Take special note of complaints of a headache. Although geriatric patients get tension headaches, they are far less common in the older population. Consider any headache as potentially serious.

As with the general population, older people can experience seizures. Remember, seizures are not necessarily caused by epilepsy. Consider and assess for the possibility of a drug overdose, stroke, heart rhythm problem, head injury, or central nervous system infection, particularly if there is no prior history of seizures. Status epilepticus in a geriatric patient increases the risk of hypoxia, irregular heart rhythm, hypotension, elevated body temperature, low blood glucose level, and, if the patient vomits, aspiration.

Remember, geriatric patients are at a higher risk for central nervous system illnesses and injuries, including brain injury, TIA, stroke, and seizures. Do not be surprised to find a serious head injury from what you might consider a simple bump on the head.

benefit may extend as long as 24 hours after the time at which the patient was last seen to be normal.[17] These therapies may not work for all patients and are not options for patients with bleeding-type (hemorrhagic) strokes. Because hospital personnel will ultimately make these treatment decisions, you should proceed under the assumption that the affected area of the brain may be saved. The sooner the treatment is begun, the better the prognosis for the patient.

Spend as little time on scene as possible. Remember, stroke is an emergency and "time is brain." Treatment may be available for the patient at the hospital, and rapid transport is essential to maximize the possibility of recovery. If you have a choice of hospitals, transport the patient to one that is a designated stroke center.

Seizure

Most patients who have had a seizure will be in a postictal state on your arrival. For those patients who are still experiencing a seizure, continue to assess and treat the ABCs. It may be necessary to maintain the patient's airway with manual airway positioning and insertion of a nasopharyngeal airway. Use suction to clear the airway of any excessive secretions or vomitus. Oxygen is rapidly consumed by the body during seizure activity, so you should monitor the patient's oxygen saturation level with a pulse oximeter and apply high-flow oxygen to maintain an oxygen saturation of 94% to 98%. Administer oxygen if the seizure persists even if you are unable to get an accurate pulse oximetry reading because of the patient's seizure activity, shaking, or tremors. Obtain a blood glucose reading when possible. Provide emotional support.

It is difficult to safely prepare a patient for transport when the individual is experiencing a seizure. Assess the patient for trauma and restrict movement of the spine if indicated. Protect the patient from the surroundings. Never attempt to tightly restrain a patient experiencing a seizure. Injury could result from tonic-clonic movement. Use soft materials for padding, and move any objects out of the way that may harm your patient.

Not every patient who has had a seizure wants to be transported, but it is usually in the best interest of the patient to be evaluated by a physician in the ED after a seizure. Your goal is to encourage the patient to be seen by a physician. Should the patient refuse transport, be prepared to discuss the situation with the hospital staff on the radio before releasing the patient. Ask yourself the following questions if a patient who was in a postictal state now refuses transport:

- Is the patient fully awake and completely oriented after the seizure (GCS score of 15)?
- Does your assessment reveal no indication of trauma or complications from the seizure?
- Has the patient ever had a seizure before?
- Was this seizure the "usual" seizure in every way (length, activity, recovery)?
- Is the patient currently being treated with medications and receiving regular evaluations by a physician?

If the answer to all of these questions is "yes," you can consider agreeing to a patient's refusal for transport if the patient can be released to a responsible person and monitored. If the patient responds "no" to any questions, strongly encourage the patient to be transported and evaluated. In all cases where a patient refuses transport after a seizure, contact online medical direction and ask them to speak directly to the patient to encourage the patient to consent to transport. Follow your local protocols for patients who refuse care and transport.

If the patient experienced a febrile seizure and fully regained normal mental status after the seizure stopped, consider administering acetaminophen or ibuprofen (for infants older than 6 months) under the guidance of medical oversight. Consider removing excess layers of clothing and apply cool compresses to the body as indicated in your protocols.[9]

Altered Mental Status

The signs and symptoms of altered mental status can vary widely, from simple confusion to coma. No matter what the cause, consider altered mental status to be an emergency that requires immediate attention, even when it appears that it may be caused by alcohol intoxication or minor head trauma. Determine the cause (mechanism of injury versus nature of illness) and provide spinal motion restriction as indicated, airway and ventilation support, and transport to the appropriate facility.

YOU are the EMT SUMMARY

1. On the basis of the dispatch information, what type of seizure is the patient most likely experiencing?

Given the patient's age (58 years), loss of consciousness, and the fact that the convulsions affect her extremities and torso, the patient is most likely experiencing a generalized seizure.

2. What are some common causes of seizures in this patient's age group?

Seizures in adults are typically caused by one of three underlying problems: epilepsy, structural brain problems (eg, brain tumors and abscesses, head trauma, stroke), or metabolic derangements (eg, cerebral hypoxia, hypoglycemia, hyperglycemia, drug overdose, poisoning, alcohol withdrawal). Febrile seizures are rare in adults. However, fever may be a sign of brain infection, such as meningitis.

3. What additional questions should you ask the patient's sister?

Important questions that need to be answered include: What was the patient doing and what position was she in when the seizure began? Was she sitting or standing? Did she hit her head during the episode? Did the patient describe experiencing an aura? If neither the patient nor her sister mentioned an aura, this does not rule out a seizure.

How long did the seizure last? Was the patient unconscious following the seizure? If so, how long was she unconscious? Does the patient have a history of recent head trauma?

4. What prehospital assessments can you perform to determine the possible cause of the patient's seizure?

In most cases, you will not be able to determine the underlying cause of the patient's seizure in the prehospital setting. However, there are a few assessments you can perform and observations you can make that may increase your index of suspicion. Assess the patient's blood glucose level to rule out hypoglycemia as the cause of her seizure. If the patient is conscious and able to follow commands, test the patient by using a stroke scale, such as the Cincinnati Prehospital Stroke Scale. You should also assess and closely monitor the patient's vital signs and assess her neurologic status using the GCS. In some cases, taking a temperature may help to uncover an underlying illness that may have caused the seizure.

5. What treatment is indicated at this point?

Unless the patient was injured during the seizure or you have identified an underlying cause of her seizure that can be treated in the prehospital setting (eg, hypoglycemia), additional treatment is mainly supportive. Maintaining a patent airway and ensuring adequate oxygenation and ventilation are your highest priorities. Provide a calm, quiet environment; reassure and reorient the patient as needed; avoid any loud or bright stimuli, which may cause another seizure; and safely transport her to the hospital. Continuously monitor the patient's ABCs, level of consciousness, and vital signs.

6. What is your field impression of this patient? Why?

From the sister's description, it is likely that the patient experienced a seizure. Her present signs and symptoms (confusion; sudden, severe headache; nausea; left-sided weakness) and medical history (poorly controlled hypertension) should make you suspicious that she is experiencing a hemorrhagic stroke, which likely caused the seizure. Signs of increased ICP include changes in level of consciousness, nausea and vomiting, seizures, and high blood pressure, among others; your patient is experiencing all of these signs and symptoms.

7. On the basis of your field impression, you should monitor the patient for which additional signs and symptoms?

Your patient's present condition suggests that a cerebral artery may be leaking and blood is slowly accumulating in her brain tissue, which will increase ICP. As the ICP increases, the patient's level of consciousness will deteriorate; therefore, the level of consciousness is the single most important assessment parameter to monitor. Because of the cerebral ischemia caused by the increased ICP, the patient may experience another seizure. As the ICP increases further, the blood pressure often increases and the heart rate commonly decreases. Pressure on the brainstem may cause irregular and ineffective breathing; therefore, assisted ventilation may be necessary. It is important to continuously monitor your patient's condition and be prepared to intervene if her condition deteriorates.

8. What should be your most immediate action?

Airway, airway, airway! Snoring respirations indicate partial obstruction of the airway by the tongue.

YOU are the EMT SUMMARY continued

Performing the head tilt–chin lift maneuver is the quickest way to correct the problem. The patient is now unconscious and unresponsive; insert an airway adjunct (eg, oral or nasal airway) to help maintain airway patency. Patients with increased ICP often vomit; remain alert to this possibility and have suction readily available. Regardless of the situation, you must ensure the patient's airway remains patent at all times. No airway, no patient—it's that simple!

9. What additional treatment does this patient require?

After establishing a patent airway, your next priority is to assist the patient's breathing. A slow (6 breaths/min), irregular breathing pattern will not support adequate minute volume; therefore, deliver positive-pressure ventilation with a bag-mask device. Be sure to attach 100% oxygen to the ventilation device you will be using.

10. What do unequal pupils indicate?

In the context of a traumatic brain injury or hemorrhagic stroke, unequal pupil size is an ominous sign. It indicates significantly increased ICP and compression of one of the oculomotor nerves (the nerves that control the pupillary response). The affected pupil is often fully dilated (blown) and does not constrict when a light source is shone into it.

11. On the basis of your last assessment, what is the patient's GCS score?

The GCS assesses three parameters: eye opening, verbal response, and motor response. Your last assessment revealed that the patient was unconscious and unresponsive (she did not open her eyes and was unresponsive to all stimuli) and was exhibiting decorticate (abnormal flexion) posturing. Therefore, she would receive a GCS score of 5, based on the following values (the numeric value for each component is in bold):

Eye opening:
- Spontaneous: 4
- Responsive to speech: 3
- Responsive to pain: 2
- **None: 1**

Best verbal response:
- Oriented conversation: 5
- Confused conversation: 4
- Inappropriate words: 3
- Incomprehensible sounds: 2
- **None: 1**

Best motor response:
- Obeys commands: 6
- Localizes pain: 5
- Withdraws from pain: 4
- **Abnormal flexion: 3**
- Abnormal extension: 2
- None: 1

Prep Kit

Ready for Review

- The cerebrum, the largest part of the brain, is divided into right and left cerebral hemispheres, each controlling the opposite side of the body.
- Different areas of the brain control different functions. The front part of the cerebrum controls emotion and thought; the middle part controls touch and movement; and the back part of the cerebrum is involved with vision. In most people, speech is controlled on the left side of the brain, near the middle of the cerebrum.
- Many different disorders can cause brain or other neurologic symptoms. In general, if the problem is primarily in the brain, only part of the brain will be affected. If the problem is in the heart or lungs, the whole brain will be affected.
- Stroke is a common brain disorder and is a leading cause of death and disability. The most effective treatment is time dependent. Seizures and altered mental status are also common brain disorders. You must learn to recognize the signs and symptoms of each condition.

Prep Kit continued

- Other causes of neurologic dysfunction include coma, infections, and tumors.
- Strokes occur when part of the blood flow to the brain is suddenly cut off; within minutes, brain cells begin to die.
- Signs and symptoms of stroke include receptive and/or expressive aphasia, slurred speech, muscle weakness or numbness on one side of the body, facial droop, abnormal balance, vision problems, and sometimes high blood pressure.
- Always perform at least three neurologic tests on a patient you suspect of experiencing a stroke: testing speech, facial movement, and arm movement. Also observe the patient's balance and ask about vision changes.
- In a TIA, normal body processes break up the blood clot, restoring blood flow and ending symptoms in less than 24 hours. However, patients experiencing a TIA are at a higher risk for a repeat episode or a more serious stroke.
- Because current treatments for stroke must be administered within 3 hours of the onset of symptoms to be most effective, provide prompt transport.
- Always notify the hospital as soon as possible that you are bringing in a patient with a possible stroke, so staff can prepare to test and treat the patient without delay.
- Generalized seizures are usually characterized by unconsciousness and generalized jerking or twitching of all or part of the body.
- Most generalized seizures last less than 5 minutes and are followed by a postictal state in which the patient may be unresponsive and have labored breathing or hemiparesis. The patient may have a loss of bladder or bowel control as a result of the seizure.
- Recognize the signs and symptoms of seizures so you can provide the ED staff with information as you transport the patient.
- Syncope may be confused with seizure. In the case of syncope, the patient recovers quickly. Assess for serious underlying causes.
- Altered mental status is a common neurologic disorder that you will encounter as an EMT. Signs and symptoms vary widely, as do the causes for this condition.
- Among the most common causes of altered mental status are hypoglycemia, intoxication, drug overdose, and poisoning.
- Do not always assume intoxication when you assess a patient with an altered mental status; hypoglycemia is just as likely a cause. Prompt transport with close monitoring of vital signs en route is indicated.

Vital Vocabulary

altered mental status Any deviation from alert and oriented to person, place, time, and event, or any deviation from a patient's normal baseline mental status.

aneurysm A swelling or enlargement of a part of an artery, resulting from weakening of the arterial wall.

aphasia The inability to understand and/or produce speech.

atherosclerosis A disorder in which cholesterol and calcium build up inside the walls of blood vessels, eventually leading to partial or complete blockage of blood flow.

aura A sensation experienced before a seizure; serves as a warning sign that a seizure is about to occur.

cerebrovascular accident (CVA) An interruption of blood flow to the brain that results in the loss of brain function; also called a stroke.

coma A state of profound unconsciousness from which the patient cannot be roused.

delirium A temporary change in mental status characterized by disorganized thoughts, inattention, memory loss, disorientation, striking changes in personality and affect, hallucinations, delusions, or a decreased level of consciousness.

Prep Kit continued

dementia A slow, progressive decline in cognitive function that impairs memory function and leads to behavior change.

dysarthria Slurred speech.

embolism A condition in which a blood clot or other substance (embolus) in the circulatory system travels to a blood vessel where it causes a blockage of blood flow.

epilepsy A disorder in which abnormal electrical discharges occur in the brain, causing seizures and possible loss of consciousness.

febrile seizure A seizure that results from sudden high fever; most often seen in children.

focal seizure A seizure affecting a limited portion of the brain.

generalized seizure A seizure characterized by severe twitching of all of the body's muscles that may last several minutes or more; formerly known as a grand mal seizure.

hemiparesis Weakness on one side of the body.

hemorrhagic stroke A type of stroke that occurs as a result of bleeding inside the brain.

hyperglycemia An abnormally high blood glucose level.

hypoglycemia An abnormally low blood glucose level.

incontinence Loss of bowel and/or bladder control; may be the result of a generalized seizure.

ischemia A lack of oxygen that deprives tissues of necessary nutrients, resulting from partial or complete blockage of blood flow; potentially reversible because permanent injury has not yet occurred.

ischemic stroke A type of stroke that occurs when blood flow to a particular part of the brain is cut off by a blockage (eg, a blood clot) inside a blood vessel.

postictal state The period following a seizure that lasts 5 to 30 minutes; characterized by labored respirations and some degree of altered mental status.

seizure A neurologic episode caused by a surge of electrical activity in the brain; can be a convulsion characterized by generalized, uncoordinated muscular activity, and can be associated with loss of consciousness.

status epilepticus A condition in which seizures recur every few minutes or last longer than 30 minutes.

stroke An interruption of blood flow to the brain that results in the loss of brain function; also called a cerebrovascular accident (CVA).

syncope A fainting spell or transient loss of consciousness.

thrombosis A condition in which a blood clot, either in the arterial or venous system, forms at the site of a damaged blood vessel (referred to as a thrombus) and obstructs blood flow.

transient ischemic attack (TIA) A disorder of the brain in which brain cells temporarily stop functioning because of insufficient oxygen, causing strokelike symptoms that resolve completely within 24 hours of onset.

References

1. Let's talk about FAST. American Stroke Association website. https://www.stroke.org/en/help-and-support/resource-library/lets-talk-about-stroke/fast. Accessed December 30, 2024.
2. McCance brain care score. Frontiers website. https://www.frontiersin.org/files/Articles/1373797/fpsyt-15-1373797-HTML-r2/image_m/fpsyt-15-1373797-g001.jpg. Published 2020. Accessed December 30, 2024.
3. When to call 911 about high blood pressure. American Heart Association website. https://www.heart.org/en/health-topics/high-blood-pressure/understanding-blood-pressure-readings/hypertensive-crisis-when-you-should-call-911-for-high-blood-pressure. Reviewed May 6, 2024. Accessed December 30, 2024.
4. Ischemic stroke (clots). American Stroke Association website. https://www.stroke.org/en/about-stroke/types-of-stroke/ischemic-stroke-clots. Accessed December 30, 2024.

Prep Kit continued

5. Hemorrhagic stroke. American Stroke Association website. https://www.stroke.org/en/about-stroke/types-of-stroke/hemorrhagic-strokes-bleeds. Accessed December 30, 2024.
6. Transient ischemic attack (TIA). American Stroke Association website. https://www.stroke.org/en/about-stroke/types-of-stroke/tia-transient-ischemic-attack. Accessed December 30, 2024.
7. Epilepsy facts and stats. Centers for Disease Control and Prevention website. https://www.cdc.gov/epilepsy/data-research/facts-stats/. Published May 15, 2024. Accessed December 30, 2024.
8. Trinka E, Cock H, Hesdorffer D, et al. A definition and classification of status epilepticus—report of the ILAE Task Force on Classification of Status Epilepticus. *Epilepsia*. 2015;56(10):1515–1523.
9. National Association of State EMS Officials. *National Model EMS Clinical Guidelines: Version 3.0.* https://nasemso.org/wp-content/uploads/National-Model-EMS-Clinical-Guidelines_2022.pdf. Updated March 2022. Accessed December 30, 2024.
10. Shen WK, Sheldon RS, Benditt DG, et al. 2017 ACC/AHA/HRS guideline for the evaluation and management of patients with syncope: a report of the American College of Cardiology/American Heart Association Task Force on Clinical Practice Guidelines and the Heart Rhythm Society [published correction appears in *Circulation*. 2017 Oct 17;136(16):e271–e272. doi:10.1161/CIR.0000000000000537]. *Circulation*. 2017;136(5):e60–e122. doi:10.1161/CIR.0000000000000499
11. European Delirium Association; American Delirium Society. The DSM-5 criteria, level of arousal and delirium diagnosis: inclusiveness is safer. *BMC Med*. 2014;12:141.
12. Dementia. Mayo Clinic website. https://www.mayoclinic.org/diseases-conditions/dementia/symptoms-causes/syc-20352013. Published September 25, 2024. Accessed January 15, 2025.
13. Gomperts SN. Lewy body dementias: dementia with Lewy bodies and Parkinson disease dementia. *Continuum (Minneap Minn)*. 2016;22(2 Dementia):435-463.
14. Helpline. Alzheimer's Association website. https://www.alz.org/help-support/resources/helpline. Accessed January 15, 2025.
15. Febrile seizures. National Institute of Neurological Disorders and Stroke website. https://www.ninds.nih.gov/health-information/disorders/febrile-seizures. Reviewed November 22, 2024. Accessed February 25, 2025.
16. Shafer PO, Sirven JI. Facts and statistics about epilepsy. Epilepsy Foundation website. http://www.epilepsy.com/learn/epilepsy-statistics. Published October 2013. Reviewed February 27, 2019. Accessed December 30, 2024.
17. Meloni S, Mastenbjörk M. *Advanced Cardiovascular Life Support: Provider Manual*. Medical Creations; 2021.
18. Aroor S, Singh R, Goldstein LB. BE-FAST (balance, eyes, face, arm, speech, time): reducing the proportion of strokes missed using the FAST mnemonic. *Stroke*. 2017;48(2):479–481
19. Prehospital/EMS care. American Stroke Association website. https://www.stroke.org/en/professionals/stroke-resource-library/pre-hospitalems. Accessed December 30, 2024.
20. Summers D. Prehospital stroke assessment tools and benefits. American Stroke Association website. https://www.stroke.org/-/media/Files/Affiliates/BiState-Stroke-Symposium/Prehospital-Stroke-Assessment-Tools-and-Benefits.pdf/. Accessed December 30, 2024.
21. Chen X, Zhao X, Xu F, et al. A systematic review and meta-analysis comparing FAST and BEFAST in acute stroke patients. *Front Neurol*. 2022;12:765069. doi:10.3389/fneur.2021.765069
22. Crowe RP, Myers JB, Fernandez AR, Bourn S, McMullan JT. The Cincinnati Prehospital Stroke Scale compared to stroke severity tools for large vessel occlusion stroke prediction. *Prehosp Emerg Care*. 2021;25(1):67–75.
23. Mo H, Chung SJ, Rozen TD, Cho SJ. Oxygen therapy in cluster headache, migraine, and other headache disorders. *J Clin Neurol*. 2022;18(3):271–279.
24. Powers WJ, Rabinstein AA, Ackerson T, et al. Guidelines for the early management of patients with acute ischemic stroke: 2019 update to the 2018 Guidelines for the Early Management of Acute Ischemic Stroke: a guideline for healthcare professionals from the American Heart Association/American Stroke Association. *Stroke*. 2019;50(12):e344–e418. doi:10.1161/STR.0000000000000211

Additional Resources

National Highway Traffic Safety Administration. *National Emergency Medical Services Education Standards*. https://www.ems.gov/assets/EMS_Education-Standards_2021_FNL.pdf. EMS.gov website. Published January 2021. Accessed December 30, 2024.

Oliveira-Filho J, Mullen TM. Initial assessment and management of acute stroke. UpToDate website. https://www.uptodate.com/contents/initial-assessment-and-management-of-acute-stroke. Updated October 11, 2023. Accessed December 30, 2024.

Wirrell E. ILAE classification of seizures and epilepsy. UpToDate website. https://www.uptodate.com/contents/ilae-classification-of-seizures-and-epilepsy. Updated April 12, 2024. Accessed December 30, 2024.

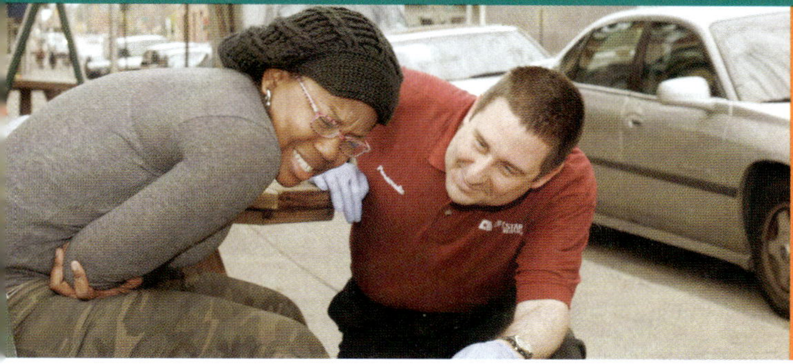

Chapter 19

Gastrointestinal and Urologic Emergencies

NATIONAL EMS EDUCATION STANDARD COMPETENCIES

Medicine

Applies knowledge to provide basic emergency care and transportation based on assessment findings for an acutely ill patient.

Abdominal and Gastrointestinal Disorders

- Acute and chronic gastrointestinal hemorrhage (pp 768–773)

Genitourinary/Renal

- Complications related to renal dialysis (pp 781–783)
- Complications related to urinary catheter management (not insertion) (p 783)
- Kidney stones (pp 773–774)
- Sexual assault (female and male) (Chapter 35, *Patients With Special Challenges*)

KNOWLEDGE OBJECTIVES

1. Describe the basic anatomy and physiology of the gastrointestinal (GI), genital, and urinary systems. (pp 764–766)
2. Define the term *acute abdomen*. (p 766)
3. Explain the concept of referred pain. (p 767)
4. Describe pathologic conditions of the GI, genital, and urinary systems. (pp 766–776)
5. Describe other organ systems that can cause abdominal pain. (pp 770–771, 773–774)
6. Identify the signs and symptoms, and common causes, of an acute abdomen. (pp 768–773)
7. Describe the assessment and management of conditions that cause acute abdomen. (pp 776–780)
8. Describe the assessment and management of emergencies associated with the urinary system. (pp 776–780)
9. Describe the procedures to follow when caring for a patient with shock associated with abdominal emergencies. (pp 776–780)
10. Describe special considerations when caring for a child or older adult experiencing a GI or urologic emergency. (pp 774–776)
11. Explain the principles of kidney dialysis. (pp 781–783)

SKILLS OBJECTIVE

1. Demonstrate the assessment of a patient's abdomen. (pp 778–780)

Introduction

Abdominal pain is a common complaint; however, the cause is often difficult to identify, even for a physician. As an EMT, you do not need to determine the exact cause of acute abdominal pain, but it is helpful for you to understand the pathophysiology and the signs and symptoms of common illnesses. You need to be able to recognize a life-threatening problem and act swiftly in response. Remember, the patient is in pain and is probably anxious, requiring your skills of rapid assessment and emotional support.

Anatomy and Physiology

The abdominal cavity contains solid and hollow organs that make up the gastrointestinal (GI), genital, and urinary systems (**FIGURE 19-1**). Solid organs include the liver, spleen, pancreas, kidneys, and ovaries (in women). Technically, organs such as the kidneys, ovaries, and the pancreas are retroperitoneal (behind the peritoneum). However, because they lie next to the peritoneum, they can cause abdominal pain. An injury to a solid organ can cause bleeding and shock because of the amount of blood vessels contained in the organ.

Hollow organs include the gallbladder, stomach, small intestine, large intestine, and urinary bladder. If there is a perforation of these hollow organs, the contents of the organ will leak and contaminate the abdominal cavity, causing serious illness.

The GI System

The GI system is responsible for the digestion process. Digestion begins when food is put into the mouth and chewed; the salivary glands secrete saliva and begin to break down the food, then it is swallowed. The food travels down the esophagus to the stomach. The stomach is the main organ of the digestive system. Absorption of nutrients occurs at various places along the digestive tract. Sugars start to be absorbed while in the mouth. Most digestion takes place in the stomach, where gastric juices break down food to a form that can be used by the body.

The liver secretes bile, which aids in the digestion of fats. The liver also filters toxic substances produced by digestion, creates glucose stores, and produces substances necessary for blood clotting and immune function. The gallbladder is a hollow pouch located beneath the liver that acts as a reservoir for bile.

From the stomach, food travels down into the small intestine, which consists of three sections: the duodenum, jejunum, and ileum. This is where absorption of most nutrients occurs. The duodenum is where digestive juices from the pancreas and liver mix together. The pancreas secretes juice containing

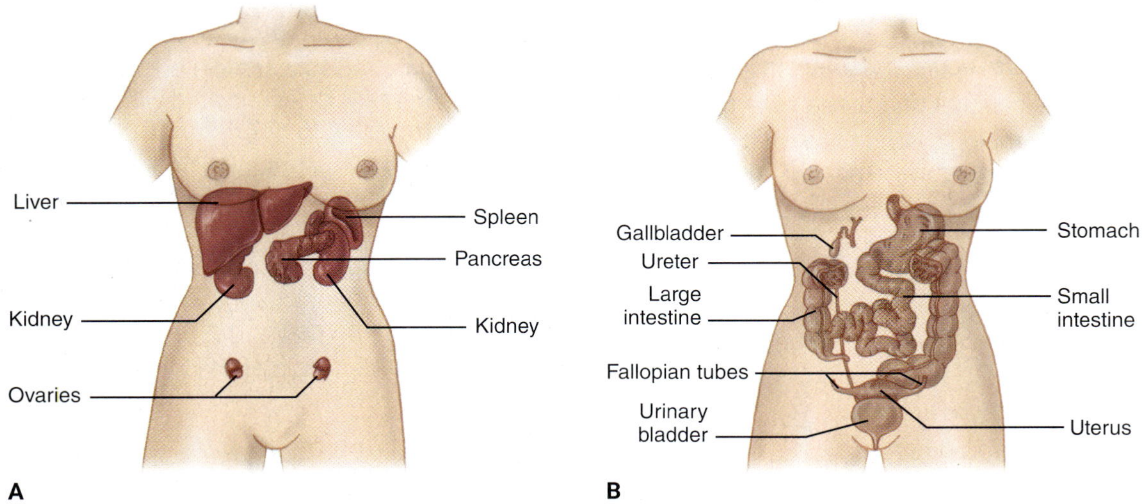

FIGURE 19-1 The solid and hollow organs of the abdomen. **A.** Solid organs include the liver, spleen, pancreas, kidneys, and ovaries (in women). **B.** Hollow organs include the gallbladder, stomach, small intestine, large intestine, and bladder.

enzymes that help break down starches, fats, and proteins. Amylase, which breaks down starches into sugar, is one enzyme the pancreas secretes. The pancreas also produces bicarbonate, insulin, and glucagon. Bicarbonate neutralizes the stomach acid in the duodenum. Insulin and glucagon help regulate the levels of glucose in the bloodstream.

The jejunum, the next part of the small intestine, plays a major role in the absorption of digestive products. The jejunum comprises a large amount of the surface area of the small intestine and does much of the work. The final part of the small intestine is the ileum, which absorbs the remaining nutrients. It also absorbs bile acids so they can be returned to the liver for future use and vitamin B_{12} for making nerve cells and red blood cells.

The food that was not broken down and used as nutrients then moves into the colon, or large intestine, as waste products. A wavelike contraction of smooth muscle called peristalsis moves the waste matter through the entire digestive system. Water and electrolytes are absorbed from the large intestine and feces are formed. The feces pass through the rectum to the anus, where it is defecated.

Additional Abdominal Organs

The spleen is also located in the abdomen but has no digestive system function. The spleen is part of the lymphatic system and plays a significant role in relation to red blood cells and the immune system. It assists in the filtration of blood, removes old red blood cells, recycles iron, and serves as a blood reservoir. The spleen also produces antibodies to help the body fight off disease and infection.

The Genital System

The abdominal space also holds the male and female reproductive organs. The male reproductive system consists of the testicles, epididymides, vasa deferentia (singular: vas deferens), seminal vesicles, prostate gland, and penis. The female reproductive system includes the ovaries, fallopian tubes, uterus, cervix, and vagina.

The Urinary System

The urinary system controls the discharge of certain waste materials filtered from the blood by the kidneys. In the urinary system, the kidneys are solid organs, and the ureters, bladder, and urethra are hollow organs (**FIGURE 19-2**). Ordinarily, the urinary and genital systems are referred to jointly as the genitourinary system because they share many organs. One system can directly affect the other. For example, if the prostate gland in the male genital system enlarges, then the urethra will narrow, impairing the emptying of the bladder, and eventually leading to urinary retention.

The body contains two kidneys, one on each side, which lie on the posterior muscular wall of the abdomen behind the peritoneum in the retroperitoneal space. The kidneys play an important role in regulating the body's acid–base balance (pH level) and blood pressure. Blood pressure regulation is associated with the kidney's ability to remove sodium chloride from the body. Kidney disease is a common cause of secondary hypertension. Most patients with chronic kidney disease (CKD) also have hypertension. The kidneys also rid the body of toxic wastes, control the body's balance of fluid and electrolytes, produce a hormone that stimulates red blood cell production, and activate vitamin D, which is essential for bone and muscle health.

Blood flow in the kidneys is high. Almost 20% of the output of blood from the heart passes through the kidneys each minute. Large vessels attach the kidneys directly to the aorta and the inferior vena

YOU are the EMT

At 0320 hours, you and your partner are dispatched to 1500 East River Road, Apartment 5, for a 79-year-old man with abdominal pain. You proceed to the scene, which is approximately 8 miles from your station. The weather is clear, the temperature is 67°F (19.4°C), and the traffic is light.

1. What is the definition of an acute abdomen?
2. What is your role as an EMT in treating a patient with abdominal pain?

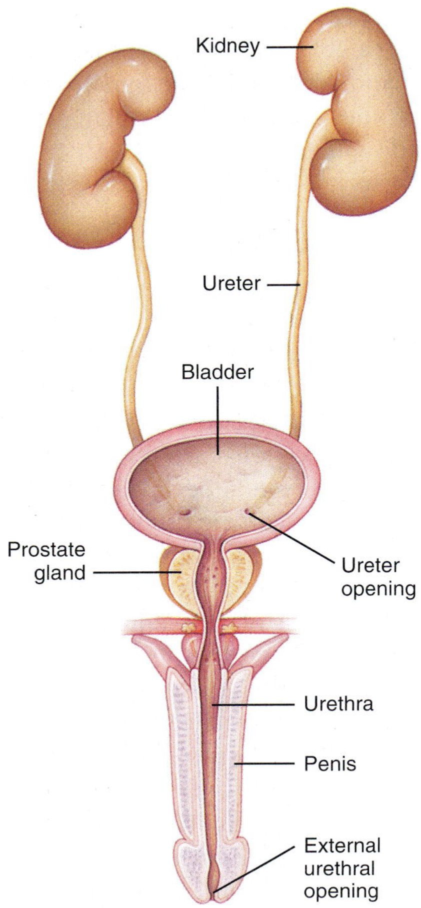

FIGURE 19-2 The urinary system lies in the retroperitoneal space behind the organs of the digestive system. The urinary system in men and women includes the kidneys, ureters, bladder, and urethra. This diagram shows the male urinary system.

cava. Waste products and water are constantly filtered from the blood to form urine. The kidneys continuously concentrate this filtered urine by reabsorbing the water as it passes through a system of specialized tubes within them. The tubes eventually unite to form the renal pelvis, a cone-shaped collecting area that connects the ureter and the kidney.

A ureter passes from the renal pelvis of each kidney along the surface of the posterior abdominal wall behind the peritoneum to drain into the urinary bladder. The ureters are small (0.2 inch [5 mm] in diameter), hollow, muscular tubes. Peristalsis occurs in these tubes to move the urine to the bladder.

The urinary bladder is located immediately behind the pubic symphysis in the pelvic cavity and is composed of smooth muscle with a specialized lining membrane. The two ureters enter posteriorly at its base on either side. The bladder empties to the outside of the body through the urethra. In the male body, the urethra passes from the anterior base of the bladder through the penis. In the female body, the urethra opens at the front of the vagina. The healthy adult forms 1.5 to 2 liters of urine every day, which is held in the urinary bladder until it is excreted through the urethra.

Pathophysiology

The abdominal cavity is lined by a membrane called the **peritoneum**. The peritoneum also covers the organs of the abdomen. The parietal peritoneum lines the walls of the abdominal cavity, and the visceral peritoneum covers the organs themselves. The abdominal space normally contains a small amount of peritoneal fluid to bathe and lubricate the organs in the abdominal cavity. Any foreign material, such as blood, pus, bile, pancreatic juice, or amniotic fluid, can cause irritation of the peritoneum, called **peritonitis**.

Acute abdomen is a medical term referring to the sudden onset of abdominal pain, often associated with severe, progressive problems that require medical attention. Peritonitis is usually associated with the acute abdomen, which, if not treated, can be fatal.

Peritonitis typically causes **ileus**, or paralysis of the muscular contractions that normally propel material through the intestine. The retained gas and feces, in turn, cause abdominal distention and tenderness. Distention usually begins after the muscular contractions cease. In the presence of such paralysis, nothing that is eaten can pass normally out of the stomach or through the bowel. In this situation, the only way the stomach can empty itself is by **emesis**, or vomiting. For this reason, peritonitis is frequently associated with nausea and vomiting. These symptoms do not point to a particular cause because they can accompany almost every type of GI disease or injury.

Peritonitis can be associated with a loss of body fluid into the abdominal cavity. The loss of fluid usually results from abnormal shifts of fluid from the bloodstream into body tissues. This fluid shift decreases the volume of circulating blood and may lead to decreased blood pressure or even shock.

The patient may have normal vital signs or, if the peritonitis has progressed further, the patient may present with tachycardia and hypotension. When peritonitis is accompanied by hemorrhage, the signs of shock are much more apparent.

Fever may or may not be present, depending on the cause of the peritonitis. Patients with **diverticulitis** (inflammation in small pockets at weak areas in the muscle walls of the intestines) or **cholecystitis** (inflammation of the gallbladder) may have a substantial elevation in body temperature. However, patients with acute appendicitis may have a temperature within normal limits until the appendix ruptures and contaminates the peritoneal cavity.

Abdominal Pain

Abdominal pain can have different qualities because two different types of nerves supply the peritoneum. The nerves from the spinal cord that supply the skin of the abdomen also supply the parietal peritoneum. Therefore, the parietal peritoneum and the skin of the abdomen can perceive much the same sensations: pain, touch, pressure, heat, and cold. These sensory nerves can easily identify and localize a point of irritation. In contrast, the visceral peritoneum is supplied by the autonomic nervous system. These nerves are far less able to localize sensation. This means that your patient will not be able to describe exactly where the pain is located. The visceral peritoneum is stimulated when distention or contraction of the hollow abdominal organs activates the stretch receptors. Patients sometimes describe it as a deep pain. Other painful sensations that occur because of an irritated visceral peritoneum may be perceived at a distant point on the surface of the body, such as the back or shoulder. This phenomenon is called **referred pain**.

Referred pain is the result of connections between the body's two separate nervous systems. The nerves connecting the somatic nervous system and autonomic nervous system cause the stimulation of the autonomic nerves to be perceived as stimulation of the spinal sensory nerves. For example, acute cholecystitis may cause pain in the right shoulder because the autonomic nerves serving the gallbladder lie near the spinal cord at the same anatomic level as the spinal sensory nerves that supply the skin of the shoulder (**FIGURE 19-3**).

The most common abdominal emergencies, with the most common locations of direct and referred pain, are listed in **TABLE 19-1**.

YOU are the EMT

When you arrive at the scene and enter the patient's residence, you find him lying on the couch on his side in obvious discomfort. He is notably diaphoretic (sweaty) and pale and is in obvious severe discomfort. You introduce yourself and begin your assessment.

Recording Time: 0 Minutes	
Appearance	Lying on his side, diaphoretic, in obvious pain
Level of consciousness	Conscious and alert; restless
Airway	Open; clear of secretions or foreign bodies
Breathing	Rapid, shallow respirations; oxygen saturation (Spo_2) unobtainable
Circulation	Radial pulse weak and rapid; skin is pale (as compared to baseline tone) and diaphoretic

Your partner administers oxygen at 15 L/min via a nonrebreathing mask as you continue your assessment. The patient tells you that his abdominal pain began suddenly and has been severe from the onset. He describes the pain as like something being pulled apart and indicates that it radiates to his lower back. He denies nausea, vomiting, fever, or any other symptoms. As you examine his abdomen, your partner prepares to take vital signs.

3. What is the proper technique of assessing a patient's abdomen? What should you assess for?

4. What is the difference between radiating pain and referred pain?

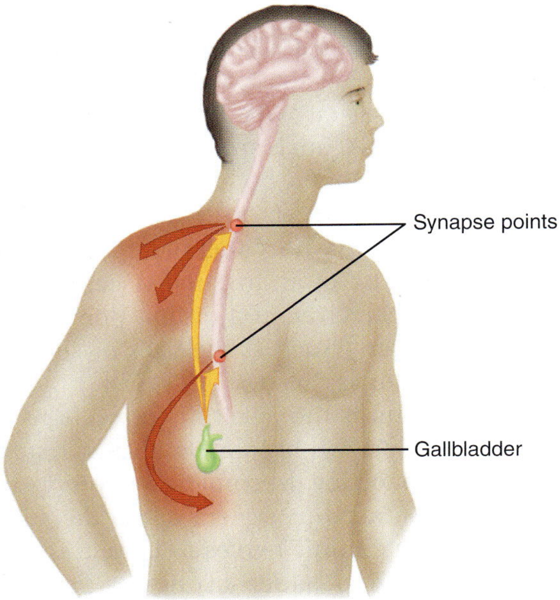

FIGURE 19-3 Acute cholecystitis causes referred pain in the right shoulder as well as in the abdomen.

TABLE 19-1 Common Abdominal Conditions

Condition	Localization of Pain
Appendicitis	Right lower quadrant (direct); around navel (referred); rebound tenderness (pain felt on the release of pressure after palpation)
Cholecystitis	Right upper quadrant (direct); right shoulder (referred)
Ulcer	Upper midabdomen or upper part of back
Diverticulitis	Left lower quadrant
Abdominal aortic aneurysm (ruptured or dissecting)	Low part of back and lower quadrants
Cystitis (inflammation of the bladder)	Lower midabdomen
Kidney infection	Bottom of ribcage on back, where the lowest (12th) rib meets the spine
Kidney stone	Right or left flank, radiating to genitalia
Pancreatitis	Upper abdomen (both quadrants); back or below left shoulder blade (radiation)
Hernia	Anywhere in the abdominal area
Peritonitis	Diffuse abdominal pain area

Causes of Acute Abdomen

Almost any problem with an abdominal organ can cause an acute abdomen. Some of the more common causes are discussed here. It is rare for the EMT to determine the exact cause. Because the visceral peritoneum is usually irritated first, early abdominal pain tends to be vague and poorly localized. As the parietal peritoneum becomes irritated, pain becomes more severe and may be more specifically located.

Ulcers

The stomach and duodenum are subjected to high levels of acidity. To prevent damage to these organs, protective layers of mucus line both organs. In peptic ulcer disease (PUD), the protective layer is eroded, allowing the acid to eat into the organ itself over the course of weeks, months, or even years.

Most peptic ulcers are the result of infection of the stomach with *Helicobacter pylori* bacteria. Another major cause is chronic use of nonsteroidal anti-inflammatory drugs (NSAIDs), such as aspirin and ibuprofen. Alcohol and smoking can also affect the severity of PUD by increasing gastric acidity.

Patients with PUD experience a classic sequence of burning or gnawing pain in the stomach that subsides or diminishes immediately after eating and then reemerges 2 to 3 hours later. The pain usually presents in the upper abdomen, but sometimes may be found below the sternum. With some patients, the pain occurs immediately after eating. Nausea, vomiting, belching, and heartburn are common symptoms. If the erosion is severe, gastric bleeding can occur, resulting in **hematemesis** (vomiting blood) and **melena** (black, tarry stools containing blood).

Some ulcers will heal without medical intervention, but often complications can occur from bleeding or perforation (a hole through the wall of the stomach). More serious ulcerative conditions can cause severe peritonitis and an acute abdomen.

Cholecystitis

The gallbladder is a storage pouch for digestive juices and waste from the liver. Cholecystitis is a condition in which the wall of the gallbladder becomes inflamed. This typically occurs when gallstones form and block the outlet of the gallbladder, causing pain. Sometimes the blockage will pass, but if not, it can lead to cholecystitis. In severe cases, the gallbladder may rupture, causing inflammation to spread and irritating surrounding structures such as the diaphragm and bowel.

This condition presents as a constant, severe pain in the right upper or midabdominal region and may refer to the right upper back, shoulder area, or flank. The pain may steadily increase for hours or may come and go. Cholecystitis commonly produces symptoms approximately 30 minutes after a particularly fatty meal and usually at night. Other symptoms include general GI distress such as nausea and vomiting, indigestion, bloating, gas, and belching. Risk factors for the development of cholecystitis include female sex, increased age, obesity, pregnancy, ethnicity (ie, Native Americans, Hispanic Americans), and rapid weight loss or gain.[1] Older adults may present without the normal symptoms described here. Localized tenderness may be the only finding.

Pancreatitis

The pancreas forms digestive juices and is also the source of insulin and glucagon. Inflammation of the pancreas is called **pancreatitis**. Pancreatitis can be caused by an obstructing gallstone, some medications, heavy alcohol use, and other diseases.[2] Severe pain may present in the upper left and right quadrants and may often radiate to the back. In addition, the patient may report that the pain is worse after eating. Other signs and symptoms accompanying the pain are nausea and vomiting, abdominal distention, and tenderness. Complications such as sepsis or hemorrhage can occur, in which case assessment may also reveal fever or tachycardia.

Street Smarts

When assessing older adults, asking questions and gathering information become even more important because they often do not present with typical signs and symptoms of abdominal emergencies. If your patient is stable, take a few extra moments to ask more questions regarding current symptoms, past medical history, and medications. Important details can be uncovered if you take a moment to look.

Appendicitis

The appendix is a small recess in the large intestine. Inflammation or infection in the appendix is called **appendicitis**, and it is a frequent cause of acute abdomen. This inflammation can eventually cause the tissues to die and/or rupture, causing an abscess, peritonitis, or shock. Initially, the pain caused by appendicitis is generalized, dull, and diffuse and may center in the umbilical area. The pain later localizes to the right lower quadrant of the abdomen. Appendicitis can also cause referred pain to the back or buttocks. The patient may also report nausea and vomiting, anorexia (lack of appetite for food), fever, and chills. Palpating the left lower quadrant of the abdomen may result in right lower quadrant abdominal pain in some patients who have appendicitis.

A classic symptom of appendicitis is rebound tenderness. Rebound tenderness is a result of peritoneal irritation. This can be assessed by pressing down gently and firmly on the abdomen and then quickly releasing the pressure. The patient will feel pain when the pressure is released. Women with appendicitis who are also pregnant may not exhibit this symptom. Another possible exam finding is pain when the supine patient raises the right leg and flexes the hip against resistance, or pain when the patient's right leg is flexed at the knee and the leg is rotated medially to laterally. Because the pain often increases when the patient's legs are straightened, the patient is often more comfortable in the fetal position.

GI Hemorrhage

Bleeding within the GI tract is a symptom of another disease, not a disease itself. GI hemorrhage can be acute, which may be shorter term and more severe, or chronic, which may be of longer duration and less severe. All complaints of bleeding should be considered serious.

A GI hemorrhage can occur in the upper or lower GI tract. Bleeding in the upper GI tract occurs from the esophagus to the first part of the upper small intestine (duodenum). In the esophagus, problems might include peptic ulcers, esophagitis, esophageal varices secondary to liver failure, or a Mallory-Weiss tear, which results from excessive retching or vomiting. Hematemesis is frequently seen in patients with upper GI bleeding. The bloody vomit is either bright red or has the appearance of coffee grounds, depending on where in the GI tract it originated and how briskly it is occurring. Melena, or dark tarry stools, may occur when there is upper GI bleeding, with dark color of the bleeding resulting from partial digestion of the blood.

Lower GI bleeding occurs between the small intestine (below the duodenum) and the anus. Bowel inflammation, diverticulosis, diverticulitis, cancer, and hemorrhoids are common causes of bleeding in the lower GI tract. When bleeding originates in the lower GI tract, the feces is often bright red or maroon in color.

Words of Wisdom

Inflammatory bowel disease (IBD) may cause lower GI bleeding. Forms of IBD include Crohn disease (which may affect the entire digestive tract), ulcerative colitis (which affects the colon and rectum), or a combination of both. IBDs cause periodic abdominal pain, diarrhea, bloody stools (especially in ulcerative colitis), and fatigue. Life-threatening complications of IBDs include cancer, bowel obstruction, bowel perforation, ulcers, and malnutrition. If a patient discloses an IBD in their medical history, consider them to be at high risk for these life-threatening conditions.

Esophagitis

Esophagitis occurs when the lining of the esophagus becomes inflamed by infection or from the acids in the stomach (**gastroesophageal reflux disease [GERD]**). GERD is a condition in which the sphincter between the esophagus and the stomach opens, allowing stomach acid to move up into the esophagus. Also referred to as acid reflux disease, this condition can cause a burning sensation within the chest (heartburn). GERD is one of the most commonly diagnosed GI disorders in the United State, affecting approximately 20% of the total population.[3] People diagnosed with GERD may use antacids, proton pump inhibitors (eg, omeprazole [Prilosec], lansoprazole [Prevacid]), and H_2 blockers (eg, nizatidine [Axid], famotidine [Pepcid]) to treat their condition.

The patient with esophagitis may report pain with swallowing and feeling as if an object is stuck in their throat. Additional symptoms include heartburn, nausea, vomiting, and sores in the mouth. In the worst cases, bleeding can occur from the small capillary vessels within the esophageal lining or the main blood vessels.

Esophageal Varices

Esophageal varices occur when the pressure within the blood vessels surrounding the esophagus increases, frequently as a result of liver failure. The esophageal blood vessels eventually drain their blood into the liver. If the liver becomes damaged and blood cannot flow through it easily, blood begins to back up into the veins that bring blood from the digestive organs to the liver so it can be filtered. This backup increases the pressure inside these veins, especially those in the esophagus. If pressure continues to build, the vessel walls may fail, causing massive upper GI bleeding and, quickly afterward, hematemesis.

In industrialized countries, alcohol is the main cause of liver damage. Long-term alcohol consumption eventually damages the interior of the liver, causing scarring (**cirrhosis**) and obstructed blood flow. In resource-limited countries, where screening and access to treatment are less readily available, viral hepatitis is the main cause of cirrhosis.[4]

Presentation of esophageal varices takes two forms. Initially, the patient shows signs of liver disease, including fatigue, weight loss, jaundice, anorexia, edema in the abdomen, right upper quadrant abdominal pain, itching, nausea, and vomiting. This gradual disease process takes months to years. The varices may be detected in routine testing, which allows for interventions to reduce the risk of rupture.

By contrast, the rupture of undetected varices is far more sudden. Patients may report sudden-onset discomfort in the epigastric region or sternum. They may have severe difficulty swallowing, vomiting of bright red blood, hypotension, and signs of shock. If the bleeding is less dramatic, hematemesis and melena are likely. Regardless of the speed of bleeding, damage to these vessels can be life threatening. Spontaneous rupture is often life threatening and significant blood loss at the scene may be evident. Major ruptures can lead to death in a matter of minutes.

Mallory-Weiss Tear

A Mallory-Weiss tear is a tear in the junction between the esophagus and the stomach, causing severe bleeding and potentially death. The leading cause of a Mallory-Weiss tear is alcohol use disorder. Other causes include eating disorders, severe vomiting related to pregnancy, and GERD.[5]

Violent coughing or vomiting is the principal cause. The extent of the bleeding can range from minor bleeding, resulting in little blood loss, to severe bleeding and extreme fluid loss. In extreme cases, patients may experience signs and symptoms of shock, upper abdominal pain, hematemesis, and melena.

Gastroenteritis

Acute gastroenteritis comprises a family of conditions revolving around a central theme of infection combined with diarrhea, nausea, and vomiting. Bacterial and viral organisms can cause this condition. These organisms typically enter the body through contaminated food or water. Patients may begin to experience an upset stomach and diarrhea as soon as several hours or several days after contact with the contaminated matter. The disease can then run its course in 2 to 3 days or continue for several weeks.

Gastroenteritis may also be caused by noninfectious conditions such as adverse reactions to medications, exposure to certain toxins, or chemotherapy. The symptoms are similar regardless of the underlying cause.

Diarrhea is the principal symptom in both infectious and noninfectious gastroenteritis. Patients may experience large dumping-type diarrhea or frequent small liquid stools. The diarrhea may contain blood and/or pus, and it may have a foul odor or be odorless. Abdominal cramping is frequently reported. Nausea, vomiting, fever, and anorexia are also present. If the diarrhea continues, dehydration will result. As the volume of fluid loss increases, the likelihood of shock increases.

Diverticulosis

Increased pressure on the weak areas of the colon will eventually create pouches, called **diverticula**. The presence of these diverticula is a condition called

YOU are the EMT

The patient's vital signs are obtained and recorded. Your assessment of his abdomen reveals that it is tender to palpation and that you are able to palpate a pulsatile mass. As your partner retrieves the stretcher from the ambulance, the patient tells you that he has high blood pressure, has depression, and had his appendix removed 30 years ago. He says he takes Toprol and Diovan for high blood pressure. You note that he is becoming more restless and is still experiencing intense pain, which he describes as a 10 on a scale of 0 to 10 (10/10).

Recording Time: 3 Minutes	
Respirations	28 breaths/min; shallow
Pulse	124 beats/min; regular
Skin	Pale (compared with patient baseline), cool, and diaphoretic
Blood pressure	98/60 mm Hg
Oxygen saturation (Spo_2)	96% (on oxygen)

5. What do the patient's vital signs indicate?
6. What do you suspect is the cause of the patient's abdominal pain?

diverticulosis. Three factors are believed to contribute to the development of diverticulosis: small areas of weakness in the colon wall, slow movement of feces through the colon, and inadequate dietary fiber.[6] Prevalence of this disease increases with age, with more than one-third of US adults experiencing diverticulosis by 60 years of age.[7]

In many cases, diverticulosis is asymptomatic throughout a person's life. However, two chief complications can develop. The first complication occurs when feces becomes trapped within these pouches and bacteria grow there, causing localized inflammation (diverticulitis) and infection. The second complication, rectal bleeding caused by a ruptured artery within a diverticulum, is the most common cause of lower GI bleeding in the United States.[8]

Because of the local infections of these pouches, scar tissue forms, causing the tissue to stick together and narrowing the diameter of the colon. The colon's decreased diameter results in constipation and bowel obstruction. In severe cases, a false channel (fistula) may form between the colon and another organ (often the bladder), or the infected diverticula may burst, causing perforation of the affected segment of colon and spilling bacteria-laden feces into the abdominal cavity. If severe enough and left untreated, infection can lead to septic shock.

The main symptom of diverticulitis is abdominal pain, which tends to be localized to the left side of the lower abdomen. Classic signs of infection include fever, malaise, body aches, chills, nausea, and vomiting. GI bleeding related to diverticulosis may be bright red (as the blood products do not have time to be digested) or dark maroon and is typically painless.

Hemorrhoids

Hemorrhoids are created by swelling and inflammation of the blood vessels surrounding the rectum. They are a common problem, with almost one-half the population having at least one hemorrhoid by age 50 years.[9] Hemorrhoids may result from conditions that increase pressure on the rectum or irritation of the rectum. Pregnancy, straining at stool, and chronic constipation cause increased pressure. Diarrhea can cause irritation.

Hemorrhoids may be internal (high in the rectum, usually not visible, often painless, and often associated with bright red, brisk bleeding) or external (low in the rectum, often clearly visible, and painful).

Hemorrhoids present as bright red blood during defecation. This bleeding tends to be minimal and is easily controlled. Additionally, patients may experience itching and a small mass on the rectum. Typically, this mass is a clot formed in response to the mild bleeding.

Abdominal Aortic Aneurysm

The aorta lies immediately behind the peritoneum. In older people, the wall of the aorta sometimes develops weak areas that swell to form an abdominal aortic aneurysm (AAA). A pulsating mass may be felt in the abdomen, although this is a rare sign and is often hard to detect. Use extreme caution when trying to assess or detect this condition. The development of an aneurysm is rarely associated with symptoms because it occurs slowly, but if the aneurysm tears and ruptures, massive hemorrhage may occur, and the patient will present with signs of acute peritoneal irritation and hemorrhagic shock. The patient may also report radiation of severe pain to the back because the peritoneum can be stripped away from the wall of the main abdominal cavity by the hemorrhage. Back pain is a common symptom when an aneurysm has started to expand and the aortic linings begin to tear. Back pain that cannot be easily explained should be investigated closely in patients who are suspected of having an AAA. The patient may describe the pain as tearing, which is different than most other descriptions of abdominal pain. The association of acute abdominal signs and symptoms of shock requires prompt transport. Because this is a fragile situation with a large, leaking artery, avoid unnecessary or vigorous palpation of the abdomen. If signs of shock develop, avoid any actions that can cause a small tear to expand. At the EMT level, aggressive treatment for shock includes administering oxygen, covering the patient with a blanket, and providing rapid transport. Remember to handle the patient gently during transport.

Hernia

A **hernia** is a protrusion of an organ or tissue through a hole or opening into a body cavity where it does not belong. Hernias can occur as a result of the following:

- A congenital defect, as around the umbilicus
- A surgical wound that has failed to heal properly
- A natural weakness in an area, such as in the groin

In adults, the risk of hernias increases with age, with the highest incidence in those between 75 and 80 years. In children, hernias are most common before 5 years of age.[10]

Hernias do not always produce a mass or lump that the patient will notice. At times, the mass will disappear back into the body cavity in which it belongs. In this case, the hernia is said to be reducible. If the mass cannot be pushed back within the body, it is said to be incarcerated. When a hernia is incarcerated, however, its contents may become seriously compressed by the surrounding tissue, eventually compromising the blood supply. This situation, called **strangulation**, is a serious medical emergency. Immediate surgery is required to remove any dead tissue and repair the hernia.

The following signs and symptoms indicate a serious hernia problem:

- Reducible mass that is no longer reducible
- Pain at the hernia site
- Tenderness when the hernia is palpated
- Red or blue skin discoloration over the hernia
- Fever and tachycardia

Any of these signs and symptoms is cause for prompt transport to the emergency department (ED).

Urinary System Dysfunction

Issues in the urinary system can cause acute abdominal pain. Bladder inflammation, called **cystitis**, is common, especially in women. This condition is generally caused by a bacterial infection and can be referred to as a **urinary tract infection (UTI)**. A bladder infection can be painful. Patients with cystitis usually have midline lower abdominal pain. They may also report blood in the urine, urgency and frequency in urination, and pressure and pain around the bladder. If the infection is severe, the urethra can become inflamed, causing urinary retention. When you are assessing a patient with cystitis, the patient may report tenderness when you are palpating the abdomen over the bladder (just above the pubic bone). Cystitis can become a serious health problem if the infection spreads to the kidneys, which, if untreated, may lead to sepsis or septic shock.

Kidney Dysfunction

The kidneys play a major role in maintaining homeostasis, or keeping all body systems in balance. The kidneys preserve this balance by eliminating waste from the blood. When the kidneys fail, the patient loses the ability to excrete waste from the body, leading to a condition called **uremia**. This means that the waste product, urea, which is normally excreted into the urine, remains in the blood.

Chemicals may crystallize in the urine and form **kidney stones** (renal calculi). Kidney stones can grow over time, and if a stone passes into the ureter, it can cause a blockage that prevents urine from passing. Pain may result from the stretching and dilating of the ureter behind the location of the stone, which causes it to spasm, and from increasing pressure in the kidney from the backup of urine. Patients may initially report vague discomfort in the flank, but the pain can become quite intense and typically will radiate to the groin or testicles. These patients are often agitated and restless as they try to get into a comfortable position to relieve the pain. They may also report nausea and vomiting. The pain from kidney stones may vary as the stone moves within the ureter. In many cases, the stone will pass on its own, moving through the ureters, into the bladder, and eventually through the urethra during urination. In other cases, it may have to be surgically removed or broken up. A slight amount of blood in the urine (hematuria) before or after the stone passes may be present because of irritation of the ureter.

Kidney (renal) failure can be acute or chronic. Acute kidney injury (AKI) is a sudden (possibly over a period of days) decrease in function. It occurs from a variety of causes, including hemorrhage, dehydration, trauma, shock, sepsis, heart failure, medications, drug use, and kidney stones. AKI very often can be reversed with prompt diagnosis and treatment.[11]

CKD is irreversible; however, with proper treatment, its progression can be slowed. It develops over months and years. Diabetes and hypertension are common causes of CKD. As the disease progresses, the kidney tissue shrinks and function diminishes. Eventually the patient requires dialysis or a kidney transplant to remove waste products from the bloodstream.[12]

Patients with untreated CKD or patients with CKD who have missed scheduled dialysis may exhibit a wide variety of symptoms, ranging from simply not feeling well to an altered level of consciousness. Additional signs and symptoms include lethargy, nausea, headaches, cramps, and edema in the extremities and face because of fluid imbalances. In later stages, seizures and coma are possible. Patients with CKD have a high incidence of heart disease, including heart failure and arrhythmias, leading to cardiac arrest.[13] These patients tend to be anemic and bleed easily, particularly when taking medications that impair clotting.

Urinary System Dysfunction in Older Adults

Although the kidneys of an older person may be capable of dealing with day-to-day demands, they may not be able to meet unusual challenges, such as those imposed by illness. For that reason, acute illness in older patients is often accompanied by derangements in fluid and electrolyte balance. Aging kidneys, for example, respond sluggishly to sodium deficiency. An older patient may experience substantial sodium loss before the kidneys halt urinary sodium excretion, a problem that is exacerbated by the markedly decreased thirst mechanism in older people. The net result may be a rapid development of severe dehydration.

Bladder continence requires an anatomically correct genitourinary tract, functioning and intact sphincters, and properly working cognitive and physical functions. Urinary incontinence (involuntary loss of urine) can have significant social and emotional effects, but relatively few people admit to the problem and even fewer seek treatment. Incontinence is not a normal part of aging and can lead to skin irritation, skin breakdown, and UTIs. As people age, the capacity of the bladder decreases. Therefore, an older person may find it difficult to postpone voiding or may have involuntary bladder contractions. An increase in nocturnal voiding is common. Two major types of incontinence are distinguished: stress and urge. Stress incontinence occurs during activities such as coughing, laughing, sneezing, lifting, and exercise. Urge incontinence occurs when you have a sudden urge to urinate. With urge incontinence, the urinary bladder contracts when it shouldn't, causing some urine to leak through the sphincter muscles holding the bladder closed. Treatment of incontinence consists of medications, physical therapy, and possibly surgery.

The opposite of incontinence is urinary retention or difficulty urinating. Patients may have difficulty voiding or absence of voiding as a result of many medical causes. Postoperative urinary retention is a common complication following surgery.[14] In men, enlargement of the prostate can place pressure on the urethra, making voiding difficult. Acute urinary retention is very painful. The patient may call 9-1-1 for transport to an ED so a urinary catheter can be inserted to relieve the pressure. Chronic urinary retention may result in bladder infections. In severe cases of urinary retention, patients may experience kidney failure. If a patient has a urinary catheter in place, it may be a source of infection.

Problems Relating to the Female Reproductive Organs

Gynecologic problems are a common cause of acute abdominal pain. Always consider that a woman with lower quadrant abdominal pain and tenderness may have a problem related to her ovaries, fallopian tubes, or uterus. Some of these conditions are life threatening, so an appropriate history and physical examination are essential. Chapter 33, *Gynecologic Emergencies*, covers gynecologic emergencies in depth.

Age-Related Considerations

GI Emergencies in the Geriatric Patient

GI issues in older people are often attributable to changes related to age or to the diseases, or medications to treat those diseases, that come with advanced age. Age-related changes in the GI system include poor muscle tone of the smooth muscle sphincter between the esophagus and stomach that can cause regurgitation and lead to heartburn and acid reflux. Other changes include a decrease in hydrochloric acid in the stomach and alterations in absorption of nutrients and slowing peristalsis, which can cause constipation. The rectal sphincter may also become weak, resulting in fecal incontinence, or lack of bowel control.

Changes in the liver predispose older people to many problems. The liver, which is responsible for removing toxins and breaking down drugs in the body, shrinks with age. Blood flow to the liver declines, and there is decreased metabolism. This has a direct effect on how medications may affect the patient.

Geriatric patients are also susceptible to acute abdomen. However, the signs and symptoms in geriatric patients might be different than in younger patients. Because of altered pain sensation, geriatric patients with an acute abdomen may not feel any discomfort or may describe the discomfort as mild, even in severe conditions. For example, a geriatric patient with cholecystitis may not present with pain, but only localized tenderness on palpation. The pain may be referred to the patient's shoulder and may mimic other conditions such as myocardial infarction. Be mindful that older patients may not exhibit rigidity or guarding as would a younger adult.

Because the older patient has decreased body temperature regulation and response, the patient with an acute abdomen, including peritonitis, may have little or no fever at all.

Also keep in mind that abdominal pain can be suggestive of other problems. It is sometimes related to cardiac conditions, and it is frequently caused by bowel impaction or obstruction. Older patients may strain while trying to have a bowel movement. This can stimulate the vagus nerve, leading to a vasovagal response, in which the heart rate drops dramatically and the patient becomes dizzy or has a syncopal episode. The patient will usually be in stable condition on your arrival but requires transport to rule out other conditions. Keep in mind that obstructions can be very serious and can lead to bowel ruptures that often are life threatening.

Because of the older patient's response to the acute abdomen, a delay in identifying the condition and seeking medical attention is possible, putting the patient at risk for complications. You should ask about the patient's medical history, especially the history of recent illness, to identify a potential illness. Ask about abdominal discomfort, when the patient last had a bowel movement, and whether the patient was constipated or had diarrhea. Inquire if the patient has had previous bowel obstructions. Inquire as to when the patient last ate, how much fluid they have consumed, and whether they have vomited. A geriatric patient may consider their daily coffee to be adequate fluid intake, but coffee and other caffeinated drinks may cause vasoconstriction and dehydration.

Quickly determining the severity of the patient's problem can hasten proper treatment and recovery. Provide transport to an appropriate facility that can meet the needs of a geriatric patient.

GI Emergencies in the Pediatric Patient

As with any injury or complaint in the abdominal region, the signs and symptoms of a GI emergency in a pediatric patient may be vague in nature. Pediatric patients may not be able to pinpoint the exact site where the pain or discomfort originates but will have complaints of diffuse tenderness. Never take a complaint of abdominal pain and discomfort lightly. Assess the child's temperature and monitor for signs and symptoms of shock, which include an altered mental status; pale (compared with patient's baseline), cool skin; tachypnea; tachycardia; and bradycardia (late sign).

Street Smarts

Some children who have pneumonia, especially in the lower lobes of the lungs, initially report abdominal pain. Be sure to note any signs of respiratory illness when you encounter this chief complaint.

Complaints of GI origin are common in the pediatric population. A common source of GI upset is the ingestion of certain foods or unknown substances, such as milk or ice cream (lactose intolerance). In most cases, you will be faced with a pediatric patient who is experiencing abdominal discomfort with nausea, vomiting, and/or diarrhea. Both vomiting and diarrhea can rapidly cause dehydration in children.

Appendicitis is also fairly common in pediatric patients and, if untreated, can lead to peritonitis (inflammation of the peritoneum, which lines the abdominal cavity) or shock. Appendicitis will typically present with a fever and pain on palpation of the right lower abdominal quadrant. Rebound tenderness is a common sign associated with appendicitis. Remember that constipation also can be a cause of abdominal pain in children. If you suspect appendicitis, promptly transport the child to the hospital for further evaluation.

Because children are sensitive to fluid loss, obtain a thorough history from the parent or primary caregiver. Specifically, ask questions such as the following:

- How many wet diapers has your child had today?

- Is your child able to tolerate liquids and keep them down?
- How many times has your child had diarrhea and for how long?
- Are tears present when your child cries?

These questions can help to determine how dehydrated the patient may be. If the child is dehydrated, transport to the hospital for further care.

Words of Wisdom

An acute abdomen usually indicates peritonitis, in which generalized signs can make it challenging to determine exactly where the problem lies, even for physicians. Knowing abdominal assessment steps well and recording your findings in detail are important early factors in reaching a diagnosis.

Patient Assessment

Scene Size-up

As always, ensure that the scene is safe and take standard precautions with a minimum of gloves and eye protection. Consider donning a face shield, gown, and covering your shoes with disposable, protective covers because there may be feces and urine on the floor and some patients may have active projectile vomiting.

Determine the number of patients at the scene. If your call involves going to the patient's home and they do not come to the door, the patient may have had a syncopal episode (fainted). Request police assistance to help you gain access to the patient. Consider the need for additional or specialized medical resources and request them early.

Be alert for clues to help you determine the nature of illness (NOI) or the mechanism of injury. Clues will help you develop an early index of suspicion for life threats. For example, a pale and sweating patient who reports tearing pain may have an AAA. Observe the scene closely and interview bystanders or family members if the NOI is not obvious. In some cases, your senses can help give you a clue as to the NOI. For example, GI bleeding often has a characteristic odor that you will learn to recognize. Keep in mind that acute abdomen can be the result of violence, such as blunt or penetrating trauma, so always be vigilant. Chapter 30, *Abdominal and Genitourinary Injuries*, discusses traumatic injuries in detail.

Primary Assessment

Begin assessing the patient by first looking for and treating any life-threatening conditions. Assess the patient's level of consciousness and ABCs; threats to airway, breathing, or circulation are considered life threatening and must be treated immediately. Rapidly observe the patient and the environment. Note the position of the patient. Commonly, the patient will have their knees drawn up to help alleviate the pain associated with acute abdomen. Consider necessary treatment and transport options and the need for early advanced life support (ALS) assistance.

If the chief complaint indicates a life-threatening problem, assess and treat it immediately. If the chief complaint is a minor problem, it should wait until you have had a chance to assess for and treat any potential life threats.

Ensure that the patient's airway is clear and that the patient's respirations are adequate. Administer oxygen to the patient when needed. As a result of the abdominal pain, the patient may show shallow or inadequate respirations because deep breaths often intensify the pain.

When you are assessing the patient's circulation, remember to assess for major bleeding. Ask the patient about amount and frequency of blood in the vomit (hematemesis); black, tarry stools (melena); or bright red, bloody stools. The patient's pulse rate and quality, as well as skin condition, may indicate shock. Because skin pallor can be difficult to detect in patients with dark skin, check for pale mucous membranes inside the inner lower eyelid or slow capillary refill. On general observation, the patient may appear ashen or gray. Ask the patient to open their mouth and assess the mucous membranes to see if they are dry or if the tongue is furrowed, which may indicate dehydration. Check the pulses in both feet because a difference in pulse strength between the arms and legs may indicate AAA. Assess for poor skin turgor, another sign of dehydration. The abdomen should be inspected for wounds or bruising. Bruising around the umbilicus or on the flanks may indicate internal abdominal bleeding.

Shock may be caused by hypovolemia or may be the result of a severe infection (septic). If evidence of shock (inadequate perfusion) is present, interventions should include high-flow oxygen, placing the patient supine, and keeping the patient warm. Ensure that you provide prompt treatment for life threats and do not delay transport.

Certain patients should be transported quickly. These include patients who have airway, breathing, or circulation problems, including problems with pulse and perfusion, and patients with suspected internal bleeding. If transport times are extended, ALS may be able to provide advanced care during transport. Included in the group to call for ALS intercept and to package quickly and transport rapidly are patients who have a poor general impression, especially pediatric and geriatric patients. Pale, cool, diaphoretic skin; tachycardia; hypotension; and altered level of consciousness are all signs of significant illness.

Ensure that the ride during transport is as gentle as possible for the patient. Drive smoothly and steadily. A rough drive can result in increased vehicle movement, potentially aggravating and possibly worsening the patient's abdominal pain.

History Taking

If the patient is responsive, begin with obtaining the SAMPLE (Signs and symptoms, Allergies, Medications, Pertinent past medical history, Last oral intake, Events leading up to the illness or injury) history. When you are obtaining the medication history, ask if the patient has taken antibiotics or pain relievers such as ibuprofen or aspirin recently. Inquire about recent use of alcohol. Ask the following questions specific to the signs and symptoms of a GI or urologic emergency:

- **Nausea and vomiting.** Do you feel nauseous? Have you vomited? How many times? Over what period of time? Was there red blood? Did it look like coffee grounds?
- **Changes in bowel habits.** Has there been any change in your bowel habits? Have you been constipated? Did the stool look dark and tarry? Have you had diarrhea? How many times and over what period of time? Was there any red blood in it?
- **Urination.** Have you been urinating more or less often? Is there pain when you urinate? Is the color dark or unusual? Is there an unusual odor?
- **Weight loss.** Have you had unexplained weight loss or weight gain recently? How many pounds?
- **Belching or flatulence.** Have you experienced belching or flatulence? For how long?
- **Pain.** What does the pain feel like? How long have you had this pain? Is the pain constant or intermittent? Have you had similar pain in the past? Have you done anything to relieve the pain? For any abdominal discomfort, use the OPQRST (Onset, Provocation/palliation, Quality, Region/radiation, Severity, Timing)

YOU are the EMT

After providing further assessment, you place the patient onto the stretcher, load him into the ambulance, and proceed to the closest appropriate hospital, which is located 20 miles away. En route, you reassess the patient.

Recording Time: 12 Minutes	
Level of consciousness	Conscious and alert; restless
Respirations	28 breaths/min; shallow
Pulse	130 beats/min; weak and regular
Skin	Cool, pale, and diaphoretic
Blood pressure	100/62 mm Hg
Oxygen saturation (Spo_2)	98% (on oxygen)

7. Are there any special considerations for this patient? If so, what are they?

mnemonic, with a focus on the *P*, by asking the patient what makes the pain better or worse.

- **Other.** Ask about any other signs or symptoms related to this complaint, such as "Are there any changes you have noted recently that may be contributing to your pain?" "Have you had a fever?"
- **Concurrent chest pain.** If the patient reports chest pain, again use the OPQRST mnemonic, with a focus on *P*, and ask the patient what makes the pain better or worse.

Continue with the SAMPLE history. If the patient is a woman of childbearing age, determine the date of the last menstrual period. This will determine if the patient could possibly be pregnant or raise the suspicion of other obstetric emergencies.

Ask the patient about their last oral intake. It is important to determine whether the patient has ingested any substance that could be causing the acute abdomen. If eating causes pain, discomfort, vomiting, or diarrhea, the patient will eat less frequently or stop eating altogether. Do not give the patient anything by mouth. Food or fluid may only aggravate many of the symptoms. Also, the presence of food in the stomach increases the risk of aspiration.

Words of Wisdom

Consider and document pertinent negatives, which are normal findings that warrant no care or intervention. It is important to know and document, for example, that the patient denies shortness of breath or radiation of abdominal pain.

Finally, determine the events that led up to the patient's present illness. If you suspect gastroenteritis, ask if other close contacts have been ill. Question the patient about any recent trauma.

The SAMPLE history may not affect the interventions you perform, but it will help provide needed information for the physician in the ED to aid in determining the cause of the acute abdomen.

Secondary Assessment

In some situations, patients are comfortable only when lying in one particular position, which tends to relax muscles adjacent to the inflamed organ and thus lessen the pain. Therefore, the position of the patient may provide you with an important clue. For example, a patient with appendicitis may draw up the right knee. A patient with pancreatitis may lie curled up on one side.

Information gathered in the history-taking portion of the patient assessment may be used to focus your physical examination of the abdomen. A normal abdomen is soft and not tender to the touch. Pain and tenderness are the most common symptoms of an acute abdomen. The pain may be sharply localized or diffuse and will vary in its severity. Localized pain gives a clue to the problem organ or area causing it. Tenderness may be minimal or so great that the patient will not allow you to touch the abdomen. In some instances, the muscles of the abdominal wall become rigid in an involuntary effort to protect the abdomen from further irritation. This boardlike muscle spasm, called **guarding**, can be seen with major problems such as a perforated ulcer or pancreatitis.

Remember, the patient with peritonitis usually has abdominal pain, even when lying quietly. The patient may have difficulty breathing and may take rapid, shallow breaths because of the pain. Usually, you will find tenderness on palpation of the abdomen or when the patient moves. The degree of pain and tenderness is usually related directly to the severity of peritoneal inflammation.

Use the following steps to assess the abdomen:

1. Explain to the patient how you will assess the abdomen.
2. Position the patient. Place the patient in a supine position with the legs drawn up and flexed at the knees to relax the abdominal muscles, unless there is any trauma, in which case the patient will remain supine and stabilized. Determine whether the patient is restless or quiet, and whether motion causes pain.
3. Perform a visual assessment. Expose the abdomen and visually assess it. Does the abdomen appear distended (enlarged)? Do you see any pulsating masses (possibly indicating an AAA)? Is there bruising to the abdominal wall? Are there any surgical scars?
4. Palpate the abdomen.
   - Ask the patient where the pain is most intense. Palpate all four quadrants, proceeding in a clockwise direction. Palpate

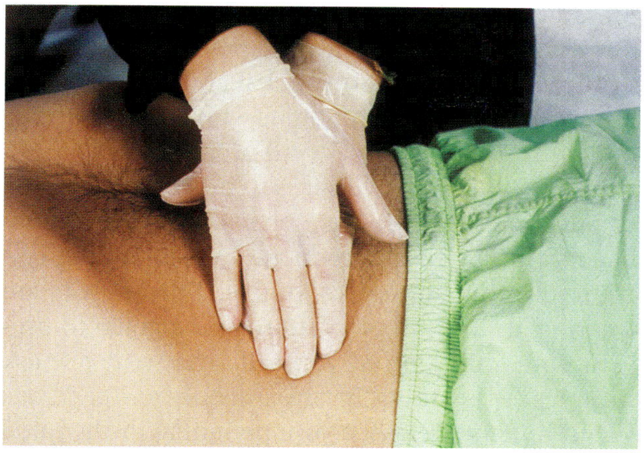

FIGURE 19-4 Check for tenderness or rigidity by gently palpating the abdomen.

gently to determine whether each quadrant is tense (guarded) or soft when palpated (**FIGURE 19-4**). Avoid palpating the painful quadrant first. If the most painful area is palpated first, the patient may guard against further examination, making your assessment more difficult and less reliable.

- Remember to be very gentle when palpating the abdomen. Occasionally, an organ within the abdomen will be enlarged and fragile. Rough palpation could cause further damage. If you see a pulsating mass, do not touch it; manipulating an aortic aneurysm could cause it to rupture.

5. Interpret the patient's response.
   - Note whether the pain is localized to a particular quadrant or diffuse (widespread).
   - Observe how the patient responds as you palpate, looking for a facial grimace or a verbal "ouch." Do not ask the patient, "Does it hurt here?" as you palpate.
   - Note any rebound tenderness, which may present as discomfort when direct pressure is applied, but extreme pain when pressure is released. This finding is an indicator of appendicitis. Use extreme caution when palpating for rebound tenderness.
   - Determine whether the patient can relax the abdominal wall on command. Guarding or rigidity may be present, which can indicate peritoneal irritation.

Findings of a high respiratory rate with a normal pulse rate and blood pressure may indicate the patient is unable to ventilate properly because deep breathing causes pain. A high respiratory rate and pulse rate with signs of shock, such as pallor and diaphoresis (profuse sweating), may indicate septic or hypovolemic shock. When treating a patient who has a dialysis shunt or fistula in their arm, it is important not to obtain a blood pressure reading in the same arm as the shunt to avoid damaging the fistula.

Words of Wisdom

Metabolic conditions such as high blood glucose (hyperglycemia) may present with abdominal pain and vomiting. In some cases, this emergency may be the first indication a patient has diabetes. When children or adults who have not yet been diagnosed with diabetes have this presentation, it can be life threatening. Consider evaluation of blood glucose levels as a component of your assessment, as allowed by your protocols. More information in diabetes is found in Chapter 20, *Endocrine and Hematologic Emergencies*.

Reassessment

Because it is often difficult to determine the cause of an acute abdominal emergency, it is extremely important to reassess your patient frequently to determine whether the patient's condition has changed. Remember, the condition of a patient with an acute abdomen can change rapidly from stable to unstable.

Vital signs must be reassessed and compared with the patient's baseline vital signs. If anything changes en route to the hospital, manage the problem and document any changes or additional treatment.

Reassess the patient and then ask the following questions (where appropriate):

- Has the patient's level of consciousness changed?
- Has the patient become more anxious?
- Has the appearance of the skin changed?
- Has the pain gotten better or worse?
- Has bleeding increased or decreased?
- Is current treatment improving the patient's condition?

- Has an already identified problem gotten better or worse?
- What is the nature of any newly identified problems?

Interventions generally include treating for shock, providing emotional support, and keeping the patient as comfortable as possible. Administer oxygen if the patient is hypoxemic, cover the patient with a blanket for warmth, and provide gentle transport for the patient without delay. Place the patient in a position of comfort. You will find that patients often want to be supine with their knees drawn up. If the patient wants to lie on their side, try to make that possible. Be sure that you can observe and maintain the patient's airway because vomiting is common. If the patient's pain is extreme or the patient is showing significant signs of shock, consider the use of ALS assistance (if available) for intravenous fluids and management of pain, nausea, or vomiting. If transport time is extended and rapid transport is needed, consider air medical transport if available.

Emergency Medical Care

Although you cannot treat the causes of acute abdomen, you can take steps to provide comfort and lessen the effects of shock by reassuring the patient and providing treatment that is appropriate for the presenting condition. Loosen restrictive clothing and transport the patient gently in a position of comfort.

Treat the patient for shock if any signs of shock are apparent. Position patients who are vomiting to maintain a patent airway and prepare to suction if needed. Contain the vomitus to prevent the spread of infections (by using a biohazard bag). Airborne bacteria and viruses produced from vomiting can be easily transmitted to others. Ensure you are wearing gloves, eye protection, and a gown to prevent contamination of yourself, and wear a mask to prevent breathing in any infectious organisms. When you have released your patient to the hospital staff, clean the ambulance and any equipment you have used, preferably with an antibacterial cleaner. Do not forget to wash your hands even though you were wearing gloves.

Constantly reassess your patient's condition for signs of deterioration.

Safety Tips

Infection from the bacterium *Clostridioides difficile* (commonly referred to as *C diff)* can present with GI symptoms such as diarrhea. To avoid the spread of *C difficile*, clinicians must wash their hands with soap and water and decontaminate equipment after each call.

YOU are the EMT

With an estimated time of arrival at the hospital of 22 minutes, you reassess the patient and then call in your radio report. The patient remains conscious and alert, but restless, and is still experiencing 10/10 abdominal pain.

Recording Time: 17 Minutes	
Level of consciousness	Conscious and alert; restless
Respirations	28 breaths/min; shallow
Pulse	128 beats/min; weak and regular
Skin	Cool, clammy, and diaphoretic
Blood pressure	96/58 mm Hg
Oxygen saturation (Spo_2)	97% (on oxygen)

The patient's condition is unchanged on arrival at the hospital. You give your verbal report to the charge nurse. After further assessment and treatment in the ED, the patient is taken to surgery. You later learn that he had an expanding AAA, which was successfully repaired.

8. Could you have done anything definitively for this patient in the field? Why or why not?

Dialysis Emergencies

Patients with end-stage renal disease (ESRD), also referred to as CKD, are treated with either kidney transplantation or dialysis, whether peritoneal dialysis (PD) or hemodialysis.[15] In dialysis, the patient's blood is filtered and cleansed of the toxins and then returned to the body. The treatment eliminates waste, normalizes the blood chemistry, and reduces excess fluid. If a patient misses a dialysis treatment, weakness and pulmonary edema can be the first in a series of conditions that can become progressively more serious if normal balance is not returned to the patient's body.

In the past, hemodialysis required the patient to make trips to a dialysis center several times a week for treatment. Now, patients and their care partner have the option to receive training and perform hemodialysis in the comfort of their home (**FIGURE 19-5**). This method allows the patient flexibility over their dialysis schedule. Occasionally, complications are encountered in this setting that require an EMS response.

In hemodialysis, the patient's blood circulates through a dialysis machine that functions in much the same way as the normal kidneys. Most patients undergoing long-term hemodialysis have some sort of fistula or graft, sometimes referred to as an access port, which is a surgically created connection between a vein and an artery. This fistula or graft creates a large vessel that will permit high blood flow into and out of the dialysis machine. The patient is connected to the dialysis machine through a large needle inserted into the arterial end of the fistula or graft and another needle placed in the venous end to return the cleaned blood from the dialysis machine to the body. The fistula or graft is usually located in the forearm or upper arm; less commonly, it is located in the leg. Another option for dialysis until a fistula or graft is created is a central venous catheter located in the chest, neck, or groin; however, the risk of infection or clotting is higher with this method, so it is typically temporary (**FIGURE 19-6**).

Dialysis machines are programmed to detect pressure changes in the lines. If the machine malfunctions and fails to detect a change in pressure caused by dislodgement of the needle at the venous end of the patient's shunt/fistula, blood will be pumped into the bed or onto the floor rather than back into the patient's venous system and the patient can lose 2 L of blood (approximately 40% of their blood volume) within a few minutes.[16] While this situation is rare, hypovolemic shock occurs quickly and mortality is high. If your basic life support (BLS) unit is dispatched to this emergency, you should request an ALS unit immediately, ideally one with the ability to transfuse blood.

In PD, fluid circulates within the peritoneal cavity. Urea and other toxins diffuse across the peritoneum into the dialysis fluid, which is then drained from the peritoneum, allowing the peritoneum to essentially function as a kidney. Patients on home PD will have a catheter in their abdomen that they use to connect to a PD machine, typically at night.

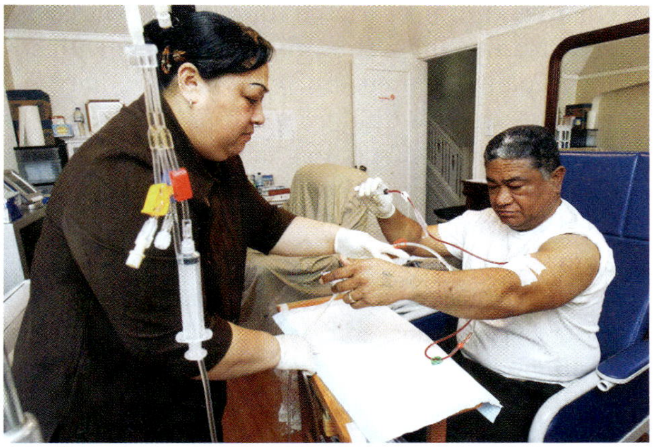

FIGURE 19-5 Patient connected to a dialysis machine at home.

Words of Wisdom

Contact local dialysis centers and inquire about home hemodialysis programs. They may be able to provide training to your department, which will help you care for home dialysis patients more effectively if an emergency arises.

In PD, large amounts of specifically formulated dialysis fluid are infused into (and back out of) a large catheter in the abdominal cavity. This fluid stays in the cavity for 1 to 2 hours, allowing equilibrium to occur. With proper training, PD can be performed in the home (**FIGURE 19-7**). PD is effective but carries a small risk of peritonitis. Peritonitis can

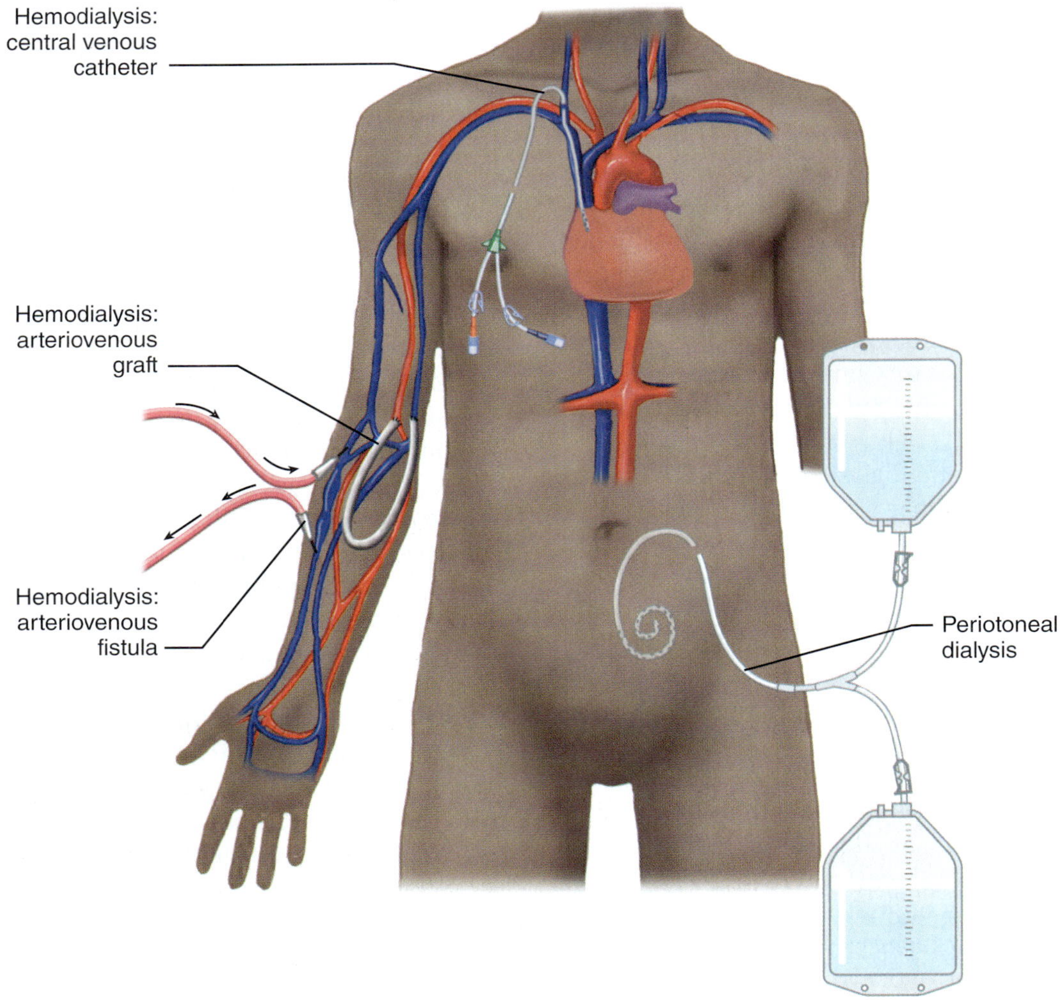

FIGURE 19-6 Types of dialysis access.

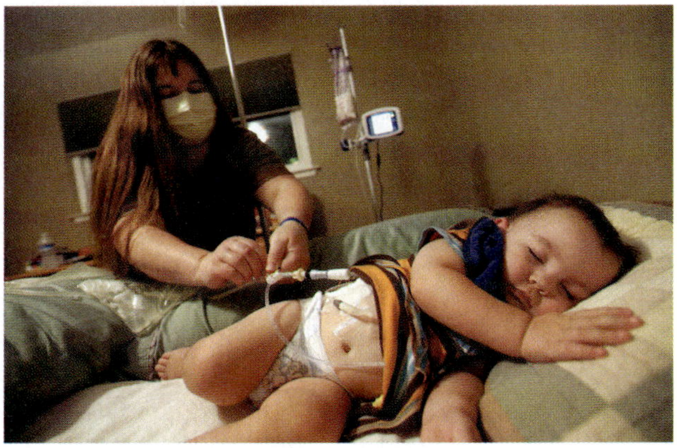

FIGURE 19-7 A mother administering peritoneal dialysis to her child at home.

occur due to bacteria contaminating the dialysis site. A patient with peritonitis may present with abdominal pain, hypotension, fever, nausea, diarrhea, and cloudy dialysis fluid.[17]

The adverse effects of dialysis include hypotension, dysrhythmias, chest pain, muscle cramps, nausea and vomiting, altered mental status, electrolyte imbalances, hemorrhage from the access site, and infection at the access site. If your call involves a patient on dialysis, start with the XABCs: control life-threatening hemorrhage (exsanguination), and assess and manage the airway, breathing, and circulation. Provide high-flow oxygen if indicated. Position the patient sitting up in cases of pulmonary edema or supine if the patient is in shock, and transport promptly.

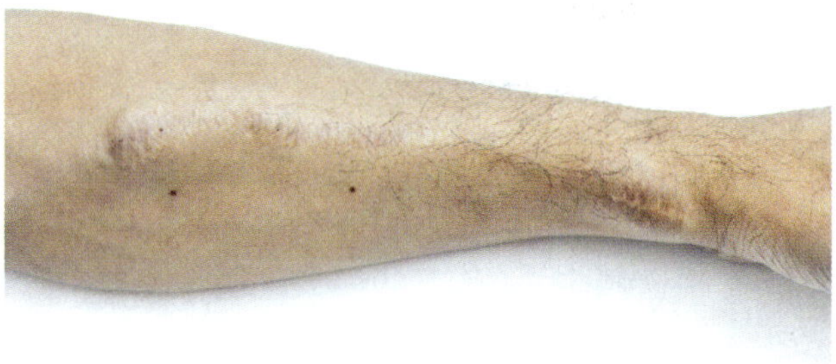

FIGURE 19-8 A healthy dialysis fistula in the patient's forearm.

Remember, when assessing vital signs in a patient with a dialysis shunt or fistula, do not place a blood pressure cuff over the site. Doing so may damage the shunt or fistula or cause a blood clot to form. If possible, avoid using the arm with the shunt or fistula for vital signs; instead, use the patient's other arm. Examine the fistula when you are assessing the patient to observe for redness or other signs of infection such as pus (**FIGURE 19-8**). When gently palpating the healthy fistula, you will feel a vibration, called a thrill, that is caused by the high pressure of blood flowing through the area when the shunt is functioning well. Note that because of this high blood flow, trauma that disrupts the shunt may cause serious hemorrhage requiring a tourniquet.

Life-threatening bleeding can occur if a patient's port does not stop bleeding after the dialysis needles are removed or if there is trauma to the site. Bleeding from a fistula that cannot be controlled with pressure after the dialysis needle is removed may be difficult to manage. If bleeding is brisk, firm pressure with two fingertips should be applied over the bleeding site with one hand while pressure is applied proximal to the bleeding area with the fingers of the other hand for 15 to 30 minutes. If hemostatic gauze (a dressing that is designed to stop bleeding quickly) is available, place the gauze between your fingers and the bleeding area.[18] Massive bleeding that cannot be immediately controlled in this manner may require application of a tourniquet to prevent exsanguination.

When you arrive on the scene, some patients may have applied a bottlecap keyring (a commercial device that is shaped like the cap of a milk container and can be carried on a keyring) over the bleeding area to control the bleeding. Research on the effectiveness of this device is limited, but if the patient is using the device when you arrive and the bleeding appears to be controlled, do not remove it during transport.[18,19]

If the patient misses a scheduled dialysis session, other emergencies can arise because of the buildup of fluid and other waste products in the body. Possible emergencies include cardiac arrhythmia from electrolyte imbalances, pulmonary edema due to fluid overload, and even cardiac arrest. When responding to a medical call for a patient whose history includes CKD, it is critical to ask what type of dialysis they undergo, how many days per week they have dialysis, when their last dialysis session occurred, and whether they have missed any dialysis sessions.

Some dialysis patients also have urinary catheters. The catheter is placed in the bladder so the urine can run into a bag. These catheters can often be a source of infection. The patient may report fever and general malaise (illness) in addition to any symptoms specific to kidney failure. Leave the device in place, and do not elevate the bag higher than the patient. Treat any signs and symptoms, and transport the patient for further evaluation.

Another option available to some patients who have CKD is kidney transplantation. The donated kidney is transplanted into the abdomen or pelvis of the recipient.[20] This location affords less protection and can be injured more easily in the event of blunt trauma. If a patient who has had a kidney transplantation complains of abdominal pain, it may be a sign of rejection or infection. The drugs used to prevent rejection of the new kidney suppress the immune system, so other signs of a serious abdominal infection may be subtle or absent. These patients require immediate transport.

During transport, unless there is a life-threatening event, make all attempts to deliver the patient to a hospital with dialysis capability.

YOU are the EMT SUMMARY

1. What is the definition of an acute abdomen?

Acute abdomen is a term used to describe the sudden (acute) onset of abdominal pain that is not caused by a traumatic injury. It is generally associated with severe, progressive symptoms that require medical attention. Acute abdominal pain can be caused by dysfunction of one or more of the abdominal organs, such as the liver, spleen, gallbladder, stomach, pancreas, kidneys, large or small intestines, or appendix. It can also be due to an irritation or infection of the lining of the abdominal cavity: the peritoneum.

2. What is your role as an EMT in treating a patient with abdominal pain?

The underlying cause of a patient's abdominal pain, acute or chronic, is often difficult to identify, even for a physician. As an EMT, it is far more important for you to recognize life-threatening conditions and provide prompt emergency care than it is to identify the underlying cause of the patient's pain. It is important to watch for signs of shock and treat it quickly. Patients who are in pain, especially when the pain occurs suddenly, are often very anxious and scared; providing emotional support is an important part of your role. Allowing the patient to assume a position of comfort may also help.

3. What is the proper technique of assessing a patient's abdomen? What should you assess for?

Although assessment of the abdomen may help localize the source of a patient's pain, it should not be prolonged. During the exam, place the patient supine with the legs drawn up and flexed at the knees; this position will relax the abdominal muscles and may alleviate some pain. Look at the abdomen first; does it appear distended (enlarged)? Do you see any pulsating masses (suggests an AAA)? Is there bruising of the abdominal wall (suggests internal hemorrhage)? Ask the patient where the pain is most intense and assess that area last. If the most painful area is palpated first, the patient may guard against further examination, making your assessment more difficult and less reliable. Gently palpate the four abdominal quadrants to determine whether each quadrant is rigid or soft or if there is tenderness, and note the presence of any masses. Pay particular attention to the patient's facial expressions when palpating each abdominal quadrant; this may yield valuable information. Note whether the pain is localized to a particular quadrant or diffuse (widespread). Determine whether the patient can relax the abdominal wall on command; if not, the abdomen is said to be rigid. Avoid vigorous palpation of the abdomen; doing so will only cause the patient more pain and can worsen their condition, especially if one of the abdominal organs is enlarged and fragile.

4. What is the difference between radiating pain and referred pain?

Radiating pain moves from its point of origin to other parts of the body, such as the pain from pancreatitis, which may radiate to the back, or the pain from a kidney stone blockage, which may radiate to the groin. With radiating pain, there is pain at point A and point B, with a trail of pain in between the two points.

Referred pain originates in a particular organ but is described or perceived by the patient as pain in a different location or pain at the point of origin and another location. For example, the origin of pain associated with cholecystitis (inflammation of the gallbladder) is usually the right upper quadrant of the abdomen. However, the patient commonly reports pain in the right shoulder. In some cases, the patient reports pain in both the right upper quadrant and the right shoulder. Unlike with radiating pain, there is no pain in between the two points.

5. What do the patient's vital signs indicate?

The patient's vital signs indicate shock. His respirations are rapid (tachypnea); he has a rapid heart rate (tachycardia); his skin is cool, pale (compared with baseline), and diaphoretic; and his blood pressure—considering the fact that he has a history of hypertension—is low. Whether the patient has an intra-abdominal infection (peritonitis) or intra-abdominal bleeding, the end result, if untreated, will be the same—death!

It is more important to recognize life-threatening conditions (eg, shock) than it is to determine the exact cause of a patient's abdominal pain, or any pain for that matter. You must begin immediate treatment aimed at maintaining adequate perfusion, such as applying high-flow oxygen when indicated (your partner has already done this), keeping him warm, and rapidly preparing for transport.

6. What do you suspect is the cause of the patient's abdominal pain?

The lack of fever, vomiting, or diarrhea makes an infectious cause less likely in this patient.

YOU are the EMT SUMMARY continued

Although only a physician can determine the exact cause of the patient's pain, a severe abdominal pain that radiates to the lower back is characteristic of an AAA.

The typical patient with an AAA is a male in his late 60s or older. As long as the aneurysm is not expanding, the patient usually will be asymptomatic. When the aneurysm starts to expand, however, the patient has a sudden onset of abdominal pain, which is classically described as a ripping or searing sensation in the abdomen that radiates to the back. When an AAA starts expanding and producing symptoms, rupture may be imminent. If aortic rupture occurs, the patient often bleeds to death (exsanguinates) very quickly. If the aneurysm is leaking, however, blood will accumulate in the retroperitoneal space and cause signs of shock; this is what may be happening to your patient.

7. Are there any special considerations for this patient? If so, what are they?

As with any patient exhibiting signs of shock, your priority is to provide transport to an appropriate medical facility with surgical capability without delay. Patients with a suspected aortic aneurysm must be handled carefully; avoid rough driving and unnecessary bumps in the road. Because this is a potentially a fragile situation, with a large, leaking artery, avoid further palpation of the abdomen. Some patients with an abdominal aortic aneurysm have a pulsating mass that can be palpated (and sometimes seen) near the umbilicus. If you see a pulsating mass, do *not* touch it; manipulating an aortic aneurysm could cause it to rupture. However, if you do not see or feel a pulsating mass, it does not necessarily rule out the patient having an abdominal aneurysm, so the same precautions in assessment and treatment should be considered.

Avoid anything that will make the patient more anxious; anxiety causes increases in heart rate and blood pressure. An acute increase in blood pressure, even a slight one, may be all that is needed to cause an aortic rupture. In this particular patient, you should avoid elevating the patient's legs. Elevating the lower extremities may cause a surge of blood back to the heart, resulting in an increase in blood pressure.

8. Could you have done anything definitively for this patient in the field? Why or why not?

No. Definitive care (eg, surgically repairing the aneurysm) can be provided only at the hospital. Although paramedics can start intravenous lines and give pain medications, these interventions are simply aimed at controlling pain and partially treating shock, not fixing the aneurysm. Your role as an EMT is to recognize that the patient's condition is serious, provide emergency medical treatment, and transport without delay.

Prep Kit

Ready for Review

- The acute abdomen is a medical emergency, requiring prompt but gentle transport.
- The pain, tenderness, and abdominal distention associated with an acute abdomen may be signs of peritonitis, which may be caused by any condition that allows pus, blood, feces, urine, gastric juice, intestinal contents, bile, pancreatic juice, amniotic fluid, or other foreign material to lie within or adjacent to the peritoneum.
- You should be able to recognize and provide emergency care and transport of patients experiencing an acute abdominal emergency. These conditions include appendicitis, cholecystitis, ulcer, diverticulosis, abdominal aortic aneurysm, cystitis, kidney infection, kidney stone, pancreatitis, hernia, GI hemorrhage, esophagitis, and Mallory-Weiss tear.
- Signs and symptoms of acute abdomen include pain, nausea, vomiting, and a tense, distended abdomen.
- Pain is common directly over the inflamed area of the peritoneum, or it may be referred

Prep Kit continued

to another part of the body. Referred pain occurs because of the connections between the two different nervous systems supplying the parietal peritoneum and the visceral peritoneum.
- Do not give the patient with an acute abdomen anything by mouth.
- A patient in shock or with any life-threatening condition should be transported without delay. Call for advanced life support assistance if your patient's condition deteriorates during transport.
- You should be familiar with the equipment and general principles of dialysis in the event you must care for or transport a patient experiencing a dialysis-related emergency.

Vital Vocabulary

acute abdomen A condition of sudden onset of pain within the abdomen, usually indicating peritonitis; immediate medical or surgical treatment is necessary.

appendicitis Inflammation or infection of the appendix.

cholecystitis Inflammation of the gallbladder.

cirrhosis A chronic and progressive disease in which normal liver cells are replaced by fibrotic scar tissue.

cystitis Inflammation of the bladder.

diverticula Pouches that bulge out through weak places in the wall of the colon.

diverticulitis Inflammation in small pockets at weak areas in the muscle walls of the intestines.

diverticulosis A condition in which diverticula develop in the colon.

emesis Vomiting.

gastroesophageal reflux disease (GERD) A condition in which the sphincter between the esophagus and the stomach opens, allowing stomach acid to move up into the esophagus, usually resulting in a burning sensation within the chest; also called acid reflux.

guarding Involuntary muscle contractions (spasm) of the abdominal wall; an effort to protect the inflamed abdomen.

hematemesis Vomiting blood.

hernia The protrusion of an organ or tissue through an abnormal body opening.

ileus Paralysis of the bowel, arising from any one of several causes; stops contractions that move material through the intestine.

kidney stones Solid crystalline masses formed in the kidney, resulting from an excess of insoluble salts or uric acid crystallizing in the urine; may become trapped anywhere along the urinary tract.

melena Black, foul-smelling, tarry stool containing digested blood.

pancreatitis Inflammation of the pancreas.

peritoneum The membrane lining the abdominal cavity (parietal peritoneum) and covering the abdominal organs (visceral peritoneum).

peritonitis Inflammation of the peritoneum.

referred pain Pain felt in an area of the body other than the area where the cause of pain is located.

strangulation Complete obstruction of blood circulation in a given organ as a result of compression or entrapment; an emergency situation causing death of tissue.

uremia Severe kidney failure resulting in the buildup of waste products within the blood. Eventually, brain functions will be impaired.

urinary tract infection (UTI) An infection, usually of the lower urinary tract (urethra and bladder), that occurs when normal flora bacteria enter the urethra and grow.

Prep Kit continued

References

1. Acute cholecystitis. MedlinePlus website. https://medlineplus.gov/ency/article/000264.htm. Reviewed August 7, 2023. Accessed March 11, 2025.
2. Symptoms and causes of pancreatitis. National Institute of Diabetes and Digestive and Kidney Diseases website. https://www.niddk.nih.gov/health-information/digestive-diseases/pancreatitis/symptoms-causes. Reviewed November 2017. Accessed January 2, 2025.
3. Antunes C, Aleem A, Curtis S. Gastroesophageal reflux disease. *StatPearls*. National Library of Medicine website. https://www.ncbi.nlm.nih.gov/books/NBK441938//. Published July 3, 2023. Accessed January 2, 2025.
4. Gonzalez-Chagolla A, Olivas-Martinez A, Ruiz-Manriquez J, et al. Cirrhosis etiology trends in developing countries: transition from infectious to metabolic conditions. Report from a multicentric cohort in central Mexico. *Lancet Reg Health Am*. 2021;7:100151. doi:10.1016/j.lana.2021.100151
5. Rawla P, Devasahayam J. Mallory-Weiss syndrome. *StatPearls*. National Library of Medicine website. https://www.ncbi.nlm.nih.gov/books/NBK538190/. Updated July 31, 2023. Accessed January 2, 2025.
6. Matrana MR, Margolin DA. Epidemiology and pathophysiology of diverticular disease. *Clin Colon Rectal Surg*. 2009;22(3):141–146.
7. Diverticulosis and diverticulitis. MedlinePlus website. https://medlineplus.gov/diverticulosisanddiverticulitis.html. Updated February 21, 2024. Accessed January 2, 2025.
8. Strate, S. Etiology of lower gastrointestinal bleeding in adults. UpToDate website. https://www.uptodate.com/contents/etiology-of-lower-gastrointestinal-bleeding-in-adults#H1. Updated January 30, 2023. Accessed January 2, 2025.
9. Definitions and facts of hemorrhoids. National Institute of Diabetes and Digestive and Kidney Disease website. https://www.niddk.nih.gov/health-information/digestive-diseases/hemorrhoids/definition-facts. Reviewed October 2016. Accessed January 2, 2025.
10. Inguinal hernia. National Institute of Diabetes and Digestive and Kidney Diseases website. https://www.niddk.nih.gov/health-information/digestive-diseases/inguinal-hernia#common. Reviewed September 2019. Accessed January 2, 2025.
11. Goyal A, Daneshpajouhnejad P, Hashmi MF, et al. Acute kidney injury. *StatPearls*. National Library of Medicine website. https://www.ncbi.nlm.nih.gov/books/NBK441896/. Updated November 25, 2023. Accessed January 2, 2025.
12. Berns J. Patient education: chronic kidney disease (beyond the basics). UpToDate website. https://www.uptodate.com/contents/chronic-kidney-disease-beyond-the-basics?topicRef=4426&source=see_link#H1. Updated March 7, 2023. Accessed January 2, 2025.
13. Cozzolino M, Mangano M, Stucchi A, Ciceri P, Conte F, Galassi A. Cardiovascular disease in dialysis patients. *Nephrol Dial Transplant*. 2018;33(suppl_3):iii28–iii34.
14. Cambise C, De Cicco R, Luca E, et al. Postoperative urinary retention (POUR): a narrative review. *Saudi J Anaesth*. 2024;18(2):265–271.
15. Krause R. Dialysis complications of chronic renal failure. Medscape website. https://emedicine.medscape.com/article/1918879-overview#a1. Updated November 29, 2023. Accessed January 2, 2025.
16. Frinak S, Kennedy J, Zasuwa G, Passalacqua KD, Yee J. Detection of hemodialysis venous needle dislodgment using venous access pressure measurements: a simulation study. *Kidney360*. 2023;4(4):e476–e485. doi:10.34067/KID.0000000000000093
17. Burkhart J. Patient education: peritoneal dialysis (beyond the basics). UpToDate website. https://www.uptodate.com/contents/peritoneal-dialysis-beyond-the-basics#H15. Updated October 24, 2023. Accessed January 2, 2025.
18. Greenstein R, Nawrocki P, Nesbit C. Bottle it up: prehospital management of an AV fistula bleed using a bottle cap. *Am J Emerg Med*. 2023;67:197.e1–197.e2. doi:10.1016/j.ajem.2023.03.011
19. Milosevic E, Forster A, Moist L, Rehman F, Thomson B. Non-surgical interventions to control bleeding from arteriovenous fistulas and grafts inside and outside the hemodialysis unit: a scoping review. *Clin Kidney J*. 2024;17(5):sfae089. doi:10.1093/ckj/sfae089
20. De Guzman JM, Kitch BB. Renal failure and dialysis. In: Cone DC, Brice JH, Delbridge TR, Myers JB, eds. *Emergency Medical Services: Clinical Practice and Systems Oversight*. 3rd ed. John Wiley & Sons; 2021:199–207.

Additional Resources

Home dialysis. National Kidney Foundation website. https://www.kidney.org/atoz/content/homehemo. Accessed January 2, 2025.

Kapoor V. Acute cholecystitis clinical presentation. *Medscape*. https://emedicine.medscape.com/article/171886-clinical#b1. Updated July 13, 2022. Accessed January 2, 2025.

Prep Kit continued

Mann J. Overview of hypertension in acute and chronic kidney disease. UpToDate website. https://www.uptodate.com/contents/overview-of-hypertension-in-acute-and-chronic-kidney-disease#H17855060. Updated March 23, 2022. Accessed January 2, 2025.

National Association of State EMS Officials. *National Model EMS Clinical Guidelines*. https://nasemso.org/wp-content/uploads/National-Model-EMS-Clinical-Guidelines_2022.pdf. Revised March 2022. Accessed January 2, 2025.

National Highway Traffic Safety Administration. *National Emergency Medical Services Education Standards*. https://www.ems.gov/assets/EMS_Education-Standards_2021_FNL.pdf. EMS.gov website. Published January 2021. Accessed January 2, 2025.

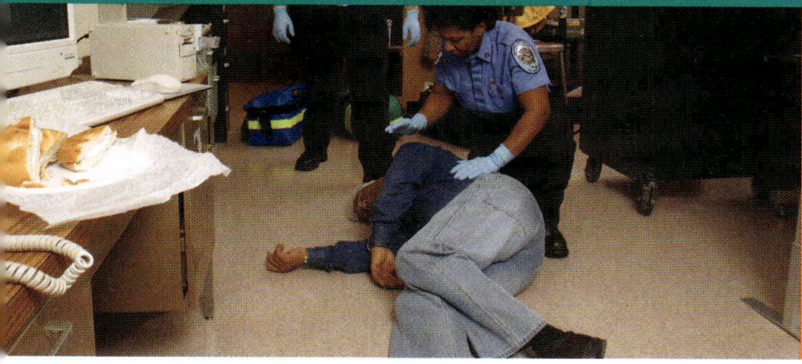

Chapter 20

Endocrine and Hematologic Emergencies

NATIONAL EMS EDUCATION STANDARD COMPETENCIES

Medicine

Applies knowledge to provide basic emergency care and transportation based on assessment findings for an acutely ill patient.

Endocrine Disorders

- Diabetic emergencies (pp 792–795, 803–805)

Hematology

- Sickle cell crisis (pp 807–808)
- Clotting disorders (pp 808–811)

KNOWLEDGE OBJECTIVES

1. Describe the anatomy and physiology of the endocrine system and its main function in the body. (pp 790–792)
2. Discuss the role of glucose as a major source of energy for the body and its relationship to insulin. (pp 790–792)
3. Define the terms diabetes mellitus, hyperglycemia, and hypoglycemia. (pp 792–793)
4. Distinguish between the types of diabetes and how their onset and presentations are different. (pp 793–799)
5. Describe the differences and similarities between hyperglycemic and hypoglycemic diabetic emergencies, including their onset, signs and symptoms, and management considerations. (pp 795–803)
6. Describe the interventions for providing emergency medical care to both a conscious and an unconscious patient with an altered mental status and a history of diabetes who is having symptomatic hyperglycemia. (pp 796–798, 805–806)
7. Describe the interventions for providing emergency medical care to both a conscious and an unconscious patient with an altered mental status and a history of diabetes who is having symptomatic hypoglycemia. (pp 798–806)
8. Explain ways to differentiate hyperglycemia from hypoglycemia. (pp 793–794)
9. Explain some age-related considerations when caring for a pediatric patient who is experiencing symptomatic hypoglycemia. (p 799)
10. Explain when it is appropriate to obtain medical direction when providing emergency medical care to a patient with diabetes. (pp 799–805)
11. Explain some age-related considerations when assessing and caring for an older adult who has undiagnosed diabetes. (p 802)

12. Provide the forms, dose, administration, indications, and contraindications for giving oral glucose to a patient with a decreased level of consciousness who has a history of diabetes. (pp 803–805)
13. Discuss the composition and functions of blood. (pp 806–807)
14. Describe the pathophysiology, complications, and management of sickle cell disease. (pp 807–808)
15. Describe two types of blood clotting disorders, and the risk factors, characteristics, and management of each. (pp 808–809)
16. Describe anemia and how the condition can affect patients and patient assessment. (p 809)

SKILLS OBJECTIVES

1. Demonstrate the assessment and care of a patient with hypoglycemia and a decreased level of consciousness. (pp 798–802, 805–806)

Introduction

The endocrine system directly or indirectly influences almost every cell, organ, and function of the body. Consequently, patients with an endocrine disorder often are seen with a multitude of signs and symptoms that require a thorough assessment and immediate treatment.

This chapter discusses the endocrine disorder of diabetes mellitus and associated emergent conditions. You will gain an understanding of the role of the pancreas in hormone production and release. Further discussion focuses on the signs and symptoms of hypoglycemia versus hyperglycemia and the adverse effects of chronically high blood glucose levels.

This chapter also discusses common hematologic emergencies that may be seen in emergency medical services (EMS) patients. Although hematologic disorders can be difficult to assess and treat in a prehospital setting, your actions may save a patient's life.

Endocrine Emergencies

Anatomy and Physiology

The **endocrine system** is a regulatory system that works with the other systems to maintain the body's homeostasis. **Endocrine glands** produce and secrete messenger chemicals called **hormones**. Hormones travel through the blood to the organs, tissues, or cells that they are intended to affect. When the hormone arrives, the cell, tissue, or organ receives the message and an action or cellular process takes place.

Endocrine disorders are caused by problems regulating the production, secretion, or reception of hormones. If a gland is not functioning normally, it may produce more hormone (hypersecretion) than is needed or not produce enough hormone (hyposecretion). A gland may function correctly, but the receiving organ may not respond because the receiving organ is less responsive to the hormone required to initiate the desired action or cellular

YOU are the EMT

A call for service comes in at 1500 hours. The call details from dispatch describe a 23-year-old man with weakness and nausea. You arrive on scene to find an adult man who states he has been weak for the past 6 days. He reports recent weight loss, unquenchable thirst, unrelenting hunger, and increased frequency of urination. The patient's other medical history is unremarkable. Your interview reveals that he has two family members with diabetes.

1. What processes are being described by the patient?
2. What hormone is not produced by the body in type 1 diabetes?

response. The most common disorder of glucose regulation by the endocrine system that EMS systems respond to is **diabetes mellitus**, commonly referred to simply as diabetes.

Glucose is important to all cells in the body. Cells metabolize glucose with oxygen to make adenosine triphosphate (ATP), which is a cell's energy source. **Insulin** is necessary for glucose to enter most cells. The brain does not need insulin to use glucose, but cells in the rest of the body require sufficient insulin, and a proper response to insulin, to make the ATP they need.

The endocrine organ primarily responsible for glucose regulation is the pancreas. The islets of Langerhans represent a small area in the pancreas that produces and stores two hormones that play a major role in glucose metabolism: glucagon, made in alpha cells, and insulin, made in beta cells.

In a person without diabetes, the pancreas stores and secretes insulin and glucagon in response to the level of glucose in the blood (**FIGURE 20-1**). When a person eats, the glucose level in their blood rises. In response, the pancreas secretes insulin into the blood. Insulin moves the glucose from the blood into tissues and cells to be used for energy. It also promotes storage of excess glucose in the form of glycogen in the liver and skeletal muscles for later use. As blood glucose levels drop to normal, insulin stops being secreted.

Between meals, the pancreas maintains consistent glucose levels by secreting glucagon, which prompts the glycogen stored previously to convert

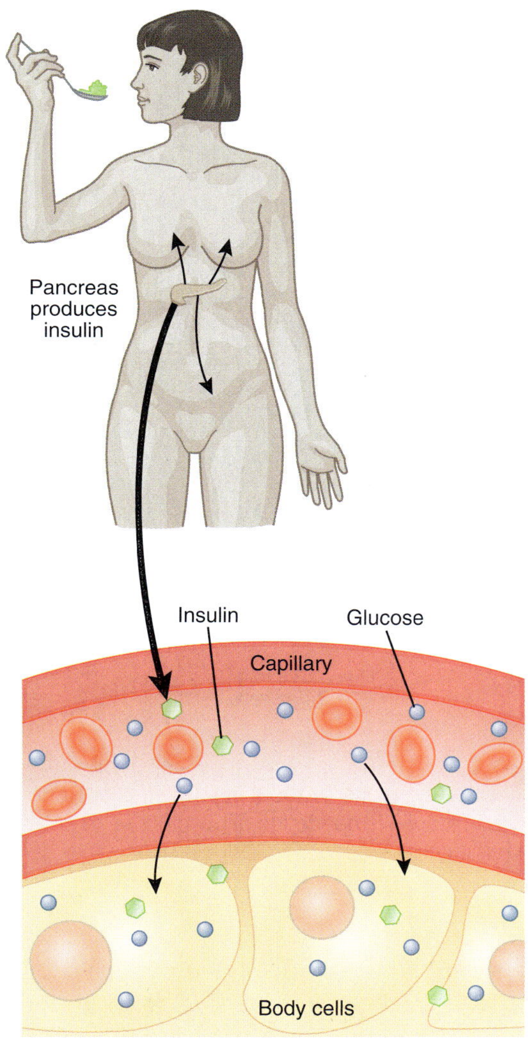

A

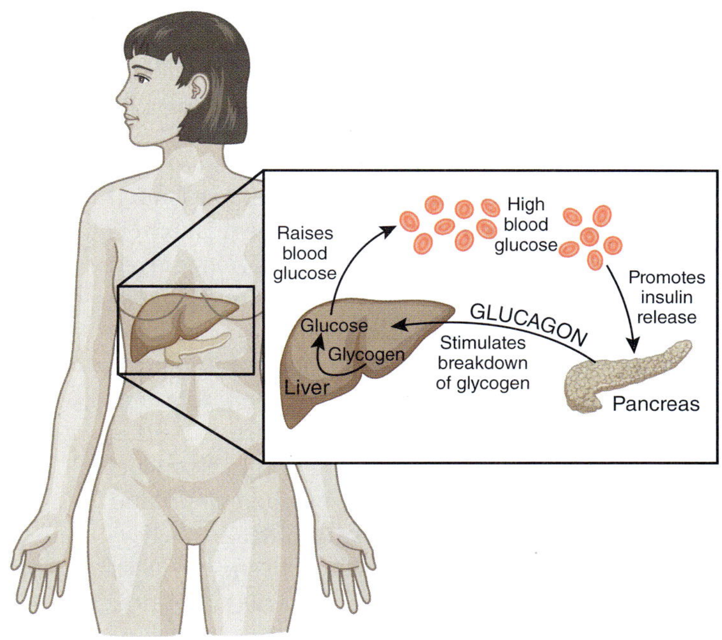

B

FIGURE 20-1 Glucose metabolism in a person without diabetes. **A.** Person eats. The blood glucose level rises and the pancreas secretes insulin into the blood. Glucose enters the body's cells and is used for energy. Glucose is also stored as glycogen in the liver and skeletal muscles for later use. Blood glucose levels return to normal and insulin stops being secreted. **B.** The body needs glucose, but the person does not eat. A message is sent to the pancreas to secrete glucagon, and glucagon stimulates the liver and skeletal muscles to release glycogen, which converts back to glucose for use as cellular fuel.

back into glucose. Regular intake of food allows the pancreas to replace glycogen stores.

Pathophysiology

According to the American Diabetes Association, each year in the United States, diabetes is diagnosed in 1.2 million people.[1] In 2021, approximately 11.6% of the US population had diabetes.[1] Diabetes includes disorders of insulin production and insulin sensitivity. Impaired insulin production or insulin resistance by the cells can prevent glucose from moving into cells and tissues. The glucose level in the blood remains high and continues to rise while cells are left without adequate glucose for ATP production (**FIGURE 20-2**).

There are multiple types of diabetes, including diabetes mellitus type 1, diabetes mellitus type 2, gestational diabetes, and, more rarely, genetically linked types. A more detailed discussion of gestational diabetes can be found in Chapter 34, *Obstetrics and Neonatal Care*.

Treatments for diabetes include medications and injectable hormones that lower the patient's blood glucose level, help maintain consistent levels, and/or help cells become more sensitive to insulin so they can use glucose. Managing diabetes can be extremely challenging, even with newer, more advanced medications and monitoring devices. These hormones and medications, whether administered correctly or incorrectly, can create a medical emergency for the patient with diabetes. If unrecognized and untreated, emergencies relating to blood glucose levels can be life threatening. You must recognize the signs and symptoms of glucose-related emergencies so you can provide the appropriate treatment and deliver the patient to the next level of care.

Hyperglycemia is when the blood glucose level is above normal. **Hypoglycemia** is when the blood glucose level is below normal (**FIGURE 20-3**). Hyperglycemia and hypoglycemia can occur with all diabetes types. In the field, you will encounter many patients displaying the signs and symptoms of high and low blood glucose levels.

Hyperglycemia and hypoglycemia have some similarities in their presentation. As an EMT, you must look for the differences that define one disorder from the other (**TABLE 20-1**). Patients at both extremes, with extremely low and extremely high blood glucose levels, can present with altered mental status. Patients with severe hypoglycemia are more likely to have a depressed level of consciousness than patients with hyperglycemia. These patients are sometimes mistakenly judged to be intoxicated. Altered mental status related to diabetic emergencies can often mimic alcohol intoxication, and intoxicated patients often have abnormal glucose levels. Be thorough and check a fingerstick glucose level for all patients who have altered mental status or a history of diabetes.

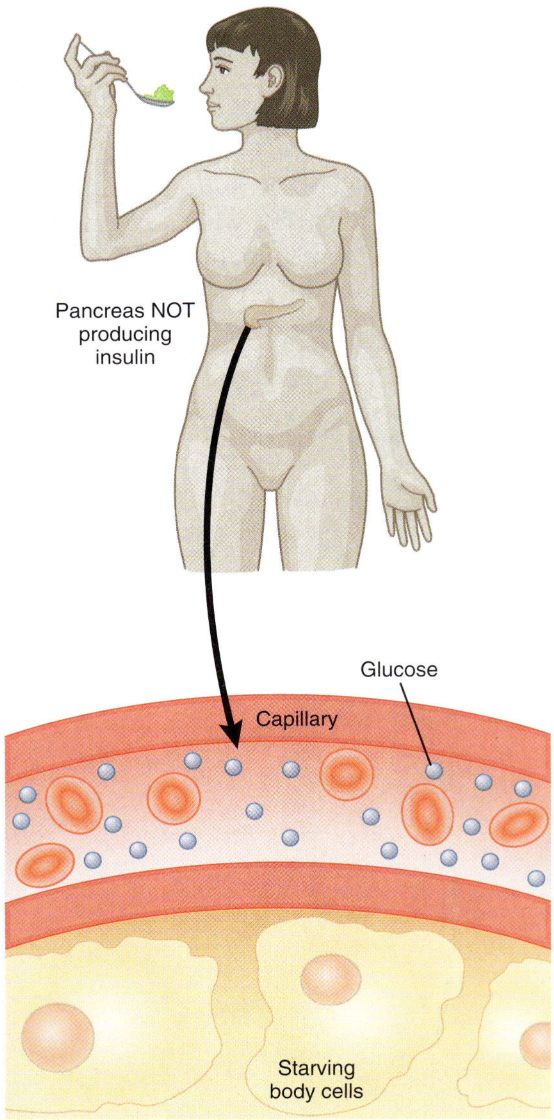

FIGURE 20-2 Diabetes is defined as the lack of or ineffective action of insulin. Without insulin, cells begin to starve because insulin is needed to allow glucose to enter and nourish the cells.

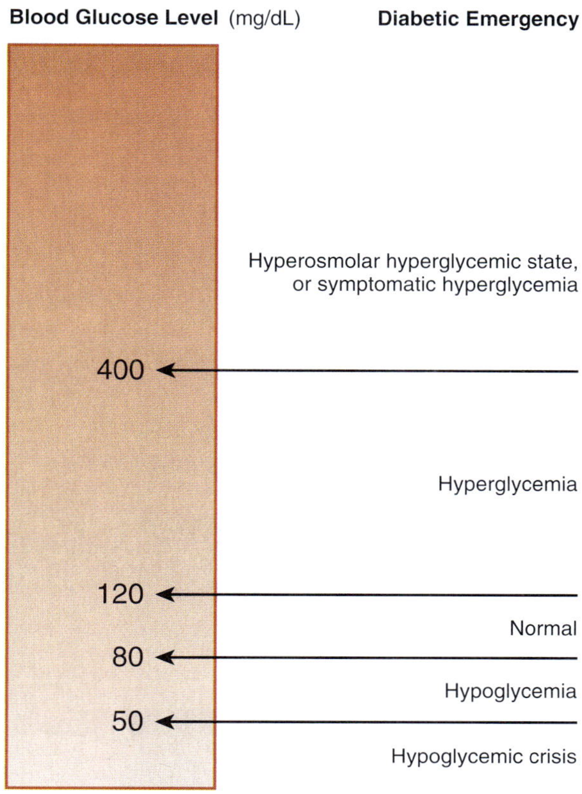

FIGURE 20-3 The left column illustrates blood glucose levels; the right column illustrates the conditions associated with that particular level of blood glucose. Notice that the normal range is rather small.

Diabetes Mellitus Type 1

Diabetes mellitus type 1, more commonly referred to as **type 1 diabetes**, is an autoimmune disorder in which the individual's immune system produces antibodies against the pancreatic beta cells. The immune system destroys the beta cells and the body can no longer produce insulin. Without insulin, glucose cannot enter most cells, and the cells cannot produce energy effectively.

The onset of type 1 diabetes usually happens from early childhood through the fourth decade of life; it is the most common metabolic disease of childhood. The patient's immune system progressively destroys the pancreas's ability to produce insulin and the patient must obtain insulin from an external source. Patients with type 1 diabetes cannot survive without insulin. Patients who inject insulin often need to check their blood glucose levels up to six times per day or more using a lancet and a small capillary blood sample, which is read by using a glucometer (**FIGURE 20-4**).

Advances in technology now allow patients to track their blood glucose in real time using wearable sensors (eg, Dexcom, FreeStyle). These devices allow for continuous glucose monitoring throughout the day and night. They have a small disposable sensor inserted under the skin that can estimate glucose levels between cells, which are

TABLE 20-1 Hyperglycemia Versus Hypoglycemia

Assessment Finding	Hyperglycemia	Hypoglycemia
Onset	Gradual (hours to days)	Rapid (within minutes)
Skin	Warm and dry	Pale (compared with patient baseline), cool, and moist
Infection	Common	Less common
Thirst	Intense	Absent
Dehydration	Often present	Dry mucous membranes
History of increased urination	Present	Not present
Hunger	Present and increasing	Present
Nausea/vomiting/abdominal pain	Common, especially in children	Uncommon

(continues)

TABLE 20-1 Hyperglycemia Versus Hypoglycemia (*continued*)

Assessment Finding	Hyperglycemia	Hypoglycemia
Breathing	With DKA there are rapid, deep (Kussmaul) respirations	Normal; may become shallow or ineffective if hypoglycemia is severe and mental status is depressed
Odor of breath	With DKA there may be a sweet, fruity odor	Normal
Blood pressure	Normal to low	Normal to low
Pulse	Rapid, weak, and thready	Rapid, weak
Consciousness	Lethargy, blurry vision, at very high levels slowed responses progressing to coma	Irritability, confusion, weakness, palpitations, seizure, or coma; unsteady gait
Response	Gradual, within 6 to 12 hours following medical treatment	Immediate improvement after administration of glucose

Abbreviation: DKA, diabetic ketoacidosis

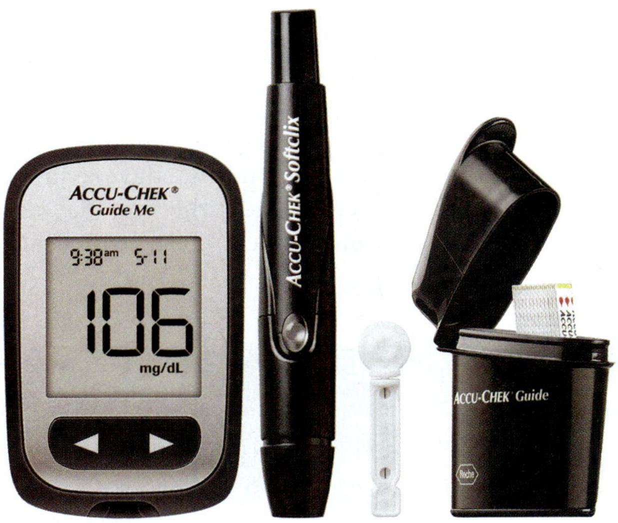

FIGURE 20-4 The blood glucose self-monitoring kit with digital meter is a device used by patients at home and by EMTs in the field in many EMS systems.

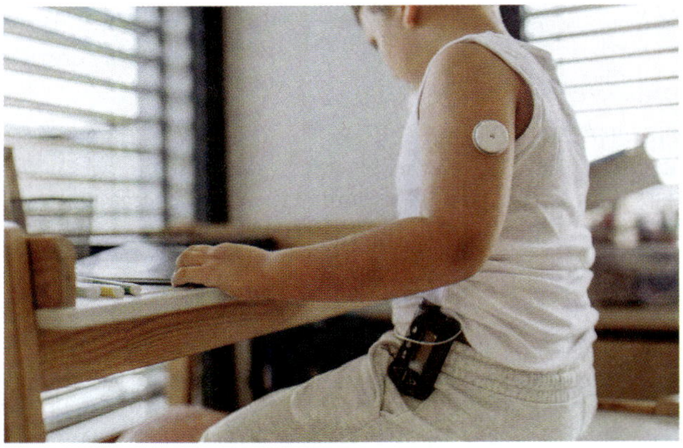

FIGURE 20-5 Patients can track their blood glucose in real time by wearing a sensor that sends information via Bluetooth to their phone.

similar to glucose levels in the blood. The disposable sensor wirelessly transmits the information to a receiver, usually in a smartphone or insulin pump. Continuous glucose monitoring can help patients make more accurate decisions about their glucose requirements and need to adjust medication use (**FIGURE 20-5**).

Many people with type 1 diabetes have an insulin pump. Some of these devices continuously measure the body's glucose levels and provide an (adjustable) infusion of insulin and correction doses of insulin based on carbohydrate intake at mealtimes. The presence of an insulin pump that automatically measures blood glucose limits the number of times patients have to check their fingerstick glucose level. Some insulin pumps do not measure blood glucose automatically, but rather, deliver a continuous baseline dose of insulin that may be supplemented by an additional bolus dose depending on the blood glucose measurement the patient takes at mealtimes. Unfortunately, insulin pumps can malfunction and hyperglycemic or hypoglycemic diabetic emergencies can develop. Always inquire about the presence of an insulin pump, particularly in patients with type 1 diabetes, and ask the patient if it is working properly. If you suspect hypoglycemia in an unconscious patient with an insulin pump, you should disconnect the insulin pump if possible.

Normal blood glucose level is between 80 and 120 mg/dL in adult patients. Levels are typically slightly lower in newborns. The body's metabolism is sensitive to the levels of particular substances, such as glucose, in the blood. The kidneys filter the blood and thus manage all substances present in the blood. At normal levels, glucose remains in the blood as it is filtered.

When a patient's blood glucose level is above normal, the kidney's filtration system tries to offload glucose into the urine. The increased amount of glucose in the urine causes more water to be pulled out of the bloodstream into the urine. This results in more frequent urination, or **polyuria**. In a young child who is already toilet trained, polyuria may manifest as bedwetting.

Increased urine production and urination also cause increased thirst and dehydration, which can lead to severe electrolyte abnormalities. An increase in fluid consumption, called **polydipsia**, occurs in an attempt to quench this thirst.

In the early phase of diabetes, patients may report severe hunger and increased food intake, a condition known as **polyphagia**. They may even lose weight despite the increased food intake.

The autoimmune destruction of the pancreatic beta cells takes time to progress. For this reason, initial symptoms are typically subtle and not readily apparent to the patient or their parent. As the lack of insulin becomes more profound, the patient will notice increasing fatigue and malaise along with vague symptoms of generalized illness. If untreated, type 1 diabetes places the patient at risk for diabetic ketoacidosis, a specific type of hyperglycemic emergency discussed later in this chapter.

Diabetes Mellitus Type 2

Diabetes mellitus type 2, more commonly referred to as **type 2 diabetes**, is caused by resistance to the effects of insulin at the cellular level and relative impairment in insulin secretion. Insulin resistance means cells are less able to uptake glucose. As a review, in type 1 diabetes, no insulin is produced in the beta cells. In type 2 diabetes, there may be fewer insulin receptors in tissues and less insulin production in the beta cells; however, the primary problem is reduced sensitivity to insulin. In this condition, the cells do not respond to insulin properly and therefore do not use it effectively for cellular functions.

Obesity predisposes patients to type 2 diabetes; there is an association between obesity and increased resistance to the effects of insulin.[2] As the number of individuals with obesity continues to rise, so does the number of patients with type 2 diabetes. There are also complex genetic factors that can make people more susceptible to type 2 diabetes.

When type 2 diabetes begins, the individual's pancreas produces more insulin to make up for the increased levels of blood glucose and dysfunction of cellular insulin receptors. Over time this response becomes inefficient. The blood glucose levels continue to rise and do not respond when the pancreas secretes insulin, a process called insulin resistance. Additionally, beta cells become damaged and unable to produce insulin effectively. In some cases, insulin resistance can be improved by exercise and dietary modification.

In many instances, diet and exercise alone cannot control insulin resistance, and medications must be started to better control blood glucose levels. Medications used to treat type 2 diabetes vary widely and include oral and injectable medications. Some of them increase the secretion of insulin and create a high risk of hypoglycemic reaction, whereas others do not (**TABLE 20-2**). Various insulin preparations are also used for type 2 diabetes when other medications alone will not regulate blood glucose.

Insulin is a hormone that is destroyed when taken by mouth, so it must be injected (although research is being conducted with nasal insulin preparations to supplement other therapies and potentially improve cognitive function[3]). Many of the oral medications listed in Table 20-2 either encourage the pancreas to produce more insulin or the cells to stimulate receptors for insulin. Other medications decrease the effects of glucagon, decrease the release of glucose stored in the liver (glycogen),

TABLE 20-2 Common Medications Used to Treat Type 2 Diabetes

Canagliflozin (Invokana), empagliflozin (Jardiance)
Glipizide (Glucotrol, Glucotrol XL)[a]
Glyburide (DiaBeta, Glynase, Micronase)[a]
Metformin (Glumetza, Glucophage, Glucophage XR)
Pioglitazone (Actos), rosiglitazone (Avandia)
Exenatide (Byetta, Bydureon), liraglutide (Victoza), semaglutide (Ozempic)
Sitagliptin (Januvia), saxagliptin (Onglyza), alogliptin (Nesina)

[a]These medications increase the risk of hypoglycemia.

and prevent increased blood glucose levels during sleep or sedentary periods. None of the available medications is the perfect solution for every patient, and many have unpleasant side effects such as diarrhea and nausea.

Hyperglycemia related to type 2 diabetes does not always result in a crisis event, so it is often diagnosed at a yearly medical examination. In some cases, the patient's physician discovers type 2 diabetes when treating the patient for a complaint related to hyperglycemia. Individuals who have hyperglycemia for a prolonged time may experience secondary conditions, including wounds that do not heal, numbness in the hands and feet, blindness, kidney failure, and gastric motility problems, to name a few.

Words of Wisdom

The patient with diabetes needs to be vigilant about maintaining a proper glucose level through diet, exercise, and, often, taking medication. If patients with diabetes have prolonged hyperglycemia or other associated conditions, serious long-term complications may develop. Patients with diabetes take a blood test called the A1C several times per year to estimate their average blood glucose level over time. The A1C level helps patients with diabetes and their physicians know how well they have been managing their blood glucose levels over 2 to 3 months.[4]

Symptomatic Hyperglycemia

Symptomatic hyperglycemia occurs when blood glucose levels are very high. Early signs and symptoms include frequent urination, increased thirst, blurred vision, and fatigue.[5] If the high blood glucose levels go untreated, the patient may present with abdominal pain, nausea and vomiting, shortness of breath, dry mouth, weakness, or altered mental status. Altered mental status can result from several combined problems, but dehydration is the most common cause. Hyperglycemia leads to dehydration due to excess urination.

There are two types of hyperglycemic emergencies: diabetic ketoacidosis and hyperosmolar hyperglycemic state.

Diabetic Ketoacidosis

In type 1 diabetes (and very advanced type 2 diabetes) the patient is dependent on an external source of insulin. Without insulin, the body's cells do not receive the glucose they require for energy and the body resorts to burning fat for energy while glucose builds up in the blood. When the body burns fat rather than glucose, acid waste is produced. These acids are called ketones. As ketone levels increase in the blood, the ketones also begin to spill into the urine (as does the excess glucose). The kidneys become saturated with glucose and ketones, and are unable to eliminate a sufficient amount of these acids, leading to acidosis (a decrease in the body's pH level). **Diabetic ketoacidosis (DKA)** is the specific type of metabolic acidosis caused by insufficient insulin. In response to the metabolic acidosis, the body begins to breathe faster and deeper to release more carbon dioxide and increase the body's pH level. This breathing pattern of fast and deep respirations is known as **Kussmaul respirations**.

DKA may present as generalized illness, accompanied by the following signs and symptoms:

- Abdominal pain
- Body aches
- Nausea
- Vomiting
- Altered mental status or unconsciousness (if severe)
- Blood glucose levels over 350 mg/dL
- Kussmaul respirations
- Fruity odor on the breath (related to ketones)

If DKA is not rapidly recognized and treated, it can result in death.

Street Smarts

Do not attempt to coach the patient to slow their breathing if you suspect Kussmaul respirations. This rapid, deep breathing is helping the patient compensate for acidosis. If breathing is slowed, more acids can accumulate and the patient's condition will worsen.

When a patient with DKA has an altered mental status, ask the family and friends about the patient's history and presentation. Obtain a glucose level with a fingerstick using a lancet and a glucometer. The patient with DKA will generally have a fingerstick glucose level higher than 350 mg/dL. The procedure for checking a patient's glucose level is covered in Chapter 10, *Patient Assessment*.

DKA does not occur only when there is an absolute lack of insulin. It may also present in cases of a relative lack of insulin, which may result from an acute illness, an untreated infection, or other stressor on the body that leaves the patient with type 1 diabetes in a weakened condition.

Hyperosmolar Hyperglycemic State

Hyperosmolar hyperglycemic state (HHS), formerly called hyperosmolar hyperglycemic nonketotic syndrome (HHNS), is a diabetic complication that occurs more often in people with type 2 diabetes than in those with type 1 diabetes.[6] Unlike DKA, the resulting high blood glucose level does not cause ketosis; instead, it leads to increased urination that results in dehydration because the excess glucose in the blood pulls fluids from the tissues into the blood vessels, and subsequently, into the urine.

HHS can present similarly to the DKA seen in patients with type 1 diabetes. The onset of this disorder is commonly associated with a profound infection or illness. Key signs and symptoms of HHS include the following:

- Hyperglycemia
- Altered mental status, drowsiness, lethargy
- Severe dehydration, thirst, dark urine
- Visual or sensory deficits
- Partial paralysis or muscle weakness
- Seizures
- Very high glucose levels, above 600 mg/dL

Higher glucose levels in the blood cause the excretion of glucose and water in the urine. Patients respond by increasing their fluid intake precipitously (polydipsia), causing an equally large increase in

YOU are the EMT

You perform a primary assessment of the patient. You attempt to obtain more information from the patient, but he is slow to answer your questions and is slightly confused. He can tell you that he has been getting progressively worse over the past 3 to 5 days. The patient's friends and wife tell you he has been experiencing weight loss for the past month, but he seems to be eating more and more.

Recording Time: 0 Minutes	
Appearance	Weak and confused
Level of consciousness	Conscious, slow to respond, and confused
Airway	Open; clear of secretions or foreign bodies
Breathing	Increased rate and depth
Circulation	Radial pulses rapid and weak; skin warm and dry with poor turgor

The patient's wife tells you that he has been urinating frequently and has been drinking large quantities of water, soda, and milk. Your partner assesses his blood glucose level using the glucometer.

3. What should you expect the patient's blood glucose level to read? Why?

4. What is causing the patient's frequent urination and deep, rapid breathing?

urination (polyuria). In HHS, however, the patient cannot drink enough fluid to keep up with the exceedingly high glucose levels in the blood. The kidneys become overwhelmed and the patient's blood becomes much more concentrated than normal. As HHS progresses, the urine becomes rather dark and concentrated. The term *hyperosmolarity* describes very concentrated blood as a result of relative dehydration. As HHS progresses, the patient may become unconscious or have seizure activity due in part to the resulting severe dehydration.

Symptomatic Hypoglycemia

Symptomatic hypoglycemia is an acute emergency in which a patient's blood glucose level drops and must be corrected swiftly. Patients who inject insulin or use oral medications that stimulate the pancreas to produce more insulin are at higher risk for hypoglycemia. When insulin levels remain high, glucose is rapidly taken out of the blood to fuel the cells. If glucose levels fall too low, there may be an insufficient amount to supply the brain. The mental status of the patient declines quickly, and they may become confused or aggressive, or may display other unusual behavior. If blood glucose remains low, unconsciousness and permanent brain damage can quickly follow.

Symptomatic hypoglycemia can occur for many different reasons. While administering more insulin than necessary can result in a lower blood glucose level, even when an appropriate dose is delivered, the following factors can contribute to hypoglycemia:

- The patient has had a change in routine (eg, exercised more, consumed a meal later than usual, or skipped the meal).
- The patient did not eat enough food.
- The patient is experiencing an acute illness.

Hypoglycemia can develop if a person with diabetes takes their medications (pills or insulin) as prescribed but fails to ingest enough glucose or has an unanticipated change in their body's glucose demand. For example, a patient with diabetes who has taken their standard insulin dose and missed lunch may have symptomatic hypoglycemia before dinner. Alternatively, a person with diabetes may take too much medication, resulting in low blood glucose levels despite normal dietary intake. All hypoglycemic patients require prompt treatment. As an EMT, you can administer oral glucose if the patient is able to protect their airway; advanced life support (ALS) clinicians can administer glucose (dextrose) or glucagon by injection. Glucagon is also prescribed to patients as an emergency kit for self-administration or administration by a bystander, similar to epinephrine auto-injectors or by the intranasal route.

Hypoglycemia develops much more quickly than hyperglycemia. In some instances, it can occur in a matter of minutes. Hypoglycemia can be associated with the following signs and symptoms:

- Normal to shallow or rapid respirations
- Pale (compared with patient baseline), moist (clammy) skin
- Diaphoresis (sweating)
- Dizziness, headache
- Rapid pulse
- Normal to low blood pressure
- Altered mental status (aggressive, confused, lethargic, or unusual behavior)
- Anxious or combative behavior
- Seizure, fainting, or coma
- Weakness on one side of the body (may mimic stroke)
- Rapid changes in mental status

Hyperglycemia is a complex metabolic condition that usually develops over time and involves all the tissues of the body. Correcting this condition may take many hours in a well-controlled hospital setting. Hypoglycemia, however, is an acute condition that can develop rapidly.

Street Smarts

If a patient who has type 2 diabetes becomes hypoglycemic, even when taking medications such as metformin that do not typically cause the blood glucose level to drop, be sure to ask them if they have started taking any new medications recently. Along with other medications that decrease blood glucose levels, some antibiotics, hormones, antihypertensives (eg, beta blockers, such as metoprolol), or drugs used to treat gastroesophageal reflux can cause symptomatic hypoglycemia in patients who take oral hypoglycemic medications. If the patient has started a new medication, report this information to the emergency department (ED) clinicians to help them determine the cause of the drop in blood glucose and prevent further episodes.

Words of Wisdom

Always remember when caring for a patient with hypoglycemia: minutes count. Without glucose, a patient can sustain permanent brain damage. The condition may be quickly reversed by giving the patient glucose.

Special Populations

HYPOGLYCEMIA IN THE PEDIATRIC PATIENT

Low blood glucose level events are not uncommon in pediatric patients. Most children adapt well to the routine of managing their diabetes, but during periods of growth, their blood glucose may be more difficult to regulate. Some toxic ingestions and overdoses cause hypoglycemia in children. Children cannot store excess glucose as effectively as adults; therefore, the blood glucose level can drop in children even in the absence of diabetes or medication. As an EMT, you must have a high index of suspicion for a low glucose level when you encounter a child who has an altered mental status or depressed level of consciousness.

Special Populations

LONG-TERM EFFECTS OF DIABETES IN THE GERIATRIC PATIENT

Older adults are at greater risk for hyperglycemia and the complications associated with long-term damage from diabetes. The risk of impaired vision, vascular disease (eg, stroke, heart attack, poor peripheral circulation), and kidney disease, among other conditions, increases as patients with diabetes age, especially when their blood glucose has not been well controlled over time.

Patient Assessment of Diabetes

Scene Size-up

Evaluate scene safety as you arrive on scene and as you approach the patient. Make sure all hazards are addressed. Remember that patients with diabetes often use syringes to administer insulin. It is possible you may be stuck by a used needle that was not disposed of properly. Noticing items on the scene such as insulin syringes on the nightstand, insulin bottles in the refrigerator, a plate of food, or a glass of orange juice may help you decide what is possibly wrong with your patient. Evaluate each situation quickly, and make sure necessary personal protective equipment is readily available. Take standard precautions. As you approach, question bystanders about events leading to your arrival.

Although your report from dispatch may be for a patient with an altered mental status, consider the possibility that trauma may have occurred because of a medical incident. Determine the mechanism of injury and/or nature of illness. Do not let your guard down, even on what appears to be a routine call.

Primary Assessment

Perform a primary assessment to form a general impression of the patient. How does the patient look? Does the patient appear anxious, restless, or listless? Is the patient apathetic or irritable? Is the patient interacting appropriately with their environment? These initial observations may lead you to suspect high or low blood glucose values. Identify life threats, and provide lifesaving interventions, particularly airway management. Determine the patient's level of consciousness using the AVPU (Awake and alert, responsive to Verbal stimuli, responsive to Pain, Unresponsive) scale. If a patient whom you suspect has diabetes is unresponsive, call for ALS immediately. An unconscious patient may have undiagnosed diabetes. In patients with altered mental status, you may be able to determine whether a diabetic emergency exists by assessing the patient's blood glucose level. At the ED, diabetes and its complications can be quickly diagnosed.

Remember that even though a person has diabetes, the diabetes may not be causing the current problem; heart attack, stroke, or another medical emergency may be the cause. For this reason, you must always carry out a thorough, careful primary assessment.

While forming your general impression, assess the patient's airway and breathing. Patients showing signs of inadequate breathing or a pulse oximetry level less than or equal to 94% on room air should receive high-flow oxygen to achieve an oxygen saturation of 94% to 98%. A patient who is hyperglycemic may have rapid, deep respirations (Kussmaul respirations) and sweet, fruity breath. A patient who is hypoglycemic will have normal or shallow to rapid respirations. If the patient is not breathing or is having difficulty breathing, open the airway and insert an airway adjunct, administer oxygen, and assist ventilations. Continue to monitor the airway while you provide care.

Once you have assessed the airway and breathing and have performed the necessary lifesaving interventions, check the patient's circulatory status. Skin that is dry and warm suggests hyperglycemia, whereas skin that is moist and pale indicates hypoglycemia. Because skin pallor can be difficult to detect in patients with dark skin, instead check for pale mucous membranes inside the inner lower eyelid or slow capillary refill. The patient with symptomatic hypoglycemia will have a rapid, weak pulse.

Whether you decide to transport at this stage of the assessment will depend on the patient's level of consciousness and ability to swallow. Patients with an altered mental status and impaired ability to swallow should be transported promptly. Patients who are able to swallow and are conscious enough to maintain their own airway may be further evaluated and treated on scene, if appropriate. If the patient has prescribed glucagon that has not yet been administered, help administer it, if appropriate, or encourage a family member to administer it.

History Taking

Investigate the chief complaint or the history of the present illness. Responsive patients usually are able to provide their own medical history. If the patient has eaten but has not taken insulin, it is more likely that hyperglycemia is developing. If the patient has taken insulin but has not eaten, the problem is more likely to be hypoglycemia. A patient with diabetes will often know (or strongly suspect) what is wrong. If the patient is not thinking or speaking clearly (or is unconscious), ask a family member or bystander the same questions.

Physical signs such as tremors, abdominal cramps, vomiting, a fruity breath odor, or a dry mouth may guide you in determining whether the patient is hypoglycemic or hyperglycemic.

You will need to obtain a SAMPLE (Signs and symptoms, Allergies, Medications, Pertinent past medical history, Last oral intake, Events leading up to the illness or injury) history from your patient or the family or bystanders if the patient is unable to speak. In addition, be sure to ask the following questions of a patient known to have diabetes:

- Do you take insulin or any pills that lower your blood sugar?
- Do you wear an insulin pump? Is it working properly?
- Have you taken your usual dose of insulin (or pills) today?
- Have you eaten normally today?
- Have you had any illness, unusual amount of activity, or stress?

When you are assessing a patient who might have diabetes, check whether the patient has an emergency medical identification device, such as a wallet card, necklace, or bracelet, or ask the patient or a family member. Remember that the environment, bystanders, and medical identification devices may provide important clues about your patient's condition.

Secondary Assessment

In some instances where the patient is critically ill or injured or the transport time is short, you may not have time to conduct a secondary assessment. In other instances, the secondary assessment may occur on scene or en route to the ED.

First, assess unresponsive patients from head to toe with a secondary assessment of the entire body, looking for clues to their condition. The patient may have experienced trauma resulting from dizziness (causing a fall) or from changes in level of consciousness resulting in a vehicle crash.

As with every call, you should perform a secondary assessment when time permits. With unconscious patients or patients with an altered mental status, you must assume the role of detective and look for problems or injuries that are not obvious because the patient is unable to communicate these to you. Although an altered mental status may be caused by a blood glucose level that is too high or too low, the patient may have sustained trauma or have another metabolic problem. An altered mental status may also be caused by something else, such as intoxication, poisoning, or a head injury. A systematic examination of the patient may provide you with information essential to proper patient care.

When you suspect a diabetes-related problem, a secondary assessment should focus on the patient's mental status and ability to swallow and protect the airway. Obtain a Glasgow Coma Scale score to track the patient's neurologic status. The Glasgow Coma Scale is described in Chapter 18, *Neurologic Emergencies*.

Obtain a complete set of vital signs, including a measurement of the patient's blood glucose level using a glucometer. The portable blood glucose monitor measures the glucose level in whole blood using either capillary or venous samples. It should be easier for you to recognize that abnormal vital signs are associated with a diabetic emergency when you know the blood glucose level is too high or too low. Remember, the patient may have abnormal vital signs and a normal blood glucose value. When this is the case, something else may be causing the patient's altered mental status, vomiting, or other complaints.

It is important to read and understand the operator's manual before using a portable glucometer because the specifications of the device may vary depending on the manufacturer. Some glucometers indicate low ("Lo") when they detect a glucose reading less than 20 mg/dL, whereas others display Lo when they detect a reading less than 30 mg/dL. The same is true with a high ("Hi") reading; some glucometers read Hi at 550 mg/dL and some at 600 mg/dL; therefore, it is important to know both the upper and lower ranges at which your glucometer functions.

The normal range for glucose levels in blood in nonfasting adults and children is 80 to 120 mg/dL; the blood glucose level in neonates should be above 70 mg/dL. Your index of suspicion for a glucose-related emergency should be high when the symptomatic patient's blood glucose level is below 60 mg/dL or above 250 mg/dL.[7]

Reassessment

It is important to reassess a patient with diabetes frequently to monitor for changes. Is there any improvement in the patient's mental status? Are the ABCs (Airway, Breathing, Circulation) still intact? How is the patient responding to the interventions performed? How must you adjust or change the interventions? In many patients with diabetes, you will note marked improvement with appropriate treatment. Document each assessment, your findings, the time of the interventions, and any changes in the patient's condition. Base your administration of glucose on serial glucometer readings. If a glucometer is not available, a deteriorating level of consciousness indicates that you need to provide more glucose.

Determining whether the blood glucose level is too high or too low in a patient in whom diabetes

YOU are the EMT

Your partner reports that the patient's blood glucose reading on the glucometer is 456 mg/dL. You continue to assess the patient while your partner obtains his vital signs. The patient's wife calls his doctor, who requests that you transport him to the closest hospital. A community hospital is located about 15 miles away.

Recording Time: 5 Minutes	
Respirations	30 breaths/min; deep
Pulse	120 beats/min; weak radial pulses
Skin	Baseline color, warm, and dry; poor turgor
Blood pressure	112/54 mm Hg
Oxygen saturation (Spo_2)	97% (on room air)

5. What other factors can cause hyperglycemia in patients with diabetes?

6. How can you distinguish symptomatic hyperglycemia from symptomatic hypoglycemia?

is diagnosed can be difficult when signs and symptoms are confusing and you have no way to test for a blood glucose value. In these situations, perform a thorough assessment and contact the hospital to help sort out the signs and symptoms. The hospital should be a resource for you to help problem-solve situations and provide guidance on how to care for your patient.

Safety Tips

Managing problems related to diabetes and altered mental status poses minimal risk to you because exposure to body fluids is generally very limited. However, some patients can become confused and even aggressive at times. Take standard precautions, as you would with any other patient. Always use gloves, a mask, and appropriate eye protection and carefully wash your hands after obtaining and checking a blood sample or coming in contact with any airway secretions.

Communication with hospital staff is important for continuity of care. Hospital personnel need to be informed about the patient's history, the present situation, your assessment findings, and your interventions and their results.

Document your assessment findings clearly, because they represent the basis for your treatment. Patients who refuse transport because their symptoms improve after taking oral glucose may require even more thorough documentation. Patients who receive treatment in the field for hypoglycemia are at great risk for development of symptomatic hypoglycemia in the near future and should be strongly discouraged from refusing further treatment or transportation to the hospital. Many long-acting forms of insulin and most oral diabetic medications remain in the bloodstream far longer than the glucose used to treat these patients. Follow your local protocols for patients who refuse treatment or transport.

Special Populations

UNDIAGNOSED DIABETES IN THE GERIATRIC PATIENT

You may encounter an older adult who has undiagnosed diabetes. The patient is likely to report that they have not been feeling well for a while but have not seen a physician. A patient with undiagnosed diabetes or one who is in denial or ignores the advice of their physician may call 9-1-1 when the signs and symptoms become pronounced. Nonhealing wounds (which can lead to infection), blindness, kidney failure, atypical (silent) myocardial infarction presentation, and other complications are associated with longstanding poorly controlled or uncontrolled diabetes. As an EMT, you may be the first to recognize and suggest medical treatment to an older adult. It is important that you recognize the signs and symptoms of diabetes.

YOU are the EMT

Because of the patient's signs and symptoms, history, and a glucometer reading that indicates a high blood glucose level, you determine that oral glucose is not indicated. The patient is moved onto the stretcher and loaded into the ambulance. Shortly after departing the scene, you reassess his mental status and vital signs.

Recording Time: 11 Minutes	
Level of consciousness	Conscious but confused
Respirations	30 breaths/min; deep
Pulse	124 beats/min; weak radial pulses
Skin	Baseline color, warm, and dry; poor turgor
Blood pressure	108/56 mm Hg
Oxygen saturation (Spo_2)	97% (on room air)

7. What additional treatment should you provide to this patient?

Street Smarts

Your patient may not be aware of the long-term effects of diabetes. Take a moment and share information with your patient. Your patient's life may one day depend on it!

Emergency Medical Care for Diabetic Emergencies

When there is any doubt about whether a conscious patient with diabetes is going into symptomatic hypoglycemia or symptomatic hyperglycemia, most protocols will err on the side of giving glucose, even though the patient may have hyperglycemia or DKA. Untreated hypoglycemia will result in loss of consciousness and can quickly cause significant brain damage or death. The condition of a patient with symptomatic hypoglycemia is far more critical and far more likely to cause permanent problems than the condition of a patient with hyperglycemia or DKA. Furthermore, the amount of sugar that is typically given to a patient with symptomatic hypoglycemia is unlikely to make a patient with DKA significantly worse. When in doubt, consult medical control.

Words of Wisdom

If the blood glucose reading is high but all signs and symptoms point to hypoglycemia, assess it again on another finger (and with a different glucose monitor if it is available). On rare occasions, the first reading is inaccurate and you may fail to detect and treat a critically low blood glucose level.

Administering Glucose

A patient who is hypoglycemic, conscious, and able to swallow without the risk of aspiration should be given glucose. There are three types of oral glucose preparations available commercially. The most common for EMS clinicians is a rapidly dissolving gel (**FIGURE 20-6**). The second preparation comes in a chewable tablet; this is the least preferred because it is the slowest acting. The third preparation is a liquid formulation.

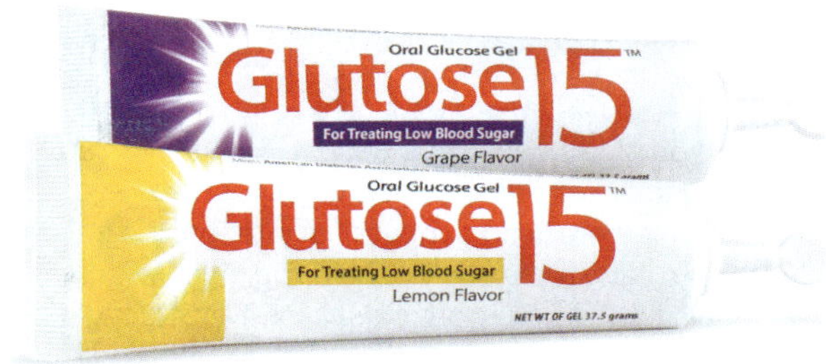

FIGURE 20-6 Oral glucose is commercially available in gel and tablet form. One tube of gel equals one 15-gram dose.

If authorized by your system, you should administer glucose gel to any patient with a decreased level of consciousness who has a history of diabetes. The only contraindications to oral glucose are an inability to swallow and unconsciousness; risk of aspiration (inhalation of the substance) is high in a patient who does not have a gag reflex. Oral glucose itself has no side effects if it is administered properly. A conscious patient (even if confused) who does not really need glucose will not be harmed by it. Therefore, do not hesitate to give glucose under these circumstances.

Be sure to wear gloves before placing anything into a patient's mouth. After you have confirmed that the patient is conscious and able to swallow and have obtained an online or off-line order, administer it: Open the glucose pouch. Either you or the patient can squeeze the glucose into the patient's mouth, either under the tongue or into the buccal space. The patient should then swallow.

Some patients may have prescribed glucagon emergency kits that they or their family can administer. You may also have local protocols that allow you to assist with administration of a patient's own glucagon or carry your own emergency glucagon kit.

Another option is to use household sources of glucose, such as juice or other drinks that contain sugar. Some ambulances even carry cake icing to treat hypoglycemia. Give sugar and do not be afraid to give too much. Do not give sugar-free drinks that are sweetened with saccharin or other synthetic sweetening compounds, because they will have little or no effect.

Safety Tips

Before you give a conscious patient glucose tablets, anything to eat or drink, or instant glucose, you must ensure that there is no danger of aspiration. In general, if patients can lift the cup or squirt the glucose into their own mouths, they are most likely not in danger of aspiration. Watch them carefully!

If your patient with hypoglycemia is unconscious, or if there is any risk of aspiration, the patient will need intravenous (IV) glucose, or intramuscular or intranasal glucagon. Intramuscular or intranasal glucagon works like glucagon secreted by the pancreas, causing a release of glucose stored in the liver in the form of glycogen. If the patient does not have adequate glycogen stores, it will not be effective.

Words of Wisdom

Intranasal glucagon was made available to patients in 2019 to treat symptomatic hypoglycemia and is now widely used, although the cost is a barrier to its use in patients who have a low socioeconomic status.[8] It has the advantage of not requiring injection, yet still achieving rapid absorption even in patients with markedly decreased levels of consciousness. Be aware of this medication and understand your local protocols regarding its use and indications.

Transporting the Patient

If the patient's blood glucose cannot be quickly increased on scene, your responsibility is to provide prompt transport to the hospital, where the proper care can be given. If you are working in a tiered system, you may want to request an ALS intercept so that an AEMT or paramedic can start an IV line and administer IV glucose.

A patient with symptomatic hypoglycemia (rapid onset of altered mental status, hypoglycemia) needs glucose immediately. A patient with symptomatic hyperglycemia (**acidosis**, dehydration, hyperglycemia) needs insulin and IV fluid therapy. These patients need prompt transport to the hospital for appropriate medical care.

Reassessing the Patient After Administering Glucose

As an EMT, you know the importance of reassessment. The patient with diabetes experiencing an altered mental status event that you treat with a glucose product is one of the most important patients to reassess frequently. As rapidly as you may see a response to your treatment, you also can see a deterioration. Monitor the airway when giving an oral medication such as a glucose product, checking for airway obstruction by the medication and remaining mindful of the potential to vomit and aspirate the glucose.

Street Smarts

If the patient's mental status, vital signs, and blood glucose level become normal after administering glucose, encourage the patient to eat a meal or snack containing carbohydrates and protein such as eggs or a peanut butter sandwich. Although the oral glucose is essential to quickly raise the patient's blood glucose level, the snack will help to prevent the glucose level from dropping again.

Words of Wisdom

Diabetes is a systemic disease affecting all tissues of the body, especially the kidneys, eyes, small arteries, and peripheral nerves. Therefore, you are likely to be called to treat patients with a variety of complications of diabetes, such as heart disease, visual disturbances, kidney failure, stroke, and ulcers or infections of the feet or toes. Except for heart attack and stroke, most of these will not be acute emergencies. Considering that diabetes is a major risk factor for cardiovascular disease, patients with diabetes should always be suspected of having a potential for heart attack, particularly older adults, even when they do not present with classic symptoms such as chest pain and shortness of breath.

Any time you change a patient's mental status with a drug, a thorough reassessment must be provided to ensure that the patient returns to their normal mental status. In some cases, you will recommend the patient be transported to the hospital, especially if the patient is a child, is newly diagnosed with diabetes, has signs of other illness, or has an underlying condition that is causing their blood sugar issues. However, you should not be surprised if your patient is familiar with hypoglycemia and does not want to be transported. In this event, document the refusal according to your protocols and consult medical direction if you are concerned about the patient's refusal of care. Refusal of care is discussed further in Chapter 3, *Medical, Legal, and Ethical Issues*.

The Presentation of Hypoglycemia

Recognizing that the patient has hypoglycemia requires an intuitive approach. There are many classic, by-the-book presentations of hypoglycemia. However, each of the altered mental status presentations is identified in much the same way. The discovery comes from a rapid examination utilizing a list of possible conditions to rule out, leading to the ultimate identification of hypoglycemia.

Seizures

Although seizures are rarely life threatening, you should consider them to be very serious, even in patients with a history of chronic seizures. Seizures, which may be brief or prolonged, are often caused by infections, poisoning, hypoglycemia, trauma, or decreased levels of oxygen, or they may be idiopathic (of unknown cause). In children, they may be caused by fever or epilepsy. Although brief seizures are not harmful, they may indicate a more dangerous and potentially life-threatening underlying condition. Because seizures can be the result of a head injury, consider trauma as a cause. In the patient with diabetes, you should also consider hypoglycemia.

Emergency medical care of seizures includes ensuring that the airway is clear and placing the patient on their side. Do not attempt to place anything in the patient's mouth (eg, a bite stick or an oral airway). Be sure to have suctioning equipment ready in case the patient vomits. Provide oxygen or artificial ventilation if the patient is cyanotic or appears to be breathing inadequately, and provide prompt transport.

Altered Mental Status

Although altered mental status is often caused by complications of diabetes, it may also be caused by a variety of other conditions, including poisoning, infection, head injury, part of the postictal state (period following a seizure), and decreased perfusion to the brain. In diabetes, altered mental status can be caused by hypoglycemia and by ketoacidosis.

The mnemonic AEIOU-TIPS is easily remembered and covers a multitude of conditions that can lead to altered mental status. As such, many of the conditions covered by the mnemonic can be confused, resulting in a misdiagnosis when the patient's blood glucose level is not assessed. AEIOU-TIPS stands for the following conditions:

A Alcohol
E Epilepsy, endocrine, electrolytes
I Insulin
O Opioids and other drugs
U Uremia (kidney failure)
T Trauma, temperature
I Infection
P Poisoning, psychogenic causes
S Shock, stroke, seizure, syncope, space-occupying lesion, subarachnoid hemorrhage

Most of the items on the preceding list can be associated with or can cause hypoglycemia. A patient might have a seizure due to hypoglycemia. A patient with an altered mental status after a heroin overdose might also be hypoglycemic. Remember to consider diabetic emergencies in patients who present with any of these emergencies, which can alter or depress mental status. Also remember that patients who present with trauma and are unconscious may have become unconscious as a result of a low blood glucose level and may secondarily became injured. Always suspect and check for low blood glucose in a patient with altered mental status.

Begin emergency medical care of altered mental status by ensuring that the airway is clear. Be prepared to provide artificial ventilation and suctioning in case the patient vomits, and provide prompt transport.

Misdiagnosis of Neurologic Dysfunction

Occasionally, patients with hypoglycemia or hyperglycemia are thought to be intoxicated, especially if their condition has caused a motor vehicle crash or other incident. Confined by police at a police station, a patient with diabetes is at risk. In such situations, an emergency medical identification bracelet, necklace, or card may help to save the patient's life. Often, only a blood glucose test performed at the scene or in the ED will identify the real problem. In many EMS systems, you will be trained and allowed to perform blood glucose testing at the scene. Regardless, until proven otherwise, you must always suspect hypoglycemia in any patient with an altered mental status.

Certainly, diabetes and alcohol intoxication can coexist in a patient. You must be alert to the similarity in symptoms of acute alcohol intoxication and diabetic emergencies. Likewise, hypoglycemia and a head injury can coexist, and you must appreciate the potential for hypoglycemia even when the head injury is obvious.

Street Smarts

Don't judge a book by its cover. What may appear to be a patient under the influence of alcohol may be a patient with hypoglycemia. Be a patient advocate and check the glucose level before making a judgment.

Relationship to Airway Management

Patients with an altered mental status, particularly those who are difficult to awaken, may not have a gag reflex. When the gag reflex is not working, patients cannot expel foreign materials in their mouths (including vomit), and their tongues will often relax and obstruct the airway. Therefore, you must carefully monitor the airway in patients with hyperglycemia, hypoglycemia, or a complication related to diabetes such as stroke or seizure. Place the patient in a lateral recumbent position, and make sure suction is readily available.

Hematologic Emergencies

Hematology is the study of blood-related diseases. This section begins by explaining the composition of blood. It then focuses on five disorders that may be seen in a prehospital emergency:

- Sickle cell disease
- Hemophilia
- Thrombophilia
- Deep vein thrombosis
- Anemia

Words of Wisdom

Diabetic complications frequently require care by EMS clinicians; however, there are other endocrine diseases that cause emergencies in rare situations. In the context of excessive or inadequate thyroid hormones, critical signs and symptoms can occur. Likewise, if the adrenal glands produce insufficient hormones, shock may occur. Rare tumors on the adrenal glands can cause tachycardia and hypertension that could ultimately cause stroke. Whenever you encounter puzzling signs and symptoms, manage the patient's ABCs and consult with medical direction for further advice.

Anatomy and Physiology

Blood and Its Parts

Blood is made up of four components:

- Erythrocytes (red blood cells)
- Leukocytes (white blood cells)
- Platelets
- Plasma

Each component serves a purpose in maintaining a person's homeostatic balance. Each of the body's other systems provides for and utilizes the blood in a specific way. In turn, the blood transports oxygen and carbon dioxide into and out of tissues to sustain the function of the organ system and tissues.

Red blood cells (RBCs) make up 42% to 47% of a person's total blood volume. RBCs contain an important protein, hemoglobin, which carries 97% of the oxygen in the blood and some of the carbon dioxide.

White blood cells (WBCs) make up 0.1% to 0.2% of a person's blood cell volume. In a healthy person, WBCs collect dead cells and provide for their correct disposal. In times of health, WBC levels are low. When an infection develops, WBCs and all of their complementary defense systems are activated and their numbers grow.

Platelets make up 4% to 7% of a person's blood cell volume and are essential for clot formation. When damage occurs to your skin or to a blood vessel, platelets are sent to the site of injury to assist in forming a blood clot to stop the bleeding. Without this protective response, bleeding from a simple cut could be uncontrollable.

Plasma serves as the transportation medium for all blood components as well as proteins and minerals.

Pathophysiology

Sickle Cell Disease

Sickle cell disease, also called hemoglobin S disease, is an inherited blood disorder that affects the RBCs. The name sickle cell comes from the first case report of the disease in 1910, when Dr. James Herrick wrote that the RBCs looked like a sickle (**FIGURE 20-7**).[9] The oddly shaped cells protect the individual from contracting malaria. This protection is useful to people who live in regions where malaria is common, and while malaria is still widely present worldwide, its protection is less helpful in regions where malaria has been eradicated.

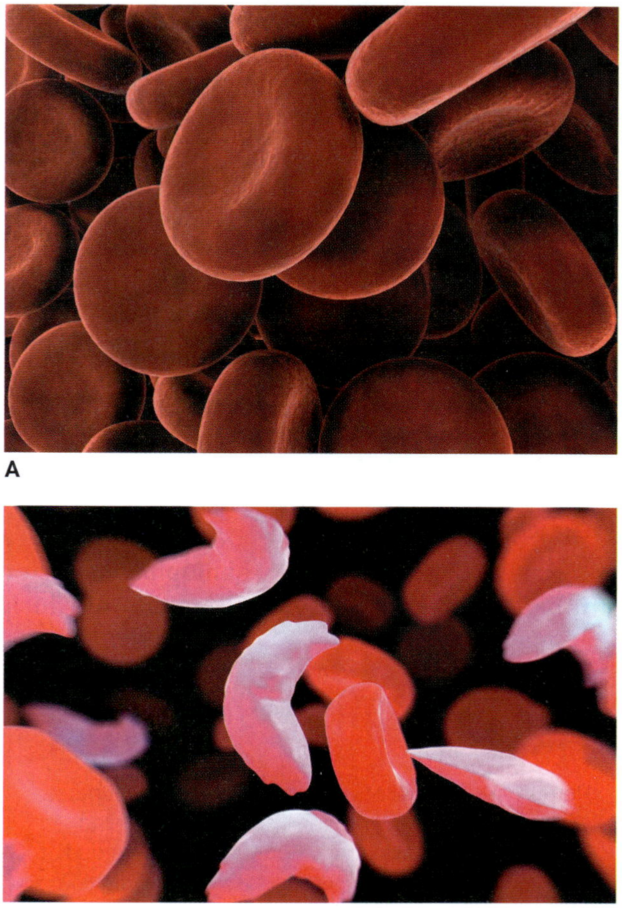

A

B

FIGURE 20-7 A. Normal red blood cells. **B.** Sickle cells.

A: © Sebastian Kaulitzki/Shutterstock; B: © Science Picture Co/Science Source.

Words of Wisdom

In the United States, most newborns have been screened for sickle cell disease. You may encounter patients who were not born in a hospital or who immigrated to the United States from a different country and are not aware they have the disease.

There are several variants that make up this genetic disease. It is sufficient to simply understand that the issues of sickle cell can happen with any of the variants. This disease is more common among people with African; Central or South American; and Middle Eastern, Asian, Indian, or Mediterranean ancestry.[10] However, individuals of any race or ethnicity can experience this condition.[11] All newborns in the United States are tested for sickle cell disease shortly after birth, regardless of their reported race or ethnic background.

The sharp and misshapen sickled cells lead to dysfunction in oxygen binding and unintentional clot formation. These unintentional clots may result in a blockage known as **vasoocclusive crisis**, which can result in tissue hypoxia. The tissue hypoxia may, in turn, produce substantial pain and organ damage, which can trigger calls to EMS for help.

The life span of normal RBCs is approximately 110 to 120 days; sickled cells have a much shorter life span. This results in more cellular waste products in the bloodstream, which can contribute to sludging (clumping) of the blood. Insufficient hydration leads to increased clumping of cells, so it is important that these patients stay hydrated and maintain their general health.

Complications associated with sickle cell disease include the following:

- Anemia
- Gallstones
- Jaundice
- Splenic dysfunction

- Vascular occlusion with ischemia, which may contribute to the following:
  - Acute chest syndrome (hypoxia, dyspnea, chest discomfort, and fever)
  - Stroke
  - Bone necrosis (avascular necrosis; specifically the head of the femur and the humerus)
  - Pain crises
  - Acute and chronic organ dysfunction/failure
  - Retinal hemorrhages

Many of these complications are very painful and potentially life threatening. Further, they increase the patient's susceptibility to infections.

Hemophilia

Hemophilia, also called classic hemophilia or factor VIII deficiency, is a hereditary condition in which the patient lacks one or more of the blood's normal clotting factors. This disorder is rare, affecting approximately 33,000 people in the United States. It is usually diagnosed at a young age.[12]

Hemophilia A is genetically passed on through the X chromosome and disproportionately affects males. Males inherit the condition from a mother who is a carrier but does not have the disease; females inherit the condition only if their mother is a carrier and their father has the disease.

The blood of a healthy individual will clot in as little as 13 seconds after a paper cut and not longer than approximately 7 minutes following a more serious injury that requires direct pressure. In people with hemophilia A, the blood clots less readily after an injury. Having an extended bleeding time from the inability to clot can be life threatening.

A patient who is otherwise healthy but has hemophilia A can have a serious reaction to a minor trauma, such as a simple ankle sprain while playing soccer. Most people would ignore the sprain and continue playing. The patient with hemophilia A would begin to experience swelling from uncontrolled internal bleeding in the region of the injury; this swelling would continue, making the seemingly minor injury a significant problem.

Acute bleeding from any source may be life threatening, depending on where the bleeding occurs. Patients with hemophilia A can be prescribed

Words of Wisdom

Remember that pallor, cyanosis, flushing, or jaundice will present differently among patients depending on their baseline skin color. For patients with a dark baseline skin tone, you may need to look for signs of abnormal perfusion in places such as the oral mucosa, conjunctiva, nail beds, or palms.

YOU are the EMT

You reassess the patient and then call your radio report to the receiving hospital. The patient is still conscious, but confused. Your estimated time of arrival at the hospital is 8 minutes.

Recording Time: 17 Minutes	
Level of consciousness	Conscious, but confused
Respirations	28 breaths/min; deep
Pulse	118 beats/min; weak radial pulses
Skin	Baseline color, warm, and dry; poor turgor
Blood pressure	110/58 mm Hg
Oxygen saturation (Spo_2)	97% (on room air)

You arrive at the hospital and transfer patient care to the attending physician. After further assessment and treatment in the ED, the patient is admitted to the medical intensive care unit.

8. What treatment is provided at the hospital for patients with symptomatic hyperglycemia that cannot be provided in the prehospital setting?

medications to replace the missing clotting factors, release the clotting factors that are stored in the patient's body, or prevent the breakdown of blood clots.

Common complications of hemophilia A include the following:

- Long-term joint problems, which may require a joint replacement
- Bleeding in the brain (intracerebral hemorrhage)
- **Thrombosis** due to treatment

Thrombophilia

Thrombophilia is a disorder that increases the risk of blood clotting. In thrombophilia, the concentration of some elements in the blood, such as clotting factors or proteins, creates conditions favorable for clots to form.

Thrombophilia has many different causes. It may be inherited (genetic) or may result from other medical conditions (eg, autoimmune disorders), use of certain medications, pregnancy, or prolonged immobility. It can develop in patients with cancer, increasing their risk of forming blood clots and life-threatening conditions such as heart attack, stroke, and pulmonary embolism. Whatever the risk factors, the common theme is that clots can spontaneously develop in the patient's blood. Most people with thrombophilia are asymptomatic until a clot forms.[13]

Deep Vein Thrombosis

Deep vein thrombosis (DVT) is a common medical problem in sedentary patients and in patients who have had recent injury or surgery. Although several risk factors increase the chance that a DVT will develop, there are several methods to prevent blood clot formation, including blood-thinning medications, compression stockings, and mechanical devices, all of which you may encounter in the field.

DVT is a particularly worrisome risk for patients who have had joint replacement surgery. Be suspicious of this in a patient with a recent history of joint replacement who complains of leg swelling. Travelers, truck and long-distance bus drivers, and bedridden nursing home patients are at higher risk for DVT because they are sedentary for long periods. Oral birth control medications, pregnancy, obesity, and smoking can also increase the risk for DVT.[14]

If DVT develops in an individual, anticoagulation therapy may be administered. A patient with DVT may be treated in the hospital with IV medications and then transitioned to oral medications or self-administered subcutaneous injectable medications to treat or prevent DVT. Patients who have been prescribed medications such as heparin, warfarin (Coumadin), dabigatran (Pradaxa), or rivaroxaban (Xarelto) to treat DVT are at increased risk of bleeding complications (ie, gastrointestinal bleeding or stroke), and minor trauma is more likely to produce severe internal or external hemorrhage.

A life threat can develop if the clot from the DVT travels from the patient's lower extremity to the lung, causing a pulmonary embolus. Pulmonary emboli can cause chest pain, difficulty breathing, or, if the clots are large, sudden cardiac arrest. Pulmonary embolism is discussed in Chapter 16, *Respiratory Emergencies*.

Anemia

Anemia is an abnormally low number of RBCs. RBCs contain hemoglobin, an iron-containing pigment that is responsible for 97% of the transport of oxygen from the lungs to the cells of the body. Each hemoglobin molecule is able to bind to and carry four molecules of oxygen. Anemia may be the result of either chronic or acute bleeding, a deficiency in certain vitamins or minerals, or an underlying disease process. Heavy menstrual bleeding can cause anemia, and it is also common in pregnancy. If anemia is present, tissues may become hypoxic because the blood is unable to deliver adequate amounts of oxygen to the tissues, even though the available hemoglobin is fully saturated with oxygen and the lungs are delivering enough oxygen to the blood. In this situation, a pulse oximeter may indicate that there is adequate saturation, even though the tissues are hypoxic.

Patient Assessment of Hematologic Disorders

Scene Size-up

Although your report from dispatch may be for a patient with an unknown medical problem, most patients presenting with a sickle cell crisis have had a crisis before and will relay that information to the dispatcher. As you approach the scene, ensure your safety by assessing for hazards. Standard precautions should consist of gloves, mask, and eye protection at a minimum.

Determine whether this is your only patient and whether trauma was involved. Decide whether you will need any additional resources. Patients experiencing a vasoocclusive crisis are often in extreme pain and would benefit from ALS clinicians being able to administer analgesics.

Remember that trauma may have occurred because of a medical incident. Determine the mechanism of injury and/or nature of illness.

Primary Assessment

Perform a primary assessment to form an initial general impression of the patient. How does the patient look? Does the patient appear anxious, restless, or listless? Is the patient apathetic or irritable? Determine the patient's level of consciousness.

While you are forming your general impression, assess the patient's airway and breathing. Patients showing signs of inadequate breathing or altered mental status should receive oxygen to maintain an oxygen saturation of greater than 94%. A patient who is experiencing a sickle cell crisis may have increased respirations as a result of severe pain or pneumonia. If the patient is having difficulty breathing, assess breath sounds, and manage the airway, oxygenation, and ventilation. Continue to monitor the airway as you provide care.

Once you have assessed the airway and breathing and have performed the necessary interventions, check the patient's circulatory status. An increased heart rate in a patient who has sickle cell disease may relate to anemia, pain, or an effort to force blood through vessels that are partially occluded by the sickled cells.

In patients with suspected hemophilia, be alert for signs of acute blood loss such as pallor, weak pulse, and hypotension. Note any bleeding, such as nosebleeds, bloody sputum, swollen joints, and blood in the urine or stool. Because of blood loss, patients with hemophilia may exhibit signs of hypoxia.

Whether you decide to rapidly transport the patient will depend on the severity of the patient's pain and the patient's wishes. Patients with a history of sickle cell disease, but who have not had a crisis in some time, may refuse transport. However, transport to an ED should always be recommended to any patient who is experiencing a sickle cell crisis or hemophilia with uncontrolled bleeding. These patients may require emotional support.

History Taking

If the patient is conscious, determine the chief complaint or history of present illness. Responsive medical patients are able to provide their own medical history to help you identify a cause for their severe pain. It is also important to ascertain whether the pain is isolated to a single location or if pain is felt throughout the entire body. Is the patient having any visual disturbances? Is the patient experiencing any gastrointestinal problems, such as nausea, vomiting, or abdominal cramping? Is the patient reporting any chest pain or shortness of breath?

In a patient with known sickle cell disease, ask the following questions in addition to obtaining a SAMPLE history:

- Have you had a crisis before?
- When was the last time you had a crisis?
- How did your last crisis resolve?
- Have you had any illness, unusual amount of activity, or stress lately?

Secondary Assessment

Obtain a complete set of vital signs, including a measurement of the patient's oxygen saturation level. In patients experiencing a sickle cell crisis, respirations are normal to rapid, pulse is weak and rapid, skin is typically pale and clammy, and blood pressure is low.

Use pulse oximetry, if available. However, keep in mind that the oxygen saturation reading you obtain may be inaccurate as a result of the patient's anemic state.

Next, systematically examine the patient, focusing on major joints at which sickled cells congregate. Evaluate and document mental status using the AVPU scale. Physical signs, such as swelling of the fingers and toes, priapism, and jaundice, may guide you in determining whether the patient is experiencing a sickle cell crisis.

Reassessment

Reassess the patient frequently to determine if there have been changes in the patient's condition. For example, are there changes in the patient's mental status? Are the ABCs still intact? How is the patient responding to the interventions performed? Should you adjust or change the interventions? Document each assessment, your findings, the time of the interventions, and any changes in the patient's condition.

At the hospital, care for patients with sickle cell disease can include analgesics for pain, antibiotics to treat infection, IV fluid for hydration, and, depending on the severity of the crisis, a blood transfusion.

Distinguishing a true sickle cell crisis from other nonspecific causes of pain can be difficult. Remember to perform a thorough assessment and consult with medical control as soon as feasible.

Hospital care for a patient with hemophilia may include IV therapy to treat hypotension and a transfusion of plasma. Analgesics may also be appropriate.

Communication with hospital staff is important for continuity of care. Inform hospital personnel about the patient's history, the current situation, your assessment findings, and your interventions and their results.

Document your assessment findings clearly, as they represent the basis for your treatment. Follow your local protocols for patients who refuse treatment or transport.

Emergency Medical Care for Hematologic Disorders

Emergency care for patients with hematologic disorders is mainly supportive and symptomatic. Patients showing signs of inadequate breathing or decreased oxygen saturation should receive oxygen to maintain an oxygen saturation greater than 94% and should be placed in a position of comfort and transported rapidly to the hospital.

Remember that some hematologic disorders cause extreme pain. If possible, you should try to manage the pain through interventions such as positioning, application of ice or heat packs, extremity elevation, distraction, or pharmacologic means if within your local protocol.

YOU are the EMT SUMMARY

1. What processes are being described by the patient?

This presentation can be typical of many illnesses until you ask the correct questions. The 3- to 5-day, subtle flulike presentation is often how type 1 diabetes presents. People must eat to have energy, but the lack of insulin deprives cells of the fuel they need, and therefore no energy is produced.

The onset of type 1 diabetes takes some time to progress. For this reason, symptoms are initially subtle and are overlooked by the patient or their parents. As the lack of insulin becomes more profound, the patient will notice increasing fatigue and malaise along with weight loss.

The patient is also experiencing (1) polydipsia, (2) polyuria, and (3) polyphagia.

Without insulin, glucose accumulates in the blood. Glucose spills into the urine until it reaches the kidney's maximum level to excrete. The glucose in the urine pulls a substantial amount of water with it, resulting in large amounts of urination (*polyuria*), causing dehydration. The patient experiences thirst, causing the patient to drink large amounts of fluid; this is called *polydipsia*. Finally, eating in excess (*polyphagia*) occurs in the face of weight loss. Polyphagia develops because of the starvation of the patient at the cellular level.

Often, the patient does not recognize these symptoms, but family and friends might, especially if they have had previous experience with diabetes.

2. What hormone is not produced by the body in type 1 diabetes?

The missing hormone is insulin. Insulin is the key to the door of the cell. Without insulin, nutrition in the form of glucose cannot get into the cell and the cell cannot function normally.

3. What should you expect the patient's blood glucose level to read? Why?

Based on the description of increased food intake with weight loss, increased fluid intake, and

YOU are the EMT SUMMARY continued

increased urination, this patient appears to be hyperglycemic and may be in DKA. In these cases, the blood glucose level will be in the mid 400s to 500s or even higher. This level is much higher than the normal blood glucose level of 80 to 120 mg/dL.

4. What is causing the patient's frequent urination and deep, rapid breathing?

Urination is frequent because an increase in his blood glucose level resulted in glucose spilling into the urine. He is excreting large amounts of urine because glucose in the urine pulls water out with it. This secondarily causes him to experience excessive thirst and to drink large amounts of fluid.

Deep, rapid breathing, known as Kussmaul respirations, is caused by the ketones that are accumulating in the blood and are being eliminated from the lungs during exhalation. Kussmaul respirations often have a fruity or sweet odor.

5. What other factors can cause hyperglycemia in patients with diabetes?

Changing mealtimes, insulin dosage changes, or a variation in exercise can result in a hyperglycemic or hypoglycemic event. An infection or other major stressors to the body could easily put an otherwise well-regulated patient with type 1 diabetes into DKA. Noncompliance with medication use can also result in hyperglycemic episodes. The patient in this chapter's scenario has new-onset diabetes and is in DKA. Noncompliance with medication use can also result in hyperglycemic episodes.

6. How can you distinguish symptomatic hyperglycemia from symptomatic hypoglycemia?

A key to distinguishing a hyperglycemic emergency from a hypoglycemic emergency is the time of symptom onset. Hyperglycemia, ketoacidosis, and dehydration typically progress over hours to days. By contrast, hypoglycemia has an acute onset: often over a period of a few minutes.

Symptomatic hyperglycemia and symptomatic hypoglycemia also present with relatively different signs and symptoms. Signs and symptoms of symptomatic hyperglycemia may include tachycardia; signs of dehydration (warm, dry skin; poor skin turgor; and sunken eyes); deep, rapid breathing (Kussmaul respirations), which indicates the respiratory system is attempting to eliminate ketones from the body; a sweet or fruity (acetone) breath odor; and mental status changes ranging from confusion to coma.

Symptomatic hypoglycemia presents with signs and symptoms similar to hypoxemia and shock that may include rapid, shallow respirations; pale (compared with baseline), cool, clammy (diaphoretic) skin; tachycardia; weakness, which may be confined to one side of the body and mimic a stroke; and varying degrees of mental status change, including confusion, irritability, combativeness, seizures, and coma.

7. What additional treatment should you provide to this patient?

The patient's signs and symptoms clearly point to symptomatic hyperglycemia and DKA. Symptomatic hyperglycemia requires definitive care that can only be provided at the hospital. Prehospital treatment at the EMT level is aimed at providing supportive care (ie, maintaining the ABCs) and promptly transporting the patient to the hospital. En route, closely monitor the patient's mental status and breathing adequacy; if his respirations become slow and/or shallow, especially if his mental status deteriorates further, assist his ventilations with a bag-mask device.

Some patients with symptomatic hyperglycemia become so dehydrated that hypovolemic shock develops; therefore, it is important to closely monitor the patient's perfusion status (eg, heart rate, peripheral pulse quality, blood pressure, mental status). If signs of shock are observed, keep the patient warm and in a supine position and administer oxygen if not already applied. Although the patient is extremely thirsty, do not give him anything to drink; doing so increases the risk of aspiration if he vomits.

8. What treatment is provided at the hospital for patients with symptomatic hyperglycemia that cannot be provided in the prehospital setting?

Symptomatic hyperglycemia is a complex medical problem that causes numerous complications; it cannot be treated in the prehospital setting, and it cannot be changed quickly. Insulin is needed to restore circulating blood glucose to a normal level, and IV fluids are needed to correct dehydration. This situation underscores the importance of performing a rapid assessment, initiating treatment without delay, and promptly transporting the patient to the hospital. If your transport time will be prolonged, consider an intercept with an ALS unit, if available; AEMTs and paramedics are trained to start IV lines and administer fluids.

Prep Kit

Ready for Review

- Diabetes is a disorder of glucose metabolism or difficulty metabolizing carbohydrates. There are different types of diabetes. Type 1 diabetes typically develops in childhood and requires daily insulin to control blood glucose. Type 2 diabetes typically develops in middle age and often can be controlled with diet, activity, and oral medications.
- Both type 1 and type 2 diabetes are serious systemic diseases, especially affecting the kidneys, eyes, small arteries, and peripheral nerves.
- Patients with diabetes have chronic complications that place them at risk for other diseases, such as heart attack, stroke, and infections. Most often, however, you will be called on to treat the acute complications of blood glucose imbalance. These include hyperglycemia (excess blood glucose) and hypoglycemia (insufficient blood glucose).
- Hyperglycemia is typically characterized by excessive urination and resulting thirst, in conjunction with the deterioration of body tissues. It is usually associated with dehydration and ketoacidosis and can result in marked rapid (often deep) respirations; warm, dry skin; a weak pulse; and a fruity breath odor. Hyperglycemia must be treated in the hospital with insulin and IV fluids.
- Symptoms of hypoglycemia classically include confusion; rapid respirations; pale, moist skin; diaphoresis; dizziness; fainting; and even coma and seizures. This condition is rapidly reversible with the administration of glucose or sugar. Without treatment, however, permanent brain damage and death can occur.
- Because a blood glucose level that is either too high or too low can result in altered mental status, you must perform a thorough history and patient assessment to determine the nature of the problem. When the problem cannot be determined, it is best to treat the patient for hypoglycemia.
- Be prepared to give oral glucose to a conscious patient who is confused or has a slightly decreased level of consciousness; however, do not give oral glucose to a patient who is unconscious or otherwise unable to swallow properly or protect their own airway.
- In all cases, providing emergency medical care and prompt transport is your primary responsibility.
- Sickle cell disease is a blood disorder that affects the shape of RBCs.
- Symptoms of sickle cell disease are pain in the joints, fever, respiratory distress, and abdominal pain.
- Patients with sickle cell disease have chronic complications that place them at risk for other diseases, such as heart attack, stroke, and infection. Most often, however, you will be called on to treat the acute complications of severe pain.
- Patients with hemophilia are not able to control bleeding because clots do not develop as they should.
- Emergency care in the prehospital setting is supportive for patients with sickle cell disease or a clotting disorder such as hemophilia.

Vital Vocabulary

acidosis The buildup of excess acid in the blood or body tissues that can result from a primary illness.

anemia A condition in which the blood contains an abnormally low number of red blood cells, resulting in a decreased ability to transport oxygen throughout the body via the bloodstream.

diabetes mellitus A metabolic disorder in which the ability to metabolize carbohydrates (sugars) is impaired, usually because of a lack of insulin.

Prep Kit continued

diabetic ketoacidosis (DKA) A form of hyperglycemia in uncontrolled diabetes in which certain acids accumulate when insulin is not available.

endocrine glands Glands that secrete or release chemicals that are used inside the body.

endocrine system The complex message and control system that integrates many body functions, including the release of hormones.

glucose One of the basic sugars; it is the primary fuel, in conjunction with oxygen, for cellular metabolism.

hematology The study and prevention of blood-related disorders.

hemophilia A hereditary condition in which the patient lacks one or more of the blood's normal clotting factors.

hormones Substances formed in specialized organs or glands and carried to another organ or group of cells in the same organism; they regulate many body functions, including metabolism, growth, and body temperature.

hyperglycemia An abnormally high blood glucose level.

hyperosmolar hyperglycemic state (HHS) A life-threatening condition resulting from high blood glucose that typically occurs in older adults and that causes altered mental status, dehydration, and organ damage; formerly called hyperosmolar hyperglycemic nonketotic syndrome.

hypoglycemia An abnormally low blood glucose level.

insulin A hormone produced by the islets of Langerhans (endocrine glands located throughout the pancreas) that enables glucose in the blood to enter cells; used in synthetic form to treat and control diabetes mellitus.

Kussmaul respirations Deep, rapid breathing; usually the result of an accumulation of certain acids when insulin is not available in the body.

polydipsia Excessive thirst that persists for long periods despite reasonable fluid intake; often the result of excessive urination.

polyphagia Excessive eating; in diabetes, the inability to use glucose properly can cause a sense of hunger.

polyuria The passage of an unusually large volume of urine in a given period; in diabetes, this can result from the wasting of glucose in the urine.

sickle cell disease A hereditary disease that causes normal, round red blood cells to become oblong, or sickle shaped.

symptomatic hyperglycemia A hyperglycemic state resulting from several problems, including ketoacidosis, dehydration because of excessive urination, and hyperglycemia.

symptomatic hypoglycemia Severe hypoglycemia resulting in changes in mental status.

thrombophilia A tendency toward the development of blood clots as a result of an abnormality of the system of coagulation.

thrombosis A blood clot, either in the arterial or venous system.

type 1 diabetes An autoimmune disorder in which the individual's immune system produces antibodies to the pancreatic beta cells, and therefore the pancreas cannot produce insulin; onset in early childhood is common.

type 2 diabetes A condition in which insulin resistance develops in response to increased blood glucose levels; can be managed by exercise and diet modification, but is often managed by medications.

vasoocclusive crisis Ischemia and pain caused by sickle-shaped red blood cells that obstruct blood flow to a portion of the body.

Prep Kit continued

References

1. Statistics about diabetes. American Diabetes Association website. https://diabetes.org/about-diabetes/statistics/about-diabetes. Updated November 2, 2023. Accessed January 24, 2025.
2. Eckel RH, Kahn SE, Ferrannini E, et al. Obesity and type 2 diabetes: what can be unified and what needs to be individualized? *Diabetes Care.* 2011;34(6):1424–1430.
3. Gaddam M, Singh A, Jain N, et al. A comprehensive review of intranasal insulin and its effect on the cognitive function of diabetics. *Cureus*. 2021;13(8):e17219. doi:10.7759/cureus.17219
4. Type 2 diabetes. Mayo Clinic website. https://www.mayoclinic.org/diseases-conditions/type-2-diabetes/diagnosis-treatment/drc-20351199. Updated March 14, 2023. Accessed January 24, 2025.
5. Hyperglycemia in diabetes: symptoms. Mayo Clinic website. https://www.mayoclinic.org/diseases-conditions/hyperglycemia/symptoms-causes/syc-20373631. Updated August 20, 2022. Accessed January 24, 2025.
6. Adeyinka A, Kondamudi NP. Hyperosmolar hyperglycemic syndrome. *StatPearls*. National Library of Medicine website. https://www.ncbi.nlm.nih.gov/books/NBK482142/. Updated August 12, 2023. Accessed January 24, 2025.
7. National Association of State EMS Officials. *National Model EMS Clinical Guidelines: Version 3.0.* https://nasemso.org/wp-content/uploads/National-Model-EMS-Clinical-Guidelines_2022.pdf. Updated March 2022. Accessed January 24, 2025.
8. Benning TJ, Heien HC, Herges JR, Creo AL, Nofal AA, McCoy RG. Glucagon fill rates and cost among children and adolescents with type 1 diabetes in the Unites States, 2011–2021. *Diabetes Res Clin Pract.* 2023;206:111026.
9. Savitt TL, Goldberg MF. Herrick's 1910 case report of sickle cell anemia: the rest of the story. *JAMA.* 1989;261(2):266–271.
10. Sickle cell disease. American Society of Hematology website. https://www.hematology.org/education/patients/anemia/sickle-cell-disease. Accessed January 24, 2025.
11. Pokhrel A, Olayemi A, Ogbonda S, Nair K, Wang JC. Racial and ethnic differences in sickle cell disease within the United States: from demographics to outcomes. *Eur J Haematol*. 2023;110(5):554–563.
12. Data and statistics on hemophilia. Centers for Disease Control and Prevention website. https://www.cdc.gov/hemophilia/data-research/. Published May 15, 2024. Accessed January 24, 2025.
13. Thrombophilia. National Health Service website. https://www.nhs.uk/conditions/thrombophilia/. Reviewed August 14, 2023. Accessed January 24, 2025.
14. McLendon K, Goyal A, Attia M. Deep venous thrombosis risk factors. *StatPearls*. National Library of Medicine website. https://www.ncbi.nlm.nih.gov/books/NBK470215/. Updated March 17, 2023. Accessed January 24, 2025.

Additional Resources

National Association of State EMS Officials. *National EMS Scope of Practice Model 2019.* Washington, DC: National Highway Traffic Safety Administration; February 2019. Report No. DOT HS 812-666. https://www.ems.gov/assets/National_EMS_Scope_of_Practice_Model_2019.pdf. Accessed January 24, 2025.

National Highway Traffic Safety Administration. *National Emergency Medical Services Education Standards*. EMS.gov website. https://www.ems.gov/assets/EMS_Education-Standards_2021_FNL.pdf. Published January 2021. Accessed January 24, 2025.

Chapter 21

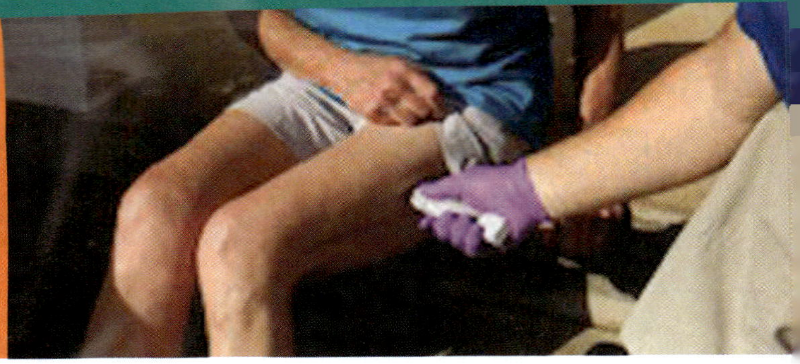

Allergy and Anaphylaxis

NATIONAL EMS EDUCATION STANDARD COMPETENCIES

Medicine

Applies knowledge to provide basic emergency care and transportation based on assessment findings for an acutely ill patient.

Immunology

- Allergic and anaphylactic reactions (pp 817–820)
- Other immunologic emergencies to be determined locally (pp 819–820)

KNOWLEDGE OBJECTIVES

1. Define the terms *allergic reaction* and *anaphylaxis*. (pp 817–818)
2. Explain the difference between a local response and a systemic response to allergens. (pp 817–819)
3. List the categories of stimuli that could cause an allergic reaction or an extreme allergic reaction. (pp 818–819)
4. Differentiate the primary assessment for a patient with a systemic allergic or anaphylactic reaction from that of a patient with a local reaction. (pp 820–821)
5. Explain the importance of managing the airway, breathing, and circulation of a patient who is having an allergic reaction. (p 820)
6. Discuss the steps in the primary assessment that are specific to a patient who is having an allergic reaction. (pp 820–825)
7. Explain the factors involved when making a transport decision for a patient having an allergic reaction. (pp 820–821)
8. Review the process for providing emergency medical care to a patient who is experiencing an allergic reaction. (pp 824–825)
9. Explain the rationale, including communication and documentation considerations, when determining whether to administer epinephrine to a patient who is having an allergic reaction. (pp 825–831)
10. Describe some special considerations in using epinephrine to treat an allergic reaction in a geriatric patient. (p 830)

SKILLS OBJECTIVES

1. Demonstrate how to use an EpiPen auto-injector. (p 827, Skill Drill 21-1)
2. Demonstrate how to use a Neffy intranasal device. (p 829, Skill Drill 21-2)

Introduction

Allergies are common. In 2021, one-third of the adult US population experienced an allergic reaction, including seasonal allergies, food allergies, and eczema.[1] Diagnosis of allergic conditions in children has increased over time. Approximately one-quarter of children in the United States have at least one allergic condition.[1] The most common type of allergic condition is seasonal allergies. Fortunately, death from allergy or anaphylaxis is rare. The fatality rate in the United States is well under 1 per million,[2] and fatality rates for those reaching the hospital emergency department (ED) in anaphylaxis are less than 0.3%.[3] Most deaths from anaphylaxis are related to allergies to medications.

As an EMT, you will often respond to calls involving an allergic reaction. When managing allergy-related emergencies, you must be aware of the possibility of acute airway obstruction and cardiovascular collapse and be prepared to treat these life-threatening complications. Your ability to recognize and manage the many signs and symptoms of allergic reactions may be the only thing standing between a patient's life and imminent death.

This chapter describes **immunology**, the study of the body's immune system, and the categories of stimuli that may provoke allergic reactions. You will learn what to look for in assessing patients who may be having an allergic reaction and how to care for them, including administration of epinephrine.

Anatomy and Physiology

The **immune system** protects the human body from foreign substances and organisms. The body is constantly exposed to multiple types of invaders, such as bacteria or viruses, that want to make your body a home. Fortunately, most people have immune systems that are well equipped to detect unauthorized visits or invading attacks by foreign substances. Once a foreign substance invades the body, the body goes on alert and initiates a series of responses to disable the invader.

Pathophysiology

Many conditions are related to the immune system, but an allergic reaction is the most common immunologic emergency you will treat as an EMT. An **allergic reaction** is an exaggerated and inappropriate **immune response** to an **allergen**. An allergen is a substance that is normally harmless to humans, such as food or pollen. In an allergic reaction, the body's normal system for defending against invaders overreacts to the allergen.

Given the right person and the right circumstances, almost any substance can become an allergen. However, some people do not experience allergic reactions the first time they are exposed to an allergen. First, individuals become *sensitized* (exposed for the first time) to the substance. During sensitization, their immune system classifies the substance as an allergen and produces antibodies to recognize it and attack it on the next exposure. The antibodies typically involved in allergic reactions are called immunoglobulin E (IgE). When the patient is exposed to the substance again, an allergic reaction occurs. As a result of the time interval in this process, some patients may not have any idea what is causing their allergic reaction or even realize they are having one. You must be able to recognize the signs and symptoms and maintain a high index of suspicion.

When exposed to an allergen, antibodies react and release chemicals, including **histamines** and

YOU are the EMT

You and your partner respond to a call involving a 33-year-old man experiencing shortness of breath. On arrival, you observe a conscious patient in obvious respiratory distress, breathing rapidly with audible wheezing. His skin is flushed, appearing red, and covered in hives. When you attempt to question the patient, you find he can speak only in two- to three-word sentences.

1. What, if any, additional resources should you request?
2. What intervention or interventions should you perform without delay?

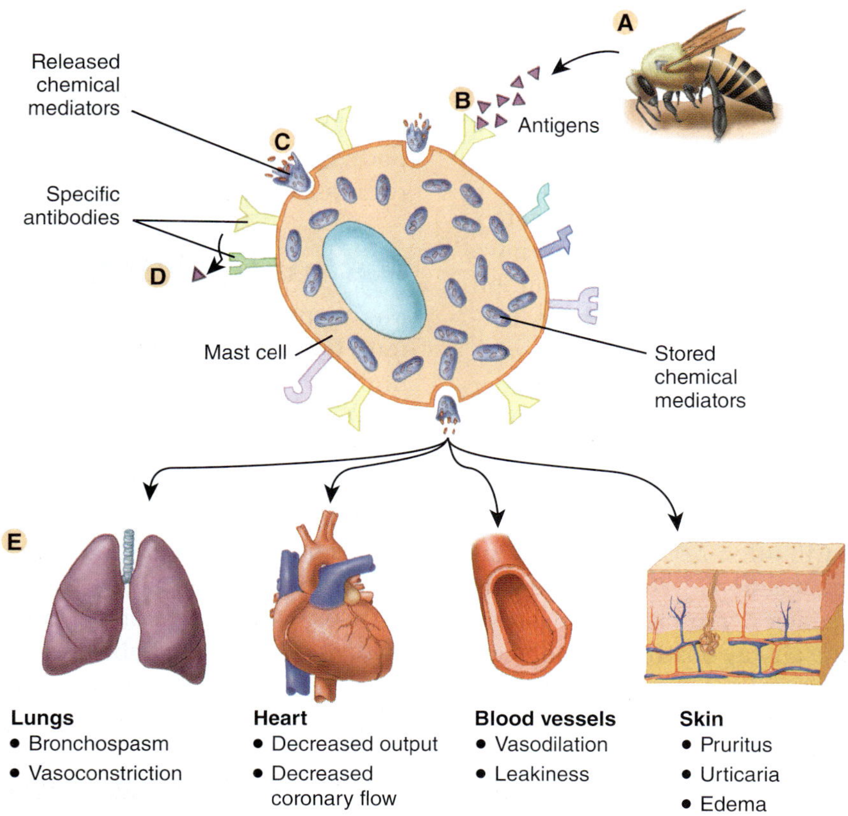

FIGURE 21-1 The sequence of events in anaphylaxis. **A.** The antigen is introduced into the body. **B.** The antigen–antibody reaction at the surface of a mast cell. **C.** The release of mast cell chemical mediators. **D.** Specific antibody reacts with its corresponding antigen. **E.** Chemical mediators exert their effects on end organs.

leukotrienes. These chemicals signal tissues such as the nasal mucosa, skin, lungs, and blood vessels, causing the signs and symptoms observed in the patient. An allergic reaction may be mild and local, characterized by itching, redness, or tenderness, or it may be severe and systemic, a condition known as **anaphylaxis** (**FIGURE 21-1**).

Anaphylaxis is an extreme allergic reaction that is life threatening and involves multiple organ systems. In severe cases, anaphylaxis can rapidly result in shock and death. Because anaphylaxis is a multisystem syndrome, it can present with various combinations of many signs and symptoms. Two of the most common signs of anaphylaxis are widespread **urticaria**, or hives, small areas of generalized itching or burning that appear as multiple small, raised areas on the skin (**FIGURE 21-2**), and **angioedema**, areas of localized swelling (**FIGURE 21-3**). These skin

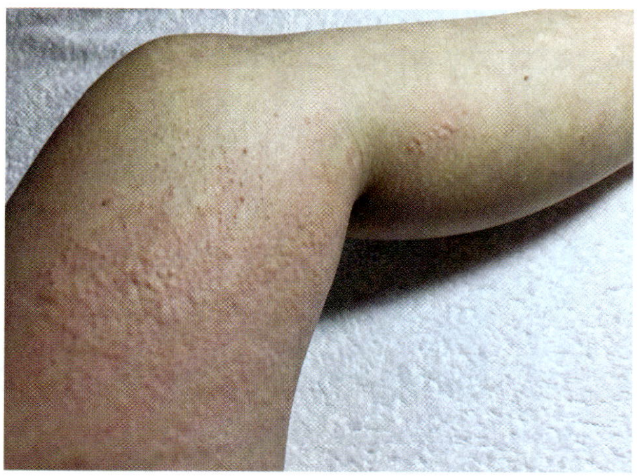

FIGURE 21-2 Urticaria, or hives, may appear following exposure to an allergen and is characterized by multiple small, raised areas on the skin. It may be one of the warning signs of an impending anaphylactic reaction.

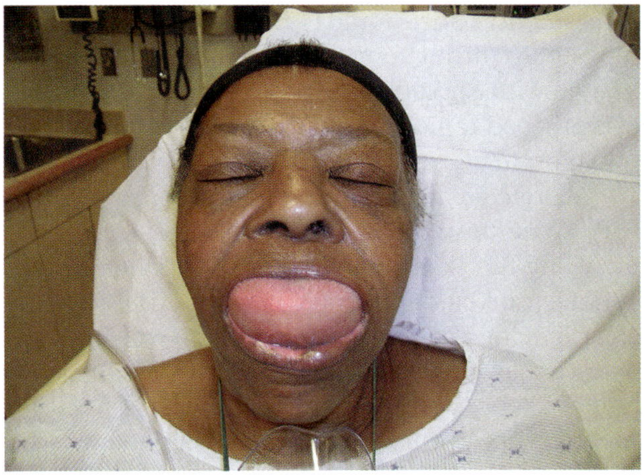

FIGURE 21-3 Angioedema is localized swelling associated with allergic reactions. If the site of swelling includes the lips, tongue, larynx, or other such structures, airway obstruction may occur.

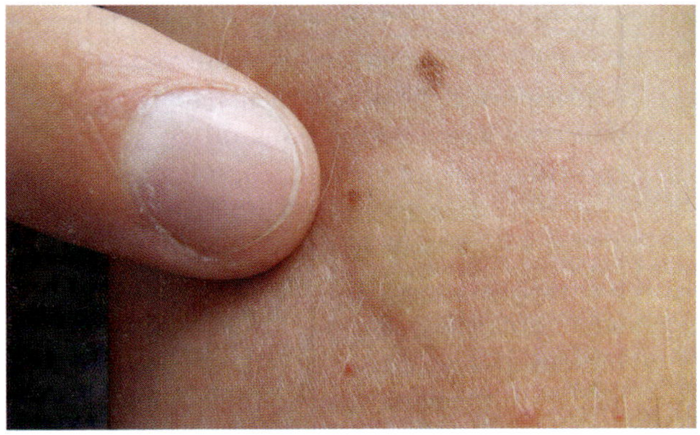

FIGURE 21-4 A wheal is a whitish, firm elevation of the skin that occurs after an insect sting or bite.

and mucosal symptoms occur in approximately 90% of anaphylaxis cases.[4] Respiratory signs and symptoms such as wheezing, stridor, runny or congested nose, and sneezing are also common. Nearly one-half of cases involve gastrointestinal dysfunction (eg, nausea, vomiting, abdominal cramps). Cardiovascular signs and symptoms such as hypotension, syncope, dizziness, and tachycardia also occur in approximately one-half of cases. Histamines cause vasodilation as well as increased capillary permeability (causing fluid from the bloodstream to seep into the tissues), which can lead to airway obstruction and profound shock.

Common Allergens

The most common allergens fall into several categories:

- **Medication.** The most common source of anaphylactic reactions is medication, particularly antibiotics (eg, penicillin, cephalosporins) and nonsteroidal anti-inflammatory drugs (NSAIDs).[5] The reaction may be immediate (within 30 minutes) or delayed. Medications are the most common cause of fatal reactions.
- **Food.** Fish, shellfish, and peanuts are common triggers of anaphylaxis.[6] Other food triggers for allergy and anaphylaxis are tree nuts (eg, walnuts, cashews), eggs, wheat, soybeans, and sesame. Cow's milk is also a common allergen and anaphylaxis trigger in infants and children. Peanuts and tree nuts account for most of the deaths from food-induced anaphylaxis, most commonly in adolescents and young adults.[7]
- **Insect bites and stings.** When an insect bites or stings, the act of injecting its venom is called **envenomation**. Envenomation by a Hymenoptera species, which include honeybees, wasps, fire ants, yellow jackets, and hornets, is another common cause of fatal anaphylactic reactions.[8] These bites and stings may produce a localized reaction, causing swelling and itching at the site, or a severe and systemic reaction (ie, anaphylaxis). Bites and stings sometimes produce a **wheal**, which is a raised, swollen, well-defined area on the skin (**FIGURE 21-4**). The swelling associated with an insect bite may be dramatic and sometimes frightening to the patient or to you. However, as long as these signs remain localized, they are not usually serious. Emergencies relating to bites and stings from insects and other animals are discussed in Chapter 32, *Environmental Emergencies.*
- **Plants and organic material.** People who inhale dust, pollen, mold, mildew, or other organic materials to which they are sensitive may experience an allergic reaction. Common plant allergens include ragweed, ryegrass, maple, and oak. Many of these allergens are seasonal. Seasonal allergies are the most common

type of allergy in both children and adults but are not common causes of anaphylaxis.[9,10]

- **Chemicals.** Certain chemicals, makeup, soap, hair dye, latex, and various other substances can cause severe allergic reactions. Latex is of particular concern to health care clinicians, and the increases in latex allergy can be attributed to health care practices, especially the advent of universal precautions in the 1990s.[11] Increased exposure is linked to increased sensitization for health care clinicians. To reduce sensitization rates, powder-free, lower allergen, or nitrile alternatives are the preferred type of gloves. It is important to remember that natural rubber latex is also found in other products, such as balloons and dental dams.

Patient Assessment of an Immunologic Emergency

Scene Size-up

First and foremost, ensure the scene is safe. The patient's environment or recent activity may indicate the source of the reaction, such as a sting or bite from an insect, a food allergy at a restaurant, or a new medication. Remember, allergic reactions have a wide variety of presentations: a respiratory problem reported by dispatch may be an allergic reaction, but a patient experiencing anaphylaxis could also have a primary complaint of vomiting. Do not neglect the possibility that traumatic injury may also be present, secondary to the medical emergency. Take standard precautions and consider the need for additional resources, such as advanced life support (ALS) personnel, who can provide advanced airway management and additional medications if needed.

Primary Assessment

When a patient presents with an allergic reaction, you should quickly identify and treat any immediate or potential life threats. It is essential that you pay careful attention to the patient's Airway, Breathing, and Circulation (ABCs), as deterioration can occur at almost any time and with little warning. This is not only paramount during the primary assessment; ABCs should continue to be reassessed repeatedly throughout transport to the ED. If untreated with epinephrine, an anaphylactic reaction can proceed rapidly to death. Rapid treatment and transport are essential.

Allergic reactions most commonly present with acute (minutes to hours) onset of symptoms involving the skin (hives, flushing, itching) and respiratory or cardiovascular compromise. Patients experiencing a severe allergic reaction will often appear very anxious. If your general impression is potential allergy or anaphylaxis, immediately call for ALS backup, if available. Sometimes patients who are known to have severe allergies wear a medical identification tag (eg, necklace or bracelet). Such clues could provide crucial information in situations where the patient is found unresponsive or is otherwise unable to answer questions about medical history.

Words of Wisdom

Note that "flushed" does not always mean "red" or "pink" skin. In a patient with dark baseline skin tone, the increased flow of blood to the skin may be difficult to detect and may present as skin coloration that is uncharacteristically dark for that patient.

Anaphylaxis can cause rapid swelling of the upper airway and constriction in the lower airways. You may have only a few minutes to assess the airway and provide lifesaving measures. Anaphylaxis can also cause profound hypotension, resulting in loss of consciousness. However, not all allergic reactions are anaphylactic reactions. Work quickly to assess the patient to determine the severity of the symptoms and the number of body systems affected.

Quickly assess for signs of impending airway obstruction, such as swollen lips or tongue, hoarseness, or stridor. Listen to the lungs on each side of the chest for wheezing. Dyspnea may present with increased work of breathing, use of accessory muscles, head bobbing, tripod positioning, nostril flaring, and abnormal breath sounds. Early on, the patient may have more subtle complaints that suggest airway swelling, such as a feeling of fullness in their neck or a lump in their throat, and you may note that they are frequently clearing their throat.[12] Wheezing occurs because of narrowing of the lower air passages and increased mucus production. The fluid in the air passages and the constricted bronchi together produce the wheezing sound. As the patient's condition worsens, breath sounds may diminish to the point of being almost silent. Stridor, a harsh, high-pitched sound heard on inspiration, occurs when swelling in the upper airway (near the vocal cords and throat) begins to close off the airway.

As the patient with respiratory failure attempts to compensate by breathing more rapidly, and as respirations become more difficult, the patient may eventually fatigue and may even stop breathing. In the latter case, cardiac arrest will shortly follow respiratory arrest.

Assist the patient into a comfortable position, generally a high Fowler position, in an effort to maximize ventilations. However, if signs of shock emerge, the patient should immediately be placed in the supine position as tolerated. Do not hesitate to initiate high-flow oxygen therapy when indicated. For a patient in severe respiratory distress, you may have to assist ventilations using a bag-mask device attached to high-concentration oxygen.

Assess for a rapid pulse rate; pale, cool, cyanotic, moist skin; and delayed capillary refill, all of which may indicate hypoperfusion. Because pallor can be difficult to detect in patients with dark skin, instead check for pale mucous membranes inside the inner lower eyelid or slow capillary refill. Remember, allergic reactions most commonly affect the skin. Flushing, hives, and edema might complicate your assessment of pallor, capillary refill, or other assessments for shock. Treatment for shock includes oxygen administration, proper positioning (ie, recumbent or supine as tolerated), and efforts to prevent heat loss. The definitive treatment for anaphylaxis is epinephrine. It should be the treatment priority in any patient with a suspected severe allergic reaction or anaphylaxis. Do not wait for signs of shock to develop.

If anaphylaxis is suspected, or if a relatively mild allergic reaction appears to be worsening, immediate transport is warranted after epinephrine is given. Before leaving the scene, be sure to take along the patient's medications (eg, auto-injectors and inhalers). If the patient is calm and does not exhibit severe signs and symptoms, consider continuing the assessment at the scene. However, if in doubt, always err on the side of urgently initiating transport.

Words of Wisdom

While flushed skin and hives are common in anaphylaxis, these findings are absent in approximately 40% of anaphylaxis cases. You must assess the physical findings in the context of a thorough patient history.[13]

Distinguishing Anaphylaxis and Nonanaphylactic Allergic Reactions

Because the interventions required for an allergic reaction may differ from those required for anaphylaxis, it is important for the EMT to distinguish between the two. Anaphylaxis can be distinguished from milder allergic reactions using the following criteria.

- Anaphylaxis
  - Acute onset that involves the skin (rash, flushing) *with* either respiratory compromise or decreased blood pressure and signs of shock, or
  - Hypotension after exposure to a known allergen, or
  - *Two or more* of the following after exposure to a known allergen:
    - Hives, itching, swollen tongue or lips
    - Dyspnea, wheezing, stridor, low oxygen saturation level
    - Persistent vomiting, abdominal pain, diarrhea
    - Hypotension or signs of shock (syncope, weakness, chest tightness, incontinence)
- Nonanaphylactic allergic reaction
  - Signs that involve just one organ system, such as itching and hives, or swelling around the eyes only

Remember that if the patient is experiencing hypotension and/or respiratory compromise associated with allergies (whether the condition is considered anaphylaxis or a nonanaphylactic allergic reaction), epinephrine is lifesaving.

Words of Wisdom

A condition that closely resembles anaphylaxis can occur in patients who are treated with a class of antihypertensive drugs known as angiotensin-converting enzyme (ACE) inhibitors. The reaction is considered an adverse side effect to the medication and is triggered by a different physiologic mechanism than anaphylaxis. It causes sudden swelling of the skin or mucous membranes, most often in the face, lips, or tongue. The patient may complain of difficulty swallowing or breathing. In some cases, the swelling can cause a complete airway obstruction.

When caring for patients with this presentation who are taking ACE inhibitors, be mindful of the distinction between anaphylaxis and this drug reaction. You can identify ACE inhibitors by their generic drug names, which end in *pril* (eg, captopril). Typically, this reaction occurs after the patient has been taking the drug for a long time and is more common in patients of African descent.

Epinephrine is still indicated for patients experiencing an adverse reaction to ACE inhibitors but may not be effective. Rapid transport is indicated, with ALS intercept if the hospital distance is far.

History Taking

Investigate the patient's chief complaint or history of the present illness. Identify signs and symptoms (**TABLE 21-1**).

If the patient is responsive, begin by obtaining the SAMPLE (Signs and symptoms, Allergies, Medications, Pertinent past medical history, Last oral intake, Events leading up to the illness or injury) history (including OPQRST [Onset, Provocation/palliation, Quality, Region/radiation, Severity, Timing]) and the following information specific to allergic reactions:

- **Have any interventions already been completed?** Prior to your arrival, the patient may have begun self-treatment with a prescribed or over-the-counter medication, such as an epinephrine auto-injector or intranasal device (Neffy), a bronchodilator inhaler, or antihistamines such as chlorpheniramine (Chlor-Trimeton), cetirizine (Zyrtec), or diphenhydramine (Benadryl).
- **Has the patient experienced a severe allergic reaction in the past?** If so, what happened? The patient's answers may indicate how severe the present reaction may become. For example, if the patient was hospitalized or required intubation and prolonged mechanical ventilation due to a previous reaction, you should perceive this as an ominous sign and assume that the patient may have another reaction of equal or even greater severity. In such cases, rapid transport and treatment, as well as ALS care, are among the highest priorities. History of severe reactions may help identify anaphylaxis

YOU are the EMT

The closest hospital is 15 minutes away, while the closest ALS ambulance is over 1 hour away. You perform a primary assessment of the patient and note the following:

Recording Time: 0 Minutes	
Appearance	Anxious; widespread hives
Level of consciousness	Conscious and alert, but mildly confused
Airway	Open, clear of obstructions or foreign bodies
Breathing	Rapid with audible wheezing
Circulation	Radial pulse rapid rate and strong; skin flushed and warm, covered with hives

The patient reports dyspnea and states that his entire body is itching. Your partner applies high-concentration oxygen via a nonrebreathing mask.

3. Is this patient experiencing a local reaction or anaphylaxis?
4. What body system or systems should you focus your secondary assessment on and why?

TABLE 21-1 Additional Signs and Symptoms of an Allergic Reaction

Respiratory System	Cardiovascular System	Skin and Mucous Membranes	Other Findings
• Sneezing or an itchy, runny nose (early sign) • Shortness of breath (dyspnea) • Tightness in the chest or throat • Irritating, persistent dry cough • Hoarseness • Rapid, labored, or noisy respirations • Wheezing and/or stridor (which may progress to a silent chest with anaphylaxis; late sign)	• Increase in pulse rate (tachycardia; early sign) • Flushed, warm skin (early sign) or pale, cyanotic, cool skin (late sign) as the vascular system fails • Decrease in blood pressure (hypotension) as the blood vessels dilate (late sign)	• Flushing, itching, or burning skin, especially common over the face and upper chest • Hives over large areas of the body; may be internal or external • Swelling, especially of the face, neck, hands, feet, and/or tongue, either local (angioedema) or generalized • Cyanosis or pallor around the lips • Warm, tingling feeling in the face, mouth, chest, feet, and hands	• Decreasing mental status (early sign of hypoperfusion), from mild confusion or lethargy to loss of consciousness or coma • Anxiety; a sense of impending doom • Gastrointestinal problems, including nausea, vomiting, or abdominal cramps • Headache • Itchy, watery eyes • Dizziness

risk quickly, but remember that most fatal anaphylaxis cases do not involve a history of previous reactions. Patients with food-induced anaphylaxis will likely have a history, although most reactions are mild and patients are not typically prescribed epinephrine rescue devices. Patients with venom- or medication-induced anaphylaxis typically have no history of any severe or systemic reaction.

- **Does the patient report eating any foods that commonly cause allergic reactions?** What was the patient doing, or what was the patient exposed to, before the onset of symptoms? This information may be the key to effective treatment, regardless of any prior history of allergic reactions. Remember that the time from exposure to onset of symptoms can vary. Allergies to medications tend to produce symptoms in 5 to 20 minutes, while food-induced allergies might not cause symptoms for 30 minutes or longer.
- **Does the patient have a history of other medical conditions that are associated with allergic reactions?** Some populations are at higher risks for fatal allergic reactions. History of asthma is a significant risk factor for fatal food-induced anaphylaxis. It is also common in other types of anaphylaxis. You should increase your index of suspicion for a severe reaction in patients with asthma or taking medications for bronchospasm. Other underlying conditions such as chronic obstructive pulmonary disease and heart disease can increase mortality risk.

Also inquire about complaints that are common during an allergic or anaphylactic emergency, including nausea and vomiting.

Street Smarts

If the patient self-administered epinephrine before you arrived and does not seem to be responding, check the expiration date. Patients may not fill their prescriptions because of the high cost of these devices.

Secondary Assessment

If indicated, perform a rapid full-body scan or conduct a physical examination focused on the area or areas of chief complaint.

If the patient is unconscious or otherwise unable to communicate, remove clothing as necessary, and observe for the presence of stingers, signs of contact with chemicals, and other clues suggestive of a reaction. Remember to look for a medical alert tag, which could indicate a severe allergy to a particular substance.

If you have not already done so, auscultate for abnormal breath sounds such as stridor or wheezing, and carefully inspect the skin for swelling, rashes, or hives. A rapidly spreading rash can indicate a systemic reaction. The skin (or mucous membranes) may appear pale (compared with baseline) or cyanotic and cool; however, red, warm skin is typical in the early stages, suggesting a systemic reaction as the blood vessels lose their ability to constrict and blood moves outward and closer to the skin. If a systemic reaction continues, the body will have difficulty supplying blood and oxygen to the vital organs. One of the first signs that this has occurred will be altered mental status, as the brain becomes relatively deprived of oxygen and glucose.

Vital signs help determine whether the body is compensating for the stress imposed by the reaction. Assess baseline vital signs, including the pulse and respiratory rate, blood pressure, pupillary response, and oxygen saturation.

In a patient experiencing an allergic reaction, pulse oximetry can be a useful method to assess the patient's oxygenation status. However, it is important to remember that pulse oximetry is just another tool in your toolbox. The decision to apply oxygen to a patient experiencing an allergic reaction should be based on a careful assessment of the patient's airway patency, work of breathing, and abnormal lung sounds on auscultation, not solely on the pulse oximetry readings.

Reassessment

The patient experiencing a suspected allergic reaction should be monitored with vigilance. Deterioration of the patient's condition can be rapid and fatal, so special attention should be given to any signs of airway or cardiovascular compromise. The patient's anxiety level and mental status should be monitored as well, as they may provide additional information about the course of the reaction. Monitor for signs of shock, and, if present, treat immediately.

To treat allergic reactions, you must first identify the severity of the reaction. Mild nonanaphylactic reactions may require only supportive care and monitoring. However, anaphylaxis can produce

YOU are the EMT

The patient's wife brings his medications, which include an EpiPen and albuterol inhaler, just before you begin rapid transport to the ED. As you move him to the ambulance, you obtain a SAMPLE history and learn that the patient is allergic to peanuts and that he was eating dinner 20 minutes before his symptoms began. Since then, his symptoms have intensified and he wonders if his meal contained or came into contact with peanuts or peanut oil. He also tells you he has been hospitalized in the past for a severe peanut reaction. He was prescribed an EpiPen but could not get to it in the upstairs bathroom. You reassess his vital signs.

Recording Time: 5 Minutes	
Respirations	28 breaths/min; labored
Pulse	120 beats/min; weak at the radial artery
Skin	Pale compared with baseline and cool; widespread hives; angioedema of the lips
Blood pressure	88/60 mm Hg
Oxygen saturation (Spo_2)	88% (on oxygen)

During the secondary assessment, you note increased swelling of the patient's face and lips. He is having greater difficulty speaking but tries to say he feels like he has a lump in his throat. Auscultation reveals worsening wheezes on exhalation and decreased air movement. As you reach the ambulance your partner removes the nonrebreathing mask and begins assisting the patient's respirations using a bag-mask device attached to high-flow oxygen.

5. During the primary assessment, why did the patient first present with warm skin? What is the significance of the changes in his skin color and temperature to pale and cool?

6. What are the therapeutic effects of epinephrine if given for anaphylaxis, and would you administer it to this patient?

severe or rapidly progressing signs and symptoms, requiring more aggressive treatment, including epinephrine and ventilatory support. If you are not sure, always treat for potential anaphylaxis. In either situation, the patient should be transported to a medical facility for further evaluation.

Recheck your interventions. If you administered epinephrine, what was the effect? Has the patient's condition improved? Does the patient need a second dose? If so, remember to consult medical control before administering any subsequent doses for which you have not already obtained authorization. Also, keep in mind that even if the patient experiences relief following the administration of epinephrine, transport to the ED is still warranted, as the medication's effect will wear off and the symptoms may return.

Your documentation should not only include the signs and symptoms found during your assessment, but should also clearly show *why* you chose the care you provided. Finally, be certain to record the patient's response to your treatment.

Emergency Medical Care of Immunologic Emergencies

The first and most important intervention in treating anaphylaxis and severe allergy is administering epinephrine. Your priority should be determining if epinephrine is indicated and minimizing time to delivery. If the patient appears to be having a severe allergic or anaphylactic reaction, you should provide basic life support (BLS) care and administer epinephrine if available and within your protocols. If epinephrine is not readily available, you should provide prompt transport to the hospital or request an ALS intercept.

Be alert for signs of airway swelling and other signs of anaphylaxis such as nausea, vomiting, and abdominal cramps, and do not give the patient anything by mouth. Provide BLS care focusing on managing the ABCs. See Chapter 32, *Environmental Emergencies*, for treatment of allergic reactions caused by an insect sting.

Epinephrine

The body normally produces epinephrine (**TABLE 21-2**). **Epinephrine** is a sympathomimetic hormone. This means it mimics the sympathetic nervous system's fight-or-flight response. Epinephrine has various properties that cause the blood vessels to constrict, which reverses vasodilation and hypotension; this, in turn, elevates the diastolic pressure and improves coronary blood flow. Other properties of epinephrine increase cardiac contractility and relieve bronchospasm in the lungs. Because epinephrine has immediate action, it can rapidly reverse the effects of anaphylaxis. There are no absolute contraindications to epinephrine

YOU are the EMT

Per standing orders, you have authorization to administer epinephrine. After confirming that the EpiPen is prescribed to the patient and is not beyond its expiration date, you administer it in the lateral aspect of his thigh. Then, as you continue transport, you reassess the patient and note the following:

Recording Time: 10 Minutes	
Level of consciousness	Conscious and alert
Respirations	22 breaths/min; less labored; wheezing continues
Pulse	124 beats/min; stronger at the radial artery
Skin	Baseline color, warm, and dry; hives are still present
Blood pressure	104/66 mm Hg
Oxygen saturation (Spo_2)	95% (on oxygen)

7. In addition to the patient's vital signs, what else should you reassess?

8. How often should you reassess this patient?

TABLE 21-2 Intramuscular Epinephrine

Indications	Severe allergic reaction causing airway, breathing, or circulatory compromise or an anaphylactic reaction
Contraindications	None in a life-threatening emergency
Actions	Vasoconstriction and increased cardiac contractility, bronchodilation
Side effects	Tachycardia, sweating, pale skin, dizziness, headache, palpitations
Typical dose	Adults: 0.3 mg (EpiPen) IM Children: 0.15 mg (EpiPen Jr) IM

Abbreviation: IM, intramuscular

if anaphylaxis is suspected. Epinephrine is prescribed by a physician and most commonly comes predosed in an auto-injector (EpiPen).

Other allergy kits may contain oral or intramuscular (IM) antihistamines, agents that block the effect of histamine. These work relatively slowly, within several minutes to 1 hour. Your protocols may also include albuterol to treat bronchospasm associated with allergic reactions and anaphylaxis. These medications can supplement treatment but do not replace epinephrine and should be given only if wheezing persists after epinephrine administration. Delay in epinephrine administration is associated with worse outcomes and increased mortality. *EMS clinicians should always consider epinephrine as first-line treatment for any suspected anaphylaxis.* The National Association of EMS Physicians released a position statement on prehospital epinephrine use,[14] emphasizing the importance for all levels of EMS clinicians to promptly identify anaphylaxis and treat with epinephrine. You should be aware of your local protocol and method for providing epinephrine.

Because epinephrine can mimic the fight-or-flight response, you may note signs and symptoms such as anxiety, restlessness, headache, dizziness, pallor, and palpitations after administration. Rarely, epinephrine can cause hypertension, cardiac dysrhythmias, chest pain, or serious side effects. The potentially concerning effects of epinephrine

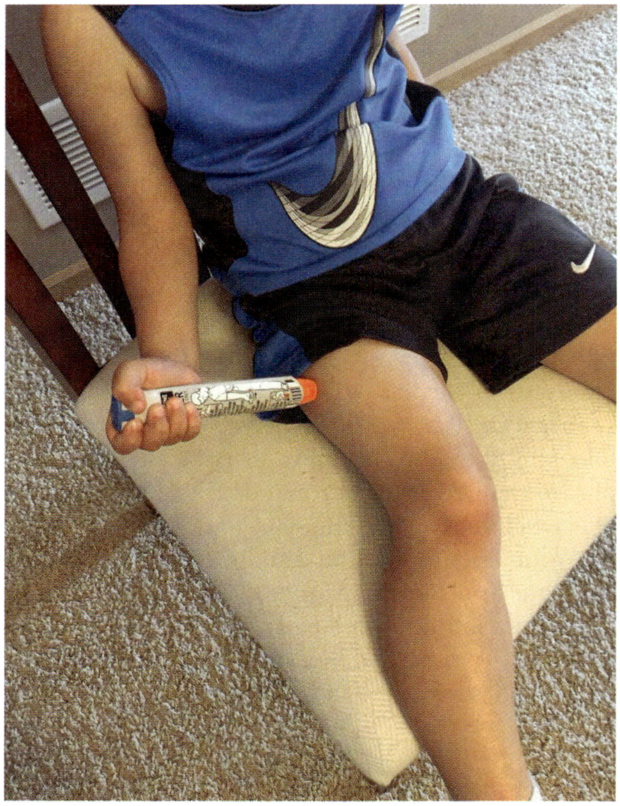

FIGURE 21-5 Patients who experience severe allergic reactions often carry their own prescription epinephrine, which comes predosed in an auto-injector or a prefilled syringe.

are also caused by untreated anaphylaxis. In a life-threatening situation, the administration of epinephrine outweighs the risk of side effects.

Administering Epinephrine via Auto-injector

All allergy emergency kits should contain a prepared, auto-injectable syringe of epinephrine, ready for IM injection, along with instructions for its use.

The adult EpiPen system delivers 0.3 mg of epinephrine via a spring-loaded needle and syringe system; the infant–child system (EpiPen Jr) delivers 0.15 mg. The spring-loaded needle automatically injects the epinephrine when the user firmly presses the device into the lateral thigh (thus the term *auto-injector*). Patients with a known allergy may carry their own EpiPen (**FIGURE 21-5**). If the patient can use the auto-injector, your role should be to assist the patient, if needed.

Take standard precautions, and make sure the medication has been prescribed specifically for that patient. If it has expired or is discolored, do not give the medication. In such an instance, you should inform medical control, use your own epinephrine if available, and continue to provide emergency care and transport.

To use an EpiPen auto-injector, follow the steps in **SKILL DRILL 21-1**.

1. Remove the safety cap from the auto-injector, and, if possible, quickly wipe the patient's thigh with alcohol or some other antiseptic (**Step 1**). (Note: Although it is best practice to

Skill Drill 21-1 Using an EpiPen Auto-injector

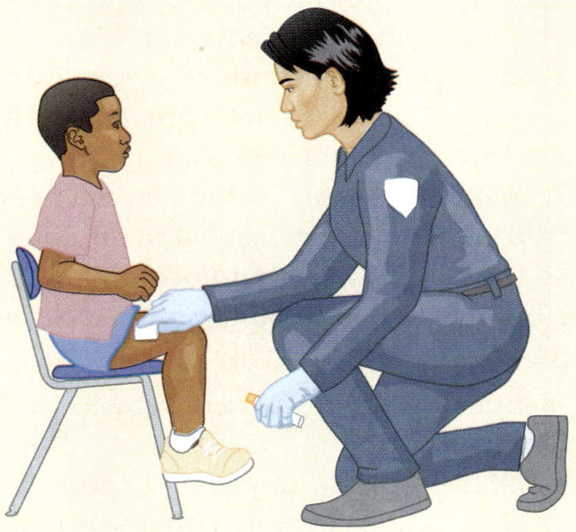

Step 1

Remove the auto-injector's safety cap, and quickly wipe the thigh with antiseptic,

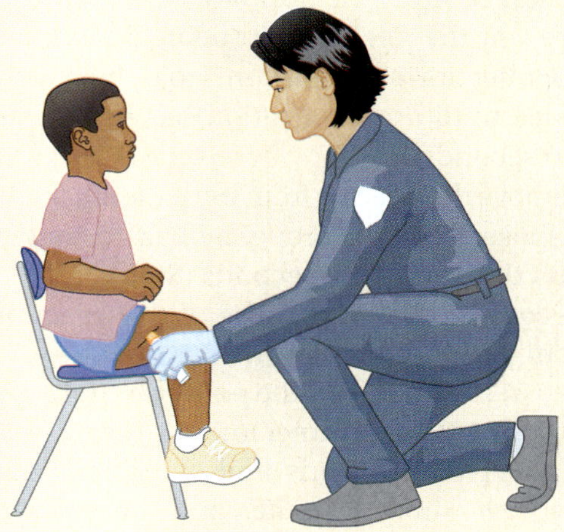

Step 2

Place the tip of the auto-injector against the lateral part of the thigh. Push the auto-injector firmly against the thigh until a click is heard. Hold it in place until all the medication has been injected (10 seconds).

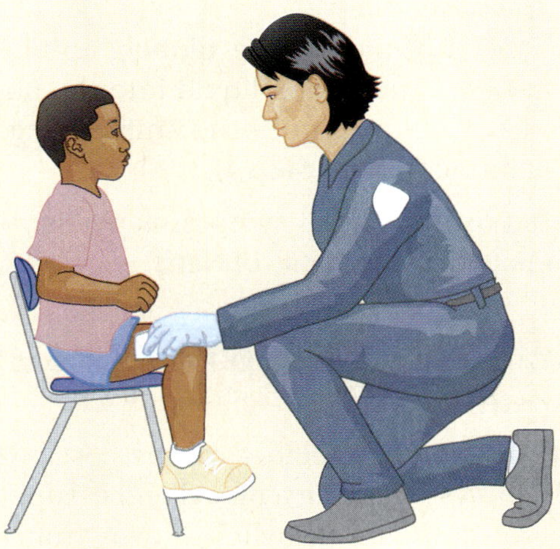

Step 3

Rub the area for 10 seconds.

clean the site, do not delay administration of the drug to do so.) If the patient is displaying signs of life-threatening anaphylaxis, it is possible to administer the auto-injector directly through the patient's clothing.

2. Place the tip of the auto-injector against the lateral part of the patient's thigh, midway between the groin and the knee (**Step 2**).
3. Push the injector firmly against the thigh until a click is heard. This indicates that the injector has activated and medication is being administered. Maintain steady pressure to prevent kickback from the spring in the syringe, and prevent the needle from being pushed out of the injection site too soon. Hold the injector in place until the medication has been injected (10 seconds).
4. Remove the injector from the patient's thigh and dispose of it in the proper biohazard container.
5. Rub the area for 10 seconds (**Step 3**).
6. Record the time and dose of the injection on your patient care report.
7. Reassess and record the patient's vital signs after using the auto-injector.
8. If the patient's signs and symptoms do not improve after 5 minutes and the patient has another auto-injector, consider assisting the patient with the administration of a second (and final) dose of epinephrine.

In addition to the EpiPen, you may encounter an Auvi-Q device, another type of epinephrine injector. The Auvi-Q injector is rectangular and offers electronic voice instructions for users. It is available in an additional dose of 0.1 mg for young children who weigh 17 to 33 pounds (7.5 to 15 kg); a dose of 0.15 mg for children weighing 33 to 66 pounds (15 to 30 kg); and a dose of 0.3 mg for teenagers and adults weighing more than 66 pounds (30 kg). Many states allow EMTs to draw up and administer epinephrine from vials and ampules in addition to using auto-injectors. Evidence suggests that this practice is safe when strict protocols are followed.[15,16]

Administering Epinephrine via Intranasal Spray

In 2024, intranasal epinephrine spray (Neffy) was approved for use in patients weighing more than 66 pounds (30 kg).[17] The Neffy device, similar to naloxone nasal spray, delivers epinephrine medication in a very fine spray through the nostril. The medication is absorbed by the mucous membranes and passes into the bloodstream, even when the patient has nasal congestion or hypotension. The medication is the same as that delivered intramuscularly; however, the dosage is significantly higher (2 mg) to compensate for the less efficient delivery method.

Epinephrine nasal spray has demonstrated the same lifesaving properties as IM administration. It offers the advantages of being more cost effective than an epinephrine autoinjector and of being more user friendly for patients who are reluctant to self-administer an injection.[18,19] A disadvantage is that presently there is no Neffy preparation for children who weigh less than 66 pounds (30 kg).

If a patient presents with their own prescribed epinephrine nasal spray instead of an EpiPen, you should use it if your local protocols allow. To use a Neffy intranasal device, follow the steps in **SKILL DRILL 21-2**.

1. Remove the Neffy device from its packaging (**Step 1**).
2. Hold the device with your thumb on the lower plunger and a finger on either side of the nozzle. Each device has only one dose, so do not prime or inadvertently depress the plunger (**Step 2**).
3. Insert the nozzle into the patient's nostril until your fingers touch the patient's nose. Keep the nozzle in line with the nostril (ie, do not angle the nozzle toward the septum or outer wall of the nose) (**Step 3**).
4. Press upward on the plunger until it snaps upward and sprays liquid into the nostril. Instruct the patient not to sniff during or after administration (**Step 4**).

If liquid drips out and symptoms persist, you may administer another dose of Neffy.

Administering IM Epinephrine via Ampule or Vial

Epinephrine autoinjectors can be cost prohibitive for EMS systems. Current evidence supports the safety of epinephrine when drawn from an ampule or vial and injected by trained EMS clinicians

Skill Drill 21-2 Using a Neffy Intranasal Device

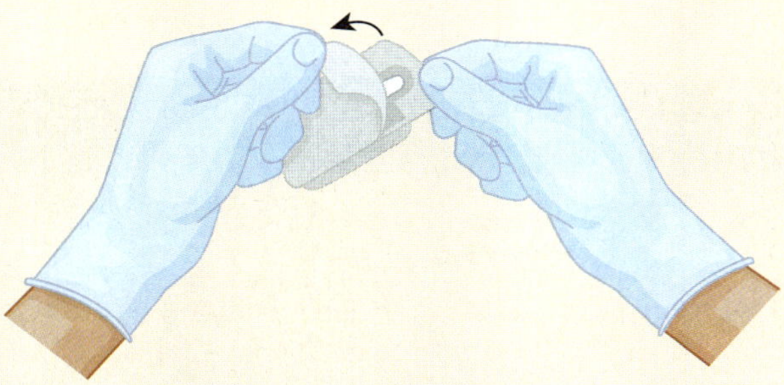

Step 1

Remove the device from its packaging.

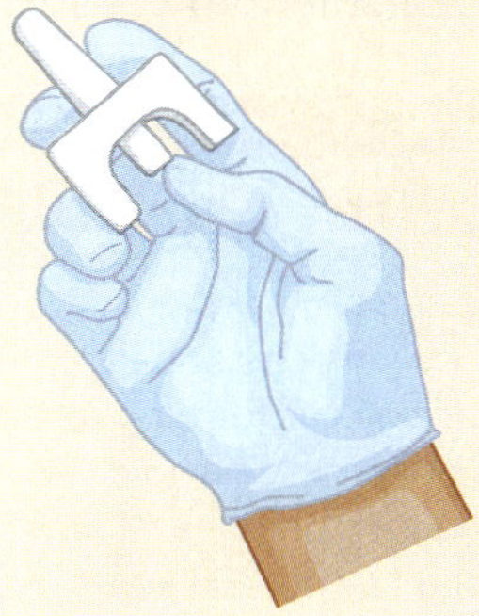

Step 2

Hold the device with your thumb on the lower plunger and a finger on either side of the nozzle.

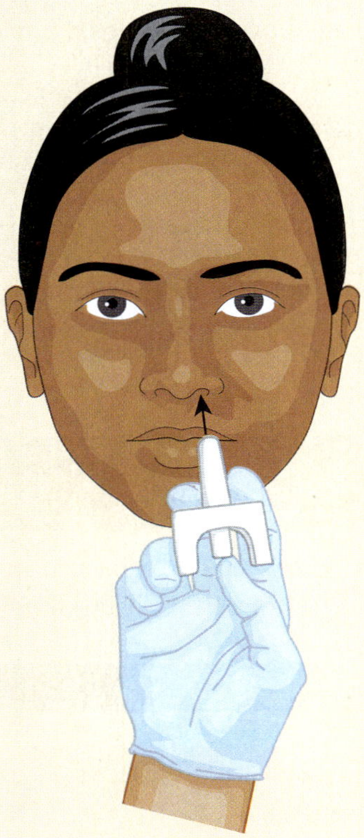

Step 3

Insert the nozzle into the nostril until your fingers touch the patient's nose, keeping the nozzle in line with the nostril.

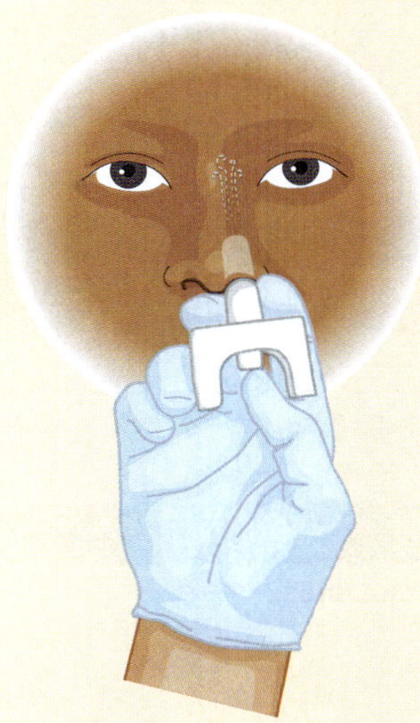

Step 4

Press upward on the plunger until it snaps upward and sprays liquid into the nostril.

of any certification level.[20] Some areas may allow administration of epinephrine by IM injection, using a vial or ampule of 1:1,000 concentration (1 mg/mL) epinephrine along with a needle and syringe. The Model Clinical Guidelines of the National Association of State EMS Officials recommend weight-based dosing. For adults (ie, individuals weighing more than 55 pounds [25 kg]), they

Words of Wisdom

Allergic reactions can progress quickly to life threats. With good care, severe signs and symptoms may subside just as quickly. Performing a multisystem examination and documenting your findings are important steps to take before and after treatment. Give particular attention to skin signs and respiratory, circulatory, gastrointestinal, and mental functioning. If the patient's symptoms seem to resolve and the individual no longer desires to go to the hospital, explain that the effects of epinephrine can wear off before the underlying allergic reaction has fully resolved, and life-threatening symptoms may recur.

Street Smarts

If the patient has received epinephrine prior to your arrival, try to determine the time. If there is no improvement in their signs and symptoms or their condition is worsening, you can give a second dose 5 to 15 minutes after the first.

Special Populations

EPINEPHRINE ADMINISTRATION IN GERIATRIC PATIENTS

Previously, caution was advised regarding administration of epinephrine in some populations. This concern potentially contributed to undertreatment of anaphylaxis in the prehospital environment. The available evidence strongly supports administration of epinephrine in all age groups and populations.[21] The risk of death or serious injury from inadequately treated anaphylaxis outweighs risks of epinephrine. Studies in older adults with underlying cardiovascular disease support IM epinephrine use. In fact, these populations are more at risk from anaphylactic-mediated damage to the heart. Cardiovascular disease can increase the amount of histamine released in the heart during an allergic reaction and allergic reactions can cause myocardial infarction and/or arrhythmias even without epinephrine administration. If you suspect anaphylaxis, administer epinephrine.

YOU are the EMT

Following standing orders, you administer a dose of albuterol from the patient's metered-dose inhaler in order to treat the bronchospasm responsible for his wheezing. A few minutes later, you call the receiving hospital and supply your radio report, including the most recent set of vital signs.

Recording Time: 20 Minutes	
Level of consciousness	Conscious and alert
Respirations	18 breaths/min; unlabored; wheezing improved
Pulse	114 beats/min; strong and regular
Skin	Baseline color, warm, and dry; scattered hives
Blood pressure	128/72 mm Hg
Oxygen saturation (Spo_2)	97% (on oxygen by nonrebreathing mask; patient no longer requires positive-pressure assistance)

You deliver the patient to the ED, where the attending physician asks you how much epinephrine the patient has received when you give her your report.

9. What is the dose and concentration of epinephrine contained in an adult EpiPen?

recommend a dose of 0.3 mg. For pediatric patients weighing less than 55 pounds [25 kg]), the dose is 0.15 mg. The route is the same in both adults and children: IM in the anterolateral thigh. It is critical to remember that with IM epinephrine injection, the concentration must be 1 mg/mL. Other concentrations are available but are not used in IM injections for anaphylaxis. Doses can be repeated every 5 to 15 minutes as needed. Know whether your protocols allow for epinephrine IM injection.

YOU are the EMT SUMMARY

1. What, if any, additional resources should you request?

You should consider requesting the response of an ALS unit. Consider the time it will take to reach the nearest hospital versus the time needed to rendezvous with an ALS unit, the feasibility of requesting transport by helicopter, etc. Understand and follow your local protocols. If those resources are not quickly available, transport to the hospital as quickly as is safely possible for more advanced care.

2. What intervention or interventions should you perform without delay?

Because the patient's respiratory distress is an immediate life threat, providing high-concentration oxygen is the first action you should take.

3. Is this patient experiencing a local reaction or anaphylaxis?

The presence of signs and symptoms from multiple systems, including the skin (hives) and respiratory system (dyspnea), indicates that the patient is experiencing anaphylaxis.

A local reaction is characterized by tenderness, redness, itching, and swelling at and immediately adjacent to a bite or sting. In many cases, the reaction is not "allergic" in nature; it is simply irritation and inflammation that is caused by the bite or sting itself. Local reactions do not involve respiratory or cardiovascular compromise or multiple systems.

It is important to perform a careful and thorough assessment of patients showing signs of an allergic reaction, whether they have a confirmed allergy or not. A seemingly local and mild reaction can become systemic and severe within a matter of minutes. Additionally, reaction to something that is ingested may take longer to have its full effects than something that is injected or inhaled, so the route of exposure to a possible allergen can make a difference in the progression of symptoms.

4. What body system or systems should you focus your secondary assessment on and why?

Further assessment of the patient should focus on body systems that are commonly affected by an allergic reaction: the respiratory, gastrointestinal, and circulatory systems and the skin. In most cases, a severe allergic reaction occurs within minutes of exposure; however, it may be delayed for multiple hours in some patients.

Your primary assessment revealed significant respiratory distress with wheezing and widespread rash, indicating anaphylaxis. As you continue to assess the patient, look for clinical signs that indicate a worsening reaction and be prepared to assist ventilations and treat for shock.

Signs of respiratory system involvement include respirations that become rapid, labored, or noisy; wheezing; stridor; an irritating, persistent dry cough; hoarseness; and tightness in the chest or throat.

Signs of circulatory system involvement include tachycardia (initially), followed by pallor, dizziness, and hypotension. A decreasing level of consciousness indicates a decrease in cerebral blood flow; this is usually secondary to vascular dilation causing hypotension.

The patient already has widespread hives, and his skin is flushed. However, you should further assess the skin by looking for swelling, especially of the face, tongue, neck, hands, and feet. If the patient reports a warm, tingling feeling in the face, mouth, chest, feet, and hands, this should also be cause for concern. You should also assess for gastrointestinal symptoms that are common with allergy and anaphylaxis.

5. During the primary assessment, why did the patient first present with warm skin? What is the significance of the changes in his skin color and temperature to pale and cool?

When vasodilation and increased capillary permeability occur in the early stages of an allergic reaction, fluid leaks out of the bloodstream and into the subcutaneous (fatty) layer of the skin. This causes swelling, redness, warmth, and hives of the skin. As the reaction progresses, bronchoconstriction impairs oxygenation and ventilation, producing hypoxemia. Clinical signs of hypoxemia include altered mental status, tachycardia, cyanosis, and a low oxygen saturation level.

Tachycardia indicates that the body is attempting to compensate for decreased perfusion and

YOU are the EMT SUMMARY continued

hypoxemia by releasing more epinephrine (adrenaline) into the bloodstream to pump more blood to the body's organs, tissues, and cells.

Hypotension occurs because of widespread vasodilation and a decrease in arterial pressure—again, in response to the body's massive release of histamines. As the blood pressure falls, the brain and other vital organs are deprived of oxygen.

6. What are the therapeutic effects of epinephrine if given for anaphylaxis, and would you administer it to this patient?

Epinephrine is a hormone that is normally produced by the body. When used to treat anaphylaxis, it does not stop the allergic reaction itself; instead, it reverses the negative effects of bronchoconstriction and vasodilation, which are caused by the reaction. Therefore, when epinephrine is administered to the patient, it dilates the bronchioles, which improves breathing, and constricts the blood vessels, which reduces swelling in the upper airway, increases the blood pressure, and improves perfusion. Epinephrine is lifesaving and should be administered to this patient as soon as possible.

7. In addition to the patient's vital signs, what else should you reassess?

Ask him if he still feels as if he has a lump in his throat; this was likely the result of mild upper airway swelling caused by angioedema and *must* be reassessed. Even though he did not present with obvious external angioedema, you should still reassess his face, lips, tongue, neck, and other parts of his body for swelling.

If bronchoconstriction worsens, the patient may have decreased lung sounds as less air is moved through the narrowed airways. If the epinephrine sufficiently dilates the bronchioles, scattered wheezing may still be heard, even though the patient is not exhibiting any outward signs of respiratory distress.

Reassess his skin to determine if his hives are resolving or if they are still present. In most cases, hives will persist, at least to some degree, following the administration of epinephrine. You will usually notice improvement in the patient's breathing and perfusion status (eg, mental status, blood pressure, peripheral pulse quality) before you see resolution of hives.

8. How often should you reassess this patient?

This patient should be considered high priority or critical and, therefore, should be reassessed every 5 minutes en route to the receiving facility.

9. What is the dose and concentration of epinephrine contained in an adult EpiPen?

The adult EpiPen contains 0.3 mg of a 1-mg/mL concentration for IM injection. Also sometimes referred to as a 1:1,000 concentration, this contains 1 mg of epinephrine per 1 mL. Therefore, 0.3 mL contains 0.3 mg of epinephrine, all of which is injected into the patient's thigh. Be sure to hold the injector against the thigh for at least 10 seconds to ensure the whole dose has been administered.

Prep Kit

Ready for Review

- An allergic reaction is a response to chemicals the body releases to combat certain stimuli, called allergens.
- Allergic reactions occur most often in response to these stimuli: food, medication, plants, chemicals, and insect bites and stings.
- The reaction may be mild and local, involving itching, redness, and tenderness, or it may be severe and systemic, including shock and respiratory failure.
- Anaphylaxis is a life-threatening allergic reaction mounted by multiple organ systems after exposure to an allergen. This emergency must be treated with epinephrine. Anaphylaxis can have many varied presentations.
- When assessing a person who may be having an allergic reaction, you should check for flushing, itching, and swelling skin or tongue; hives; wheezing and stridor; a persistent cough; a decrease in blood pressure; a weak

Prep Kit continued

pulse; dizziness; abdominal cramps; and headache.

- All patients with suspected anaphylaxis require epinephrine and oxygen. Epinephrine is the primary way to save the life of someone having a severe anaphylactic reaction.
- You may help a patient to administer epinephrine via auto-injector or an intranasal device, or you may draw it up from an ampule or vial and administer it intramuscularly.
- Always provide prompt transport to the hospital for any patient who is having an allergic reaction. Remember that signs and symptoms can rapidly become more severe. Carefully monitor the patient's vital signs en route; be especially alert for airway or cardiovascular compromise.

Vital Vocabulary

allergen A substance that causes an allergic reaction.

allergic reaction The body's exaggerated immune response to an internal or surface agent.

anaphylaxis An extreme, life-threatening, systemic allergic reaction that may include shock and respiratory failure.

angioedema Localized areas of swelling beneath the skin, often around the eyes and lips, but can also involve other body areas.

envenomation The act of injecting venom.

epinephrine A substance produced by the body (commonly called adrenaline), and a drug produced by pharmaceutical companies that increases pulse rate and blood pressure; the drug of choice for an anaphylactic reaction.

histamines Chemical substances released by the immune system in allergic reactions that are responsible for many of the symptoms of anaphylaxis, such as vasodilation.

immune response The body's response to a substance perceived by the body as foreign.

immune system The body system that includes all of the structures and processes designed to mount a defense against foreign substances and disease-causing agents.

immunology The study of the body's immune system.

leukotrienes Chemical substances that contribute to anaphylaxis; released by the immune system in allergic reactions.

urticaria Small areas of generalized itching and/or burning that appear as multiple raised areas on the skin; also known as hives.

wheal A raised, swollen, well-defined area on the skin resulting from an insect bite or allergic reaction.

References

1. More than a quarter of US adults and children have at least one allergy. Centers for Disease Control and Prevention website. https://www.cdc.gov/nchs/pressroom/nchs_press_releases/2022/20220126.htm. Published January 26, 2023. Accessed January 24, 2025.
2. Bock SA. Fatal anaphylaxis. UpToDate website. https://www.uptodate.com/contents/fatal-anaphylaxis. Updated April 27, 2024. Accessed January 24, 2025.
3. Pflipsen MC, Vega Colon KM. Anaphylaxis: recognition and management. *Am Fam Physician*. 2020;102(6):355–362.
4. Campbell R. Anaphylaxis: acute diagnosis. UpToDate website. https://www.uptodate.com/contents/anaphylaxis-acute-diagnosis. Updated May 14, 2024. Accessed January 24, 2025.
5. Turner PJ, Jerschow E, Umasunthar T, Lin R, Campbell DE, Boyle RJ. Fatal anaphylaxis: mortality rate and risk factors. *J Allergy Clin Immunol Pract.* 2017;5(5):1169–1178.
6. Mayo Clinic staff. Anaphylaxis. Mayo Clinic website. https://www.mayoclinic.org/diseases-conditions/anaphylaxis/symptoms-causes/syc-20351468. Published October 2, 2021. Accessed January 24, 2025.

Prep Kit continued

7. Anagnostou A, Sharma V, Herbert Ln, Turner PJ. Fatal food anaphylaxis: distinguishing fact from fiction. *Immunol Pract*. 2022;10(1):11–17.
8. Freeman T. Bee, yellow jacket, wasp, and other Hymenoptera stings: reaction types and acute management. UpToDate website. https://www.uptodate.com/contents/bee-yellowjacket-wasp-and-other-hymenoptera-stings-reaction-types-and-acute-management. Updated June 10, 2024. Accessed January 24, 2025.
9. Ng AE, Boersma P. Diagnosed allergic conditions in adults: United States, 2021. *NCHS Data Brief*. 2023;(460):1–8.
10. Kerr M. Pollen library: plants that cause allergies. Healthline website. https://www.healthline.com/health/allergies/pollen-library. Updated March 4, 2024. Accessed January 24, 2025.
11. Wu M, McIntosh J, Liu J. Current prevalence rate of latex allergy: why it remains a problem. *J Occup Health*. 2016;58(2):138–144.
12. McLendon K, Sternard BT. Anaphylaxis. *StatPearls*. National Library of Medicine website. https://www.ncbi.nlm.nih.gov/books/NBK482124/. Updated January 26, 2023. Accessed January 24, 2025.
13. National Association of State EMS Officials. *National Model EMS Clinical Guidelines: Version 3.0.* https://nasemso.org/wp-content/uploads/National-Model-EMS-Clinical-Guidelines_2022.pdf. Updated March 2022. Accessed January 24, 2025.
14. Jacobsen RC, Millin MG. The use of epinephrine for out-of-hospital treatment of anaphylaxis: resource document for the National Association of EMS Physicians position statement. *Prehosp Emerg Care*. 2011;15(4):570–576.
15. Latimer AJ, Husain S, Nolan J, et al. Syringe administration of epinephrine by emergency medical technicians for anaphylaxis. *Prehosp Emerg Care*. 2018;22(3):319–325.
16. Use of epinephrine for out-of-hospital treatment of anaphylaxis. *Prehosp Emerg Care*. 2019;23(4):592.
17. FDA approves first nasal spray for treatments of anaphylaxis. US Food and Drug Administration website. https://www.fda.gov/news-events/press-announcements/fda-approves-first-nasal-spray-treatment-anaphylaxis. Published August 9, 2024. Accessed January 24, 2025.
18. Ellis AK, Casale TB, Kaliner M, et al. Development of Neffy, an epinephrine nasal spray, for severe allergic reactions. *Pharmaceutics*. 2024;16(6):811.
19. Christianson E. Neffy versus EpiPen: clinical comparison. Med Ed 101 website. https://www.meded101.com/neffy-versus-epipen-clinical-comparison/. Published September 18, 2024. Accessed January 24, 2025.
20. Lyng JW, White CC 4th, Peterson TQ, et al. Non-autoinjector epinephrine administration by basic life support providers: a literature review and consensus process. *Prehosp Emerg Care*. 2019;23(6):855–861.
21. Kawano T, Scheuermeyer FX, Stenstrom R, Rowe BH, Grafstein E, Grunau B. Epinephrine use in older patients with anaphylaxis: clinical outcomes and cardiovascular complications. *Resuscitation*. 2017;112:53–58.

Additional Resources

National Association of State EMS Officials. *National EMS Scope of Practice Model 2019*. Washington, DC: National Highway Traffic Safety Administration; February 2019. Report No. DOT HS 812-666. https://www.ems.gov/assets/National_EMS_Scope_of_Practice_Model_2019.pdf. Accessed January 24, 2025.

National Highway Traffic Safety Administration. *National Emergency Medical Services Education Standards*. EMS.gov website. https://www.ems.gov/assets/EMS_Education-Standards_2021_FNL.pdf. Published January 2021. Accessed January 24, 2025.

Wesley K, Wesley K. Is epinephrine safe for older patients with anaphylaxis? *JEMS* website. https://www.jems.com/patient-care/emergency-medical-care/is-epinephrine-safe-for-older-patients-with-anaphylaxis/. Published June 1, 2017. Accessed January 24, 2025.

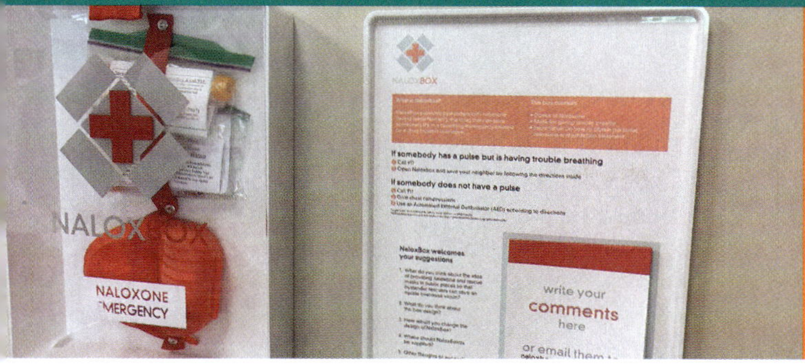

Chapter 22

Toxicology

NATIONAL EMS EDUCATION STANDARD COMPETENCIES

Medicine

Applies knowledge to provide basic emergency care and transportation based on assessment findings for an acutely ill patient.

Toxicology

- Carbon monoxide poisoning (pp 839–841)
- Nerve agent poisoning (pp 857–858)
- Opioid toxicity (pp 851–853)
- Poisons
  - Inhaled (pp 839–841, 853–854)
  - Ingested (pp 842–843)
  - Injected (pp 843–844)
  - Absorbed (pp 841–843)
- Alcohol intoxication and withdrawal (pp 849–850)

KNOWLEDGE OBJECTIVES

1. Define toxicology, poison, toxin, and overdose. (pp 836–837)
2. Identify the common signs and symptoms of poisoning or toxic exposure. (pp 837–838)
3. Describe how poisons and toxins can enter the body. (pp 838–844)
4. Describe the assessment and treatment of a patient with a suspected poisoning or toxic exposure. (pp 844–848)
5. Describe the assessment and treatment of a patient with a suspected overdose. (pp 844–848)
6. Discuss scene safety considerations for working at a scene with a potentially hazardous material or violent patient. (p 845)
7. Understand the role of airway management in a patient experiencing poisoning or overdose. (pp 845–846)
8. Explain the use of activated charcoal, including indications, contraindications, and the need to obtain approval from medical direction before administration. (pp 846–848)
9. Identify the main types of toxins and poisons and their effects, including alcohol, opioids, sedative-hypnotic drugs, inhalants, hydrogen sulfide, sympathomimetics, synthetic cathinones, marijuana, hallucinogens, anticholinergic agents, and cholinergic agents. (pp 848–859)
10. Discuss how to care for a patient who has overdosed on an opioid and who has gone into cardiac or respiratory arrest. (pp 850–853)
11. Describe the assessment and treatment of a patient with suspected food poisoning. (pp 859–860)
12. Describe the assessment and treatment of a patient with suspected plant poisoning. (pp 860–862)
13. Explain the special considerations when assessing and treating an older adult who is experiencing a toxicologic emergency. (p 862)
14. Explain the special considerations when assessing and treating a child who is experiencing a toxicologic emergency. (pp 862–864)

SKILLS OBJECTIVES

1. Demonstrate how to assess and treat a patient with a suspected poisoning. (pp 844–847)
2. Demonstrate how to assess and treat a patient with a suspected overdose. (pp 844–847)
3. Demonstrate how to administer activated charcoal. (pp 847–848)
4. Demonstrate how to administer intranasal naloxone. (pp 851–853)

Introduction

Every day, each of us comes in contact with things that are potentially poisonous. This is not surprising when you consider that almost any substance may be a poison in certain circumstances. Different doses can turn even a remedy into a poison. Consider a common medication such as acetaminophen. When taken in recommended doses, it is a safe and effective pain reliever (analgesic). However, too much acetaminophen can cause serious medical conditions, including liver dysfunction.[1]

According to the National Poison Data System, more than 2 million people contact a poison control center each year for guidance following exposure to a dangerous substance.[2] Chronic poisoning, often caused by the long-term use of medications, tobacco, and alcohol, is more common. Fortunately, deaths caused by acute poisoning are fairly rare. Rates of death as the result of acute poisoning in children have decreased steadily since the late 1960s, when child-resistant caps were introduced for drug bottles and containers. However, deaths caused by chronic poisoning in adults have risen in the past few years, primarily as the result of drug misuse.

In this chapter, the term *poisoning* includes acute and chronic poisonings. As an EMT, you must recognize that patients with either type of condition may have a variety of symptoms. You may be able to prevent death caused by the acute effects of a poison simply by providing airway management and symptomatic care during transport.

This chapter discusses how to identify a patient who has been poisoned or exposed to a toxin, and how to gather clues about the substance. Also described are the different ways in which a poison or toxin is introduced into the body. The chapter then discusses the signs, symptoms, and treatment of specific poisons. Hazardous materials exposure, food poisoning, and plant poisoning are also discussed.

Words of Wisdom

Drugs interact with one another. Food, alcohol, vitamins, over-the-counter (OTC) medications, homeopathic agents, and other substances can prevent a drug from working as expected. These interactions can alter the effectiveness of the drug and increase the risk of adverse (harmful) effects.

Identifying the Patient and the Poison

Toxicology is the study of toxic or poisonous substances. A **poison** is any substance whose chemical action can damage body structures or impair body function. A **toxin** is a poisonous substance produced by bacteria, animals, or plants that acts by changing the normal metabolism of cells or by destroying them. Toxins can have acute effects

Street Smarts

As a key health advocate in your community, be mindful of the words you use to describe substance use disorders. Words that negatively characterize a person, such as "addict," "alcoholic," or "substance abuser," can reinforce a person's feelings of shame. Individuals who do not feel worthy of treatment or who fear the social judgment that might result from seeking treatment are less likely to receive the help they need. Moreover, when these biased words are used in legal proceedings, the person is more likely to be deemed a criminal and punished more severely.[3] Using nonjudgmental wording, such as "substance use disorder," "substance misuse," and "addiction to alcohol," has been shown to decrease stigma around these disorders and improve a person's likelihood of seeking treatment. Choose your words carefully, and encourage your coworkers and other members of your community to do likewise.

(eg, loss of consciousness after high-level exposure to carbon monoxide, an injection of heroin may cause respiratory arrest) and chronic effects (eg, years of substance use may lead to a weakened immune system). **Substance misuse** is the use of any substance in a manner other than its intended design to produce a desired effect (eg, use of fentanyl to achieve intoxication). A common complication of substance misuse is **overdose**, when a patient takes a toxic or lethal dose of a substance.

Your primary responsibility to the patient who has been poisoned is to recognize that a poisoning has occurred. Your own safety plays a key role here as well; pay attention to your surroundings (**FIGURE 22-1**).

The where, what, and how of the exposure is important. Keep in mind that very small amounts of some poisons or toxins can cause considerable harm or death. Never let your guard down and allow yourself to become exposed to the same substance.

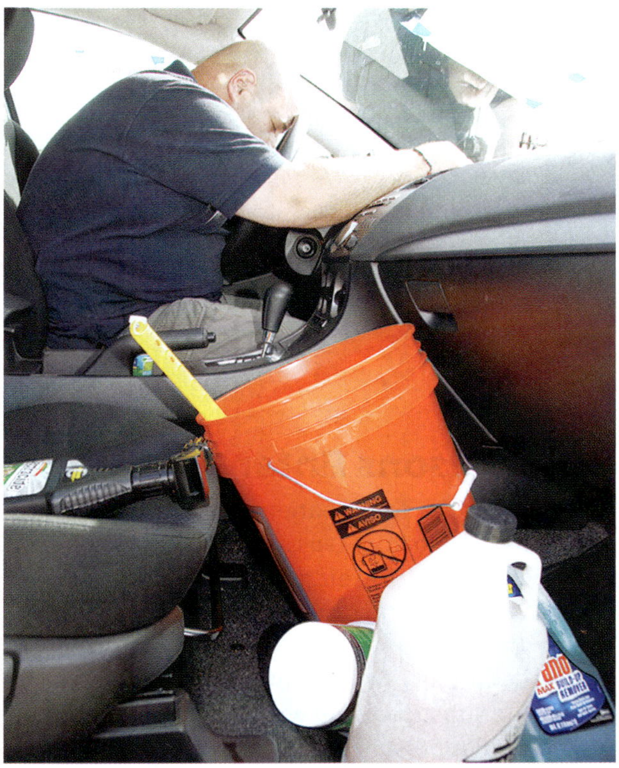

FIGURE 22-1 Never open a door or approach a scene until you have ascertained that the area is safe to enter. Keep in mind that very small amounts of some poisons or toxins can cause considerable harm or death.

Courtesy of Darin Dowe/*Law and Order Magazine*/Hedon Media Group.

If you have even the slightest suspicion that a person has been exposed to a toxic substance, notify medical direction and begin emergency treatment immediately. A discussion of issues relating to substance use disorder and suicide is presented in Chapter 23, *Behavioral Health Emergencies*.

Symptoms and signs of poisoning or overdose vary according to the specific agent, as shown in **TABLE 22-1**. Some poisons cause the pulse to speed up, whereas others cause it to slow down; some poisons cause the pupils to dilate, whereas others cause the pupils to constrict. If respiration is depressed or difficult, cyanosis may occur. Some chemical compounds will irritate or burn the skin or mucous membranes, resulting in burning or blistering. The presence of such injuries at the patient's mouth strongly suggests the ingestion of a poison, such as lye.

The overall constellation of signs and symptoms is referred to as a **toxidrome**. Understanding toxidromes can help responders identify the toxin to which a person has been exposed.

Be extremely careful when caring for a child who has ingested a poisonous substance. Although such incidents usually do not lead to death, family members may be distraught, and your calm, professional attitude will help to ease the tension. Remember, however, that a single swallow or single pill of some substances can kill a child.

Street Smarts

Do not judge the patient for becoming exposed to a poisonous substance, including if the exposure was an incident of self-harm. Similarly, do not judge a parent or caregiver if the victim was a child. Always treat the patient and others with respect and compassion.

Try to determine the nature of the poison. Look around the immediate area for objects that may provide clues: an overturned bottle, a needle or syringe, scattered pills, chemicals, the remains of food or drink items, or even an overturned or damaged plant. Place any suspicious material in a plastic bag and take it with you to the hospital, along with any containers you find.

Drug containers at the scene can provide critical information. In addition to the name and

TABLE 22-1 Typical Signs and Symptoms of Specific Overdoses

Agent	Signs and Symptoms
Opioids (Examples: heroin, fentanyl, methadone, oxycodone, morphine, codeine)	• Hypoventilation or respiratory arrest • Pinpoint pupils • Sedation or coma • Hypotension
Stimulants/sympathomimetics (Examples: mephedrone, cocaine, methamphetamine, mixed amphetamine salts [Adderall])	• Hypertension • Tachycardia • Dilated pupils • Agitation or seizures • Hyperthermia
Sedative-hypnotics (Examples: diazepam, alprazolam, temazepam, midazolam)	• Slurred speech • Sedation or coma • Hypoventilation • Hypotension
Anticholinergics (Examples: atropine, diphenhydramine, chlorpheniramine, doxylamine, *Datura stramonium* [jimsonweed])	• Tachycardia • Hyperthermia • Hypertension • Dilated pupils • Dry skin and mucous membranes • Sedation, agitation, seizures, coma, or delirium • Decreased bowel sounds

Cholinergics (Examples: organophosphates, pilccarpine, nerve gas)	• Airway compromise
	• SLUDGEM:
	  • **S** Salivation, sweating
	  • **L** Lacrimation (excessive tearing of the eyes)
	  • **U** Urination
	  • **D** Defecation, drooling, diarrhea
	  • **G** Gastric upset and cramps
	  • **E** Emesis (vomiting)
	  • **M** Muscle twitching/miosis (pinpoint pupils)

concentration of the drug, a pill bottle label may list specific ingredients, the number of pills that were originally in the bottle, the name of the manufacturer, and the dose that was prescribed. This information can help emergency department (ED) physicians determine how much has been ingested and what specific treatment may be required. For certain food poisonings, a food container that lists the name and location of the restaurant or vendor may help save the life of the patient and possibly other customers.

If the patient vomits, examine the contents for pill fragments. Wear proper personal protective equipment (PPE) for this activity. Note and document anything unusual that you see.

How Poisons Enter the Body

Emergency care for a patient who has been poisoned may range from reassuring an anxious parent or caregiver to performing CPR. For these patients, definitive treatment can only be provided at the ED, so transport promptly whenever poisoning is involved. Often, you will not administer a specific **antidote** (a substance that will counteract the effects of a particular poison) because most poisons do not have one. Depending on local protocols, the antidote most commonly available to EMTs is naloxone (Narcan), which is used to reverse the effects of an opioid overdose. Naloxone is discussed later in the chapter. If you work in a tiered system, advanced life support (ALS) backup may also be appropriate, because these clinicians can administer additional medications and therapies.

In general, the most important treatment you can perform for a poisoning is to dilute and/or physically remove the poisonous agent. How you do this depends on how the poison entered the patient's body in the first place. The four routes to consider are as follows:

- Inhalation (**FIGURE 22-2A**)
- Absorption (surface contact) (**FIGURE 22-2B**)
- Ingestion (**FIGURE 22-2C**)
- Injection (**FIGURE 22-2D**)

All four routes of poisoning can lead to serious and possibly life-threatening conditions. Take care to treat these patients appropriately and to keep yourself safe from harm. If you are uncertain how to treat a patient who has been poisoned or exposed to a specific substance, find the container if possible, and contact medical direction and/or the poison control center before you proceed. Always assess the situation and determine whether the scene is safe before you approach the patient.

Inhaled Poisons

Patients who have inhaled poison, including natural gas, sewer gas, certain pesticides, carbon monoxide, and chlorine, should be moved to fresh air immediately. Depending on the length of exposure, the patient may require supplemental

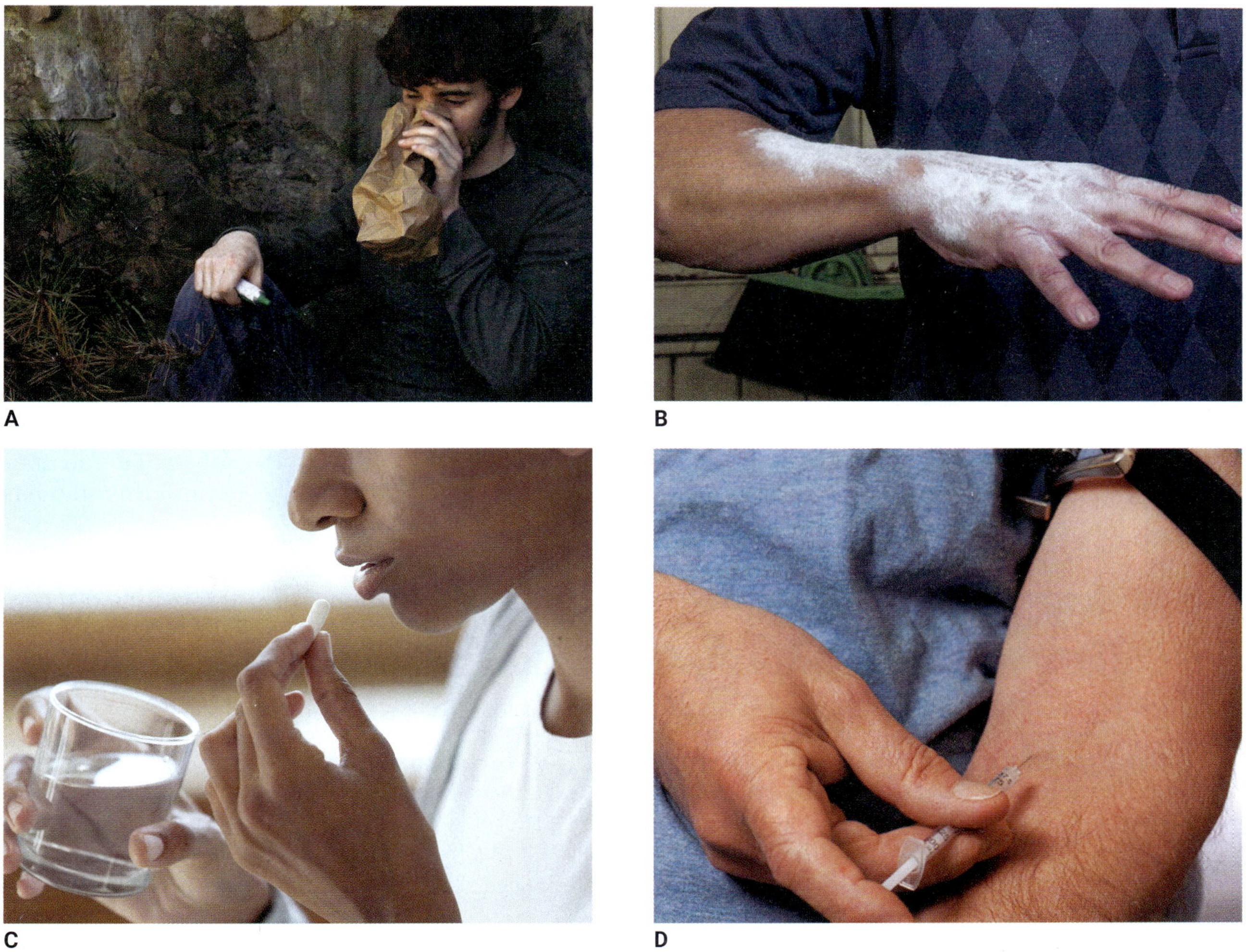

FIGURE 22-2 There are four routes by which a poison can enter the body. **A.** Inhalation. **B.** Absorption (surface contact). **C.** Ingestion. **D.** Injection.

A: © Science History Images/Alamy Stock Photo; B: © Jones & Bartlett Learning; C: © fizkes/Shutterstock; D: © Cate Frost/Shutterstock.

Words of Wisdom

The American Association of Poison Control Centers (AAPCC) supports the nation's 55 poison control centers in their efforts to prevent and treat poison exposures. The telephone number of your regional poison center is on the AAPCC website (www.aapcc.org). It should be programmed into your department mobile phone. You can also call the Poison Help hotline at 1-800-222-1222 (available 24/7, 365 days per year), or visit an interactive online tool, www.poisonhelp.org, to receive confidential expert medical advice. Staff members at every center have access to information about virtually all of the commonly used medications, chemicals, and substances that could possibly be poisonous. These experts know the appropriate emergency treatment for each, including the antidote, if there is one.

If you believe a patient has been poisoned, immediately provide the poison center with all relevant information: when the poisoning occurred; evidence found at the scene; a description of the suspected poison, including the amount involved; and the patient's size, weight, and age. If necessary, medical direction can contact the regional poison center for you and relay specific instructions back to you. The poison control personnel will provide treatment advice and relay information to the receiving facility. Follow your local protocols.

A medical toxicologist is a physician who specializes in caring for patients who have been poisoned. These specialists work in special facilities called medical toxicology treatment centers, located throughout the United States. At times, your medical direction may divert a patient who meets certain poisoning criteria to one of these centers instead of to the closest hospital.

You and your medical oversight center should know the telephone number of your regional poison center and have it available in the event you encounter an unexpected case of poisoning.

oxygen (**FIGURE 22-3**). During the scene size-up, if you suspect the presence of a toxic gas, call for specialized resources such as the hazardous materials (hazmat) team. Never approach a contaminated patient unless you have specialized hazmat training and are using the appropriate PPE (not all patients exposed to toxic gases will have contaminants on them). It will be necessary to use a self-contained breathing apparatus for protection from poisonous fumes if they are present. If you are not specifically trained in the use of this apparatus or do not have appropriately fit-tested equipment available, defer to appropriately trained and equipped personnel. Some patients may need to be decontaminated by the hazmat team after they are removed from the toxic environment. The patient's clothing should be removed in this process because it may contain trapped gases that can be released, exposing you to the substance. You cannot administer emergency care until this step has

YOU are the EMT

It is 0220 hours. Your unit is dispatched to a prominent gated community. A security guard meets you and fire department personnel at the gate and escorts you to 1968 Holly Creek Place. Dispatch advises you the patient had an acute onset of "flulike symptoms." As you arrive, you notice several police cars on scene. You and your EMT partner enter the home and find a 17-year-old female slouched on the couch. There is a strong odor of vomit and the patient appears sleepy.

The patient's mother is present and there is a basin with vomit on the floor. The father reports he was awakened when the teenager and friends came home from a party and were making a lot of noise. He found his daughter on the front porch and had to assist her inside.

1. In addition to providing immediate lifesaving treatment, what else should you do when you arrive at this scene?
2. How can knowledge of various signs and symptoms caused by different types of medications improve the care you provide to a patient?

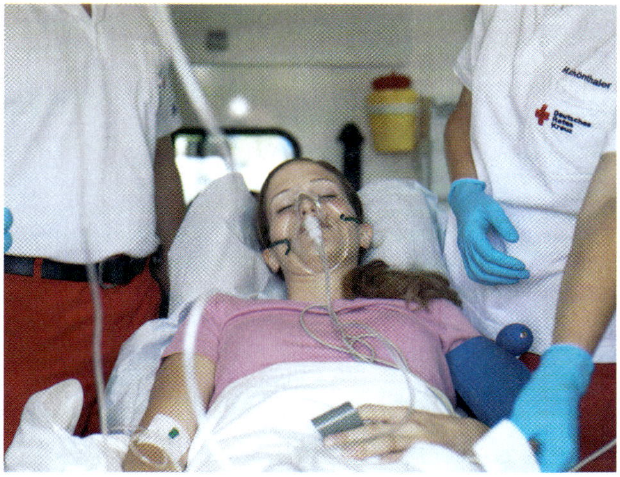

FIGURE 22-3 Patients who have inhaled poisons may need supplemental oxygen and prompt transport to the emergency department.

been completed and there is no danger of the poison contaminating you.

Some inhaled poisons, such as carbon monoxide, are colorless and odorless and produce severe hypoxia without damaging or even irritating the lungs. Others, such as chlorine, are very irritating to the tissues and cause airway obstruction and pulmonary edema. The patient may have the following signs and symptoms: dyspnea, burning eyes, sore throat, cough, chest pain, hoarseness, wheezing, respiratory distress, dizziness, confusion, headache, or stridor in severe cases. The patient may also have seizures or an altered mental status. Most inhaled toxins can be treated by removing the patient from the exposure and applying oxygen. However, some inhaled agents cause progressive lung damage, even after the patient has been removed from direct exposure; this damage may not be evident for several hours. Meanwhile, it may take 2 or 3 days or more of intensive care to restore normal lung function. Therefore, all patients who have inhaled poison require prompt transport to an ED. Be prepared to use supplemental oxygen via a nonrebreathing mask and/or ventilatory support with a bag-mask device, if necessary. Remember that pulse oximetry readings may be inaccurate with some inhaled poisons such as carbon monoxide. Make sure a suction unit is available in case the patient vomits.

Words of Wisdom

During the winter months, the increased use of alternative heating systems in poorly ventilated spaces may lead to an increase in carbon monoxide poisonings. If there is a prolonged power outage, carbon monoxide poisonings often occur when gas-powered generators are located in or close to the home.

Some patients use inhaled poisons to attempt suicide. A common method is for the patient to sit inside a vehicle with the engine running in an enclosed garage. The exhaust fumes from the vehicle contain high levels of carbon monoxide that will cause the patient to become unconscious and eventually stop breathing.

Words of Wisdom

Any time there is more than one ill patient and no evidence of the mechanism of injury (MOI) or nature of illness (NOI), be suspicious. This is especially true when you encounter patients with changes in level of consciousness, especially at an industrial site or in an enclosed space. Toxic fumes may be odorless and colorless or may seem harmless, such as in the case of sewer gas. If the substance is in the atmosphere, it will affect the emergency clinicians as well as the patients. An EMT who is incapacitated is no help to anyone.

Absorbed and Surface Contact Poisons

Poisons that come in contact with the surface of the body can affect the patient in many ways. Many corrosive substances will damage the skin, mucous membranes, or eyes, causing chemical burns, rashes, or lesions. Acids, alkalis, and some petroleum (hydrocarbon) products are very destructive. Other substances are absorbed into the bloodstream through the skin and have systemic effects, just like medications or drugs taken via the oral or injectable routes. Other substances, such as poison ivy or poison oak, may cause an itchy rash without being dangerous to the patient's health. It is important, therefore, to distinguish between contact burns and contact absorption.

> **Words of Wisdom**
>
> Absorption of toxic substances through the skin is a common problem in the agriculture and manufacturing industries. Most solvents, insecticides, herbicides, and pesticides are toxic and can be readily absorbed through the skin.

Signs and symptoms of absorbed poisons include a history of exposure, liquid or powder on a patient's skin, burns, itching, irritation, redness of the skin in light-skinned people, or typical odors of the substance.

Emergency treatment for a typical contact poisoning includes the following two steps:

1. Wear appropriate PPE to avoid contaminating yourself or others.
2. While protecting yourself from exposure, remove the irritating or corrosive substance from the patient as rapidly as possible.

Remove all clothing that has been contaminated with poisons or irritating substances. If a dry powder has been spilled, thoroughly brush off the chemical (avoid creating a dust cloud), flush the skin with clean water for 15 to 20 minutes, and then wash the skin with soap and water. If liquid material has been spilled on a patient, flood the affected part for 15 to 20 minutes. If the patient has a chemical agent in the eyes, irrigate them quickly and thoroughly. To avoid contaminating the other eye as you irrigate the affected eye, make sure the fluid runs from the bridge of the nose outward (**FIGURE 22-4**). Initiate this action on the scene and continue it during transport. Keep in mind that you may have to help patients keep their eyes open.

Many chemical burns occur in industrial settings, where safety showers and specific protocols for handling surface burns are available. If you are called to such a scene, a hazmat team should be available to assist you. Always ensure you, your team members, and the exposed patient are thoroughly decontaminated prior to transport. Failure to do so will result in the risk of contaminating the entire ED and staff. After effective decontamination has occurred, promptly transport to the ED for definitive care. Obtain a **safety data sheet (SDS)** (formerly called material safety data sheet [MSDS])

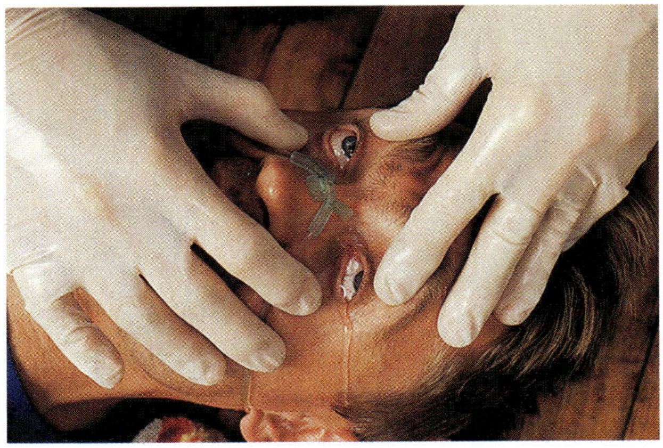

FIGURE 22-4 If chemical agents are in the patient's eyes, irrigate the eyes quickly and thoroughly, ensuring that the irrigation fluid runs from the bridge of the nose outward. (Use of a nasal cannula is shown.)

from industrial sites and transport it with the patient. If the SDS is not immediately available, ask the company to send it to the receiving hospital while you are en route. This will help to identify and quickly make available specific interventions and potential antidotes. Chapter 38, *Incident Management*, discusses hazardous materials and decontamination in detail.

> **Words of Wisdom**
>
> Be aware that some chemicals react with water. Although small amounts can usually be flushed safely with large quantities of water, larger amounts of such chemicals can give off toxic fumes or explode when wet. Be sure to check the relevant warnings and placards, and avoid potential injury to your patient and yourself by calling for additional resources (hazmat team) when in doubt.

Ingested Poisons

Most poisonings occur by mouth (**ingestion**). Ingested poisons include liquids, household cleaners, contaminated food, plants, and, in most cases, drugs. Ingested poisoning is usually accidental in children and, except for contaminated food, deliberate in adults. Plant poisonings are common among children, who like to explore and often bite the leaves of various bushes or shrubs.

Words of Wisdom

It is not uncommon for a child to ingest pills, cleaning supplies (eg, detergent solution), and other household items (eg, button batteries), mistaking them for candies and flavored drinks.

The signs and symptoms of ingested poisons vary greatly with the type of poison, the age of the patient, and the time that has passed since the ingestion. Small children may respond by crying if the poison is an acid or alkaline, and these types of poisons often cause burns around the mouth. Gastrointestinal pain may be present in some cases, and patients may vomit before or after your arrival. If the patient has an altered mental status, it is critical that you protect the patient from aspirating if they vomit. Other signs and symptoms depend on the substance involved; for example, some poisons may cause cardiac dysrhythmias, whereas others may cause seizures. It is important to treat these signs and symptoms and notify the poison center and medical direction of the patient's condition. Consider whether there is unabsorbed poison remaining in the gastrointestinal tract and whether you can safely and effectively prevent its absorption.

When the patient has ingested a toxin, some EMS systems allow EMTs to administer activated charcoal by mouth. Activated charcoal is discussed later in the chapter.

Although every poison will result in a specific set of symptoms and signs, always immediately assess the Airway, Breathing, and Circulation (ABCs) of every patient who has been poisoned. Many patients have died as a result of conditions related to the ABCs that might have been managed easily. Be prepared to provide aggressive ventilatory support and cardiopulmonary resuscitation (CPR), if necessary, to a patient who has ingested an opioid, a sedative, or a barbiturate, each of which can depress the central nervous system (CNS) and slow breathing.

Injected Poisons

Exposure by injection includes intravenous (IV) drug misuse and envenomation by insects, arachnids, and reptiles. Injected poisons cannot be diluted or removed from the body in the field because they are usually absorbed quickly into the body or cause intense local tissue destruction. When people become ill from an injected poison, their condition can be life threatening and you must act quickly (**FIGURE 22-5**). Envenomation is discussed further in Chapter 32, *Environmental Emergencies.*

Signs and symptoms of poisoning by injection depend on the toxin that was injected. They include weakness, dizziness, fever, chills, slow breathing,

YOU are the EMT

You approach the patient, and the mother tells you she vomited up some pills. You glance down at the basin of vomit on the floor and note several different colors of pill fragments. You also notice a vomit stain on the patient's shirt is speckled with different colors. As you begin your assessment of the patient, you note that respirations are very slow.

Recording Time: 0 Minutes	
Appearance	Slouched into the couch with head down, motionless
Level of consciousness	Sleepy and not responding without stimulation; constricted pupils
Airway	Oral secretions; snoring respirations
Breathing	Slow rate; shallow depth; breath sounds diminished to absent
Circulation	Radial pulses rapid and weak; skin cool, pale, and wet; no gross bleeding

3. On the basis of your initial assessment, what is the most appropriate treatment for this patient?

4. On the basis of the patient's initial presentation, what type of drug should you suspect she overdosed on?

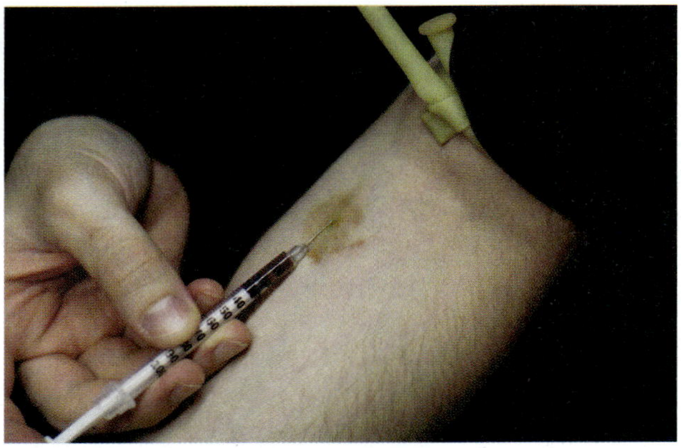

FIGURE 22-5 Injected poisons are impossible to dilute or remove from the body in the field; therefore, prompt transport to the emergency department is critical.

and unresponsiveness, or the patient may be easily excited.

If you suspect that rapid absorption has occurred, monitor the patient's airway, provide high-flow oxygen for any patient with respiratory distress or signs of hypoxia (ie, oxygen saturation level of less than 94%, cyanosis), and be alert for nausea and vomiting. Remove rings, watches, and bracelets from areas around the injection site if swelling occurs. Prompt transport to the ED is essential. Take all containers, bottles, and labels with the patient to the hospital.

Words of Wisdom

Take time at the scene to make thorough notes about the nature of the poisoning. You can then use this information to state the type and amount of substance and the time and route of exposure in your radio, verbal, and written reports. The busy ED staff will also appreciate clear notes that can quickly be handed over on arrival.

Patient Assessment

Scene Size-up

When you have a situation that involves a toxicologic emergency, a well-trained dispatcher can obtain important information pertaining to

YOU are the EMT

The patient's respirations continue to slow and then stop completely. You, your partner, and the fire crew begin to treat the patient. She is placed supine on the floor. One of the firefighters inserts an oropharyngeal airway and begins ventilation with a bag-mask device and oxygen.

Recording Time: 6 Minutes	
Respirations	Apneic; assisted ventilations
Pulse	116 beats/min; weak and regular
Skin	Cool, pale, and wet
Blood pressure	96/50 mm Hg
Oxygen saturation (Spo_2)	99% (on oxygen)

As you treat the patient, a law enforcement officer brings inside one of the friends who brought the patient home. He reports they went to a "Skittles party" earlier that night. He explains the teenagers took prescription pills from their parents' medicine cabinets, mixed them up in a bowl, and then took turns selecting pills to get high. They were also drinking beer and liquor.

You check the patient's pupils. You and your partner agree they are and the patient needs naloxone, which your partner prepares to administer. You then check the patient's blood glucose level. The glucometer registers a fingerstick glucose level of 112 mg/dL.

5. Would activated charcoal benefit this patient? Why or why not?

6. Why is naloxone being given to this patient?

a poisoning call that will help you anticipate the proper protection needed to ensure your safety. The dispatcher may be able to obtain information pertaining to the MOI/NOI, the number of patients involved, whether additional resources are needed, and whether trauma is involved. If this information has been obtained before your arrival, you must assess the scene nevertheless to ensure your safety and to determine the accuracy of the dispatcher's information.

Because of the risk of possible cross-contamination by poisons that can be inhaled, absorbed, ingested, and injected, you must take appropriate standard precautions. As you approach the scene, think like a detective and look for clues that might indicate the substance involved. Ask yourself the following questions:

- Is there an unpleasant or odd odor in the room? If so, is the scene safe? (This could indicate an inhaled poison.)
- Are there medication bottles near the patient or at the scene? If so, is there medication missing that might indicate an overdose?
- Are there alcoholic beverage containers present?
- Are there syringes or other drug paraphernalia on the scene?
- Is there a suspicious odor and/or drug paraphernalia present that may indicate the presence of an illegal drug laboratory? Drug laboratories can be volatile, so ensure scene safety (**FIGURE 22-6**).

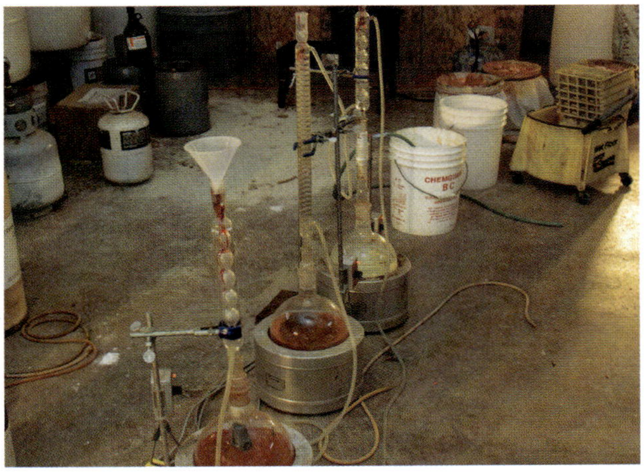

FIGURE 22-6 An illegal laboratory capable of producing large quantities of methamphetamine.

Courtesy of DEA.

The location of the patient may help contribute to identifying a suspected poisoning, and other clues such as empty pill bottles or open bottles of household cleaners near the patient may provide further information to help you determine what happened. Keep a constant eye on the surroundings, and keep an open mind when questioning the patient or bystanders to avoid incorrect conclusions.

Primary Assessment

To best determine the severity of the patient's condition, first obtain a general impression of the patient, assess level of consciousness, and determine any life threats. When responding to a toxicologic emergency, do not assume a conscious, alert, and oriented patient who is in stable condition has no apparent life threats. The patient may have a harmful or even lethal amount of poison in their system that has not had time to produce systemic reactions. A primary assessment that reveals a patient with signs of distress and/or altered mental status gives you early confirmation that the poisonous substance is causing systemic reactions.

Quickly ensure that the patient has an open airway and adequate ventilation. If the patient is hypoxic, begin oxygen therapy. In situations where a patient may have an inhalation injury (typically carbon monoxide and/or cyanide poisoning), place the patient on high-flow oxygen regardless of the pulse oximetry reading. If the patient is unresponsive to painful stimuli, consider inserting an airway adjunct to ensure an open airway. Have suction available; these patients are susceptible to vomiting. You may also have to assist a patient's ventilations with a bag-mask device because some substances act as depressants on the body's systems.

ALS Assist

If your ALS partner is preparing to intubate, be alert to situations that indicate the need to have suction immediately available, such as calls involving overdoses or accidental ingestions. These patients are at high risk to vomit, and the suction unit will not help you or your patient if it is not with you when you need it.

Once the airway and breathing have been assessed and appropriate interventions performed, assess the patient's circulatory status. You will find variations in a patient's circulatory status depending on the substance involved. Assess the pulse and skin condition. Although pallor can be difficult to detect in patients with dark skin, it may be observed by examining mucous membranes inside the inner lower eyelid and capillary refill. On general observation, the patient may appear ashen or gray.

Some poisons are stimulants, and others are depressants. Some poisons will cause vasoconstriction and others vasodilation. Although bleeding may not be obvious, alterations in consciousness may have contributed to trauma and bleeding.

Consider prompt transport for patients with obvious alterations in the ABCs or for patients you have determined have a poor general impression. Some industrial settings may have specific decontamination stations and antidotes available at the site. Remember, everyone who is exposed to the hazardous material must be thoroughly decontaminated by the hazmat team before leaving the scene.

Street Smarts

Do not rule out the possibility of an overdose or an exposure when assessing a patient who has sustained trauma. Patients who are intoxicated with drugs or alcohol are at risk for falls and other mechanisms for trauma. Medications that promote vasodilation or bleeding can speed up the development of shock due to hypovolemia. Also, identifying an overdose or exposure can help the medical team prepare for unforeseen complications.

History Taking

After you have managed the life threats during the primary assessment, investigate the chief complaint or history of present illness. Obtain the patient's medical history. In many situations, you can perform this in the ambulance en route to the hospital. If your patient is responsive and can answer questions, begin with an evaluation of the exposure and the SAMPLE (Signs and symptoms, Allergies, Medications, Pertinent past medical history, Last oral intake, Events leading up to the injury or illness) history. If the patient is unresponsive, attempt to obtain the history from coworkers, bystanders, friends, or family members. Medical identification jewelry and wallet cards may also provide information about the patient's medical history.

In these situations, the SAMPLE history guides you in what to focus on as you continue to assess the patient's complaints, and the physical examination and vital signs tell you what is happening to the patient's body. These three assessments give you direction in the interventions your patient might need.

In addition to the SAMPLE history, ask the following questions:

- **What is the substance involved?** If you know the substance involved, you will be better able to access the appropriate resource, such as the poison center, to determine lethal doses, time before adverse effects begin, effects of the substance at toxic levels, and appropriate interventions.
- **When did the patient ingest or become exposed to the substance?** This will let you know if and when the adverse effects will begin. This will also let the emergency physician know what adverse effects can be reversed and which ones cannot because of the length of time the patient has been exposed to the substance.
- **How much did the patient ingest or what was the level of exposure?** With this information, the poison center will be able to inform you whether the patient has had a harmful or lethal dose.
- **Over what period did the patient take or was the patient exposed to the substance?** Did the exposure occur all at once or over minutes or hours?
- **Has the patient or a bystander performed any intervention on the patient? Has the intervention helped?** The patient's or bystander's intervention may cause complications. The emergency physician will need to know this information to be able to adjust interventions accordingly.
- **How much does the patient weigh?** If activated charcoal is indicated and permitted by local protocols, you will need to determine the dose based on the patient's weight. The

antidote or neutralizing agent given by the emergency physician may be based on the patient's weight as well.

Secondary Assessment

In some instances, such as a critically ill patient or a short transport time, you may not have time to conduct a secondary assessment.

Your physical examination should focus on the area of the body involved with the route of exposure and the particular drug or chemical the patient was exposed to. For example, if you suspect a person has ingested a poison, inspect the mouth for indications of poisoning. Are there burns from caustic chemicals? Are there plant or pill fragments? If the person's skin came in contact with a poison, is there a rash or burns? How large an area is involved? If a respiratory exposure occurred, auscultate the lungs. Is there good air movement in and out of the lungs? Do you hear any wheezing or crackles? Learn about the effects of general classes of drugs and chemicals so that you will be familiar with specific and common poisons.

Your priority is to manage the ABCs during the primary assessment. These interventions take precedence over a thorough physical examination. However, once the ABCs have been addressed and managed, conducting a thorough physical examination will often provide additional information on the exposure the patient experienced. A general review of all body systems may help to identify systemic problems. Perform this review, at a minimum, on patients with extensive chemical burns or other significant trauma and on patients who are unresponsive.

A complete set of baseline vital signs, including oxygen saturation and blood glucose levels, is important. Many poisons have no outward indications of the seriousness of the exposure. Alterations in the level of consciousness, pulse, respirations, blood pressure, and skin are more sensitive indicators that something serious is wrong. Assessing temperature can add important information following certain ingestions or if the patient has been unresponsive for an extended time. In addition, medical direction may ask you to acquire and transmit a 12-lead electrocardiogram if doing so is appropriate and possible.

Reassessment

The condition of patients exposed to poisons may change suddenly and without warning. Continually reassess the adequacy of the patient's ABCs. Repeat the vital signs, and compare them with the baseline set obtained earlier in your assessment. Evaluate the effectiveness of interventions you have provided. If your assessment has provided necessary information about the poisonous substance, you may be able to anticipate changes in the patient's condition. If the patient has consumed a harmful or lethal dose of a poisonous substance, reassess the vital signs at least every 5 minutes. If the patient is in stable condition and there are no life threats, reassess every 15 minutes. If the poison or the level of exposure (eg, the number and type of pills taken) is unknown, careful and frequent reassessment is mandatory.

The treatment you provide for poisoned patients depends a great deal on what they were exposed to, how they were exposed, and other signs and symptoms found in your assessment. Remember, supporting the ABCs is your most important task. Contact your medical direction or a poison center to discuss treatment options for particular poisonings. Manage airborne exposures with oxygen if indicated, remove contact exposures with large amounts of water unless contraindicated, and consider activated charcoal for ingested poisons (if permitted by local protocol).

Once you have completed your primary assessment, history taking, and secondary assessment, contact medical direction to request necessary interventions. Report to the hospital as much information as you have about the poison or chemical to which the patient was exposed. If an SDS is immediately available in a work setting, take it with you to the hospital.

Emergency Medical Care

First, ensure scene safety by taking standard precautions and performing external decontamination. Suction tablet or pill fragments from the patient's mouth, and wash or brush dry poison from the patient's skin. Treatment focuses on support. Assess and maintain the patient's ABCs. Provide oxygen to the patient, and assist ventilations if necessary.

Keep the patient warm, treat for shock as necessary, and transport promptly to the nearest appropriate hospital.

In certain cases, some EMS systems allow EMTs to give activated charcoal by mouth. Activated charcoal binds to specific toxins, such as pills that have been ingested, and prevents their absorption by the body. The toxins are then carried out of the body in the stool.

Activated charcoal is not indicated, nor will it be effective, for patients who have ingested alkali poisons, cyanide, ethanol, iron, lithium, methanol, mineral acids, or organic solvents. If the patient has a decreased level of consciousness and cannot protect their airway, do not give activated charcoal because the risk of aspiration is great.

If local protocol permits, your ambulance will likely carry plastic bottles of premixed suspension, each containing up to 50 g of activated charcoal (**FIGURE 22-7**). Some common trade names for the suspension form are InstaChar, Actidose, and LiquiChar. The usual dosage for an adult or child is 1 g of activated charcoal per kilogram of body weight (more if food is present). Thus, the usual adult dose is 30 to 100 g, and the usual pediatric dose is 15 to 30 g for children younger than 13 years.

Before you give a patient charcoal, obtain approval from medical direction. Consider the amount and type of the toxin and the patient's condition. In most cases, the activated charcoal should be used within 1 hour of ingestion. Next, shake the bottle vigorously to mix the suspension. The medication looks like mud, so it is best to cover the outside of the container so that the fluid is not visible and ask the patient to drink it with a straw. Some patients may not tolerate the medication due to its gritty texture. You might need to convince the patient why this intervention is important, particularly if the patient is a child, but never force the patient. If the patient takes a long time to drink the mixture, you will have to shake the container frequently to keep the medication mixed. Once the patient has finished, discard the container from which the charcoal was administered. Be sure to record the time when you administered the activated charcoal. If the patient refuses the activated charcoal, document the refusal and your attempts to counsel the patient, and transport the patient for further evaluation.

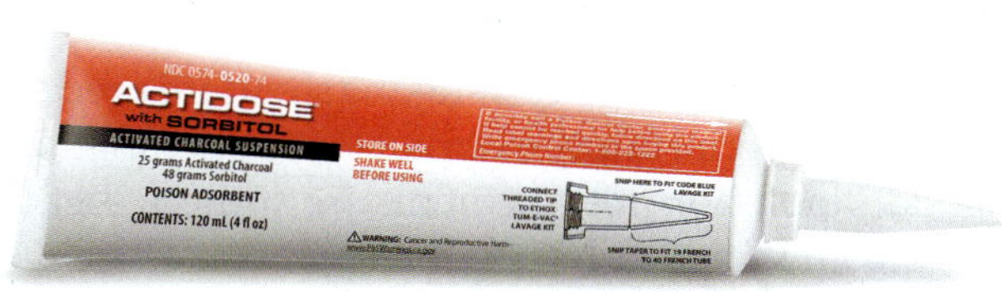

FIGURE 22-7 Activated charcoal comes as a premixed suspension.

Used with permission from Padagis US LLC.

The adverse effects of ingesting activated charcoal include constipation and black stools. A patient who has ingested a poison that causes nausea may vomit after taking activated charcoal, and the dose will have to be repeated. As you reassess the patient, be prepared for vomiting, nausea, and possible airway conditions.

> **Words of Wisdom**
>
> While one EMT explains the activated charcoal treatment to the patient, the other EMT can prepare a large plastic garbage bag to hang on the patient as a bib. This will help contain the charcoal suspension if the patient vomits.

Specific Poisons

Over time, **tolerance** may develop in a person who routinely uses a substance, meaning increasing amounts of it are required to produce the same result. A person with an **addiction** has an overwhelming desire or need to continue using the substance, at whatever cost, with a tendency to increase the dose. Addiction does not happen only with the classic drugs of misuse, such as cocaine, fentanyl, or heroin. Many substances can result in an addiction, including laxatives, nasal decongestants, vitamins, and food. You should be familiar with the concepts of tolerance, addiction, and substance use/misuse and the differences between the terms.

The importance of safety awareness when caring for people experiencing a drug-related emergency cannot be overemphasized. Individuals who use certain drugs have a relatively high incidence of serious and undiagnosed infections, including human immunodeficiency virus and hepatitis. These patients, when intoxicated, may bite, spit, hit, or otherwise injure you, causing you to come in contact with their blood and other body fluids. Always wear appropriate PPE. A calm, professional approach can defuse frightening situations, but keep your safety and that of your team uppermost in mind. Expect the unexpected and remember: The drug user, not the drug, can pose the greatest threat.

Alcohol

As a new EMT, you will notice that many calls for service have a connection to alcohol use. Alcohol can damage the liver, whether thorough chronic overuse or occasional excessive use (binge drinking). Many people dismiss the dangers of drinking and do not understand that binge use can be more damaging than chronic use, depending on the frequency of the binging and the surrounding circumstances. Binge drinking is a serious health concern in the United States, contributing to nearly 180,000 deaths each year.[4] The Centers for Disease Control and Prevention (CDC) defines it as consumption of five or more drinks during a single occasion for males, and four or more drinks for females.

Alcohol is a powerful CNS depressant. It is a **sedative**, a substance that decreases activity and excitement, and a **hypnotic**, meaning it induces sleep. In general, alcohol dulls the sense of awareness, slows reflexes, and increases reaction time (**FIGURE 22-8**). It may also cause aggressive and inappropriate behavior and lack of coordination. However, a person who appears intoxicated may have other medical conditions as well. Look for signs of head trauma, mental illness, toxic reactions, or uncontrolled diabetes. Severe acute alcohol ingestion may cause hypoglycemia, which may contribute to the symptoms. In most states, patients who are impaired and lack decision-making capacity, whether by mental illness, medical condition, or intoxication, cannot legally refuse transport. Always consult with your supervisor, law enforcement, or medical direction in these situations. Chapter 23, *Behavioral Health Emergencies*, covers this topic in more detail.

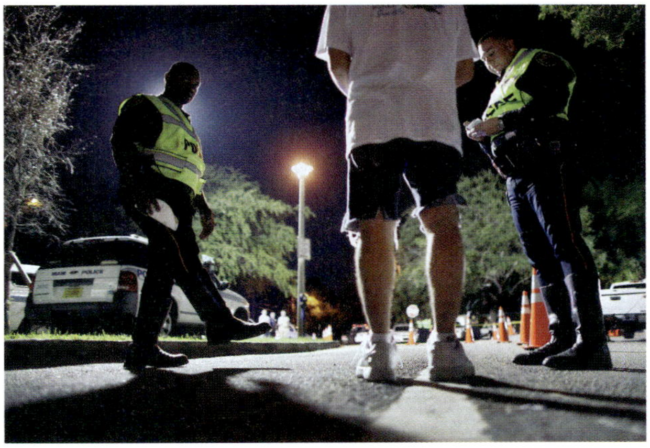

FIGURE 22-8 Alcohol intoxication causes altered mental status, slowed reflexes, and impaired reaction time.

YOU are the EMT

Your partner administers the naloxone intranasally. After about a minute, the patient starts moving, spits out the oral airway, and pushes the bag mask away. You apply a nonrebreathing mask at 15 L/min, which the patient tolerates. You reassess the patient's condition and vital signs and prepare for transport.

Recording Time: 11 Minutes	
Level of consciousness	Conscious, but sleepy
Respirations	12 breaths/min; adequate depth
Pulse	84 beats/min; regular and stronger
Skin	Cool; color is returning to baseline
Blood pressure	108/52 mm Hg
Oxygen saturation (Spo_2)	100% (on oxygen)

7. What other issues about this patient should concern you?

8. How would this patient's presentation have differed had she overdosed on a sympathomimetic?

Alcohol increases the effects of many drugs and is often taken with other substances. OTC drugs, including antihistamines and diet medications, can cause serious complications when combined with alcohol.

If a patient exhibits signs of serious CNS depression, provide respiratory support. This may be difficult, however, because depression of the respiratory system can also cause vomiting (**emesis**). The vomiting may be forceful or even bloody (**hematemesis**) because large amounts of alcohol irritate the stomach. Internal bleeding should also be considered if the patient appears to be in shock (hypoperfusion) because blood might not clot effectively in a patient who has a prolonged history of alcohol use disorder.

Special Populations

DRUG AND ALCOHOL MISUSE AMONG TEENAGERS

Drug and alcohol misuse among teenagers is an ongoing social problem in the United States. Teenagers are often encouraged to experiment with drugs through peer pressure. Many teenagers will do things they know are not safe just to gain acceptance. These experiments are often poorly controlled, resulting in an overdose. For example, individuals with drug tolerance may give too large of a dose to a first-time user. In other instances, a teenager may be given a combination of drugs, or drugs that are believed to be "pure" but that actually contain unknown types or quantities of a different drug. These situations can be fatal.

When caring for teenagers experiencing a drug-related emergency, keep in mind that they may lie about having taken drugs, or what they have taken, out of fear of being arrested. Reassure them that your intent is only to give them the best treatment possible.

Recurrent use can become a problem in this age group as well. In 2020, almost 10 million US children ages 12 to 17 years met diagnostic criteria for a substance use disorder.[5]

Also be aware that some teenagers use drugs to attempt suicide. According to the CDC, suicide is the second leading cause of death for children and young adults ages 10 to 24 years.[6] Do not be judgmental with these teenagers, and treat them as you would any other patient, with empathy and patience.

A patient in alcohol withdrawal may experience frightening hallucinations, or **delirium tremens (DTs)**. Approximately 1 to 7 days after a person stops drinking or when alcohol consumption levels are decreased suddenly, DTs may develop. Alcoholic hallucinations come and go. A patient with an otherwise clear mental state may see fantastic shapes or figures or hear odd voices. Such auditory and visual hallucinations often precede DTs, which are a more severe complication.

Patients may experience one or more of the following signs and symptoms:

- Agitation and restlessness
- Fever
- Sweating
- Tremors
- Confusion and/or disorientation
- Delusions and/or hallucinations
- Seizures

Provide prompt transport after you have completed your assessment and given necessary care. A person who is experiencing hallucinations or DTs is extremely ill. Should seizures develop, treat them as you would any other seizure. Protect the patient from self-injury, but do not restrain the patient. If the patient has difficulty breathing, provide supplemental oxygen and watch carefully for vomiting; have suction ready. Hypovolemia may develop because of sweating, fluid loss, insufficient fluid intake, or vomiting associated with DTs. If you see signs of hypovolemic shock, clear the airway and turn the patient's head to one side to minimize the chance of aspiration during transport. These patients may not respond appropriately to suggestions or conversation; they are often confused and frightened. Therefore, use a calm and relaxed approach. Reassure the patient, and provide emotional support.

Safety Tips

In situations that involve toxic substances, your safety is paramount. Always be aware of the environment. When responding to patients who have taken illegal drugs, be cautious and be prepared for unexpected violence. Do not hesitate to call for law enforcement support.

Opioids

An **opioid** is a drug that acts as a CNS depressant and produces insensibility or stupor. An opioid can be a natural product derived from the opium or poppy plant such as heroin (referred to more specifically as an opiate) or a synthetic product such as fentanyl designed to produce similar effects.

Words of Wisdom

The term *narcotic* originally referred to a substance that dulled the senses and relieved pain. In everyday speech, it is often used to mean all illegal drugs, but technically, it refers only to opioids. To avoid confusion, *opioid* is the preferred term in the medical community.

Some people become physically dependent on opioids after taking an appropriate medical prescription. These drugs include fentanyl, hydromorphone, oxycodone, hydrocodone, and methadone (**TABLE 22-2**). In 2022, approximately 82,000 people died from opioid overdose in the United States.[7] The incidence of fentanyl overdose in particular continues to rise. Fentanyl is approximately 100 times stronger than morphine and relatively inexpensive.

Words of Wisdom

In recent years, street use of incredibly potent drugs such as carfentanil and desomorphine has increased. Carfentanil is an animal tranquilizer used for large mammals, such as elephants. It is far more potent than morphine or fentanyl, and its use by persons with a substance use disorder seeking a quick opioid high can be fatal.

TABLE 22-2 Common Opioids

- Butorphanol (Stadol)
- Codeine
- Fentanyl (Sublimaze)
- Heroin
- Hydrocodone (Vicodin)
- Hydromorphone (Dilaudid)
- Methadone (Dolophine)
- Morphine
- Oxycodone hydrochloride (OxyContin)
- Oxymorphone (Opana)

These agents are CNS depressants and can cause severe respiratory depression. Tolerance develops rapidly, so users typically require larger and larger doses to experience the same high. In general, emergency medical conditions related to opioids are caused by respiratory depression, including a decreased volume of inspired air and decreased respirations. This can lead to respiratory and then cardiac arrest if not treated promptly. These drugs often cause nausea and vomiting and may lead to hypotension. Although seizures are uncommon, they can occur and an overdose can result in the patient entering a comatose condition. Patients typically appear sedated or unconscious and exhibit cyanosis, frequently with pinpoint pupils. Whereas all of these signs and symptoms may be present with other drugs, the pinpoint pupils are a classic sign of opioid use.

Words of Wisdom

Some patients who use opioids via IV injection are at high risk for hepatitis C and human immunodeficiency virus. Be aware of your surroundings and practice bloodborne precautions. Be alert for improperly discarded or stored needles.

Naloxone (Narcan) is an antidote that reverses the effects of opioid overdose. This medication can be given IV, intramuscularly, or intranasally. The intranasal route is becoming a preferred route for the administration of naloxone due to its ease of administration and rapid effects. Intranasal administration is safer than IV or intramuscular injection because a needle is not required to administer the medication.

EMTs are permitted to administer prefilled naloxone by the intramuscular route or by the intranasal route. Naloxone is indicated when a patient suspected of having experienced an opioid overdose presents with very slow respirations or apnea. Ensure an adequate airway (oropharyngeal or nasopharyngeal) and ventilate the patient using a bag-mask device while preparing to administer naloxone. Providing adequate ventilation while you prepare to administer naloxone decreases the risk of permanent brain damage related to hypoxia. Watch the patient closely as the level of consciousness rises. If you previously inserted an oropharyngeal airway, you will have to remove it to prevent vomiting and aspiration.

In most areas, laypeople are permitted to administer naloxone (**FIGURE 22-9**). Be aware that it may have been administered prior to your arrival. Find out from bystanders what has occurred and who was given naloxone.

Special Populations

OPIOID OVERDOSE IN OLDER ADULTS

When a geriatric patient has altered mental status, consider and assess for opioid overdose as a possible cause. Between 2000 and 2020, the federal government reported a significant increase in deaths from opioids, particularly synthetic opioids such as fentanyl, in people 65 years and older.[8]

When a patient goes into cardiac arrest, follow the algorithm shown in **FIGURE 22-10**, including administration of naloxone if it is available. However,

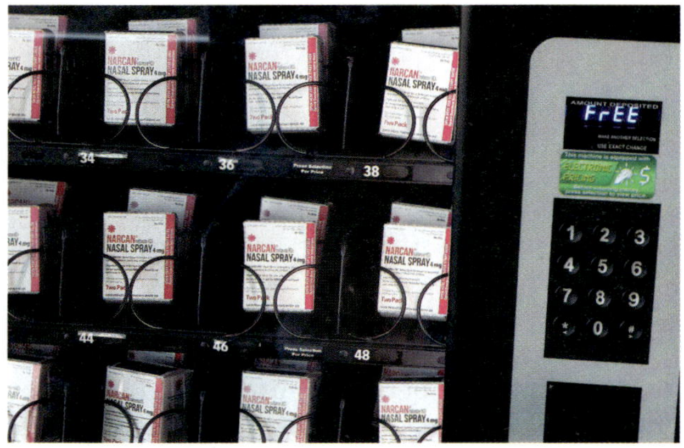

FIGURE 22-9 In some cities, vending machines that dispense naloxone at no cost are accessible to the public.

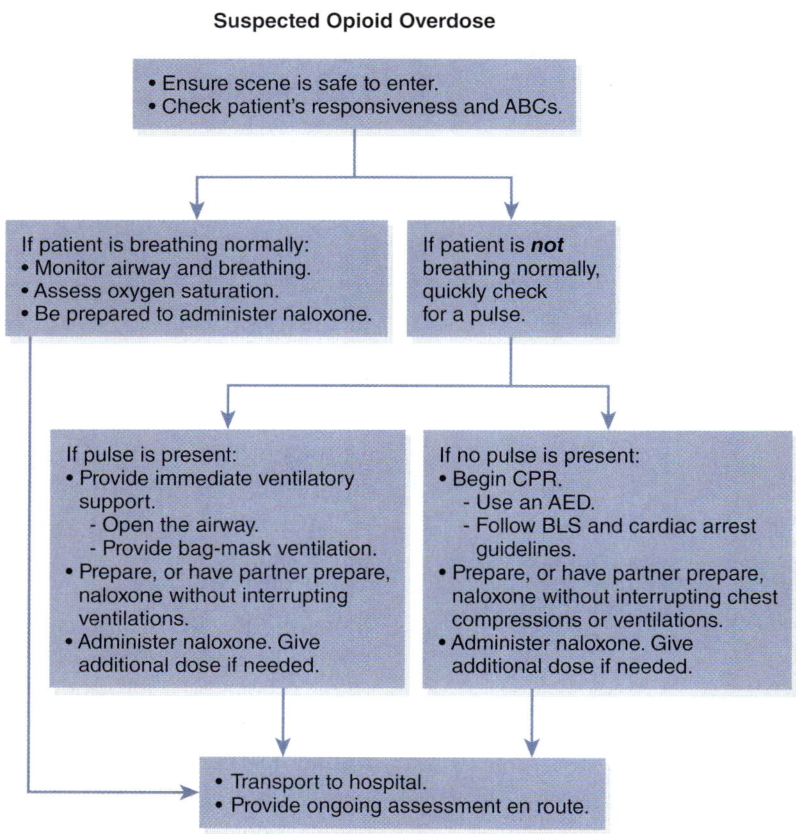

FIGURE 22-10 EMT response to suspected opioid overdose.

Abbreviations: ABCs, airway, breathing, and circulation; AED, automated external defibrillator; BLS, basic life support; CPR, cardiopulmonary resuscitation providing bag-mask ventilations is a critical treatment for these patients as well. Whether or not naloxone is available, provide ventilations and rapid transport.

Sedative-Hypnotic Drugs

Barbiturates and benzodiazepines have been a part of legitimate medicine for a long time. They are easy to obtain and relatively cheap. People sometimes solicit prescriptions from several physicians for the same hypnotics or a variety of sedative-hypnotics (**TABLE 22-3**). These drugs are CNS depressants and alter the level of consciousness, with effects similar to those of alcohol so that the patient may appear drowsy, peaceful, or intoxicated. By themselves, these drugs do not relieve pain, nor do they produce a specific high, although users often take alcohol or an opioid at the same time to boost their effects.

In general, these agents are taken by mouth. Occasionally, however, contents of capsules are suspended or dissolved in water and injected to produce a sudden state of ease and contentment. Use of IV sedative-hypnotic drugs quickly induces tolerance, so the person requires increasingly larger doses. You are less likely to be called to treat an acute overdose in someone who chronically uses these drugs; however, you may be called to a scene of an attempted suicide in which the patient has taken large quantities of these drugs. In these situations, patients will often have marked respiratory depression and may be in a coma.

Sedative-hypnotic drugs such as chloral hydrate may also be given to people as a "knock-out" drink, or "Mickey Finn," to incapacitate them without their knowledge. Date rape or club drugs such as flunitrazepam (Rohypnol or roofies) and ketamine (Ketalar or Special K) are often colorless, tasteless, and odorless. They cause an unwary person to become sedated and even unconscious, which may facilitate sexual assault or rape. The person later awakens, confused and unable to remember what happened. Chapter 35, *Patients With Special Challenges*, discusses this topic in more detail.

In general, your treatment of patients who have overdosed with sedative-hypnotics and have respiratory depression is to ensure the airway is patent, assist ventilations, and give supplemental oxygen when appropriate. Provide prompt transport and closely monitor the patient's mental status. You may attempt to stimulate the person by speaking loudly or gently shaking the person; remember to watch for vomiting.

As multidrug use becomes more common, you may find it increasingly difficult to determine what agent or agents patients have taken. Your best approach is to treat any obvious injuries or illnesses, keeping in mind that drug use may complicate the picture and make full life support necessary. Focus on the ABCs, especially the possibility of airway problems (relaxation of the tongue, causing

TABLE 22-3 Examples of Sedative-Hypnotic Drugs

Barbiturates	Benzodiazepines	Others
Amobarbital (Amytal)	Alprazolam (Xanax)	Carisoprodol (Soma)
Butabarbital (Butisol)	Chlordiazepoxide (Librium)	Chloral hydrate ("Mickey Finn")
Pentobarbital (Nembutal)	Diazepam (Valium)	Cyclobenzaprine (Flexeril)
Phenobarbital (Luminal)	Flunitrazepam (Rohypnol)	Eszopiclone (Lunesta)
Secobarbital (Seconal)	Lorazepam (Ativan)	Ethchlorvynol (Placidyl)
	Oxazepam (Serax)	Ethyl alcohol (drinking alcohol)
	Temazepam (Restoril)	Isopropyl alcohol (rubbing alcohol)
		Ketamine (Ketalar)

obstruction), vomiting, respiratory depression, and, in severe cases, cardiac arrest.

Inhalants

Inhalants are volatile substances that are primarily found in household products. Many misused inhalants produce several of the same CNS effects as do other sedative-hypnotics, but these agents are inhaled instead of ingested or injected. This practice is known as bagging or sniffing when the fumes are sprayed into a paper or plastic bag, then inhaled; it is known as huffing when an inhalant-soaked rag is stuffed into the mouth or nitrous oxide gas is inhaled from a balloon.[9] Some of the more commonly used agents include acetone, toluene, xylene, and hexane, which are found in glues, cleaning compounds, paint thinners, and lacquers. Similarly, gasoline and various halogenated hydrocarbons, such as Freon or difluoroethane (used as propellants in aerosol sprays such as compressed air to dust off electronics), are also used as inhalants. None of these inhalants are medications; rather, these substances briefly displace oxygen in the brain and cause a rush of euphoria. Because these are inexpensive products that can be bought in hardware stores, they are commonly used by teenagers and curious adults seeking an alcohol-like high. The intoxicating dose and the lethal dose are very close, making these extremely dangerous drugs. Long-term use can lead to permanent brain damage.

The effects of inhalants have a rapid onset but also dissipate within minutes, so users often inhale many times over a period of hours. Effects of inhalants range from mild drowsiness to coma, but unlike most other sedative-hypnotics, these agents often cause seizures. Inhalants can cause asphyxia when the inhaled substance takes the place of oxygen in the lungs. The lack of oxygen to the brain may cause a loss of brain function. Aspiration can occur if the patient vomits. Also, halogenated hydrocarbon solvents can make the heart hypersensitive to the patient's own adrenaline, putting the patient at high risk for sudden cardiac death because of ventricular fibrillation; even the action of walking may release enough adrenaline to cause a fatal ventricular dysrhythmia. This effect, sometimes referred to as sudden sniffing death, can occur from a single use and is usually linked to butane, propane, and aerosol chemicals. You must try to keep these patients from struggling with you or exerting themselves. Give supplemental oxygen for patients with respiratory distress or signs of hypoxia, and use a stretcher to move the patient. Prompt transport to the hospital is essential; monitor vital signs en route.

Hydrogen Sulfide

Hydrogen sulfide is a highly toxic, colorless, and flammable gas with a distinctive rotten-egg odor. Poisoning by hydrogen sulfide usually occurs by inhalation. Hydrogen sulfide affects all organs, but it has the most impact on the lungs and CNS.

Hydrogen sulfide occurs naturally in sewers, swamps, volcanoes, and crude petroleum. Hydrogen sulfide poisoning is also a method used to attempt suicide, referred to as chemical or detergent suicide because household chemicals are mixed together to create the toxin. According to the Chemical Hazards Emergency Medical Management database, this method of self-inflicted exposure to toxic gas originated in Japan and reached the United States via the Internet.[10] The patient may obtain a warning sign to place near the area of the suicide, such as an enclosed vehicle, to warn responders of the deadly gas. If you approach an enclosed vehicle with an unconscious patient inside, be alert for warning signs, as well as containers, buckets, or pots. Remember, do not enter a scene where a toxic gas may be present. Be aware of your surroundings as you approach, and if you suspect the presence of a toxic gas, wait for a hazmat team to tell you the scene is safe.

Workers in industrial settings may experience low-level exposure to hydrogen sulfide over a long period, leading to eye, nose, and throat irritation, as well as headaches and bronchitis. Chronic exposure to this gas may cause an inability to smell the gas. When patients are exposed to high concentrations of the gas, they will experience nausea and vomiting, confusion, dyspnea, and a loss of consciousness. Seizures, shock, coma, and cardiopulmonary arrest may also result.

There is no antidote for hydrogen sulfide poisoning. Therefore, a hazmat team must quickly remove the patient from the contaminated area. Once the patient has been decontaminated, treatment is largely supportive. Monitor and assist the patient's respiratory and cardiovascular functions and provide rapid transport.

Street Smarts

Fire departments often carry four-gas meters. Using these meters, fire personnel can check the environment for dangerous levels of oxygen, carbon monoxide, hydrogen sulfide, and combustible gas to ensure it is safe for you to enter.

Sympathomimetics

Sympathomimetics are CNS stimulants that mimic the effects of the sympathetic (fight-or-flight) nervous system. These stimulants frequently cause hypertension, tachycardia, and dilated pupils. A **stimulant** is an agent that produces an excited state. Examples include amphetamine and methamphetamine (also called meth or ice), which are commonly taken by mouth or smoked. They are also injected in many cases. Sympathomimetic drugs are typically taken to make the user "feel good," improve task performance, suppress appetite, or prevent sleepiness. They may also produce irritability, anxiety, fear, lack of concentration, or seizures. Paranoia and delusions are common symptoms of sympathomimetic use.

Other examples include phentermine hydrochloride, an appetite suppressant, and amphetamine sulfate, taken for weight control (short term), narcolepsy, and attention deficit/hyperactivity disorder. Caffeine and phenylpropanolamine (a nasal decongestant) are mild sympathomimetics. So-called designer drugs such as MDMA (3,4-methylenedioxymethamphetamine, also known as ecstasy or Molly) are also frequently used in the United States.

Sympathomimetic drugs are known by various street names that change often (**TABLE 22-4**).

TABLE 22-4 Examples of Street Names for Sympathomimetics

Street Name	Drug Name
Adam	3,4-Methylenedioxymethamphetamine (MDMA)
Angel dust	Phencyclidine (PCP)
Bennies	Amphetamines
Coke	Cocaine
Crank	Crack cocaine, heroin, amphetamine, methamphetamine, methcathinone
DOM	4-Methyl-2,5-dimethoxyamphetamine
Ecstasy	MDMA
Eve	MDMA
Golden eagle	4-Methylthioamphetamine
Ice	Cocaine, crack cocaine, smokable methamphetamine, methamphetamine, MDMA, PCP
MDA	Methaqualone
Meth	Methamphetamine
Molly	MDMA
Speed	Crack cocaine, amphetamine, methamphetamine
Uppers	Amphetamines

Cocaine, also called crystal, snow, freebase, rock, gold dust, blow, and lady, is one of the most addictive substances known. It may be taken several different ways. Classically, it is inhaled into the nose and absorbed through the nasal mucosa, damaging tissue, causing nosebleeds, and ultimately destroying the nasal septum. It can also be injected IV or subcutaneously (skin popping). Cocaine can be absorbed through all mucous membranes and even across the skin. In any form, the immediate effects of a given dose, including excitement and euphoria, last less than 1 hour.

Cocaine may also be smoked. Crack is pure cocaine. It melts at 93°F (33.9°C) and vaporizes at a slightly higher temperature. Therefore, crack is easily smoked. In this form, it reaches the capillary network of the lungs and can be absorbed into the body in seconds. The immediate outflow of blood from the heart speeds the drug to the brain, so its effect is felt at once. Smoked crack produces the most rapid means of absorption and, therefore, the most potent effect.

Acute cocaine overdose is a genuine emergency because patients are at high risk for seizures, cardiac dysrhythmias, and stroke. You may see blood pressure measurements as high as 250/150 mm Hg. Chronic cocaine use may cause hallucinations; patients experiencing "cocaine bugs" think that bugs are crawling out of their skin.

Be aware that patients who have been poisoned by a sympathomimetic may be paranoid, putting you and other health care clinicians in danger. Law enforcement officers should be at the scene to restrain the patient, if necessary. Do not leave the patient unattended and unmonitored during transport.

All of these patients need prompt transport to the ED. Give supplemental oxygen if necessary and be ready to provide suctioning. If the patient is already having a seizure, protect against self-injury.

Words of Wisdom

Some medications used to treat attention-deficit/hyperactivity disorder, such as amphetamines (eg, Adderall) and methylphenidate (eg, Ritalin, Concerta), also have sympathetic effects. While they may be safely prescribed by a physician, illicit use of these drugs, especially when smoked or injected intravenously, is associated with heart attack, stroke, and cardiac arrest.[11]

Synthetic Cathinones (Bath Salts)

Bath salts, or synthetic cathinones, are an emerging class of drugs similar to MDMA. The drug commonly includes the chemical methylenedioxypyrovalerone (MDPV). Bath salts should not be confused with products such as Epsom salt (magnesium sulfate), although selling them under this umbrella label has allowed their manufacturers and users to escape the legal restrictions imposed on illicit drugs. Brand names include Ivory Wave and Cloud Nine. Many states are working to make it illegal to manufacture or possess this drug.

Bath salts produce euphoria, increased mental clarity, and sexual arousal. Most users of this drug snort or insufflate the powder nasally. The effects reportedly last as long as 48 hours. Adverse effects include teeth grinding, appetite loss, muscle twitching, lip-smacking, confusion, gastrointestinal conditions, paranoia, headache, elevated heart rate, and hallucinations.

Keep the patient calm and transport. Consider ALS assistance; some of these patients may require chemical restraint to facilitate safe transport.

Cannabis

The flowering hemp plant, *Cannabis sativa*, from which hash, hash oil, and marijuana are derived, is used throughout the world. Tetrahydrocannabinol, or THC, is the chemical in the cannabis plant that produces its high. Smoking or vaping hashish or marijuana can produce euphoria, relaxation, and drowsiness. It also impairs short-term memory and the capacity to do complex thinking and work. In some people, the euphoria progresses to depression and confusion. An altered perception of time is common, and anxiety and panic can occur. With very high doses, some patients may experience hallucinations or become very anxious or paranoid. In these cases, keep the patient calm and provide transport. However, be aware that marijuana may be used as a vehicle to get other drugs into the body. For example, it may be laced with crack, fentanyl, or PCP.

More than one-half of the US population now resides in states that have legalized the recreational use of marijuana, and many other states have legalized the medical use of marijuana and products that contain THC.[12] As the move toward legalization has continued and as people have become more aware of the health risks associated with smoking, delivery methods have evolved. Many medical users opt against smoking marijuana and instead obtain THC in the form of edibles or baked goods, candies, and other food additives that have been infused with THC. The ingestion of marijuana can also lead to *cannabinoid hyperemesis syndrome*, characterized by chronic marijuana use and extreme nausea and vomiting that is relieved only by a hot shower or bath. Bathing can become compulsive in these patients. The definitive treatment for this condition is to stop using marijuana; however, these users often believe that more marijuana will help the nausea and continue to consume it.

Special Populations

ACCIDENTAL THC INGESTION IN CHILDREN

Edible products containing THC, such as infused gummies or chocolates, are attractive to children, leading to a dramatic increase in ED visits related to THC ingestion in children.[13] Common findings in young children include drowsiness, tachycardia, loss of balance, and vomiting. More serious effects are possible, depending on the amount consumed, and include hypotension, coma, seizures, and respiratory depression.

Synthetic Marijuana

Synthetic marijuana, or "spice," refers to a variety of herbal incense or smoking blends that resemble THC and produce a similar high. Synthetic marijuana is often marketed as a safe alternative to that drug under brand names such as K2 and Skunk. However, the chemicals commonly found in spice products have no medical benefit and have a high potential for misuse.[14] Powerful and unpredictable effects may result, ranging from simple euphoria to complete loss of consciousness.

Words of Wisdom

Both cannabidiol (CBD) and THC are derived from the *Cannabis sativa* plant; however, CBD comes from a variety called hemp that has very little THC. CBD does not have any of the psychoactive effects of THC and does not produce the same high. Further, it is not believed to have the potential for abuse and addiction and is therefore legal federally. Some research suggests that some forms of CBD may be helpful to treat anxiety, inflammation, and nerve pain.[15] The Food and Drug Administration (FDA) has approved one drug containing CBD (Epidiolex) to treat seizures related to several rare conditions. Because other CBD products are not regulated by the FDA, consumers cannot be assured of their purity.

Hallucinogens

A **hallucinogen** alters a person's sensory perceptions (**TABLE 22-5**). The classic hallucinogen is lysergic acid diethylamide (LSD). Use of another hallucinogen, phencyclidine (PCP, or angel dust), is relatively uncommon among young adults. PCP is a dissociative anesthetic that is easily synthesized and highly potent. Its effectiveness by oral, nasal, pulmonary, and IV routes makes it easy to add to other street drugs. It is dangerous because it causes severe behavioral changes in which people often inflict injury on themselves.

All of these agents cause visual hallucinations, intensify vision and hearing, and generally separate the user from reality. The user, of course, expects that the altered sensory state will be pleasurable. Often, however, it can be terrifying. At some point, you are bound to encounter patients who are having a "bad trip." They will usually have hypertension, tachycardia, anxiety, and paranoia.

TABLE 22-5 Common Hallucinogens

- Bufotenine (toad skin)
- *Datura stramonium* (jimsonweed)
- Dextromethorphan (DXM)
- Dimethyltryptamine (DMT)
- Ketamine
- LSD
- Mescaline (peyote)
- 3,4-Methylenedioxymethamphetamine (MDMA)
- Morning glory
- Nutmeg
- PCP
- Psilocybin (mushrooms)
- Salvia

Many hallucinogens have sympathomimetic properties. Your care for a patient who is having a bad reaction to a hallucinogenic agent is the same as that for a patient who has taken a sympathomimetic. Use a calm, professional manner, and provide emotional support. Do not use restraints unless you or the patient is in danger of injury. Follow the guidelines specified by local authorities. These patients may suddenly experience hallucinations or odd perceptions, so watch them carefully throughout transport. Never leave a patient who has taken a hallucinogen unattended and unmonitored. Request ALS assistance when appropriate.

Anticholinergic Agents

Anticholinergic agents are medications that block the parasympathetic nerves. The classic picture of a person who has taken too much of an anticholinergic medication is "hot as a hare, blind as a bat, dry as a bone, red as a beet, and mad as a hatter." In other words, the patient will exhibit hyperthermia, dilated pupils, dry skin and mucous membranes, reddened skin, and agitation or delirium. Common drugs with a significant anticholinergic effect include atropine, antihistamines such as diphenhydramine (Benadryl), *Datura stramonium* (jimsonweed), and certain tricyclic antidepressants such as amitriptyline (Elavil). With the exception of jimsonweed, these agents usually are not misused for recreational purposes; however, they may be taken as an intentional overdose. It is often difficult to distinguish between an anticholinergic overdose and a sympathomimetic overdose. Both groups of patients may be agitated and have tachycardia and dilated pupils.

In addition to its anticholinergic effects, a tricyclic antidepressant overdose may cause more serious and life-threatening effects because the medication may block the electrical conduction system in the heart, leading to lethal cardiac dysrhythmias. Patients with acute tricyclic antidepressant overdose must be transported immediately to the ED; they may appear "normal," but seizure and death can occur within 30 minutes. The seizures and cardiac dysrhythmias caused by a severe tricyclic antidepressant overdose are best treated in the hospital. If you work in a tiered system, consider calling for ALS backup when you are en route to the scene.

Cholinergic Agents

Cholinergic agents are medications that overstimulate the normal body functions controlled by the parasympathetic nervous system. These agents have been used for chemical warfare, such as during the sarin gas attack on the Tokyo subway system in 1995. These agents also occur in organophosphate insecticides, which are commonly used for lawn and garden care. A patient who has been poisoned by a cholinergic agent will exhibit excessive salivation or drooling, excessive mucus secretions, excessive urination, excessive tearing of the eyes, uncontrolled diarrhea, and an abnormal heart rate. The signs and symptoms of cholinergic drug poisoning are easy to remember using the mnemonic DUMBELS:

- **D** Diarrhea
- **U** Urination
- **M** Miosis (constriction of the pupils), muscle weakness
- **B** Bradycardia, bronchospasm, bronchorrhea (discharge of mucus from the lungs)
- **E** Emesis (vomiting)
- **L** Lacrimation (excessive tearing of the eyes)
- **S** Seizures, salivation, sweating

Alternatively, you can use the mnemonic SLUDGEM:

- **S** Salivation, sweating
- **L** Lacrimation (excessive tearing)
- **U** Urination
- **D** Defecation, drooling, diarrhea
- **G** Gastrointestinal upset and cramps
- **E** Emesis (vomiting)
- **M** Muscle twitching/miosis (pinpoint pupils)

Patients who have been poisoned will have excessive body secretions. In addition, patients may have bradycardia.

The most important consideration in caring for a patient who has been exposed to a cholinergic agent is to avoid exposure yourself. Because these agents may cling to a patient's clothing and skin, decontamination will take priority over prompt transport to the ED. In many jurisdictions, the hazmat team will provide decontamination and contain the exposure chemical.

To care for the exposed patient, hospital staff or paramedics can use the anticholinergic drug atropine to dry up the patient's secretions, followed by the use of pralidoxime to reverse the nerve agent's effect on the patient's nervous system. In the meantime, your priorities after decontamination are to decrease the secretions in the mouth and trachea that threaten to suffocate the patient and provide airway support.

The military has developed antidotes to nerve gas agents that responders can self-administer if the agents are available. In some areas across the country, these kits are issued to emergency medical clinicians depending on local protocols. The most common kit is the DuoDote Auto-Injector. The Antidote Treatment Nerve Agent Auto-Injector (ATNAA) is the military form of the DuoDote Auto-Injector.

The DuoDote Auto-Injector is a single auto-injector containing 2 mg of atropine and 600 mg of pralidoxime. If a known exposure to nerve agents or organophosphates with manifestation of signs and symptoms has occurred, use the antidote kit only on yourself. If your service carries these antidote kits, you should receive training on their proper use prior to administering them.

Miscellaneous Drugs

Accidental or intentional overdose with cardiac medications has become common because there are so many patients who have these medications prescribed for them. For example, children may ingest these medications at their grandparent's house, thinking they are candy. Another common scenario is older patients who have forgotten they have already taken their medication and take a second dose. Occasionally, people attempting suicide will take an overdose of cardiac medications if that is all they have available. The signs and symptoms of cardiac medication overdose depend on the medication ingested. These drugs may cause bleeding, cardiac dysrhythmias, unconsciousness, and even cardiac arrest. Most of these medications are powerful, so contact the poison center as soon as possible. Depending on local protocol, you may be ordered to administer activated charcoal, but check with the poison center first.

Aspirin poisoning is a potentially lethal condition. Ingesting too many aspirin tablets, acutely or chronically, is an emergency that may result in nausea, vomiting, hyperventilation, and ringing in the ears. Patients with this condition frequently have anxiety, confusion, tachypnea, and hyperthermia, and are in danger of having seizures. Rapidly transport these patients to the hospital.

When consumed in excess, acetaminophen becomes toxic. Overdosing with acetaminophen and combination medications containing acetaminophen is also common. Acetaminophen overdose is the leading cause of acute liver failure and a leading cause of death from acute liver failure in the United States.[16,17]

It is essential to determine what medications the patient takes or has taken, including OTC medications. Acetaminophen overdose, unintentional or intentional, must be treated promptly and aggressively.

Accidental acetaminophen overdose is as serious as intentional overdose. In fact, its effects can be worse because the patient is unaware of the continuous exposure to the toxin. For example, massive liver failure may not be apparent for a full week. In addition, patients may not provide the information necessary for a correct diagnosis. For this reason, gathering information at the scene is very important. By finding an empty acetaminophen bottle, you may save a patient's life. If a specific antidote is given early enough (before liver failure occurs), liver damage may be reduced or prevented.

Some alcohols, including methyl alcohol and ethylene glycol, are even more toxic than ethyl alcohol (drinking alcohol). Methyl alcohol is found in dry gas products and stove kits (Sterno); ethylene glycol is found in some antifreeze products. Both cause a feeling of intoxication. Left untreated, both will also cause severe tachypnea, blindness (methyl alcohol), kidney failure (ethylene glycol), and eventually death. Even ethyl alcohol can stop a patient's breathing if taken in too high a dose or too fast, particularly in children. Although methyl alcohol or ethylene glycol may be used as a substitute by a person with alcohol use disorder who is unable to obtain ethyl alcohol, they are more often taken by someone attempting suicide. In either case, prompt transport to the ED is essential.

TABLE 22-6 lists the poisonous substances that most commonly result in fatality when ingested.

Food Poisoning

Food poisoning is almost always caused by eating food that is contaminated by bacteria. The food may appear normal, with little or no decay or odor to suggest danger.

There are two main types of food poisoning. In one, the organism itself causes disease; in the other, the organism produces toxins that cause disease (**TABLE 22-7**).

TABLE 22-6 Common Fatal Ingested Poisons

- Acetaminophen
- Sedative-hypnotics (eg, alprazolam, diazepam, zolpidem) and antipsychotics
- Alcohols
- Opioids (eg, heroin, fentanyl, oxycodone)
- Stimulants and street drugs
- Calcium channel blockers (verapamil, nifedipine, diltiazem)
- Beta blockers (metoprolol, atenolol)
- Miscellaneous antidepressants (eg, bupropion, amitriptyline)
- Hypoglycemics (eg, insulin)
- Sedating antihistamines

Data from Gummin DD, Mowry JB, Beuhler MC, et al. 2023 Annual Report of the National Poison Data System (NPDS) from America's Poison Centers: 41st Annual Report. *Clin Toxicol (Phila)*. 2024;62(12):793–1027.

TABLE 22-7 Common Causes of Food Poisoning

- *Campylobacter*
- *Clostridium botulinum* toxin
- *Clostridium perfringens*
- *Cryptosporidium*
- *Cyclospora*
- *Escherichia coli*
- *Giardia lamblia*
- *Listeria monocytogenes*
- Norovirus
- Rotavirus
- *Salmonella*
- *Shigella*
- *Staphylococcus* toxin
- *Vibrio parahaemolyticus*
- *Yersinia enterocolitica*

One organism that produces direct effects of food poisoning is the *Salmonella* bacterium. Salmonellosis is a condition characterized by severe gastrointestinal symptoms within 72 hours of ingestion, including nausea, vomiting, abdominal pain, and diarrhea. In addition, patients with salmonellosis may be systemically ill with fever and generalized weakness. Some people are carriers of certain bacteria; although they may not become ill themselves, they may transmit diseases, particularly if they work in the food services industry. Usually, proper cooking kills bacteria, and proper cleanliness in the kitchen prevents the contamination of uncooked foods.

The more common cause of food poisoning is the ingestion of powerful toxins produced by bacteria, often in leftovers. The bacterium *Staphylococcus*, a common culprit, is quick to grow and produce toxins in foods that have been prepared in advance and kept too long, even in the refrigerator. Foods left unrefrigerated are a common vehicle for the development of staphylococcal toxins. Usually, staphylococcal food poisoning results in sudden gastrointestinal symptoms, including nausea, vomiting, and diarrhea. Although time frames may vary from person to person, these symptoms usually start within 2 to 3 hours after ingestion or as long as 8 to 12 hours after ingestion.

Although rare in the United States, the most severe result of food poisoning is botulism. This potentially fatal disease usually results from eating improperly canned food, in which the spores of *Clostridium* bacteria have grown and produced a toxin. The symptoms of botulism are neurologic: blurring of vision, weakness, and difficulty in speaking and breathing. Botulism can also cause muscle paralysis and is typically fatal when it reaches the muscles of respiration. Symptoms of botulism may develop as long as 4 days after ingestion or as early as the first 24 hours.

In general, do not try to determine the specific cause of acute gastrointestinal conditions. After all, severe vomiting may be a sign of food poisoning, a bowel obstruction requiring surgery, or poisoning by substances such as copper, arsenic, zinc, cadmium, scombrotoxin (fish poison), or *Clitocybe* or *Inocybe* mushrooms. Instead, gather as much history as possible from the patient and transport promptly to the hospital. When two or more people in one group have the same illness, take along some of the suspected food to the hospital. In advanced cases of botulism, you may have to assist ventilation and give basic life support.

Plant Poisoning

According to the National Poison Data System, tens of thousands of cases of poisoning from plants occur each year, some severe. Many household plants are poisonous if ingested; children have been known to nibble on the leaves (**TABLE 22-8**). Some poisonous plants cause local irritation of the skin; others can affect the circulatory system, the gastrointestinal tract, or the CNS. It is impossible for you to memorize every plant and poison, let alone their

TABLE 22-8 Common Toxic Plants

Scientific Name	Common Name
Abrus precatorius	Jequirity bean/rosary pea
Cicuta species	Water hemlock/wild carrot
Colchicum autumnale	Autumn crocus
Conium maculatum	Poison hemlock
Convallaria majalis	Lily of the valley
Datura species	Jimsonweed/stinkweed
Dieffenbachia	Dumbcane
Digitalis purpurea	Foxglove
Nerium oleander	Oleander or rose laurel
Nicotiana glauca	Tree tobacco
Phoradendron	Mistletoe
Phytolacca americana	Pokeweed
Rheum rhabarbarum	Rhubarb
Rhododendron	Rhododendron or azalea
Ricinus communis	Castor bean
Solarium nigrum	Nightshade
Zygadenus species	Death camas

effects (**FIGURE 22-11**). You can and should do the following:

1. Assess the patient's airway and vital signs.
2. Notify the regional poison center for assistance in identifying the plant.
3. Take the plant to the ED. If this is not possible, take a photo of the plant.
4. Provide prompt transport.

Irritation of the skin and/or mucous membranes is a problem with the common houseplant

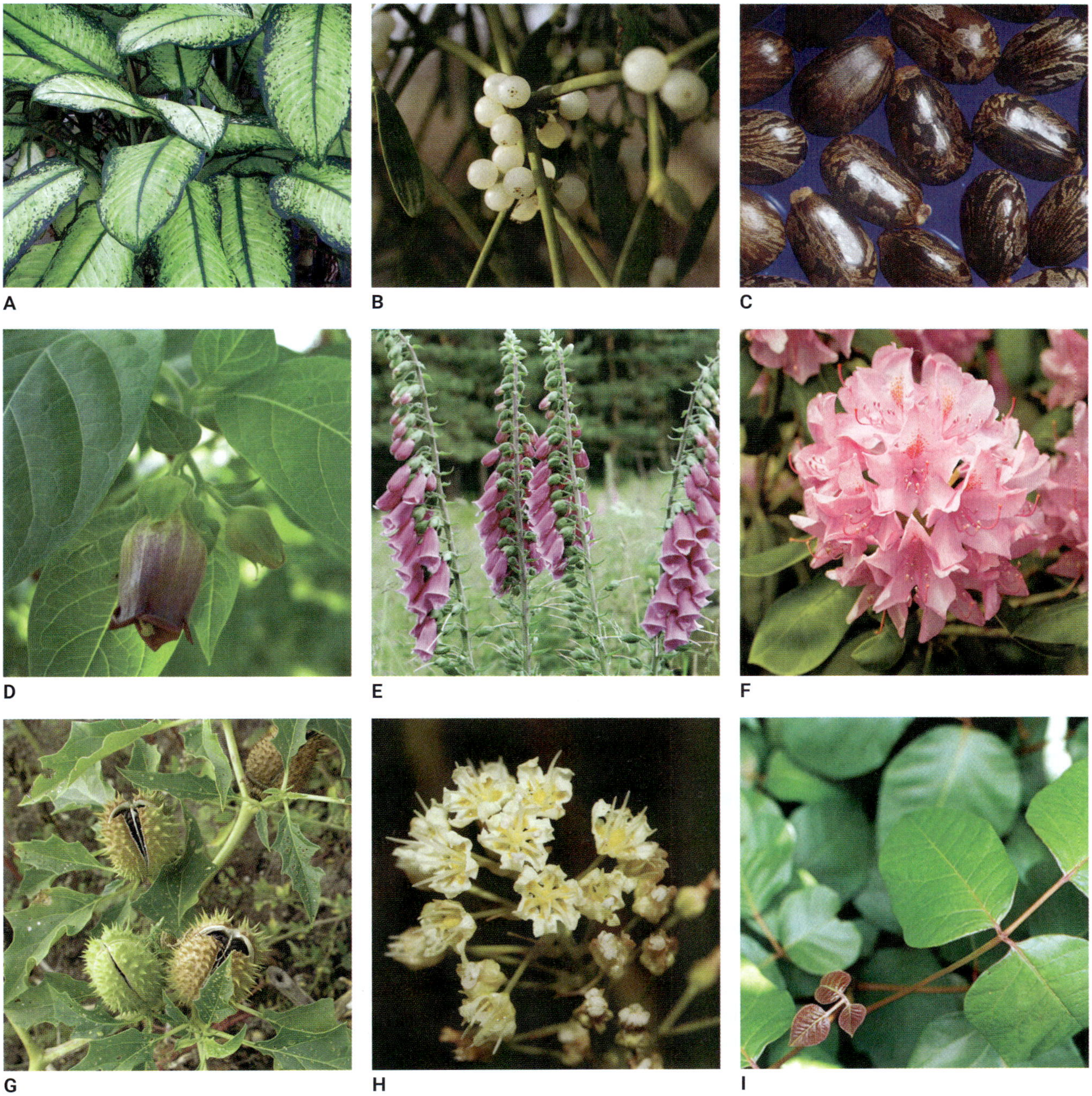

FIGURE 22-11 The toxins in these common poisonous plants are often ingested or absorbed through the skin. **A.** Dieffenbachia. **B.** Mistletoe. **C.** Castor bean. **D.** Nightshade. **E.** Foxglove. **F.** Rhododendron. **G.** Jimsonweed. **H.** Death camas. **I.** Poison ivy.

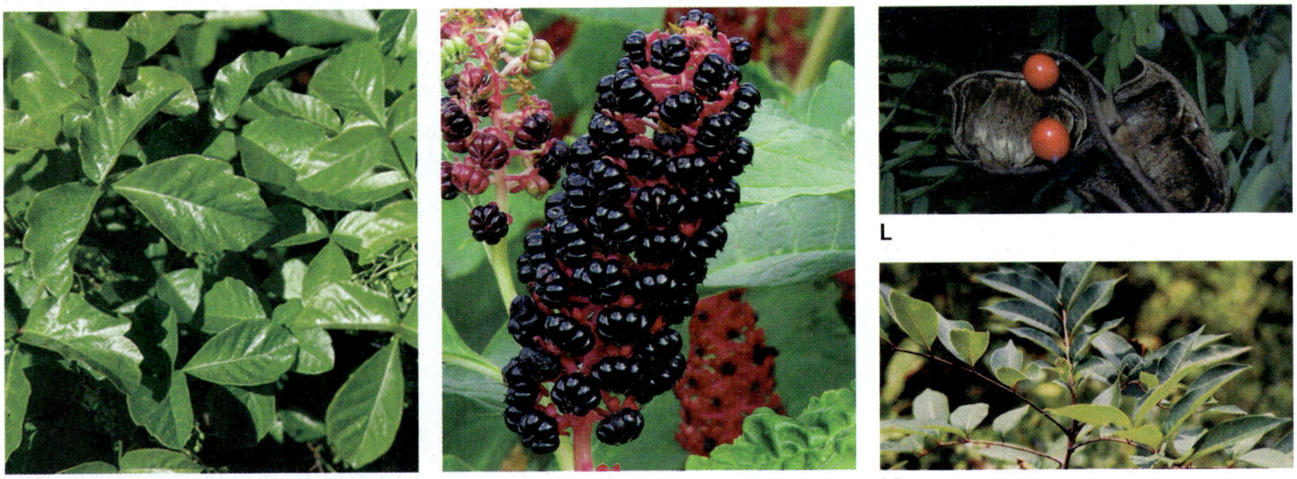

FIGURE 22-11 **J.** Poison oak. **K.** Pokeweed. **L.** Rosary pea. **M.** Poison sumac.

called dieffenbachia, which resembles elephant ears. When chewed, a single leaf may irritate the lining of the upper airway enough to cause difficulty swallowing, breathing, and speaking. For this reason, dieffenbachia has been called "dumb cane." In rare circumstances, the airway may be completely obstructed. Emergency medical treatment of dieffenbachia poisoning includes maintaining an open airway, giving oxygen when necessary, and transporting the patient promptly to the hospital for respiratory support. Assess the patient for airway difficulties throughout transport. If necessary, provide positive-pressure ventilation.

Special Populations

Considerations for Geriatric Patients

Geriatric patients are susceptible to toxicity for several reasons. Consider the case of an accidental overdose or poisoning. The older patient may have forgotten that the medication had been taken and take repeated doses. Alcohol use disorder can make a patient more likely to make medication mistakes. Many older patients take multiple prescriptions (**polypharmacy**) that may negatively interfere with each other, resulting in increased effects or unwanted drug interactions. The aging process may also impair the older patient's ability to metabolize or excrete the poison. The drug could quickly accumulate to toxic levels and become fatal in lesser doses than in a younger person.

If an older person inhales a poison, even in tiny quantities, lung damage can be severe. Consider the decreased lung capacity and ability to exchange oxygen and carbon dioxide in an older patient's lungs. Pulmonary function could be worsened to potentially fatal levels with the inhalation of minute amounts of poison. For poisons that are absorbed by or injected into the skin, reduced circulation to the skin can decrease or delay absorption into the body. Watch for an increased reaction or irritation at the skin site.

A geriatric patient may also intentionally overdose in a suicide attempt. Be alert for any indication of an intentional overdose or poisoning, even though the patient might deny an attempted suicide.

Considerations for Pediatric Patients

As mentioned previously, accidental poisoning is common among children. The most common fatal ingestions in children younger than 5 years are related to analgesics, stimulants, street drugs, batteries, alcohols, and antidepressants. The most frequently reported sources of poisoning in children are listed in **TABLE 22-9**. Accidental poisoning in children usually occurs at home.

The signs and symptoms of poisoning vary widely, depending on the substance and the age and weight of the pediatric patient. The child may appear normal at first, even in serious cases, or may be confused, sleepy, or unconscious. With some substances, one pill may be enough to cause death in a small child.

TABLE 22-9 Common Sources of Poisoning in Children

- Household cleaning products (eg, bleach, furniture polish)
- Analgesics
- Cosmetics and personal care products
- Foreign bodies, toys, and similar objects (eg, button batteries, water beads)
- Dietary supplements/herbals
- Antihistamines
- Vitamins
- Topical preparations (eg, ointments, oils)
- Pesticides
- Plants

Gummin DD, Mowry JB, Beuhler MC, et al. 2023 Annual Report of the National Poison Data System (NPDS) from America's Poison Centers: 41st Annual Report. *Clin Toxicol (Phila)*. 2024;62(12):793–1027.

Infants may be poisoned as a result of being fed a harmful substance by a sibling, parent, or caregiver, or as a result of child abuse. Infants can be exposed to drugs and poisons left on floors and carpeting. They can also be exposed in a setting in which harmful drugs are being smoked. Toddlers are curious and often ingest poisons when they find them in the home or garage (**FIGURE 22-12**). Adolescents are more likely to have ingested alcohol and street drugs while partying or during a suicide attempt.

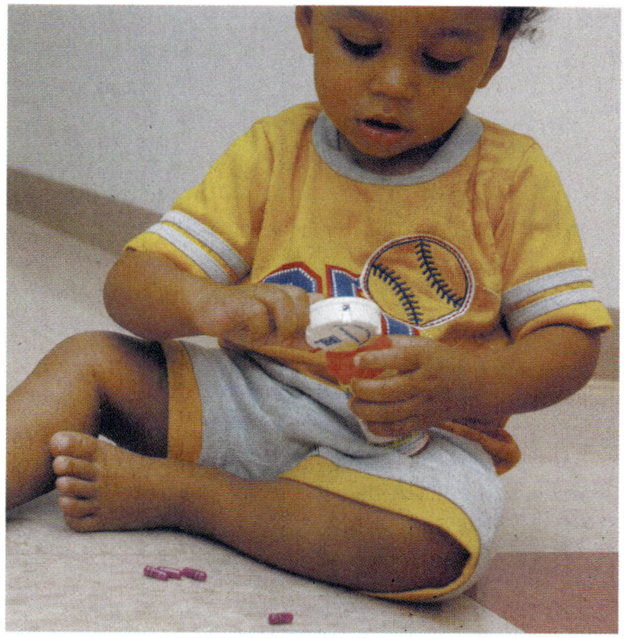

FIGURE 22-12 A curious child will try to taste or swallow almost any substance. A common victim of accidental ingestion of dangerous compounds is the unwatched toddler.

After you have completed your primary assessment, ask the parent or caregiver the following questions:

- What is the substance or substances involved?
- Approximately how much of the substance was ingested or involved in the exposure (eg, number of pills, amount of liquid)?
- What time did the incident occur?
- Are there any changes in behavior or level of consciousness?

YOU are the EMT

You begin transport to the hospital, which is located a short distance away. You and your partner monitor the patient's airway carefully. The patient's vital signs remain normal. You call in your radio report to the hospital. The estimated time of arrival is 6 minutes.

Recording Time: 17 Minutes	
Level of consciousness	Conscious, but sleepy
Respirations	14 breaths/min; adequate depth
Pulse	72 beats/min; strong and regular
Skin	Baseline color, warm, and dry
Blood pressure	108/60 mm Hg
Oxygen saturation (Spo_2)	100% (on oxygen)

9. What additional treatment is required for this patient?

10. What information should you relay to the hospital staff during your verbal report?

- Was there any choking or coughing after the exposure? (These can be signs of airway involvement.)

Treatment of a pediatric patient exposed to a poisonous substance is similar to that for an adult. First perform an external decontamination. Remove tablets or fragments from the patient's mouth, and wash or brush poison from the skin. Treatment is supportive: Assess and maintain the child's ABCs and monitor breathing. Provide oxygen and perform ventilations if necessary. If the patient demonstrates signs and symptoms of shock, position the child supine, keep the child warm, and transport promptly to the nearest appropriate hospital.

When you respond to a poisoning of a pediatric patient, remember to remain calm and control the scene. Poisonings can be emotional for the parents or caregivers involved because of the potential for self-blame.

Words of Wisdom

Calling Poison Control early is especially important when the call involves an infant or child. Some substances that are not typically considered lethal, such as baby oil, are potentially lethal if the child vomits and aspirates the oil into their lungs. Early steps in the care of the poisoned patient can be essential to their recovery.

Street Smarts

Consider initiating a community program to help make homes safer for children. Identifying cleaning agents that resemble children's drinks and placing them out of reach, placing child locks on cabinets, identifying poisonous plants, and educating parents about the potential for accidental poisoning or exposure could save a life.

YOU are the EMT SUMMARY

1. In addition to providing immediate lifesaving treatment, what else should you do when you arrive at this scene?

Never make assumptions about the scene. Although the home is located in an affluent neighborhood with law enforcement officers available at the scene, always remember that your safety is of the utmost importance. If possible, obtain information from family members or bystanders at the scene. This information is essential to the proper treatment of your patient. In this case, the father reported that he was awakened when the patient and her friends came home from a party and were making a lot of noise. A full secondary assessment may reveal injuries or symptoms that are not immediately apparent. It may also be useful to ask if others are having the same symptoms: Could there be an environmental exposure risk or other group exposure? Because both parents are available, obtain a full SAMPLE history.

2. How can knowledge of various signs and symptoms caused by different types of medications improve the care you provide to a patient?

When you assess a patient who has overdosed on a medication or other substance, a careful assessment may help you identify a series of signs and symptoms that indicate a particular type of toxic exposure, thereby allowing you to direct your treatment accordingly. For some toxins (eg, barbiturate-type sedative drug overdose), only supportive treatment such as oxygen or ventilation might be done, whereas for others, an antidote (eg, oral glucose for an insulin or oral diabetes medication overdose) may be available. In some cases, activated charcoal may be useful, if permitted by local protocols. Knowing that a patient has taken or been exposed to certain types of overdoses (eg, stimulant-type drugs) may make you better prepared if agitation, hallucinations, or even seizures develop.

3. On the basis of your initial assessment, what is the most appropriate treatment for this patient?

Your patient is sleepy and not responding without stimulation. She has vomited but her airway is currently patent. Her ventilation status is inadequate and requires immediate attention.

With the help of your partner and the members of the fire crew, position the patient supine. Ensure the patient and other clinicians are not injured in the process. You have assigned a firefighter to manage her airway with a bag-mask device and an airway adjunct as she does not have a gag reflex. Blood glucose level should be determined. This patient requires aggressive treatment and monitoring.

YOU are the EMT SUMMARY continued

4. On the basis of the patient's initial presentation, what type of drug should you suspect she overdosed on?

On the basis of the patient's initial presentation—unconsciousness, hypoventilation, and pinpoint pupils—you should suspect that she has overdosed on an opioid.

As an EMT, your job is to recognize the signs and symptoms that are associated with these types of drugs, begin immediate treatment to support the ABCs, administer naloxone, and transport the patient to the hospital without delay.

5. Would activated charcoal benefit this patient? Why or why not?

There are several reasons why activated charcoal is not indicated for this patient. First, the patient is unconscious, is unable to protect her own airway, and clearly cannot swallow. Pouring anything into her mouth would lead to aspiration, thus substantially increasing her chance of death.

On the basis of the patient's clinical presentation, it is clear that at least some of the medications she ingested are no longer in her stomach. Therefore, it may be too late for charcoal, even if she was alert enough to safely swallow it. She is now experiencing systemic effects that are causing compromise of her breathing and circulatory status. Activated charcoal can only absorb toxins in the gastrointestinal tract, so it has no effect on the drug or drugs already absorbed into the system. There are also many drugs/toxins that are not neutralized by charcoal.

6. Why is naloxone being given to this patient?

Naloxone blocks opioid receptors in the body and reverses the effects of an opioid overdose. The patient's presentation indicates that one (or many) of the unknown ingested medications are opioids, based on the patient's pinpoint pupils, level of sedation, and decreased ventilation; therefore, naloxone is indicated.

7. What other issues about this patient should concern you?

Although the patient's condition has improved following the administration of naloxone, the fact remains that the patient also ingested an unknown quantity of unknown medications. Because the drugs were taken orally, they may be absorbed or metabolized over a longer period and the symptoms could return. Also, other drugs that may have been ingested could take longer to be absorbed and have maximum effect. Other ingested medications may have temporarily had their effects decreased by the opioids (eg, stimulants). These medications may begin to produce symptoms as time passes. By no means is the patient out of danger.

8. How would this patient's presentation have differed had she overdosed on a sympathomimetic?

Unlike CNS depressants, sympathomimetics are CNS stimulants. A sympathomimetic is any substance that mimics the effects of the sympathetic (fight-or-flight) nervous system. When the sympathetic nervous system is stimulated, it releases epinephrine and norepinephrine, resulting in hypertension, tachycardia, and restlessness or agitation.

Had the patient overdosed on a sympathomimetic, her clinical presentation would have been the exact opposite. Her vital functions, such as breathing, heart rate, and blood pressure, would have significantly increased. Furthermore, she would likely have experienced paranoia, delusions, and disorganized behavior. She may even have experienced heart dysrhythmias or seizures.

9. What additional treatment is required for this patient?

Further treatment for this patient is mainly supportive; closely monitor her ABCs and be alert for the recurrence of CNS depression (eg, decreased level of consciousness, hypoventilation, hypotension). Monitor her vital signs at regular intervals.

Naloxone is a short-acting reversal agent compared with most opioids. Assisted ventilation and additional naloxone may be required if the patient lapses back into CNS depression.

10. What information should you relay to the hospital staff during your verbal report?

Your verbal (handoff) report at the hospital should be more in-depth than what was provided over the radio. Advise the receiving nurse or physician of how you found the patient and the suspected circumstances leading up to the onset of her symptoms, what you initially did to treat her, and how she responded to your treatment.

Inform the hospital staff of the patient's condition en route to the hospital, and advise them of any changes, good or bad, that may have occurred after you gave your radio report.

Prep Kit

Ready for Review

- Poisons act acutely or chronically to destroy or impair body cells.
- If you believe a patient may have taken a poisonous substance, support the ABCs and notify medical direction.
- Treatment of the patient may also entail collecting any evidence of the type of poison that was used and taking it to the hospital; diluting and physically removing the poisonous agent; providing respiratory support; and transporting the patient promptly to the hospital.
- Emergency treatment may include administration of an antidote, usually at the hospital, if an antidote exists.
- A poison can be introduced into the body in one of four ways:
  - Inhalation
  - Absorption (surface contact)
  - Ingestion
  - Injection
- It is impossible to remove or dilute injected poisons from the body, making these cases especially urgent.
- Consult medical direction and/or poison control for advice on the care of the poisoned patient based on local protocols.
- Move patients who have inhaled poison to fresh air; be prepared to use supplemental oxygen via a nonrebreathing mask and/or ventilatory support via a bag-mask device if necessary.
- With absorbed or surface contact poisons, avoid contaminating yourself. Remove all contaminated substances and clothing from the patient, and flood the affected part.
- Most poisonings occur by ingestion, including plants, contaminated food, and most drugs. Consider activated charcoal for ingested toxins, as permitted by local protocol.
- One of the most commonly used drugs in the United States is alcohol. It can depress the CNS and can cause respiratory depression. You must support the airway in such cases and be prepared for the patient to vomit.
- Opioids, sedative-hypnotic drugs, and inhalants can also depress the CNS and can cause respiratory depression.
- Naloxone is an antidote that reverses the effects of opioid overdose. Indications for this drug include agonal respirations or apnea. To minimize the risk of hypoxia, ventilate the patient while preparing to administer naloxone.
- Take special care with patients who have used inhalants due to the risk of seizures or sudden death.
- Sympathomimetics, including cocaine, stimulate the CNS, causing hypertension, tachycardia, seizures, and dilated pupils. Patients who have taken these drugs may be paranoid, as may patients who have taken hallucinogens.
- Anticholinergic medications, often taken in suicide attempts, may cause the patient to present with hyperthermia, dilated pupils, dry skin and mucous membranes, reddened/darkened skin, and agitation or delirium. An overdose of tricyclic antidepressants can lead to cardiac dysrhythmias.
- The symptoms of cholinergic medications, which include organophosphate insecticides, can be remembered by the mnemonic DUMBELS (Diarrhea; Urination; Miosis [constriction of the pupils], muscle weakness; Bradycardia, bronchospasm, bronchorrhea [discharge of mucus from the lungs]; Emesis [vomiting]; Lacrimation [excessive tearing of the eyes]; Seizures, salivation, sweating) or SLUDGEM (Salivation, sweating; Lacrimation [excessive tearing of the eyes]; Urination; Defecation, drooling, diarrhea; Gastrointestinal upset and cramps; Emesis [vomiting]; Muscle twitching/miosis [pinpoint pupils]).
- Two main types of food poisoning cause gastrointestinal symptoms.

Prep Kit continued

- In one type, bacteria in the food directly cause disease, such as salmonellosis.
- In the other type, bacteria such as *Staphylococcus* produce powerful toxins, often in leftover food. The most severe form of toxin ingestion is botulism; the first neurologic symptoms may appear as late as 4 days after ingestion.

- Plant poisoning can affect the circulatory system, the gastrointestinal system, and the CNS. Some plants, such as dieffenbachia, irritate the skin or mucous membranes and may cause obstruction of the airway.
- When caring for older adults, keep in mind the possibility of multiple drug interactions and dosing errors.
- Children may ingest poisons while exploring their household environment. They may also be exposed to poisons deliberately (ie, abuse) or accidentally by others.
- Always remember the importance of scene safety.

Vital Vocabulary

addiction A state of overwhelming obsession or physical need to continue the use of a substance.

antidote A substance that is used to neutralize or counteract a poison.

delirium tremens (DTs) A severe withdrawal syndrome seen in alcoholics who are deprived of ethyl alcohol; characterized by restlessness, fever, sweating, disorientation, agitation, and seizures; can be fatal if untreated.

emesis Vomiting.

hallucinogen An agent that produces false perceptions in any one of the five senses.

hematemesis Vomiting blood.

hypnotic A sleep-inducing effect or agent.

ingestion Swallowing; taking a substance by mouth.

opioid A synthetically produced medication, drug, or agent that acts as a central nervous system depressant and produces insensibility or stupor; used to relieve pain.

overdose An excessive quantity of a drug that, when taken or administered, can have toxic or lethal consequences.

poison A substance whose chemical action could damage structures or impair function when introduced into the body.

polypharmacy The use of multiple medications on a regular basis.

safety data sheet (SDS) A form, provided by manufacturers and compounders (blenders) of chemicals, containing information about chemical composition, physical and chemical properties, health and safety hazards, emergency response, and waste disposal of a specific material; formerly known as a material safety data sheet (MSDS).

sedative A substance that decreases activity and excitement.

stimulant An agent that produces an excited state.

substance misuse The use of any substance in a manner other than its intended design to produce a desired effect.

tolerance The need for increasing amounts of a drug to obtain the same effect.

toxicology The study of toxic or poisonous substances.

toxidrome A collection of signs and symptoms associated with a class of poison; aids in the identification of certain toxins.

toxin A poison or harmful substance.

Prep Kit continued

References

1. Agrawal S, Khazaeni B. Acetaminophen toxicity. *StatPearls*. National Library of Medicine website. https://www.ncbi.nlm.nih.gov/books/NBK441917/. Updated June 9, 2023. Accessed January 24, 2025.
2. National Poison Data System. America's Poison Centers website. https://www.aapcc.org/national-poison-data-system. Accessed January 24, 2025.
3. Volkow ND, Gordon JA, Koob GF. Choosing appropriate language to reduce the stigma around mental illness and substance use disorders. *Neuropsychopharmacology*. 2021;46(13):2230–2232.
4. Alcohol use and your health. Centers for Disease Control and Prevention website. https://www.cdc.gov/alcohol/about-alcohol-use/. Published January 14, 2025. Accessed January 24, 2025.
5. Simon KM, Levy SJ, Bukstein OG. Adolescent substance use disorders. *NEJM Evid*. 2022;1(6). doi:10.1056/EVIDra2200051
6. Health disparities in suicide. Centers for Disease Control and Prevention website. https://www.cdc.gov/suicide/facts/disparities-in-suicide.html#age. Published May 16, 2023. Accessed January 24, 2025.
7. Understanding the opioid overdose epidemic. Centers for Disease Control and Prevention website. https://www.cdc.gov/overdose-prevention/about/understanding-the-opioid-overdose-epidemic.html. Published November 1, 2024. Accessed January 24, 2025.
8. Kramarow EA, Tejada-Vera B. Drug overdose deaths in adults aged 65 and over: United States, 2000–2020. *NCHS Data Brief*. 2022;(455):1–8.
9. Inhalants. US Drug Enforcement Administration website. https://www.dea.gov/factsheets/inhalants. Accessed January 24, 2025.
10. Chemical suicides: the risk to emergency responders. Chemical Hazards Emergency Medical Management website. https://chemm.hhs.gov/chemicalsuicide.htm. Updated December 26, 2024. Accessed January 24, 2025.
11. Nissen SE. ADHD drugs and cardiovascular risk. *N Engl J Med*. 2006;354(14):1445–1448.
12. Center for Behavioral Health Statistics and Quality, Substance Abuse and Mental Health Services Administration (SAMSHA). *Key Substance Use and Mental Health Indicators in the United States: Results From the 2023 National Survey on Drug Use and Health* (HHS Publication No. PEP24-07-021, NSDUH Series H-59). SAMSHA website. https://www.samhsa.gov/data/report/2023-nsduh-annual-national-report. Published 2024. Accessed January 24, 2025.
13. Pepin LC, Simon MW, Banerji S, Leonard J, Hoyte CO, Wang GS. Toxic tetrahydrocannabinol (THC) dose in pediatric cannabis edible ingestions. *Pediatrics*. 2023;152(3):e2023061374. doi:10.1542/peds.2023-061374
14. Drug facts: spice (synthetic marijuana). National Institute on Drug Abuse website. https://nida.nih.gov/sites/default/files/spice_1.pdf. Published December 2012. Accessed January 24, 2025.
15. Grinspoon P. Cannabidiol (CBD): what we know and what we don't. Harvard Health Publishing website. https://www.health.harvard.edu/blog/cannabidiol-cbd-what-we-know-and-what-we-dont-2018082414476. Published April 4, 2024. Accessed January 24, 2025.
16. US Food and Drug Administration. Prescription drug products containing acetaminophen: actions to reduce liver injury from unintentional overdose. Regulations.gov website. https://www.regulations.gov/document/FDA-2011-N-0021-0001. Published January 14, 2011. Accessed January 24, 2025.
17. Farrell SE. Acetaminophen toxicity. Medscape website. https://emedicine.medscape.com/article/820200-overview?form=fpf. Updated February 2, 2024. Accessed January 24, 2025.

Additional Resources

Acetaminophen. US Food and Drug Administration website. https://www.fda.gov/drugs/information-drug-class/acetaminophen. Updated June 9, 2022. Accessed January 24, 2025.

Alcohol facts and statistics. National Institute on Alcohol Abuse and Alcoholism website. https://www.niaaa.nih.gov/publications/brochures-and-fact-sheets/alcohol-facts-and-statistics. Updated June 2024. Accessed January 24, 2025.

Drug overdose deaths: facts and figures. National Institute on Drug Abuse website. https://www.drugabuse.gov/related-topics/trends-statistics/overdose-death-rates. Published August 2024. Accessed January 24, 2025.

National Association of State EMS Officials. *National EMS Scope of Practice Model 2019*. Washington, DC: National Highway Traffic Safety Administration; February 2019. Report No. DOT HS 812-666. https://www.ems.gov/assets/National_EMS_Scope_of_Practice_Model_2019.pdf. Accessed January 24, 2025.

National Highway Traffic Safety Administration. *National Emergency Medical Services Education Standards*. EMS.gov website. https://www.ems.gov/assets/EMS_Education-Standards_2021_FNL.pdf. Published January 2021. Accessed January 24, 2025.

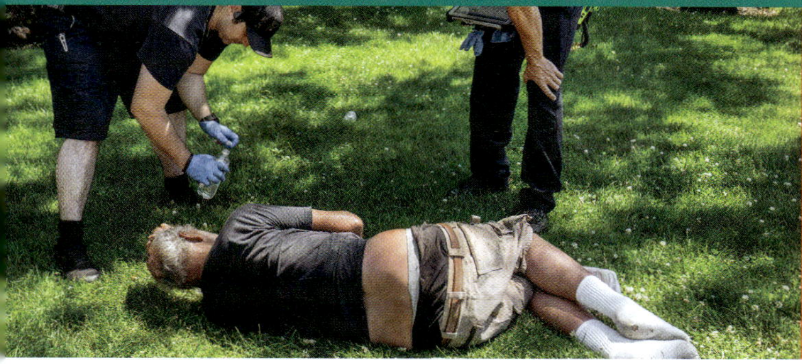

Chapter 23

Behavioral Health Emergencies

NATIONAL EMS EDUCATION STANDARD COMPETENCIES

Medicine

Applies knowledge to provide basic emergency care and transportation based on assessment findings for an acutely ill patient.

Psychiatric or Behavioral Emergencies

- Basic principles of the mental health system (p 871)
- Patterns of violence, abuse, and neglect (Chapter 35, *Patients With Special Challenges*)
- Acute psychosis (pp 877–878)
- Suicide ideation (pp 873–875)
- Delirium with agitation (also called *hyperactive delirium with severe agitation*; formerly referred to as *excited delirium*) (p 877)
- Anxiety (pp 871–872, 875–876)
- Depression (pp 871–872)
- Medical fear (Chapter 4, *Communications and Documentation*)
- Substance use disorder (p 877, Chapter 22, *Toxicology*)
- Posttraumatic stress disorder (pp 875–876)

KNOWLEDGE OBJECTIVES

1. Distinguish between patients with a mental illness and a behavioral health emergency. (p 870)
2. Know the main principles of how the mental health care system functions. (p 871)
3. Explain how the signs and symptoms of medical and trauma emergencies may overlap those of a behavioral health emergency. (p 871)
4. Describe patient assessment and care relating to depression. (pp 871–872)
5. Describe patient assessment and care relating to a bipolar disorder. (p 872)
6. Describe patient assessment and care relating to schizophrenia. (p 873)
7. Explain how to recognize the behavior of a patient at risk of suicide and how to care for this patient. (pp 873–875)
8. Recognize issues specific to posttraumatic stress disorder. (pp 875–876)
9. Describe patient assessment and care relating to dementia. (p 876)
10. Describe patient assessment and care relating to delirium. (p 877)
11. Describe patient assessment and care relating to a substance use disorder. (p 877)
12. Describe patient assessment and care relating to acute psychosis. (pp 877–878)

13. Describe situations that may pose a greater risk of violence and measures the emergency medical technician (EMT) should take to remain safe. (p 879)
14. Explain special considerations for assessing and treating patients with a behavioral crisis or behavioral health emergency. (pp 880–884)
15. Describe methods used to restrain patients. (pp 886–888)
16. Discuss the medical and legal aspects of caring for patients with a behavioral health emergency. (p 890)

SKILLS OBJECTIVE

1. Demonstrate the techniques used to restrain a patient. (p 888, Skill Drill 23-1)

Introduction

Behavior can be defined as the way in which individuals interact with their environment. As an EMT, you will frequently care for patients experiencing behavioral health emergencies. Abnormal behavior may result from an acute medical condition, mental illness, mind-altering substances, stress, or myriad other causes. In this chapter, you will learn how to recognize, assess, and treat a person who exhibits signs and symptoms of a behavioral health emergency.

Mental Illness Versus Behavioral Health Emergency

Although this chapter addresses a select few forms of mental illness, it is important to understand that many behavioral emergency calls do not involve patients with a mental illness. Often, the behavioral health emergency arises when an otherwise healthy person has an extreme or dangerous reaction to a stressor. It is important to understand the distinctions between these situations.

Defining Mental Illness

In general, a **mental illness** (sometimes referred to as a psychiatric illness) is a chronic health condition involving changes in behavior, thinking, and/or emotion that significantly interferes with the patient's ability to function in daily life. In most cases, to be diagnosed with a mental illness, the patient must present with the signs and symptoms for several weeks or longer. Many of these conditions are thought to have a biologic cause, and without treatment, the patient may have trouble relating to people, holding a job, or caring for their most basic needs. Examples of mental illness include schizophrenia, bipolar disorder, major depressive disorder, eating disorders, anxiety disorders, and substance use disorders.

Defining a Behavioral Health Emergency

Throughout life, people experience various emotional stressors, such as the death of a loved one, the end of a relationship, academic struggles, or the loss of a job. Usually, they cope with these stressors in reasonable ways over a reasonable time. However, think of the stress bucket analogy: when the bucket overflows with stressors, the person's coping strategies have been overwhelmed and negative health consequences may occur. (Chapter 2, *Workforce Safety and Wellness*, describes the stress bucket analogy in greater detail.) A **behavioral health emergency**, sometimes referred to as a behavioral health crisis, is any situation in which a person's behavior poses a threat to themselves or others or prevents them from caring for themselves or functioning effectively in their community.[1]

Mental Health Crisis Care Systems

In many communities across the United States, the lack of adequate and well-integrated mental health crisis care often leaves emergency medical services (EMS) and law enforcement to act as the default crisis response system. Connecting patients with appropriate mental health care requires strong partnerships between EMS, law enforcement, and crisis care systems within a community. Without comprehensive crisis care systems, mental illness is often criminalized, leading to tragic outcomes for patients, clinicians, and law enforcement personnel. Integrated systems can improve patient outcomes, reduce justice system involvement, and end the practice of psychiatric boarding in emergency departments (EDs).

The three core elements of a crisis system include a crisis call center, **mobile integrated health care (MIH)**, and crisis receiving and stabilization facilities.[2] In 2020, Congress designated the 9-8-8 dialing code to be operated through the National Suicide Prevention Line; 9-8-8 is specifically designed to assist people with behavioral crises, including emotional distress, suicidal ideation, or problematic substance use.[3] In some systems, EMTs may be part of an MIH program that offers community-based intervention to patients in need wherever they are. These programs help avoid unnecessary contact with the ED and justice system. MIH teams consist of licensed or credentialed clinicians capable of assessing the needs of the patient as well as peers. Because the ED is not always the best resource for every patient, specialized crisis receiving facilities have been established in some communities. They offer a "no wrong door" access to mental health and substance use care, accepting referrals from EMS, law enforcement, other health care professionals, or walk-ins. EMS systems are beginning to include these alternative destinations within their transport protocols. As an EMT, become familiar with the systems and resources available for patients with behavioral health crises in your community and expect these resources to continue evolving.

Conditions That Resemble Behavioral Health Emergencies

When assessing any patient presenting with altered, bizarre, or otherwise abnormal behavior, always remember that the person may be experiencing an underlying medical emergency or traumatic injury. Never assume that a person's behavior is caused by a mental illness. Perform a thorough patient assessment to rule out underlying causes of **altered mental status**, such as the following:

- Stroke
- Hypo- or hyperglycemia
- Traumatic brain injury
- Brain tumor
- Seizure (postictal)
- Drug or alcohol intoxication
- Poisoning or exposure to toxins
- Sepsis (ie, systemic infection)
- Urinary tract infection (particularly in geriatric patients)
- Electrolyte imbalance
- Any condition that reduces the delivery of blood or oxygen to the brain

As an EMT, your priority when caring for the patient is addressing any potentially life-threatening emergency, such as giving glucose to treat hypoglycemia. A psychiatric diagnosis is not made until alternative causes of altered behavior have been ruled out. This diagnosis typically requires evaluation by a physician. Maintain a high index of suspicion that a life-threatening condition is responsible for the unusual behavior.

Common Behavioral Health Emergencies

Depression

Depression (officially known as major depressive disorder) is a **psychiatric disorder** that negatively affects a person's mood, with feelings of sadness, despair, and hopelessness interfering with their normal daily functioning. People who have been diagnosed with depression have at least five of the following symptoms over a 2-week period that are not explained by other medical conditions[4]:

- Depressed mood (feeling sad, empty, hopeless)
- Greatly decreased interest or pleasure in activities they usually enjoy
- Significant weight loss or gain
- Insomnia or excessive sleeping
- Motor agitation or slowing
- Fatigue or loss of energy
- Feelings of worthlessness or excessive/inappropriate guilt
- Decreased ability to think, concentrate, or make decisions
- Thoughts of suicide (with or without planning or attempting suicide)

Often, when assessing the patient who has a major depressive disorder, the EMT will observe a person who appears sad and tearful, or who displays little emotion, even when describing profound sadness or hopelessness. Although most patients who have depression are not suicidal, this disease does increase the risk of suicide, so it is important to ask the patient if they have thought about hurting or killing themselves as you obtain their history.

While treatment options for depression, including psychotherapy, medications, and applied energy to the brain (eg, electroconvulsive therapy, deep brain stimulation, transcranial magnetic stimulation), are not within the EMT's scope of practice, you may be able to guide these patients to further help. People with depression may not realize there are resources available to help them through a difficult time. Keep a list of helpful numbers, such as the local crisis center, psychiatric centers, and suicide and crisis lifeline (9-8-8), to provide to patients. Your simple act of caring may save a life.

Words of Wisdom

Changes in endocrine function, such as those that occur during menopause, can be a contributing factor to depression.

Depression Among Older Adults

Depression is not part of normal aging, but rather a medical disease. This common, often debilitating psychiatric disorder affects millions of older adults. Older adults residing in long-term care facilities are even more likely to experience depression.[5] In contrast with the normal emotional experiences of sadness, grief, loss, and temporary bad moods, depression is extreme and persistent and can interfere significantly with an older adult's ability to function.

The good news is that depression is treatable with medication and therapy. For many older adults, simply reestablishing relationships with the community or with family will lessen the severity of the illness. The bad news is that if depression goes unrecognized or untreated in adults 75 years and older, it is associated with a higher suicide rate than in any other age group.[6] Depression in older patients can mimic the effects of many other medical problems (such as dementia). Risk factors for depression in older people include a history of depression, chronic disease, and loss of function, independence, or significant others.

It is impossible to predict which older adults will have depression, but studies indicate that substance use disorder, isolation, prescription medication use, and chronic medical conditions all contribute to the onset of significant depression.[7]

Keep in mind that only a small percentage of older people pursue medical treatment for behavioral issues. Not only do many older adults fail to seek care, but they also frequently deny the problem when asked about it. When assessing the patient who is displaying signs of depression, it is appropriate to ask if they are considering suicide. If the answer is yes, proceed to ask the additional questions included in this chapter relating to assessing suicide risk. It is vital that hospital staff be aware of these issues and take appropriate steps to ensure the patient's and their own safety.

Bipolar Disorders

Bipolar disorders are another group of major psychiatric disorders that, when untreated, impair a person's ability to work, go to school, or continue their normal daily activities. A **bipolar disorder** is a type of mental illness characterized by alternating periods of depression and manic episodes. Patients who are in the depressive phase display the same features as a person diagnosed with depression. During a **manic episode**, the patient may display behaviors lasting a week or more in which their mood appears abnormally elevated and their activity and energy levels are markedly increased. In one type of bipolar disorder, the patient typically has several of the following symptoms:

- Exaggerated feelings of self-importance
- Little need for sleep or food
- Talkativeness, or disjointed or racing thoughts
- Distractibility
- Increased activity (eg, work, sexual, or meaningless activities)
- Increased impulsivity and reckless behaviors (eg, spending too much, having indiscriminate sexual relations)
- If severe, delusions or hallucinations

Treatment for bipolar disorders typically includes medications and psychotherapy. These patients, like those with depression, are at much higher risk than the general population for suicide.

Schizophrenia

Schizophrenia is a complex disorder that is not easily defined or treated. It affects how a person thinks, feels, and behaves, and it is characterized by recurrent episodes of psychotic behavior. Symptoms of the illness become more prominent over time. The typical age of onset is between adolescence and early adulthood, between the ages of 16 and 30 years.[8] However, in certain instances, some signs may appear during early childhood.

Schizophrenia is thought to be caused by a complex combination of factors, including genetics, brain chemistry or structure, and social influences.[9] In addition to hallucinations and delusions, patients with schizophrenia may experience paranoia, a lack of interest in everyday activities or relationships with others, and erratic, disorganized speech. They may exhibit a rapid shifting of subjects, often perceived as disjointed rambling. Patients may exhibit a flat or blunted affect, meaning they appear to lack the normal range of feelings, perhaps to the point of seeming devoid of emotions altogether.

Suicide

Suicide can happen in any family, regardless of socioeconomic class, culture, race, or religious affiliation. Suicide rates are about four times higher among men.[6] Among women, the suicide rate is highest between ages 45 and 64 years.[10] Non-Hispanic American Indian/Alaskan Native and non-Hispanic White individuals are at the highest risk of suicide.[6]

When assessing any patient in crisis, you should evaluate their suicide risk. Gather as much information as you can, as these details may help hospital staff gauge the severity of the risk and determine the best course of action. During your assessment, consider the following and remain alert for warning signs of suicide:

- Is the environment safe? Note any unsafe objects in the patient's hands or nearby, such as a sharp knife, glass, poisons, or a gun. Also note situations that could facilitate suicide, such as an open window in a high-rise building.
- Does the patient have an air of tearfulness, sadness, deep despair, or hopelessness that suggests depression?
- Does the patient avoid eye contact, speak slowly or haltingly, and project a sense of vacancy?
- Does the patient seem unable to talk about the future? Ask the patient whether they have any vacation plans. People at risk of suicide often will not invest in detailed plans for the future, or may consider the future so uninteresting that they do not think about it; people with serious depression consider the future so distant that they may not be able to think about it at all.
- Is there any suggestion of suicide? Even vague suggestions should not be taken lightly, even if presented as a joke. If you think that suicide is a possibility, do not hesitate to bring up the subject. You will not give the patient ideas if you ask directly, "Are you considering suicide?"
- Does the patient have any specific plans related to death? If so, does the patient have access to the means in the plan? For example, if the plan is to use a handgun, does the person have access to this weapon? How detailed is the plan? For example, does it include the "when" and "where"?
- Has the patient recently prepared a will? Has the patient given away significant possessions, told close friends what they would like done with them, or arranged for a funeral service? These are critical warning signs.
- Is there evidence of self-destructive behavior (eg, partially cut wrists, excessive alcohol or drug use)? Has the patient already taken steps? For example, has the person collected pills, purchased a gun, or written a suicide note?
- Is there an underlying medical problem? Has the patient experienced any recent trauma?
- Does the patient have any cultural, religious, or social beliefs that promote suicide?

Factors associated with suicide are listed in **TABLE 23-1**.

On the basis of your observations and conversations with the patient, you may need to determine if interventions such as restraints are needed. Although not common, a patient who is suicidal may be homicidal as well. Do not jeopardize your life or the lives of your partners. If you have reason to believe that you are in danger, you must obtain police intervention. In the meantime, try not to frighten the patient or make them suspicious. Remember, the most important service you can provide for a suicidal patient is compassionate transport to a medical facility where they can receive proper treatment.

TABLE 23-1 Factors Associated With Suicide Risk

Category	Factors That Increase Risk	Factors That Protect Against Risk
Individual	• Previous suicide attempt • History of depression and other mental illnesses • Serious illness such as chronic pain • Criminal/legal problems • Job/financial problems or loss • Impulsive or aggressive tendencies • Substance use disorder • Current or prior history of adverse childhood experiences • Sense of hopelessness • Violence victimization and/or perpetration	• Effective coping and problem-solving skills • Reasons for living (eg, family, friends, pets) • Strong sense of cultural identity
Relationship	• Bullying • Family/loved one's history of suicide • Loss of relationships • High-conflict or violent relationships • Social isolation	• Support from partners, friends, and family • Feeling connected to others
Community	• Lack of access to health care • Suicide cluster in the community • Stress of acculturation • Community violence • Historical trauma • Discrimination	• Feeling connected to school, community, and other social institutions • Availability of consistent and high-quality physical and behavioral health care
Societal	• Stigma associated with help-seeking and mental illness • Easy access to lethal means of suicide among people at risk • Unsafe media portrayals of suicide	• Reduced access to lethal means of suicide among people at risk • Cultural, religious, or moral objections to suicide

"Risk and Protective Factors for Suicide." Centers for Disease Control and Prevention. Accessed January 17, 2025. https://www.cdc.gov/suicide/risk-factors/index.html.

Suicide Risk Among Adolescents

According to the Centers for Disease Control and Prevention, suicide is the second leading cause of death for people 10 to 24 years of age.[10] Although we sometimes tend to view a teenager's problems as minor, problems often appear insurmountable to them. Never discount a teenager's comments about suicide as being "just an attempt to get attention."

Common factors that lead to suicide attempts in adults are often also found in teenagers. One of them is dealing with the end of a relationship. Teenagers are just beginning to relate to others in an intimate way, so when a relationship ends, they often do not know how to handle the apparent rejection. Adults who attempt suicide may have a drug or alcohol use disorder, and this is common among teenagers as well. Other factors that increase the risk of suicide include a history of disciplinary problems and an unstable home life. Social pressures are also an important factor in this population. Peer approval is one of the most important aspects of a teenager's life, and teenagers who seem to have poor relationships with their peers may be at a higher risk for suicide. In other cases, teenagers can be influenced by peers to attempt suicide either individually or as part of a pact. Another risk factor to consider is that children of parents who died from suicide are more likely to attempt it themselves.[11]

Expression of thoughts of suicide and attempts at suicide by teenagers should always be taken seriously. Never disregard suicidal comments, even if a parent insists the child is "faking." Take action to ensure that teenagers are evaluated by a professional after attempting or considering suicide because it is very important for their long-term emotional well-being.

Safety Tips

Patients with suicidal thoughts, especially patients who have made a threat or previous attempt, may not be thinking clearly and may behave in unpredictable ways. Some recognize that if they get into the ambulance or enter the hospital, they will not have the opportunity to complete their threat or intent. In some situations, a patient in acute suicidal crisis may behave unpredictably and may act aggressively toward responders if they perceive them as a barrier to their intent. Be careful how you assess the situation; make certain you, your team, and the patient are safe.

Suicide Risk Among Older Adults

Unlike younger people, geriatric patients typically do not make suicidal gestures or attempts that might prompt help to interrupt the attempt. Many see no other way out when they have a terminal illness or debilitating cardiac or neurologic condition (eg, severe heart disease, stroke).

As with younger patients, do not assume an older adult who threatens suicide will not actually carry it out. Immediate intervention is necessary.

Street Smarts

A geriatric patient who has taken too much of a medication may have simply made an error, but it is possible that the patient was attempting suicide. Consider the possibility of depression and suicidal thoughts when conducting your assessment.

Posttraumatic Stress Disorder

Posttraumatic stress disorder (PTSD) can occur after exposure to, or injury from, a traumatic event. Such events may include experiencing or witnessing sexual or physical assault, child abuse, a serious accident, a natural disaster, war, loss of a loved one, or stressful life changes. It can also be related to repeated exposure to very unpleasant situations such as repeatedly hearing details of abuse or repeated exposure to dead bodies.

It is estimated that approximately 7% of the general population will experience signs of PTSD at some point in their lives.[12] Military personnel who experienced combat have a far higher incidence of PTSD, with studies suggesting 20% to 30% of those who served in Operations Iraqi Freedom or Enduring Freedom or the Persian Gulf War will experience PTSD at some point in their lives.[13] The risk is higher among female veterans, and studies are ongoing for transgender veterans and those who identify as nonbinary.[13] For health care workers returning from a warfare environment, which could include disaster workers, threat of personal harm increases the person's likelihood of experiencing PTSD.[14]

Street Smarts

PTSD is more prevalent in those working in EMS than in the general public.[15,16] In a 2016 report published by the National Association of EMTs, *National Survey on EMS Mental Health Services*, the majority of EMS clinicians surveyed felt affected personally by mental health issues.[15,17] Cumulative stress in EMS clinicians is also prevalent and can lead to compassion fatigue and a higher incidence of considering suicide.[17] Take care of yourself, and watch those you work with for signs of depression and other mental illness. Helpful resources on this subject include EMS Week (emsweek.org) and the Code Green Campaign (codegreencampaign.org). Chapter 2, *Workforce Safety and Wellness*, discusses strategies to help reduce the risk of PTSD among EMS clinicians.

Signs and Symptoms of PTSD

Symptoms of PTSD include feelings of helplessness, anxiety, anger, and fear. People with PTSD may avoid things that remind them of the trauma, including loud noises or smells, and sometimes avoid interactions with other people. This emotional and physical distancing from others can have a negative effect on one's quality of life. Memories of the trauma linger and continue to be disruptive. Symptoms of PTSD may be made worse in the context of other mental health challenges.

The sympathetic nervous system provides the fight-or-flight mechanism (also called the fight, flight, or freeze response) to help protect us in a perceived dangerous situation. It is not intended to last any longer than required to mitigate the threat. People with PTSD experience nervous system arousal that continues and is not easily suppressed. The heart rate increases to channel blood into the heart, lungs, and brain; pupils dilate; and systolic blood pressure is increased. Senses are sharpened and mental acuity is heightened. The person may feel numb or be hypervigilant, have trouble sleeping, or display an exaggerated startle response to perceived danger.

People with PTSD may relive the traumatic event through intrusive thoughts, nightmares, or even flashbacks. *Flashbacks* are uncontrollable events triggered by a sound, sight, or smell. In children they may be seen as reenactments during play. The patient may experience the same visceral response as when they initially encountered the stress. These episodes can last seconds or hours and can occur at any time, even years after the exposure. The person fears this inability to control a flashback and worries that it will present as irrational behavior. Recent traumatic events may also trigger old memories and create a reflex reaction of preparing for the worst. A person who has experienced flashbacks may become preoccupied with the perception of danger.

Dissociative PTSD occurs when the person attempts to escape from constant internal distress or a particularly disturbing event. The person's altered consciousness allows them to continue functioning under negative conditions. Some people may undergo an out-of-body experience. Others experience delusions. Other psychological conditions such as personality disorders and increased functional impairment can develop in those with a dissociative subtype of PTSD.

Guilt, shame, paranoia, hostility, and depression are not uncommon for patients who have PTSD. Alcohol and/or drug use is a common way to suppress the sympathetic nervous system activity. This can lead to substance use disorders. Suicide is sometimes sought to end the pain.

PTSD is also associated with a higher risk of certain secondary medical conditions.[18] High cholesterol levels and hypertension are not uncommon and are often undiagnosed or misdiagnosed.

PTSD and the Combat Veteran

Veterans are much more likely to harm themselves or try to harm themselves.[19] They also sustain a host of physical conditions, some from injuries sustained in combat, and sometimes vague, unfocused pain not associated with any specific part of the body. This perception of physical pain may be a sign of their anguish. In particular, combat veterans may have heart disease at a younger age than expected, a higher incidence of type 2 diabetes, and a loss of gray matter in the brain.

Try to eliminate excess noise. Do not touch or do anything to the veteran without first providing an explanation. Because military vehicles are often diesel fueled, diesel fumes can be a trigger for combat veterans.[20] Keep this in mind if you are operating diesel equipment in the vicinity of a combat veteran.

Combat veterans tend to show respect for authority but may be reluctant to talk to you about PTSD. They may not be aware that they have it or may not want to be considered "mental." They might have trouble asking for help. Asking, "How do you want me to help you?" or "What is it you need right now?" is a good way to open the conversation.

Dementia

The growth of the older adult population in the United States has resulted in an increasing proportion of geriatric calls for EMS systems.[21] Behavioral or psychiatric symptoms that are more common in this population include depression, delirium, and **dementia**.

In the older adult population, dementia is a common cause of abnormal behavior. Dementia is a slow, progressive decline in cognitive function that impairs memory function and leads to behavior change. Alzheimer disease is the most common form of dementia.[22] According to the Alzheimer's Association, nearly 7 million people, and approximately 1 in 9 older US adults, are afflicted with this condition; it is the fifth leading cause of death in the United States. Populations at increased risk include women and older individuals who are Black or Hispanic.[23] Currently, there is no cure for Alzheimer disease, but there are medications that can slow the disease's progression.

Openly hostile behavior, including kicking, yelling, pinching, and hitting, can develop in patients with Alzheimer disease. If a patient must be restrained, ensure the process is handled gently and only to the point at which the violent behavior is controlled.

Delirium

Delirium is an acute state of confusion that occurs suddenly and may fluctuate over short periods. This impairment in attention, awareness, and cognitive function may present with disorientation, hallucinations, delusions, or agitation (behavior characterized by restless and irregular physical activity). Delirium is not a disease itself, but rather a sign of any number of underlying problems. Because of its sudden, rapid onset, you should consider a new case of delirium to be a true emergency. Although patients experiencing delirium are generally not dangerous, those experiencing agitation may inadvertently or irrationally strike out. Therefore, responders must maintain focus on personal safety.

You may hear the term "excited delirium" used to describe patients who have extreme agitation. This term should not be confused with the description of delirium provided here. This term is no longer used clinically because it lacks a clear, evidence-based definition and has been associated with misuse, particularly in law enforcement contexts. Current medical practice emphasizes identifying and treating underlying conditions, such as substance use, psychiatric disorders, or medical emergencies, rather than using this outdated and controversial term. Terms such as *delirium with agitation* and *hyperactive delirium with severe agitation* are now used to describe the presenting condition rather than assign a diagnosis to these patients.

Words of Wisdom

In 2023, the American College of Emergency Physicians released a position statement recognizing the existence of hyperactive delirium syndrome with severe agitation as a potentially life-threatening clinical condition characterized by a combination of vital sign abnormalities (eg, elevated temperature and blood pressure), pronounced agitation, altered mental status, and metabolic derangements.[24]

Substance Use Disorders

Substance use disorders (SUDs) are chronic, treatable medical conditions characterized by the uncontrolled use of substances such as alcohol, opioids, stimulants, or other drugs, despite harmful consequences. EMTs often encounter patients experiencing medical emergencies related to SUDs, including overdoses, withdrawal symptoms, or complications such as respiratory depression and altered mental status. Recognizing the signs of substance use and responding with empathy and professionalism are critical.

Treatment includes stabilizing the patient, administering interventions such as naloxone for opioid overdoses when appropriate, and connecting patients to long-term care resources. Understanding SUDs as medical conditions, not moral failings, helps reduce stigma and improve patient outcomes. See Chapter 22, *Toxicology*, for discussion of assessing and treating a patient with a suspected overdose.

Words of Wisdom

MIH teams at some EMS agencies have developed policies and partnered with community resources to provide an additional layer of support to individuals in need of behavioral health services. MIH teams can help by providing telehealth consultation on the scene and transport from the scene to alternative destinations, such as treatment facilities for mental health or substance use disorders. They can also provide on-scene treatment, follow-up care, or referral services for patients who have been revived after an opioid overdose by specially trained advanced life support (ALS) clinicians with medications such as buprenorphine (Suboxone). MIH teams can play a key role in enrolling these patients in a rehabilitation program and preventing withdrawal symptoms until enrollment is possible.

Acute Psychosis

Psychosis is a disruption to a person's thoughts and perceptions that make it difficult for them to recognize what is real and what is not.[25] Psychosis is a symptom, not an illness, and psychotic episodes occur for many reasons. The use of mind-altering substances is one cause, and in such cases, the experience may resolve on its own once the substance has been eliminated from the patient's body. Other causes of psychosis include genetics, intense stress, sleep deprivation, use of certain medications (eg, stimulants, hallucinogens), infection, traumatic brain injury, dementia, and other mental health conditions such as schizophrenia, bipolar disorder, or severe depression. Some psychotic episodes are relatively brief, while others last a lifetime.[26]

The patient may experience hallucinations, delusions, or both. **Hallucinations** are false perceptions involving the senses of sight, sound, taste, smell, or touch. A person who hears voices no one else can hear or sees objects no one else can see may be experiencing hallucinations. By contrast, **delusions** are, in the most basic sense, false beliefs that persist despite incontrovertible evidence to the contrary. Delusions can come in many forms. A few examples include delusions of persecution (feeling conspired against), grandeur (having an inflated sense of power or importance), thought-broadcasting (believing other people can read your thoughts), or thought-insertion (believing others are putting ideas into your mind). As the saying goes, "perception is reality."

Objectively, these faulty perceptions and beliefs are entirely false, but to the person experiencing them, hallucinations and delusions seem all too real. Therefore, it should come as no surprise when these patients behave in accordance with their "reality." When the line between reality and fantasy is blurred, the patient may become frightened, belligerent, or angry. They may also seem unusually silent and withdrawn, because they are giving all of their attention to the voices and feelings within.

Scene Safety Considerations

Even though most patients with a mental illness or behavioral health crisis are not dangerous, there may be an increased potential for violence in certain situations, especially in settings involving drug or alcohol intoxication, acute psychosis, and involuntary treatment and transport situations. Additionally, as an EMT, you are more likely to be exposed to aggressive or uncooperative patients because you are seeing people who are in the midst of a behavioral crisis severe enough that someone felt it was necessary to call 9-1-1. Perhaps family members or friends felt unable to manage the patient's behavior on their own. Therefore, it is critical that you remain vigilant.

Words of Wisdom

A study published in 2006 found that over 70% of restrained patients were suspected to have drug or alcohol intoxication, with alcohol accounting for over 90% of these instances. Only 37% of the patients who were restrained had a known psychiatric history of anxiety disorder, bipolar disorder, unipolar depression, psychosis/schizophrenia, PTSD, or suicidal ideation.[27]

If at any time signs of danger become apparent during the patient encounter, move to a safe location immediately and wait for law enforcement to intervene. Fleeing an unsafe scene where the patient poses a danger to responders is *not* patient abandonment. In such instances, your duty to that patient ends until the scene has been rendered safe. Remember, your safety must come first. See **TABLE 23-2** for additional strategies to stay safe when responding to a behavioral health emergency.

Street Smarts

Family members often experience an emotional response to the patient's actions. They may be frustrated or feel like they are the cause of the patient's behavior. Be sensitive to their feelings and concerns.

YOU are the EMT

At 1920 hours, you are dispatched to 517 East Bandera Road for a man who, according to a neighbor, is sitting in his yard "acting bizarre." Law enforcement is en route to the scene but has not yet arrived. You and your partner acknowledge the call, get into the ambulance, and proceed to the scene. The weather is clear, the temperature is 70°F (21°C), and the traffic is moderate.

1. How should you and your partner proceed to this call?
2. Other than an underlying psychiatric condition, what other conditions can affect a person's behavior?

TABLE 23-2 Safety Guidelines for Responding to Patients With a Behavioral Health Emergency

- **Continuously assess the scene for threats to your safety.** *Do not remain on an unsafe scene!* If signs of danger become apparent before, or even during, the patient encounter, move to a safe location immediately and wait for law enforcement to intervene.
- **Ensure you have a means of communication, such as a radio.** If there is an unexpected problem, you may need to immediately contact help. Do not leave your partner alone on scene.
- **Know where the exits are and keep them clear.** Park your ambulance in a location that allows you a safe and easy way to retreat quickly if it becomes necessary. When possible, avoid parking in a way that would require you to turn the vehicle around before you could drive away. Inside the patient's home, maintain a clear path to the exit. Do not let the patient, bystanders, or any significant obstacle get between you and the door.
- **Have a plan for patient restraint.** If restraint is needed, how will it be accomplished? This process should be preplanned, approved by the medical director, and coordinated with law enforcement prior to this type of call so roles are clearly defined. National guidelines recommend having at least five rescuers present to perform physical restraint. Therefore, the best time to apply restraints is prior to transport, when additional personnel are available. When appropriate, consider requesting ALS assistance for sedation.
- **Attempt to de-escalate.** Often, effective communication skills can keep an agitated patient from becoming a violent one. Remove any stimulus that distresses the patient.
- **Calmly identify yourself.** Sometimes, patients may not distinguish you from law enforcement. Ensure the patient knows you are there to provide medical care.
- **Present a calm, confident presence.** Be friendly, but not patronizing. Ask questions in a low, calm voice. Clearly explain what you are doing and what you need from the patient. Maintain good eye contact and open body language.
- **Be patient.** These calls may require more time on scene than normal. This is often due to communication challenges.
- **Stay with the patient.** Unless the patient becomes aggressive or violent, do not leave them alone.
- **Do not get too close to a potentially volatile patient.** Avoid immediately approaching and squatting down beside the patient. Instead, maintain a safe distance (6–8 feet) until you are confident it is safe and necessary to get closer for assessment purposes. Respect the patient's personal space and avoid unnecessary physical contact. Be prepared to move quickly if the patient becomes violent; otherwise do not make sudden movements. Do not wear any items around your neck, such as a stethoscope, that the patient could easily grasp.
- **Show interest in the patient's story.** Listening and showing empathy can be your best defense on a potentially volatile scene. Let the patient "vent." If you can respond with empathy to the feelings the patient is expressing, whether the feeling is anger or fear or desperation, you may be able to gain the person's cooperation. However, do not make statements like, "I know exactly what you're going through." Such statements can cause a patient to become less communicative, perhaps even angry. Likewise, do not offer advice. Your goal should be to let the patient know you *want* to understand, not that you already *do* understand.
- **Do not argue or retaliate.** Be nonconfrontational. Do not talk down to the patient. Do not match threats. If the patient verbally attacks you, do not take it personally. Remember, the patient is not responding to you in a normal manner. They may be wrestling with internal forces over which neither of you has control. If possible, try to involve a friend or family member whom the patient trusts. However, do not speak with family in a hushed or secretive manner, especially when the patient has already shown signs of paranoia.
- **Be careful how you respond to patients with psychosis or paranoia.** Remember, these misperceptions are very real to the person experiencing them. Do not minimize the effect these thoughts may have on the individual. However, do not play along either. For example, if the patient asks you if you can hear the voices in their head, respond with something like, "No. I don't hear them, but that must be very frightening for you." If the patient is hearing voices, it is important to know what those voices are saying. If the voices are commanding the person to harm someone (including you), you need to be aware of it.
- **Be honest and reassuring.** If the patient asks whether they need to go to the hospital, the answer should be, "Yes, that is where you can receive help." Also, do not make promises you cannot keep. If, for example, the patient describes plans of suicide, you have a legal and ethical responsibility to share that information with receiving hospital staff. If they ask you to keep their plans secret, calmly explain why you cannot. If the patient realizes later that you have misled them, they may become angry, which could create a safety threat to you and others, including those caring for the patient after you.

Patient Assessment

Scene Size-up

The first things for you to consider at the scene of a patient experiencing a behavioral health crisis are your safety and the patient's response to the environment. Is the situation potentially dangerous for you and your partner? Should you stage until law enforcement personnel have secured the scene? Be vigilant and avoid tunnel vision.

Determine the mechanism of injury and/or nature of illness. Remember, certain injuries and medical conditions can cause altered behavior that can be mistaken for a behavioral health emergency. Note any medications or substances that may have contributed to the patient's current mental status or that may have been prescribed for the treatment of a relevant medical condition.

Primary Assessment

Having taken appropriate standard precautions, begin your assessment from the doorway or from a distance. How does the patient appear? Calm or agitated? Awake or sleepy? Is the patient's attire appropriate for the situation? For example, is the patient out in the cold wearing only shorts? Does the patient's behavior seem typical or normal given the circumstances? Are there any indications that the scene is or might become unsafe? Do you see any weapons? Pay attention to the patient's body language, tone of voice, and other cues.

When you approach the patient, introduce yourself, and explain you are there to help. Note whether the patient is alert and oriented. Until you have assessed the situation, maintain a safe distance and stand at a 45° angle to the patient, making sure there is a clear exit path. If indicated, attempt to perform a rapid physical exam, looking for signs of trauma and other findings that could explain the patient's presentation. If the patient is not responsive, it is especially important to rule out head trauma. Inspect for hidden life threats and treat them accordingly.

If your patient is in physical distress, assess the airway to make sure it is patent and adequate. Next, evaluate the patient's breathing and obtain rate and effort. Use pulse oximetry if available. Provide the appropriate interventions based on your assessment findings. Some behavioral situations will involve a compromised airway or inadequate breathing if a patient has ingested prescription medications, drugs, or alcohol.

Next, you will need to assess the pulse rate, quality, and rhythm. Assessing a patient's circulation includes an evaluation for the presence of shock and bleeding. Assess the patient's perfusion by evaluating skin color, temperature, and capillary refill. Because pallor can be difficult to detect in patients with dark skin, instead check for pale mucous membranes inside the inner lower eyelid or slow capillary refill.

Unless your patient is unstable from a medical problem or trauma, prepare to spend time with your patient. It may take time and patience to gain the patient's trust if they are fearful or unwilling to cooperate with you. Note their posture for signs of aggression, and listen to the tone and rate of their speech. Observe for any abnormal body movements such as facial tics, tremors, or spastic motions.

During these calls, it is important to consider how your observations compare to the patient's baseline daily behavior and cognitive function. Try to determine, possibly with the help of someone on scene who knows the patient, whether the patient's current behavior is normal for *them.* For example, if your patient has Alzheimer disease, finding them to be markedly confused might not be especially worrisome if that level of disorientation has been the patient's baseline status for several months. By contrast, a sudden, severe decline in cognitive function may signal an emergency condition, such as a stroke or accidental drug overdose.

Street Smarts

When you visit the home of an older adult, especially one who lives alone, assess whether the person is living in a safe and healthy environment. Do they have food and medications? Is the home sanitary, or is it overrun with bugs or rodents? Is there hoarding behavior? Is the person's mental status in question? If you have concerns, call adult protective services.

History Taking

If the patient is conscious and without traumatic injury, the next step is to investigate the chief complaint and then obtain a SAMPLE (Signs and symptoms, Allergies, Medications, Pertinent past medical history, Last oral intake, Events leading up to the illness or injury) history. Obtain relevant medical information from the patient or family. Ask specifically about previous episodes, treatments, hospitalizations, and medications related to behavioral symptoms. Determining the patient's baseline mental status will be essential in guiding your treatment and transport decisions and will also be extremely helpful to hospital personnel.

As you conduct the interview, consider not only the information you receive but also the nature of the patient's responses and behavior:

- Does the patient appropriately answer your questions?
- Does the patient's behavior seem appropriate?
- Does the patient seem to understand you?
- Is the patient withdrawn or detached? Hostile or friendly? Happy or depressed?
- Are the patient's vocabulary and expressions what you would expect under the circumstances?
- Does the patient seem aggressive or dangerous to you or others?
- Is the patient's memory intact? Check orientation to time, place, person, and event.
- Does the patient express disordered thoughts, delusions, or hallucinations?

As mentioned previously, when trying to determine the underlying source of the patient's abnormal behavior, consider the possibility that something other than a purely psychiatric cause is to blame. Even if you learn the patient does indeed have a history of mental illness, keep in mind that you have not entirely ruled out the possibility that a

Street Smarts

It is easy to assume the patient having a behavioral crisis does not understand the situation or the message you are trying to convey. However, especially during an acute crisis, many patients still have awareness and understanding. Communication is key. In some cases, patients will de-escalate once a level of trust has been established. Never make disparaging or inappropriate statements. It is not only poor patient care, but inappropriate comments could escalate an already tense situation. Effective communication skills can be among the best self-defense tactics in your repertoire.

YOU are the EMT

Law enforcement personnel arrive at the scene and inform you that it is safe for you to enter. One of the police officers informs you that the patient allowed them to check him for any weapons and that he does not have any.

You find the patient, a 44-year-old man, sitting on the lawn in front of his house; one of the police officers is trying to talk to him. He appears sad and withdrawn and is rocking back and forth. You introduce yourself to the patient and perform a primary assessment.

Recording Time: 0 Minutes	
Appearance	Sad, withdrawn appearance
Level of consciousness	Conscious and alert
Airway	Open; clear of secretions and foreign bodies
Breathing	Normal rate; adequate depth
Circulation	Normal pulse rate; skin baseline color and moist; no obvious bleeding

The patient tells you he "has a lot of problems," but nobody will listen to him.

3. What should be your most immediate concern with this patient?

4. How should you proceed with your assessment of this patient?

coexisting emergency is present. Could this patient with a mental illness also have hypoglycemia or an injury?

If the patient has been diagnosed with a mental illness, are they currently under the care of a physician? Has the physician prescribed medication to treat the condition? Is the patient taking these prescriptions as directed? An unfortunate reality in the treatment of functional behavioral health conditions is that establishing an effective medication regimen is often a trial-and-error process. The patient may be required to change medications several times before the most effective course of treatment is finally discovered. These changes often come with unexpected or undesirable effects. A related problem can occur when a patient, against the physician's advice, suddenly stops taking a psychiatric medication. Patients may stop taking a medication for many reasons. For example, they may find the side effects unpleasant, they may begin feeling better and believe they no longer need the medication, they may not be able to afford the medication, or their condition may make adherence to a medication regimen challenging. Unfortunately, sudden cessation of these medications can cause a return of previous symptoms as well as other, possibly worse, consequences.

Reflective listening is a technique frequently used by behavioral health professionals to gain insight into a patient's thinking. It involves repeating, in question form, what the patient has said, encouraging the patient to expand on their thoughts. Although it often requires more time to be effective than is available in an EMS setting, it may be a helpful tool for you to use when other techniques are unsuccessful at gathering the patient's history. For a more in-depth discussion of therapeutic communication techniques, see Chapter 4, *Communications and Documentation.*

Street Smarts

When attempting to determine the cause of altered behavior in a patient with a behavioral health history, the patient may not know the cause of their own behavior. This lack of insight can be frustrating to EMS clinicians attempting to help. Demonstrate patience when assessing and talking with these patients. The unexplained behavior is confusing and frustrating to the patient as well. In these situations, consider gathering information separately from a relative or caregiver. Doing so may yield valuable information and can help reduce tension.

Secondary Assessment

If you are able to do so without worsening your patient's emotional state, obtain vital signs. Pay special attention to signs of conditions that could explain alterations in mental status (eg, blood glucose level, oxygen saturation level, pupil size and reactivity). If possible, administer high-concentration oxygen by mask when a patient is too agitated for you to obtain an oxygen saturation reading.[28]

Words of Wisdom

If an older adult experiences a sudden cognitive or behavioral change, assess their temperature to help detect a possible medical condition. Urinary tract and lung infections account for almost 50% of delirium cases in older adults.[29]

Sometimes, even a conscious patient in the middle of a behavioral health emergency will not respond to your questions. In those cases, you may be able to tell a lot about the patient's emotional state by observing facial expressions, pulse rate, and respirations. Also, look at the patient's eyes; a patient who has a blank gaze or rapidly moving eyes may be experiencing central nervous system dysfunction (**FIGURE 23-1**). However, be aware

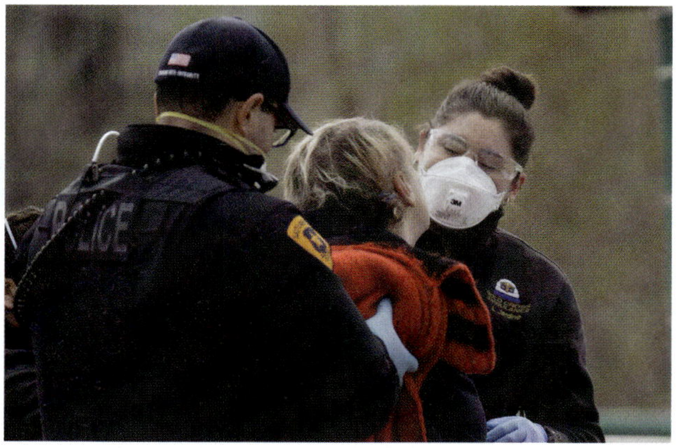

FIGURE 23-1 Making appropriate eye contact with a patient can provide useful clues about a patient's emotional state.

that for some patients with autism or autism spectrum disorder, eye contact may be very stressful and could provoke agitation. Similarly, making persistent eye contact with an aggressive individual can be perceived as a challenge, escalating the risk of violence. Finally, certain cultures find persistent eye contact offensive. Therefore, make appropriate eye contact, but do not force it beyond what is necessary. Be cognizant of how your behavior is affecting your patient.

Your area may have a specific facility equipped to care for patients with behavioral health emergencies. Try to make the patient comfortable but require that they ride on the stretcher with all straps secured. Placing the stretcher in a Fowler or high Fowler position helps prevent aspiration and reduces physical exertion by relaxing the abdominal muscles.

Reassessment

Never let your guard down. Most patients you treat and transport with emotional complaints pose no danger to you or others. However, it is not always possible to predict on scene whether a patient may become violent during transport. Be prepared to intervene quickly. If a patient becomes a threat to your safety, it is not patient abandonment to remove yourself from the danger. For a lone EMT to attempt to restrain a violent person in the back of a moving ambulance is incredibly unsafe. You and your partner should have a plan in place for such events. That may include pulling over to the side of the road and radioing for law enforcement assistance.

Words of Wisdom

In many cases, EMS clinicians do not have as much training to subdue and restrain physically aggressive individuals as law enforcement. Law enforcement officers may receive hundreds of hours of instruction on restraint, constitutional law, defensive tactics, and the lawful use of force. Therefore, when EMS clinicians have reason to believe a patient will become violent, law enforcement officers should be involved and should oversee the application of physical restraints if necessary. Remember that EMS is in the business of providing patient *care*, not taking *custody*. It is the EMT's responsibility to advocate for the patient's medical care, ensuring the patient receives safe, appropriate assessment and treatment.[28] Do not allow the lines separating law enforcement from EMS to become blurred. Know your role!

YOU are the EMT

The patient tells you his wife was killed in a car accident 1 year ago today, and even though he has been to numerous counseling sessions over the past year, they have not seemed to help. He further tells you his employer does not seem to care about his problems and has threatened to fire him unless he "snaps out of it." He allows your partner to take his vital signs but refuses to allow you to perform any other assessment or treatment.

Recording Time: 9 Minutes	
Respirations	16 breaths/min; adequate depth
Pulse	88 beats/min; strong and regular
Skin	Baseline color, warm, and moist
Blood pressure	144/84 mm Hg
Oxygen saturation (Spo_2)	98% (on room air)

The patient denies chest pain, shortness of breath, or any other physical symptoms. He tells you it is extremely difficult for him to even get out of bed and face each day and he feels as though his life no longer serves any purpose.

5. What is your field impression of this patient?

6. What care can you provide to this patient in the field?

Give the receiving hospital advance warning when a patient experiencing a behavioral health emergency is coming in. Many hospitals require extra preparation to ensure the appropriate staff and rooms are available. Report whether restraints will be required when the patient arrives. Communicate anything that may help explain the patient's situation, and include behaviors or items you observed in the prehospital setting, such as medications or weapons. The hospital personnel will not know about these important facts unless you tell them.

Describing what took place on the scene of a behavioral crisis can be challenging, but it is important for readers of your patient care report to understand the actions you took and why they were appropriate. Because there are serious legal concerns in matters involving involuntary transport and patient restraint, it is especially important to document the details factually and clearly. If restraints were necessary, explain why. If you believed the patient was a threat to self or others, what observations brought you to that conclusion? If someone on the scene stated the patient had expressed suicidal intentions, clearly document the witness's name and relationship with the patient. Use direct quotes when possible. This information is essential to determine if the patient's condition warrants an involuntary admission or to provide insight if the case is ever reviewed for medicolegal reasons.

De-escalation and Restraint

Before you consider physical restraint, attempt verbal de-escalation techniques. Often, effective de-escalation can reduce the need for physical restraint. If it is helpful, consider asking the family to assist you in calming and reasoning with the patient. Effective de-escalation includes showing empathy, practicing active listening, using open body language, controlling the volume and tone of your voice, and validating the patient's feelings. Even when your attempts to de-escalate prove ineffective, the fact that you tried shows you made a good-faith effort to avoid having to apply restraints. Be sure to document these attempts and their outcomes. Verbal de-escalation is discussed further in Chapter 4, *Communications and Documentation*.

Street Smarts

When on the scene with an agitated patient, bystander, or family member, avoid telling the person to "calm down." This statement implies that the person does not have a valid reason to be upset, which can escalate their behavior. Instead, you might consider saying, "I can tell you are upset. Can you slow down and help me understand the situation?"

If a situation requires use of physical restraint, it is crucial that EMS clinicians follow local protocol and involve properly trained personnel. As ever, personal safety must be your top priority

The National Association of Emergency Medical Services Physicians (NAEMSP) recommends that every EMS agency have specific protocols for managing situations in which the patient is agitated, violent, or combative.[28] Such protocols should offer guidance in making the decision to apply restraints, specify the types of restraints to be used, and list actions expected of the EMT following the application of restraints. Well-written guidelines will consider both federal and state laws governing the use of restraint and involuntary transport (**TABLE 23-3**).

While restraint types vary, most can be classified as either soft or hard. Soft restraints include those constructed from nylon and neoprene or any other soft material. In most cases, you can identify a soft restraint as one that could be cut with relative ease, such as by using trauma shears. By contrast, hard restraints cannot be removed so easily, often requiring a key. Examples include handcuffs, leather

Safety Tips

If the patient's condition does not indicate high-flow oxygen by mask and the patient is spitting, place a surgical mask or commercial spit mask loosely over their mouth,[30] and make sure you are wearing appropriate personal protective equipment (PPE), including adequate eye protection and a mask. However, keep in mind that placing a mask on the patient's face may hinder your ability to monitor their airway; therefore, you must be extra vigilant and monitor oxygen saturation and, if available, end-tidal carbon dioxide continuously.

TABLE 23-3 Example of a Restraint Protocol

Clinical Indications

For the protection of the patient, the crew, and/or a third party, the patient may be physically restrained and/or sedated when the crew has a reasonable belief that the patient poses a risk of harm to self or others.

Procedure

1. Request law enforcement assistance early.
2. If at any time the scene becomes unsafe, the crew should immediately retreat and await confirmation from law enforcement that the scene has been rendered safe. The crew may use reasonable force to defend themselves against an attack, but their priority should be to retreat.
3. The crew should not attempt any "takedown" maneuvers or in any way force the patient to comply by causing pain. EMS clinicians must not use weapons to help restrain a patient. Any attempt to physically subdue an aggressive or violent person should be performed by law enforcement personnel only.
4. Whenever possible, less restrictive means of managing the patient's behavior should be attempted before physical and/or medical restraint is used. These attempts and their outcomes, whether successful or unsuccessful, must be documented in the patient care report (PCR).
5. When using physical restraints, all four extremities (not just one or two) should be secured.
6. Ensure that sufficient personnel are present to physically restrain the patient safely. A minimum of five people is recommended for safe restraint application.
7. **ALS only:** Unless contraindicated, physical restraint may be accompanied by the administration of medication(s) to control the person's behavior, in accordance with protocol. Medical restraint, also called pharmacologic management, should be considered early and may be required prior to physical restraint to make physical restraint application safer for the patient and crew.
8. The restrained patient should be positioned supine with the head of the stretcher elevated by at least 30°. Devices such as backboards and splints should not be placed on top of the patient, and the patient must never be restrained in a prone position, in a position with their hands and feet tied together behind their back, or in any other position that may lead to **positional asphyxia** (ie, a position in which the patient's physical position restricts chest wall movement or causes airway obstruction, potentially resulting in sudden death).
9. A clinician must maintain continuous visual observation of the patient, keeping an unobstructed view of all restrained extremities, all restraint devices, and all signs indicative of the patient's respiratory, circulatory, and neurologic function.
10. If available, cardiac function (electrocardiography), pulse oximetry, and waveform capnography should be monitored throughout transport.
11. Distal circulation in restrained extremities must be assessed at a minimum frequency of every 15 minutes. The first of these assessments should be conducted no more than 5 minutes following restraint application. All assessments must be documented in the PCR.
12. The PCR must contain a clear explanation for why physical restraint and/or sedation was necessary, the type of restraint device(s) used, and the time of their application.
13. Once applied, unless contraindicated by patient condition, physical restraints should not be removed until after arrival at the receiving facility, when an adequate number of personnel are present to ensure safe patient transfer. This should occur inside the facility, not in the back of the ambulance.
14. If the patient is transported in handcuffs or flex cuffs, a law enforcement officer must accompany the patient in the ambulance during transport.

Adapted from EMSrestraint.com website [homepage]. https://emsrestraint.com. Accessed January 14, 2025; Kupas DF, Wydro GC, Tan DK, Kamin R, Harrell AJ, Wang A. Clinical care and restraint of agitated or combative patients by emergency medical services practitioners. *Prehosp Emerg Care.* 2021;25(5):721–723; and Levy MK, Tan DK, McArdle DQ, et al. Consensus statement of the National Association of EMS Physicians International Association of Fire Chiefs and the International Association of Chiefs of Police: best practices for collaboration between law enforcement and emergency medical services during acute behavioral emergencies. *Prehosp Emerg Care.* 2024;28(8):1058–1062.

restraints, and flex cuffs (plastic ties). When possible, hard restraints should be avoided as they are more likely to cause patient injury. Further, devices that can be removed only with a key are discouraged because if the key is not immediately available during an emergency (eg, the device may need to be removed to manage the airway), the patient's safety could be placed in jeopardy. Even soft restraints that incorporate keyed locks should be used with caution; although these devices could be cut with trauma shears in an emergency, the agency should make every effort to ensure spare keys are readily available (eg, fastened to the ambulance's ignition key ring).

Street Smarts

Be aware of the message conveyed by your body language and tone of voice. Closed body language, such as standing rigidly with your arms crossed, can communicate a lack of empathy. A bladed stance (feet spread and body turned sidewise to the person, such as a boxer may stand) may convey aggression. Used properly, nonverbal communication can help you establish rapport and gain the patient's cooperation. Used unwisely, it can cause the patient to become more withdrawn or even hostile.

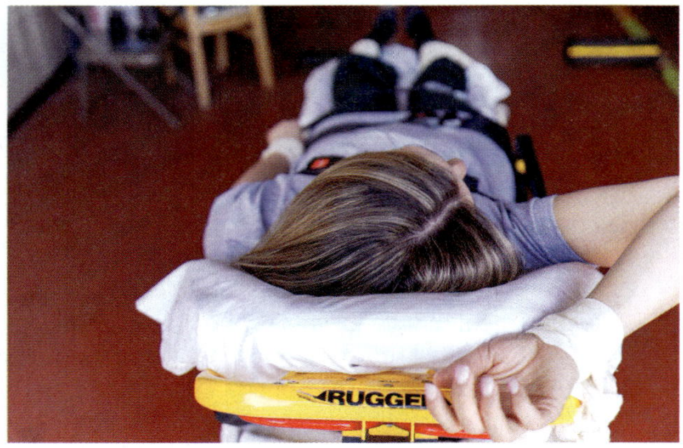

FIGURE 23-2 One wrist may be secured above the patient's head while the other is secured downward along the patient's side.

Courtesy of Aura Prep/Rescue Training International.

The Process of Restraining a Patient

Once the decision has been made to restrain a patient, you should carry it out as quickly and safely as possible. Ideally, five rescuers should be present to carry out the restraint, each being responsible for one extremity and the head. There should be a team leader who directs the restraining process, as well as a person designated to securing the restraints to the patient and stretcher. Before you begin, discuss the plan of action. Have the stretcher close by, in its lowest position, with the brakes locked and handrails lowered.

Throughout the process, remain mindful of the guidelines previously discussed. Important considerations include the following:

- At no time should any weight be placed on the patient's chest, face, neck, or groin.
- Avoid manipulating any joint beyond its normal range of motion.
- No team member should release their assigned extremity until all restraints have been secured.
- The team member at the patient's head should carefully grasp the sides of the patient's head and speak calmly to the patient throughout the process. This person should also ensure the patient does not bite other members.
- Apply restraint devices in accordance with the manufacturer's instructions.
- One wrist may be secured above the patient's head while the other is secured downward along the patient's side (**FIGURE 23-2**).
- Whenever possible, to prevent the restraints from sliding up or down the stretcher frame and creating slack, they should be anchored to "T-joints" along the stretcher's upper frame. Avoid anchoring to handrails or other moveable parts.
- Elevate the head of the stretcher to at least 30°.
- Secure all stretcher seat belts, being careful not to overtighten the chest straps. Chest wall movement should never be impaired.
- To prevent kicking and unwanted movement, one seat belt should be positioned across the thighs, just above the patient's knees. This method is more effective at controlling leg movements than securing the ankles alone.
- Immediately after the patient has been restrained, assess the patient's respiratory and cardiovascular status, along with motor, sensory, and circulatory function in all four extremities. At a minimum, reassess every 15 minutes. Document your findings in each instance.
- High-flow oxygen by mask should be applied early.
- At all times, treat the patient with dignity and respect. Your speech should never be punitive or aggressive.
- Restraints applied in the field should not be removed until the patient is evaluated at the receiving facility. Release en route only if

necessary to provide emergency patient care and only if you have assistance.
- Document the reason for the restraint, the type of restraint used, and the technique used.

Respiratory and circulatory problems have been known to occur in patients struggling against restraints. Some of these patients can experience severe acidosis or a fatal dysrhythmia. Patients with drug or alcohol intoxication and those with a severe psychiatric disorder may be at greater risk. Therefore, continuous vigilance and reassessment are crucial. Be alert for vomiting and other airway obstructions, respiratory and circulatory decline (eg, hypotension), and changes in the patient's level of consciousness. Reassess distal circulation frequently (**FIGURE 23-3**).

SKILL DRILL 23-1 provides an example of a patient restraint technique.

Words of Wisdom

The medical condition of patients who persistently struggle against their restraints may rapidly decline, up to and including sudden cardiac arrest. To avoid this outcome, if ALS is available and protocol allows, you should consider requesting their assistance. They may be able to provide pharmacologic management/sedation, which could prove to be a lifesaving intervention.[31]

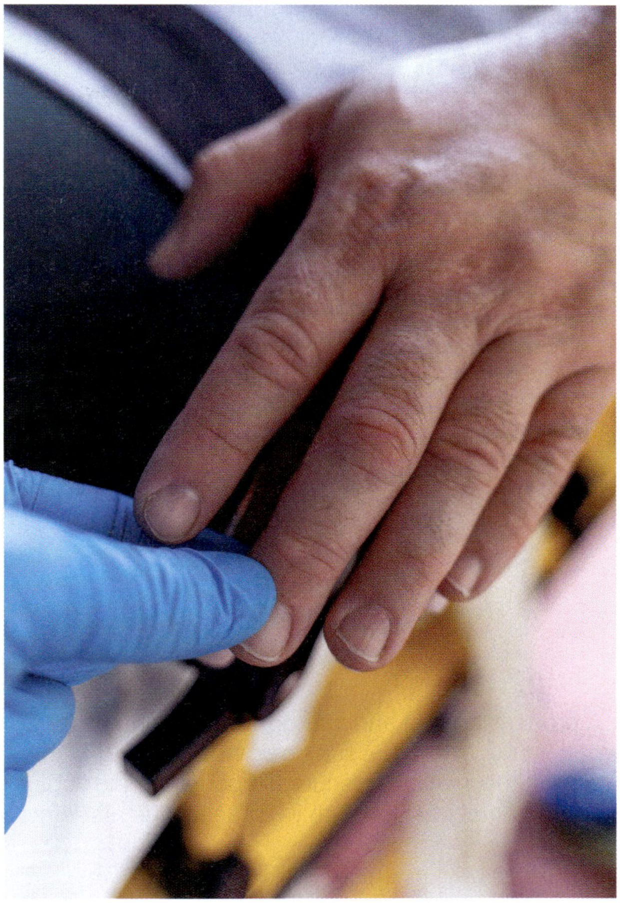

FIGURE 23-3 Frequently assess circulation while a patient is restrained.

YOU are the EMT

The patient is initially reluctant to allow you to transport him to the hospital. However, after you express your concern about his safety and well-being, he consents to transport. Other than allowing you to reassess his vital signs, he tells you he would prefer to just be taken to the hospital; he does not want to be physically assessed.

Recording Time: 20 Minutes	
Level of consciousness	Conscious and alert
Respirations	16 breaths/min; adequate depth
Pulse	76 beats/min; strong and regular
Skin	Baseline color, warm, and moist
Blood pressure	138/86 mm Hg
Oxygen saturation (Spo_2)	98% (on room air)

7. Should you perform a physical assessment of this patient even though he requested that you not? Why or why not?

Skill Drill 23-1 Restraining a Patient

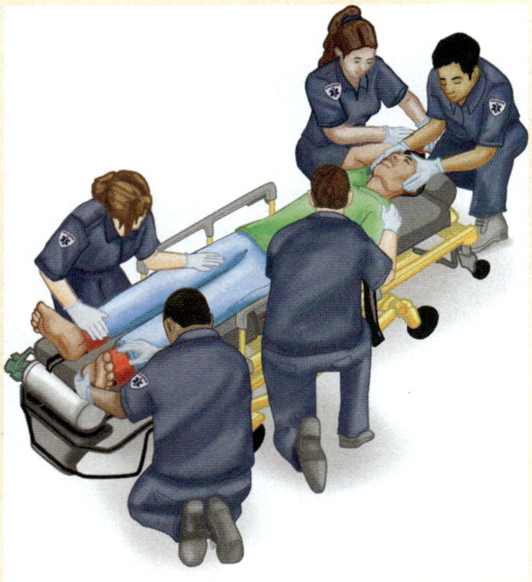

Step 1

A properly trained and authorized crew brings the patient down into the supine position. Acting at the same time, rescuers secure the patient in the supine or left lateral position with wrist and ankle restraints.

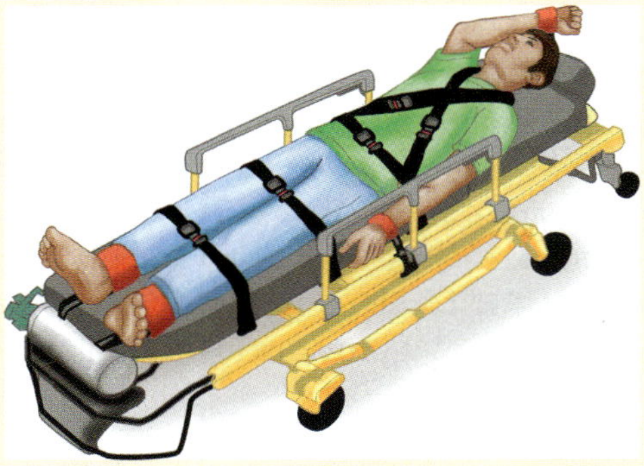

Step 2

The stretcher straps are then applied to the patient.

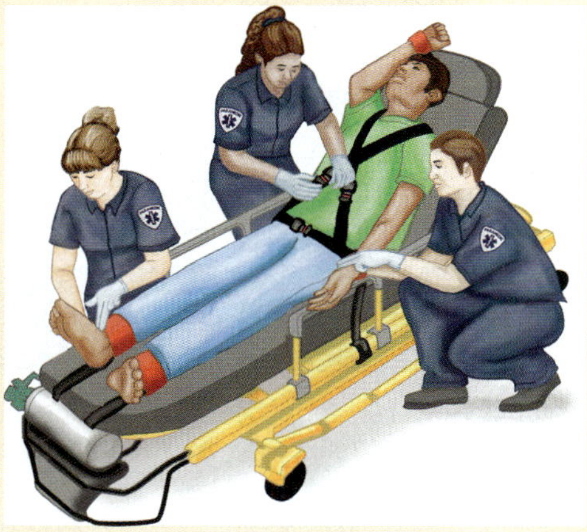

Step 3

Rescuers continue to verbally reassure and calm the patient following physical restraint and/or sedation. Circulation to the extremities is continually rechecked.

Words of Wisdom

EMTs have been accused of sexual misconduct and other physical abuse in circumstances that involve involuntary transport or restraint. To protect against false accusations, it is extremely helpful to have (and document the presence of) any witnesses on scene or in the ambulance during transport.

The Potentially Violent Patient

Violent patients account for only a small percentage of the patients experiencing a behavioral crisis. However, the potential for violence should always be a critical consideration for you (**FIGURE 23-4**).

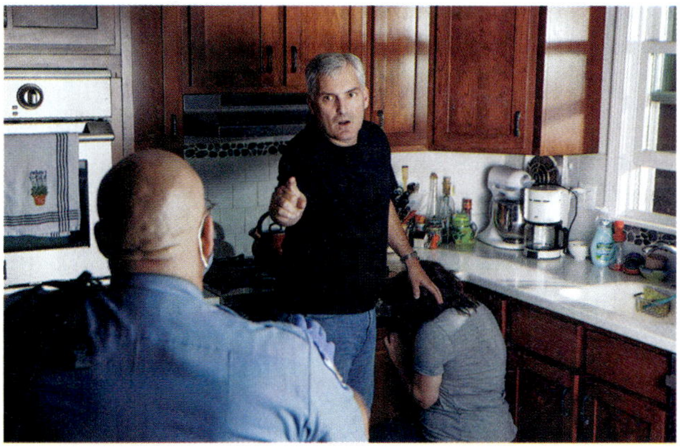

FIGURE 23-4 Watch for indicators of potential violence when approaching the scene.

Use the following list of risk factors to assess the level of danger:

- **History.** Has the patient previously exhibited hostile, overly aggressive, or violent behavior? Ask people at the scene, or request this information from law enforcement personnel or family. Has the patient become violent in the past under similar circumstances? Is the patient suspected to have ingested alcohol or stimulants?
- **Posture.** How is the patient sitting or standing? Is the patient tense, rigid, or sitting on the edge of their seat? Do you observe clenched fists, a targeting stare, or other aggressive body language? Such observations may signal impending hostility.
- **Weapons.** Is the patient holding or near a weapon (eg, knife, gun) or an object that can be used as a weapon (eg, baseball bat)?
- **Vocal activity.** How is the patient speaking? Loud, obscene, erratic, and bizarre speech patterns usually indicate emotional distress. Someone using quiet, ordered speech is not as likely to strike out as someone who is yelling and screaming.
- **Physical activity.** The motor activity of a person experiencing a behavioral emergency may be the most telling factor of all. A patient who has tense muscles, clenched fists, or glaring eyes; is pacing or cannot sit still; or is fiercely protecting their personal space requires careful observation.

YOU are the EMT

You depart the scene and begin transport to a hospital located 8 miles away. The patient remains conscious and alert but is still withdrawn and sad. You ask him additional questions about his present situation, but he does not answer you; he briefly looks up at you and then looks back down. You reassess his vital signs and then call in your report to the receiving facility.

Recording Time: 30 Minutes	
Level of consciousness	Conscious and alert
Respirations	16 breaths/min; adequate depth
Pulse	72 beats/min; strong and regular
Skin	Baseline, warm, and dry
Blood pressure	130/80 mm Hg
Oxygen saturation (Spo_2)	99% (on room air)

You arrive at the destination hospital and give your verbal report to the charge nurse. After transferring patient care to the hospital staff, you return to service.

8. What factors should you consider before transporting a patient with a behavioral health emergency?
9. If the patient does not answer your questions, should you continue to encourage him to talk? Why or why not?

Words of Wisdom

When encountering a potentially hostile individual, if a family member who has a positive influence on the patient is present, you may consider allowing this person to stay and help. Otherwise, remove everyone from the scene who is not needed. This may ease the tension and prevent injuries to bystanders.

Medicolegal Considerations

The medical and legal aspects of emergency medical care become more complicated when the patient is experiencing a behavioral health emergency. Legal challenges are greatly reduced when the patient consents to care. In situations that are not immediately life threatening, medical care or transport may be delayed until the proper authorization is obtained.

In emergencies requiring restraint and involuntary transport, improper restraint is a major liability concern for EMS systems. It is imperative that you familiarize yourself with both state and federal laws governing the use of restraint and involuntary transport. For further discussion of these legal concepts, see Chapter 3, *Medical, Legal, and Ethical Issues.*

YOU are the EMT SUMMARY

1. How should you and your partner proceed to this call?

The patient's reported behavior, "acting bizarre," is a broad description that could indicate any number of conditions. In the interest of your safety, you should assume that the patient is a danger to self or others. This is not a scene that you should enter without the protection of law enforcement. Never approach a scene of actual or potential violence until law enforcement personnel have arrived and deemed the scene safe for you to enter. In this case, you and your partner should stage a few blocks away from the scene and wait for law enforcement personnel to arrive. Proceed to the scene *only* after they have notified you and given you the all clear.

2. Other than an underlying psychiatric condition, what other conditions can affect a person's behavior?

A multitude of factors can affect a person's behavior; the presence of an underlying psychiatric condition is only one. Conditions such as hypoxemia, hypoglycemia, metabolic disorders, drug- or alcohol-related problems, stress-related issues, head trauma, and brain tumors (among others) can profoundly affect a person's behavior; these conditions may even cause the patient to become violent.

3. What should be your most immediate concern with this patient?

Personal safety should be your primary concern when caring for *any* patient. This is especially true when caring for patients who are displaying abnormal or bizarre behavior. When caring for a patient who is experiencing a behavioral crisis, you must always consider the potential for violence. There are certain behaviors and risk factors that you should look for when assessing a patient's potential for violence: patient history, posture, and verbal and physical activity.

Does the patient have a history of hostile, overly aggressive, or violent behavior? Observe the patient's speech. Loud, obscene, erratic, or bizarre speech patterns are clear indicators of emotional distress.

Your patient is sitting on the ground, rocking back and forth; this could indicate a general state of nervousness or increasing agitation.

4. How should you proceed with your assessment of this patient?

The patient has something to say; he states he "has a lot of problems," but also notes that nobody will listen to him. Therefore, use the most important assessment tool you have: listening. Actively listen to what the patient is saying. It may give you clues as to the underlying cause of his behavior; it also reassures him that you *are* listening.

Express sincere interest in what the patient is saying. Let him tell you in his own words what happened or what is going on. Do not interrupt him. Allow him to finish what he is saying before you ask him any questions, just as you would with any other patient.

When you are caring for a patient with a behavioral crisis, you must be prepared to spend extra time with the patient. It often takes longer to assess, listen to, and prepare the patient for transport.

5. What is your field impression of this patient?

The field impression of the patient is based on many factors, including physical assessment, medical

YOU are the EMT SUMMARY continued

history, and chief complaint. On the basis of your field impression, you can begin the treatment most appropriate for the situation.

Your patient is displaying clear signs of depression. Despite attending counseling sessions, he is unable to cope with the loss of his wife; this has brought him to the point of lacking the desire to even get out of bed in the morning. He no longer feels as though he has a purpose in life. He has experienced emotional distress for a year, and today, the anniversary of his wife's death, has precipitated an acute emotional crisis.

6. What care can you provide to this patient in the field?

Although the patient does not appear to be experiencing any physical problems, clearly he is emotionally overwhelmed. The fact that your patient has severe depression places him in a high-risk category for suicide. He should *not* be left alone! Patients who are experiencing a behavioral crisis require a great deal of emotional support and active listening.

7. Should you perform a physical assessment of this patient even though he requested that you not? Why or why not?

The patient, despite his severe depression, still has decision-making capacity. He is conscious and alert, is able to answer your questions appropriately, and is not displaying any psychotic behavior (eg, hallucinations, delusions). Therefore, he maintains the legal right to refuse a physical examination; touching him without his consent could lead to allegations of assault against you.

Unless there is an accompanying physical complaint, a detailed physical exam is rarely indicated in a patient with an emotional crisis; in fact, it may be detrimental to your gaining the patient's trust.

8. What factors should you consider before transporting a patient with a behavioral health emergency?

On arriving at the scene of a patient with a behavioral health emergency, you must assess the patient for signs of potential violence. These observations should continue throughout the *entire* patient encounter. Even though this patient is calm right now, this could easily change and he could become acutely violent. The worst time for this to happen is in the back of the ambulance, where you will be the only EMT. Do not let your guard down when caring for a patient with an emotional crisis; continuously monitor the individual's behavior. Stay attentive at all times.

If you have reason to believe that the patient is at an increased risk for becoming violent, you should have other authorized personnel, such as a police officer or firefighter, ride in the back of the ambulance. If it is necessary to restrain the patient, use just enough force to effectively accomplish the task. Unless it is absolutely necessary to provide patient care, do not release the restraints, regardless of any promises the patient makes to calm down. Never hesitate to call for ALS assistance, if available, for consideration of using medical restraint.

9. If the patient does not answer your questions, should you continue to encourage him to talk? Why or why not?

Some patients who are experiencing a behavioral health emergency talk excessively, while others talk little or not at all (as in depression). If the patient wants to talk, you should encourage them to do so. Many patients find relief, even if it is only temporary, by simply having someone to talk to. If the patient prefers not to talk, *do not force the issue.*

Patients with depression are typically withdrawn and not very talkative. Instead of persistently encouraging a patient to talk, you should continue to monitor the patient's behavior.

Prep Kit

Ready for Review

- During a behavioral crisis, the patient experiences a sudden change in behavior that threatens their own or others' safety. By contrast, with a mental illness, such as major depressive disorder, the patient may be unable to function in daily life for no discernable reason or for a disproportionately long period.
- According to the National Institute of Mental Health, mental health disorders are common throughout the United States, affecting tens

Prep Kit continued

of millions of people each year. Psychiatric disorders are illnesses with psychological or behavioral symptoms that may result in impaired functioning.

- Behavioral health emergencies have many possible underlying causes, including social or situational stress, such as divorce or death of a loved one; mental illnesses, such as schizophrenia; physical illnesses, such as diabetic emergencies; chemical problems, such as alcohol or drug use; and biologic disturbances, such as electrolyte imbalances. Sometimes these conditions can be compounded by noncompliance with prescribed medication regimens.
- You may be called to assist a person experiencing psychosis, schizophrenia, delirium, dementia, or other mental health condition. As an EMT, you are not responsible for diagnosing the underlying cause of a behavioral health emergency. Your job is to defuse and control the situation and safely transport your patient to the hospital. Intervene only as much as it takes to accomplish these tasks. Be caring and careful.
- When responding to a behavioral health emergency, if at any time signs of danger become apparent, move to a safe location immediately and wait for law enforcement to intervene.
- Always consult medical direction and contact law enforcement personnel for help if restraints are required. Use the minimum force necessary. Assess the airway and circulation frequently while the patient is restrained.
- The threat of suicide requires immediate intervention. You should be able to recognize the unique signs and risk factors of suicidal thought in various patient populations, including adolescents and older adults.
- A patient with PTSD has experienced feelings of helplessness, anxiety, anger, and fear. In PTSD, memories of the trauma linger and continue to be disruptive. The condition can be made worse with the existence of concurrent mental illness.

Vital Vocabulary

altered mental status A change in the way a person thinks and behaves that may signal disease in the central nervous system or elsewhere in the body.

behavior The way in which individuals interact with their environment.

behavioral health emergency A situation in which a person's behavior poses a threat to themselves or others or prevents them from caring for themselves or functioning effectively in their community.

bipolar disorder A type of mental illness characterized by alternating periods of depression and manic episodes.

delirium An acute state of confusion, which occurs suddenly and may fluctuate over short periods. Rather than a disease itself, it is a sign of any number of underlying problems.

delusions False beliefs that persist despite incontrovertible evidence to the contrary.

dementia A slow, progressive decline in cognitive function that impairs memory function and leads to behavior change.

depression A persistent mood of sadness, despair, and discouragement; may be a symptom of many different mental and physical disorders, or may be a disorder on its own.

hallucinations False perceptions involving the senses of sight, sound, taste, smell, or touch.

manic episode A period of markedly elevated mood and increased activity and energy levels, often lasting a week or longer.

mental illness A chronic health condition involving changes in behavior, thinking, and/or emotion, which significantly interferes with the patient's ability to function in daily life.

Prep Kit continued

mobile integrated health care (MIH) A method of delivering health care that involves providing care within the community rather than at a physician's office or hospital.

positional asphyxia Restriction of chest wall movements and/or airway obstruction; can rapidly lead to sudden death.

posttraumatic stress disorder (PTSD) A delayed reaction to a prior incident. Often the result of one or more conditions concerning the incident, and may relate to an incident that involved physical harm or the threat of physical harm.

psychiatric disorder An illness with psychological or behavioral symptoms and/or impairment in functioning caused by a social, psychological, genetic, physical, chemical, or biologic disturbance.

psychosis A mental disorder characterized by the loss of contact with reality; may be evidenced by hallucinations and/or delusions.

schizophrenia A complex, difficult-to-identify mental disorder whose onset typically occurs during early adulthood. Symptoms typically become more prominent over time and include delusions, hallucinations, a lack of interest in pleasure, and erratic speech.

substance use disorders (SUDs) Chronic, treatable medical conditions characterized by the uncontrolled use of substances such as alcohol, opioids, stimulants, or other drugs, despite harmful consequences.

References

1. Navigating a mental health crisis: a NAMI resource guide for those experiencing a mental health emergency. National Alliance of Mental Illness website. https://www.nami.org/wp-content/uploads/2023/07/Navigating-A-Mental-Health-Crisis.pdf. Published 2018. Accessed January 14, 2025.
2. National guidelines for behavioral health crisis care: a best practice toolkit. Substance Abuse and Mental Health Services Administration website. https://www.samhsa.gov/sites/default/files/national-guidelines-for-behavioral-health-crisis-care-02242020.pdf. Published 2020. Accessed January 14, 2025.
3. Advising people on using 988 versus 911: practical approaches for healthcare providers. Substance Abuse and Mental Health Services Administration website. https://store.samhsa.gov/sites/default/files/988-vs-911-practical-guide-pep24-06-009.pdf. Published 2024. Accessed January 14, 2025.
4. DSM-5 criteria for major depressive disorder. MDCalc website. https://www.mdcalc.com/calc/10195/dsm-5-criteria-major-depressive-disorder. Accessed January 14, 2025.
5. Thakur M, Blazer DG. Depression in long-term care. *J Am Med Dir Assoc*. 2008;9(2):82–87.
6. Suicide data and statistics. Centers for Disease Control and Prevention website. https://www.cdc.gov/suicide/facts/data.html#cdc_data_surveillance_section_4-suicide-rates. Published October 29, 2024. Accessed January 14, 2025.
7. Schaakxs R, Comijs HC, van der Mast RC, Schoevers RA, Beekman ATF, Penninx BWJH. Risk factors for depression: differential across age? *Am J Geriatr Psychiatry*. 2017;25(9):966–977.
8. Schizophrenia. National Institute of Mental Health website. https://www.nimh.nih.gov/health/topics/schizophrenia/index.shtml. Reviewed January 2025. Accessed January 14, 2025.
9. Schizophrenia. Mayo Clinic website. https://www.mayoclinic.org/diseases-conditions/schizophrenia/. Published October 16, 2024. Accessed January 14, 2025.
10. Suicide. National Institute of Mental Health website. https://www.nimh.nih.gov/health/statistics/suicide. Accessed January 14, 2025.
11. McManama O'Brien KH, Salas-Wright CP, Vaughn MG, LeCloux M. Childhood exposure to a parental suicide attempt and risk for substance use disorders. *Addict Behav*. 2015;46:70–76.
12. Post-traumatic stress disorder (PTSD). National Institute of Mental Health website. https://www.nimh.nih.gov/health/statistics/post-traumatic-stress-disorder-ptsd. Accessed January 14, 2025.
13. PTSD: National Center for PTSD. How common is PTSD in veterans? US Department of Veterans Affairs website. https://www.ptsd.va.gov/understand/common/common_veterans.asp. Accessed January 14, 2025.
14. Hoell A, Kourmpeli E, Dressing H. Work-related posttraumatic stress disorder in paramedics in comparison to data from the general population of working age. A systematic review and meta-analysis. *Front Public Health*. 2023;11:1151248. doi:10.3389/fpubh.2023.1151248
15. Petrie K, Milligan-Saville J, Gayed A, et al. Prevalence of PTSD and common mental disorders amongst

Prep Kit continued

ambulance personnel: a systematic review and meta-analysis. *Soc Psychiatry Psychiatr Epidemiol*. 2018;53:897–909.

16. Hatcher S, Sinyor M, Edgar NE, et al. A comparison of suicides in public safety personnel with suicides in the general population in Ontario, 2014 to 2018 [published correction appears in *Crisis*. 2024;45(5):364]. *Crisis*. 2024;45(5):355–363.
17. Renkiewicz GK, Hubble MW. Secondary Traumatic Stress in Emergency Services Systems (STRESS) project: quantifying and predicting compassion fatigue in emergency medical services personnel. *Prehosp Emerg Care*. 2022;26(5):652–663.
18. Pietrzak RH, Goldstein RB, Southwick SM, Grant BF. Physical health conditions associated with posttraumatic stress disorder in US older adults: results from wave 2 of the National Epidemiologic Survey on Alcohol and Related Conditions. *J Am Geriatr Soc*. 2012;60(2):296–303.
19. Saulnier KG, Brabbs S, Szymanski BR, Harpaz-Rotem I, McCarthy JF, Sripada RK. Suicide risk among veterans who receive evidence-based therapy for posttraumatic stress disorder. *JAMA Network Open*. 2024;7(12):e2452144–e2452144. doi:10.1001/jamanetworkopen.2024.52144
20. Tips for veterans to manage sensory overload and triggers. Wounded Warrior Project website. https://newsroom.woundedwarriorproject.org/Tips-for-Veterans-to-Manage-Sensory-Overload-and-Triggers. Accessed January 14, 2025.
21. Evans CS, Platts-Mills TF, Fernandez AR, et al. Repeated emergency medical services use by older adults: analysis of a comprehensive statewide database. *Ann Emerg Med*. 2017;70(4):506–515.e3. doi:10.1016/j.annemergmed.2017.03.058
22. About Alzheimer's. Centers for Disease Control and Prevention website. https://www.cdc.gov/alzheimers-dementia/about/alzheimers.html. Published August 15, 2024. Accessed January 14, 2025.
23. Alzheimer's disease facts and figures. Alzheimer's Association website. https://www.alz.org/alzheimers-dementia/facts-figures. Published 2024. Accessed January 14, 2025.
24. ACEP reaffirms positions on hyperactive delirium. American College of Emergency Physicians website. https://www.acep.org/news/acep-newsroom-articles/aceps-position-on-hyperactive-delirium. Published October 12, 2023. Accessed January 14, 2025.
25. Psychosis. National Alliance of Mental Illness website. https://www.nami.org/about-mental-illness/mental-health-conditions/psychosis/. Accessed January 14, 2025.
26. Understanding psychosis. National Institute of Mental Health website. https://www.nimh.nih.gov/health/publications/understanding-psychosis. Revised 2023. Accessed February 3, 2025.
27. Cheney PR, Gossett L, Fullerton-Gleason L, Weiss SJ, Ernst AA, Sklar D. Relationship of restraint use, patient injury, and assaults on EMS personnel. *Prehosp Emerg Care*. 2006;10(2):207–212.
28. Kupas DF, Wydro GC, Tan DK, Kamin R, Harrell AJ, Wang A. Clinical care and restraint of agitated or combative patients by emergency medical services practitioners. *Prehosp Emerg Care*. 2021;25(5):721–723.
29. Dutta C, Pasha K, Paul S, et al. Urinary tract infection induced delirium in elderly patients: a systematic review. *Cureus*. 2022;14(12):e32321. doi:10.7759/cureus.32321
30. Zewe JA, Castillo EM, Cronin AO, et al. Physiological effects of a spit restraint device saturated with artificial saliva. *J Emerg Med*. 2023;64(4):464–470.
31. Levy MK, Tan DK, McArdle DQ, et al. Consensus statement of the National Association of EMS Physicians, International Association of Fire Chiefs, and the International Association of Chiefs of Police: best practices for collaboration between law enforcement and emergency medical services during acute behavioral emergencies. *Prehosp Emerg Care*. 2024;28(8):1058–1062.

Additional Resources

Hsieh A. Seven tips to remember when restraining patients. EMS1.com website. https://www.ems1.com/patient-handling/articles/7-tips-to-remember-when-restraining-patients-HXtosXLkeKvR1pDm/. Published December 23, 2010. Accessed January 14, 2025.

Kupas DF, Wydro GC. Patient restraint in emergency medical services systems. *Prehosp Emerg Care*. 2002;6(3):340–345.

McGuire JM. The incidence of and risk factors for emergence delirium in US military combat veterans. *J Perianesth Nurs*. 2012;27(4):236–245.

National Association of State EMS Officials. *National Model EMS Clinical Guidelines: Version 3.0.* https://nasemso.org/wp-content/uploads/National-Model-EMS-Clinical-Guidelines_2022.pdf. Updated March 2022. Accessed January 14, 2025.

National Highway Traffic Safety Administration. *National Emergency Medical Services Education Standards*. https://www.ems.gov/assets/EMS_Education-Standards_2021_FNL.pdf. EMS.gov website. Published January 2021. Accessed January 14, 2025.

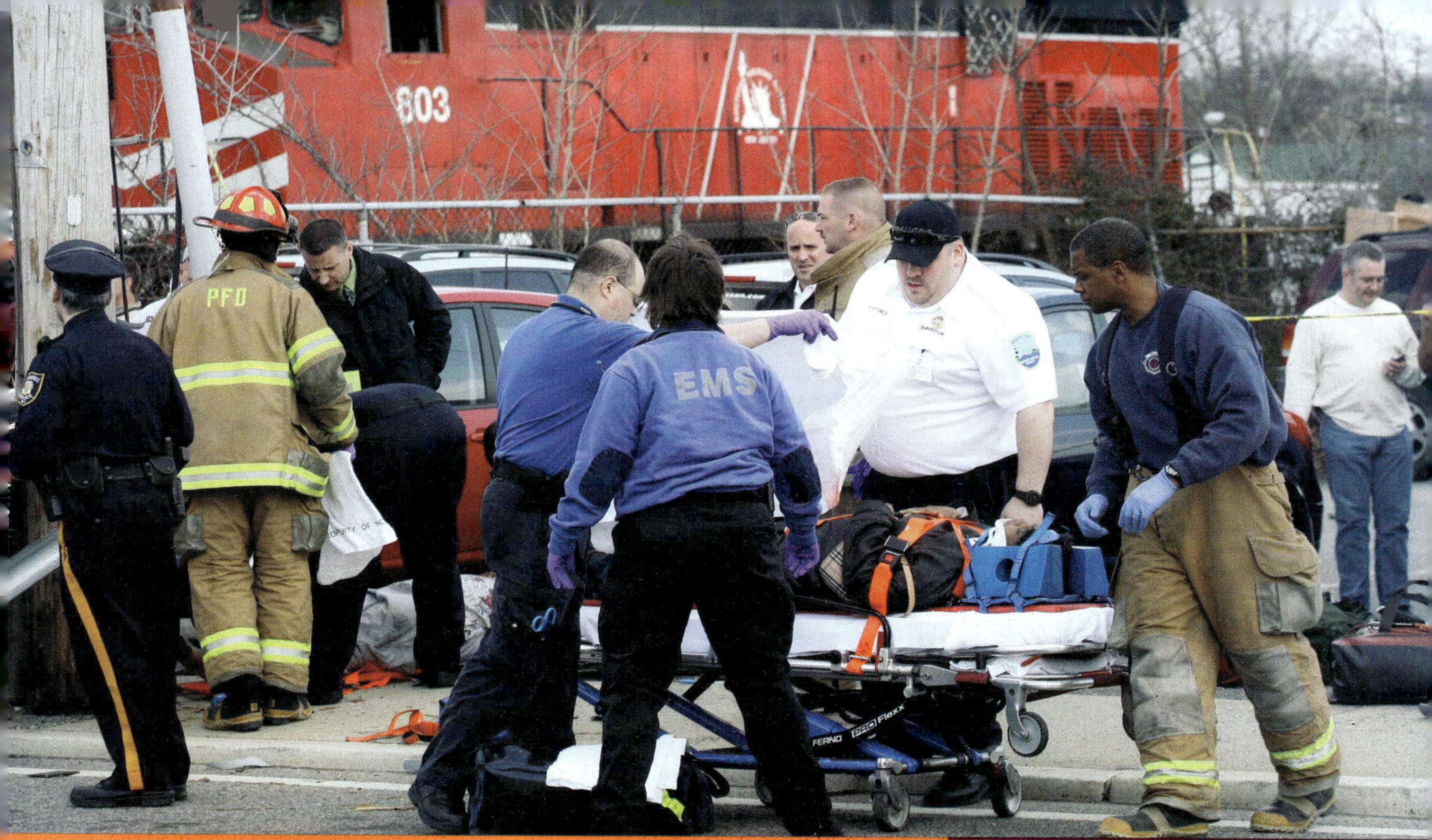

SECTION 7

Trauma

24 Trauma Overview

25 Bleeding

26 Soft-Tissue Injuries

27 Face and Neck Injuries

28 Head and Spine Injuries

29 Chest Injuries

30 Abdominal and Genitourinary Injuries

31 Orthopaedic Injuries

32 Environmental Emergencies

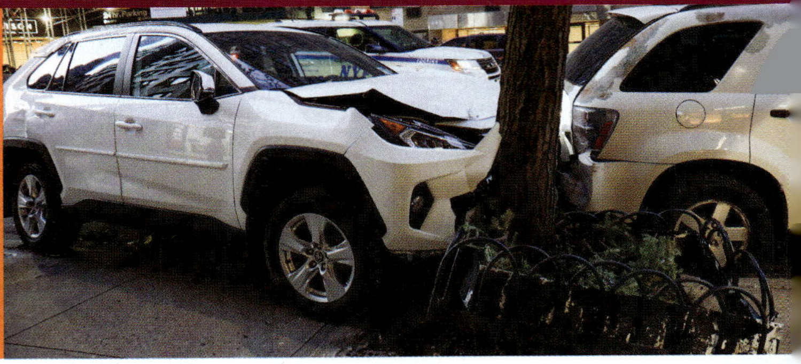

Chapter 24

Trauma Overview

NATIONAL EMS EDUCATION STANDARD COMPETENCIES

Trauma

Applies knowledge to provide basic emergency care and transportation based on assessment findings for an acutely injured patient.

Trauma Overview

- Trauma scoring (pp 918–921)
- Transport and destination issues (pp 916–918)
- Transport mode (p 918)

Multisystem Trauma

- Multisystem trauma (p 914)
- Blast injuries (pp 911–914)

KNOWLEDGE OBJECTIVES

1. Explain the relationship of the MOI to potential energy, kinetic energy, and work. (pp 897–900)
2. Define the terms mechanism of injury (MOI), blunt trauma, and penetrating trauma. (p 900)
3. Provide examples of the MOI that would cause blunt and penetrating trauma to occur. (pp 900–911)
4. Describe the different types of motor vehicle crashes (frontal, rear-end, lateral, rollover, and rotational), the injury patterns associated with each one, and how each relates to the index of suspicion of life-threatening injuries. (pp 901–907)
5. Discuss the specific factors to consider during assessment of a patient who has been injured in a fall, plus additional considerations for pediatric and geriatric patients. (pp 908–909)
6. Discuss the effects of high-, medium-, and low-velocity penetrating trauma on the body and how an understanding of each type helps emergency medical technicians (EMTs) form an index of suspicion about unseen life-threatening injuries. (pp 909–911)
7. Discuss primary, secondary, tertiary, quaternary, and quinary blast injuries and the anticipated damage each one will cause to the body. (pp 911–914)
8. Describe multisystem trauma and the special considerations that are required for patients who fit this category. (p 914)
9. Explain the major components of trauma patient assessment; include considerations related to whether the MOI was significant or nonsignificant. (p 914)
10. Discuss the special assessment considerations related to a trauma patient who has injuries in each of the following areas: head, neck and throat, chest, and abdomen. (pp 914–916)
11. Provide a general overview of multisystem trauma management. (pp 914–916)
12. Explain trauma patient care in relation to scene time and transport selection. (pp 916–918)

13. List the criteria for the appropriate use of helicopter emergency medical services. (p 918)
14. Discuss the American College of Surgeons Committee on Trauma classification of trauma centers. (pp 917–920)
15. Explain the 2021 National Guideline for the Field Triage of Injured Patients as it relates to making an appropriate destination selection for a trauma patient. (pp 917–920)

SKILLS OBJECTIVE

There are no skills objectives for this chapter.

Introduction

According to the Centers for Disease Control and Prevention (CDC), traumatic injuries and unintentional injuries, including vehicle crashes, violence, and suicide, are the leading causes of death in the United States among people from 1 to 44 years of age.[1] Proper prehospital evaluation and care has the capability to reduce a patient's suffering, long-term disability, and risk of death from trauma. Patients who need emergency medical services (EMS) assistance are generally categorized as either a medical or trauma emergency, although one may result from the other or both may exist.

Trauma emergencies occur as a result of physical forces applied to the body. **Medical emergencies** include illnesses or conditions; these are not caused by an outside force. Traumatic injuries may be caused by underlying medical conditions (a patient has a stroke and veers off the road, striking a tree). Similarly, medical illnesses may result from recent or remote traumatic injuries (pneumonia develops in a patient a few days after a fall that fractured the patient's ribs). This chapter introduces the basic physical concepts that dictate how traumatic injuries occur and how they affect the human body.

Energy and Trauma

Traumatic injury occurs when the body's tissues are exposed to energy levels beyond their tolerance (**FIGURE 24-1**). The **mechanism of injury (MOI)** is the way in which traumatic injuries occur; it describes how energy, acting on a human body, can cause injury. Kinetic energy (energy transferred from an external source to the body) is the most common mechanism associated with injury. Other forms of energy that are mechanisms of injury are thermal (heat), chemical, electrical, and radiation. These

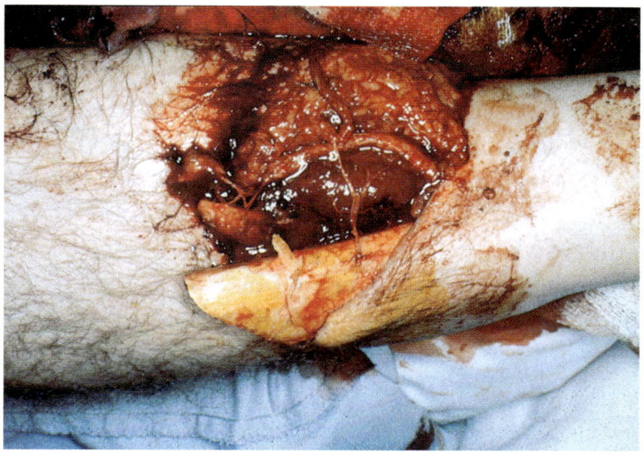

A

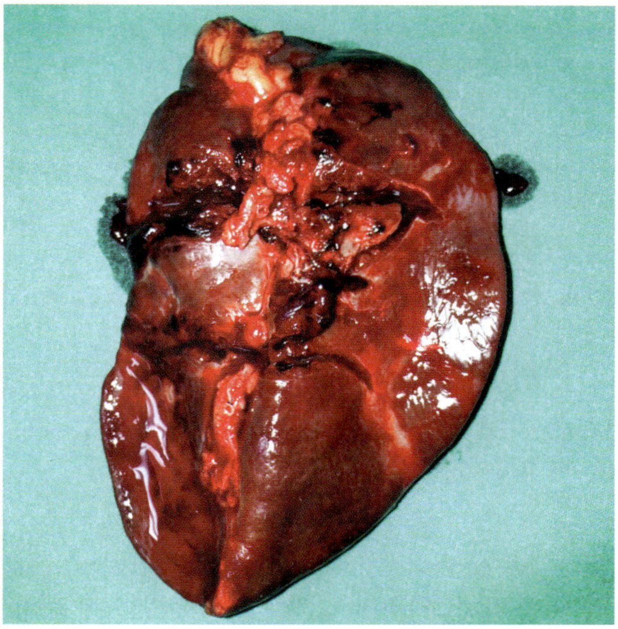

B

FIGURE 24-1 Traumatic injury occurs when the body's tissues are exposed to energy levels beyond their tolerance. **A.** Some injuries, such as this open fracture of the tibia and fibula, are easy to recognize. **B.** Other injuries, such as this ruptured spleen, will not be visible in the field.

mechanisms are discussed in Chapter 26, *Soft-Tissue Injuries,* and Chapter 39, *Terrorism Response and Disaster Management.*

When considering the effects of energy on the human body, it is important to remember that energy can be neither created nor destroyed: it can only be transformed. At the completion of this chapter, you should understand how energy transforms from one type to another and how energy causes trauma to the human body. The **index of suspicion** is your awareness of potentially serious injuries based on your understanding of how energy causes trauma. For example, when assessing a patient who has fallen, it is important to estimate the height from which the patient fell, as well as the surface they landed on, to fully appreciate the potential injuries they may have sustained.

The energy of a moving object is called **kinetic energy**. Kinetic energy is calculated as follows:

$$\text{Kinetic energy} = \tfrac{1}{2}\,\text{mass} \times \text{velocity}^2, \quad \text{or KE} = \tfrac{1}{2}\,\text{mv}^2$$

The velocity (speed) of an object will often have a much greater effect on the amount of energy than will the object's mass (size). Likewise, an increase in velocity will have a greater effect than will an increase in mass. Consider, for example, the kinetic energy if an object's mass is 140 and velocity is 10 (to illustrate the concept, we will not define the units of mass or velocity here):

$$140(\tfrac{1}{2}) \times 10^2 = 7{,}000$$

Now, consider the kinetic energy if mass is doubled and velocity remains the same:

$$280(\tfrac{1}{2}) \times 10^2 = 14{,}000$$

Finally, consider the kinetic energy if velocity is instead doubled and mass remains the same:

$$140(\tfrac{1}{2}) \times 20^2 = 28{,}000$$

Thus, we can see that doubling the object's mass doubles the total kinetic energy, whereas doubling its velocity quadruples the total kinetic energy.

Remember, energy cannot be created or destroyed, only converted. In the case of a motor vehicle crash, the kinetic energy of the speeding vehicle is converted into the work of stopping the vehicle, usually by crushing the vehicle's exterior (**FIGURE 24-2**).

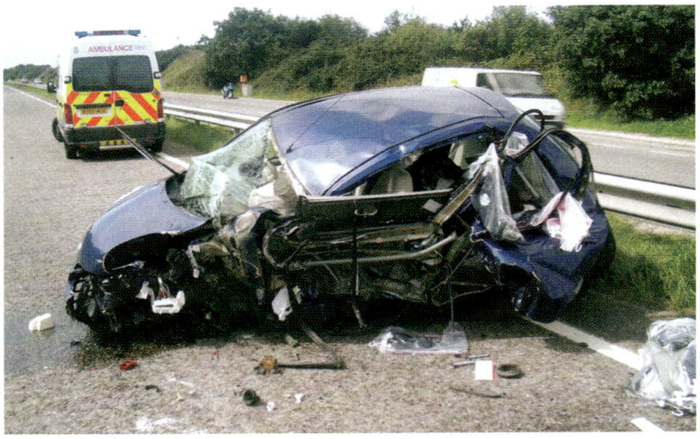

FIGURE 24-2 The kinetic energy of a speeding car is converted into the work of stopping the car, usually by crushing the car's exterior and damaging the point of impact.

Courtesy of Mark Woolcock.

Similarly, the passengers of the vehicle have kinetic energy because they were traveling at the same speed as the vehicle. Their kinetic energy is converted to the work of bringing them to a stop. It is this work on the passengers that results in injury.

Notice that, according to the equation for kinetic energy, when a car's speed increases from 50 to 70 mph, the energy that is available to cause injury nearly doubles. This point is even more clear when considering gunshot wounds. The speed of the bullet (high-velocity compared with low-velocity) has a greater impact on producing injury than the mass (size) of the bullet. Therefore, it is important to report to the hospital the type of firearm that was used in a shooting, if possible. The amount of kinetic energy that is converted to do work on the body dictates the severity of the injury. High-energy injuries often produce such severe damage that patients require immediate transport to an appropriate facility to have any hope of survival.

Potential energy is the product of mass (weight), force of gravity, and height:

$$\text{Potential energy} = \text{Mass} \times \text{Gravity} \times \text{Height} \quad \text{or PE} = \text{mgh}$$

This type of energy can be thought of as stored energy that is ready to be released and is primarily associated with the energy of falling objects. A worker on a scaffold has potential energy because they are some height above the ground. If the worker falls, potential energy is converted into kinetic energy. As the worker hits the ground, the kinetic energy is converted into work—that is, the work of bringing the body to a stop and thereby fracturing bones and damaging tissues.

While understanding the concepts of kinetic energy, work energy, and potential energy can help focus your patient assessment, it is important to remember that the priority is to assess for injury, regardless of the mechanism of injury.

Newton's Laws of Motion

Mathematician Isaac Newton defined three physical laws that allow us to predict the effects of motion and gravity on objects.

Newton's First Law

Newton's first law of motion states that objects at rest tend to stay at rest and objects in motion tend to stay in motion unless acted on by an outside force. For example, an object such as an empty soda can will not move spontaneously unless some force, such as a gust of wind, acts on it. Once in motion, it will continue until stopped by an external force. That force could be a person placing a foot on the can, or the simple forces of Earth's gravity and friction acting on it.

Newton's Second Law

Newton's second law of motion states that force equals mass times acceleration:

$$F = m \times a,$$

where acceleration is the change in velocity (speed) that occurs over time. Therefore, it is not so much speed, in itself, that causes injuries, but the sudden change in velocity. Simply put, it is not the fall, but the sudden stop at the bottom, that causes the injury.

For example, it takes approximately 3 seconds for a car traveling at 30 mph to come to a stop when the driver applies the brakes smoothly. If the car is stopped not by braking but by hitting a large tree, the deceleration now occurs in approximately 0.01 second. Because the period of deceleration is 300 times less, the average force of impact is 300 times greater.

Now consider the driver's experience within the vehicle. If the driver is restrained with a shoulder and lap belt, the driver is essentially tied to the car and stops during the same period the car stops. It takes some time, although brief, to crush the front of the car and bring it to a halt. The car comes to a stop in approximately 0.05 second. The change in the driver's velocity is the same (30 to 0 mph), but the longer period of deceleration results in a *g* force of 30 times that of gravity (one *g* force is the normal acceleration due to gravity). Moreover, the vehicle is a large object and is designed to efficiently distribute impact. The restrained driver still experiences a substantial force, but it is much less than the force experienced by an unrestrained driver. An unrestrained body would stay in motion at 30 mph until it is stopped by an external force, such as a steering wheel, windshield, dashboard, or pavement.

In a final example, the car and driver, as before, are traveling at 30 mph, and the driver is properly restrained with a three-point seat belt. This time, the car is also equipped with an airbag. When the car hits the tree and suddenly stops, the driver's upper body, though partially slowed by the lap and shoulder belts, initially continues forward. The body is finally brought to rest by the airbag. The upper body compresses the airbag, which stops the body's forward motion in approximately 0.1 second. Thanks to the airbag, the force of impact is applied over a much larger area. The dual action of the airbag (distributing the force of impact over a greater area and increasing the duration of impact) results in less severe injuries.

Newton's Third Law

Newton's third law of motion states that for every action, there is an equal and opposite reaction. Therefore, if you push on a door, the door pushes back (reacts) with an equal force but in the opposite direction. In the case of a vehicle crash with a dented A-pillar (the pillar supporting the roof between the front side windows and the windshield), you should consider that the force of the driver's head was sufficient to dent the strong metal. But in terms of patient assessment, the more important point is the reaction force of the pillar on the head. Newton's third law states that the two forces are equal but occur in opposite directions. In other words, the head was essentially hit by an A-pillar traveling at 30 mph (the velocity of the unrestrained driver in the preceding example). Similarly, it takes a substantial force to collapse a steering wheel. When you notice a collapsed steering wheel during scene size-up, suspect serious chest injuries even if the driver initially has no visible signs of chest injury. Often, reading the scene and understanding the basic principles of energy transfer will give you as clear a picture of the patient's potential injuries and injury severity as the actual physical patient assessment.

It is important to understand that these examples are simply illustrations to help you picture these concepts in energy transfer and injuries. Engineers designing automobiles also understand these concepts and design modern vehicles in ways to transfer energy around the passengers and slow the passengers in the event of a crash by using supplemental restraint systems. A patient's injuries should be assessed directly whenever possible, not simply presumed based on the vehicle's speed or the exterior damage it sustained.

MOI Profiles

Different MOIs will produce different types of injuries. Examples of significant MOIs include the following[2]:

- Falls from heights (>10 feet [3 m])
- Motor vehicle crash involving a partial or complete ejection, significant intrusion requiring extrication, death in the passenger compartment, unrestrained occupant or child younger than 9 years, or vehicle telemetry that indicates potential for severe injury
- A crash in which the rider was separated from the transport vehicle (eg, motorcycle, all-terrain vehicle, horse), causing significant impact
- Car-versus-pedestrian/bicycle crash in which the pedestrian/rider was thrown, was run over, or sustained significant impact

Traumatic injuries can be considered in two categories: blunt trauma and penetrating trauma. **Blunt trauma** is the result of force (or energy transmission) to the body that causes injury without anything penetrating the soft tissues or internal organs and cavities. **Penetrating trauma** results in injury by objects that pierce the surface of the body, cutting through the underlying soft tissues, internal organs, and body cavities. Either type of trauma may occur from a variety of MOIs. It is important to consider unseen as well as visible injuries with either type of trauma. Damage to the underlying deeper tissues is often more significant.

Words of Wisdom

Vehicle telemetry or vehicle crash notification systems use sensors to automatically detect a crash and notify 911 call centers. In some cases, additional information such as potential severity of the collision and vehicle occupant communications can be relayed. The global positioning system (GPS) in these systems can also pinpoint the location of the crash. The system will not work if there is no cellular or GPS signal reception or if the vehicle owner has not subscribed to the service.[3]

Blunt Trauma

Motor vehicle crashes and falls are two of the most common MOIs for blunt trauma. When providing care for your patient, be alert to skin discoloration, bone deformation, or reports of pain because these

YOU are the EMT

At 1520 hours, you and your partner are dispatched to a motor vehicle crash in which a passenger vehicle reportedly struck a tree head-on at an unknown rate of speed. The emergency medical dispatcher (EMD) reports that the driver is the only patient and is still in the vehicle. It is unknown if the driver is trapped. Law enforcement personnel and a rescue company have also been dispatched.

1. On the basis of the information provided by the EMD, can you predict the potential types of injuries the patient may have? If so, how?
2. Why is it important to estimate the approximate speed at which a vehicle was traveling at the time of impact?

may be the only signs of blunt trauma. During assessment, maintain a high index of suspicion for hidden (internal) injuries in patients with blunt trauma.

Vehicular Crashes

Motor vehicle crashes are traditionally classified as frontal (head-on), rear-end, lateral (T-bone), rollover, and rotational (spins). The principal difference among these crash types is the direction of the force of impact. With spins and rollovers there is a significant possibility of multiple impacts. Motor vehicle crashes typically consist of a series of three collisions. Understanding the events that occur during each of these three collisions will help you be alert for certain types of injury patterns.

The three collisions in a typical impact are as follows:

1. The collision of the car against another car, a tree, or some other object. Damage to the car is perhaps the most dramatic part of the collision, but it does not directly affect patient care, except possibly to make extrication difficult (**FIGURE 24-3**). However, it does provide information about the severity of the collision, and therefore has an indirect effect on patient care. If damage is significant enough to require extrication or cause intrusion into the passenger compartment, tear seats from their mountings, and collapse steering wheels, maintain a high index of suspicion for the presence of high-energy trauma.
2. The collision of the passenger against the interior of the car. Just as the kinetic energy produced by the vehicle's mass and velocity is converted into the work of bringing the vehicle to a stop, the kinetic energy produced by the passenger's mass and velocity is converted into the work of stopping their body (**FIGURE 24-4**). Just like the obvious damage to the exterior of the car, the injuries that result are often dramatic and usually immediately apparent during your scene size-up or primary assessment. Common passenger injuries include lower extremity fractures (knees into the dashboard), rib fractures (rib cage into the steering wheel), and head trauma (head into the windshield). Such injuries occur more frequently if the passenger is not restrained. But even when the passenger is restrained with a properly adjusted seat belt, injuries can occur, especially in lateral and rollover impacts.
3. The collision of the passenger's internal organs against the solid structures of the body. The injuries that occur during the third collision may not be as obvious as external injuries, but they are often the most life threatening. For example, as the passenger's head hits the

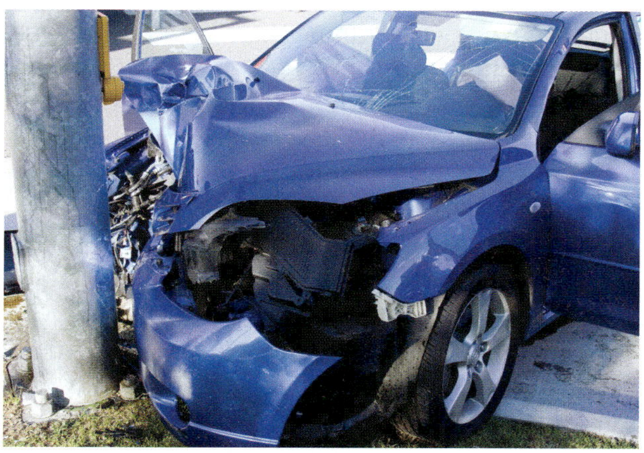

FIGURE 24-3 The first collision in a typical impact is that of the vehicle against another object (in this case, a utility pole). The appearance of the vehicle can provide you with critical information about the severity of the crash. The greater the damage to the vehicle, the greater the energy that was involved.

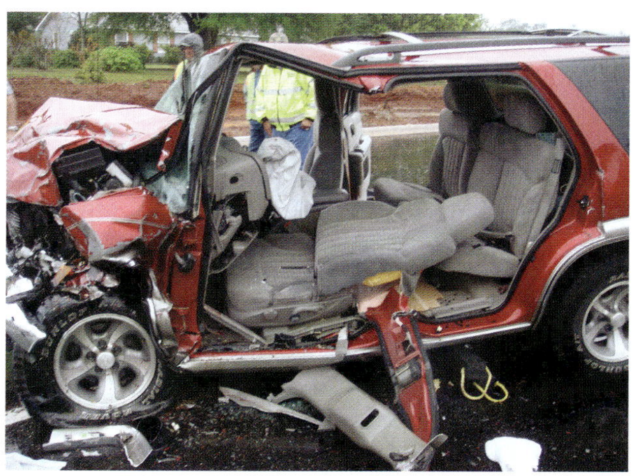

FIGURE 24-4 The second collision in a typical impact is that of the passenger against the interior of the car. The appearance of the interior of the car can provide you with information about the severity of the patient's injuries.

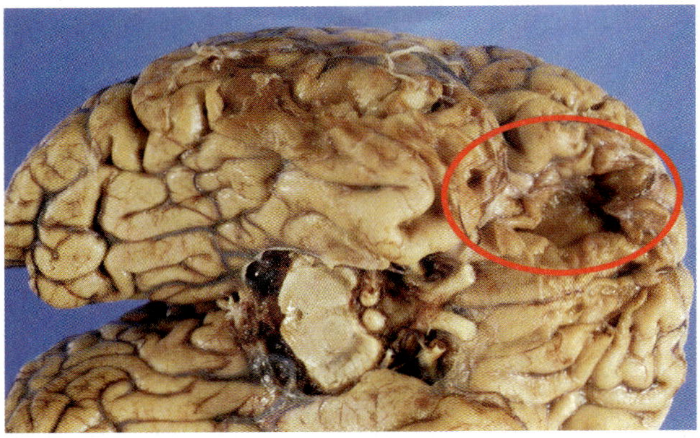

FIGURE 24-5 The discolored spots show injuries (contusions) in this brain.

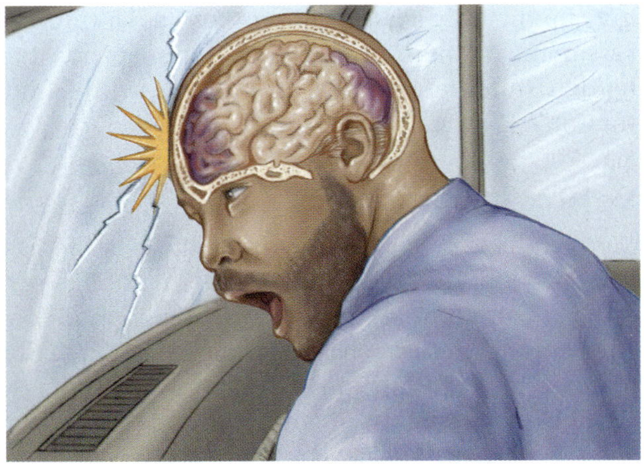

FIGURE 24-6 The third collision in a typical impact is that of the passenger's internal organs against the solid structures of the body. A coup–contrecoup injury occurs when the brain continues its forward motion and strikes the inside of the skull (the coup), resulting in a compression injury to the anterior portion of the brain, and a secondary injury on rebound (the contrecoup), when the posterior portion of the brain is stretched or strikes the opposite side of the skull.

windshield, the brain continues forward until it strikes the inside of the skull, resulting in a compression injury (or bruising) to the anterior portion of the brain (**FIGURE 24-5**). Injury to the posterior portion of the brain may also occur as the result of a tension injury (stretching) or as the result of the brain striking the opposite side of the skull after it rebounds from the first impact, referred to as a **coup–contrecoup brain injury** (**FIGURE 24-6**).[4,5] Similarly, traumatic aortic transection or rupture is associated with a sudden and rapid deceleration of the heart and the aorta within the thoracic cavity, which may rupture the aorta and cause fatal bleeding.

The amount of damage considered significant varies, depending on the type of crash, but deformity of the vehicle is considered after the patient's injury patterns, mental status, and vital signs are assessed. These factors determine the need to transport the patient to a trauma center. In addition to the patient's presentation, some protocols may identify specific mechanisms that warrant transport to a trauma center.

Damage to the vehicle that was involved and information obtained during the scene size-up are not the only clues you can use to determine crash severity. Clearly, if one or more of the passengers are dead, you should suspect that the other passengers have sustained serious injuries, even if the injuries are not obvious. Therefore, focus on treating life-threatening injuries and providing rapid care and transport to a trauma center, because these passengers have likely experienced the same amount of force that caused the death of the others.

Restraint Systems and Airbags

Properly used restraint systems are proven to reduce injuries and deaths related to vehicular crashes. According to the National Highway Traffic Safety Administration, most front seat passengers (91.9%) wear safety restraints. Yet, approximately 50% of the individuals who die in vehicle crashes were not wearing a seat belt, demonstrating the disproportionate risk to those who do not buckle up.[6]

When properly applied, seat belts are successful in restraining the passengers in a vehicle and preventing a second collision inside the motor vehicle. Seat belts may also decrease the severity of the third collision, that of the passenger's organs with the chest or abdominal wall. The protective abilities of seat belts are further enhanced by deployment of the airbags. Airbags provide supplemental protection that, with seat belts, provide the final capture point of the passengers and decrease the severity of **deceleration** injuries by allowing seat belts to be more compliant and by gently cushioning the occupant as the body slows, or decelerates.

Note that supplemental restraint systems can cause harm if not used properly. For example, in some older vehicle models, the seat belts buckle automatically at the shoulder but require the passengers to buckle the lap portion; not buckling the lap portion can cause the occupant to travel down and under the shoulder strap as the body continues forward, resulting in the lower body striking the dashboard. This movement of the body can cause the lower extremities and the pelvis to crash into the dashboard because that part of the body is unrestrained. Seat belts may also cause unseen abdominal injuries, particularly in pediatric patients. Seat belts are designed to be worn over the iliac crests of the pelvis to distribute the force over the bony surface. Hip dislocations may result if seat belts are worn too low. Internal injuries can occur when the belt is worn too high, resulting in damage to abdominal organs (**FIGURE 24-7**). Lumbar spine fractures are also possible, particularly in children and older adults.

Airbags were first developed to prevent or reduce injuries in frontal collisions and have been standard equipment in most motor vehicles since 1999. They reduce the forces applied to the body during deceleration by slowing the stopping distance. Because the airbag deflates in less than 1 second after impact, they are less effective in crashes that involve multiple impacts such as rollover collisions. The addition of side-impact airbags and more recently rear-window and far-side airbags in some vehicles has reduced injuries in rear-end, lateral, and rollover crashes as well.[8]

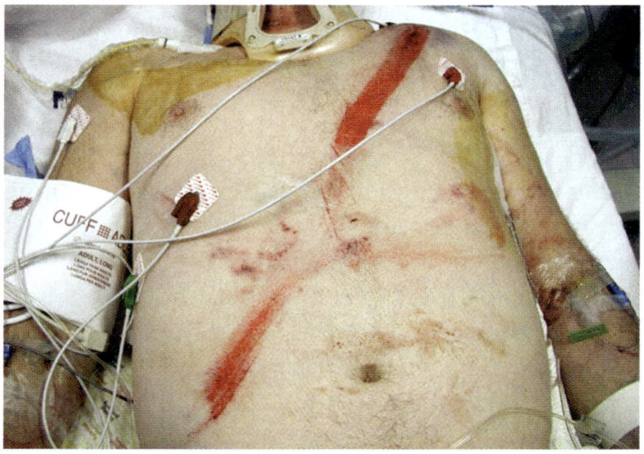

FIGURE 24-7 Injuries can result if the seat belt is worn too high or too low across the waist. Although less common, injuries can also result from seat belts worn in the correct position across the torso.

Courtesy of ED, Royal North Shore Hospital/NSW Institute of Trauma & Injury.

Special Populations

PEDIATRIC AND PREGNANT PATIENTS

Vehicle occupants are at increased risk of injury when seat belts are applied inappropriately or when occupants are seated at an improper distance from airbags. Populations at particular risk are pregnant persons and children. Pregnant individuals often wear seat belts too high, or not at all.[7] If the seat belt is worn too high, the force transferred during a rapid deceleration does not go to the bony structure of the hips as designed, but instead is distributed to the abdominal organs and developing fetus. Pregnant persons should wear the lap belt under their stomach and across their thighs and hip bones, and the shoulder belt between their breasts and to the side of their stomach. They can adjust the seat and steering wheel to improve comfort.

Because the car is designed around adult proportions, infants and children must use a child safety seat. These seats, when secured properly to the vehicle using seat belts or lower anchors, are designed to absorb the injury of sudden deceleration without displacing that force onto the child.

Remember that airbags decrease many injuries effectively. However, you should still suspect that other serious injuries to the extremities (resulting from the second collision) and to internal organs (resulting from the third collision) may have occurred.

Airbag deployment is associated with injuries such as abrasions and foreign body or eyeglass injuries to the face and eyes. Typically, airbag-related injuries are minor when the driver is positioned at least 10 inches (25 cm) from the steering wheel airbag cover and the front seat passenger is at least 18 inches (45 cm) away from the airbag cover.[5] When passengers are riding in vehicles equipped with airbags but are not restrained by seat belts, they are often thrown forward in the act of emergency braking. As a result, they come into contact with the airbag and/or the doors at the time of deployment, which may cause serious injuries. This MOI is also responsible for some severe injuries to children who are riding unrestrained in the front seats of vehicles, unrestrained passengers, and those sitting too close to the airbag. Because a rear-facing car seat is in proximity to the dashboard, rapid inflation of the airbag could cause serious injury or death to an infant. All children who are shorter than 4 feet 9 inches (145 cm) should ride in the rear seat, or, in the case of a pickup truck or other single-seated vehicle, the airbag should be turned off.[5]

When providing care to an occupant inside a motor vehicle, it is important to remember that if the airbag did not inflate during the accident, it may deploy during extrication. If this occurs, you may be seriously injured. Extreme caution must be used when extricating a patient in a vehicle with an airbag that has not deployed. See Chapter 37, *Vehicle Extrication and Special Rescue*, for further discussion.

Safety Tips

Although rare, ambulance collisions do occur. Safety precautions include wearing seat belts, securing all patients with the proper restraint device, securing medical equipment, and ensuring cabinets are closed appropriately. See Chapter 36, *Transport Operations*, for more information about ambulance safety restraints.

Frontal Crashes

Understanding the MOI after a frontal crash first involves evaluation of the supplemental restraint system, including seat belts and airbags. Determine whether the passenger was restrained by a full and properly applied three-point restraint (lap and shoulder belts). Also determine whether the airbag was deployed. Identifying the types of restraints used and whether airbags were deployed will help you identify injury patterns related to the supplemental restraint systems.

When properly applied, seat belts are successful in restraining the passengers in a vehicle and preventing a second collision inside the motor vehicle. If restraint systems are not used or not used properly, contact points are often obvious as you perform a simple, quick evaluation of the interior of the vehicle. If there is no intrusion into the passenger compartment, you might see that an unrestrained front-seat passenger in a frontal crash has come into contact with the dashboard or the instrument panel at the knees, thus transferring loads from the knees through the femur to the pelvis and hip joint (**FIGURE 24-8A**). The chest and/or abdomen may also hit the steering wheel (**FIGURE 24-8B**). In addition, the passenger's face often hits the steering wheel, or the passenger may launch forward and upward, hitting the windshield and/or the roof header in the area of the visors (**FIGURE 24-8C**). Signs of most of these injuries can be found by inspecting the interior of the vehicle during extrication of the patient.

Rear-End Crashes

Rear-end impacts are known to cause whiplash injuries, which are strain injuries to the neck and spine due to sudden forces. This injury is particularly likely when the passenger's head and/or neck is not restrained by an appropriately placed headrest (**FIGURE 24-9**). On impact, the passenger's body and torso move forward. As the body is propelled forward, the head and neck are left behind because the head is relatively heavy, and they appear to be whipped back relative to the torso. As the vehicle comes to rest, an unrestrained passenger will move forward, striking the dashboard. In this type of crash, the cervical spine and surrounding area may be injured. The cervical spine is less tolerant of damage when it is bent back. Properly positioned headrests decrease extension of the head and neck during a crash and, therefore, help reduce injury. Other parts of the spine and the pelvis may also be at risk for injury. In addition, the patient may sustain an acceleration injury to the brain (ie, the third collision of the brain within the skull).

Lateral Crashes

Lateral or side impacts (commonly called T-bone crashes) are a common cause of death associated with motor vehicle crashes. When a vehicle is struck from the side, it is typically struck above its center of gravity and begins to rock away from the side of the impact. This results in the passenger sustaining a lateral whiplash injury (**FIGURE 24-10**). The movement is to the side, and the passenger's shoulders and head whip toward the intruding vehicle. This action may thrust the shoulder, thorax, and upper extremities, and, more important, the skull against the doorpost or the window. The cervical spine has little tolerance for lateral bending.

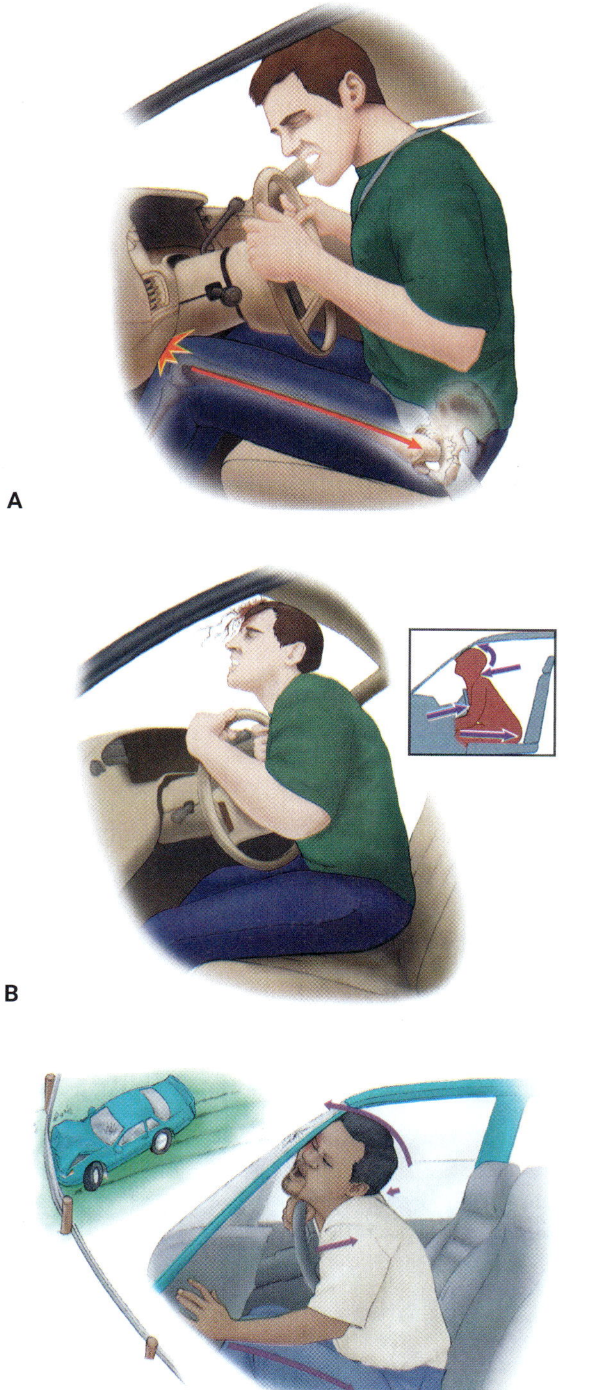

FIGURE 24-8 Mechanism of injury and condition of the vehicle interior suggest likely areas of injury. **A.** The knees can strike the dashboard, resulting in a hip fracture or dislocation. **B.** Serious chest and abdominal injuries can result from striking the steering wheel. **C.** Head and spinal injuries can result when the face and head strike the windshield.

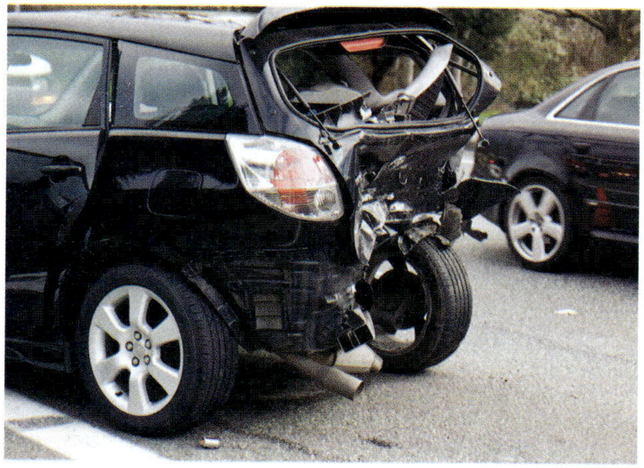

FIGURE 24-9 Rear-end impacts often cause whiplash injuries, particularly when the head and/or neck is not restrained by a headrest.

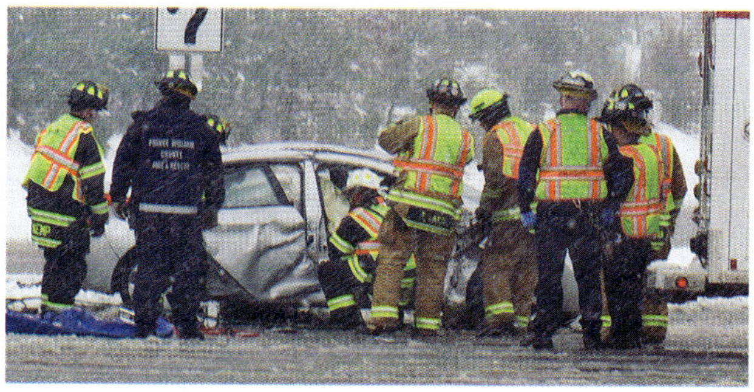

FIGURE 24-10 In a lateral crash, the car is typically struck above its center of gravity and begins to rock away from the side of impact. This causes a type of lateral whiplash in which the passenger's shoulders and head whip toward the intruding vehicle.

If there is substantial intrusion into the passenger compartment, suspect your patient to have lateral chest and abdomen injuries on the side of the impact, as well as possible fractures of the lower extremities, pelvis, and ribs. In addition, the organs within the abdomen are at risk because of a possible third collision. Side-curtain airbags can reduce the incidence and severity of head injuries and death in this type of collision.[8]

Rollover Crashes

Certain vehicles, such as large trucks, ambulances, and some sport utility vehicles, are more susceptible to rollover crashes because of their high center of gravity. Injury patterns that are commonly associated with rollover crashes differ, depending on whether the passenger was restrained, whether airbags deployed, vehicle speed, impact angle, and location of the occupants at the time of the crash. The most unpredictable types of injuries are caused by rollover crashes in which an unrestrained passenger may have sustained multiple strikes within the interior of the vehicle as it rolled one or more times.

The most common life-threatening event in a rollover is ejection or partial ejection of the passenger from the vehicle. Passengers who are ejected may strike the interior of the vehicle many times before ejection. They may also strike several objects, such as trees, a guardrail, or the vehicle's exterior, before or after striking the ground. Passengers who have been completely ejected have been shown to be six times more likely to die.[5] Passengers who have been partially ejected may have struck both the interior and the exterior of the vehicle and may have been sandwiched between the exterior of the vehicle and the environment as the vehicle rolled. Ejection and partial ejection are significant MOIs; in these cases, prepare to care for life-threatening injuries.

Even when restrained, passengers can sustain severe injuries during a rollover crash, although the patterns of injury tend to be more predictable, and when the restraint system is properly used, ejection from the vehicle is less likely. A passenger on the outboard side of a vehicle that rolls over is at high risk for injury because of the centrifugal force (the patient is pinned against the door of the vehicle). Rollover crashes can also cause injury when the roof of the vehicle hits the ground during the rollover; a passenger who is restrained can still move far enough toward the roof to make contact and sustain a spinal cord injury. Therefore, rollover crashes are dangerous for both restrained and, to a greater degree, unrestrained passengers because these crashes provide multiple opportunities for second and third collisions.

Safety Tips

Ambulances have a high center of gravity, predisposing them to rollover crashes.

Rotational Crashes

Rotational crashes (spins) are conceptually similar to rollovers. The rotation of the vehicle as it spins

YOU are the EMT

When you arrive at the scene, fire and law enforcement personnel are already present. An air transport helicopter is available with a 10-minute estimated time of arrival (ETA) upon dispatch. The front of the vehicle has been crushed all the way up to the windshield. The driver, a young man, was unrestrained and is still in the driver's seat; he appears to be unconscious and his face is covered with blood. As your partner accesses the patient from the backseat and manually stabilizes his head, you perform a primary assessment.

Recording Time: 0 Minutes	
Appearance	Bleeding from the head, face, and mouth; pale skin (as compared to baseline color); labored breathing
Level of consciousness	Responsive only to pain
Airway	Blood in the nasopharynx and oropharynx
Breathing	Rapid and labored
Circulation	Radial pulses weak and rapid; skin cool, pale, and clammy

Despite the severity of exterior damage to the vehicle, the patient is not entrapped and there is no interior intrusion into the passenger compartment. You suction the patient's mouth, apply a cervical collar, and prepare to rapidly extricate him from the vehicle. Responders from one of the engine companies have prepared a backboard to move him to the stretcher.

3. What damage in the vehicle's interior may have caused the patient's signs and symptoms?

provides opportunities for the vehicle to strike other vehicles or objects such as utility poles. For example, as a vehicle spins and strikes a pole, the passengers experience not only the rotational motion, but also a lateral impact.

Car Versus Pedestrian

Car-versus-pedestrian crashes often result in patients who have graphic and apparent injuries, such as broken bones; however, even when no serious external injuries are evident, this type of crash can cause serious injuries to underlying body systems. Therefore, you must maintain a high index of suspicion for unseen injuries. A thorough evaluation of the MOI is critical. First, estimate the speed of the vehicle that struck the patient; next, determine whether the patient was thrown (and how far), what surface the patient landed on, and if the patient was subsequently run over. Evaluate the vehicle that struck the patient for structural damage that might indicate contact points with the patient and alert you to potential injuries. Multisystem injuries are common after this type of event. If available, consider summoning advanced life support (ALS) backup for any patients who have or are thought to have sustained a significant MOI.

Car Versus Bicycle

In a car-versus-bicycle crash, evaluate the MOI in much the same manner as car-versus-pedestrian crashes. However, additional evaluation of damage to and the position of the bicycle is warranted. If the patient was wearing a helmet, inspect the helmet for damage and suspect potential injury to the head (**FIGURE 24-11**). If the patient was ejected from the bicycle, run over, or sustained significant impact, presume that they meet trauma triage criteria. These patients should undergo cervical spine assessment and have a cervical collar placed if indicated, and you should maintain appropriate spinal motion restriction during the encounter. When practical, roll the patient onto their side to allow for an appropriate assessment of the posterior side of the body.

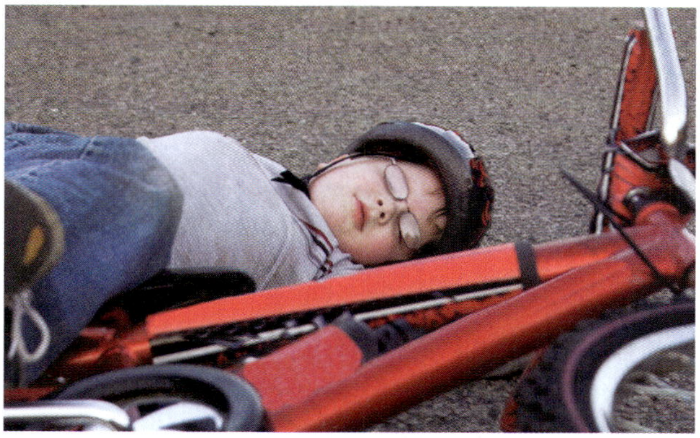

FIGURE 24-11 If the patient's bike helmet is damaged, suspect head and spine injuries.

Motorcycle Crash

Motorcyclists have a higher incidence of crashes, injuries, and death than those driving enclosed vehicles.[9] In a motorcycle crash, any structural protection afforded to the victim is not derived from a steel cage, as is the case in an automobile, but from protective devices worn by the rider. These protective items include a helmet, leather or abrasion-resistant clothing, and boots. Although helmets are designed to protect against impact forces to the head, they do not protect from cervical spinal injury. Patients who have experienced a motorcycle crash should undergo cervical spine assessment and have a cervical collar placed if indicated. Leather and synthetic gear worn over the body was initially designed to protect professional riders in competition, where falls tend to be controlled and result in long sliding mechanisms on hard surfaces rather than multiple collisions against road objects and other vehicles. Leather clothing will mostly protect against road abrasion but offers no protection against blunt trauma from secondary impacts. In a street crash, collisions usually occur against other larger vehicles or stationary objects.

When assessing the scene of a motorcycle crash, look for deformity of the motorcycle, the side of most damage, the distance of skid in the road, the deformity of stationary objects or other vehicles, and the extent and location of deformity in the helmet. These findings can be helpful in estimating the extent of trauma sustained by a patient. If a helmet was not worn, report this to the emergency department. The incidence of moderate to severe head injuries increases threefold when no helmet is worn, which is more common in states that do not require their use.[10]

Words of Wisdom

If possible, bring the helmet to the hospital for the trauma staff to see. The helmet may offer critical information about the type and extent of potential head injury.

There are four types of motorcycle impacts.

- **Head-on crash.** The motorcycle strikes another object and stops its forward motion while the rider and parts of the motorcycle that are broken off continue their forward motion until stopped by an outside force, such as drag from the road or another opposing force from a secondary collision. These patients are at high risk for injuries to the head, chest, abdomen, and pelvis, depending which part of the body struck the handlebars or ground.
- **Angular crash.** The motorcycle strikes an object or another vehicle at an angle so that the rider sustains direct crushing injuries to the lower extremity between the object and the motorcycle. This usually results in severe open and comminuted lower extremity injuries with severe neurovascular compromise, often resulting in traumatic amputation or otherwise requiring surgical amputation.
- **Ejection.** The rider will travel at high speed until stopped by a stationary object, another vehicle, or road drag. Severe abrasion injuries (road rash) down to bone can occur with drag. An unpredictable combination of blunt injuries can occur from secondary collisions.
- **Controlled crash.** A technique used to separate the rider from the motorcycle before crashing into an object is referred to as laying the bike down. It was developed by motorcycle racers and adapted by street bikers as a means of achieving a controlled crash. As a crash approaches, the rider tips the motorcycle toward one side and turns it at 90° to the direction of travel. With one leg sliding along the ground, the rider is able to slow at a greater rate than the motorcycle and can then let go to separate from it. If properly protected with leather or synthetic abrasion-resistant gear, injuries should be limited to those sustained by rolling over the pavement and any secondary collision that may occur. When executed properly, this maneuver prevents the rider from being trapped between the bike and the object. However, a rider unable to clear the bike will continue into the vehicle, often with devastating results.

Falls

The injury potential of a fall is related to the height from which the patient fell. Falls are common MOIs for blunt trauma. The greater the height of the fall, the greater the potential for injury. A fall from more than 10 feet (3 m) is considered significant. The patient lands on the surface just as an unrestrained passenger smashes into the interior of a vehicle. The internal organs travel at the speed of the patient's body before it hits the ground and stop by smashing into the interior of the body. Again, as in a motor vehicle crash, it is these internal injuries that are the least obvious during assessment but pose the gravest threat to life. Therefore, suspect internal injuries in a patient who has fallen from a significant height, just as you would in a patient who has been in a high-speed motor vehicle crash.

Special Populations

SIGNIFICANT MOIS IN THE PEDIATRIC PATIENT

When your patient is a child, the following constitute a significant MOI[11]:

- The child is 5 years old or younger and has sustained a low-level fall with significant head impact.
- The child is younger than 9 years old and has sustained an injury resulting in a systolic blood pressure less than 70 mm Hg + (2 × age in years).
- You suspect the injuries are the result of child abuse.
- The child has special, high-resource health care needs.

Children should be triaged preferentially to pediatric-capable centers.

Patients who fall and land on their feet may have less severe internal injuries because their legs may have absorbed much of the energy of the

Special Populations

FALLS IN THE GERIATRIC PATIENT

Falls account for the highest number of injuries in patients 65 years and older and are the leading cause of injury-related death in this population.[12] More than one-half of patients who require EMS assistance after a fall have had a previous fall-related emergency requiring EMS response.[13] There are many reasons that older adults are susceptible to falling, including the following:

- Weakness in their lower extremities
- Insufficient vitamin D levels
- Problems with balance and walking
- Use of medications that impair thinking or balance
- Impaired vision
- Foot pain or inappropriate footwear

Hazards in the home such as broken or uneven steps and throw rugs or clutter also cause falls in older adults. Many of these risk factors can be controlled or eliminated. Some EMS agencies offer fall reduction screening for older adults in their communities, and some of these programs report significant decreases in both the number of fall-related calls and the number of fall-related calls requiring transport to the hospital.[14]

Many older adults can be seriously injured from standing, low-level falls. Aside from a fall of more than 10 feet (3 m), assessment findings that indicate a high risk for serious injury requiring transport to a trauma center include systolic blood pressure of less than 110 mm Hg or a heart rate that is higher than the systolic blood pressure value. Factors that suggest a moderate risk for serious injury in the geriatric patient include having sustained a fall of less than 10 feet (3 m) that caused significant head impact, taking anticoagulant medication, or having special, high-resource health care needs.[11]

Completely assess older adults for all possible injuries, even from low-impact falls. When obtaining the patient history, ask what led up to the fall, and determine if they have any new symptoms or medications. The assessment should include a complete set of vital signs, including temperature, and a thorough head-to-toe examination, including assessments for both trauma and medical concerns. The medical assessment should include a selection of focused medical exams based on the possibility that a problem such as stroke, heart failure, or infection might have contributed to the fall.

If the patient has decision-making capacity and refuses transport despite your concerns, ask them to walk across the room. If they are unable to do so, contact medical direction and possibly social services, depending on your protocols. When explaining the risks of refusal, attempt to involve the patient's family or caregivers. The simple mnemonic MEMAW (developed by a paramedic in Rochester, New York) may help you recall elements that are important during your assessment:

M Manual vital signs
E Events leading up to the fall
M Medications
A Assessment (including stroke)
W Walk

fall (**FIGURE 24-12**). However, as a result, they may have serious injuries to the lower extremities and pelvic and spinal injuries from energy that was transmitted through the legs. Patients who impact headfirst, as in diving accidents, will likely have serious head and/or spinal injuries. In either case, a fall from a significant height is a serious event with great injury potential, and the patient should be evaluated thoroughly. Take the following factors into account:

- The height of the fall
- The type of surface struck
- The part of the body that hit first, followed by the path of energy displacement

Many falls, especially those sustained by older adults, are not the result of high-energy trauma, even though broken bones may result. Older adults can have osteoporosis, a condition in which the bones can fail under relatively low stress because they are structurally weakened. Because of this condition, an older adult can sustain a fracture as a result of a fall from a standing position. These cases do not constitute true high-energy trauma unless the patient fell from a significant height.

Penetrating Trauma

Penetrating trauma is the second leading cause of trauma death in the United States after blunt trauma. In 2022, the CDC reported more than 48,000 deaths from firearms, which is just under the number of deaths related to motor vehicles.[15] Low-energy penetrating trauma may be caused

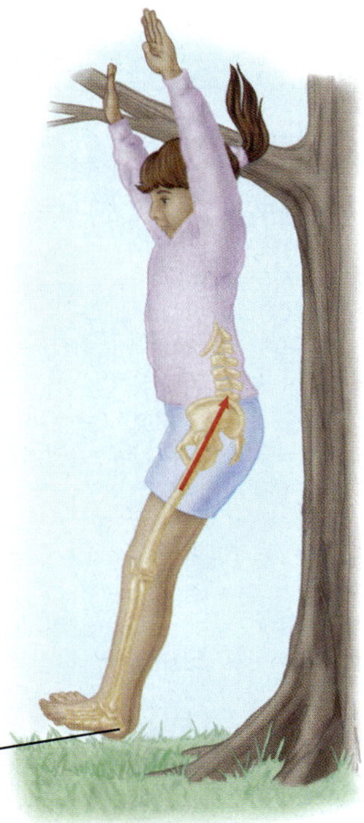

FIGURE 24-12 When a patient falls and lands on the feet, the energy is transmitted to the spine, sometimes producing a spinal injury in addition to injuries to the legs and pelvis.

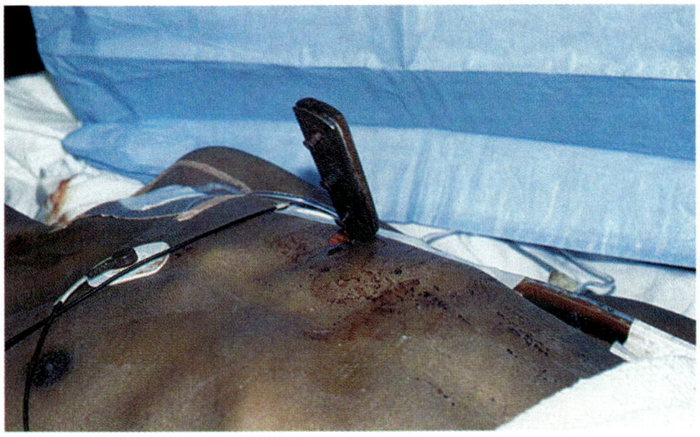

FIGURE 24-13 Injuries from low-energy penetrations, such as a stab wound, are caused by the sharp edges of the object moving through the body.

Words of Wisdom

Do not waste time trying to determine whether a penetrating wound is an entrance or exit wound; making this distinction can be difficult. Instead, focus on identifying all wounds and providing appropriate care. Document only the description and location of the wound, not your opinion about whether it was an entrance or an exit wound. Those statements can be difficult to defend if you do not have specific expertise in ballistics and wound patterns.

accidentally by impalement or intentionally by a knife, ice pick, or other weapon (**FIGURE 24-13**).

Often, it is difficult to determine the entrance and exit wounds from a **projectile** in a prehospital setting; labeling the wounds is not necessary, although it is valuable to observe whether there is an exit hole (ie, to determine if the projectile is still in the person's body). Determine the number of penetrating injuries and then combine that information with the important things you already know about the potential pathway of penetrating projectiles to form an index of suspicion about unseen life-threatening injuries. With low-energy penetrations, injuries are caused by the sharp edges of the object moving through the body and are, therefore, close to the object's path. However, weapons such as knives may have been deliberately moved around internally, causing more damage than the external wound might suggest.

In medium- and high-velocity penetrating trauma, the path of the projectile (usually a bullet) may not be as easy to predict. This is because the bullet may flatten out, tumble, or even ricochet within the body before exiting. The path the projectile takes is referred to as a **trajectory**. Fragmentation, especially frangible bullets that are designed to disintegrate into tiny particles on impact, will increase damage as multiple fragments increase the likelihood of multiple organs/vessels sustaining injury. Full metal jacket bullets cause less damage than fragmented rounds because of their tendency to pass through the body's tissues. The bullet's speed is another factor in the resulting injury pattern; there is often additional damage caused by the object moving inside the body, but not along the suspected pathway. This phenomenon, called **cavitation**, results from the rapid changes in tissue and fluid pressure that occur with the passage of the projectile, and it can result in serious injury to internal organs distant to the actual path of the bullet (**FIGURE 24-14**). Consequences of cavitation can be temporary or permanent. Temporary cavitation injury results from a stretching of the tissues that occurs with the pressure changes. Permanent cavitation injury results along the path where the projectile, such as a bullet, has passed through the tissue. Remain alert during assessment because patients will exhibit various signs and symptoms depending on the organ or organs affected.

As with motor vehicle crashes, the energy available for a bullet to cause damage is more a function of its speed than its mass (weight). Although it is not necessary for you to distinguish between medium- and high-velocity injuries, any information regarding the type of weapon that was used should be relayed to medical control. Medium-velocity injuries are generally classified as those occurring from projectiles fired at less than 2,000 feet/s (610 m/s), such as by handguns and some rifles; high-velocity injuries are caused by projectiles fired at greater than 2,000 feet/s (610 m/s), such as by military-style weapons.[16]

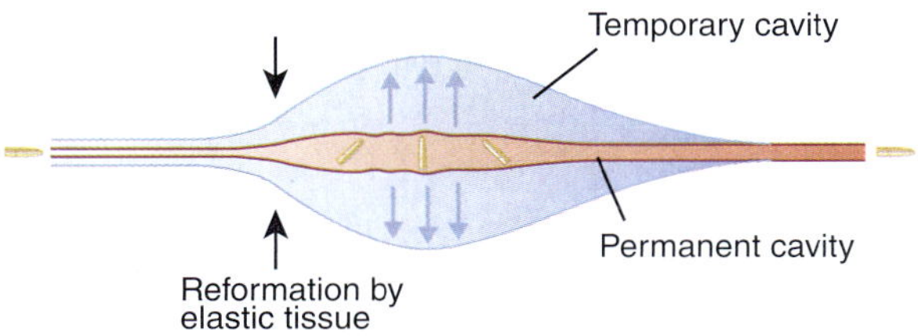

FIGURE 24-14 Two types of injury are caused by cavitation: temporary and permanent.

TABLE 24-1 summarizes how to recognize developing problems in trauma patients.

Blast Injuries

Although most commonly associated with military conflict, blast injuries are also seen in civilian practice in mines, shipyards, and chemical plants and, increasingly, in association with terrorist activities. As with any explosion, there is a risk of contamination of patients from environmental contaminants, toxic chemicals, or dirty bombs. People who are

TABLE 24-1 Recognizing Developing Problems in Trauma Patients

Mechanism of Injury	Signs and Symptoms	Index of Suspicion
Blunt or penetrating trauma to the neck	• Noisy or labored breathing • Increased respiratory rate • Swelling of the face or neck • Decreasing/low GCS score (<9 is severe) • Decreasing/low Spo_2 • Rapid, weak pulse • Decreasing/low BP • External hemorrhage • HR > SBP value	• Significant bleeding or foreign bodies in the upper or lower airway, causing obstruction • Be alert for airway compromise
Significant chest wall blunt trauma from motor vehicle, car-versus-pedestrian, and other crashes; penetrating trauma to the chest wall	• Significant chest pain • Shortness of breath • Increased respiratory rate • Asymmetric chest wall movement • Subcutaneous emphysema • Decreasing GCS score (<9 is severe) • Decreasing/low Spo_2 • Presence of jugular venous distention • Rapid, weak pulse • Decreasing BP • Narrowing pulse pressures • HR > SBP value • Loss of peripheral pulses during inspiration	• Cardiac or pulmonary contusion • Pneumothorax (accumulation of air or gas in the pleural cavity) or hemothorax (accumulation of blood in the pleural cavity) • Broken ribs, causing respiratory compromise • Aortic damage

(continues)

TABLE 24-1 Recognizing Developing Problems in Trauma Patients (*continued*)

Mechanism of Injury	Signs and Symptoms	Index of Suspicion
Any significant blunt force trauma from motor vehicle crashes or penetrating injury	• Blunt or penetrating trauma to the neck, chest, abdomen, or groin • Blows to the head sustained during motor vehicle crashes, falls, or other incidents, producing loss of consciousness, altered mental status, inability to recall events, combativeness, or changes in speech patterns • Inability to maintain airway • Difficulty moving extremities; headache, especially with nausea and vomiting • Decreasing GCS score (motor score <6 is high risk) • Decreasing/low Spo_2 • Rapid, weak pulse • Decreasing/low BP or increasing BP with slow pulse • HR $>$ SBP value	• Injuries in these regions may tear and cause damage to the large blood vessels located in these body areas, resulting in significant internal and external bleeding • Be alert to the possibility of bruising to the brain and bleeding in and around the brain tissue, which may cause excess pressure to develop inside the skull around the brain
Any significant blunt trauma, falls from a significant height, or penetrating trauma	• Severe back and/or neck pain, history of difficulty moving extremities, loss of sensation or tingling in the extremities • Decreasing GCS score (<9 is severe) • Rapid, weak pulse or slow pulse	• Injury to the bones of the spinal column or to the spinal cord • Multiple extremity fractures

Abbreviation: BP, blood pressure; GCS, Glasgow Coma Scale; HR, heart rate; SBP, systolic blood pressure; Spo_2, oxygen saturation

injured in explosions may be injured by the following mechanisms (**FIGURE 24-15**).

- **Primary blast injuries.** These injuries are due entirely to the blast itself; that is, damage to the body is caused by the pressure wave generated by the explosion. If the explosion occurs within an enclosed space such as a building, mine, or vehicle, the incidence of injury and death is higher.[17] When the victim is close to the blast, the blast wave may cause disruption of major blood vessels and rupture of eardrums and major organs, including the lungs. Hollow organs are the most susceptible to the pressure wave. In some cases, pressure wave injuries can amputate limbs.
- **Secondary blast injuries.** Damage to the body results from being struck by flying debris, such as shrapnel from the device or from glass or splinters, which have been set in motion by the explosion. Objects are propelled by the force of the blast wave and strike the victim, causing injury. These objects can travel great distances and be propelled at tremendous speeds.
- **Tertiary blast injuries.** These injuries occur when the patient is hurled by the force of the explosion against a stationary object, such as the ground. A blast wind (sudden change in the surrounding atmosphere) creates a pressure wave. This can cause the patient's body to be hurled or thrown, resulting in further injury. This physical displacement of the body is also referred to as ground shock when the body impacts the ground.
- **Quaternary blast injuries.** This category of miscellaneous injuries includes burns from hot gases or fires started by the blast, respiratory injury from inhaling toxic gases, suffocation, poisoning, medical emergencies incurred as a result of the explosion, crush injuries from the collapse of buildings, radiation injuries, and mental health emergencies. Essentially, all injuries due to the blast event that are not

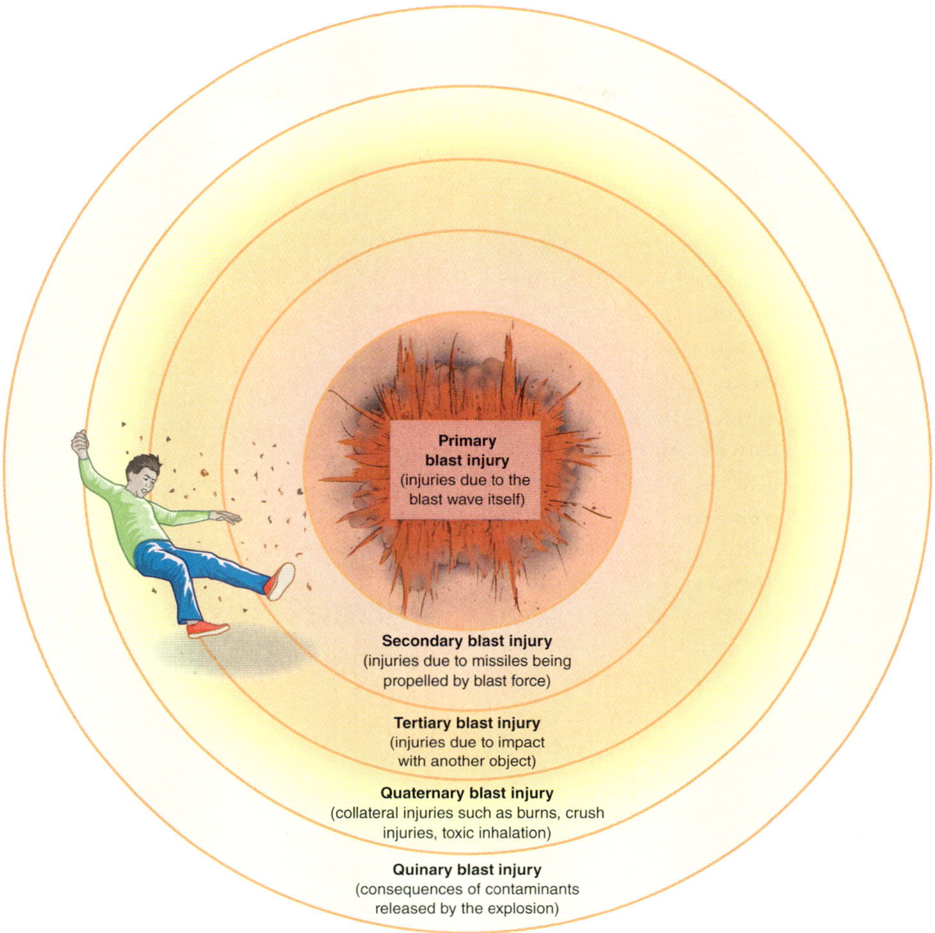

FIGURE 24-15 Mechanisms of blast injuries.

attributable directly to a primary, secondary, or tertiary mechanism are categorized as quaternary blast injuries.

- **Quinary blast injuries.** These injuries are the clinical consequences of contaminants released into the environment by an explosion. Contaminants can include hazards that were intentionally added to the explosive source, such as chemical, biologic, and radiologic substances (eg, dirty bombs). The contaminants are intended to cause damage or injury beyond those produced by the projectiles.

Most patients who survive an explosion will have some combination of the types of injuries mentioned. The remainder of the discussion will be confined to primary blast injuries because although secondary blast injuries account for most of the trauma, their treatment typically follows the procedures outlined in the respective trauma chapters of this text. Primary blast injuries are unique to this MOI and are easily overlooked if the clinician does not know what to look for or focuses solely on the subsequent injuries.

Types of Primary Blast Injury

Hollow organs (those that contain air), such as the middle ear, lungs, and gastrointestinal tract, are most susceptible to pressure changes. The junction between tissues of different densities and exposed areas such as head and neck tissues are also susceptible to injury. The ear is the organ system that is most sensitive to blast injuries. The **tympanic membrane** evolved to detect minor changes in pressure. The patient may report ringing in the ears, pain in the ears, or some loss of hearing, and blood may be visible in the ear canal.

Pulmonary blast injuries are defined as pulmonary trauma (consisting of contusions and hemorrhages) that results from short-range exposure to the detonation of explosives. When the explosion occurs in an open space, both lungs are usually injured. Primary blast injury is often characterized by a lack of external visible injuries and thus can go unrecognized. The patient may report tightness or pain in the chest and may cough up blood and have tachypnea or other signs of respiratory distress. Subcutaneous emphysema (crackling under the skin) can be palpated over the chest, indicating air in the thorax. Pneumothorax is a common injury and may require emergency decompression in the field for your patient to survive. Pulmonary edema may ensue rapidly. If there is any reason to suspect lung injury in a blast victim (even just the presence of a ruptured eardrum), administer oxygen to maintain Spo_2 of 94% to 99%. However, avoid giving oxygen under positive pressure unless absolutely essential, because doing so may simply increase the damage to the lung or increase the size of a pneumothorax.

Solid organs are relatively protected from shock wave injury but may be injured by secondary missiles or a hurled body. Hollow organs, however, may be injured by the same mechanisms that damage lung tissue. Skin injuries, ranging from petechiae (ie, pinpoint red-purple hemorrhages on the skin) to large hematomas, may be found. Perforation or rupture of the bowel and colon is a risk. Underwater explosions can result in severe abdominal injuries.

Brain injuries and head trauma are a common cause of death from blast injuries. Subarachnoid (beneath the arachnoid layer covering the brain) and subdural (beneath the outermost covering of the brain) hematomas are often seen. Permanent or transient neurologic deficits may be secondary to concussion, intracerebral bleeding, or air embolism. Instant but transient unconsciousness, with or without retrograde amnesia, may be initiated not only by head trauma but also by cardiovascular problems. Bradycardia and hypotension are common after an intense pressure wave from an explosion.

Multisystem Trauma

Multisystem trauma refers to multiple traumatic injuries involving more than one body system, such as head and spinal trauma, chest and abdominal trauma, or chest and multiple extremity trauma. You must recognize patients who fit into this classification and provide rapid treatment and transportation, and alert medical control as to the nature of the patient's injuries so that the trauma center is prepared prior to your arrival. Multisystem trauma patients have a high level of morbidity and mortality; therefore, they require teams of physicians to treat their injuries.

Words of Wisdom

Rapid transport decisions are needed for patients who have sustained significant trauma. Patients with significant traumatic injuries tend to have better outcomes the more promptly they receive definitive care at a designated trauma hospital. This care often includes surgical intervention.[18]

Patient Assessment

Identifying life-threatening illnesses and injuries as soon as possible has proven to improve patient outcomes. As an EMT, you must apply this knowledge as well as the appropriate assessment skills to assess, triage, treat, and transport patients with traumatic injuries to the most appropriate facility. The major components of patient assessment include the following:

- Scene size-up
- Primary assessment
- History taking
- Secondary assessment
- Reassessment

When you are caring for a patient who has experienced a life-threatening MOI and the patient is considered to be in serious or critical condition, you should rapidly perform a physical examination. With a patient who has experienced a non-life-threatening MOI, focus on the chief complaint while assessing the patient as a whole.

Words of Wisdom

A mnemonic sometimes used to remember priorities of trauma care is MARCH:

M Massive hemorrhage
A Airway
R Respirations
C Circulation
H Head injury, hypothermia

Injuries to the Head

The brain lies well protected within the skull. However, when the head is injured from trauma, disability and unseen injury to the brain may occur. The brain itself may tear or become bruised, causing bleeding. The blood vessels around the brain may also tear and produce bleeding. Bleeding or swelling inside the skull from brain injury is often life threatening; therefore, your assessment must include conducting frequent neurologic examinations. Neurologic assessments, coupled with the patient's level of consciousness, will often provide details on subtle changes in the patient's condition. Some patients will not have obvious signs or symptoms, such as changes in pupillary size and reactivity, of unseen brain injury until minutes or hours after the injury has occurred.

Injuries to the Neck and Throat

The neck and throat contain many structures that are susceptible to injuries from trauma that could be serious or deadly to your patients. In this region of the human body, the trachea (or windpipe) may become torn or swell after an injury to the neck or deviate after an injury to the lungs. These types of injuries may result in an airway problem that could quickly become a serious life threat because they interfere with the patient's ability to breathe; therefore, your assessment must include frequent physical examination looking for DCAP-BTLS (Deformities, Contusions, Abrasions, Punctures/penetrations, Burns, Tenderness, Lacerations, Swelling) in the neck region. In addition, you should assess for jugular venous (vein) distention and tracheal deviation (late sign of injury).

The neck also contains large blood vessels that supply the brain with oxygen-rich blood. When a neck injury occurs, swelling may prevent blood flow to the brain and cause injury to the central nervous system, even though the brain may not have been directly affected by the initial force that caused the injury to the neck. If a penetrating injury to the neck results in an open wound, the patient may have significant bleeding or air may be drawn into the circulatory system. If air enters the veins, this may result in air embolism, which may lead to cardiac arrest if the air enters the heart. Occlusive dressings must be used to keep this from happening. A crushing injury to the upper part of the neck may cause the cartilages of the upper airway and larynx to fracture. This can lead to air leaking into the soft tissue of the neck. When air is trapped in subcutaneous tissue (subcutaneous emphysema), it produces a crackling sound or feeling when palpated, called subcutaneous crepitation. Either air in the circulation or an airway cartilage fracture may cause rapid death.

Injuries to the Chest

The chest contains the heart, the lungs, and the large blood vessels of the body. When injury occurs to this area of the body, many life-threatening injuries may occur. For example, blunt trauma to the chest can fracture ribs or the sternum. When ribs are broken and the chest wall does not expand normally during breathing, this interferes with the body's ability to obtain sufficient amounts of oxygen for the cells. Bruising may occur to the heart and cause an irregular heartbeat. Depending on the severity of the trauma, the large vessels of the heart may be torn inside the chest, causing massive unseen bleeding that can quickly kill the trauma patient. In some chest injuries the lungs become bruised, thus interfering with normal oxygen exchange in the body.

In the event of a pneumothorax, air collects between the lung tissue and the chest wall. As air accumulates in this space, the lung tissue becomes compressed, again interfering with the body's ability to effectively exchange oxygen. If left untreated or unrecognized, the lung tissue becomes squeezed under pressure until the heart is also squeezed and can no longer pump blood. This condition is called a tension pneumothorax and is a life-threatening emergency. In some patients, bleeding develops in this portion of the chest. Instead of air collecting in this space, blood collects and causes interference with breathing. This condition is called a hemothorax, and it also poses a threat to the patient's life.

A penetration or perforation of the integrity of the chest is called an open chest wound. As air enters the chest cavity, the natural pressure balance within the chest cavity is no longer equal. If left untreated, shock and/or death will result. Regardless of the particular injury, it is imperative that you reassess a trauma patient's chest region every 5 minutes. The assessment should include DCAP-BTLS, lung sounds, and chest rise and fall. Some patients will not have obvious signs or symptoms such as absent breath sounds or respiratory difficulty immediately.

Injuries to the Abdomen

The abdomen is an area of the human body that contains many organs vital to body function. These organs also require a high blood flow so they can perform the functions necessary for life. The organs of the abdomen and retroperitoneum (the space immediately behind the true abdomen) can be classified into two simple categories: solid and hollow. The solid organs include the liver, spleen, pancreas, and kidneys. The hollow organs include the stomach, large and small intestines, and urinary bladder.

When injuries from trauma occur in this region of the body, serious and life-threatening problems may occur. The solid organs may tear, lacerate, or fracture. This causes serious bleeding into the abdomen that can quickly cause death. Be alert for a trauma patient who reports abdominal pain—it may be a symptom of abdominal bleeding. Also be alert to vital signs that begin to worsen; this can be a sign of serious, unseen bleeding inside the abdominal region of the body.

When the hollow organs of the body have been injured, they may rupture and leak toxic chemicals used for digestion into the abdomen. This not only causes pain, but a life-threatening infection also may eventually develop.

The abdomen also contains large blood vessels that supply the organs of this region and the lower extremities with oxygen-rich blood. Occasionally these vessels rupture or tear and cause serious unseen bleeding that may cause death. Some patients, particularly healthy young adults, are able to compensate longer than others from blood loss; therefore, you should always maintain a high index of suspicion when the MOI suggests injury to the abdominal region. This is best accomplished by reassessing the abdominal region.

Management: Transport and Destination

Caring for victims of traumatic injuries requires a solid understanding of the trauma system in the United States. You need a good working knowledge of the resources available to you, including the most optimal methods of rapid transport and trauma centers that can best provide definitive care. Call for ALS and helicopter assistance early, possibly even before you arrive on scene, to avoid delays in treatment and transport.

Scene Time

Because survival of critically injured trauma patients is time dependent, limit on-scene time to the minimum amount necessary to correct life-threatening injuries and package the patient. The following criteria will help you identify a critically injured patient:

- Dangerous MOI
- Decreased level of consciousness
- Any threats to airway, breathing, or circulation

Patients who present with these criteria or who are very young or old or have chronic illnesses should also be considered to be high risk, thus requiring rapid treatment and transport.

Destination Selection

You will often be summoned to injury scenes to transport critically ill trauma patients to definitive care. For this reason, it is important for you to be familiar with how the American College of Surgeons Committee on Trauma verifies trauma care. Trauma centers are classified into Levels I through III, with Level I having the most resources (**TABLE 24-2**).[19] Many states also designate Levels IV and V trauma centers using specific training and staffing criteria.

Because of the extensive requirements, most Level I facilities are university-based teaching hospitals. Pediatric centers have different criteria and are classified as Level I or Level II. To be classified as Level I, the pediatric trauma center must care for 200 or more injured patients younger than 15 years annually.

Level II centers are expected to provide initial definitive care, regardless of injury severity. Because of its resources, a Level II trauma center may not be able to provide the same comprehensive care as a Level I trauma center.

Level III facilities serve communities that do not have access to Level I or II facilities. Level III facilities provide assessment, resuscitation, emergency care, and stabilization. A Level III facility

TABLE 24-2 Key Elements for Adult Trauma Centers

Level	Definition	Key Elements
Level I	A comprehensive regional resource that is a tertiary care facility; capable of providing total care for every aspect of injury, from prevention through rehabilitation. Cares for at least 1,200 trauma patients per year, with at least 240 seriously injured.	**1.** 24-hour in-house coverage by general surgeons available at patient's bedside within 15 minutes 80% of the time. Board-certified or board-eligible emergency physician in the emergency department at all times[a] **2.** Rapid availability of care in specialties such as orthopaedic surgery, neurosurgery, anesthesiology, emergency medicine, radiology, internal medicine, and critical care **3.** Should also include cardiac, hand, pediatric, and microvascular surgery and hemodialysis **4.** Provides leadership in prevention, public education, and continuing education of trauma team members **5.** Committed to continued improvement through a comprehensive quality assessment program and organized research to help direct new innovations in trauma care
Level II	Able to initiate definitive care for all injured patients	**1.** 24-hour immediate coverage by general surgeons available at patient's bedside within 15 minutes 80% of the time. Board-certified or board-eligible emergency physician in the emergency department at all times[a] **2.** Availability of orthopaedic surgery, neurosurgery, anesthesiology, emergency medicine, radiology, and critical care **3.** Tertiary care needs such as cardiac surgery, hemodialysis, and microvascular surgery may be referred to a Level I trauma center **4.** Committed to trauma prevention and continuing education of trauma team members **5.** Provides continued improvement in trauma care through a comprehensive quality assessment program
Level III	Able to provide prompt assessment, resuscitation, and stabilization of injured patients and emergency operations	**1.** 24-hour immediate coverage by emergency medicine physicians and prompt availability of general surgeons and anesthesiologists **2.** Program dedicated to continued improvement in trauma care through a comprehensive quality assessment program **3.** Has developed transfer agreements for patients requiring more comprehensive care at a Level I or Level II trauma center **4.** Committed to continuing education of nursing and allied health personnel or the trauma team **5.** Must be involved with prevention and have an active outreach program for its referring communities

[a] Certain exceptions apply.

must have transfer agreements with a Level I or II trauma center and must have protocols in place to transfer patients whose needs exceed the resources of the facility.

Level IV facilities are typically found in remote outlying areas where no higher level of care is available. These facilities provide advanced trauma life support prior to transfer to a higher-level trauma center. Such a facility may be an urgent care clinic, with or without a physician.

In 2021, the American College of Surgeons led an expert panel to create an updated field triage decision scheme (**FIGURE 24-16**). These criteria are intended to help prehospital care clinicians recognize injured patients who are likely to benefit from transport to a trauma center compared with transport to an emergency department. The decision scheme is not intended to serve as a mass-casualty or disaster triage tool; it is intended to provide a recommendation for taking the patient to the most capable hospital.[11]

Type of Transport

Modes of transport ultimately come in one of two categories: ground or air. Ground transport EMS units are generally staffed by EMTs, AEMTs, and paramedics. Air transport EMS units or critical care transport units are often staffed by critical care transport clinicians such as critical care nurses and paramedics. Transport modes are discussed further in Chapter 15, *Medical Overview*.

You should be familiar with your local protocols defining indications for use of helicopter emergency medical services (HEMS) transport. In 2021, several EMS physician groups developed a position paper outlining the appropriate use of emergency air medical services.[20] They note that the use of HEMS should be integrated within the regional plan and use validated triage methods to determine the need for a trauma center. The decision to transport trauma patients by air or ground will depend on local geography, distance to a trauma center, and the skills and capability of the local ground EMS clinicians.

Words of Wisdom

When triaging patients after a blast, consider the possibility of hearing damage in individuals who do not follow verbal commands. Although hearing loss is a serious concern, you should not allow it to unduly affect your assessment or patient prioritization.

Trauma Scoring Systems

The numeric scoring of trauma patients for determining the severity of their injury is common practice in the health care profession. When the various scoring systems were created, it was thought that the implementation of the scoring system would assist in rapidly identifying the severity of the patient's injuries. There are several different trauma scoring systems.

Trauma Score

The **trauma score** calculates a number from 1 to 16, with 16 being the best possible score. It accounts

YOU are the EMT

The patient is removed from the vehicle and you perform a quick secondary assessment. Because the patient is hypoxic, your partner applies high-concentration oxygen via a nonrebreathing mask while one of the EMTs from the rescue company obtains the patient's vital signs.

Recording Time: 5 Minutes	
Respirations	22 breaths/min; labored
Pulse	120 beats/min; weak radial pulses
Skin	Cool, clammy, and pale
Blood pressure	84/64 mm Hg
Oxygen saturation (Spo_2)	97% (with supplemental oxygen)

The patient's level of consciousness is still markedly decreased; he responds only to pain. He has a large hematoma and laceration to his forehead, which is covered with a sterile dressing. He also has crepitus and bruising to his chest. A Level I trauma center is 30 miles away, but there is a Level III trauma center only 15 miles away.

4. Should the patient be transported to the Level I trauma center or the Level III trauma center? Why?

5. What other transport factors should you consider with this patient?

RED CRITERIA
High Risk for Serious Injury

Injury Patterns	Mental Status and Vital Signs
• Penetrating injuries to head, neck, torso, and proximal extremities • Skull deformity, suspected skull fracture • Suspected spinal injury with new motor or sensory loss • Chest wall instability, deformity, or suspected flail chest • Suspected pelvic fracture • Suspected fracture of two or more proximal long bones • Crushed, degloved, mangled, or pulseless extremity • Amputation proximal to wrist or ankle • Active bleeding requiring a tourniquet or wound packing with continuous pressure	**All Patients** • Unable to follow commands (motor GCS < 6) • RR < 10 or > 29 breaths/min • Respiratory distress or need for respiratory support • Room-air pulse oximetry < 90% **Age 0–9 years** • SBP < 70 mm Hg + (2 × age in years) **Age 10–64 years** • SBP < 90 mm Hg or • HR > SBP **Age 65 years** • SBP < 110 mm Hg or • HR > SBP

Patients meeting any one of the above RED criteria should be transported to the highest-level trauma center available within the geographic constraints of the regional trauma system

YELLOW CRITERIA
Moderate Risk for Serious Injury

Mechanism of Injury	EMS Judgment
• High-risk auto crash – Partial or complete ejection – Significant intrusion (including roof) • > 12 inches occupant site OR • > 18 inches any site OR • Need for extrication for entrapped patient – Death in passenger compartment – Child (age 0–9 years) unrestrained or in unsecured child safety seat – Vehicle telemetry data consistent with severe injury • Rider separated from transport vehicle with significant impact (eg, motorcycle, ATV, horse) • Pedestrian/bicycle rider thrown, run over, or with significant impact • Fall from height > 10 feet (all ages)	**Consider risk factors, including:** • Low-level falls in young children (age ≤5 years) or older adults (age ≥65 years) with significant head impact • Anticoagulant use • Suspicion of child abuse • Special, high-resource health care needs • Pregnancy > 20 weeks • Burns in conjunction with trauma • Children should be triaged preferentially to pediatric capable centers **If concerned, take to a trauma center**

FIGURE 24-16 2021 National Guideline for the Field Triage of Injured Patients.

Abbreviations: ATV, all-terrain vehicle; GCS, Glasgow Coma Scale; HR, heart rate; RR, respiratory rate; SBP, systolic blood pressure

for the **Glasgow Coma Scale (GCS) score**, respiratory rate, respiratory expansion, systolic blood pressure, and capillary refill. The GCS is an evaluation tool used to determine level of consciousness (**TABLE 24-3**). It evaluates and assigns point values (scores) for eye opening, verbal response, and motor response; these scores are then totaled and help to effectively predict patient outcomes. Note that the lower the score, the more severe the extent of brain injury.

The trauma score relates to the likelihood of patient survival. However, this scoring system does not accurately predict survivability in patients with severe head injuries because motor and verbal deficits make those criteria difficult to assess; in its place, the Revised Trauma Score, discussed next, is used.

Revised Trauma Score

The **Revised Trauma Score (RTS)** is most commonly used for patients with head trauma because it is weighted to compensate for major head injury without multisystem injury or major physiologic changes.

The RTS is a physiologic scoring system that is also used to assess the severity of a trauma patient's injuries. Objective data used to calculate the RTS include the GCS score, systolic blood pressure, and

TABLE 24-3 Glasgow Coma Scale[a]

Eye Opening		Best Verbal Response		Best Motor Response	
Spontaneous	4	Oriented conversation	5	Obeys commands	6
In response to sound	3	Confused conversation	4	Localizes to pressure	5
In response to pressure	2	Inappropriate words	3	Withdraws from pressure	4
None	1	Incomprehensible sounds	2	Abnormal flexion	3
		None	1	Abnormal extension	2
				None	1

[a]Some systems use a "Not testable (NT)" score for any element that cannot be tested. Eye opening cannot be tested in a patient whose eyes are closed due to a local factor, such as swelling; verbal response cannot be tested in a patient who has a preexisting factor interfering with communication, such as mutism; and motor response cannot be tested in a patient who has preexisting paralysis or other limiting factor.

Score: 13–15 may indicate mild dysfunction, although 15 is the score a person without neurologic disabilities would receive.

Score: 9–12 may indicate moderate dysfunction.

Score: 8 or less indicatives severe dysfunction.

YOU are the EMT

You decide to transport to a Level I trauma center. The patient is loaded into the ambulance. You continue your assessment and care while en route.

Recording Time: 10 Minutes	
Level of consciousness	Responds only to pain
Respirations	30 breaths/min; extremely labored
Pulse	130 beats/min; absent radial pulses
Skin	Cool, clammy, and pale
Blood pressure	80/50 mm Hg
Oxygen saturation (Spo_2)	89% (supplemental oxygen)

Your partner inserts an oropharyngeal airway and, using a jaw thrust, assists the patient's ventilations with a bag-mask device and high-concentration oxygen, being careful to ventilate at the appropriate rate and tidal volume. Oral suctioning is performed as needed to keep the patient's airway clear of blood. The patient flexes his arms in response to pain, but does not open his eyes or respond verbally when you talk to him. An EMT from one of the engine companies drives the ambulance to the landing zone, which is about a mile away.

6. What trauma scoring systems are commonly used to assess the severity of a trauma patient's condition? How would you apply them to this patient?

respiratory rate. In addition to assessing injury severity, the RTS has demonstrated reliability in predicting survival in patients with severe injuries. The highest RTS a patient can receive is 12; the lowest is 0. The RTS is calculated as shown in **TABLE 24-4**.

Factors to consider when determining whether the patient is seriously injured include the following:

- There is an extended period required to access or extricate a remote patient (eg, injured hiker, snowmobiler, or boater) or trapped patient (eg, passenger in a crashed car) who has evidence of serious injury, and this access/extrication depletes the time window to get the patient to the trauma center by ground.
- The patient needs medical care and stabilization at the ALS level, and there is no ALS-level ground ambulance service available within a reasonable time frame.
- Traffic conditions or hospital availability make it unlikely that the seriously injured patient will get to a trauma center via ground ambulance within the ideal time frame for best clinical outcome.
- There is a mass-casualty incident with serious injuries.

These recommendations are a guideline for local decision makers to develop more comprehensive protocols for the use of HEMS transport. Always follow your local protocols when determining what type of patient transportation is appropriate.

TABLE 24-4 Revised Trauma Score

GCS	SBP	RR	Value
13 to 15	>89 mm Hg	10 to 29 breaths/min	4
9 to 12	76 to 89 mm Hg	>29 breaths/min	3
6 to 8	50 to 75 mm Hg	6 to 9 breaths/min	2
4 to 5	1 to 49 mm Hg	1 to 5 breaths/min	1
3	0	0	0

Abbreviations: GCS, Glasgow Coma Scale; RR, respiratory rate; SBP, systolic blood pressure

Street Smarts

Most EMS professionals will experience some type of psychologically traumatic incident while on duty. Take care of yourself. Know the resources that are available to you. Seek help when needed.

YOU are the EMT

While en route to the trauma center, you call to report a trauma alert and intercept with a paramedic who joins your crew. When the paramedic arrives, you transfer care with a patient handoff report.

Recording Time: 15 Minutes	
Level of consciousness	Responds only to pain
Respirations	10 breaths/min; assisted
Pulse	140 beats/min; absent radial pulses
Skin	Cool, clammy, and pale
Blood pressure	74/50 mm Hg
Oxygen saturation (Spo_2)	95% (supplemental oxygen)

You later learn that the patient had bleeding in the brain and chest and multiple rib fractures. He was taken to surgery and was in critical condition in the surgical intensive care unit.

7. How does the level of trauma care provided by the paramedic differ from that of the EMT?

YOU are the EMT SUMMARY

1. On the basis of the information provided by the EMD, can you predict the potential types of injuries the patient may have? If so, how?

Although you will not ultimately know the type and severity of injuries the patient has until you arrive at the scene and assess the patient, information provided by the dispatch operator can influence your index of suspicion.

En route to this scene, you know that the incident involves a head-on (frontal) crash with a tree, and the patient is still in the vehicle. What you do not know is the speed of the vehicle at the time of impact, whether the patient was restrained, or whether any airbags deployed.

The patient has experienced three collisions: collision of the vehicle against another object, collision of himself against the interior of the vehicle, and collision of his internal organs against the solid structures of the body.

Damage to the vehicle (the first collision) provides information about the severity of the collision. The greater the damage is to the vehicle, the greater the energy that was involved and, therefore, the greater the potential to cause injury. If there is significant damage to the vehicle, your index of suspicion for serious injury to the patient should increase, even if injuries are not immediately apparent.

Just like the obvious damage that occurs to the exterior of the vehicle during the first collision, the injuries that result from the second collision are often obvious during the primary assessment. Common injuries that occur during the second collision include lower extremity and pelvic fractures (when the knees impact the dashboard), rib fractures, pneumothoraces (when the chest impacts the steering wheel), and head and neck trauma (when the head impacts the windshield).

The type of injury experienced by the unrestrained occupant depends on the path the person took at the time of impact. There may be injuries to the abdomen, pelvis, and lower extremities if the patient's body took the down-and-under path, causing the abdomen to impact the lower part of the steering wheel and the knees to impact the dashboard. Head, neck, or chest trauma may be present if the patient was propelled over the steering wheel. Blunt chest and/or abdominal trauma may result from direct impact with the steering wheel.

The injuries that occur during the third collision may not be as obvious as external injuries, but these injuries may be the most life threatening. For example, if the chest impacts the steering wheel, the thoracic organs continue their forward motion until they collide with the inside of the chest cavity. As a result of these forces, shearing injuries of the great vessels (eg, aorta, venae cavae) or injury to the heart as it impacts with the sternum may occur. If the occupant's head strikes the windshield, the brain continues its forward motion until it strikes the inside of the skull; this results in compression injuries to the anterior part of the brain and stretching or tearing or bruising of the posterior part of the brain.

2. Why is it important to estimate the approximate speed at which a vehicle was traveling at the time of impact?

A vehicle's speed affects the potential for injury to its occupant or occupants. According to the equation for kinetic energy ($KE = \frac{1}{2}mv^2$), the energy available to cause injury doubles when the object's weight doubles, but *quadruples* when the object's speed doubles.

The relationship between a vehicle's speed and its deceleration is best described in these terms: The faster the vehicle is traveling and the quicker it stops, the greater the potential for serious injury to any occupant.

3. What damage in the vehicle's interior may have caused the patient's signs and symptoms?

The patient's signs and symptoms indicate, at a minimum, injury to his head and chest. He is bleeding from the head, face, and mouth; his level of consciousness is markedly decreased; and his respirations are rapid and labored.

Inspection of the interior of the vehicle in this incident will most likely reveal a deformed steering wheel (top, bottom, or both) that occurred when the patient's chest, and maybe abdomen, impacted it. You will also likely find an outward bulge of the windshield with a typical starburst fracture where the patient's head and face made impact with it. You may also find some of the patient's hair caught in the windshield, and this is a clear indicator of patient impact. Keep in mind that these may not be the only contact points; they are simply the most likely areas based on the patient's injuries.

4. Should the patient be transported to the Level I trauma center or the Level III trauma center? Why?

You are caring for a multisystem trauma patient; that is, he has experienced trauma that affects more than

YOU are the EMT SUMMARY continued

one body system. The obvious trauma to his head and his level of consciousness indicate a traumatic brain injury. The bruising and crepitus to his chest and his labored breathing indicate intrathoracic trauma, and his vital signs indicate a general state of shock. He meets many requirements for transport to the highest level of trauma care available (ie, a Level I trauma center) including the following: unable to follow commands, respiratory distress, oxygen saturation <90%, systolic blood pressure <90 mm Hg, and heart rate greater than systolic blood pressure value. However, there are several reasons you may consider the Level III center. If you are unable to achieve an adequate airway to maintain ventilation throughout the transport to the Level I center, you should consider going to the Level III center first for stabilization prior to transfer to the Level I center. Similarly, if the patient's condition is otherwise sufficiently grave from the standpoint of his head injury or blood pressure, going to the Level III center first might be warranted. Be familiar with local policies, transport times, and options to minimize those times (ie, HEMS transport) in your area.

5. What other transport factors should you consider with this patient?

The patient should be transported to a Level I trauma center; however, the closest one is 30 miles away. In this scenario, you coordinated with a paramedic intercept and transport by ground to the landing zone for air transport to a Level I facility.

6. What trauma scoring systems are commonly used to assess the severity of a trauma patient's condition? How would you apply them to this patient?

The two most commonly used numeric trauma scoring systems are the GCS and the RTS.

To assess the patient in this scenario, you must first calculate his GCS. The patient does not open his eyes, even when a painful stimulus is applied; therefore, he receives a 1 for eye opening. For verbal response, he also receives a 1 because he does not respond when you talk to him. For motor response, he receives a 3; he responds to pain by flexing his arms (decorticate posturing). Currently, the patient's GCS score is 5, which indicates a severe brain injury.

To calculate the patient's RTS when you arrive at the hospital, you will use his initial GCS, along with his systolic blood pressure and respiratory rate. He has already been assigned a GCS score of 5; therefore, he is assigned a numeric value of 1. His systolic blood pressure was 84 mm Hg; therefore, he is assigned a numeric value of 3. His respiratory value was 22 breaths/min; therefore, he is assigned a numeric value of 4. Given these parameters, the patient's RTS is 8.

Note that *a single assessment of a trauma patient's GCS and RTS scores cannot reliably capture the clinical progression*. Obtain baseline scores and then frequently (at least every 5 minutes) reassess them. Document all scores you obtained in the field, including the times they were obtained.

7. How does the level of trauma care provided by the paramedic differ from that of the EMT?

The level of trauma care you provide as an EMT versus personnel with a higher level of training, such as AEMTs and paramedics, differs mainly in the emergency treatment interventions that can be performed. For example, paramedics are trained to provide advanced airway management and intravenous therapy, and to administer certain emergency medications, among others. Although these additional skills can be of great benefit to the patient, they are not definitive care interventions. Paramedics cannot repair a lacerated liver or stop bleeding in the brain; therefore, their focus on trauma care should not be significantly different from yours. Trauma care is based on identifying injuries, stabilizing the patient, and rapid transport to the appropriate medical facility, in this case, a trauma center. In many cases, you will be called on to assist the paramedic in performing advanced level skills. Depending on local protocols, you may even be able to perform additional skills as deemed necessary by the EMS system medical director.

YOU are the EMT SUMMARY continued

EMS Patient Care Report (PCR)

Date: 10-1-25	**Incident No.:** 012109 N	**Nature of Call:** Motor vehicle crash		**Location:** 642 Danbury Rd.	
Dispatched: 1520	**En Route:** 1520	**At Scene:** 1528	**Transport:** 1538	**At Hospital:** 1552	**In Service:** 1630

Patient Information

Age: 20 **Sex:** M **Weight (in kg [lb]):** estimated at 68 kg (150 lb)	**Allergies:** Unknown **Medications:** Unknown **Past Medical History:** Unknown **Chief Complaint:** Multiple traumatic injuries

Vital Signs

Time: 1533	**BP:** 84/64	**Pulse:** 120	**Respirations:** 22	**Spo_2:** 97%
Time: 1538	**BP:** 80/50	**Pulse:** 130	**Respirations:** 30	**Spo_2:** 89%
Time: 1543	**BP:** 74/50	**Pulse:** 140	**Respirations:** 10/min assisted	**Spo_2:** 95%

EMS Treatment (circle all that apply)

Oxygen @ 15 **L/min via:** **NC** **NRM** (circled) **Bag mask**		**Assisted Ventilation**	**Airway Adjunct: OPA** (circled)	**CPR**
Defibrillation	**Bleeding Control**	**Bandaging**	**Splinting**	**Other:** Thermal management, OPA, suction, spinal motion restriction

Narrative

Dispatched for a motor vehicle versus tree head-on crash. Rescue assignment and law enforcement were dispatched as well.

Chief Complaint: Multiple traumatic injuries

History: Arrived at the scene and noted that a small passenger vehicle made frontal impact with a large tree. Damage to the front of the vehicle was significant. The driver, a 20-year-old man, was still in the vehicle; however, he was unrestrained. Driver- and passenger-side airbags both deployed, and patient was not entrapped. Medevac requested after initial assessment given ground transport time and patient condition. Partner accessed patient through backseat and manually stabilized his head. Rescue 3 firefighter reported interior damage to the steering wheel and a starburst fracture to the windshield with evidence of human hair.

Assessment: Primary assessment revealed that the patient was responsive only to pain. He had blood in his oropharynx, a large hematoma and laceration with active bleeding to his forehead, and facial bleeding. His respirations were rapid and labored.

Treatment (Rx): Suctioned the patient's oropharynx, controlled the bleeding on his forehead, applied cervical collar, and rapidly extricated him from the vehicle. Applied oxygen @ 15 L/min via nonrebreathing mask and performed secondary assessment, which revealed diffuse bruising and crepitus to the chest. Breath sounds were diminished over the left side of the chest. Pelvis and upper and lower extremities were unremarkable for gross injury. Pupils were dilated to approximately 6 mm, and sluggish to react.

Transport: Applied spinal motion restriction precautions and a blanket for warmth, and loaded patient into the ambulance. Rescue 3 EMT drove ambulance to landing zone (LZ) to meet with air transport helicopter.

Reassessment: Reassessment revealed that his respiratory rate had increased, his breathing effort was more labored, and his oxygen saturation had decreased. Inserted an OPA and began assisting his ventilations with a bag-mask device at 10 breaths/min and high-flow oxygen. Continued to reassess patient every 3 to 5 minutes and noted no change in his clinical status. Contacted air medical helicopter via radio and provided patient status update. Continued to assist patient's ventilations and suctioned his oropharynx as needed to maintain airway patency. Vital signs were also reassessed, as noted above. Patient handoff report was given to the intercept paramedic, and patient care was transferred.

****End of report****

Prep Kit

Ready for Review

- Determine the mechanism of injury (MOI) as quickly as possible; this will assist you in developing an index of suspicion for the seriousness of your patient's unseen injuries.
- Three concepts of energy are typically associated with injury: potential energy, kinetic energy, and work.
- Traumatic injuries can be described as blunt trauma or penetrating trauma.
- Motor vehicle crashes are classified traditionally as frontal (head-on), lateral (T-bone), rear-end, rotational (spins), and rollover.
- In every crash, there are three collisions that occur:
  - The collision of the vehicle against some type of object
  - The collision of the passenger against the interior of the vehicle
  - The collision of the passenger's internal organs against the solid structures of the body
- Maintain a high index of suspicion for serious injury in the patient who has been involved in a motor vehicle crash with significant damage to the vehicle, has fallen from a significant height, or has sustained penetrating trauma to the body.
- Communicate MOI findings in the written patient care report and verbally to hospital staff; this will ensure that appropriate treatment of potential serious injuries continues for the patient at the hospital.
- The effects of a particular MOI can vary greatly depending on the patient; likewise, some patients are more likely to experience certain injuries. Understand how patient assessment and treatment may differ for special populations, such as children, pregnant persons, and older adults.
- The mechanisms of injury from explosions relate not just to the initial blast wave, but also to the effects of the explosion that follow. These injury mechanisms are classified as primary, secondary, tertiary, quaternary, or quinary.
- A patient who has sustained a significant MOI and is considered to be in serious or critical condition should receive a secondary assessment, including a rapid examination of the entire body. Any patient who has sustained a nonsignificant MOI should receive an assessment more focused on the chief complaint while still assessing the patient as a whole.
- Caring for patients who have sustained traumatic injuries requires a solid understanding of the trauma system in the United States. This includes transport time, transport destination, and selection of type of transport.
- The criteria for transport to a trauma center vary from system to system. Key variables define the level rating of a trauma center. The American College of Surgeons verifies three categories of trauma centers; however, states may designate five levels. Your system may include a Level I trauma center, the highest-level trauma center.
- The 2021 National Guideline for the Field Triage of Injured Patients outlines criteria to help prehospital care clinicians recognize injured patients who are likely to benefit from transport to a trauma center.

Vital Vocabulary

blunt trauma An impact on the body by objects that cause injury without penetrating soft tissues or internal organs and cavities.

cavitation A phenomenon in which speed causes a bullet to generate pressure waves, which cause damage distant from the bullet's path.

Prep Kit continued

coup–contrecoup brain injury A brain injury that occurs when force is applied to the head and energy transmission through brain tissue causes injury on the opposite side of original impact.

deceleration The slowing of an object.

Glasgow Coma Scale (GCS) score An evaluation tool used to determine level of consciousness, which evaluates and assigns point values (scores) for eye opening, verbal response, and motor response, which are then totaled; it is effective in helping predict patient outcomes.

index of suspicion Awareness that unseen life-threatening injuries may exist when determining the mechanism of injury.

kinetic energy The energy of a moving object.

mechanism of injury (MOI) The forces, or energy transmission, applied to the body that cause injury.

medical emergencies Emergencies that require EMS attention because of illnesses or conditions not caused by an outside force.

multisystem trauma Trauma that affects more than one body system.

penetrating trauma Injury caused by objects, such as knives and bullets, that pierce the surface of the body and damage internal tissues and organs.

potential energy The product of mass, gravity, and height, which is converted into kinetic energy and results in injury, such as from a fall.

projectile Any object propelled by force, such as a bullet by a weapon.

pulmonary blast injuries Pulmonary trauma resulting from short-range exposure to the detonation of explosives.

Revised Trauma Score (RTS) A scoring system used for patients with head trauma.

trajectory The path a projectile takes once it is propelled.

trauma emergencies Emergencies that result from physical forces applied to a patient's body.

trauma score A score calculated from 1 to 16, with 16 being the best possible score. It relates to the likelihood of patient survival with the exception of a severe head injury. It takes into account the Glasgow Coma Scale (GCS) score, respiratory rate, respiratory expansion, systolic blood pressure, and capillary refill.

tympanic membrane The eardrum; a thin, semitransparent membrane in the middle ear that transmits sound vibrations to the internal ear by means of auditory ossicles.

References

1. Injuries and violence are leading causes of death. Centers for Disease Control and Prevention website. https://www.cdc.gov/injury/wisqars/animated-leading-causes.html. Accessed February 4, 2025.
2. Sasser SM, Hunt RC, Faul M, et al. Guidelines for field triage of injured patients: recommendations of the National Expert Panel on Field Triage, 2011. *MMWR Recomm Rep*. 2012;61(RR-1):1–20.
3. Choksey JS. What is automatic collision notification? JD Power website. https://www.jdpower.com/cars/shopping-guides/what-is-automatic-collision-notification. Published May 3, 2024. Accessed February 4, 2025.
4. Payne WN, De Jesus O, Payne AN. Contrecoup brain injury. *StatPearls*. National Library of Medicine website. https://www.ncbi.nlm.nih.gov/books/NBK536965/. Updated May 22, 2023. Accessed February 4, 2025.
5. National Association of Emergency Medical Technicians. *PHTLS: Prehospital Trauma Life Support*. 10th ed. Burlington, MA: Jones & Bartlett Learning; 2023.
6. Seat belts. National Highway Traffic Safety Administration website. https://www.nhtsa.gov/vehicle-safety/seat-belts. Accessed February 4, 2025.
7. Redelmeier DA, May SC, Thiruchelvam D, Barrett JF. Pregnancy and the risk of a traffic crash. *CMAJ*. 2014;186(10):7427–750.
8. Airbags. Insurance Institute and Highway Safety website. https://www.iihs.org/topics/airbags. Updated January 2025. Accessed February 4, 2025.
9. Facts and statistics: motorcycle crashes. Insurance Information Institute website. https://www.iii.org/fact-statistic/facts-statistics-motorcycle-crashes. Accessed February 4, 2025.

Prep Kit continued

10. Hayes JM, Cash RE, Buzzard L, Green AM, Boland LL, Anderson MK. State-level helmet use laws, helmet use, and head injuries in EMS patients involved in motorcycle collisions. *Prehosp Emerg Care*. Published online January 31, 2025. doi:10.1080/10903127.2025.2450280
11. Trauma systems: national guideline for the field triage of injured patients. American College of Surgeons website. https://www.facs.org/quality-programs/trauma/systems/field-triage-guidelines/. Accessed February 4, 2025.
12. Older adult falls data. Centers for Disease Control and Prevention website. https://www.cdc.gov/falls/data-research/index.html. Published October 28, 2024. Accessed February 4, 2025.
13. Simpson PM, Bendall JC, Tiedemann A, Lord SR, Close JC. Epidemiology of emergency medical service responses to older people who have fallen: a prospective cohort study. *Prehosp Emerg Care*. 2014;18(2):185–194.
14. Quatman-Yates CC, Wisner D, Weade M, et al. Assessment of fall-related emergency medical service calls and transports after a community-level fall-prevention initiative. *Prehosp Emerg Care*. 2022;26(3):410–421.
15. Fast facts: firearm injury and death. Centers for Disease Control and Prevention website. https://www.cdc.gov/firearm-violence/data-research/facts-stats/index.html. Published July 5, 2024. Accessed February 4, 2025.
16. Baum GR, Baum JT, Hayward D, MacKay BJ. Gunshot wounds: ballistics, pathology, and treatment recommendations, with a focus on retained bullets. *Orthop Res Rev*. 2022;14:293–317.
17. Blast injuries: essential facts. America Trauma Society website. https://cdn.ymaws.com/www.amtrauma.org/resource/resmgr/TIIDE/Blast_InjuryEssential_Facts.pdf. Published 2009. Accessed February 4, 2025.
18. Choi J, Carlos G, Nassar AK, Knowlton LM, Spain DA. The impact of trauma systems on patient outcomes. *Curr Probl Surg*. 2021;58(1):100849. doi:10.1016/j.cpsurg.2020.100849
19. Resources for optimal care of the trauma patient. American College of Surgeons website. https://www.facs.org/quality-programs/trauma/quality/verification-review-and-consultation-program/standards/. Revised 2023. Accessed February 4, 2025.
20. Lyng JW, Braithwaite S, Abraham H, et al. Appropriate air medical services utilization and recommendations for integration of air medical services resources into the EMS system of care: a joint position statement and resource document of NAEMSP, ACEP, and AMPA. *Prehosp Emerg Care*. 2021;25(6):854–873.

Additional Resources

Duckworth R. Combating the trauma triad of death. Fire Engineering website. https://www.fireengineering.com/fire-ems/combating-the-trauma-triad-of-death/. Published January 1, 2019. Accessed February 4, 2025.

Nickson C. Trauma mortality and the golden hour. Life in the Fast Lane website. https://litfl.com/trauma-mortality-and-the-golden-hour/. Published November 3, 2020. Accessed February 4, 2025.

Selde W. Damage control resuscitation principles adapted for EMS civilian trauma. JEMS website. https://www.jems.com/patient-care/trauma/damage-control-resuscitation-principles-adapted-for-ems-civilian-trauma/. Published April 1, 2017. Accessed February 4, 2025.

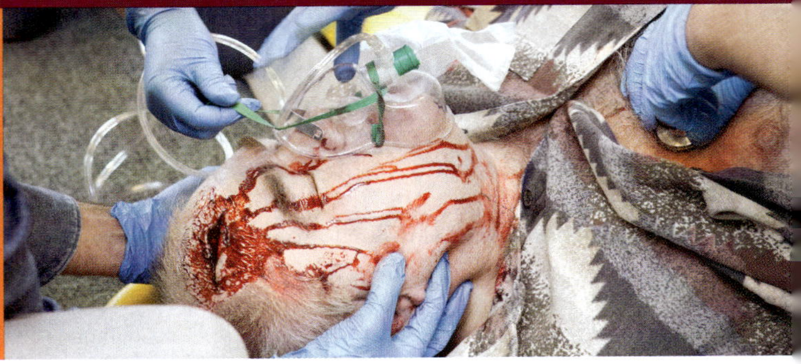

Chapter 25

Bleeding

NATIONAL EMS EDUCATION STANDARD COMPETENCIES

Trauma

Applies knowledge to provide basic emergency care and transportation based on assessment findings for an acutely injured patient.

Bleeding

- Bleeding (pp 932–936)

Pathophysiology

Applies fundamental knowledge of the pathophysiology of respiration and perfusion to patient assessment and management.

KNOWLEDGE OBJECTIVES

1. Describe the general structure of the circulatory system and the function of its parts, including the heart, arteries, veins, and capillaries. (pp 929–931)
2. Explain the significance of bleeding caused by blunt force trauma, including the importance of perfusion. (pp 931–932)
3. Discuss hypovolemic shock as a result of bleeding, including the signs of shock. (p 933)
4. Explain the importance of taking standard precautions when treating a patient with external bleeding. (p 933)
5. Describe the characteristics of external bleeding, including the identification of the following types of bleeding: arterial, venous, and capillary. (pp 932–934)
6. Explain how to determine the nature of the illness (NOI) for internal bleeding, including identifying possible traumatic and nontraumatic sources. (p 935)
7. Identify the signs and symptoms of internal bleeding. (pp 935–936)
8. Discuss internal bleeding in terms of the different mechanisms of injury (MOIs) and their associated internal bleeding sources. (p 935)
9. Explain how to conduct a primary assessment, including identification of life threats beyond bleeding, ensuring a patent airway, and making a transport decision. (pp 936–939)
10. Explain how to assess a patient with external or internal bleeding, including the physical examination, vital signs, and the use of monitoring devices. (pp 936–939)
11. Explain the emergency medical care of the patient with external bleeding. (pp 940–948)
12. Explain the emergency medical care of the patient with internal bleeding. (pp 948–951)

SKILLS OBJECTIVES

1. Demonstrate the emergency medical care of the patient with external bleeding. (p 942; Skill Drill 25-1)
2. Demonstrate the emergency medical care of the patient with external bleeding using wound packing. (pp 943–944; Skill Drill 25-2)

3. Demonstrate the emergency medical care of the patient with external bleeding using a commercial tourniquet. (p 946; Skill Drill 25-3)
4. Demonstrate emergency medical care of the patient with epistaxis, or nosebleed. (p 949; Skill Drill 25-4)
5. Demonstrate the emergency medical care of the patient who shows signs and symptoms of internal bleeding. (p 950; Skill Drill 25-5)

Introduction

In addition to airway management, two of the most important skills you will learn as an EMT are recognizing and managing life-threatening bleeding. Bleeding can be external and obvious or internal and hidden. Either type of bleeding is potentially dangerous and can lead to hypoperfusion (shock) and death. Hemorrhage is the single most preventable cause of traumatic death.[1]

This chapter will help you understand how the cardiovascular system reacts to blood loss. The chapter begins with a brief review of the anatomy and function of the cardiovascular system. It then describes the signs, symptoms, and emergency medical care of both external and internal bleeding. The chapter concludes with a discussion about the relationship between bleeding and hypovolemic shock.

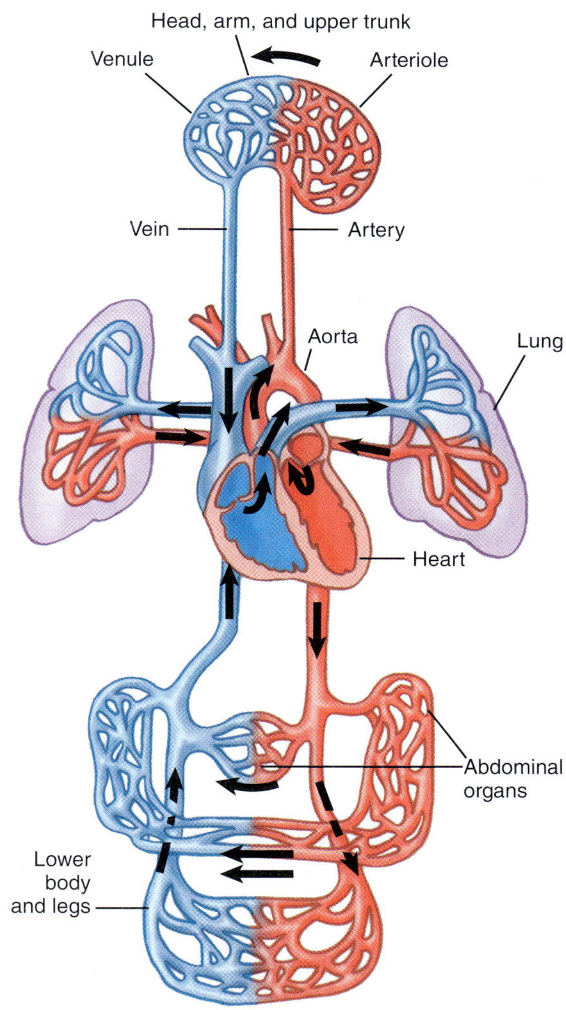

FIGURE 25-1 The cardiovascular system includes the heart, arteries, veins, and interconnecting capillaries.

Anatomy and Physiology of the Cardiovascular System

The cardiovascular system circulates blood to the body's cells and tissues, delivering oxygen and nutrients and carrying away metabolic waste products. It consists of three parts (**FIGURE 25-1**):

- The pump (the heart)
- A container (the blood vessels that reach the cells of the body)
- The fluid (blood and body fluids)

A quick review of the cardiovascular system follows. It is discussed further in Chapter 6, *The Human Body,* and Chapter 17, *Cardiovascular Emergencies.*

The Heart

All organs depend on the heart to provide an oxygen-rich blood supply. The heart works as two paired pumps (**FIGURE 25-2**). Each side of the heart has an upper chamber (atrium) and a lower chamber (ventricle). Blood leaves each chamber of a normal heart through a one-way valve, which keeps the blood moving in the proper direction by preventing backflow.

Blood Vessels and Blood

As blood flows out of the heart, it passes into the **aorta**, the largest **artery** in the body. The arteries become smaller the farther they are from the heart.

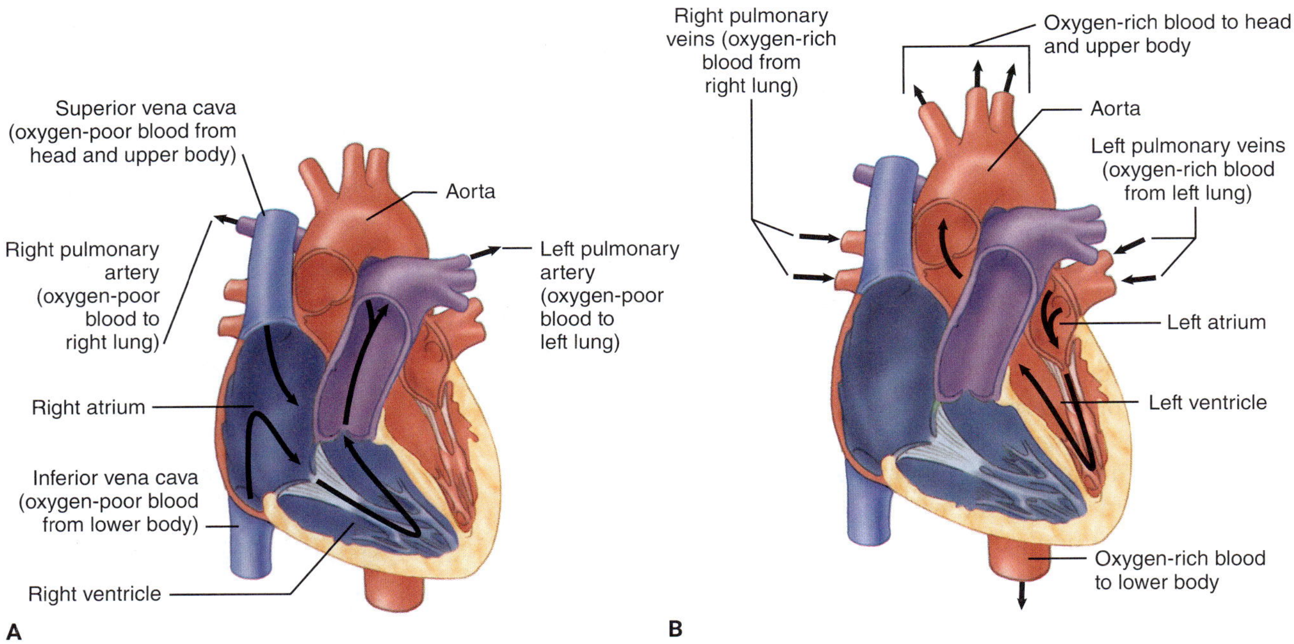

FIGURE 25-2 A. The right side of the heart circulates blood from the body to the lungs. **B.** The left side of the heart circulates oxygen-rich blood from the lungs to the rest of the body. It is the more muscular of the two pumps because it must pump blood into the aorta and arteries in order to reach all cells of the body.

The smaller blood vessels that connect the arteries and capillaries are **arterioles**. **Capillaries** are small tubes that are the diameter of a single red blood cell, which pass among all the cells in the body, linking the arterioles and the **venules**. Blood leaving the distal side of the capillaries flows into the venules. These small, thin-walled vessels empty into the **veins**, and the veins then empty into the inferior and superior venae cavae. This is the process that returns blood in the venous portion of the circulatory system to the heart. Oxygen and nutrients easily pass from the capillaries into the cells, and waste and carbon dioxide diffuse from the cells into the capillaries (**FIGURE 25-3**). This transportation system allows the body to rid itself of waste products.

Blood contains red blood cells, white blood cells, platelets, and plasma (**FIGURE 25-4**). Red blood cells transport oxygen to the cells and transport carbon dioxide (a waste product of cellular metabolism) away from the cells to the lungs, where it is removed from the body during exhalation. Platelets are the key to formation of blood clots. Blood clots are an important response from the body to control blood loss. In the body, blood clot formation depends on several factors: blood stasis, changes in the blood vessel wall (such as a wound), and the blood's ability to clot (affected by disease processes or medications). When tissues are injured, platelets begin to collect at the site of injury; this causes red blood cells to become sticky

YOU are the EMT

At 1620 hours, you are dispatched to a woodworking shop at 517 East Graham Street for a 32-year-old patient with severe bleeding from the arm. The exact mechanism of injury (MOI) is unknown. You and your partner proceed to the scene with a response time of approximately 6 minutes.

1. What are the functions of arteries? What major arteries are located in the upper extremity?
2. Why is arterial bleeding more severe than venous bleeding?

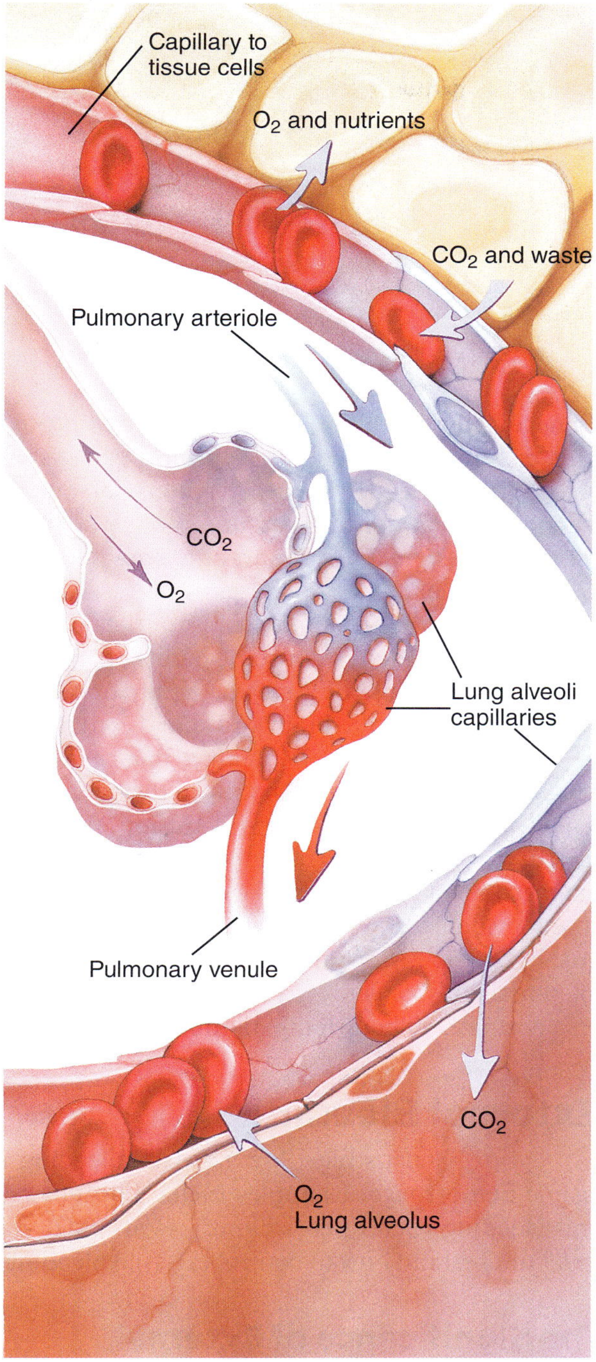

FIGURE 25-3 Oxygen (O_2) and nutrients pass easily from the capillaries into the cells, and waste and carbon dioxide (CO_2) diffuse from the cells into the capillaries (top). Oxygen and carbon dioxide pass freely between the lungs and capillaries (bottom).

and clump together. As the red blood cells begin to clump, a protein in plasma reinforces the developing clot by converting to a threadlike mesh that forms a clot. Medical conditions that interfere with

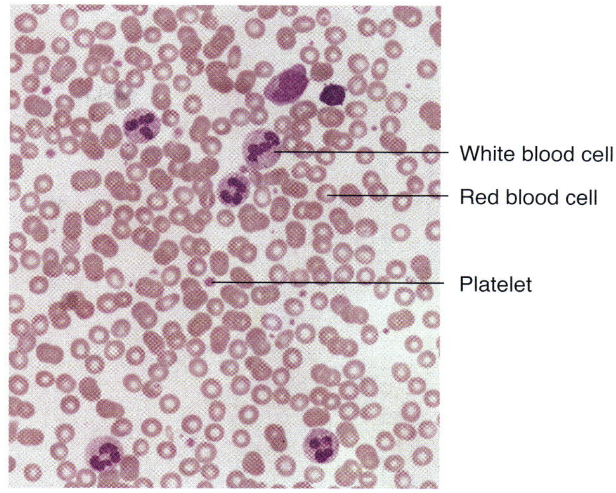

FIGURE 25-4 The microscopic appearance of the three major elements in blood: red blood cells, white blood cells, and platelets.

the normal clotting process will be discussed later in this chapter.

The autonomic nervous system monitors the body's needs and adjusts the blood flow by constricting or dilating blood vessels as required. During an emergency, the autonomic nervous system automatically redirects blood away from other organs to the heart, brain, lungs, and kidneys. Thus, the cardiovascular system adapts to changing conditions in the body to maintain homeostasis and perfusion. If blood volume is significantly diminished and the system fails to provide sufficient circulation for every body part to perform its function, then **hypoperfusion**, or **shock**, results. See Chapter 13, *Shock*, for a more detailed discussion of this process.

Pathophysiology and Perfusion

Perfusion is the circulation of blood within an organ or tissue to allow it to meet the cells' current needs for oxygen, nutrients, and waste removal. Blood enters an organ or tissue first through the arteries, then the arterioles, and finally, the capillary beds (**FIGURE 25-5**). As it passes through the capillaries, the blood delivers nutrients and oxygen to the surrounding cells and picks up the wastes they have generated.

Blood must pass through the cardiovascular system fast enough to maintain adequate circulation throughout the body and to avoid clotting, yet

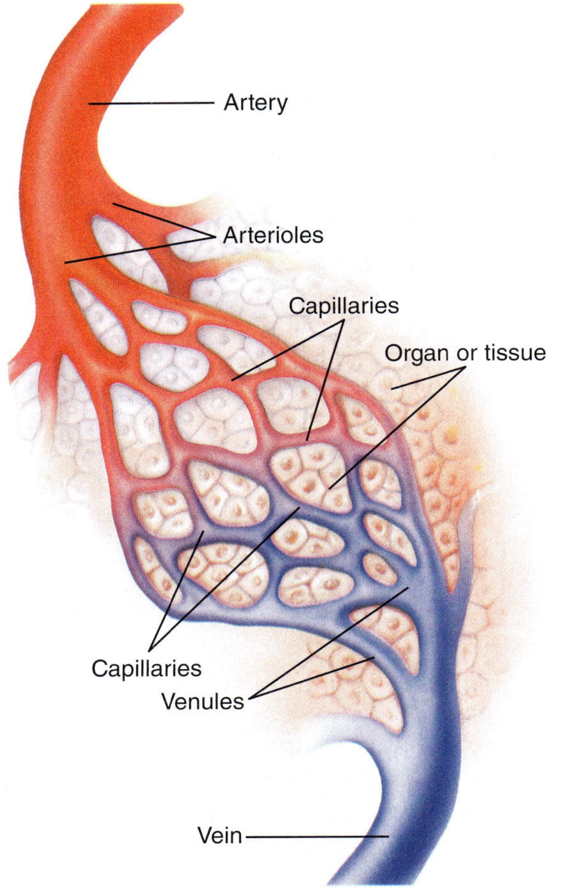

FIGURE 25-5 Perfusion occurs when blood circulates through tissues or an organ to provide the necessary oxygen and nutrients and remove waste products.

slow enough to allow each cell time to exchange oxygen and nutrients for carbon dioxide and other waste products. Although some tissues never rest and require a constant blood supply, most require a large volume of circulating blood only intermittently, with less required when at rest. For example, skeletal muscles require a minimal blood supply during sleep, as opposed to a large blood supply during exercise. Another example is the gastrointestinal tract, which requires a high flow of blood after a meal. After digestion is completed, however, the gastrointestinal tract functions well with a small fraction of that blood flow.

All organs and organ systems of the human body depend on adequate perfusion to function properly. Some organs require a rich supply of blood and do not tolerate interruption of blood supply for even a few minutes without sustaining

TABLE 25-1 Critical Organs and Corresponding Organ Systems

Organ	Organ System
Heart	Cardiovascular system
Brain	Central nervous system
Lungs	Respiratory system
Kidneys	Renal system

damage. If perfusion to these organs is interrupted, then dysfunction and failure of that organ system will occur. The death of an organ system can quickly lead to the death of the patient. Emergency medical care is designed to support adequate perfusion of these critical organs and organ systems, listed in **TABLE 25-1**, until the patient arrives at the hospital.

The heart requires constant perfusion to function optimally; without a steady supply of oxygenated blood, cells in the brain and spinal cord start to die after 4 to 6 minutes. (Remember that cells of the central nervous system do not have the capacity to regenerate.) Without adequate perfusion, the lungs can survive only 15 to 20 minutes and kidneys can be damaged after 45 minutes. Skeletal muscle demonstrates evidence of injury after 2 to 3 hours of inadequate perfusion, while the gastrointestinal tract can tolerate slightly longer periods. These times are based on a normal core body temperature (98.6°F [37.0°C]).

External Bleeding

Hemorrhage means bleeding. External bleeding is visible hemorrhage. Examples include nosebleeds and bleeding from open wounds. As an EMT, you must understand how to control external bleeding.

The Significance of External Bleeding

With serious external bleeding, it is often difficult to determine the amount of blood loss because blood will look different on different surfaces, such as when it is absorbed in clothing, when it has been diluted in water, or when the environment is dark. It is important to estimate the amount of external blood loss; however, treatment should be based on the patient's presentation and MOI.

The typical adult has an average total blood volume of 9 to 10 pints (5 to 5.5 L). The blood volume in a typical adult male is approximately 70 mL of blood per kilogram of body weight; in an adult female, it is approximately 65 mL of blood per kilogram of body weight. Therefore, an adult man weighing 175 pounds (79 kg) has a total blood volume of 5.5 L; an adult female of the same weight has a total blood volume of 5.1 L. The body cannot tolerate an acute blood loss of greater than 20% of this total blood volume, or more than 2 pints (approximately 1 L) in the average adult. With significant blood loss, adverse changes in vital signs will occur, including increased heart and respiratory rates and decreased blood pressure. Because infants and children have less blood volume compared with adults, these effects are seen with smaller amounts of blood loss. For example, a 1-year-old has a typical total blood volume of approximately 27 oz (800 mL); the child will show significant symptoms of blood loss after only 3 to 6 oz (100 to 200 mL) of blood loss, or less than one-half the volume of liquid in a 12-oz (350-mL) can of soda.

How well a patient's body can compensate for blood loss is related to how rapidly the blood loss occurs. A healthy adult can comfortably donate 1 unit, or roughly 1 pint (500 mL), of blood within 15 to 20 minutes and adapt well to this decrease in blood volume. If this volume of blood loss occurs during a much shorter period, however, symptoms of **hypovolemic shock**, a condition in which low blood volume results in inadequate perfusion and even death, might develop. The patient's age and preexisting health should also be considered.

In any situation, severe blood loss presents an immediate life threat. Your priority is to quickly control major external bleeding, even before you address airway and breathing concerns.

Safety Tips

Remember that a bleeding patient may expose you to potentially infectious body fluids; therefore, always take standard precautions when treating patients with external bleeding. Wear gloves and eye protection in all situations, and wear a gown and mask if there is a risk of blood splatter (**FIGURE 25-6**). Always keep spare gloves with you. Avoid direct contact with body fluids if possible. Take special care if you have an open sore, cut, scratch, or ulcer. Also remember that frequent, thorough handwashing between patients and after every call is a simple yet important protective measure. When you care for multiple patients, remember to wash your hands frequently and don clean gloves between patients to avoid cross-contamination of body fluids and blood. If soap and water are unavailable, use a waterless hand sanitizer, and wash with soap and water as soon as possible.

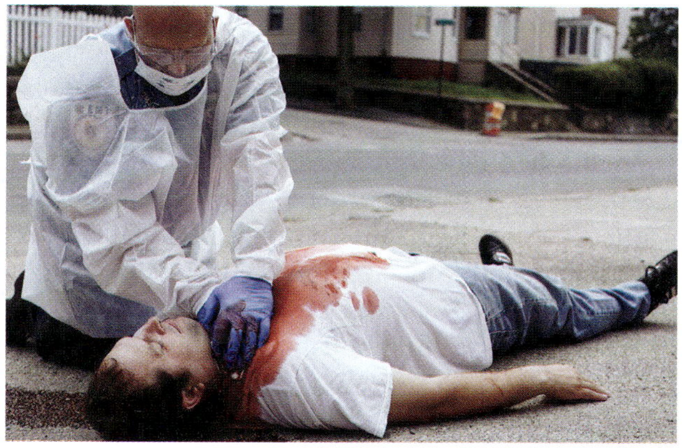

FIGURE 25-6 Your safety is paramount. Always wear proper protective equipment when caring for a patient who is bleeding.

Characteristics of External Bleeding

Injuries and some illnesses can disrupt blood vessels and cause external bleeding. You should consider bleeding to be severe if any of the following conditions exist:

- The patient has a poor general appearance and has no response to external stimuli.
- Assessment reveals signs and symptoms of shock (hypoperfusion).
- You note a significant amount of blood loss.
- The blood loss is rapid and ongoing.
- You cannot control the bleeding.
- The bleeding is associated with a significant MOI.

Typically, arterial bleeding from an open artery is bright red (because it is oxygen rich) and spurts in time with the pulse. The pressure that causes the blood to spurt also makes this type of bleeding difficult to control. As the amount of blood circulating in the body drops, so does the patient's blood pressure and, eventually, the arterial spurting.

Venous bleeding from an open wound is darker than arterial blood (because it is oxygen poor) and can flow slowly or rapidly, depending on the size of the vein. Because it is under less pressure, most venous blood does not spurt and is easier to manage; however, it can be profuse and life threatening. Capillary bleeding from damaged capillary vessels is dark red and oozes from a wound steadily but slowly. Venous and capillary blood is more likely to clot spontaneously than arterial blood (**FIGURE 25-7**).

On its own, minor bleeding tends to stop rather quickly, within approximately 10 minutes, in response to internal mechanisms and exposure to air. When a person's skin is broken, blood flows rapidly from the open blood vessel. Soon afterward, the cut ends of the blood vessel begin to narrow (**vasoconstriction**), reducing the amount of bleeding. Then a clot forms, plugging the hole and sealing the injured portions of the blood vessel. This process is called **coagulation**. With a severe injury, the damage to the blood vessel may be so great that a clot cannot completely block the hole. Bleeding will never stop if an effective clot does not form, unless the injured blood vessel is completely cut off from the main blood supply by direct pressure or a tourniquet.

Despite the efficiency of the circulatory system, it may fail in certain situations. Movement, disease process, certain medications (such as anticoagulants), removal of bandages, the external environment, or body temperature commonly affect the blood's clotting factors. Occasionally, blood loss is very rapid. In these cases, the patient might die before clotting occurs.

A small portion of the population lacks one or more of the blood's clotting factors, a condition called **hemophilia**. There are several forms of hemophilia, most of which are hereditary and some of which are severe. Sometimes bleeding occurs spontaneously in patients with hemophilia. Because the patient's blood does not clot effectively, all injuries, no matter how trivial, are potentially serious. Transport any injured patient with hemophilia immediately. See Chapter 20, *Endocrine and Hematologic Emergencies*, for further discussion of this condition.

Words of Wisdom

If a bandage has already been applied to control bleeding before your arrival on the scene, obtain a description of the wound and the amount of bleeding from the patient or bystanders. If blood has seeped through the dressing, do not remove it; most likely the clotting process has already begun and removing the dressing will disturb the clot. Instead, apply a clean dressing on top of the first one to reinforce it. You can also observe the old dressing to estimate the amount of blood loss.

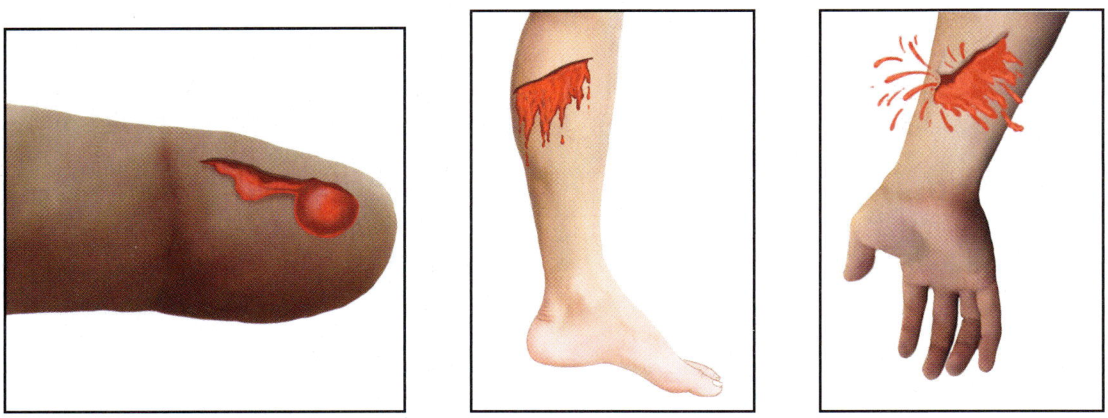

A B C

FIGURE 25-7 A. Bleeding from capillary vessels is dark red and oozes from the wound slowly but steadily. **B.** Venous bleeding is darker than arterial bleeding and flows steadily. **C.** Arterial bleeding is characteristically bright red and spurts in time with the pulse.

Internal Bleeding

Internal bleeding is any bleeding that occurs in a cavity or space inside the body. Internal bleeding can be very serious, especially because it is not easy to detect immediately. Injury or damage to internal organs commonly results in extensive internal bleeding, which can cause hypovolemic shock before you realize the extent of blood loss. A person with a bleeding stomach ulcer may sustain a large amount of blood loss very quickly. Similarly, a person who has a lacerated liver or a ruptured spleen may sustain a considerable amount of blood loss within the abdomen, yet the patient may have no outward signs of bleeding.

Broken bones also may cause serious internal blood loss. A broken femur can easily result in the loss of 2 pints (approximately 1 L) or more of blood into the soft tissues of the thigh. Often, the only signs of such bleeding are local swelling and bruising (called a **contusion** or **ecchymosis**) caused by the accumulation of blood around the ends of the broken bone. Severe pelvic fractures may result in life-threatening hemorrhage that is difficult to control.

Always be alert to the possibility of internal bleeding. Assess the patient for related signs and symptoms, particularly if the MOI is significant. If you suspect that a patient is bleeding internally, treat for shock and promptly transport the patient to the hospital.

Mechanism of Injury for Internal Bleeding

A high-energy MOI should increase your index of suspicion for the possibility of serious, unseen injuries such as internal bleeding in the abdominal cavity. Internal bleeding is possible whenever the MOI suggests that severe forces affected the body. These forces include blunt and penetrating trauma. Internal bleeding commonly occurs as a result of falls, blast injuries, motor vehicle crashes, and other blunt trauma. Remember that internal bleeding can also result from penetrating trauma.

As you assess a patient, look for signs of injury using the DCAP-BTLS (Deformities, Contusions, Abrasions, Punctures/penetrations, Burns, Tenderness, Lacerations, Swelling) mnemonic as well as any other signs of injury. Always suspect internal bleeding in a patient who has sustained a penetrating injury or blunt trauma.

Nature of Illness for Internal Bleeding

Internal bleeding is not always caused by trauma. Many illnesses can cause internal bleeding. Some of the more common causes of nontraumatic internal bleeding include bleeding ulcers, bleeding from the colon, ruptured ectopic pregnancy, and aneurysms.

Abdominal tenderness, guarding, rigidity, pain, and distention are frequent in these situations but are not always present. In older adults, dizziness, faintness, or weakness may be the first sign of nontraumatic internal bleeding. Ulcers or other gastrointestinal problems may cause **hematemesis** (vomiting of blood), bloody diarrhea, **melena** (dark, tarry stools), or vomitus that resembles coffee grounds.

It is not as important for you to know the specific organ involved as it is to recognize that the patient is in shock. When combined with prompt transport decisions and limited time spent at the scene, the rapid recognition of a patient in shock should result in the rapid administration of potentially lifesaving treatments.

Signs and Symptoms of Internal Bleeding

A common symptom of internal bleeding is pain. Significant internal bleeding will generally cause swelling in the area of bleeding, but swelling is often undetected until massive blood loss has occurred. Internal bleeding is most common in head, extremity, and pelvic injuries and is often associated with significant abdominal trauma. Intra-abdominal bleeding will often cause pain and abdominal distention. Bleeding into the chest cavity or lung may cause dyspnea, tachycardia, **hemoptysis** (the coughing up of bright red blood), and hypotension. A **hematoma**, a mass of blood that has collected in the soft tissues beneath the skin, indicates bleeding into soft tissues and may be the result of a minor or a severe injury. Bruising or ecchymosis may not be present initially, and the only sign of severe pelvic or abdominal bleeding may be redness, skin abrasions, pain, and signs of shock.

Bleeding from any body opening, however slight, is serious. It usually indicates internal bleeding that is not easy to see or control. Bright red bleeding from the mouth or rectum or blood in the urine (**hematuria**) may suggest serious internal injury or disease. Nonmenstrual vaginal bleeding is always significant.

Street Smarts

EMTs must be able to provide emotional support to patients in an emergency, especially patients who are in life-threatening situations or extreme mental distress or pain.

Signs and symptoms of internal bleeding in trauma and medical patients include the following:

- **Hematemesis.** The vomitus may be bright red or dark red. If the blood has been partially digested, the vomitus may look like coffee grounds.
- **Melena.** Melena is unusually dark, foul-smelling, tarry stool that contains digested blood.
- **Pain, tenderness, bruising, guarding, or swelling.** These signs and symptoms, particularly in an extremity, may mean that a closed fracture is bleeding.
- **Broken ribs, bruises over the lower part of the chest, or a rigid, distended abdomen.** These signs and symptoms may indicate a lacerated spleen or liver. Patients with an injury to one of these organs may have referred pain in the right shoulder (indicating the liver is injured) or left shoulder (indicating the spleen is injured). Suspect internal abdominal bleeding in a patient with referred pain.

The first sign of hypovolemic shock is a change in mental status, such as anxiety, restlessness, or combativeness. In nontrauma patients, weakness, faintness, or dizziness on standing can all be early signs. Changes in skin color, including pallor (skin that is lighter than its baseline coloration), are often seen in both trauma and medical patients with severe bleeding. Later signs of hypovolemic shock that suggest internal bleeding include the following:

- Tachycardia
- Weakness, fainting, or dizziness at rest
- Thirst
- Nausea and vomiting
- Cold, moist (clammy) skin
- Shallow, rapid breathing
- Dull eyes
- Slightly dilated pupils that are slow to respond to light
- Capillary refill time longer than 2 seconds in infants and children
- Weak, rapid (thready) pulse
- Decreasing blood pressure
- Altered level of consciousness

Patients with these signs and symptoms, particularly in the setting of significant MOI, require prompt transport, preferably to a trauma center. See Chapter 13, *Shock*, for a review of hypovolemic shock.

Patient Assessment for External and Internal Bleeding

Scene Size-Up

As you approach the patient, be alert to potential hazards to yourself and the crew, bystanders, and the patient. Take standard precautions. Place several spare pairs of gloves in your pocket for easy access in case your gloves tear or there are multiple patients with bleeding. Determine the number of patients needing care. Consider early on what additional resources you may need, and verify as you begin your assessment.

Words of Wisdom

It is best to don gloves and eye protection before you enter the scene. By the time you realize you need them, it is often too late.

Determine the nature of the illness (NOI) or the MOI by using the clues available to you; for example, bloody emesis may suggest the NOI, and a knife on the counter may suggest the MOI. Consider the need for spinal motion restriction and/or additional resources, such as an advanced life support (ALS) unit. Be sure to also consider environmental factors in your decision making. For example, caring for a sick or injured patient from a motor vehicle crash on a clear, sunny day is different from treating the same patient during a snowstorm. Extremely hot or cold weather can worsen a patient's overall condition.

Primary Assessment

When you treat a patient who has experienced significant blood loss from a visible wound or with suspected internal bleeding, do not be distracted from identifying and managing life threats, which is the focus of your primary assessment. As you approach a trauma patient, note important indicators that may signal the seriousness of the patient's condition. For example, a patient with external bleeding may have bloodstains on their clothing. Be aware of obvious signs of injury and distress, such as facial grimace.

Perform a rapid exam of the patient, look for life threats, and treat them as you find them. If the patient has obvious, life-threatening external bleeding, remember to address it *first* (the XABC [eXsanguinating hemorrhage, Airway, Breathing, Circulation] approach) by controlling it quickly; then continue assessing the ABCs, including the airway and breathing, and provide treatment. If direct pressure is ineffective in controlling massive hemorrhage from an arm or leg, apply a tourniquet immediately, even before the airway is opened. Next, assess skin color: cool, moist skin that is pale or gray suggests a perfusion problem. Because skin pallor can be difficult to detect in patients with dark skin, instead check for pale mucous membranes inside the inner lower eyelid or slow capillary refill. Determine the patient's level of consciousness using the AVPU (Awake and alert, responsive to Verbal stimuli, responsive to Pain, Unresponsive) scale. Does the patient have a patent (open) airway? If the patient is able to speak, this indicates that the airway is patent. What is the mental status of the patient? These indicators will help you assess how sick the patient is, which will help you develop an index of suspicion for serious illness or injuries related to internal bleeding.

Consider the need for spinal motion restriction. At the same time, ensure a patent airway, look for adequate breathing, and check for breath sounds. If necessary, provide the patient with high-flow oxygen via a nonrebreathing mask or assist ventilations with a bag-mask device, depending on the patient's level of consciousness and rate and quality of breathing. If the patient is unconscious, the airway may be obstructed. Insert an oropharyngeal (oral) airway to secure the airway.

Words of Wisdom

Non–life-threatening bleeding, such as from an abrasion, can be bandaged later in the assessment as necessary. However, significant and ongoing bleeding, whether internal or external, is an immediate life threat.

Quickly assess pulse rate and quality; determine the condition, color, and temperature of the skin; and check the capillary refill time to help establish the potential for internal bleeding and shock. Treat the patient for shock, if needed, by applying oxygen and maintaining a normal body temperature.

The results of your initial general impression and your assessment of the XABCs will help you decide whether to treat the patient on scene or transport immediately and treat the patient en route to the hospital. If the patient has signs and symptoms of internal bleeding or airway or breathing problems, provide rapid transport to the most appropriate facility. The condition of patients with significant bleeding may quickly become unstable. Signs such as tachycardia, tachypnea, low blood

Street Smarts

EMTs often serve as leaders and teachers within the community. Many schools and businesses have adopted Stop the Bleed programs.[2] EMTs often lead these programs and are the primary instructors. Take the opportunity to help educate those around you.

Special Populations

RECOGNIZING INTERNAL BLEEDING IN THE GERIATRIC PATIENT

Remember that in older adults, dizziness, syncope, or weakness may indicate nontraumatic internal hemorrhage.

pressure, a heart rate that is greater than the systolic blood pressure value, weak pulse, and clammy skin indicate impending circulatory collapse and the need for rapid transport.

History Taking

After the primary assessment is complete, investigate the chief complaint and be alert for signs or symptoms of other injuries based on the MOI and/or NOI. Remember, internal bleeding can be found in both medical and trauma patients. For example, ectopic pregnancy, gastrointestinal bleeding, bleeding from a dialysis shunt, and severe nosebleed are medical causes of potential bleeding. If signs and symptoms of internal bleeding are not obvious, look more carefully during the patient assessment process. In a responsive trauma patient with an isolated injury and a limited MOI, consider a detailed physical examination of the specific area after you assess vital signs and obtain a history.

When you encounter a patient with minor or superficial bleeding, avoid focusing solely on the bleeding. With significant trauma, assess the entire patient, looking for the source of the problem, any preexisting illnesses, and other issues.

If the patient is responsive, obtain a SAMPLE (Signs and symptoms, Allergies, Medications, Pertinent past medical history, Last oral intake, Events leading up to the illness or injury) history. It is important to ask patients if they take blood-thinning medications because bleeding is generally more profuse and difficult to control in patients who take blood thinners. Blood thinners or anticoagulants are often prescribed for patients with a history of stroke, pulmonary embolism, or heart attack. Common blood thinners include antiplatelets such as aspirin, clopidogrel (Plavix), and ticagrelor (Brilinta), and anticoagulants such as warfarin (Coumadin), rivaroxaban (Xarelto), dabigatran (Pradaxa), apixaban (Eliquis), and edoxaban (Savaysa).

If the patient is unresponsive, obtain medical history information from medical alert tags or ask family members or bystanders if they have any information. Look for signs and symptoms of hypoperfusion and determine how much blood loss has occurred.

Secondary Assessment

Unless you discover a life-threatening condition during the primary assessment, next conduct a secondary assessment, which is a detailed, comprehensive examination of the patient to uncover injuries or illness that may have been missed during the primary assessment. Record vital signs, complete an assessment of pain, and attach appropriate monitoring devices to quantify oxygenation and circulatory status. In some instances, such as a

YOU are the EMT

You arrive at the scene and find the patient standing outside in front of the shop. He has a towel wrapped around his left wrist; it is soaked in blood and you can see a large amount of blood on the ground. He is conscious and alert but anxious. He tells you he cut his wrist on a table saw when his arm slipped and ran into the blade.

Recording Time: 0 Minutes	
Appearance	Anxious
Level of consciousness	Conscious and alert
Airway	Open; clear of secretions or foreign bodies
Breathing	Increased rate; adequate depth
Circulation	Bleeding from the left wrist; skin is cool, pale (compared with baseline skin tone), and dry; pulse is rapid and strong

3. Is the patient effectively controlling the bleeding from his injury?

4. What should be your initial treatment priority?

critically injured patient or a short transport time, there may not be time to conduct a secondary assessment, as this is generally conducted en route to the hospital.

Assess all areas of the body for DCAP-BTLS to identify underlying or secondary injuries. For isolated injuries such as pain in the ankle, assess that area only (detailed physical examination). When examining the head, be alert for uncontrolled bleeding from large scalp lacerations; untreated, these can lead to shock, especially in infants and young children. In the abdomen, feel all four quadrants for tenderness or rigidity. In the extremities, record pulse, motor, and sensory function.

Obtain baseline vital signs; knowing these baseline values allows you to more easily identify any changes that may occur during treatment. In an adult patient, a systolic blood pressure of less than 90 mm Hg with a weak, rapid pulse; cool, moist skin that is pale or gray; and a heart rate that is greater than the systolic blood pressure value are signs of hypoperfusion that require immediate attention. In children 9 years and younger, a systolic blood pressure less than 70 mm Hg + (2 × age in years) indicates shock.[3,4] As people age, the baseline blood pressure tends to be higher and their ability to compensate decreases; as such, a systolic blood pressure less than 110 mm Hg or a heart rate that is greater than the systolic blood pressure value indicates shock.[4]

Special Populations

ASSESSMENT OF SHOCK IN GERIATRIC PATIENTS

In geriatric patients and patients who take certain blood pressure medications, the pulse rate may not increase with early shock; therefore, try to determine the patient's baseline blood pressure and quickly obtain a medical history and list of medications to help you better assess the patient's condition.

Special Populations

ASSESSMENT OF SHOCK IN PEDIATRIC PATIENTS

Pediatric patients can mask the signs and symptoms of shock until they are severely hypovolemic. Do not rule out shock in any pediatric patient who has a significant mechanism of injury or suspected dehydration from vomiting or diarrhea.

Reassessment

Because the signs and symptoms of internal bleeding are often slow to develop, it is important to reassess the patient frequently. Children especially will compensate well for blood loss and then crash quickly. The reassessment is your best opportunity to determine whether your patient's condition is improving or getting worse and to determine the effectiveness of any interventions and treatments. Reassess an unstable patient every 5 minutes and a stable patient every 15 minutes.

Whenever you suspect significant bleeding, either external or internal, and signs of shock are present, provide high-flow oxygen. If significant external bleeding is visible, control it first (shown later in Skill Drill 25-1). Using multiple methods to control external bleeding usually works best. If the patient has signs of hypoperfusion, provide aggressive treatment for shock and rapid transport to the appropriate hospital. If internal bleeding is suspected, apply high-concentration oxygen via a nonrebreathing mask and provide rapid transport to the hospital. (See Skill Drill 25-5 for additional steps.)

Do not delay transport of a patient to complete an assessment, particularly when significant bleeding is present, even if the bleeding is controlled. The assessment can be started during transport.

In patients with severe external bleeding, it is important to recognize, estimate, and report the amount of blood loss that has occurred and how rapidly or over what duration of time it occurred. For example, you may report that approximately 2 pints (approximately 1 L) of blood loss occurred if the bleeding is measurable, or you may note that the bleeding soaked through three trauma dressings. Report this information to hospital personnel during transport to allow the hospital to evaluate needed resources, such as the availability of surgical suites, surgeons, and other specialty clinicians. Your transfer report at the hospital should update hospital personnel on how your patient has responded to your care. Be sure your paperwork reflects all of the patient's injuries and the care you have provided.

Emergency Medical Care for External Bleeding

Several methods are available to control external bleeding:

- Direct pressure
- Pressure dressings and/or splints
- Tourniquets
- Junctional tourniquet
- Hemostatic dressing
- Wound packing

To control external bleeding, follow the steps shown in **FIGURE 25-8**. Begin with direct pressure, and move to the next steps if direct pressure does not control the bleeding.[5]

The most common way to control external bleeding is simple application of direct, local pressure to the bleeding site. This method is usually effective. (Previously, elevation of the extremity was also recommended, but there is no evidence that it helps control bleeding.) Pressure slows or stops the flow of blood and permits normal coagulation to occur. You may apply pressure with your gloved fingertips or hand over the top of a sterile dressing if one is immediately available. If there is an object protruding from the wound, never remove it unless it is in the cheek and blocking the patient's airway. Apply bulky dressings to stabilize the impaled object in place, and apply pressure as best you can for at least 3 minutes without interruption.[5]

In most cases, direct pressure will stop the bleeding. Once you have applied a dressing to control bleeding, create a pressure dressing to maintain the pressure by firmly wrapping a sterile, self-adhering roller bandage around the entire

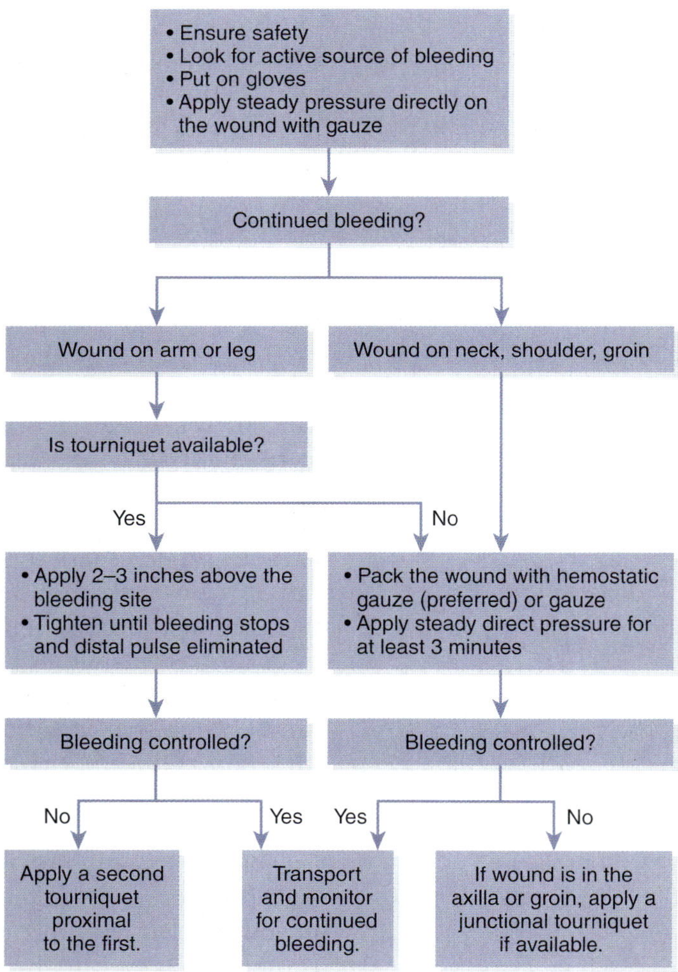

FIGURE 25-8 Steps to control life-threatening external bleeding.

Adapted from Berry C, Gallagher JM, Goodloe JM, Dorlac WC, Dodd J, Fischer PE. Prehospital hemorrhage control and treatment by clinicians: a joint position statement. *Prehosp Emerg Care.* 2023;27(5):544–551. copyright © 2023 National Association of EMS Physicians, reprinted by permission of Informa UK Limited, trading as Taylor & Francis Group, www.tandfonline.com on behalf of National Association of EMS Physicians.

wound. Use 4 × 4–inch (10 × 10–cm) sterile gauze pads for small wounds and sterile universal dressings for larger wounds.

Cover the entire dressing with the bandage above (proximal to) and below (distal to) the wound and stretch the bandage tight enough to control bleeding. If you were able to palpate a distal pulse before applying the dressing, then you should still be able to palpate a distal pulse on the injured extremity after applying the pressure dressing. If bleeding continues, then the dressing is insufficient. If the bleeding oozes slowly through the dressing, then reinforce it by applying more dressings on top of it. Do not remove a dressing until a physician has evaluated the patient.

Bleeding will almost always stop when the pressure of the dressing exceeds arterial pressure. This will assist in controlling bleeding and helping blood to clot.

If direct pressure fails to immediately stop hemorrhage on an extremity, then apply a tourniquet at least 2 to 3 inches (5 to 8 cm) proximal to the bleeding. Do not place a tourniquet over a joint, such as the elbow or knee, because you will be unable to achieve compression. If, for example, the elbow is 2 to 3 inches (5 to 8 cm) proximal to the wound, place the tourniquet more proximally on the arm. If application of a tourniquet is not possible because the bleeding is in the axilla or groin, then consider a junctional tourniquet if available. If the wound is on the neck or other location where a tourniquet is not possible, or when a junctional tourniquet is not available, pack the wound with gauze or a hemostatic dressing (preferred) if available. Follow local protocols.

SKILL DRILL 25-1 illustrates the basic techniques to control external bleeding:

1. Take standard precautions.
2. Apply direct pressure over the wound with a dry, sterile dressing (**Step 1**).
3. Apply a pressure dressing (**Step 2**).
4. If direct pressure is not immediately effective, apply a tourniquet to an extremity at least 2 to 3 inches (5 to 8 cm) proximal to the bleeding, but not over a joint (**Step 3**).
5. Tighten the tourniquet until bleeding stops (**Step 4**) and no distal pulse is palpable. Position the patient supine unless there is a reason not to, such as underlying respiratory distress.
6. Apply high-flow oxygen to maintain an oxygen saturation level of 94% to 98%, once hemorrhage is controlled. Keep the patient warm. Transport promptly.

Wound Packing and Hemostatic Dressings

Gauze can be packed into larger wounds to control hemorrhage when direct pressure is not adequate or application of a tourniquet is not possible. A

YOU are the EMT

You immediately apply direct pressure to the patient's wrist with a dry, sterile dressing, and apply a pressure dressing. This effectively controls the patient's bleeding. While you further assess the patient and apply a splint in case there are fractures, your partner applies high-concentration oxygen with a nonrebreathing mask, obtains the patient's vital signs, and inquires about his medical history. The patient denies having any medical problems and states he does not take any medications.

Recording Time: 5 Minutes	
Respirations	24 breaths/min; regular and adequate
Pulse	120 beats/min; strong and regular
Skin	Cool, pale, and dry
Blood pressure	104/60 mm Hg
Oxygen saturation (Spo_2)	94% (on oxygen)

5. What are the components of the cardiovascular system and how are they affected by the patient's injury?
6. What factors determine the severity of external bleeding?

Skill Drill 25-1 Controlling External Bleeding

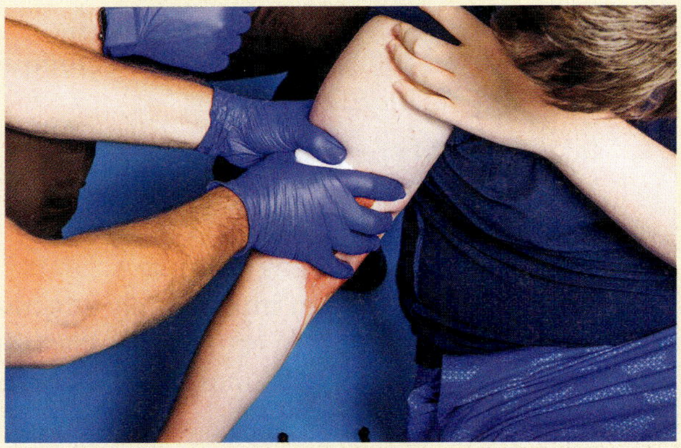

Step 1

Take standard precautions. Apply direct pressure over the wound with a dry, sterile dressing.

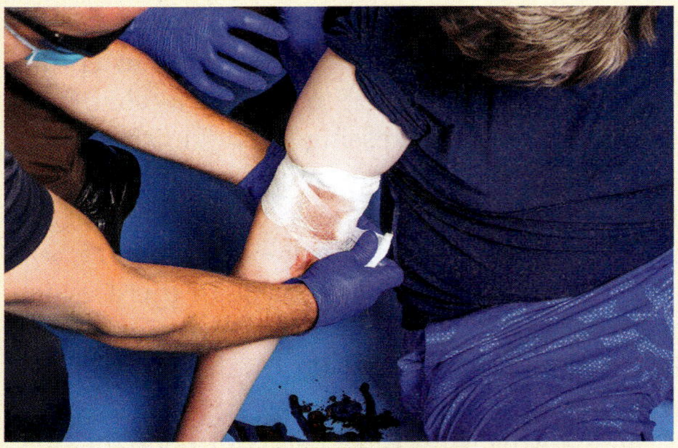

Step 2

Apply a pressure dressing.

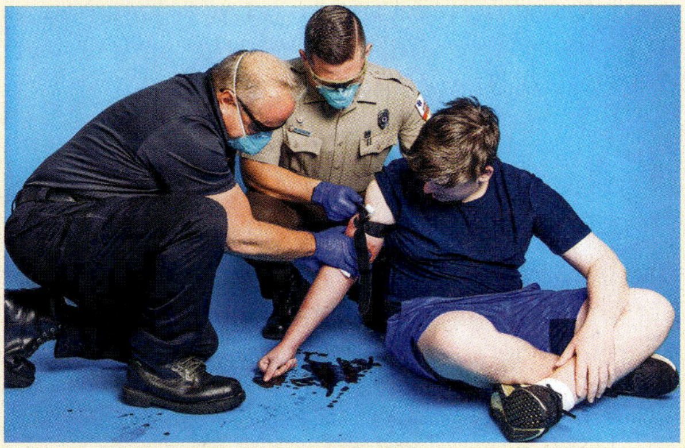

Step 3

If direct pressure with a pressure dressing does not control bleeding, apply a tourniquet at least 2 to 3 inches (5 to 8 cm) proximal to the bleeding, but not over a joint.

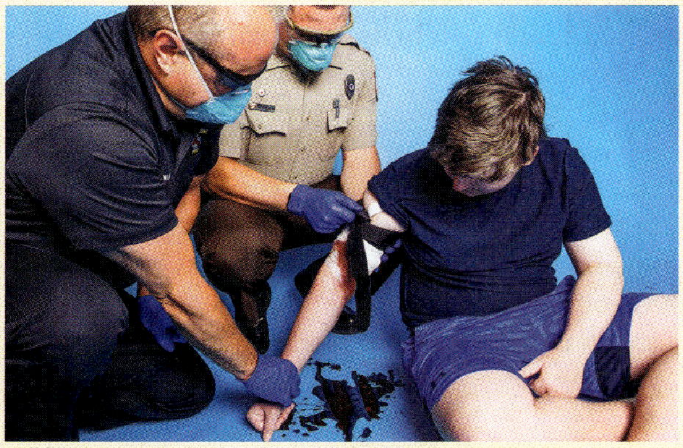

Step 4

Tighten the tourniquet until bleeding is controlled and pulses are no longer palpable distal to the tourniquet. Properly position the patient. Apply high-flow oxygen to maintain an oxygen saturation level of 94% to 98%. Keep the patient warm. Transport promptly.

hemostatic dressing is a dressing impregnated with a chemical compound that slows or stops bleeding by promoting clot formation.

Hemostatic dressings can be used together with wound packing and direct pressure when direct pressure alone is ineffective, such as with massive abdominal injuries, or when tourniquet placement is otherwise impossible (eg, on the neck). These dressings have the potential to improve prehospital bleeding control. Be aware of and follow your local protocols regarding use of wound packing and hemostatic dressings.

Words of Wisdom

Much of the bleeding associated with broken bones occurs because the sharp ends of the bones cut muscles and other tissues. As long as a fracture remains unstable, the bone ends will move and continue to injure partially clotted blood vessels. Therefore, immobilizing a fracture and decreasing movement will help control bleeding. Often, a simple splint will quickly reduce the bleeding associated with a fracture (**FIGURE 25-9**). If the patient is unstable, however, do not spend excess time splinting a fracture.

Follow your local protocols and the steps in **SKILL DRILL 25-2** to pack a wound.

1. Take standard precautions.
2. Remove or open the patient's clothing as needed to expose the wound (**Step 1**).
3. Wipe away any pooled blood.
4. Pack the wound tightly into the full depth of the wound with hemostatic gauze (preferred) or plain gauze (**Step 2**).
5. Apply steady pressure by pressing with both hands directly on top of the bleeding wound. Push down as hard as you can (**Step 3**).
6. Continue holding pressure until relieved by another prehospital clinician or the patient is delivered to definitive care.

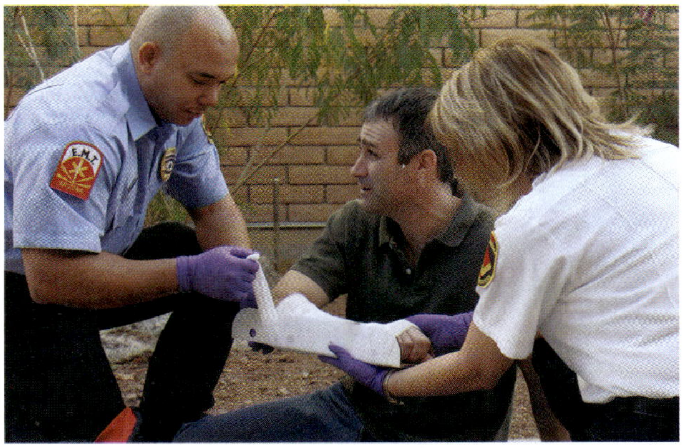

FIGURE 25-9 Use of a simple splint will often quickly control internal bleeding associated with a fracture. If a fracture is not immobilized, then the bone ends are free to move and may continue to injure partially clotted blood vessels.

Skill Drill 25-2 Packing a Wound

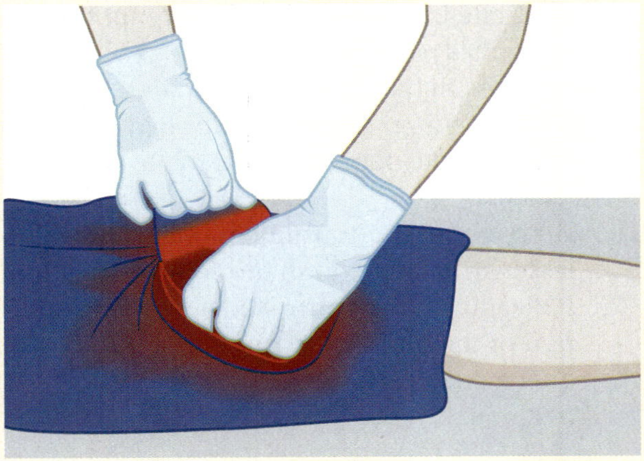

Step 1

Expose the wound and wipe away any pooled blood.

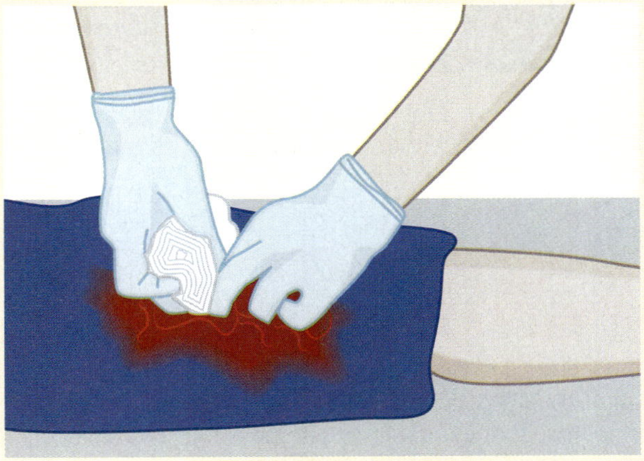

Step 2

Pack the wound tightly with hemostatic gauze (preferred), plain gauze, or a clean cloth.

(continues)

Skill Drill 25-2 Packing a Wound continued

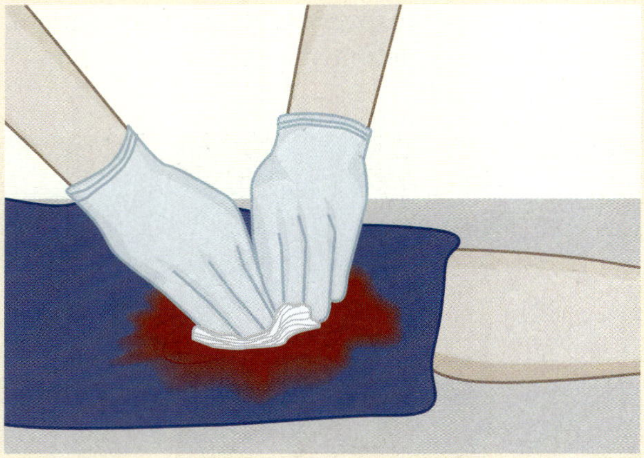

Step 3

Apply steady pressure by pressing with both hands directly on top of the bleeding wound. Push down as hard as you can.

Tourniquets

If direct pressure does not immediately control extremity bleeding, then use a **tourniquet**. The tourniquet is useful only if a patient has substantial bleeding from an extremity injury. Several different types of commercial tourniquets are available (**FIGURE 25-10**). Make sure you are familiar with the type of tourniquet used by your service.

Street Smarts

A properly applied tourniquet is painful. As you apply it, explain to the patient that it will be uncomfortable.

Words of Wisdom

It used to be taught to apply the tourniquet "high and tight," meaning close to the axilla for arm hemorrhage and close to the groin for leg hemorrhage. However, this method is now used only when the site of the bleeding cannot be easily determined or it is unsafe to take the time to do so. When the location of the wound is clear, the tourniquet should be applied at least 2 to 3 inches (5 to 8 cm) proximal to it.[5]

Follow the manufacturer's instructions for the specific type of tourniquet used by your service. Follow the steps in **SKILL DRILL 25-3** to apply a commercial tourniquet.

1. Take standard precautions.
2. Apply direct pressure over the bleeding site.
3. Place the tourniquet around the bare skin of the extremity tightly, at least 2 to 3 inches (5 to 8 cm) proximal to the bleeding site, but not over a joint (**Step 1**).
4. Click the buckle into place and pull the strap as tight as possible.
5. Turn the tightening dial or windlass clockwise until bleeding has been controlled and pulses are no longer palpable distal to the tourniquet. (**Step 2**).
6. Do not release a tourniquet once applied, unless instructed to do so by medical direction.
7. If bleeding is not controlled by proper application of the tourniquet, apply a second tourniquet 2 to 3 inches (5 to 8 cm) proximal to the first one.

Whenever you apply a tourniquet, make sure you observe the following precautions:

- Do not apply a tourniquet directly over any joint. Always place the tourniquet proximal to the injury.

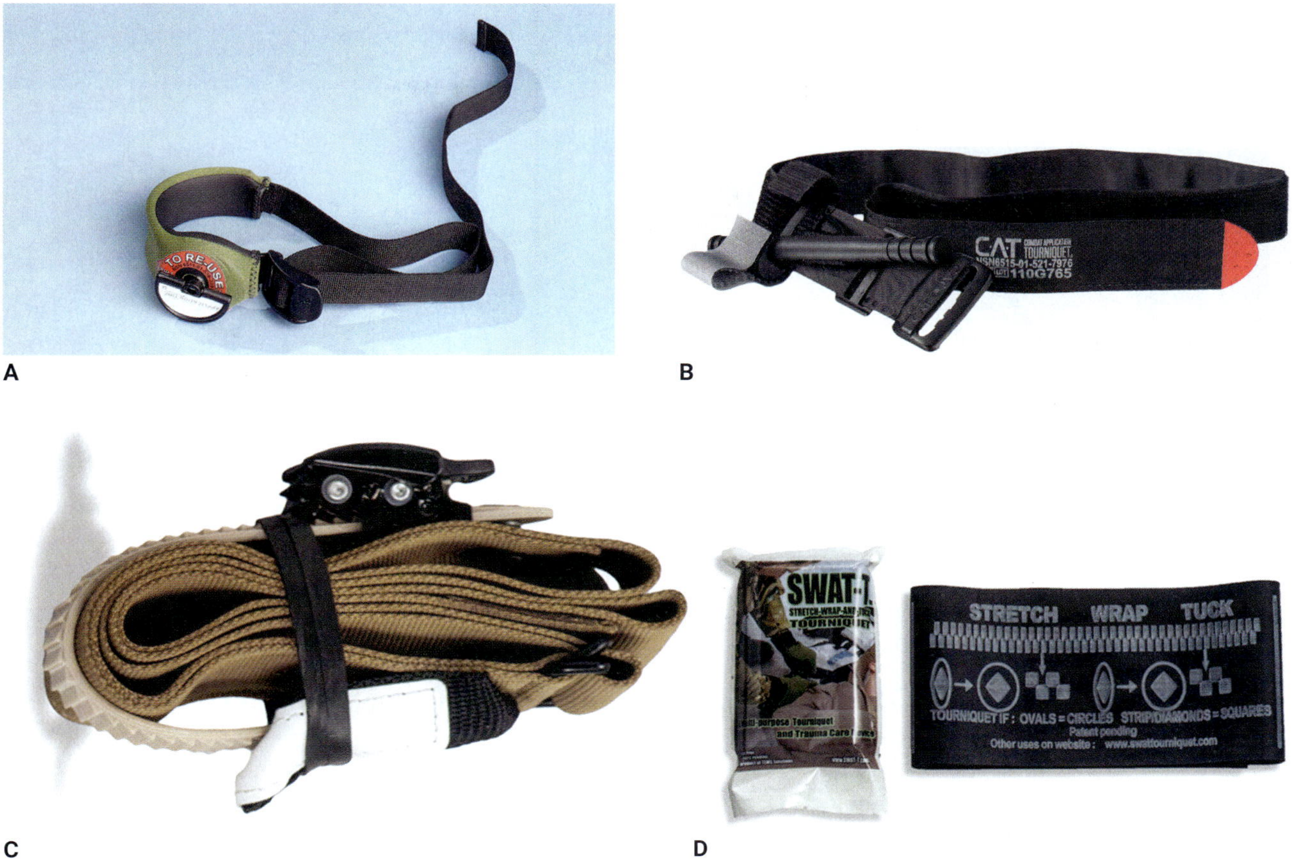

FIGURE 25-10 Different examples of commercial tourniquets. **A.** Mechanical advantage tourniquet (MAT). **B.** Combat application tourniquet (CAT). **C.** Ratcheting medical tourniquet (RMT). **D.** Special weapons and tactics tourniquet (SWAT-T).

A: © Jones & Bartlett Learning; **B:** Courtesy of North American Rescue, LLC; **C, D:** Photo by Diane Zahorodny. Courtesy of Chinook Medical Gear.

- If the tourniquet does not immediately control bleeding, apply a second one 2 to 3 inches (5 to 8 cm) proximal to the first, leaving the first one in place.
- Make sure the tourniquet is tightened securely.
- Use a commercial tourniquet rather than an improvised one when available. Never use wire, rope, a belt, or any other narrow material that could cut into the skin.
- If a tourniquet was applied by a bystander prior to your arrival, assess its effectiveness. If the bleeding continues or the pulse is still present, apply another tourniquet 2 to 3 inches (6 to 8 cm) proximal to the first one. If it appears that a tourniquet was not indicated and the bleeding has stopped, contact medical direction for instructions on how to proceed.
- Never cover a tourniquet with a bandage. Leave it in full view.
- Do not loosen the tourniquet after you have applied it, unless medical direction instructs you to do so. Hospital personnel will follow a specific procedure to release it once they are prepared to manage the bleeding.
- If the patient complains of severe pain related to the tourniquet, attempt calming measures and explain why you are unable to release the tourniquet after it has been applied.

Mark the exact time the tourniquet was applied on the tourniquet or the patient and be sure to communicate the time of application, the site of application, and the rationale for application clearly and specifically to hospital personnel on arrival.

Skill Drill 25-3 Applying a Commercial Tourniquet

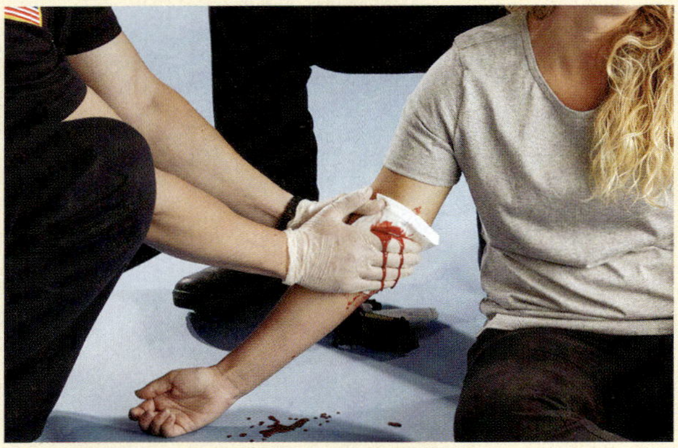

Step 1

Apply pressure over the bleeding site and place the tourniquet proximal to the injury.

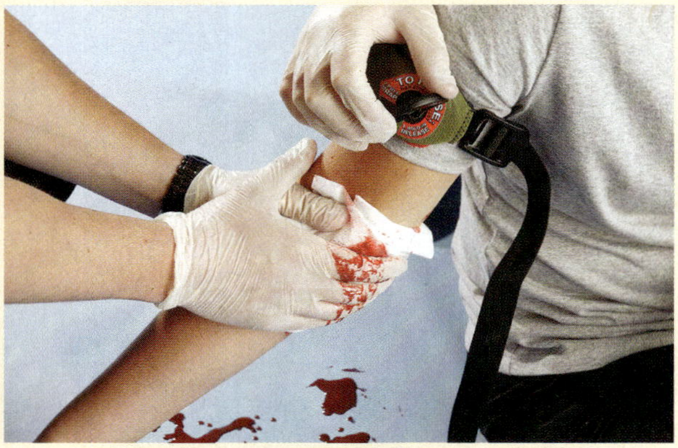

Step 2

Click the buckle into place, pull the strap tight, and turn the tightening dial clockwise until pulses are no longer palpable distal to the tourniquet and until bleeding has been controlled.

Words of Wisdom

If the patient has an open fracture of an extremity, bleeding can be substantial. Consider a tourniquet early if bleeding is not easily controlled with direct pressure. The method used to control severe external bleeding may be governed by local protocols, but regardless of the method, it must be quick and effective. Remember, uncontrolled bleeding may quickly result in shock and death. Patients can bleed to death quickly from extremity injuries. It is imperative that you use effective techniques to stop bleeding when you encounter it.

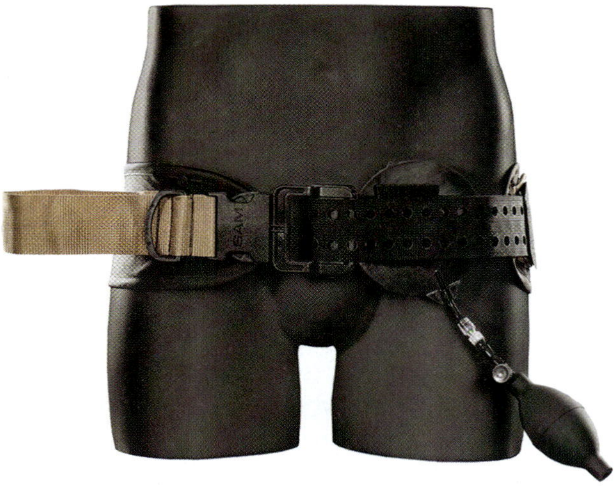

FIGURE 25-11 The SAM junctional tourniquet can be used for inguinal or axillary hemorrhage control.

Junctional Tourniquets

A **junctional tourniquet** allows for compression of life-threatening bleeding in areas where standard tourniquet application is not possible, such as the groin or the axilla (**FIGURE 25-11**). A junctional tourniquet may be indicated for severe hemorrhage at the junction of the torso with the arms (axillary area) or legs (inguinal area, or groin). Junctional tourniquets have been approved by the Food and Drug Administration for use in prehospital medicine and have been shown to be highly effective in controlling hemorrhage when used properly.[7]

Special Populations

BLEEDING CONTROL IN PEDIATRIC PATIENTS

Initial steps to manage severe bleeding in infants and children are the same as for adults. They include applying direct pressure, or wound packing with direct pressure, depending on the location of the bleeding. For most children older than 2 years, a commercial adult tourniquet can be used to stop uncontrolled extremity bleeding that cannot be managed by direct pressure,[5] whereas a stretch–wrap–tuck elastic tourniquet can be used on patients of any age.[6] Application of the tourniquet is the same as for an adult; however, additional turns of the windlass may be needed for bleeding control. If the bleeding is not controlled by tourniquet application, apply direct pressure while transporting to the closest appropriate facility.

Junctional tourniquets are presently used most commonly in military and tactical settings. Application of junctional tourniquets varies widely between types. If a junctional tourniquet is used in your emergency medical services (EMS) agency, you should be trained and credentialed to use it. While it is possible that junctional tourniquets might work on older children or adolescents, there is little research in this area.

Pelvic Binder

Use of a pelvic binder (pelvic compression device) is now common in prehospital care (**FIGURE 25-12**). A **pelvic binder** is a type of splint that may be indicated for a suspected unstable closed pelvic fracture. Research indicates that a pelvic binder is an effective method to reduce the width of and to stabilize pelvic ring injuries.[8] This helps to control internal bleeding, specifically bleeding associated with a life-threatening **open-book pelvic fracture**. It is applied when pelvic fracture is suspected and the patient has signs of shock.

To apply a pelvic binder, slide the binder under the supine patient with the device centered over the trochanters (hips). Secure and tighten the device according to manufacturer's instructions. It is important to provide the correct amount of force when applying a compression device.

Pediatric patients who weigh less than 50 pounds (23 kg) may be too small for an adult pelvic binder; however, there are commercial pediatric pelvic binders available. Follow local protocols regarding use of a pelvic binder.

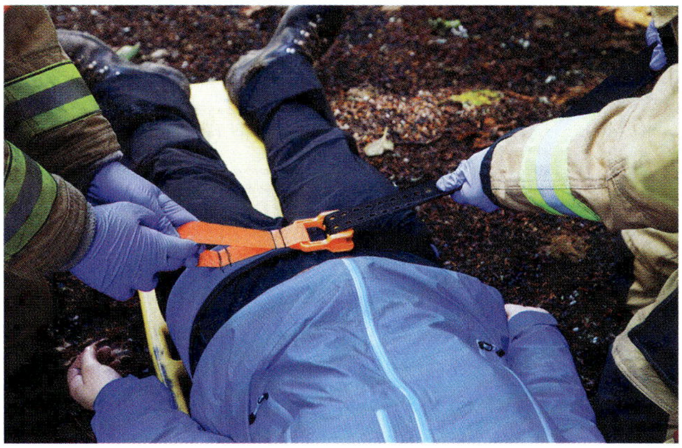

FIGURE 25-12 A pelvic compression device or binder.

ALS Assist

Competence in bleeding control is a high-priority intervention that is proven to save lives. EMTs should be thoroughly familiar with the techniques and tools available within their EMS system, including tourniquets, junctional tourniquets, and hemostatic dressings. Your ability to control hemorrhage will allow ALS clinicians to attend to other bleeding sites and then focus on other interventions and expedite patient stabilization and transport.

Bleeding From the Nose, Ears, and Mouth

Bleeding around the face always presents a risk for airway obstruction or aspiration. Maintain a clear airway by positioning the patient appropriately and using suction when indicated. Several conditions can result in bleeding from the nose, ears, and/or mouth, including the following:

- Fracture of the base of the skull
- Facial injuries, including those caused by a direct blow to the nose
- Sinusitis and infections
- Use of nose drops and intranasal use of street drugs (snorting)

- Exposure to dry air, causing dried or cracked nasal mucosa
- High blood pressure
- Coagulation disorders or use of anticoagulant medication
- Digital trauma (nose picking)
- Cancer

Epistaxis, or nosebleed, is a common emergency. Occasionally, it can cause blood loss great enough to send a patient into shock. Keep in mind that the blood that is visible may be only a small part of the total blood loss. Much of the blood may pass down the throat into the stomach as the patient swallows. A person who swallows a large amount of blood may become nauseated and start vomiting the blood, which is sometimes confused with internal bleeding. Most nontraumatic nosebleeds occur from sites in the septum (the tissue dividing the nostrils). You can usually handle this type of bleeding effectively by pinching the nostrils together. **SKILL DRILL 25-4** illustrates the basic techniques to control epistaxis.

1. Take standard precautions.
2. Help the patient to sit, leaning forward, with the head tilted forward. This position stops the blood from trickling down the throat or being aspirated into the lungs.
3. Apply direct pressure for at least 10 to 15 minutes by pinching the fleshy part of the nostrils together. This is the preferred method. This technique may also be performed by the patient (**Step 1**).
4. Keep the patient calm and quiet, especially if the patient has high blood pressure or is anxious. Anxiety tends to increase blood pressure, which could worsen the nosebleed.
5. Apply ice over the nose.
6. Maintain the pressure until the bleeding is completely controlled, usually no more than 15 minutes if this is the patient's only problem. Most often, failure to stop a nosebleed is the result of releasing the pressure too soon (**Step 2**).
7. Provide prompt transport. You can initiate transport while having the patient maintain direct pressure or while maintaining pressure yourself.
8. Assess the patient for signs and symptoms of shock and treat appropriately.

Emergency Medical Care for Internal Bleeding

Controlling internal bleeding or bleeding from major organs usually requires surgery or other procedures that must be done in the hospital. It is important for you to remain calm and reassure the patient. Keeping the patient as still and quiet as possible assists the body's clotting process. Provide

YOU are the EMT

The patient is placed onto the stretcher and loaded into the ambulance. He remains conscious and alert but is still anxious. You place him in a supine position and cover him with a blanket. Shortly before departing the scene, you reassess him and obtain another set of vital signs.

Recording Time: 10 Minutes	
Level of consciousness	Conscious and alert; anxious
Respirations	24 breaths/min; regular and adequate
Pulse	116 beats/min; strong and regular
Skin	Cool, pale, and dry
Blood pressure	112/70 mm Hg
Oxygen saturation (Spo_2)	98% (on oxygen)

7. How might a patient's outcome be affected if bleeding is internal rather than external?

8. What are the signs and symptoms of internal bleeding?

Skill Drill 25-4 Controlling Epistaxis

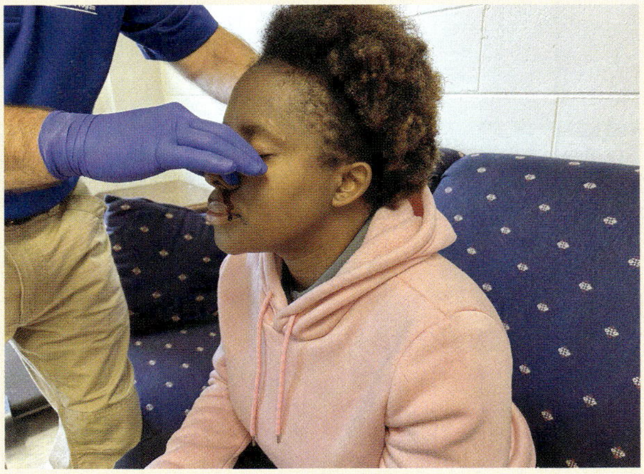

Step 1

Position the patient sitting, leaning forward. Apply direct pressure, pinching the fleshy part of the nostrils together. Calm the patient.

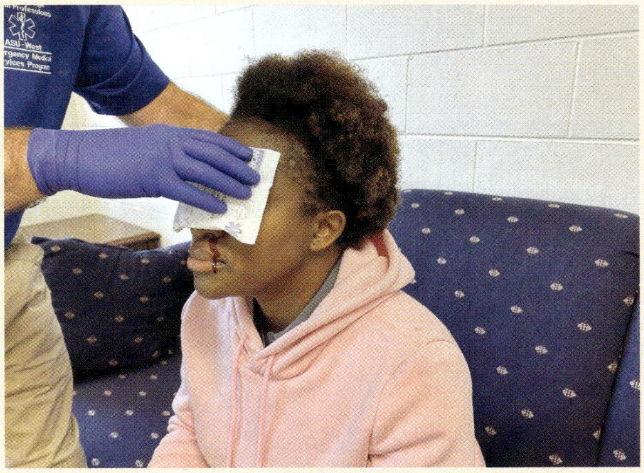

Step 2

Apply ice over the nose. Maintain pressure on the nares until bleeding is controlled. The cold helps to constrict blood vessels to slow or stop bleeding. Initiate prompt transport while you or the patient applies pressure. Assess and treat for shock, including oxygen, as needed.

All images Courtesy of Rhonda Hunt.

YOU are the EMT

You continue to monitor the patient en route to the hospital and reassess his condition as appropriate. After reassessing the patient and his vital signs, you call your radio report into the receiving facility.

Recording Time: 17 Minutes	
Level of consciousness	Conscious and alert; restless
Respirations	20 breaths/min; regular and adequate
Pulse	110 beats/min; strong and regular
Skin	Cool, pale, and dry
Blood pressure	114/68 mm Hg
Oxygen saturation (Spo_2)	97% (on oxygen)

The patient is delivered to the hospital and you give your report to the attending physician. An intravenous line is started, and the patient is given a small amount of medication to address his pain and anxiety. He is taken to the operating room for repair of severed tendons, nerves, and an artery as a result of the injury.

9. How does the body typically respond to blood loss?

high-flow oxygen, if indicated, and cover the patient with a blanket to maintain body temperature. You can usually control internal bleeding related to fractures of the extremities in the field simply by splinting the extremity. Never use a tourniquet to control the bleeding from closed, internal, soft-tissue injuries. Follow the steps in **SKILL DRILL 25-5** to care for patients with possible internal bleeding.

Skill Drill 25-5 Controlling Internal Bleeding

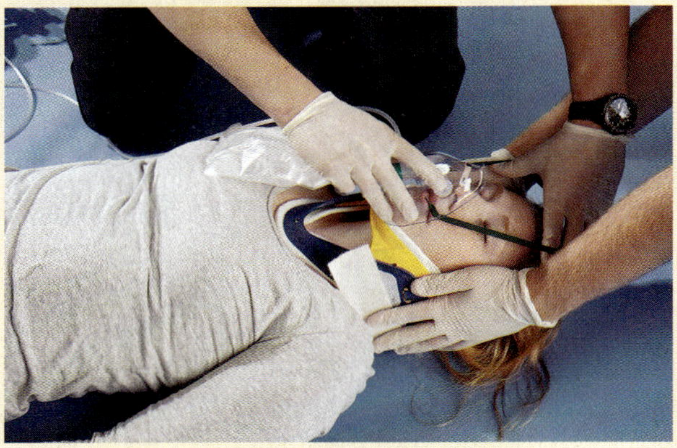

Step 1

Take standard precautions. Control obvious external bleeding and treat suspected internal bleeding using a splint. Maintain the airway and be alert for cervical spine injury. Administer oxygen if indicated and provide ventilation as necessary.

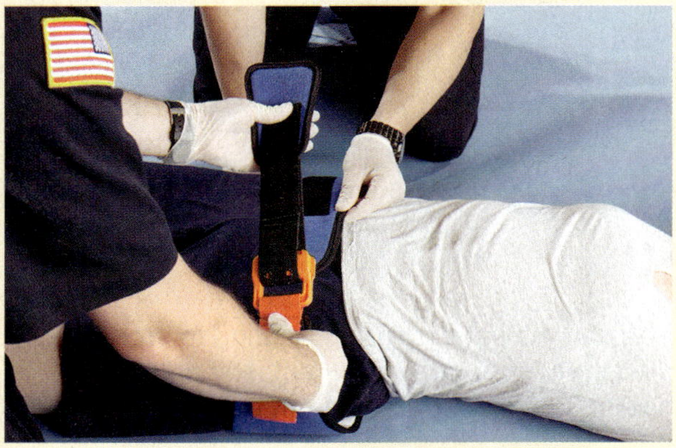

Step 2

Depending on local protocols, use a pelvic compression device or splint to control suspected internal bleeding related to possible pelvic fracture.

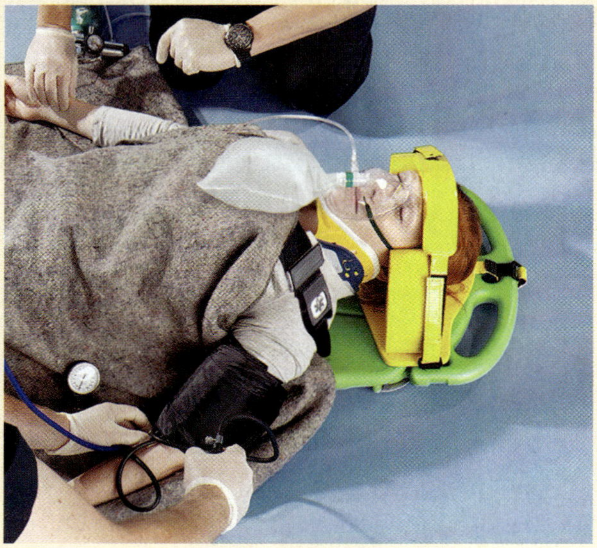

Step 3

Monitor vital signs and keep the patient warm.

1. Take standard precautions.
2. Control all obvious external bleeding. Treat suspected internal bleeding in an extremity by applying a splint.
3. Maintain the airway with spinal motion restriction if the MOI suggests the possibility of spinal injury.
4. Administer high-flow oxygen and provide artificial ventilation as necessary (**Step 1**).
5. Depending on local protocols, use a pelvic compression device or splint to control suspected internal bleeding from possible pelvic fracture (**Step 2**).
6. Monitor and record the vital signs at least every 5 minutes.
7. Keep the patient warm (**Step 3**).
8. Give the patient nothing by mouth, not even small sips of water.
9. Provide prompt transport for all patients with signs and symptoms of hypoperfusion. Report any changes in the patient's condition to emergency department personnel.

YOU are the EMT SUMMARY

1. What are the functions of arteries? What major arteries are located in the upper extremity?

Arteries are high-pressure blood vessels that distribute oxygenated blood throughout the body. The major arteries located in the upper extremity include the brachial artery, located on the inner (ulnar) aspect of the arm; the radial artery, located on the thumb-side (radial) aspect of the wrist and forearm, proximal to the hand; and the ulnar artery, located on the opposite side of the forearm from the radial artery. The radial and ulnar arteries are the two terminal branches of the brachial artery.

2. Why is arterial bleeding more severe than venous bleeding?

Blood flow through the arteries is driven by contraction of the left ventricle. Pressure in the arteries is much higher than pressure in the veins, so blood loss from an artery is generally more rapid and severe. Arterial bleeding is also more difficult to control than venous bleeding.

3. Is the patient effectively controlling the bleeding from his injury?

As evidenced by the blood-soaked towel and large amount of blood on the ground, the patient clearly is *not* effectively controlling the bleeding from his injury. Further, you do not know how much blood loss he has sustained because he is standing outside, not in the area where the injury occurred. The fact that he is anxious and has cool, pale skin suggests significant external blood loss.

4. What should be your initial treatment priority?

You must take immediate action to control the patient's bleeding. His airway is patent, as evidenced by the fact that he is conscious, alert, and talking.

In most cases, direct pressure will control both venous and arterial bleeding. If direct pressure and a pressure dressing are ineffective in immediately controlling severe external bleeding, apply a tourniquet and transport. Your partner can apply oxygen while you are attempting to manage the bleeding but if you are alone, administration of oxygen should be delayed until after the bleeding is controlled. Other treatment such as splinting the arm, would also be delayed.

5. What are the components of the cardiovascular system and how are they affected by the patient's injury?

The cardiovascular system is responsible for supplying and maintaining adequate blood flow to the body's tissues and cells. It consists of three components: the pump (the heart), the container (the blood vessels), and the fluid (blood and body fluids). These components of the cardiovascular system are interdependent; that is, they rely on each other to perform a common function. Because the patient is bleeding significantly, the intravascular volume is markedly decreased in all of the blood vessels, potentially leading to hypovolemic shock. The heart increased its rate to compensate for the decreased blood volume to keep perfusion adequate. If it was not able to compensate adequately or the bleeding could not be controlled and the blood pressure decreased further (below 90 mm Hg systolic), decompensated shock would have developed.

6. What factors determine the severity of external bleeding?

The single most influential factor is the type and size of the blood vessel that is injured. A lacerated brachial artery, for example, will bleed more severely than a small vein in the leg. The patient's blood

YOU are the EMT SUMMARY continued

pressure and heart rate can also affect the severity of external bleeding. The greater the pressure on the arterial wall and the faster the heart rate, the more rapid the bleeding tends to be. The patient's medical history also should be considered. Bleeding in patients who take blood-thinning medications or in those with a bleeding disorder tends to be more difficult to control and may result in more blood loss because it takes longer for the blood to clot.

7. How might a patient's outcome be affected if bleeding is internal rather than external?

Internal bleeding is hidden and cannot be controlled in the prehospital setting. Many patients with internal bleeding do not have signs or symptoms of shock until a significant amount of blood loss has occurred. Overall, patients with internal bleeding have a higher mortality rate than those with external bleeding. Most of these deaths are the result of intrathoracic or intra-abdominal bleeding in which surgical intervention is delayed. Internal bleeding can also be caused by multiple long bone fractures and pelvic fractures.

8. What are the signs and symptoms of internal bleeding?

Because internal bleeding is not visible, you must rely on your assessment skills and careful evaluation of the MOI. Signs and symptoms of internal bleeding are essentially those of shock: restlessness or anxiety; cool, pale, clammy skin; tachycardia; rapid, shallow breathing; and thirst. A late sign is hypotension. External indicators of internal bleeding in both medical and trauma patients include hematemesis, melena, and hemoptysis. Other indicators of internal bleeding, which are more common in trauma patients, include redness or bruising, swelling, or tenderness over the injured area. Always be alert to the possibility of internal bleeding, particularly if the MOI is significant. Remember that if a trauma patient is in shock but does not have any obvious external signs of injury, suspect internal bleeding!

9. How does the body typically respond to blood loss?

If the typical adult sustains more than approximately 2 pints (approximately 1 L) of blood loss, significant changes in vital signs will occur, including increased heart and respiratory rates (compensatory phase) and, as a later sign, decreased blood pressure (indicating decompensation).

A loss of circulating blood volume is sensed by receptors in the body that send messages to the nervous system. In response, the sympathetic nervous system releases epinephrine and norepinephrine. Norepinephrine constricts the peripheral blood vessels (vasoconstriction), thus shunting blood from areas of lesser need (eg, skin and muscles) to areas of greater need (eg, heart, brain, kidneys, liver). If blood loss continues, however, the body's compensatory mechanisms will eventually fail, the patient's blood pressure will fall, resulting in death.

Prep Kit

Ready for Review

- Perfusion is the circulation of blood in adequate amounts to meet the cells' current needs for oxygen, nutrients, and waste removal.
- The cardiovascular systems contains three main parts: a working pump (heart), a container (blood vessels), and fluid (oxygen-carrying blood).
- Hypoperfusion, or shock, occurs when one or more of these three components is not working properly and the cardiovascular system fails to provide adequate perfusion.
- Always ask patients if they take blood-thinning medications (aspirin, warfarin) because bleeding is generally more profuse and difficult to control in these patients.
- Both internal and external bleeding can cause shock. You must know how to recognize and control both.
- The methods to use to control bleeding, in order, are as follows:
  - Direct pressure
  - Pressure dressing

Prep Kit continued

- Wound packing with hemostatic gauze
- Tourniquet
- Splinting device

- Bleeding around the face always presents a risk for airway obstruction or aspiration. Maintain a clear airway by positioning the patient appropriately and using suction when indicated.
- Epistaxis can be controlled by pinching both nostrils together for 15 and applying ice over the nose.
- Promptly transport any patient you suspect of having internal bleeding or significant external bleeding.
- If the MOI is significant, be alert to signs and symptoms of internal bleeding in the chest or abdomen, such as serious bruising or complaints of difficulty breathing or abdominal pain.
- Signs of serious internal bleeding include the following:
  - Vomiting blood (hematemesis)
  - Black, tarry stools (melena)
  - Coughing up blood (hemoptysis)
  - Distended abdomen
  - Broken ribs
- The signs and symptoms of internal bleeding are often slow to develop; therefore, reassess an unstable patient every 5 minutes and a stable patient every 15 minutes.

Vital Vocabulary

aorta The main artery that receives blood from the left ventricle and delivers it to all the other arteries that carry blood to the tissues of the body.

arterioles The smallest branches of arteries leading to the vast network of capillaries.

artery A blood vessel, consisting of three layers of tissue and smooth muscle, that carries blood away from the heart.

capillaries The small blood vessels that connect arterioles and venules; various substances pass through capillary walls, into and out of the interstitial fluid, and then on to the cells.

coagulation The formation of clots to plug openings in injured blood vessels and stop blood flow.

contusion A bruise from an injury that causes bleeding beneath the skin without breaking the skin; also see *ecchymosis.*

ecchymosis A buildup of blood beneath the skin that produces a characteristic blue or black discoloration as the result of an injury; also see *contusion.*

epistaxis A nosebleed.

hematemesis The vomiting of blood.

hematoma A mass of blood that has collected within damaged tissue beneath the skin or in a body cavity.

hematuria Blood in the urine.

hemophilia A hereditary condition in which the patient lacks one or more of the blood's normal clotting factors.

hemoptysis The coughing up of blood.

hemorrhage Bleeding.

hemostatic dressing A dressing impregnated with a chemical compound that slows or stops bleeding by assisting with clot formation.

hypoperfusion A condition in which the circulatory system fails to provide sufficient circulation to maintain normal cellular functions; also called shock.

hypovolemic shock A condition in which low blood volume, due to massive internal or external bleeding or extensive loss of body water, results in inadequate perfusion.

junctional tourniquet A device that provides proximal compression of severe bleeding near the axial or inguinal junction with the torso.

Prep Kit continued

melena Dark, foul-smelling, tarry stool containing digested blood.

open-book pelvic fracture A life-threatening fracture of the pelvis caused by a force that displaces one or both sides of the pelvis laterally and posteriorly.

pelvic binder A device to splint the bony pelvis to reduce hemorrhage from bone ends, venous disruption, and pain.

perfusion The circulation of blood within an organ or tissue in adequate amounts to meet the current needs of the cells.

shock A condition in which the circulatory system fails to provide sufficient circulation to maintain normal cellular functions; also called hypoperfusion.

tourniquet The bleeding control method used when a wound continues to bleed despite the use of direct pressure; useful if a patient is bleeding severely from a partial or complete amputation.

vasoconstriction The narrowing of a blood vessel, such as with hypoperfusion or cold extremities.

veins The blood vessels that carry blood from the tissues to the heart.

venules Very small, thin-walled blood vessels.

References

1. Robaix M, Mathais Q, de Malleray H, et al. Independent factors of preventable death in a mature trauma center: a propensity-score analysis. *Eur J Trauma Emerg Surg*. 2024;50(2):477–487.
2. American College of Surgeons. Stop the Bleed [homepage] website. https://www.stopthebleed.org/. Accessed February 12, 2025.
3. National Association of Emergency Medical Technicians. *PHTLS: Prehospital Trauma Life Support*. 10th ed. Burlington, MA: Jones & Bartlett Learning; 2023.
4. Trauma systems: national guideline for the field triage of injured patients. American College of Surgeons website. https://www.facs.org/quality-programs/trauma/systems/field-triage-guidelines/. Accessed February 12, 2025.
5. Berry C, Gallagher JM, Goodloe JM, Dorlac WC, Dodd J, Fischer PE. Prehospital hemorrhage control and treatment by clinicians: a joint position statement. *Prehosp Emerg Care*. 2023;27(5):544–551.
6. National Association of State EMS Officials. *National Model EMS Clinical Guidelines: Version 3.0*. https://nasemso.org/content.aspx?page_id=22&club_id=157064&module_id=701974. Updated March 2022. Accessed February 12, 2025.
7. Smith S, White J, Wanis KN, Beckett A, McAlister VC, Hilsden R. The effectiveness of junctional tourniquets: a systematic review and meta-analysis. *J Trauma Acute Care Surg*. 2019;86(3):532–539.
8. Hsu S-D, Chen C-J, Chou Y-C, Wang S-H, Chan D-C. Effect of early pelvic binder use in the emergency management of suspected pelvic trauma: a retrospective cohort study. *Int J Environ Res Public Health*. 2017;14(10):1217.

Additional Resources

Scott I, Porter K, Laird C, Greaves I, Bloch M. The prehospital management of pelvic fractures: initial consensus statement. *Emerg Med J*. 2013;30(12):1070–1072.

Vaidya R, Roth M, Zarling B, et al. Application of circumferential compression device (binder) in pelvic injuries: room for improvement. *West J Emerg Med*. 2016;17(6):766–774.

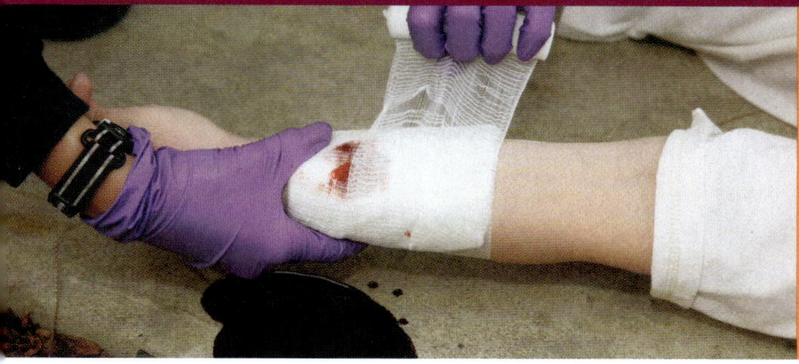

Chapter 26

Soft-Tissue Injuries

NATIONAL EMS EDUCATION STANDARD COMPETENCIES

Trauma

Applies knowledge to provide basic emergency care and transportation based on assessment findings for an acutely injured patient.

Soft-Tissue Trauma

Recognition and management of

- Wounds
  - Avulsion (pp 962–963)
  - Bite (pp 975–976)
  - Laceration (p 962)
  - Puncture (pp 963–965)
  - Incision (p 962)
- Burns
  - Electrical (pp 964–965, 989–991)
  - Chemical (pp 988–989)
  - Thermal (p 987)
  - Radiation (pp 991–992)
  - Inhalation injury (pp 987–988)
- Chemicals in the eye and on the skin (pp 988–989)
- Crush/compartment syndrome (pp 960–961, 965–972)
- High-pressure injection injury (p 965)

KNOWLEDGE OBJECTIVES

1. Describe the anatomy of the skin; include the layers of the skin. (pp 957–958)
2. Explain the major functions of the skin. (p 958)
3. Name the three types of soft-tissue injuries. (p 958)
4. Describe the types of closed soft-tissue injuries. (pp 959–961)
5. Describe the types of open soft-tissue injuries. (pp 961–965)
6. Explain patient assessment of closed and open injuries. (pp 965–972)
7. Explain patient assessment of closed and open injuries in relation to airway management. (pp 966–969)
8. Explain the emergency medical care for closed and open injuries. (pp 972–973)
9. Explain the emergency medical care for an open wound to the abdomen. (pp 973–974)
10. Explain the emergency medical care for an impaled object. (pp 974–975)
11. Explain the emergency medical care for neck injuries. (p 975)
12. Describe the steps of the emergency treatment of small animal bites, human bites, and rabies. (pp 975–976)
13. Explain how the seriousness of a burn is related to its depth and extent. (pp 977–980)
14. Define superficial, partial-thickness, and full-thickness burns; include the characteristics of each burn. (pp 978–979)
15. Explain the primary assessment of a patient with a burn. (pp 981–985)
16. Explain the emergency medical care for burn injuries. (pp 985–986)

17. Describe the emergency management of chemical, electrical, thermal, inhalation, and radiation burns. (pp 987–992)
18. Explain the functions of sterile dressings and bandages. (pp 992–993)

SKILLS OBJECTIVES

1. Demonstrate the emergency medical care of an open chest wound. (pp 965–973)
2. Demonstrate the emergency medical care of closed soft-tissue injuries. (p 972)
3. Demonstrate how to control bleeding from an open soft-tissue injury. (pp 972–973)
4. Demonstrate how to stabilize an impaled object. (p 974; Skill Drill 26-1)
5. Demonstrate how to care for a burn. (p 986; Skill Drill 26-2)
6. Demonstrate the emergency medical care of a chemical, electrical, thermal, inhalation, or radiation burn. (pp 987–992)

Introduction

As an EMT, you will commonly be called to care for victims with soft-tissue injuries. These injuries can vary from a simple cut to a burn to significant bleeding with life-threatening internal injuries. It is important to not allow yourself to become distracted by dramatic wounds and make the mistake of neglecting more life-threatening conditions such as an airway obstruction or inadequate breathing. It is your responsibility as an EMT to assess and treat each of these injuries within the current standard of care guidelines.

The soft tissues of the body can be injured through a variety of mechanisms. A blunt injury occurs when the body is impacted by an object with greater force than the tissue can withstand, but the body's surface is not penetrated. Whereas a blunt injury does not penetrate the skin, a penetrating injury occurs when an object, such as a bullet or knife, breaks through the skin and enters the body. Burns may also result in soft-tissue injuries. Mechanisms of injury are discussed in greater detail in Chapter 24, *Trauma Overview*.

Soft-tissue trauma is a common form of injury. In fact, wound care is one of the most frequently performed procedures in emergency departments (EDs) across the United States. Most of these injuries require basic interventions such as wound irrigation, dressing, bandaging, and limited suturing.

Death resulting from soft-tissue injury is often related to hemorrhage or infection. Uncontrolled hemorrhage can quickly lead to shock and death. When the skin barrier is breached, invading pathogens such as bacteria, fungi, and viruses can cause local or systemic infection. Infection can be life or limb threatening, especially in children, older adults, and people with diabetes or other conditions that may compromise the immune system.

Soft-tissue injuries and their associated complications can often be prevented by using simple protective actions. For example, wearing gloves when working with abrasive materials helps prevent skin injuries. To reduce injuries in the workplace, safety measures have been implemented that include the use of safety devices to prevent interaction between machine parts and body parts. Effective strategies that have reduced injury and death from burns include educating employees about burn prevention, using smoke alarms, controlling the temperature of hot water heaters, and enforcing building codes that regulate electrical and construction practices.

This chapter discusses the various types of soft-tissue injuries and the appropriate assessment and treatment of this classification of injuries.

Anatomy and Physiology of the Skin

The skin is our first line of defense against external forces and infection. It is also the largest organ in the body. Although it is relatively tough, skin is still quite susceptible to injury. Injuries to soft tissues range from simple bruises and abrasions to serious lacerations and amputations. Soft-tissue injury may result in exposure of deep structures such as blood vessels, nerves, and bones. In all instances, you must control bleeding, prevent further contamination to decrease the risk of infection, and protect

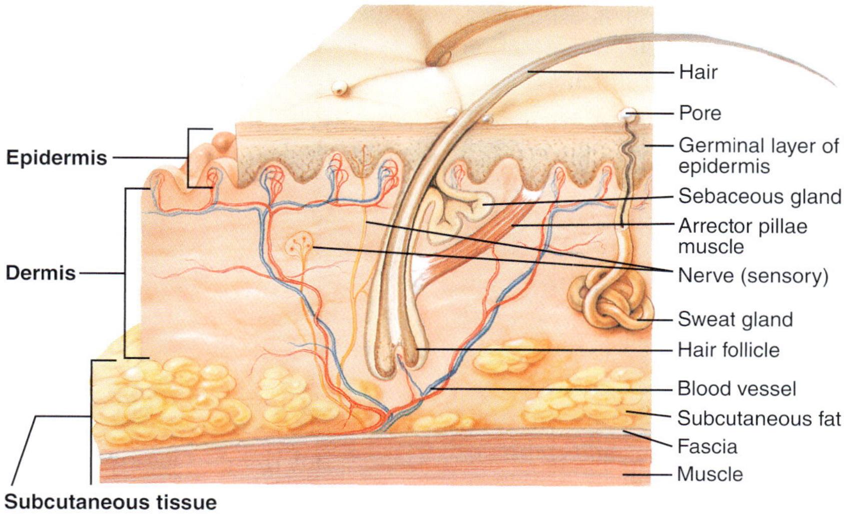

FIGURE 26-1 The skin comprises a tough external layer called the epidermis and a vascular inner layer called the dermis.

the wound from further damage. Therefore, you must know how to apply dressings and bandages to various parts of the body.

Skin varies in thickness, depending on a person's age and the area the skin covers. The skin of the very young and the very old is thinner than the skin of a young adult. The skin covering the scalp, the back, and the soles of the feet is quite thick, whereas the skin of the eyelids, lips, and ears is very thin. Thin skin is more easily damaged than thick skin.

Anatomy

The skin has two principal layers: the epidermis and the dermis (**FIGURE 26-1**). The **epidermis** is the tough, external layer that forms a watertight covering for the body. The epidermis contains several layers. The cells on the surface layer of the epidermis are constantly worn away. They are replaced by cells that are pushed to the surface when new cells form in the germinal layer at the base of the epidermis. Deeper cells in the germinal layer contain pigment granules. Along with blood vessels in the dermis, these granules produce skin color.

The **dermis** is the inner layer of the skin. It lies below the germinal cells of the epidermis. The dermis contains the skin's accessory structures: hair follicles, sweat glands, and sebaceous glands. The sweat glands' primary function is to cool the body. They discharge sweat onto the surface of the skin through small pores, or ducts, that pass through the epidermis. Sebaceous glands produce sebum, the oily material that waterproofs the skin and keeps it supple. Sebum travels to the skin's surface along the shaft of adjacent hair follicles. *Hair follicles* are small organs that produce hair. There is one follicle

YOU are the EMT

You and your partner are standing by at the scene of a house fire when firefighters bring over a 45-year-old man who was rescued from the burning structure. The patient is wrapped in a blanket. He is conscious and alert, he is in severe pain, and his face is covered with soot.

1. What should be your most immediate priority?
2. What is a thermal burn? What are the causes of thermal burns?

for each hair, each connected with a sebaceous gland and a tiny muscle. This muscle pulls the hair erect whenever a person is cold or frightened.

Blood vessels in the dermis provide the skin with nutrients and oxygen. Small branches reach up to the germinal cells, but blood vessels do not penetrate farther into the epidermis. The dermis also contains specialized nerve endings.

The skin covers all external surfaces of the body. The various openings in the body, including the mouth, nose, anus, and vagina, are not covered by skin. Instead, these openings are lined with **mucous membranes**. Similar to skin, these membranes provide a protective barrier against bacterial invasion, but mucous membranes differ from skin in that they secrete a watery substance that lubricates the openings. Therefore, mucous membranes are moist, whereas skin is generally dry.

Special Populations

AGING-RELATED SKIN CHANGES

The production of proteins that make the skin pliable declines with age. The layer of fat under the skin also becomes thinner because of the redistribution of fluids and proteins. As skin loses elasticity, bruising becomes more common because the skin can tear more easily. Exocrine (sweat) glands do not respond as readily to heat because of atrophy and because of changes to the tissues in the dermal layer of the skin. This can result in difficulty regulating body temperature.

Physiology

The skin serves many functions. It protects the body by keeping pathogens out and fluids in, and it helps regulate body temperature. The nerves in the skin report to the brain on the environment and on many sensations. It is this nerve pathway connection that allows the body to adapt to environments through responses in the skin and surrounding tissues.

The skin is the body's major organ for regulating temperature. In a cold environment, the blood vessels in the skin constrict, diverting blood away from the skin and decreasing the amount of heat that radiates from the body's surface. In hot environments, the vessels in the skin dilate. The skin becomes flushed, and heat radiates from the body's surface. In addition, sweat glands secrete sweat to help cool the body. As the sweat evaporates from the skin's surface, the body temperature drops, and the person begins to cool down.

Any break in the skin allows bacteria to enter and increases the possibilities of infection, fluid loss, and loss of temperature control. Any one of these conditions can cause serious illness and even death. Soft tissues are often injured because they are exposed to the environment. There are three types of soft-tissue injuries:

- **Closed injuries**, in which soft-tissue damage occurs beneath the skin or mucous membrane but the surface of the skin or mucous membrane remains intact.
- **Open injuries**, in which there is a break in the surface of the skin or the mucous membrane, exposing deeper tissues to potential contamination.
- **Burns**, in which the soft-tissue damage occurs as a result of thermal heat, frictional heat, toxic chemicals, electricity, or nuclear radiation.

Pathophysiology of Closed and Open Injuries

Wounds heal in a natural process that involves several overlapping stages, all directed toward the larger goal of maintaining homeostasis or balance. Ultimately, the goal is for the body to return to a functional state, although the injured area may not always be restored to its preinjury state.

Among the primary concerns in wound healing is the cessation of bleeding. Loss of blood, internal or external, hinders the provision of vital nutrients and oxygen to the affected area. It also impairs the tissue's ability to eliminate wastes. The result is abnormal or absent function, which interferes with homeostasis. To stop the flow of blood, the vessels, platelets, and clotting cascade must work in unison.

During inflammation (the next stage of wound healing), additional cells move into the damaged area to begin repair. White blood cells migrate to the area to combat pathogens that have invaded exposed tissue. Foreign products and bacteria are also removed from the body. Similarly, lymphocytes (a type of white blood cell) destroy bacteria and other pathogens. Mast cells release histamine as part of the body's response in the early stages of inflammation. Histamine dilates blood vessels, increasing blood flow to the injured area and resulting in a reddened, warm area immediately around the site. Histamine makes capillaries more permeable, and swelling may occur as fluid seeps out of these "leaky" capillaries. Inflammation ultimately leads to the removal of foreign material, damaged cellular parts, and invading microorganisms from the wound site.

In the outer layer of skin, cells are stacked in layers. To replace the area damaged in a soft-tissue injury, a new layer of cells must be moved into this region. This is the next stage of wound healing. Cells quickly multiply and redevelop across the edges of the wound. Except in cases of clean incisions, the appearance of the restructured area seldom returns to the preinjury state. For example, large wounds or injuries that result in significant disruption of the skin will often not complete this process. People with lightly pigmented skin may see a pink line of scar tissue signaling the presence of collagen, a structural protein that has reinforced the damaged tissue. Despite the changed appearance, the function of the area may be restored to near normal. Tissue injuries may be difficult to detect in individuals with dark skin.

During the next stage of wound healing, new blood vessels form as the body attempts to bring oxygen and nutrients to the injured tissue. New capillaries bud from intact capillaries that lie adjacent to the damaged skin. These vessels provide a channel for oxygen and nutrients and serve as a pathway for waste removal. Because they are new and delicate, bleeding might result from a very minor injury. It may take weeks to months for the new capillaries to be as stable as preexisting vessels.

Collagen is a tough, fibrous protein found in scar tissue, hair, bones, and other connective tissues. In the last stage of wound healing, collagen provides stability to the damaged tissue and joins wound borders, thereby closing the open tissue. Unfortunately, collagen cannot restore damaged tissue to its original strength.

Closed Injuries

Closed soft-tissue injuries are characterized by a history of blunt trauma, pain at the site of injury, swelling beneath the skin, and discoloration. Such injuries can vary from mild to quite severe.

Contusions and Hematomas

A **contusion**, or bruise, is an injury that causes bleeding beneath the skin but does not break the skin. Contusions result from blunt forces striking the body. The epidermis remains intact, but cells within the dermis are damaged, and small blood vessels are usually torn, creating discoloration of the affected skin. The depth of the injury varies, depending on the amount of energy absorbed. As fluid and blood leak into the damaged area, the patient may have swelling and pain. The buildup of blood produces a characteristic blue or black discoloration called **ecchymosis** (**FIGURE 26-2**).

A **hematoma** is a larger collection of blood than a contusion within damaged tissue or in a body cavity (**FIGURE 26-3**). A hematoma occurs whenever a blood vessel is damaged and bleeds into the surrounding tissues. When a hematoma occurs on the body's surface, a visible lump can be seen and palpated. It is often associated with extensive tissue damage. A hematoma can result from a soft-tissue injury, a fracture, or any injury to a blood vessel. In severe cases, the hematoma may contain more than 1 liter of blood.

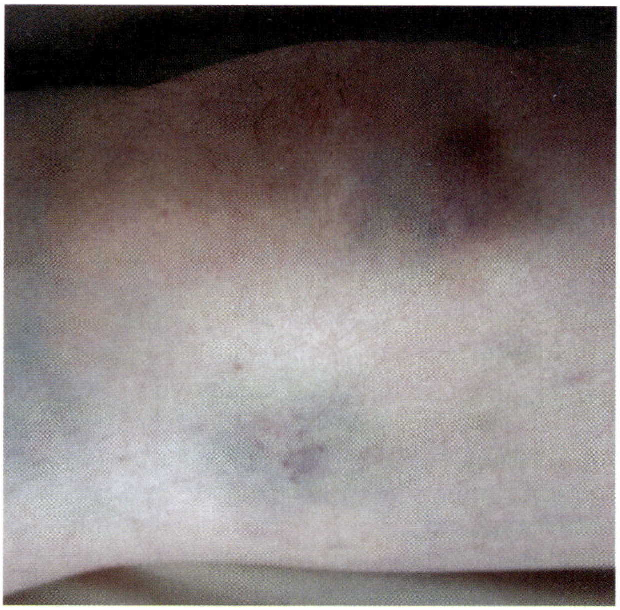

FIGURE 26-2 Contusions, more commonly known as bruises, occur as a result of a blunt force striking the body. The characteristic blue or black discoloration (ecchymosis) signifies bleeding underneath the skin.

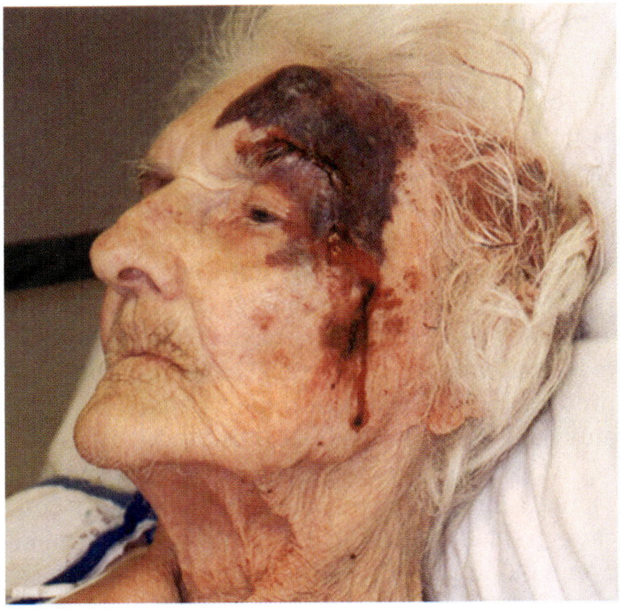

FIGURE 26-3 A hematoma develops whenever a blood vessel is damaged and bleeds into surrounding tissues.

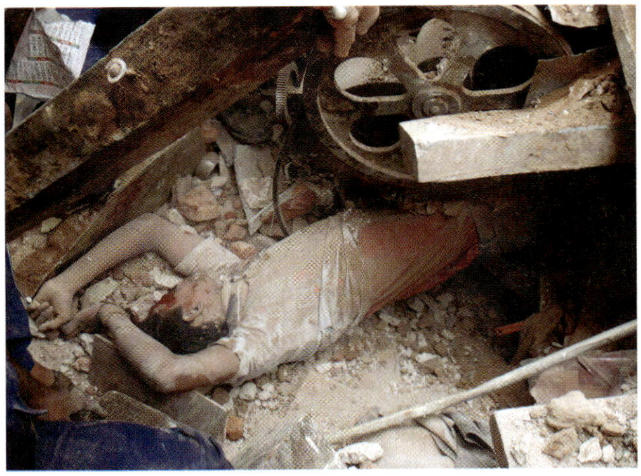

FIGURE 26-4 The damage associated with a crush or compression injury varies depending on the direct damage to the soft tissues and how long the tissue was cut off from circulation.

Crush Syndrome and Compartment Syndrome

A **crush injury** refers to trauma caused by a direct crushing force applied to the body (**FIGURE 26-4**). Crush injuries can be open or closed. The extent of the damage depends on how much force is applied and how long it is applied. In addition to the direct tissue damage, the compression force can prevent perfusion to the affected area and venous outflow from the injured area.

When an area of the body is trapped for an extended time with arterial blood flow compromised, **crush syndrome** can develop. Irreversible damage can begin to occur after just 1 hour. When a patient's tissues are crushed beyond repair, muscle cells die and release harmful substances into the surrounding tissues. The oppressive force prevents blood from returning to the injured body part, so these harmful substances are released into the body's circulation only *after* the limb is freed and blood flow is returned. For this reason, when possible, if a patient has been trapped with a crushing object for a prolonged time, advanced life support (ALS) clinicians should administer intravenous (IV) fluid *before* the crushing object is lifted off the body. Freeing the limb or other body part from entrapment results in the release of the by-products of metabolism and harmful products of tissue destruction, and as a result it can create the potential for cardiac arrest and kidney failure. Consider requesting ALS assistance for situations of prolonged entrapment prior to extrication.

Compartment syndrome develops when edema and swelling result in increased pressure within a closed soft-tissue compartment. Because tissues are limited in the amount they can stretch or expand, pressure increases within the compartment, which interferes with circulation. Compartment syndrome commonly develops in the extremities

Words of Wisdom

Compartment syndrome or crush syndrome may result from a severe thermal or electrical burn or from a traumatic event such as entrapment under a vehicle after a crash or under part of a building after an earthquake; however, it can also happen when a person is unresponsive for a long period and unable to move from one position. This situation may include unconscious patients who have had a stroke or those who have overdosed on drugs and are not discovered for several hours.

and may occur in conjunction with open or closed musculoskeletal injuries or when swelling occurs under restrictive devices such as a cast or tight dressing. Signs and symptoms of compartment syndrome include pain that seems out of proportion to the injury or pain with passive stretching, tense tissue, swelling, tightness, and, later, muscle weakness, absent pulses (late), and numbness.[1] Compartment syndrome is discussed further in Chapter 31, *Orthopaedic Injuries*.

Pressure Ulcers

Pressure ulcers, sometimes referred to as bedsores or decubitus ulcers, form when a patient is lying or sitting in the same position for a long time. The pressure from the weight of the body cuts off the blood flow to the area of skin. With no blood flow to the skin, a sore develops (**FIGURE 26-5**). These sores can develop in as little as 45 minutes. To help prevent these ulcers, take special care to pad under any bony prominences and in the voids under a patient.

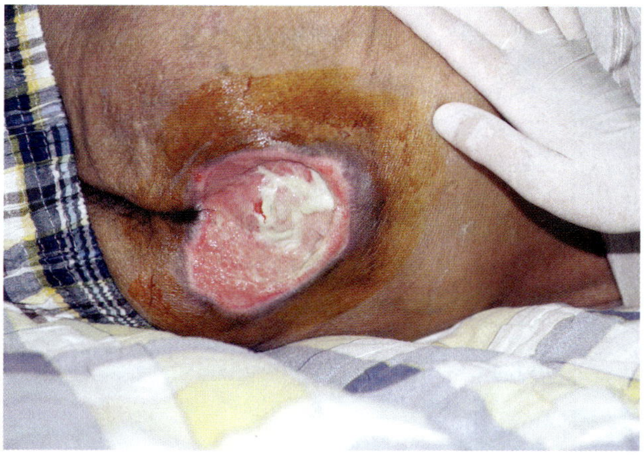

FIGURE 26-5 Pressure ulcer (stage III).

Placing a geriatric patient on a backboard can cause significant injury to the patient's skin.

You may see these ulcers in the following various stages of development (**FIGURE 26-6**):

- Stage I: Nonblanching redness/darkening with damage under the skin
- Stage II: Blister or ulcer that can affect the dermis and epidermis
- Stage III: Invasion of the fat layer through to the fascia
- Stage IV: Invasion to muscle or bone

Decubitus ulcers can be painful and cause complications such as bleeding, sepsis, and bone infection, called osteomyelitis.

Open Injuries

Open injuries differ from closed injuries in that the protective layer of skin is damaged. This can produce extensive bleeding. A break in the protective skin layer or mucous membrane also means that the wound is contaminated and may become infected. **Contamination** is the presence of infectious organisms (pathogens) or foreign bodies, such as dirt, gravel, or metal, in the wound. You must address excessive bleeding and contamination in your treatment of open soft-tissue wounds. The following are the five types of open soft-tissue wounds that you must be prepared to manage:

- Abrasions
- Lacerations
- Avulsions and amputations
- Penetrating wounds
- Open crush injuries

Abrasions

An **abrasion** is a wound of the superficial layer of the skin, caused by friction when a body part rubs

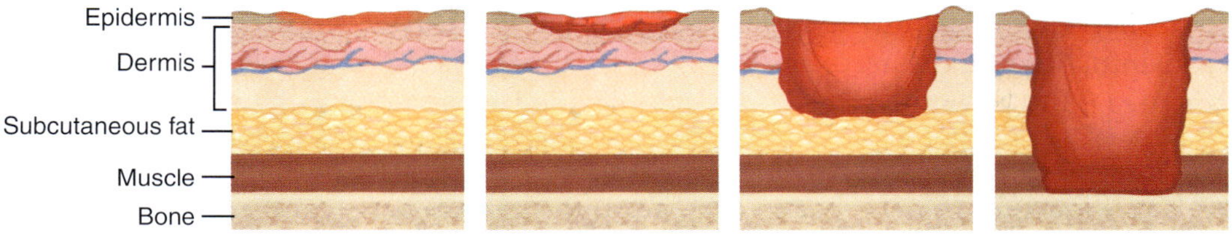

FIGURE 26-6 Pressure ulcers are described by the degree of tissue damage that has occurred.

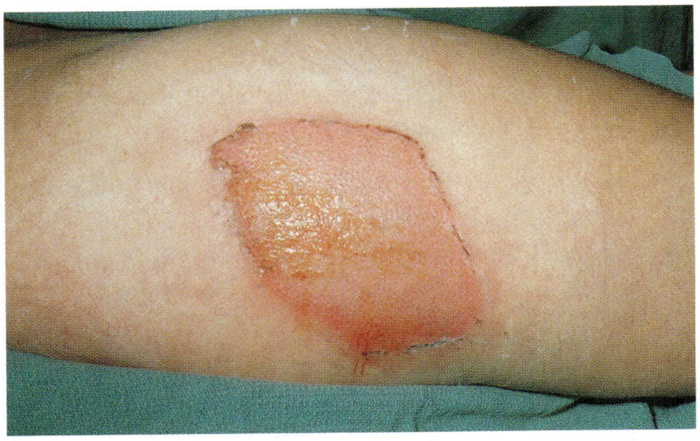

A

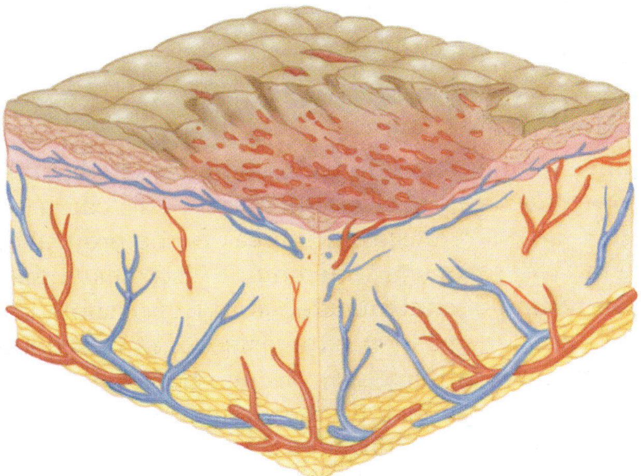

B

FIGURE 26-7 Abrasions usually do not penetrate completely through the dermis (**A**), but blood may ooze from the capillaries (**B**). These wounds are typically superficial and result from rubbing or scraping across a hard, rough surface.

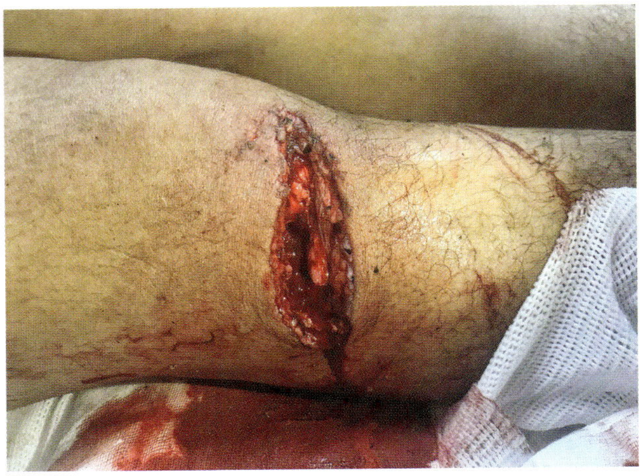

A

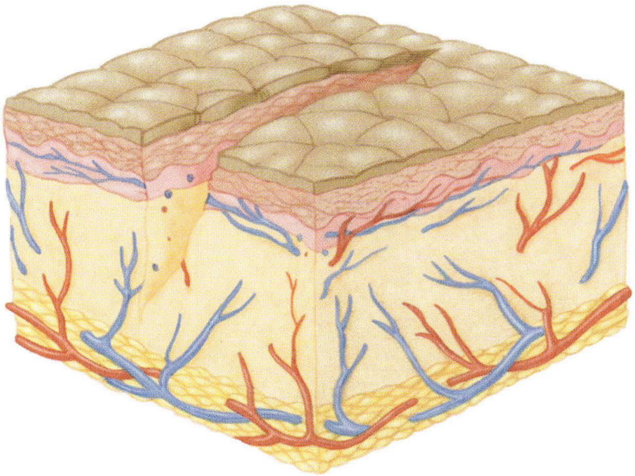

B

FIGURE 26-8 Lacerations vary in depth (**A**) and can extend through the skin and subcutaneous tissue to the underlying muscles, nerves, and blood vessels (**B**). These wounds can be smooth or jagged, depending on the object that caused the injury.

or scrapes across a rough or hard surface. An abrasion usually does not penetrate completely through the dermis, but blood may ooze from the injured capillaries in the dermis. Also known as road rash, road burn, strawberry, and rug burn, abrasions can be extremely painful because the nerve endings are located in this area (**FIGURE 26-7**).

Lacerations

A **laceration** is a jagged cut in the skin caused by a sharp object or a blunt force that tears the tissue, whereas an **incision** is a sharp, smooth cut. The depth of the injury can vary, extending through the skin and subcutaneous tissue, even into the underlying muscles and adjacent nerves and blood vessels (**FIGURE 26-8**). Lacerations and incisions may appear linear (regular) or stellate (irregular) and may occur along with other types of soft-tissue injury. Lacerations or incisions that involve arteries or large veins may result in severe bleeding.

Avulsions and Amputations

An **avulsion** is an injury that separates various layers of soft tissue (usually between the subcutaneous

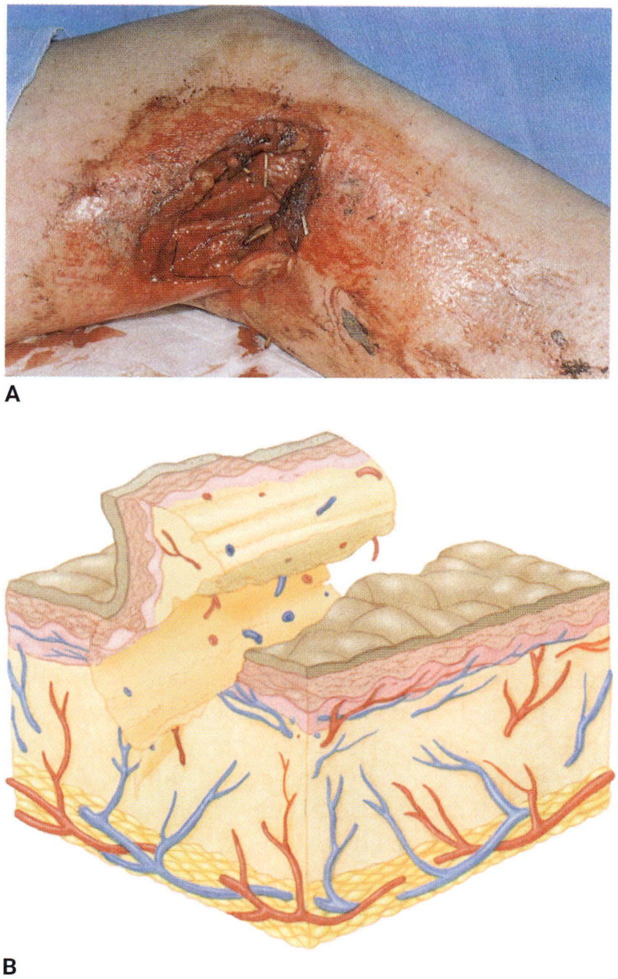

FIGURE 26-9 Avulsions are injuries characterized by complete separation of tissue (**A**) or tissue hanging as a flap (**B**). Significant bleeding is common.

layer and **fascia**) so they become either completely detached or hang as a flap (**FIGURE 26-9**). Often there is significant bleeding. If the avulsed tissue is hanging from a small piece of skin, the circulation through the flap may be at risk. If you can, replace the flat avulsed flap in its original position as long as it is not visibly contaminated with dirt and/or other foreign materials. If an avulsion is complete, you should wrap the separated tissue in dry, sterile gauze, caring for it as for amputated tissue (discussed next), and take it with you to the ED. This type of avulsion often has serious risk for infection. Never remove an avulsion skin flap, regardless of its size.

An **amputation** is an injury in which part of the body is completely severed. We usually think of amputations as involving the upper and lower extremities. But other body parts, such as the scalp, ear, nose, penis, or lips, may also be totally avulsed or amputated. You can easily control the bleeding from some amputations, such as a finger, with direct pressure and pressure dressings. If an amputation involves a large area of muscle mass, such as a thigh, there may be massive bleeding. In this situation, you should stop the bleeding, which often requires a tourniquet, and treat the patient for hypovolemic shock. Severe bleeding can also occur in truncal areas that do not allow for application of a traditional tourniquet. These wounds may require wound packing or application of a junctional tourniquet. Once bleeding is controlled, attempt to retrieve the amputated tissue.[1] You will need to keep it cool and dry during transport to the hospital. To do so, place the amputated tissue in a plastic bag, then place that bag in a cooled container. Do not allow the tissue to freeze by coming in direct contact with ice. See Chapter 31, *Orthopaedic Injuries*, for further discussion of amputation; see Chapter 25, *Bleeding*, for further discussion of tourniquets and bleeding control.

Penetrating Wounds

A **penetrating wound** (or puncture wound) is an injury resulting from a piercing object, such as a knife, ice pick, splinter, or bullet. Such objects leave relatively small entrance wounds, so there may be little external bleeding (**FIGURE 26-10**). However, these objects can damage structures deep within the body and cause unseen bleeding. If the wound is to the chest or abdomen, the injury can cause rapid, fatal bleeding. Assessing the amount of damage caused by a puncture wound is difficult and is reserved for the physician at the hospital.

Objects that penetrate the skin but remain in place are referred to as **impaled objects**. The concerns with this type of injury include the amount of damage to structures deep inside the body and the presence of foreign materials deep inside the tissue. The damage to underlying structures is difficult to determine and manage, and the presence of foreign materials inside the tissue results in a significantly higher risk of infection. An impaled object also requires specific treatments and care, described later in this chapter.

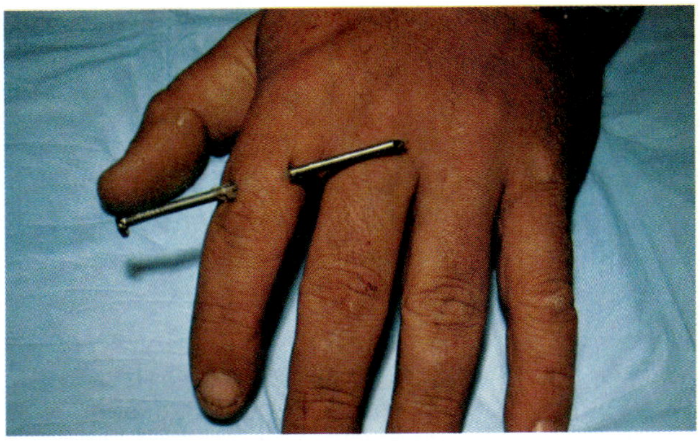

A

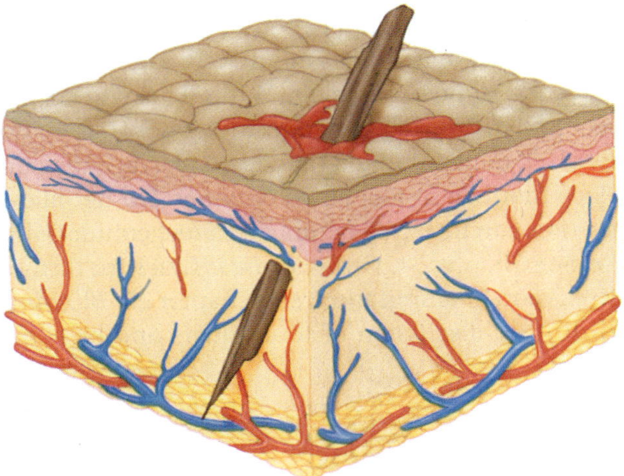

B

FIGURE 26-10 Penetrating wounds and impaled objects (**A**) may cause very little external bleeding but can damage structures deep within the body (**B**).

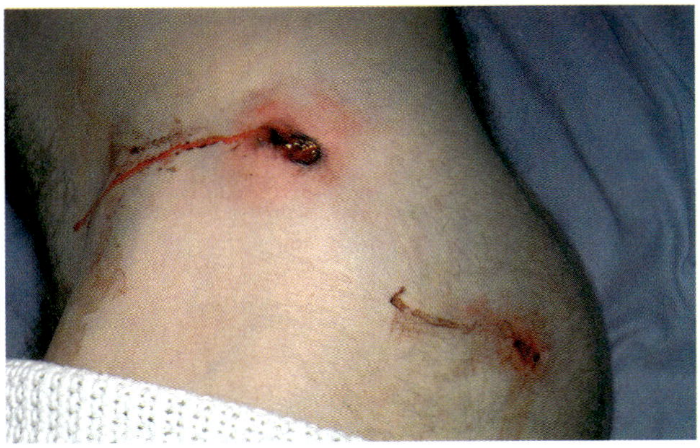

FIGURE 26-11 An entrance and exit wound from a gunshot. An entrance wound may have burns around the edges. An exit wound can be larger than an entrance wound and is associated with greater damage to soft tissues locally.

Stabbings and Shootings

Stabbings and shootings often result in multiple penetrating injuries. You must assess these patients carefully to identify all wounds. Because a penetrating object can pass completely through the body, always count the number of penetrating injuries (or holes), especially with gunshot wounds. Knowing the difference between entrance wounds and exit wounds may be difficult in a prehospital setting, especially when considering different types of ammunition. Although entrance wounds are often smaller than exit wounds (**FIGURE 26-11**), it is better to simply count the number of penetrating injuries, and leave the distinction between entrance and exit to the physician who is working in a more controlled environment. Gunshot wounds have unique characteristics that require special care. The amount of energy transmitted by a gunshot injury is directly related to the speed of the bullet. When possible, determine the type of gun used in the shooting, but do not let this delay patient transport. Sometimes, the patient or bystanders can tell you how many rounds were fired, but given the stress of the environment, their information may be unreliable; however, it may help hospital personnel to better care for the patient. Shotgun wounds create multiple paths of missiles (shot) and create a larger surface area and volume of tissue damage.

Many cases involving shootings go to court at some point, and you may be called to testify. Therefore, you must carefully document the circumstances surrounding any gunshot injury, the patient's condition, and the treatment you provide.

Conducted Electrical Weapon Injuries

In recent years, law enforcement has increased its use of conducted electrical weapons (CEWs), such as the TASER. These weapons fire two small darts (electrodes) that puncture the patient's skin. CEW injuries are generally treated as impaled objects and the electrodes are removed by a physician; however, in some jurisdictions, EMTs are permitted to remove these barbs from patients, depending on local protocol. The barbs are approximately 0.5 inch (13 mm) in length, and although they produce wounds, they are small and easily managed unless they penetrate the eye.

When a CEW is used, the patient can experience potential complications, particularly when the individual is already experiencing certain underlying disorders. Considerable attention has focused on a condition known as delirium with agitation (also called *hyperactive delirium with severe agitation* and formerly referred to as *excited delirium*), which is often characterized by extreme agitation, reduced pain sensitivity, hallucinations, persistent struggling, and elevated temperature. This condition is commonly associated with illegal drug ingestion. It is a true emergency and warrants assisted ALS response.

Previously, using a CEW in patients experiencing delirium with agitation had been associated with dysrhythmias and sudden cardiac arrest. Other studies have found that the risk of sudden death is related to the medical condition, rather than CEW use. Regardless, be aware of this possibility, and be certain you have access to an automated external defibrillator (AED) when you respond to calls for patients who have been exposed to CEW use.

High-Pressure Injection Injuries

High-pressure injection injuries are a type of puncture wound caused by injection of a substance under high pressure through the skin and deep into the underlying tissues. Equipment used for painting, lubricating, greasing, and cleaning are associated with this mechanism of injury (MOI), and the hand is the typical site of injury.[2] High-pressure injection causes direct injury to the tissue that the injected substance passes through followed by inflammation and chemical damage from the substances, some of which are highly toxic, and finally infection from bacteria introduced during the injury.

The exterior wound from a high-pressure injection injury often appears minor, with mild swelling and pain; however, the damage to the underlying tissues can be severe. Patients who have sustained these injuries should be transported even when the wound appears minor. If not treated immediately by specialized surgeons, high-pressure injection injuries may result in amputation.

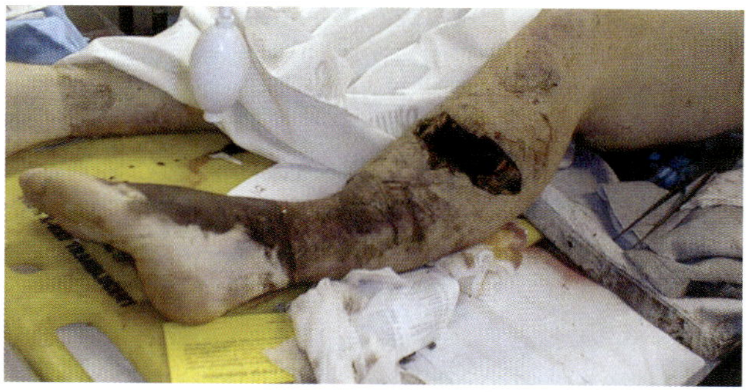

FIGURE 26-12 An open crush wound is characterized by extensive tissue damage and deformity that is often accompanied by swelling and extreme pain.

Courtesy of Andrew N. Pollak, MD, FAAOS.

Blast Injuries

Blast injuries may also result in multiple penetrating injuries. The MOI from a blast may be the blast wave itself, objects propelled by the blast wave, or other secondary impacts or conditions caused by the blast. Blast injuries are discussed further in Chapter 24, *Trauma Overview*.

Open Crush Injuries

As with closed wounds caused by crushing forces, open crush wounds may involve damaged internal organs or broken bones, as well as extensive soft-tissue damage (**FIGURE 26-12**). Whereas external bleeding may be minimal, internal bleeding may be severe, or even life threatening. The crushing force damages soft tissues as well as vessels and nerves. This frequently results in a painful, swollen, deformed area.

Patient Assessment of Closed and Open Injuries

Assessing closed injuries is often more difficult than assessing open injuries. Therefore, any time you observe bruising, swelling, or deformity, or the patient reports pain, the possibility of a closed injury should be considered.

Assessing an open injury in some ways is easier than assessing a closed injury because you can see the injury. Open wounds are defined as injuries in which there is a break in the surface of the skin or the mucous membrane, exposing deeper tissues to potential contamination. You must use caution to avoid letting a patient's non–life-threatening gruesome injury distract you from recognizing another, more serious injury.

Words of Wisdom

Extremities that are painful, swollen, or deformed should be splinted whenever time allows. When you splint these types of injuries, remember to assess the patient's pulses and motor and sensory functions before and after applying the splint. You should also evaluate the MOI. Because diffuse or generalized soft-tissue injuries can be life threatening, all patients with a significant MOI should be considered to have internal bleeding and shock until proven otherwise by the ED staff.

Scene Size-Up

As you arrive on scene, observe the scene for hazards and threats to the safety of the crew, bystanders, and the patient. Assess the effect of hazards on patient care and address the hazards. As always, ensure the scene is safe, and consider the need for additional resources.

Ensure that you and your crew have taken the necessary standard precautions before you approach the scene: a minimum of gloves and eye protection. Eye exposures may occur from splashes and droplets at a busy scene. Eye and mask protection are required when managing open injuries to avoid potential splashing. Place several pairs of gloves in your pocket for easy access in case your gloves tear or there are multiple patients with bleeding.

Open soft-tissue injuries can be very messy but should not take priority over more serious life-threatening injuries. Controlling bleeding and bloody contaminants can be difficult because of the nature of the wounds. Be careful where you put your hands or place your equipment and how you prepare the patient for transport. Because of the color of blood and how well it soaks through clothing, you can often identify patients with an open injury as you approach the scene. However, blood can be hidden under thick, dark clothing, such as denim and leather, or in the environment, such as sand, grass, or carpeting. Do not spend time trying to estimate blood loss; focus on controlling the bleeding.

As you observe the scene, look for indicators of the MOI. This helps you develop an early index of suspicion for underlying injuries in a patient who has sustained a significant MOI. Remember, the MOI alone does not necessarily describe the true extent of injuries, but it helps you understand the potential for injury. When you put together information from dispatch and your observations of the scene, consider how the MOI produced the injuries expected. Remember, medical emergencies may result in trauma, so there may be conditions to consider beyond the traumatic injuries. Your interactions with the patient and your assessment will ultimately provide you with additional information about the extent of the actual injuries. For example, in a vehicle crash, a patient who has sustained abrasions and lacerations to the face from an impact with the steering wheel or windshield may have experienced enough force to injure the cervical spine as well. In this case, spinal motion restriction should be maintained throughout your care of the patient. The MOI may also provide information about potential safety threats. For example, gunshot wounds may indicate the presence of an angry and violent offender in the area or a dangerous scene. Make sure you use all available information to evaluate scene safety and consider whether additional resources may be necessary.

Primary Assessment

The primary assessment of a patient with a closed or open injury should focus on identifying and managing life-threatening concerns and identifying transport priority.

Your general impression will help you develop an index of suspicion for serious injuries and determine how urgently your patient needs care. As you approach the patient, important indicators will alert you to the seriousness of the patient's condition, including the following:

- Is the patient awake and interacting with their surroundings, or lying still and not making sounds?
- Is the patient appropriately or inappropriately responding to you?
- Is the patient's breathing pattern rapid or slow, deep or shallow?

- What is the color and condition of the patient's skin? Pallor indicates a decrease in blood flow. In a person with light skin tone, it presents as a lighter or "white" coloration. In people with dark skin, pallor can be difficult to detect. It may be observed by examining mucous membranes inside the inner lower eyelid and capillary refill. On general observation, the patient may appear ashen or gray.
- Does the patient have any bleeding or other apparent life threats?

The answers to these questions contribute to your general impression and help to determine your treatment priorities and the urgency of care needed. A good question to ask yourself is, "How sick is my patient based on what I know right now?"

Closed soft-tissue injuries may appear to be minor but may indicate serious internal injuries. For example, a patient with a hematoma on the head and a decreased level of consciousness may have a serious brain injury. Open injuries may be obvious and significant, likely indicating a serious condition. Other injuries may not be as obvious but may still indicate a serious condition.

Check for responsiveness. If the patient is alert, ask about the chief complaint to help direct you to any apparent life threats. If the patient is not alert, determine if they respond to verbal or painful stimuli or if they are unresponsive. An unresponsive patient may indicate a life-threatening condition. Administer high-flow oxygen via a nonrebreathing mask to patients with a possible head injury whose level of consciousness is less than alert and oriented, treat for potential shock, and provide immediate transport to the ED.

Words of Wisdom

It is easy to become distracted when a patient has significant soft-tissue injuries, there is a large amount of blood, or the patient is frightened or screaming. Remain focused on the problems at hand and manage life-threatening injuries.

If significant trauma has likely affected multiple body systems, start with a rapid exam of the patient to be sure you have found all of the problems and injuries. A rapid 60- to 90-second exam may identify factors that assist you in determining whether a patient requires rapid transport. Begin with the head and neck while manually holding the head in place. When you are done, apply a cervical collar if it is indicated.

When performing the rapid exam, look for life threats and treat them as you find them. Significant bleeding is an immediate life threat and must be controlled quickly using appropriate

YOU are the EMT

The patient is ambulatory, so you immediately move him to the ambulance that is parked a short distance away and complete your primary assessment. Your partner obtains additional information from the firefighters who rescued him.

Recording Time: 2 Minutes	
Appearance	Shivering; in obvious pain
Level of consciousness	Conscious and alert
Airway	Open; clear of secretions or foreign bodies; no signs of swelling or redness
Breathing	14 breaths/min; adequate depth; unlabored
Circulation	Increased pulse rate; strong at the radial site; no obvious bleeding

You apply high-flow oxygen via a nonrebreathing mask and then carefully remove clothing that is not adhered to his skin so you can assess the severity of his burns.

3. What additional information should you obtain from the firefighters who rescued the patient?
4. How are thermal burns classified? What are the characteristics of each type of burn?

methods. A patient with massive hemorrhage may require a tourniquet *before* the airway is opened. Use the XABC assessment sequence if the patient has obvious life-threatening external (eXsanguinating) bleeding; that is, control the bleeding first, then attend to the ABCs (Airway, Breathing, and Circulation).

Words of Wisdom

As you consider the MOI and form suspicions about where bleeding is occurring, expose that part of the body. Blood flowing freely from veins in a large wound can be as much of a threat as blood spurting from an artery.

Ensure the patient has a clear and patent airway. If the airway is not patent, take the necessary steps to make it clear and patent. Protect the patient from further spinal injury as you manage the airway by preventing the head and torso from moving. If the patient is unresponsive or has a significantly altered level of consciousness, consider inserting an oropharyngeal airway or nasopharyngeal airway, and suction the airway as needed.

Providing high-flow oxygen to achieve an oxygen saturation level of 94% to 98% may help reduce the effects of shock and assist in oxygenation of damaged tissues.[1] Provide assisted ventilations using a bag-mask device as needed, depending on the patient's level of consciousness and ability to breathe adequately.

If the patient has signs of hypoperfusion, treat them aggressively for shock: Place the patient supine, prevent heat loss with a blanket, and provide rapid transport to the hospital. Request ALS as necessary to assist with more aggressive shock and airway management as needed.

Inspect and palpate the chest wall for DCAP-BTLS (Deformities, Contusions, Abrasions, Punctures/penetrations, Burns, Tenderness, Lacerations, Swelling). If a soft-tissue injury is discovered on the chest or abdomen, auscultate for clear and symmetric breath sounds, and look at the structure of the chest wall to ensure equal expansion and rise and fall of the chest.

Open soft-tissue injuries of the face and neck have the potential to interfere with the effectiveness of the airway and breathing. Evaluate the patient's voice and ability to speak to identify throat injuries. If an open injury is found on the chest, evaluate for air movement through the wound in the form of bubbling or sucking sounds, which indicate a deep, penetrating injury. Quickly place an occlusive dressing over the wound. Assess the patient's back for injuries that might need treatment. Monitor the patient for signs of increasing respiratory distress that may require you to relieve pressure that has built up under the dressing (caused by a pneumothorax).

Quickly assess the patient's pulse rate, rhythm, and quality; determine the skin condition, color, and temperature; and check the capillary refill time. These assessments will help you determine the presence of circulatory problems or shock. Closed soft-tissue injuries may not always have visible signs of bleeding because most of the bleeding is occurring inside the body. Your assessment of the pulse and skin will indicate how aggressively you need to treat your patient for shock. Severe closed injuries can also damage internal organs. The greater the amount of energy absorbed from the blunt force, the greater the risk of injury to deeper structures. Therefore, you must assess all patients with closed injuries for more serious hidden injuries. Remain alert for signs of shock or internal bleeding, and begin treatment of these conditions if necessary.

Determine whether your patient needs immediate transport or stabilization on scene. If the patient you are treating has an airway or breathing problem or signs and symptoms of shock or internal bleeding, you must consider rapid transport to the hospital for treatment or request ALS support. Also, if you identify conditions that have the potential to become unstable, such as a distended abdomen or femur fractures, the patient requires rapid and immediate transport.

You should also consider whether transport to the closest hospital is appropriate or whether the patient would be better served by transport to a trauma center that might be farther away. In some situations, it may be appropriate to request aeromedical transport to expedite transfer to a trauma or specialty center. Each consideration requires that you clearly and completely understand your local resources and protocols.

Most patients do not require immediate, rapid transportation, but there are certain conditions for which treatment is limited in the field, and, therefore, immediate transport is the better choice. The following list will help guide you in determining the types of patients who require immediate transport:

- Poor initial general impression
- Altered level of consciousness
- Dyspnea
- Abnormal vital signs
- Shock
- Severe pain

Do not delay transport of a seriously injured trauma patient to complete non-lifesaving treatments in the field, such as splinting extremity fractures or treating minor bleeding such as abrasions; instead, complete these types of treatments en route to the hospital during the secondary assessment.

Patients who have visible significant bleeding or signs of significant internal bleeding may quickly become unstable. Stay alert for signs of hypoperfusion (tachycardia; tachypnea; weak pulse; cool, moist skin), and reassess your priority and transport decision if these signs develop.

History Taking

After you manage life threats during the primary assessment, investigate the chief complaint or history of present illness. Obtain a medical history and be alert for injury-specific signs and symptoms as well as any pertinent negatives such as no pain or loss of sensation.

Make every attempt to obtain a SAMPLE (Signs and symptoms, Allergies, Medications, Pertinent past medical history, Last oral intake, Events leading up to the illness or injury) history from your patient. Using OPQRST (Onset, Provocation/palliation, Quality, Region/radiation, Severity, Timing) may provide some background on isolated extremity injuries. When you use SAMPLE, OPQRST, and DCAP-BTLS together, your assessment will be well rounded and provide significant insight into the patient's condition. You have the opportunity to interview the patient well before the ED physician's examination. Any information you receive will be valuable if the patient loses consciousness. If the patient is not responsive, attempt to obtain the

YOU are the EMT

The patient tells you he sustained the burns when he was trying to escape from the burning house. Both of the exits were blocked by fire and debris, so he ran into the bedroom. However, he was unable to exit through the window because of burglar bars he had installed; this was when the firefighters found him. He denies losing consciousness. Your partner assesses his vital signs as you perform a secondary assessment.

Recording Time: 6 Minutes	
Respirations	14 breaths/min; adequate depth; unlabored
Pulse	108 beats/min; strong and regular
Skin	Red, warm, and dry; burns to the torso and arms
Blood pressure	166/86 mm Hg
Oxygen saturation (Spo_2)	98% (on oxygen)

Your secondary assessment reveals partial-thickness burns to his anterior chest and abdomen, and partial- and full-thickness burns to both of his arms, including his hands. His face is covered with soot, and his facial hair and the hair just above his hairline are singed. You do not see any obvious skin burns to his facial area, and the remainder of your assessment does not reveal any other injuries. The patient denies having difficulty breathing or any other symptoms other than pain.

5. What percentage of the patient's body surface area has been burned?

6. What factors should you consider to determine the severity of a burn?

history from other sources, such as friends, family members, or even bystanders who might have witnessed the event.

Typical signs of an open injury include bleeding, a break in the skin, shock, hemorrhage, and disfigurement or loss of a body part. Typically, symptoms include pain and/or burning at the injury site. Chronic medical conditions such as anemia (low quantity of hemoglobin in the blood) and hemophilia (a disorder in which blood has a diminished ability to clot), as well as a host of other medical conditions, can complicate open soft-tissue injuries. Medications such as aspirin or others that impair the blood's ability to clot and are frequently taken by older adults may make it more difficult to control bleeding.

Secondary Assessment

After you evaluate the ABCs and identify and treat immediate life threats, a more detailed assessment should follow. The secondary assessment is a more systematic full-body scan or focused examination of the patient that is used to reveal injuries or medical conditions that may have been missed during the primary assessment. In some instances, such as with a critically injured patient or a short transport time, you may not have time to conduct a full secondary assessment. Typically, the secondary assessment, which includes assessing interventions and repeating vital signs, occurs en route to the ED. In other instances, your assessment will focus on the areas of the body affected by the injury. For example, if a patient has avulsed a fingertip while chopping onions, the exam will focus only on that extremity.

Listen to breath sounds with a stethoscope. Breath sounds should be clear and equal bilaterally, anteriorly, and posteriorly. Determine the patient's respiratory rate and note the pattern and quality of the respiratory effort. Assess for asymmetric chest wall movement.

Assess the neurologic system to gather baseline data on your patient. This examination should include the level of consciousness, pupil size and reactivity, and motor and sensory response.

Assess the musculoskeletal system by performing a detailed exam of the entire body. Look for DCAP-BTLS. Assess the chest, abdomen, and extremities for hidden bleeding and injuries. Log roll the patient and assess the posterior torso for injuries. Once the back has been assessed, the patient can be log rolled back down onto a backboard, followed by spinal motion restriction if indicated. Log rolling and maintaining spinal motion restriction should take into consideration injuries found during the primary assessment as well as local protocols.

Assess all anatomic regions, looking for the following signs/symptoms:

- Check the neck for jugular venous distention and tracheal deviation. Be alert for patients with a stoma or tracheostomy.
- Check the pelvis for stability.
- Check the abdomen; feel all four quadrants for tenderness or rigidity and inspect for bruising. If the abdomen is tender, expect internal bleeding.
- Check the extremities and record the pulse and motor and sensory function.

Patients who have hidden internal injuries under a closed soft-tissue injury may have internal bleeding and may rapidly become unstable. It is important to reassess the vital signs to identify how quickly the patient's condition is changing; a single vital sign will not always provide the necessary information to evaluate the patient's condition. Make sure you obtain a series of vital signs to ensure subtle changes are evident as soon as possible. Signs such as tachycardia, tachypnea, low blood pressure, weak pulse, and cool, moist, and pale skin indicate hypoperfusion and imply the need for rapid transport and treatment at the hospital. Remember that soft-tissue injuries can cause shock, even without a significant MOI. The reassessment of your patient's vital signs will give you a good understanding of how well or how poorly your patient is tolerating the injury and whether your interventions have been effective.

Reassessment

Reassessment of a patient is just as important as your original assessment and should be regularly conducted during transport to ensure your patient's condition is not declining. Repeat the primary assessment completely, but pay extra attention to areas of concern that you identified during your initial assessment and assess the effectiveness of prior treatments. Reassess vital signs and the chief complaint. Are the airway, breathing, and circulation still adequate? Recheck patient interventions.

Are the treatments you provided for problems with the ABCs still effective?

Reassessing a patient with an open soft-tissue injury is extremely important, especially if you did not put the bandage on the patient's injury. Frequently, other emergency care personnel may have dressed and bandaged the wound before your arrival. You may need to place additional dressings over the original dressing or bandages if blood soaks through the original dressing. If so, frequently reassess the effectiveness of the bandaging. If blood continues to soak through bandages, use additional methods to control bleeding as discussed later in the chapter. How is the patient's condition improving with the interventions? Identify and treat changes in the patient's condition.

Although most open soft-tissue injuries are not serious, they tend to be graphic and can be distracting. If not appropriately treated, they can lead to substantial blood loss and even shock. By appropriately treating open soft-tissue injuries, you can decrease the risk of common complications such as bleeding, shock, pain, and infection. Expose all wounds, control bleeding, and be prepared to treat the patient for shock. Consider flushing small wound surfaces *without* significant bleeding with sterile saline prior to applying a dressing. If any material is stuck in the wound, do not remove it because this may worsen bleeding and shock.

Closed soft-tissue injuries can be life threatening if not appropriately treated. Assess and manage all threats to the patient's airway, breathing, and circulation. Supplemental oxygen via a nonrebreathing mask is commonly given to all patients with traumatic injuries affecting airway or ventilation or those who have signs of shock.

Words of Wisdom

Estimating blood loss is very difficult, and even the most skilled clinicians are often not able to accurately estimate blood loss, especially when blood has been absorbed into fabrics or porous surfaces. Note that blood has soaked through a towel, an article of clothing, or the number of bandages used to control the patient's bleeding, as these are valuable descriptors for the ED staff.

Your communication and documentation must include a description of the MOI and the position in which you found the patient when you arrived on scene. This will provide key information to the hospital staff that may affect the patient care plan provided at the hospital. You should attempt to report blood loss using terms that you are comfortable with and that will be easily understood by other personnel. For example, you may say "the

YOU are the EMT

After caring for the patient's burns, you cover him with a blanket and begin transport to the hospital. You contact medical direction as soon as you leave the scene, and you are advised to provide transport to the ED because the closest burn center is 75 miles away. You reassess the patient, including his vital signs.

Recording Time: 12 Minutes	
Level of consciousness	Conscious and alert, but anxious
Respirations	22 breaths/min; becoming labored; voice is becoming hoarse
Pulse	120 beats/min; strong and regular
Skin	Red, warm, and dry
Blood pressure	158/84 mm Hg
Oxygen saturation (Spo_2)	99% (on oxygen)

7. What is the proper treatment for the patient's burns?

8. How has the patient's condition changed? What should you do now?

bleeding soaked through the patient's jeans prior to our arrival" or "the bleeding soaked through three trauma dressings during our time with the patient." Include the location and description of any soft-tissue injuries or other wounds you have located and treated. Describe the size and depth of the injury. Provide an accurate account of how you treated these injuries. Your ability to clearly and accurately communicate and document enables the physicians and nurses at the hospital to continue to deliver quality care.

Emergency Medical Care for Closed Injuries

Small contusions generally do not require special emergency medical care, but you should note their presence when trying to determine the true extent of the patient's injuries. More extensive closed injuries may involve significant swelling and bleeding beneath the skin, which could lead to hypovolemic shock. Depending on the time the injury occurred and the response time, the injuries might not have had time to cause swelling or bruising. Closely watch any area of injury throughout the time you are caring for the patient, no matter how minor it may look on initial assessment.

Treat a closed soft-tissue injury by applying the mnemonic RICES:

- **Rest.** Keep the patient as quiet and comfortable as possible.
- **Ice.** Use ice or cold packs to slow bleeding by causing blood vessels to constrict and to reduce pain.
- **Compression.** Apply pressure over the injury site to slow bleeding by compressing the blood vessels.
- **Elevation.** Raise the injured part just above the level of the patient's heart to decrease swelling.
- **Splinting.** Immobilize a soft-tissue injury or an injured extremity to decrease bleeding and reduce pain.

Extremities that are painful, swollen, or deformed should be splinted. Take great care when splinting these types of injuries. If done correctly, splinting can assist with pain management and bleeding control; if done poorly, it may cause greater harm. When splinting these types of injuries, remember to assess the patient's pulse and motor and sensory functions distal to the injury zone both before and after applying the splint. You can also apply ice packs over swollen painful areas to relieve pain and reduce swelling.

In addition to using these measures to control bleeding and swelling, you should be alert for signs of developing shock. Look for anxiety or agitation and changes in mental status, as these can be early signs of developing shock. An increased heart rate, increased respiratory rate, diaphoresis, cool or clammy skin, and eventual decreases in blood pressure may not develop until late in your care of the patient. Any or all of these signs may indicate internal bleeding resulting from injuries to internal organs. If the patient exhibits signs and symptoms of shock, treat accordingly and aggressively.

Emergency Medical Care for Open Injuries

Before you begin caring for a patient with an open wound, protect yourself by taking standard precautions. If life-threatening bleeding is observed, assign a team member to apply direct pressure over the wound to control the bleeding. Then assess the severity of the wound. If the wound is in the chest, upper abdomen, or upper back, cover it with an occlusive dressing.

Your treatment priorities are performing the primary assessment and beginning lifesaving interventions. This includes controlling the bleeding, which can be extensive and severe. Several methods are available to control open injuries or external bleeding. Start with the most commonly used; these include the following:

- Direct, even pressure and elevation
- Pressure dressings and/or splints
- Tourniquets
- Wound packing with hemostatic gauze

It will often be useful to combine these methods.

Words of Wisdom

Although most wounds can be managed with direct pressure, do not waste time with a wound in an arm or leg that is hemorrhaging profusely. Apply a tourniquet early when there is life-threatening hemorrhage.

All open wounds are assumed to be contaminated and present a risk of infection. By applying a sterile dressing, you are reducing the risk of further contamination. This keeps foreign material, such as hair, clothing, and dirt, out of the wound and decreases the risk of infection. If a wound appears to be grossly contaminated with debris, gently rinse it with normal saline before applying a dressing, if time permits. Open wounds over a fracture should be dressed with saline-moistened gauze.[1] Rubbing, brushing, or washing an open wound can cause additional bleeding, but small wound surfaces without significant bleeding can be flushed with sterile saline prior to applying a dressing. Chemical burns and contamination should be flushed to remove remaining chemicals. In most circumstances, hospital personnel, rather than EMTs, will clean open wounds. To prevent a wound from drying, you may apply sterile dressings moistened with sterile saline solution and then cover the moist dressing with a dry, sterile dressing.

In some cases, you can better control bleeding from open soft-tissue wounds by splinting the extremity, even if there is no fracture. Splinting can help you keep the patient calm and quiet, as it typically reduces pain. Splinting also keeps sterile dressings in place, minimizes damage to an already injured extremity, and makes it easier to move the patient.

Words of Wisdom

Hypovolemic shock is a risk for any patient who has had significant bleeding or bleeding that cannot be controlled. Be alert for this potential condition and treat aggressively.

Abdominal Wounds

An open wound in the abdominal cavity may expose internal organs. In some cases, the organs may even protrude through the wound, an injury called an **evisceration** (**FIGURE 26-13**). Do not touch or move the exposed organs. Instead, cover the wound with sterile gauze moistened with sterile saline solution and secure it with occlusive dressing (**FIGURE 26-14**). Because the open abdomen radiates body heat very effectively and quickly, and because exposed organs lose fluid rapidly, you must keep the organs moist and warm. If you do not have gauze compresses, you may use moist sterile dressings, covered and secured in place with a bandage and tape. Do not use any material that is adherent or loses its substance when wet, such as toilet paper, facial tissue, paper

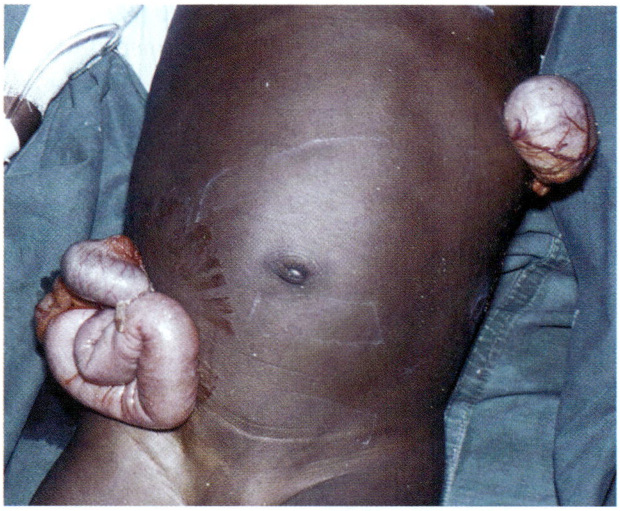

FIGURE 26-13 An abdominal evisceration is an open wound to the abdomen in which organs protrude through the wound.

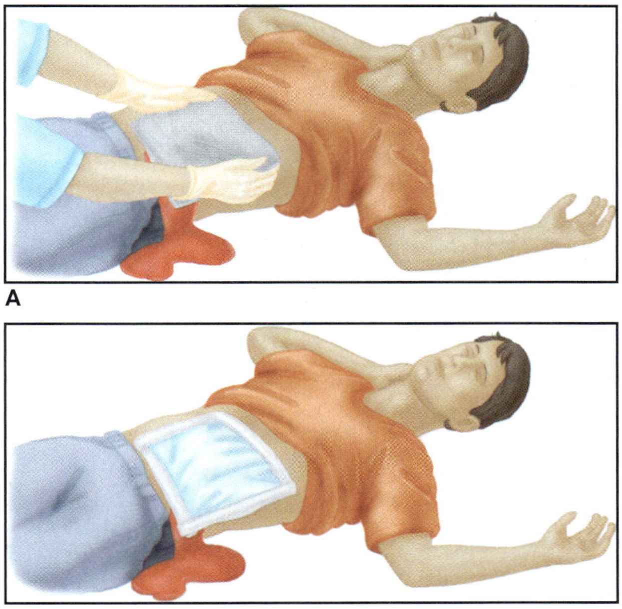

A

B

FIGURE 26-14 A. Cover exposed organs with sterile gauze compresses moistened with sterile saline solution. **B.** Place an occlusive dressing over the compresses and secure it in place by taping all four sides.

towels, or absorbent cotton. If the patient's legs and knees are uninjured, flex them to relieve pressure on the abdomen. Most patients with abdominal wounds require immediate transport to a trauma center, depending on the local protocol.

Impaled Objects

Occasionally, a patient will have an object, such as a knife, fishhook, wood splinter, or piece of glass, impaled in their body. To treat this injury, follow the steps in **SKILL DRILL 26-1**:

1. Do not attempt to move or remove the object unless it is impaled through the cheek or mouth and is causing airway obstruction, or unless the patient is pulseless and you must remove it to perform cardiopulmonary resuscitation (CPR). In most cases, a surgeon will have to remove the object; removing it in the field may cause more bleeding or damage nerves, blood vessels, or muscles within the wound. Stabilize the impaled body part (**Step 1**).
2. Remove any clothing covering the injury. Control bleeding with direct pressure on either side of the object, and apply a bulky dressing to stabilize the object. If the object is in the chest, neck, or upper back, consider applying a base layer of occlusive dressing around the

Skill Drill 26-1 Stabilizing an Impaled Object

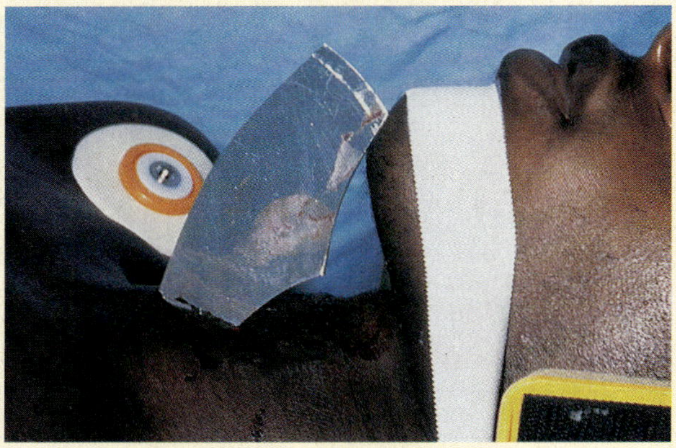

Step 1

Do not attempt to move or remove the object. Stabilize the impaled body part.

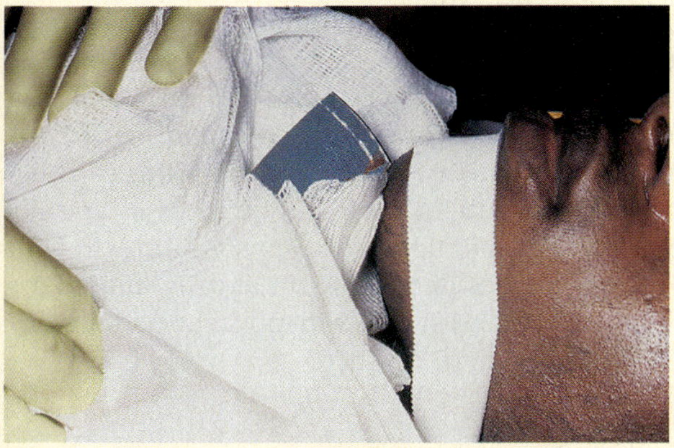

Step 2

Control bleeding, and stabilize the object in place using soft dressings, gauze, and/or tape.

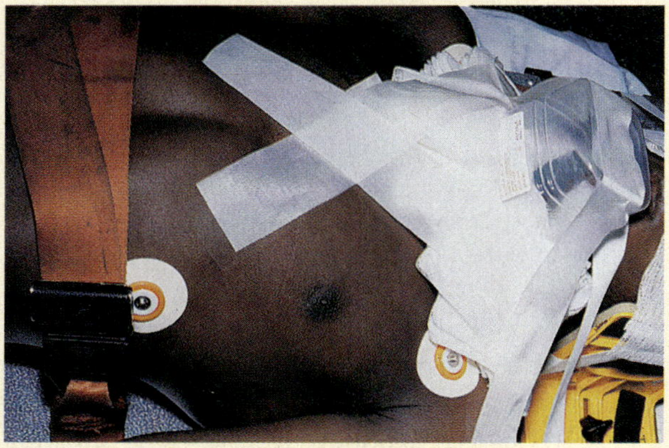

Step 3

Tape a rigid item over the stabilized object to prevent it from moving during transport.

object to prevent air from entering the wound. Some combination of soft dressings, gauze, and tape may be effective, depending on the location and size of the object. To prevent further injury, manually secure the object by incorporating it into the dressing (**Step 2**).

3. Protect the impaled object from being bumped or moved during transport by stabilizing it manually, with a commercial device, or with improvised padding and other objects (**Step 3**).

The only exceptions to the rule of not removing an impaled object are objects in the cheek or mouth that actively obstruct breathing and objects in the chest that directly interfere with performing CPR on a patient who is already in cardiac arrest. If the object is very long, cut off (shorten) the exposed portion, first securing it to minimize motion and, thus, internal damage and pain. Once the object has been properly secured and the bleeding is under control, provide prompt transport.

Neck Injuries

An open neck injury can be life threatening. If the veins of the neck are open to the environment, they may suck in air (**FIGURE 26-15**). If enough air is sucked into a blood vessel, it can block the flow of blood into the lungs and cause cardiac arrest. This condition is called air embolism. To control bleeding and prevent the possibility of air embolism, cover the wound with an occlusive dressing. Apply manual pressure, but do not compress both carotid vessels at the same time; if you do, this may impair circulation to the brain and cause a stroke. Secure a pressure dressing over the wound by wrapping roller gauze loosely around the neck and then firmly through the opposite axilla (**FIGURE 26-16**).

Use caution with patients who have sustained a neck injury, depending on the MOI involved. Restrict movement of the cervical spine if there is not a penetrating wound, including placing a cervical collar. The cervical collar may assist with holding a dressing in place over a neck wound.

Bites

Small Animal Bites and Rabies

At times you may be called to care for a person who has been bitten by a small animal such as a dog, cat, raccoon, or squirrel. Be sure to consider scene and crew safety prior to entering the environment.

Most people who are bitten by small animals do not report the incident to a physician, believing that these bites are not serious; however, they can be very serious. A small animal's mouth is heavily contaminated with bacteria. You should consider all small animal bites, even those from pets such as cats and dogs, as contaminated and potentially infected wounds that may require débridement (the removal of damaged tissue), antibiotics, and

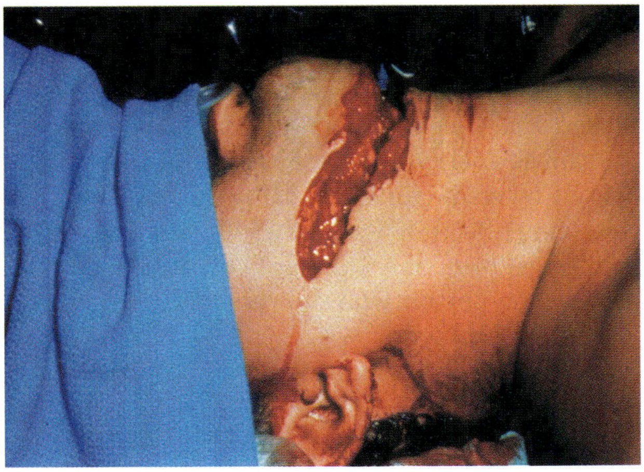

FIGURE 26-15 Open injuries to the neck can be very dangerous. If veins are open to the environment, they can suck in air, resulting in a potentially fatal condition called air embolism.

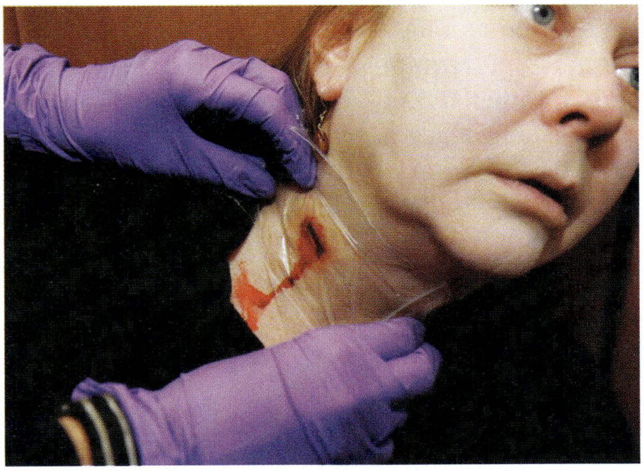

FIGURE 26-16 Cover neck wounds with an airtight dressing and apply manual pressure. Do not compress both carotid arteries at the same time, as this may impair circulation to the brain.

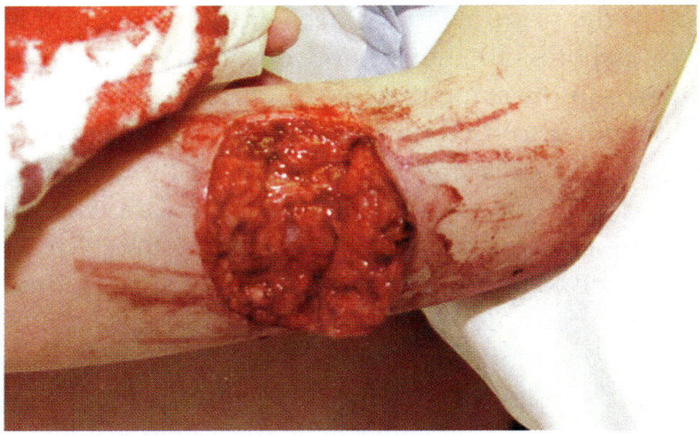

A

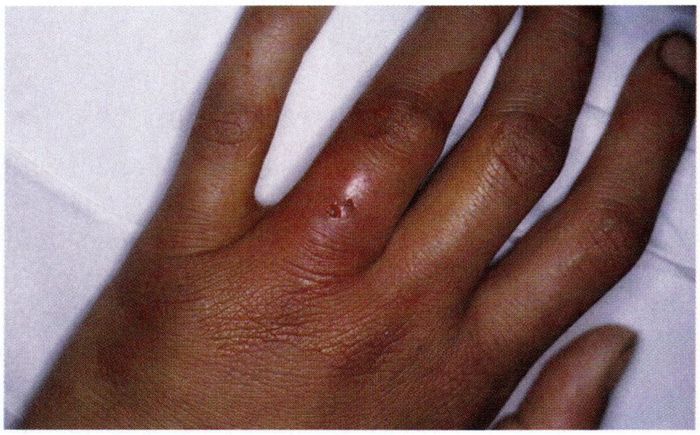

B

FIGURE 26-17 Bite wounds caused by small animals should be examined at the hospital, as these wounds are heavily contaminated with bacteria. **A.** Dog bite. **B.** Cat bite.

tetanus prophylaxis (**FIGURE 26-17**). Occasionally, small animal bites result in mangled, complex wounds that require surgical repair. For these reasons, all small animal bites should be evaluated by a physician. Place a dry, sterile dressing over the wound, and promptly transport the patient to the ED. If an arm or leg was injured, splint that extremity. Often, the patient will be extremely upset and frightened, a situation that calls for reassurance on your part.

A major concern with small animal bites is the spread of rabies, an acute, potentially fatal viral infection of the central nervous system that can affect all warm-blooded animals. Although rabies is currently extremely rare, particularly with widespread vaccination of pets, it still exists. Stray dogs that have not been vaccinated can be carriers of the disease, as can squirrels, bats, foxes, skunks, and raccoons. The virus is in the saliva of a rabid, or infected, animal and is transmitted through biting or licking an open wound. Infection can be prevented in a person who has been bitten by such an animal only by a series of special vaccine injections, a procedure that must be started soon after the bite. Because animals that have rabies do not always demonstrate symptoms immediately, a person's only chance to avoid the vaccine is to find the animal and turn it over to the health department for observation and/or testing. Refer to your local animal control procedures.

Children, particularly young ones, may be seriously injured or even killed by dogs. These dogs are not always vicious or **rabid**; sometimes a child unknowingly provokes the animal. However, you must assume the animal may turn and attack you as well. Therefore, you generally should not enter the scene until the animal has been secured. Then you may carry out the necessary emergency care and transport the child to the ED.

Words of Wisdom

In many locations, reporting animal bites to public health officials is mandatory. Based on your protocols you may need to have law enforcement respond to the scene or to the hospital.

Human Bites

The human mouth, more so than even the small animal's mouth, contains an exceptionally wide range of bacteria and viruses. For this reason, you should regard any human bite that has penetrated the skin as a serious injury. Similarly, any laceration caused by a human tooth can result in a serious, spreading infection (**FIGURE 26-18**). Remember this if you treat someone who has been punched in the mouth; the person who delivered the punch may also need treatment.

The emergency treatment of bites consists of the following steps:

1. Apply a dry, sterile dressing.
2. Promptly immobilize the area with a splint or bandage.
3. Provide transport to the ED for surgical cleansing of the wound and antibiotic therapy.

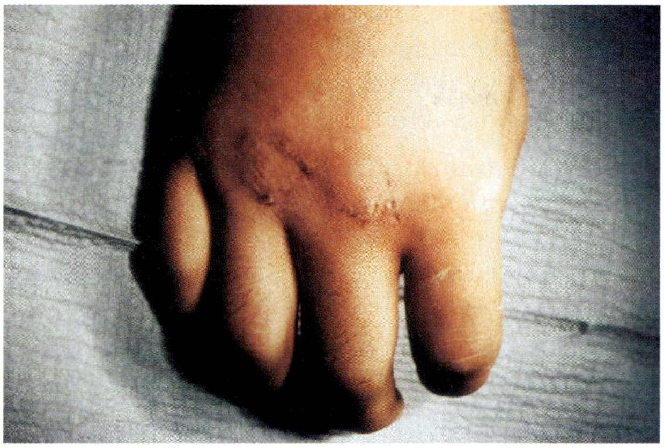

FIGURE 26-18 Human bites can result in a serious, spreading infection. Thus, patients must be evaluated at the hospital.

Burns

As an EMT, you will provide care to patients who have been burned. Often, these calls involve pediatric patients. Burns are among the most serious and painful of all injuries. A severe burn injury presents several simultaneous life threats, including hypovolemic shock, sepsis, hypothermia, and respiratory compromise and failure. Management of severe burn injuries has improved over the years, including an emphasis on the psychological challenges that survivors face. Burn units typically employ social workers, vocational counselors, and psychologists as part of a multidisciplinary approach to patient care.

A burn occurs when the body, or a body part, receives more radiant energy than it can absorb, resulting in an injury. Potential sources of this energy include heat, toxic chemicals, and electricity. The proper emergency care of a burn may increase a patient's chances of survival and decrease the risk or duration of a long-term disability. Although a burn may be the patient's most obvious injury, you should always perform a complete assessment to determine whether there are other serious injuries. Finally, keep in mind that children, older adults, and patients with chronic illnesses are more likely to experience shock from burn injuries. Be prepared to treat accordingly.

Pathophysiology of Burns

Burns are soft-tissue injuries spread out over a large area created by the transfer of radiation, thermal, or electrical energy. Thermal burns can occur when skin is exposed to temperatures higher than 111°F (44°C). In general, the severity of a thermal injury directly correlates with temperature, concentration, or amount of heat energy possessed by the object or substance and the duration of exposure. For example, solids generally have higher heat content than gases, so exposure to a hot solid (such as the rack inside an oven) typically causes a more significant burn than exposure to hot gases (such as those coming out of an oven). Burn injuries are progressive: the greater the heat energy, the deeper the wound.

Exposure time is another important factor. Thermal injury can occur to unresponsive or paralyzed patients from seemingly innocent heat sources such as heating pads or heat lamps if the patient is left unattended and exposed for long periods. It may be difficult to evaluate the amount of heat energy or the amount of exposure time in many cases. There can be a vast difference in the temperature of a fire from the floor to the ceiling. Although most people naturally limit the amount of time they are exposed to such heat, if clothing is on fire or the person is trapped or unconscious, exposure time can be extended.

Safety Tips

Many fires generate toxic compounds such as carbon monoxide and cyanides, which are produced as a result of the combustion of synthetic materials. This environment is dangerous to all responders, and use of a self-contained breathing apparatus is mandatory. You should enter only if you have been trained and are equipped to function in those areas.

Complications of Burns

Several complications can result from a burn injury, all of which can be life threatening. The skin serves as a barrier between the environment and the body. When a person is burned, this barrier is destroyed; the person is now at a high risk for infection, hypovolemia, and shock. The person is also at risk of hypothermia and acidosis, which can increase the risk of complications and death. Therefore, in the field and during transport, keep the patient warm and provide high-concentration supplemental oxygen to all patients who have been rescued from an enclosed space.[1] Monitor and maintain an oxygen saturation level of 94% to 98% in patients who have serious burn injuries.

Special Populations

RISK OF INFECTION IN CHILDREN WITH BURN INJURIES

One common problem following burn injuries in children is infection. Burned skin cannot resist infection as effectively as normal skin can. For this reason, whenever possible, sterile techniques should be used in handling the skin of children with burn wounds.[3]

Burns to the airway are of great importance because the loose mucosa in the hypopharynx can swell and result in complete airway obstruction. **Circumferential burns** (burns that go completely around a part of the body) of the chest can compromise breathing. Circumferential burns of an extremity can lead to compartment syndrome, resulting in neurovascular compromise and irreversible damage if not appropriately treated. Additionally, when the patient inhaled the hot air or smoke from the fire, they may have also inhaled toxic substances such as carbon monoxide and cyanide. If you suspect any complications, call for ALS backup if available or provide rapid transport to the ED.

Burn Assessment

Proper assessment of burn injuries will help you determine the best care and possibly treatment facility for the patient. To make this determination, you must assess the depth and extent of the burn and consider other factors specific to the patient and injury. When assessing burns, ask yourself the following questions:

- What is the depth of the burn? Burn depth is identified as superficial, partial thickness, or full thickness.
- What is the extent of the burn? The extent of the burn is identified as a percentage of the total body surface area (TBSA) that has been burned.

These first two factors are the most important. After gauging them, consider the following additional information to determine whether the burn should be considered severe:

- Are there any partial-thickness or full-thickness burns to critical areas (face, hands, genitalia, feet, perineum, or over any joints) involved? Also included in critical areas are any circumferential burns.
- Does the patient have any preexisting medical conditions or other injuries?
- Is the patient 14 years or younger, or older than 55 years?

A more detailed review of these factors follows.

Depth

Burns are first classified according to their depth (**FIGURE 26-19**). While you must be able to distinguish between superficial burns and those of greater depth, classifying the exact depth is typically not possible until after the wounds are fully cleaned at the hospital. The American Burn Association describes the following burn depths:

- **Superficial burns** involve only the top layer of skin, the epidermis. The skin turns red or darker but does not blister or burn through this top layer. The burn site is often painful and the skin blanches when fingertip pressure is applied and released. Sunburn is a good example of a superficial burn. The extent of superficial burns is not used when calculating the TBSA of the burn. Superficial burns are sometimes referred to as first-degree burns.
- **Superficial partial-thickness burns** involve the epidermis and some portion of the dermis. These burns do not destroy the entire thickness of the skin, nor is the subcutaneous tissue injured. Typically, the skin is moist, is red or darker than the patient's baseline skin color, and blanches when touched; blisters are often present. Partial-thickness burns cause intense pain. **Deep partial-thickness burns** extend farther into the dermis, destroying more of the blood vessels. They appear lighter in color than superficial partial-thickness burns and are dryer and less painful. Partial-thickness burns are sometimes referred to as second-degree burns.

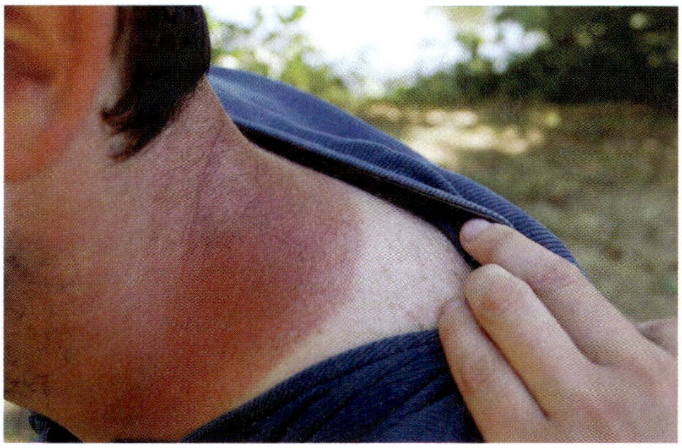

A

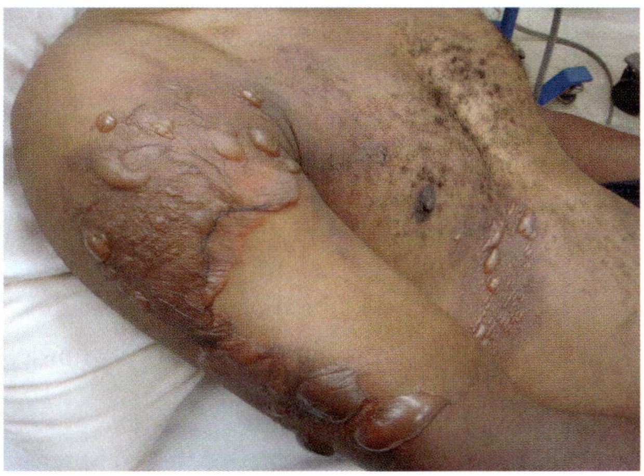

B

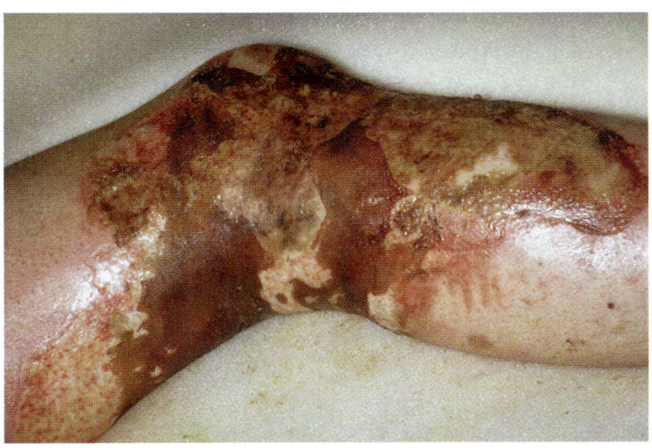

C

FIGURE 26-19 Classification of burns. **A.** Superficial burns involve only the epidermis. **B.** Partial-thickness burns involve some of the dermis, but they do not destroy the entire thickness of the skin. **C.** Full-thickness burns extend through all layers of the skin and may involve subcutaneous tissue and muscle.

- **Full-thickness burns** extend through all skin layers and may involve subcutaneous layers, muscle, bone, or internal organs. The burned area is dry and leathery and may appear white, dark brown, or even charred. Some full-thickness burns feel hard to the touch. Clotted blood vessels or subcutaneous tissue may be visible under the burned skin. The area of a full-thickness burn does not have feeling. These burns will require surgical treatment, such as skin grafting. Full-thickness burns are sometimes referred to as third-degree burns or, when they extend into deeper tissues, fourth-degree burns.

Words of Wisdom

The depth of burns can vary. A full-thickness burn may be surrounded by areas of partial-thickness and superficial burns. So, although the area of the full-thickness burn is painless, the patient can still experience pain due to the extent of damage to the surrounding tissues. Request ALS for assistance with pain management if appropriate.

A pure full-thickness burn is unusual. Severe burns are typically a combination of superficial, partial-thickness, and full-thickness burns. Superficial burns heal well without scarring. Small superficial partial-thickness burns also heal without scarring. However, deep partial-thickness burns and all full-thickness burns are prone to scarring and may be best managed surgically.

Significant airway burns are also serious. They may be associated with singed hair within the nostrils, soot around the nose and mouth, hoarseness, and hypoxia. These patients should be rapidly transported to an ED or facility capable of advanced airway management. It becomes increasingly difficult to achieve airway control once swelling begins.

It is almost impossible to accurately estimate the depth of a burn shortly after injury. Even experienced burn surgeons sometimes underestimate or overestimate the extent of a burn.

Extent

One quick way to estimate the surface area that has been burned is to compare it with the size of

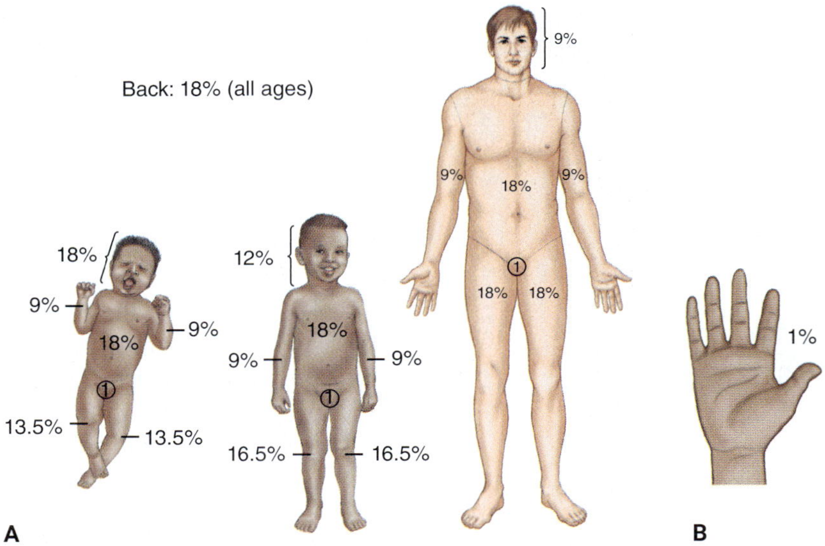

FIGURE 26-20 **A.** The rule of nines is a quick way to estimate the amount of surface area that has been burned; it divides the body into sections, each representing approximately 9% of the total body surface area (TBSA). The proportions differ for adults and infants. **B.** The rule of palms method is useful for splatter burn injuries, which are common in pediatric burn patients. The palm and fingers of the patient's hand equal approximately 1% of the TBSA.

the patient's palm, including their fingers, which is equal to almost 1% of the patient's TBSA. This technique is called the rule of palms. Another useful measurement system is the **rule of nines**, which divides the body into sections, each of which is approximately 9% of TBSA (**FIGURE 26-20**). Remember that the head of an infant or child is relatively larger than the head of an adult, and the legs are relatively smaller. When you calculate the extent of burn injury, include only partial-thickness and full-thickness burns. Document superficial burns, but do not include them in the TBSA estimation of extent of burn injury.

Severe Burns

The American Burn Association and the American College of Surgeons recommend immediate consultation and consideration for transfer to a designated burn center for all severe burns. Burns are considered severe if they meet any of the following criteria[4]:

- All full-thickness burns
- All partial-thickness burns covering 10% or more of TBSA
- Any deep partial- or full-thickness burns to the face, hands, genitalia, feet, or perineum, or over any joints
- All burns with concomitant traumatic injuries or other comorbidities
- All burns with poorly controlled pain
- All burns with suspected inhalation injury
- All chemical injuries
- All high-voltage electrical injuries
- All lightning injuries
- All burns to pediatric patients (defined as age 14 years or younger or weight less than 66 pounds [30 kg])

Follow local protocols regarding how burns should be treated in the field and where these patients should be transported.

Special Populations

PATHOPHYSIOLOGY OF BURN INJURIES IN CHILDREN

Burns to children are generally considered more serious than burns to adults. This is because infants and children have more surface area relative to total body mass, which means greater fluid and heat loss. In addition, children do not tolerate burns as well as adults do. Children are also more likely to experience shock, hypothermia, and airway problems because of the unique differences of their ages and anatomy.

Patient Assessment of Burns

As discussed, assessment of a burn injury involves consideration of the burn's depth and extent and other factors unique to the patient and MOI. The general assessment principles are otherwise similar to those applied when assessing any other trauma patient.

Scene Size-up

As you arrive on scene, observe the scene for hazards and threats to the safety of you and your crew, bystanders, and the patient. Ensure that the factors that led to the patient's burn injury do not pose a hazard to you and your crew. For example, is the electricity turned off? Is the chemical leak secure? Are any hazardous materials present? Has the fire been extinguished? Is there any potential for violence? Has the patient been decontaminated? In the case of a lightning strike, is the weather still a threat to your safety?

Regardless of the situation, always take standard precautions. Do not approach an area still engulfed in smoke without appropriate training and protective breathing apparatus.[1] Wear gloves and eye protection when treating any patient with a burn; add a gown when serious injuries are expected.

Determine the number of patients; the possibility for multiple patients grows if you are responding to a lightning strike or a vehicle crash. At vehicle crashes, ensure the scene is safe from energized electrical lines or leaking fuel in the area where you will be working. If you determine the power company, the fire department, or ALS units are needed, call for additional resources early.

Primary Assessment

The primary assessment includes a rapid exam of the patient to identify and manage life-threatening concerns and to assist with transport decisions. The primary assessment begins when you approach the patient and form a general impression.

As you approach the burn trauma patient, simple clues can help identify how serious the injuries are and how quickly you need to assess and treat them. If the patient or their clothing is burning when you reach them, stop the burning process immediately.

If you see significant bleeding, take the necessary steps to control it. Significant bleeding is an immediate life threat. If the patient has obvious life-threatening external hemorrhage, control the bleeding first (before airway and breathing); then treat the patient for shock as quickly as possible.

If your patient greets you with a hoarse voice or reports being in an enclosed space with a fire or intense heat source, these should be indications of a significant MOI. The presence of stridor means your patient's airway is significantly swollen and can signal impending complete airway obstruction. Summon ALS responders immediately. Similarly, if the patient has singed facial hair, eyebrows, or nasal

Special Populations

BURN INJURIES SUGGESTIVE OF PHYSICAL ABUSE

When you are treating older adults, pediatric patients, or special needs patients with burns, it is important to be alert for the possibility of abuse. Burns that appear in a pattern are suspicious for intentional injuries. Multiple small, circular burns may be indicative of cigarette or cigar injuries. Other patterns may indicate irons, stovetops, or other hot surfaces not easily encountered accidentally. Scalding injuries to the buttocks, hands, or feet may indicate abuse. Signs of abuse not necessarily specific to burns include evidence of multiple injuries in various stages of healing (eg, multiple bruises of different colors, new and old fractures involving more than one extremity), injuries that do not seem to correspond to the history provided by caregivers, and injuries associated with a suspicious history.

Older adult patients who are institutionalized, disoriented, or incapable of clear communication are particularly susceptible to abuse. Remember, their injuries are often inflicted in areas not readily seen. If you are suspicious that an older adult has been abused, fully examine the patient under their clothing for signs of abuse.

Children may sustain burns from a variety of sources. The most common cause of an abuse-related burn in children is scalding, such as by exposure to hot water in a bathtub.[5] Exposure to other hot sources, such items on a stove, and exposure to caustic substances, such as cleaning solvents or paint thinners, can also produce burn injuries (**FIGURE 26-21**).

As always, your priority is to provide appropriate support and transport the patient in a timely manner. Report any information about your suspicions to the appropriate authorities.

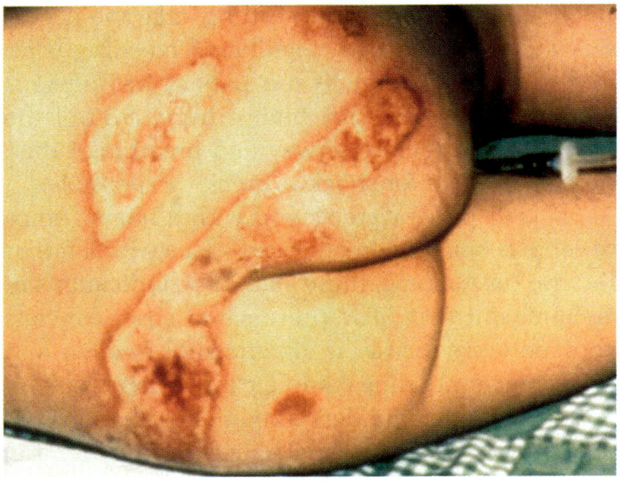

FIGURE 26-21 Some burns in children involve exposure to hot surfaces. This child's buttocks were placed against a hot heating grate.

hair, your initial general impression might be that the patient has a potential airway and/or breathing problem.

The burned patient you encounter may have graphic injuries. It is easy to become overwhelmed by the sights, sounds, and smells of burn victims. However, stay focused on the primary assessment. As you begin, always assess for uncontrolled bleeding if there are other traumatic injuries and consider the need for manual spinal stabilization.

Check for responsiveness using the AVPU scale (Awake and alert, responsive to Verbal stimuli, responsive to Pain, Unresponsive). Assess a patient's mental status by asking the patient about their chief complaint. If the patient is alert, this should help direct you to any apparent life threats. If the patient is not alert, determine if they respond to verbal or painful stimuli or if they are unresponsive. An unresponsive patient may very well have a life-threatening condition. In all patients whose level of consciousness is less than alert and oriented, you should administer high-flow oxygen via a nonrebreathing mask and provide immediate transport to the ED.

Ensure the patient has a clear and patent airway. If the patient is unresponsive or has a significantly altered level of consciousness, consider inserting the proper-size oropharyngeal or nasopharyngeal airway. Be alert to signs that the patient has inhaled hot gases or vapors, such as singed facial hair or soot present in or around the airway. Heavy amounts of secretions and frequent coughing may also indicate a respiratory burn.

Street Smarts

Being burned is a scary experience for most patients. They experience pain, odors associated with burning flesh and hair, and the fear of disfigurement. In your interaction with these patients, be supportive and empathetic. Do your best to make them comfortable while managing life-threatening injuries and transporting them to the closest appropriate facility.

Words of Wisdom

An isolated burn injury should not cause an altered level of consciousness in your patient. If your patient with a burn has an altered level of consciousness, you should suspect other potential complications, such as toxic inhalation, hypoperfusion, hypoxia, hypoglycemia, or head injury.

Quickly assess for adequate breathing. Inspect and palpate the chest wall for DCAP-BTLS. Check for clear and symmetric breath sounds and the presence of abnormal breath sounds such as wheezing if smoke was inhaled. Provide high-flow oxygen to all patients rescued from a confined space or who may have inhaled smoke. Assist ventilations using a bag-mask device as needed, depending on the level of consciousness and breathing rate/quality of your patient.

Remember, the patient with a burn is a trauma patient. Evaluate and treat these patients for spinal injuries and airway problems concurrently. How you open the airway depends on whether a neck injury is suspected. Consider whether the MOI suggests a possible spinal injury. Could the patient have fallen? Was there an explosion?

Quickly assess the pulse rate and quality, and determine perfusion based on the patient's skin condition, color, temperature, and capillary refill time. Shock rarely develops in patients with burns. If you observe signs of shock within the first hour of the burn injury, it is likely due to other trauma or cyanide toxicity, not the burn itself. Burn shock develops over several hours. Call for ALS and treat the shock by preventing heat loss. This is important because the damaged skin has only a limited ability to regulate body temperature. After the burning process has stopped, cover the patient with a blanket to prevent heat loss.

If the patient you are treating has an airway or breathing problem, significant burn injuries, significant external bleeding, or signs and symptoms of internal bleeding, consider rapid transport to the nearest hospital, trauma center, or burn center for treatment. Consulting with ALS clinicians may be appropriate for patients with severe burns and burns of the airway or inhalation injury. ALS clinicians can treat these patients with endotracheal intubation and intravenous fluids to support airway, breathing, and circulation (shock) difficulties. These can progress so rapidly that immediate ALS assistance can make the difference between life and death. ALS clinicians also have additional means to treat the patient's pain.

Words of Wisdom

More fire victims die from smoke inhalation than from skin burns.[6] A patient who has facial burns or has inhaled smoke or fumes may experience respiratory distress.

History Taking

Investigate the chief complaint or history of present illness. Next, be alert for signs or symptoms of other injuries due to the MOI. If the patient was burned in a confined space, suspect an inhalation injury. When burns result from explosive forces, be alert for other internal injuries and fractures.

Obtain a medical history and be alert for injury-specific signs and symptoms as well as any pertinent negatives such as no pain. Typical signs of a burn are pain, redness, swelling, blisters, or charring. Typically, symptoms include pain and/or burning at the injury site. Regardless of the type of burn injury, it is important to stop the burning process, apply dressings to prevent contamination, and treat the patient for shock.

Obtain a SAMPLE history from your patient. In addition, ask the following questions of a patient with a burn:

- Are you having any difficulty breathing?
- Are you having any difficulty swallowing?
- Are you having any pain?

The information reported by the patient will often help you estimate the extent of the injury.

When you assess a patient with a burn, check whether the patient has an emergency medical identification device (ie, a wallet card, necklace, or bracelet), or ask the patient or a family member about preexisting conditions that may increase the

YOU are the EMT

You reassess the patient and then call your radio report to the receiving facility. The patient is still experiencing respiratory distress, but he is moving air adequately. Your estimated time of arrival at the hospital is 6 minutes.

Recording Time: 17 Minutes	
Level of consciousness	Conscious and alert, but anxious
Respirations	22 breaths/min; labored; hoarse voice
Pulse	116 beats/min; strong and regular
Skin	Red, warm, and dry
Blood pressure	160/80 mm Hg
Oxygen saturation (Spo_2)	99% (on oxygen)

9. What, if any, additional treatment is indicated for this patient?

risk of a poor outcome. Remember that the environment, bystanders, and medical identification devices may provide important clues about your patient's condition.

Secondary Assessment

The secondary assessment is a more detailed, comprehensive, or focused examination of the patient that is conducted to reveal injuries that may have been missed during the primary assessment. In some instances where the patient is critically injured or the transport time is short, you may not have time to conduct a secondary assessment. In other instances, the secondary assessment may occur en route to the ED.

After you complete the primary assessment, remove any wet or smoldering clothing and jewelry from the patient and then examine the entire body. Quickly assess the patient from head to toe looking for DCAP-BTLS to ensure you have found all of the problems and injuries. Make a rough estimate, using the rule of nines, of the extent of the burned area to report to medical direction. Determine what classification of burns the victim has sustained. The patient may report pain depending on the amount of nerve damage. Before you package your patient, determine the severity of the burns the victim has sustained. Severity is calculated by considering what caused the burn, the body region that is burned, the depth and extent of the burn, the patient's age, and preexisting illness or injuries. Follow your local protocols for criteria for transport to a burn center. Package the patient for transport based on your findings. Remember to immobilize your patient for spinal injuries as appropriate.

Assessing the respiratory system involves looking, listening, and feeling. A patient who is conscious, alert, and talking does not have immediate airway or breathing difficulties. When you assess the respiratory system of a patient with a burn, look specifically for the following findings:

1. Soot around the mouth
2. Soot around the nose
3. Singed nasal hairs

If any of these findings are present, open the patient's mouth and examine for burns or swelling of the tongue. Ask the patient to cough, and assess for black sputum, which indicates smoke inhalation.

Next, listen to breath sounds with a stethoscope. Stridor indicates impending airway obstruction that will require ALS interventions. Wheezing may indicate inhalation of toxic gases. Determine the patient's rate and quality of respiration. Finally, assess the chest for circumferential burns that may restrict breathing by limiting chest wall movement. Patients with burns who present with any type of airway problem should be considered critical.

Quickly assess pulse rate and quality; determine the skin condition, color, and temperature; and check the capillary refill time. If the patient has obvious life-threatening bleeding, quickly control it and treat for shock as quickly as possible. Non–life-threatening bleeding, such as in abrasions, can be bandaged later in your assessment as necessary.

Assess the patient's neurologic system to formulate baseline data for further decisions on patient care. This examination should include assessing for the following:

- Level of consciousness (using the AVPU scale)
- Pupil size and reactivity
- Motor response
- Sensory response

Assess the musculoskeletal system by performing a detailed full-body scan. Assess all anatomic regions looking for DCAP-BTLS. Specifically look for the following features:

- In the head, check for singed nasal or facial hair, burns or swelling of the face or ears, or burns or swelling in the mouth. If the patient sustained an electrical injury, examine the scalp for signs of an entrance or exit wounds.
- In the neck, check for burns, especially if they encircle the entire neck, which can impair the airway.
- In the chest, check for burns that encircle the entire chest, which can impair normal chest rise.
- In the abdomen and pelvis, feel all four quadrants for tenderness or rigidity. If the abdomen is tender, expect internal bleeding. Look for burns of the genitalia, as burns to this area are considered high risk.
- Look for burns that encircle an extremity, as they can impair circulation. If the patient sustained an electrical injury, assess thoroughly for entry or exit burn wounds. This should include the axilla and the area between digits. Record the pulse and motor and sensory function.

- Examine the posterior surface of the body, as large burns or electrical exit burns may be located in this body area.

A systematic examination helps you understand what has happened to the outside of your patient. Vital signs are a good indication of how your patient is doing on the inside. If you obtain an early set of vital signs, you will know how your patient is tolerating the injuries while en route to the hospital. Because shock develops over time in a patient with a large burn, blood pressure, pulse, and skin assessment for perfusion are important vital signs to reassess often.

In addition to hands-on assessment, use monitoring devices, including oxygen saturation monitors and carbon monoxide monitors, to quantify oxygenation and circulatory status.

Reassessment

Repeat the primary assessment and reassess the patient's vital signs. Reassess the patient's chief complaint. Reevaluate interventions and treatment you have provided to the patient, particularly those used to treat shock. Identify and treat any changes in the patient's condition.

Do not delay transport of a seriously injured patient to complete non-lifesaving treatments in the field such as splinting extremity fractures. Instead, complete these types of treatment en route to the hospital.

Provide hospital personnel with a description of how the burn occurred. Often, the ED staff can determine the appropriate diluent for chemical burns or calculate appropriate treatments for other types of burns with enough advance notice. Report and document the extent of the burns. This should include the total amount of body surface area involved, the depth of the burns, and the location. For example, you may say "approximately 40% TBSA burns, with full-thickness burns and partial-thickness burns to the chest, abdomen, and left lower extremity." If special areas are involved (genitalia, feet, hands, face, or circumferential), they should be specifically mentioned and documented.

Emergency Medical Care for Burns

The goals in treating patients with burns are to stop the burning process, assess and treat breathing, support circulation, and provide rapid transport. When caring for a patient with a burn, follow the steps in **SKILL DRILL 26-2**:

1. Take standard precautions. Because a burn destroys the patient's protective skin layer, always wear gloves and eye protection when treating a patient with a burn.
2. Move the patient away from the burning area. Stop the burning process. If any clothing is on fire, wrap the patient in a blanket or follow the specific guidelines outlined by your local fire department protocol to put out the flames, and then remove any smoldering clothing and/or jewelry.
3. Briefly immerse the burning area in room temperature, sterile water or saline solution. This not only stops the burning, but also relieves pain. Prolonged immersion, however, may increase the risk of infection and hypothermia. If the burning has stopped before you arrive, do not immerse the affected part at all (**Step 1**).
4. Provide high-flow oxygen if the patient was burned in an enclosed space or has signs of inhalation injury. If carbon monoxide toxicity is present, pulse oximetry values may not be accurate. Maintain an oxygen saturation level between 94% and 98% in all burn patients. Keep in mind that a patient who appears to be breathing well at first may suddenly experience severe respiratory distress. Continually assess the airway for possible problems (**Step 2**).
5. Rapidly estimate the burn's severity. Cover the burned area with a dry, sterile dressing to prevent further contamination. Sterile gauze is best if the area is not too large. Never use ointments, lotions, or antiseptics of any kind and do not intentionally break any blisters. To help reduce the risk of infection, cover large (>10% of TBSA) burns with a dry nonadherent dressing, such as a clean sheet, Mylar blanket, or sterile burn sheet.[1]
6. Check for traumatic injuries or other medical conditions that may be immediately life threatening. Most patients who have been burned do not have signs of shock in the first hour after the burn and can communicate at first, which will make your assessment easier (**Step 3**).
7. If the patient has signs of hypoperfusion, treat aggressively for shock, and look for the source of the shock.

Skill Drill 26-2 Caring for Burns

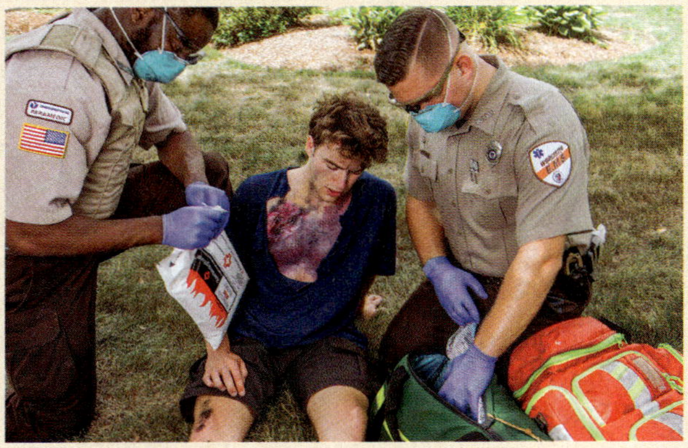

Step 1

Take standard precautions to help prevent infection. Remove the patient from the burning area; extinguish or remove hot clothing and jewelry as necessary. If the wound is still burning or hot, immerse the hot area in cool, sterile water, or cover with a wet, cool dressing.

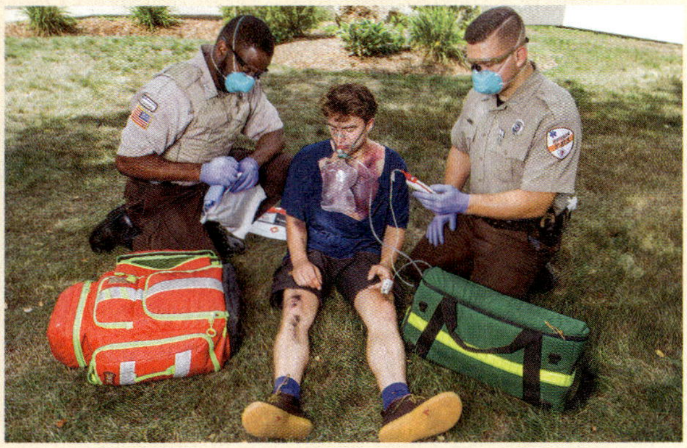

Step 2

Provide high-flow oxygen, and continue to assess the airway.

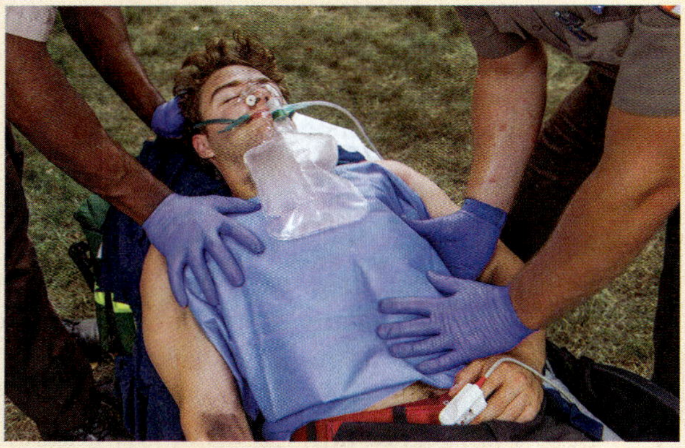

Step 3

Estimate the severity of the burn and then cover the area with a dry, sterile dressing or clean sheet. Assess and treat the patient for any other injuries.

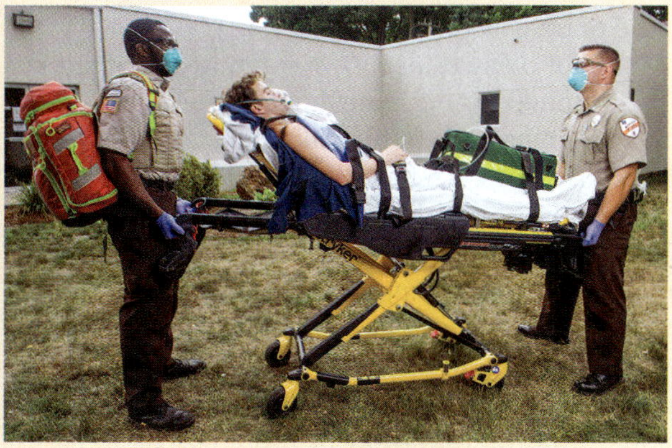

Step 4

Prepare for transport. Treat for shock. Cover the patient with blankets to prevent loss of body heat. Transport promptly.

8. An extensive burn can produce hypothermia (loss of body heat). Prevent further heat loss by covering the patient with warm blankets.
9. Provide prompt transport by local protocol. Do not delay transport to perform a prolonged assessment or to apply coverings to burns in a critical patient (**Step 4**).

Management of Specific Burns

Thermal Burns

A **thermal burn** is caused by heat (as opposed to electricity, chemicals, or radiation). Many different situations can cause thermal burns, and all pose a safety hazard to responding emergency care clinicians. Most commonly, thermal burns are caused by scalds or an open flame.[8] A **flame burn** is very often a deep burn, especially if a person's clothing catches fire. Hot liquids produce scald injuries. A **scald burn** is most commonly seen in children and handicapped adults but can happen to anyone, particularly while cooking. Scald burns often cover large surface areas of the body because liquids can spread quickly. Coming in contact with hot objects produces a **contact burn**. Ordinarily, reflexes protect a person from prolonged exposure to a very hot object, so contact burns are rarely deep unless the patient was prevented from drawing away from the hot object (eg, unconscious, intoxicated, restrained, or impaired).

> **Words of Wisdom**
>
> Some military and wilderness medical directors, in cooperation with local burn centers, may approve the use of high-concentration antimicrobial-coated dressings for prehospital burn care.[7]

> **Words of Wisdom**
>
> The key to initial burn treatment is to stop the burning process. Using room-temperature water, not cold water, is crucial. Using cold water or ice can cause further injury to the tissue. Once you have stopped the burning process, you must remember to immediately prevent heat loss to reduce the risk of hypothermia.

A **steam burn** can produce a topical (scald) burn. Minor steam burns are common when uncovering the plastic wrap from microwaved food. When the plastic is peeled away, hot steam escapes directly onto the person's hand. Steam (ie, gaseous water) may also cause airway burns.

Another important source of thermal burns is the **flash burn** produced by an explosion, which may briefly expose a person to very intense heat. Lightning strikes can also cause a flash burn. These injuries are usually minor compared with the potential for trauma from whatever caused the flash.

Manage thermal burns mostly the same as you would manage any other burn. Stop the burning source, cool the burned area if appropriate, and remove all jewelry. Maintain a high index of suspicion for inhalation injuries. Increased exposure time will increase damage to the patient. The larger the burn, the more likely the patient will be susceptible to hypothermia and/or hypovolemia. All patients with large surface burns should have dry dressings (sterile, if possible) applied to the burned areas to help maintain body temperature, prevent infection, and provide comfort.

Inhalation Burns

Inhalation injuries can occur when burning takes place in enclosed spaces without ventilation. When the upper airway is exposed to excessive heat, the patient can experience rapid and serious airway compromise. The heat can be an irritant to the lungs and the airway, causing coughing, wheezing, and rapid swelling or edema of the mucosa of the upper airway tissues, often evidenced first by hoarseness; as swelling increases, stridor may be heard. Upper airway damage is often associated with the inhalation of superheated gases. Lower airway damage is more often associated with the inhalation of chemicals (eg, acids, aldehydes) and particulate matter. When treating a patient for inhalation injuries, you may encounter severe upper airway swelling that requires immediate intervention. Sometimes airway swelling and compromise will develop more slowly and not manifest until transport. You should consider requesting ALS backup if the patient has signs or symptoms of edema, such as stridor, a hoarse voice, singed nasal hairs, singed facial hairs, burns of the face, or carbon particles in the sputum. Alternatively, expediting transport to the nearest ED capable of advanced airway management should be considered if it would be faster than waiting for ALS

> **Words of Wisdom**
>
> Burns of 20% of TBSA or more will likely require IV fluid resuscitation. Burns of 30% of TBSA or more (less than 15% in older adults) may be fatal without appropriate treatment. Inhalation injury can double the risk of death from a burn injury.

arrival at the scene. Remember that these patients can deteriorate quickly. Administer humidified oxygen (if available) until additional ALS interventions are available.

Inhalation of Toxic Gases

The combustion process produces a variety of toxic gases. The less efficient the combustion process, the more toxic the gases (eg, carbon monoxide, cyanide) that may be created. Whenever a patient has inhaled smoke or hot air from a fire, consider the possibility that they also inhaled carbon monoxide or cyanide. Chapter 22, *Toxicology*, discusses these situations in greater depth.

Chemical Burns

A chemical burn can occur whenever a toxic substance contacts the body. Most chemical burns are caused by strong acids or strong alkalis. The eyes are particularly vulnerable to chemical burns (**FIGURE 26-22**). Sometimes the fumes alone from strong chemicals can cause burns, especially to the respiratory tract. The severity of the burn is directly related to the type of chemical, the concentration of the chemical, and the duration of the exposure.

In cases of severe chemical burns or exposure, consider mobilizing a hazardous materials (hazmat) team, if appropriate. To prevent exposure to hazardous materials, determine if you can safely approach the patient. In some cases, you will need to wait to provide care until hazmat technicians have decontaminated the patient. You must wear the appropriate chemical-resistant gloves and eye protection whenever you are caring for a patient with a chemical burn. Be particularly careful not to get any chemical, dry or liquid, on yourself or on your uniform; consider wearing a protective gown when this is a possibility. Remember that exposure risk is also present when you are cleaning up after a call.

Treatment of chemical burns can be specific to the chemical agent. If available, read all of the labels of the chemical agent. Do not risk exposure while attempting to gather information on the chemical. If the exposure occurs at an industrial site, such as a chemical manufacturing plant, an expert should be on site and should be able to provide you with valuable information about the chemical. You may also contact a poison control center for advice.

The emergency care of a chemical burn is basically the same as that for a thermal burn, discussed earlier in the chapter. The severity of the burn will depend on the type of chemical, its strength, the duration of exposure, and the area of the body exposed. To stop the burning process, remove any chemical from the patient. A dry chemical that is activated by contact with water may damage the skin more when it is wet than when it is dry. Therefore, always brush off dry chemicals from the skin and clothing before flushing the patient with water (**FIGURE 26-23**). Remove the patient's clothing,

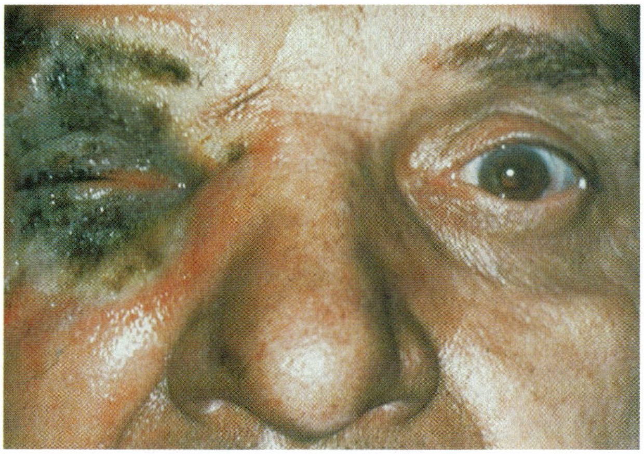

FIGURE 26-22 The eyes are particularly vulnerable to chemical burns.

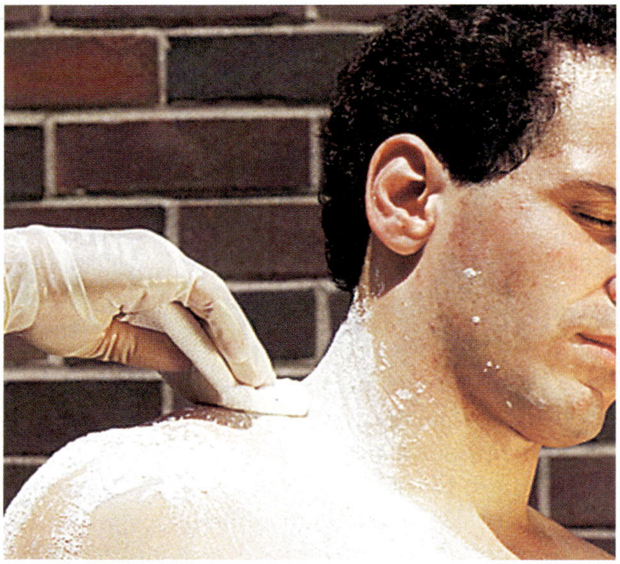

FIGURE 26-23 Brush off dry chemicals before you flush the burned area with water.

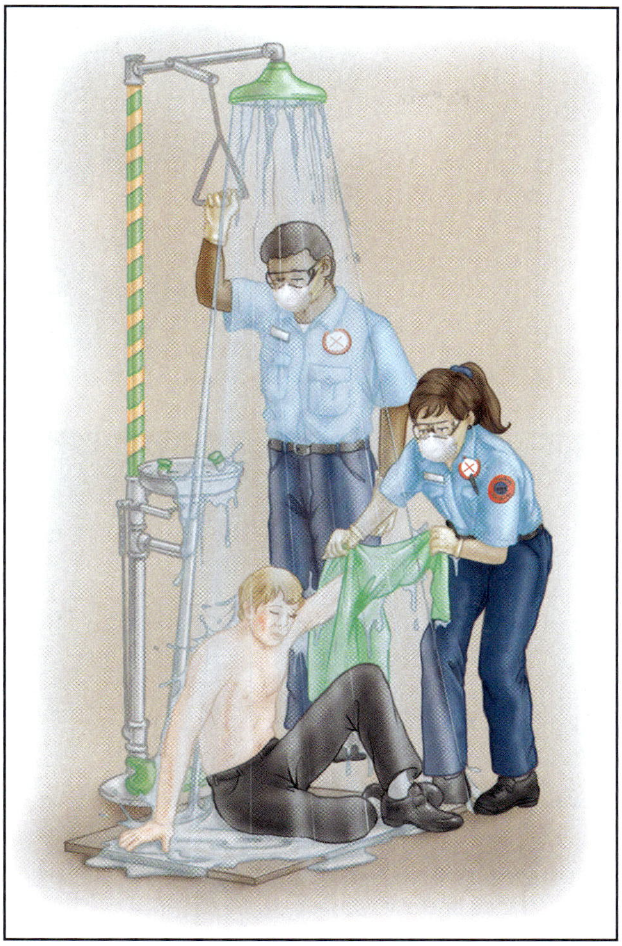

FIGURE 26-24 Flush the burned area with large amounts of water for 15 to 20 minutes after the patient says that the burning pain has stopped. Avoid contaminating uninjured areas.

including shoes, stockings, gloves, and any jewelry or eyeglasses, because there may be small amounts of chemicals in the creases. Take great care to ensure you do not come in contact with the chemical. The patient should be properly decontaminated by properly trained personnel.

For liquid chemicals, immediately flush the burned area with large amounts of water (**FIGURE 26-24**). Take care not to contaminate uninjured areas or make the patient hypothermic. Never direct a forceful stream of water from a hose at the patient; the extreme water pressure may mechanically injure the burned skin. Continue flooding the area with gallons of water for 15 to 20 minutes after the patient says the burning pain has stopped. If the patient's eye has been burned, hold the eyelid open

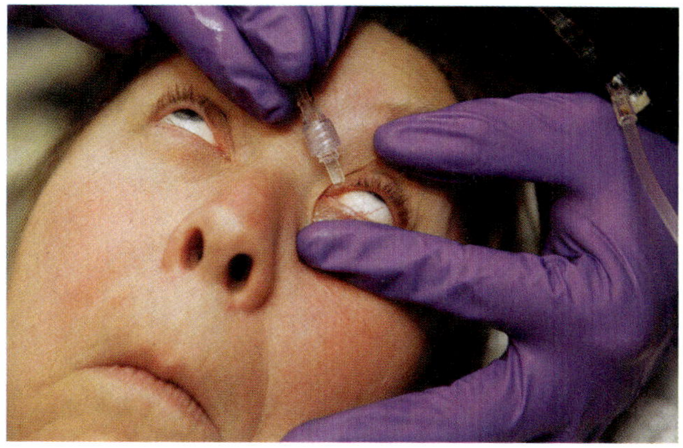

FIGURE 26-25 Flood the affected eye with a gentle stream of water. Hold the eyelids open, a challenging task because the patient's reflex is to keep the eye shut. Take care to prevent any of the chemical from getting into the other eye during flushing.

(without applying pressure over the globe of the eye) while flooding the eye with a gentle stream of water or normal saline (**FIGURE 26-25**). Flush the eyes from the inside corners to the outside to prevent cross contamination. If only one eye has been affected, turn the patient's head to that side and flush. If both eyes are affected, consider hooking up a nasal cannula to a bag of saline to flush both eyes simultaneously. The prongs can be placed on the bridge of the nose to flush from the inside corners of the eyes to the outside corners. Be careful not to touch the prongs to the eye or surrounding tissue. Continue flushing the contaminated area en route to the hospital. As much as 5 L of fluid may be needed.[7]

As with any substance, once the fluid has been contaminated with the chemical, collect it and properly dispose of it. Conduct a proper decontamination prior to loading any patient into the ambulance and again prior to entering a hospital.

Words of Wisdom

You should suspect possible internal injuries from chemical ingestion when you see a child who has burns, particularly around the face and mouth.

Electrical Burns

Electrical burns may be the result of contact with high- or low-voltage electricity. High-voltage burns

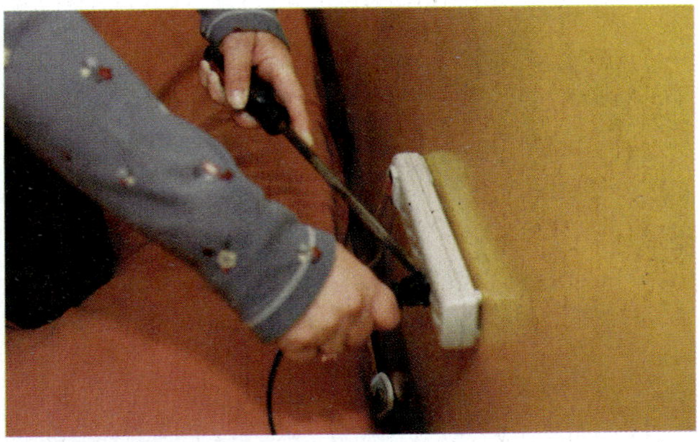

FIGURE 26-26 The human body is a good conductor of electricity. An electrical burn usually occurs when the body, acting as a conductor, completes a circuit.

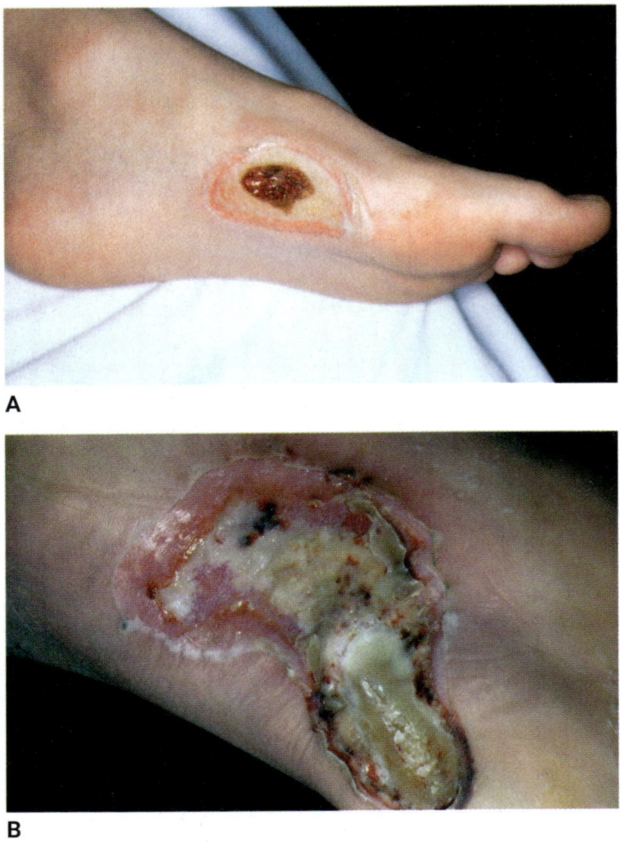

FIGURE 26-27 Electrical burns, like gunshot wounds, have entrance and exit wounds. **A.** An entrance wound is often quite small. **B.** The exit wound can be extensive and deep.

may occur when utility workers make direct contact with power lines. Ordinary household current is still powerful enough to cause severe burns as well as cardiac dysrhythmias.

There must be a complete circuit between the electrical source and the ground for electricity to flow. Any substance that prevents this circuit from being completed, such as rubber, is called an insulator. Any substance that allows a current to flow through it is called a conductor. The human body, which is primarily water, is a good conductor. Thus, electrical burns occur when the body, or a part of it, completes a circuit connecting a power source to the ground (**FIGURE 26-26**).

The type of electric current, magnitude of current (amperage), and voltage have effects on the seriousness of burns. When an electric current enters the body, the skin is burned at the entrance wound as well as everywhere along the path until the current grounds and exits the body. In addition to tissues damaged by the heat, significant chemical changes take place in the nervous, cardiovascular, and muscular systems of the body, causing disruption of the body's normal functions and/or even system failure.

Your safety is particularly important when you are called to the scene of an emergency involving electricity. Obviously, you can be fatally injured by coming into contact with power lines. But you can also be fatally injured by touching a patient who is still in contact with a live power line or any other electrical source. For this reason, never attempt to remove someone from an electrical source unless you are specially trained to do so. Likewise, never move a downed power line unless you have the special training and equipment necessary for the job. Before even approaching someone who may still be in contact with a power line or an electrical appliance, make certain the power is turned off. Always assume that any downed power line is live.

A burn injury appears where the electricity enters (an entrance wound) and exits (an exit wound) the body. The entrance wound may be quite small (**FIGURE 26-27A**), but the exit wound can be extensive and deep (**FIGURE 26-27B**). Always look for both entrance and exit wounds. There are two dangers specifically associated with electrical burns. First, there may be a large amount of deep tissue injury. Electrical burns are often more severe than the external signs indicate. The patient may have only a small burn to the skin but may have massive damage to the deeper tissues, organs, and the nervous

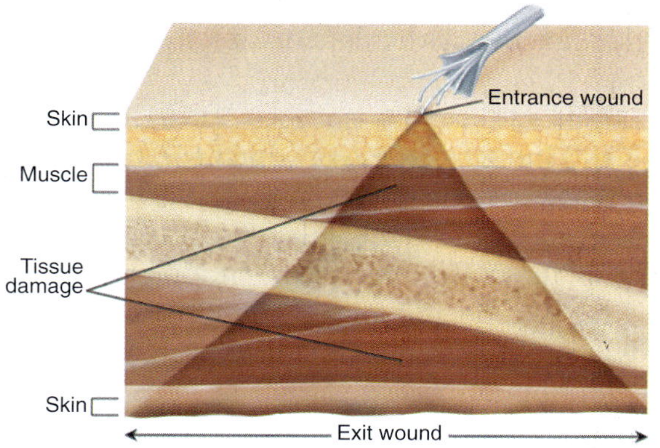

FIGURE 26-28 External signs of an electrical burn may be deceiving. The entrance wound may be a small burn, whereas the damage to deeper tissue may be massive.

system (**FIGURE 26-28**). The force of the electrical energy can also cause fractures or joint dislocations. Second, the patient may go into cardiac or respiratory arrest from the electric shock.

Electrical current can cross the chest and cause cardiac arrest or dysrhythmias. Cardiac arrest can also occur after a lightning strike, which is a form of an electrical burn. If indicated, begin CPR on the patient and apply the AED. Although CPR may need to be quite prolonged in patients with electrical burns, it has a high success rate if started promptly. Be prepared to defibrillate, if necessary. If neither CPR nor defibrillation is indicated, give supplemental oxygen if needed to maintain an oxygen saturation level between 94% and 98%, and monitor the patient closely for respiratory and cardiac arrest. Treat the soft-tissue injuries by placing dry, sterile dressings on all burn wounds and splinting suspected fractures. Assess for other trauma if the patient was thrown from the electrical contact point after the electrical shock. Provide prompt transport; all electrical burns are potentially severe injuries that require further treatment in the hospital. Monitor pulse, movement, and sensation in burned extremities; signs of compartment syndrome may develop. Report as many details as possible regarding the electrical source to the receiving hospital.

Radiation Burns

Acute radiation exposure has become more than a theoretical issue because the use of radioactive materials has increased in industry and medicine; therefore, you must understand it to effectively treat patients exposed to radiation. Potential threats include incidents related to the use and transportation of radioactive isotopes and intentionally released radioactivity in terrorist attacks. To be effective, first determine if there has been a radiation exposure, and then determine whether ongoing exposure continues to exist. Increasingly, special response units are equipped with pager-size radiation detectors, or such detection devices may be provided by other public safety services.

There are three types of ionizing radiation: alpha, beta, and gamma. Alpha particles have little penetrating energy and are easily stopped by the skin. Beta particles have greater penetrating power and can travel much farther in air than alpha particles. They can penetrate the skin but can be blocked by simple protective clothing designed for this purpose. The threat from gamma radiation is directly proportional to its wavelength. This type of radiation is highly penetrating and easily passes through the body and solid materials.

Radiation is measured in units of radiation absorbed dose (rad), the amount of radiation absorbed by an object or person, where 100 rad = 1 gray (Gy). The radiation equivalent man (rem) unit is used to account for the effects of different types of radiation on human tissue.[9] Small amounts of everyday background radiation are measured in rad; the amount of radiation released in a major incident may be measured in gray. The average human exposure from background radiation is 0.31 rem per year. Mild radiation sickness can be expected with exposures of 1 to 2 Gy (100 to 200 rad), moderate sickness at 2 to 5 Gy, and severe sickness at 4 to 6 Gy. Exposure to more than 10 Gy may result in death within 2 to 4 weeks.

Most ionizing radiation accidents involve gamma radiation, or x-rays. People who have been

Words of Wisdom

Know the "Five Ps of compartment syndrome": Pain, Pulselessness; Pallor, Paresthesia, and Paralysis. Do not wait for all five signs and symptoms to appear, as some of them are late findings. Pain and paresthesia (tingling) occur early, whereas pulselessness, pallor, and paralysis are late findings.

exposed to radiation generally do not pose a risk to the people around them. However, in some types of incidents, particularly those involving explosions, patients may be contaminated with radioactive particulate matter. It is speculated that after a nuclear explosion, most patients will have sustained some type of trauma in addition to the radiation exposure.

Being exposed to a radiation source does not make a patient contaminated or radioactive. However, when patients have a radioactive source on their body (such as debris from a bomb that dispersed radioactive material), they are contaminated and must be initially cared for by a hazmat responder. Maintain a safe distance and wait for the hazmat team to decontaminate the patient before initiating care. Once decontaminated by the hazmat team, care is often transferred to the EMT. Most contaminants can be removed by simply removing the patient's clothes. Call for additional resources to manage this situation. Once the patient is decontaminated and there is no threat to you, begin treating the ABCs and treat the patient for any burns or trauma.

Irrigate open wounds. Washing should be gentle to avoid further damage to the skin, which could result in additional internal radiation absorption. Irrigate the head and scalp the same way. The ED should be notified as soon as practical if you are transporting a potentially contaminated patient. In contrast with other types of contamination, radioactive particulate matter probably poses a relatively small risk to the clinician. Consider providing basic care to the patient before decontamination if you are wearing protective clothing.

Increasing your and the patient's distance from the source by even a few feet may dramatically decrease your exposure. One law of physics, the inverse square law, states that doubling the distance from the radiation source reduces the source's intensity by one-fourth of its original strength. Therefore, it is important to identify the radioactive source and the length of the patient's exposure to it, if this information is available without putting you or your patient at risk for exposure. If not readily available, rely on the hazmat team to obtain this information. Limit your duration of exposure, increase your distance from the source, and attempt to place shielding between yourself and sources of gamma radiation.

With contact radiation burns, decontaminate the wound as if it were a chemical burn to remove any radioactive particulate matter, then treat it as a burn.

Many radioactive isotopes are used in medicine and industry, some of which can be absorbed or have their toxic effects blunted by another substance. Like their radioactive effects, the toxic effects of these isotopes vary. Antidotes may help bind an isotope, enhance its elimination from the body, or reduce the toxic effects on other organs. Such antidotal therapy should be considered only under the guidance of a knowledgeable physician or public health agency.

Dressing and Bandaging

All wounds require bandaging. In most instances, splints help to control bleeding and provide firm support for the dressing. There are many different types of dressings and bandages (**FIGURE 26-29**). You should be familiar with the function and proper application of each.

In general, dressings and bandages have three primary functions:

- To control bleeding
- To protect the wound from further damage
- To prevent further contamination and infection

Sterile Dressings

Universal dressings, conventional 4 × 4–inch (10 × 10–cm) and 4 × 8–inch (10 × 20–cm) gauze pads, and assorted small adhesive-type dressings and soft self-adherent roller dressings will cover most wounds. The universal dressing measures 9 × 36 inches (23 × 91 cm), is made of thick, absorbent material, and is ideal for covering large open wounds. It also makes an efficient pad for rigid splints. These dressings are available in compact, commercially sterilized packages.

Gauze pads are appropriate for smaller wounds, and adhesive-type dressings are useful for minor wounds. Hemostatic gauze contains a chemical agent that speeds up blood clotting. An **occlusive dressing**, made of petroleum jelly–based (Vaseline) gauze, aluminum foil, or plastic, prevents air and liquids from entering (or exiting) the wound. These

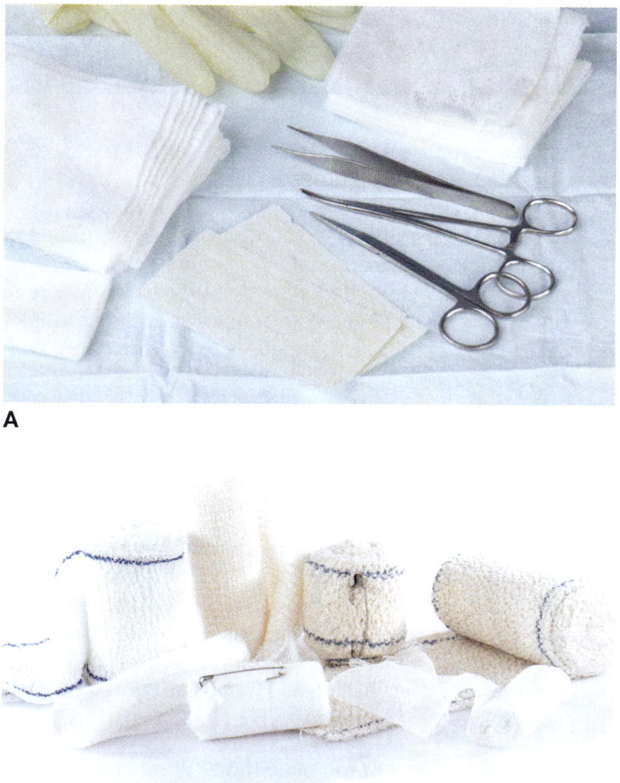

A

B

FIGURE 26-29 A. Many types of sterile dressings are used for covering open wounds, including universal dressings, gauze pads, adhesive dressings, and occlusive dressings. **B.** Bandages keep dressings in place and include soft roller bandages, triangular bandages, and adhesive tape. Splints may also be used to hold dressings in place.

dressings are used to cover sucking chest wounds, abdominal eviscerations, penetrating back wounds, and neck injuries.

Bandages

To keep dressings in place during transport, you can use soft roller bandages, rolls of gauze, triangular bandages, or adhesive tape. The self-adherent, soft roller bandages are probably easiest to use. They are slightly elastic, which makes them easy to apply, and you can tuck the end of the roll into a deeper layer to secure it in place. The layers adhere somewhat but should not be applied too tightly to one another.

Adhesive tape holds small dressings in place and helps secure larger dressings. Some people, however, are allergic to adhesive tape. If you know your patient is allergic, use paper or plastic tape instead.

Do not use elastic bandages to secure dressings. If the injury swells, the bandage may become a tourniquet and cause further damage. Any improperly applied bandage that impairs circulation can result in additional tissue damage or even the loss of a limb. Always check a limb distal to a bandage for signs of impaired circulation and loss of sensation. Air splints and vacuum splints are useful in stabilizing broken extremities, and they can be used with dressings to help control bleeding from soft-tissue injuries.

If a wound continues to bleed vigorously despite the use of direct pressure, quickly use a tourniquet. Use of a tourniquet is rarely harmful. If you cannot control bleeding from a major vessel in an extremity, a properly applied tourniquet may save a patient's life. Specifically, the tourniquet is useful if a patient is bleeding severely from any limb injury. Furthermore, the tourniquet is most effective as a lifesaving measure if applied prior to the onset of shock from blood loss. Tourniquets are discussed further in Chapter 25, *Bleeding*.

ALS Assist

Calls involving burns may require several ALS procedures. You can assist your ALS partner by being familiar with the setup of IV lines, cardiac monitors, and the equipment necessary to establish an advanced airway.

YOU are the EMT SUMMARY

1. What should be your most immediate priority?

As with any patient, your first priority is to prevent further harm. Although the patient was brought to you wrapped in a blanket, this does not mean that his skin or clothing have stopped burning. First, remove the blanket to ensure that his clothes are not smoldering and that the burning process has stopped.

If the patient's clothes are still smoldering or if there is any other evidence to indicate the burning process is ongoing, pour room-temperature sterile water or saline over the affected areas. Doing so not only stops the burning process, but also helps relieve pain. If the burning process has stopped, do not apply any water, saline, or dressings until you further assess the patient.

Once you have stopped the burning process, airway and breathing assessment is essential, as the soot on the patient's face indicates a strong risk of smoke or toxic gas inhalation or potential airway injury from inhaling heated air.

2. What is a thermal burn? What are the causes of thermal burns?

A thermal burn is a burn caused by heat, as opposed to radiation, chemicals, or electricity; however, many different situations can cause thermal burns.

Most commonly, thermal burns are caused by an open flame (flame burn), but thermal burns can result whenever the skin is exposed to temperatures higher than 111°F (44°C), which can occur even from prolonged exposure to sunlight. In general, the severity of a thermal burn correlates directly with the temperature of the heat source, the amount of heat energy possessed by the object or substance, and the duration of exposure.

Sources of heat energy other than fire include scald burns, which occur from exposure to boiling liquids; contact burns, which occur when a person comes in contact with a heated surface; steam burns, which occur when the body is exposed to superheated gaseous water; and flash burns, which occur when a person is briefly exposed to very intense heat (eg, explosion).

3. What additional information should you obtain from the firefighters who rescued the patient?

It has already been established that the patient was trapped in an enclosed space, because the firefighters rescued him from the structure. However, you should determine an approximate length of exposure; this is usually a gross estimate at best.

Determine if the patient was conscious or unconscious when he was found. Conscious patients are often able to extinguish themselves unless they are completely engulfed in flames. Patients who are unconscious, however, do not have control over the duration of exposure to the fire itself or the quantity of superheated air that they inhale.

Determine how the patient was found. For example, was the patient in an open area of a room or trapped beneath a collapsed ceiling beam or other heavy structure? Although you should always assess the patient for traumatic injuries, information provided by the firefighters regarding any MOI can help you focus on a particular area (or areas) of the body. Do not assume the patient's injuries are limited to skin burns and toxic gas exposure; the patient may have experienced other injuries (eg, blunt trauma with internal bleeding, head injury) that could also be life threatening.

4. How are thermal burns classified? What are the characteristics of each type of burn?

Burns are classified according to their depth—that is, how far the burn injury extends through the layers of the skin (ie, epidermis, dermis). The types of burns you must be able to identify are superficial, partial-thickness (superficial and deep), and full-thickness.

Superficial burns involve only the outer layer of the skin (the epidermis). The skin turns red and is often painful, but it does not blister or the burn does not extend below the epidermis.

Superficial partial-thickness burns involve the epidermis and some portion of the dermis. These burns do not destroy the entire thickness of the skin, nor is the subcutaneous (fatty) tissue injured. Usually these burns are very painful and have blisters that may or may not be intact. Deep partial-thickness burns have destroyed more of the dermis and its accessory structures. The skin is often dryer and the area less painful than with superficial partial-thickness burns.

Full-thickness burns extend through all layers of the dermis and epidermis and may involve the subcutaneous skin layers, muscle, bone, or internal organs. The burned area may appear dry and leathery and may appear white, dark brown, or even charred. However, because the nerve endings in the dermis have been destroyed, the areas of full-thickness burn are painless.

YOU are the EMT SUMMARY continued

5. What percentage of the patient's body surface area has been burned?

After you identify the depth of a burn, you must rapidly estimate the extent of the burns (ie, the percentage of the patient's TBSA that is burned). Your patient has experienced burns to the anterior torso (chest and abdomen); this represents 18% of TBSA. Additionally, both upper extremities are burned, which represents 18% (9% per extremity) of TBSA. Therefore, *your patient has burns that cover approximately 36% of the TBSA*.

6. What factors should you consider to determine the severity of a burn?

When determining the severity of a burn, the two most important factors to consider initially are the depth and extent of the burn. In addition to the depth and extent of the burn, you must determine if the burns are located in any critical areas of the body. Critical areas of the body include the face, hands, genitalia, feet, perineum, or over any joints. Also, airway burns or circumferential burns (ie, burns that completely go around an extremity) are considered critical burns. Circumferential burns can cause compartment syndrome, with the edema compressing and decreasing blood flow distal to the burn, or if they go around the chest can cause decreased chest expansion and diminished ventilation. The same burn that this patient has would be considered critical in infants, children 14 years or younger, or older adults. Additional trauma or other comorbidities may also elevate the patient's severity and need for immediate consultation and consideration for transfer to a burn center.

7. What is the proper treatment for the patient's burns?

Large (greater than 10% of TBSA) burns should be covered with a dry, sterile, nonadherent dressing or a clean sheet; ***your patient has burns that cover approximately 36% of TBSA***. Other than for the purpose of stopping the burning process, do not apply water or saline to large surface area burns. The larger the burn area, the greater the risks of hypothermia, hypovolemia, and infection.

Dry, sterile dressings applied to large surface area burns help maintain body temperature (reduce the risk of hypothermia), prevent further contamination of the burn (reduce the risk of infection), and provide comfort.

Use further treatment to prevent hypothermia (cover the patient with a blanket); closely monitor the patient's airway and ventilation status and monitor for signs of shock. An ALS clinician, if available, can provide pain management and treat complications such as airway swelling.

8. How has the patient's condition changed? What should you do now?

The patient's breathing is becoming labored. Respiratory distress in a patient with a burn, especially in a patient without other injuries that would cause breathing difficulties (eg, blunt chest trauma), indicates upper airway swelling secondary to inhaling excessive heat (inhalation injury).

Patients who are trapped in an enclosed space with poor ventilation, especially if they have a loss of consciousness, are at highest risk for an inhalation injury. Although your patient denies a loss of consciousness, you should still suspect some degree of upper airway swelling because he was in an enclosed space.

If the patient is breathing adequately, continue to administer high-flow oxygen and closely observe the patient. Cool mist or aerosol therapy may help reduce mild airway swelling. If the patient is not breathing adequately (eg, shallow breathing [reduced tidal volume], labored respirations, falling oxygen saturation, decreasing level of consciousness), assist ventilations with a bag-mask device.

Depending on your transport time to the closest appropriate hospital and the availability of ALS resources in your area, you should consider an intercept with an ALS unit. Some patients with inhalation injuries require advanced airway management, such as endotracheal intubation, to protect the airway before it closes completely.

9. What, if any, additional treatment is indicated for this patient?

Continuous, careful monitoring of this patient is essential. Although the patient's condition does not seem to have worsened, it also has not improved. Continue to administer high-flow oxygen, closely monitor the adequacy of breathing, and be prepared to assist ventilations. Monitor him for altered mental status and signs of shock and treat accordingly.

Any patient who is experiencing respiratory distress will be anxious. Provide emotional support and let the patient assume a position of comfort; this is usually a full Fowler (90° angle) position.

Prep Kit

Ready for Review

- The skin protects the body by keeping pathogens out and water in and assisting in body temperature regulation.
- There are three types of soft-tissue injuries:
  - Closed injuries (Soft-tissue damage occurs beneath the skin or mucous membrane but the surface remains intact.)
  - Open injuries (There is a break in the surface of the skin or the mucous membrane, exposing deeper tissue to potential contamination.)
  - Burns (The soft tissue receives more energy than it can absorb without injury; the source of this energy can be thermal, toxic chemicals, electricity, or radiation.)
- Closed soft-tissue injuries are characterized by a history of blunt trauma, pain at the site of injury, swelling beneath the skin, and discoloration. Contusions, hematomas, and crush injuries are classified as closed injuries. Treat a closed soft-tissue injury by applying the mnemonic RICES: Rest, Ice, Compression, Elevation, and Splinting.
- Open injuries differ from closed injuries in that the protective layer of skin is damaged. Abrasions, lacerations, avulsions, and penetrating wounds are classified as open injuries. Treat an open soft-tissue injury by applying direct pressure with a sterile bandage using a roller bandage, and splint the extremity. Use a tourniquet when necessary to control bleeding.
- It is generally easier to assess an open injury than it is to assess a closed injury because you can see the injury.
- Small animal and human bites can lead to serious infection and must be evaluated by a physician. Small animals can carry rabies.
- Burns are serious and painful soft-tissue injuries caused by heat (thermal), chemicals, electricity, and radiation.
- Burn severity is assessed primarily by the depth and extent of the burn injury and the body area involved.
- Burns are considered to be superficial, superficial partial-thickness, deep partial-thickness, or full-thickness based on the depth of tissue involved. Superficial burns are not included in the calculation of total body surface area burned.
- When treating older adults, pediatric patients, or special needs patients with burns, be alert for the possibility of physical abuse.
- When providing emergency care for burns, do the following:
  - Take standard precautions to protect yourself from potentially contaminated body fluid and to protect the patient from potential infection.
  - Cool the burned area to prevent further cellular damage.
  - Remove jewelry and constrictive clothing; never attempt to remove any synthetic material that may have melted into the burned skin.
  - Ensure an open and clear airway, provide high-flow oxygen, and be alert to signs and symptoms of inhalation injury such as difficulty breathing, stridor, or wheezing.
  - Place sterile dressings over the burn areas; to prevent hypothermia, cover the patient with a clean blanket. Provide prompt transport.
- Dressings and bandages are designed to control bleeding, protect the wound from further damage, prevent further contamination, and prevent infection.

Vital Vocabulary

abrasion Loss or damage of the superficial layer of skin as a result of a body part rubbing or scraping across a rough or hard surface.

amputation An injury in which part of the body is completely severed.

Prep Kit continued

avulsion An injury in which soft tissue is torn completely loose or is hanging as a flap.

burns Injuries in which soft-tissue damage occurs as a result of thermal heat, frictional heat, toxic chemicals, electricity, or nuclear radiation.

circumferential burns Burns that go completely around a body part, such as an arm, a foot, or the chest.

closed injuries Injuries in which damage occurs beneath the skin or mucous membrane but the surface of the skin remains intact.

compartment syndrome Swelling in a confined space that produces dangerous pressure; may cut off blood flow or damage sensitive tissue.

contact burn A burn caused by direct contact with a hot object.

contamination The presence of infective organisms or foreign bodies such as dirt, gravel, or metal.

contusion A bruise from an injury that causes bleeding beneath the skin without breaking the skin.

crush injury An injury that occurs when a great amount of force is applied to the body.

crush syndrome Significant metabolic derangement that develops when crushed extremities or body parts remain trapped for prolonged periods. This can lead to kidney failure and death.

deep partial-thickness burns Burns that extend deeper into the dermis, destroying more of the blood vessels. They appear lighter in color than superficial partial-thickness burns and are dryer and less painful. Partial-thickness burns are also referred to as second-degree burns.

dermis The inner layer of the skin, containing hair follicles, sweat glands, nerve endings, and blood vessels.

ecchymosis A buildup of blood beneath the skin that produces a characteristic blue or black discoloration as the result of an injury.

epidermis The outer layer of skin, which is made up of cells that are sealed together to form a watertight protective covering for the body.

evisceration The displacement of organs outside the body.

fascia The fiber-like connective tissue that covers arteries, veins, tendons, and ligaments.

flame burn A burn caused by an open flame.

flash burn A burn caused by exposure to very intense heat, such as in an explosion.

full-thickness burns Burns that affect all skin layers and may affect the subcutaneous layers, muscle, bone, and internal organs, leaving the area dry, leathery, and white, dark brown, or charred; often referred to as third-degree burns.

hematoma A mass of blood that has collected within damaged tissue beneath the skin or in a body cavity.

impaled objects Objects that penetrate the skin but remain in place.

incision A sharp, smooth cut in the skin.

laceration A deep, jagged cut in the skin.

mucous membranes The linings of body cavities and passages that communicate directly or indirectly with the environment outside the body.

occlusive dressing An airtight dressing that protects a wound from air and bacteria; a commercial vented version allows air to passively escape from the chest, while an unvented dressing may be made of petroleum jelly–based (Vaseline) gauze, aluminum foil, or plastic.

open injuries Injuries in which there is a break in the surface of the skin or the mucous membrane, exposing deeper tissue to potential contamination.

penetrating wound An injury resulting from a sharp, piercing object.

rabid Infected with the rabies virus.

rule of nines A system that assigns percentages to sections of the body, allowing calculation of the amount of skin surface involved in the burn area.

scald burn A burn caused by hot liquids.

steam burn A burn caused by exposure to hot steam.

Prep Kit continued

superficial burns Burns that affect only the epidermis, characterized by skin that is red/darker but not blistered or actually burned through; also referred to as first-degree burns.

superficial partial-thickness burns Burns that affect the epidermis and some portion of the dermis but not the subcutaneous tissue, characterized by blisters and skin that is discolored (ranging from lighter to red/darker compared to baseline skin color), moist, and mottled. Partial-thickness burns are also referred to as second-degree burns.

thermal burn A burn caused by heat.

References

1. National Association of State EMS Officials. *National Model EMS Clinical Guidelines: Version 3.0.* https://nasemso.org/content.aspx?page_id=22&club_id=157064&module_id=701974. Updated March 2022. Accessed February 25, 2025.
2. Hadeed A, Anthony JH, Hoffler CE. Hand high pressure injury. *StatPearls*. National Library of Medicine website. https://www.ncbi.nlm.nih.gov/books/NBK542210/. Updated June 26, 2023. Accessed February 25, 2025.
3. Rodgers GL, Mortensen J, Fisher MC, Lo A, Cresswell A, Long SS. Predictors of infectious complications after burn injuries in children. *Pediatr Infect Dis J*. 2000;19(10):990–995.
4. Guidelines for burn patient referral. American Burn Association website. https://ameriburn.org/wp-content/uploads/2024/04/one-page-guidelines-for-burn-patient-referral-1.pdf. Published 2022. Accessed February 25, 2025.
5. Hamza Hermis A, Tehrany PM, Hosseini SJ, et al. Prevalence of non-accidental burns and related factors in children: a systematic review and meta-analysis. *Int Wound J*. 2023;20(9):3855–3870.
6. Lafferty KA. Smoke inhalation injury. Medscape website. https://emedicine.medscape.com/article/771194-overview?form=fpf. Updated October 15, 2021. Accessed February 25, 2025.
7. National Association of Emergency Medical Technicians. *PHTLS: Prehospital Trauma Life Support*. 10th ed. Burlington, MA: Jones & Bartlett Learning; 2023.
8. Schaefer TJ, Szymanski KD. Burn evaluation and management. *StatPearls*. National Library of Medicine website. https://www.ncbi.nlm.nih.gov/books/NBK430741/. Updated August 8, 2023. Accessed February 25, 2025.
9. Measuring radiation. US Nuclear Regulatory Commission website. https://www.nrc.gov/about-nrc/radiation/health-effects/measuring-radiation.html. Updated March 20, 2020. Accessed April 10, 2025.

Additional Resources

Emergency medical services. US Fire Administration website. https://www.usfa.fema.gov/ems/. Reviewed November 26, 2024. Accessed February 25, 2025.

Statistics. US Fire Administration website. https://www.usfa.fema.gov/statistics/. Reviewed February 18, 2025. Accessed February 25, 2025.

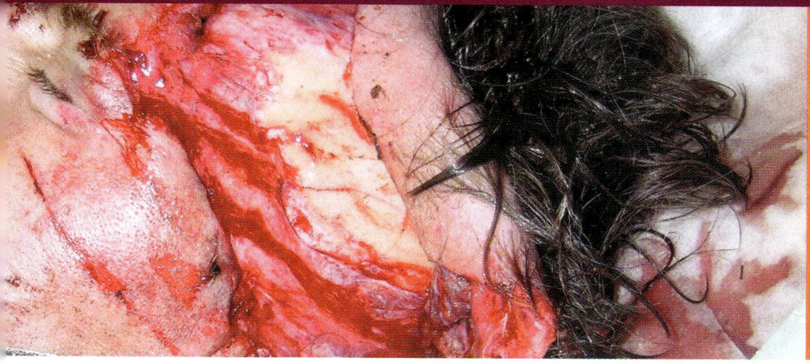

Chapter 27

Face and Neck Injuries

NATIONAL EMS EDUCATION STANDARD COMPETENCIES

Medicine

Applies knowledge to provide basic emergency care and transportation based on assessment findings for an acutely ill patient.

Diseases of the Eyes, Ears, Nose, and Throat

- Epistaxis (pp 1020–1021)

Trauma

Applies knowledge to provide basic emergency care and transportation based on assessment findings for an acutely injured patient.

Head, Facial, Neck, and Spine Trauma

- Life threats (pp 1017–1019, 1025–1026)
- Spine trauma (Chapter 28, *Head and Spine Injuries*)
- Penetrating neck trauma (pp 1003–1004, 1025–1026)
- Laryngotracheal injuries (p 1025)
- Shaken baby syndrome (Chapter 35, *Patients With Special Challenges*)
- Facial fractures (pp 1003–1004)
- Skull fractures (Chapter 28, *Head and Spine Injuries*)
- Foreign bodies in the eyes (pp 1010–1014)
- Globe rupture (p 1018)
- Dental trauma (p 1024)
- Severe epistaxis (pp 1020–1021)

KNOWLEDGE OBJECTIVES

1. Describe the anatomy and physiology of the head, face, and neck; include major structures and specific important landmarks of which EMTs must be aware. (pp 1000–1003)
2. Describe the factors that may cause obstruction of the upper airway following a facial injury. (pp 1003–1004)
3. Discuss the different types of facial injuries and the patient care considerations related to each one. (pp 1003–1004)
4. Explain emergency medical care of a patient with soft-tissue wounds of the face and neck. (pp 1008–1009)
5. Explain the emergency medical care of a patient with an eye injury based on the following scenarios: foreign object, impaled object, burns, lacerations, blunt trauma, closed head injuries, and blast injuries. (pp 1010–1020)
6. Describe the three different causes of a burn injury to the eye and the patient care considerations related to each one. (pp 1014–1016)
7. Explain emergency medical care of a patient with injuries of the nose. (pp 1020–1021)
8. Explain the emergency medical care of a patient with injuries of the ear, including lacerations and foreign body insertions. (pp 1021–1022)
9. Explain the physical findings and emergency care of a patient with a facial fracture. (pp 1023–1024)

10. Explain the emergency medical care of the patient with dental and cheek injuries. (p 1024)
11. Explain the emergency medical care of a patient with an upper airway injury caused by blunt trauma. (pp 1025–1026)
12. Explain the emergency medical care of the patient with a penetrating injury to the neck. (pp 1025–1026)

SKILLS OBJECTIVES

1. Demonstrate the removal of a foreign object from under a patient's upper eyelid. (pp 1011–1012; Skill Drill 27-1)
2. Demonstrate the stabilization of a foreign object that has been impaled in a patient's eye. (p 1013; Skill Drill 27-2)
3. Demonstrate irrigation of a patient's eye using a nasal cannula, bottle, or basin. (pp 1014–1015)
4. Demonstrate the care of a patient who has a penetrating eye injury. (pp 1016–1017)
5. Demonstrate how to control bleeding from a neck injury. (p 1026; Skill Drill 27-3)

Introduction

The face and neck are particularly vulnerable to injury because of their relatively unprotected positions on the body. Soft-tissue injuries and fractures to the bones of the face are common and vary greatly in severity. Some are potentially life threatening, and many leave disfiguring scars if not treated properly. Penetrating trauma to the neck may cause severe bleeding or compromise the airway. An open injury may allow an air embolism to enter the circulatory system. If a hematoma forms in this area, it may stop or slow blood flow to the brain, causing permanent brain damage. Appropriate prehospital and hospital care can sometimes allow a seemingly devastating injury to result in a surprisingly good outcome.

As an EMT, your objectives when treating a patient with face and neck injuries include preventing further injury, particularly to the cervical spine; managing any acute airway problems; and controlling bleeding. This chapter first reviews the anatomy of the head and neck and then examines the factors that can produce upper airway obstruction. A discussion follows that includes emergency medical care of soft-tissue wounds of the face, nose, and ear; facial fractures; penetrating injuries of the neck; and dental injuries.

Anatomy and Physiology

The head is divided into two parts: the cranium and the face. The cranium, or skull, contains the brain, which connects to the spinal cord through the foramen magnum, a large opening at the base of the skull. The most posterior portion of the cranium is called the occiput. On each side of the cranium, the lateral portions are called the temples or temporal regions. Between the temporal regions and the occiput lie the parietal regions. The forehead is called the frontal region. Just anterior to the ear, in the temporal region, you can feel the pulse of the superficial temporal artery.

The face comprises the eyes, ears, nose, mouth, and cheeks. Its structure includes six major bones: the nasal bone, the two maxillae (upper jawbones), the two zygomas (cheekbones), and the mandible (lower jawbone) (**FIGURE 27-1**).

The orbit of the eye is composed of the lower edge of the frontal bone of the skull, the zygomas, the maxilla, and the nasal bone. The bony orbit

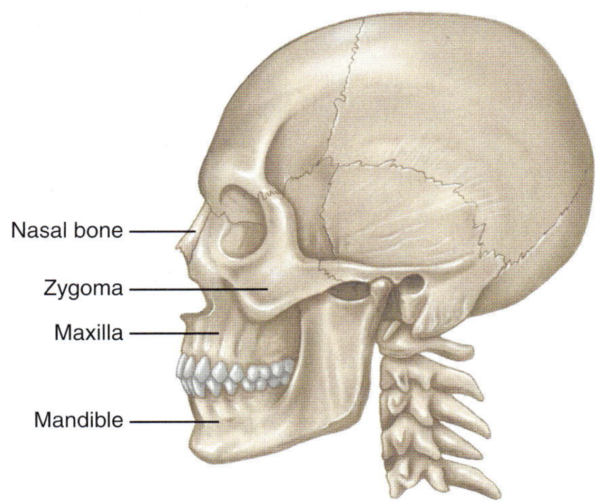

FIGURE 27-1 The face is composed of six bones: the nasal bone, two maxillae, two zygomas, and the mandible.

protects the eye from injury. By viewing the face from the side, you can see the eyeball recessed in the orbit. Only the proximal third of the nose (the bridge) is formed by bone. The remaining two-thirds is composed of cartilage.

The exposed portion of the ear is composed entirely of cartilage that is covered by skin. The external, visible part of the ear is called the pinna (**FIGURE 27-2**). The ear lobes are the fleshy portions at the bottom of each ear. The **tragus** is a small, rounded, fleshy bulge immediately anterior to the ear canal. The superficial temporal artery can be palpated just anterior to the tragus. Approximately 1 inch (2.5 cm) posterior to the external opening of the ear is a prominent bony mass at the base of the skull called the **mastoid process**.

The mandible forms the jaw and chin. The jaw is the lower border of the mouth, where the tongue and 32 teeth are located. Motion of the mandible occurs at the **temporomandibular joint**, which lies just in front of the ear on either side of the face. Below the ear and anterior to the mastoid process, the angle of the mandible is easily palpated.

The neck also contains many important structures. It is supported by the cervical spine, or the first seven vertebrae in the spinal column (C1 through C7). The spinal cord exits from the foramen magnum and lies within the spinal canal formed by the vertebrae. The upper part of the esophagus and the trachea lie in the midline of the neck. The carotid arteries are found on either side of the trachea, along with the jugular veins and several nerves.

Several useful landmarks can be palpated and seen in the neck (**FIGURE 27-3**). The most obvious is the firm prominence in the center of the anterior surface, commonly known as the Adam's apple. Specifically, this prominence is the upper part of the larynx, formed by the thyroid cartilage. It tends

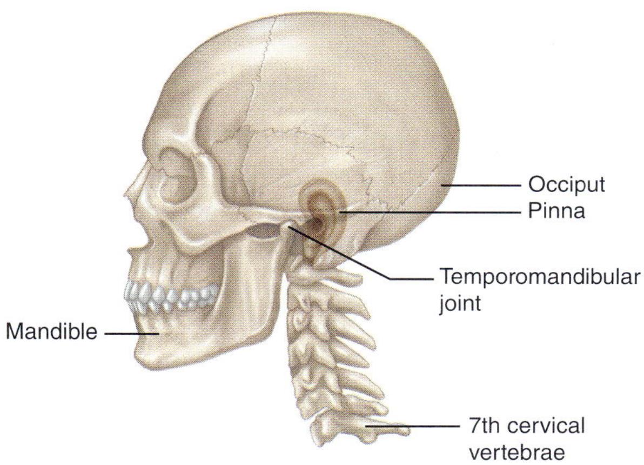

FIGURE 27-2 Specific landmarks of the head and neck include the pinna, the mandible, the occiput, the seventh cervical vertebra, and the temporomandibular joint.

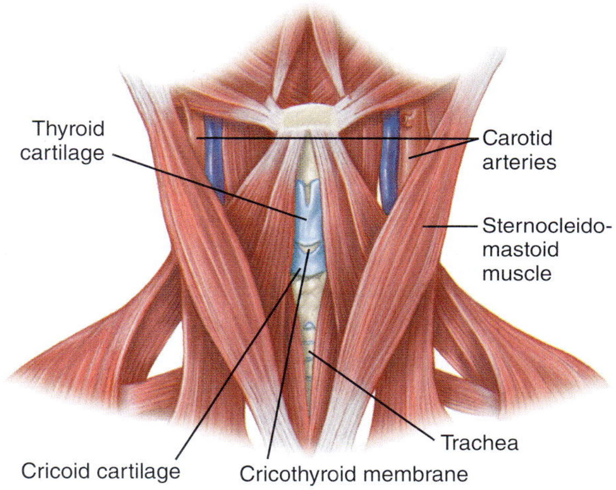

FIGURE 27-3 Important landmarks in the neck include the cricoid cartilage, the thyroid cartilage, the carotid arteries, the cricothyroid membrane, and the sternocleidomastoid muscles.

YOU are the EMT

At 1926 hours, you are dispatched to the parking lot of a convenience store at 1505 Eagle Rock Drive for a patient who was assaulted. You and your partner respond to the scene, which is located approximately 3 miles (4.8 km) away. Law enforcement personnel, who are on scene, advise you that the scene has been secured and that your patient, a young man, is conscious but has sustained severe trauma to his face.

1. What should be your most immediate concern after receiving this initial patient information?
2. What should your initial actions consist of when you arrive at the scene?

to be more prominent in men than in women. The other portion of the larynx is the cricoid cartilage, a firm ridge of cartilage (the only complete circular cartilage structure of the trachea) below the thyroid cartilage, which is somewhat more difficult to palpate. Between the thyroid cartilage and the cricoid cartilage in the midline of the neck is a soft depression, the cricothyroid membrane. This is a thin sheet of connective tissue (fascia) that joins the two cartilages (**FIGURE 27-4**). The cricothyroid membrane is covered at this point only by skin.

Below the larynx, several additional firm ridges are palpable in the anterior midline. These ridges are the cartilage rings of the trachea. The trachea connects the oropharynx and the larynx with the main air passages of the lungs (the bronchi). On either side of the lower larynx and the upper trachea lies the thyroid gland. Unless it is enlarged, this gland is usually not palpable.

Pulsations of the carotid arteries are easily palpable in a groove approximately 0.5 inch (13 mm) lateral to the larynx. Lying immediately adjacent to these arteries, but not palpable, are the internal jugular veins and several important nerves. Lateral to these vessels and nerves lie the **sternocleidomastoid muscles**. These muscles originate from the mastoid process of the cranium and insert into the medial border of each collarbone and the sternum at the base of the neck. They allow movement of the head.

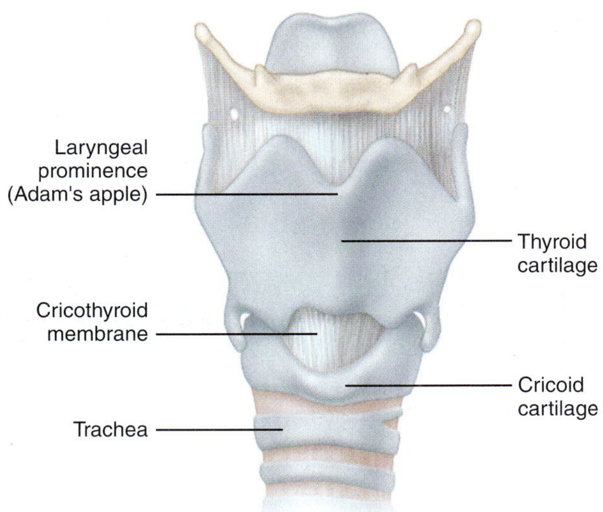

FIGURE 27-4 The larynx.

A series of bony prominences lie posteriorly, in the midline of the neck. They are the spines of the cervical vertebrae. The lower cervical spines are more prominent than the upper ones. They are more easily palpable when the neck is in flexion. At the base of the neck posteriorly, the most prominent spine is the seventh cervical vertebra.

The Eye

The eye is globe-shaped, approximately 1 inch (2.5 cm) in diameter, and located within a bony socket in the skull called the orbit **FIGURE 27-5**. The orbit is composed of the adjacent bones of the face and skull; the orbit forms the base of the floor of the cranial cavity, and directly above it are the frontal lobes of the brain. In the adult, more than 80% of the eyeball is protected within this bony orbit. Between and below the orbits are the nasal bone and the sinuses, respectively. Therefore, any severe injury to the face or head can potentially damage the eyeball or the muscles attached to the eyeball that cause the eye to move.

The eyeball, or **globe**, keeps its global shape as a result of the pressure of the fluid contained within its two chambers. The clear, jellylike fluid near the back of the eye is called the vitreous humor. In front of the lens is a clear fluid called the aqueous humor, named for its watery appearance; in Latin, aqua means water. In penetrating injuries of the eye, aqueous humor can leak out, but with time and appropriate medical treatment, the body can make more.

The inner surface of the eyelids and the exposed surface of the eye itself, which are covered

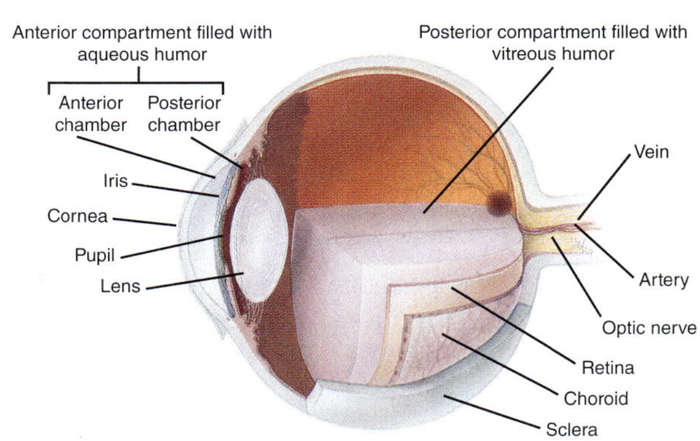

FIGURE 27-5 The major structures of the eye.

by a delicate membrane, the **conjunctiva**, are kept moist by fluid produced by the **lacrimal glands**, often called tear glands (**FIGURE 27-6**). Humans blink unconsciously many times per minute. This action sweeps fluid from the lacrimal glands over the surface of the eye, cleaning it. The tears drain on the inner side of the eye through two lacrimal (tear) ducts into the nasal cavity. This is why people sometimes need to blow their nose when they cry.

The white of the eye, called the **sclera**, extends over the surface of the globe. This extremely tough, fibrous tissue helps maintain the eye's globular shape and protects the more delicate inner structures. On the front of the eye, the sclera is replaced by a clear, transparent membrane called the **cornea**, which allows light to enter the eye. A circular muscle lies behind the cornea with an opening in its center. Like the shutter in a camera, this muscle adjusts the size of the opening to regulate the amount of light that enters the eye. This circular muscle and surrounding tissue are called the **iris**. The iris is pigmented, giving the eye its characteristic brown, green, or blue color.

The opening in the center of the iris, which allows light to move to the back of the eye, is called the **pupil**. Normally, the pupil appears black. Like the opening in a camera, the pupil becomes smaller in bright light and larger in dim light. The pupil also becomes smaller when the person is looking at objects near at hand and larger when looking at objects farther away; these adjustments occur almost instantaneously. Normally, the pupils in both eyes are equal in size. Some people are born with pupils that are not equal (**anisocoria**); however, particularly in unconscious patients, unequal pupil size may indicate serious illness or injury of the brain or eye.

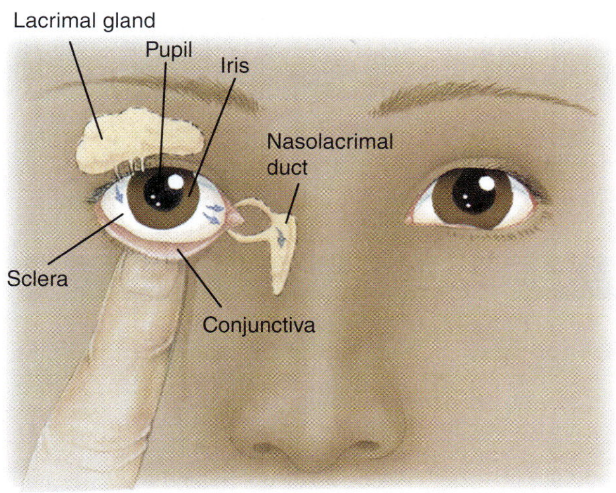

FIGURE 27-6 The lacrimal system consists of tear glands and ducts. Tears act as a lubricant and keep the front of the eye from drying out.

Behind the iris is the **lens**. Like the lens of a camera, this lens focuses images on the light-sensitive area at the back of the globe, called the **retina**. Within the retina are numerous nerve endings that respond to light by transmitting nerve impulses through the **optic nerve** to the brain. In the brain, the impulses are interpreted as vision.

The retina is nourished by a layer of blood vessels between it and the sclera at the back of the globe. This layer is called the choroid. If, as sometimes happens, the retina detaches from the underlying choroid and sclera, the nerve endings will not be nourished and the patient will experience complete or partial blindness, depending on how much of the retina is separated. This condition is called **retinal detachment**.

Injuries of the Face and Neck

Injuries involving the face and neck can often lead to partial or complete obstruction of the upper airway. Several factors may contribute to the obstruction. Bleeding from facial injuries can be heavy, producing large blood clots in the upper airway. These clots can lead to complete obstruction, particularly in a patient who is not fully conscious. In particular, direct injuries to the nose and mouth, the larynx, or the trachea are often the source of significant bleeding and/or respiratory compromise. You may need to suction the airway if you are unable to control the bleeding. In addition, the injuries may cause loosened teeth or dentures to become dislodged into the throat, where they may be swallowed or aspirated. The swelling that often accompanies direct and indirect injury to the soft tissues in these areas can also contribute to airway obstruction.

The airway may also be partially obstructed when the patient's head is turned to the side, which often occurs when the patient is not actively controlling the head's position, such as when the patient has an altered level of consciousness. Other factors that interfere with normal respirations include possible injuries to the brain and/or cervical spine that may be associated with facial injuries. If the great vessels in the neck are injured, significant bleeding and pressure on the upper airway are common, which can result in airway obstruction as well.

Depending on the mechanism of injury (MOI), there may be a cervical spine injury. If there is significant impact to the face, suspect accompanying cervical spine injury and follow your agency's protocol for spinal motion restriction.

Soft-Tissue Injuries

Soft-tissue injuries of the face and neck are common. Because the face and neck are extremely vascular, swelling from soft-tissue injuries in this area may be more severe than in other injured parts of the body. The skin and underlying tissues in these areas have a rich blood supply, so bleeding from penetrating injuries may be heavy. Even minor soft-tissue wounds of the face and neck may bleed profusely. A blunt injury that does not break the skin may cause a break in a blood vessel wall, causing blood to collect under the skin; this is called a hematoma (**FIGURE 27-7**). In some situations, a flap of skin may become peeled back, or avulsed, from the underlying muscle and fascia. See Chapter 26, *Soft-Tissue Injuries*.

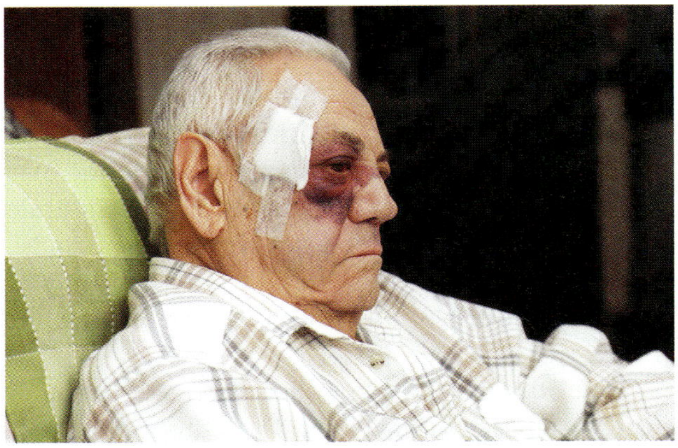

FIGURE 27-7 Facial hematoma.

Patient Assessment

Scene Size-Up

As you arrive on the scene, observe for hazards and threats to the safety of the crew, bystanders, and the patient. Assess the effect of hazards on patient care, and address those hazards. Assess for the potential for violence and for environmental hazards.

Patients who are conscious and supine and have oral or facial bleeding may protect their airway by coughing, projecting the blood at you. Therefore,

YOU are the EMT

When you arrive at the scene, you find the patient, a 30-year-old man, sitting on the ground. He is conscious and alert and tells you, "They hurt me bad!" His face is swollen and covered with blood, he keeps spitting out small amounts of blood from his mouth, and his voice is hoarse. As your partner manually stabilizes his head, you perform a primary assessment.

Recording Time: 0 Minutes	
Appearance	Face is covered with blood; appears anxious
Level of consciousness	Conscious and alert
Airway	A small amount of blood in the mouth, which he is spitting out
Breathing	Increased rate; adequate depth
Circulation	Radial pulses increased rate and strong; skin baseline color, warm, and dry

3. Does this patient have a patent airway? How can you tell?

4. What should be your initial treatment priorities for this patient?

standard precautions require eye protection and a face mask. Also, put several pairs of gloves in your pocket for easy access in the event your gloves tear or there are multiple patients with bleeding.

If your response is to a motor vehicle crash, you may be confronted with more than one patient in a vehicle. Determine the number of patients and consider whether you will need additional or specialized resources on the scene.

As you observe the scene, look for indicators of the MOI. This assessment helps you develop an early index of suspicion for underlying injuries in the patient who has sustained a significant MOI. As you put together information from dispatch and your observations of the scene, consider how the MOI produced the injuries expected. Common MOIs for face and neck injuries include motor vehicle collisions (especially when the passenger is not restrained), sports participation, falls, penetrating trauma, and blunt trauma. In motor vehicle collisions, the probability of injury increases if the vehicle rolled over or came to an abrupt stop when striking an immovable object, such as a tree. During sports participation, injuries can occur in a player who is struck by another object or another player.

Primary Assessment

The primary assessment focuses on identifying and managing life-threatening concerns. Threats to airway, breathing, or circulation (ABCs) must be treated immediately. When there is obvious, active, life-threatening external hemorrhage (exsanguination), it should be addressed before airway and breathing. In this case, the ABC mnemonic should be thought of as XABC, where *X* represents exsanguination.

As you approach the patient, look for important indicators to alert you to the seriousness of the patient's condition. Is the patient interacting with the environment or lying still, making no sounds? Does the patient have any apparent life threats such as significant bleeding? How is the patient's skin color? The general impression will help you develop an index of suspicion for serious injuries and determine your sense of urgency for medical intervention.

Injuries to the face and throat, such as bleeding and significant swelling, may be obvious but may also be hidden under collars and hats. Because of the likelihood of respiratory distress with these injuries, they should be recognized as early as possible.

As with any injury with life-threatening bleeding, control the blood loss with direct pressure. Always consider the need for manual spinal stabilization and check for responsiveness using the AVPU (Awake and alert, responsive to Verbal stimuli, responsive to Pain, Unresponsive) scale.

Ensure that the patient has a clear and patent airway. If the patient is unresponsive or has a significantly altered level of consciousness, consider inserting the proper-size oropharyngeal airway. The use of a nasopharyngeal airway is controversial, because many consider that the insertion of a nasopharyngeal airway into the nares of a patient with facial or head trauma carries the risk of introducing the device into the cranial vault and brain tissue. While some research suggests this risk is extremely small, the nasopharyngeal airway should be avoided if you suspect a nasal fracture or severe maxillofacial trauma.[1] As always, be aware of and follow your local protocols.

When a patient who has a mandibular fracture is positioned supine, their tongue may occlude the airway because its bony support has been compromised. Observe the patient carefully.

Street Smarts

Because a patient who has an unstable mandibular fracture may have difficulty swallowing, suction should be immediately available. When your assessment does not indicate the need for spinal motion restriction, position this patient sitting, with an emesis basin to spit into.[2] If the patient is alert and their condition permits, allow them to hold the rigid suction catheter so they can suction at will. Doing so gives them more control of their airway, thus reducing their anxiety. This can also be done for alert patients who have significant bleeding in their mouths.

Quickly assess the pulse rate and quality; determine the skin condition, color, and temperature; and check the capillary refill time. Significant bleeding is an immediate life threat. If the patient has obvious life-threatening bleeding, you must control it quickly.

If the patient you are treating has an airway or a breathing problem or significant bleeding, you must consider quickly transporting the patient to the hospital for treatment or requesting an advanced life support (ALS) unit if that will result in faster access to someone who will be able to intubate the patient. Stabilization and maintenance of airway and breathing and controlling bleeding can be difficult in patients with facial or neck injuries. Avoid delays in transport and consider ALS rendezvous if the transport time is long.

A patient with signs and symptoms of internal bleeding must be transported quickly to the appropriate hospital for treatment by a physician. Internal bleeding in face and throat injuries may compromise blood flow to the brain. Bleeding from major vessels of the throat can have a serious effect on the patient's airway. The condition of a patient with visible significant bleeding or signs of significant internal bleeding may quickly become unstable. Treatment is directed at quickly addressing life threats and providing rapid transport to the closest appropriate hospital. Signs such as tachycardia, tachypnea, low blood pressure, weak pulse, and cool, moist, and pale (compared with the patient's baseline color) skin suggest hypoperfusion and the need for rapid transport. The patient who has a significant MOI but whose condition appears stable should also be transported promptly to the closest appropriate hospital. Remember that any significant blow to the face or throat should increase your suspicion of spinal or brain injury. Be alert to these signs and reconsider your priority and transport decision if they develop.

Words of Wisdom

Face and throat injuries increase the need for airway and breathing maintenance, so do not hesitate to place a nonrebreathing mask over facial injuries, if indicated. The seal may not be as easy to maintain, but airway and breathing take priority over soft-tissue injuries.

Even if the patient has no signs of hypoperfusion or other life-threatening injuries, if the patient has an injury involving the eye, it should be considered potentially serious. Consider transporting a patient with serious, isolated eye injuries to an eye care specialty center, depending on local protocol. Do not delay transport of a seriously injured patient, particularly one with significant bleeding, even if it is controlled, to take a patient's history or perform a secondary assessment. Further assessment can continue during transport.

History Taking

After the life threats have been managed during the primary assessment, investigate the chief complaint or history of present illness. Obtain a medical history and be alert for injury-specific signs and symptoms, as well as any pertinent negatives such as no pain or no loss of sensation.

Next, obtain a SAMPLE (Signs and symptoms, Allergies, Medications, Pertinent past medical history, Last oral intake, Events leading up to the illness or injury) history from your patient or their family. Specifically ask if the patient takes any blood thinners or antiplatelet medications.

In an unresponsive patient, you will be able to observe only the signs of the patient's injuries. Any other information will need to be obtained by someone who is knowledgeable about the patient. The person providing the information may not be able to give you the actual names of the patient's medications but might be able to provide some pertinent medical history and possibly known allergies.

Secondary Assessment

If there is significant trauma that likely affects multiple systems, start with an assessment of the entire body looking for DCAP-BTLS (Deformities, Contusions, Abrasions, Punctures/penetrations, Burns, Tenderness, Lacerations, Swelling) to be sure you have found all life threats and injuries. When this is completed, perform a detailed examination of specific areas. However, do not delay transport to complete a thorough physical examination.

In the responsive patient who has an isolated injury with a limited MOI, consider focusing your physical examination on the isolated injury, the patient's chief complaint, and the body region affected, which, in this case, is the face and throat. Ensure that control of bleeding is maintained and note the location of the injury. Inspect open wounds for any foreign matter and stabilize impaled objects if they do not obstruct the airway.

During the physical examination, use your eyes and your hands. Your eyes will be looking for swelling, deformities of the bones, contusions, and discoloration, whereas your hands will be gently palpating the face, looking and feeling for any abnormalities such as deformity or tenderness. Ask yourself the following questions:

1. Do the facial bones seem to be in alignment?
2. Does the nasal bone seem to deviate from the midline?
3. Note any variations from the normal facial examination; is there any facial drooping?
4. Does one eye appear to be lower than the other? If so, this is an indication of an orbital fracture.
5. Does the patient report having any visual disturbances following the injury?
6. Does the mandible appear to deviate toward one side or the other?
7. Is there any drainage from the nose or ears?

If your patient is responsive, explain exactly what you are doing and what you are looking for. Your discovery of what you consider to be an abnormality may actually be an old injury that the patient can tell you more about.

Assess all underlying systems. This should include the neurologic system, including the brain and major nerves; sensory organs, including the eyes and nose; the respiratory system, including the mouth, nose, sinuses, and airway; and the circulatory system, particularly focusing on the carotid arteries and jugular veins.

When you are evaluating the eyes, start at the outer aspect of the eye and work your way in toward the pupils. Examine the eye for any obvious foreign matter. Your patient may relay this information to you ("I have something in my eye"). Visual acuity, or the clarity of the patient's vision in each eye, is considered the vital sign of the eye. Quickly assess the patient's visual acuity by gently covering one eye and holding fingers up at arm's length in front of the open eye. Test for the ability to see fingers in both the injured and uninjured eyes and document your findings. Note any discoloration of the eye, bleeding in the iris area, or redness. Look for eye symmetry because asymmetry is a possible indication of a brain injury.

Look at each pupil for equal size and reaction to light. If the pupils are not symmetric, ask the patient if they have undergone any previous eye surgeries, sustained any previous injuries, or have a history of unequal pupils. Previous surgery or injury, rather than brain injury, may be the root cause of the pupils not appearing the same. Cataract surgery can cause unequal pupils, but when you have a patient with a suspected head injury or ocular injury, unequal pupils in dim light may be present. Determine whether the unequal pupils are caused by physiologic or pathologic issues. Use of over-the-counter eye drops can change pupil size, and certain asthma inhalers can have the same effect if inadvertently sprayed into the eye. Brain injury, nerve disease, glaucoma, and meningitis are all possible causes of unequal pupils.

Is the patient able to follow your finger to the right, then up and down, and then to the left and up and down in an H pattern? The inability to do so can signal direct trauma to the eye or a brain injury. Can the patient read normal print? Does the patient report blurry vision in either eye? Is there a new sensitivity to light? Does the patient report seeing "floaters" in their vision from either eye?

Assess vital signs to obtain a baseline so that you can observe any changes a patient may display during treatment. In a patient who may have significant bleeding, a systolic blood pressure reading of less than 90 mm Hg, or a heart rate that exceeds the systolic blood pressure value, and cool, moist skin that is pale or gray (compared with the patient's baseline skin color) should alert you to hypoperfusion. Remember, you must be concerned with both visible bleeding and unseen bleeding inside a body cavity. With facial and throat injuries, baseline information about the rate and quality of respirations and pulse is very important, as is monitoring throughout patient care.

In addition to hands-on assessment, use monitoring devices to quantify your patient's oxygenation and circulatory status.

Reassessment

Repeat the primary assessment. Reassess vital signs and the chief complaint. Continually reassess the adequacy of the patient's airway, breathing, and circulation. Recheck patient interventions. Are the treatments you provided for problems with ABCs still effective? This is particularly important in patients with facial or neck injuries because of the ease with which injuries can affect associated systems, such as the respiratory (airway and breathing), circulatory, and nervous systems. The patient's condition should be reassessed at least every 5 minutes.

If you suspect possible spinal injury, follow local protocols regarding spinal motion restriction precautions. Spinal injuries should be suspected any time there is significant trauma to the face or neck. Maintain an open airway, be prepared to suction the patient, and consider an oropharyngeal airway if the patient becomes unresponsive. Whenever you suspect significant bleeding, provide oxygen to maintain an oxygen saturation level of 94% to 98%. Adequate oxygenation and airway maintenance are important for all patients with face and neck injuries. If needed, provide assisted ventilation using a bag-mask device with high-flow oxygen.

Control any significant visible bleeding. If the patient has signs of hypoperfusion, treat the patient aggressively for shock and provide rapid transport to the appropriate hospital. Do not delay transport of a seriously injured trauma patient to complete non-lifesaving treatments in the field, such as splinting extremity fractures. Instead, complete these treatments en route to the hospital. If there is no cervical spine injury suspected, the patient may be more comfortable in the sitting position during transport.

In your documentation, describe the MOI and the position in which you found the patient when you arrived at the scene. Inform the hospital personnel about all injuries involving the patient's head and neck.

Emergency Medical Care

The emergency care of soft-tissue injuries to the face and neck is the same as treatment of soft-tissue injuries elsewhere on the body. You should assess the ABCs and care for any life threats first. Remember also to take standard precautions in all cases.

In the absence of life-threatening bleeding, your first step is to open and clear the airway. Securing and maintaining a patent airway is paramount. Remember that blood draining into the throat can cause nausea in the patient, resulting in vomiting and airway obstruction; therefore, the patient may need frequent suctioning. Avoid moving the neck if you suspect that the patient may have sustained a cervical spine injury. Use the jaw-thrust maneuver to open the patient's airway if their injuries do not prohibit that maneuver, and then suction the mouth. Once spinal motion restriction is achieved, you can tilt the patient to one side to allow any blood or vomitus to drain out of the mouth rather than pool in the pharynx and obstruct the airway.

Control external bleeding by applying direct manual pressure with a dry, sterile dressing. Use roller gauze, wrapped around the circumference of the head, to hold a pressure dressing in place (**FIGURE 27-8**). Do not apply excessive pressure if there is a possibility of an underlying skull fracture. When an injury exposes the brain, eye,

YOU are the EMT

As your partner continues to manually stabilize the patient's head, you perform a secondary assessment of the entire body, which reveals bruising and mild swelling to the anterior part of the neck, directly over the trachea. The remainder of your assessment does not reveal any obvious injuries. You apply a cervical collar and assess his vital signs.

The patient tells you that he was struck in the face with a steel pipe. After he fell to the ground, he was kicked in the face and throat several times. His face is severely swollen, three of his front teeth are missing, and he tells you that it "doesn't feel right" when he closes his mouth.

Recording Time: 5 Minutes	
Respirations	22 breaths/min; adequate depth
Pulse	118 breaths/min; strong and regular
Skin	Baseline color, warm, and dry
Blood pressure	132/68 mm Hg
Oxygen saturation (Spo_2)	97% (on room air)

5. On the basis of the MOI, what type of injuries should you suspect and assess for?

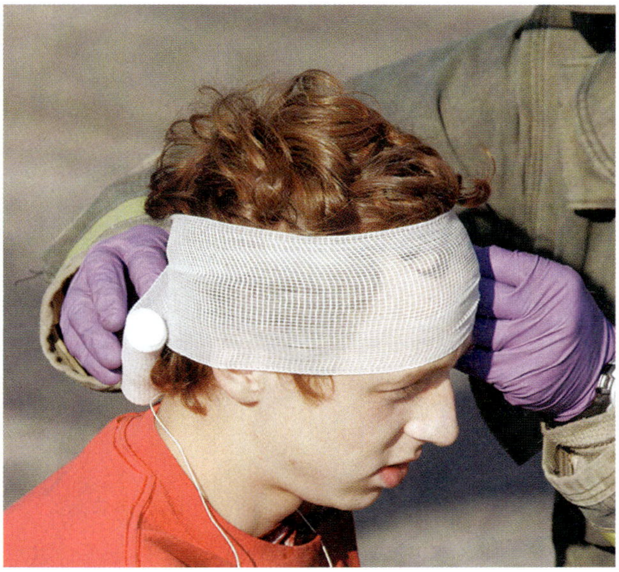

FIGURE 27-8 Use roller gauze, wrapped around the circumference of the head, to hold a pressure dressing in place.

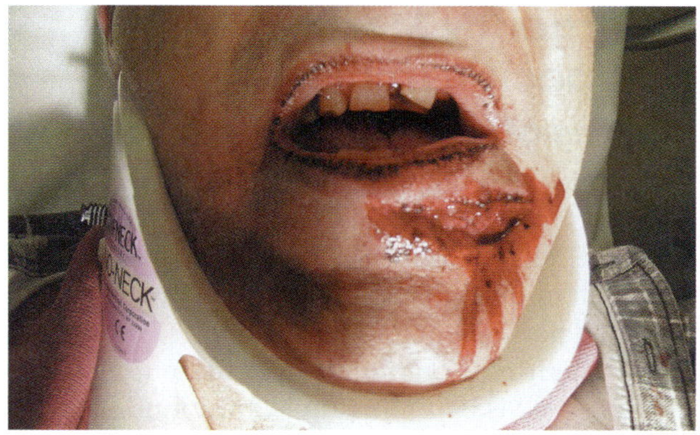

FIGURE 27-9 Soft-tissue injuries around the mouth can be associated with profuse bleeding inside the mouth and obstruction of the airway.

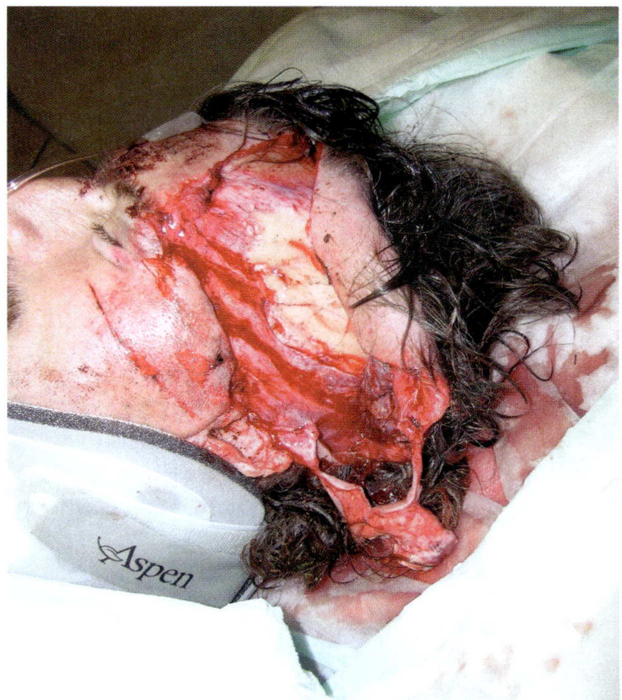

FIGURE 27-10 If avulsed skin is still attached, place the flap in a position that is as close to normal as possible, and hold it in place with a dry, sterile dressing.

or other structures, cover the exposed parts with a moist, sterile dressing to protect them from further damage. For injuries in which the skin is not broken, apply ice or a cold pack locally to help control the swelling of bruised tissues. Place a towel or gauze between the cold pack and the skin to avoid tissue injury caused by the cold.

For soft-tissue injuries around the mouth, always check for bleeding inside the mouth. Broken teeth and lacerations to the tongue may cause profuse bleeding and obstruction of the upper airway (**FIGURE 27-9**). Often, the patient will swallow the blood from lacerations inside the mouth, so the hemorrhage may not be apparent. You should also inspect the inside of the mouth for bleeding and hidden injuries in patients who have sustained facial trauma. Remember that patients who swallow significant amounts of blood may begin vomiting.

Often, physicians will be able to graft a piece of avulsed skin back into the appropriate position. For this reason, if you find portions of avulsed skin, such as the nose or ear, that have become separated, wrap them in a dry sterile dressing, place them in a plastic bag, and keep the bag cool by placing it on ice or a cold pack.[2] Never place tissue directly on ice because freezing will cause further injury to the tissue and make it unusable. Deliver the bag labeled with the patient's name to the emergency department (ED) along with the patient. In many avulsion injuries, the skin will still be attached in a loose flap (**FIGURE 27-10**). Place the flap in a position that is as close to normal as possible, and hold it in place with a dry, sterile dressing. These steps will help to increase the patient's chances of having their normal appearance restored.

Emergency Medical Care for Specific Injuries

Injuries of the Eyes

Eye injuries are common, particularly in sports. An eye injury can produce severe, lifelong complications, including blindness. Proper emergency treatment will minimize pain and may very well help to prevent a permanent loss of vision.

In a normal, uninjured eye, the entire circle of the iris is visible. The pupils are round, usually equal in size, and react equally when exposed to light (**FIGURE 27-11**). Both eyes move together in the same direction when following your moving finger. After an injury, pupil reaction or shape and eye movement are often disturbed. Any of these conditions should cause you to suspect an injury of the globe or its associated tissues. Remember, though, in patients who are unconscious or who have a significantly altered mental status, abnormal pupil reactions sometimes are a sign of brain injury rather than eye injury.

Treatment starts with a thorough examination to determine the extent and nature of any damage. Perform your examination taking standard precautions, taking care to avoid aggravating any problems. You are looking for specific abnormalities or conditions that may suggest the nature of the injury (**FIGURE 27-12**). For example, blunt or penetrating injuries can produce swollen or lacerated eyelids. Bleeding soon after irritation or injury can result in a bright red conjunctiva. A damaged cornea quickly loses its smooth, wet appearance.

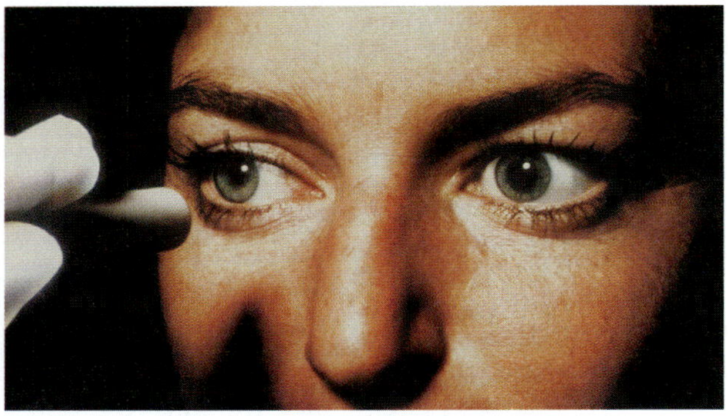

FIGURE 27-11 Normally, the pupils are round, equal in size, and equally reactive when exposed to light. The pupils shown here appear unequal.

Foreign Objects

Large objects are prevented from penetrating the eye by the protective orbit that surrounds it. However, moderate-size and smaller foreign objects of many different types can enter the eye and cause significant damage. Even a tiny foreign object, such

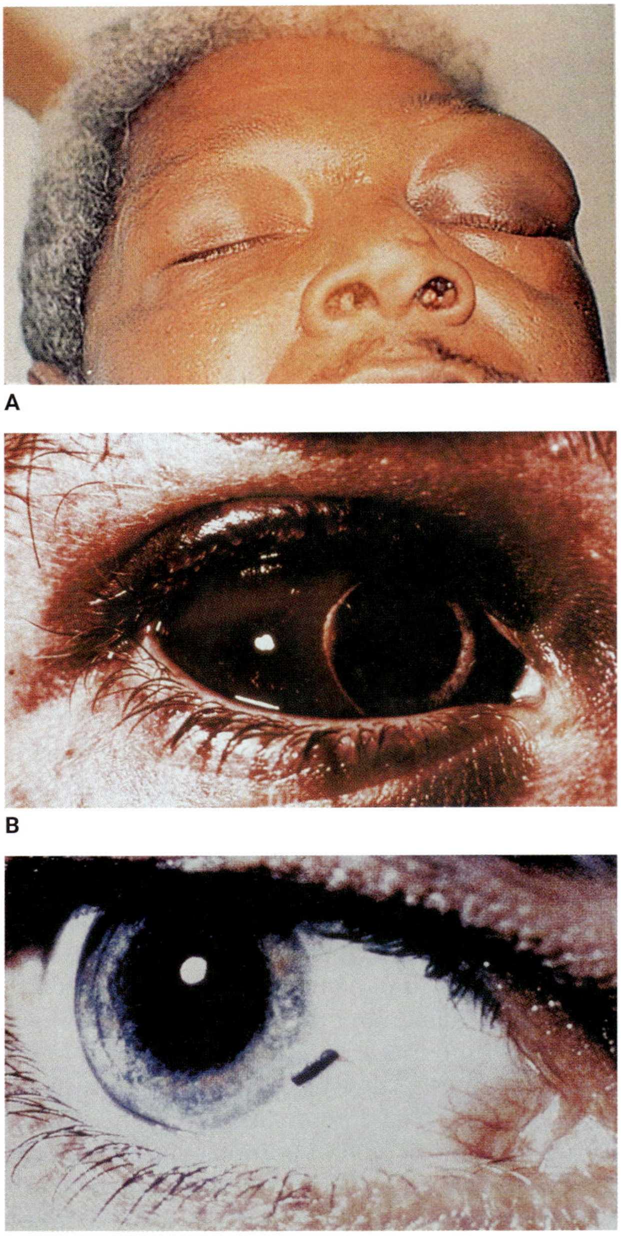

A

B

C

FIGURE 27-12 Injuries to the eyes are easily detected by swelling (**A**), bleeding (**B**), and the presence of foreign objects in the eye (**C**).

as a grain of sand lying on the surface of the conjunctiva, may produce severe irritation (**FIGURE 27-13**). The conjunctiva becomes inflamed and red, a condition known as **conjunctivitis**, almost immediately, and the eye begins to produce tears to flush out the object. Irritation of the cornea or conjunctiva causes intense pain. The patient may have difficulty keeping the eyelids open, because the irritation is further aggravated by bright light.

If a small foreign object is lying on the surface of the patient's eye, you should use a normal saline solution to gently irrigate the eye. Irrigation with a sterile saline solution will frequently flush away loose, small particles. If a small bulb syringe is available, you can use this, or a nasal airway or cannula, to direct the saline into the affected eye. Always flush from the nose side of the eye toward the outside (laterally) to avoid flushing material into the other eye. After it has been flushed away, a foreign body will often leave a small abrasion on the surface of the conjunctiva. For this reason, the patient will report irritation even when the particle itself is gone. It is always a good idea to transport the patient to the hospital for further assessment to ensure appropriate medical care to the affected eye.

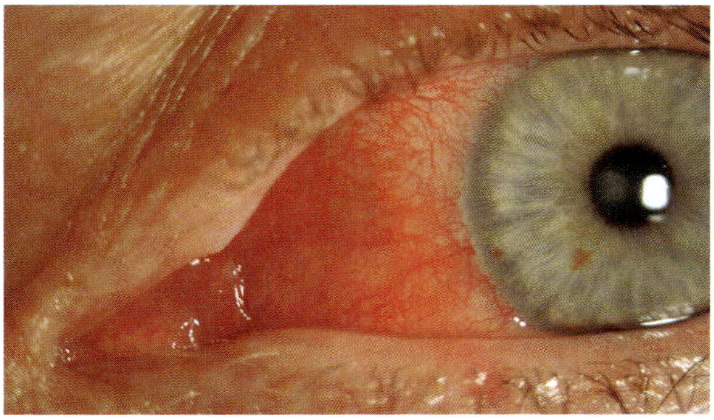

FIGURE 27-13 Conjunctivitis can result from the presence of a foreign object in the eye.

Gentle irrigation usually will not wash out foreign bodies that are stuck to the cornea or lying under the upper eyelid. To examine the undersurface of the upper eyelid, pull the lid upward and forward. If you spot a foreign object on the surface of the eyelid, you may be able to remove it with a moist, sterile cotton-tipped applicator (**SKILL DRILL 27-1**). Never attempt to remove a foreign body that is stuck to the cornea.

1. Tell the patient to look down while you grasp the lashes of the upper eyelid with your thumb and index finger. Gently pull the eyelid away from the eyeball (**Step 1**).

Skill Drill 27-1 Removing a Foreign Object From Under the Upper Eyelid

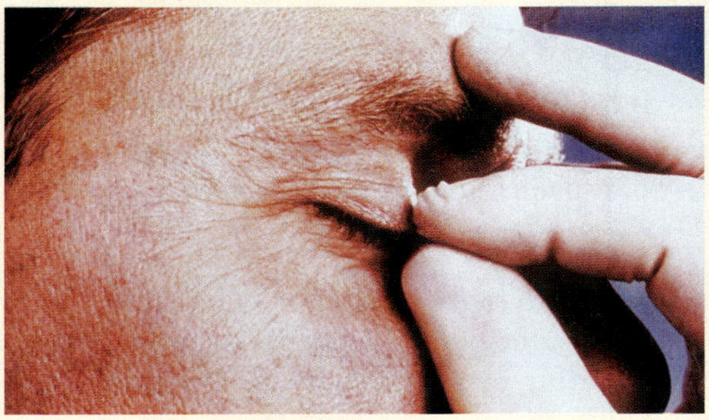

Step 1

Have the patient look down, then grasp the upper lashes and gently pull the lid away from the eye.

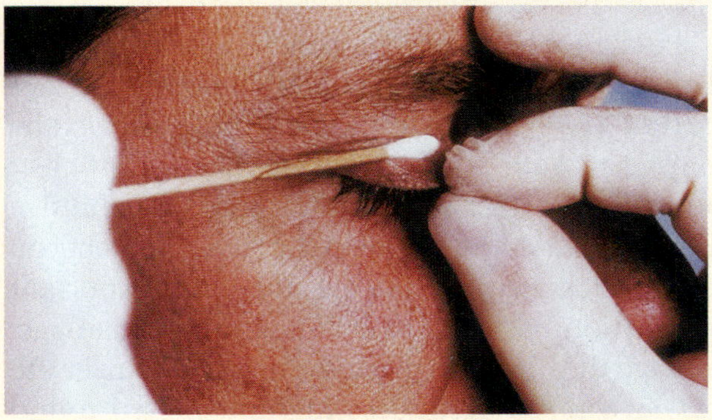

Step 2

Place a cotton-tipped applicator on the outer surface of the upper lid.

(continues)

Skill Drill 27-1 Removing a Foreign Object From Under the Upper Eyelid continued

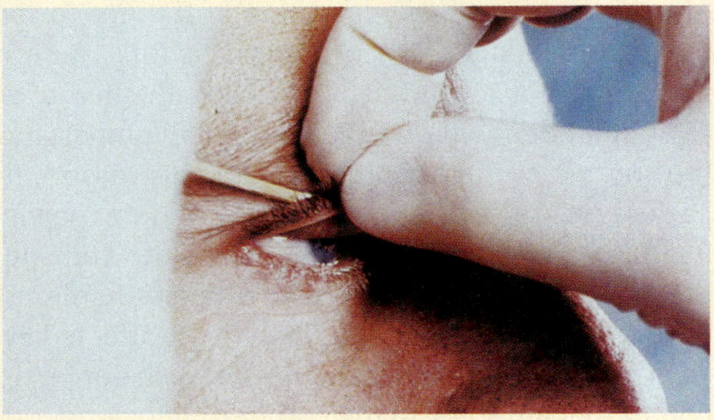

Step 3

Pull the lid forward and up, folding it back over the applicator.

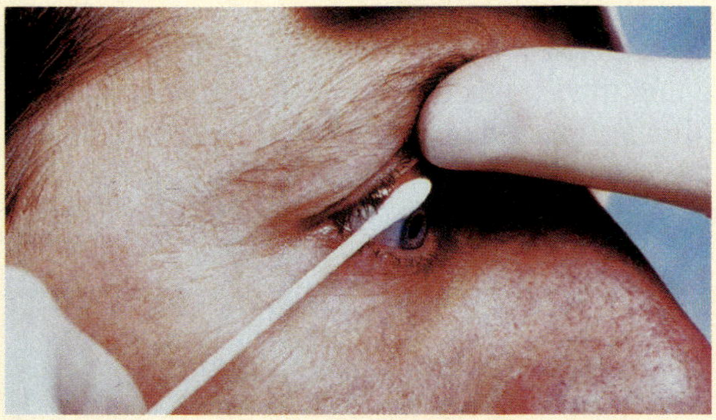

Step 4

Gently remove the foreign object from the eyelid with a moistened, sterile cotton-tipped applicator.

2. Gently place a cotton-tipped applicator horizontally along the center of the outer surface of the upper eyelid (**Step 2**).
3. Pull the eyelid forward and up, which causes it to roll or fold back over the applicator, exposing the undersurface of the eyelid (**Step 3**).
4. If you see a foreign object on the surface of the eyelid, gently remove it with a moistened, sterile cotton-tipped applicator (**Step 4**).

Foreign bodies ranging in size from a pencil to a sliver of metal may be impaled in the eye (**FIGURE 27-14**). These objects must be removed by a physician. Your care involves stabilizing the object and preparing the patient for transport to definitive care. The greater the length of the foreign object you can see sticking out of the eye, the more important stabilization becomes in avoiding further damage. Bandage the object in place to support it. Cover the eye with a moist, sterile dressing, and then surround the object with an eye shield or doughnut-shaped collar made from roller gauze or a small gauze pack. Follow the steps in **SKILL DRILL 27-2**:

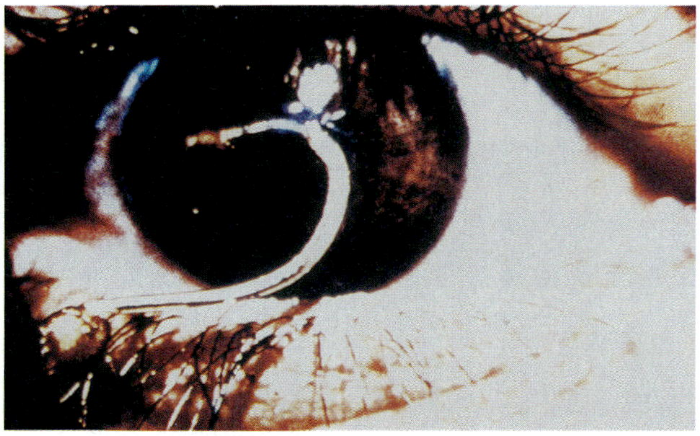

FIGURE 27-14 Any number of objects, such as the fishhook shown here, can become impaled in the eye.

1. Begin to prepare the doughnut ring by wrapping a 2-inch (5-cm) gauze roll circumferentially around your fingers and thumb enough times to make a thick dressing layer. You can adjust the inner diameter of what will become the ring by spreading your fingers or squeezing them together (**Step 1**).
2. Remove the gauze from your hand and wrap the remainder of the gauze roll radially around the ring that you have created (**Step 2**).
3. Work your way around the ring until you have wrapped all the way around it and finished the doughnut (**Step 3**).

Skill Drill 27-2 Stabilizing a Foreign Object Impaled in the Eye

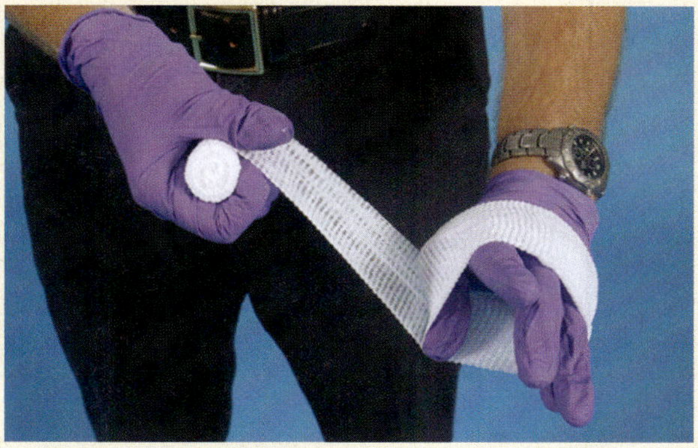

Step 1

To prepare a doughnut ring, wrap a 2-inch (5-cm) gauze roll around your fingers and thumb seven or eight times. Adjust the diameter by spreading your fingers or squeezing them together.

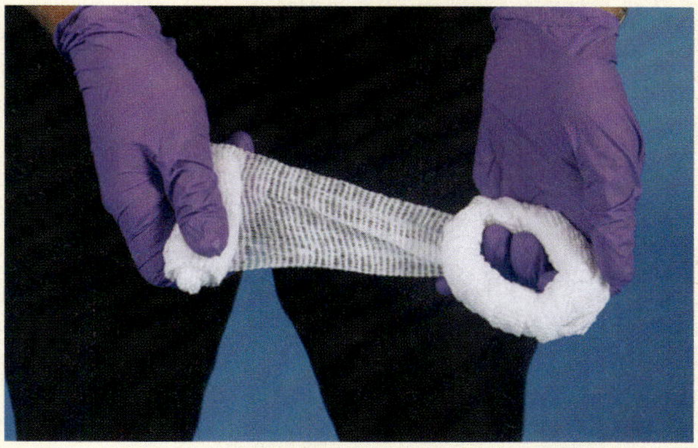

Step 2

Remove the gauze from your hand and wrap the remainder of the gauze roll radially around the ring that you have created.

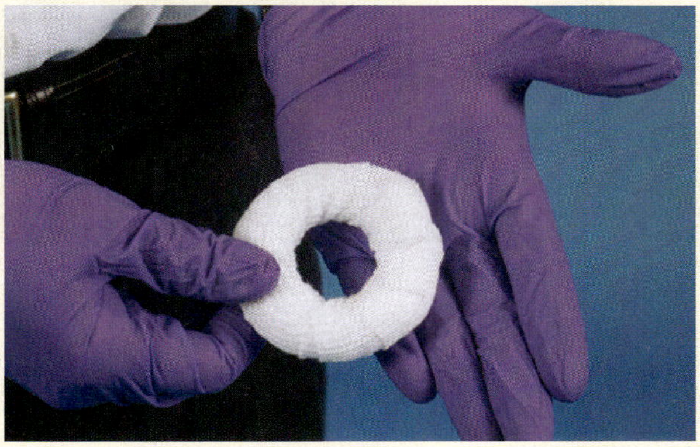

Step 3

Work around the entire ring to form a doughnut.

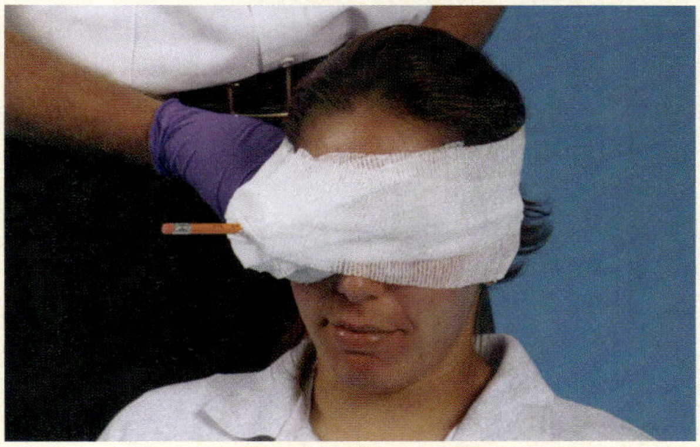

Step 4

Place the dressing over the eye with a protective barrier to hold the impaled object in place, and then secure it with a roller bandage.

4. Carefully place the ring over the eye and impaled object, without bumping the object. You can then stabilize the object with a cup or other protective barrier over the object, and secure the object with a roller bandage surrounding the head. Cover the injured eye and either bandage the uninjured eye or ask the patient to close that eye to minimize eye movement and prevent further damage to the globe because when one eye moves, so does the other. Transport to an appropriate medical facility for treatment (**Step 4**).

> **Words of Wisdom**
>
> While some sources suggest covering or having the patient close the uninjured eye, other sources do not. These latter sources argue that the eyes move more when closed, because people, particularly children, react to sound and other stimuli. Follow your EMS protocols.

Various types of large and small foreign bodies, particularly small metal fragments, can become completely embedded within the eye itself. The patient may not even be aware of the cause of the problem. Suspect such an injury when the history includes metal work (such as hammering, exposure to splinters, grinding, vigorous filing) and when there are other signs of ocular injury. When you see or suspect an impaled object in the eye, or any other significant eye injury, place an eye shield over the affected eye and then bandage both eyes with soft, bulky dressings to prevent further injury to the affected eye. Your bandage should be tight enough to hold the eyelid closed but not cause pressure on the eye itself. Bandaging both eyes prevents sympathetic motion (the movement of one eye causing both eyes to move), which may cause additional damage to the injured eye. This type of injury must be handled by an ophthalmologist on an urgent basis. Radiographs and special equipment may be required to find the foreign body.

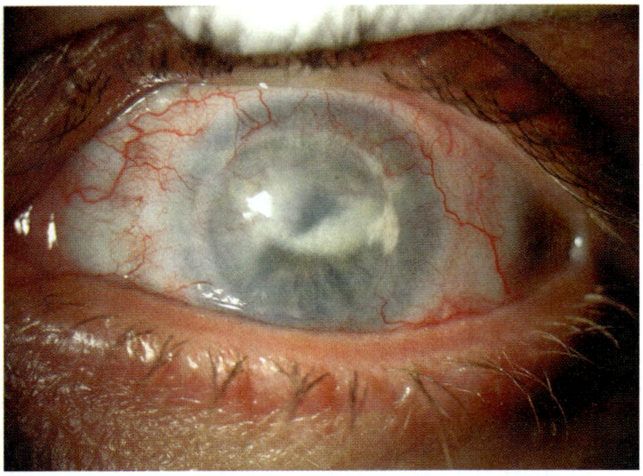

A

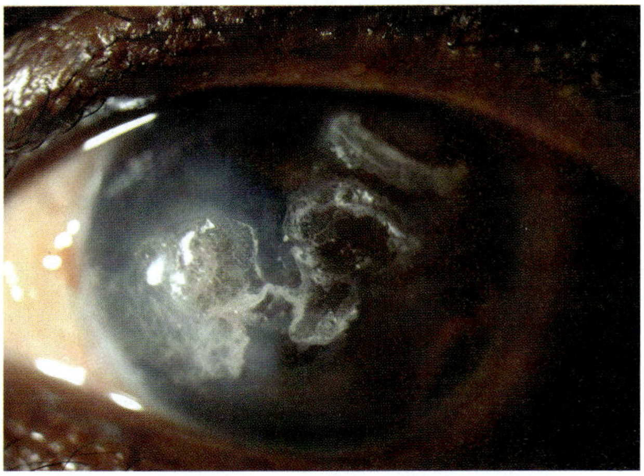

B

FIGURE 27-15 A. Chemical burns typically occur when an acid or alkali is splashed into the eye. **B.** This figure shows a chemical burn from lye, an alkaline solution. Because lye can continue to damage the eye even when diluted, fast action is needed.

Burns of the Eye

Chemicals, heat, and light rays all can burn the delicate tissues, such as the cornea, often causing permanent damage. Your role is to stop the burn and prevent further damage.

Chemical Burns

Chemical burns, usually caused by acid or alkaline solutions, require immediate emergency care (**FIGURE 27-15**). This consists of flushing the eye with water or a sterile saline irrigation solution. If sterile saline is not available, you can use any clean water.

The idea is to direct the greatest amount of irrigating solution or water into the eye as gently as possible (**FIGURE 27-16**). Because opening the eye spontaneously may cause the patient pain, you may have to force the lids open to irrigate the eye adequately. Ideally, you will use a bulb or irrigation syringe, a nasal cannula, or some other device that will allow you to control the flow. In some circumstances, you may have to resort to pouring water into the eye by holding the patient's head under a gently running faucet. You can even have the patient immerse their face in a large pan or basin of water and rapidly blink the affected eyelid. If only one eye is affected, care must be taken to avoid contaminated water from getting into the unaffected eye.

As when removing a foreign body, when removing chemicals from the eye, be sure to flush from the

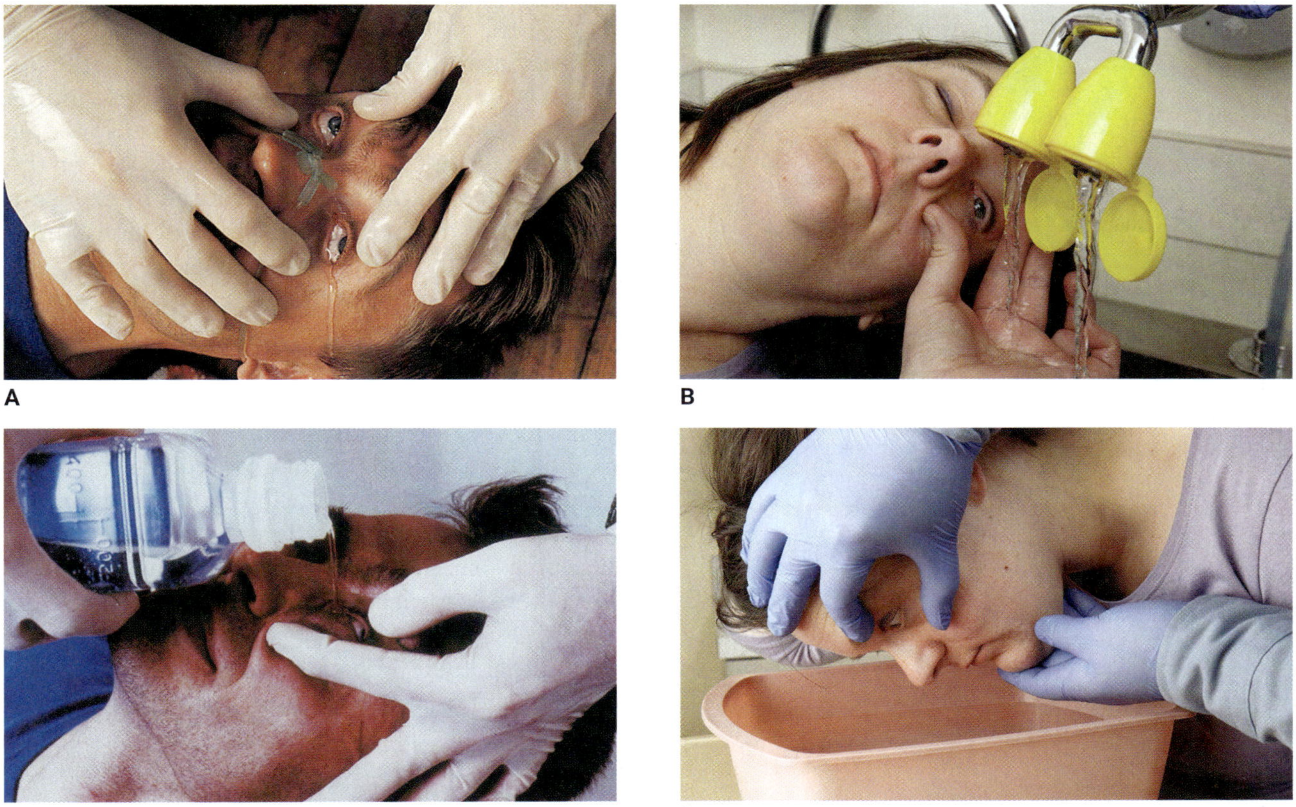
A
B
C
D

FIGURE 27-16 The eye may be effectively irrigated by using a nasal cannula (**A**), a faucet (**B**), a bottle (**C**), or a basin (**D**). Remember, you must protect the uninjured eye from the irrigating solution to prevent exposure of the unaffected eye to the substance.

inner corner of the affected eye toward the outside corner. Never flush from the outside corner, as doing so may cause the substance to contaminate the unaffected eye. If the burn was caused by an alkali or a strong acid, irrigate the eye continuously for at least 20 minutes. Follow local protocols or consult with medical direction regarding whether to try to irrigate while transporting or to stay on scene until flushing is complete. Strong acids and all alkaline solutions can penetrate deeply, requiring a prolonged flush. Again, always take care to protect the uninjured eye and prevent irrigation fluid from running into it.

After you have completed irrigation, apply a clean, dry dressing to cover the eye, and transport the patient promptly to the hospital for further care (**FIGURE 27-17**). If the irrigation can be carried out satisfactorily in the ambulance, it should be done during transport to save time.

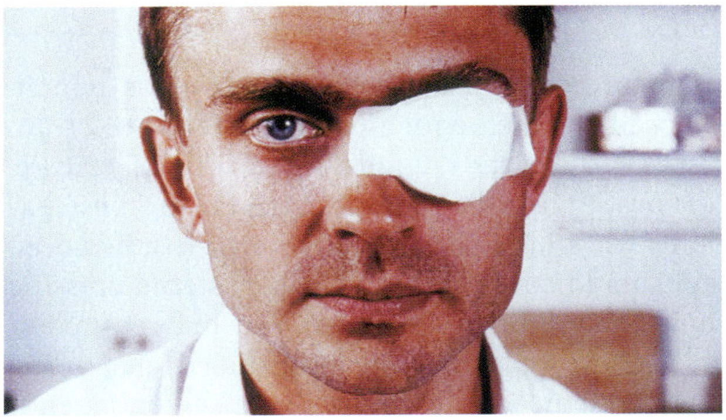

FIGURE 27-17 Apply a clean, dry dressing to cover the eye after you have finished irrigation.

Thermal Burns

When a patient is burned on the face during a fire, the eyes usually close rapidly because of the heat. This reaction is a natural reflex to protect the eye

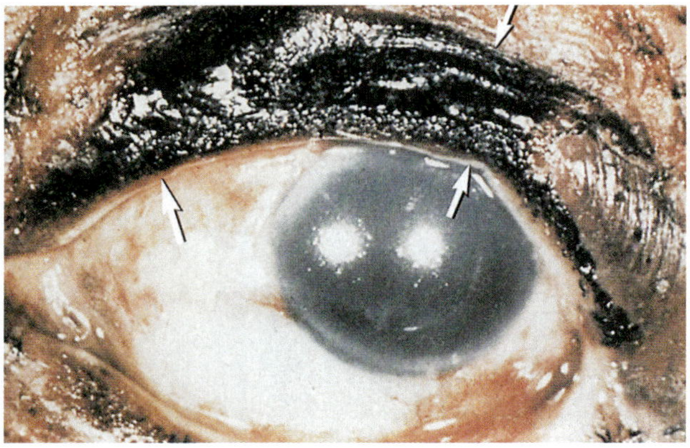

A

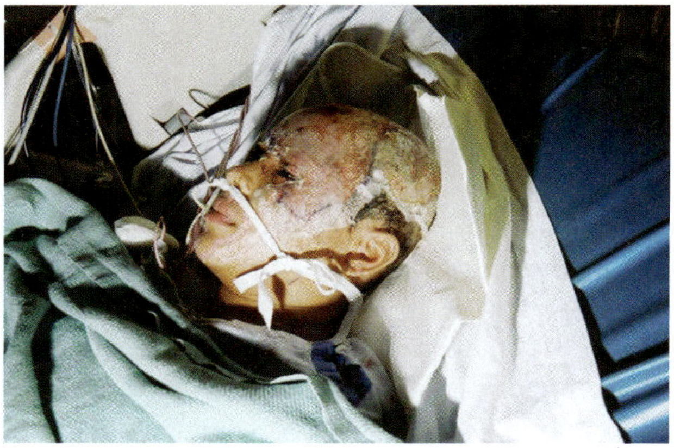

B

FIGURE 27-18 Thermal burns occasionally cause significant damage to the eyelids. **A.** Arrows show some full-thickness burns. **B.** Burns of the eyelids require immediate hospital care.

from further injury. However, the eyelids remain exposed and are frequently burned (**FIGURE 27-18**). Burns of the eyelids require highly specialized care. It is best to provide prompt transport for these patients without further examination. First, however, you should cover both eyes with a sterile dressing moistened with sterile saline. You may apply eye shields over the dressing. Consider transporting these patients to a designated burn center depending on local protocol or medical direction.

Words of Wisdom

A patient who has sustained thermal burns to the face may also have experienced inhalation burns.

Light Burns

Infrared rays, the light from a solar eclipse (if the patient has looked directly at the sun), and laser burns all can cause significant damage to the sensory cells of the eye when rays of light become focused on the retina. Retinal injuries that are caused by exposure to extremely bright light are generally not painful but may result in permanent damage to vision.

Superficial burns of the eye can result from ultraviolet rays from an arc welding unit, light from prolonged exposure to a sun lamp, or reflected light from a bright, snow-covered area (snow blindness). This kind of burn often is not painful at first but may become so 3 to 5 hours later, when the damaged cornea responds to the injury. Severe conjunctivitis usually develops, with redness, swelling, and excessive tear production. You can ease the pain from these corneal burns by covering each eye with a sterile, saline-moistened pad and an eye shield. Have the patient lie down during transport to the hospital and protect them from further exposure to bright light.

The patient should be examined by a physician as soon as possible.

Lacerations

Lacerations of the eyelids require careful repair to restore appearance and function (**FIGURE 27-19**). Bleeding may be heavy, but it usually can be controlled by gentle, manual pressure. If there is a laceration of the globe itself, apply no pressure to the eye. Compression can interfere with the blood supply to the back of the eye and result in loss of vision from damage to the retina. Furthermore, pressure may squeeze the vitreous humor, iris, lens, or even the retina out of the eye and cause irreparable damage or blindness.

Follow these three important guidelines in treating penetrating injuries of the eye:

1. Never exert pressure on or manipulate the injured eye (globe) in any way.
2. If part of the eyeball is exposed, gently apply a sterile, saline-moistened dressing to prevent drying.
3. Cover the injured eye with a protective metal eye shield or cup. Apply soft dressings to both eyes, and provide prompt transport to the hospital.

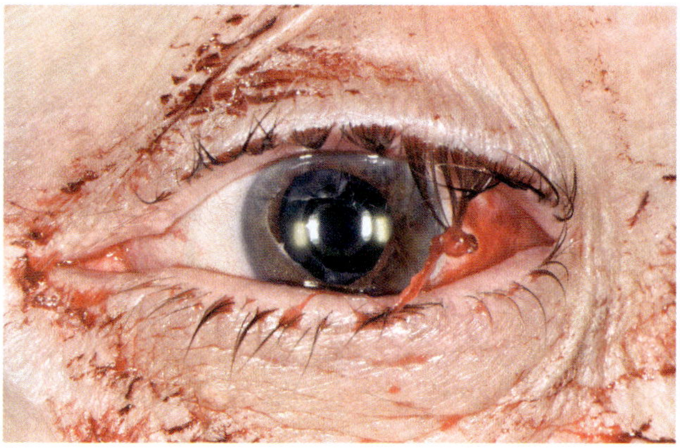

A

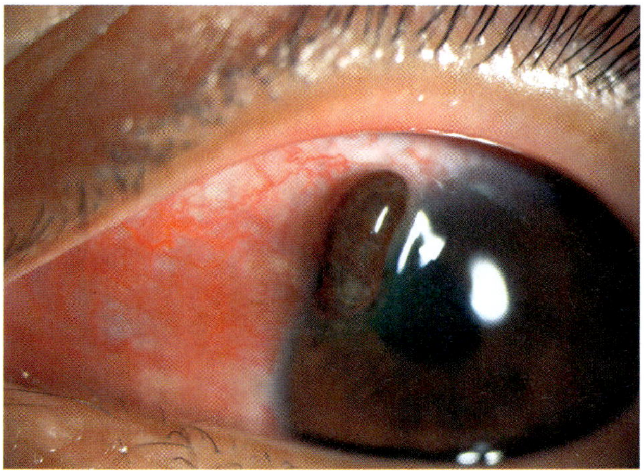

B

FIGURE 27-19 Lacerations are serious injuries that require prompt transport. **A.** Although bleeding can be heavy, never exert pressure on the eye. **B.** Pressure may squeeze the vitreous humor, iris, lens, or even the retina out of the eye.

On rare occasions following a serious injury, the eyeball may be displaced out of its socket. Do not attempt to reposition it. Simply cover the eye with a moist, sterile dressing. Have the patient lie in a supine position en route to the hospital to prevent further loss of fluid from the eye.

Blunt Trauma

Blunt trauma can cause serious eye injuries. These range from the ordinary black eye, a result of bleeding into the tissue around the orbit, to a severely damaged globe (**FIGURE 27-20**). You may see an injury called hyphema, or bleeding into the anterior chamber of the eye, that obscures part or all

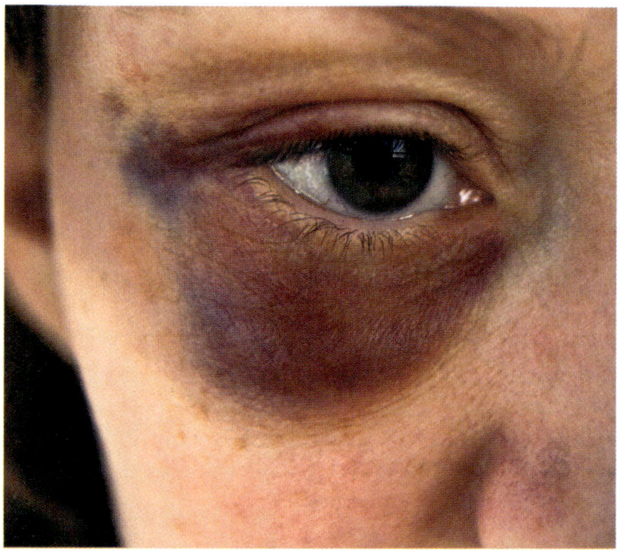

FIGURE 27-20 The typical "black eye" is caused by bleeding into the tissue around the orbit.

of the iris (**FIGURE 27-21**). This injury is common in blunt trauma and may seriously impair vision. Approximately 70% of hyphemas occur in children and result from sports or recreational injury.[3] They are often associated with underlying globe injuries, which are a serious injury to the eye. Cover the eye to protect it from further injury, and transport the patient to the hospital for further medical evaluation.

Blunt trauma can also cause a fracture of the orbit, specifically of the bones that form its floor and support the globe. When associated with displacement, this injury is sometimes referred to as a **blow-out fracture**. The fragments of fractured bone can entrap some of the muscles that control eye movement, causing double vision (**FIGURE 27-22**). Any patient who reports pain, double vision, or decreased vision following a blunt injury in the area of the eye should be placed on a stretcher and promptly transported to the ED. Protect the eye from further injury with a metal shield; cover the other eye to minimize sympathetic eye movement.

Another possible result of blunt eye injury is retinal detachment. This injury is often seen in sports, especially boxing. It is painless but produces flashing lights, specks, or floaters in the field of vision and a cloud or shade over the patient's vision. Because the retina is separated from the nourishing

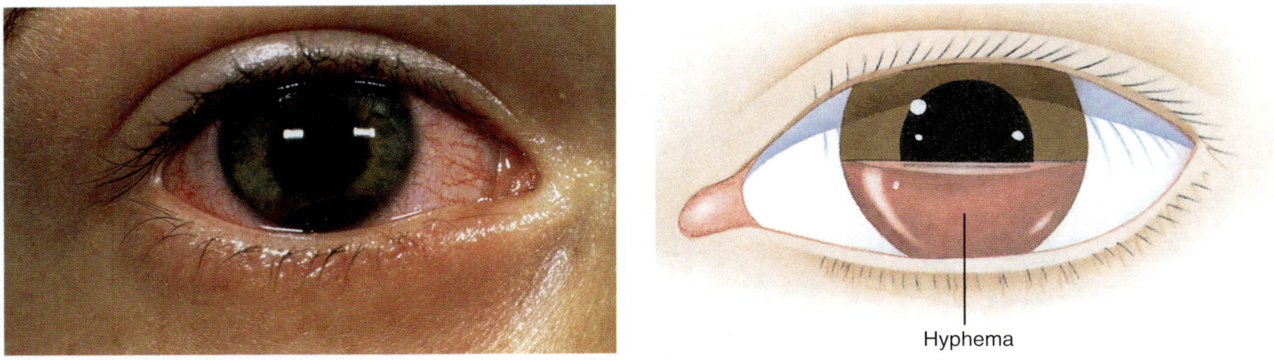

A **B**

FIGURE 27-21 A. A hyphema, characterized by bleeding into the anterior chamber of the eye, is common following blunt trauma to the eye. This condition may seriously impair vision and should be considered a sight-threatening emergency. **B.** Illustration of hyphema.

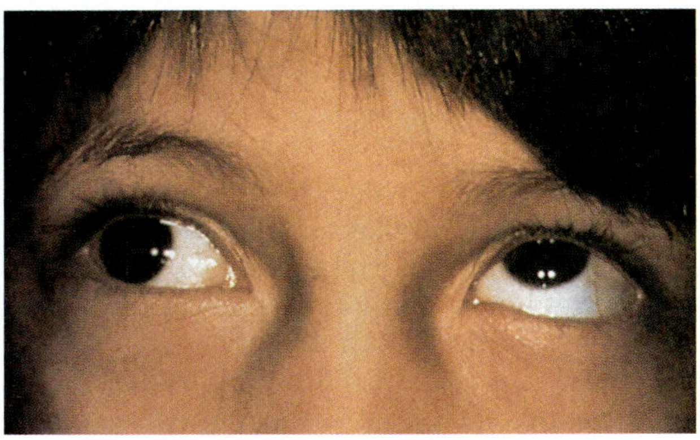

FIGURE 27-22 A patient with a blow-out fracture may not move their eyes together because of muscle entrapment. Therefore, the patient sees double images of any object.

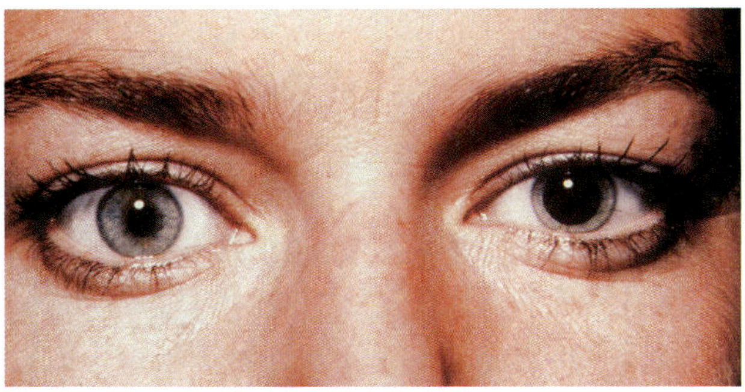

FIGURE 27-23 Variation of pupil size may indicate a brain injury.

choroid, this injury requires prompt medical attention to preserve vision in the eye.

Globe Rupture

A globe rupture is an injury in which the protective layer of the eye is disrupted. This injury can be caused by penetrating or blunt trauma to the eye and is often associated with other eye injuries. Assessment may reveal significant pain, decreased vision, impaired extraocular movements, hyphema, and abnormal or absent pupillary reflexes. It may be possible to recognize this injury when you first look at the eye if there is an obvious laceration to the eye, gel-like substance on the surface of the eye, or penetration of the eye, or if the pupil is teardrop-shaped. If these signs are observed, no further eye exam is indicated. Cover the eye with an eye shield, and initiate transport with the head of the stretcher elevated 30° to 45° if not contraindicated.[4]

Eye Injuries Following Head Injury

Abnormalities in the appearance or function of the eyes often occur following a brain injury. Any of the following eye findings should alert you to the possibility of a head injury:

- One pupil larger than the other in an unconscious patient (**FIGURE 27-23**)
- The eyes not moving together or pointing in different directions
- Failure of the eyes to follow the movement of your finger as instructed
- Bleeding under the conjunctiva, which obscures the sclera (white portion) of the eye
- Protrusion or bulging of one eye

Record any of these observations, along with the time that you make them. Normal tears will keep the tissues moist.

Blast Injuries

The signs and symptoms of blast injuries range from severe pain and loss of vision to foreign bodies within the globe. Before responding to patients after the blast, first ensure that the scene is safe.

Management of blast injuries to the eye depends on the severity of the injury. If there is a foreign body within the globe, do not attempt to remove it. Use a clean cup or similar item to protect the area. If only one eye is injured, follow local protocols, which may include covering the other eye to eliminate sympathetic motion. Patients with a sudden loss or decrease of vision will need to be verbally instructed on what actions are taking place around them. If the patient has severe swelling or a hematoma to the eyelid, do not attempt to force the eyelid open to examine the eye because this increases the pressure already present within the globe.

Contact Lenses and Artificial Eyes

Small, hard contact lenses usually are tinted, making them relatively easy to see. Large, soft contact lenses are clear and can be very difficult to see. In general, you should not attempt to remove either type of lens from a patient's eye. You should never attempt to remove a lens from an eye that has been, or may have been, injured because manipulating the lens can aggravate the problem. The only time that contact lenses should be removed immediately in the field is in the case of a chemical burn of the eye. In this situation, the lens can trap the chemical and make irrigation difficult.

If it is necessary to remove a hard contact lens, use a small suction cup, moistening the end with saline (**FIGURE 27-24A**). To remove soft lenses, place one to two drops of saline in the eye (**FIGURE 27-24B**), gently pinch the lens between your gloved thumb and index finger, and lift it off the surface of the eye (**FIGURE 27-24C**). Place the contact lens in a container filled with sterile saline solution to prevent damage to the contact lens. Always advise the ED staff if a patient is wearing contact lenses.

Occasionally, you may find yourself caring for a patient who is wearing an eye prosthesis (an artificial eye). Many people are surprised to find that it can be difficult to distinguish a prosthesis from a natural eye. You should suspect that an eye is artificial when it does not respond to light, move in

YOU are the EMT

After taking appropriate spinal precautions, you place the patient onto the stretcher and load him into the ambulance. You recovered his teeth and placed them in a commercial tooth-saver container. While you reassess the interventions you have performed thus far, your partner reassesses the patient's vital signs.

Recording Time: 11 Minutes	
Level of consciousness	Conscious and alert
Respirations	20 breaths/min; adequate depth
Pulse	108 beats/min; strong and regular
Skin	Baseline color, warm, and dry
Blood pressure	128/62 mm Hg
Oxygen saturation (Spo_2)	98% (on room air)

Reassessment of the patient's mouth reveals that it is clear of blood. You begin transport to a trauma center, which is located 15 miles away. En route, the patient tells you that he is becoming nauseated. You call in your radio report and give an estimated time of arrival of 18 to 20 minutes.

6. What should you do if this patient begins to vomit?

7. How should you treat a patient with active oral bleeding and inadequate ventilation?

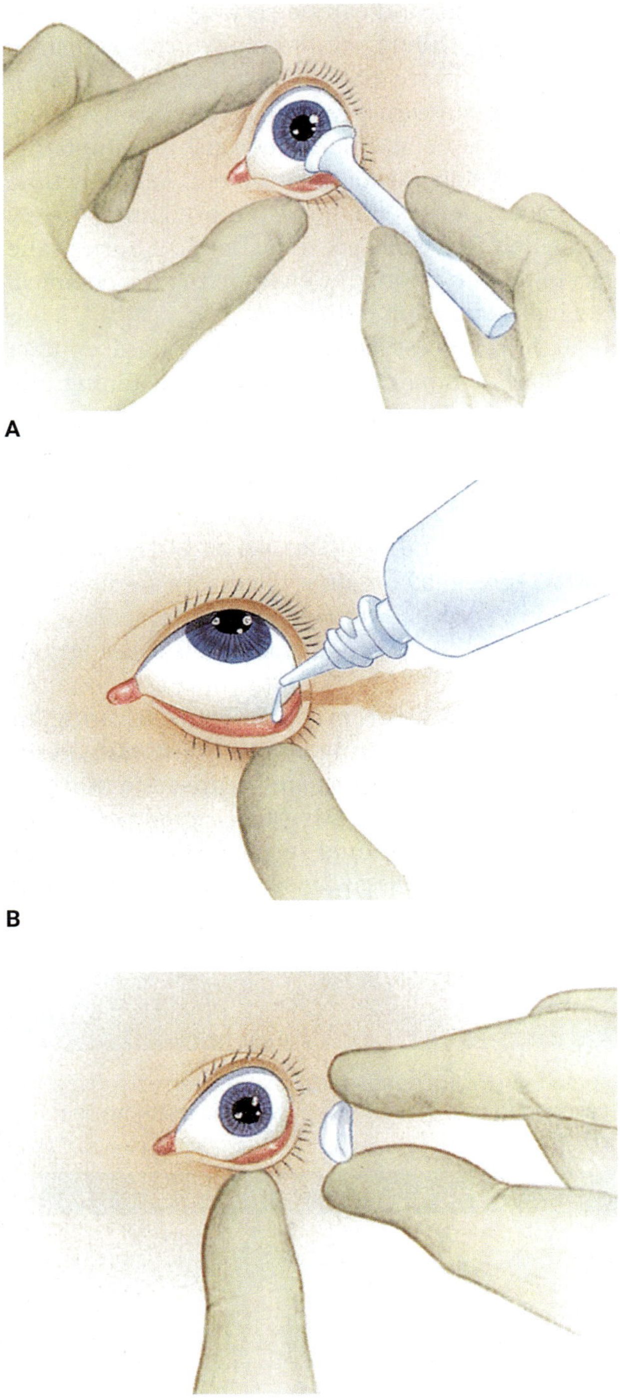
A
B
C

FIGURE 27-24 Removing contact lenses should be limited to patients with chemical burn injuries to the eye. **A.** To remove hard contact lenses, use a specialized suction cup moistened with sterile saline solution. **B.** To remove soft contact lenses, instill one or two drops of saline or irrigating solution. **C.** Next, pinch off the lens with your gloved thumb and index finger.

concert with the opposite eye, or appear quite the same as the opposite eye. If you think a patient may have an artificial eye but are not sure, go ahead and ask about it. Although no harm will be done if you care for an artificial eye as you would a normal one, you need to clearly understand the patient's eye function.

Epistaxis and Injuries of the Nose

Epistaxis, typically referred to as a nosebleed, is a common problem that can occur spontaneously or from trauma. Common causes of nosebleeds include digital trauma (picking the nose with a finger) and dry air. Nosebleeds are further classified into anterior and posterior epistaxis. Anterior nosebleeds usually originate from the area of the septum and bleed slowly. They are usually self-limited and resolve quickly. Posterior nosebleeds are usually more severe and often cause the patient to swallow blood, which can lead to nausea and vomiting. Trauma to the face and skull that results in a basilar skull fracture can cause the posterior wall of the nasal cavity to become unstable. Due to this risk, attempting to place a nasopharyngeal airway in a patient with significant facial trauma, or a suspected basilar skull fracture, is avoided. Follow local protocols regarding insertion of a nasopharyngeal airway in a patient with head or facial trauma.

When you are assessing injuries involving the nose, it helps to picture the inside of the nose itself (**FIGURE 27-25**). The nasal cavity is divided into two sections or chambers by the nasal septum, which is made of cartilage. Within each nasal chamber, there are layers of bone called the **turbinates**, which are covered with a moist lining. Both chambers have a superior turbinate, a middle turbinate, and an inferior turbinate. As a person breathes, air moves through the nasal chambers and is humidified as it passes over the turbinates. Directly above the nose are the frontal sinuses and, on either side, the orbit of the eye.

In patients with severe nasal injury, there may also be injury to the cervical spine. Keep in mind that cerebrospinal fluid (CSF) may escape down through the nose (or ears) following a fracture at the base of the skull. If blood or drainage contains CSF, a characteristic staining of the dressing will occur. This can be seen by using a piece of gauze to absorb

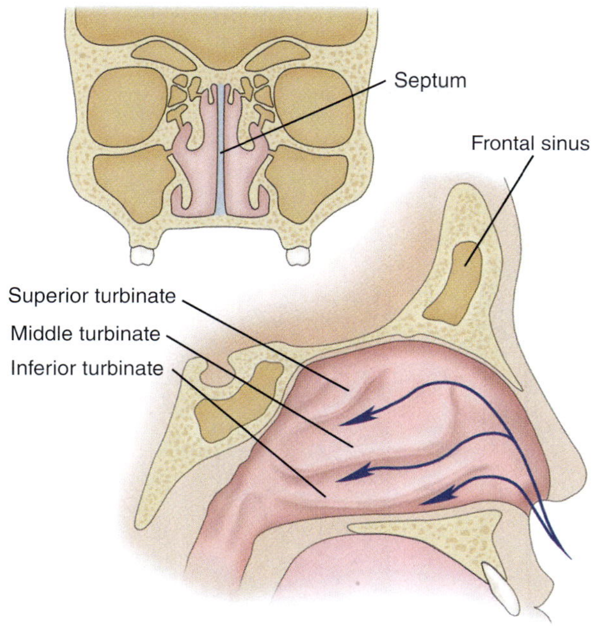

FIGURE 27-25 The nose has two chambers, divided by the septum. Each chamber is composed of layers of bone called turbinates. Above the nose are the frontal sinuses and, on either side, the orbits of the eyes.

blood that is flowing from the nose or ears. If CSF is present, the blood will be surrounded by a lighter ring of fluid. This is often called the halo test. Do not delay care or transport of a priority patient to perform the halo test.

You can control bleeding from abrasions and lacerations to the nose by applying pressure with a sterile dressing. When there are nasal fractures, blood may drain posteriorly down the patient's throat, requiring frequent suctioning. If the patient is bleeding heavily from the nose, this is most likely caused by significant trauma, and you must consider cervical spine injury. The patient should not be moved if the airway can be managed in the patient's current position. For a nontrauma patient who is bleeding from the nose, one effective way to control bleeding is to place the patient in a sitting position, leaning forward, and pinch the nostrils together for 10 to 15 minutes. For a detailed discussion of the care for epistaxis, see Chapter 25, *Bleeding*.

Words of Wisdom

Patients diagnosed with hemophilia, hypertension, or liver problems or who take anticoagulant drugs (eg, aspirin, warfarin, apixaban, rivaroxaban) have a significantly increased risk of severe epistaxis. This bleeding will be difficult to control even if there is no trauma. In these cases, minimize scene time and consider an ALS intercept if there is a long transport distance.

Injuries of the Ear

The ear is a complex organ that is associated with hearing and balance. The ear is divided into three parts (**FIGURE 27-26**). The external ear is composed of the **pinna**, or auricle, which is the part lying outside of the head, and the **external auditory canal**, which leads in toward the **tympanic membrane**, or eardrum. The middle ear contains three small bones (the hammer, anvil, and stirrup) that move in response to sound waves hitting the tympanic membrane. This is the mechanism by which sounds are heard and differentiated. The middle ear is connected to the nasopharynx by the **eustachian tube**. This connection permits equalization of pressure in the middle ear when external atmospheric pressure changes. The inner ear is composed of bony chambers filled with fluid. As the head moves, so does the fluid. In response, fine nerve endings within the fluid send impulses to the brain indicating the position of the head and the rate of change of position.

Ears are often injured, but they usually do not bleed very much. If local pressure does not control the bleeding, you can apply a roller dressing (**FIGURE 27-27**). First, however, you should place a soft, padded dressing between the back of the ear and the scalp because bandaging the ear against the tender underlying scalp can be extremely painful for the patient. In the case of an ear avulsion, you should wrap the avulsed part in a dry sterile dressing and put it in a plastic bag labeled with the patient's name, then float the bag in ice water, without allowing the tissue to come in direct contact with the ice. Transport the avulsed part to the hospital with the patient. Often, avulsed tissue from the ear can be reattached.

Sudden changes in pressure created by a blast wave may rupture one or both tympanic membranes. Patients with a ruptured tympanic membrane will often report severe ear pain, difficulty hearing, or ringing in the affected ear. The tympanic

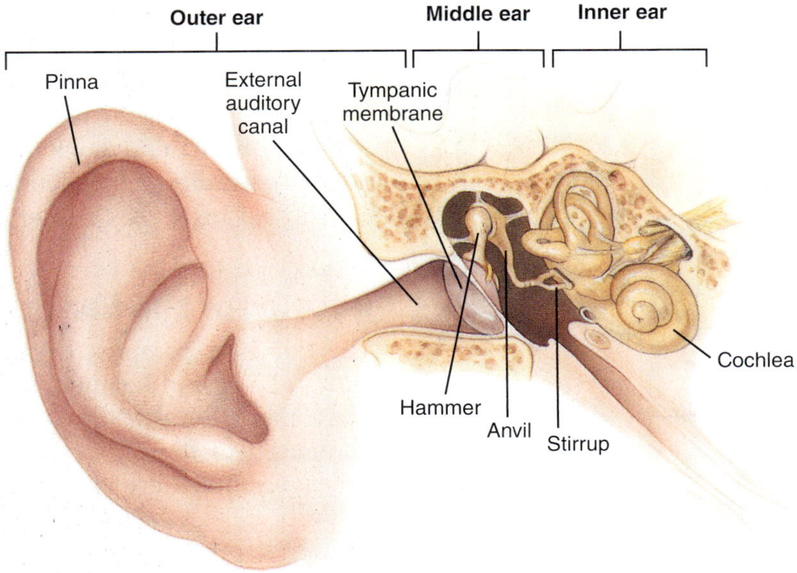

FIGURE 27-26 The ear has three principal parts: the external, or outer, ear, composed of the pinna, external auditory canal, and tympanic membrane; the middle ear, including the hammer, anvil, and stirrup; and the inner ear, composed of bony chambers filled with fluid.

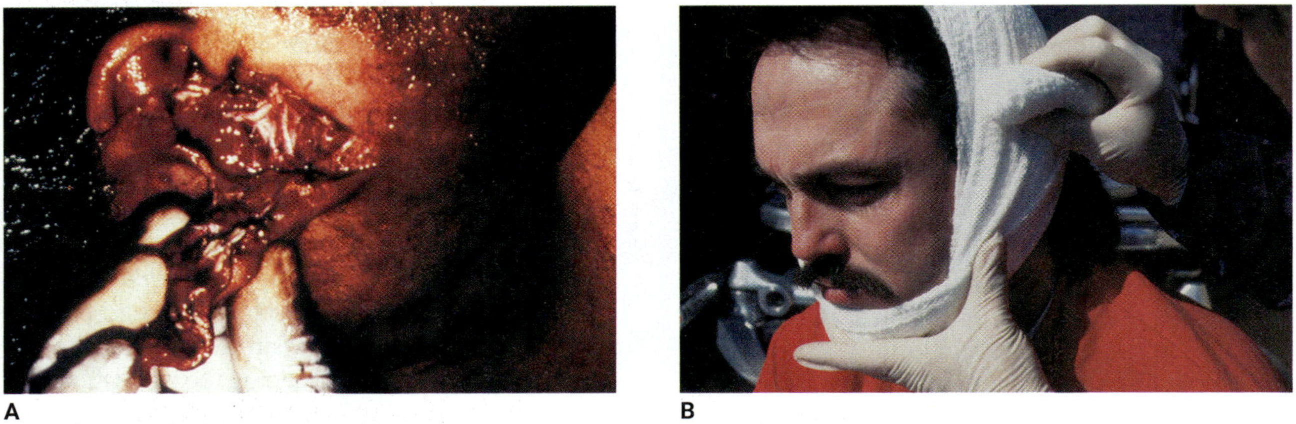

FIGURE 27-27 A. A major laceration of the ear. **B.** Proper treatment includes use of a soft, sterile pad behind the ear, between it and the scalp. Then wrap a roller gauze dressing around the head to include the entire ear.

membrane may also be perforated by insertion of objects (such as a cotton swab) too far into the ear. Any patient with a suspected tympanic membrane injury should be transported to the hospital for a more detailed evaluation.

The external auditory canal is a favorite place for children to place foreign bodies such as crayons or food. All such items should be removed by a physician in the ED. Never try to manipulate the foreign body because you may press it further into the auditory canal and cause permanent damage to the tympanic membrane.

Again, note any clear fluid coming from the ear of a severely injured patient because this may indicate a fracture at the base of the skull with communication to the brain.

Facial Fractures

Fractures of the facial bones typically result from blunt impact. For example, the patient's head collides with a steering wheel or windshield in an automobile crash or is hit by a baseball bat or pipe in an assault. You should assume that any patient who has sustained a direct blow to the mouth or nose has a facial fracture. Other clues to the possibility of fracture include bleeding in the mouth, inability to swallow or talk, absent or loose teeth, and/or loose or movable bone fragments. Patients may also report that "it doesn't feel right" when they close their jaw, signaling an irregularity of bite.

Facial fractures alone are not acute emergencies unless there is airway compromise or serious bleeding; however, they are an indication of significant blunt force trauma applied to that region of the body. Serious bleeding from a facial fracture can be life threatening. In addition to external hemorrhage, there is the danger of blood clots lodging in the upper airway and causing an obstruction (**FIGURE 27-28**). Another source of potential airway obstruction is swelling, which can be extreme within the first 24 hours after injury. If you notice swelling during assessment or at any time while the patient is in your care, check for airway obstruction.

Mandible (lower jaw) fractures are relatively common because of the prominence of the mandible itself. These fractures are second only to nasal fractures in frequency.[5] Most of these fractures are the result of vehicle collisions and assaults. If your patient has a mandibular fracture, then consider the major force necessary to cause that fracture; there

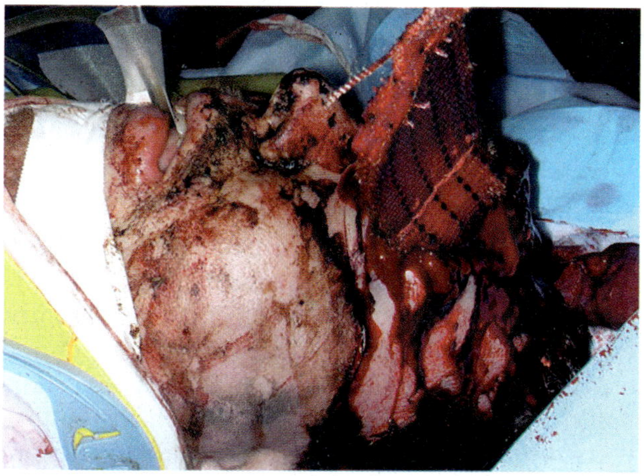

FIGURE 27-28 Bleeding following a crushing injury to the face can be life threatening because, in addition to the external hemorrhage, blood clots in the airway can cause a complete obstruction.

YOU are the EMT

You reassess the patient en route, including his vital signs, and note that his breathing is becoming increasingly labored. His airway remains clear of secretions and blood, but his neck appears to be more swollen than it was during previous assessments.

Recording Time: 16 Minutes	
Level of consciousness	Conscious and alert; anxious
Respirations	26 breaths/min; labored
Pulse	124 beats/min; strong and regular
Skin	Cool and moist; perioral cyanosis is developing
Blood pressure	122/58 mm Hg
Oxygen saturation (Spo_2)	88% (on room air)

The hospital staff are notified of the change in the patient's condition. The nurse tells you to bring him straight to the trauma room on your arrival.

8. What is the most likely cause of your patient's labored breathing?

9. What adjustments, if any, should you make to your current treatment?

is a strong probability your patient will have additional facial trauma and/or cervical injuries. Signs of a mandibular fracture include a misalignment of the teeth, numbness of the chin, and an inability to open the mouth. The patient will most likely have swelling, bruising, and loosened or missing teeth.

Maxillary fractures are predominantly found after blunt-force, high-energy impacts such as an unrestrained driver striking the steering wheel, a fall, or a direct blow from an object such as a pipe. The signs include massive facial swelling, instability of the facial bones, and misalignment of the teeth.

Dental Injuries

Fractured and avulsed teeth are common following facial trauma. Dental injuries may be associated with motor vehicle crashes or an assault. Always assess the patient's mouth following a facial injury, especially if your examination reveals fractured or avulsed teeth. Teeth fragments (or even whole teeth) can become an airway obstruction. Remove them or bone fragments from the mouth; it is often possible to reimplant them. Also remove any loose dentures or dental bridges to protect against airway obstruction. Note that the removal of dentures will affect the shape of the patient's jaw, making it more difficult to get a mask seal when performing bag-mask ventilation. Bleeding will occur whenever a tooth is violently displaced from its socket; therefore, apply direct pressure to stop the bleeding.

Street Smarts

Dental injuries can be traumatic to a patient. Not only is the injury itself traumatic, but the patient's permanent teeth may also be lost, affecting everything from eating to smiling. Keep this in mind when providing care.

When managing an avulsed tooth, handle it by its crown and not by the root. Do not wipe off the tooth if it is dirty; instead, rinse it under cold water. When transporting the patient, bring along the tooth, placing it in a special tooth storage solution if available in your supplies, or in cold milk or sterile saline. There are also commercially available kits that may be used. If none of these options is available, a patient who is alert and cooperative without other serious injuries can hold the tooth in their mouth, where their saliva will provide an appropriate storage medium (**FIGURE 27-29**). Notify the receiving facility about the avulsed tooth because reimplantation is recommended within 1 hour after the trauma.

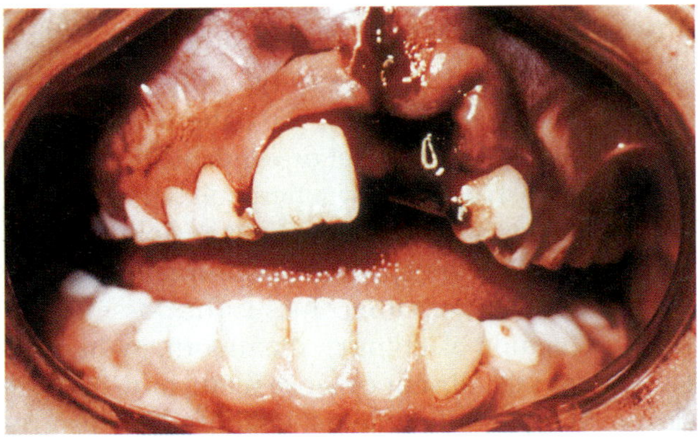

A

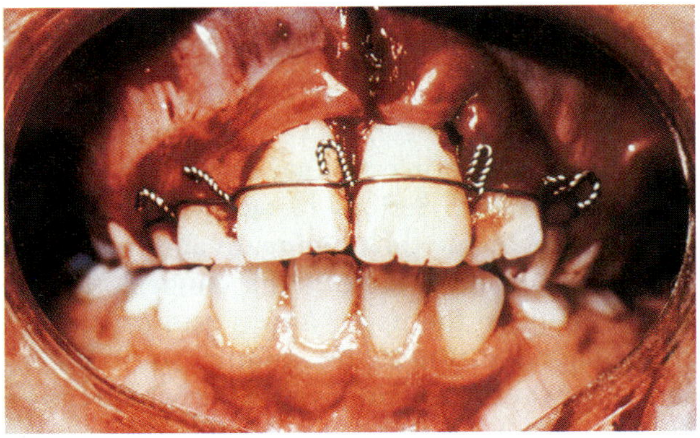

B

FIGURE 27-29 A. Save any lost teeth or bone fragments following an injury to the mouth. **B.** Even with traumatic loss of a tooth, the possibility of successful reimplantation is very good, especially if the tooth is stored in an appropriate tooth-storage solution, cold milk, or sterile saline.

Injuries of the Cheek

You may encounter an object that is impaled in the patient's cheek. If you are unable to control the bleeding and it is compromising the patient's airway, remove the impaled object if possible and provide direct pressure on the inside and outside of the cheek. The amount of bandaging should not be so overwhelming that it occludes the mouth and makes it difficult for the patient to breathe.

Injuries of the Neck

The neck contains many structures that are vulnerable to injury by blunt trauma, such as from a steering wheel in a car crash, or by penetrating injury, such as a stab or gunshot wound. These structures include the upper airway, the esophagus, the carotid arteries and jugular veins, the thyroid cartilage or Adam's apple, the cricoid cartilage, and the upper part of the trachea. Any injury to the neck is serious and should be considered life threatening until proven otherwise in the ED.

Blunt Injuries

Any crushing injury of the upper part of the neck has the potential to involve the larynx or trachea. In blunt-force injuries, such as a collision with a steering wheel or a clothesline injury sustained while riding a bicycle, the larynx becomes crushed against the cervical spine, resulting in soft-tissue injury, fractures, and/or separation of the fascia that connects the thyroid and cricoid cartilages. These strangulation injuries can also be found in either intentional or unintentional hangings. Once the cartilages of the upper airway and larynx are fractured, they do not spring back to their normal position. This type of fracture can lead to loss of voice, difficulty swallowing, severe and sometimes fatal airway obstruction, and leakage of air into the soft tissues of the neck (**FIGURE 27-30**).

The presence of air in the soft tissues produces a characteristic crackling sensation called **subcutaneous emphysema**. If you feel this sensation when you palpate the neck, you should maintain the airway as best you can and provide immediate transport. Be aware that complete airway obstruction can develop rapidly in these patients as a result of swelling or bleeding into the underlying tissues. Recall that a hoarse voice is a sign of airway swelling, and stridor indicates impending airway obstruction.

To manage a laryngeal injury, secure the patient's airway and provide oxygenation and ventilation as needed. It may be difficult to manage the airway in patients with these injuries; therefore, ALS should be considered early if available. An incident involving an injury to the throat may also have caused a cervical spinal injury; therefore, spinal motion restriction may be indicated. Follow local protocols regarding use of spinal precautions.

> **Words of Wisdom**
>
> When laryngeal injury is suspected, unless doing so is contraindicated, elevate the head of the stretcher and allow the patient to assume the position that allows them to breathe most easily.

Penetrating Injuries

Penetrating injuries to the neck can cause profuse bleeding from laceration of the great vessels in the neck: the carotid arteries or the jugular veins (**FIGURE 27-31**). Injuries to the carotid and jugular

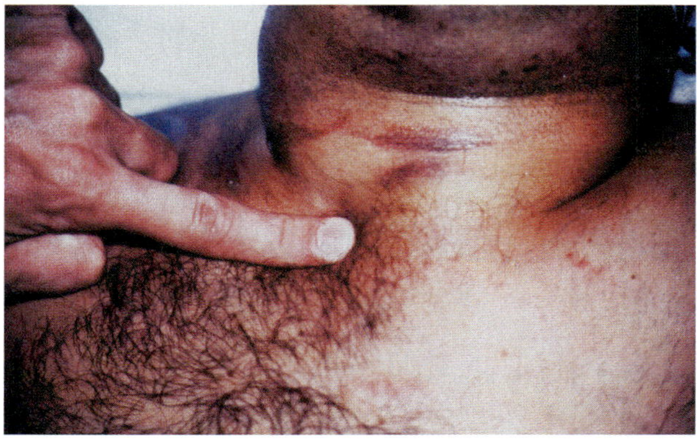

FIGURE 27-30 Fractures of the larynx or trachea can cause air to leak from the airway into the subcutaneous tissues. The presence of air in the soft tissues produces a crackling sensation called subcutaneous emphysema.

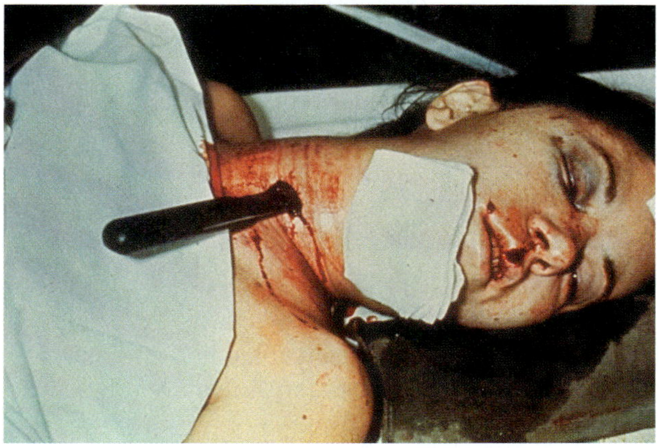

FIGURE 27-31 Penetrating injuries to the neck can result in profuse bleeding if a carotid artery or jugular vein is damaged.

vessels in the neck can cause the body to bleed out. Injuries to these large vessels may also allow air to enter the circulatory system. If a vein has been punctured, air may be sucked through it to the heart, a clinical situation called an **air embolism**. A large amount of air in the right atrium and right ventricle of the heart can lead to cardiac arrest. The airway, the esophagus, and even the spinal cord can be damaged by a penetrating injury.

Open injuries to the larynx can result from a knife stabbing or penetration by a similar object. Penetrating and impaled objects should not be removed unless they interfere with cardiopulmonary resuscitation (CPR). Stabilize all impaled objects if they are not obstructing the airway. See Chapter 26, *Soft-Tissue Injuries*.

Direct pressure over the bleeding site will control most neck bleeding. Follow the steps in **SKILL DRILL 27-3**:

1. Apply direct pressure to the bleeding site using a gloved fingertip, if necessary, to control bleeding (**Step 1**).
2. Apply a sterile occlusive dressing to ensure that air does not enter a vein (**Step 2**).
3. Secure the dressing in place with roller gauze, adding more dressings if needed.
4. Wrap the gauze around and under the patient's shoulder. To avoid possible airway and circulation problems, do not wrap the gauze around the neck.

Despite the use of these measures, the tissues within the neck may continue to bleed and compress the upper airway, so you should look for signs of airway obstruction.

You might find it necessary to apply pressure both above and below the penetrating wound to control life-threatening bleeding from the carotid artery (above) and the jugular vein (below). You may also need to treat the patient for shock.

If indicated, initiate spinal motion restriction precautions and provide prompt transport. Ensure that the airway remains open en route and apply high-flow oxygen.

Skill Drill 27-3 Controlling Bleeding From a Neck Injury

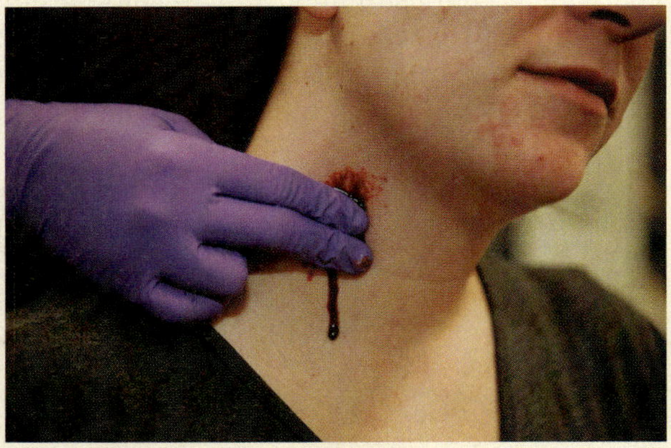

Step 1

Apply direct pressure to the bleeding site using a gloved fingertip, if necessary, to control bleeding.

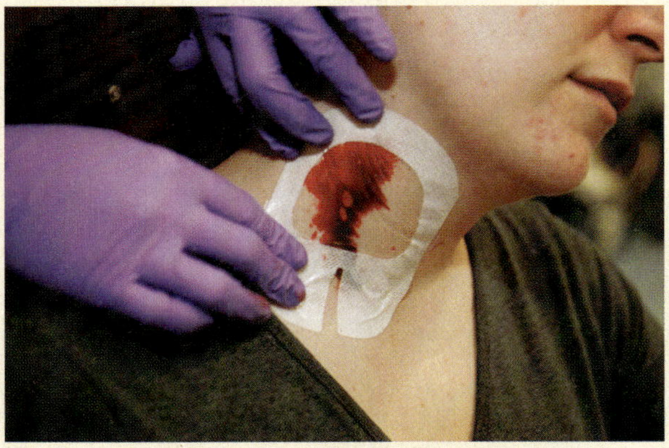

Step 2

Apply a sterile occlusive dressing to ensure that air does not enter a vein.

YOU are the EMT SUMMARY

1. What should be your most immediate concern after receiving this initial patient information?

The presence of severe facial trauma should immediately increase your index of suspicion for potential airway and ventilation compromise, including partial or complete upper airway obstruction. Direct trauma to the nose and mouth can be a source of significant bleeding. Severe swelling and bleeding can occur in the oropharynx. Crushing injuries to the larynx and trachea are associated with a high incidence of airway and ventilation compromise. The risk of upper airway obstruction is significantly higher if the patient has a decreased level of consciousness and is unable to expel blood from the mouth on their own. Also, if the patient swallows large amounts of blood, the risk of vomiting and subsequent aspiration is high.

Dislodged teeth can fall to the back of the throat and be aspirated into the lungs or cause complete obstruction of the upper airway.

Crushing injuries to the throat should increase your index of suspicion for a spinal injury. In addition, when trauma is severe enough to fracture facial bones, the possibility of an underlying brain injury should be considered as well.

2. What should your initial actions consist of when you arrive at the scene?

First, conduct a scene size-up. Although law enforcement personnel have advised you that the scene is secure, you must remain aware of your surroundings at all times. Your patient has been assaulted, which means that the perpetrator, if not in custody, could return to the scene. Ascertain the total number of patients and call for additional resources if you think you will need them.

As you are approaching the patient, form a general impression.

As you make physical contact with the patient, introduce yourself and manually stabilize his head. Next, assess the status of the patient's airway. If he can talk to you, he has no *immediate* airway problems, although this can quickly change. If there is any blood in his oropharynx, remove it with suction. If he is conscious and alert, consider allowing him to suction his own mouth. Take standard precautions, including facial protection.

After ensuring a patent airway, assess the quality of the patient's breathing and intervene at once. If he is breathing adequately, monitor his oxygen saturation and administer high-flow oxygen via a nonrebreathing mask if he becomes hypoxic. If he has signs of inadequate breathing (eg, fast or slow rate, shallow breathing [reduced tidal volume]), assist his ventilations.

Complete your primary assessment by assessing the rate and quality of his radial and carotid pulses and looking for and immediately controlling any severe external bleeding. If signs of shock are present, begin immediate shock treatment.

3. Does this patient have a patent airway? How can you tell?

Because the patient is conscious, alert, and talking, he has a patent airway—at least, for the time being. Although he has blood in his mouth, he is able to keep his airway clear by spitting it out. The patient's voice is hoarse; this should concern you because it could indicate upper airway swelling or a crushing injury to the structures of the anterior neck (ie, trachea, larynx).

At this point in the primary assessment, you have not yet determined if he has any injuries that could affect his level of consciousness, such as a closed head injury. Therefore, you must pay meticulous attention to his mental status and be prepared to suction the blood from his mouth. If he has a loss of consciousness, he will not be able to maintain his airway and you need to be prepared to intervene immediately. *Regardless of the situation, a patient's airway must remain patent at all times!*

4. What should be your initial treatment priorities for this patient?

The goal of the primary assessment is to *find and quickly treat* problems associated with the ABCs. Further assessment and treatment must focus on injuries or conditions that will kill your patient *first*.

Your patient has severe facial trauma and his voice is hoarse. Although he is able to maintain his own airway right now, do not assume that he will be able to continue to do this until you get him to a hospital. Closely monitor his airway and ventilation status!

Your partner is providing manual stabilization of the patient's head based on the assumption that trauma significant enough to cause massive facial trauma can just as easily fracture or dislocate a spinal vertebra.

Closely monitor his airway for continued oral bleeding. If he remains conscious and can easily follow commands, you can allow him to hold the rigid suction catheter and suction the blood from his mouth himself.

Carefully monitor the patient's level of consciousness and breathing adequacy, keep his airway clear

YOU are the EMT SUMMARY continued

of blood, and be prepared to assist his ventilations if his condition deteriorates.

5. On the basis of the MOI, what type of injuries should you suspect and assess for?

On the basis of your assessment, the patient's injuries appear to be isolated to his face and anterior part of the neck. However, a more in-depth assessment by a physician is needed to rule out occult injuries. Facial swelling, which is common following blunt force facial trauma, can make assessment difficult.

On the basis of the MOI, you should be suspicious for facial bone fractures and injury to his trachea and/or larynx. Indicators of facial fractures include oropharyngeal bleeding, loose or absent teeth, difficulty talking or swallowing, and loose or obviously movable bone fragments. Your patient's report that it "doesn't feel right" when he tries to close his mouth signals an irregular bite (dental malocclusion) and is a sign of a mandibular fracture. This is a significant finding because it takes *a lot* of force to fracture the mandible!

Any crushing injury to the anterior part of the neck is likely to involve the larynx or trachea. During your assessment, you detected bruising and swelling of the throat, and the patient's voice is hoarse. These are red-flag indicators of significant anterior neck trauma. Suspect fracture of the cartilage of the larynx or trachea if you detect subcutaneous emphysema, a crackling sensation that is felt when palpating the soft tissues of the neck.

Fractures of the zygomas (cheekbones) often present with a flattened appearance of the cheekbones; however, if the face is severely swollen, this may not be grossly apparent.

When caring for a patient with blunt facial trauma, assess the ability of the patient to move their eyes in all directions. Inability of the patient to look up (paralysis of upward gaze) suggests an orbital (blowout) fracture, in which case a bone fragment has entrapped one of the oculomotor nerves.

A brain injury cannot be ruled out. During your assessment, you should look in and behind the ears. Bruising over the mastoid bone (Battle sign) indicates a basilar skull fracture. Blood that is draining from the ears may contain CSF. This is also an indicator of a basilar skull fracture. Blood or clear fluid drainage from the nose is also a sign of an underlying skull fracture.

Sudden hyperextension of the head during trauma can cause fractures or dislocations of the vertebrae of the cervical spine. Initiate spinal motion restriction precautions when caring for a patient with significant blunt facial trauma.

6. What should you do if this patient begins to vomit?

If aspiration occurs, the risk of mortality increases significantly, so you *must* have a plan of action to prevent aspiration while transporting a patient who is secured in the supine position.

If the patient begins to vomit, *immediately* place him on his side to allow vomitus to drain from his mouth. It is imperative that you protect the patient's airway, but as you turn the patient onto his side, you must also avoid aggravating any possible spinal injury by ensuring that spinal alignment and motion restriction are properly maintained.

While the patient is on his side, suction his mouth to remove any remaining vomitus that did not drain with gravity. Before returning the patient to a supine position, make sure *all* vomitus and other secretions are removed from his mouth!

7. How should you treat a patient with active oral bleeding and inadequate ventilation?

Not only is the patient's airway in immediate jeopardy from obstruction from blood clots and aspiration, but inadequate ventilation will result in hypoxia and may lead to respiratory or cardiopulmonary arrest. Therefore, you must treat both problems simultaneously.

If blood has pooled in the patient's mouth, immediately place the patient onto his side to allow the blood to drain from his mouth. Suction the airway for up to 15 seconds. Then assist the patient's ventilations if they are not adequate.

Continue this alternating pattern of suctioning and assisting ventilations as needed, until the bleeding in the oropharynx is minimal or stops altogether. The patient's airway must remain patent at all times and adequate ventilation must be ensured.

Patients with this type of airway and ventilation predicament would benefit from advanced airway management, especially if they are unconscious. Paramedics can intubate the patient, thus isolating the trachea and preventing aspiration, while manually ventilating the patient with a bag-mask device attached to the endotracheal tube. Request ALS, if possible, when caring for patients with this type of complex airway and breathing problem.

8. What is the most likely cause of your patient's labored breathing?

Reassessment reveals that his airway remains clear of blood. However, the anterior part of his neck is more swollen, so you should suspect that

YOU are the EMT SUMMARY continued

the swelling in his upper airway is increasing, most likely because of injury to his trachea or larynx, thus making it increasingly difficult for him to breathe. His oxygen saturation of 88% reflects significant hypoxemia, and perioral cyanosis (cyanosis around the mouth) is developing.

It is important to note that not all patients with significant injuries deteriorate at the scene. Many of them deteriorate en route to the hospital or shortly after you arrive at the hospital. Therefore, it is critical to *frequently reassess* any patient with injuries that could jeopardize airway patency and impair ventilation.

9. What adjustments, if any, should you make to your current treatment?

Your patient's ventilation status has clearly deteriorated. You should administer oxygen by nonrebreathing mask and consider assisting his ventilations with a bag-mask device and high-flow oxygen. Try to assist the patient's breathing, but do not be too aggressive. If he becomes combative and pushes the bag-mask device away from his face, apply a nonrebreathing mask and carefully monitor his breathing.

If he tolerates assisted ventilation, use extreme caution. Although you must maintain adequate minute volume, a tracheal or laryngeal injury can be exacerbated by aggressive positive-pressure ventilation. Squeeze the bag-mask device just enough to improve the amount of tidal volume with each breath; observe for visible chest rise.

You should *not* use any type of mechanical ventilation device, such as a flow-restricted, oxygen-powered ventilation device, when ventilating a patient with tracheal or laryngeal trauma. These devices deliver oxygen under high pressure and can cause further injury to patients with fractures of the trachea or larynx.

Prep Kit

Ready for Review

- Soft-tissue injuries and fractures of the bones of the face and neck are common and vary in severity.
- For face and neck injuries, your priorities are to prevent further injury to the cervical spine, manage the airway and ventilation of the patient, and control bleeding.
- Airway compromise may be caused by heavy bleeding into the airway, swelling in and around the structures of the airway located in the face and neck, and injuries to the central nervous system that interfere with normal respiration.
- To control heavy bleeding from soft-tissue injuries to the face, use direct pressure with a dry, sterile dressing. If brain tissue is exposed, use a moist, sterile dressing.
- Check for bleeding inside the mouth because this may produce airway obstruction.
- Open the airway using the jaw-thrust maneuver (when indicated), and clear the airway in all patients with facial injuries.
- Save avulsed pieces of skin and tissue, and transport them with the patient for possible reattachment at the hospital.
- Maintain a high index of suspicion for unconscious patients with unequal pupils; this sign may indicate an illness or an injury to the brain. Remember, unequal pupil size is not an abnormal finding in some individuals.
- Foreign bodies on the surface of the eye should be irrigated gently with normal saline solution. Always flush from the region of the eye closest to the nose toward the outside, away from the midline.
- If a foreign body is on the underside of the eyelid, remove it gently with a cotton-tipped

Prep Kit continued

applicator. Never remove foreign bodies stuck to the cornea.
- Chemicals, heat, and light rays all can cause burn injury to the eyes, resulting in permanent damage.
- Be alert to clear fluid draining from the ears or nose. This may indicate a basilar skull fracture.
- Blunt and penetrating trauma to the neck can produce life-threatening injuries. Palpate the neck for signs of subcutaneous emphysema.

In patients with this sign, complete airway obstruction may develop in minutes.
- If bleeding is present from a penetrating injury, direct pressure over the site will usually control most forms of bleeding.
- Be alert to the possibility of an air embolism from an open neck injury. Place an occlusive dressing over the site, and provide direct pressure.

Vital Vocabulary

air embolism The presence of air in the veins, which can lead to cardiac arrest if it enters the heart.

anisocoria Uneven pupil size.

blow-out fracture A fracture of the orbit or of the bones that support the floor of the orbit.

conjunctiva The delicate membrane that lines the eyelids and covers the exposed surface of the eye.

conjunctivitis Inflammation of the conjunctiva.

cornea The transparent tissue layer in front of the pupil and iris of the eye.

epistaxis A nosebleed.

eustachian tube A tube that connects the middle ear to the oropharynx.

external auditory canal The ear canal; leads to the tympanic membrane.

globe The eyeball.

iris The muscle and surrounding tissue behind the cornea that dilate and constrict the pupil, regulating the amount of light that enters the eye; pigment in this tissue gives the eye its color.

lacrimal glands The glands that produce fluids to keep the eye moist; also called tear glands.

lens The transparent part of the eye through which images are focused on the retina.

mastoid process The prominent bony mass at the base of the skull approximately 1 inch (2.5 cm) posterior to the external opening of the ear.

optic nerve A cranial nerve that transmits visual information to the brain.

pinna The external, visible part of the ear.

pupil The circular opening in the middle of the iris that admits light to the back of the eye.

retina The light-sensitive area of the eye where images are projected; a layer of cells at the back of the eye that changes the light image into electric impulses, which are carried by the optic nerve to the brain.

retinal detachment Separation of the retina from its attachments at the back of the eye.

sclera The tough, fibrous, white portion of the eye that protects the more delicate inner structures.

sternocleidomastoid muscles The muscles on either side of the neck that allow movement of the head.

subcutaneous emphysema A characteristic crackling sensation felt on palpation of the skin, caused by the presence of air in soft tissues.

temporomandibular joint The joint formed where the mandible and cranium meet, just in front of the ear.

tragus The small, rounded, fleshy bulge that lies immediately anterior to the ear canal.

turbinates Layers of bone within the nasal cavity.

tympanic membrane The eardrum; a thin, semi-transparent membrane in the middle ear that transmits sound vibrations to the internal ear by means of auditory ossicles.

Prep Kit continued

References

1. National Association of Emergency Medical Technicians. *PHTLS: Prehospital Trauma Life Support*. 10th ed. Burlington, MA: Jones & Bartlett Learning; 2023.
2. National Association of State EMS Officials. *National Model EMS Clinical Guidelines: Version 3.0 https://nasemso.org/content.aspx?page_id=22&club_id=157064&module_id=701974*. Updated March 2022. Accessed February 12, 2025.
3. Gragg J, Blair K, Baker MB. Hyphema. *StatPearls*. National Library of Medicine website. https://www.ncbi.nlm.nih.gov/books/NBK507802/. Updated December 26, 2022. Accessed February 12, 2025.
4. Hawkins E, Mills MD. Ocular trauma. In: Cone D, Brice JH, Delbridge TR, eds. *Emergency Medical Services: Clinical Practice and Systems Oversight*. John Wiley & Sons, Ltd; 2021:316–320.
5. Chang EW. General principles of mandible fracture and occlusion. Medscape website. https://emedicine.medscape.com/article/868375-overview?form=fpf. Updated December 6, 2021. Accessed February 12, 2025.

Chapter 28

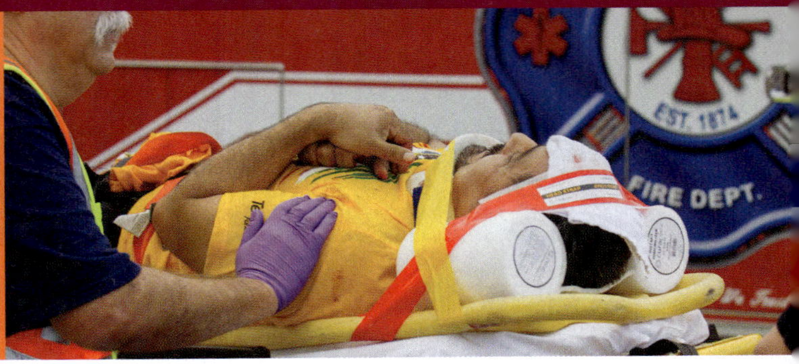

Head and Spine Injuries

NATIONAL EMS EDUCATION COMPETENCIES

Trauma

Applies knowledge to provide basic emergency care and transportation based on assessment findings for an acutely injured patient.

Head, Facial, Neck, and Spine Trauma

- Life threats (pp 1050–1060)
- Spine trauma (pp 1045–1049, 1053–1055)
- Penetrating neck trauma (Chapter 27, *Face and Neck Injuries*)
- Laryngotracheal injuries (Chapter 27, *Face and Neck Injuries*)
- Shaken baby syndrome (Chapter 35, *Patients With Special Challenges*)
- Facial fractures (Chapter 27, *Face and Neck Injuries*)
- Skull fractures (pp 1039–1043)
- Foreign bodies in the eyes (Chapter 27, *Face and Neck Injuries*)
- Globe rupture (Chapter 27, *Face and Neck Injuries*)
- Dental trauma (Chapter 27, *Face and Neck Injuries*)
- Severe epistaxis (Chapter 27, *Face and Neck Injuries*)

Nervous System Trauma

- Traumatic brain injury (pp 1041–1045)
- Spinal cord injury (pp 1045–1046, 1057–1062)

KNOWLEDGE OBJECTIVES

1. Describe the anatomy and physiology of the nervous system, including its divisions into the central nervous system (CNS) and peripheral nervous system (PNS) and the structures and functions of each. (pp 1033–1038)
2. Explain the functions of the somatic and autonomic nervous systems. (pp 1036–1037)
3. Discuss the major bones of the skull and spinal column and their related structures as they relate to the nervous system. (pp 1037–1038)
4. Explain the different types of head injuries, their potential mechanism of injury (MOI), and general signs and symptoms of a head injury that EMTs should consider when performing a patient assessment. (pp 1038–1045)
5. Describe the assessment process to determine if the patient has a traumatic brain injury (TBI). (p 1041)
6. Explain the difference between a primary (direct) injury and a secondary (indirect) injury. (pp 1041–1042)
7. Describe the different types of brain injuries and their corresponding signs and symptoms, including increased intracranial pressure, concussion, contusion, and injuries caused by medical conditions. (pp 1038–1045)
8. Describe the different types of injuries that may damage the cervical, thoracic, or lumbar spine. (p 1045)
9. Explain the steps in the patient assessment process for a person who has a suspected head or spine injury, including variations that may be required as related to the type of injury. (pp 1046–1055)

10. List the MOIs that cause a high index of suspicion for the possibility of a head or spinal injury. (pp 1048–1049)
11. Explain emergency medical care of a patient with a head injury, including the three general principles designed to protect and maintain the critical functions of the CNS. (pp 1055–1057)
12. Explain emergency medical care of a patient with a spinal injury, including the implications of not properly caring for patients with injuries of this nature, the steps for performing manual in-line stabilization, proper use of a cervical collar, and key symptoms that contraindicate in-line stabilization. (pp 1057–1062)
13. Explain the process of preparing patients who have suspected head or spinal injuries for transport, including the use of a long backboard, vacuum mattress, short backboard, and other devices to minimize movement of the patient's cervical and thoracic spine. (pp 1062–1074)
14. Discuss age-related variations in the care of pediatric patients suspected of having head or spine trauma. (pp 1072–1074)
15. Explain the circumstances in which a helmet should be left in place or removed from a patient with a possible head or spinal injury. (pp 1074–1079)
16. List the steps EMTs must follow to remove a helmet. (pp 1074–1079)

SKILLS OBJECTIVES

1. Demonstrate how to perform a jaw-thrust maneuver on a patient with a suspected spinal injury. (p 1048)
2. Demonstrate how to perform manual in-line stabilization on a patient with a suspected spinal injury. (p 1059; Skill Drill 28-1)
3. Demonstrate how to apply a cervical collar to a patient with a suspected spinal injury. (pp 1060–1061; Skill Drill 28-2)
4. Demonstrate how to secure a patient with a suspected spinal injury to a long backboard. (pp 1063–1064; Skill Drill 28-3)
5. Demonstrate how to secure a patient with a suspected spinal injury using a vacuum mattress. (pp 1066–1069; Skill Drill 28-4)
6. Demonstrate how to secure a patient with a suspected spinal injury who was found in a sitting position. (pp 1070–1072; Skill Drill 28-5)
7. Demonstrate how to perform spinal motion restriction for pediatric patients. (pp 1073–1074; Skill Drill 28-6)
8. Demonstrate how to perform spinal motion restriction for a child in a car seat. (p 1075; Skill Drill 28-7)
9. Demonstrate how to remove the face mask of a sports helmet from a patient with a suspected head or spinal injury. (pp 1076–1077)
10. Demonstrate how to remove an entire helmet from a patient with a suspected head or spinal injury. (pp 1077–1079; Skill Drill 28-8)

Introduction

The nervous system is a complex network of nerve cells that enables all parts of the body to function. It includes the brain, the spinal cord, and several billion nerve fibers that carry information to and from all parts of the body. Because the nervous system is so vital, it is well protected. The brain lies within the skull, and the spinal cord is inside the bony spinal canal. Despite this protection, serious injuries can damage the nervous system.

This chapter briefly reviews the anatomy and function of the central and peripheral nervous systems and of the skeletal system. Discussion of specific head, brain, and spinal injuries follows, including signs, symptoms, assessment, and treatment. Management of possible spinal injuries and removal of helmets are also discussed.

Anatomy and Physiology

Nervous System

The nervous system is divided into two major anatomic parts: the central nervous system (CNS) and the peripheral nervous system (PNS) (**FIGURE 28-1**). The CNS is composed of the brain and the spinal cord, including the nuclei and cell bodies of most nerve cells. Long nerve fibers link these cells to the body's various organs through openings in the spinal column. These fibers constitute the PNS.

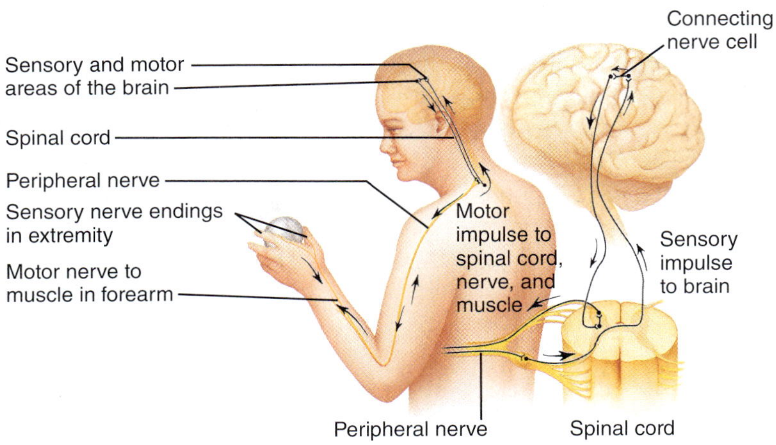

FIGURE 28-1 The nervous system has two anatomic components: the central nervous system and the peripheral nervous system. The central nervous system is composed of the brain and the spinal cord. The peripheral nervous system conducts sensory impulses from the skin and other organs to the spinal cord, and motor impulses from the spinal cord to the muscles.

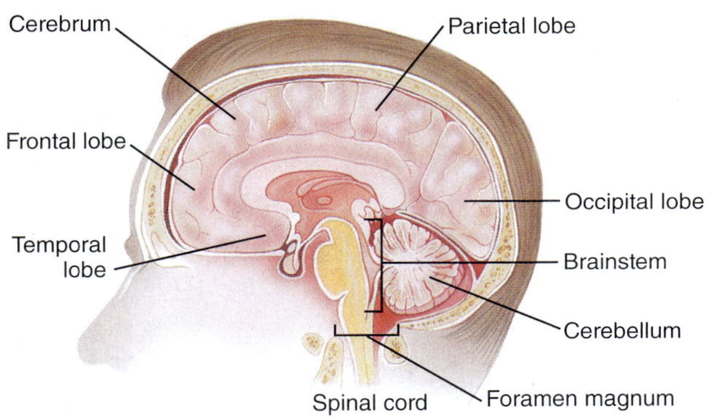

FIGURE 28-2 The brain is part of the central nervous system and is the organ that controls the body. It is divided into three major areas: the cerebrum, the cerebellum, and the brainstem.

Central Nervous System

The CNS is composed of the brain and spinal cord. The brain controls the body and is the center of consciousness. It is divided into three major areas: the cerebrum, the cerebellum, and the brainstem (**FIGURE 28-2**).

Of these segments, the cerebrum is the largest, accounting for approximately 75% of the brain's total volume. Divided into right and left hemispheres, the cerebrum is responsible for most voluntary motor functions and conscious thought. Beneath the cerebrum lies the cerebellum, which coordinates balance and body movements. The most primitive part of the CNS, the brainstem, controls virtually all involuntary functions, including those of the cardiac and respiratory systems. Located deep within the cranium, the brainstem is the best-protected part of the CNS.

The spinal cord, the other major portion of the CNS, is mostly made up of fibers that extend from the brain's nerve cells. The spinal cord carries messages between the brain and the body via the gray and white matter of the spinal cord. Gray matter is composed of neural cell bodies and synapses, which are connections between nerve cells. White matter consists of fiber pathways.

Protective Coverings

Without a protective framework of skin, muscle, bone, and other tissues, the fragile brain and spinal cord would be incredibly vulnerable to devastating injury and infection. In addition to these protective layers, the superficial fascia connecting the muscle to the skin contains white blood cells that destroy pathogens attempting to enter through an open wound.

The brain and spinal cord are further protected by three distinct membranes called the **meninges**: the dura mater, arachnoid mater, and the pia mater (**FIGURE 28-3**).

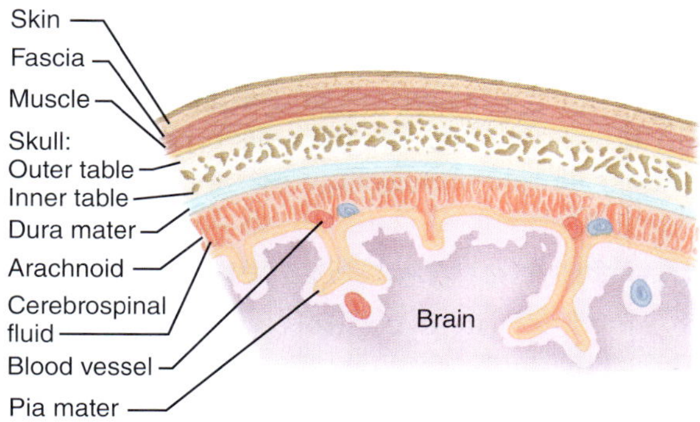

FIGURE 28-3 The central nervous system has several layers of protective coverings: the skin, muscles and their fascia, bone, and the meninges. The three layers of the meninges are the dura mater, the arachnoid mater, and the pia mater.

Special Populations

THE NERVOUS SYSTEM OF CHILDREN

Compared with the adult nervous system, the pediatric nervous system is immature, underdeveloped, and not well protected. The head-to-body ratio of an infant and young child is disproportionately larger, making this population more susceptible to head injuries from falls or motor vehicle crashes. The occipital region of the head is larger, which increases the momentum of the head during a fall. The subarachnoid space is relatively smaller, resulting in less cushioning for the brain. The brain tissue and the cerebral vasculature are fragile and susceptible to bleeding from shearing forces, such as during an incident of shaken baby syndrome. See Chapter 35, *Patients With Special Challenges*.

The brain has a limited store of glucose and relies on a steady supply from the bloodstream to meet its energy needs. In children, the brain demands a relatively greater amount of glucose than in adults. The demand is particularly high during the early developmental period, such as infancy.[1] These special needs mean the pediatric brain is at risk for secondary brain damage from hypotension and hypoxic events.

Spinal cord injuries are less common in pediatric patients when compared to adults, with less than 5% of these injuries occurring in children.[2] If a child's cervical spine is injured, it is most likely to be an injury to the ligaments as the result of a fall. If you suspect a neck injury, apply spinal motion restriction according to your protocols.

The outermost meningeal layer, the dura mater, is a tough, fibrous tissue resembling leather. Ordinarily, there is no gap between the dura mater and the inner surface of the skull. However, a traumatic injury could cause bleeding into this potential space. Beneath the dura mater is the arachnoid mater, so named because it is often described as having a spiderweb appearance. Between the dura mater and the arachnoid mater is a space referred to as the subdural space, which contains blood vessels called bridging veins. Beneath the arachnoid mater is the innermost meningeal layer, the pia mater, which adheres to the brain tissue. Between the arachnoid mater and the pia mater is a thin space referred to as the subarachnoid space, which contains cerebral blood vessels and cerebrospinal fluid (CSF), which bathes, nourishes, and cushions the brain and spinal cord. CSF is produced within ventricular chambers inside the brain itself. At any given time, there is approximately 125 to 150 mL of CSF surrounding the CNS.

If an injury disrupts the meningeal layers, CSF may leak from the nose, the ears, or an open skull fracture. Because CSF appears as a clear, watery fluid, its leakage may be mistaken for a runny nose. Therefore, the EMT should be suspicious any time a patient with a head injury presents with a runny nose or reports having a salty taste at the back of the throat. Because such leaks indicate that a pathway has been opened between the brain and the outside environment, the risk of infection and meningitis is especially concerning.

Peripheral Nervous System

The PNS has two anatomic parts: 31 pairs of spinal nerves and 12 pairs of cranial nerves (**FIGURE 28-4**).

The 31 pairs of spinal nerves conduct sensory impulses from the skin and other organs to the spinal cord. They also conduct motor impulses from the spinal cord to the muscles. Because the arms and legs have so many muscles, the spinal nerves serving the extremities are arranged in complex networks. The brachial plexus controls the arms, and the lumbosacral plexus controls the legs.

Twelve pairs of cranial nerves emerge from the brainstem and transmit information directly to or from the brain. For the most part, they perform special functions in the head and face, related to sight, smell, taste, hearing, and facial movements.

There are two major types of peripheral nerves. The sensory nerves, with endings that perceive only one type of information, carry that information from the body to the brain via the spinal cord. The motor nerves, one for each muscle, carry information from the CNS to the muscles. The connecting nerves, found only in the brain and spinal cord, connect the sensory and motor nerves with short fibers, which allow the cells on either end to exchange simple messages.

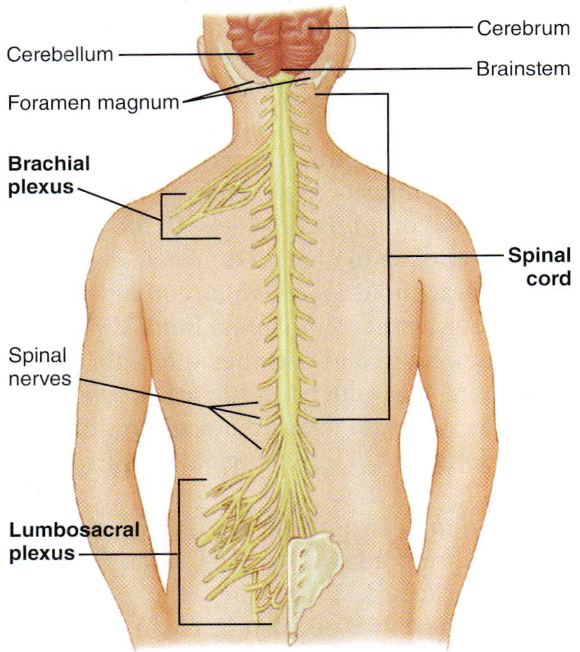

FIGURE 28-4 The peripheral nervous system is a complex network of motor and sensory nerves. The brachial plexus controls the arms, and the lumbosacral plexus controls the legs.

How the Nervous System Works

The nervous system controls virtually all of the body's activities, including reflex, voluntary, and involuntary activities.

In connecting the sensory and motor nerves of the limbs, the connecting nerves in the spinal cord form a reflex arc. If a sensory nerve in this arc detects an irritating stimulus, such as heat, it will bypass the brain and send a message directly to a motor nerve, causing a response such as pulling away from the heat (**FIGURE 28-5**).

Voluntary activities are the actions that we consciously perform, in which sensory input determines the specific muscular activity; for example, reaching across the table for a salt shaker or to pass a dish. **Involuntary activities** are the actions that are not under our conscious control, such as breathing; in most instances, we inhale and exhale without consciously thinking about it. Many of our body's functions occur independently of thought, or involuntarily.

The part of the nervous system that regulates or controls our voluntary activities, including almost all coordinated muscular activities, is called the somatic (voluntary) nervous system. The mechanism

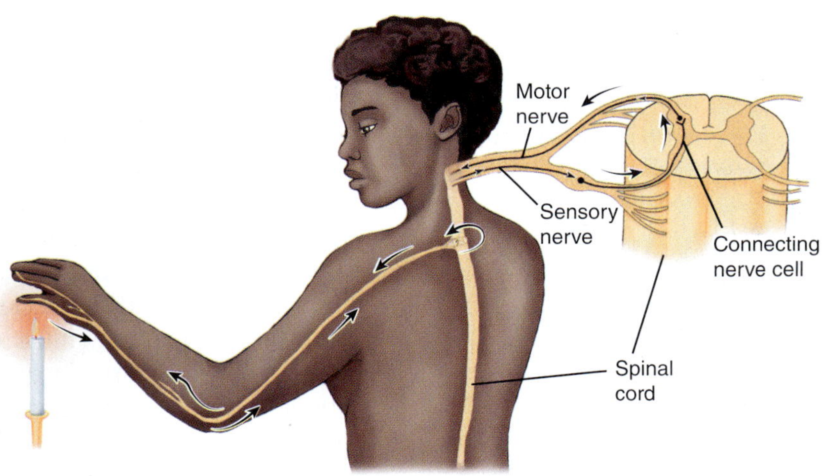

FIGURE 28-5 The connecting nerves in the spinal cord form a reflex arc. If a sensory nerve in this arc detects an irritating stimulus, it will bypass the brain and send a direct message to a motor nerve.

> **Words of Wisdom**
>
> CNS structures, whose bony enclosures protect them quite well, are also very fragile. Protecting them from further damage is vital to the patient's future ability to live a normal life. Lean toward caution and overprotection in assessing and treating possible brain and spinal cord injuries.

of the somatic nervous system is simple. The brain interprets the sensory information that it receives from the peripheral and cranial nerves and responds by sending signals to the voluntary muscles.

The body functions that occur without conscious effort are regulated by the much more primitive autonomic (involuntary) nervous system. The autonomic nervous system controls the functions of many of the body's vital organs, over which the brain has no voluntary control.

The autonomic nervous system is divided into two sections: the sympathetic nervous system and the parasympathetic nervous system. When confronted with a threatening situation, the sympathetic nervous system reacts to the stress with the fight-or-flight response. This response causes the pupils to dilate, smooth muscle in the lungs to dilate, heart rate to increase, and blood pressure to rise. This response also causes the body to shunt blood to vital organs and to skeletal muscle. During this time of stress, a hormone called epinephrine (also known as adrenaline) is released, which is responsible for much of these activities inside the body. The parasympathetic nervous system has the opposite effect on the body, causing blood vessels to dilate, slowing the heart rate, and relaxing the muscle sphincters. When this portion of the autonomic nervous system is activated, the body shunts blood to the organs of digestion. As the body attempts to maintain homeostasis (balance), these two divisions of the autonomic nervous system tend to balance each other so that basic body functions remain stable and effective.

Skeletal System

Skull

The skull is composed of two groups of bones: the cranium, which protects the brain, and the facial bones (**FIGURE 28-6**). The cranium is composed of several thick bones that fuse together to form a shell above the eyes and ears that holds and protects the brain. It is occupied by 80% brain tissue, 10% blood supply, and 10% CSF. The brain connects to the spinal cord through a large opening at the base of the skull called the foramen magnum.

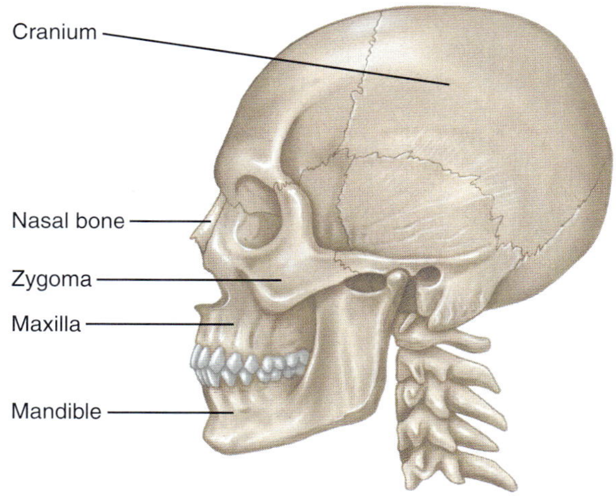

FIGURE 28-6 The skull includes two large structures: the cranium and the face.

The bones of the cranial vault divide the cranium into distinct portions. The most posterior portion of the cranium is called the occiput. On each side of the cranium, the lateral portions are called the temples or temporal regions. Between the temporal regions and the occiput lie the parietal regions. The forehead is called the frontal region.

Spinal Column

The spinal column is the body's central supporting structure. It has 33 bones, called vertebrae, and is divided into five sections: cervical, thoracic, lumbar, sacral, and coccygeal (**FIGURE 28-7**). Injury to the vertebrae, depending on the level at which the injury occurs, may result in paralysis if the underlying spinal cord or nervous structures are also damaged.

The front part of each vertebra consists of a round, solid block of bone called the vertebral body; the back part forms a bony arch. From one vertebra to the next, the series of arches form a tunnel running the length of the spinal column. This tunnel is the spinal canal, which encases and protects the spinal cord (**FIGURE 28-8**).

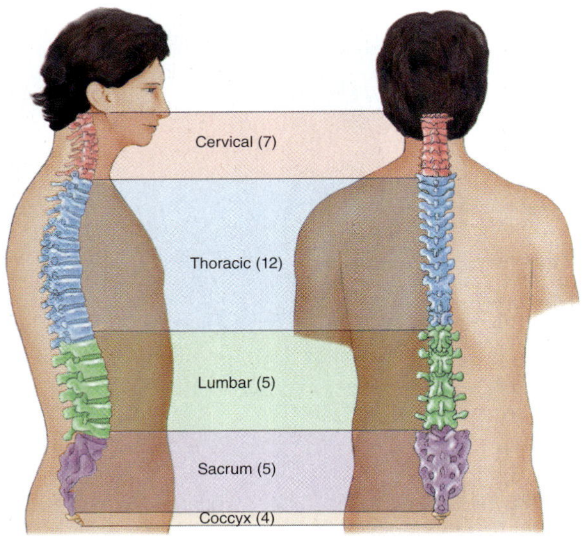

FIGURE 28-7 The spinal column is the body's central supporting system and consists of 33 bones divided into five sections. Injury to the vertebrae may cause paralysis.

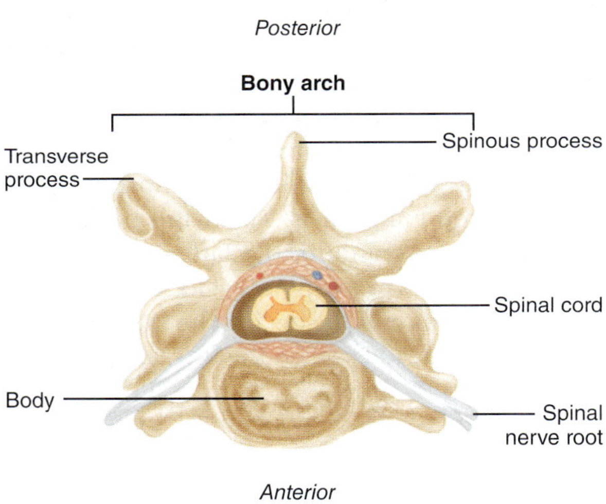

FIGURE 28-8 The spinal canal is formed by the vertebral body in the front (or anteriorly) and the bony arch in the back (or posteriorly).

The vertebrae are connected by ligaments and separated by cushions, called **intervertebral disks**. These ligaments and disks allow the trunk to bend forward and back, but they also limit motion so that the spinal cord is not injured. When the spine is injured or fractured, the spinal cord and its nerves are left unprotected. Therefore, keep the spine aligned throughout transport, using manual stabilization, as necessary. The spinal column itself is almost entirely surrounded by muscles. However, you can usually palpate the posterior spinous processes of some of the vertebrae, which lie just under the skin in the midline of the back. The most prominent and most easily palpable spinous process is at the seventh cervical vertebra at the base of the neck.

Head Injuries

A head injury is a traumatic insult to the head that may result in injury to soft tissue, bony structures, or the brain. These injuries resulted in almost 70,000 deaths in 2021. People 75 years or older are particularly at risk, accounting for approximately one-third of hospitalizations and deaths relating to these injuries.[3] When head injuries are fatal, invariably, the cause is associated injury to the brain. In addition to the head injury, and dependent on the mechanism of injury (MOI), you should be alert to the fact that the patient may have sustained additional trauma such as cervical spine injuries, pelvic injuries, and chest injuries.

There are two types of head injuries. In a **closed head injury**, the brain has been injured but there is no opening to the brain. For example, a severe blow that fractures the skull but does not create an open wound would be considered a closed head injury. In an **open head injury**, an opening exists from the outside world to the brain. Obvious skull deformity with a break in the skin is a sign of an open head injury, which is often caused by penetrating trauma. There may be bleeding and exposed brain tissue.

Falls and motor vehicle crashes are among the most common MOIs resulting in head and brain injuries. Head injuries also occur commonly in victims of assault, during sports-related incidents, and as a result of child abuse.

Words of Wisdom

The possibility of physical abuse should be considered in all children who have signs and symptoms of mild to moderate head injury.[4]

Any head injury is potentially serious. If not properly treated, those injuries that seem minor at first may become a life-threatening brain injury

TABLE 28-1 General Signs and Symptoms of a Head Injury

Following a head injury, any patient who exhibits one or more of these signs or symptoms has potentially sustained a very serious underlying brain injury:

- Lacerations, contusions, or hematomas to the scalp
- Soft area or skull depression on palpation
- Visible fractures or deformities of the skull
- Decreased mentation, confusion
- Irregular breathing pattern
- Widening pulse pressure
- Slow heart rate
- Ecchymosis around the eyes or behind the ear over the mastoid process
- Clear or pink CSF leakage from a scalp wound, the nose, or the ear
- Failure of the pupils to react to light
- Unequal pupil size
- Loss of sensation and/or motor function
- A period of unconsciousness
- Amnesia
- Seizures
- Numbness or tingling in the extremities
- Dizziness
- Visual complaints
- Combative or other abnormal behavior
- Nausea or vomiting
- Posturing: decorticate (arms rigidly flexed and drawn in toward the body; legs extended with pointed toes) or decerebrate (limbs rigidly extended away from the body)

(**TABLE 28-1**). Conversely, severe lacerations of the scalp or fractures of the skull may occur with little or no brain injury and may lead to minimal or no long-term consequences.

Scalp Lacerations

Scalp lacerations can be minor or very serious, particularly in children. Because both the face and the scalp have unusually rich blood supplies, even small lacerations can quickly lead to significant blood loss (**FIGURE 28-9**). Occasionally, this blood loss may be severe enough to cause hypovolemic shock, particularly in children. In any patient with multiple injuries, bleeding from scalp or facial lacerations may contribute to hypovolemia. In addition, because scalp lacerations are usually the result of direct blows to the head, they are often an indicator of deeper, more serious injuries.

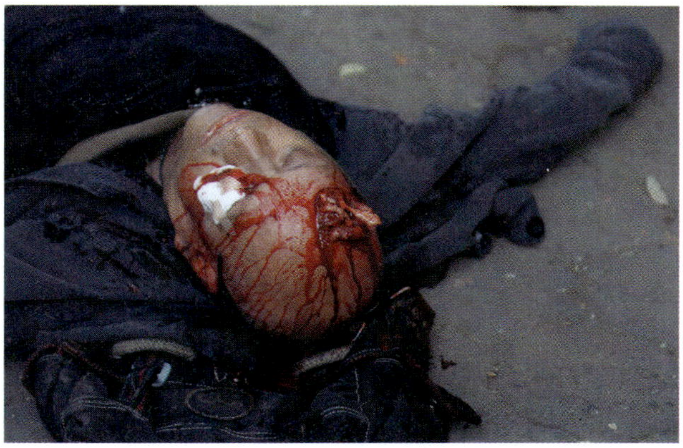

FIGURE 28-9 Because scalp lacerations are usually the result of direct blows to the head, they are often an indicator of deeper, more serious injuries.

Skull Fracture

Significant force applied to the head may cause a skull fracture. As with any fracture, a skull fracture may be open or closed, depending on whether there is an overlying laceration of the scalp. Injuries from bullets or other penetrating weapons frequently result in fracture of the skull. The diagnosis of a skull fracture is usually made in the hospital with a computed tomography (CT) scan, but maintain a high index of suspicion that a fracture is present if the patient's head appears deformed or if there is a visible crack in the skull within a scalp laceration. Additional signs of skull fracture that you may see include ecchymosis (bruising) that develops under the eyes (**raccoon eyes**) (**FIGURE 28-10A**) or behind one ear over the mastoid process (**Battle sign**) (**FIGURE 28-10B**). These signs may be less obvious in patients with dark skin.

Linear Skull Fractures

Linear skull fractures (nondisplaced skull fractures) are the most common type of fracture to the skull (**FIGURE 28-11A**). Radiographs are required to diagnose a linear skull fracture because there are often no physical signs such as deformity. If the brain is uninjured and there are no scalp lacerations, then linear fractures are not life threatening. However, if there is a scalp laceration with the linear fracture, making it an open fracture, there is a risk of infection and bleeding inside the brain.

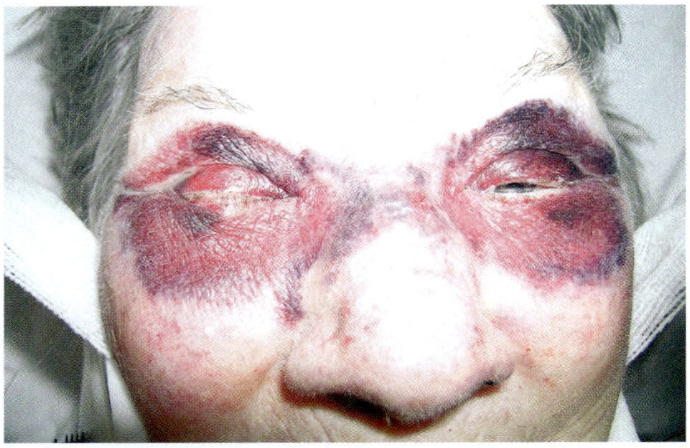

A

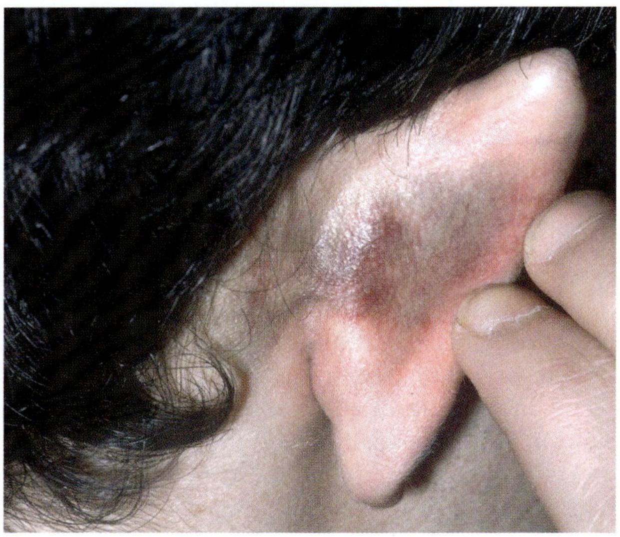

B

FIGURE 28-10 Signs of skull fracture include ecchymosis under the eyes (raccoon eyes) (**A**) or behind one ear over the mastoid process (Battle sign) (**B**).

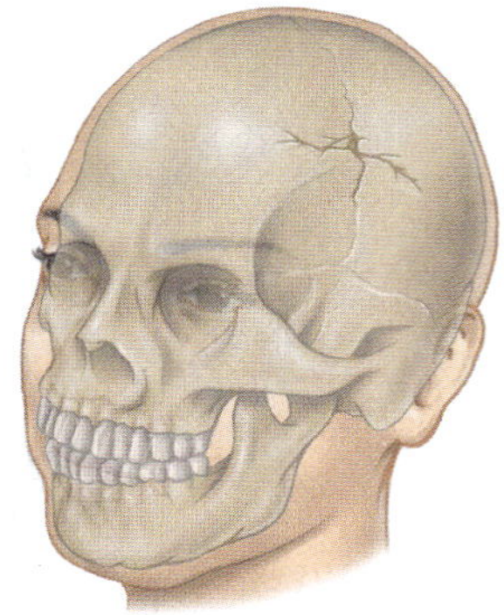

A

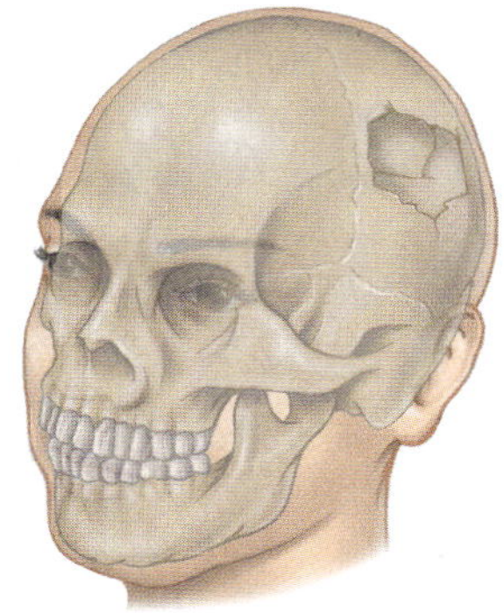

B

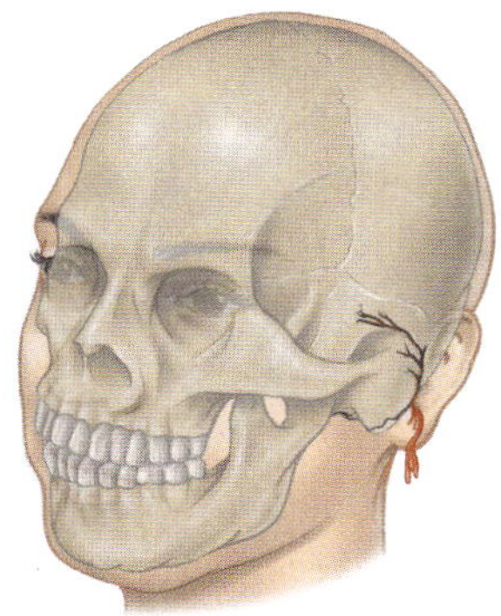

C

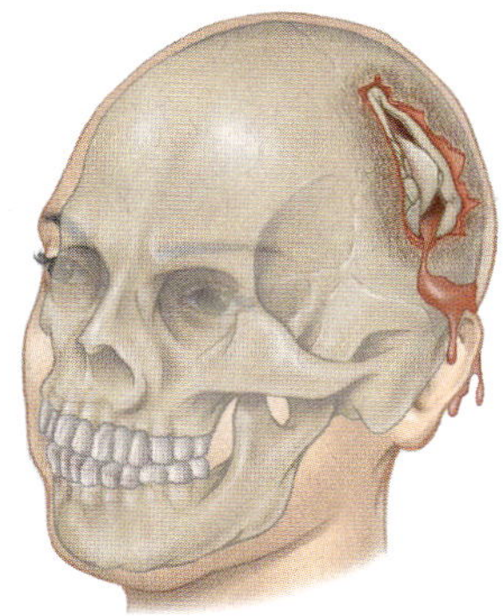

D

FIGURE 28-11 Types of skull fractures. **A.** Linear. **B.** Depressed. **C.** Basilar. **D.** Open.

Depressed Skull Fractures

Depressed skull fractures result from high-energy direct trauma to the head with a blunt object (such as a baseball bat) (**FIGURE 28-11B**). The frontal and parietal bones of the skull are most susceptible to these types of fractures because the bones in these areas are relatively thin. Consequently, bony fragments may be driven into the brain, resulting in injury. The scalp may or may not be lacerated. Patients with depressed skull fractures often present with signs of neurologic injury (such as loss of consciousness).

Basilar Skull Fractures

Basilar skull fractures are also associated with high-energy trauma, but they usually occur following diffuse impact to the head (eg, falls, motor vehicle crashes). These injuries generally result from extension of a linear fracture to the base of the skull and are usually diagnosed with a CT scan of the head (**FIGURE 28-11C**).

Signs of a basilar skull fracture include CSF drainage from the nose or the ears, which indicates rupture of the tympanic membrane in the ear. Patients with leaking CSF from either the nose or the ear are at risk for bacterial meningitis.

Other signs of a basilar skull fracture include raccoon eyes or Battle sign. Depending on the extent of the damage, raccoon eyes and Battle sign may appear relatively quickly, but in many patients, they may not appear until up to 24 hours following the injury, so their absence in the field does not rule out a basilar skull fracture.

Open Skull Fractures

Open fractures of the cranial vault result when severe forces are applied to the head and are often associated with trauma to multiple body systems (**FIGURE 28-11D**). Brain tissue may be exposed to the environment, which significantly increases the risk of a bacterial infection (such as bacterial meningitis). Open cranial vault fractures have a very high mortality rate.

Traumatic Brain Injuries

Traumatic brain injury (TBI) refers to physical damage to the brain caused by an external force. This damage can result in cognitive, movement, communication, behavioral, and emotional changes in the person.[5] TBIs may be mild (such as concussion) or moderate to severe. Suspect a moderate to severe TBI when the Glasgow Coma Scale (GCS) score is less than 15, the patient has lost consciousness, there is multisystem trauma that requires airway interventions, or the patient reportedly had a seizure after the traumatic event.[6]

TBIs are classified into two broad categories: **primary (direct) injury** and **secondary (indirect) injury**. Primary brain injury is injury to the brain and its associated structures that results instantaneously from impact to the head. Secondary brain injury refers to a multitude of processes that increase the severity of a primary brain injury and, therefore, negatively affect the outcome. Secondary injuries may be caused by cerebral edema, intracranial hemorrhage, increased intracranial pressure, cerebral ischemia, and infection; however, hypoxia and hypotension are the two most common causes. When caring for patients in the emergency medical services (EMS) setting, it is critical to note that hypertension, hyperventilation, hypothermia, hyperthermia, and particularly hypoxia or hypotension significantly increase the risk of death and disability in a patient with a head injury.[6–8] It is important to monitor for and address all of these issues when they are detected. Secondary brain injury may occur anywhere from a few minutes to several days following the initial head injury.

The brain can be injured directly by a penetrating object, such as a bullet, knife, or other sharp object. More commonly, brain injuries occur indirectly, as a result of external forces exerted on the skull. Consider the most common cause of brain injury, the motor vehicle crash. When the passenger's head hits the windshield on impact with a fixed object, the brain continues to move forward until it comes to an abrupt stop by striking the inside of the skull. This rapid deceleration results in compression injury (or bruising) to the anterior portion of the brain along with stretching or tearing of the posterior portion of the brain. As the brain strikes the front of the skull, the body begins its path of moving backward. The head falls back against the headrest and/or seat, and the brain slams into the rear of the skull. This type of front-and-rear injury is known as a **coup–contrecoup injury**. The same type of injury may occur on opposite sides of the brain in a lateral collision. See Chapter 24, *Trauma Overview*, for further discussion of this MOI.

Words of Wisdom

Based on the mechanism involved with a coup–contrecoup injury, it is possible for a patient to receive a brain injury without a direct impact to the head. A rapid change in direction of movement of the head can cause the brain to move forward and then back with such force that it impacts the inside of the skull. Do not exclude the possibility of brain injury simply because the patient has no external head injuries.

The injured brain starts to swell, initially because of cerebral vasodilation. An increase in cerebral water then contributes to further brain swelling (**cerebral edema**). Note that cerebral edema may not develop until several hours following the initial injury.

Low oxygen levels in the blood aggravate cerebral edema. Therefore, patients with cerebral edema may be at particular risk if hypoxemia is not adequately corrected. In fact, the brain consumes more oxygen than any other organ in the body. For this reason, you must make sure that the airway is open and that adequate ventilations and high-flow oxygen are given to any patient with significant head injury. This is especially true if the patient is unconscious. Do not wait for cyanosis or other obvious signs of hypoxia to develop. Similarly, do not wait for pulse oximetry to confirm hypoxia. Early airway positioning and oxygen administration to achieve an oxygen saturation level greater than 90% is essential for patients suspected to have a moderate or severe TBI.[6]

It is not uncommon for the patient with a head injury to have a convulsion, or seizure.[9] This is the result of excessive excitability of the brain, caused by direct injury or the accumulation of fluid within the brain (edema). Be prepared to manage seizures in all patients who have had a head injury because the brain may have sustained an injury as well.

Words of Wisdom

Another consideration for the combat veteran is the higher incidence of a TBI sustained from trauma secondary to explosion of an improvised explosive device. In some cases, the TBI may go undiagnosed due to similarities with the symptoms of posttraumatic stress disorder or because the patient downplays the symptoms. People with TBI can sustain sensory dysfunction, confusion headaches, memory loss, and general disorientation.

Intracranial Pressure and Herniation

Accumulations of blood within the skull or swelling of the brain itself can rapidly lead to an increase in **intracranial pressure (ICP)**, the pressure within the cranial vault. Increased ICP can squeeze the brain against bony prominences within the cranium or down toward the foramen magnum, a large opening at the base of the skull where the brainstem connects with the spinal cord. If enough pressure is applied to the brainstem, it may protrude (herniate) through the foramen magnum. Because the brainstem regulates vital functions such as heart rate, breathing, and consciousness, pressure applied against the brainstem may produce abnormal changes in the patient's vital signs.

Words of Wisdom

A bulging anterior fontanelle in a non-crying infant is one indicator of increased ICP.

Respiratory indicators of herniation may include Cheyne-Stokes respirations (respirations that are fast and then become slow, with intervening periods of apnea), ataxic (Biot) respirations (characterized by irregular rate, pattern, and volume of breathing with intermittent periods of apnea), and **central neurogenic hyperventilation** (deep, rapid breathing pattern similar to Kussmaul respirations seen in diabetic ketoacidosis, but without an acetone breath odor). Other signs and symptoms of increasing ICP include headache; nausea; vomiting; decreasing alertness; asymmetric, sluggish pupils; decerebrate or decorticate posturing or flaccidity; and increased or widened pulse pressure (the difference between the systolic and diastolic blood pressures). Signs and symptoms will increase in number and severity as ICP continues to rise until herniation occurs.[6]

The triad of increased systolic blood pressure, decreased heart rate, and irregular respirations in the setting of TBI is called the **Cushing triad**. It is a cardinal sign of active herniation of the brain. Other cardinal signs include GCS score of less than 9, posturing or lateralizing signs, progressive neurologic deterioration, and a fixed dilated pupil in one or both eyes.[6]

Intracranial Hemorrhage

For adults, the skull is a rigid, unyielding globe that allows little, if any, expansion of the intracranial contents. It also provides a hard and somewhat

YOU are the EMT

At 0220 hours, you receive a call for a man who was assaulted outside a nightclub. Law enforcement personnel are present and have secured the scene. While you are en route, a police officer radios you and informs you the patient was struck on the side of the head with a baseball bat and is unconscious. Your response time to the scene is less than 5 minutes.

1. What are the potential concerns surrounding the structure of the cranium and potential brain swelling?
2. What is the difference between a primary and a secondary brain injury?

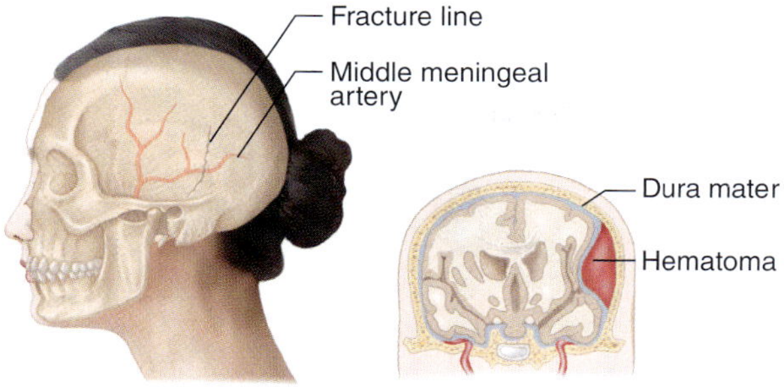

FIGURE 28-12 An epidural hematoma is usually the result of a blow to the head that produces a linear fracture of the temporal bone and damages the middle meningeal artery. Blood accumulates between the dura mater and the skull.

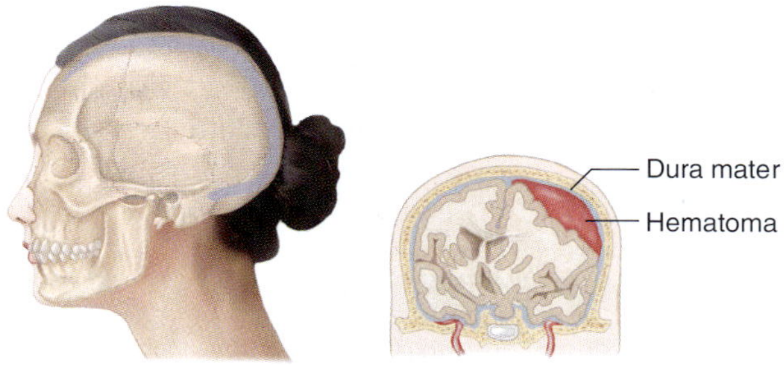

FIGURE 28-13 In a subdural hematoma, venous bleeding occurs beneath the dura mater but outside the brain.

irregular surface against which brain tissue and its blood vessels can be injured when the head sustains trauma.

Epidural Hematoma

An **epidural hematoma** is an accumulation of blood between the skull and dura mater (**FIGURE 28-12**). It is nearly always the result of a blow to the head that produces a linear fracture of the thin temporal bone. The middle meningeal artery runs along a groove in that bone; therefore, it is vulnerable to rupture when the temporal bone is fractured.

Because epidural hemorrhage is usually arterial, symptoms of ICP may progress rapidly. As with many other forms of TBI, the patient may experience an immediate loss of consciousness at the time of injury. Sometimes, this is followed by a brief period of consciousness (lucid interval), during which the patient may be oriented or confused and may complain of nothing more than a worsening headache. However, if such a lucid interval does occur, the person will rapidly lapse back into unconsciousness. Meanwhile, as ICP increases, the pupil on the affected side may become fixed and dilated. Without early surgical intervention to evacuate the hematoma, mortality is approximately 20%. However, when recognized and treated quickly, mortality may be as low as 2%.[10]

Subdural Hematoma

A **subdural hematoma** is an accumulation of blood between the dura mater and the arachnoid mater (**FIGURE 28-13**). It usually occurs after falls or injuries involving strong deceleration forces. Subdural hematomas are more common than epidural hematomas and may or may not be associated with a skull fracture. Bleeding within the subdural space typically results from rupture of the veins that bridge the cerebral cortex and dura.

Because subdural hematomas are associated with venous bleeding, the signs of increasing ICP typically develop more gradually than they do in the setting of an epidural hematoma. However, this can vary depending on the severity of the injury and factors such as the patient's age, medical history, and medications. Signs and symptoms may not develop for hours, days, or even weeks following injury. Older adults may be at greater risk for a variety of reasons. First, due to brain atrophy, the subdural space is enlarged, allowing the brain to move more freely inside the cranium, potentially causing bridging veins to stretch and tear more easily. The increased size of the subdural space also allows for more bleeding to occur before pressure on the brain increases and signs and symptoms become obvious. These patients are also frequently prescribed blood-thinning (anticoagulant) medications, which decrease the blood's ability to clot, and they are more susceptible to falls. Combined, these factors make geriatric patients more susceptible to intracranial hemorrhage from seemingly minor MOIs. Other persons at greater risk are those with clotting deficiencies (eg, hemophilia, alcohol use disorder). Therefore, you must be especially suspicious when assessing these patients, even when their injuries appear minor.

In some cases, the patient with a subdural hematoma presents with signs and symptoms less dramatic than those found in patients experiencing an epidural hemorrhage. These patients may present with complaints of headache, fluctuations in their level of consciousness, or slurred speech. Regardless, these patients require evaluation in the hospital.

> **Street Smarts**
>
> If you are called for symptoms such as headache, dizziness, and vomiting in an older adult or patient with chronic alcohol use disorder, ask if they have fallen recently and look for signs of trauma on their head. Even if the injuries show signs of healing or aging, these findings may indicate that a subdural hematoma has formed. The patient may not make the connection between the current symptoms and a previous injury if the trauma occurred days or even weeks before the onset of their symptoms.

Subarachnoid Hemorrhage

In a **subarachnoid hemorrhage**, bleeding occurs in the subarachnoid space, where the CSF circulates. Common causes of a subarachnoid hemorrhage include trauma or rupture of an aneurysm. A hallmark of subarachnoid hemorrhage is a sudden, severe headache. Other signs may include nausea, vomiting, dizziness, sensitivity to bright lights, and neck rigidity or pain.

In severe cases, as bleeding into the subarachnoid space increases, the patient may display signs and symptoms of increased ICP: decreased level of consciousness, pupillary changes, and seizures. A sudden, severe subarachnoid hemorrhage often results in death. People who survive often have permanent neurologic impairment.

Intracerebral Hematoma

An **intracerebral hematoma** involves bleeding within the brain tissue itself (**FIGURE 28-14**). This type of injury is rare, typically resulting from penetrating trauma to the head; however, when it occurs, mortality is high even with surgery. Further, the location of the bleed may preclude surgical intervention. The progression of increased ICP depends on several factors, including the presence of other brain injuries, the region of the brain involved (frontal and temporal lobes are the most common locations), and the size of the hemorrhage. Once symptoms appear, the patient's condition often deteriorates quickly.

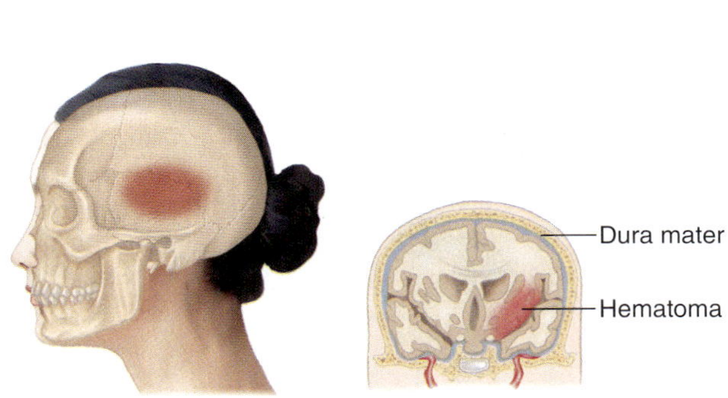

FIGURE 28-14 An intracerebral hematoma involves bleeding within the brain tissue itself.

Concussion

A blow to the head or face may cause **concussion** of the brain. Concussions are also known as mild TBIs. There is no universal definition of a concussion, but in general, it is a TBI with a temporary loss or alteration of part or all of the brain's abilities to function without demonstrable physical damage to the brain. For example, a person who "sees stars" after being struck on the head has sustained a concussion that affects the occipital portion of the brain. A concussion may result in unconsciousness and even the inability to breathe for short periods of time; however, over 90% of patients who sustain a concussion do not experience a loss of consciousness.[11] A concussion is a functional change, not a structural change that could be detected, in the brain. The signs and symptoms are usually transient, resolving on their own without specific interventions.

A patient with a concussion may be confused or have amnesia (loss of memory). Occasionally, the patient can remember everything but the events leading up to the injury; this is called **retrograde amnesia**. Inability to remember events after the injury is called **anterograde (posttraumatic) amnesia**.

Usually, acute signs and symptoms of a concussion last only a short time. In fact, they have often resolved by the time EMS arrives on the scene. Nevertheless, you should ask about symptoms of concussion in any patient who has sustained an injury to the head because a concussive injury may exist; these symptoms include dizziness, weakness, visual changes, or changes in mood. Additional signs and symptoms you may encounter with a patient who has sustained a concussion may include nausea or vomiting, and the patient may report ringing in the ears. Slurred speech and the inability to focus may also be present. Depending on the severity of the concussion, you may also notice that the patient has a lack of coordination, has delayed motor functions, displays inappropriate emotional responses, or reports feeling "in a fog" or "just not right." Patients may also report a temporary headache and may appear to be disoriented.

Patients with symptoms consistent with concussion may also have more serious underlying brain injury. A CT scan is necessary to differentiate between these conditions. Always assume that a patient with signs or symptoms of concussion has a more serious injury until proven otherwise. All patients with signs or symptoms of a concussion should be evaluated by a physician or other qualified health care clinician.

Words of Wisdom

Be aware that all athletes who sustain a concussion should be evaluated by a qualified health care clinician prior to being allowed to return to play. Some of the tools these health care clinicians use are specific, commercially available computerized tests to assess concussion and recovery from it. Often the results of the test are compared to baseline evaluations conducted prior to injury. EMTs are not qualified to conduct these types of assessments or to determine when it is safe to return to play after a concussion. A history of severe or repeated concussions, particularly in athletes, has been associated with decrease in brain function and severe dementia in later life and death.[12]

Brain Contusion

Like any other soft tissue in the body, the brain can sustain a contusion, or bruise. A contusion is often far more serious than a concussion because it involves physical injury to the brain tissue, which may sustain long-lasting and even permanent damage. As with contusions that occur elsewhere in the body, there is associated bleeding and swelling from injured blood vessels. Injury of brain tissue or bleeding inside the skull causes an increase of pressure within the skull. A patient who has sustained a brain contusion may exhibit any or all of the signs of brain injury.

Other Brain Injuries

Brain injuries are not always a result of trauma. Certain medical conditions, such as blood clots or hemorrhages, can also cause brain injuries that produce significant bleeding or swelling. Problems with the blood vessels themselves, high blood pressure, or any number of other problems may cause spontaneous bleeding into the brain, producing an altered mental status. The signs and symptoms of nontraumatic injuries are often the same as those of TBIs, except that there is no obvious history of MOI or any external evidence of trauma. Altered mental status is discussed in Chapter 18, *Neurologic Emergencies*.

Spine Injuries

The cervical, thoracic, and lumbar portions of the spine can be injured in a variety of ways. In **axial loading injuries**, also referred to as axial compression injuries, force is applied along the vertical or longitudinal axis of the spine, which results in load being transmitted along the entire length of the vertebral column. This type of injury can occur one of two ways. It can result when the head strikes a stationary object and the weight of the body continues moving toward the head (eg, shallow diving accident), or it can occur when a person falls from a height and lands on their feet in a standing position, driving the weight of the entire body down into the lumbar spine. These forces can cause herniation of intervertebral disks, compression of the spinal cord and nerve roots, and fragmentation of the vertebrae into the spinal canal.

Other forces that may produce spinal injuries include **hyperflexion** (excessive flexion), **hyperextension** (excessive extension), **hyper-rotation** (excessive rotation), excessive **lateral bending** (such as might occur during a side-impact motor vehicle collision), and **distraction** (pulling apart of the vertebrae along the vertical axis, such as might occur in a hanging). Any one of these unnatural motions can produce fractures and neurologic deficits from damage to the spinal cord or any number of nerves passing through the spinal column.

Patients may complain of pain and tenderness on palpation of the spine. You may rarely even feel or observe a displaced or damaged vertebra under the skin, a deformity sometimes referred to as a "step-off." Other signs and symptoms may include numbness and tingling or paralysis below the level of the injury. However, it is critical to note that a patient with a severe spinal fracture may present with no indications of spinal injury whatsoever. This may occur because the patient has a distracting injury or trauma in another part of the body that produces such severe pain that the patient is unable to notice pain in the spine.

If you suspect these types of injuries, **spinal motion restriction (SMR)** is indicated. SMR refers to patient positioning and moving techniques that minimize unwanted movement of the potentially injured spine.[13] SMR techniques include both manual control and use of adjuncts, such as cervical collars and full-body devices (eg, scoop stretchers, vacuum splints, long spine boards).

Words of Wisdom

While SMR measures limit movement of the spine, they do not completely eliminate those movements; thus, the previously used term spinal *immobilization* is no longer recommended.

Words of Wisdom

When assessing the spine, be aware of the possibility of open wounds from the associated trauma. These open wounds can be penetrating injuries or lacerations. If you follow the mnemonic DCAP-BTLS (Deformities, Contusions, Abrasions, Punctures/penetrations, Burns, Tenderness, Lacerations, Swelling), you will discover any open wounds prior to securing the patient to a backboard. SMR is not indicated in patients with penetrating trauma injuries.[13] Taking the time to do this may delay lifesaving care.

Patient Assessment

You should suspect a possible head or spinal injury anytime you encounter one of the following MOIs:

- Motor vehicle crashes (including motorcycles, snowmobiles, and all-terrain vehicles)
- Pedestrian–motor vehicle crashes
- Fall of greater than 10 feet (3 m) (all ages)
- Blunt trauma to the head or neck
- Penetrating trauma to the head, neck, back, or torso
- Rapid deceleration injuries
- Hangings (distraction)
- Axial loading injuries
- Diving accidents

Motor vehicle crashes, direct blows, falls from heights, assaults, and sports injuries are common causes of head and spinal trauma. A deformed windshield or dented helmet may indicate a major blow to the head, which is likely to have caused TBI (**FIGURE 28-15**). It is especially important to evaluate and monitor the level of consciousness in patients with suspected head injuries, paying particular attention to any changes that may occur.

Scene Size-Up

Evaluate every scene for hazards to your health and the health of your team or bystanders. Motor vehicle crashes are a common cause of head and spinal injuries. These situations have the potential to cause injury to rescuers and bystanders as well. Be prepared with appropriate standard precautions before you approach the patient. You will be spending a great deal of time at the head of the patient. Gloves, a mask, and eye protection should be the minimum standard precautions that you use. Because these patients can have very complicated

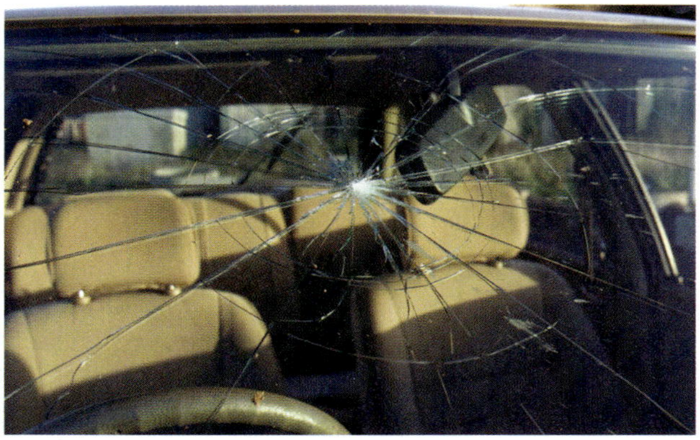

FIGURE 28-15 The classic "star" on the windshield after an automobile crash is a significant indicator of head injury. Be alert for the signs and symptoms of head injury, as well as spinal trauma from axial loading.

injuries, call for advanced life support (ALS) as soon as possible when initial assessment reveals triage criteria indicating high risk for serious injury. Law enforcement may be needed to control traffic or unruly people.

Safety Tips

Many MOIs that cause head and spine injuries may also pose a risk to EMTs. Before you approach the patient, get the "big picture" of scene safety and take any actions necessary to ensure your own well-being. Do not rely entirely on assistance from fire or police personnel; maintain your own awareness of the scene.

As you observe the scene, look for indicators of the MOI. This helps you develop an early index of suspicion for underlying injuries in the patient who has sustained a significant MOI. As you put together information from dispatch and your observations of the scene, consider how the MOI produced the injuries suspected. For example, if you respond to a baseball field for a patient who was knocked unconscious by a foul ball, you may begin to suspect that the patient may have a depressed skull fracture and perform a neurologic assessment during the physical examination. Continue to consider the MOI while assessing a patient.

Words of Wisdom

Proper care of a patient with a possible spinal injury requires assessment of motor and sensory functions both before and after stabilizing the patient. Likewise, careful observation of level of consciousness at different stages of your care for a head-injured patient can provide crucial information. Document your detailed findings of these repeated neurologic examinations to make the information available to hospital personnel and to help establish that your care has been thorough and appropriate.

Primary Assessment

The primary assessment should focus on identifying and managing life-threatening concerns. Threats to the ABCs (Airway, Breathing, and Circulation) are considered life threatening and must be treated immediately to prevent mortality. If life-threatening external hemorrhage exists, follow the XABC sequence (with *X* representing eXsanguination) by controlling the bleeding before addressing airway and breathing concerns.

Most head injuries are considered mild and result in no or limited permanent disability. A small percentage of head injuries are considered moderate, and the patient is left with some permanent disabilities. Even fewer head injuries are considered severe, and many patients with severe head injury die before reaching the hospital. Some patients with head or spine injuries will not require much intervention other than a thorough assessment, appropriate SMR, and continued observation during transport to the hospital. In patients who have airway, breathing, and circulation problems or have other conditions for which you decide a rapid transport to the closest appropriate hospital is needed, SMR and quick loading into the ambulance may be indicated. Reduction of on-scene time and recognition of a critical patient increase the patient's chances for survival and may reduce the amount of irreversible damage.

SMR Considerations

When assessing a patient with suspected head and/or spine injuries, be aware that any unnecessary

Special Populations

ASSESSMENT OF HEAD INJURIES IN CHILDREN

Head injuries are common in children. This is because the size of a child's head, in relation to the body, is larger than that of an adult. An infant also has a softer, thinner skull, which may result in injury to the underlying brain tissues. The signs and symptoms of head injury in a child are similar to those in an adult, but there are some important differences. A common response to head injuries, even among children with only very slight head injuries, is nausea and vomiting. These symptoms are sometimes the result of increased ICP. It is easy to mistake nausea and vomiting for an abdominal injury or illness. You should suspect a serious head injury in any child who experiences nausea and vomiting after a traumatic event. In managing such vomiting, pay particular attention to protecting the patient's airway.

movement of the patient can cause additional injury. Assess the patient in the position found. After determining and correcting any life-threatening injuries, determine whether a cervical collar needs to be applied. Begin by assessing the scene and the MOI, then form a general impression of your patient based on their level of consciousness and the chief complaint, followed by an assessment of the need for SMR. The following factors indicate the need for SMR following blunt trauma[13]:

- GCS score less than 15 or evidence of intoxication
- Midline neck or back pain or tenderness
- Numbness or motor weakness affecting one area of the body (eg, leg or arm weakness or weakness on one side of the body)
- Visible or palpable deformity of the spine
- Other distracting injuries (eg, long bone fracture, degloving or crush injuries, large burns)
- Other circumstances that interfere with the patient's ability to give reliable exam information (eg, communication barriers, emotional distress)

The protocol may also indicate that caution is advised in patients at the extremes of age.

Words of Wisdom

Place padding around the head to stabilize the neck of injured patients who have ankylosing spondylitis (a type of severe arthritis that fuses spinal bones in some cases) rather than applying a cervical collar. Because the spine is so rigid in these patients, moving the neck to apply the collar could cause further injury.

Assessing for Signs and Symptoms of a Head or Spine Injury

Patients with head injuries frequently have spinal injuries, and vice versa. Confused or slurred speech, repetitive questioning, or amnesia in responsive patients suggests a head injury. Whereas other problems may produce similar signs and symptoms (eg, hypoglycemia, stroke), in the setting of trauma, you should assume the cause is TBI until proven otherwise.

For unresponsive trauma victims and those presenting with a decreased level of responsiveness on the AVPU (Awake and alert, responsive to Verbal stimuli, responsive to Pain, Unresponsive) scale, you should suspect spinal injury, as it cannot be reliably ruled out in such patients. Family members, bystanders, and responders who were on scene prior to your arrival may have helpful information, including when the patient lost consciousness or whether the person is displaying a change in their baseline mental status.

ABC Considerations

In patients with head and spinal injuries, airway and breathing problems are common and may result in death if not recognized and treated immediately. Failure to open the airway can result in a poor outcome, including death. When a spinal injury is suspected, how you open and assess the airway is important. Begin by manually holding the patient's head still while you assess the airway. Use a jaw-thrust maneuver to open the airway. When performed correctly, this will prevent movement of the cervical spine. The head tilt–chin lift technique is contraindicated in trauma victims who are suspected to have a spinal injury. However, because a patient cannot survive without a functioning airway, a head tilt–chin lift may be considered as a last resort. An oropharyngeal or nasopharyngeal airway may assist in maintaining an open airway. In most cases, basic life support (BLS) techniques will suffice in protecting the patient's airway. However, if they prove ineffective or too difficult to maintain, the advanced airway methods used by AEMTs and paramedics may be necessary. Airway interventions are discussed further in Chapter 11, *Airway and Ventilation Management.*

Vomiting may occur in patients who have head injuries. Therefore, keeping the airway clear is of great concern. Although log rolling patients with potential spinal trauma is not ideal, if you are unable to keep the airway clear by suctioning, large amounts of emesis may leave you with no other alternative. In cases when suction is inadequate or unavailable, roll the patient while keeping the spine as straight as possible to minimize secondary spinal injuries.

In TBIs that result in increasing ICP, compressive forces may affect the brainstem, which regulates breathing. Dysfunction of the brainstem can lead to irregular breathing patterns, such as Cheyne-Stokes respirations, Biot respirations, or even apnea. Regardless, it is imperative that you closely monitor and manage the patient's breathing. Are respirations present? Are they adequate? All patients who have a suspected severe TBI should have their airway positioned appropriately and be placed on oxygen by a nasal cannula or nonrebreathing mask. Pulse oximeter values should not fall below 90% and, ideally, should be between 95% and 99%. If the patient's oxygen saturation level remains below 90% despite administration of oxygen or if their breathing becomes ineffective, reposition the airway while maintaining spinal alignment, insert an airway adjunct, and begin positive-pressure ventilation using a bag-mask device. A single episode of hypoxia in a patient with a head injury nearly doubles the risk of death or permanent disability.[14]

Use the ventilatory rates established for BLS guidelines: 10 breaths/min for an adult, 20 to 30 breaths/min for children. The end-tidal carbon dioxide ($ETCO_2$) level should be maintained between 35 and 45 mm Hg; values less than 35 mm Hg should be avoided. Routine hyperventilation of patients with head injuries is discouraged because rapid ventilatory rates can cause cerebral blood vessels to constrict, reducing blood flow to the brain and worsening hypoxic injury. If signs of imminent brainstem herniation have been identified, *mild* hyperventilation is acceptable, but only when capnography is available and only to achieve an $ETCO_2$ level of between 30 and 35 mm Hg.

After ensuring the airway is patent and the patient's breathing is adequate, you should check to see if the pulse is weak or strong and determine the rate. A pulse that is too slow in the setting of a head injury can indicate a serious condition in your patient, whereas a rapid pulse may indicate shock. If the pulse is present and adequate, continue your evaluation of the patient.

A single episode of hypoperfusion in a patient with a head injury can lead to significant brain damage and even death. Assess for signs and symptoms of shock and treat appropriately. Shock relating to spinal injury (neurogenic shock) is discussed in Chapter 13, *Shock*.

Bleeding not found or deemed life threatening in the primary survey may also be present from the same injury that caused the spine and/or head injury. That injury may involve blunt or penetrating forces. Consider again the MOI and the effects it has had on your patient. Control bleeding as previously discussed, following the XABC sequence if life-threatening bleeding is present. When bandaging the head, be careful that you do not move the neck if spinal injuries are suspected, and do not apply pressure if a skull fracture is suspected. Remember that head and spine injuries often occur together; however, be aware that bleeding from the scalp should be controlled, as it can lead to a large volume loss over time if not addressed early.

Manner of Transport

Several transport considerations should be kept in mind for patients with head trauma. Patients with impaired airways, open head wounds, or abnormal vital signs and patients who do not respond to painful stimuli may need to be rapidly extricated from a motor vehicle and transported. During transport, providing the patient with a patent airway and high-flow oxygen is paramount. Because of the potential for increasing ICP, there is an increased risk of vomiting and seizures, so suction should be readily available. A patient with head trauma may

Special Populations

TRANSPORT DETERMINATION FOR CHILDREN WITH HEAD INJURIES

Children who have sustained a head injury should be transported if the MOI was severe or if they exhibit any of the following signs or symptoms at the scene or within 72 hours of injury[4]:

- Seizure
- Visual disturbances, ataxia, or gait abnormality
- Loss of consciousness or any change in normal consciousness
- Weakness or tingling in the arms or legs
- Signs of a skull fracture
- Vomiting
- Severe headache
- Abnormal behavior such as increased drowsiness or agitation; restlessness or combativeness; or, in children younger than 2 years, any other uncharacteristic behavior reported by the parent or caregiver
- Hematoma on the occipital, parietal, or temporal scalp in children younger than 2 years

deteriorate rapidly, thus requiring aeromedical transport depending on your local protocols. In supine patients, the head should be elevated 30°, if possible, to help reduce ICP.[15] A blanket or one or two towels placed under the long backboard will elevate the head. Maintain SMR if indicated.

History Taking

After immediate life threats have been managed during the primary assessment, investigate the chief complaint. Obtain a medical history and be alert for injury-specific signs and symptoms as well as any pertinent negatives, such as no pain or no loss of sensation.

You have the opportunity to interview the patient well in advance of the emergency physician. Any information you receive will be valuable if the patient loses consciousness. When assessing a patient for possible head or spinal injury, begin by asking the responsive patient the following questions to determine the chief complaint:

- What happened?
- Where does it hurt?
- Does your neck or back hurt?
- Can you move your hands and feet?
- Did you hit your head?
- Did you lose consciousness?

A patient's inability to recall events is an important finding in patients with head injuries.

If the patient is not responsive, attempt to obtain the history from other sources, such as friends or family members. Medical identification jewelry and cards in wallets may also provide information about the patient's medical history (follow local protocols regarding the removal of items from a patient's wallet). Does the patient have a recent or previous history of unresponsiveness? These key indicators may lead you to suspect a developing TBI.

Make every attempt to obtain a SAMPLE (Signs and symptoms, Allergies, Medications, Pertinent past medical history, Last oral intake, Events leading up to the illness or injury) history from your patient. History may be difficult to obtain when a person is confused from a head injury or frightened from a spinal injury. Whereas the prehospital environment is an excellent place to obtain important history, do not delay rapid transport for patients who need hospital intervention. Gather as much SAMPLE history as you can while preparing for transport. In less urgent situations, you should have enough time to gather a complete SAMPLE history without compromising patient care.

Secondary Assessment

Remember that the ability to walk, move the extremities, or feel sensation does not necessarily rule out a spinal cord or spinal column injury. Similarly, the absence of pain does not always indicate that a spinal injury has not occurred. Do not ask patients with possible spinal injuries to move their necks as a test for pain. Instead, instruct the patient to keep still and not to move the head or neck.

The physical examination may be a systematic full-body scan or a systematic assessment that focuses on a certain area or region of the body, often determined through the chief complaint or MOI. Patients with moderate or severe head injuries associated with a significant MOI should receive lifesaving medical or surgical intervention at the closest appropriate trauma hospital without delay. If time allows, perform a secondary assessment to identify and treat injuries that may have been missed during the primary assessment en route to the emergency department (ED). Extremities can be stabilized using the backboard and splinted individually while in the back of the ambulance, as time and conditions permit.

Obtaining a complete set of baseline vital signs is essential in patients with head and spine injuries. Significant head injuries may cause the pulse to slow and the blood pressure to rise. With neurogenic shock from spinal cord injury, the blood pressure and heart rate may both decrease. Head and spine injuries can cause respirations to become erratic or absent.

Words of Wisdom

Patients who have neurogenic shock often have associated findings, such as paralysis below the level of their injury, impaired respiration due to paralysis of muscles of breathing, inability to regulate their body temperature, and loss of bowel and bladder control. The key indicators of neurogenic shock associated with high spinal cord injury include hypotension, slow or normal heart rate, and warm skin below the level of the injury.

If available, use monitoring devices to quantify your patient's oxygenation and circulatory status. Pulse oximetry and $ETCO_2$ monitoring should be used to ensure the patient is not hypo- or hyperventilating. If herniation is suspected, maintain a target $ETCO_2$ reading between 35 and 40 mm Hg and a pulse oximetry reading greater than 90% (optimal targets may be higher).[6] When obtaining a blood pressure, take the first reading manually with a sphygmomanometer (blood pressure cuff) and stethoscope rather than relying solely on an automatic blood pressure device.

Assess the blood glucose level and body temperature. Report abnormal values during the patient handoff. If the patient is hypothermic, take measures to warm the patient to a target temperature of 98°F to 99°F (36.7°C to 37.2°C).[6]

Physical Examination Considerations

Examine the entire body using DCAP-BTLS. Check perfusion, motor function, and sensation in all extremities prior to moving the patient.

A decreased or altered level of consciousness is the most reliable sign of a head injury. Monitor the patient for changes in level of consciousness, including signs of confusion, disorientation, or deteriorating mental status. Is the patient unresponsive or repeating questions? Experiencing seizures? Nauseous or vomiting?

Determine whether there is decreased movement and/or numbness and tingling in the extremities. Is there any posturing? Is the patient able to perform motor functions such as squeezing your hands appropriately and equally? Determine whether the strength in each extremity is equal by asking the patient to squeeze your hands and to gently push each foot against your hands (**FIGURE 28-16**).

Part the patient's hair and inspect the scalp for bruising. Look for blood or CSF leaking from the ears, nose, or mouth and for bruising around the eyes and behind the ears.

To establish a baseline, assess pupil size, symmetry, and reaction to light as soon as possible. Compare the size of the pupils to detect a difference in diameter of more than 1 mm. Observe for the presence of fixed and dilated pupils, which is defined as a response to bright light of less than 1 mm. Reassess periodically to monitor for changes en route to the hospital, as such changes may indicate progressively worsening brain injury. The brain controls the diameter and reactivity of the pupils. Unequal pupil size after a head injury in an unconscious patient often signals a serious problem, such as herniation from dangerously high ICP. If an injury is isolated to just one side of the brain, the pupil on the same side may dilate. However, as pressure continues to build, both pupils may become affected.

YOU are the EMT

When you arrive at the scene you find a 22-year-old man lying supine on the ground; he is motionless and his head is lying in a large pool of blood. Your partner manually stabilizes his head in a neutral position and opens his airway with the jaw-thrust maneuver as you perform a primary assessment.

Recording Time: 0 Minutes	
Appearance	Motionless; large pool of blood under his head
Level of consciousness	Responsive only to deep painful stimuli
Airway	Open; clear of secretions or foreign bodies
Breathing	Slow and irregular
Circulation	Radial pulses slow and bounding; skin warm and dry; bleeding from a large laceration to the right side of his head

3. What are your most immediate treatment priorities for this patient?
4. Where should you focus your secondary assessment of this patient?

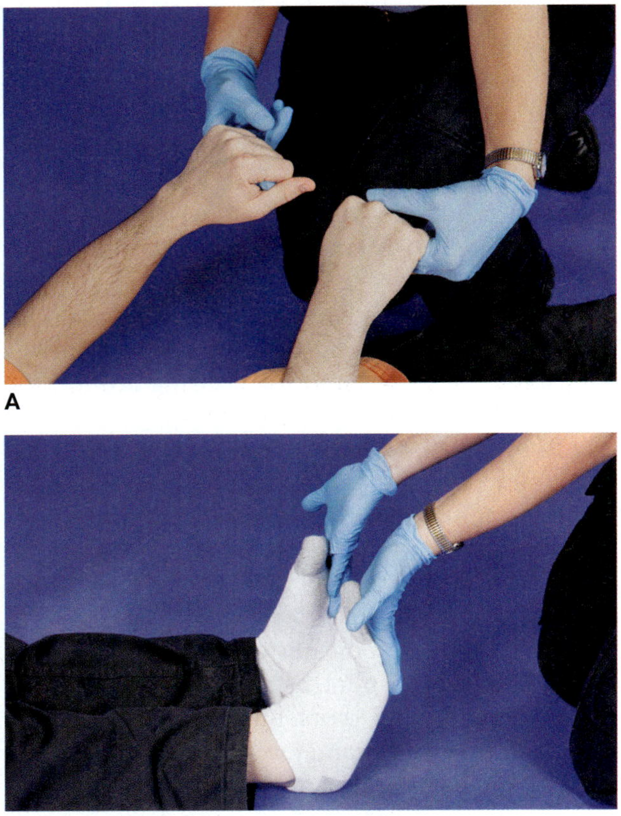

FIGURE 28-16 A. Assess the equality of strength in each extremity by asking the patient to squeeze your hands. **B.** Next, ask the patient to gently push each foot against your hands.

Do not palpate an obvious cranial deformity or probe an open scalp laceration, as doing so may push bone fragments into the brain. If an impaled object is present, do not attempt to remove it unless it prevents you from providing lifesaving airway interventions.

Neurologic Examination

For a patient with a head injury, perform a neurologic examination after life threats are assessed during the initial assessment, after any change in mental status, and at least every 30 minutes. Perform a baseline assessment using the GCS, and record the time (**TABLE 28-2**). Use the adult scale for patients older than 2 years and the pediatric scale for those 2 years and younger.[6] The GCS helps you to identify the patient's speech and ability to follow commands. Always use simple, easily understood

TABLE 28-2 Glasgow Coma Scale (GCS) for Adult and Pediatric Patients[a]

Adult GCS		Pediatric GCS	
Eye Opening			
Spontaneous	4	Spontaneous	4
In response to sound	3	In response to sound	3
In response to pressure	2	In response to pressure	2
None	1	None	1
Best Verbal Response			
Oriented conversation	5	Coos, babbles	5
Confused conversation	4	Irritable cry	4
Inappropriate words	3	Cries to pain	3
Incomprehensible sounds	2	Moans to pain	2
None	1	None	1
Best Motor Response			
Obeys commands	6	Spontaneous movement	6
Localizes to pressure	5	Withdraws to touch	5
Withdraws from pressure	4	Withdraws from pressure	4
Abnormal flexion	3	Abnormal flexion	3
Abnormal extension	2	Abnormal extension	2
None	1	None	1
Total		**Total**	

[a]Some systems use a "Not testable (NT)" score for any element that cannot be tested. Eye opening cannot be tested in a patient whose eyes are closed due to a local factor, such as swelling; verbal response cannot be tested in a patient who has a preexisting factor interfering with communication, such as mutism; and motor response cannot be tested in a patient who has preexisting paralysis or other limiting factor.

Score: 13–15 may indicate mild dysfunction, although 15 is the score a person with no neurologic disabilities would receive.

Score: 9–12 may indicate moderate dysfunction.

Score: 8 or less is indicative of severe dysfunction.

terms when reporting the level of consciousness, such as "does not remember events immediately before the injury" or "confused about date and time." Terms such as "obtunded" or "dazed" have different meanings to different people and should not be used in either written or verbal reports.

If your jurisdiction uses the Revised Trauma Score, then the findings from the GCS will be used to determine the Revised Trauma Score value. See Chapter 24, *Trauma Overview*, for a discussion of this scoring system.

Frequently, the level of consciousness will fluctuate: improving, deteriorating, and improving again over time. On other occasions, there may be a gradual, progressive deterioration in the patient's response to stimuli; this usually indicates serious brain injury that may need aggressive medical and/or surgical treatment. The physicians who treat the patient will need to know when a loss of consciousness occurred. They will want to compare their neurologic evaluation with the one you performed in the field.

As you proceed with your assessment, ask yourself these questions: Is the patient's speech clear and appropriate? Does the patient answer in a logical manner, and is the patient able to make decisions? Is the patient aware of their current location? Is the patient alert to person, place, time, and why you are at the scene? Can the patient recall the events leading up to the incident, or is there a period of memory lapse? Can the patient recall major current events?

Any person with a head injury that has resulted in a change in level of consciousness, progressive development of signs or symptoms of a concussion, or other causes of concern should be evaluated. This evaluation should occur soon after injury and must be conducted by a qualified health care clinician. EMTs are not qualified to conduct these evaluations in the field.

Words of Wisdom

A change in the level of consciousness is the single most important observation that you can make in assessing the severity of brain injury. Level of consciousness usually corresponds to the extent of loss of brain function.

Spine Examination

If there is a potential spine injury, examine the spine. To start, inspect for overt signs of injury or deformity and check the extremities for circulation, motor, or sensory problems. If there is impairment, note the level. You do not need to know the exact nerve impairment because this will not change your treatment.

Pain or tenderness when you palpate the spinal area is a warning sign that a spinal injury may exist. Patients with spinal injuries may report constant or intermittent pain along the spinal column or in the extremities. A spinal cord injury may also produce pain independent of movement or palpation.

Other signs and symptoms of spinal injury include an obvious deformity as you gently palpate the spine; numbness, weakness, or tingling in the extremities; and soft-tissue injuries in the spinal region. Patients with severe spinal injury may lose sensation or experience paralysis below the suspected level of injury or be incontinent (loss of urinary or bowel control) (**FIGURE 28-17**). However,

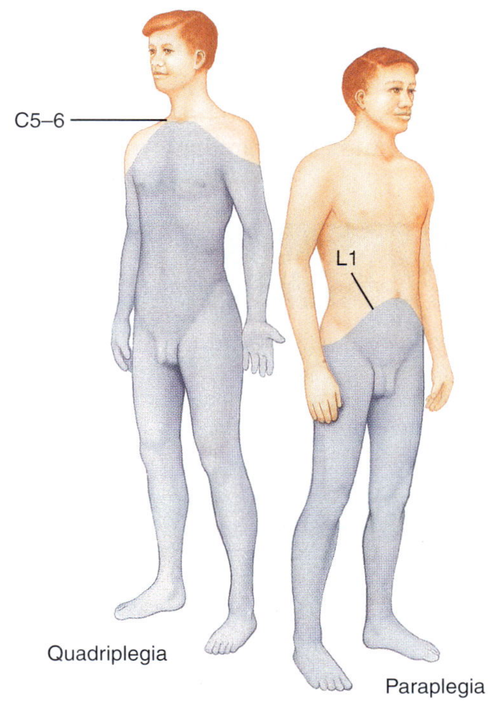

FIGURE 28-17 With severe spinal injuries, patients may lose sensation or experience paralysis below the level of the injury. A patient who sustains a spinal cord injury below the level of C5 and is paralyzed can still breathe spontaneously because the phrenic nerves, which cause the diaphragm to contract, originate at the C3, C4, and C5 levels.

be aware that some patients with spinal injuries may present without obvious signs or symptoms, perhaps due to distracting injuries or intoxication.

Injuries to the cervical area may cause damage to the phrenic nerve, which is responsible for innervation of the diaphragm. If the diaphragm is unable to function properly, respirations can be significantly impaired, resulting in inadequate breathing and severe fatigue as the patient tries to compensate using other muscles. These patients need ventilatory assistance urgently. Spinal cord injuries at T1–T11 levels interfere with normal intercostal muscle function. Although they will not completely disrupt ventilation as high cervical injuries can, the tidal volume will often decrease, which, coupled with other chest injuries, can interfere with the ability to breathe effectively. Additional signs of spinal cord trauma include priapism (a prolonged erection), a loss of bowel or bladder control, and a diminished ability to maintain body temperature.

Street Smarts

Patients who are paralyzed by a spinal cord injury but are conscious and aware of the inability to move their limbs need to be offered emotional support. Remember that it can be traumatizing for patients to realize they may have a debilitating and life-altering injury; therefore, you need to be careful in your choice of words. A patient may ask you difficult questions, such as "Will I be able to walk?" It is best to tell the patient that you are providing immediate care and you cannot predict the outcome.

Patients suspected to have a moderate to severe TBI should be transported to a trauma center with immediate access to CT scan and neurosurgical critical care. Pediatric patients who have a suspected TBI should be treated in a pediatric trauma center, if possible, or in an adult trauma center that is qualified to treat children.

Reassessment

The patient's condition should be reassessed at least every 5 minutes. Repeat the primary assessment. Reassess vital signs and the chief complaint. Are the airway, breathing, and circulation still adequate? Recheck patient interventions. Are the treatments you provided still effective? Are additional interventions needed? The effectiveness of positive-pressure ventilations, SMR, and treatments for shock may be determined only with both immediate and continuous observation after providing the intervention. Multiple interventions may be necessary in patients

YOU are the EMT

Your secondary assessment reveals an area of depression to the right side of the patient's head over the temporal bone and dilated and sluggishly reactive pupils. The rest of his body is unremarkable for gross injury. He opens his eyes in response to pain, is making unrecognizable sounds, and his arms are flexed and drawn in toward his body. An engine company arrives at the scene to provide assistance. You ask them to prepare the backboard and straps while you quickly assess the patient's vital signs.

Recording Time: 5 Minutes	
Respirations	6 breaths/min and irregular (baseline); ventilations are being assisted
Pulse	60 beats/min; regular and bounding
Skin	Baseline color, warm, and dry
Blood pressure	190/104 mm Hg
Oxygen saturation (Spo_2)	94% (on oxygen)

There are numerous bystanders present; however, no one knows the patient. During your physical assessment, you did not find any medical alert bracelets or any other evidence of a past medical history.

5. What is this patient's GCS score?

6. What is the likely explanation for the patient's vital signs?

with head and spinal injuries. If something is not working, try something else.

Following a head injury, the patient may experience a rapid deterioration of neurologic function. Alterations in the patient's mental status may be the earliest indication that a problem exists. You may observe a deterioration in a conscious patient's awareness of time, place, and person, in that order. Trauma patients with signs and symptoms of head injury may also show signs of shock. This may signal the presence of internal bleeding in another region of the body. If the spinal cord is damaged, neurogenic shock can produce hypotension in the absence of hemorrhage. Recall that if an epidural hematoma develops, the patient who was reportedly "knocked out" at the time of injury and was alert when you arrived may deteriorate to the point of herniation very quickly.

As discussed earlier, the appearance of clear or pink watery CSF from the nose, the ear, or an open scalp wound may indicate that the dura and the skull have both been penetrated. Do not attempt to pack the wound, ear, or nose in these instances. Cover the scalp wound, if there is one, with sterile gauze to prevent further contamination, but do not bandage it tightly.

Your local protocol for treatment of a suspected head injury should include the administration of high-flow oxygen and the application of a cervical collar, if indicated, as part of SMR. Reassessment should take place as the patient is transported to an appropriate trauma facility. Monitor the patient's condition and vital signs and relay this information to the receiving facility, especially if there is a significant or noteworthy change.

When providing care for patients with suspected head and spinal injuries, maintain good communication with other clinicians and give complete and detailed information to the destination facility. Key observations that you relay will help hospitals better prepare for seriously injured patients and additional resources can be made available when you arrive. For example, a helicopter may be standing by for transport from a smaller hospital to a Level I trauma center. Larger hospitals may have trauma specialists or neurosurgeons available to meet you on arrival.

Your documentation should include the history you were able to obtain at the scene, your findings during your assessment, treatments you provided, and how the patient responded to them. How frequently you document repeat vital signs depends on the condition of your patient. More seriously injured patients should have documented vital signs every 5 minutes, whereas more stable patients should have documented vital signs every 15 minutes. Always follow local protocols. Take time after your verbal handoff to hospital staff to sit and make a complete and accurate record of the situation. This will be your only accepted legal memory of the call.

Many events that cause spinal or head injuries may eventually result in some type of litigation. As with all responses, proper documentation of what you observed and the treatment provided will be beneficial as time passes. You may be requested to testify years later in court as a witness to the incident, and proper and complete documentation recorded at the time of the incident will lay the framework for answering questions.

Emergency Medical Care of Head Injuries

Treat the patient with a head injury according to three general principles that are designed to protect and maintain the critical functions of the CNS:

1. Control bleeding and provide adequate circulation to maintain cerebral perfusion. Begin cardiopulmonary resuscitation (CPR) if necessary. Be sure to take standard precautions.
2. Establish an adequate airway. If necessary, begin and maintain ventilation and provide supplemental oxygen to maintain an oxygen saturation level of greater than 90%. Avoid hyperventilation. Maintain the $ETCO_2$ level at a target value of 40 mm Hg (between 35 and 45 mm Hg). If signs of herniation appear, maintain the $ETCO_2$ level between 30 and 35 mm Hg.
3. Assess the patient's baseline level of consciousness, and continuously monitor it.

As you continue to treat the patient, place a sterile dressing over an open skull injury; however, do not apply pressure over an open or compressed skull injury. In addition, you must assess and treat other injuries, dress and bandage open wounds as indicated in the treatment of soft-tissue injuries, splint fractures, anticipate and manage vomiting to prevent aspiration, be prepared for convulsions and changes in the patient's condition, and transport the patient promptly and with extreme care.

Managing the Airway

The most important step in the treatment of patients with head injury, regardless of the severity, is to establish an adequate airway. If the patient has an airway obstruction, perform the jaw-thrust maneuver to open the airway. Once the airway is open, maintain the head and cervical spine in a neutral, in-line position until you have placed a cervical collar and stabilized the patient on a backboard, scoop stretcher, ambulance cot, or other SMR device (**FIGURE 28-18**). Remove any foreign bodies, secretions, or vomitus from the airway. Make sure a suctioning unit is available, because you will often need to clear blood, saliva, or vomitus from the airway.

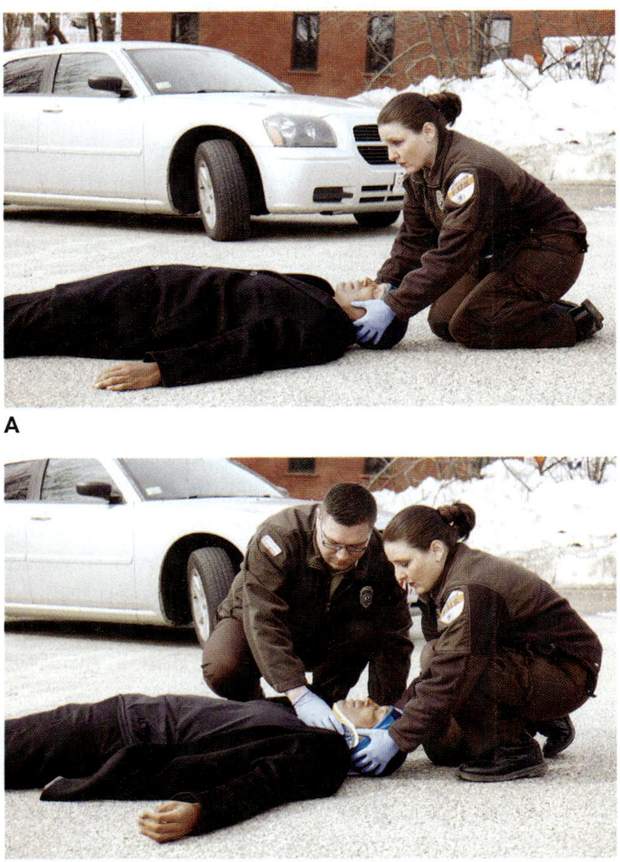

A

B

FIGURE 28-18 A. Maintain the head and cervical spine in a neutral in-line position. **B.** Apply a cervical collar as you finish the primary assessment.

Once you have cleared the airway, check ventilation. If the respiratory control center of the brain has been injured, the rate and/or depth of breathing may be ineffective. Ventilation may also be limited by chest injuries or, if the spinal cord is injured, by paralysis of some or all of the muscles of respiration. Give supplemental oxygen by nasal cannula or nonrebreathing mask to any patient with suspected head injury, particularly anyone who is having trouble breathing, and ensure the oxygen saturation level remains higher than 90%. This reduces hypoxia and possible cerebral edema. Evaluate the patient's rate and depth of breathing. If the patient is breathing too slowly or too shallowly, use a bag-mask device to assist ventilations. Placement of an oropharyngeal airway, supraglottic airway, or endotracheal tube may be necessary to maintain an open airway. Consider calling for ALS if the patient's airway is compromised. An injured brain is even less tolerant of hypoxia than a healthy brain, and studies have shown that supplemental oxygen can reduce the risk of hypoxic episodes; to be effective, however, it must be started as soon as possible.[6] Do not wait until the patient's oxygen saturation level drops below 90% or the patient becomes cyanotic. Continue to assist ventilations and administer supplemental oxygen until the patient reaches the hospital. Avoid hyperventilation.

Managing Circulation

If the heart is not beating, begin CPR.

Active blood loss aggravates hypoxia by reducing the available number of oxygen-carrying red blood cells. Control bleeding from a scalp laceration by applying direct pressure over the wound. Remember to follow standard precautions. Use a dry, sterile dressing, folding any torn skin flaps back down onto the skin bed before applying pressure (**FIGURE 28-19A**). In some instances, you will have to apply firm compression for several minutes to control bleeding (**FIGURE 28-19B**). If you suspect a skull fracture, do not apply excessive pressure to the open wound. Otherwise, you may increase the ICP or push bone fragments into the brain. If the bandage covers the patient's ears, remember that communication may become difficult because the patient's ability to hear will be decreased. To avoid limiting access to the patient's airway, do not cover the patient's mouth, nose, or jaw.

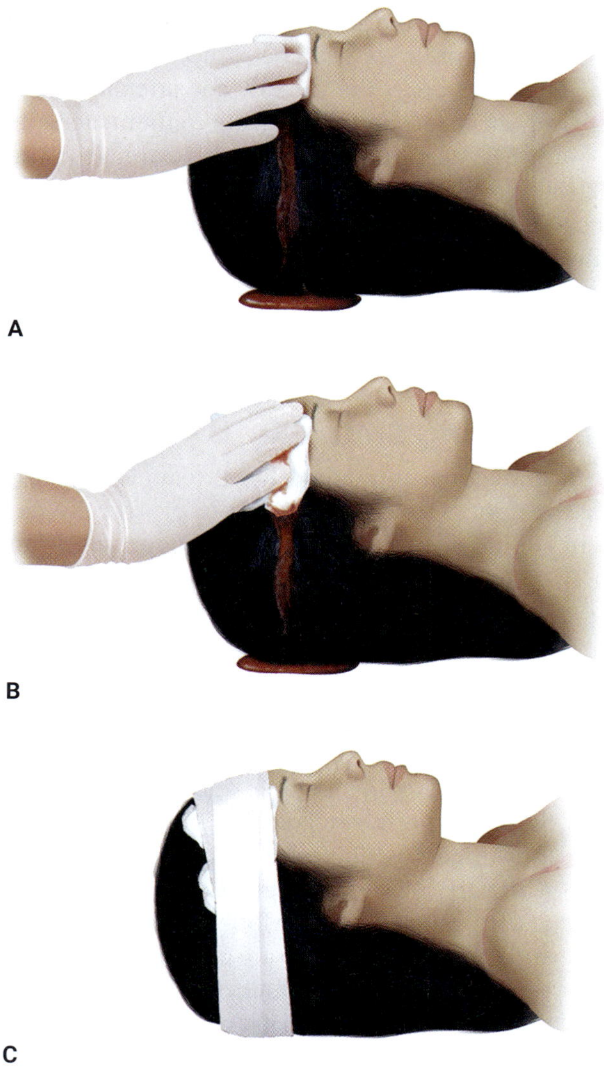

FIGURE 28-19 A. Use a dry sterile dressing to fold torn skin flaps back down onto the skin bed before applying pressure. **B.** If you do not suspect an open brain injury or skull fracture, apply firm compression for several minutes to control the bleeding. **C.** Secure the compression dressing in place with a soft, self-adhering roller bandage.

If the dressing becomes soaked, do not remove it. Instead, place a second dressing over the first. Continue applying manual pressure until the bleeding has been controlled, then secure the dressing in place with a soft, self-adhering roller bandage (**FIGURE 28-19C**).

Shock that develops in a patient with a head injury is usually the result of hypovolemia caused by bleeding from other injuries. As with other trauma patients, shock in these cases indicates that the situation is critical. Such patients must be transported immediately to a trauma center. Maintain the airway while you protect the patient's cervical spine, ensure adequate ventilation, administer 100% oxygen, control obvious sites of bleeding with direct pressure, place the patient supine with appropriate SMR, keep the patient warm, and provide immediate transport.

If the patient becomes nauseated or begins to vomit, elevate one side of the backboard to prevent aspiration. Be sure to maintain the head in the in-line neutral position, with the cervical collar in place. You should also have a suctioning unit available.

Cushing Triad

If the patient's head injuries are significant enough to cause a TBI, the patient may begin to exhibit the signs of the Cushing triad: increased blood pressure (hypertension), decreased heart rate (bradycardia), and irregular respirations. The Cushing triad identifies the effects seen as the pressure in the skull increases secondary to brain swelling or bleeding. As the pressure in the skull increases, the brainstem and the midbrain may be pushed through the foramen magnum, the hole at the base of the skull. If this process is allowed to continue, the patient will die. Manage shock, administer oxygen, and ventilate as appropriate. If $ETCO_2$ monitoring is available, mild hyperventilation (guided by a target $ETCO_2$ reading between 30 and 35 mm Hg) should be reserved only for those patients showing clear signs of herniation; do not exceed ventilatory rates of 20 breaths/min for adults, 25 breaths/min for children, and 30 breaths/min for infants younger than 1 year. Patients without evidence of herniation should be ventilated normally.

Words of Wisdom

Hypoxemia is one of the key factors, along with hypotension, of a poor outcome in patients with TBIs.

Emergency Medical Care of Spinal Injuries

Emergency medical care of a patient with a possible spinal injury begins, as does all patient care, with your protection; therefore, you must remember to take standard precautions. Next, you must maintain the patient's airway while manually keeping the spine in the proper position, assess respirations, and give supplemental oxygen.

Managing the Airway

Knowing that improper handling of a spinal injury can leave a patient permanently paralyzed must not prevent you from properly and promptly addressing an airway obstruction. Remember, all patients without an airway will die. If a patient with a spinal injury has an airway obstruction, perform the jaw-thrust maneuver to open the airway (**FIGURE 28-20**). Do not use the head tilt–chin lift maneuver because it extends the neck and may further damage the cervical spine. If the patient is unconscious, you can lift or pull the tongue forward so that you do not have to move the neck. Once the airway is open, hold the head still in a neutral, in-line position until SMR can be completed.

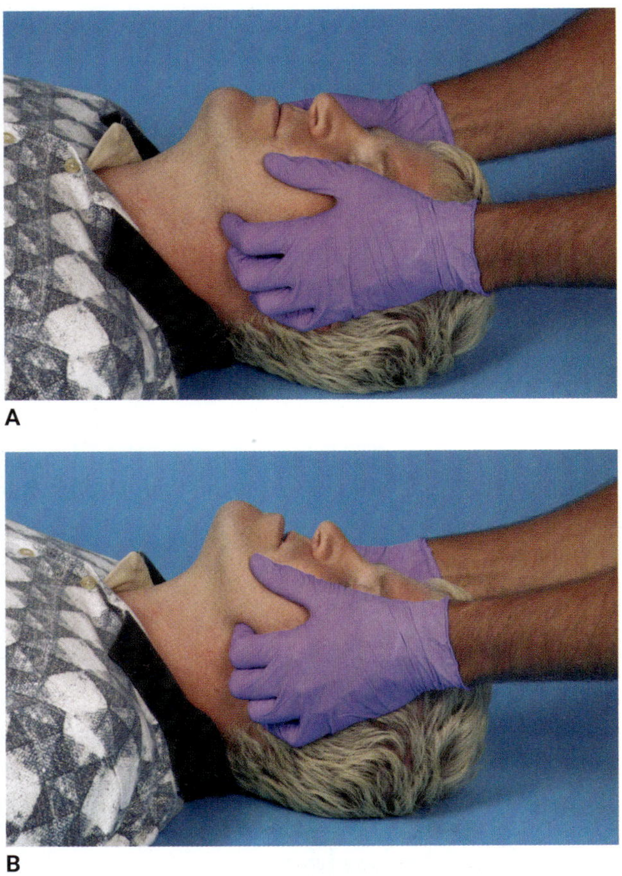

FIGURE 28-20 Jaw-thrust maneuver. **A.** Stabilize the neck in a neutral, in-line position. **B.** Push the angle of the lower jaw upward.

After you open the airway, consider inserting an oropharyngeal airway. If your patient accepts an oropharyngeal airway, be sure to monitor the airway closely. Have a suctioning unit available because you will often need to clear away blood, saliva, or vomitus. Provide supplemental oxygen. Continuously monitor the patient's airway and be prepared for any changes in the patient's condition based on your treatment.

Performing SMR

After managing immediate life threats and securing the patient's airway, attempt to protect the patient's spine from further damage. Follow the steps in **SKILL DRILL 28-1**:

1. Take standard precautions. Begin manual in-line stabilization by holding or having someone firmly hold the head with both hands. Whenever possible, kneel at the head of the patient, and place your hands around the base of the skull on either side (**Step 1**).
2. Support the lower jaw with your index and long fingers, while you are supporting the head with your palms. Then gently lift the head until the patient's eyes are looking straight ahead and the head and torso are in line. This neutral **eyes-forward position** makes SMR easier. Align the nose with the navel. Never twist, flex, or extend the head or neck excessively (**Step 2**).
3. Manually maintain this position as you continue to maintain the airway. Have your partner place a rigid cervical collar around the neck to provide more stability. As described previously, take appropriate steps to limit the patient's motion as you move them to the stretcher for transport. Once positioned on the ambulance cot, you may remove transfer or extrication devices, being careful to minimize unnecessary movement, while leaving the cervical collar in place.[13] SMR should be maintained until the patient has been evaluated by a physician (**Step 3**).

You should never force the head into a neutral, in-line position. Do not move the head any farther if the patient reports any of the following symptoms:

- Muscle spasms in the neck
- Substantial increased pain

Skill Drill 28-1 Performing Manual In-Line Stabilization

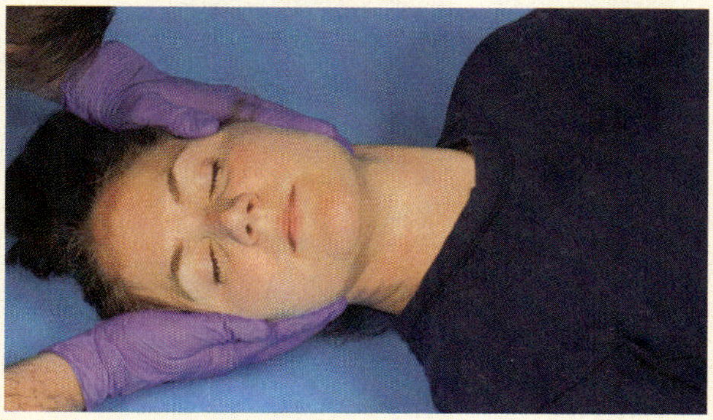

Step 1

Take standard precautions. Kneel behind the patient and firmly place your hands around the base of the skull on either side.

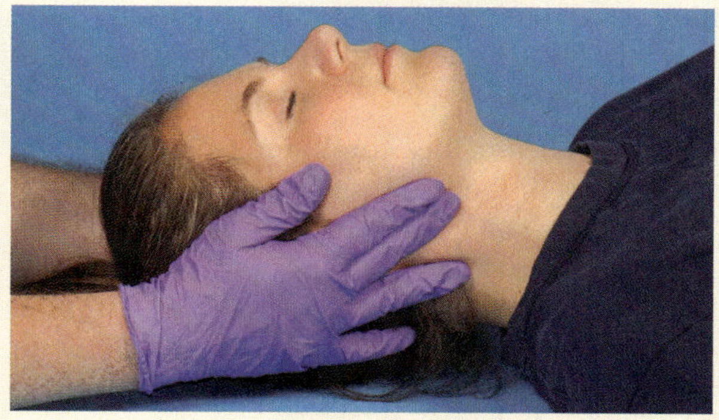

Step 2

Support the lower jaw with your index and long fingers, and the head with your palms. Gently lift the head into a neutral, eyes-forward position, aligned with the torso. Do not move the head or neck excessively, forcefully, or rapidly.

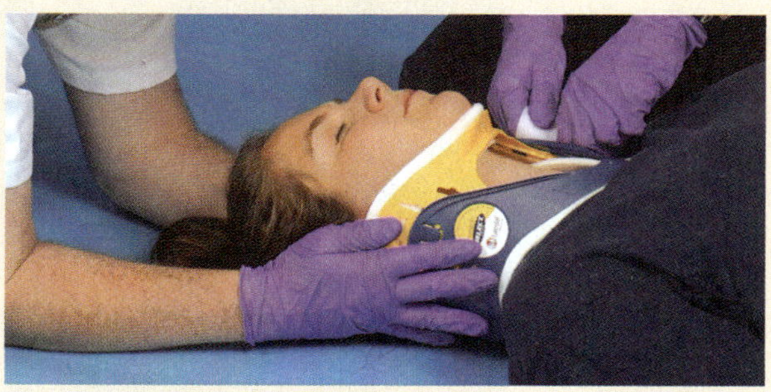

Step 3

Continue to manually support the head while your partner places a rigid cervical collar around the neck. Maintain manual support until SMR precautions for transport have been completed.

- Numbness, tingling, or weakness in the arms or legs
- Compromised airway or ventilations

In these situations, stabilize the patient in their current position.

Applying a Cervical Collar

Rigid cervical collars provide preliminary, partial support. When SMR is indicated, apply a cervical collar as soon as you have addressed any immediate life threats such as severe bleeding and airway or breathing problems. At all times, even before a collar is placed, make every effort to maintain in-line stabilization of the cervical spine throughout the encounter. Once the collar has been applied, do not remove it unless it interferes with airway management or the patient shows signs of increasing ICP. If you must remove the cervical collar, you will have to maintain manual stabilization of the cervical spine until it can be reapplied.

Keep in mind, however, that cervical collars are only one element of SMR. You must maintain manual support until the patient has been secured to a backboard, vacuum mattress, scoop stretcher, or ambulance stretcher for transport.

To be effective, a rigid cervical collar must be the correct size for the patient. An improperly fitting collar could do more harm than good. The method for determining the correct size is provided by the manufacturer. Make sure you are familiar with the types of collars your service carries. The cervical collar should rest on the shoulder girdle and provide firm support under both sides of the mandible, without obstructing the airway or ventilation efforts in any way (**FIGURE 28-21**). To apply a cervical collar, follow the steps in **SKILL DRILL 28-2**:

1. One EMT provides continuous manual in-line support of the head while the other EMT prepares the collar (**Step 1**).
2. Determine the correct collar according to the manufacturer's specifications. It is essential that the cervical collar fits properly. If you do not have the correct-size collar, use a rolled towel or head blocks secured to the transport device to limit movement of the patient's head (**FIGURE 28-22**) (**Step 2**).

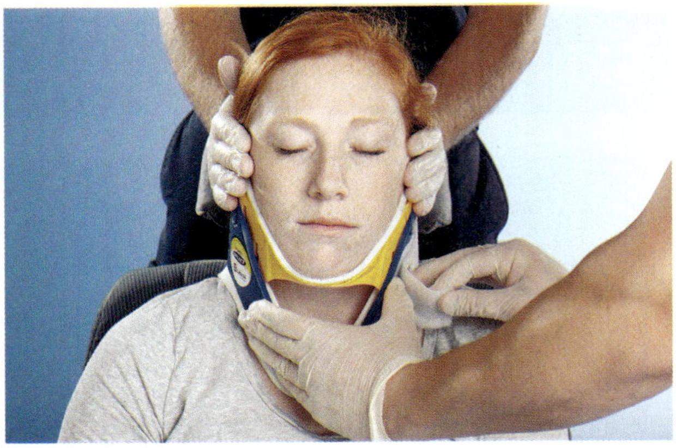

FIGURE 28-21 Proper fit is essential in applying a cervical collar. The collar should rest on the shoulder girdle and provide firm support under both sides of the mandible without obstructing the airway or any ventilation efforts.

Skill Drill 28-2 Applying a Cervical Collar

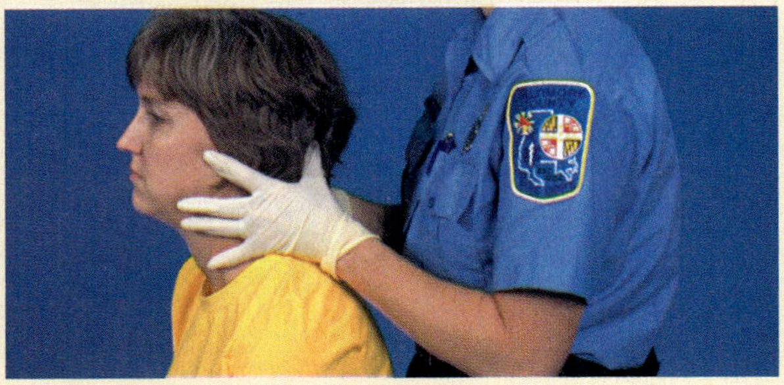

Step 1

Apply in-line stabilization.

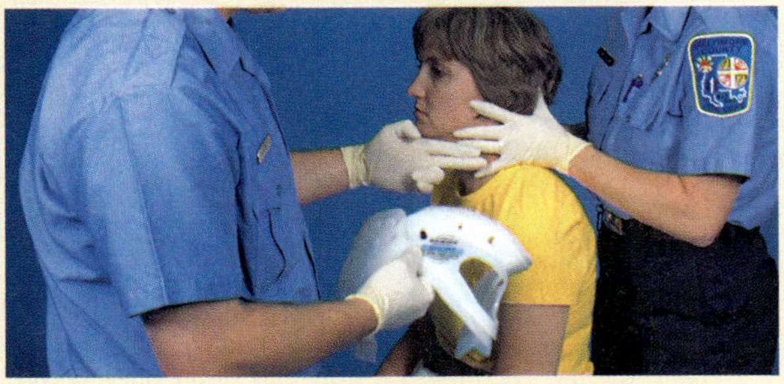

Step 2

Determine the proper collar size.

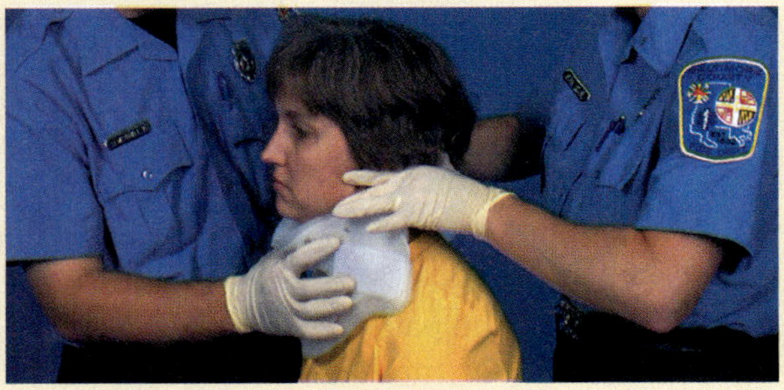

Step 3

Place the chin support first.

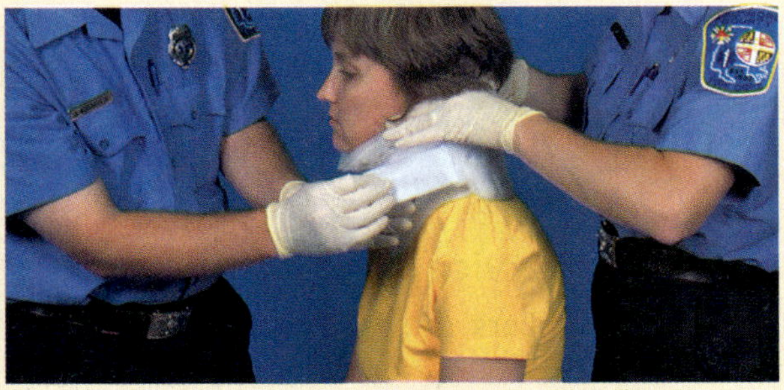

Step 4

Wrap the collar around the neck, and secure the collar.

Skill Drill 28-2 Applying a Cervical Collar continued

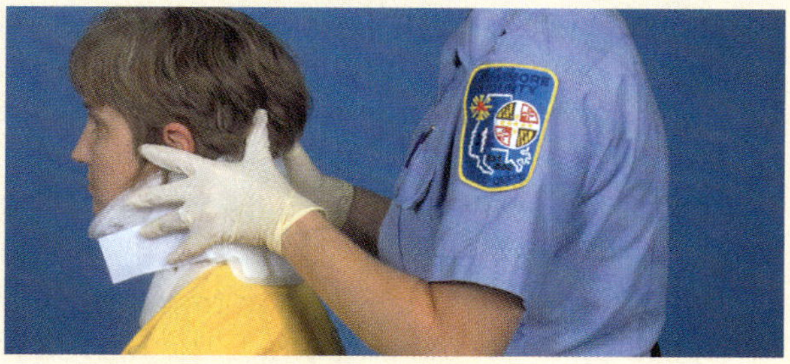

Step 5

Ensure proper fit, and maintain neutral, in-line stabilization until the patient is secured to the transport device.

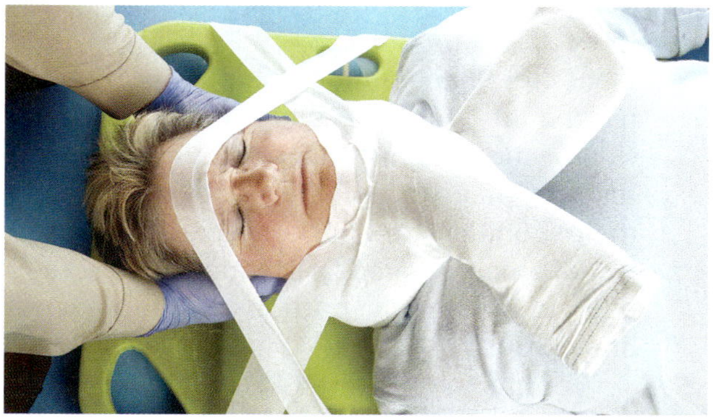

FIGURE 28-22 If you do not have an appropriate-size cervical collar, you may use a rolled towel around the patient's head. Tape the towel to the backboard or mattress and provide continuous manual support.

3. Begin by placing the chin support snugly under the chin (**Step 3**).
4. Maintain head stabilization and neutral neck alignment, wrap the collar around the neck, and secure the collar to the far side of the chin support (**Step 4**).
5. Ensure that the collar fits properly, and recheck that the patient is in a neutral, in-line position. Maintain in-line stabilization until the patient has been completely secured to the transport device (**Step 5**).

Once the patient's head and neck have been manually stabilized, assess the pulse, motor, and sensory function in all extremities. Then assess the cervical spine area and neck.

YOU are the EMT

Full SMR is established, assisted ventilations are continued, and the patient is loaded into the ambulance. An EMR from the engine company drives the ambulance so your partner can help you with the patient in the back. You begin transport to a local trauma center and reassess the patient's vital signs en route.

Recording Time: 11 Minutes	
Level of consciousness	Responsive only to deep painful stimuli
Respirations	6 breaths/min and irregular (baseline); ventilations are being assisted
Pulse	64 beats/min; regular and bounding
Skin	Baseline color, warm, and dry
Blood pressure	192/100 mm Hg
Oxygen saturation (Spo_2)	96% (on oxygen)

7. What further treatment is indicated for this patient?

8. What should you specifically monitor this patient for during transport?

> **Words of Wisdom**
>
> Be aware that a cervical collar is not a benign tool. When measured or applied incorrectly, it may actually have a detrimental effect. Research has demonstrated that even experienced emergency personnel, when asked to apply cervical collars to training manikins, rarely apply the collars correctly.[16]
>
> There is some concern that a cervical collar secured too tightly may compress the veins in the neck, impeding blood return from the head to the heart, resulting in an increase in ICP.[17] If disruption of blood flow is suspected, the collar should be loosened. Impaired blood flow could be particularly harmful to patients with TBIs.[10] A cervical collar may also make airway management more difficult or hide areas on the neck where rescuers might otherwise note signs of a developing problem (eg, tracheal deviation, jugular venous distention, expanding hematoma). Ensure that the collar permits downward movement of the mandible and opening of the mouth. If this is not possible and the patient vomits, aspiration may occur.[10] Another potential adverse effect of inappropriate cervical collar application may occur when a responder uses a collar that is too tall for the patient's neck. In the presence of an unstable cervical spine injury, it may pull the vertebrae above and below the injury site apart, worsening spinal cord trauma.[18] For all of these reasons, care must be taken to ensure that cervical collars are measured, applied, and monitored properly.

Preparation for Transport

Supine Patients

The scoop stretcher (clamshell stretcher) minimizes movement of the patient's spine and is ideal for transferring a patient from the supine position to the ambulance stretcher with minimal spinal movement. If use of a scoop stretcher is not an option, one procedure for moving a patient from the ground to an appropriate SMR device is the **four-person log roll**. In other cases, you may choose instead to slide the patient onto a backboard or vacuum mattress. The patient's condition, the scene, available resources, and local guidelines will dictate the method you choose. Using a scoop stretcher and performing the four-person log roll are described in Chapter 8, *Lifting and Moving Patients.*

You should first take the necessary precautions and then direct the team from a kneeling position at the patient's head so that you can maintain manual in-line cervical stabilization. Your job is to ensure that the head, torso, and pelvis move as a unit, with your teammates controlling the movement of the body. If necessary, you may recruit bystanders to assist the team, but be sure to instruct them fully before moving the patient. If using a backboard, follow the steps in **SKILL DRILL 28-3**:

1. Maintain in-line stabilization from a kneeling position at the patient's head. The EMT at the head will direct the log roll.
2. Assess motor, sensory, and circulatory function in each extremity (**Step 1**).
3. Apply an appropriate-size cervical collar (**Step 2**).
4. The other team members should position the backboard and place their hands on the far side of the patient to increase their leverage. Instruct them to use their body weight and their shoulders and back muscles to ensure a smooth, coordinated pull, concentrating their pull on the heavier portions of the patient's body (**Step 3**).
5. On command from the EMT at the head, the rescuers roll the patient toward themselves. One rescuer quickly examines the back while the patient is rolled on the side, and then slides the backboard behind and under the patient. The team rolls the patient back onto the backboard, avoiding independent rotation of the head, shoulders, or pelvis (**Step 4**).
6. Ensure the patient is centered on the backboard (**Step 5**).
7. Secure the upper torso to the backboard (without restricting the patient's breathing with the straps) once the patient is centered on the backboard (**Step 6**). Consider padding voids between the patient and the backboard to make transport more comfortable and protect the patient.
8. Secure the pelvis and upper legs, using padding as needed. For the pelvis, use straps over the iliac crests and/or groin loops (**Step 7**).
9. Begin to secure the head to the backboard by positioning a commercial securing device or towel rolls (**Step 8**).
10. Secure the head by taping the towels across the forehead. To prevent airway problems and

Skill Drill 28-3 Securing a Patient to a Long Backboard

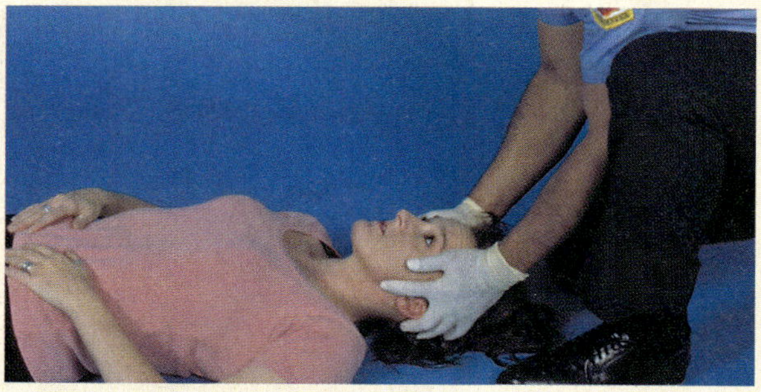

Step 1

Apply and maintain manual cervical stabilization. Assess distal functions in all extremities.

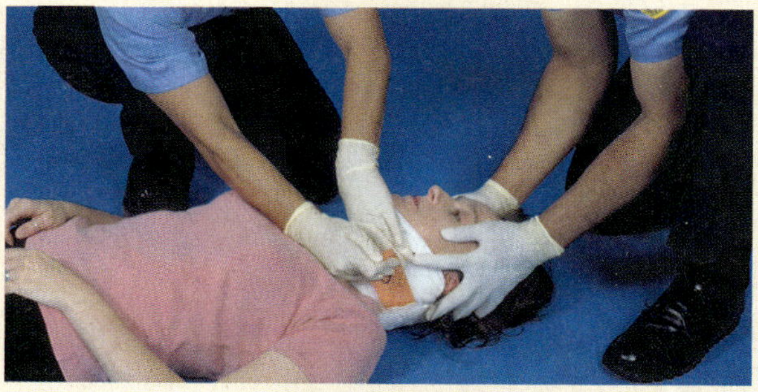

Step 2

Apply a cervical collar.

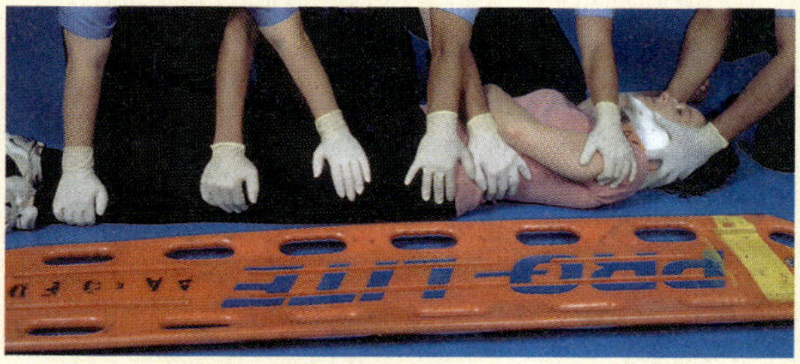

Step 3

Rescuers kneel on one side of the patient and place hands on the far side of the patient.

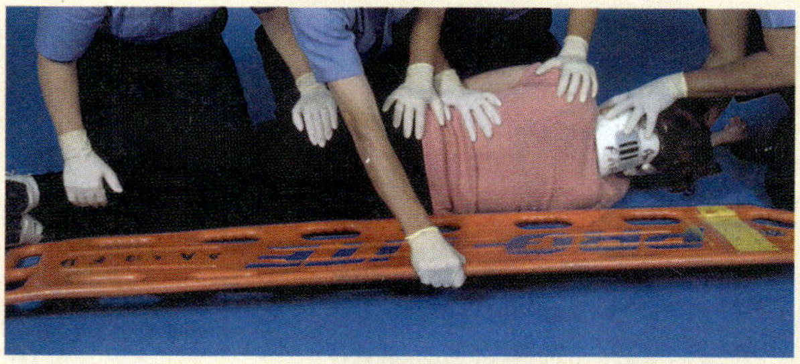

Step 4

On command, rescuers roll the patient toward themselves, quickly examine the back, slide the backboard under the patient, and roll the patient onto the backboard.

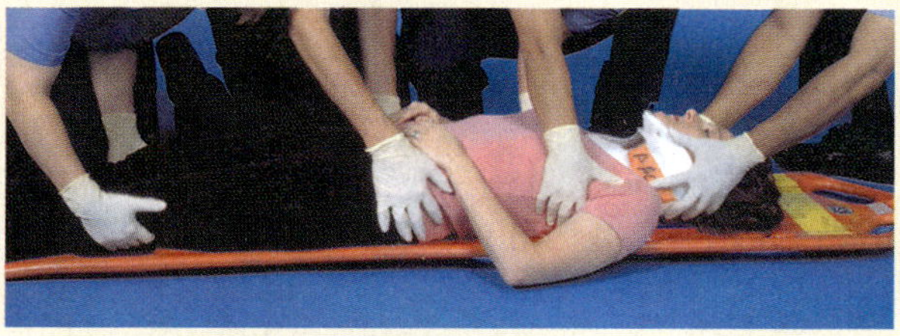

Step 5

Center the patient on the backboard.

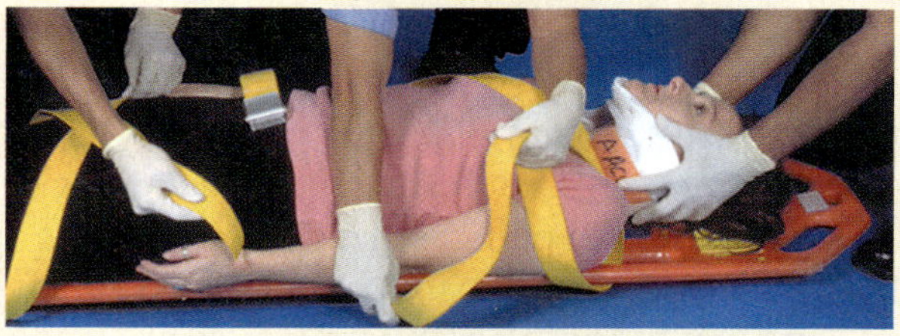

Step 6

Secure the upper torso first.

(continues)

Skill Drill 28-3 Securing a Patient to a Long Backboard continued

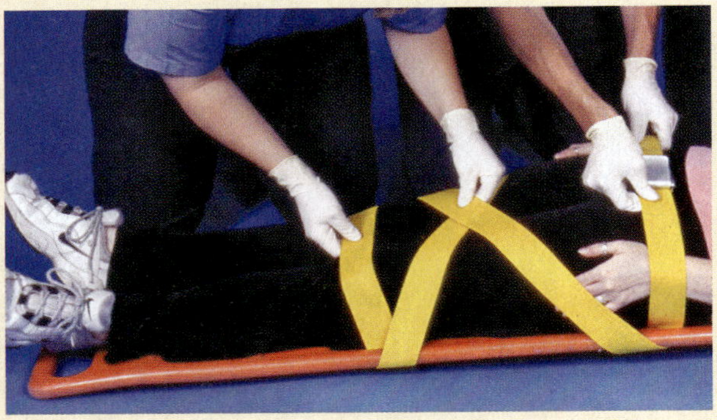

Step 7

Secure the pelvis and upper legs.

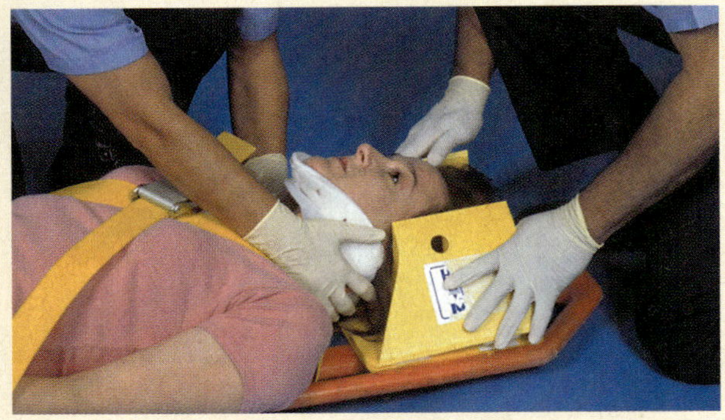

Step 8

Begin to secure the patient's head using a commercial securing device or rolled towels.

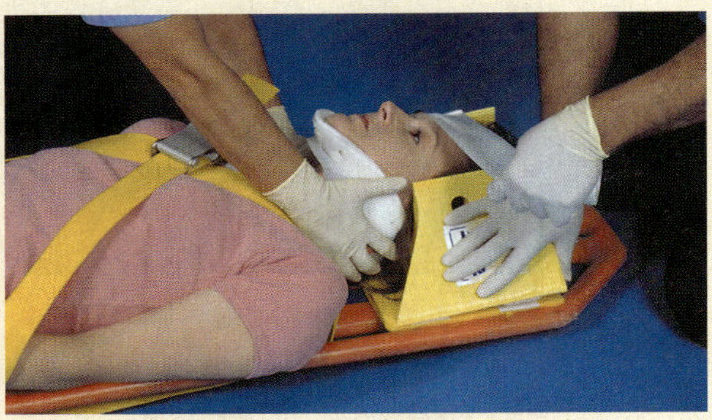

Step 9

Place tape or a soft strap across the patient's forehead to secure the commercial device or towel rolls (do *not* place the adhesive side of medical duct tape directly onto the patient's skin or eyebrows). Check all straps and readjust as needed. Reassess distal functions in all extremities.

leave access to the airway, do not tape over the throat or chin. Avoid placing the sticky side of the tape on the patient's head (**Step 9**).

11. Check and readjust straps as needed to ensure that the entire body is snugly secured and will not slide during patient movement, but breathing is not restricted.
12. Reassess motor, sensory, and circulatory function in each extremity, and continue to do so periodically.

An alternative to the long backboard or scoop stretcher is to place the patient on a vacuum mattress. The vacuum mattress molds to the specific contours of the patient's body, reducing pressure point tenderness and therefore providing better comfort. The mattress also provides thermal insulation, potentially decreasing the risk of hypothermia. In some areas, such as Germany, it is routinely used for spinal stabilization.[19] It is an excellent alternative to a backboard for older adults or patients with abnormal curvature of the spine. A drawback to the device is its thickness, requiring careful patient movement to maintain spinal stabilization during the application procedure. The vacuum mattress cannot be used for patients who weigh more than 350 pounds (159 kilograms).

Like a backboard, a vacuum mattress can be used on a supine, sitting, or standing patient.

Words of Wisdom

The backboard is rigid and often places the patient in an anatomically incorrect and uncomfortable position for a long time. The discomfort that results from lying on a hard surface may provoke patients to reposition themselves, causing the kind of unwanted movement that SMR is intended to inhibit. Another complication is that while the back is pressed against the board, circulation to compressed skin may be compromised. If this compression lasts long enough (usually several hours), decubitus ulcers can develop.

Some patients may experience respiratory compromise while lying flat. In one study, perfectly healthy volunteers experienced a 15% to 20% reduction in respiratory effectiveness when secured to a backboard.[20,21] Presumably this was provoked by a combination of the supine position on a rigid surface plus the application of chest straps. The pulmonary restrictive effects are even more pronounced at extremes of age and in patients with obesity. Clinicians should ensure that the straps are tight enough to secure the patient but not so tight as to limit the movement of the patient's chest. Pulling the straps too tight may result in hypoventilation.

Another potential complication of the backboard is the risk of aspiration in patients restricted in the supine position. In general, while the board may be a useful tool for extricating or moving patients who cannot safely walk to the ambulance stretcher, there is no proven benefit to leaving patients on the board during transport.[22–25] However, if transport duration is relatively short, your agency may opt to leave the patient on the board.

Another commonly cited complication of backboard use is a potential increase in mortality in patients with life-threatening injuries.[25] The process of extricating and securing a patient to a backboard takes time, and even a delay on scene of a few minutes could prove fatal in patients who have significant injuries requiring surgical intervention (eg, internal bleeding, intracranial hemorrhage).

National consensus documents suggest there are viable alternatives to the backboard in achieving SMR, including using the ambulance stretcher alone with application of a cervical collar.[13] However, the EMS crew must first get the patient to the stretcher. If the patient is conscious and can follow commands, and if the patient is able to self-extricate or is already standing when you arrive on scene, it may be best to simply apply a cervical collar and instruct the patient to lie down on the ambulance stretcher. However, when patients are unconscious or cannot move to the stretcher safely by themselves, alternative devices may be indicated. Although using the long backboard to move the patient from the ground to the stretcher is certainly an acceptable option, there may be benefits to using a scoop stretcher or vacuum mattress instead. The scoop stretcher is a favored option for lifting patients from the ground because it lessens the need to perform a log roll maneuver, which has been shown to cause greater displacement of the spine than a simple lift technique using the scoop stretcher.[26] The vacuum mattress is an attractive option because it conforms to the natural curvature of the patient's spine and may therefore be more comfortable.

Regardless of which device you use to move the patient to the stretcher, it is important to weigh the risks and benefits of having the patient remain on the device during transport. If SMR during transport can be accomplished by simply having the patient lie supine on the stretcher with a cervical collar in place, and if the patient can follow commands, then your role may simply be to coach the patient to remain still. If the patient has an altered level of consciousness, head blocks may be used to maintain in-line positioning of the cervical spine. Regardless, leaving a patient on a backboard throughout transport to the hospital should be avoided when possible.

A patient can be moved onto the vacuum mattress with a scoop stretcher or a log roll. For the scoop stretcher method, the mattress does not need to be partially rigid.

It is important to secure the patient sufficiently but without restricting breathing. Failure to sufficiently secure the patient can cause excessive movement, increasing the risk of subsequent spinal cord injury.

Follow the steps in **SKILL DRILL 28-4** to use a vacuum mattress:

1. Place the mattress on a flat surface near the patient. Make sure the head end of the mattress is at the patient's head (**Step 1**).
2. Allow air to enter the mattress (**Step 2**). The valve stem can remain open until the mattress is soft and pliable.

3. Smooth the mattress so that it is flat and level. Remove any sharp or bulky items that may damage the vacuum mattress (**Step 3**).
4. Connect the pump to the mattress (**Step 4**).
5. Determine which method you will use to move the patient onto the mattress, then prepare the patient and equipment as follows:
   a. Log roll method: Evacuate the mattress until it is partially rigid. (This step is not needed if using the scoop stretcher method.) The surface should be smooth and the beads inside the mattress should be spread out as evenly as possible (**Step 5A**).
   b. Scoop stretcher method: For this method, the mattress does not need to be partially rigid. Apply the scoop stretcher to the patient (**Step 5B**).
6. Move the patient onto the vacuum mattress using the selected method (**Step 6**).

Skill Drill 28-4 Placing a Patient on a Full-Body Vacuum Mattress

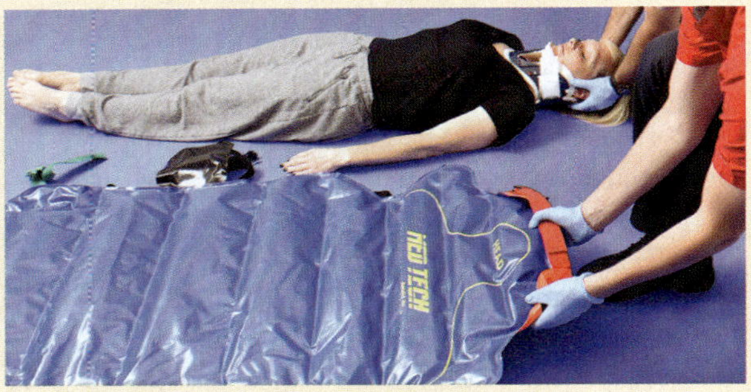

Step 1

Place the mattress on a flat surface near the patient, with the head end of the mattress at the patient's head.

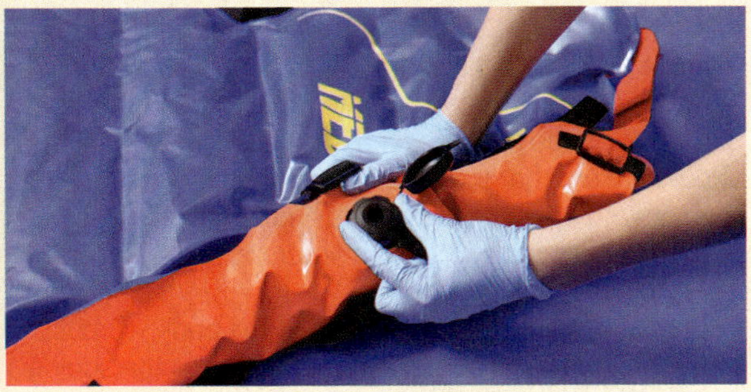

Step 2

Allow air to enter the mattress. Keep the valve stem open until the mattress is soft and pliable.

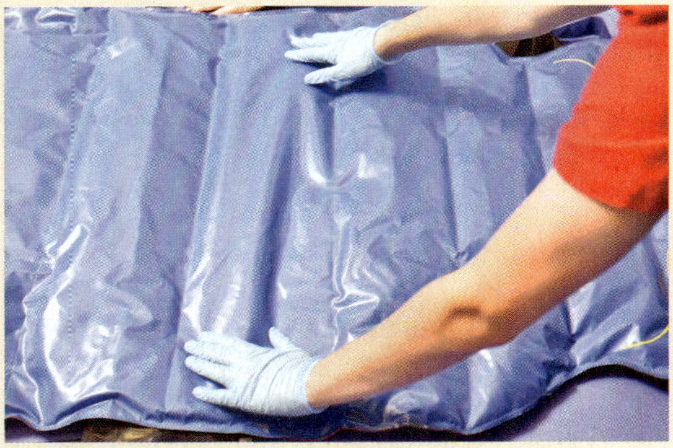

Step 3

Smooth the mattress. Remove any sharp or bulky items that may damage the mattress.

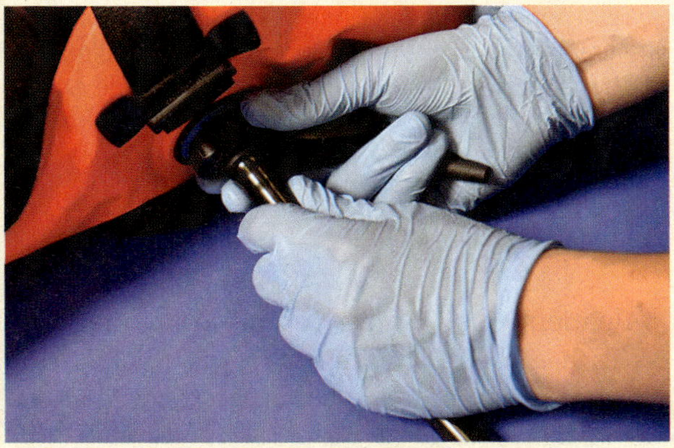

Step 4

Connect the pump to the mattress.

Skill Drill 28-4 Placing a Patient on a Full-Body Vacuum Mattress continued

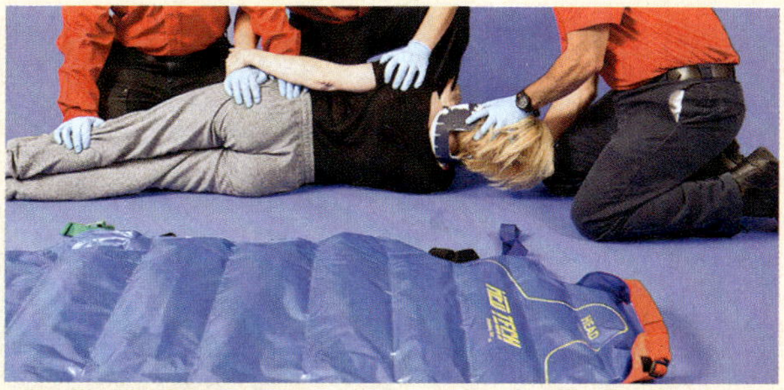

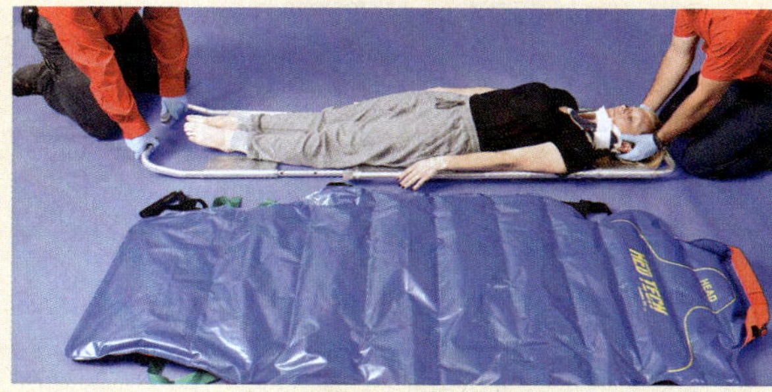

Step 5

Determine which method you will use to move the patient onto the mattress. If you use the log roll method, evacuate the mattress until it is partially rigid (this step is not needed if using the scoop stretcher method). The surface should be smooth and the beads should be spread out as evenly as possible.

If using a scoop stretcher, you do not need to partially evacuate the mattress at this stage.

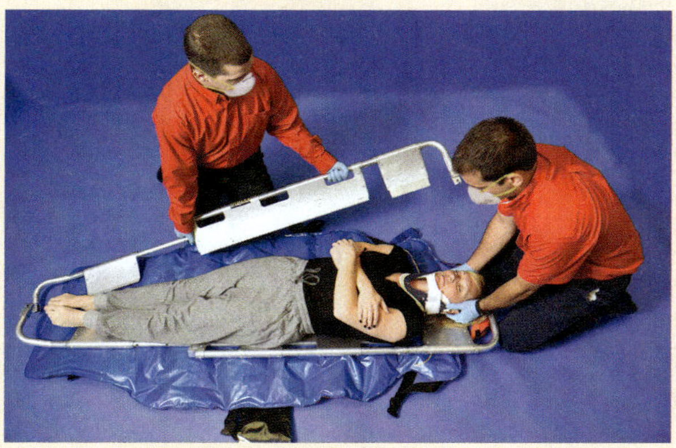

Step 6

Move the patient onto the vacuum mattress using the method you determined during the previous step. Maintain spinal alignment.

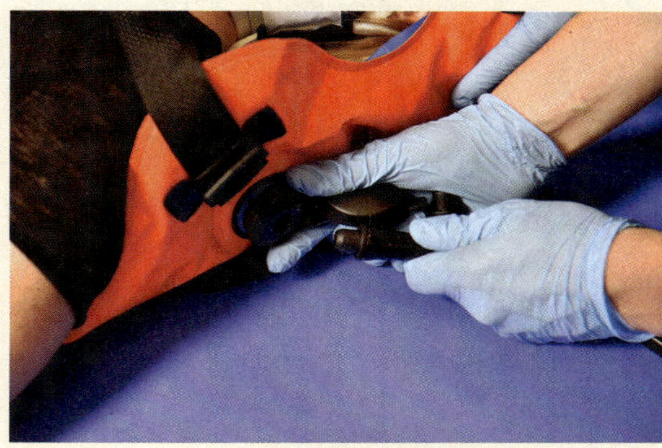

Step 7

If the vacuum mattress is partially rigid, open the valve to allow air to enter. Keep the valve open until the mattress is pliable.

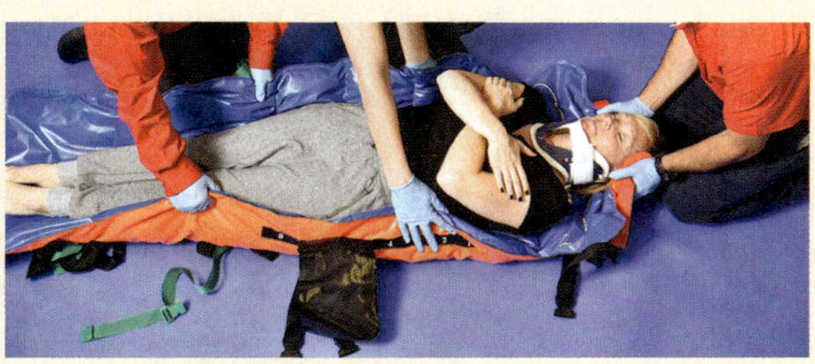

Step 8

Conform the mattress to each side of the patient's head, close to the shoulders but not the top of the head. Continue to hold these "head blocks" that you have formed and have a second person hold up the sides of the mattress to the patient's hips until the mattress is evacuated of air completely.

(continues)

Skill Drill 28-4 Placing a Patient on a Full-Body Vacuum Mattress continued

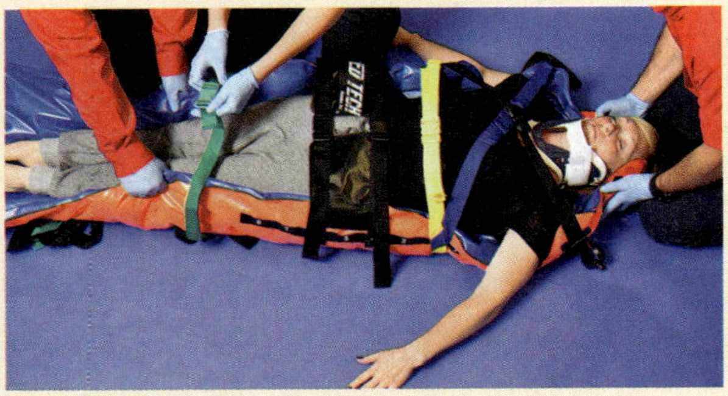

Step 9

Secure the patient's chest, hips, and legs.

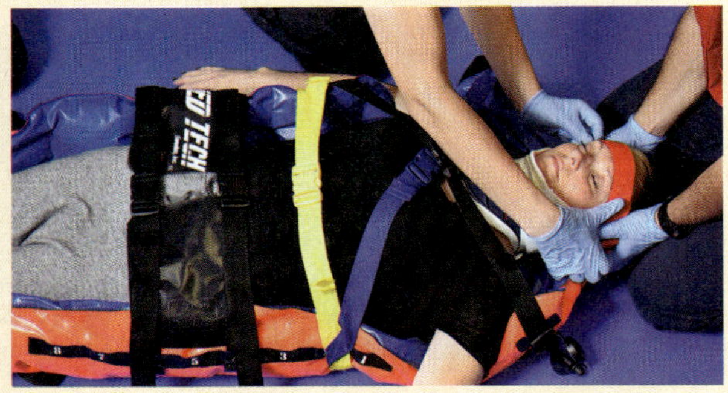

Step 10

Secure the patient's head. Pad any voids at the top of the shoulders.

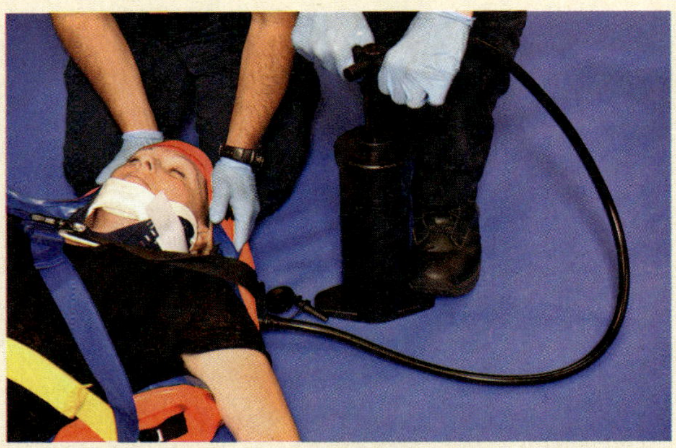

Step 11

Ensure the patient is as comfortable as possible, then evacuate the remaining air to achieve effective SMR.

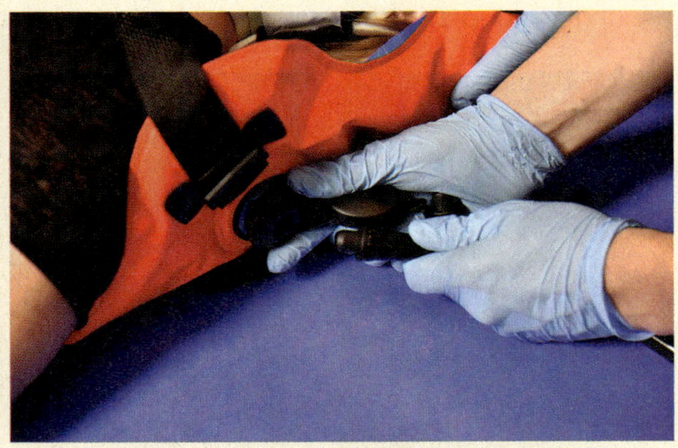

Step 12

Disconnect the vacuum pump and ensure that the valve is closed or secured.

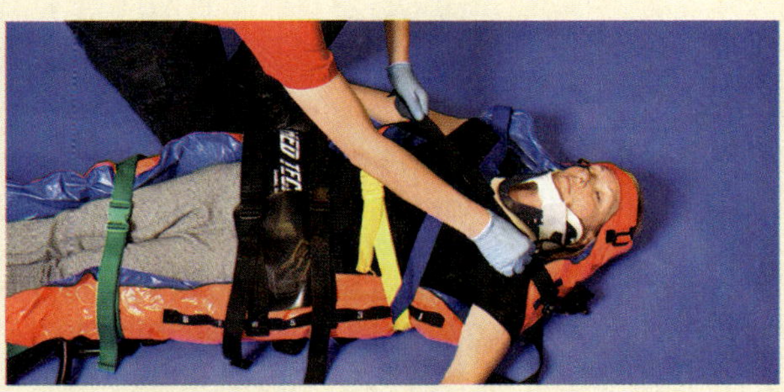

Step 13

Reassess and adjust the straps around the chest, hips, and legs.

Skill Drill 28-4 Placing a Patient on a Full-Body Vacuum Mattress continued

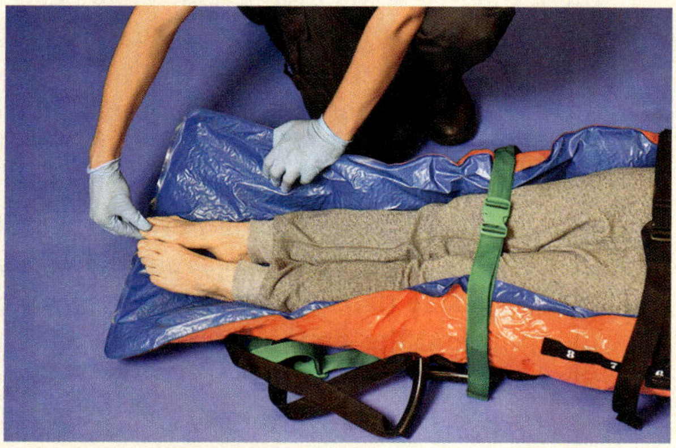

Step 14

Check the patient's neurovascular status and recheck all straps prior to lifting or moving the patient.

Throughout this procedure, maintain spinal alignment.

a. Log roll method: Place the mattress on a backboard or transfer device. Hold the mattress in place on the backboard, and log roll the patient onto the backboard with the mattress on top of it. (The long backboard is used only for stabilization.) Position the patient so their head is very close to the top edge.

b. Scoop stretcher method: Lift and transfer the patient onto the mattress. Position the patient so their head is in the head area of the mattress or very close to the mattress's top edge. Remove the scoop stretcher from around the patient and proceed with application of the vacuum mattress.

7. If the vacuum mattress is partially rigid, open the valve to allow air to enter (**Step 7**). Keep the valve open until the mattress is pliable.
8. Conform the mattress to each side of the patient's head close to the shoulders, but not the top of the head (**Step 8**). Continue to hold these "head blocks" that you have formed and have a second person hold up the sides of the mattress to the patient's hips until the mattress is evacuated of air completely. Always form the mattress to meet the needs of the patient. Use additional rescuers if needed. Some patients may be more comfortable with their knees slightly bent.
9. Secure the patient's chest, hips, and legs in the mattress (**Step 9**).
10. Secure the patient's head with medical tape (**Step 10**). Pad any voids at the top of the shoulders.
11. If the patient is as comfortable as possible, evacuate the remaining air from the mattress to achieve rigid SMR (**Step 11**). (A portable suction unit can be used to evacuate some mattresses; see the manufacturer's recommendations.)
12. Disconnect the vacuum pump and ensure that the valve is closed or secured so the mattress does not accidentally lose its rigidity (**Step 12**).
13. Reassess and adjust the straps around the chest, hips, and legs (**Step 13**).
14. Check the patient's neurovascular status and recheck all straps prior to lifting or moving the patient (**Step 14**).

Words of Wisdom

Patients who have kyphosis, a condition that causes the upper part of the spine to have an exaggerated outward curve giving them a hunchback appearance, will need extra padding under their head when placed in SMR.

Sitting Patients

If the patient who is at risk of spinal injury is in a vehicle and is alert and able, apply a cervical collar and allow them to get out of the vehicle on their own and onto the ambulance stretcher. This includes children in booster seats.[15]

The short spine board and Kendrick extrication device (KED) have been used to move stable patients who had neck or back pain from a vehicle to an SMR device. In some EMS systems this procedure is not used often because some evidence suggests that the use of these devices creates more movement than applying a cervical collar and allowing the conscious patient to self-extricate.[27] When needed, the device is placed behind the seated patient after a cervical collar has been applied and the straps secured, as indicated in Skill Drill 28-2. The patient is then removed and placed supine on the stretcher. After releasing the groin straps, the patient is secured to the appropriate SMR surface and secured for transport.

Rapid extrication is indicated in cases of life-threatening or limb-threatening injury. Follow the steps in **SKILL DRILL 28-5** to secure a sitting patient's cervical spine using a commercial device.

1. Take standard precautions. As with the supine patient, you must first stabilize the head and then maintain manual in-line stabilization until the patient has been secured to the long backboard or vacuum mattress.
2. Assess pulse, motor, and sensory function in each extremity.
3. Apply the cervical collar (**Step 1**).
4. Insert an extrication device between the patient's upper back and the seat back (**Step 2**).
5. Open the side flaps (if present), and position them around the patient's torso and snug to the armpits (**Step 3**).
6. Once the extrication device has been properly positioned, secure the upper torso straps and then the midtorso straps (**Step 4**).
7. Position and fasten both groin (leg) straps. Check all torso straps to make sure they are secure. Make any adjustments necessary without excessive movement of the patient (**Step 5**).
8. Pad any space between the patient's head and the extrication device as necessary.

Skill Drill 28-5 Securing a Patient Found in a Sitting Position

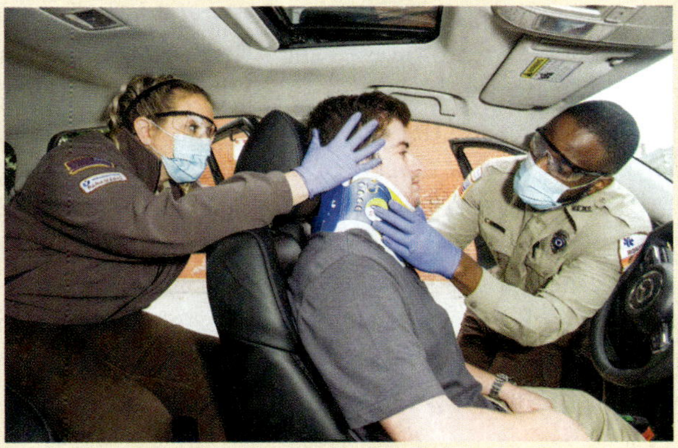

Step 1

Take standard precautions. Stabilize the head and neck in a neutral, in-line position. Assess pulse, motor, and sensory function in each extremity. Apply a cervical collar.

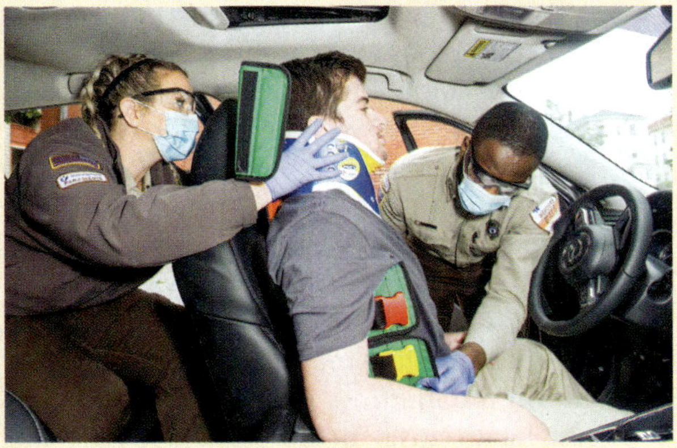

Step 2

Insert a SMR device between the patient's upper back and the seat.

Skill Drill 28-5 Securing a Patient Found in a Sitting Position

continued

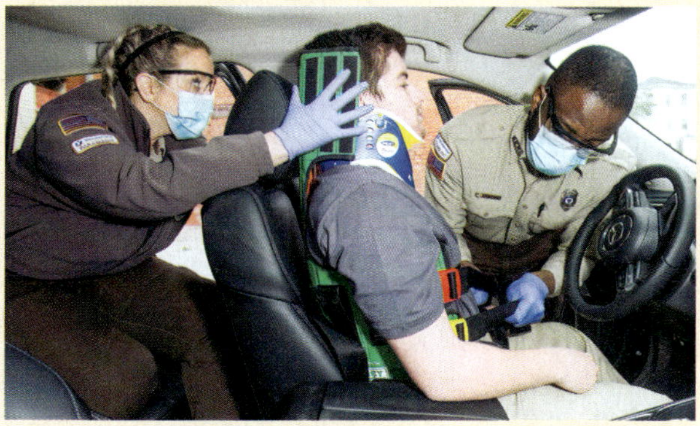

Step 3

Open the side flaps, and position them around the patient's torso, snug around the armpits.

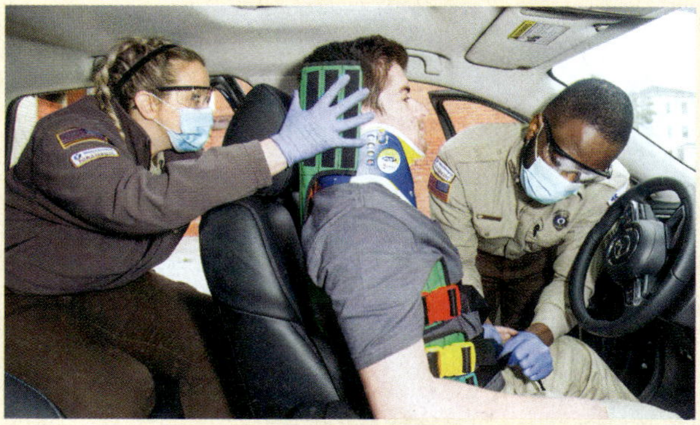

Step 4

Secure the upper torso flaps, then the mid-torso flaps.

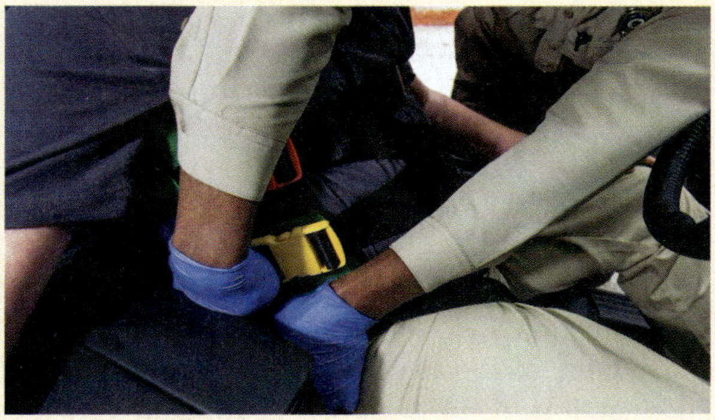

Step 5

Secure the groin (leg) straps. Check and adjust the torso straps.

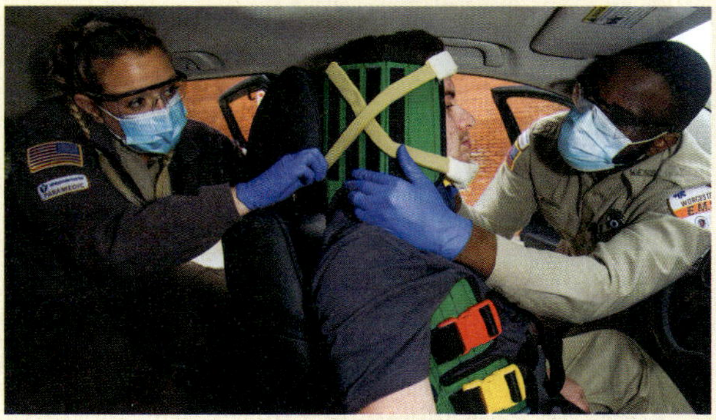

Step 6

Pad between the head and the device as needed. Secure the forehead strap and fasten the lower head strap around the cervical collar.

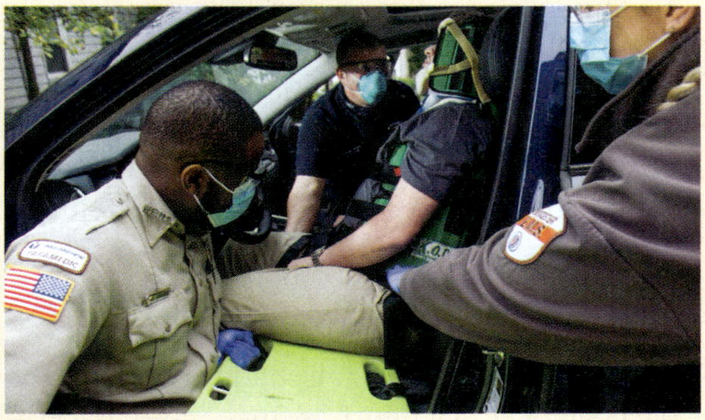

Step 7

Place a long backboard next to the patient's buttocks, perpendicular to the trunk.

(continues)

Skill Drill 28-5 Securing a Patient Found in a Sitting Position

continued

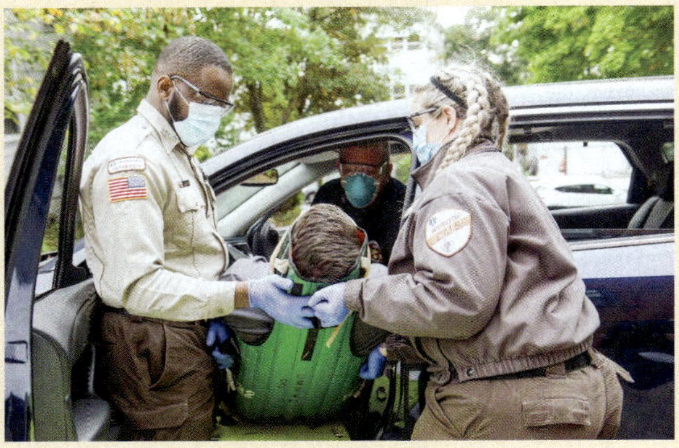

Step 8

Turn and lower the patient onto the long backboard. Lift the patient and slip the long backboard under the securing device.

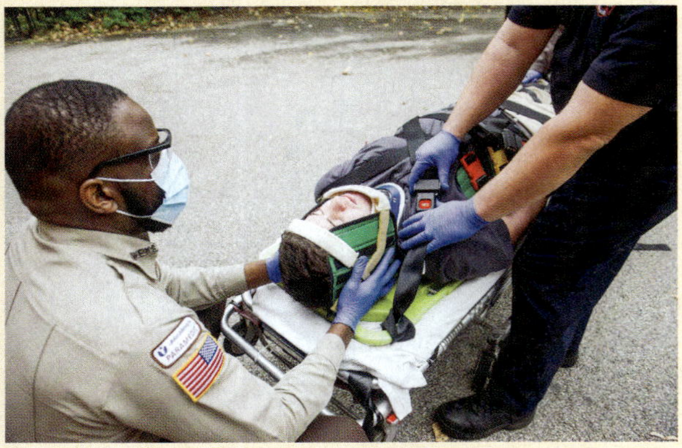

Step 9

Secure the spinal precaution device and long backboard to each other. Loosen or release the groin straps. Reassess pulse, motor, and sensory function in each extremity.

9. Secure the forehead strap, and then fasten the lower head strap around the cervical collar (**Step 6**).
10. Place the long backboard next to the patient's buttocks, perpendicular to the trunk (**Step 7**).
11. Turn the patient parallel to the long backboard, and slowly lower the patient onto it.
12. Lift the patient (without rotating them), and slip the long backboard under the short board (**Step 8**).
13. Secure the extrication device and long backboard together. Loosen or release the groin straps.
14. Reassess the pulse, motor, and sensory function in all four extremities. Document your findings, and prepare for immediate transport (**Step 9**).

Standing Patients

You may arrive at a scene in which you find a patient standing or wandering around after a crash or injury. If this patient reports neck pain, apply a cervical collar and have the patient sit and then carefully lie down on the stretcher, minimizing movement of the head and neck. Manual in-line stabilization of the neck is not indicated in these patients.[15]

If the MOI and clinical indications suggest spinal injury or the patient's inability to protect the spine, establish SMR. Clinical indications may include the following:

- Spinal tenderness or pain
- An altered level of consciousness
- Neurologic deficits
- Obvious anatomic deformity of the spine
- High-energy trauma in a patient intoxicated from drugs, alcohol, or a distracting injury

SMR in Children

SMR is recommended for all children who have possible head or spinal injuries after a traumatic event. If an infant or toddler who is strapped into a car seat with a built-in harness requires extrication from a vehicle, extricate them while strapped into the car seat. Remember that infants and small children may require additional padding under the torso to maintain the in-line neutral position. They have smaller airways and proportionately larger heads, so padding is important to maintain the airway. Pad under the shoulders to the toes, as needed, to avoid excessive neck flexion (**FIGURE 28-23**). Beginning at ages 8 to 10 years, children no longer require padding under the torso to create a neutral position. Instead, they can simply lie supine on the SMR device.

Another complication may occur if a child is secured to an adult-size backboard. A child's body is narrower than an adult's; therefore, padding (eg, blanket rolls) will be required along the sides of the adult-size backboard to prevent the child from slipping to one side or the other. Backboards designed for children are also available.

Follow these steps to perform SMR for children (**SKILL DRILL 28-6**):

1. Maintain the child's head in a neutral position by placing a towel under the shoulders and torso (**Step 1**).
2. Place an appropriate-size cervical collar on the pediatric patient (**Step 2**).
3. Carefully log roll the child onto the short backboard or pediatric transport device (**Step 3**).
4. Secure the pediatric patient's torso to the device first (**Step 4**).
5. Secure the child's head to the device (**Step 5**).
6. Ensure that the child is strapped in properly (**Step 6**).

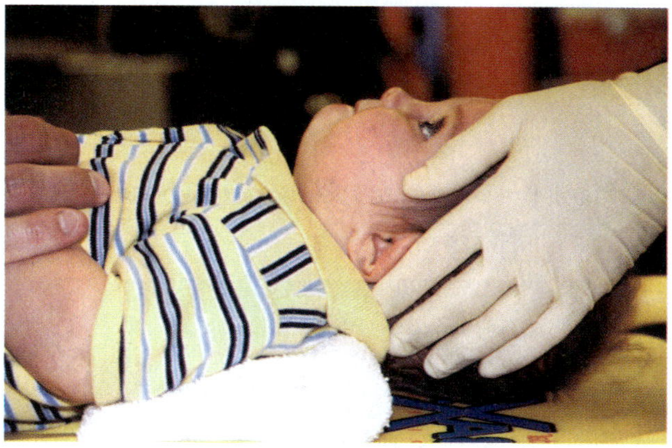

FIGURE 28-23 Children have proportionately larger heads than adults, so you may need to place padding under the shoulders to avoid excessive flexion of the head.

Skill Drill 28-6 Performing SMR for a Pediatric Patient

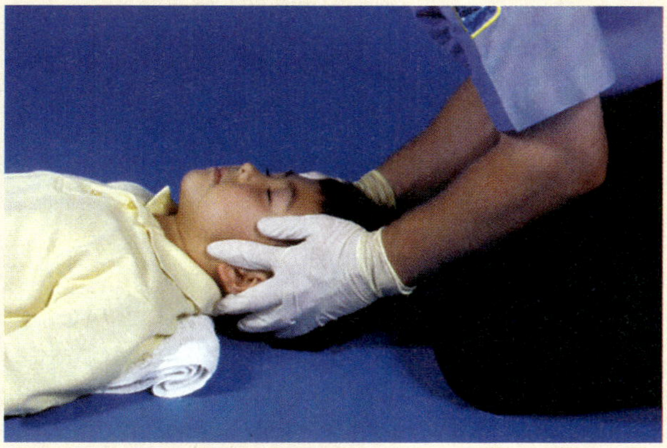

Step 1

Use a towel under the back, from the shoulders to the hips, to maintain the head in a neutral position.

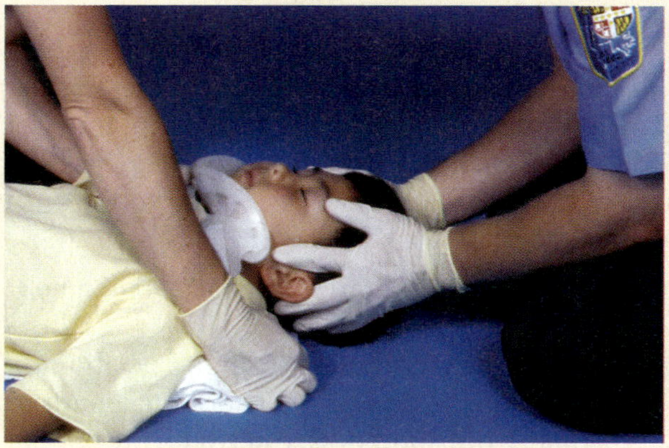

Step 2

Apply an appropriate-size cervical collar.

(continues)

Skill Drill 28-6 Performing SMR for a Pediatric Patient continued

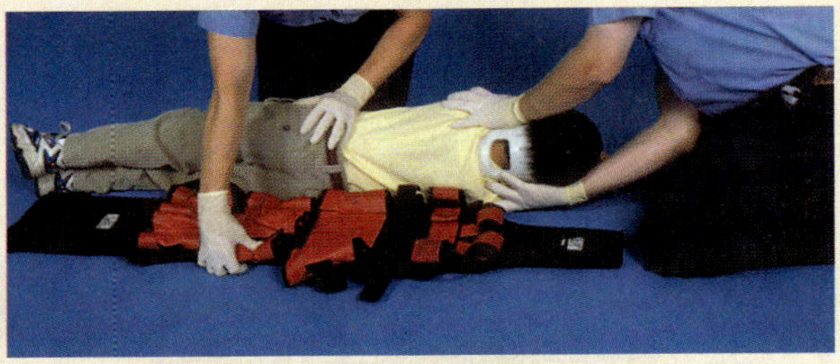

Step 3

Log roll the child onto the short backboard or pediatric transport device.

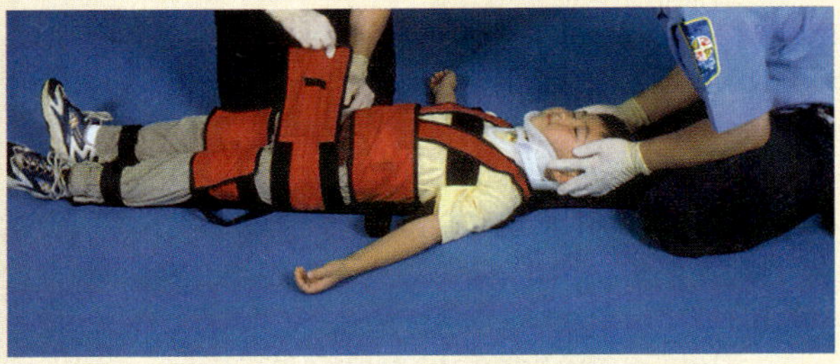

Step 4

Secure the torso first.

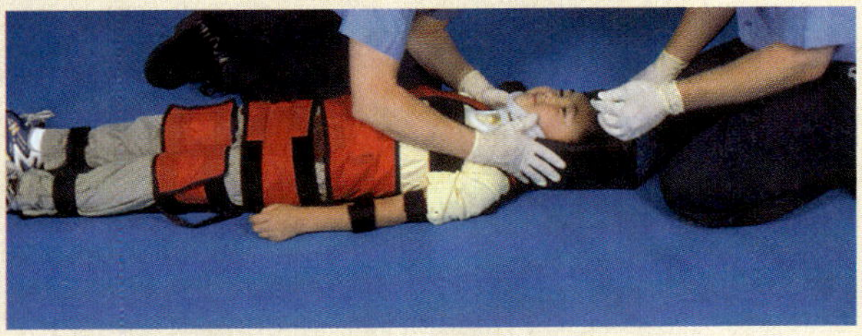

Step 5

Secure the head.

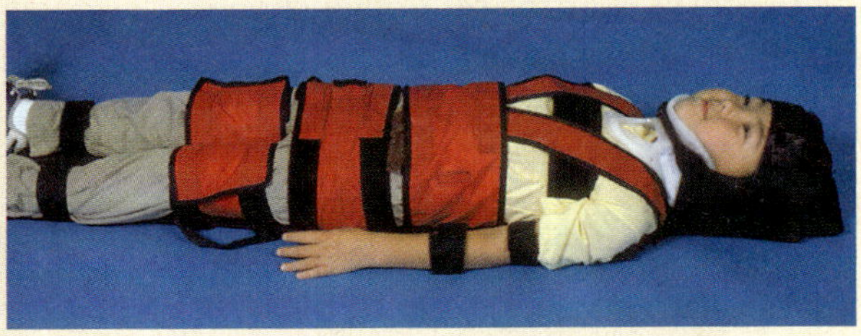

Step 6

Ensure that the child is strapped in properly.

Many infants and small children will be in a car seat when you approach them. The patient must be removed to a short backboard or pediatric device prior to transport. Follow these steps to perform SMR for a patient in a car seat (**SKILL DRILL 28-7**):

1. Carefully stabilize the patient's head in a neutral position (**Step 1**).
2. Lay the seat down into a reclined position on a hard surface. Position a short backboard or pediatric transport device between the patient and the surface on which the patient is resting (**Step 2**).
3. Carefully slide the patient into position on the device (**Step 3**).
4. Make sure the patient's head is in a neutral position by placing a towel under the back, from the shoulders to the hips (**Step 4**).
5. Secure the torso first and place padding to fill any voids (**Step 5**).
6. Secure the patient's head to the device (**Step 6**).

Helmet Removal

When caring for a patient wearing a helmet, you will need to determine whether it is appropriate to remove it. In weighing the risks and benefits, ask yourself the following questions:

- Is the patient's airway clear?
- Is the patient breathing adequately?
- Can you maintain the airway and assist ventilations if the helmet remains in place?
- Can the face guard be easily removed to allow access to the airway without removing the helmet?

Skill Drill 28-7 Performing SMR for a Patient in a Car Seat

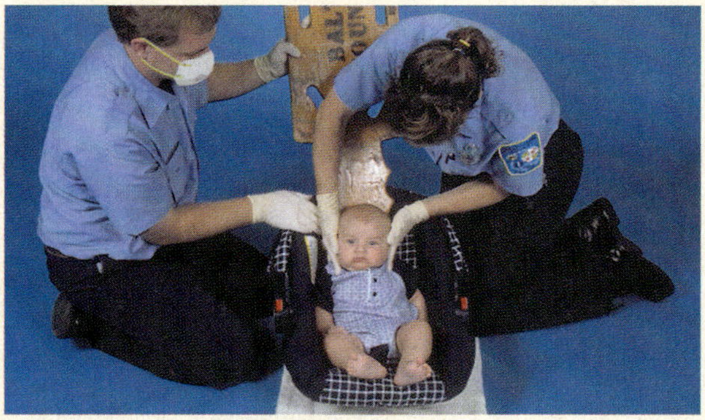

Step 1

Stabilize the head in neutral position.

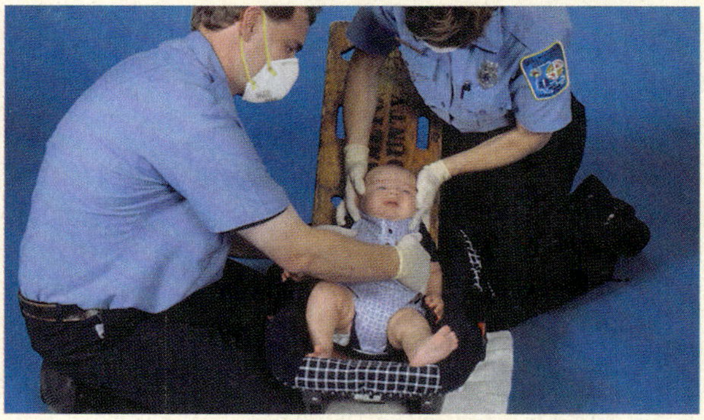

Step 2

Place a short backboard or pediatric transport device between the patient and the surface on which the patient is resting.

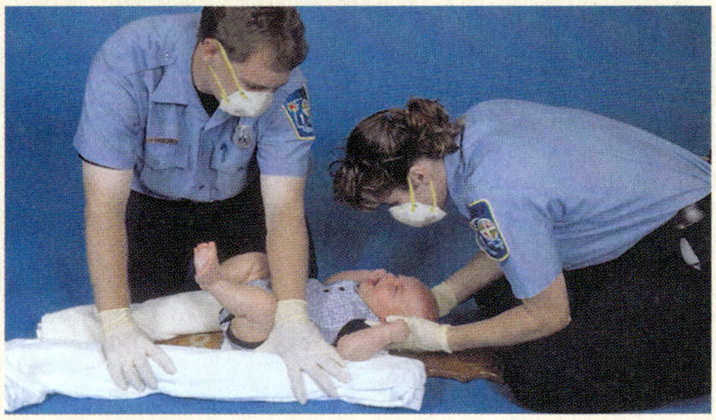

Step 3

Slide the patient onto the device.

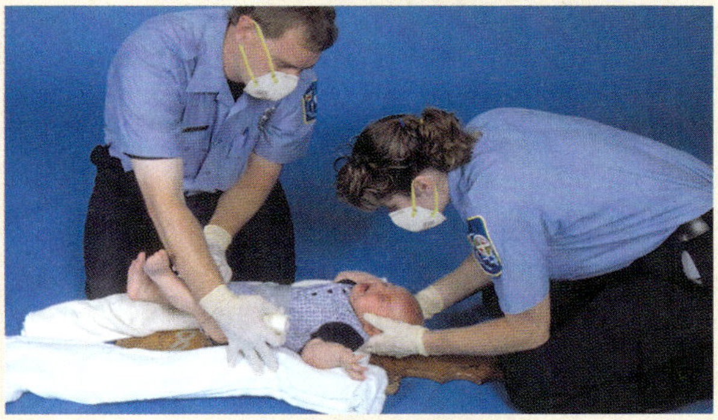

Step 4

Place a towel under the back, from the shoulders to the hips, to ensure neutral head position.

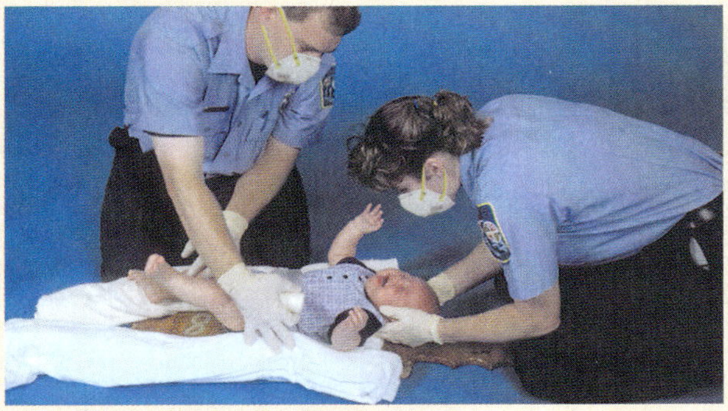

Step 5

Secure the torso first; pad any voids.

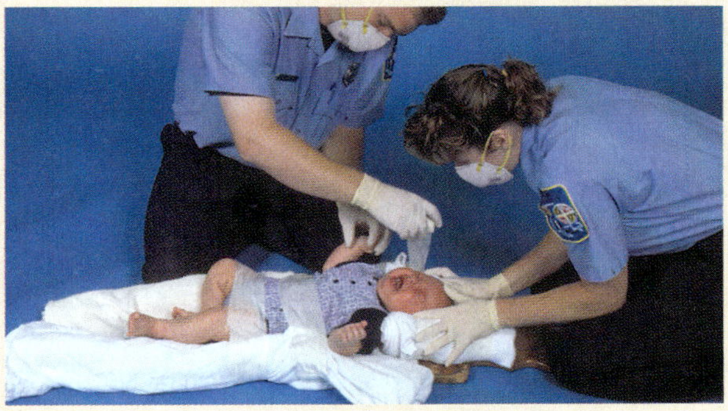

Step 6

Secure the head to the device.

- How well does the helmet fit?
- Can the patient move within the helmet?
- Can SMR in a neutral position be accomplished with the helmet on?

A helmet that fits well prevents the patient's head from moving and should be left on, given the following circumstances:

1. There are no impending airway or breathing problems.
2. The helmet does not interfere with assessment and treatment of airway or ventilation problems.
3. You can perform SMR.

You should also leave on the helmet if there is any chance that removing it will further injure the patient.

Remove a helmet if any of the following conditions exist:

1. It is a full-face helmet (**FIGURE 28-24**).
2. It makes assessing or managing airway problems difficult and removal of a face guard to improve airway access is not possible.
3. It prevents you from performing SMR.
4. It allows excessive head movement.

Finally, always remove a helmet from a patient who is in cardiac arrest.

Sports helmets are typically open in the front and may or may not include an attached face mask. The mask can be removed without affecting helmet position or function by simply removing or cutting the straps that hold it to the helmet, thus allowing easy access to the airway (**FIGURE 28-25**). A patient who is involved in full-contact sports may be wearing bulky pads to protect various body regions, such as shoulder pads. Leaving a helmet in place whenever possible is preferred because it helps the body maintain an in-line neutral position. If the helmet is removed, be sure to remove the shoulder pads also or to provide padding to compensate for the shoulder pads and maintain in-line positioning of the body.

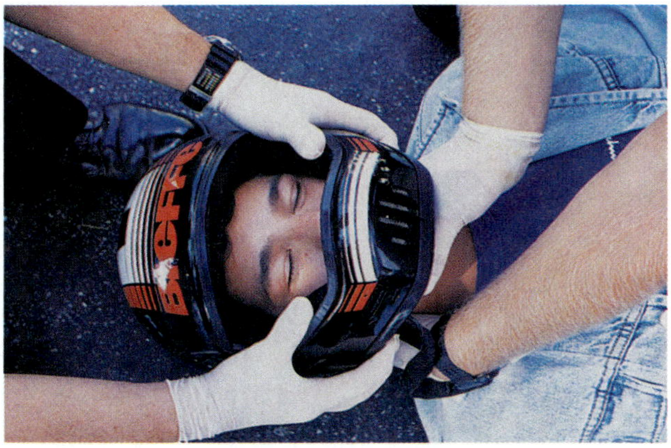

FIGURE 28-24 A full-face helmet, such as this motorcycle helmet, should be removed from the patient.

YOU are the EMT

Your partner continues to assist the patient's ventilations while you reassess his condition and vital signs. His GCS score remains unchanged from the previous readings. You call the trauma center to give your radio report and advise the center of your estimated time of arrival.

Recording Time: 16 Minutes	
Level of consciousness	Responsive only to deep painful stimuli
Respirations	6 breaths/min and irregular (baseline); ventilations are being assisted
Pulse	70 beats/min; regular and bounding
Skin	Baseline color, warm, and dry
Blood pressure	188/98 mm Hg
Oxygen saturation (Spo_2)	98% (on oxygen)

You deliver the patient to the ED and give your verbal report to the attending physician. After further assessment and treatment in the ED, the patient is taken to radiology for CT scanning, which reveals an epidural hematoma.

9. What is an epidural hematoma?

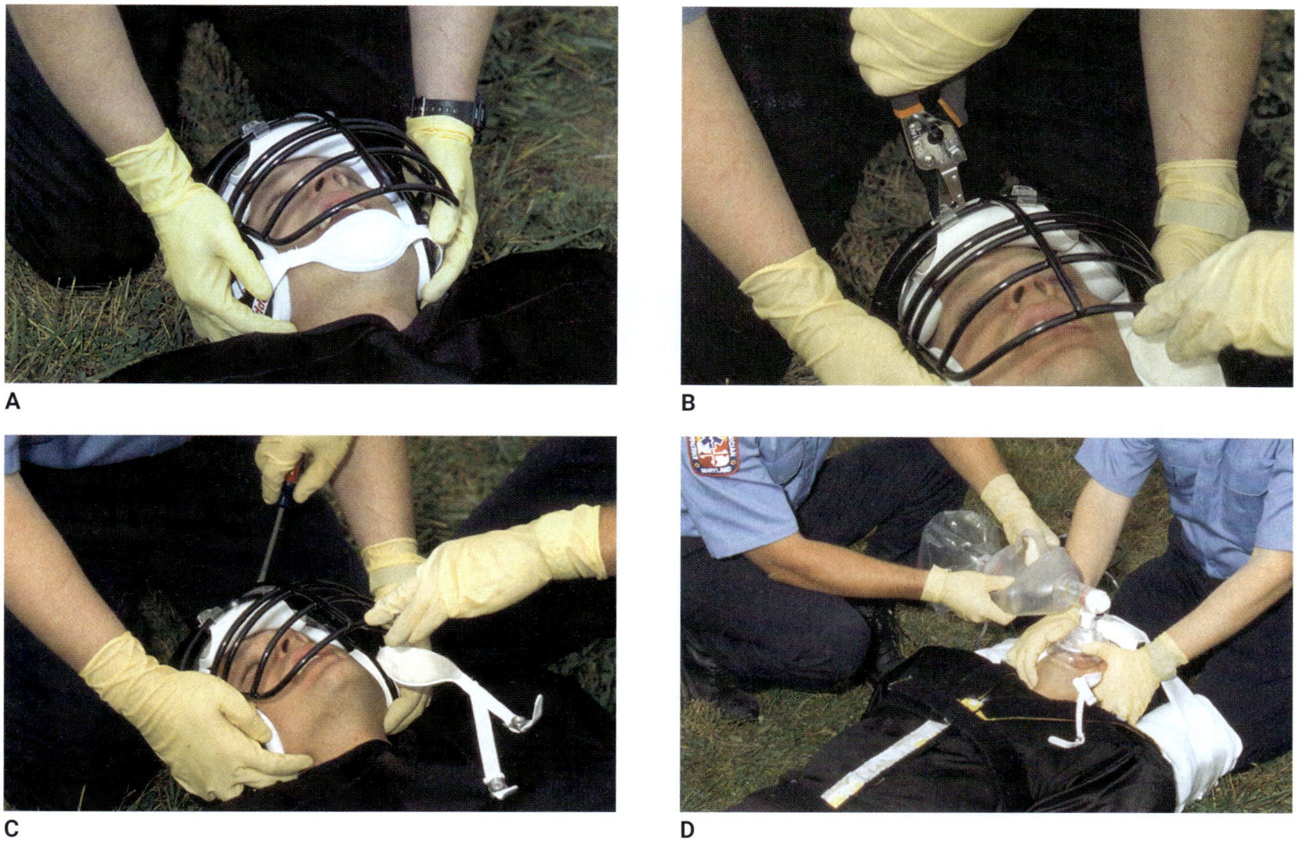

FIGURE 28-25 The face mask on most sports helmets can be removed without affecting helmet position or function. **A.** Stabilize the patient's head and helmet. Remove the face mask in one of two ways: Use a trainer's tool designed for cutting retaining clips (**B**), or unscrew the retaining clips from the face mask (**C**). **D.** After the face mask is removed, the helmet can be secured against the backboard and a bag-mask device can be used effectively.

Removing a helmet should always be at least a two-person job; however, the technique for helmet removal depends on the actual type of helmet worn by the patient. One EMT provides constant in-line support as the other EMT performs the various moves; you and your partner should not move at the same time. You should first consult with medical direction, if possible, about your decision to remove a helmet. When you decide to do so, follow the steps in **SKILL DRILL 28-8**:

1. Begin by kneeling at the patient's head. Your partner should kneel on one side of the patient, at the shoulder area.
2. Open the face shield, if there is one, and assess the patient's airway and breathing. Remove eyeglasses if the patient is wearing them (**Step 1**).
3. Stabilize the helmet by placing your hands on either side of it, with your fingers on the patient's lower jaw to prevent movement of the head. Once your hands are in position, your partner can loosen the face strap (**Step 2**).
4. Once the strap has been loosened, your partner should place one hand on the patient's lower jaw at the angle of the jaw and the other behind the head at the occipital region. Once your partner's hands are in position, you may pull the sides of the helmet away from the patient's head (**Step 3**).
5. Gently slip the helmet halfway off the patient's head, stopping when the helmet reaches the halfway point (**Step 4**).
6. Your partner then slides a hand from the occiput to the back of the head. This will prevent

the head from snapping back once the helmet has been completely removed (**Step 5**).

7. With your partner's hand in place, remove the helmet, and stabilize the cervical spine.
8. Apply the cervical collar and then secure the patient to the backboard.
9. With large helmets or small patients, you may need to pad under the shoulders to prevent flexion of the neck. If shoulder pads or heavy clothing are in place, you may need to pad behind the patient's head to prevent extension of the neck (**Step 6**).

Skill Drill 28-8 Removing a Helmet

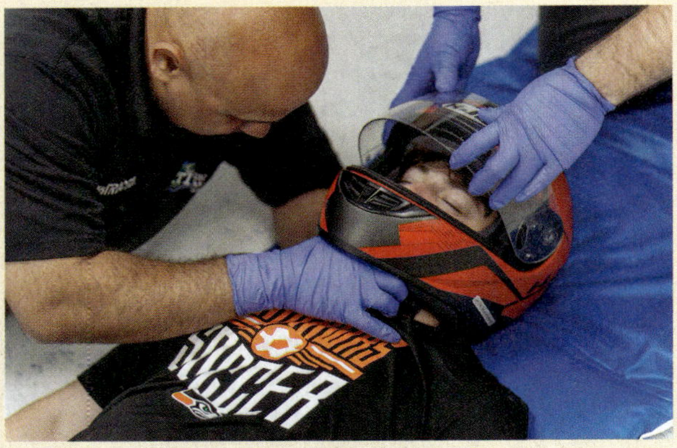

Step 1

Kneel at the patient's head with your partner at one side. Open the face shield to assess airway and breathing. Remove eyeglasses if present.

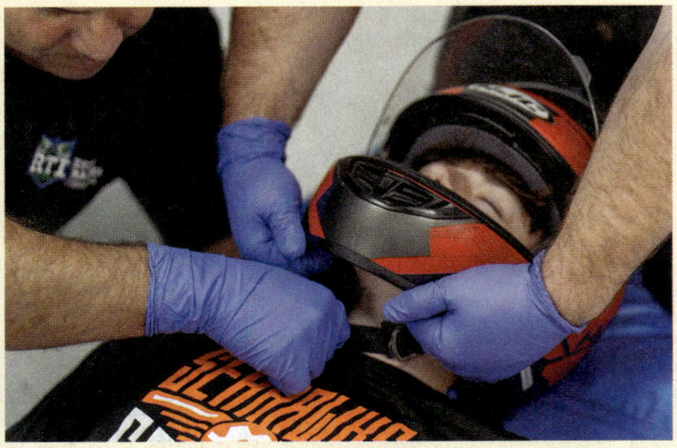

Step 2

Prevent head movement by placing your hands on either side of the helmet and fingers on the lower jaw. Have your partner loosen the strap.

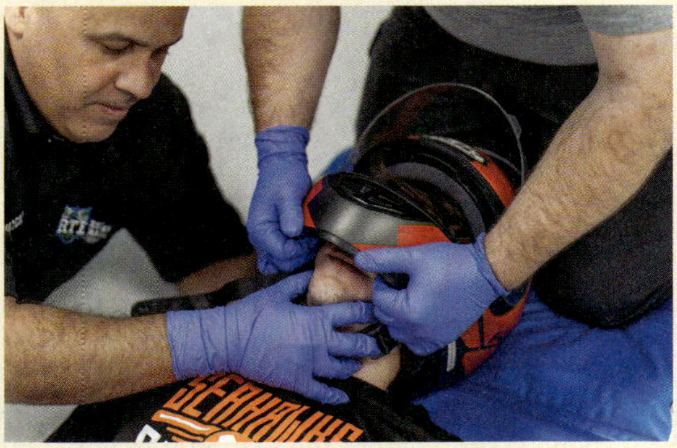

Step 3

Have your partner place one hand at the angle of the lower jaw and the other at the occiput.

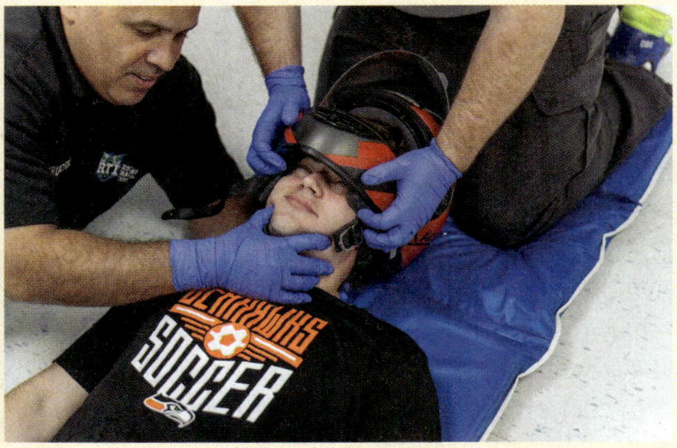

Step 4

Gently slip the helmet about halfway off, then stop.

Skill Drill 28-8 Removing a Helmet continued

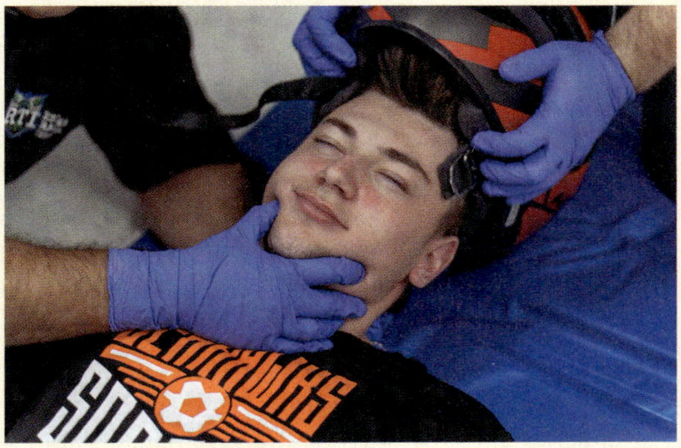

Step 5

Have your partner slide the hand from the occiput to the back of the head to prevent the head from snapping back.

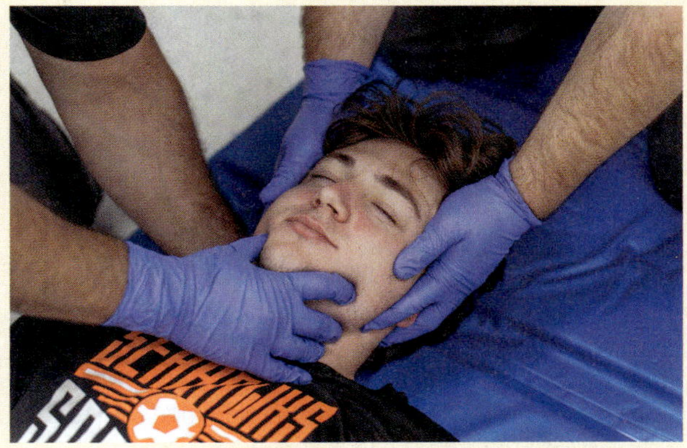

Step 6

Remove the helmet and stabilize the cervical spine. Apply a cervical collar and secure the patient to a long backboard. Pad as needed to prevent neck flexion or extension.

All images Courtesy of Aura Prep/Rescue Training International.

YOU are the EMT SUMMARY

1. What are the potential concerns surrounding the structure of the cranium and potential brain swelling?

The cranium does an excellent job of protecting the brain from direct trauma following minor injuries. The hard shell of the cranium provides protection for the brain from the bumps and blows that occur as a part of everyday life. However, the very fact that the cranium is a hard shell makes it a mixed blessing following a significant head injury. The cranium's rigid, unyielding structure allows little, if any, expansion of the brain if swelling or bleeding occurs. Furthermore, its hard and somewhat irregular internal surface can injure the brain and its blood vessels following significant deceleration injury.

2. What is the difference between a primary and a secondary brain injury?

A TBI can be classified into one of two categories: primary (direct) injury and secondary (indirect) injury.

Primary brain injury is injury to the brain and its associated structures that occurs immediately on impact to the head. It can occur following a penetrating injury, such as a stabbing or a gunshot wound, or if a bone fragment is driven into the brain following a skull fracture; however, it more commonly occurs following blunt-force trauma.

Secondary brain injury refers to damage to the brain as a result of complications from the primary head injury. It may result from abnormal processes such as cerebral edema, increased ICP, cerebral

YOU are the EMT SUMMARY continued

ischemia and hypoxia, and infection. Secondary brain injury can occur anywhere from a few minutes to several days following the initial head injury.

3. What are your most immediate treatment priorities for this patient?

As with any patient, your initial treatment must focus on what could cause death *first*. Your patient's breathing rate and quality, slow and irregular, is not adequate and requires immediate treatment. You should instruct your partner to maintain in-line spinal position while he assists the patient's ventilations with a bag-mask device and high-flow oxygen. If a law enforcement officer is available, ask them to stabilize the patient's head while your partner assists his ventilations.

Consider inserting a simple airway adjunct. If the patient does not have a gag reflex, insert an oropharyngeal (oral) airway. Use of a nasopharyngeal (nasal) airway should be avoided in patients with significant facial injuries or possible basilar skull fracture, especially if you observe fluid drainage from the nose. If a simple airway adjunct is not an option, keep the airway open with the jaw-thrust maneuver and maintain the patient's head in a neutral position.

While your partner is managing the patient's airway, you should control the bleeding from the laceration to his head. Use just enough pressure to control the bleeding; if a skull fracture is present, too much pressure could drive fractured bone fragments into his brain. Quickly scan the rest of the patient's body for any other external bleeding, and control that as well. Remember the objective of the primary assessment: to find life threats, fix them, and move on.

4. Where should you focus your secondary assessment of this patient?

When the patient is unconscious or has experienced a significant MOI, the entire body should be assessed to look for life-threatening injuries that were not grossly apparent in the primary assessment. If immediate threats to the patient's life are found, they should be treated immediately.

Emphasis should be placed on the patient's head and face because this area appears to be where the patient experienced the most injury. Assess the integrity of the skull by *gently* palpating it and noting any areas of deformity, crepitus, or instability. Although you have already bandaged the laceration on the patient's head, you should reassess the bandage to ensure that the bleeding is controlled.

Look in the ears for fluid drainage and look behind the ears for bruising (Battle sign). Fluid or blood drainage from the ears may contain CSF, which would indicate a basilar skull fracture.

Assess the size, equality, and reactivity of the patient's pupils. The nerves that control the dilation and constriction of the pupils are extremely sensitive to increased ICP. Normally, both pupils should briskly constrict when a light is shone into either of the eyes. Pupils that are sluggish (slow) to react could indicate early increased ICP and/or cerebral hypoxia. Unequal or bilaterally fixed and dilated (blown) pupils are later, more ominous signs of increased ICP and indicate pressure on one or both oculomotor nerves. Also observe if there is any sign of blood in the eyes or bruising under the eye orbits (raccoon eyes—another sign of potential basilar skull fracture).

Palpate the facial bones for stability and note any deformities or crepitus.

Patients with a significant head injury should also be assumed to have a cervical spine injury until proven otherwise. Blunt-force trauma that is significant enough to render the patient unconscious could easily fracture a cervical vertebra. Palpate the cervical spine for obvious deformities and then apply a cervical collar. Manually stabilize the patient's head until other SMR precautions have been completed (eg, cervical collar, backboard, scoop stretcher, or other spinal motion restricting devices).

Your secondary assessment of *any* critically injured patient should not take long. Address only life-threatening injuries and remain focused on preparing the patient for immediate transport.

5. What is this patient's GCS score?

Your patient opens his eyes in response to painful stimuli; therefore, you should assign a score of 2 for eye opening. He is making unrecognizable sounds; therefore, you should assign a score of 2 for verbal response. You noted that his arms were flexed and drawn in toward his body (decorticate posturing); therefore, you should assign a score of 3 for motor response. Based on these findings, the patient's current GCS score is 7, which indicates a severe TBI.

6. What is the likely explanation for the patient's vital signs?

Your patient's current vital signs represent a classic trio of findings in patients with a TBI and increased ICP: hypertension, bradycardia, and irregular respirations. These findings, called the Cushing triad, indicate significant cerebral edema and increased ICP.

A predictable response of the injured brain is swelling. Cerebral edema decreases cerebral perfusion pressure (CPP) because there is little room

YOU are the EMT SUMMARY continued

in the cranium for the brain to swell, causing compression of cerebral blood vessels and decreased blood flow. In an attempt to maintain cerebral blood flow, and thus CPP, arterial blood pressure increases, which presents with hypertension, and the cerebral blood vessels attempt to dilate against the exterior pressure from compression of the vessels. Bradycardia occurs as a reflex response to the increase in the patient's blood pressure.

Pressure on the respiratory centers of the brainstem causes a variety of abnormal respiratory patterns. Irregular respirations, slow or fast, are the third component of the Cushing triad. Cheyne-Stokes respirations are characterized by a pattern of rapid breathing (tachypnea), followed by slow breathing (bradypnea) and periods of apnea. Central neurogenic hyperventilation is characterized by deep, rapid breathing; this pattern is similar to Kussmaul respirations, but without an acetone breath odor. Biot respirations, also called ataxic respirations, are characterized by an irregular rate, pattern, and depth of breathing with intermittent periods of apnea.

7. What further treatment is indicated for this patient?

Continue to ensure adequate oxygenation and ventilation, and take steps to decrease the ICP and maximize cerebral blood flow.

Continue to assist the patient's ventilations; however, do *not* hyperventilate him. Hyperventilation with high-flow oxygen constricts the blood vessels in the brain, and although this *may* cause a slight decrease in the ICP, it also pushes oxygenated blood away from the brain, potentially causing a decrease in CPp and further brain injury.

Consider elevating the head of the backboard to a 30° angle to reduce the ICP. However, elevating the backboard greater than 30° may cause blood (and oxygen) to leave the brain by gravity, thus causing a decrease in cerebral perfusion, and should be avoided.

Notifying the receiving facility early is critical in the treatment of a patient with a TBI. Report your findings, any treatment that you provided, the patient's response to your treatment, and your estimated time of arrival. This will allow the receiving facility adequate time to prepare to receive the patient.

8. What should you specifically monitor this patient for during transport?

The importance of reassessing the brain-injured patient cannot be overemphasized.

Patients with increased ICP commonly vomit and experience seizures. Be prepared to turn the patient onto the side and suction the patient's airway if vomiting occurs. If the patient experiences a seizure, continue to assist his ventilations and do not attempt to restrain him.

Carefully and frequently monitor the patient's vital signs, specifically the blood pressure and oxygen saturation. A *single* episode of hypotension (a systolic blood pressure of less than 90 mm Hg) in the adult with a TBI is associated with a significant increase in mortality because it causes a decrease in cerebral perfusion. A *single* drop in the patient's oxygen saturation to below 90% is also associated with a significant increase in mortality; ensure the continual delivery of high-flow oxygen and adequate ventilation!

Frequently reassess the patient's GCS score and pupils and observe for signs of brain herniation. If directed by local protocol or online medical direction, ventilate the patient at a rate of 20 breaths/min (targeting an $ETCO_2$ of 30 to 35 mm Hg) if signs of brain herniation are observed.

If possible, request an ALS ambulance at the scene to assist with airway management or seizure control as needed, if it does not delay your scene time, or consider an ALS intercept during transport, if it does not cause a delay in transport. The most important intervention for the patient with a TBI, however, is to rapidly transport the patient to a definitive care facility as soon as possible.

9. What is an epidural hematoma?

Your patient has an epidural hematoma, which is an accumulation of blood between the skull and dura mater. An epidural hematoma is almost always the result of a blow to the head that produces a fracture of the thin temporal bone (recall that the patient had a compressed area over the temporal region of his skull). The middle meningeal artery courses along the groove in the temporal bone, so it is susceptible to laceration or rupture when the temporal bone is fractured. When this occurs, brisk arterial bleeding will result in rapidly progressing symptoms. The patient with an epidural hematoma typically has an immediate loss of consciousness; this may be followed by a brief return of consciousness (lucid interval), after which the level of consciousness rapidly declines and signs and symptoms of increasing ICP present. *This is consistent with how your patient presented.*

Prep Kit

Ready for Review

- The nervous system of the human is divided into two anatomic parts: the CNS and the PNS.
- The CNS is composed of the brain and the spinal cord; the PNS includes a network of nerve fibers, like cables, that transmit information between the body's organs and the brain.
- The CNS is well protected by bony structures; the brain is protected by the skull, and the spinal cord is protected by the bones of the spinal column.
- The CNS is also covered and protected by three layers of tissue called the meninges. The layers are called the dura mater, the arachnoid, and the pia mater.
- A head injury is a traumatic injury to the head that may result in injury to soft tissue, bony structures, or the brain.
- A TBI is a severe head injury that can be a life threat or leave the patient with life-altering injuries.
- The cervical, thoracic, and lumbar portions of the spinal column can be injured through compression such as in a fall, unnatural motions such as overextension from trauma, pulling forces such as from a hanging, or a combination of mechanisms. Each of these may also cause injury to the spinal cord encased in these regions of bone, causing permanent neurologic injury or death.
- Motor vehicle crashes, falls from heights greater than 10 feet (3 m), and axial loading injuries to the spine are common causes of spinal injury. A patient who has experienced any of these events may have also sustained a head injury.
- Treat the patient with a head injury according to three general principles that are designed to protect and maintain the critical functions of the CNS: control bleeding, establish an adequate airway, and reassess the patient's baseline level of consciousness.
- Treat the patient with a spinal injury by maintaining the airway while keeping the spine in proper alignment, assess respirations, and give supplemental oxygen to maintain an oxygen saturation level greater than 90%.
- Infants and young children are more susceptible to shock. Provide oxygen, monitor the airway, treat for shock, and provide immediate transport.
- Older people are at higher risk for a subdural hematoma developing. Signs and symptoms of the condition may not occur for several hours, days, or weeks. Be sure to get a thorough history of any previous trauma.
- When the patient's condition indicates the need for rapid transport to the hospital, management of the ABCS with SMR precautions and quick loading into the ambulance may be lifesaving and may reduce irreversible damage.
- Safely transporting children with possible spinal injury requires unique considerations, such as additional padding and possibly specialized equipment.

Vital Vocabulary

anterograde (posttraumatic) amnesia Inability to remember events after an injury.

axial loading injuries Injuries in which load is applied along the vertical or longitudinal axis of the spine, which results in load being transmitted along the entire length of the vertebral column (eg, shallow-water diving accident, fall from height with feetfirst landing).

basilar skull fractures Fractures that usually occur following diffuse impact to the head (eg, falls, motor vehicle crashes); generally result from extension of a linear fracture to the base of the skull.

Prep Kit continued

Battle sign Bruising behind an ear over the mastoid process that may indicate a skull fracture.

central neurogenic hyperventilation An abnormal breathing pattern associated with increased ICP that is characterized by deep, rapid breathing; this pattern is similar to Kussmaul respirations, but without an acetone breath odor.

cerebral edema Swelling of the brain.

closed head injury Injury in which the brain has been injured but the skin has not been broken and there is no obvious bleeding.

concussion A temporary loss or alteration of part or all of the brain's abilities to function without actual physical damage to the brain.

coup–contrecoup injury A brain injury that occurs when force is applied to the head and energy transmission through brain tissue causes injury on the opposite side of original impact.

Cushing triad Increased systolic blood pressure, decreased heart rate, and irregular respirations that result from increased intracranial pressure.

distraction A spinal injury in which adjacent vertebrae are pulled apart from one another, such as may occur in hanging victims.

epidural hematoma An accumulation of blood between the skull and the dura mater.

eyes-forward position A head position in which the patient's eyes are looking straight ahead and the head and torso are in line.

four-person log roll The recommended procedure for moving a patient with a suspected spinal injury from the ground to a long backboard or other spinal precaution device.

hyperextension Excessive extension of the spine.

hyperflexion Excessive flexion of the spine.

hyper-rotation Excessive rotation of the spine.

intervertebral disks Tough, elastic structures between adjoining vertebrae that act as shock absorbers.

intracerebral hematoma Bleeding within the brain tissue (parenchyma) itself; also referred to as an intraparenchymal hematoma.

intracranial pressure (ICP) The pressure within the cranial vault.

involuntary activities Actions of the body that are not under a person's conscious control.

lateral bending A mechanism of injury whereby a segment of the spine is suddenly or excessively bent laterally.

linear skull fractures Fractures that commonly occur in the temporoparietal region of the skull and that are not associated with deformities to the skull; also referred to as nondisplaced skull fractures.

meninges Three distinct layers of tissue that surround and protect the brain and the spinal cord within the skull and the spinal canal.

open head injury Injury to the head often caused by a penetrating object in which there may be bleeding and exposed brain tissue.

primary (direct) injury An injury to the brain and its associated structures that is a direct result of impact to the head.

raccoon eyes Bruising under the eyes that may indicate a skull fracture.

retrograde amnesia The inability to remember events leading up to a head injury.

secondary (indirect) injury The aftereffects of the primary injury; includes abnormal processes such as cerebral edema, increased intracranial pressure, cerebral ischemia and hypoxia, and infection; onset is often delayed following the primary brain injury.

spinal motion restriction (SMR) Patient positioning and moving techniques that minimize unwanted movement of the potentially injured spine.

subarachnoid hemorrhage Bleeding into the subarachnoid space, where the cerebrospinal fluid circulates.

Prep Kit continued

subdural hematoma An accumulation of blood beneath the dura mater but outside the brain.

traumatic brain injury (TBI) Physical damage to the brain caused by an external force; can result in cognitive, movement, communication, behavioral, and emotional changes.

voluntary activities Actions that we consciously perform, in which sensory input or conscious thought determines a specific muscular activity.

References

1. Ritter S. Monitoring and maintenance of brain glucose supply: importance of hindbrain catecholamine neurons in this multifaceted task. In: Harris RBS, editor. *Appetite and Food Intake: Central Control*. 2nd edition. Boca Raton, FL: CRC Press/Taylor & Francis; 2017. Chapter 9. Available from: https://www.ncbi.nlm.nih.gov/books/NBK453140/doi: 10.1201/9781315120171-9
2. Parent S, Mac-Thiong JM, Roy-Beaudry M, Sosa JF, Labelle H. Spinal cord injury in the pediatric population: a systematic review of the literature. *J Neurotrauma*. 2011;28(8):1515–1524.
3. TBI in the United States. Centers for Disease Control and Prevention website. https://www.cdc.gov/traumatic-brain-injury/data-research/index.html. Published October 29, 2024. Accessed February 27, 2025.
4. Babl FE, Tavender E, Ballard DW, et al. Australian and New Zealand guideline for mild to moderate head injuries in children. *Emerg Med Australas*. 2021;33(2):214–231.
5. National Institute of Neurological Disorders and Stroke. Traumatic brain injury (TBI). National Institutes of Health website. https://www.ninds.nih.gov/health-information/disorders/traumatic-brain-injury-tbi. Reviewed October 15, 2024. Accessed February 27, 2025.
6. Lulla A, Lumba-Brown A, Totten AM, et al. Prehospital guidelines for the management of traumatic brain injury: 3rd edition. *Prehosp Emerg Care*. 2023;27(5):507–538.
7. Spaite DW, Hu C, Bobrow BJ, et al. The effect of combined out-of-hospital hypotension and hypoxia on mortality in major traumatic brain injury. *Ann Emerg Med*. 2017;69(1):62–72.
8. Spaite DW, Bobrow BJ, Keim SM, et al. Association of statewide implementation of the prehospital traumatic brain injury treatment guidelines with patient survival following traumatic brain injury: the Excellence in Prehospital Injury Care (EPIC) study. *JAMA Surgery*. 2019;154(7):e191152–e191152. doi:10.1001/jamasurg.2019.1152
9. Nehring SM, Tadi P, Tenny S. Cerebral edema. *StatPearls*. National Library of Medicine website. https://www.ncbi.nlm.nih.gov/books/NBK537272/. Updated July 3, 2023. Accessed February 27, 2025.
10. National Association of Emergency Medical Technicians. *PHTLS: Prehospital Trauma Life Support*. 10th ed. Burlington, MA: Jones & Bartlett Learning; 2023.
11. Ferry B, DeCastro A. Concussion. *StatPearls*. National Library of Medicine website. https://www.ncbi.nlm.nih.gov/books/NBK537017/#. Updated January 9, 2023. Accessed February 27, 2025.
12. Committee on Sports-Related Concussions in Youth; Board on Children, Youth, and Families; Institute of Medicine; National Research Council; Graham R, Rivara FP, Ford MA, et al., eds. *Sports-Related Concussions in Youth: Improving the Science, Changing the Culture*. Washington, DC: National Academies Press; 2014.
13. Fischer PE, Perina DG, Delbridge TR, et al. Spinal motion restriction in the trauma patient: a joint position statement. *Prehosp Emerg Care*. 2018;22(6):659–661.
14. Assele DD, Lendado TA, Awato MA, Workie SB, Faltamo WF. Incidence and predictors of mortality among patients with head injury admitted to Hawassa University Comprehensive Specialized Hospital, Southern Ethiopia: A retrospective follow-up study. *PLoS One*. 2021;16(8):e0254245. Published 2021 Aug 19. doi:10.1371/journal.pone.0254245
15. National Association of State EMS Officials. *National Model EMS Clinical Guidelines: Version 3.0*. https://nasemso.org/content.aspx?page_id=22&club_id=157064&module_id=701974. Updated March 2022. Accessed February 27, 2025.
16. Kreinest M, Goller S, Rauch G, et al. Application of cervical collars: an analysis of practical skills of professional emergency medical care providers. *PLoS One*. 2015;10(11):e0143409. doi:10.1371/journal.pone.0143409
17. Bazaie N, Alghamdi I, Alqurashi N, Ahmed Z. The impact of a cervical collar on intracranial pressure in traumatic brain injury patients: a systematic review and meta-analysis. *Trauma Care*. 2022;2(1):1–10.
18. Ben-Galim P, Dreiangel N, Mattox KL, Reitman CA, Kalantar SB, Hipp JA. Extrication collars can result in abnormal separation between vertebrae in the presence of a dissociative injury. *J Trauma*. 2010;69(2):447–450.
19. Ms R, Riffelmann M, Kunze-Szikszay N, et al. Vacuum mattress or long spine board: which method of spinal stabilisation in trauma patients is more time consuming? A simulation study. *Scand J Trauma Resusc Emerg Med*. 2021;29(1):46.
20. Ay D, Aktaş C, Yeşilyurt S, et al. Effects of spinal immobilization devices on pulmonary function in healthy volunteer individuals. *Ulus Travma Acil Cerrahi Derg*. 2011;17:103–107.

Prep Kit continued

21. Totten VY, Sugarman DB. Respiratory effects of spinal immobilization. *Prehosp Emerg Care*. 1999;3:347–352.
22. Abram S, Bulstrode C. Routine spinal immobilization in trauma patients: what are the advantages and disadvantages? *Surgeon*. 2010;8:218–222.
23. Platzer P, Hauswirth N, Jaindl M, et al. Delayed or missed diagnosis of cervical spine injuries. *J Trauma*. 2006;61:150–155.
24. Davis JW, Phreaner DL, Hoyt DB, et al. The etiology of missed cervical spine injuries. *J Trauma*. 1993;34:342–346.
25. Hauswald M, Ong G, Tandberg D, et al. Out-of-hospital spinal immobilization: its effect on neurologic injury. *Acad Emerg Med*. 1998;5:214–219.
26. Hyldmo K, Horodyski M, Conrad B, et al. Does the novel lateral trauma position cause more motion in an unstable cervical spine injury than the logroll maneuver? *Am J Emerg Med*. 2017;35(11):1630–1635.
27. Dixon M, O'Halloran J, Cummins NM. Biomechanical analysis of spinal immobilisation during prehospital extrication: a proof of concept study. *Emerg Med J*. 2014;31(9):745–749.

Additional Resources

Frequently asked questions. Brain Trauma Foundation website. https://www.braintrauma.org/faq. Accessed February 27, 2025.

Kane E, Braithwaite S. Spinal motion restriction. *StatPearls*. National Library of Medicine website. https://www.ncbi.nlm.nih.gov/books/NBK557714/. Updated October 31, 2022. Accessed February 27, 2025.

Nuanprom P, Yuksen C, Tienpratarn W, Jamkrajang P. Traditional spinal immobilization versus spinal motion restriction in cervical spine movement: a randomized crossover trial. *Arch Acad Emerg Med*. 2024;12(1):e36. doi:10.22037/aaem.v12i1.2263

Ward CE, Browne LR, Rogers AJ, et al. Prevalence and indications for applying prehospital spinal motion restriction in children at risk for cervical spine injury. *Prehosp Emerg Care*. Published online March 12, 2025. doi:10.1080/10903127.2025.2472269

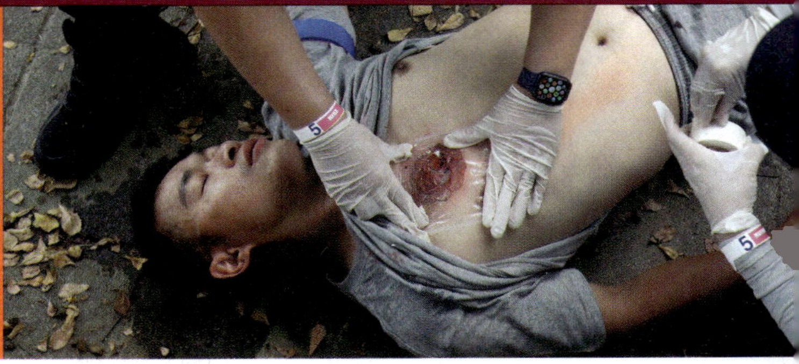

Chapter 29

Chest Injuries

NATIONAL EMS EDUCATION STANDARD COMPETENCIES

Trauma

Applies knowledge to provide basic emergency care and transportation based on assessment findings for an acutely injured patient.

Chest Trauma

- Blunt versus penetrating mechanisms (pp 1089–1105)
- Open chest wound (pp 1089–1099)
- Impaled object (pp 1089–1091)
- Hemothorax (p 1100)
- Pneumothorax (pp 1097–1100)
- Cardiac tamponade (pp 1100–1102)
- Rib fractures (p 1102)
- Flail chest (pp 1102–1103)
- Commotio cordis (p 1105)

KNOWLEDGE OBJECTIVES

1. Explain the mechanics of ventilation in relation to chest injuries. (p 1089)
2. Describe the differences between an open and closed chest injury. (pp 1089–1092)
3. Recognize the signs of chest injury. (pp 1091–1092)
4. Describe the treatment of a patient with a suspected chest injury, including pneumothorax, hemothorax, cardiac tamponade, rib fractures, flail chest, pulmonary contusion, traumatic asphyxia, blunt myocardial injury, commotio cordis, and laceration of the great vessels. (pp 1097–1105)
5. Recognize the complications that can accompany chest injuries. (pp 1097–1105)
6. Explain the complications of a patient with an open pneumothorax (sucking chest wound). (pp 1097–1099)
7. Differentiate between a pneumothorax (open, simple, and tension) and a hemothorax. (pp 1097–1100)
8. Describe the complications of cardiac tamponade. (pp 1100–1102)
9. Describe the complications of rib fractures. (p 1102)
10. Describe the complications of a patient with a flail chest. (pp 1102–1103)

SKILLS OBJECTIVES

1. Demonstrate the assessment of a patient with a suspected chest injury. (pp 1092–1096)
2. Demonstrate the treatment of a patient with a sucking chest wound. (pp 1097–1099)

Introduction

EMTs commonly encounter chest injuries. In the United States, chest trauma results in approximately 1 million emergency department (ED) visits every year.[1] It accounts for as many as 25% to 35% of trauma-related deaths annually.[2,3] Given the location of the heart, lungs, and great blood vessels within the chest cavity, potentially serious injuries may occur. Chest injuries may be the result of blunt trauma, penetrating trauma, or both. Blunt trauma most often results from motor vehicle crashes (approximately 80% of incidents) but may result from mechanisms such as falls or sports activities.[3] Penetrating trauma may result from shootings, stabbings, or other mechanisms, such as industrial or construction incidents. Shootings and stabbings alone account for 20% of major trauma events in the United States.[3]

Any injury that interferes with breathing must be treated without delay to minimize or prevent permanent damage to tissues that depend on a continuous supply of oxygen. Another major problem with chest injuries may be internal bleeding. Blood from lacerations of the thoracic organs or major blood vessels can collect in the chest cavity, compressing the lungs or heart. This may also occur when air collects in the chest and prevents the lungs from expanding. Your ability to act quickly to care for patients with these injuries can make the difference between a successful outcome and death.

This chapter begins with a review of the anatomy of the chest and the physiology of respiration. It then describes the common signs and symptoms of chest injuries and the proper emergency medical treatment for specific injuries.

Anatomy and Physiology

To understand and evaluate chest injuries in the prehospital setting, you must first understand the anatomy of the chest and the mechanism by which gases are exchanged during breathing. A quick review will help you understand the logic in the emergency treatment of chest injuries and the potential complications of that treatment.

A key point to remember is the difference between ventilation and oxygenation. Ventilation is the body's ability to move air in and out of the chest and lung tissue. This is described in the section on mechanics of ventilation. Any injury that affects the patient's ability to move air in and out of the chest is serious and may be life threatening. Oxygenation is the process of delivering oxygen to the blood by diffusion from the alveoli following inhalation into the lungs. Oxygen must be delivered to the cells, and carbon dioxide (a waste product of cell function) must be removed from the body for proper organ system function.

The chest (thoracic cage) extends from where the neck and chest meet to the diaphragm (**FIGURE 29-1**). In a person who is lying supine or who has just completed exhalation, the diaphragm may rise as high as the nipple line. Thus, a penetrating injury to the chest, such as a gunshot or stab wound, may also penetrate the lung and diaphragm and injure the liver, spleen, or stomach.

The skin, muscle, and bones of the thoracic region have some unique features to allow for the ventilation process. Just under the normal three layers of skin, the epidermis, dermis, and subcutaneous layers, lies striated, or skeletal muscle. This muscle extends between the ribs, forming the intercostal muscles. These muscles, innervated from the spinal nerves originating in the lower cervical

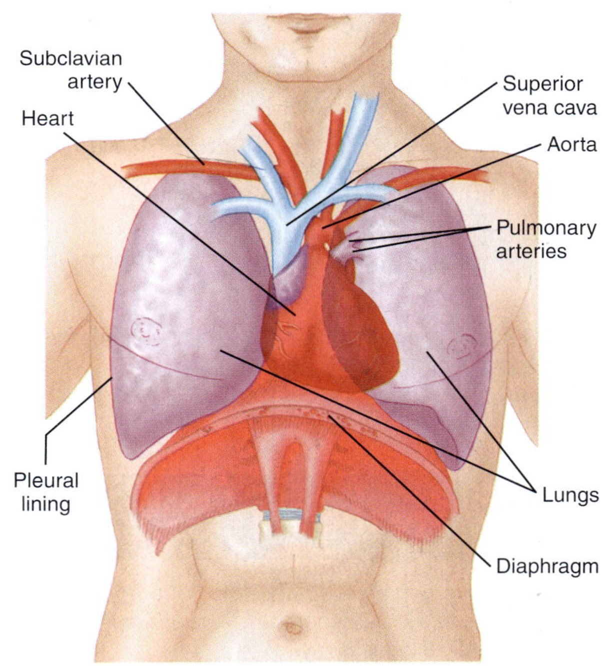

FIGURE 29-1 A view of the anterior aspect of the chest shows the major organs beneath the surface.

or upper thoracic region, contract to expand the rib cage during inhalation. In very young children, the intercostal muscles are not yet developed. Children therefore tend to breathe with their diaphragm, referred to as belly breathing, which is normal for their age group.

Lying on the inferior and slightly posterior part of each rib is the neurovascular bundle, composed of a network of nerves, arteries, and veins. When punctured by fractured ribs, bleeding from these vessels can cause a hemothorax. The ribs themselves create a protective and functional cage around the vital organs. Each side of the chest (hemithorax) contains lung tissue that is separated into lobes. The right lung has three lobes, and the left lung has two lobes. The left lobe formation allows space for the heart to reside; this is called the cardiac notch. A thin membrane called the pleura covers each of the lungs and the thoracic cavity. The inner chest wall has a lining called the parietal pleura, and a lining called the visceral pleura covers the lung. Between these two linings is a small amount of pleural fluid that allows the lungs to move freely against the inner chest wall as a person breathes. Pleural fluid also creates surface tension to allow the lungs to adhere to the rib cage, thus allowing the mechanics of ventilation to occur.

The contents of the chest are partially protected by the ribs, which are connected in the back to the vertebrae and in the front, through the costal cartilages, to the sternum (**FIGURE 29-2**). The trachea, in the middle of the neck, divides into the left and right mainstem bronchi, which supply air to the lungs. The thoracic cage also contains the heart and the great vessels: the aorta, the right and left subclavian arteries and their branches, the pulmonary arteries, and the superior and inferior venae cavae. The esophagus runs through the back of the chest, connecting the pharynx above with the stomach and the abdomen below. The esophagus, trachea,

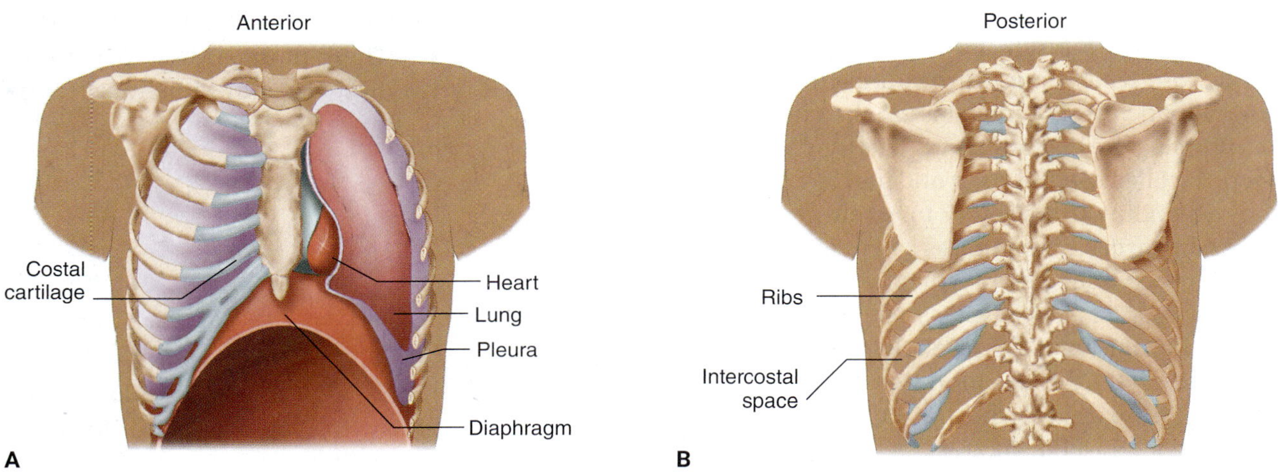

FIGURE 29-2 The organs within the chest are protected by the ribs, which are connected in front (**A**) to the sternum and in back (**B**) to the vertebrae.

YOU are the EMT

At 1020 hours, you are dispatched to 7100 Douglas Avenue for a woman with a chest injury. The caller is unsure what has occurred but reports that the address is a construction site. You respond to the scene, which is located approximately 5 miles away.

1. What major organs and structures lie within the chest cavity?
2. What injuries commonly result from blunt chest trauma? Penetrating chest trauma?

and great vessels lie in the mediastinum, a cavity or space centrally located in the thorax. At the bottom of the chest, the diaphragm is a muscle that separates the thoracic cavity from the abdominal cavity.

Mechanics of Ventilation

When you inhale, the intercostal muscles between the ribs contract, elevating and expanding the rib cage. At the same time, the diaphragm contracts or flattens, increasing the inferior-superior diameter of the chest. The intrathoracic pressure inside the chest decreases, creating a negative pressure differential. Air then enters the lungs through the nose and mouth, which is the path of least resistance from the ambient air space to the upper and lower airway. When you exhale, the intercostal muscles and diaphragm relax, and the tissues move back to their normal positions, forcing the air out (**FIGURE 29-3**). In a normal respiratory system, relaxation of the thoracic muscles and the diaphragm is a relatively passive function. When you are assessing the patient, you should be able to recognize when there is an increase in the work of breathing and equate that with respiratory distress.

Tidal volume is the amount of air moved into or out of the lungs during a single breath. The average tidal volume is approximately 500 mL. If you multiply this amount of air by the number of breaths/min, the result is called the minute ventilation or minute volume. Changing either of these numbers (increasing or decreasing the rate or volume) affects the amount of air moving through the system. For example, if you ventilate a patient with 500 mL at the normal rate of 12 breaths/min, then the minute volume is 6,000 mL (6 L). If you increase the ventilation rate by four extra breaths per minute, then the minute volume increases to 8,000 mL (8 L). Conversely, if the amount of tidal volume decreases, then the minute volume will drop. Tidal volume is discussed further in Chapter 11, *Airway and Ventilation Management*.

This information is important because a patient who can inhale only small amounts of air (in the case of a chest injury) will need to exceed the normal respiratory rate of 12 to 20 breaths/min to make up the difference in the minute volume. If you need to ventilate the patient, remember that an adult bag-mask device consists of a self-inflating bag that usually contains 1,200 to 1,600 mL of air. This device can quickly overinflate the lungs, causing gastric distention, and increase intrathoracic pressure (pressure inside the chest), reducing venous return to the chest and secondarily reducing cardiac output. It can also potentially worsen chest injuries such as pneumothorax. In addition, there is the risk of causing acid–base imbalance by blowing off too much carbon dioxide if the rate of artificial ventilation is too high.

Injuries of the Chest

Recall the discussion of kinematics in Chapter 24, *Trauma Overview*. There are two basic types of chest injuries: open and closed. As the name implies, a

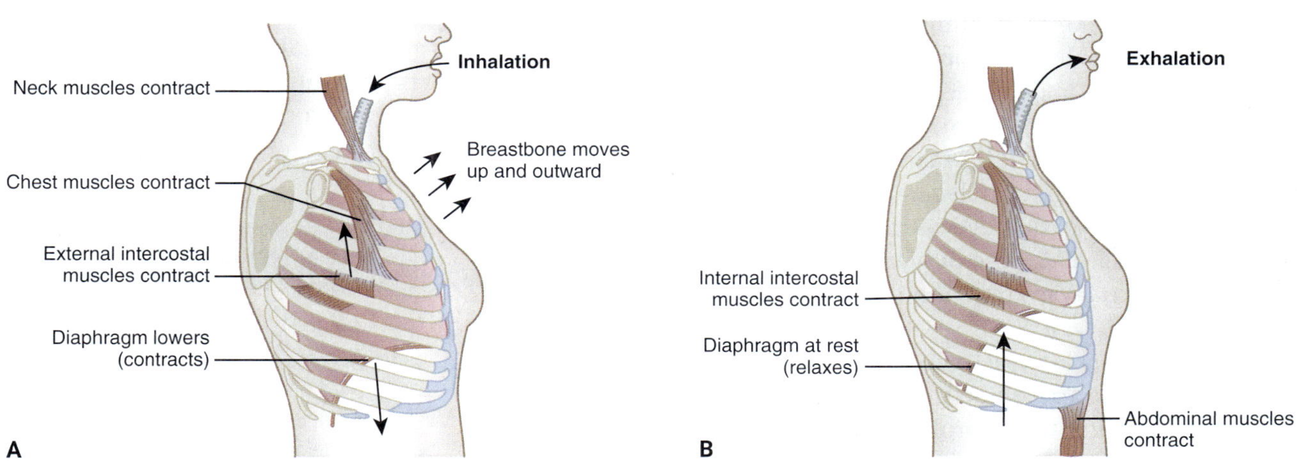

FIGURE 29-3 The mechanics of inhalation (**A**) and exhalation (**B**).

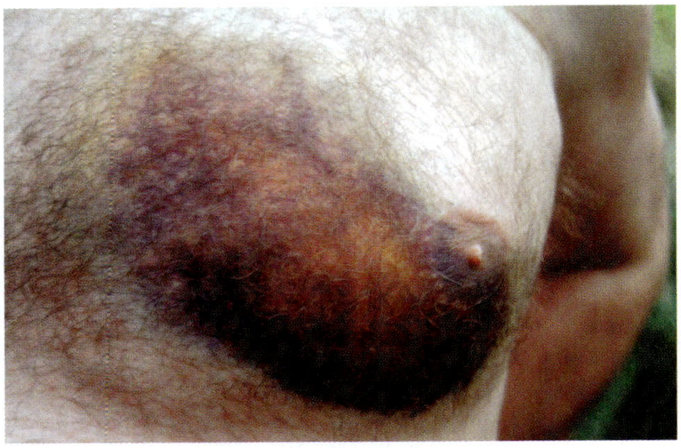

FIGURE 29-4 Closed chest injuries usually result from blunt trauma, such as when a patient strikes the steering wheel or an airbag in a motor vehicle crash, or is struck by a falling object. A closed chest injury can occur even when a seat belt is worn.

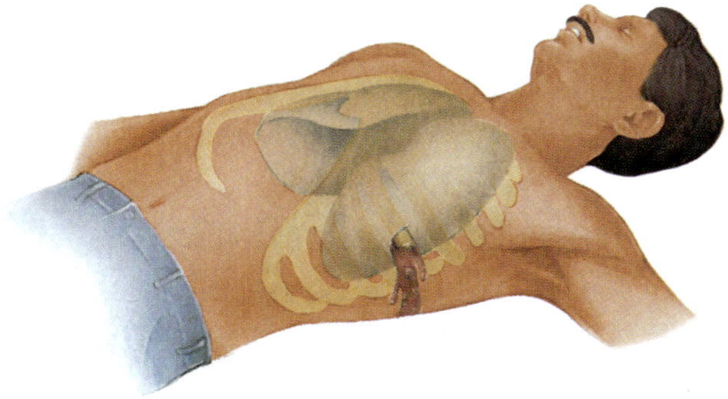

FIGURE 29-5 Open chest injuries can occur when an external object or the broken end of a fractured rib penetrates the chest wall.

closed chest injury is one in which the skin is not broken. This type of injury is generally caused by blunt trauma, such as when a person strikes a steering wheel or an airbag in a motor vehicle crash, is struck by a falling object, or is struck in the chest by some object during a fight (**FIGURE 29-4**). These types of injuries may cause fractures, pneumothorax, or significant contusions in both the cardiac muscle (cardiac contusion) and the lung tissue (pulmonary contusion), thus impairing the function of those organs.

If the heart is damaged in this manner, it may not be able to refill with blood or may not be able to pump blood with enough force, creating a form of inadequate tissue oxygenation called cardiogenic shock. Any bruising of the lung tissue may result in the affected alveoli not functioning. This impairment can cause a decrease in available oxygen (hypoxia) and an increase in carbon dioxide in the blood (hypercapnia). Rib fractures create sharp broken bone ends that can lacerate lung tissue and cause further vessel damage with every movement of the chest wall. This type of bleeding can be hidden from external view and rapidly lead to hypovolemic shock.

An **open chest injury** is generally caused by penetrating trauma. Some objects, such as a knife, a bullet, a piece of metal, or the broken end of a fractured rib, penetrate the chest wall itself (**FIGURE 29-5**). The damage occurring from this type of trauma typically is instant. However, the symptoms of these injuries may take time to develop as the damaged vessels continue to bleed or the lung collapses from a puncture that results in an expanding pneumothorax. Occasionally, the object that penetrates and creates an open chest injury remains in place. This is referred to as an impaled object. When you have a patient with an impaled object, do not attempt to move or remove the object because it may be occluding the hole in the vessel that has been punctured. Removing the object can lead to severe bleeding. Another reason not to remove the impaled object from the chest is that the objects that cause tissue damage on entry will likely cause damage on removal, resulting in further injury. The removal is best left to a surgeon. Any alteration from this standard, such as for a patient who requires CPR, should come directly from online medical direction.

In blunt trauma, a blow to the chest may fracture the ribs, the sternum, or whole areas of the chest wall; bruise the lungs and the heart; and even damage the aorta. Traumatic rupture of the aorta, a condition in which the aorta is torn from its attachment to the chest cavity, is a chief cause of death in patients who

Street Smarts

If the patient's oxygen saturation was normal initially and begins to drop rapidly, suspect tension pneumothorax and immediately communicate your suspicions to the team. This life threat must be treated rapidly by a paramedic or physician. Rapid transport or intercept with an advanced life support (ALS) unit is essential.

are killed immediately in car crashes. Although the skin and chest wall are not penetrated in a closed injury, broken ribs may lacerate the contents of the chest. Damage to the chest wall structures may impair patients' ability to ventilate on their own.

Signs and Symptoms of Chest Injury

Important signs and symptoms of chest injury include the following:

- Pain at the site of injury
- Pain localized at the site of injury that is aggravated by or increased with breathing
- Bruising to the chest wall
- **Crepitus** (the sensation felt when broken bone ends grind together) with palpation of the chest
- Any penetrating injury to the chest
- Dyspnea (difficulty breathing, shortness of breath)
- Hemoptysis (coughing up blood)
- Failure of one or both sides of the chest to expand normally with inspiration
- Rapid, weak pulse and low blood pressure
- Cyanosis around the lips or fingernails
- Diminished breath sounds on one side
- Low oxygen saturation

After a chest injury, any change in normal breathing is a particularly important sign. A healthy, uninjured adult usually breathes at a rate from 12 to 20 breaths/min without difficulty and without pain. The chest should rise and fall in a symmetric pattern with each breath. Respirations of fewer than 10 breaths/min or of more than 20 breaths/min may indicate inadequate breathing. Patients with chest injuries often have **tachypnea** (rapid respirations) and shallow respirations because it hurts to take a deep breath. Shallow breathing or chest wall trauma may interfere with the actual ability to move air. Check the respiratory rate and see if there is actual air movement from the mouth and/or nose. This is best accomplished through visualizing the chest wall for rise and fall.

As with any other injury, pain and tenderness are common at the point of impact as a result of a bruise or fracture. The normal process of breathing usually aggravates pain. Irritation or damage to the pleural surfaces causes a characteristic sharp or sticking pain with each breath when these normally smooth surfaces slide on one another. This sharp pain is called *pleuritic pain* and is typical of chest injuries.

In an injured patient, dyspnea, or difficulty breathing, has many causes, including airway obstruction, damage to the chest wall, poor chest

YOU are the EMT

You arrive at the scene and ensure it is safe. You are directed to the patient by a coworker. The patient, a 19-year-old woman, was struck on the left side of the chest by a piece of lumber that was thrown from a piece of equipment operated by a coworker. You find the patient sitting on the ground; she is conscious and alert, but restless and is experiencing respiratory distress. She tells you that it hurts to take a breath.

Recording Time: 0 Minutes	
Appearance	Restless; obvious respiratory distress
Level of consciousness	Conscious and alert, but restless
Airway	Open; clear of secretions and foreign bodies
Breathing	Increased rate; labored
Circulation	Radial pulses strong and rapid; skin is baseline color and moist; no obvious external bleeding

Your partner applies high-flow oxygen via nonrebreathing mask as you perform a secondary assessment. The patient denies any other injuries, and coworkers confirm that she did not lose consciousness.

3. How should you proceed with your secondary assessment?

expansion because of the loss of normal control of breathing, or lung compression because of accumulated blood or air in the chest cavity.

Hemoptysis, the spitting or coughing up of blood, usually indicates that the lung itself or the air passages have been damaged. With a laceration of the lung tissue, blood can enter the bronchial passages and is coughed up as the patient tries to clear the airway.

A rapid, weak pulse and low blood pressure are the principal signs of hypovolemic shock, which can result from extensive bleeding from lacerated structures within the chest cavity. Shock following a chest injury may also result from an increase in intrathoracic pressure from air or blood in the chest, or from direct injury to the heart itself.

Cyanosis in a patient with a chest injury is a sign of inadequate respiration. The classic blue or ashen gray appearance around the lips and fingernails indicates that blood is not being oxygenated sufficiently. Patients with cyanosis are unable to provide a sufficient supply of oxygen to the blood through the lungs and require immediate ventilation and oxygenation.

Many of these signs and symptoms occur simultaneously. When any one of these develops as a result of a chest injury, the patient requires prompt hospital care.

Words of Wisdom

Cyanosis may be difficult to identify in the prehospital setting, especially in patients who have darker skin tones. In patients with a light skin tone, cyanosis presents as a dark bluish tint to the skin and mucous membranes. However, in patients with dark skin, it may present as gray or white (not blue) skin around the mouth, and the conjunctivae may appear gray or blue. In patients with a more yellow skin tone, cyanosis may cause a gray-green skin coloration.

Patient Assessment

Scene Size-Up

As you arrive on the scene, observe for hazards and threats to the safety of the crew, bystanders, and the patient. Ensure that the police are on scene at incidents involving violence, such as assaults or gunshot wounds. Begin the encounter with scene safety as the highest priority. If you determine the power company, fire department, or ALS units are needed, call for them early.

Ensure that you and your crew take standard precautions; at a minimum, put on gloves and eye protection. Because of the color of blood and the fact that it easily soaks through clothing, you can often identify patients with bleeding as you approach the scene. However, darker clothing may mask signs of bleeding, so you must remain vigilant when the mechanism of injury (MOI) suggests the patient may be bleeding.

As you observe the scene, look for indicators and significance of the MOI. This helps you develop an early index of suspicion for underlying injuries in a patient who has sustained a significant MOI. Chest injuries are common in motor vehicle crashes, falls, industrial incidents, and assaults. Determine the number of patients and consider spinal stabilization. Keep in mind the unique safety considerations when responding to vehicle crashes, such as risks posed by electric vehicle batteries and undeployed airbags, described in Chapter 37, *Vehicle Extrication and Special Rescue*.

Words of Wisdom

The dashboard or steering wheel can cause significant chest injuries in patients who are not wearing seat belts or who are in older vehicles without airbags.[4] Maintain a high degree of suspicion for severe injuries in unrestrained patients when an airbag has deployed.

Primary Assessment

During your primary assessment, you must quickly identify and treat potential life threats and determine priority of patient care and transport. Life-threatening hemorrhage, when present, should be addressed immediately, even before airway concerns.

As you approach, note the patient's level of consciousness. Responsive patients may be able to tell you their chief complaint. Note not only what they say, but also how they say it. Difficulty speaking may indicate several problems, and chest injury is an important one. Perform a rapid physical examination of the patient. Look for obvious injuries, the appearance of blood, and difficulty breathing. Look for cyanosis, irregular breathing, and chest rise and fall on only one side. The initial general impression will help you develop an index of suspicion for serious injuries and determine your sense of urgency for medical intervention. A good question to ask yourself is, "How sick is this patient?" Patients with significant chest injuries will look sick and are often frightened or anxious. Keep in mind that you are rapidly searching for life threats and you will repeat the physical examination in a more detailed manner later in the assessment if time and patient condition allow.

Addressing life threats follows the ABCs (Airway, Breathing, and Circulation) approach, unless life-threatening uncontrolled bleeding is seen, in which case the sequence becomes XABC (with *X* representing eXsanguination). Ensure that the patient has a clear and patent airway. Normal breathing should be effortless, and any deviation from this pattern should be cause for concern. How you assess and manage the airway depends a great deal on whether you suspect a spinal injury. Be suspicious, and protect the spine early in your care if indicated. Further measures to ensure spinal motion restriction can be performed after you have secured the ABCs and completed your secondary assessment.

Words of Wisdom

Be sure to assess the neck before applying the cervical collar. Jugular venous distention (JVD) cannot be observed after the collar is applied. The presence of JVD may indicate tension pneumothorax (significant ongoing air accumulation in the pleural space) or pericardial tamponade, an injury to the heart that results in blood accumulating in the pericardial sac.

Once you have determined the patient has a patent airway, determine whether breathing is present and adequate. With chest injuries, begin by inspecting for DCAP-BTLS (Deformities, Contusions, Abrasions, Punctures/penetrations, Burns, Tenderness, Lacerations, Swelling), and look for equal expansion of the chest wall. Listen with a stethoscope to each side of the chest. Absent or decreased breath sounds on one side usually indicate significant damage to a lung, preventing it from expanding properly. Be alert to the pattern of symmetric rise and fall of the patient's chest wall. If the chest wall does not expand on each side when the patient inhales, the chest muscles may have lost their ability to work appropriately. Loss of muscle function may be the result of a direct injury to the chest wall, or it may be related to an injury of the nerves that control those muscles. Check for **paradoxical chest motion**, an abnormality associated with multiple fractured ribs, in which the chest moves in a direction opposite its normal movement. Normally the chest expands (moves outward) when a person inhales, but during paradoxical chest motion, it instead retracts (moves inward). This paradoxical motion may occur in a single part of the chest if multiple ribs have been fractured in more than one place, creating a condition called flail chest (discussed later in the chapter). In this case, only the part of the chest underlying the fractures moves in a paradoxical motion.

If you determine the patient has penetrating trauma, address this life threat at once. This condition may interfere with the normal mechanics of breathing and can cause the patient's condition to worsen quickly. For quick initial care, you can use your gloved hand to occlude an open chest wound. When further dressings can be applied, use a **vented chest seal** or an **occlusive dressing** for all penetrating injuries to the chest. There are numerous commercial occlusive dressings on the market that provide a ventilated chest seal. Management of open chest wounds is discussed later in this chapter.

Words of Wisdom

Penetrating wounds on the patient's back are easy to miss. Be sure to assess both the anterior surface and the posterior surface of the chest so you do not miss a potentially lethal wound.

Assess the patient's pulse. Determine whether it is present and adequate. If the pulse is too fast or too slow, or if the skin is pale, cool, or clammy, consider your patient to be in shock. Note that because skin pallor can be difficult to detect in patients with dark skin, you may need to check for pale mucous membranes inside the inner lower eyelid or slow capillary refill. You need to treat aggressively to reverse the cause of shock and support the patient's circulatory system. In the early stage of shock, the body compensates for blood loss by increasing the heart rate. Be alert for this change, especially if tachycardia is still present beyond a few minutes after the initial adrenaline rush from the incident or injury. External bleeding may or may not be significant, but if it is considered life threatening, address this threat immediately. Bleeding inside the chest can be significant and, as discussed earlier, can rapidly cause death. Control external bleeding with direct pressure and a bulky trauma dressing.

Priority patients are considered patients who have a problem with their ABCs. Sometimes the priority is obvious, and the decision to transport quickly is also easy. At other times, what is happening outside the body may not provide obvious clues to the seriousness of what is happening inside the body. Pay attention to subtle clues such as the appearance of the skin, level of consciousness, or a sense of impending doom in the patient. When you find signs of poor perfusion or inadequate breathing, transport quickly and perform the remainder of the assessment en route to the ED. A delay on the scene to perform a lengthy assessment will reduce your patient's chances of survival. With chest injuries, when in doubt, transport rapidly to a trauma center. **TABLE 29-1** lists the "deadly dozen" chest injuries.

TABLE 29-1 Deadly Dozen Chest Injuries

1. Airway obstruction
2. Bronchial disruption
3. Diaphragmatic tear
4. Esophageal injury
5. Open pneumothorax
6. Tension pneumothorax
7. Massive hemothorax
8. Flail chest
9. Cardiac tamponade
10. Thoracic aortic dissection (leakage from a traumatic aneurysm of the portion of the aorta that lies within the chest)
11. Myocardial contusion
12. Pulmonary contusion

History Taking

Once you have identified and treated life threats, you can gather the patient's history. If you have not yet done so, determine and investigate the patient's chief complaint and further investigate the MOI. Identify any associated signs and symptoms and pertinent negatives. If the patient was assaulted with a blunt object such as a bat, further evaluate the spinal region for injury because the force may have been transferred through the body from the point of impact. If the patient fell from a great height and is reporting chest discomfort or dyspnea, this may distract the patient from recognizing the presence of fractures or bleeding from the extremities. Palpation of the chest will typically cause direct pain at the site of the fracture. When a patient reacts to the pain, verify where the pain was located relative to the area being touched.

Pertinent negatives when examining the chest include no associated shortness of breath, no rapid breathing, no absent or abnormal breath sounds, and no areas of deformity or abnormal movement.

A SAMPLE history (Signs and symptoms, Allergies, Medications, Pertinent past medical history, Last oral intake, Events leading up to the illness or injury) should be completed when time allows. The evaluation of past medical history may reveal respiratory or cardiovascular disease. Questions about the events leading to the emergency should focus on the MOI: the speed of the vehicle or height of the fall; the use of safety equipment such as a helmet, airbag, seat belt, or life jacket; the type of weapon used; the number of penetrating wounds; and so on. A SAMPLE history can be obtained quickly in most situations and can certainly be obtained while accomplishing other tasks. However, if the patient has a loss of consciousness, it will no longer be possible to obtain the information directly. Interviewing witnesses briefly in these circumstances is important.

Secondary Assessment

In a patient who has an isolated injury to the chest with a limited MOI, such as in a stabbing, after performing a quick body scan to ensure there are no other injuries, you should focus your assessment on the isolated injury, the patient's chief complaint, and the body region affected. Ensure that wounds are identified and that any bleeding is controlled. Note the location and extent of the injury. Assess all underlying systems. Examine the anterior and posterior aspects of the chest wall, and be alert to changes in the patient's ability to maintain adequate respirations.

It is important in patients with a chest injury not to focus only on a chest wound. With significant trauma, you should quickly assess the entire patient from head to toe. If there is significant trauma (such as a blunt trauma or gunshot wound) likely affecting multiple systems, start with a rapid physical examination of the body, looking for DCAP-BTLS to determine the nature and extent of thoracic injury. This examination will help to determine all injuries and the extent of these injuries. Inspection or visualization of the region looking for deformities, such as asymmetry of the left and right sides of the chest or shoulder girdle, may reveal the presence of multiple rib fractures, crush injuries, or significant chest wall injury. Identification of discrete areas of contusion or abrasion may pinpoint a specific point of impact. The presence of puncture wounds or other penetrating injuries indicates a possible open chest injury that should be managed accordingly. Be alert for burns that encircle the chest, which may alter respiratory mechanics. Palpate for tenderness to localize the injury and the presence of fractures. Look for lacerations and local swelling. Application of this systematic approach to patient assessment minimizes the chance of missing a significant injury.

Once you have stabilized the ABCs and have checked the patient from head to toe to identify injuries, obtain a baseline set of vital signs. This activity should include assessment of pulse, respirations, blood pressure, skin condition, oxygen saturation, and pupils. Each of these is considered a sign indicating how your patient is tolerating the injuries. Consider these signs as a window to the functioning of the vital organs. This baseline set of vital signs will be used to evaluate changes in the patient's condition. Because patients with chest injury have so much potential for rapid deterioration, they should be reevaluated every 5 minutes. This

Special Populations

CHEST INJURY IN THE GERIATRIC PATIENT

In adults aged 65 and older with reduced bone density or more fragile bones, even minor trauma to the chest wall can cause rib fractures with significant injury to the underlying tissues and organs. Be alert for these injuries and for signs and symptoms of respiratory compromise, even in lower-energy MOIs. Older adults also have a decreased amount of physiologic reserve and are likely to decompensate more quickly following an injury. Recall that triage to a trauma center is indicated when the systolic blood pressure of a patient 65 years or older is less than 110 mm Hg or the heart rate is greater than the systolic blood pressure value.[5,6]

YOU are the EMT

Your secondary assessment reveals bruising and crepitus on the left side of the chest and diminished breath sounds over that same side; no paradoxical chest motion is noted. The trachea is midline, and the jugular veins are nondistended. Abdominal exam is unremarkable. Your partner obtains the patient's vital signs and reports them to you.

Recording Time: 5 Minutes	
Respirations	24 breaths/min; labored
Pulses	110 beats/min; strong and regular
Skin	Baseline color, warm, and moist
Blood pressure	138/88 mm Hg
Oxygen saturation (Spo_2)	95% (on oxygen)

4. On the basis of your assessment findings, what injury or injuries should you suspect?

5. How should you proceed with your treatment of this patient?

will allow you to quickly recognize changes in the vital sign numbers or trends.

If you find an accelerated pulse rate or respiratory rate, the chest injury may be causing either a decrease in available oxygen (hypoxia) or blood loss that results in a decreased number of red blood cells that can carry oxygen (hypoxemia). The increased respiratory rate is often associated with an obvious increase in work of breathing. This can be identified by noting increased use of the accessory muscles in the face, neck, and chest to assist in the movement of air. In the later stages of injuries, as respiratory failure develops, the pulse rate may slow as the myocardium becomes starved for oxygen and the body is no longer able to keep up with the demands. The respiratory rate may drop as the brain becomes starved for oxygen and overloaded with carbon dioxide and other waste products. These are usually signs of impending cardiopulmonary arrest if appropriate interventions are not provided immediately. In the case of increasing pressure on the heart from air in the pleural space or blood in the pericardial space, the blood pressure may exhibit a narrowing pulse pressure as the systolic and diastolic pressures come closer together. This is a result of the inability of the heart to fill with an adequate volume of blood and contract normally.

Reassessment

The reassessment identifies how your patient's condition is changing. It should focus on repeating the primary assessment, reassessing the chief complaint, and reassessing interventions performed. Reevaluate the patient's airway, breathing, pulse, perfusion, and bleeding. Has breathing improved now that the wound is sealed, or has it become more difficult? If assisting ventilations with a bag-mask device, is it becoming increasingly difficult to deliver breaths to the patient? Other interventions should also be assessed to determine if they are effective. For example, are pulse oximeter values rising now that the patient is receiving oxygen? Reassess vital signs and compare them to vital signs taken earlier. Vital signs are a snapshot in time. Reassessing them frequently allows you to trend the patient's status and determine if the patient is compensating versus decompensating. Many chest injuries will worsen during transport to the hospital because of the seriousness of the injuries. An astute reassessment will help identify worsening conditions in a timely manner so that they can be addressed.

If the patient's shortness of breath is worsened in the supine position, consider placing the patient in a position of comfort by elevating the head 30° while maintaining spinal motion restriction, if necessary (**FIGURE 29-6**).[7] Maintain an open airway, be prepared to suction the patient, and consider an oropharyngeal or nasopharyngeal airway. Whenever you suspect significant bleeding, provide high-flow oxygen. If needed, provide assisted ventilation using a bag-mask device with high-flow oxygen. If significant bleeding is visible, you must control the bleeding. If you find penetrating trauma to the chest wall, place a vented chest seal or semiocclusive dressing over the wound. Be prepared to provide positive-pressure ventilation if the patient's breathing efforts are not effective. If the patient has signs of hypoperfusion, treat aggressively for shock and provide rapid transport to the appropriate hospital. Do not delay transport of a seriously injured trauma patient to complete non-lifesaving treatments such as splinting extremity fractures; instead, complete these types of treatments en route to the hospital.

Communicating with hospital staff early when your patient has a significant MOI to the chest can help them be prepared with appropriate equipment and personnel when you arrive. If a penetrating injury is present, describe it in your report, along with what you have done to care for it. Your documentation should be complete and thorough. Describe all injuries and the treatment given. Remember, your documentation is your legal record of what happened.

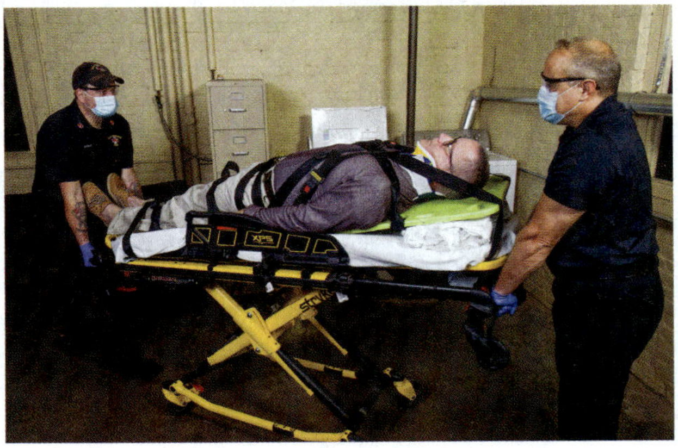

FIGURE 29-6 If a patient's shortness of breath is worsening, elevate the patient's head.

Special Populations

CHEST INJURY IN THE PEDIATRIC PATIENT

In young children, the rib cage is very flexible and does not provide the same level of protection that the adult rib cage provides. This flexibility can allow any significant injury or compression of the rib cage to be masked because the ribs give way to the pressure and do not fracture as easily as those of adults. Because the ribs do not often fracture, which would help dissipate the force from the blunt object, the force transfers more directly to the organs beneath the ribs. It is important to remember that the organs that underlie the rib cage have been exposed to that force and are likely injured. This flexibility of the ribs may result in injuries that are hidden on examination, and the only indication you may have of compromise is increased work of breathing or evidence of shock (**FIGURE 29-7**). When rib fractures do occur in children, they are frequently associated with serious underlying injuries.[8]

This age group is often injured in pedestrian or bicycle collisions that involve vehicles. In car-versus-pedestrian crashes, children often turn toward the vehicle instead of away as adults do, thus resulting in direct impact to the chest by the bumper or hood. Children also may not be cognizant of height or distances and, therefore, may be prone to falls from distances greater than twice their height, resulting in severe trauma.

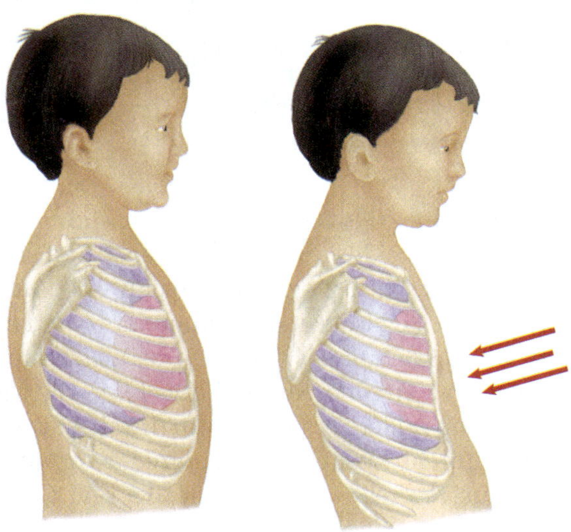

FIGURE 29-7 A child's ribs are softer and more flexible than an adult's. As a result, they may compress the lungs and heart if there is blunt trauma, causing serious injury with no obvious external damage.

Complications and Management of Chest Injuries

Pneumothorax

In any chest injury, damage to the heart, lungs, great vessels, and other organs in the chest can be complicated by the accumulation of air in the pleural space. This is a dangerous condition called a **pneumothorax** (commonly called a collapsed lung). In this condition, air enters through a hole in the chest wall or the surface of the lung as the patient attempts to breathe, causing the lung on that side to collapse (**FIGURE 29-8**). As a result, any blood that passes through the collapsed portion of the lung is not oxygenated, and hypoxia can develop. If the lung is collapsed beyond 30% to 40%, you may hear diminished breath sounds on that side of the chest. Absent breath sounds are a significant finding in chest trauma and may indicate the development of a tension pneumothorax, discussed later. Depending on the size of the hole and the rate at which air fills the cavity, the lung may collapse in a few seconds or a few hours. In the uncommon situation

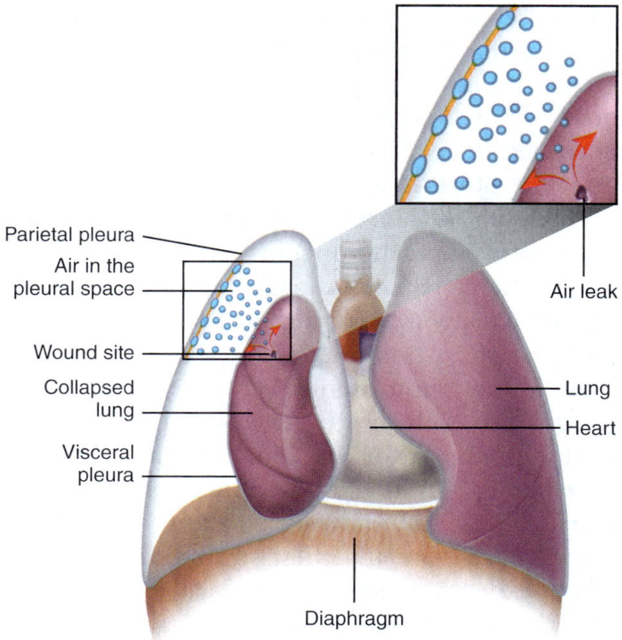

FIGURE 29-8 Pneumothorax occurs when air leaks into the space between the pleural surfaces from an opening in the chest wall or the surface of the lung. Air in the pleural space causes the lung to collapse.

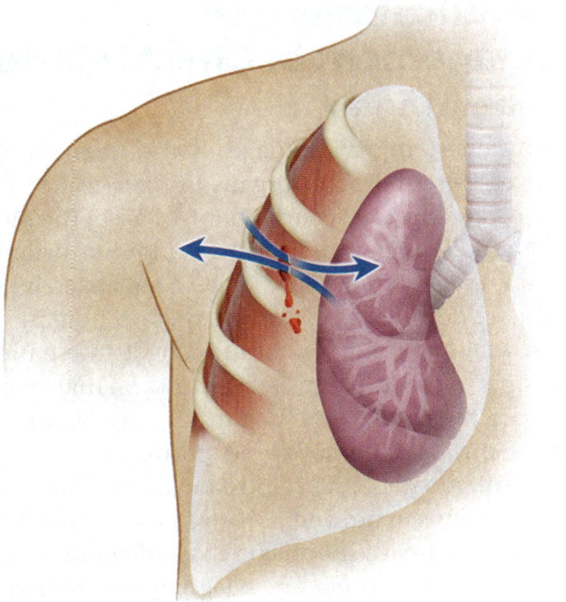

FIGURE 29-9 With a sucking chest wound, air passes from the outside into the pleural space and back out with each breath, creating a sucking sound.

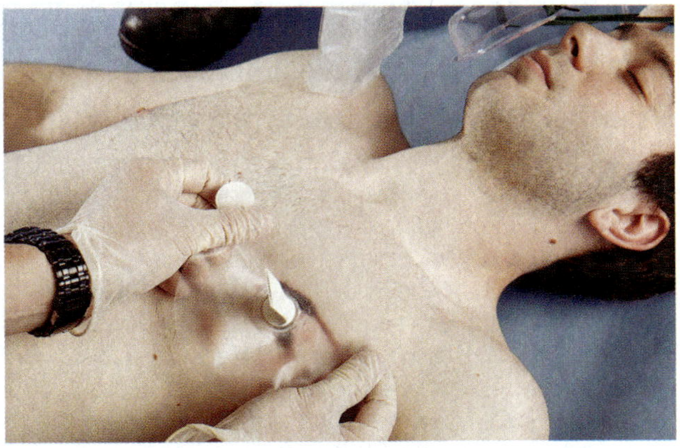

FIGURE 29-10 A commercial occlusive dressing may be used to seal all four sides of a sucking chest wound. An Asherman Chest Seal, which is vented, is shown in the figure.

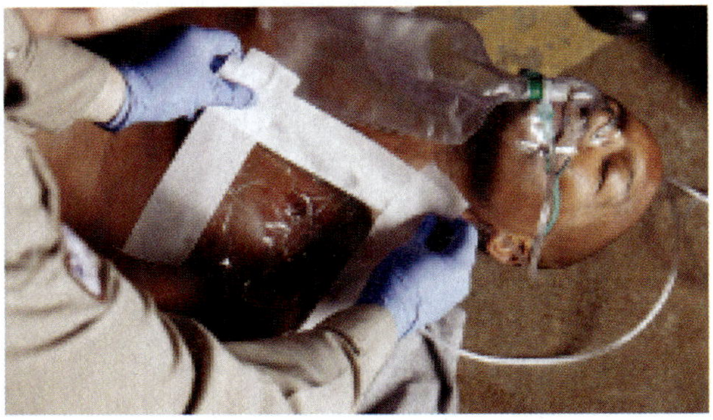

FIGURE 29-11 An improvised vented occlusive dressing seals three sides of a sucking chest wound, with the fourth left open to allow air to escape.

when the hole is in the chest wall, you may hear a sucking sound as the patient inhales and the sound of rushing air as they exhale. For this reason, an open or penetrating wound to the chest wall is often called an **open pneumothorax** or a **sucking chest wound** (**FIGURE 29-9**).

This type of injury is a true emergency requiring immediate emergency medical care and transport. Initial emergency care, after clearing and maintaining the airway, is to rapidly seal the open wound and prevent air from being sucked into the pleural space through the wound. Vented chest seals are designed to allow air to escape through the dressing but not be sucked back in, thus preventing the development of a tension pneumothorax. They contain a one-way valve, called a **flutter valve**, that allows air to leave the chest cavity but not return (**FIGURE 29-10**). Follow local protocol and the manufacturer's guidelines if you use such a dressing.

In the absence of a vented chest seal, a semiocclusive dressing can be created by taping an occlusive dressing over the wound. In the past, EMTs were taught to seal three sides of the dressing over the open chest wound, allowing air to leak from the fourth side to prevent development of a tension pneumothorax (**FIGURE 29-11**). Some sources now say to tape all sides and briefly release one side to allow air to escape if signs of tension pneumothorax develop. Regardless, a commercial vented chest seal, when available, is preferred by all sources. In all instances, use a dressing that is large enough to avoid being pulled or sucked into the chest cavity.

Careful observation is required after placing an occlusive dressing. The occlusive seal or a clot in the injury may prevent the escape of excess air from the chest and allow a tension pneumothorax to develop. If signs of a tension pneumothorax develop, it is suggested that the occlusive dressing be partially removed by lifting one corner and allowing air to escape (ie, "burping") and then be resecured on three sides. You may hear a sudden release of air pressure when you remove one side of the dressing. This situation can develop even after a flutter valve has been applied.

Words of Wisdom

When a vented chest seal is not available, plastic wrap, foil, or petrolatum gauze can be used to create the semiocclusive dressing. If the wound is very large and no suitable material is available, a defibrillation pad can work as an occlusive dressing. When you use an occlusive dressing to seal an open chest wound, record the type of material used and any changes noted afterward: skin color, vital signs, breath sounds, and particularly the patient's level of anxiety.

Simple Pneumothorax

Any pneumothorax that does not result in major changes in the patient's cardiac physiology is referred to as a **simple pneumothorax**. These are commonly the result of blunt trauma that results in fractured ribs. As in the spontaneous pneumothorax, the simple pneumothorax is often difficult to diagnose. The lung has to collapse significantly before the effects will be heard as decreased breath sounds. The more common findings are similar to those of other types of pneumothoraces: pleuritic chest pain, dyspnea or increased work of breathing exhibited as tachypnea and accessory muscle use, and decreasing oxygen saturation on the pulse oximeter. Another sign of pneumothorax can be a crackling sensation felt on palpation of the skin (called **subcutaneous emphysema**), which indicates that air escaping from a lacerated lung is leaking into the tissues of the chest wall. Late findings can be decreased breath sounds on the injured side as well as lethargy and cyanosis. Be vigilant because the simple pneumothorax can often worsen or deteriorate into a tension pneumothorax or develop complications such as bleeding or hemothorax. The treatment for a simple pneumothorax is much like any treatment for respiratory compromise; provide a high concentration of oxygen. Monitor oximeter readings and breath sounds, and treat underlying causes of the injury. As in all pneumothorax treatment, adding positive-pressure ventilation may cause the pathology to advance rapidly and possibly cause a tension pneumothorax to develop. However, you should not withhold positive-pressure ventilation if the patient needs the support. Simply be aware of the risk, and plan on how to resolve complications. Most patients with this problem require ALS intervention, so call for it early or transport rapidly to the nearest hospital or trauma center, depending on which is the fastest way to get your patient to a higher level of care.

Tension Pneumothorax

A potential complication that may develop following chest injuries with pneumothorax is a **tension pneumothorax** (**FIGURE 29-12**). This can occur when there is significant ongoing air accumulation in the pleural space. This air gradually increases the pressure in the chest, first causing the complete collapse of the affected lung and then pushing the mediastinum (the central part of the chest containing the heart and great vessels) into the opposite pleural cavity. This prevents blood from returning through the venae cavae to the heart, decreasing cardiac output, causing shock, and ultimately, leading to death.

Words of Wisdom

The conscious, spontaneously breathing patient in whom tension pneumothorax is developing may exhibit a slower onset of signs and symptoms of tension pneumothorax. In this patient, complaints of chest pain, increasing dyspnea, and dropping oxygen saturation levels, despite administration of oxygen, may be noted before the blood pressure drops.

Tension pneumothorax occurs more commonly as a result of closed, blunt injury to the chest in which a fractured rib lacerates a lung or bronchus. A patient with a tension pneumothorax will have chest pain, tachycardia, marked respiratory distress, low or rapidly dropping oxygen saturation, and absent or severely decreased lung sounds on the affected side, with signs of shock such as hypotension or altered mental status. Because the increased pressure in the chest may force air into the subcutaneous tissues, crepitus related to subcutaneous emphysema is also a frequent finding.[8] The patient may also exhibit JVD, cyanosis, or tracheal deviation, but these signs are not always present.

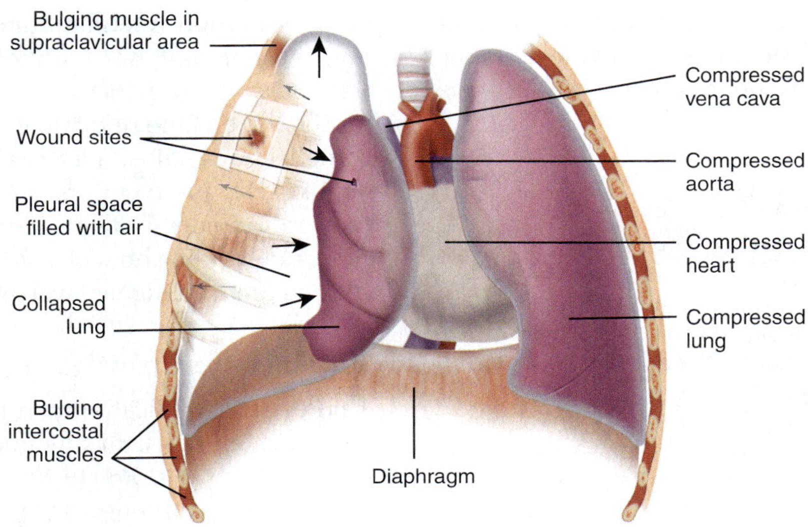

FIGURE 29-12 A tension pneumothorax can develop if a penetrating chest wound is bandaged tightly (such as with the unvented occlusive dressing shown here) and air from a damaged lung cannot escape. The air then accumulates in the pleural space, eventually causing compression of the heart and great vessels. If a dressing sealed on four sides with no vent is used, monitor for signs of tension pneumothorax developing and prepare to vent one side of the dressing.

JVD is best assessed for with the patient sitting at a 45° angle. Tracheal deviation away from the affected side, if seen, is a late and grave finding and is a sign that the patient requires immediate intervention.

Relieving a tension pneumothorax that is the result of blunt trauma is often done by inserting a needle through the rib cage into the pleural space, called a needle thoracotomy; however, this procedure typically is performed by ALS personnel or ED staff, depending on local protocols. A tension pneumothorax is a life-threatening condition. Be prepared to support ventilation with high-flow oxygen, and request ALS support or transport immediately to the closest hospital.

ALS Assist

When ventilating a patient with chest trauma, it is important to avoid hyperventilation and to continuously monitor the patient for changes. If the patient becomes harder to ventilate (poor bag-mask compliance), the oxygen saturation level falls, the patient's color changes, JVD develops, or you note a change in chest rise, immediately notify your ALS partner and reassess lung sounds.

Hemothorax

In blunt and penetrating chest injuries, blood can collect in the pleural space from bleeding around the rib cage or from a lung or great vessel. This condition is called a **hemothorax** (**FIGURE 29-13**). Suspect a hemothorax if the patient has signs and symptoms of shock without any obvious external bleeding or apparent reason for the shock state, or decreased breath sounds on the affected side, an indication that the lung is being compressed by the blood in the cavity. Because the bleeding is typically caused by severe damage within the chest cavity, there is virtually no way to control the bleeding in the prehospital setting. The only person who can treat this condition is often a surgeon. The presence of air and blood in the pleural space is known as a **hemopneumothorax**. Again, because the injury has occurred within the walls of the chest, the treatment involves providing rapid transport to the nearest facility capable of inserting a chest tube and potentially performing surgery.

Cardiac Tamponade

Cardiac tamponade (pericardial tamponade) occurs when the pericardial sac, the space between the protective membrane around the heart (**pericardium**) and the heart, fills with blood or fluid, perhaps from a ruptured, torn, or lacerated coronary artery or vein (**FIGURE 29-14**). The pericardial sac can also fill with fluid as a result of cancer, pericarditis, or an autoimmune disease such as lupus. As the amount of blood or fluid increases, the heart is less able to fill with blood during each relaxation phase. As a result, the heart cannot pump an adequate amount of blood and the patient experiences a decrease in systemic blood flow, or cardiac output. The signs of this condition are often subtle until the situation is dire. Along with shock, the signs and symptoms, referred to as the Beck triad, include distended or engorged jugular veins seen on both sides of the trachea, a narrowing pulse pressure (the difference between the systolic and diastolic blood pressure numbers), and muffled heart sounds. Because the heart cannot pump sufficiently, the jugular veins fill with blood and, thus, blood backs up. The narrowing pulse pressure occurs as the diastolic pressure increases but the systolic pressure cannot, because the heart cannot stretch to contract harder. An associated and more commonly noticed sign is a decrease in mental status as blood flow decreases to the brain. The heart muscle is unique in that it needs to be stretched to generate an effective contraction to pump blood out of the ventricles. This mechanism can fail because of tamponade and can be directly related to a decrease in blood returning to the heart.

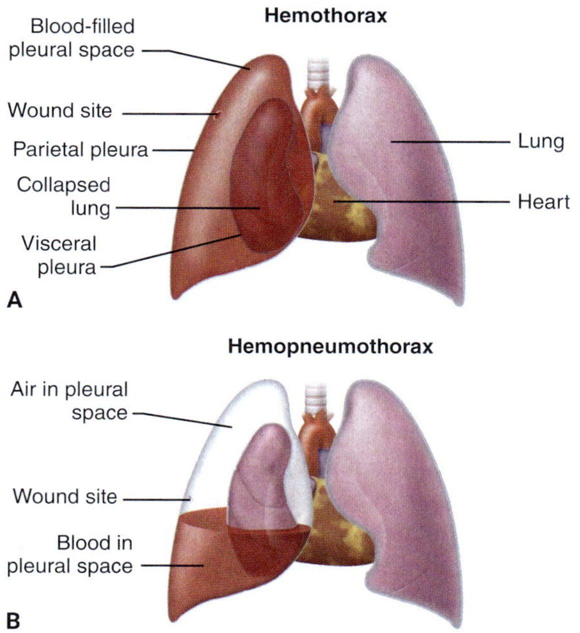

FIGURE 29-13 A. A hemothorax is a collection of blood in the pleural space produced by bleeding within the chest. **B.** When both blood and air are present, the condition is a hemopneumothorax.

Field treatment for this condition involves recognition and supportive care. Administer oxygen

YOU are the EMT

The patient is placed onto the stretcher and loaded into the ambulance. While continuing to provide high-flow oxygen via nonrebreathing mask, you reassess her condition and vital signs shortly before departing the scene.

Recording Time: 10 Minutes	
Level of consciousness	Conscious, but confused and restless
Respirations	28 breaths/min; labored and shallow
Pulse	124 beats/min; weak at the radial artery
Skin	Cool, clammy, and pale; cyanosis around the mouth
Blood pressure	104/58 mm Hg
Oxygen saturation (Spo_2)	88% (on oxygen)

Breath sounds are now inaudible on the entire left side of the patient's chest, and you note that cyanosis is developing around her mouth. Her jugular veins appear somewhat distended, and her trachea is midline. The closest appropriate facility is approximately 10 minutes away, so you instruct your partner to begin transport at once.

6. What is most likely happening to your patient?

7. Should you adjust your current treatment? If so, how?

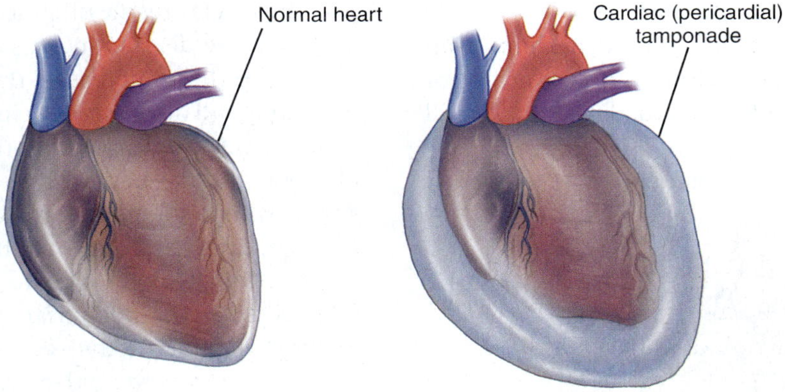

FIGURE 29-14 Cardiac tamponade, also known as pericardial tamponade, is a potentially fatal condition in which fluid or blood builds up within the pericardial sac, causing compression of the heart's chambers and dramatically impairing its ability to pump blood to the body.

and provide positive-pressure ventilation to any patient who is hypoventilating or apneic. Rapidly transport the patient to a facility that is capable of intervention.

Words of Wisdom

In a trauma situation, even a small amount of fluid or blood in the pericardial sac is enough to cause fatal pericardial tamponade. Occasionally, fluid in surprisingly large amounts may collect slowly in the pericardial sac as a result of chronic medical conditions, such as cancers and autoimmune diseases or due to infection. Fluid that builds up over time is tolerated much better than fluid from injury that accumulates rapidly within the pericardial sac.

Rib Fractures

Rib fractures are very common, particularly in older people, whose bones can be more brittle. Because the upper four ribs are well protected by the bony girdle of the clavicle and scapula, a fracture of one of these upper ribs is unusual; when it occurs, it suggests a substantial MOI. Other factors that predict the potential for serious complications after rib fractures include the total number of ribs fractured, the presence of bilateral rib fractures, and patient age greater than 65 years.

Be aware that a fractured rib that penetrates into the pleural space may lacerate the surface of the lung, causing a pneumothorax, a tension pneumothorax, a hemothorax, or a hemopneumothorax.

Patients with one or more cracked ribs will report localized tenderness and pain when breathing. The pain is the result of broken ends of the fracture rubbing against each other with each inspiration and expiration. Patients will tend to avoid taking deep breaths, and their breathing will be rapid and shallow instead. They will often hold the affected portion of the rib cage to minimize the discomfort. Patients with rib fractures should receive supplemental oxygen during assessment and transport if they are experiencing any respiratory distress to maintain an oxygen saturation level of 94% to 98%.

Flail Chest

Ribs may be fractured in more than one place. If two or more adjacent ribs are fractured in two or more places, a segment of chest wall may be detached from the rest of the thoracic cage[8] (**FIGURE 29-15**). As mentioned previously, this condition is known as **flail chest**. Flail chest can also occur if the sternum is fractured along with several ribs.

Flail chest may cause paradoxical chest motion, and breathing may be painful and ineffective, especially if there is a large flail segment. Hypoxemia easily results as air is circulated between the lungs due to the flail segment. A flail segment seriously interferes with the body's normal mechanics of ventilation and must be treated quickly. Paradoxical

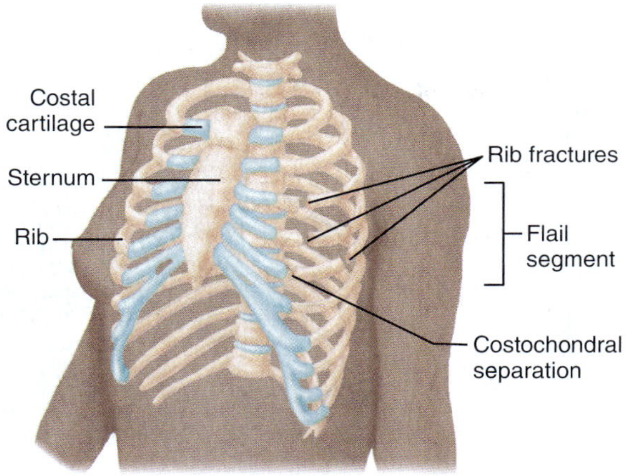

FIGURE 29-15 When two or more adjacent ribs are fractured in two or more places, a flail chest results. A flail segment will move paradoxically when the patient breathes.

chest motion is a late sign of flail segment; therefore, an absence of paradoxical motion does not mean the patient does not have a flail segment.

Management of a flail chest must include maintaining adequate ventilation, pain management, and management of the unstable chest wall. Maintain the airway, and provide supplemental oxygen and respiratory support if necessary. Perform ongoing assessments for possible pneumothorax or other respiratory complications. Positive-pressure ventilation with a bag-mask device is always indicated for any patient with signs of inadequate ventilation. Historically, other treatments have been recommended, including splinting the flail segment; however, these treatments are not evidence-based and are not appropriate interventions for a patient suspected of having a flail chest.[8]

Special Populations

FLAIL CHEST RISK IN PEDIATRIC AND GERIATRIC PATIENTS

Older adults are at an increased risk of flail chest injury.[9] It does not take significant trauma to cause a flail chest injury in this population. Conversely, children rarely experience a flail chest injury due to the increased pliability of their chest wall. If a child does present with a flail chest injury, it indicates that the child was exposed to a significant traumatic force.

Keep in mind that although flail chest itself is a serious condition, it also suggests an injury that was forceful enough to cause other serious internal damage and possible spinal injury.

Other Chest Injuries

Pulmonary Contusion

In addition to fracturing ribs, any severe blunt trauma to the chest can injure or bruise the lung. The pulmonary alveoli become filled with blood, and fluid accumulates in the injured area, which interferes with the movement of oxygen from the lungs to the capillaries, leaving the patient hypoxic. Severe **pulmonary contusion** should always be suspected in patients with a flail chest and usually develops over a period of hours following the injury. If you believe that a patient may have a pulmonary contusion, provide supplemental oxygen and positive-pressure ventilation as needed to ensure adequate oxygenation and ventilation.

Other Fractures

In addition to the rib fractures you have already learned about, there are other types of fractures that should be discussed.

Sternal Fractures

Any suspected fracture of the sternum should increase your index of suspicion for injuries to the underlying organs because the amount of force required to break the sternum is significant. There may be involvement of the lungs, great vessels, and the heart.

Clavicle Fractures

Whereas this fracture is also covered under skeletal injuries, it is important to mention here that the clavicle overlies the first rib and protects a large neurovascular bundle (nerve, artery, and vein) that can be significantly damaged or disrupted should injury to the clavicle occur. The pain, deformity, and swelling that accompany a clavicle fracture can also detract from assessment of the first and second ribs in proximity to the fracture. Suspect upper rib fractures in medial clavicle fractures, and be alert to possible signs of pneumothorax development.

Traumatic Asphyxia

Sometimes a patient will experience a sudden, severe compression of the chest, which produces a rapid increase in pressure within the chest. This may occur in a pedestrian who is compressed between a vehicle and a wall, or a patient who is pinned under a vehicle. The sudden increase in intrathoracic pressure results in a characteristic appearance, including distended neck veins, cyanosis in the face and neck, and hemorrhage into the sclera of the eye, signaling the bursting of small blood vessels (**FIGURE 29-16**). This is called **traumatic asphyxia**. These findings suggest an underlying injury to the heart and possibly a pulmonary contusion. Provide ventilatory support with supplemental oxygen and monitor the patient's vital signs as you provide immediate transport.

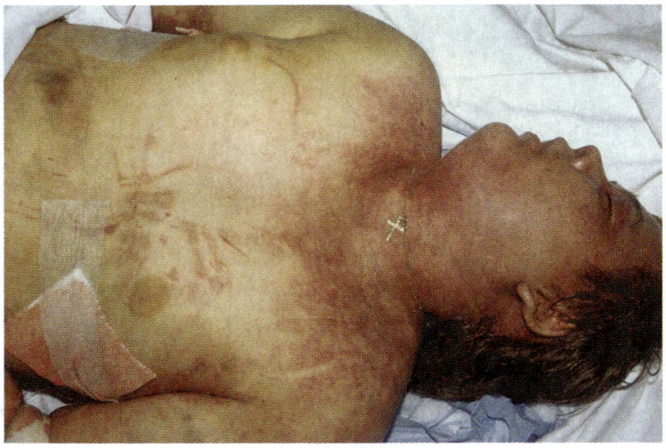

FIGURE 29-16 Traumatic asphyxia.

Blunt Myocardial Injury

Blunt trauma to the chest may injure the heart itself, causing arrythmias (most frequently sinus tachycardia), or rarely, causing enough damage to the heart muscle that it is unable to maintain adequate blood pressure. The patient who has a **myocardial contusion**, or bruising of the heart muscle, may have a rapid or irregular pulse, and although dangerous rhythms such as ventricular tachycardia and ventricular fibrillation may be encountered, they are uncommon. Prehospital treatment is supportive in nature. Still, you should suspect myocardial contusion in all cases of severe blunt injury to the chest, especially if evidence of

YOU are the EMT

You promptly call for ALS, but it is 15 minutes away, so you elect to continue treatment and transport. After reassessing the patient's condition, you call a radio report to the receiving facility.

Recording Time: 15 Minutes	
Level of consciousness	Conscious, but confused and restless
Respirations	28 breaths/min; labored and shallow
Pulse	128 beats/min; weak at the radial artery
Skin	Cool and clammy; cyanosis around the mouth
Blood pressure	90/60 mm Hg
Oxygen saturation (Spo_2)	85% (on oxygen, 15 L/min by nonrebreathing mask)

You arrive at the hospital and find a physician and nurse waiting for you in the ambulance bay. The patient is quickly taken into a treatment room, where further assessment is performed. After the physician performs a needle decompression, the patient's condition improves. After returning to service, you follow up with the hospital and learn that the patient had a tension hemopneumothorax that required a chest tube. They report the patient will likely recover after a stay in the intensive care unit.

8. What is a tension hemopneumothorax?

9. Should you attempt to distinguish a tension pneumothorax from a tension hemopneumothorax? Why or why not?

sternal fracture, such as crepitus on palpation, is noted. Note any change in blood pressure because this can be a direct result of the injury to the myocardium. The patient may report chest pain or discomfort that is similar in nature to cardiac symptoms. Provide supplemental oxygen to achieve an oxygen saturation level of 94% to 98%, and transport immediately.

Commotio Cordis

Commotio cordis is a blunt chest injury caused by a sudden, direct blow to the chest (over the heart) that occurs during a critical portion of a person's heartbeat, causing ventricular fibrillation and immediate cardiac arrest. This phenomenon has occurred after patients were struck with softballs, baseballs, bats, football helmets, snowballs, fists, and even kicks during kickboxing. The incidence of commotio cordis is most frequent in young male athletes, with most cases occurring between the ages of 11 and 20 years.[10] The force of the blow to the chest is commonly at speeds of 35 to 40 miles per hour. The ventricular fibrillation is often responsive to defibrillation and early initiation of cardiopulmonary resuscitation (CPR). While commotio cordis is more commonly associated with sports-related injuries, it should be suspected in all cases in which the person is unconscious and unresponsive after a blow to the chest. These patients present in cardiac arrest that should be treated as any other cardiac arrest. Early defibrillation is crucial for these patients. In recent years, the widespread availability of AEDs has significantly improved their outcome, with more than 50% of patients now surviving commotio cordis. However, it is imperative that responders recognize the nature of this emergency and apply the AED within 3 to 5 minutes.[11]

Street Smarts

When dispatched to a youth sporting event for a child who has "passed out," consider commotio cordis as a possible cause. Early treatment with effective CPR and defibrillation is the key to survival if this is the cause of their collapse.

Laceration of the Great Vessels

The chest contains several large blood vessels: the superior vena cava, the inferior vena cava, the pulmonary arteries, four main pulmonary veins, and the aorta, with its major branches distributing blood throughout the body. Injury to any of these vessels may be accompanied by massive, rapidly fatal hemorrhage. Any patient with a chest wound who shows signs of shock may have sustained an injury to one or more of these vessels. Frequently, significant blood loss is unseen because it remains within the chest cavity. Remain alert to signs and symptoms of shock and to changes in the baseline vital signs, such as tachycardia and hypotension.

Emergency treatment in these cases includes ventilatory support and supplemental oxygen. Immediate transport to the trauma center is critical. The overwhelming majority of injuries to the great vessels in the chest are rapidly fatal, and the survival rate is low.

Words of Wisdom

Transection of the aorta is a significant contributor to on-scene fatalities following motor vehicle crashes. Given that the body's entire blood volume passes through this vessel, the high mortality rate associated with such an injury comes as no surprise. Many aortic injuries are rapidly fatal, often causing cardiac arrest prior to hospital arrival, or even prior to arrival of EMS. Local protocols are specific to when CPR should *not* be started in traumatic arrests. Because the survival rate is very low in trauma patients who are pulseless and apneic, national guidelines suggest that for patients whose cause of cardiac arrest is likely traumatic, resuscitation efforts should be withheld when EMS arrives on the scene and encounters any of the following conditions[7]:

- There is presence of an obviously fatal injury (eg, decapitation), dependent lividity, rigor mortis, or decomposition.
- In cases of blunt trauma, the patient was pulseless and apneic and without organized electrical activity on the electrocardiogram.
- In cases of penetrating trauma, the patient was pulseless, apneic, and without other signs of life (ie, no pupil response, no movement, no organized electrical activity on the electrocardiogram).

YOU are the EMT SUMMARY

1. What major organs and structures lie within the chest cavity?

Critical organs and structures in the chest cavity include the trachea, large bronchi, lungs, great vessels (eg, aorta, venae cavae), heart, and left and right subclavian arteries and their branches. The heart, trachea, great vessels, and a portion of the esophagus reside within the mediastinum, the space between the lungs.

A thin lining called the visceral pleura covers the lungs, and the parietal pleura covers the inner chest wall. A small amount of pleural fluid is found between the pleurae. The space in between the visceral and parietal pleurae (the pleural space) is only a potential space because the two pleural layers are in direct contact with each other in normal circumstances. However, if trauma occurs to the chest wall, the layers can separate, creating an actual space that becomes filled with air, blood, or both.

2. What injuries commonly result from blunt chest trauma? Penetrating chest trauma?

Blunt (closed) chest trauma occurs when an object strikes the chest (eg, a steel pipe during an assault) or when the chest strikes an object (eg, chest impacts the steering wheel during a car crash). The severity of the injury depends on the amount of energy that the chest wall absorbs. Although the skin and chest wall are not penetrated by blunt force trauma, injury to the intrathoracic organs may be severe.

Rib fractures are common injuries associated with blunt chest trauma. In some cases, a single rib is fractured; in other cases, several adjacent ribs are fractured in more than one place (flail chest). A flail chest can impair ventilation because the section of fractured ribs collapses and puts pressure on the lung during inhalation. A fractured rib can also perforate an internal chest organ, such as the lung, causing air to leak out of the lung and into the pleural space (pneumothorax). If air moves freely between the pleural space and lung, the injury is called a simple pneumothorax. In a tension pneumothorax, the lung is completely collapsed, and the heart and great vessels (eg, aorta, venae cavae) are compressed as pressure shifts across the mediastinum. This causes further ventilatory compromise, decreased cardiac output, shock, and death if untreated. A hemothorax, which may be caused by blunt or penetrating chest trauma, occurs when blood, rather than air, fills the pleural space.

Blunt force chest trauma can also cause bruising of the lung (pulmonary contusion) or the heart muscle (myocardial contusion). Other injuries include shearing injuries of the aorta, traumatic asphyxia, and commotio cordis.

In a penetrating (open) chest injury, the chest wall itself is penetrated by an object such as a knife or bullet, resulting in injury to vital organs in the thoracic cavity. A common injury associated with penetrating chest trauma is a sucking chest wound (open pneumothorax). Sucking chest wounds cause various degrees of ventilatory compromise, depending on the size of the hole in the chest wall.

3. How should you proceed with your secondary assessment?

For patients with an isolated injury, your secondary assessment should focus on that area of the body—in this case, the chest and adjacent structures. However, remember that even with an isolated injury, the patient may have other injuries worthy of a head-to-toe trauma assessment.

Expose the patient's chest, and assess for obvious signs of injury, such as bruising, lacerations, or abrasions. Observe the chest wall for symmetry. Asymmetric chest movement indicates decreased airflow into one lung. Look for any sections of the rib cage that collapse during inhalation and bulge during exhalation (paradoxical chest motion); this is an indication of flail chest injury.

Palpate the chest wall to determine if it is stable, if there are any deformities, or if you feel crepitus (the sensation felt when broken bone ends grind together). Chest wall crepitus is a clear indicator of one or more fractured ribs.

Auscultate the apices (top) and bases (bottom) of both lungs. Decreased or absent breath sounds over the injured side of the chest indicate decreased or absent airflow into that lung and should immediately increase your index of suspicion for a pneumothorax.

Based on the MOI of blunt chest trauma, you should also assess the trachea and jugular veins. Note whether the trachea is in the midline position or if it appears to be deviated to one side or the other. Bear in mind that if the patient has a tension pneumothorax, tracheal deviation is a relatively late sign; a midline trachea does not rule out such an injury. Observe the jugular veins to determine if they appear to be normal, distended, or flat. JVD is best assessed with the patient sitting at a 45° angle. Do not move the patient to this position solely for the purpose of assessing JVD. Remember that patients who lie flat may naturally have JVD. The presence of JVD in the

YOU are the EMT SUMMARY continued

context of chest trauma suggests a tension pneumothorax or cardiac tamponade, although it is often not present until the injury is well progressed. In addition, collapsed jugular veins suggest shock.

Chest injuries, especially if located below the nipple line, often also involve abdominal injuries. Abdominal assessment therefore may be beneficial, especially as the signs and symptoms of abdominal injury may appear later and the pain from the chest injury may distract from any pain from the abdominal injury. Further assessment beyond that discussed is based on any other symptoms the patient may report and any obvious injuries that you observe.

4. On the basis of your assessment findings, what injury or injuries should you suspect?

On the basis of the MOI, blunt trauma to the chest, and the findings of your primary and secondary assessments, you should suspect that your patient has rib fractures and a pneumothorax. She has obvious chest wall bruising, labored breathing, crepitus on palpation, and diminished breath sounds on the same side that the injury occurred.

Depending on the size of the lung perforation and the rate at which air fills the pleural space, the lung may collapse in a few seconds. Breath sounds on the injured side are diminished because the collapsing lung is not fully expanding during inhalation.

Because a pneumothorax impairs oxygenation and ventilation, begin treatment immediately and prepare for rapid transport to the hospital. If the lung on the injured side collapses totally, pressure will shift to the opposite side of the chest—compressing the heart, aorta, and venae cavae in the process—and begin collapsing the unaffected lung; this condition is called a tension pneumothorax and is an immediately life-threatening condition that can result in profound shock and cardiac arrest.

5. How should you proceed with your treatment of this patient?

Patients with a pneumothorax need high-flow oxygen, continual close monitoring, and prompt transport to the hospital.

Be especially concerned about the adequacy of the patient's breathing, and continuously monitor it. Your patient is tachypneic, which is common in patients with chest injuries; her respirations are labored, and it hurts when she breathes. Patients with chest injuries often take shallow breaths to minimize the pain. You should consider calling for ALS, particularly if it leads to intervention that is faster than transporting the patient to the hospital, as ALS clinicians can administer pain medication that can ease the patient's pain and potentially allow the patient to breathe more easily.

If her respirations become too shallow, she will not move adequate amounts of air into her lungs during inhalation; this will only worsen any hypoxemia that already exists from the pneumothorax itself. If this occurs, begin assisting her ventilations with a bag-mask device attached to high-flow oxygen. Other signs of inadequate breathing, which may also necessitate assisted ventilations, include a falling oxygen saturation (despite administration of high-flow oxygen), cyanosis, and a decreasing level of consciousness.

Continue to monitor the patient's level of consciousness and vital signs. If she begins experiencing signs of shock, suspect a developing tension pneumothorax.

6. What is most likely happening to your patient?

Compared with previous assessments, your patient's clinical condition has obviously deteriorated. She is now confused and more tachypneic; her respirations are still labored, but are now shallow; cyanosis is developing around her mouth (perioral cyanosis); her radial pulses are weak; and her oxygen saturation has fallen to 88% despite high-flow oxygen via nonrebreathing mask. Although her systolic blood pressure is still above 100 mm Hg, compared with your previous reading of 138/88 mm Hg, this is a significant decrease. The patient's signs and symptoms indicate she is deteriorating and is in respiratory failure.

The additional signs of inaudible (absent) breath sounds on the injured side of her chest and the appearance of cyanosis indicate that the left lung has collapsed or is filling with blood and air, and pressure is now shifting across the mediastinum toward the unaffected lung. You should suspect your patient has a tension pneumothorax and will continue to deteriorate until she can receive definitive treatment.

7. Should you adjust your current treatment? If so, how?

A tension pneumothorax is an immediate life threat and requires aggressive treatment.

The patient now has clear evidence of respiratory failure (decreased level of consciousness [confusion]), which is causing inadequate oxygenation and ventilation. Begin assisting her ventilations with a bag-mask device. Avoid hyperventilating the patient, as doing so may worsen the pneumothorax and ultimately decrease cardiac output. You must also

YOU are the EMT SUMMARY continued

initiate treatment for shock. At a minimum, cover the patient with a blanket to keep her warm. Patients with any injury or condition that impairs their ability to breathe are often resistant to being placed in a supine position; this is especially true if they are conscious. Elevating the head of the stretcher while maintaining spinal motion restriction as indicated may result in an improved ability of the patient to exchange air. If the patient becomes unconscious, however, place her in a supine position and continue to assist her ventilations.

Patients with a tension pneumothorax need an immediate needle thoracentesis (chest decompression). If it will not delay your transport time, intercept an ALS unit, if possible. Otherwise, notify the receiving facility, continue assisting ventilations and treating for shock, and get the patient to the ED as soon as possible.

8. What is a tension hemopneumothorax?

In some cases, when a fractured rib perforates a lung, blood from the injured lung also accumulates in the pleural space; this is called a hemopneumothorax because the pleural space contains both blood and air. The amount of blood that accumulates in the pleural space depends on the size and severity of the lung injury.

As blood and air continue to accumulate in the pleural space, the lung on the injured side collapses and pressure shifts across the mediastinum toward the uninjured lung. In a tension hemopneumothorax, the patient experiences respiratory impairment from both blood and air in the pleural space, but also experiences internal blood loss of varying severity.

9. Should you attempt to distinguish a tension pneumothorax from a tension hemopneumothorax? Why or why not?

It is impractical to attempt to distinguish a tension pneumothorax from a tension hemopneumothorax in the prehospital setting. Both conditions cause impaired ventilation and perfusion; this is what you should focus on when treating the patient. Provide high-flow oxygen, assist ventilations as needed, initiate treatment for shock, and transport without delay. Attempting to distinguish one injury from the other may only delay treatment and transport, thereby increasing the chance of a negative outcome.

Prep Kit

Ready for Review

- A penetrating chest injury has the potential to penetrate the lung and diaphragm and injure the liver or stomach.
- Chest injuries are classified as closed or open. Closed injuries are often the result of blunt force trauma, and open injuries are the result of an object penetrating the skin and/or chest wall.
- Blunt trauma may result in fractures to the ribs and the sternum.
- Life-threatening external hemorrhage must be addressed immediately during the primary assessment, even before airway or breathing concerns.
- During the primary assessment, if an injury is encountered that interferes with the ability of the patient to oxygenate or ventilate, the injury must be addressed quickly.
- Any penetrating injury to the chest may result in air entering the pleural space and may cause pneumothorax. A vented chest seal should be placed on this injury as soon as it is identified.
- When a penetrating injury creates a hole in the chest wall, you may hear a sucking sound as the patient inhales. This is called an open pneumothorax.
- A simple pneumothorax is a result of blunt trauma, such as fractured ribs.
- A pneumothorax may progress to a tension pneumothorax and potentially cause cardiac arrest.

Prep Kit continued

- Hemothorax is the result of blood accumulating in the pleural space after a traumatic injury when the vessels of the lung are lacerated and leak blood.
- A flail chest segment is two or more adjacent ribs broken in two or more places. Positive-pressure ventilation may be particularly important for the patient with a flail chest that compromises ventilation.
- All patients with chest injuries should receive high-flow oxygen or ventilation with a bag-mask device.
- Pulmonary contusion, which is bruising of or injury to lung tissue after traumatic injury, may interfere with oxygen exchange in the lung tissue.
- Myocardial contusion is bruising of the heart muscle after traumatic injury. This condition may have the same signs and symptoms as a heart attack, including an irregular pulse. Remember that this is an injury to the heart muscle from trauma, not from a heart attack.
- Commotio cordis occurs from a direct blow to the chest during a critical portion of the patient's heartbeat. It may result in immediate cardiac arrest.
- Cardiac tamponade is when blood collects in the space between the pericardial sac and the heart. This condition results in pressure building up inside the pericardial sac until the heart cannot pump effectively; cardiac arrest may occur quickly.
- The great vessels of the body are located in the mediastinum. These large vessels may be lacerated or tear after traumatic injury and cause heavy, unseen bleeding inside the patient's chest cavity.
- For a patient with a chest injury who has signs of shock, even if bleeding is not visible, suspect life-threatening bleeding inside the chest cavity.

Vital Vocabulary

cardiac tamponade (pericardial tamponade) Compression of the heart as the result of buildup of blood or other fluid in the pericardial sac, leading to decreased cardiac output.

closed chest injury An injury to the chest in which the skin is not broken, usually caused by blunt trauma.

commotio cordis A blunt chest injury caused by a sudden, direct blow to the chest that occurs only during the critical portion of a person's heartbeat.

crepitus A grating or grinding sensation caused by fractured bone ends or joints rubbing together.

flail chest A condition in which two or more adjacent ribs are fractured in two or more places or in association with a fracture of the sternum so that a segment of the chest wall is effectively detached from the rest of the thoracic cage.

flutter valve A one-way valve that allows air to leave the chest cavity but not return; may be part of a commercial vented occlusive dressing.

hemopneumothorax The accumulation of blood and air in the pleural space of the chest.

hemothorax A collection of blood in the pleural cavity.

myocardial contusion Bruising of the heart muscle.

occlusive dressing An airtight dressing that protects a wound from air and bacteria; a commercial vented version allows air to passively escape from the chest, while an unvented dressing may be made of petrolatum gauze, aluminum foil, or plastic.

open chest injury An injury to the chest in which the chest wall itself is penetrated by a fractured rib or, more frequently, by an external object such as a bullet or knife.

Prep Kit continued

open pneumothorax An open or penetrating chest wall wound through which air passes during inspiration and expiration, creating a sucking sound; also referred to as a sucking chest wound.

paradoxical chest motion Respirations in which the chest moves inward during inhalation and outward during exhalation, opposite of the chest wall's normal motion during breathing.

pericardium The fibrous sac that surrounds the heart.

pneumothorax An accumulation of air or gas in the pleural cavity.

pulmonary contusion Injury or bruising of lung tissue that results in hemorrhage.

simple pneumothorax Any pneumothorax that is free from significant physiologic changes and does not cause drastic changes in the vital signs of the patient.

subcutaneous emphysema A crackling sensation felt on palpation of the skin indicating that air has become trapped beneath the skin.

sucking chest wound An open or penetrating chest wall wound through which air passes during inspiration and expiration, creating a sucking sound. See also *open pneumothorax*.

tachypnea Rapid respirations.

tension pneumothorax An accumulation of air or gas in the pleural cavity that progressively increases pressure in the chest that interferes with cardiac function with potentially fatal results.

traumatic asphyxia A pattern of injuries seen after a severe force is applied to the chest, forcing blood from the great vessels back into the head and neck.

vented chest seal An occlusive dressing designed to allow air to escape through the dressing but not be drawn back in.

References

1. US Department of Health and Human Services, Centers for Disease Control and Prevention (CDC), National Center for Health Statistics. National Hospital Ambulatory Medical Care Survey: 2021 emergency department summary tables. CDC website. https://www.cdc.gov/nchs/data/nhamcs/web_tables/2021-nhamcs-ed-web-tables-508.pdf. Revised October 11, 2023. Accessed March 7, 2025.
2. Tobey N, Lopez RA, Waseem M. EMS chest injury. *StatPearls*. National Library of Medicine website. https://www.ncbi.nlm.nih.gov/books/NBK539743/. Updated March 4, 2024. Accessed March 7, 2025.
3. Edgecombe L, Sigmon DF, Galuska MA, et al. Thoracic trauma. *StatPearls*. National Library of Medicine website. https://www.ncbi.nlm.nih.gov/books/NBK534843/. Updated May 23, 2023. Accessed March 7, 2025.
4. Khouzam RN, Al-Mawed S, Farah V, Mizeracki A. Next-generation airbags and the possibility of negative outcomes due to thoracic injury. *Can J Cardiol*. 2014;30(4):396–404.
5. Egodage T, Ho VP, Bongiovanni T, et al. Geriatric trauma triage: optimizing systems for older adults—a publication of the American Association for the Surgery of Trauma Geriatric Trauma Committee. *Trauma Surg Acute Care Open*. 2024;9(1):e001395. doi:10.1136/tsaco-2024-001395
6. Trauma systems: national guideline for the field triage of injured patients. American College of Surgeons website. https://www.facs.org/quality-programs/trauma/systems/field-triage-guidelines/. Accessed
7. National Association of State EMS Officials. *National Model EMS Clinical Guidelines: Version 3.0.* https://nasemso.org/content.aspx?page_id=22&club_id=157064&module_id=701974. Updated March 2022. Accessed March 7, 2025.
8. National Association of Emergency Medical Technicians. *PHTLS: Prehospital Trauma Life Support*. 10th ed. Burlington, MA: Jones & Bartlett Learning; 2023.
9. Perera T, King K. Flail chest. *StatPearls*. National Library of Medicine website. https://www.ncbi.nlm.nih.gov/books/NBK534090/. Updated July 17, 2023. Accessed March 7, 2025.
10. Commotio cordis. American Heart Association website. https://www.heart.org/en/health-topics/commotio-cordis. Reviewed April 17, 2023. Accessed March 7, 2025.
11. Commotio cordis. American Heart Association website. https://www.heart.org/en/health-topics/commotio-cordis. Reviewed April 17, 2023. Accessed April 28, 2025.

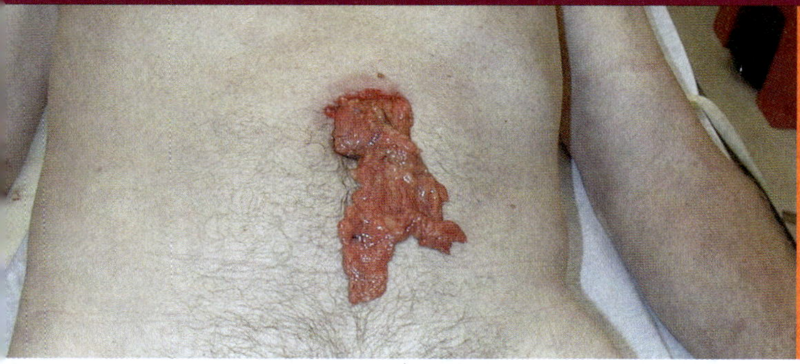

Chapter 30

Abdominal and Genitourinary Injuries

NATIONAL EMS EDUCATION STANDARD COMPETENCIES

Trauma

Applies knowledge to provide basic emergency care and transportation based on assessment findings for an acutely injured patient.

Abdominal and Genitourinary Trauma

- Blunt versus penetrating mechanisms (pp 1113–1114, 1115–1119, 1124–1126, 1127–1129)
- Evisceration (pp 1117, 1125)
- Impaled object (pp 1122, 1132)
- Solid and hollow organ injuries (pp 1117–1119)
- Injuries to the internal or external genitalia (p 1129)

KNOWLEDGE OBJECTIVES

1. Describe the anatomy and physiology of the abdomen, including the abdominal quadrants and boundaries and the difference between hollow and solid organs. (pp 1112–1115)
2. Explain some special considerations related to the care of pediatric patients and geriatric patients who have experienced abdominal trauma. (pp 1113, 1115)
3. Describe closed abdominal injuries and the mechanisms of injury (MOIs) likely to cause this type of trauma. (pp 1115–1116)
4. Explain the emergency medical care of a patient who has sustained a closed abdominal injury, including blunt trauma caused by a seat belt or airbag. (pp 1115, 1124)
5. Describe open abdominal injuries and the MOIs that would cause this type of trauma. (pp 1116–1117)
6. Describe the different ways hollow and solid organs of the abdomen can be injured and the common signs and symptoms relating to the specific organs involved. (pp 1117–1119)
7. Explain assessment of a patient who has experienced an abdominal injury. (pp 1119–1124)
8. Explain the emergency medical care of a patient who has sustained an open abdominal injury, including penetrating injuries and abdominal evisceration. (pp 1125–1126)
9. Describe the anatomy and physiology of the female and male genitourinary systems. (pp 1126–1127)
10. Discuss the types of traumatic injuries sustained by the genitourinary system, including the kidneys, urinary bladder, and internal and external genitalia. (pp 1127–1129)

11. Explain assessment of a patient who has experienced a genitourinary injury. (pp 1130–1132)
12. Explain the emergency medical care of a patient who has sustained a genitourinary injury to the kidneys, urinary bladder, external male genitalia, female genitalia, or rectum. (pp 1132–1133)

SKILLS OBJECTIVES

1. Demonstrate proper emergency medical care of a patient who has experienced a blunt abdominal injury. (pp 1124–1125)
2. Demonstrate proper emergency medical care of a patient who has a penetrating abdominal injury with an impaled object. (pp 1125–1126)
3. Demonstrate how to apply a dressing to an abdominal evisceration wound. (pp 1125–1126)

Introduction

The abdomen is the major body cavity extending from the diaphragm to the pelvis. It contains organs from the digestive, urinary, and genitourinary systems. Although any of these organs can be injured, some are better protected than others. Being well acquainted with the anatomy and positions of abdominal and pelvic organs is important for emergency medical services (EMS) clinicians. In the presence of traumatic injury to these areas, clinicians must understand the functions of these organs if they are to determine the severity.

Significant abdominal trauma can arise from blunt and/or penetrating forces. In the absence of obvious external trauma, internal injuries in this region may be overlooked. Indeed, unrecognized and untreated abdominal injuries are a leading cause of traumatic death. Despite the fact that 10% of all trauma patients have some form of genitourinary injury, such injuries are frequently missed.[1] These oversights may increase the patient's risk for incontinence, infertility, impotence, or other life-altering consequences. Therefore, when assessing patients with a mechanism of injury (MOI) capable of causing abdominal or genitourinary injury, the EMT must maintain a high index of suspicion. Relevant findings should be relayed to the receiving hospital expeditiously to ensure prompt delivery of definitive care.

Anatomy and Physiology of the Abdomen

Abdominal Quadrants

By visualizing two imaginary lines (one horizontal and one vertical) that intersect at the umbilicus, the abdomen can be divided into four quadrants (**FIGURE 30-1**): the right upper quadrant (RUQ), left upper quadrant (LUQ), right lower quadrant (RLQ), and left lower quadrant (LLQ). Remember, "right" and "left" are from the *patient's* point of view.

Bruising or pain in one of these quadrants can help the EMT ascertain which organs are most likely to have been affected. For example, the RUQ

YOU are the EMT

You and your partner are working a special event: the annual rodeo. While on standby, you witness a rider being thrown and trampled by a bull. After a rodeo clown distracts and corrals the bull, the rider, a 20-year-old man, slowly gets up and begins to walk. He is clutching his abdomen with one hand and rubbing his lower back with the other hand.

1. How do hollow organ injuries differ from solid organ injuries?

2. How should you focus your assessment of a patient with potential intra-abdominal bleeding?

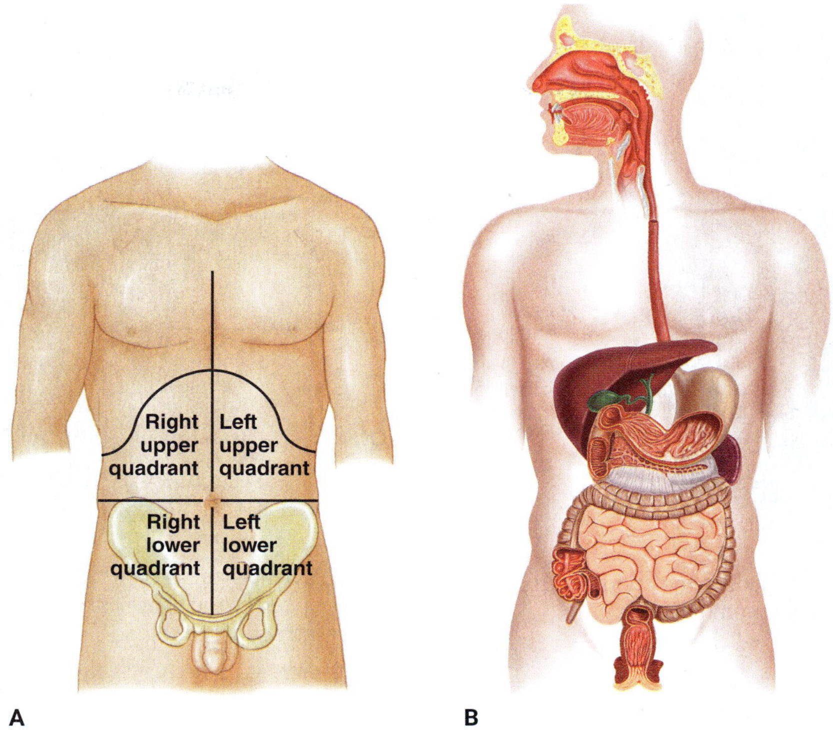

FIGURE 30-1 A. Locations on the abdomen are often designated according to four quadrants. **B.** Many organs lie in more than one quadrant.

contains the gallbladder, the duodenum of the intestines, most of the liver, and a small portion of the pancreas. The LUQ contains the spleen, most of the stomach, and the larger portion of the pancreas.

Special Populations

INJURY CONSIDERATIONS RELATING TO PEDIATRIC ANATOMY

The abdominal muscle structures are less developed in children, which results in less protection from blunt or penetrating trauma. The internal organs, such as the liver and the spleen, are proportionally larger and situated more anteriorly. Moreover, the soft, flexible ribs of infants and young children do not protect these two organs very well and may allow injury to underlying organs, even without fracturing the ribs. Because the internal organs are positioned in closer proximity to each other, there is a higher risk for multiple organ injury caused by minimal direct impact to this region, such as from a lap belt in a motor vehicle. The liver, spleen, and kidneys are more frequently injured in children than in adults.

The LLQ contains portions of the large and small intestines (most notably, the descending colon and the left half of the transverse colon). The RLQ also contains large portions of the large and small intestines (including the ascending colon and the right half of the transverse colon), as well as the appendix, which is situated at the proximal end of the ascending colon.

Hollow and Solid Organs

The abdomen contains hollow and solid organs. **Hollow organs** include the stomach, large and small intestines, gallbladder, ureters, and urinary bladder (**FIGURE 30-2**). It is through these hollow structures that an assortment of materials pass, with most containing food in various stages of digestion. Exceptions include the urinary bladder and ureters, through which urine passes for release, and the gallbladder, which plays a supportive role in the breakdown of fats passing through the intestine.

When ruptured or lacerated, these organs may spill their contents into the abdominal cavity, resulting in intense inflammation and possible

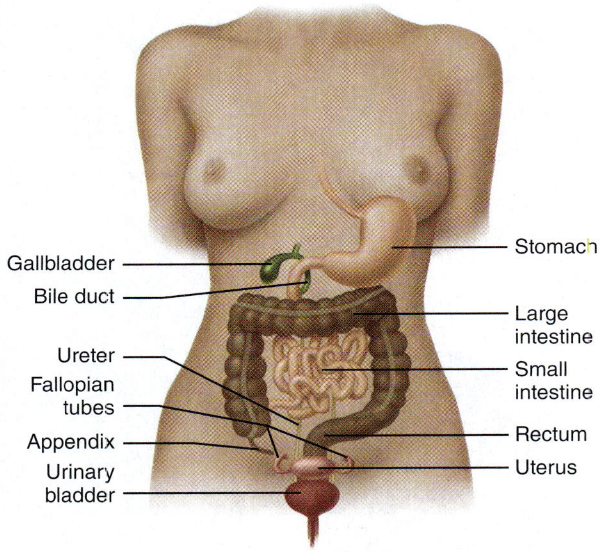

FIGURE 30-2 The hollow organs in the abdominal cavity are structures through which materials pass.

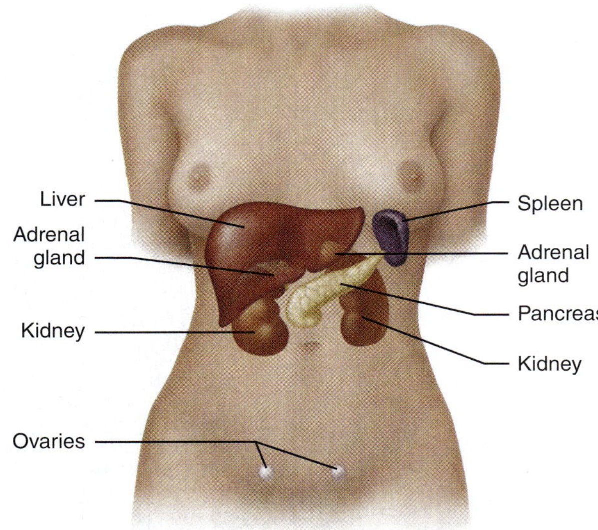

FIGURE 30-3 The solid organs are solid masses of tissue that do much of the chemical work in the body and receive a large, rich supply of blood.

infection. For example, the intestines and stomach contain acidic substances that aid in digestion, but when leaked into the abdominal cavity, these substances may irritate the lining of the cavity (called the **peritoneum**), resulting in inflammation and pain. This condition, called **peritonitis**, is a potentially life-threatening emergency. The first signs of peritonitis are severe abdominal pain, tenderness, and muscular spasm. Later, bowel sounds diminish or disappear, because bowel functioning has been impaired. The patient may complain of nausea and vomiting, the abdomen may become distended and rigid, and signs of infection may be present.

The small intestine comprises the duodenum, the jejunum, and the ileum. The large intestine includes the cecum, the colon, and the rectum. Intestinal blood supply comes from the mesentery. The term *mesentery* refers to any fold of tissue that attaches an organ to the body wall. However, the majority of the time this term is used specifically in reference to the intestinal mesentery: a fold of tissue that contains a web of vessels, both arteries and veins, as well as nerves and lymphatic tissues. It connects the small intestine to the posterior of the abdominal wall. Both blunt and penetrating abdominal injuries can affect this vasculature, and patients with injuries to the mesentery can bleed significantly into the **peritoneal cavity**. Although abdominal distention and rigidity may be indicative of inflammation, they can also alert the attentive EMT to the possibility that the patient is bleeding internally into the peritoneal cavity. Occasionally, bruising or ecchymosis may appear around the umbilicus (periumbilical bruising).

As the name implies, **solid organs** are solid masses of tissue. Solid organs such as the liver, spleen, pancreas, and kidneys carry out numerous chemical processes in the body, including enzyme production, blood cleansing, endocrine functions, and energy production (**FIGURE 30-3**). Because these organs have a rich blood supply, their injury can result in severe unseen hemorrhage. The same holds true for the aorta and inferior vena cava. And similar to contents spilled from hollow organs, blood that has escaped solid organs can cause peritoneal irritation, resulting in abdominal pain; however, this is not always the case. Therefore, the absence of abdominal pain and tenderness does not necessarily rule out the possibility of major bleeding in the abdomen.

Along with the abdominal aorta and a portion of the inferior vena cava, many solid organs are considered *retroperitoneal* (*retro-* means "behind"), because they are situated primarily in the posterior aspect of the abdominal cavity and behind the peritoneum. This region is referred to as the

retroperitoneum. It also houses the kidneys, ureters, and urinary bladder. The majority of the pancreas is located in this region, which is why the pancreas is referred to as a retroperitoneal organ. The last portion of a hollow organ, the colon, occupies the lowest portion of the retroperitoneal space.

Special Populations

FALL INJURIES IN GERIATRIC PATIENTS

Falls are the most common MOI in geriatric patients. The trauma sustained in a fall is not limited to musculoskeletal injuries. For a number of reasons, the EMT should maintain a high index of suspicion for internal injuries, even in patients who have experienced relatively "minor" falls. With advancing age, the abdominal organs lose some of their elasticity, making them more prone to injury when exposed to the forces present in a fall. The aorta, liver, and spleen are particularly vulnerable. Furthermore, if the geriatric patient's bones are brittle, they can fracture even with falls from standing height. The sharp edges of broken bones, such as the ribs, have the potential to puncture internal organs.

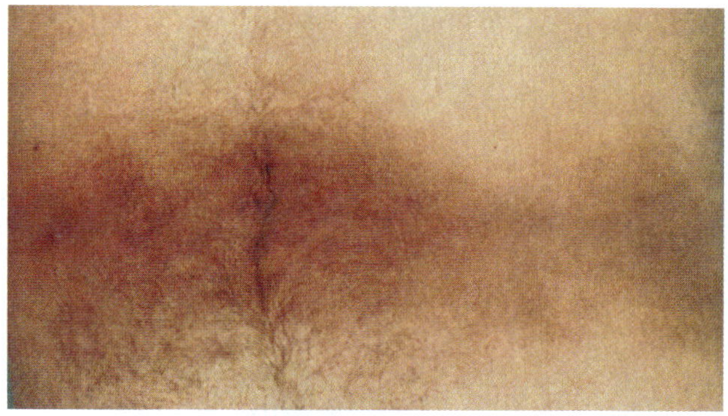

FIGURE 30-4 Blunt trauma to the abdomen can occur when a patient strikes the steering wheel of a vehicle as a result of a crash.

Words of Wisdom

Rib fractures are common traumatic injuries. When your assessment leads you to suspect lower rib fractures, remember that any trauma forceful enough to break the ribs may also have damaged underlying internal organs.

Abdominal Injuries

Abdominal injuries can be as obvious as loops of intestines protruding from an open wound, or they can be as covert as a liver laceration, hidden beneath unbroken skin.

Closed Abdominal Injuries

When a traumatic injury to the abdomen occurs without breaking the skin, it is considered a **closed abdominal injury**. Examples include an assault victim struck in the abdomen by a baseball bat or a rapid deceleration injury from a fall or front-end motor vehicle collision (**FIGURE 30-4**). MOIs capable of causing closed injuries include the following:

- Motor vehicle collisions
- Motorcycle crashes
- Falls
- Blast injuries (barotrauma)
- Pedestrian versus vehicle
- Rapid deceleration
- Compression

Closed abdominal injuries may initially appear as abrasions to the surface of the skin, depending on the MOI, such as a physical assault or a pedestrian struck by a motor vehicle. In some circumstances, depending on how deep in the abdomen the injury occurs, it may take several minutes to hours for the contusion or hematoma to become visible on the surface. Therefore, an EMT cannot rule out the possibility of injury merely on the basis of absence of these findings.

Injuries From Seat Belts and Airbags

Seat belts have prevented countless injuries and deaths, protecting against ejections from motor vehicles involved in collisions. Despite the undeniable benefits, seat belts occasionally contribute to blunt trauma to abdominal organs. Worn properly, a lap seat belt lies below the anterior superior iliac spines of the pelvis and against the hip joints (**FIGURE 30-5A**). Positioned too high, it can squeeze abdominal organs or great vessels against the spine when the vehicle rapidly decelerates or comes to a sudden stop. Fractures of the lumbar spine have also been reported. The diagonal (shoulder) belt should lie across the chest and the top of the

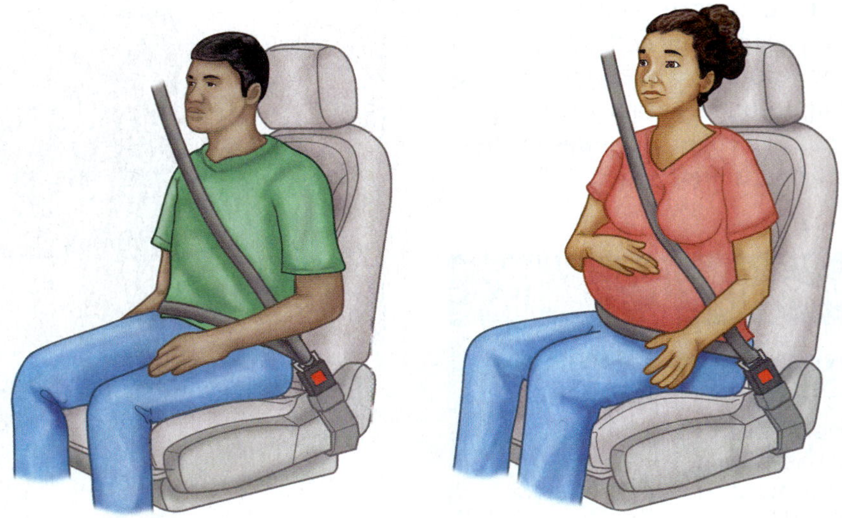

FIGURE 30-5 A. When properly positioned, the lap seat belt should lie across the upper thighs and hip joints, and the shoulder belt should lie across the chest and shoulder. **B.** For a pregnant person, the lap belt should be worn below the stomach and across the thighs and hip bones, and the shoulder belt should be worn between the breasts and to the side of the stomach.

shoulder. It should never be placed behind the person or under the arm. Note that the position of the shoulder belt is slightly different for persons in the later stages of pregnancy (**FIGURE 30-5B**). Further, because the gravid uterus displaces the urinary bladder to the anterior, making it more susceptible to injury, pregnant patients who adjust the lap belt for comfort as opposed to functionality can sustain additional injuries.

In all current-model vehicles, the lap and shoulder safety belts are combined into one so that they may not be used independently. Of course, people can still place the shoulder belt behind their back, significantly reducing the effectiveness of this design. Remember to inspect beneath the airbag for signs of damage to the steering column.

Words of Wisdom

Hospital personnel depend on you to record scene findings that explain the MOI. For example, thoroughly document your observations about the vehicle the patient was driving or riding in as a passenger. Notes about deployment of airbags and the condition of the exterior and the steering column help in the assessment of possible internal injuries.

Open Abdominal Injuries

As the name implies, in an **open abdominal injury**, the peritoneal cavity has been opened to the outside. Penetrating traumatic injuries such as stab wounds and gunshot wounds are examples of open injuries. Although some open wounds may not extend any deeper than the muscular wall of the abdomen, this cannot be reliably determined in the prehospital setting. Therefore, the EMT should maintain a high index of suspicion for unseen injuries and potential life threats and expedite transport to the nearest appropriate hospital, usually a designated trauma center.

A major determining factor in the severity of a penetrating MOI is the velocity of the object that penetrated the abdominal wall. The velocity correlates to the amount of energy transmitted to the tissues and therefore to the amount of damage incurred. The following are three levels of velocity commonly used in the discussion of traumatic injuries:

- **Low velocity.** Caused by handheld or hand-powered objects such as knives and other edged weapons
- **Medium velocity.** Caused by small-caliber handguns and shotguns

- **High velocity.** Caused by more powerful weapons such as high-powered rifles and handguns of higher caliber

In addition to entrance and exit wounds, medium- and high-velocity projectiles create temporary wound channels or cavities. Cavitation occurs as the pressure wave from the projectile is transferred to the tissues. This causes microscopic tears to blood vessels and nerves, expanding the width and length of the wound beyond what can be seen on physical examination. Depending on the velocity of the projectile, cavitation can produce significant tissue destruction and bleeding. The higher the velocity, the larger the cavity created and, subsequently, the greater the extent of damaged tissue.

Despite the absence of cavitation, low-velocity penetrations can cause substantial damage to underlying organs. A visual inspection of the entry wound does not necessarily convey the severity of the internal damage. This is an especially important consideration when treating patients with penetrating trauma in the region of the diaphragm, the muscle that separates the thoracic cavity from the peritoneal cavity. Because the diaphragm rises and falls as we breathe, its location is somewhat variable from one moment to the next. For that reason, it should be assumed that any penetrating abdominal injury at or below the xiphoid process may have punctured the diaphragm. The resulting opening could create a passageway through which abdominal contents might pass, or *herniate*, into the thoracic cavity, potentially hindering chest expansion and causing respiratory complications.

An open abdominal injury that goes through the skin and muscle layer and through the fascia or the interior covering of the abdomen, such that organs now protrude from the peritoneum, is an **evisceration**. This visually shocking injury can be extremely painful. Do not push down on the patient's abdomen, and perform only a visual assessment when there is any suspicion of this type of injury. If there is clothing close to the wound, carefully cut the clothing around the wound, leaving a border of intact cloth outside the injured area. Always be certain you can see exactly where the tips of your scissors are when cutting clothing. The risk of injury to the underlying exposed abdominal contents is extremely high. Never pull, even gently, on any clothing stuck to or inside the wound channel because doing so may remove even more of the abdominal contents.

Hollow Organ Injuries

Injuries that involve the hollow organs often have delayed signs and symptoms. The hollow organs commonly spill their contents into the abdomen and then an infection occurs, which can take a few hours to days to develop. When the stomach and the intestines are injured, they can spill gastrointestinal

YOU are the EMT

When you reach the patient, he is lying supine on the ground outside of the arena area. The scene is safe, and the bull has been penned up. The patient is conscious but restless. He reports pain over his entire abdomen, both flank areas, and the back of his head. Your partner manually stabilizes his head while you perform a primary assessment.

Recording Time: 0 Minutes	
Appearance	In obvious pain; restless
Level of consciousness	Conscious and alert; restless
Airway	Open, clear of secretions or foreign bodies
Breathing	Increased rate; adequate depth
Circulation	Radial pulses rapid and weak; skin pale compared with baseline, cool, and moist; no obvious bleeding

3. How should you interpret your primary assessment findings?

4. What immediate treatment is indicated for this patient?

contents such as food, waste, and digestive liquids that are highly toxic and acidic. These substances cause significant tissue damage to the entire peritoneum.

Both blunt and penetrating trauma can cause injuries to the hollow organs. Blunt trauma causes the organ to "pop," thus releasing fluids or air. Penetrating trauma causes direct injury such as laceration and punctures. In open wounds, patients typically report an intense pain that can be out of character for the size of the injury. Patients may also report intense pain with open wounds of the stomach or small bowel.

Words of Wisdom

The signs of abdominal injury are usually more definite than the symptoms, including firmness on palpation of the abdomen, obvious penetrating wounds, bruises, and altered vital signs, such as increased pulse rate, increased respiratory rate, decreased blood pressure, and shallow respirations (although these signs might not appear until later). Common symptoms include abdominal tenderness, particularly localized tenderness and difficulty moving because of pain.

The gallbladder and the urinary bladder, which are filled with bile and urine, are two additional hollow organs whose contents are potentially irritating and damaging to the tissues of the abdomen if ruptured by injury. These fluids move via gravity into the loose spaces and voids in the peritoneal cavity, eventually leading to infection.

Free air in the peritoneal cavity is abnormal, and it usually indicates that a hollow organ or loop of bowel has perforated. Perforation with free air is usually very painful. If the site of perforation is not rapidly identified and repaired, severe infection and septic shock may develop. Any air in the peritoneal cavity seeks the most superior space or void; thus, the location of the air can change with positioning of the patient.

Solid Organ Injuries

Solid organs (liver, spleen, diaphragm, kidneys, and pancreas) can bleed significantly and cause rapid blood loss that can be hard to identify from a physical examination, because the patient is not experiencing significant pain. Conversely, solid organs can slowly ooze blood into the peritoneal cavity, causing pain to increase slowly over time and increasing the chance for inflammation to develop. Blood in the peritoneal cavity irritates tissue and fills any voids or spaces, which can make it difficult for you to determine the exact source of the bleeding. Because of the structures in the retroperitoneal space (the kidneys, adrenal gland, pancreas, nerve roots, lymph nodes, abdominal aorta, and inferior vena cava) and the spaces in the abdominal cavity, the peritoneal cavity can hold a large volume of blood following traumatic injuries of solid organs and major blood vessels.

The liver is the largest organ in the abdomen. It is very vascular; therefore, it can contribute to hypoperfusion if it is injured. It is often injured by a fractured lower right rib or a penetrating injury, such as a stab wound. A common finding during assessment of patients with an injured liver is referred pain to the right shoulder.

Like the liver, the pancreas and especially the spleen are very vascular. Both organs are prone to heavy bleeding when fractured by blunt force or lacerated or punctured by penetrating injury. The spleen is often injured during motor vehicle crashes, especially in the cases of improperly placed seat belts or impact from the steering wheel, falls from heights or onto sharp objects, and bicycle and motorcycle crashes where the patient hits the handlebars on impact. Referred left shoulder pain also occurs often in cases of splenic injury.

If the diaphragm is penetrated or ruptured, loops of bowel may herniate into the thoracic cavity. Because the bowel will now be displacing lung tissue and vital capacity, patients will exhibit dyspnea or feel short of breath. Patients with a ruptured diaphragm after a motor vehicle crash may become very anxious and short of breath if placed in the supine position on a backboard. Change in position from upright to supine results in more abdominal contents spilling into the thoracic cavity and compressing the lungs, prohibiting the lungs from fully expanding.

In the retroperitoneal space, the kidneys can be impacted or penetrated by trauma. The kidneys are filtration organs; therefore, they are supplied with large quantities of blood. They can be sheared from their base, crushed, or fractured, causing significant blood loss. If a kidney is injured, a common finding is **hematuria**, or blood in the urine. This may be obvious to the naked eye or impossible to detect in the field. You may find drops of blood or blood-tinged urine on the patient's underwear, leading you to inspect the exterior of the genitals. Blood visible on inspection of the urinary meatus (opening of the urethra situated on the glans penis in men and in the vulva in women) indicates significant trauma to the genitourinary system. If blood is not present, do not take this as a sign that the patient is free from injury; the blood may not be visible yet. Other findings related to kidney injury from blunt trauma include severe flank pain, bruising of the flank or lower back, and signs of shock.

Patient Assessment of Abdominal Injuries

The assessment findings in patients with potential abdominal injuries can be challenging to interpret. Some abdominal injuries are obvious and graphic; however, many are subtle and easy to overlook. On the surface, injuries may appear minor (eg, abrasions, bruising) when in fact these outward signs may be the only visible clues that a more severe internal injury exists. Sometimes, coexisting injuries, such as a fractured bone, may cause so much pain that the patient is distracted from perceiving the abdominal discomfort. Other times, the pain may begin subtly and worsen gradually over time. In some cases, the traumatic event may have occurred hours or even days prior to your receiving the call to respond, because the pain has only recently grown severe enough to drive the patient to seek help.

Scene Size-Up

Your scene size-up begins at the time of dispatch. The initial information you receive may be vague or incomplete, but it still provides a place to start your mental preparation en route to the scene. Is the patient injured or ill? What equipment should you bring to the patient's side? Are additional resources, such as law enforcement, hazardous materials personnel, or an advanced life support (ALS) unit, necessary? As always, standard precautions should be in place prior to exiting the ambulance.

As you inspect the scene, consider the MOI and the need for spinal motion restriction. The MOI may supply you with clues as to what underlying injuries are most likely. If the MOI is a motor vehicle collision, inspect the inside and outside of the vehicle. Is the windshield starred? Is the dashboard deformed? Was the patient wearing a seat belt?

In the case of an assault, your first priority is to ensure that law enforcement has rendered the scene safe. Do not approach a questionable scene; your safety must come first. Once the scene has been secured, gather more detailed information about the assault. For blunt trauma, where and how many times was the patient struck? If a weapon was used, was it low-, medium-, or high-velocity? If an edged weapon was used, was it serrated, smooth, or jagged? Was it clean or dirty? How long was it? Such specifics can be especially helpful to hospital staff; however, do not delay transport for the sake of locating a weapon, and be careful not to contaminate evidence in the process.

Special Populations

ABDOMINAL TRAUMA IN PEDIATRIC PATIENTS

In pediatric patients, a common MOI is a motor vehicle versus pedestrian or motor vehicle versus bicycle. In young children, the chest and abdomen are less protected by bony structures than in the adult. The pediatric patient may experience significant transfer of energy on impact. In the pediatric patient, the rib cage is so flexible that the chest can be compressed deeply before rib fractures occur. This extensive compression can involve not only the organs of the chest, but also the abdomen. The ribs then recoil to their normal position, and the patient is left with very few outward signs that an injury has occurred.

Primary Assessment

As you approach the patient, quickly form a general impression of the person's condition and note their level of consciousness. Is the patient awake and alert, interacting with surroundings, or is the patient lying motionless and silent?

The purpose of the primary assessment is to quickly evaluate the patient's ABCs (Airway, Breathing, and Circulation) and mental status, while treating all immediate life threats. In the event of severe external hemorrhage, the sequence should become XABC, where *X* represents control of eXsanguinating bleeding immediately on discovery. Next, ensure the patient has a clear and patent airway. Patients experiencing nausea and/or vomiting may be at risk for aspiration, especially if their level of consciousness is diminished. Have suction ready, and be prepared to turn these patients onto their side should sudden vomiting occur.

Trauma to the kidneys, liver, and spleen can cause profound internal bleeding, posing a substantial risk for shock. One of the earliest signs of shock is tachycardia, as the heart attempts to compensate for the loss of blood. Later signs include hypotension; skin that is pale compared with patient baseline, cool, and moist; and an altered mental status. In people with dark skin, pallor may present as ashen or gray skin, compared to the baseline skin tone; it may be easier to detect by examining the mucous membranes inside the inner lower eyelid and assessing capillary refill.

In some cases, the abdomen may become distended from a large accumulation of blood. If present, shock must be treated aggressively by administering oxygen, positioning the patient supine, and keeping the patient warm.

Remember that children can compensate for significant blood loss better than adults without signs or symptoms of shock developing (**FIGURE 30-6**). They can also have a serious injury

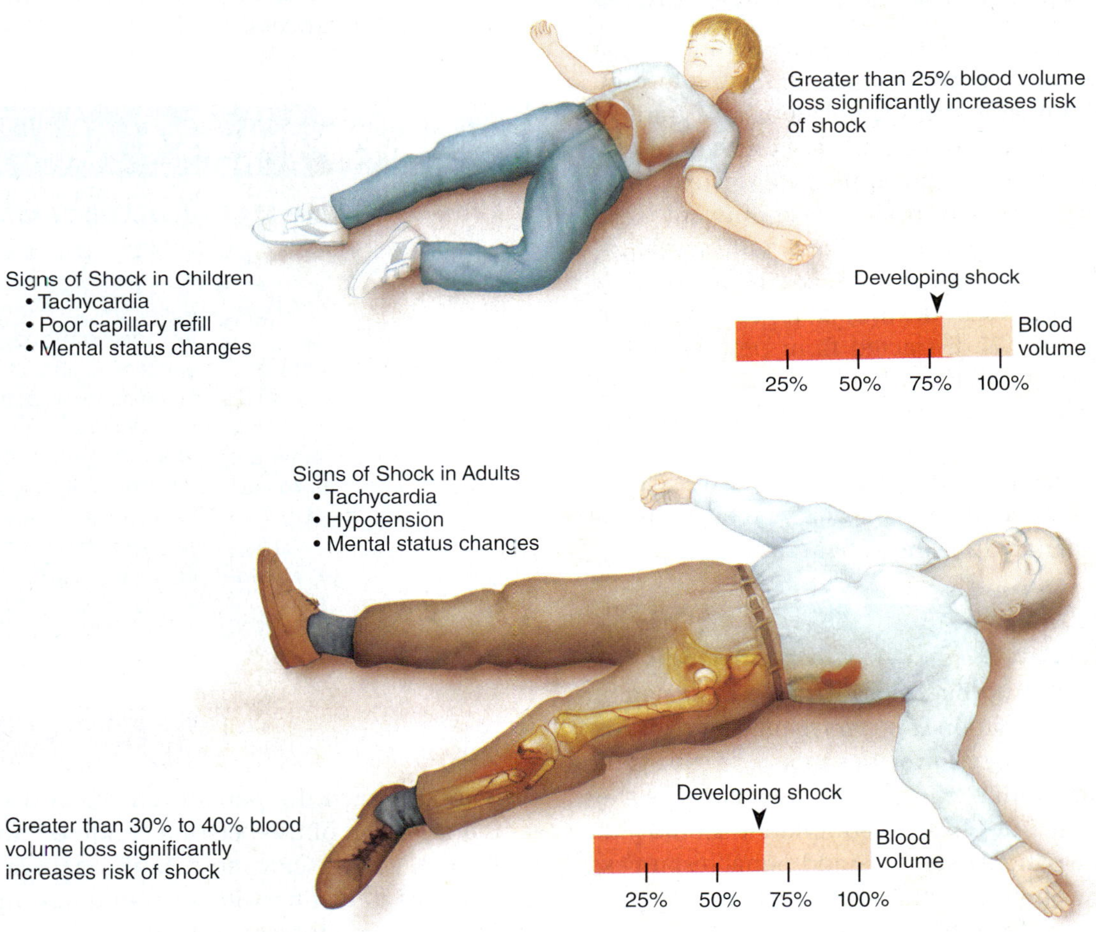

FIGURE 30-6 All children with abdominal injuries should be monitored closely for signs of shock. Although children may compensate for significant blood loss better than adults, shock develops in children after proportionally smaller blood losses.

without early external evidence of a problem. All children with abdominal injuries should be monitored for signs and symptoms of shock, including a weak, rapid pulse; cold, clammy skin; decreased capillary refill time (an early sign); confusion; and decreased systolic blood pressure (a late sign). Even in the absence of signs and symptoms of shock, or with only very few signs and symptoms, you should remain cautious about the possibility of internal injuries.

For critical patients, quickly scan the body from head to toe for additional injuries and initiate rapid transport to the closest appropriate facility without further delay. If the patient's condition is stable, you may opt to gather additional information prior to departure.

History Taking

Once you have identified and treated immediate life threats, attempt to gather more information from the patient (eg, SAMPLE [Signs and symptoms, Allergies, Medications, Pertinent past medical history, Last oral intake, Events leading up to the illness or injury] history). Building on the chief complaint, apply the OPQRST mnemonic (Onset, Provocation/palliation, Quality, Region/radiation, Severity, Timing) as you seek details about the patient's symptoms. Specifically, have the patient describe the pain in their own words. Ask if the pain travels (ie, radiates) to any other part of the body. Has the patient experienced nausea, vomiting, or diarrhea? If the answer is yes, how many times has the patient vomited or had an unusual stool? How long has this problem persisted? And what did it look like? As an example, a patient who describes having black and tarry stools (**melena**) may be experiencing gastrointestinal bleeding. Coffee-ground emesis could be the result of partially digested blood. If the patient is unresponsive or otherwise unable to answer your questions, collect as much information as you can from friends and family.

Unfortunately, a patient's complaint of pain in the abdomen can be deceiving. Injured organs tend to irritate surrounding tissues. As a result, the pain is often diffuse, making it difficult for the patient to pinpoint a specific spot on the abdomen where the pain is felt. Instead, the patient may report having pain "all over" the abdomen. To further complicate matters, it is not uncommon for patients with abdominal trauma to report pain coming from an altogether different part of the body. This referred pain is the result of interconnecting sensory neurons that serve multiple tissues. When the nerves from one part of the body converge with those coming from another site, the result is essentially a distortion in the patient's perception of the pain's location. However, the relationship between a given injury site and the location where pain is perceived often can provide the attentive clinician with valuable insight. For example, bleeding from an injury to the spleen frequently presents with pain referred to the left shoulder. A patient who complains of tearing pain that travels from the abdomen to the back could be experiencing a dissecting abdominal aneurysm. Pain that radiates from the lateral hip to the midline of the groin might be a sign of damage to the kidneys or ureter. Pain located predominantly in the RLQ might be indicative of an inflamed or ruptured appendix. When the gallbladder is injured or inflamed, the patient may report having pain just under the margin of the ribs on the right side or pain between the shoulder blades.

As blood and fluid from damaged organs flow into the peritoneal cavity, the common response is acute pain that gradually spreads across the entire abdomen. The resulting peritonitis can result in pain provoked by removal of pressure, a finding commonly referred to as rebound tenderness. It is often discovered while rescuers are in the process of moving the patient onto the stretcher or while palpating the abdomen during the physical examination. If you suspect rebound tenderness, do not attempt to reproduce it. Note the finding but then refrain from aggravating the site further.

Making your assessment even more challenging is that the patient may present with voluntary or involuntary **guarding**. Voluntary guarding occurs when the patient tenses up or stiffens the abdominal muscles in a conscious effort to splint the area, *guarding* against movements that would provoke additional pain. By contrast, involuntary guarding persists even when the patient is distracted; it is the result of muscle spasms from peritonitis. Additionally, the patient with abdominal pain may prefer to lie still with the knees drawn up toward the chest. If taking a deep breath causes the pain to intensify, the patient's breathing may be rapid and shallow.

If the patient has been subjected to a significant MOI, an exam of the entire body is warranted.

Moving from head to toe, quickly but thoroughly survey for additional injuries. If a life-threatening injury is discovered, the EMT must treat it immediately. Assess the patient's need for spinal motion restriction and apply it in accordance with local protocol. Immobilizing a patient with penetrating trauma is not indicated. Spinal column instability after gunshot wounds is uncommon, whereas delaying transport to a trauma center could prove fatal. Do not delay the transport of seriously injured trauma patients for the sake of completing nonlifesaving treatments, such as splinting extremity fractures or dressing superficial wounds. Secondary injuries should be managed en route to the hospital.

Secondary Assessment

In some instances, whether due to a short transport time or the need to manage life-threatening injuries en route to the hospital, the EMT may not have sufficient time to complete a secondary assessment. However, when time and circumstances permit it, perform a systematic physical examination:

- As much as practical, protect the patient's dignity and privacy. If the patient's condition permits, wait until you are in the back of the ambulance before removing clothing.
- Unless spinal injury is suspected, transport the patient in a position of comfort. For some, the fetal position may provide the greatest degree of comfort, as it reduces abdominal tension and subsequently provides measure of pain relief.
- For a patient with a suspected spinal injury, place padding such as blankets or pillows under the knees to help alleviate tension on the abdominal wall.
- Remove or loosen clothing to expose the injured regions of the body. Use care in situations where blood may have adhered to the material, and avoid causing further damage to exposed tissues, such as in the case of an evisceration.

Inspect and palpate the abdomen, looking for signs of injury (DCAP-BTLS [Deformities, Contusions, Abrasions, Punctures/penetrations, Burns, Tenderness, Lacerations, Swelling]). Palpation should be systematic, assessing each of the four abdominal quadrants individually, preferably beginning with an area in which the patient does not report having pain. This approach allows you to investigate the possibility of radiation and extension of the pain into other quadrants without causing the patient to voluntarily guard the rest of the abdomen. Palpation should begin with light touch, slowly progressing deeper into the tissues. The objective is to pinpoint the pain's location, not to increase its intensity. If a light touch produces pain, deep palpation is unnecessary and may actually aggravate the underlying trauma. Likewise, if the abdomen is obviously injured (eg, impaled object, evisceration), palpation is unlikely to yield information of value and may therefore be bypassed.

Words of Wisdom

For a number of reasons, bowel sounds are not typically auscultated in the field. The noise often found at an out-of-hospital scene makes it incredibly difficult to hear and interpret these sounds. Even in a relatively quiet environment, those trained in the performance of this skill will rarely have sufficient time to do it properly. Ultimately, bowel sounds are of limited value in the prehospital evaluation of trauma patients.

Closed injuries from blunt trauma may be evidenced by bruises (often reddened areas of skin at this early stage), abrasions, or other visible marks. The location or locations of these indicators should guide you to consider the underlying structures (**FIGURE 30-7**). For example, bruises in the RUQ, LUQ, or **flank** (the region below the rib cage and above the hip) might suggest an injury to the

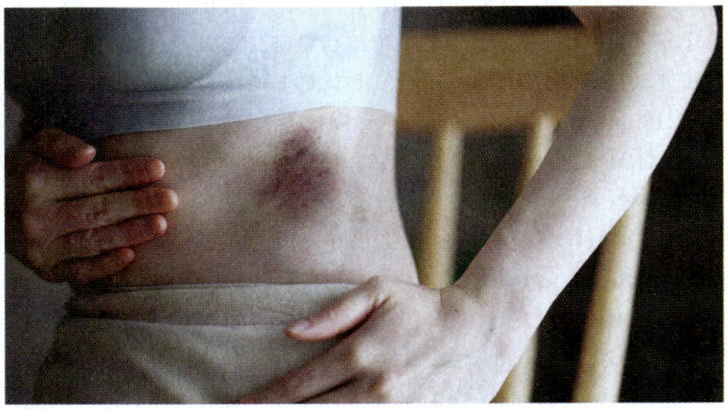

FIGURE 30-7 Bruising on the abdomen can provide clues to the possible injury of underlying organs.

liver, spleen, or kidney, respectively (**FIGURE 30-8**). Bruises around the umbilicus may signify severe internal bleeding in the abdomen (**FIGURE 30-9**).

Obtain and record the patient's vital signs early, and repeat them every 5 minutes in the patient whom you suspect has a serious injury. This regular monitoring will help you to quickly identify changes in the patient's condition, including signs of decompensation from blood loss. Patients experiencing external or internal hemorrhaging should be monitored closely. Generally, the first blood pressure reading should be obtained manually with a sphygmomanometer (blood pressure cuff) and stethoscope. Subsequent blood pressure values may be assessed using an automated device. Remember that hypotension is a late sign of shock. Therefore, be on the alert for earlier signs, such as tachycardia and pale, cool, clammy skin.

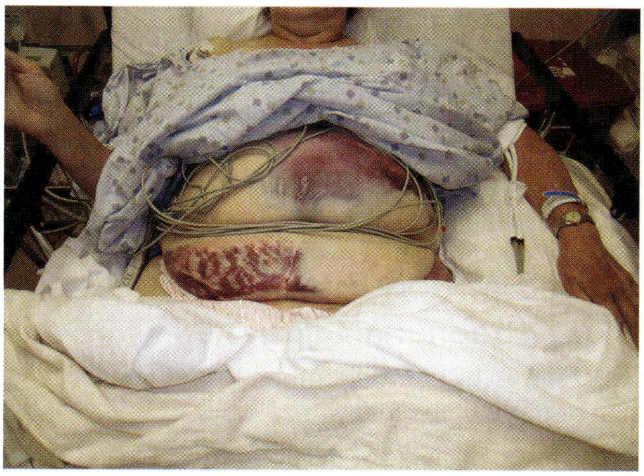

FIGURE 30-8 Bruises in the right upper quadrant, left upper quadrant, or flank suggest an injury to the liver, spleen, or kidney, respectively.

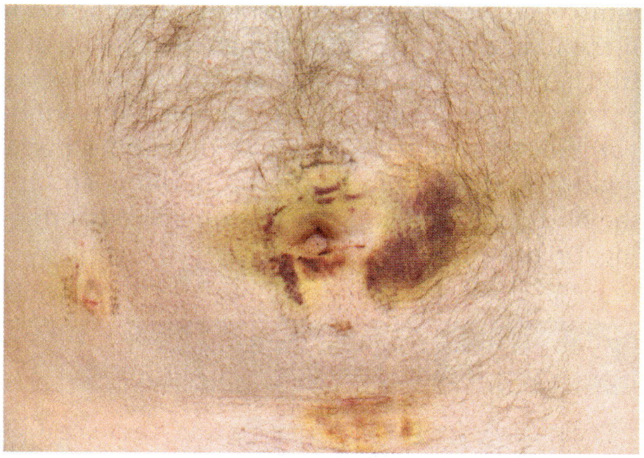

FIGURE 30-9 Bruising around the umbilicus indicates the possibility of significant bleeding inside the abdomen.

YOU are the EMT

After applying oxygen to the patient at 15 L/min by nonrebreathing mask, you perform a secondary assessment. Your partner continues to manually stabilize the patient's head in a neutral position. During your physical examination, you find numerous abrasions to his anterior abdomen and flanks, and he has pain to palpation of his RUQ. The rest of your secondary assessment is unremarkable for gross injuries. An off-duty EMT from your agency, who was a spectator at the rodeo, provides assistance and obtains a set of vital signs.

Recording Time: 6 Minutes	
Respirations	24 breaths/min; adequate depth
Pulse	120 beats/min; weak and regular
Skin	Pale, cool, and clammy
Blood pressure	104/54 mm Hg
Oxygen saturation (Spo_2)	97% (on oxygen, 15 L/min by nonrebreathing mask)

Spinal motion restriction is maintained and the patient is loaded into the ambulance. He is conscious and alert, but is restless and reports being very thirsty. You begin transport to the hospital while continuing to assess and treat the patient en route.

5. What are some common bruising patterns and clinical signs associated with intra-abdominal bleeding?

Assessment of an Isolated Abdominal Injury

If the evidence suggests the injury is isolated to the abdomen, you may limit the focus of your physical examination to the affected area. Visually inspect the abdomen for penetrating wounds (eg, gunshots, stabbings). As mentioned previously, you should not be deceived by a seemingly small wound; the outward appearance does not necessarily reflect the extent of the underlying injuries. If an entry wound is discovered, check for a corresponding exit wound. If the injury was caused by a high-velocity missile from a rifle, you may see a small, harmless-looking entrance wound with a large, gaping exit wound. For patients who have a knife or other object embedded in the abdomen, control bleeding around the object and stabilize it with supportive bandaging. Do not attempt to remove it.

Street Smarts

Occasionally, you will have a patient who is extremely sensitive to palpation or is ticklish. This can make the physical examination process more difficult. Because it is unlikely that patients will tickle themselves, use the technique of placing the patient's hand on the surface of the abdomen and then palpate and compress the abdomen with the patient's hand between your hand and the patient's skin.

Words of Wisdom

Roll patients onto their side to examine the back for signs of injury. Avoid log rolling a patient with an evisceration; doing so may cause more abdominal contents to protrude from the wound. Keep such patients supine. When safe to do so, allow them to flex their knees to reduce tension in the abdominal muscles.

Reassessment

Repeat the primary assessment, and reassess the vital signs. Evaluate the status of interventions performed as well as the patient's response to treatment. Note trends in the patient's mental status, pain level, and vital signs, and determine whether the patient's condition is improving or deteriorating. Adjust care as needed.

Contact the receiving hospital and outline the patient's MOI, injuries, and relevant vital signs. Use approved medical and anatomic terminology correctly, but when in doubt, avoid jargon and simply describe what you see. Include pertinent negatives and details about the scene.

Emergency Medical Care of Abdominal Injuries

Your recognition of the MOI and understanding of the patient's immediate needs will guide your treatment and transport decisions.

Closed Abdominal Injuries

Blunt Abdominal Injuries

A patient with blunt abdominal trauma may have one or more of the following:

- Severe bruising of the abdominal wall
- Laceration of the liver and spleen
- Rupture of the intestine
- Tears in the mesentery, the membranous folds that attach the intestines to the walls of the body, and injury to blood vessels within them
- Kidney rupture or avulsion from its arteries and veins
- Rupture of the urinary bladder, especially in a patient who had a full and distended bladder at the time of the injury
- Severe intra-abdominal hemorrhage
- Peritoneal irritation and inflammation in response to the rupture of hollow organs

A patient who has sustained blunt abdominal trauma should be monitored closely and evaluated for progression into shock. The patient with blunt abdominal trauma may experience nausea and vomiting. Be prepared to protect the airway with suctioning as needed. Administer oxygen to patients who are unconscious or who are in shock. Cover patients with a blanket to keep them warm. In a patient with a ruptured diaphragm, the anterior abdominal wall may appear sunken because abdominal contents have shifted up into the chest cavity. The added pressure on the lungs may lead to impaired lung expansion and difficulty breathing, necessitating positive-pressure ventilation by bag-mask device. Consider calling ALS for placement of an oral or nasal gastric tube. Minimize scene time and transport to an appropriate hospital.

Open Abdominal Injuries

Penetrating Abdominal Injuries

Patients with penetrating injuries generally have obvious wounds and external bleeding (**FIGURE 30-10A**). For example, a large wound may have protrusions of bowel, fat, or other structures. However, not all open injuries will present with significant external bleeding. The EMT should maintain a high index of suspicion that these patients have substantial, albeit unseen, internal hemorrhage.

In caring for a patient with a penetrating wound to the abdomen, follow the general procedures previously described for care of a blunt abdominal injury as well as following the specific steps for the penetrating wound. Inspect the patient's back and sides for exit wounds, and apply a dry, sterile dressing to any open wounds. If the penetrating object is still in place, apply a stabilizing bandage around it to control external bleeding and to minimize movement of the object (**FIGURE 30-10B**).

Abdominal Evisceration

Severe lacerations of the abdominal wall may produce an evisceration, a wound from which internal organs protrude (**FIGURE 30-11**). If an evisceration is discovered, place a sterile dressing moistened with normal saline over the wound, apply a bandage, and transport. Never attempt to push eviscerated tissue or organs back into the abdominal cavity. Because body heat escapes quickly from open abdominal wounds, and because exposed organs lose fluid rapidly, the affected area should be kept warm and moist (**FIGURE 30-12**). Avoid using adherent materials and those that lose substance when wet, such as toilet/tissue paper, paper towels, or absorbent cotton. Protocols in some EMS systems direct that an occlusive dressing be placed over the top of the moistened dressing.

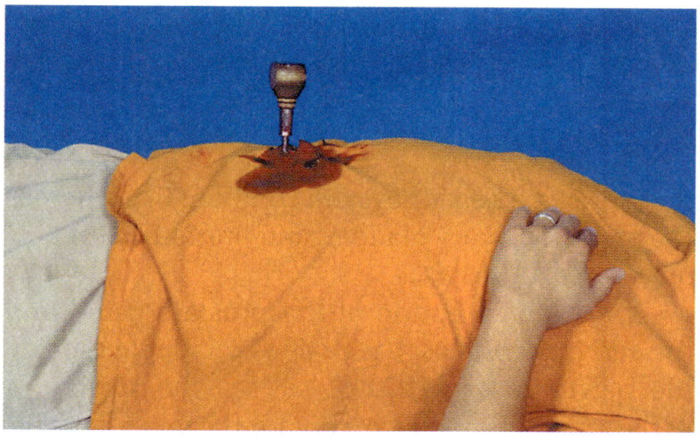

A

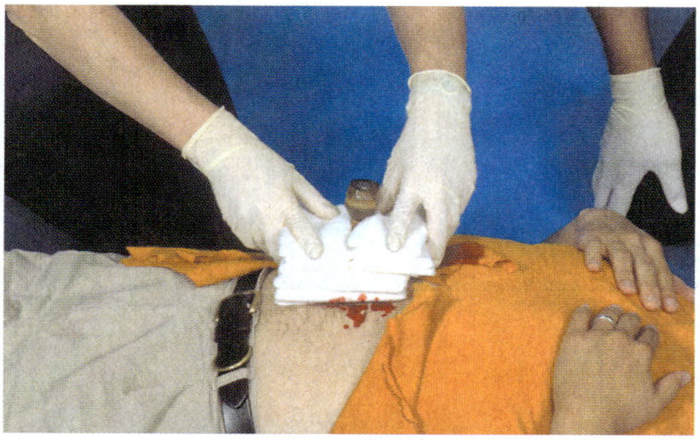

B

FIGURE 30-10 A. Penetrating injuries have obvious wounds and may also have external bleeding. **B.** If the penetrating object is still in place, use a roller bandage to stabilize the object and to control bleeding.

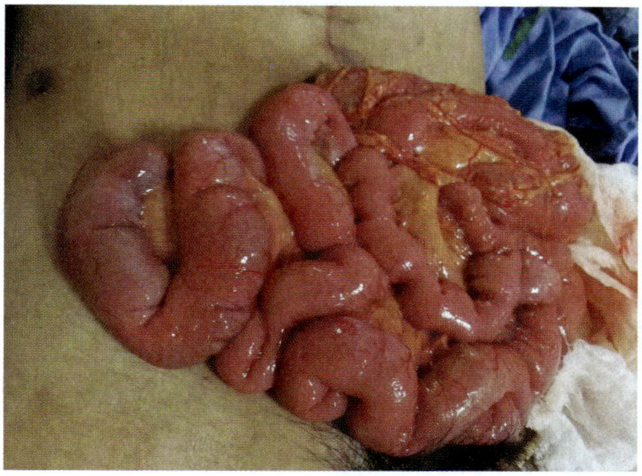

FIGURE 30-11 An abdominal evisceration is an open abdominal wound from which internal organs protrude.

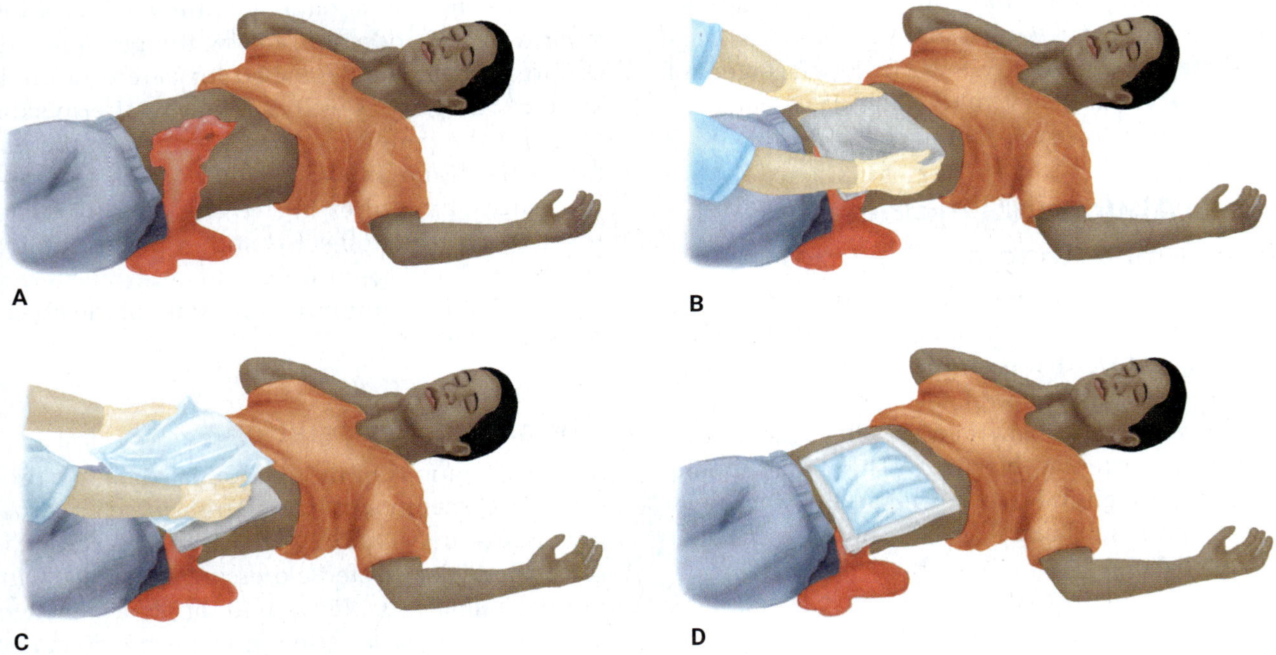

FIGURE 30-12 A. The open abdomen radiates body heat rapidly and must be covered. **B.** Cover the wound with moistened, sterile dressings and with an occlusive dressing, depending on local protocol. **C.** Secure the dressing with a bandage. **D.** Secure the bandage with tape.

Anatomy of the Genitourinary System

The organs of the genitourinary system play a role in waste removal and sexual reproduction.

The urinary system controls the discharge of certain waste materials filtered from the blood by the kidneys. The kidneys are solid organs, whereas the ureters, urinary bladder, and urethra are hollow organs (**FIGURE 30-13**).

With the exception of the prostate gland and the seminal vesicles, the male genitalia lie outside the pelvic cavity (**FIGURE 30-14**). The structures of the female genitalia, except for the vulva, clitoris,

YOU are the EMT

You reassess the patient en route and note that his clinical status has deteriorated. You ask your driver to notify the receiving facility as you continue to treat the patient. Given your relatively short transport time to the hospital, you determine that ALS rendezvous would not result in earlier appropriate care for the patient.

Recording Time: 12 Minutes	
Level of consciousness	Responsive to pain only
Respirations	28 breaths/min; shallow
Pulse	134 beats/min; absent radial pulses
Skin	Cool, pale, and clammy
Blood pressure	82/54 mm Hg
Oxygen saturation (Spo_2)	88% (on oxygen, 15 L/min by nonrebreathing mask)

6. Why is your patient's condition deteriorating? How should you modify your treatment?

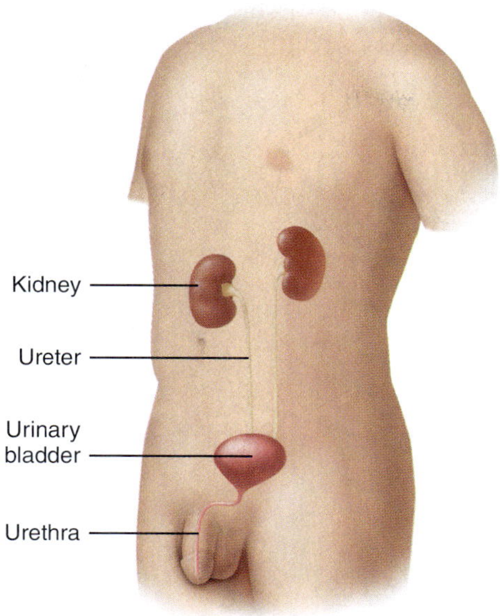

FIGURE 30-13 The urinary system lies behind the digestive tract. The kidneys are solid organs; the ureter, urinary bladder, and urethra are hollow organs.

and labia, are contained entirely within the pelvis (**FIGURE 30-15**). The male and female reproductive organs have certain similarities and, of course, basic differences. They allow for the production of sperm and egg cells and their respective hormones, the act of sexual intercourse, and, ultimately, reproduction.

Injuries of the Genitourinary System

Injuries of the Kidneys

Injuries of the kidneys are not uncommon, and they rarely occur in isolation. This is because the kidneys lie in such a well-protected area of the body that for them to sustain damage from blunt or penetrating mechanisms, the structures that surround them would almost certainly have to be damaged as well. Less significant injuries to the kidneys may result from a smaller yet concentrated direct blow or from something as innocuous as being tackled while playing football (**FIGURE 30-16**). Suspect kidney

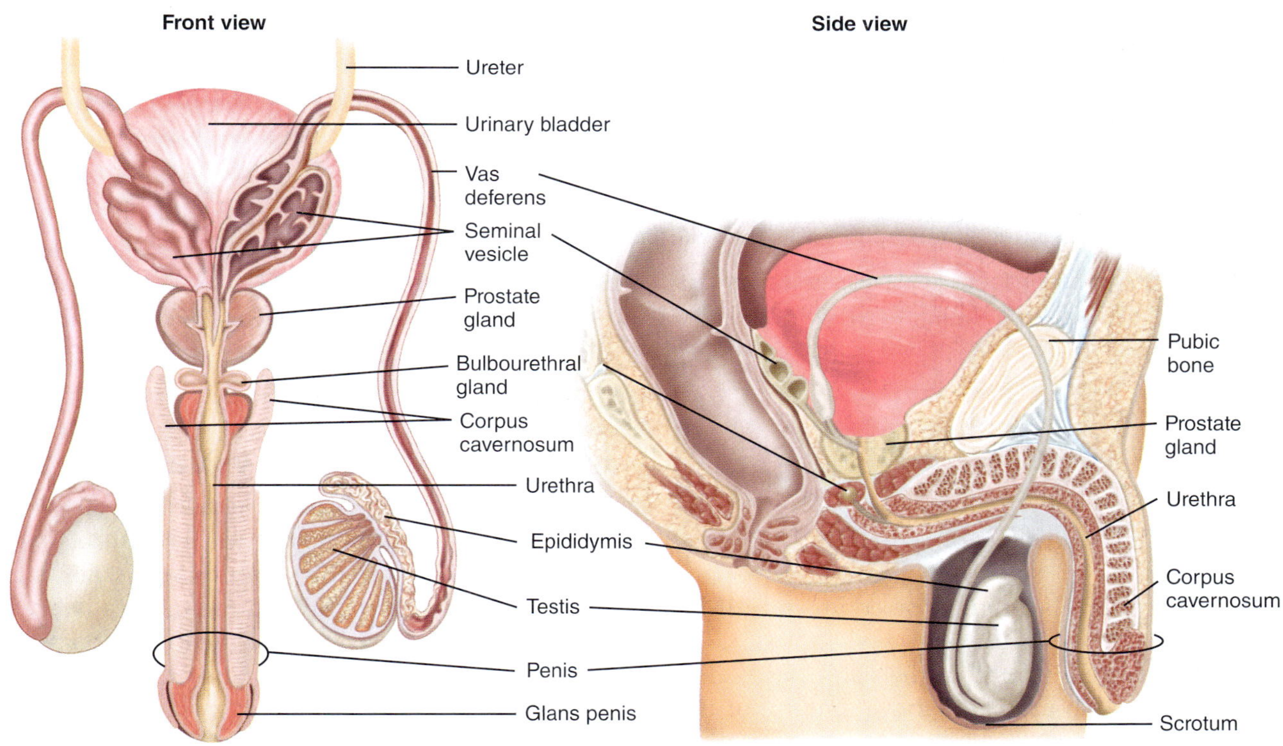

FIGURE 30-14 The male reproductive system includes the testicles, vas deferens, seminal vesicles, prostate gland, urethra, and penis.

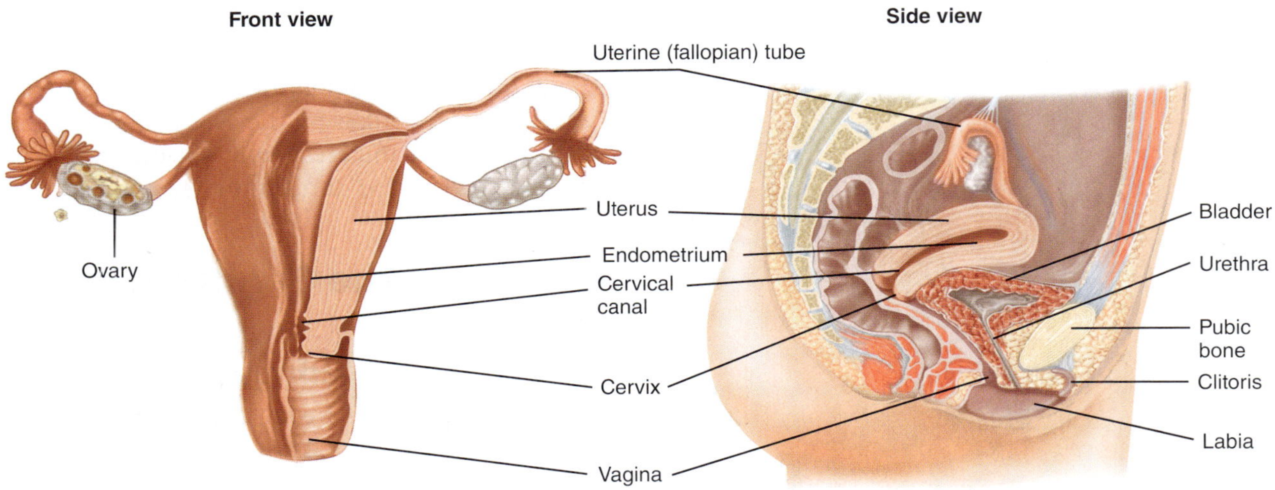

FIGURE 30-15 The female reproductive system includes the ovaries, fallopian tubes, uterus, cervix, and vagina.

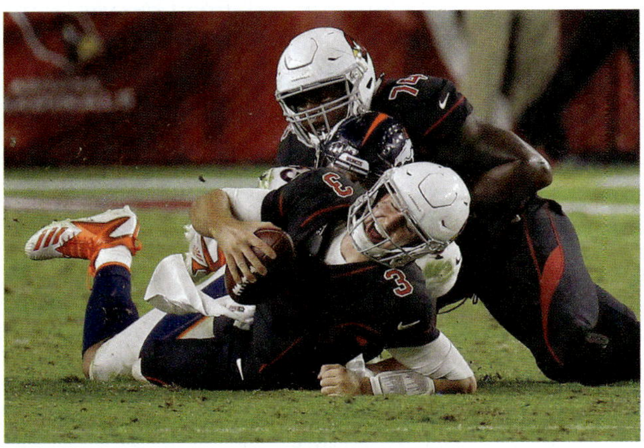

FIGURE 30-16 A tackle in football that results in blunt trauma to the lower rib cage or the flank can cause kidney injury.

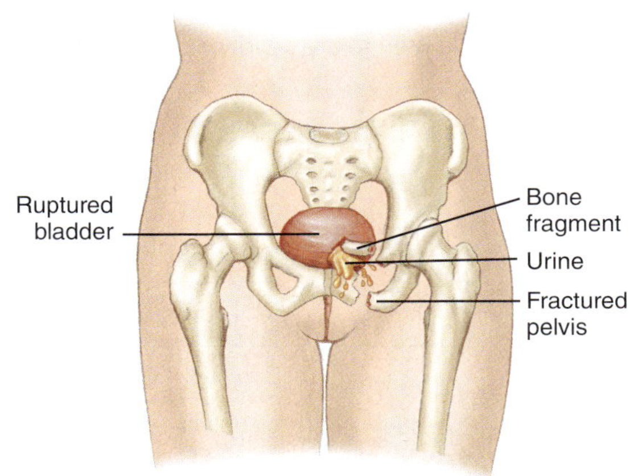

FIGURE 30-17 Fracture of the pelvis can result in perforation of the bladder by the bony fragments. Urine then leaks into the pelvis.

damage if the patient has a history or physical evidence of any of the following:

- Complaint of flank pain
- Hematuria
- An abrasion, laceration, or contusion in the flank
- A penetrating wound in the flank (the region below the rib cage and above the hip) or the upper abdomen
- Fractures on either side of the lower rib cage or of the lower thoracic or upper lumbar vertebrae
- A hematoma in the flank region

Injuries to the Urinary Bladder

Injury to the urinary bladder, either blunt or penetrating, may result in its rupture. When this happens, urine spills into the surrounding tissues, and any urine that passes through the urethra is likely to be bloody. Blunt injuries of the lower abdomen or pelvis often cause rupture of the urinary bladder, particularly when the bladder is full and distended. Sharp, bony fragments from a fracture of the pelvis may perforate the urinary bladder (**FIGURE 30-17**). Penetrating wounds of the lower midabdomen or the perineum (the area of skin between the vagina and the anus) can directly involve the urinary bladder. In men, sudden deceleration from a motor vehicle or motorcycle crash can literally shear the bladder from the urethra. In women, remember that in the second and third trimesters of pregnancy, the incidence of injury to the urinary bladder is increased due to displacement by the uterus.

Injuries of the External Male Genitalia

Injuries of the external male genitalia include all types of soft-tissue wounds. Although these injuries are uniformly painful and generally a source of great concern to the patient, they are rarely life threatening. They should not be given priority over other, more severe wounds, unless the rich blood supply causes significant bleeding. It is important to know that pain from an injury to the testicles or another cause, such as infection or cancer, may be referred to the lower abdomen. As a result, when assessing men with lower abdominal pain, you should also consider injury or other causes of pain to the testicles.

Injuries of the Female Genitalia

Internal Female Genitalia

The uterus, ovaries, and fallopian tubes are subject to the same types of injuries as any other internal organ. However, they are rarely damaged because they are small, deep in the pelvis, and well protected by the pelvic bones. Unlike the urinary bladder, which lies adjacent to the bony pelvis, they are usually not injured as a result of a pelvic fracture.

An exception is the uterus during pregnancy. As pregnancy progresses, the uterus enlarges substantially and rises out of the pelvis, becoming vulnerable to both penetrating and blunt injuries. These injuries can be particularly severe because the uterus has a rich blood supply during pregnancy. In addition, you must keep in mind that the fetus is also at risk. Ask these patients if they have abdominal pain or contractions or have vaginal bleeding. You can expect to see the signs and symptoms of shock with these patients; be prepared to provide all necessary support and prompt transport. Note also that contractions may begin. If possible, ask when the patient is due to deliver and report this information to the hospital staff.

In the third trimester of pregnancy, the uterus is large and may obstruct the inferior vena cava, leading to a decrease in the amount of blood returning to the heart if the patient is placed in a supine position (supine hypotensive syndrome). As a result, blood pressure may decrease. The patient should be carefully placed on the left side so that the uterus will not lie on the inferior vena cava. If the patient is secured to a backboard, tilt the board to the left. Chapter 33, *Gynecologic Emergencies*, and Chapter 34, *Obstetrics and Neonatal Care*, cover gynecologic emergencies and the special considerations for pregnant trauma patients in detail.

External Female Genitalia

The external female genitalia include the vulva, the clitoris, and the major and minor labia (lips) at the entrance of the vagina. Injuries of the external female genitalia can include all types of soft-tissue injuries. Because these genital parts have a rich nerve supply, injuries are very painful. Vaginal bleeding may occur because of penetrating or blunt trauma. These injuries can be accidental, as in the case of straddle injuries from bicycles or motorcycles; or they can be intentional, as in the case of assaults. Determining the MOI will assist you in deciding if you need to call for additional resources, as in the case of sexual assault.

In any case of trauma, it is important to determine the possibility of pregnancy. Ask the patient the date of the last known menstrual period or whether the patient has been sexually active. Assume all women of childbearing age are possibly pregnant. This information is medically relevant because some medications and diagnostic imaging may be harmful for a fetus, and there is the potential for another source of blood loss in the gravid uterus.

In cases of external bleeding and trauma, a sterile absorbent sanitary napkin or pad may be applied to the labia. Do not insert instruments, gloved fingers, or a tampon into the vagina because doing so can cause further damage.

Patient Assessment of the Genitourinary System

Being examined after sustaining a genitourinary injury can be embarrassing for the patient. Therefore, the EMT should maintain a professional presence at all times when interacting with these patients. As much as is practical, provide the patient with privacy during the assessment process. Be sure to explain to the patient what you are doing and the reason it is necessary. Obtain consent from the patient before the assessment. Often, the patient may prefer to be examined by a clinician of the same gender, but this is not always possible in the prehospital setting. Be professional and respectful.

Scene Size-Up

Assess the scene for anything that could jeopardize the safety of the crew, the patient, or bystanders. Do not approach until all threats have been mitigated by the appropriate personnel (eg, law enforcement, hazmat). Apply standard precautions to minimize your direct exposure to body fluids. Be aware that while visible blood on the patient's clothing or surroundings can be apparent as you approach, blood can also be hidden under thick clothing such as denim and leather. In addition to gloves, eye protection is required whenever treating a patient with open injuries. Determine the number of patients and consider if you need additional or specialized resources on the scene.

By integrating the information supplied by dispatch with your observations of the scene and the MOI, you may be able to anticipate the presence of certain injuries. Be cognizant that the patient may be reluctant to discuss injuries or consent to a physical examination. The patient may also withhold or understate the details of the MOI for fear of embarrassment. Only by maintaining a professional demeanor, respecting the patient's privacy, and protecting the patient's dignity will you be able to gain the patient's trust. Having that trust increases the likelihood that the patient will disclose important pieces of information that may affect the care you provide.

Primary Assessment

On reaching the patient, quickly identify and treat immediate life threats, establish the priority level of the patient's condition, and prepare for transport. The genitourinary system is highly vascular. Consequently, genitourinary injuries can precipitate a substantial loss of blood. Because life-threatening

YOU are the EMT

The patient is becoming combative and resists your attempts to assist his ventilations, but he will tolerate oxygen via a nonrebreathing mask. During your reassessment, you note blood on the front of the patient's underwear, which was not there during previous assessments. You examine the area more carefully but do not see any open injuries to the genitalia or adjacent areas. You call your radio report in to the receiving facility.

Recording Time: 17 Minutes	
Level of consciousness	Responsive to pain only
Respirations	28 breaths/min; shallow
Pulse	128 beats/min; weak and regular
Skin	Cool, pale, and clammy
Blood pressure	90/58 mm Hg
Oxygen saturation (Spo_2)	93% (on oxygen, 15 L/min by nonrebreathing mask)

The patient begins vomiting bright red blood. You quickly turn the backboard to the side to allow the vomitus to drain and then suction his mouth to ensure that his airway remains clear.

7. On the basis of your reassessment, what additional injuries should you suspect?

8. How will your reassessment findings change your current treatment plan?

hemorrhage must be addressed immediately, even before airway or breathing concerns, do not circumvent examining this area of the body. Look externally at the patient's undergarments for signs of bleeding and injury. Make every effort to protect the patient's privacy and dignity as you inspect the exterior genitalia for visible signs of injury.

Once severe bleeding has been controlled, ensure the patient has a clear and patent airway. Consider the need for spinal motion restriction, and use caution to avoid excessive manipulation of the cervical spine as you manage the patient's airway. If the patient is unresponsive or has a significantly altered level of consciousness, consider inserting an oropharyngeal or nasopharyngeal airway. Ensure the patient is breathing adequately. Provide assisted ventilations using a bag-mask device as needed.

Check the patient's pulse rate and quality; determine the skin condition, color, and temperature; and assess the capillary refill time. If signs of shock are present, treat accordingly. Remember that because internal bleeding may be well hidden in patients with closed injuries, you must have a high index of suspicion for shock in such cases.

Also during the primary assessment, note the patient's level of alertness. Is the patient awake and interacting with surroundings? By contrast, is the patient lying motionless and silent? If so, does the patient respond when you say their name? If not, will the patient react to physical stimuli such as a sternal rub?

A patient with a genitourinary system injury should be taken to a trauma center for evaluation and treatment. Even when these injuries do not become life-*ending*, they can nevertheless be life-*altering*; often dramatically so, requiring specialized medical care. When possible and when protocol permits, these patients should be transported to a facility capable of treating this subset of injuries.

History Taking

When attempting to ascertain the chief complaint, your goal is to understand why the patient felt the need for medical assistance. Why did the person call 9-1-1? Ask about associated complaints, but avoid putting words in the patient's mouth by asking closed-ended questions. For example, when asking the patient to describe discomfort, do not ask, "Is it a stabbing pain?" or "Do you also have pain in your shoulder?" Instead, ask open-ended questions such as "How would you describe the discomfort?" or "Is anything else bothering you?" Common associated complaints with genitourinary injuries are nausea, vomiting, diarrhea, hematuria, and abnormal bowel and bladder habits such as an increase in frequency or the absence of the need to void.

You can use the SAMPLE history to gain further insight into the specifics of the chief complaint. Use OPQRST to learn more about the patient's pain experience. Inquire about urine output; specifically, did the patient notice the presence of blood in the urine? Note, however, that occult bleeding into the urine may still exist even though it was not severe enough for the patient to see it with the naked eye. Therefore, just because bleeding has not been obvious, that fact alone does not preclude the possibility that your patient has internal genitourinary injuries.

Ask patients if they are allergic to any medications and other triggers. Medications may mask the signs and symptoms of injuries or make them more severe, so it is important to know what your patient takes, whether prescribed, over-the-counter, or "natural" (eg, herbal remedies). The importance of past medical history cannot be overstated. The incidence of previous injuries or illnesses affecting the genitourinary system may be a key element to understanding the patient's present condition. The last oral intake is important to ascertain as well, as this information may inform physicians about the risk of aspiration if surgery is indicated. Finally, addressing the events that led to the injury may supply you with valuable clues.

Secondary Assessment

The secondary assessment is a more thorough physical examination used to uncover injuries that may have been missed during the primary assessment. As previously mentioned, there are times when the EMT is unable to conduct a secondary assessment. Most often, this is due to one of two conditions: (1) the need to provide ongoing lifesaving treatment to a patient with critical injuries or (2) an especially short duration of transport to the emergency department (ED).

Generally, when your patient's injuries are isolated to the genitourinary system and the MOI is relatively minor, you can forego a full head-to-toe exam and instead focus solely on the affected region. By contrast, if trauma is extensive, likely affecting multiple systems, the physical exam should include the entire body. Applying a systematic approach while assessing for DCAP-BTLS reduces the risk that a significant injury will be missed.

Finally, obtain the patient's vital signs and reassess them frequently, observing for trends in the patient's condition. As previously mentioned, signs such as tachycardia, tachypnea, low blood pressure, weak pulse, and cool, moist, and pale skin should lead you to suspect shock. Treat accordingly.

Reassessment

Repeat the primary assessment, and obtain additional sets of vital signs. Reassess all interventions performed and determine how the patient is responding to care. Adjust interventions as necessary. As early as possible, communicate your suspicions, concerns, and assessment findings to receiving facility staff. Giving timely advance notice ensures ED staff are prepared.

Emergency Medical Care of Genitourinary Injuries

Kidneys

Damage to the kidneys may not be obvious on inspection of the patient. You may or may not see bruises or lacerations on the overlying skin. However, if the injury is associated with significant blood loss, you will see signs of shock. Another potential sign of kidney damage is hematuria. Treat shock and associated injuries in the appropriate manner. Provide rapid transport to the hospital, keeping the patient warm and carefully monitoring the patient's vital signs en route.

Urinary Bladder

If you discover blood at the urethral opening or physical signs of trauma on the lower abdomen, pelvis, or perineum, the urethra or urinary bladder may be damaged. There may be blood at the tip of the penis or a bloodstain on the patient's underwear.

External Male Genitalia

A few general rules apply to the treatment of injuries involving the external male genitalia:

- Because these injuries can be very painful, do whatever possible to make the patient comfortable.
- Cover abrasions with sterile, moist compresses.
- To control bleeding, apply direct pressure with dry, sterile gauze dressings.
- Never remove or manipulate objects impaled through or embedded in the urethra.
- If possible, retrieve avulsed skin and transport it along with the patient. However, any search for missing tissue should not delay transport, and it should never distract the clinicians from providing emergency care.

After controlling serious bleeding, the EMT who encounters a patient with an avulsion of the skin of the penis should wrap the tissue in a soft, sterile dressing moistened with sterile saline solution, place it in a bag, place that bag in a cool container (but not directly in contact with ice), label the container with the patient's name, and rapidly transport it along with the patient.

When caring for a patient who has sustained an amputation of the penile shaft, whether partial or complete, the EMT's first concern must be bleeding control. Using a sterile dressing, apply direct pressure to the site. Constricting devices (ie, tourniquets) are not appropriate for the control of penile bleeding. As with avulsions, a completely amputated penis should be retrieved, as surgical reconstruction is possible. Wrap it in a moist, sterile dressing, place it in a plastic bag, and transport it along with the patient if possible. It should be kept cool but not placed into direct contact with ice.

When an erect penis is bent sharply, the shaft can be severely damaged, sometimes requiring surgical repair. This injury is associated with intense pain and bleeding into the tissues, and it can be quite frightening for the patient. Provide rapid transport to the ED.

Accidental laceration of the skin around the head of the penis usually occurs when the penis is erect and is associated with heavy bleeding. Local pressure with a sterile dressing is usually sufficient to stop the hemorrhage.

It is not uncommon for the skin of the shaft of the penis or the foreskin to get caught in the zipper of pants. If a small segment of the zipper is involved (one or two teeth), you can try to unzip the pants. However, if a longer segment is involved, or if the patient is agitated, do not attempt to unzip the pants. Instead, use heavy scissors to cut the zipper out of the pants to make the patient more comfortable during transport. Prior to cutting, explain to the patient what you are about to do. Be particularly careful not to cause injury to the scrotum while cutting the zipper away. Always be certain that you are able to see exactly what you are cutting with your scissors.

Urethral injuries in men are not uncommon. Lacerations of the urethra can result from straddle injuries, pelvic fractures, or penetrating wounds of the perineum. These injuries may bleed profusely; however, the bleeding may not be apparent externally. Direct pressure with a dry, sterile dressing usually controls any external hemorrhage. Because the urethra is the channel for urine, it is very important to know whether the patient can urinate and whether hematuria is present. For this reason, you should save any voided urine for later examination at the hospital. Any foreign bodies that may be protruding from the urethra will have to be removed in a surgical setting.

Avulsion of the skin of the scrotum may damage the scrotal contents. If possible, preserve the avulsed skin in a moist, sterile dressing for possible use in reconstruction. Wrap the scrotal contents or the perineal area with a sterile, moist compress, and use a local pressure dressing to control bleeding. Promptly transport the patient to the ED.

Direct blows to the scrotum can result in the rupture of a testicle or significant accumulation of blood around the testes. In either case, you should apply an ice pack to the scrotal area while transporting the patient.

Female Genitalia

Lacerations, abrasions, and avulsions should be treated with moist, sterile compresses. Use local pressure to control bleeding and a sanitary napkin or a diaper-type bandage to hold dressings in place. Under no circumstances should you pack or place dressings into the vagina. Leave any foreign bodies in place after you stabilize them with bandages.

In general, although these injuries are painful, they are seldom life threatening. Bleeding may be heavy but is usually controllable with local compression. Contusions and other blunt injuries all require careful in-hospital evaluation. However, the urgency for transport will be determined by associated injuries, the amount of hemorrhage, and the presence of shock.

Rectal Bleeding

Rectal bleeding is a common complaint and something that you may hear as a chief complaint or secondary to abdominal or pelvic complaints. Bleeding from the rectum may present as bloodstains or blood soaking through underwear, or patients may report blood in the toilet after a bowel movement or attempted bowel movement. Rectal bleeding can be caused by a sexual assault, rectal foreign bodies, hemorrhoids, colitis, or ulcers of the digestive tract. Significant rectal bleeding can occur after hemorrhoid surgery and can lead to significant blood loss and shock.

Street Smarts

As health care professionals trained in the management of life-threatening emergencies, EMTs and paramedics have learned how to respond in situations others would find terrifying. Over time, what you consider to be an "emergency" and what that word means to a layperson may differ greatly. What has become a routine sight for you may be unfamiliar and frightening for patients and their family. In fact, your routine day may be the worst day of their lives. For this reason, we in EMS must continually remind ourselves to put ourselves in our patients' shoes. Of all the types of care we provide, one of the most meaningful is often overlooked: empathy.

Sexual Assault and Rape

Sexual assault and rape are all-too-common crimes. In the United States, an average of 463,634 individuals 12 years or older become victims of rape or sexual assault each year.[2] Patients, who include both males and females, can sustain various abdominal and genitourinary injuries during these attacks. Treatment for these patients is discussed in Chapter 35, *Patients With Special Challenges.*

YOU are the EMT SUMMARY

1. How do hollow organ injuries differ from solid organ injuries?

Hollow organs, such as the stomach, intestines, and urinary bladder, are structures through which materials pass. When hollow organs are ruptured or lacerated, they release their contents into the pelvis or peritoneal (abdominal) cavity. The release of hollow organ contents into the peritoneal cavity causes an intense inflammatory response (peritonitis), which can result in a life-threatening infection. Hollow organ injury may be associated with some internal bleeding; however, the major cause of death is sepsis, which typically occurs later in the hospital.

Solid organs, such as the liver, spleen, pancreas, and kidneys, are highly vascular and tend to bleed profusely when injured by blunt or penetrating trauma. Unlike hollow organ injury, the major cause of death following injury to the solid organs is internal hemorrhage, which can very quickly lead to death.

2. How should you focus your assessment of a patient with potential intra-abdominal bleeding?

When caring for a patient with blunt or penetrating abdominal trauma, focus on recognizing signs and symptoms of shock, initiating treatment without delay, and providing rapid transport to the hospital.

If your patient sustained blunt abdominal trauma, has external evidence of injury (eg, bruising, distention, rigidity), or signs of shock—all signs that clearly suggest intra-abdominal bleeding—does the origin of the hemorrhage affect the treatment that you provide in the field? The answer, of course, is no. What *does* matter is that *the patient is bleeding from a source that you cannot control* and that the patient's outcome depends on you recognizing the situation, initiating prompt treatment, and providing rapid transport.

3. How should you interpret your primary assessment findings?

Rarely do EMS clinicians actually witness the injury when it occurs; this is why it is so important for you to pay attention to clues that suggest a particular MOI. However, in this situation you did witness the patient being trampled by a bull and were able to see that his injuries appear to be to the abdomen and flanks.

On the basis of the MOI and your primary assessment findings, your initial impression should be that your patient is in shock, which is likely the result of intra-abdominal bleeding. Although you will need to perform a head-to-toe secondary assessment to identify any other injuries, intra-abdominal bleeding is the most plausible field impression given the information that you have. You should quickly identify this patient as a "load and go," begin immediate treatment, and arrange for rapid transport to the hospital.

4. What immediate treatment is indicated for this patient?

Apply oxygen via a nonrebreathing mask at 15 L/min. Oxygen is a critical treatment for any patient with signs and symptoms of shock and should be administered as soon as possible. Carefully monitor the patient's breathing, and be ready to assist his ventilations if signs of inadequate breathing (eg, shallow breaths [reduced tidal volume], decreased mental status) are observed.

Cover the patient with a blanket to keep him warm. Some body functions, such as blood clotting, are negatively affected by decreased body temperature; therefore keeping the patient warm is essential. Patients in shock are also less able to maintain body temperature because heat production requires energy, and energy requires oxygen, so diminished heat production is made worse by a lack of oxygen. In this case, oxygen is also needed as the loss of oxygen-carrying red blood cells reduces perfusion to the vital organs.

5. What are some common bruising patterns and clinical signs associated with intra-abdominal bleeding?

As blood accumulates in the abdominal cavity, the abdomen typically becomes distended and rigid. Palpation of the patient's abdomen can be challenging in the presence of abdominal guarding. Guarding is a conscious (voluntary) or unintentional (involuntary) response to abdominal trauma, and it is characterized by stiffening of the rectus abdominis muscles in an attempt to minimize the pain. Although guarding may be seen in patients who do not have significant intra-abdominal injury, *any abdominal rigidity following trauma should be assumed to be the result of internal bleeding*.

If bruising is observed following abdominal trauma, there are several patterns that you should look for during your assessment of the abdomen.

YOU are the EMT SUMMARY continued

Periumbilical (around the umbilicus) bruising is an indicator of blood in the peritoneal cavity. Bruising to the flank area is an indicator of blood behind the peritoneal cavity and suggests injury to the kidneys, pancreas, pelvis, or bladder.

Injury to the liver or spleen may present with referred pain to the shoulder on the same side. Unlike radiating pain, which is characterized by pain that "moves" from one area of the body to another, referred pain is characterized by pain in two separate locations.

It is important to note that some patients with intra-abdominal bleeding may not present with external signs of injury. The retroperitoneal space is a common location for hidden bleeding and can accommodate a large volume of blood.

6. Why is your patient's condition deteriorating? How should you modify your treatment?

Your patient was exhibiting signs of shock on initial contact with him. His level of consciousness has decreased, he is hypotensive, his breathing is inadequate, and his oxygen saturation is falling despite the use of high-flow oxygen. This indicates that he is now in decompensated shock; the compensatory mechanisms that help maintain adequate perfusion to the tissues and cells of the body are failing.

Any deterioration in a patient's clinical status should prompt you to immediately repeat the primary assessment. His oxygen saturation is falling, which is likely the result of the combined effects of internal bleeding and inadequate breathing. At this point, you should begin assisting his ventilations with a bag-mask device attached to high-flow oxygen. Consider inserting a nasopharyngeal airway; his level of consciousness has decreased to the point that he may not be able to completely maintain his own airway.

Patients who have experienced trauma and who are in shock should be transported in the supine position.

As you continue to treat the patient, you must continuously monitor his ABCs. His condition is critical, and he is at high risk for cardiac arrest. If he becomes apneic and pulseless, begin cardiopulmonary resuscitation and ask your partner to update the receiving facility. An ALS unit would be beneficial for airway management and intravenous (IV) fluid administration if it could be arranged without delaying transport.

7. On the basis of your reassessment, what additional injuries should you suspect?

Bloodstains on the front of the patient's underwear without evidence of any open genitalia injuries indicates that he has blood in his urine (hematuria) and suggests injury to his kidneys, urinary bladder, or both. Remember, the patient had diffuse abdominal pain and abrasions to *both* the anterior part of his abdomen and flanks. In addition to injury to his liver or spleen, which is likely the cause of his shock, it is clearly possible that he experienced injury to his genitourinary organs as well.

As you will recall from your evaluation of the patient, he had pain and abrasions of his flanks; this indicates direct trauma to that area, which overlies the kidneys. Injury to the kidneys may not be obvious during your assessment. If anything, you may see only abrasions or redness over the flanks; flank bruising typically does not manifest until later. Because one of the functions of the kidney is the formation of urine, another sign of kidney injury is hematuria.

Hematuria can also indicate rupture of the urinary bladder. Blood at the urethral opening should also make you suspicious for urinary bladder rupture.

Hematemesis, the vomiting of blood, indicates bleeding within the gastrointestinal tract. More specifically, vomiting bright red blood indicates injury to some part of the upper gastrointestinal tract. You should suspect injury to the patient's stomach.

8. How will your reassessment findings change your current treatment plan?

Despite the presence of indicators that suggest injury to both solid and hollow abdominal and genitourinary organs, you should concentrate on maintaining the patient's airway, ensure adequate oxygenation and ventilation, and treat for shock. There are no other prehospital treatments for the patient's suspected specific injuries. Rapid transport to a trauma center is critical! If the scene location is a distance from the hospital, air transport should be considered. Blunt trauma with internal bleeding is often more likely to be fatal than penetrating abdominal trauma with external bleeding. Blunt trauma with internal bleeding is often more significant than penetrating abdominal trauma with external bleeding. Open injuries are obvious, whereas internal injuries are often hidden and may be missed. In the absence of obvious external injury, a trauma patient with signs of shock should be assumed to be bleeding into the abdomen.

Prep Kit

Ready for Review

- Abdominal injuries are categorized as either open (penetrating wounds and evisceration) or closed (blunt force trauma).
- Either classification of injury can result in injury to the hollow or solid organs of the abdomen and cause significant life-threatening bleeding.
- Blunt force trauma that causes closed injuries results from an object striking the body without breaking the skin, such as when the abdomen is struck with a baseball bat or when the patient's body strikes the steering wheel during a motor vehicle crash.
- Penetrating trauma is often a result of a gunshot wound or stab wound. Other MOIs such as a fall on an object can also cause penetrating trauma to the abdomen.
- Injury to the solid organs often causes significant internal bleeding that can be life threatening.
- Injury to the hollow organs of the abdomen may cause irritation and inflammation to the peritoneum as caustic digestive juices leak into the peritoneum. A serious infection may also occur over several hours.
- Always maintain a high index of suspicion for serious intra-abdominal injury in the trauma patient, particularly in the patient who exhibits unexplained signs of shock.
- Assess the abdomen for signs of bruising, rigidity, penetrating injuries, and pain.
- Never remove an impaled object from the abdominal region. Secure it in place with a large bulky dressing and provide rapid transport. When the MOI is penetrating trauma, spinal motion restriction is usually not indicated (follow local protocol).
- Be prepared to treat the patient for shock. Place the patient supine, keep the patient warm, and provide high-flow oxygen.
- If an organ protrudes from an open injury to the abdomen (evisceration), do not attempt to place the organ back inside the abdomen. Instead, keep the organ moist and warm. Cover the injury site with a large, sterile, moist, bulky dressing and an occlusive dressing, if specified by local protocol.
- Injuries to the kidneys may be difficult to detect because they are located in the well-protected region of the body. Be alert to bruising or a hematoma in the flank region.
- Injury to the external male or female genitalia is very painful for patients but is usually not life threatening.

Vital Vocabulary

closed abdominal injury An injury in which there is soft-tissue damage inside the body but the skin remains intact.

evisceration The displacement of organs outside of the body.

flank The region below the rib cage and above the hip.

guarding Muscle contractions of the abdominal wall to minimize the pain of abdominal movement. It may occur through conscious effort of the patient or involuntarily, in which case it is a sign of peritonitis.

hematuria Blood in the urine.

hollow organs Structures through which materials pass, such as the stomach, small intestines, large intestines, ureters, and urinary bladder.

melena Black, foul-smelling, tarry stool containing digested blood.

open abdominal injury An injury in which there is a break in the surface of the skin or mucous membrane, exposing deeper tissue to potential contamination.

peritoneal cavity The abdominal cavity.

peritoneum The membrane lining the abdominal cavity (parietal peritoneum) and covering the abdominal organs (visceral peritoneum).

Prep Kit continued

peritonitis Inflammation of the peritoneum.

retroperitoneum The potential space located posterior to the peritoneal cavity of the abdomen.

solid organs Solid masses of tissue where much of the chemical work of the body takes place (eg, liver, spleen, pancreas, kidneys).

References

1. McGready JB, Breyer BN. Current epidemiology of genitourinary trauma. *Urol Clin North Am*. 2013;40(3): 323–334.
2. Victims of sexual violence: statistics. RAINN website. https://www.rainn.org/statistics/victims-sexual-violence. Accessed March 3, 2025.

Additional Resources

National Association of Emergency Medical Technicians. *PHTLS: Prehospital Trauma Life Support*. 10th ed. Burlington, MA: Jones & Bartlett Learning; 2023.

National Association of State EMS Officials. *National Model EMS Clinical Guidelines: Version 3.0*. https://nasemso.org/content.aspx?page_id=22&club_id=157064&module_id=701974. Updated March 2022. Accessed March 3, 2025.

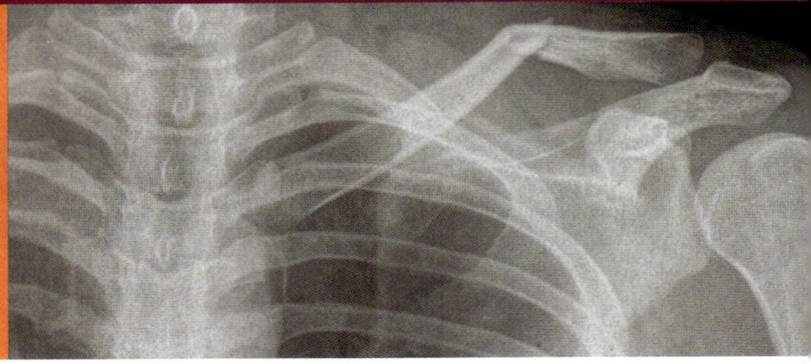

Chapter 31

Orthopaedic Injuries

NATIONAL EMS EDUCATION STANDARD COMPETENCIES

Trauma

Applies knowledge to provide basic emergency care and transportation based on assessment findings for an acutely injured patient.

Orthopaedic Trauma

- Open fractures (pp 1146–1149, 1156–1157)
- Closed fractures (pp 1146–1149, 1156–1157)
- Dislocations (pp 1149–1150, 1181–1183)
- Amputations/replantation (pp 1151, 1176, 1185)
- Upper and lower extremity orthopaedic trauma (pp 1167–1171, 1174–1185)
- Sprains/strains (pp 1150–1154, 1184–1185)
- Pelvic fractures (pp 1172–1173)

Medicine

Applies knowledge to provide basic emergency care and transportation based on assessment findings for an acutely ill patient.

Nontraumatic Musculoskeletal Disorders

- Nontraumatic fractures (pp 1144–1145)

KNOWLEDGE OBJECTIVES

1. Describe the anatomy and physiology of the musculoskeletal system. (pp 1139–1143)
2. Recognize the unique risk factors for musculoskeletal injury and disease common in pediatric and geriatric patients. (pp 1143–1145)
3. Explain the different mechanisms of musculoskeletal injury. (pp 1145–1146)
4. Describe the different types of musculoskeletal injuries, including fractures, dislocations, amputations, sprains, and strains. (pp 1145–1151)
5. Recognize the characteristics of specific types of musculoskeletal injuries. (pp 1145–1151)
6. Differentiate between open and closed fractures. (pp 1146–1149)
7. Explain how to assess the severity of an injury. (p 1154)
8. Describe the emergency medical care of the patient with an orthopaedic injury. (pp 1156–1162)
9. Describe the emergency medical care of the patient with a swollen, painful, deformed extremity (fracture). (pp 1156–1157)
10. Discuss the need for, general rules of, and possible complications of splinting. (pp 1157–1159)
11. Explain the reasons for splinting fractures, dislocations, and sprains at the scene versus transporting the patient immediately. (pp 1157–1159)
12. Describe the emergency medical care of the patient with an amputation. (pp 1185–1186)

SKILLS OBJECTIVES

1. Demonstrate how to apply a rigid splint. (p 1160; Skill Drill 31-1)
2. Demonstrate how to apply a vacuum splint. (p 1162; Skill Drill 31-2)
3. Demonstrate how to splint the hand and wrist. (p 1171; Skill Drill 31-3)
4. Demonstrate how to apply a Hare traction splint. (pp 1177–1178; Skill Drill 31-4)
5. Demonstrate how to apply a Slishman traction splint. (pp 1179–1180; Skill Drill 31-5)
6. Demonstrate how to splint the clavicle, the scapula, the shoulder, the humerus, the elbow, and the forearm. (pp 1163–1170)
7. Demonstrate how to care for a patient with an amputation. (pp 1185–1186)

Introduction

The musculoskeletal system is fundamental to human form, posture, and movement. It also helps protect the body's vital internal organs from external forces. This system of bones, voluntary muscles, tendons, cartilage, and ligaments is designed to allow people to enjoy a healthy, active lifestyle. When it is injured, however, a person may struggle with mobility limitations and chronic pain.

Musculoskeletal injuries are among the most common reasons patients seek medical attention. In the United States, approximately 8% of emergency department (ED) visits relate to musculoskeletal complaints, and some research estimates that 30% of ED and urgent care visits result from musculoskeletal injury.[1] As an EMT, you will regularly encounter injuries to this body system.

Musculoskeletal system injuries are often easily identified because of pain, swelling, and deformity. Although these injuries are less frequently fatal than injuries to vital organs, they often result in short- and long-term disability. By providing prompt assessment and treatment such as splinting, EMTs may not only help relieve pain, but also reduce disability. Although these injuries can appear dramatic, do not focus solely on a musculoskeletal injury without first determining that no life-threatening injuries exist. Never forget the XABCs (Exsanguinating hemorrhage, Airway, Breathing, and Circulation).

This chapter begins with a review of the musculoskeletal anatomy. Various types and causes of musculoskeletal injuries in general are identified, and the assessment and treatment process for each is explained, followed by a detailed discussion of splinting. The chapter then focuses on specific musculoskeletal injuries, beginning at the clavicle and ending at the feet.

Anatomy and Physiology of the Musculoskeletal System

Muscles

The muscular system includes three types of muscles: skeletal, smooth, and cardiac.

Skeletal muscle, also called striated muscle because of its characteristic stripes, attaches to the bones and usually crosses at least one joint. This type of muscle is also called voluntary muscle because it is under direct voluntary control of the brain, responding to commands to move specific body parts (**FIGURE 31-1**). Usually, movement is the result of several muscles contracting and relaxing simultaneously. Skeletal muscle makes up the largest portion of the body's muscle mass. Its primary functions are movement and posture.

All skeletal muscles are supplied with arteries, veins, and nerves. Blood from the arteries brings oxygen, glucose, and nutrients to the muscles (**FIGURE 31-2**). Waste products, including carbon dioxide and lactic acid, are carried away in the veins. Disease or trauma can result in the loss of a muscle's nervous supply; this, in turn, can lead to weakness and eventually atrophy, or a decrease in the size of the muscle and its inherent ability to function. Skeletal muscle tissue is directly attached to the bone by tough, ropelike structures known as **tendons**. **Fascia** (fibrous tissue) surrounds and supports the muscles and neurovascular structures.

Smooth muscle, also called involuntary muscle because it is not under voluntary control of the brain, performs much of the automatic work of the body. This type of muscle is found in the walls of most tubular structures of the body, such as the gastrointestinal tract and the blood vessels. Smooth muscle contracts and relaxes to control the

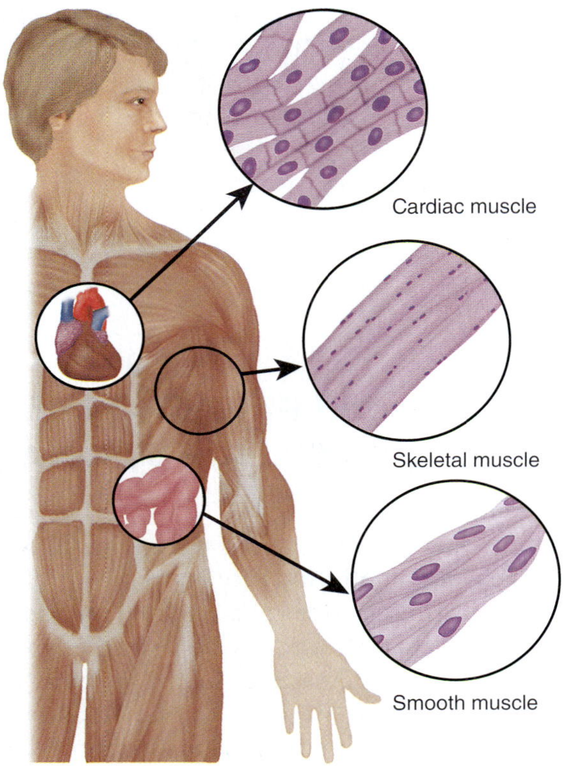

FIGURE 31-1 For musculoskeletal injuries, the major muscle type involved is skeletal muscle.

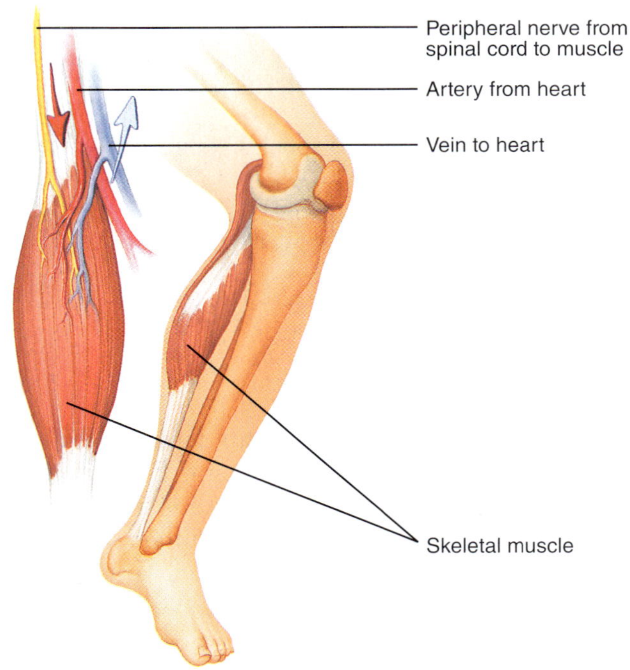

FIGURE 31-2 Skeletal muscles are supplied by arteries, veins, and nerves that respectively bring oxygen and nutrients, carry away waste products, and conduct nervous stimuli.

movement of the contents within these structures (**FIGURE 31-3**).

The heart neither looks nor acts like skeletal or smooth muscle. It is composed largely of cardiac muscle, a specifically adapted involuntary muscle with its own regulatory system. The remainder of this chapter is concerned exclusively with skeletal muscle.

The Skeleton

The skeleton, which gives us our recognizable human form, protects our vital internal organs, and allows us to move, is composed of approximately 206 bones (**FIGURE 31-4**). The bones in the skeleton also produce blood cells (in the bone marrow) and serve as a reservoir for important minerals and electrolytes.

The skull is a solid, vaultlike structure that surrounds and protects the brain. The thoracic cage protects the heart, lungs, and great vessels; the lower ribs protect the liver and spleen. The bony spinal canal encases and protects the spinal cord.

The pectoral girdle, also referred to as the shoulder girdle, consists of two scapulae and two clavicles (**FIGURE 31-5**). The scapula (shoulder blade) is a flat, triangular bone held to the rib cage by powerful

YOU are the EMT

At 1620 hours, you are dispatched to a soccer field for a player with a possible broken leg. You and your partner proceed to the scene, with a response time of approximately 5 minutes. En route, dispatch advises you that the patient is conscious, alert, and breathing. The weather is overcast, the temperature is 88°F (31°C), and the traffic is moderate.

1. Under which circumstances can orthopaedic injuries pose a threat to a patient's life?
2. Given the information you have, can you rule out a critical injury?

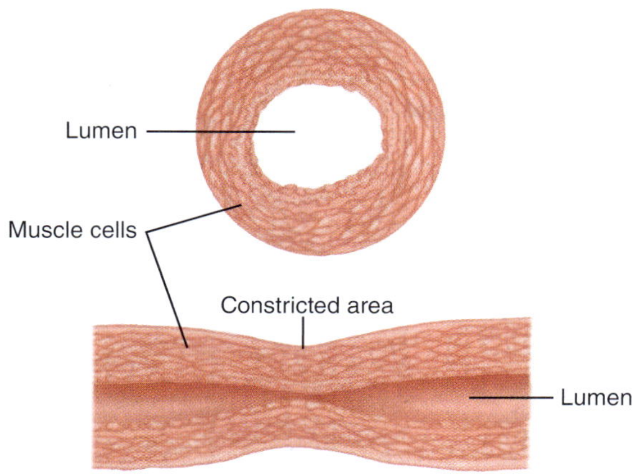

FIGURE 31-3 Smooth muscle is found in the walls of most tubular structures in the body. These muscles contract and relax to control the movement of the contents within these structures.

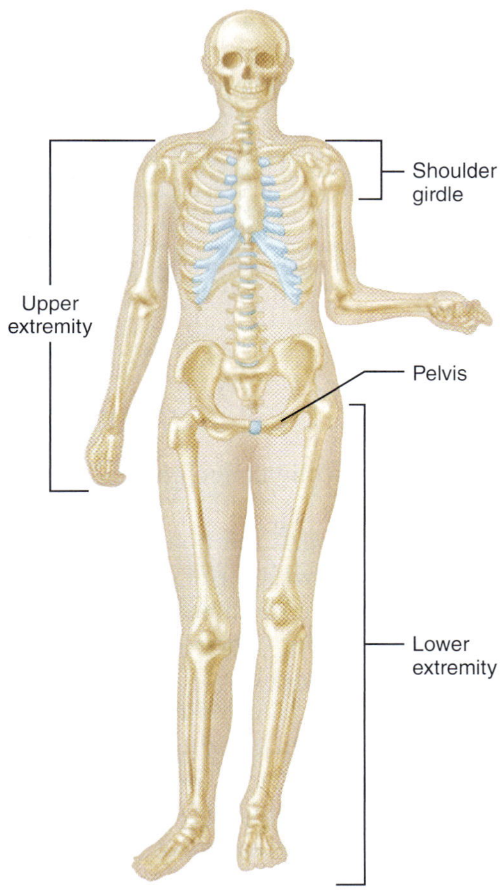

FIGURE 31-4 The human skeleton, consisting of approximately 206 bones, gives us our form and protects our vital organs.

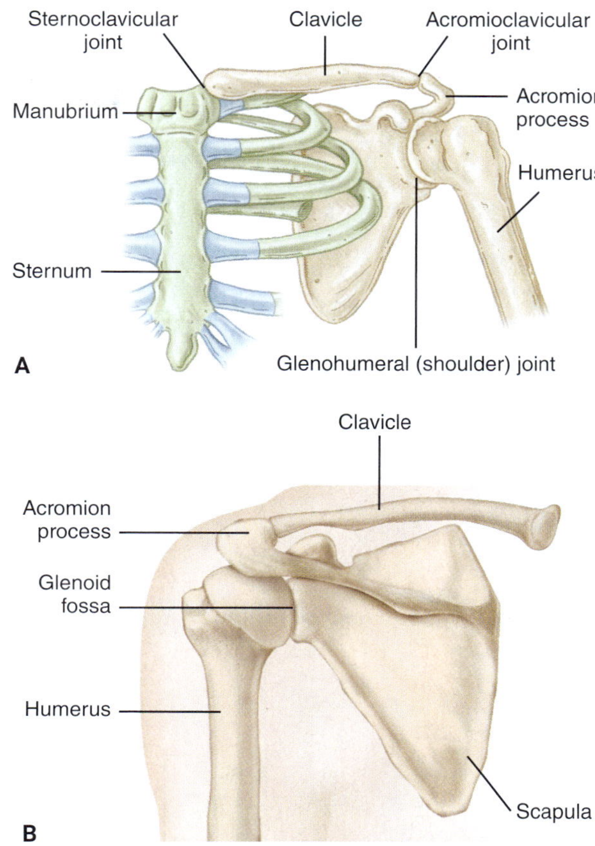

FIGURE 31-5 The pectoral girdle. **A.** Anterior view, including the clavicle. **B.** Posterior view, including the scapula.

muscles that buffer it against injury. The clavicle (collarbone) is a slender, S-shaped bone attached by ligaments to the sternum on one end and to the acromion process on the other. The clavicle acts as a strut to keep the shoulder propped up; however, because it is slender and very exposed, this bone is vulnerable to injury.

The upper extremity extends from the shoulder to the fingertips. The arm is composed of the upper arm (humerus), elbow, and forearm (radius and ulna) (**FIGURE 31-6**). The upper extremity joins the shoulder girdle at the glenohumeral joint. The upper extremity begins with the humerus. The humerus connects with the bones of the forearm, the radius and ulna, to form the hinged elbow joint.

The radius and ulna make up the forearm. The radius, the larger of the two forearm bones, lies on the thumb side of the forearm. The ulna is narrow and is on the little finger side of the forearm.

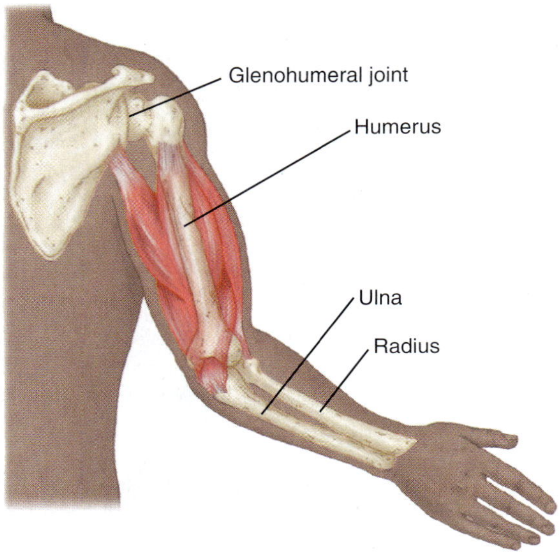

FIGURE 31-6 The anatomy of the arm.

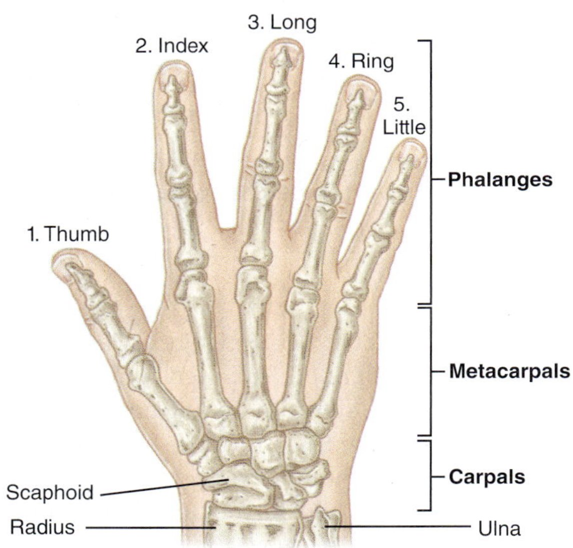

FIGURE 31-7 The anatomy of the wrist and hand.

Because the radius and the ulna are connected by relatively stiff ligaments at both ends, when one is broken, the other is often broken as well.

The hand contains three sets of bones: carpals (wrist bones), metacarpals (hand bones), and phalanges (finger bones) (**FIGURE 31-7**). The carpals are vulnerable to fracture when a person falls on an outstretched hand. Phalanges are more apt to be injured by a crush injury, such as being slammed in a door.

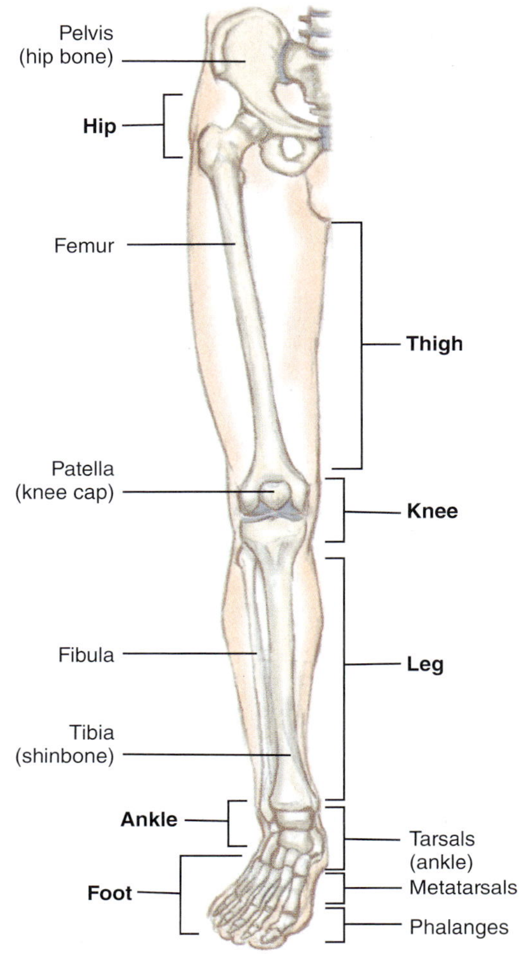

FIGURE 31-8 The bones of the thigh, leg, and foot.

The pelvis supports the body weight and protects the structures within the pelvis: the bladder, rectum, and female reproductive organs. The pelvic girdle is three separate bones—the ischium, ilium, and pubis—fused together to form the innominate (or hip) bone. The two iliac bones are joined posteriorly by tough ligaments to the sacrum at the sacroiliac joints; the two pubic bones are connected anteriorly by equally tough ligaments at the pubic symphysis. These joints allow very little motion so that the pelvic ring is strong and stable.

The lower extremity consists of the bones of the thigh, leg, and foot (**FIGURE 31-8**). The femur (thighbone) is a long, powerful bone that connects in the ball-and-socket joint of the hip and in the hinge joint of the knee. The femoral *head* is the ball-shaped part that fits into the acetabulum (hip socket). It is connected to the *shaft* (diaphysis), or long tubular portion of the femur, by the femoral *neck*. The femoral neck is a common site for fractures, generally referred to as hip fractures, especially in the older population. The greater trochanter and lesser trochanter are the names given to the respective lateral and medial bony protuberances below the femoral neck and just above the shaft of the femur.

The lower leg consists of two bones, the tibia and the fibula. The **tibia** (shinbone) is the larger of the two leg bones and is responsible for supporting the major weight-bearing surfaces of the knee and ankle. The tibia connects to the patella (kneecap) via the patellar tendon just below the knee joint and runs down the front of the lower leg. The tibia is vulnerable to direct blows and can be felt just beneath the skin. The much smaller **fibula** runs along the lateral side of the tibia and slightly posterior to it. The fibula is an important anchor for ligaments surrounding the knee joint, and it forms the lateral side of the ankle joint.

The foot consists of three types of bones: tarsals (ankle and hindfoot bones), metatarsals (foot and forefoot bones), and phalanges (toe bones) (**FIGURE 31-9**). The largest of the tarsal bones is the heel bone, or **calcaneus**, which is subject to injury with axial loading, such as when a person jumps from a height and lands on their feet.

The bones of the skeleton provide a framework to which the muscles and tendons are attached. Bone is a living tissue that contains nerves and receives oxygen and nutrients from the arterial system. Therefore, when a bone breaks, a patient

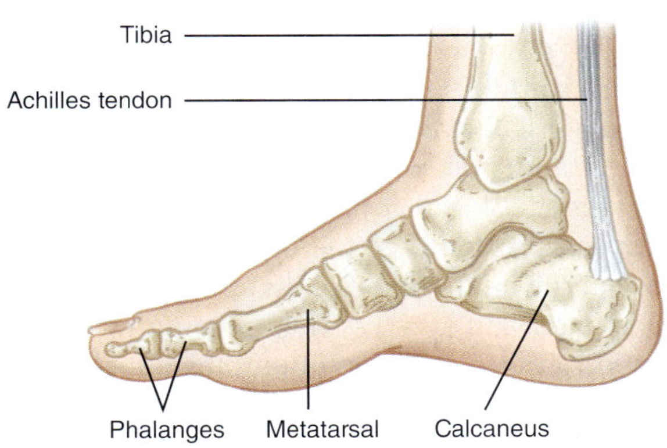

FIGURE 31-9 The bones of the foot and ankle.

typically experiences severe pain and bleeding. Bone marrow, located in the center of each bone, produces red and white blood cells and platelets.

A **joint** is formed wherever two bones come into contact. The sternoclavicular joint, for example, is where the sternum and the clavicle come together. Most joints are held together in a tough, fibrous structure known as a capsule, which is supported and strengthened in certain key areas by bands of fibrous tissue called **ligaments**. In moving joints, the ends of the bones are covered with a thin layer of cartilage known as **articular cartilage**. This cartilage is a pearly white substance that allows the ends of the bones to glide easily. Most joints are bathed and lubricated by synovial (joint) fluid.

Some joints, such as the shoulder, allow motion to occur in a circular manner. Other joints, such as the knee and elbow, act as hinges. Still other joints, including the sacroiliac joint in the lower back and the sternoclavicular joints, allow only a minimum amount of motion. Certain joints, such as the sutures in the skull (present until approximately 18 months of age), fuse together during growth to create a solid, immobile, bony structure (**FIGURE 31-10**).

Pathophysiology of the Musculoskeletal System

A person's risk of having a musculoskeletal disorder or sustaining an injury relates to many factors, including the person's overall health and nutrition, comorbid conditions, and hereditary and congenital conditions. In particular, the body's physical development during childhood and the effects of aging during later adulthood present unique considerations relating to the musculoskeletal system.

Children

Children have immature bones with active growth centers. Growth of long bones occurs from the ends at specialized growth plates. Growth plate injuries in children are common, especially around the wrist, elbow, knee, and ankle. Injuries tend to occur through these cartilaginous growth centers because they are inherently weaker than the surrounding bone. In general, children's bones bend more easily than adults' bones. As a result, greenstick fractures (described later in the chapter) can occur.

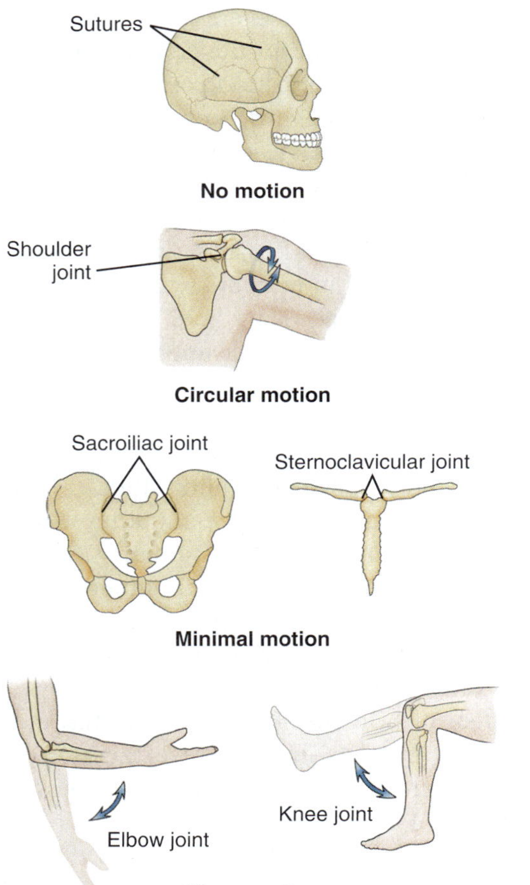

FIGURE 31-10 Joints have many functions. Some joints allow for motion to occur in a circular manner; others act as hinges. Still others allow only minimal motion or none at all.

Older Adults

Aging brings a widespread decrease in bone mass in men and women. Bones become more brittle and tend to break more easily. The disks between the vertebrae of the spine begin to narrow, and a decrease in height of between 2 and 3 inches (5 and 8 cm) may occur through the lifespan, along with changes in posture. Joints lose their flexibility and motion may be further affected by arthritic changes. In fact, more than one-half of all older people have some form of arthritis. A decrease in the amount of muscle mass often results in less strength.

The older adult's muscle system atrophies and weakens with age. Muscle fibers become smaller and fewer, motor neurons decline in number, and strength declines. The ligaments and cartilage of the joints lose their elasticity. Cartilage also goes through degenerative changes with aging, contributing to arthritis.

The stooped posture of older people comes from atrophy of the supporting structures of the body. Two of every three older adult patients will show some degree of **kyphosis** (a forward curving of the upper spine, also called humpback or hunchback). A loss of height in older adults generally results from compression in the spinal column, first in the disks and then from the process of osteoporosis in the vertebral bodies.

Osteoporosis, a condition that affects both men and women, but especially postmenopausal women, is characterized by a decrease in bone mass leading to reduction in bone strength and greater susceptibility to fracture. The extent of bone loss that a person undergoes is influenced by numerous factors, including the person's physical activity level, genetics, smoking, diet, alcohol consumption, hormonal factors, and body weight. Because rapid bone loss may occur in women during the years following menopause, calcium and vitamin D supplementation is encouraged, and many other medications, such as bisphosphonates, may be prescribed by the woman's physician to improve bone strength. Older people should remain active and engage in a low-impact exercise program to maintain bone and muscle strength.

Osteoarthritis is a progressive disease of the joints that destroys cartilage, promotes the formation of bone spurs in joints, and leads to joint stiffness. This type of arthritis is thought to result from "wear and tear" and, in some cases, from repetitive trauma to the joints. It affects approximately 10% of US adults, nearly one-half of whom are 65 years or older. Its prevalence is trending upward as the population continues to age and more individuals experience risk factors such as diabetes and obesity.[2] Women and non-Hispanic White patients represent higher risk categories. Typically, osteoarthritis affects several joints of the body, most commonly those in the hands, knees, hips, and spine. Patients report pain and stiffness that become worse with exertion. The end result is often substantial disability and disfigurement. Patients are typically treated first with anti-inflammatory medications and physical therapy to improve the range of motion. Joint replacement surgery is often effective for arthritis of the hip, knee, ankle, and shoulder when nonsurgical treatment fails.

The effects of these conditions can be both physical, such as decreased balance, coordination, and mobility, as well as psychological, such as fear of engaging in certain activities or depression regarding lost function. Moreover, recovering from musculoskeletal injuries can be complicated for an older adult, especially one with a compromised immune system or diabetes. The fact that the person may be bedridden for a considerable amount of time may inhibit their ability to continue to live independently.

Musculoskeletal Injuries

Injury to bones and joints is often associated with injury to the surrounding soft tissues, especially to the adjacent nerves and blood vessels. The entire area is known as the **zone of injury** (**FIGURE 31-11**). Depending on the amount of kinetic energy the tissues absorb from forces acting on the body, the zone may extend to a distant point. For this reason, you should not become distracted by a patient's obvious injury; you must first complete a primary assessment to check for life-threatening injuries. This is especially true in assessing damage from high-energy trauma, which is discussed next.

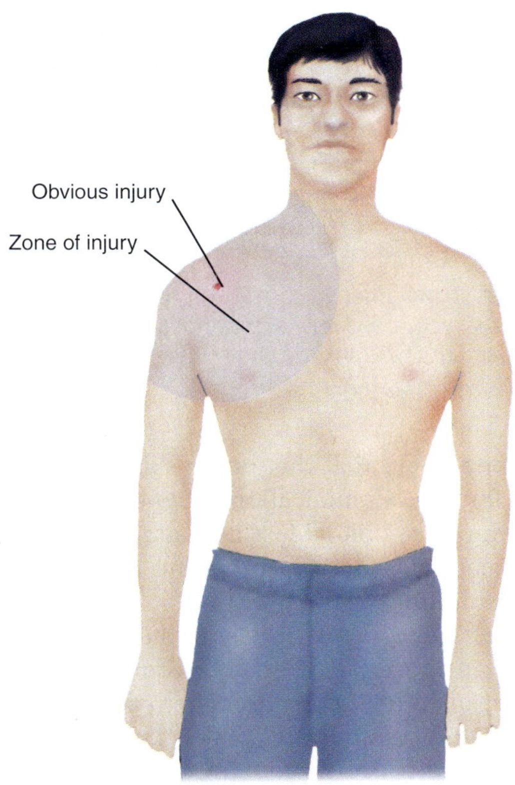

FIGURE 31-11 The zone of injury is the area of soft tissue, including the adjacent nerves and blood vessels, that surrounds the obvious injury of a bone or joint.

Mechanism of Injury

Significant force is generally required to cause fractures and dislocations. This force may be applied to the limb in any of the following ways (**FIGURE 31-12**):

- Direct blows
- Indirect forces
- Twisting forces
- High-energy injuries

A direct blow can result in fracture of the bone at the point of impact. An example is the patella (kneecap) that fractures when it strikes the dashboard in a motor vehicle crash.

Alternatively, the resultant force may cause a fracture or dislocation at a distant point, as when a person falls and lands on an outstretched hand. The direct impact may cause a wrist fracture, but the resultant force can also cause dislocation of the elbow or a fracture of the forearm, humerus, or even clavicle. Therefore, when you are caring for patients who have fallen, immediately identify the point of contact and the mechanism of injury (MOI) so that you decrease the risk of overlooking any associated injuries.

Twisting forces are a common cause of musculoskeletal injury, especially to the anterior cruciate ligament (ACL) or the medial cruciate ligament (MCL) in the knee. Skiing injuries often happen because of twisting: A ski becomes caught and the skier falls, applying a twisting force to the lower extremity.

High-energy injuries, such as those that result from motor vehicle crashes, falls from heights, gunshot wounds, and other extreme forces, produce severe damage to the skeleton, surrounding soft tissues, and vital internal organs. A patient may have multiple injuries to many body parts, including more than one fracture or dislocation in a single limb.

A significant MOI is not always necessary to fracture a bone. A slight force can easily fracture a bone that is weakened by a tumor, infection, or

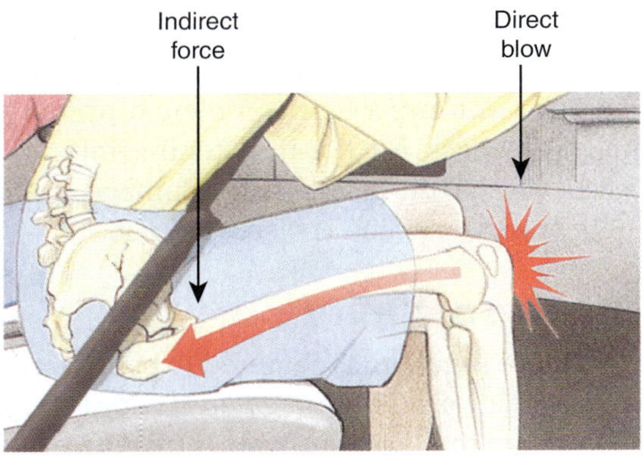

A

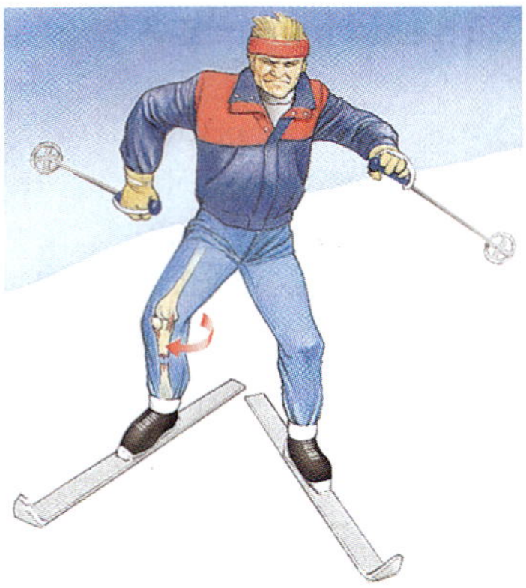

B

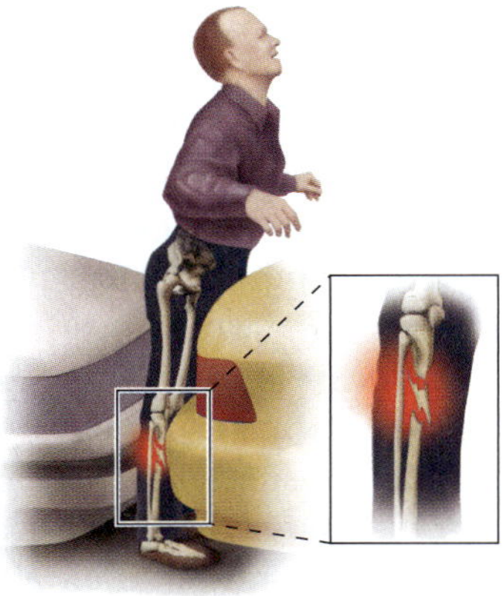

C

FIGURE 31-12 Significant force is required to cause fractures or dislocations. Among these are (**A**) direct blows and indirect forces, (**B**) twisting forces, and (**C**) high-energy crush injuries.

osteoporosis. In geriatric patients with osteoporosis, minor falls or simple twisting injuries can cause a fracture, most often of the wrist, spine, or hip. You should suspect the presence of a fracture in any older adult who reports pain and has sustained even a mild injury.

Fractures

A **fracture** is a broken bone. More precisely, it is a break in the continuity of the bone, often occurring as a result of an external force. The break can occur anywhere on the surface of the bone and in many different types of patterns. Contrary to a common misconception, there is no difference between a broken bone and a fractured bone. A potential complication of fractures is compartment syndrome (discussed later in the chapter), which refers to elevated pressure within a fascial compartment.

Fractures are classified as either closed or open. In assessing and treating patients with possible fractures or dislocations, your first priority is to determine whether the overlying skin is damaged. If it is not, the patient has a **closed fracture**. However, making this determination is not always as easy as it sounds. With an **open fracture**, there is an external wound, caused either by the same blow that fractured the bone or by the broken bone ends lacerating the skin (**FIGURE 31-13**). The wound may vary in size from a small puncture to a gaping tear that exposes bone and soft tissue. Regardless of the extent and severity of the damage to the skin, you should treat any injury that breaks the skin as a possible open fracture. Complications of open fractures include increased blood loss and a higher likelihood of infection. Be sure to wear gloves if there are any open wounds.

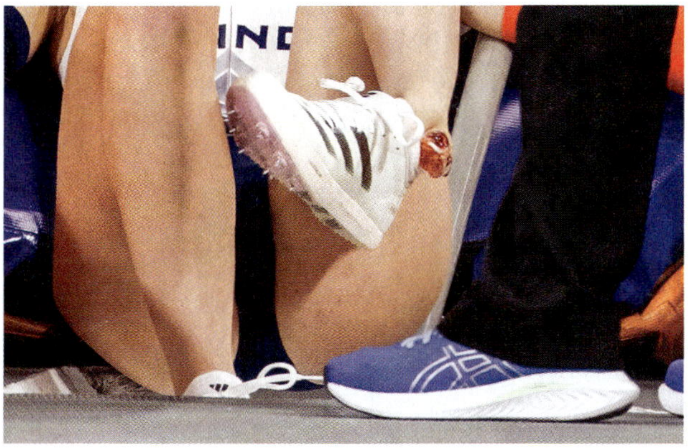

FIGURE 31-13 A fracture can occur anywhere on the surface of a bone and may or may not break the skin. An open fracture of the ankle is shown here.

Fractures are also described by whether the bone is moved from its normal position. A **nondisplaced fracture** (sometimes called a hairline fracture) is a simple crack of the bone that may be difficult to distinguish from a sprain or simple contusion. Radiographic examinations are required for physicians to diagnose a nondisplaced fracture. A **displaced fracture** produces actual deformity, or distortion, of the limb by shortening, rotating, or

Words of Wisdom

The terms *fracture* and *break* mean the same thing. If a bone is fractured, it is by definition broken, and if it is broken, it is by definition fractured. As an EMT, you should understand that regardless of which term the patient or another clinician uses, they are describing the same injury.

angulating it. Often, the deformity is obvious and can be associated with crepitus. However, in some cases the deformity is minimal. Be sure to look for differences between the injured limb and the opposite uninjured limb in any patient with a suspected fracture of an extremity (**FIGURE 31-14**).

Medical clinicians use special terms to describe specific types of fractures (**FIGURE 31-15**):

- **Comminuted.** A fracture in which the bone is broken into more than two fragments.
- **Epiphyseal.** A fracture that occurs in a growth section of a child's bone and may result in growth abnormalities.
- **Greenstick.** An incomplete fracture that passes only partway through the shaft of a bone but may still cause substantial angulation; occurs in children.
- **Incomplete.** A fracture that does not run completely through the bone; a nondisplaced partial crack.
- **Oblique.** A fracture in which the bone is broken at an angle across the bone. This is usually the result of a sharp, angled blow to the bone.
- **Pathologic.** A fracture of weakened or diseased bone, seen in patients with osteoporosis, infection, or cancer; often produced by minimal force. Osteogenesis imperfecta, commonly referred to as brittle bone disease, is a rare genetic condition seen most commonly in children.
- **Spiral.** A fracture caused by a twisting or spinning force, causing a long, spiral-shaped break in the bone. This is sometimes the result of abuse in young children.
- **Transverse.** A fracture that occurs straight across the bone. This is usually the result of a direct and relatively high-energy blow.

Suspect a fracture if any of the following signs are present in a patient who has a history of injury and reports pain.

Deformity

The limb may appear to be shortened, rotated, or angulated at a point where there is no joint (**FIGURE 31-16**). Always use the opposite, uninjured limb as a mirror image for comparison.

Tenderness

Point tenderness on palpation in the zone of injury is the most reliable indicator of an underlying fracture, although it does not tell you the type of fracture (**FIGURE 31-17**).

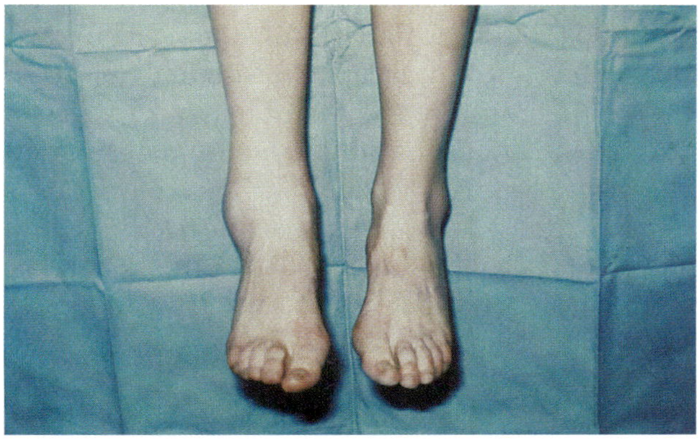

FIGURE 31-14 Always compare the injured limb with the uninjured limb when checking for deformity.

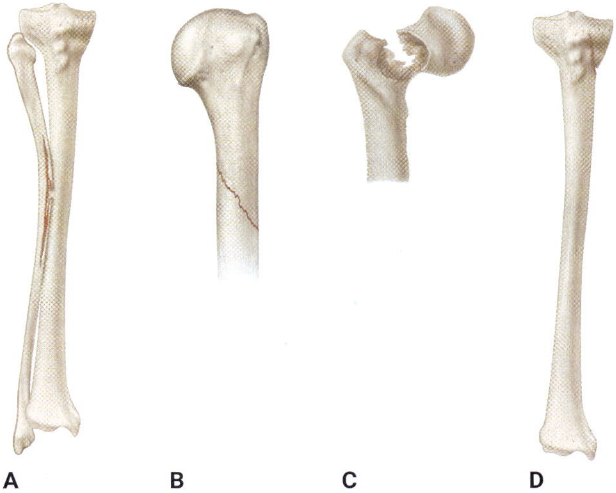

FIGURE 31-15 Special terms to describe fractures. **A.** Greenstick fracture. **B.** Oblique fracture. **C.** Pathologic fracture. **D.** Incomplete fracture.

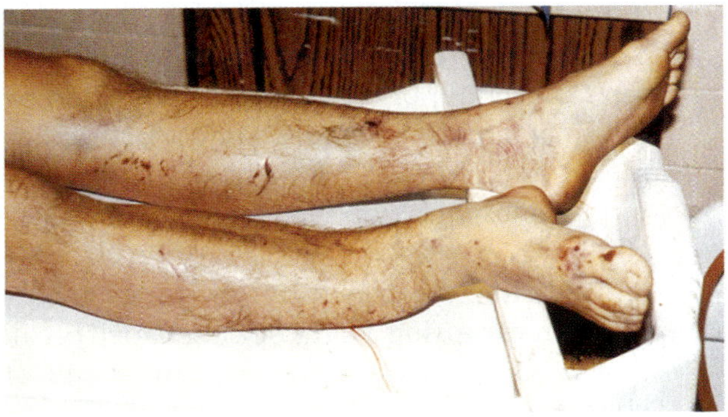

FIGURE 31-16 Obvious deformity, shortening, rotation, or angulation should increase your index of suspicion for a fracture.

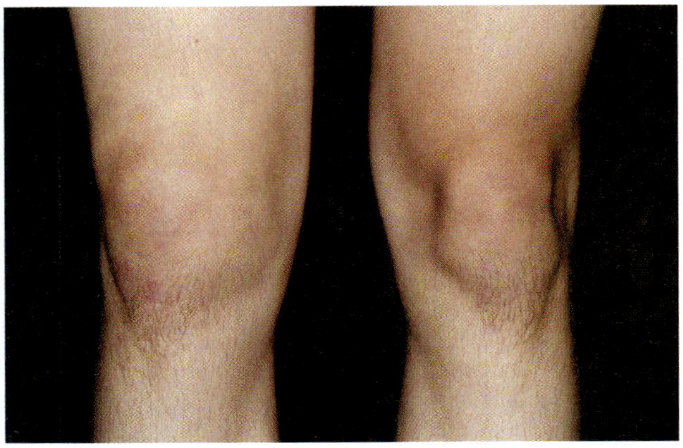

FIGURE 31-18 Swelling that occurs in association with a fracture can often mask deformity of the limb.

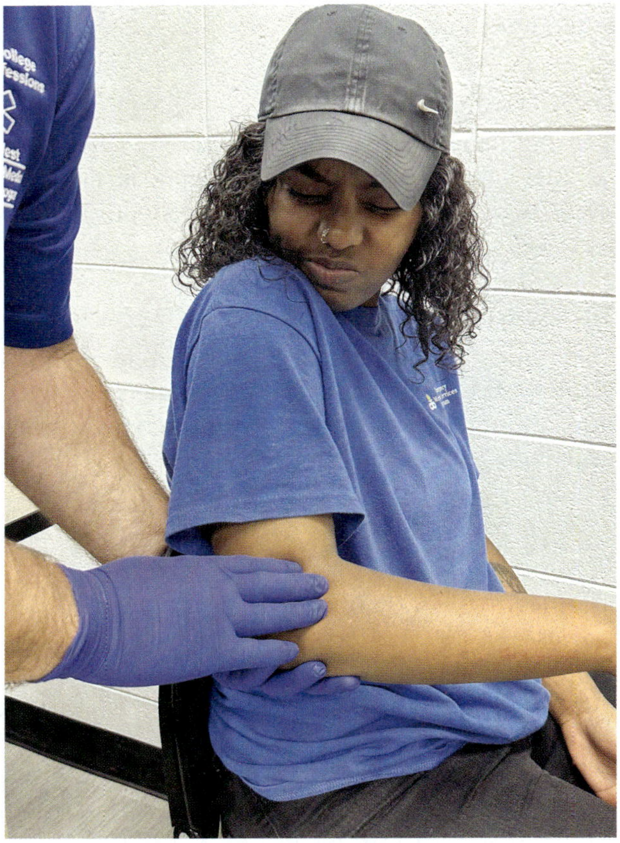

FIGURE 31-17 Point tenderness is pain elicited by palpation with a finger at the site of an injury.

Guarding

In the context of bone fractures, guarding (or muscle guarding) refers to the involuntary contraction of muscles around a fracture to prevent any movement. This restriction of the bone's movement is the body's way of minimizing pain. Guarding does not occur with all fractures; some patients may continue to use the injured part for a time. Occasionally, nondisplaced fractures are less painful, and there is minimal soft-tissue damage.

Swelling

Rapid swelling usually indicates bleeding from a fracture or significant soft-tissue injury and is typically followed by substantial pain. Often, if the swelling is severe, it may mask deformity of the limb (**FIGURE 31-18**). Generalized swelling from fluid buildup may occur several hours after an injury.

Bruising

Fractures are almost always associated with **ecchymosis** (discoloration) of the surrounding soft tissues (**FIGURE 31-19**). Bruising may be present after almost any injury and may take hours to develop; it is not specific to bone or joint injuries. The discoloration associated with acute injuries is usually redness, as you may have seen with someone who has been punched. Within hours or days, blue, purple, and black discoloration will appear, followed by yellow and green.

Crepitus

A grating or grinding sensation known as **crepitus** can be felt and sometimes even heard when fractured bone ends rub together.

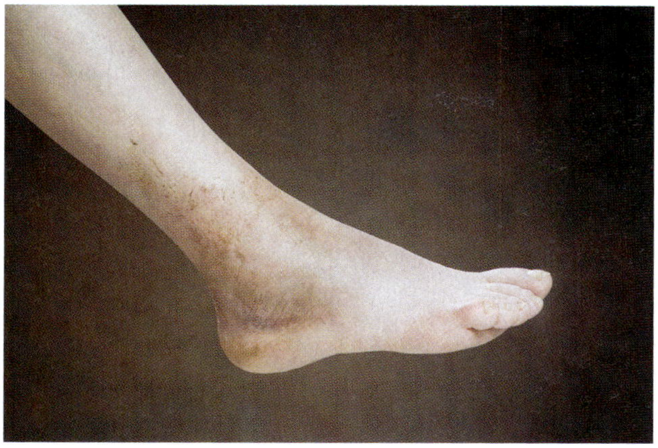

FIGURE 31-19 Fractures almost always have associated bruising into the surrounding soft tissue.

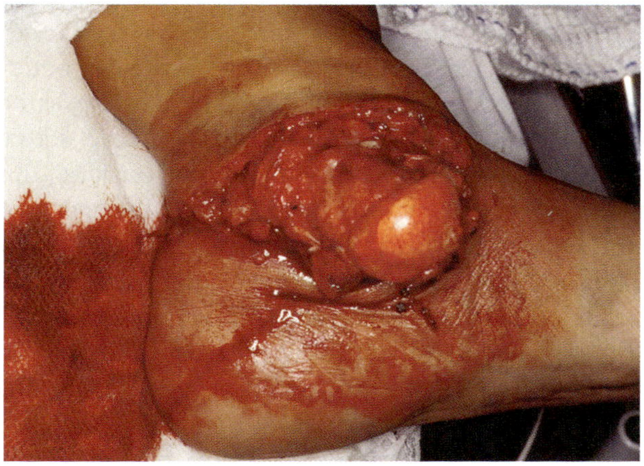

FIGURE 31-20 Bone ends may protrude through the skin or be visible within the wound of an open fracture.

False Motion

Also called free movement, **false motion** is any motion at a point in the limb where there is no joint and therefore motion is not expected to occur. It is an indication of a fracture.

Exposed Fragments

In open fractures, bone ends may protrude through the skin or be visible within the wound (**FIGURE 31-20**). *Never* attempt to push the end of a protruding bone back into place. Doing so could increase the risk for infection.

Pain

Pain, along with tenderness, bruising, and bleeding, commonly occurs in association with fractures. Remember to use the OPQRST mnemonic to assess pain: Onset, Provocation/palliation, Quality, Region/radiation, Severity, and Timing.

Locked Joint

A joint that is locked into position is difficult and painful to move. Do not manipulate the limb excessively in an effort to elicit these signs. This sign is more commonly the result of a soft-tissue injury within the joint (typically the knee or elbow), but the presence of a locked joint should alert you to the possibility of an underlying fracture or cartilage injury.

Dislocations

A **dislocation** is a disruption of a joint in which the bone ends are no longer in contact. The supporting ligaments are often torn, usually completely, allowing the bone ends to separate from each other (**FIGURE 31-21**). A fracture–dislocation is a combination injury at the joint, in which the joint is dislocated and there is a fracture of the end of one or more of the bones.

A dislocated joint may sometimes spontaneously **reduce**, or return to its normal position, before your assessment. In this situation, you will be able to confirm the dislocation only by taking a patient history. However, the joint surfaces often remain completely separated from one another. A dislocation that does not spontaneously reduce is a serious problem. The ends of the bone can be locked in a displaced position, making any motion of the joint difficult and painful. Commonly dislocated joints include the fingers, shoulder, elbow, hip, and knee.

The signs and symptoms of a dislocated joint are similar to those of a fracture (**FIGURE 31-22**):

- Marked deformity
- Swelling
- Pain that is aggravated by any attempt at movement
- Tenderness on palpation
- Loss of normal joint motion
- Numbness or impaired circulation to the limb or digit

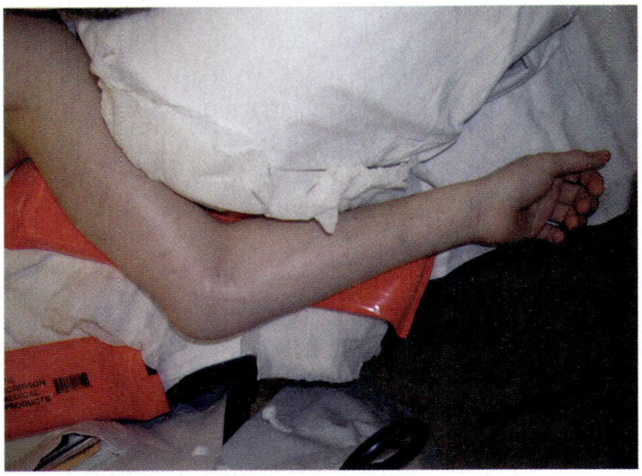

A

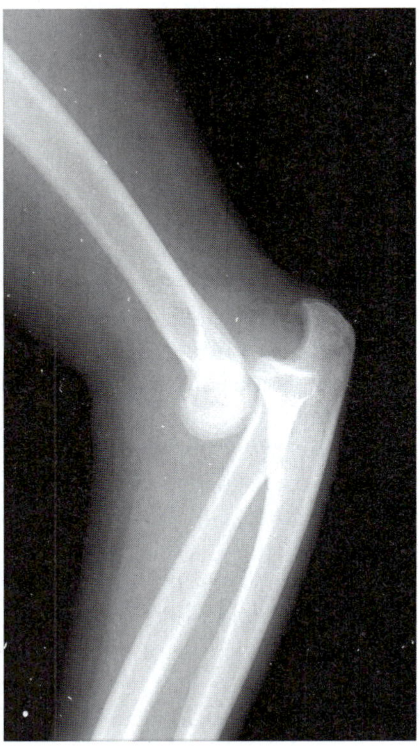

B

FIGURE 31-21 A dislocation is a disruption of a joint in which the bone ends are no longer in contact. **A.** The clinical appearance of an elbow dislocation. **B.** Radiographic appearance of the same elbow.

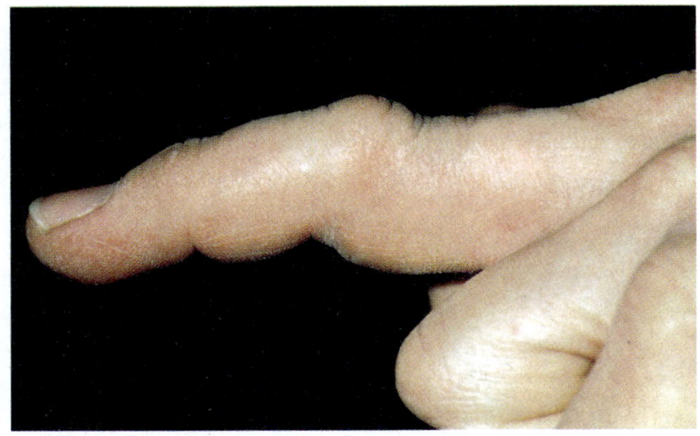

FIGURE 31-22 Joint dislocations, such as the one shown in this finger, are characterized by deformity, swelling, pain with any movement, tenderness, locking, and impaired circulation.

Sprains

A **sprain** occurs when a joint is twisted or stretched beyond its normal range of motion. As a result, the supporting capsule and ligaments are stretched or torn, resulting in injury to the ligaments, articular capsule, synovial membrane, and tendons crossing the joint.

Sprains can range from mild to severe, depending on the amount of damage done to the supporting ligaments. The most severe sprains involve actual tearing of the ligament and may allow transient joint dislocation. Mild sprains are caused by ligament stretching rather than tearing. A sprain can occur in any joint, but they most often occur in the knee, shoulder, and ankle. Many sprains occur after a person misjudges a step or landing. Evasive moves, such as those done during a sporting event, commonly cause sprains in athletes. Some patients might report hearing a "snap" when the injury occurred.

After the injury, the joint alignment generally returns to a somewhat normal position, so the joint is not significantly displaced. In contrast with fractures and dislocations, sprains usually do not involve deformity, and joint mobility is usually limited by pain, not by joint incongruity. The following signs and symptoms often indicate that the patient may have a sprain:

- The patient is unwilling to use the limb (guarding).
- Swelling and ecchymosis are present at the injured joint as a result of torn blood vessels.
- Pain prevents the patient from moving or using the limb normally.
- Instability of the joint is indicated by increased motion, especially at the knee; however, this may be masked by severe swelling and guarding.

A fracture can look like a sprain, and vice versa. You will frequently not be able to distinguish a nondisplaced fracture from a sprain. Therefore, it is important to document the MOI, because certain sprains and fractures occur more consistently with certain mechanisms. Your approach should always be to determine the MOI. The basic principles of prehospital management for sprains, dislocations, and fractures are essentially the same and are discussed later in the chapter.

Strains

A **strain** (pulled muscle) is a stretching or tearing of the muscle and/or tendon, causing pain, swelling, and bruising of the soft tissues in the area. It occurs because of an abnormal contraction or from excessive stretching. Strains may range from minute separation to complete rupture. Unlike with a sprain, no ligament or joint damage typically occurs.

Often, no deformity is present and only minor swelling is noted at the site of the injury. Some patients may report a "snap" when a muscle tears. Some may report increased sharp pain with passive movement of the injured extremity. Patients may report severe weakness of the muscle. Many patients also have some tenderness. The prehospital treatment of strains is similar to the prehospital management for sprains, dislocations, and fractures.

Amputations

A limb **amputation** is an injury in which an extremity is completely severed from the body. This injury is associated with every aspect of the musculoskeletal system, from bone to ligament to muscle. Amputations can occur as a result of trauma or a surgical intervention.

Patient Assessment

As an EMT, your assessments, attempts to splint, and efforts to stabilize the patient's condition are very important. However, always look at the big picture, evaluating the overall complexity of the situation to determine and treat any life threats. For example, overlooking an obstructed airway to splint a lower leg fracture could be deadly for the patient. Always carefully assess the MOI to try to determine the amount of kinetic energy that an injured limb has absorbed, and maintain a high index of suspicion for associated injuries.

It is not important to distinguish among fractures, dislocations, sprains, and contusions. In most cases, your assessment will be reported as an extremity injury. However, you must be able to distinguish mild injuries from severe injuries because some severe injuries may compromise neurovascular function, which could threaten long-term function.

YOU are the EMT

When you arrive at the scene, you find the patient, a 21-year-old woman, sitting on the ground with an ice pack over her left tibia. She is conscious and alert and tells you that another player fell against her leg.

Recording Time: 0 Minutes	
Appearance	Anxious; in obvious pain; no sign of severe bleeding
Level of consciousness	Conscious and alert
Airway	Open; clear of secretions and foreign bodies
Breathing	Increased rate; adequate depth
Circulation	Radial pulses increased rate, strong and regular

The patient denies having any other injuries and tells you that she heard a "snap" when the other player fell against her leg. She is in severe pain.

3. What initial treatment should you provide to this patient?

4. What are some indicators of a fractured bone?

Scene Size-up

Information from dispatch may indicate the MOI, the number of patients involved, and any first aid procedures used prior to your arrival. This will be useful information for you to think about as you travel to the scene. Remember, the information given by the dispatcher is only as accurate as the patient's or bystander's report. In addition, the situation may change prior to your arrival at the incident. Dispatch information can still be used to help you consider whether spinal motion restriction will be needed, the equipment you may need, and whether hazards might be present.

As you arrive at the scene, try to identify the forces associated with the MOI. Could they have produced injuries other than the musculoskeletal injuries reported by dispatch? Consider the possibility of hidden bleeding; internal injuries that you cannot see and closed fractures of the femur are examples. Standard precautions may be as simple as wearing gloves. With a severe MOI or other risk factors, a mask, gown, and eye protection may be necessary. Evaluate the need for law enforcement support, advanced life support (ALS), or additional ambulances, and request them early based on your initial scene assessment.

When you assess a patient who has experienced a significant MOI, look for indicators of the MOI and be alert for both primary and secondary injuries. Primary injuries occur as a result of the MOI, whereas secondary injuries are the result of what happens after the initial injury. For example, being hit by a motor vehicle will often result in a primary pelvic injury and often a secondary head injury when the patient rolls onto the hood of the car. As you put together information from dispatch and your observations of the scene, consider what injuries the MOI would lead you to expect. For example, when you approach a call for a person who has fallen off a ladder, you should suspect head, neck, and extremity injuries.

Primary Assessment

The primary assessment should focus on identifying and managing life threats. Treating the patient according to their level of consciousness and the ABCs is always the priority. Threats to airway, breathing, and circulation are considered life threatening and must be treated immediately to prevent mortality. Significant bleeding, internal or external, is an immediate life threat. If the patient has obvious life-threatening external hemorrhage, the ABC sequence should be modified to XABC, where control of eXsanguination comes before airway and breathing interventions. Efforts to prevent shock or address its underlying causes should begin as quickly as possible. For example, if you are unable to control arterial bleeding from extremities by using direct pressure, apply a **tourniquet** (if possible). Arterial bleeding from an open fracture should be treated prior to giving oxygen.

When evaluating the patient's level of consciousness and orientation, check for responsiveness using the AVPU (Awake and alert, responsive to Verbal stimuli, responsive to Pain, Unresponsive) scale, and assess mental status by asking the patient about their chief complaint. If the patient is alert, this should help direct you to any apparent life threats. An unresponsive patient may have an underlying life-threatening condition. You should administer high-flow oxygen via a nonrebreathing mask (or a bag-mask device, if indicated) to all patients whose level of consciousness is less than alert and oriented if signs of respiratory distress are evident.

Perform a primary assessment of the patient and ask about the MOI. Was it a direct blow, indirect force, twisting force, or high-energy injury? In many situations, the musculoskeletal complaints will be simple and usually not life threatening; however, some situations, such as those with a significant MOI, will include multiple problems that include musculoskeletal injuries. The initial interaction with your patient will provide you with a starting point and help you to distinguish the simple from the complex injuries. If there was significant trauma and multiple body systems were affected, the musculoskeletal injuries may be a lower priority. Scene time should not be wasted on prolonged

Words of Wisdom

Medical emergencies can result in falls and fractures. For example, a cardiac event or stroke can cause a fall and fractured hip in an older person.

musculoskeletal assessment or splinting fractures that are otherwise not life threatening. The expression "splinting to death" is used to describe a situation in which the responder is so involved in splinting fractures that the patient dies from other injuries.

Fractures and sprains usually do not create airway and breathing problems. Other problems, such as injuries to the head, intoxication, or other related illnesses and injuries, may cause inadequate breathing. Evaluating the chief complaint and MOI will help you to identify whether the patient has an open airway and whether breathing is present and adequate. In a conscious patient, this is as simple as noting whether the patient can speak normally. In an unconscious patient, it is as simple as opening the airway using the appropriate technique to check for breathing. Remember, little else matters if the patient's airway and breathing are inadequate.

Your circulatory assessment should focus on determining whether the patient has a pulse, has adequate perfusion, or is bleeding. If the patient is unconscious, make sure there is a pulse by palpating the carotid artery. Hypoperfusion (shock) and bleeding problems will most likely be your primary concern. If the skin is pale, cool, or clammy and capillary refill time is slow, immediately treat your patient for shock. Maintain a normal body temperature, because trauma patients can rapidly become hypothermic even in warm environments. If musculoskeletal injuries in the extremities are suspected, they must be at least initially stabilized, if not splinted, prior to moving. This cause of shock may need to be eliminated later in your assessment.

If the patient has an airway or breathing problem, or significant bleeding, provide rapid transport to the hospital after quickly treating these life threats. A patient who has a significant MOI but whose condition appears otherwise stable should also be transported promptly to the closest appropriate hospital. You must become skilled at quickly and accurately assessing the severity of an injury. The Golden Period (the time from injury to definitive care) is critical not only for life, but also for preserving limb viability. Patients with bilateral fractures of the long bones (humerus, femur, or tibia) have been subjected to a high amount of kinetic energy, which should dramatically increase your index of suspicion for serious unseen injuries. When a decision for rapid transport is made, you can use a long backboard as a splinting device to splint the whole body rather than splinting each extremity individually. If you take time to splint the patient's arms and legs individually, you may delay the prompt surgical intervention that may be needed for other injuries when a significant MOI has occurred. Individual splints should be applied en route if the ABCs are stable and time permits.

Words of Wisdom

Prolonged hypoperfusion to an extremity can cause significant damage. Therefore, any injury that may compromise blood flow is considered an emergency. In a patient who has multisystem trauma, any additional bleeding can increase problems with underlying injuries or overall perfusion.

Patients with a simple MOI, such as twisting of an ankle or dislocating a shoulder, may be further assessed and their condition stabilized on scene prior to transport if no other problems exist. Remember that most injuries are not critical. You can estimate the severity of isolated extremity injuries using the criteria shown in **TABLE 31-1** as a guideline.

History Taking

After the life threats have been managed during the primary assessment, investigate the chief complaint. Obtain a medical history and be alert for injury-specific signs and symptoms and for any pertinent negatives, such as no pain or loss of sensation.

Obtain a SAMPLE history (Signs and symptoms, Allergies, Medications, Pertinent past medical history, Last oral intake, Events leading up to the illness or injury) for all trauma patients. How much and in what detail you explore this history depends on the patient's condition and how quickly you need to transport the patient to the hospital. For patients with simple fractures, dislocations, or sprains, it is easier to obtain a SAMPLE history. At the scene you may have access to family members and others who have information about the patient's history. Attempt to obtain this history without delaying time to definitive care.

OPQRST can be of limited use in cases of severe injury and is usually too lengthy when matters

TABLE 31-1 Musculoskeletal Injury Severity

Minor Injuries
- Minor sprains
- Fractures or dislocations of digits

Moderate Injuries
- Open fractures of digits
- Nondisplaced long bone fractures
- Nondisplaced pelvic fractures
- Major sprains of a major joint

Serious Injuries
- Displaced long bone fractures
- Multiple hand and foot fractures
- Open long bone fractures
- Displaced pelvic fractures
- Dislocations of major joints
- Multiple digit amputations
- Laceration of major nerves or blood vessels

Severe, Life-Threatening Injuries (Survival Is Probable)
- Multiple closed fractures
- Limb amputations
- Fractures of both long bones of the legs (bilateral femur fractures)

Critical Injuries (Survival Is Uncertain)
- Multiple open fractures of the limbs
- Suspected pelvic fractures with hemodynamic instability

of exsanguinating hemorrhage, airway, breathing, circulation, and rapid transport require immediate attention. However, OPQRST may be useful when the MOI is unclear, the patient's condition is stable, or details of the injury are uncertain. This more detailed questioning for simple trauma may help you and the hospital staff to better understand the specific injury.

Secondary Assessment

If significant trauma may have affected multiple systems, start with a secondary assessment of the entire body to be sure you have identified all problems and injuries. Begin with the head and work systematically toward the feet, checking the head, chest, abdomen, extremities, and back. The goal is to identify hidden and potentially life-threatening injuries. This secondary assessment will also help you to prepare for packaging and rapid transport. Knowing if an arm or leg is broken will be important when log rolling and securing the patient prior to transport.

Words of Wisdom

Keep in mind that there is a patient attached to the injured extremity! For example, pregnant patients who sustain pelvic fractures tend to have higher mortality rates. Therefore, it is imperative to treat not only the fracture, but also the other needs of the patient and fetus.

Use the DCAP-BTLS approach (Deformities, Contusions, Abrasions, Punctures/penetrations, Burns, Tenderness, Lacerations, Swelling) to assess the musculoskeletal system. Identify any extremity deformities that likely represent significant musculoskeletal injury, and stabilize them appropriately. Contusions and abrasions may overlie more subtle injuries and should prompt you to carefully evaluate the stability and neurovascular status of the limb. The presence of puncture wounds or other signs of penetrating injury should alert you to the possibility of an open fracture. Associated burns must be identified and treated appropriately. Palpate for tenderness, which, like contusions or abrasions, may be the only significant sign of an underlying musculoskeletal injury.

When lacerations are present in an extremity, an open fracture must be considered, bleeding controlled, and dressings applied. Careful inspection for swelling and comparison with the opposite limb may also reveal otherwise occult musculoskeletal injury. You may find a hematoma in the zone of injury during the assessment.

If your assessment reveals no external signs of injury, ask the patient to move each limb carefully, stopping immediately if a movement causes pain. Skip this step in your evaluation if the patient reports neck or back pain; excess motion could cause permanent damage to the spinal cord.

When nonsignificant trauma has occurred and you suspect that your patient has a simple strain, sprain, dislocation, or fracture, take the time to focus your secondary assessment on that specific injury. Look for DCAP-BTLS. Be sure to assess the entire zone of injury by removing clothing from the area and looking and palpating for injuries. In musculoskeletal injuries, this zone generally extends from the joint above (proximal) to the joint below (distal), front and back.

Words of Wisdom

If the patient has two or more injured extremities, treat the patient as a significant trauma patient and provide rapid transport to the hospital. The likelihood of other more severe injuries is greater when two or more bones have been broken.

Remember to evaluate the circulation, motor function, and sensation distal to the injury. Many important blood vessels and nerves lie close to the bone, especially around the major joints. Therefore, any injury or deformity of the bone may be associated with vessel or nerve injury. For this reason, you must assess neurovascular function every 5 to 10 minutes during the assessment, depending on the patient's condition, until the patient is at the hospital. Always recheck the neurovascular function before and after you splint or otherwise manipulate the limb. Manipulation can cause a bone fragment to press against or compress a nerve or vessel. Failure to restore circulation in this situation can lead to death of the limb. Always give priority to patients with impaired circulation that develops or remains present after a manipulation.

Because many of the steps require patient cooperation, you will not be able to assess sensory and motor functions in an unconscious patient, but you can evaluate the limb for deformity, swelling, ecchymosis, false motion, and crepitus.

Evaluation of the injured limb should include the 6 Ps of musculoskeletal assessment: pain, paralysis, paresthesia (numbness or tingling), pulselessness, pallor, and pressure. Assess neurovascular status. This process is described in Chapter 10, *Patient Assessment*.

Determine a baseline set of vital signs, including pulse rate, rhythm, and quality; respiratory rate, rhythm, and quality; blood pressure; skin condition; oxygen saturation level; and pupil size and reaction to light. These need to be obtained as

Words of Wisdom

Extremity injuries that impair circulation or nerve function in distal tissues are urgent conditions. Patients with these injuries need careful assessment, prompt transport, and frequent reassessment of distal functions. It is also valuable to report this information in your initial radio contact with the hospital to allow personnel to prepare.

soon as possible. Administer oxygen if indicated to achieve an oxygen saturation of 94% to 98%. Your patient may appear to be tolerating the injury well until you reassess these vital signs and they indicate otherwise. Trending these vital signs helps you to understand whether your patient's condition is improving or worsening over time, particularly during long transports. Shock or hypoperfusion is possible in musculoskeletal injuries; therefore, this baseline information is a very important part of your initial assessment.

Street Smarts

Long-term disability is one of the most devastating consequences of an orthopaedic injury. In many cases, a severely injured limb can be repaired and made to look almost normal. Unfortunately, many patients cannot return to work for long periods because of the extensive rehabilitation required and because of pain. As an EMT, you have a critical role in mitigating the risk of long-term disability by preventing further injury, reducing the risk of wound infection, and transporting patients with orthopaedic injuries to an appropriate hospital.

Reassessment

Repeat the primary assessment to ensure your interventions are working as they should. Perform a reassessment every 5 minutes for an unstable patient and every 15 minutes for a stable patient.

Because trauma patients often have multiple injuries, you must assess their overall condition, stabilize the ABCs, and control any serious bleeding before further treating the injured area. In a critically injured patient who has multiple injuries, secure the patient to a backboard to restrict movement of the spine, pelvis, and extremities, and provide prompt transport to a trauma center. In this situation, a secondary assessment with extensive evaluation and splinting of limb injuries in the field is a waste of valuable time. Perform the primary assessment and transport, reassessing the patient en route to the ED.

If the patient has no life-threatening injuries, you may take extra time at the scene to stabilize the patient's overall condition and more completely evaluate the injury. If time permits, remove or cut away the patient's clothing to look for open fractures or dislocations, severe deformity, swelling, and/or ecchymosis.

When you have finished assessing the extremity and removed any jewelry or constrictive clothing from that limb, apply a secure splint to stabilize the injury prior to transport. The joints above and below the site of injury should be included in the splint. To minimize the potential for complications, the splint should be well padded. A comfortable and secure splint will reduce pain, reduce shock, and minimize compromised circulation. A good rule is to check the patient's circulation, motor function, and sensation before and after splinting. Splint application will be discussed later in the chapter.

The main goal in providing care for musculoskeletal injuries is stabilization in the most comfortable position that allows for maintenance of good circulation distal to the injury. This should be done whether you are preparing the patient for rapid transport or you have as much time as you need to assess and treat the patient.

Your radio report to the hospital should include a description of the problems found during your assessment. Particularly, you should report problems with the patient's ABCs, open fractures, and compromised circulation that occurred before or after splinting. Often, the hospital staff can arrange for specialists or consider antibiotics early if they are aware of problems. How much information you include in your radio report will depend on your local protocols. Additional details, such as the mandated reporting of situations involving elder or child abuse, can be given during your verbal report at the hospital when you transfer care to the nursing staff or physician.

It is important to document the presence or absence of circulation, motor function, and sensation distal to the injury before you move an extremity, after manipulation or splinting of the injury, and on arrival at the hospital. Hospital staff may refer to your notes to clarify confusing situations or communication problems. Your careful documentation becomes part of the patient's permanent medical record and may protect you from legal action that the patient may pursue later. Do not rely on your memory for details about situations; your memory is unreliable. Always document your findings.

Emergency Medical Care

Your first steps in providing care for any patient are the primary assessment and management of the patient's ABCs. If needed, perform a secondary assessment of either the entire body or the specific area of injury. Always take standard precautions and be alert for signs and symptoms of internal bleeding. Internal bleeding should be suspected whenever the MOI suggests that severe forces have impacted the body.

The general steps of caring for patients with musculoskeletal injuries are as follows. These steps are discussed in greater detail in the sections that follow.

1. Remove jewelry, including rings, bracelets, and piercings, that may cause damage as the extremity swells. Expose the entire zone of injury by removing or cutting away clothing. Cover open wounds with saline-moistened, sterile dressings, and apply direct pressure to control bleeding. If heavy bleeding cannot be controlled, quickly apply a tourniquet. Assess distal motor, sensory, and circulatory function. Once dressed, open fractures may be managed in the same manner as a closed fracture.
2. Apply the appropriate splint and elevate the extremity. For fractures, it is essential to splint the joints above and below the injury to ensure adequate stabilization. Position injured limbs slightly above the level of the heart. Patients with lower extremity injuries should lie supine with the affected limb elevated approximately 6 inches (15 cm) to minimize swelling. Never allow the injured limb to flop about or dangle from the edge of the backboard. Always reassess distal motor, sensory, and circulatory

function following the application of splints. Evaluate motor function by asking the patient to move their fingers and toes. Assess sensation by having the patient close their eyes and state which finger or toe you are touching. Examine circulatory status by palpating the distal pulse and checking capillary refill time. Additionally, note the color and condition of the patient's skin.

3. If swelling is present, apply cold packs to the affected area. However, cold packs should never be placed directly on exposed skin or other tissues.
4. Prepare for transport. A patient with an isolated upper extremity injury will likely prefer to sit in the semi-Fowler position than lie supine on the stretcher. Assuming there is no risk of spinal injury, either position is acceptable. Continue to keep the extremity elevated above the level of the heart, and secure it so that it does not dangle from the edge of the backboard or stretcher.
5. Transport your patient to the most appropriate facility and consider the need to request ALS for pain management.
6. Advise hospital personnel of the patient's injuries and all interventions performed.

Words of Wisdom

When an arm or leg is broken, the distal extremity may swell. Rings on fingers and toes should be removed. If the ring cannot be easily slipped off the digit, a ring cutter may be used if allowed in your system after you have received the proper training in its use (**FIGURE 31-23**).

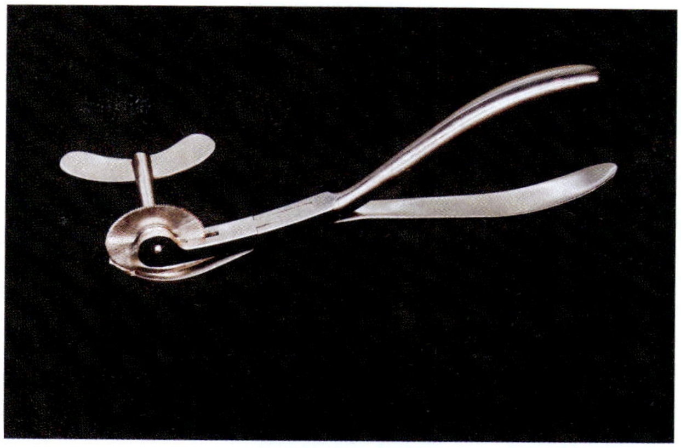

FIGURE 31-23 A ring cutter for removing jewelry from the finger or toe.

Handling Injured Extremities

Recall that fractures can break through the skin and cause external bleeding or damage blood vessels beneath the skin and cause internal bleeding. This may occur during the initial injury or during manipulation of the extremity while preparing for splinting or transport. Careful handling of the extremity minimizes this risk.

Contamination is also a concern when managing an open fracture. Brush away any obvious debris on the skin surrounding an open fracture before applying a sterile dressing moistened with saline. Do not enter or probe the open fracture site to retrieve debris because doing so may cause further contamination. If external bleeding is present, bandage the extremity quickly to control bleeding. The dressings that cover the wound and bone should be kept clean to reduce the potential for bone infection. The bandage should be secure enough to control bleeding without restricting circulation distal to the injury. Monitor bandage tightness by assessing the circulation, sensation, and movement distal to the bandage. Swelling from fractures and internal bleeding may cause bandages to become too tight. If heavy bleeding cannot be controlled, quickly apply a tourniquet.

Splinting

A **splint** is any flexible or rigid device used to prevent motion in an injured bone or joint (**FIGURE 31-24**). Unless the patient's life is in immediate danger, the EMT should splint all fractures, dislocations, and sprains prior to moving the patient. By preventing movement of bone fragments, joint dislocations, and soft-tissue trauma, splinting reduces pain and makes it easier to transfer and transport the patient. In addition, splinting will help to prevent the following:

- Further damage to muscles, the spinal cord, peripheral nerves, and blood vessels from broken bone ends
- Laceration of the skin by broken bone ends. One of the primary indications for splinting is

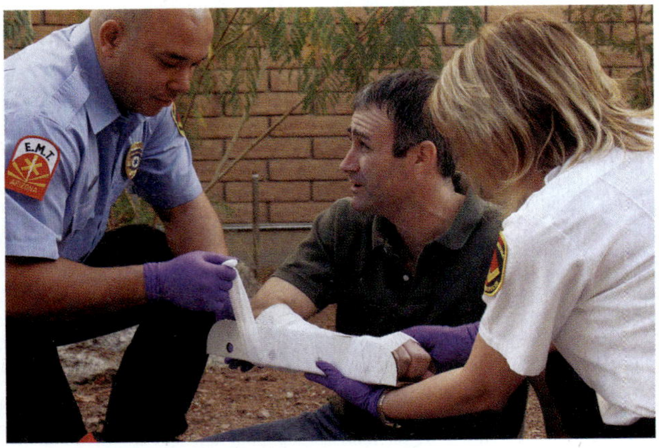

FIGURE 31-24 Splinting reduces pain and prevents additional damage to the injured extremity.

to prevent a closed fracture from becoming an open fracture (conversion).

- Restriction of distal blood flow resulting from compression of blood vessels
- Excessive bleeding of the tissues at the injury site caused by broken bone ends
- Increased pain from movement of bone ends

Special Populations

SPLINTING FRACTURES IN PEDIATRIC PATIENTS

Extremity injuries in pediatric patients are generally managed in the same manner as those in adults. Painful, deformed limbs with evidence of broken bones should be splinted. Specialized splinting equipment, such as a traction splint for fractures of the femur, should be used only if it fits the pediatric patient. Do not attempt to use adult devices on a pediatric patient unless the child is large enough to properly fit in the device.

General Principles of Splinting

The following principles of splinting apply to most situations:

1. Remove clothing from the area of any suspected fracture or dislocation so that you can inspect the extremity for DCAP-BTLS.
2. Note and record the patient's neurovascular status distal to the site of the injury, including pulse, sensation, and movement. Continue to monitor the neurovascular status until the patient reaches the hospital.
3. Cover open wounds with a saline-moistened, sterile dressing before splinting. Be sure to take standard precautions. Do not intentionally replace protruding bones. Notify the receiving hospital of all open wounds.
4. Do not move the patient before splinting an extremity unless there is an immediate danger to the patient or you, or unless there are threats defined in the primary assessment of the ABCs that you are unable to correct.
5. In a suspected fracture of the shaft of any bone, stabilize the joints above and below the fracture.
6. With injuries in and around the joint, stabilize the bones above and below the injured joint.
7. Pad all rigid splints to prevent local pressure and patient discomfort.
8. While applying the splint, maintain manual stabilization to minimize movement of the limb and to support the injury site.
9. If fracture of a long bone shaft has resulted in severe deformity, use constant, gentle manual traction to align the limb so that it can be splinted. This is especially important if the distal part of the extremity is cyanotic or pulseless.
10. If you encounter resistance to limb alignment, splint the limb in its deformed position.
11. If spinal injury is suspected, perform spinal motion restriction, using a collar and backboard or other device (eg, vacuum mattress, scoop stretcher) to secure the patient in a neutral in-line position. See Chapter 28, *Head and Spine Injuries*, for discussion of spinal motion restriction.

Words of Wisdom

Straightening or splinting an injured limb can compromise distal functions, as can the initial injury. Record the status of distal circulation and nervous function (neurovascular status) before and after straightening or splinting. At a minimum, your written record should describe these functions before splinting and confirm whether they were normal immediately after splinting and on hospital arrival. For all but the shortest transports, also indicate the results of reassessments while en route.

12. If the patient has signs of shock (hypoperfusion), align the limb in the normal anatomic position, take measures to restrict patient movement, and provide transport.
13. When in doubt, splint.

Types of Splints

Although a splint can be improvised using a variety of materials, the EMT must be competent in utilizing the commercial devices on the ambulance that are frequently used. The basic types of splints are rigid splints, formable splints, pelvic binders, and traction splints. The first three types are described next, and traction splints are described later in the chapter because of their unique role in managing femur fractures.

Rigid Splints

Rigid (nonformable) splints are made from firm material and are applied to the sides, front, and/or back of an injured extremity to prevent motion at the injury site. Common examples of rigid splints include padded board splints, molded plastic and metal splints, padded wire ladder splints, and folded cardboard splints. As always, be sure to take standard precautions. It takes two people to apply a rigid splint. Follow the steps in **SKILL DRILL 31-1**:

1. Gently support the limb at the site of injury as your partner prepares and begins to position the equipment. Apply steady, in-line traction if necessary. Maintain this support until the splint is completely applied (**Step 1**). Assess distal pulse and motor and sensory function.
2. Place the rigid splint under or alongside the limb.
3. Place padding between the limb and the splint to make sure there is even pressure and even contact. Look for bony prominences, and pad them (**Step 2**).
4. Apply bindings to hold the splint securely to the limb (**Step 3**).
5. Check and record the distal nervous and circulatory (neurovascular) function (**Step 4**).

There are two situations in which you must splint the limb in the position of deformity: when the deformity is severe, as is the case with many dislocations, and when you encounter resistance or extreme pain when applying gentle traction to the fracture of a shaft of a long bone. In either situation, apply padded board splints to each side of the limb and secure them with soft roller bandages (**FIGURE 31-25**). Most dislocations should be splinted as found, but follow local protocols. Attempts to realign or reduce dislocations may lead to more damage.

Formable Splints

The formable splints you are most likely to use as an EMT are structural aluminum malleable splints and vacuum splints. Other formable splints include

YOU are the EMT

A nurse present at the scene assists by stabilizing the leg above the ankle and below the knee while you expose the injury. The patient has an obvious deformity in the midshaft area of her tibia/fibula; however, there are no open wounds. As you further assess the injury, your partner obtains the patient's vital signs.

Recording Time: 5 Minutes	
Respirations	22 breaths/min; adequate depth
Pulse	112 beats/min; strong and regular
Skin	Baseline color, warm, and moist
Blood pressure	130/78 mm Hg
Oxygen saturation (Spo_2)	98% (on ambient air)

5. How should you proceed with your assessment of this patient's injury?

6. How should you treat an injured extremity in which distal perfusion is absent?

Skill Drill 31-1 Applying a Rigid Splint

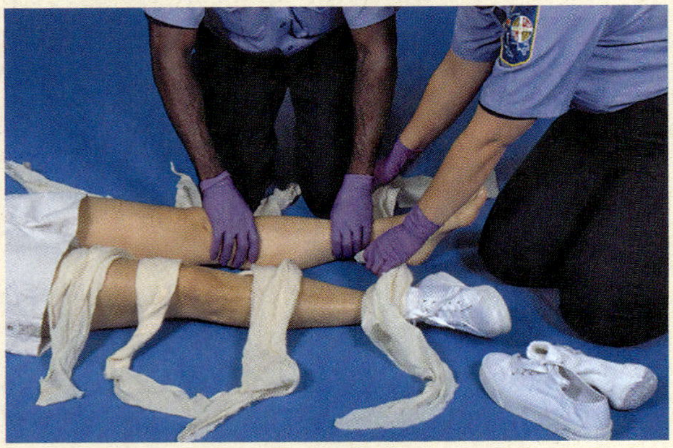

Step 1

Provide gentle support and in-line traction for the limb. Assess distal pulse and motor and sensory function.

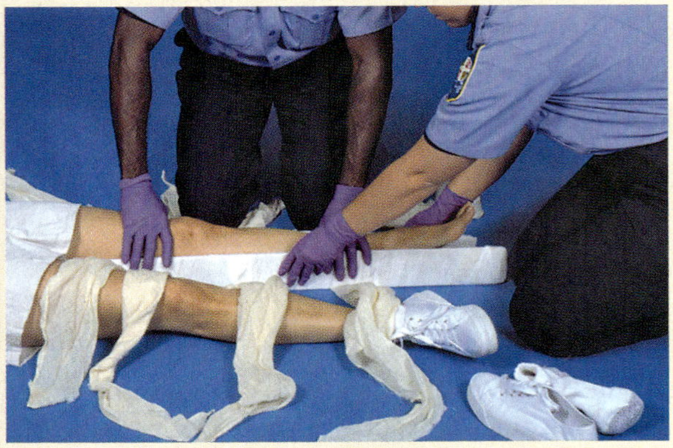

Step 2

Place the splint alongside or under the limb. Pad between the limb and the splint as needed to ensure even pressure and contact.

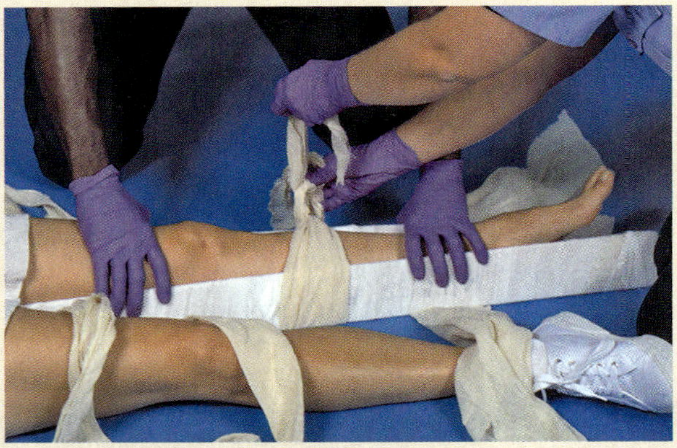

Step 3

Secure the splint to the limb with bindings.

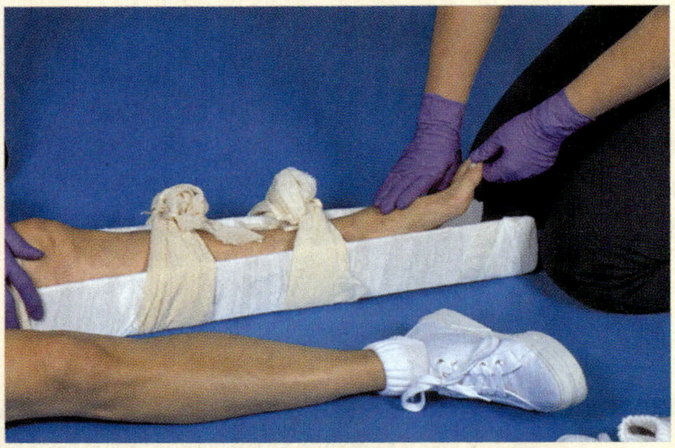

Step 4

Assess and record distal neurovascular function.

air splints, pillow splints, and sling and swathe bandages. Technically, pelvic binders are also a type of formable splint; however, they are discussed as a distinct type of splint later in this section.

Common brand names of structural aluminum malleable splints are the SAM splint and the C-Splint. These products consist of a moldable aluminum core encased in layers of foam padding. They usually come packaged in a roll and can quickly be shaped, folded, or cut to serve numerous splinting needs. When curved or molded into a *C* or *T* shape (SAM splint) or a *U* shape (C-Splint),

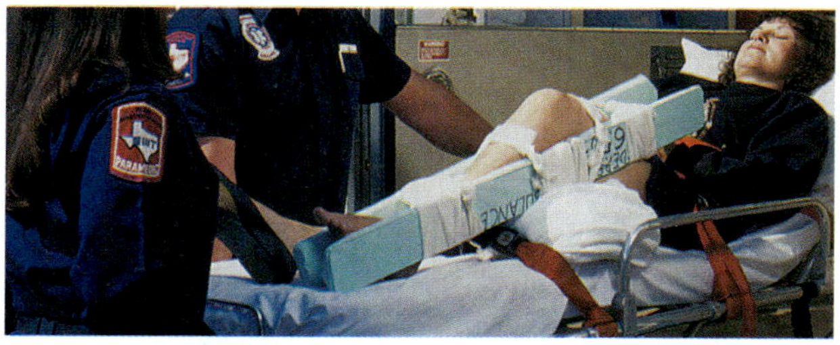

FIGURE 31-25 If you encounter resistance or extreme pain when applying traction to a long bone, apply padded board splints to each side of the limb, and secure them with soft roller bandages, stabilizing the limb in its deformed position.

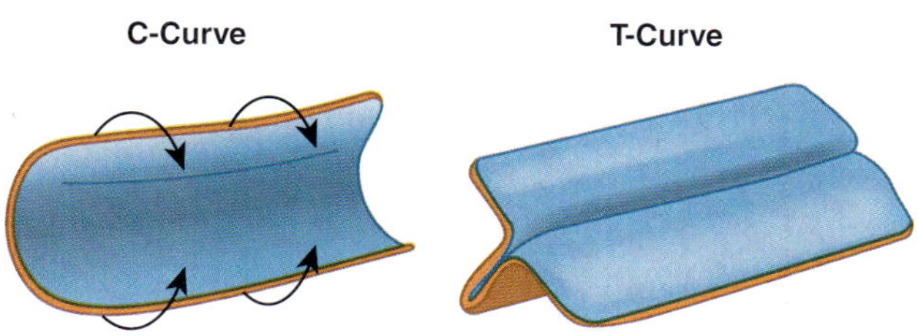

FIGURE 31-26 A structural aluminum malleable splint becomes rigid after it is molded into the desired shape.

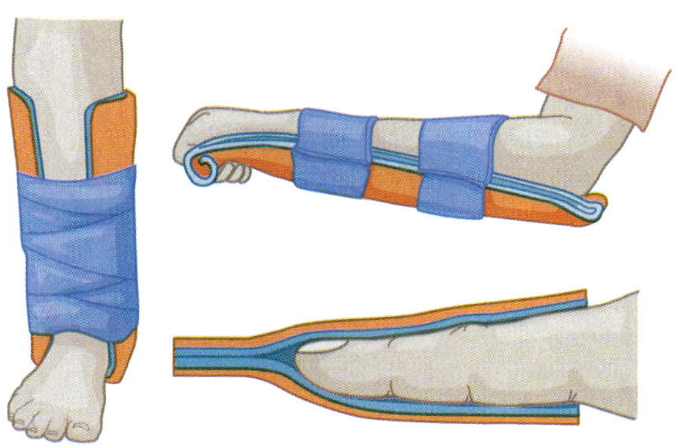

FIGURE 31-27 Structural aluminum malleable splints can be used in various ways.

the splint becomes rigid (**FIGURE 31-26**). It can be molded and remolded as needed. Because there are several ways to use the splint, depending on the area to be stabilized, the EMT must be familiar with its application in a variety of scenarios (**FIGURE 31-27**).

Words of Wisdom

Test your problem-solving skills. Practice using the structural aluminum malleable splint for a variety of injuries. With a partner, try splinting fractures and dislocations of sites such as a thumb, finger, wrist, forearm, elbow, humerus, shoulder, ankle, lower leg, knee, and cervical spine. Remember to follow the basic rules of splinting discussed earlier in this chapter.

A vacuum splint can be easily shaped to fit around a deformed limb. Instead of pumping air in, however, you can use a hand pump to pull the air out through a valve. Follow the steps in **SKILL DRILL 31-2** to apply a vacuum splint:

1. Assess distal pulse and motor and sensory function.
2. Your partner supports and stabilizes the injured limb, applying traction if needed (**Step 1**).
3. Gently place the injured limb onto the vacuum splint and wrap the splint around the limb (**Step 2**).
4. Draw the air out of the splint through the suction valve, and then seal the valve. Once the air has been drawn out, the vacuum splint becomes rigid, conforming to the shape of the deformed limb and stabilizing it. The splint will remain rigid as long as the valve remains closed (**Step 3**).
5. Check distal circulation and nervous functions and monitor them en route.

Pelvic Binders

A **pelvic binder** is used to splint the bony pelvis to reduce hemorrhage from bone ends, venous disruption, and pain (**FIGURE 31-28**). Generally, pelvic binders are lightweight, made of soft material, easily applied by one EMT, and should allow access to the abdomen, perineum, anus, and groin for examination and diagnostic testing. Because multiple manufacturers produce pelvic binder devices, you should be familiar with the manufacturer's instructions for your specific device.

Skill Drill 31-2 Applying a Vacuum Splint

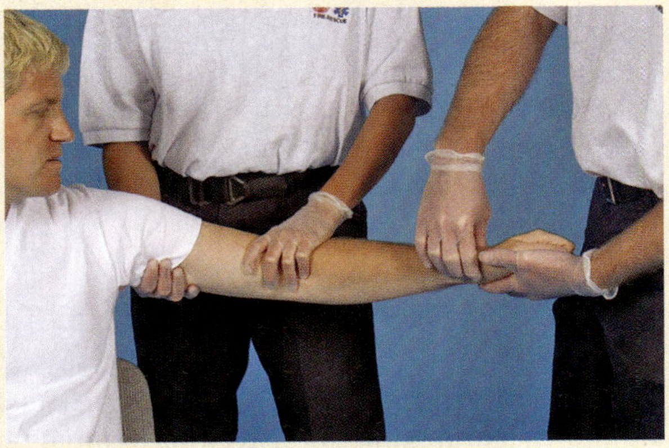

Step 1

Assess distal pulse and motor and sensory function. Your partner stabilizes and supports the injury.

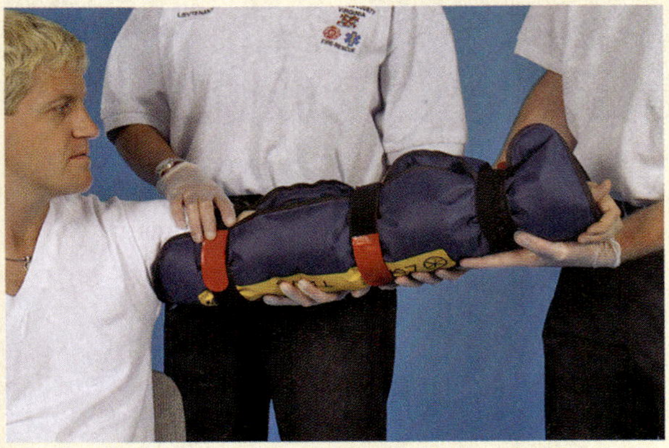

Step 2

Place the splint, and wrap it around the limb.

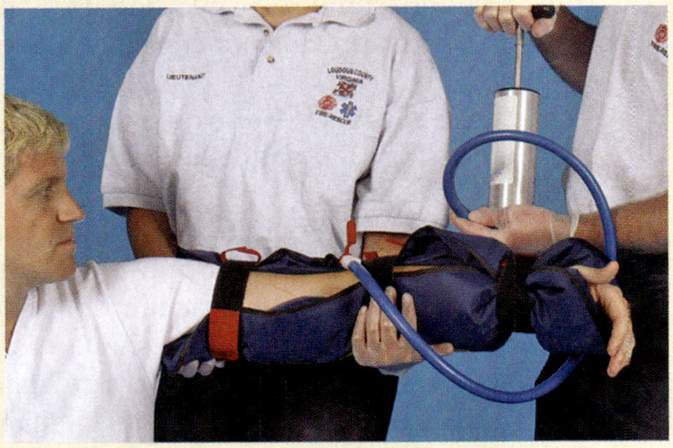

Step 3

Draw the air out of the splint through the suction valve, and then seal the valve. Assess distal pulse and motor and sensory function.

Hazards of Improper Splinting

You must be aware of the hazards associated with the improper application of splints, including the following:

- Compression of nerves, tissues, and blood vessels
- Delay in transport of a patient with a life-threatening injury
- Reduction of distal circulation
- Aggravation of the injury
- Injury to tissue, nerves, blood vessels, or muscles as a result of excessive movement of the bone or joint

Transport

Once an injured limb is adequately splinted, the patient is ready to be transferred to a backboard, scoop stretcher, vacuum mattress, or stretcher and transported.

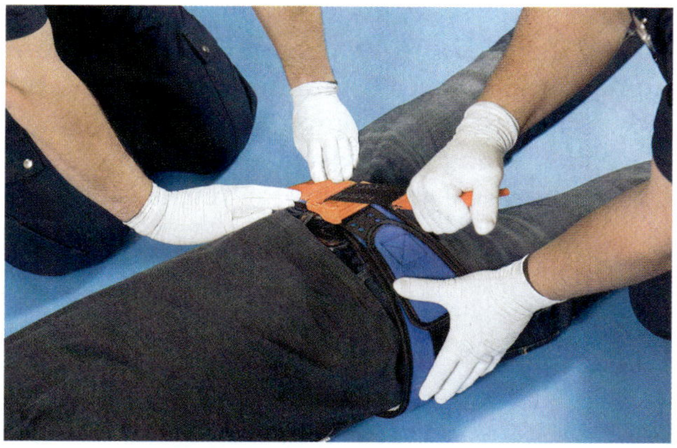

FIGURE 31-28 Pelvic binders are meant to provide temporary stabilization until spinal motion restriction can be achieved. Note: On a real patient, the clothing would be cut away prior to application of the splint.

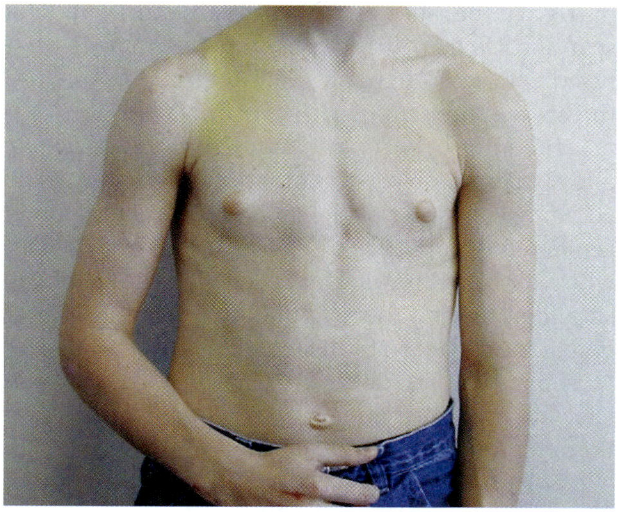

FIGURE 31-29 A patient with a fracture of the clavicle will usually hold the arm across the front of their body.

Very few, if any, musculoskeletal injuries justify the use of excessive speed during transport. The limb will be stable once a dressing and splint have been applied. However, a patient with a pulseless limb must be given a higher priority. Still, if the hospital is only a few minutes away, speeding to the ED will not make an important difference to the patient's time to definitive treatment. If the treatment facility is a more substantial distance away, a patient with a pulseless limb should be transported by helicopter or urgent ground transportation. If circulation in the distal limb is impaired, always notify medical oversight so that proper steps can be taken quickly once the patient arrives in the ED.

Specific Musculoskeletal Injuries

Injuries of the Clavicle and Scapula

Fractures of the clavicle occur commonly in children when they fall on an outstretched hand. They can also occur with crush injuries of the chest. A patient with a fracture of the clavicle will report pain in the shoulder and will usually hold the arm across the front of their body (**FIGURE 31-29**). A young child often reports pain throughout the entire arm and is unwilling to use any part of that limb. These complaints may make it difficult to localize the point of injury, but, generally, swelling and point tenderness occur over the clavicle. Because the clavicle is subcutaneous (just beneath the skin), the skin will occasionally tent over the fracture fragment. The clavicle lies directly over major arteries, veins, and nerves; therefore, fracture of the clavicle may lead to neurovascular compromise.

Words of Wisdom

Point tenderness and severe pain with or without gross instability are the most reliable indicators of an underlying fracture.

Fractures of the scapula, or shoulder blade, occur much less frequently because this bone is well protected by many large muscles. Fractures of the scapula are almost always the result of a forceful, direct blow to the back, directly over the scapula, which may also injure the thoracic cage, lungs, and heart. For this reason, you must carefully assess the patient for signs of breathing problems. Provide supplemental oxygen and prompt transport for patients who are having difficulty breathing. Remember, it is the associated chest injuries, not the fractured scapula itself, that pose the greatest threat of long-term disability.

Abrasions, contusions, and significant swelling may also occur, and the patient will often limit use of the arm because of pain at the fracture site. The scapula also has bony projections that may be fractured with less force than that required to fracture the body of the scapula.

The joint between the outer end of the clavicle and the acromion process of the scapula is called the **acromioclavicular (AC) joint**. This joint is frequently separated during sports, such as football or hockey, when a player falls and lands on the point of the shoulder, driving the scapula away from the outer end of the clavicle. This dislocation is often called an AC separation. The distal end of the clavicle will often stick out, and the patient will report pain, including point tenderness over the AC joint (**FIGURE 31-30**).

Fractures of the clavicle and scapula and AC separations can all be splinted effectively with a sling and swathe. A **sling** is any bandage or material that helps support the weight of an injured upper extremity, relieving the downward pull of gravity on the injured site. To be effective, a sling must apply gentle upward support to the olecranon process of the ulna. The knot of the sling should be tied to one side of the neck so that it does not press uncomfortably on the cervical spine and the hand positioned slightly higher than the elbow to prevent swelling (**FIGURE 31-31A**).

To fully stabilize the shoulder region, a **swathe**, a bandage that passes completely around the chest, must be used to bind the arm to the chest wall. The swathe should be tight enough to prevent the arm from swinging freely, but not so tight as to compress the chest and compromise breathing. Leave the patient's fingers exposed so that you can assess neurovascular function at regular intervals (**FIGURE 31-31B**).

Commercially available shoulder stabilizers or slings will provide adequate splinting for injuries of the shoulder region, as will triangular bandage slings.

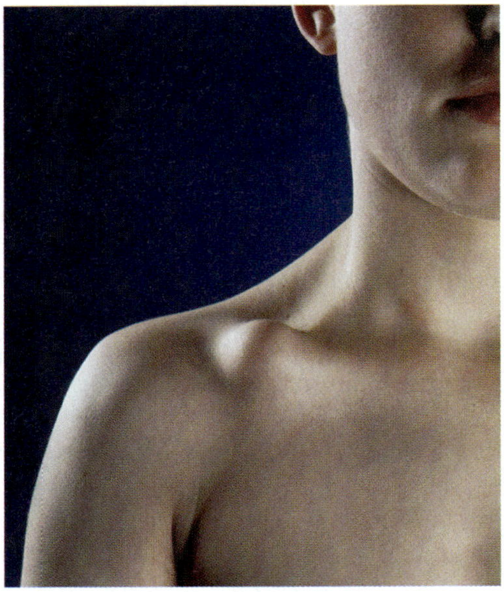

FIGURE 31-30 With acromioclavicular separations, the distal end of the clavicle usually sticks out.

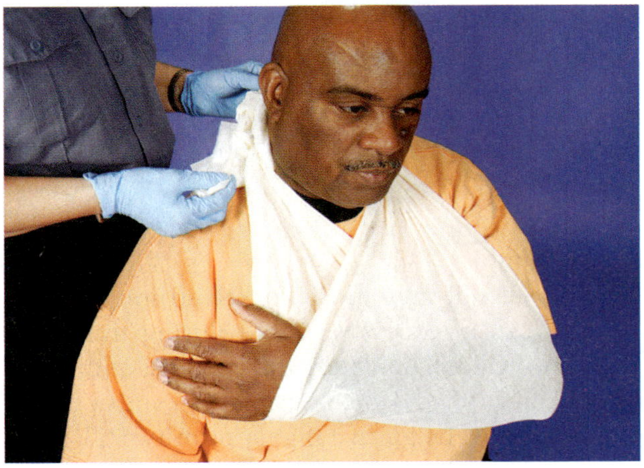

A

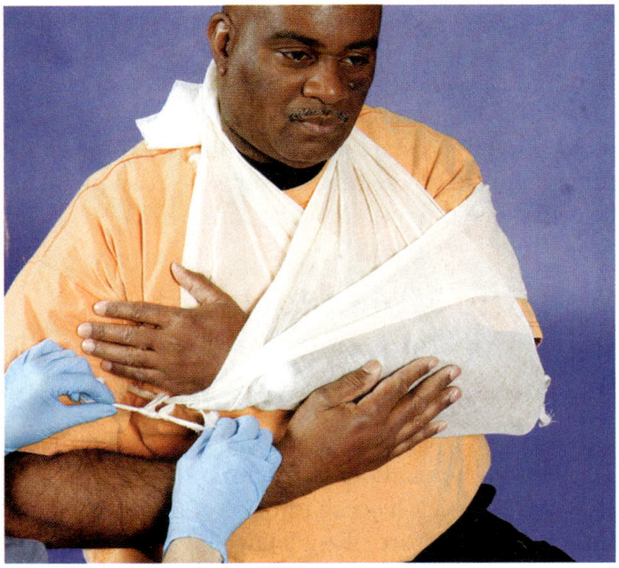

B

FIGURE 31-31 A. Apply a sling so that the knot is tied to one side of the neck. **B.** Bind the arm to the chest wall with a swathe so that the arm cannot swing freely. Leave the patient's fingers exposed so that you can assess distal circulation.

Dislocation of the Shoulder

The glenohumeral joint (shoulder joint) is where the head of the humerus, the supporting bone of the upper arm, meets the **glenoid fossa** of the scapula. The glenoid fossa joins with the humeral head to form the glenohumeral joint. In shoulder dislocations, the humeral head most commonly dislocates anteriorly, coming to lie in front of the scapula as a result of forced abduction (away from the midline) and external rotation of the arm (**FIGURE 31-32**).

Shoulder dislocations are extremely painful. The patient will guard the shoulder and try to protect it by holding the dislocated arm in a fixed position away from the chest wall (**FIGURE 31-33**). The shoulder joint will usually be locked, and the shoulder will appear squared off or flattened. The humeral head will protrude anteriorly underneath the pectoralis major on the anterior chest wall. As a result, the axillary nerve may be compressed, causing a numb patch on the outer aspect of the shoulder. Be sure to document this finding. Some patients may also report some numbness in the hand because of either nervous or circulatory compromise.

Stabilizing an anterior shoulder dislocation is difficult because any attempt to bring the arm in toward the chest will produce pain. You must splint the joint in whatever position is most comfortable for the patient. If necessary, place a pillow or rolled blankets or towels between the arm and chest to fill up the space between them (**FIGURE 31-34**). Once the arm has been stabilized in this way, the elbow can usually be flexed to 90° without causing further pain. At this point, you can apply a sling to

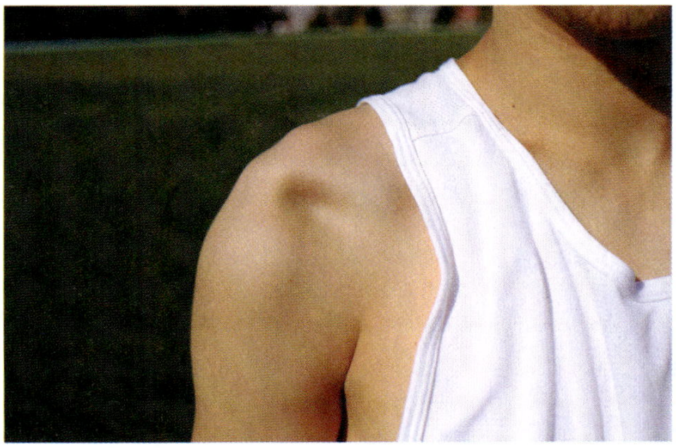

FIGURE 31-32 Most shoulder dislocations are anterior. Note the absence of the normal rounded appearance of the shoulder.

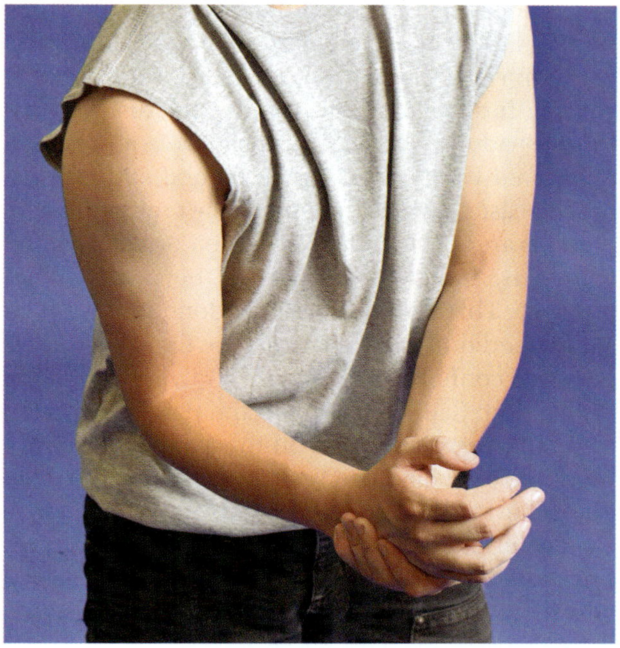

FIGURE 31-33 A patient with a dislocated shoulder will guard the shoulder, trying to protect it by holding the arm in a fixed position away from the chest wall.

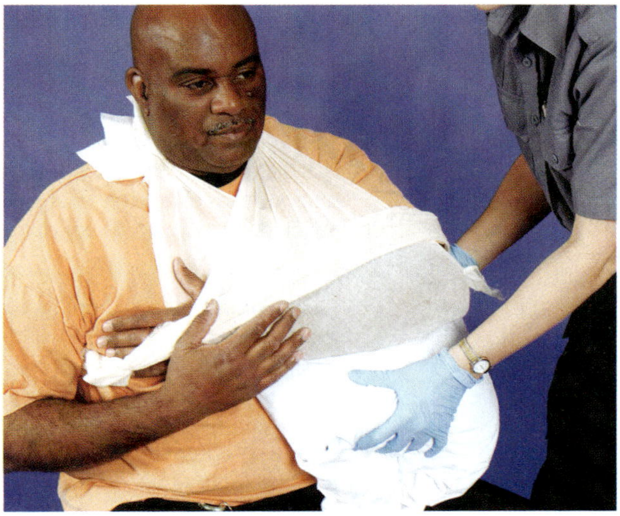

FIGURE 31-34 Splint the shoulder joint in a position of comfort, and place a pillow or towel between the arm and the chest wall to stabilize the arm, after which the elbow can be flexed to 90°. Apply a sling and secure the arm to the chest with a swathe.

the forearm and wrist to support the weight of the arm. Finally, secure the arm in the sling to the pillow and chest with a swathe. Transport the patient in a seated or semiseated position.

Dislocation of the shoulder disrupts the supporting ligaments. In children especially, these ligaments may fail to heal properly, so dislocation recurs, causing further joint injury with each dislocation.[3] In older adults, shoulder dislocation is more often associated with rotator cuff tears and stiffness.[4] In certain cases, surgical repair may be required. Some patients are able to reduce (set) their own dislocated shoulders. However, discourage the patient from doing so. This maneuver is best done in a hospital setting and only after radiographic films have been obtained confirming the nature and direction of the dislocation. Remember that if the patient was able to reduce the dislocation on their own, you would most likely not have been called. Recommend transport for evaluation and treatment.

Posterior dislocation is less common than anterior shoulder dislocation. Football players, especially linemen, are susceptible to this injury due to repeated impact during blocking when the shoulder is flexed and rotated inward.[5] Seizures can also lead to posterior dislocations of the shoulder. The arm will often be locked in adduction (toward the midline), so it cannot be rotated. Reducing dislocated shoulders usually requires medical supervision.

Words of Wisdom

When you assess a patient with a possible shoulder dislocation, position yourself behind the patient and compare the shoulders. The dislocated side is often lower than the uninjured side.

Fracture of the Humerus

Fractures of the humerus occur either proximally, in the midshaft, or distally at the elbow (**TABLE 31-2**). Fractures of the proximal humerus resulting from

TABLE 31-2 Characteristics and Treatment of Fractures of the Humerus

Type	Characteristics	Treatment
Proximal humeral fractures	• Significant swelling, but no significant deformity of the upper arm • Neurovascular compromise uncommon • If neurologic compromise present, any or all of the brachial plexus may be affected, depending on the degree of displacement • Concurrent soft-tissue injuries possible • Possible rotator cuff injury (If radiograph films show no fracture, a tear of the rotator cuff is possible, especially if the patient cannot rotate the arm.)	• Stabilize in a sling and swathe or a shoulder stabilizer. • Use the chest wall as a splint, and secure the injured arm to the chest wall. • Place a short, padded board splint on the lateral side of the arm under the sling and swathe for additional support.
Midshaft fractures	• Gross angulation of the arm • Marked instability and crepitus of fracture fragments • Possible neurovascular compromise • Possible entrapment of the radial nerve (The patient cannot extend or dorsiflex the wrist or fingers and may report numbness on the dorsum of the hand; classic wrist drop.)	• Stabilize with a sling and swathe or a shoulder stabilizer. • Use the chest wall as a splint, and secure the injured arm to the chest wall. • Place a short, padded board splint on the lateral side of the arm under the sling and swathe for additional support.
Distal humeral fractures	• Significant swelling at the elbow • Possible neurovascular compromise • Possible injury to the ulnar or median nerve (Document nerve status before and after any attempt to reduce or stabilize the fracture.)	• Stabilize in a splint, in addition to a sling and swathe or a shoulder stabilizer.

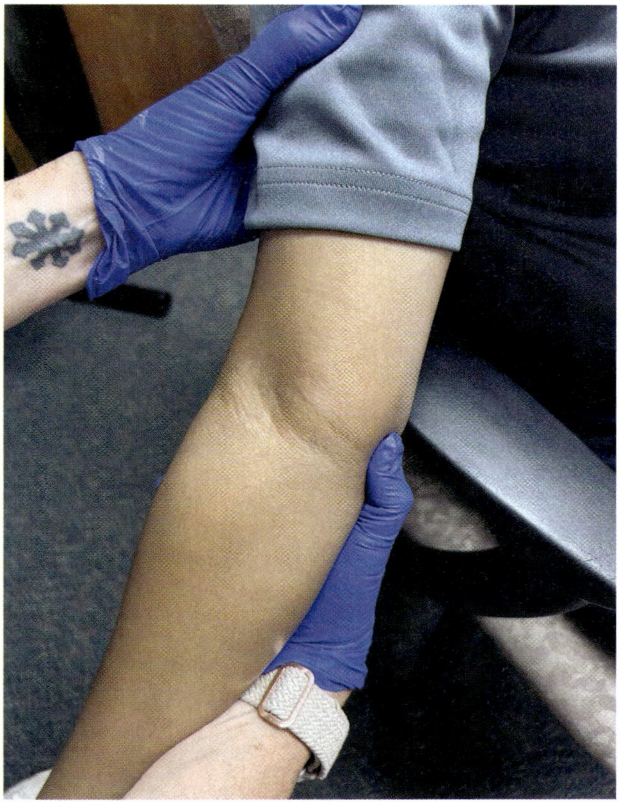

FIGURE 31-35 To align a severe deformity associated with a humeral shaft fracture, apply gentle pressure to the humeral condyles, as shown in this uninjured arm.

falls are common among older people. Fractures of the midshaft occur more often in young patients, usually as the result of a violent injury.

With any severely angulated fracture, consider applying traction to realign the fracture fragments before splinting them. Check your local protocols for indications and techniques for applying traction to a severely angulated fracture. Support the site of the fracture with one hand, and with the other hand, grasp the two humeral condyles (its lateral and medial protrusions) just above the elbow. Pull gently in line with the normal axis of the limb (**FIGURE 31-35**). Once you achieve gross realignment of the limb, splint the arm with a sling and swathe, supplemented by a padded board splint on the lateral aspect of the arm (**FIGURE 31-36**). If the patient reports significant pain or resists gentle traction, splint the fracture in the deformed position with a padded wire ladder or a padded board splint, using pillows to support the injured limb. Note that compartment syndrome, discussed later in this chapter,

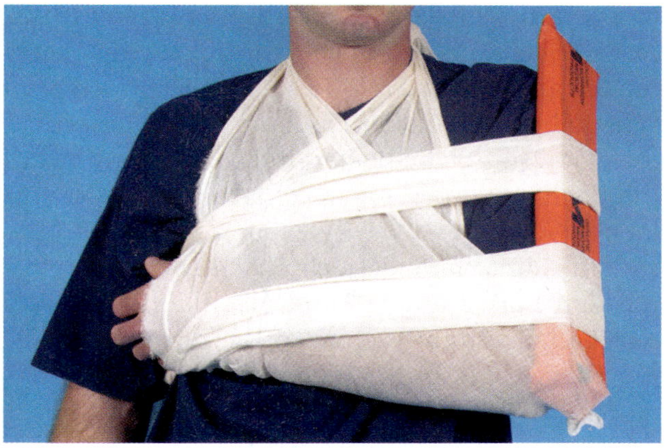

FIGURE 31-36 Splint a humeral shaft fracture with a sling and swathe supplemented by a padded board splint on the lateral aspect of the arm.

can develop in the forearm in children with these fractures. When compartment syndrome occurs, it typically begins to develop several hours after injury and can evolve over the course of days. Once present, it represents a surgical emergency requiring emergent surgical treatment to avoid catastrophic and permanent muscle and nerve damage in the arm.

Elbow Injuries

Fractures and dislocations often occur around the elbow, and the different types of injuries are difficult to distinguish without radiographic examinations. However, they all produce similar limb deformities and require the same emergency care. Injuries to nerves and blood vessels are quite common in this region. Such injuries can be worsened or even caused by inappropriate emergency care, particularly by excessive manipulation of the injured joint.

Fracture of the Distal Humerus

This type of fracture, also known as a supracondylar or intercondylar fracture, depending on its location, is common in children. Frequently, the fracture fragments rotate significantly, producing deformity and causing injuries to nearby vessels and nerves. Swelling occurs rapidly and is often severe.

Dislocation of the Elbow

This type of injury typically occurs in athletes and rarely in young children. The ulna and radius are most often displaced posteriorly relative to the humerus. The ulna, the bone on the little finger side of the forearm, and the radius, the bone on the thumb side of the forearm, both join the distal humerus at the elbow joint. The posterior displacement makes the olecranon process of the ulna much more prominent (**FIGURE 31-37**). The joint is usually locked, with the forearm moderately flexed on the arm; this position makes any attempt at motion extremely painful. As with a fracture of the distal humerus, there is swelling and significant potential for vessel or nerve injury.

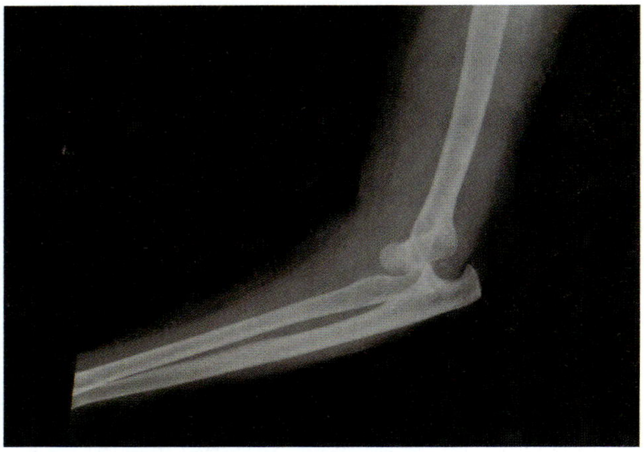

FIGURE 31-37 Radiograph showing posterior dislocation of the elbow, which makes the olecranon process of the ulna much more prominent.

Words of Wisdom

Toddlers can sustain an injury similar to an elbow dislocation when they are lifted or pulled by the arm. This injury, which is sometimes called nursemaid's elbow, is actually a soft-tissue impingement condition, not a joint dislocation.

Elbow Joint Sprain

This diagnosis is often mistakenly applied to an occult, nondisplaced fracture, because it can be difficult to distinguish between sprains and fractures.

Fracture of the Olecranon Process of the Ulna

This fracture can result from direct or indirect forces and is often associated with lacerations and abrasions. The patient will be unable to actively extend the elbow.

Fractures of the Radial Head

Often missed during diagnosis, this fracture generally occurs as a result of a fall on an outstretched arm or a direct blow to the lateral aspect of the elbow. Attempts to rotate the forearm will cause discomfort.

YOU are the EMT

As the nurse continues to manually stabilize the patient's leg, you retrieve the splinting supplies from the ambulance, and your partner reassesses her vital signs.

Recording Time: 13 Minutes	
Level of consciousness	Conscious and alert
Respirations	22 breaths/min; adequate depth
Pulse	110 beats/min; strong and regular
Skin	Mucous membranes in inner lower eyelid and capillary refill normal; warm and moist
Blood pressure	134/80 mm Hg
Oxygen saturation (Spo_2)	99% (on ambient air)

7. How should you splint this patient's injury?

8. What are some methods for providing pain relief from orthopaedic trauma?

Care of Elbow Injuries

All elbow injuries are potentially serious and require careful management. Always assess distal neurovascular functions periodically in patients with elbow injuries. If you find strong pulses and good capillary refill, splint the elbow injury in the position in which you found it, adding a wrist sling if this seems helpful. Two padded board splints, one applied to each side of the limb and secured with soft roller bandages, usually are enough to stabilize the arm (**FIGURE 31-38A**). Make sure the board extends from the shoulder joint to the wrist joint, stabilizing the entire bone above and below the injured joint. Alternatively, you can mold a padded wire ladder splint or a structural aluminum malleable splint to the shape of the limb (**FIGURE 31-38B**). If necessary, you may add further support to the limb with a pillow.

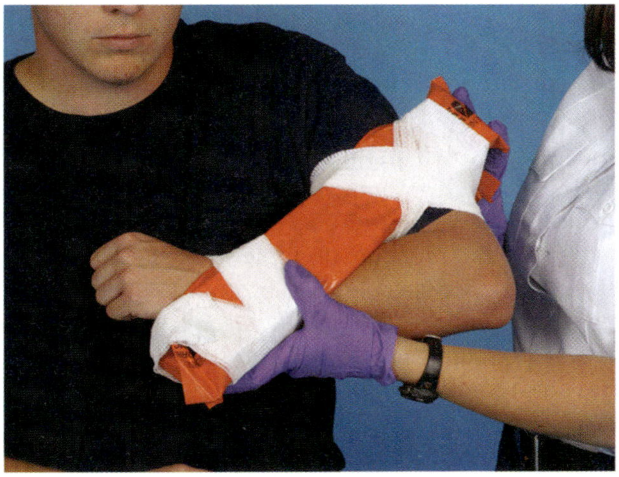

A

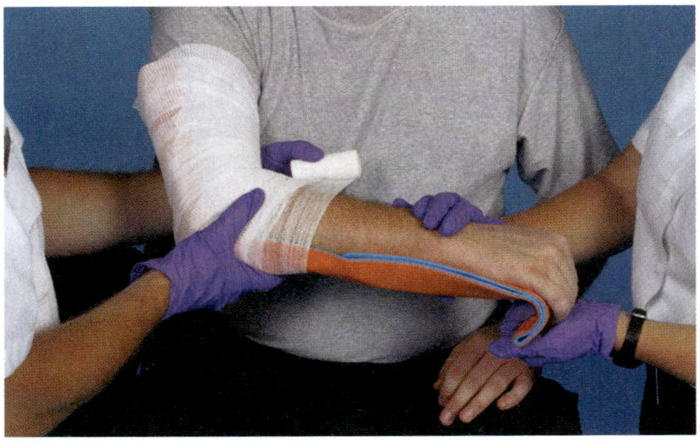

B

FIGURE 31-38 A. Two padded board splints provide adequate stabilization for an injured elbow. **B.** A structural aluminum malleable splint can be molded to the shape of the limb so that you can splint it in the position in which it was found.

A cold, pale hand or a weak pulse and poor capillary refill indicate that the blood vessels have likely been injured. Further care of this patient must be dictated by a physician. Notify medical oversight immediately. They may direct you to try to realign the limb to a normal anatomic position to improve circulation in the hand.[6]

If the limb is pulseless and significantly deformed at the elbow, apply gentle manual traction in line with the long axis of the limb to decrease the deformity. This maneuver may restore the pulse. Be careful, because excessive manipulation may only worsen the vascular problem. If no pulse returns after one attempt, splint the limb in the most comfortable position for the patient. If the pulse is restored by gentle longitudinal traction, splint the limb in whatever position allows the strongest pulse. Provide prompt transport for all patients with impaired distal circulation.

Special Populations

GROWTH PLATE INJURIES IN CHILDREN

Because longitudinal growth of the limb depends on the function of the growth plate, it is extremely important to recognize the possibility of growth plate injuries, stabilize the injured limb, and transport the patient in a timely manner to an appropriate center. Proper functioning of the injured growth plate throughout the remainder of skeletal growth may depend on timely anatomic reduction of the fracture and close follow-up by a pediatric orthopaedic surgeon. Any deformity close to a joint in children younger than 16 years should be assumed to be a growth plate injury. Treat and transport the patient appropriately.

Fractures of the Forearm

Fractures of the shaft of the radius and ulna are common in people of all age groups but are seen most often in children and older people. Usually, both bones break at the same time when the injury is the result of a fall on an outstretched hand (**FIGURE 31-39**). An isolated fracture of the shaft of

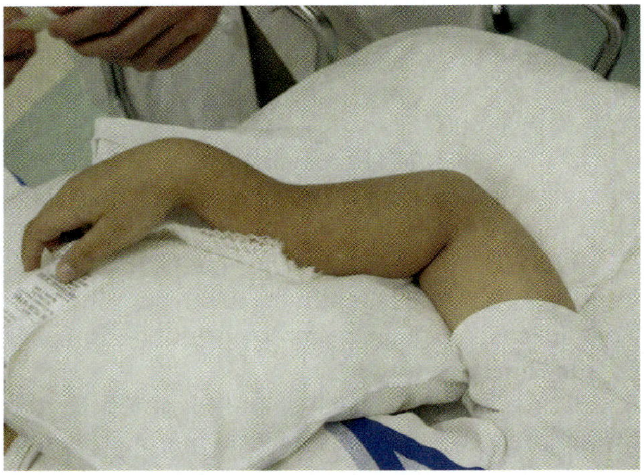

FIGURE 31-39 Fractures of the forearm often occur in children as a result of a fall on an outstretched hand.

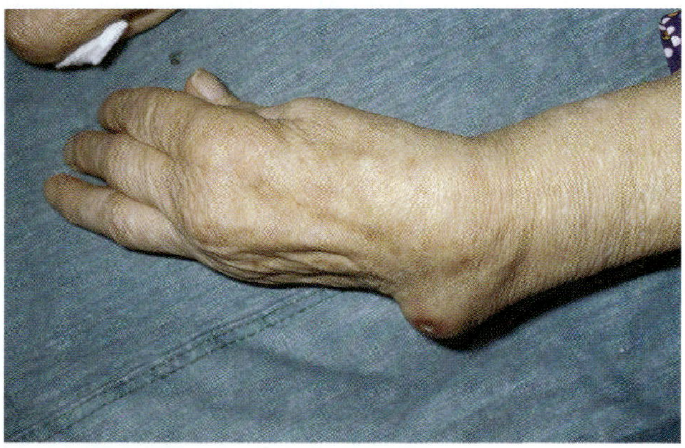

FIGURE 31-40 Fracture of the distal radius.

the ulna may occur as the result of a direct blow to it; this is known as a nightstick fracture.

Fractures of the distal radius are especially common in older adults with osteoporosis (**FIGURE 31-40**). One type is the Colles fracture. This injury may cause the arm to appear angulated in a manner that resembles a dinner fork. In children, this fracture may occur through the growth plate and can have long-term consequences.

To stabilize fractures of the forearm or wrist, you can use a padded board, structural aluminum malleable, vacuum, or pillow splint. If the shaft of the bone has been fractured, be sure to include the elbow joint in the splint. Splinting of the elbow joint is not essential with fractures near the wrist; however, the patient will be more comfortable if you add a sling or pillow for more support. If possible, elevate the injured extremity above the heart to help alleviate swelling.

Special Populations

DISTAL RADIAL FRACTURES IN OLDER ADULTS

In people older than 65 years, distal radial fractures are the second most common type of fracture, after hip fractures, accounting for 18% of fractures.[7] Osteoporosis increases the likelihood that even low-energy mechanisms (ie, falling a distance of standing height or less) will cause this injury.

Injuries of the Wrist and Hand

Injuries of the wrist, ranging from dislocations to sprains, are common after falls. A dislocation may occur subsequent to a fracture (ie, a fracture–dislocation). Another wrist injury is the isolated, nondisplaced fracture of a carpal bone, especially the scaphoid. Any questionable wrist sprain or fracture should be splinted and evaluated in the ED or an orthopaedic surgeon's office.

Hand injuries vary widely, and some may have potentially serious consequences. Industrial, recreational, and home accidents often result in dislocations, fractures, lacerations, burns, and amputations. Because the fingers and hands are required to function in intricate ways, any injury that is not treated properly may result in permanent disability, as well as deformity. For this reason, all injuries to the hand, including simple lacerations, should be evaluated by a physician. For example, do not attempt to "pop" a dislocated finger joint back in place (**FIGURE 31-41**).

A malleable structural aluminum or board splint makes an effective splint for any hand or wrist injury. Follow the steps in **SKILL DRILL 31-3**:

1. Take standard precautions.
2. Cover open wounds with a moist, sterile dressing.
3. Assess distal pulse and motor and sensory function.
4. Supporting the injured limb, form the injured hand into the **position of function**, with the wrist slightly bent down and all finger joints

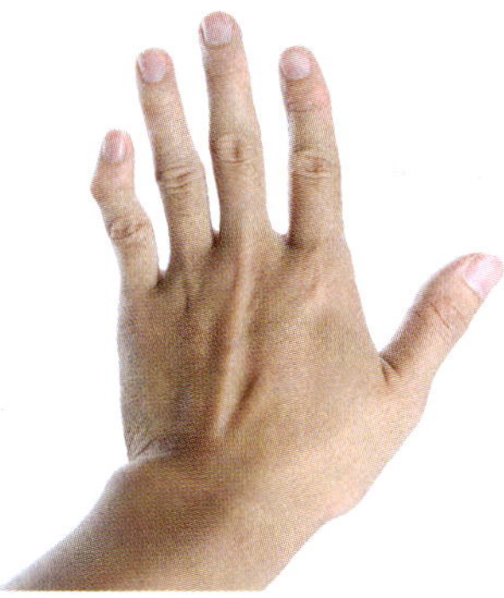

FIGURE 31-41 Dislocation of the finger joint. Do not try to "pop" the joint back into place.

moderately flexed. This is the position that is used to hold a can most comfortably.

5. Place a soft roller bandage into the palm of the hand (**Step 1**).
6. Apply a malleable structural aluminum or padded board splint to the palmar side of the wrist, leaving the fingers exposed (**Step 2**).
7. Secure the entire length of the splint with a soft roller bandage (**Step 3**). Assess distal pulse and motor and sensory function.
8. Apply a sling and swathe, or prop the splinted hand and wrist on a pillow or on the patient's chest during transport to the hospital.

Skill Drill 31-3 Splinting the Hand and Wrist

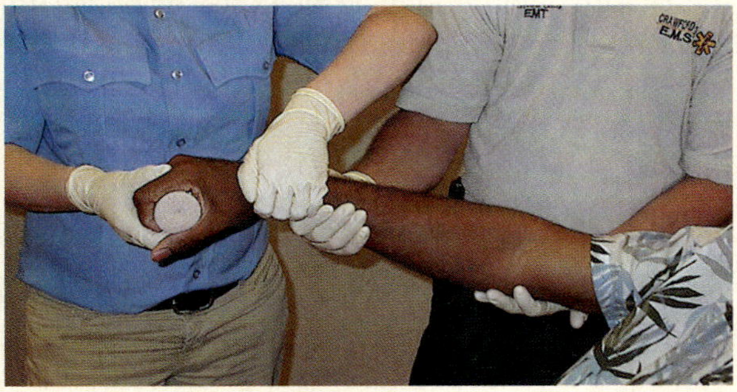

Step 1

Support the injured limb and move the hand into the position of function. Place a soft roller bandage in the palm.

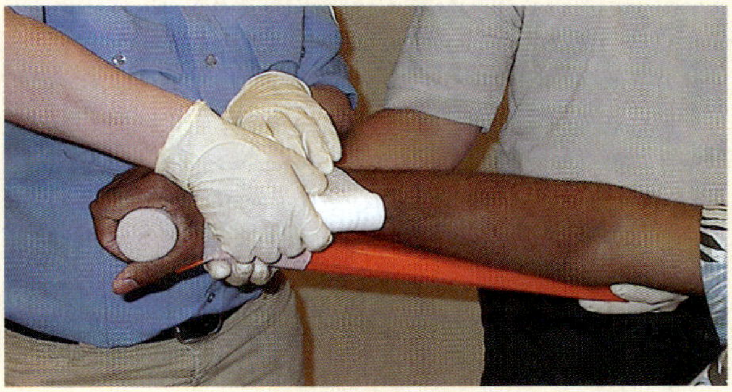

Step 2

Apply a padded board splint on the palmar side with fingers exposed.

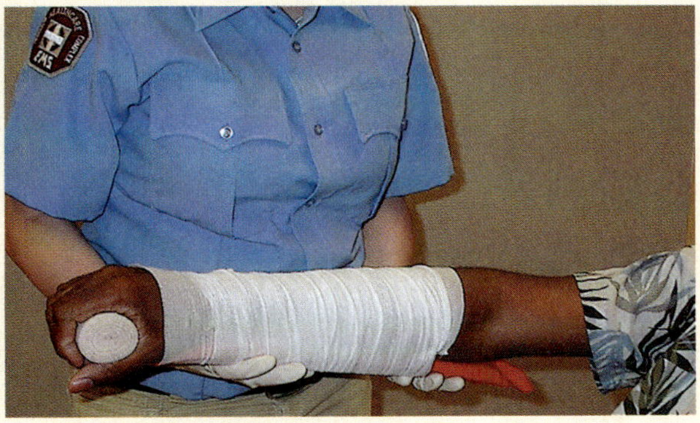

Step 3

Secure the splint with a roller bandage.

Fractures of the Pelvis

Fractures of the pelvis often result from direct compression in the form of a heavy blow that literally crushes the pelvis. The blow may be from a motor vehicle crash, a weapon, a falling object, or a fall from a height. Injuries to the pelvis can also be caused by indirect forces. For example, when the knee strikes the dashboard in a motor vehicle crash, the impact of the force is transmitted along the line of the femur (thighbone), which is the longest and largest bone in the body. The head of the femur is driven into the pelvis, causing a fracture of the acetabulum, the portion of the pelvis that forms the socket of the hip joint.

However, keep in mind that not all pelvic fractures result from violent trauma. Even a low-energy mechanism or a standing fall can produce a fracture of the pelvis, especially in older adults with osteoporosis (**FIGURE 31-42**). The person may sustain this injury when getting out of the bathtub or descending stairs. These injuries do not usually damage the structural integrity of the pelvic ring but may fracture an individual bone.

Certain types of pelvic fractures may be accompanied by life-threatening loss of blood from the laceration of blood vessels affixed to the pelvis at certain key points. Up to several liters of blood may drain into the pelvic space and the **retroperitoneal space**, which lies between the abdominal cavity and the posterior abdominal wall. The result is significant hypotension, shock, and sometimes death. For this reason, you must take immediate steps to treat shock, even if there is no visible swelling. Often, there is no evidence of bleeding until severe blood loss has occurred. Be prepared to resuscitate the patient rapidly if this becomes necessary.

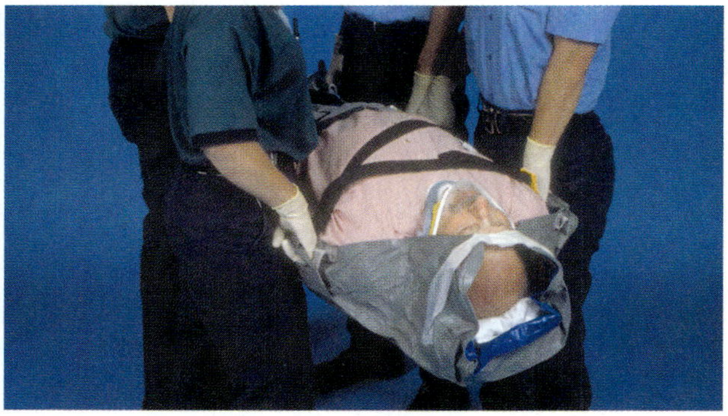

FIGURE 31-42 Vacuum mattresses that conform to body contours can be a good choice for restricting body movement of geriatric patients with possible pelvic fractures.

Words of Wisdom

Remember that fractures can result in substantial bleeding. The inability of the blood to clot normally can be a significant problem in patients, such as older adults who take warfarin (Coumadin), apixaban (Eliquis), or other blood-thinning medications.

Because the pelvis is surrounded by heavy muscle, open fractures of the pelvis are uncommon. However, pelvis fracture fragments can lacerate the rectum and vagina, creating an open fracture that is often overlooked. Once the protective pelvic ring is broken, the structures it is designed to protect, including the urinary bladder, are more susceptible to injury. The bladder may be lacerated by pelvic bone fragments, or it may tear as a result of direct pressure on the bladder itself or tension on the urethra. Fractures of the pelvic ring area are often accompanied by other serious internal injuries.

You should suspect a fracture of the pelvis in any patient who has sustained a high-velocity injury and reports discomfort in the lower back or abdomen. Because the area is covered by heavy muscle and other soft tissue, deformity or swelling may be difficult to see. The most reliable sign of pelvic fracture is simple tenderness or instability on firm compression and palpation. Firm compression on the two iliac crests will produce pain at a fracture site in the pelvic ring. Once tenderness over the pelvic bones or other signs of fracture are identified, further palpation is not indicated. Assess for tenderness by taking the following steps (**FIGURE 31-43**):

1. Place the palms of your hands over the lateral aspect of each iliac crest, and apply firm but gentle inward pressure on the pelvic ring.
2. With the patient lying supine, place a palm over the anterior aspect of each iliac crest, and apply firm downward pressure.
3. Use the palm of your hand to firmly but gently palpate the pubic symphysis, the firm cartilaginous joint between the two pubic bones. This area will be tender if there is injury to the anterior portion of the pelvic ring.

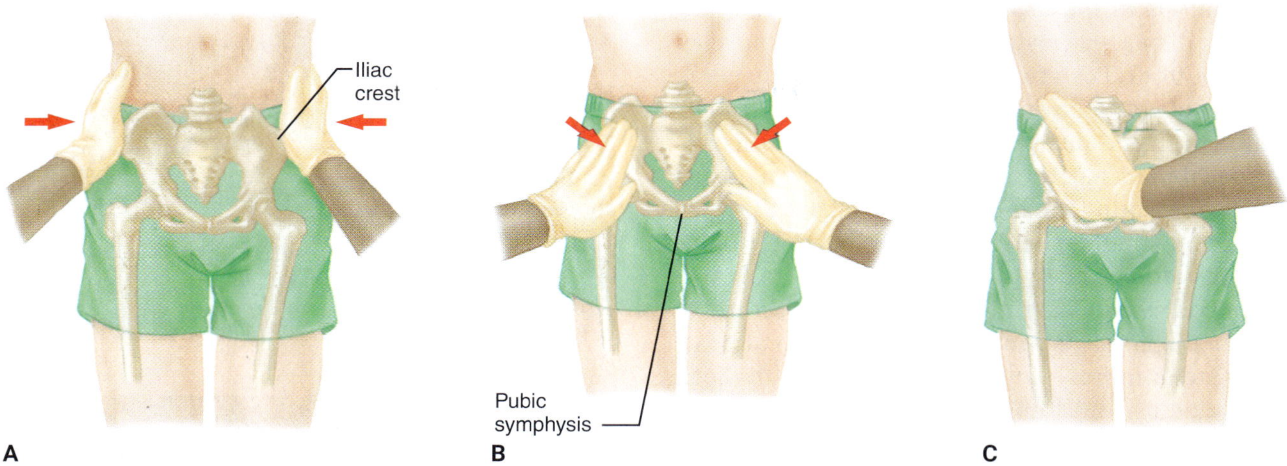

FIGURE 31-43 A. To assess for tenderness or instability in the pelvic region, place your hands over the lateral aspect of each iliac crest, and gently compress the pelvis. **B.** With the patient in a supine position, place your palms over the anterior aspect of each iliac crest, and apply firm but gentle downward pressure. **C.** Palpate the pubic symphysis with the palm of your hand.

If there has been injury to the bladder or the urethra, the patient will have lower abdominal tenderness and may have evidence of **hematuria** (blood in the urine) or blood at the urethral opening.

Perform the primary assessment, and carefully monitor the general condition of any patient whom you suspect has a pelvic fracture, because the patient is at high risk for hypovolemic shock. Patients in stable condition can be secured to a backboard or a scoop stretcher to stabilize isolated fractures of the pelvis.

Dislocation of the Hip

The hip joint is a stable ball-and-socket joint that dislocates only after significant injury. Most

YOU are the EMT

After properly splinting the patient's leg, you place her onto the stretcher, load her into the ambulance, and begin transport to the hospital. You reassess her condition and vital signs en route and note that her condition remains stable. You call your radio report in to the receiving facility; your estimated time of arrival is 8 minutes.

Recording Time: 23 Minutes	
Level of consciousness	Conscious and alert
Respirations	20 breaths/min; adequate depth
Pulse	115 beats/min; strong and regular
Skin	Mucous membranes in inner lower eyelid and capillary refill normal; warm and dry
Blood pressure	128/76 mm Hg
Oxygen saturation (Spo_2)	98% (on ambient air)

During transport, the patient reports numbness and tingling in her left foot. Your reassessment reveals that her pedal pulse is weaker than it was before and that her foot looks pale and feels cool.

9. What is the most likely cause of the patient's complaint? What can you do to remedy the situation?

10. What factors increase the risk of complications following orthopaedic trauma?

dislocations of the hip are posterior. The femoral head is displaced posteriorly to lie in the muscles of the buttock. Posterior dislocation of the hip commonly occurs as a result of a motor vehicle crash in which the knee meets with a direct force, such as the dashboard, and the entire femur is driven posteriorly, dislocating the hip joint (see Figure 31-12A). Thus, you should suspect a hip dislocation in any patient who has been in a motor vehicle crash and has a contusion, laceration, or obvious fracture in the knee region. Very rarely does the femoral head dislocate anteriorly; in this circumstance, the legs are suddenly and forcibly spread wide apart and locked in this position.

Posterior dislocation of the hip is frequently complicated by injury to the sciatic nerve, which is located directly behind the hip joint. The **sciatic nerve** is the largest peripheral nerve in the body; it controls the activity of muscles in the posterior thigh and below the knee and the sensation in most of the leg and foot. When the head of the femur is forced out of the hip socket, it may compress or stretch the sciatic nerve, leading to partial or complete paralysis of the nerve. The result is decreased sensation in the leg and foot and frequently weakness in the foot muscles. Generally, only the dorsiflexors, the muscles that raise the toes or foot, are involved, causing the foot drop that is characteristic of damage to the peroneal portion of the sciatic nerve.

Patients with a posterior dislocation of the hip typically lie with the hip joint flexed (the knee joint drawn up toward the chest) and the thigh rotated inward toward the midline of the body over the top of the opposite thigh (**FIGURE 31-44A**). With the less common anterior dislocation, the limb is in the opposite position, extended straight out, externally rotated, and pointing away from the midline of the body.

Dislocation of the hip is associated with distinctive signs. The patient will have severe pain in the hip and will strongly resist any attempt to move the joint. The lateral and posterior aspects of the hip region will be tender on palpation. With some thin patients, you can palpate the femoral head deep within the muscles of the buttock. The leg on the side of the dislocated hip will appear shorter than the other leg, and the foot may appear to rotate inward or outward. Check for a sciatic nerve injury by carefully assessing sensation and motor function in the lower extremity. Occasionally,

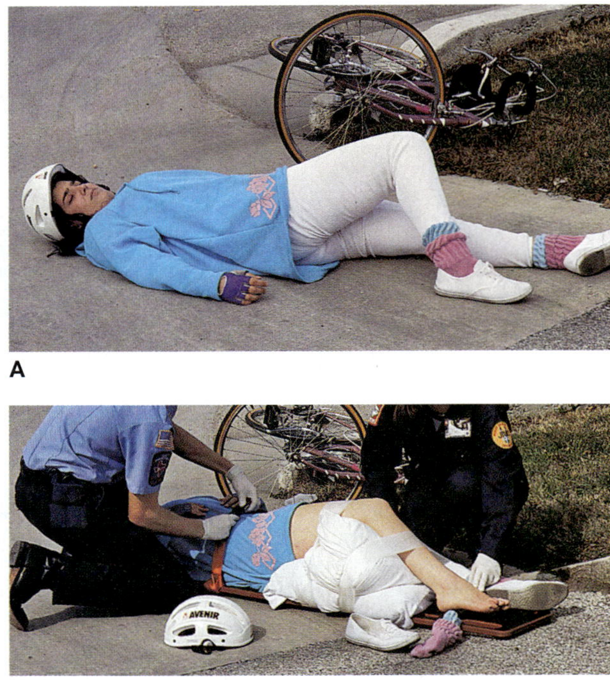

FIGURE 31-44 A. The usual position of a patient with a posterior dislocation of the hip. The hip joint is flexed, and the thigh is rotated inward and adducted across the midline of the body. **B.** Support the affected limb with pillows and blankets, particularly under the flexed knee. Secure the entire limb to a backboard with long straps to prevent movement during transport.

sciatic nerve function will be normal at first and then slowly diminish.

As with any other extremity injury, do not attempt to reduce the dislocated hip in the field. Splint the dislocation in the position of the deformity, and place the patient supine on a backboard. Support the affected limb with pillows and rolled blankets, particularly under the flexed knee (**FIGURE 31-44B**). Then secure the entire limb to the backboard with long straps so that the hip region will not move, and provide prompt transport.

Fractures of the Proximal Femur

Fractures of the proximal (upper) end of the femur are common, especially in older people and patients with osteoporosis. Although these fractures are usually called hip fractures, they rarely involve the hip joint. Instead, the break goes through the neck of the femur, the intertrochanteric (middle) region, or across the proximal shaft of the femur (subtrochanteric fractures). These three fracture types may also be a result of high-energy injuries in younger patients.

> **Words of Wisdom**
>
> People with osteoporosis may fracture a hip as a result of a fall from a standing position. Contributing factors to osteoporosis and the risk of fracture include vitamin D and calcium deficiencies, metabolic bone diseases, and tumors. Injuries to the hip can also be recurring. A previous fracture increases the likelihood of a future injury.

Patients with displaced fractures of the proximal femur display a very characteristic deformity. They lie with the leg externally rotated, and the injured leg is usually shorter than the opposite, uninjured limb. When the fracture is not displaced, this deformity is not present. With any kind of hip fracture, patients typically are unable to walk or move the leg because of pain in the hip region or in the groin or inner aspect of the thigh. The hip region may be tender on palpation, and gentle rolling of the leg will cause pain but will not do further damage. On occasion, the pain is referred to the knee; it is not uncommon for a geriatric patient with a hip fracture to report knee pain after a fall. Assess the pelvis for any soft-tissue injury and bandage appropriately. In addition, assess pulses and motor and sensory functions, looking for signs of vascular and nerve damage. Once your assessment is complete, splint the lower extremity of an older adult who has fallen and reports pain in either the hip or the knee, even if there is no deformity, and then transport the patient to the ED.

The age of the patient and the severity of the injury will dictate how you splint the fracture. You can effectively stabilize such a fracture by placing the patient on a backboard, vacuum mattress, or scoop stretcher, using pillows or rolled blankets to support the injured limb in the deformed position. Then secure the injured limb carefully to the device with long straps.

Patients with hip fractures may have a significant amount of blood loss. Therefore, you should treat with high-flow oxygen if indicated, monitor vital signs frequently, and be alert for signs of shock.

> **Words of Wisdom**
>
> A traction splint is used only for midshaft femur fractures and is therefore not indicated when there are injuries above or below the fracture. For these reasons, a traction splint is not indicated in pelvic, proximal femur (hip), or distal (knee) fractures.[8]

Femoral Shaft Fractures

Fractures of the femur can occur in any part of the shaft, from the hip region to the femoral condyles just above the knee joint. Following a fracture, the large muscles of the thigh spasm to "splint" the unstable limb. The muscle spasm often produces significant deformity of the limb, with severe angulation or external rotation at the fracture site. Usually, the limb also shortens significantly. Fractures of the femoral shaft may be open, and fragments of bone may protrude through the skin. As with any other open fracture, never attempt to push the bone or bones back into the skin.

There is often a significant amount of blood loss, as much as 500 to 1,000 mL, after a fracture of the femoral shaft. With open fractures, the amount of blood loss may be even greater. However, it is rare for hypovolemic shock to develop in unilateral, closed femur fractures. The presence of shock in these patients suggests other injuries.[8]

Because of the severe deformity that occurs with these fractures, bone fragments may impinge on important nerves and vessels and produce significant damage. For this reason, you must carefully and periodically assess the distal neurovascular function in patients who have sustained a fracture of the femoral shaft. Remove the clothing from the affected limb so that you can adequately inspect the injury site for any open wounds. Remember to take standard precautions when any blood or body fluids are present. Monitor the patient's vital signs closely, and continue to watch for the onset of hypovolemic shock. You must provide rapid transport in this situation.

Cover any open wound with a saline-moistened, sterile dressing. If the foot or leg below the level of the fracture shows signs of impaired circulation (is pale, cold, or pulseless), apply gentle longitudinal traction to the deformed limb in line with the long axis of the limb. Gradually turn the leg from the deformed position to restore the limb's overall alignment. Often, this restores or improves circulation to the foot. If it does not, the patient may have sustained a serious vascular injury and may be in need of prompt medical attention.

A fracture of the femoral shaft is stabilized with a static (rigid) splint, a vacuum splint or spine board, or a traction splint, such as a Sager or Slishman splint.[8]

Traction Splints

Application of in-line **traction** is the act of pulling on a body structure in the direction of its normal alignment. It is an effective way to realign a fracture of the shaft of a long bone so that the limb can be splinted more effectively. Traction splints are used to secure fractures of the midshaft of the femur, which are characterized by pain, swelling, and deformity of the midthigh. These splints should not be used if there is damage to the ankle, knee, pelvis, or hip.

Excessive traction can be harmful to an injured limb. When applied correctly, however, traction stabilizes the bone fragments and improves the overall alignment of the limb. Do not attempt to force the bone fragments back into alignment. In the field, the goals of in-line traction are as follows:

1. Stabilize the fracture fragments to prevent excessive movement.
2. Align the limb sufficiently to allow it to be placed in a splint.
3. Avoid potential neurovascular compromise.

Several different types of lower extremity traction splints are commercially available, such as the Hare traction splint, the Sager splint, the Slishman splint, and the Kendrick splint (**FIGURE 31-45**). Each has its own unique method of application; therefore, it is important to practice using the device or devices your agency carries.

Traction splints are not suitable for use on the upper extremity because the major nerves and blood vessels in the axilla cannot tolerate countertraction forces.

Do not use traction splints for injuries of the upper extremity or in the presence of any of the following conditions:

- Injuries close to or involving the knee
- Injuries of the pelvis
- Partial amputations or avulsions with bone separation
- Lower leg, foot, or ankle injuries

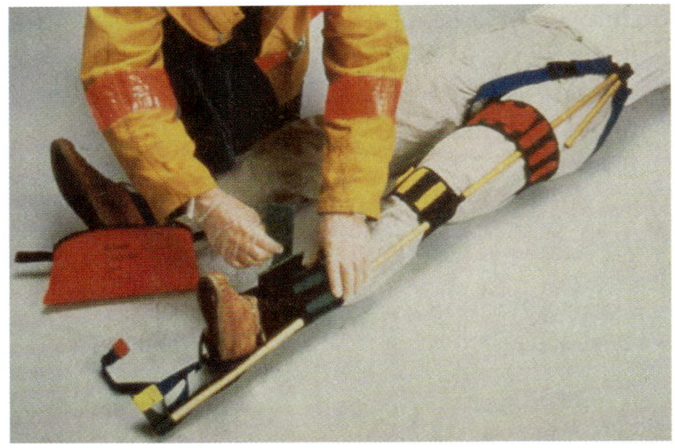

FIGURE 31-45 The Kendrick traction splint.

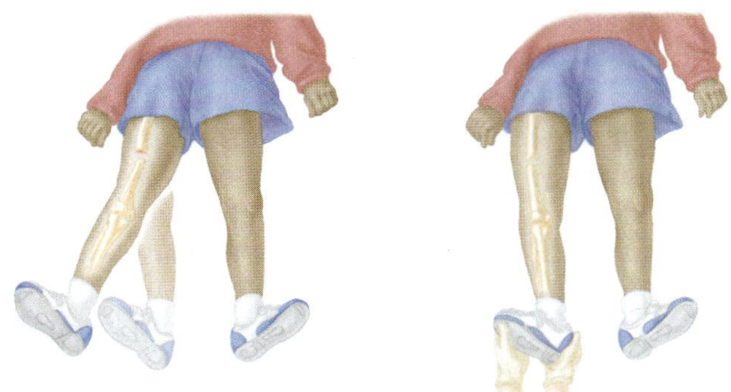

FIGURE 31-46 To apply traction, imagine the position where the uninjured limb would lie, and then gently pull along that line until the injured limb is in that position. Do not release traction once you have applied it.

Proper application of a traction splint requires a minimum of two EMTs. Before you apply a traction splint, be sure to control any external bleeding. The amount of traction that is required varies but often does not exceed 15 pounds (7 kg) or 10% of the patient's body weight, whichever is less. Use the least amount of force necessary. Grasp the foot at the end of the injured limb firmly; once you start pulling, do not stop until the limb is fully splinted. Releasing manual traction before the limb is secured will allow the muscles to contract, allowing the bone fragments to cause more damage to surrounding tissue. Always apply traction along the long axis of the limb. Imagine where the uninjured limb would lie, and pull gently along the line of that imaginary limb until the injured limb is in approximately that position (**FIGURE 31-46**). Grasping the foot and applying the initial pull of traction usually cause the patient some discomfort as the bone fragments move. A second EMT should support the injured limb directly under the site of the fracture. This initial discomfort quickly subsides, and you can then apply further gentle traction. However, if the patient strongly resists the traction or if it causes more pain that persists, stop and splint the limb in the deformed position.

To apply a Hare traction splint, follow the steps in **SKILL DRILL 31-4**:

1. Cut open the patient's pant leg, or otherwise expose the injured lower extremity. Remove the patient's shoe. Take standard precautions as needed. Be sure to assess and record the pulse and motor function and sensation distal to the injury.

Skill Drill 31-4 Applying a Hare Traction Splint

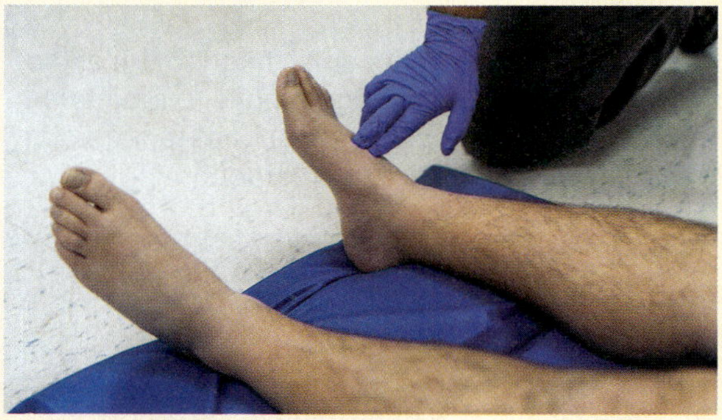

Step 1

Expose the injured limb and check pulse and motor and sensory function. Place the splint beside the uninjured limb, adjust the splint to the proper length, and prepare the straps.

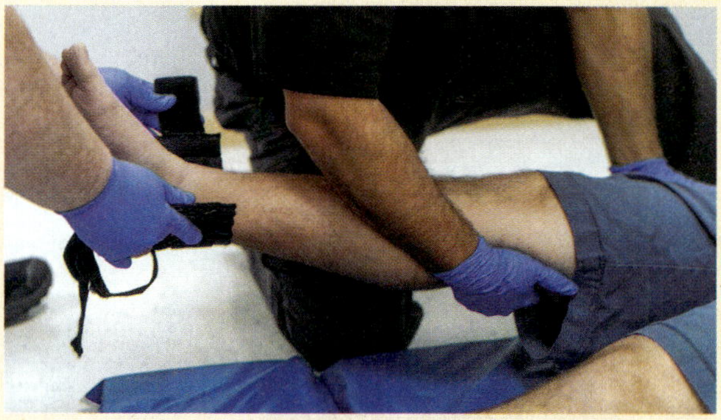

Step 2

Support the injured limb as your partner fastens the ankle hitch around the foot and ankle.

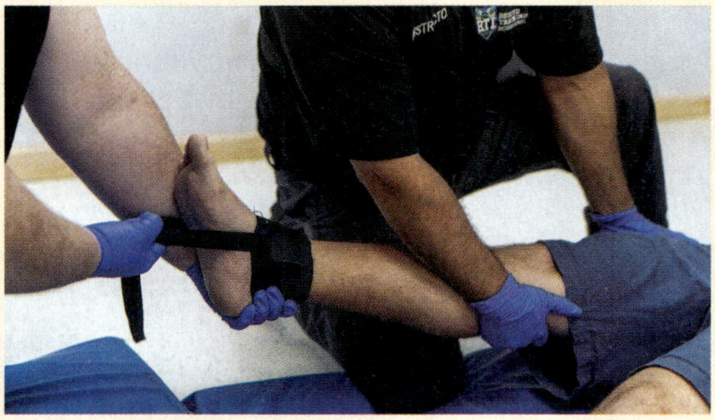

Step 3

Continue to support the limb as your partner applies gentle in-line traction to the ankle hitch and foot.

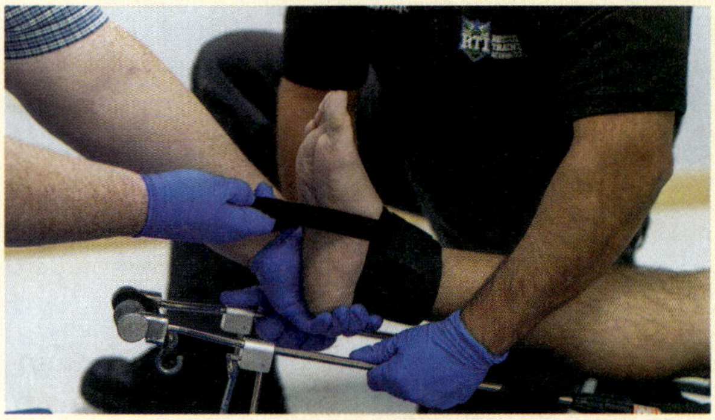

Step 4

Slide the splint into position under the injured limb.

(continues)

Skill Drill 31-4 Applying a Hare Traction Splint continued

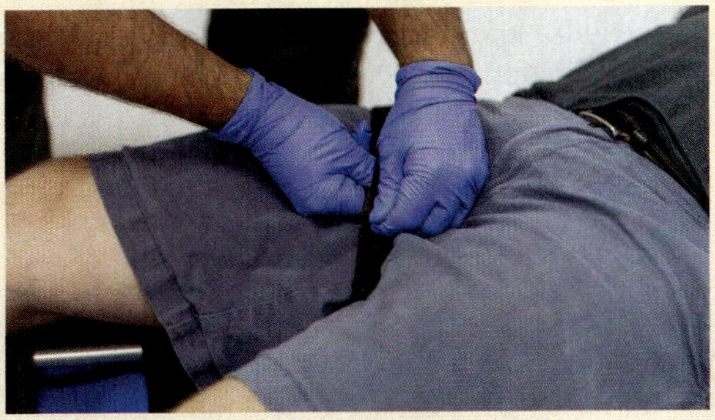

Step 5

Pad the groin and fasten the ischial strap.

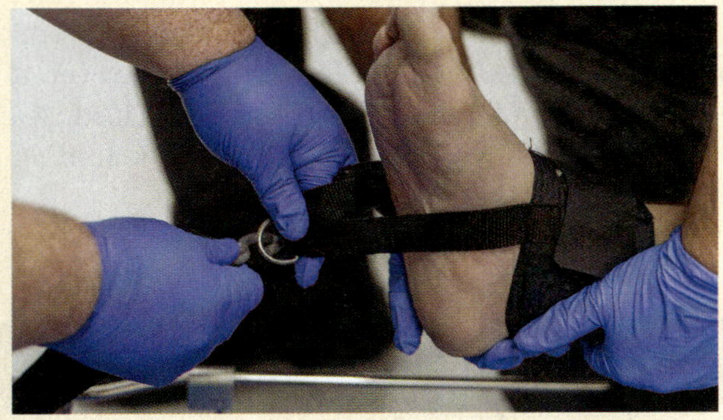

Step 6

Connect the loops of the ankle hitch to the end of the splint as your partner continues to maintain traction. Carefully tighten the ratchet to the point that the splint holds adequate traction.

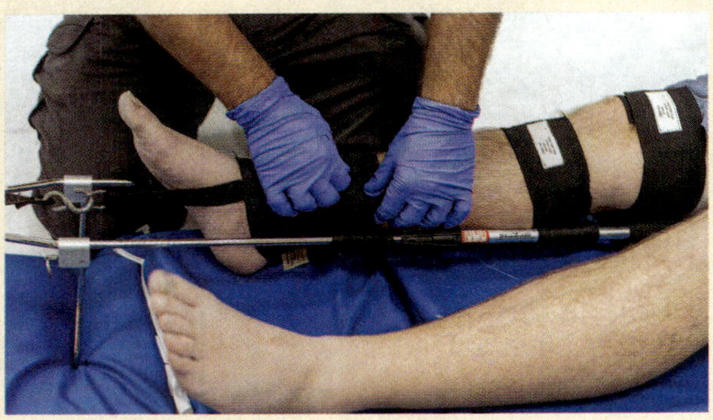

Step 7

Secure and check support straps.

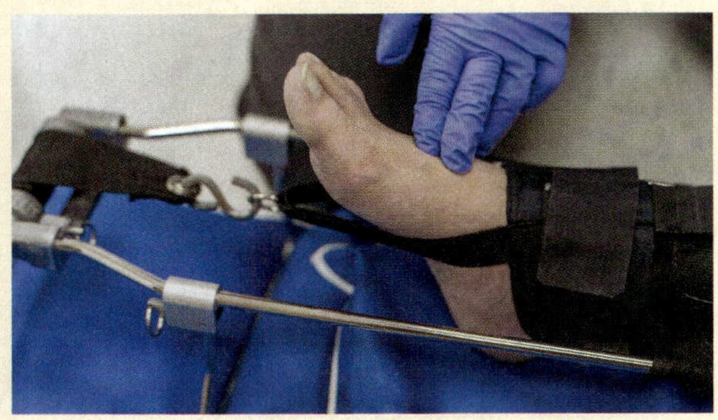

Step 8

Assess pulse and motor and sensory functions. Secure the patient and splint to the backboard in a way that will prevent movement of the splint during patient movement and transport.

2. Place the splint beside the patient's uninjured leg, and adjust it to the proper length, with the ring at the ischial tuberosity and the splint extending 12 inches (30 cm) beyond the foot. Open and adjust the four Velcro support straps, which should be positioned at the midthigh, above the knee, below the knee, and above the ankle (**Step 1**).
3. Manually support and stabilize the injured limb so that no motion will occur at the fracture site while your partner fastens the appropriate-size ankle hitch around the patient's ankle and foot (**Step 2**).
4. Support the leg at the site of the suspected injury while your partner manually applies gentle longitudinal traction to the ankle hitch and foot. Use only enough force to align (reposition) the limb so that it will fit into the splint; do not attempt to align the fracture fragments anatomically (**Step 3**).

5. Slide the splint into position under the patient's injured limb, making certain that the ring is seated well on the ischial tuberosity (**Step 4**).
6. Pad the groin area, and gently apply the ischial strap (**Step 5**).
7. While your partner continues to maintain traction, connect the loops of the ankle hitch to the end of the splint. Then apply gentle traction to the connecting strap between the ankle hitch and the splint, just strongly enough to maintain limb alignment. Use caution. This splint comes with a ratchet mechanism to tighten the strap. Overtightening can theoretically overstretch the limb and further injure the patient. Adequate traction has been applied when the leg is the same length as the other leg and the patient feels relief (**Step 6**).
8. Once proper traction has been applied, fasten the support straps so that the limb is securely held in the splint. Check all proximal and distal support straps to make sure they are secure.
9. At this point, reassess distal pulses and motor function and sensation (**Step 7**).
10. Place the patient securely on a backboard or other stabilization device for transport to the ED. You may need to load the patient feetfirst into the ambulance so that you do not shut the door against the splint (**Step 8**).

Because the traction splint stabilizes the limb by producing countertraction on the ischium and in the groin, pad these areas well. Avoid excessive pressure on the external genitalia. Always use commercially available padded ankle hitches rather than pieces of rope, cord, or tape. Such improvised hitches can sometimes be painful and can potentially impair circulation in the foot.

Some services use other traction splints, such as the Sager traction splint or the Slishman traction splint. These devices are lightweight, easy to store, and apply a measurable amount of traction. Unlike the Hare device, they can be applied by a single rescuer when necessary. As with any splint, in addition to knowing the precise sequence of steps to apply the splint properly, you must practice the splinting technique frequently to remain competent. Follow these steps to apply a Slishman traction splint (**SKILL DRILL 31-5**):

1. Having taken standard precautions, expose the injured extremity. Assess distal motor, sensory, and circulatory function in the injured leg (**Step 1**).

Skill Drill 31-5 Applying a Slishman Traction Splint

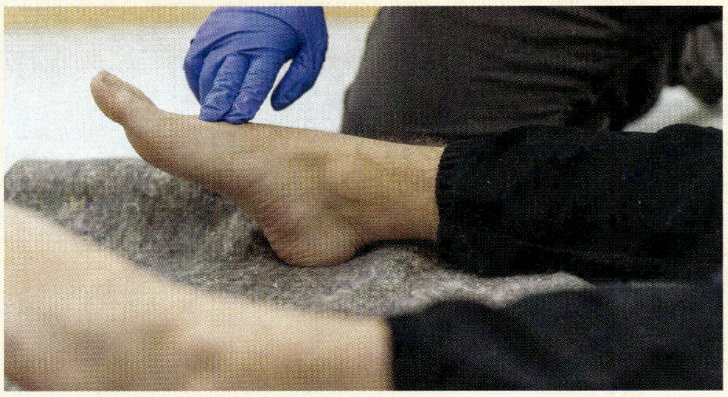

Step 1

After exposing the injured area (exposure of the leg is not shown here), assess distal motor, sensory, and circulatory function.

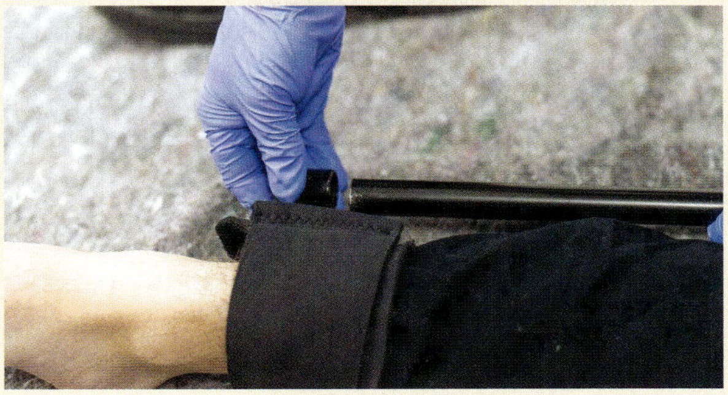

Step 2

Place the ankle strap around the ankle of the injured leg with the end cap on the outside of the leg and facing up to receive the splint pole. Secure the Velcro fastener.

(continues)

Skill Drill 31-5 Applying a Slishman Traction Splint *continued*

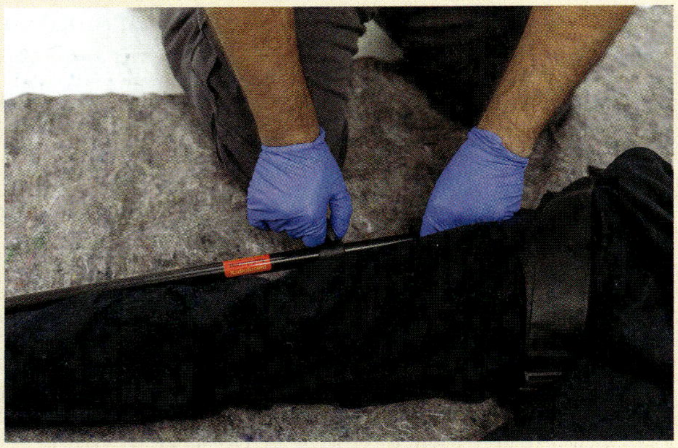

Step 3

Place the female portion of the groin strap to the outside of the thigh. Wrap the male buckle and strap around the thigh, then fasten the buckle. Place the pole in the ankle strap, adjust it to the length of the patient's leg, then tighten the thumb screw on the black pole.

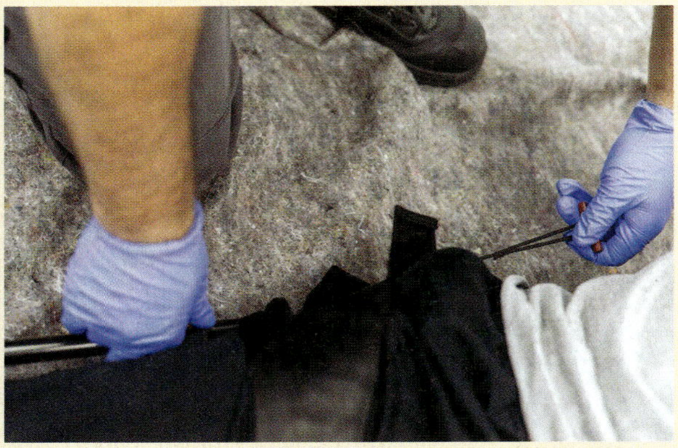

Step 4

Release the thumb screw on the red pole clamp, pull on the cord to apply traction, tighten the thumb screw, and release the cord.

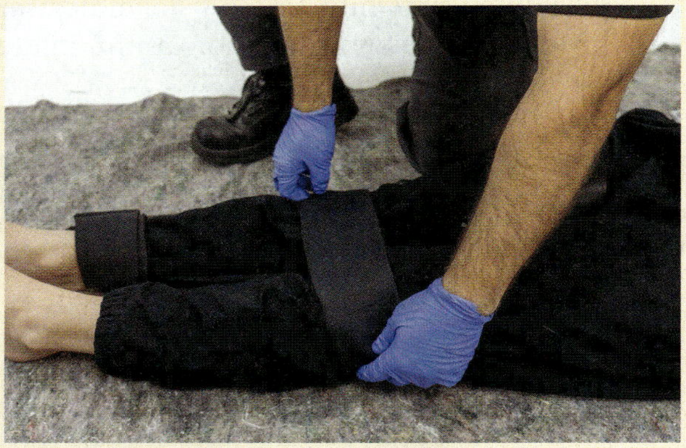

Step 5

For rotational stability, attach a leg strap over one or both knees.

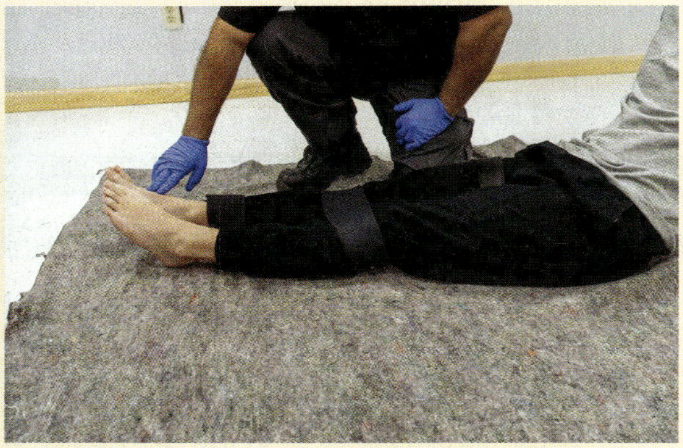

Step 6

Reassess distal motor, sensory, and circulatory function.

All images courtesy of Aura Prep/Rescue Training International.

2. Place the ankle strap around the ankle of the injured leg. The end cap should be on the outside of the leg and facing up to receive the splint pole. Secure the Velcro fastener (**Step 2**). Note that if necessary, the ankle strap can be applied above the calf to avoid placement over an injury to the lower leg.
3. Place the female portion of the groin strap to the outside of the thigh. Wrap the male buckle and strap around the thigh, then snap the female and male ends of the buckle together.
4. Release the thumb screw on the black pole and extend the pole into the ankle strap. Once the pole is adjusted to approximately the length

of the patient's leg, tighten the thumb screw (**Step 3**).

5. Release the thumb screw on the red pole clamp, then pull on the cord to achieve the desired amount of traction. Traction is typically considered sufficient when the injured leg is equal in length to the uninjured leg or when pain is relieved. Once achieved, tighten the thumb screw and release the cord (**Step 4**).
6. For rotational stability, attach a leg strap over one or both knees (**Step 5**).
7. Move the patient to a stretcher. First secure the patient to a backboard if indicated.
8. Assess distal motor, sensory, and circulatory function in the injured leg (**Step 6**).

Injuries of Knee Ligaments

The knee is very vulnerable to injury; therefore, many different types of injuries occur in this region. Ligament injuries, for example, range from mild sprains to complete dislocation of the joint. The patella can also dislocate. In addition, all the bony elements of the knee (distal femur, upper tibia, and patella) can fracture.

The knee is especially susceptible to ligament injuries, which occur when abnormal bending or twisting forces are applied to the joint. Such injuries are often seen in both recreational and competitive athletes. The ligaments on the medial side of the knee are most frequently injured, typically when the foot is fixed to the ground and the lateral aspect of the knee is struck by a heavy object, such as when a football player is tackled from the side.

Usually, a patient with a knee ligament injury will report pain in the joint and be unable to use the extremity normally. When you examine the patient, you will generally find swelling, occasional ecchymosis, point tenderness at the injury site, and a joint effusion (excess fluid in the joint).

Splint all suspected knee ligament injuries. The splint should extend from the hip joint to the foot, stabilizing the bone above the injured joint (the femur) and the bone below it (the tibia). A variety of splints can be used, including a padded rigid long leg splint or two padded board splints securely applied to the medial and lateral aspects of the limb. Applying a backboard or pillow splint, or simply binding the injured limb to its uninjured mate, is an acceptable but less effective splinting technique. The patient will usually be able to straighten the knee to allow you to apply the splint. However, if you encounter resistance or pain when trying to straighten the knee, splint it in the flexed position. Then continue to monitor the distal neurovascular function until the patient reaches the hospital.

Dislocation of the Knee

Dislocations of the knee are true emergencies that may be associated with vascular occlusion or injury that may threaten the limb. When the knee is dislocated, the ligaments that provide support to it may be damaged or torn. When this happens, the proximal end of the tibia completely displaces from its juncture with the lower end of the femur, usually producing a significant deformity. Although substantial ligament damage always occurs with a knee dislocation, the more urgent injury is often to the popliteal artery, which is frequently lacerated or compressed by the tibia, which typically displaces posteriorly. When gross deformity, severe pain, and an inability to move the joint cause you to suspect a dislocation of the knee, always check the distal circulation carefully before taking any other step. If the distal pulses are absent, contact medical oversight immediately for further stabilization and transport instructions.

The direction of dislocation refers to the position of the tibia with respect to the femur. Anterior knee dislocations, which result from extreme hyperextension of the knee, are the most common, occurring in almost one-half of all cases. Commonly, the anterior and posterior cruciate ligaments are damaged, and there is a high risk of nerve damage. Posterior knee dislocations account for approximately 30% to 40% of these injuries and are caused by direct pressure (axial loading) onto a flexed knee. The anterior knee dislocation presents the highest risk of damage to the popliteal artery.[9] Lateral and medial dislocations happen far less commonly and are less likely to injure the popliteal artery.

Patients with a knee dislocation will typically report pain in the knee and report that the knee "gave out." If the knee did not spontaneously reduce, there may be evidence of significant deformity and decreased range of motion. Complications may include limb-threatening popliteal artery disruption, injuries to the nerves, and joint instability. Do not confuse this injury with a relatively minor patella dislocation, discussed later.

If adequate distal pulses are present, splint the knee in the position in which you found it, and transport the patient promptly. Do not attempt to manipulate or straighten any severe knee injury if there are good distal pulses. If the limb is straight, apply standard rigid long leg splints to at least two sides of the limb to stabilize it (**FIGURE 31-47A**). If the knee is bent and the foot has a good pulse, splint the joint in the bent position, using parallel padded board splints secured at the hip and ankle joint to provide a stable A-frame (**FIGURE 31-47B**). Secure the limb to a backboard or stretcher with pillows and straps to eliminate any motion during transport.

On rare occasions, and depending on local protocol in the context of a very prolonged anticipated transport time to the hospital, the medical director may instruct you to attempt to realign a deformed, pulseless limb to reduce compression of the popliteal artery and, thus, restore distal circulation. Only make one attempt to do this. First, straighten the limb by applying gentle longitudinal traction in the axis of the limb. Once you apply manual traction, maintain it until the limb is fully splinted; otherwise, the limb might return to its deformed position. If traction significantly increases the patient's pain, do not continue. As you apply traction, monitor the posterior tibial pulse to see whether it returns. Splint the limb in the position in which you feel the strongest pulse. If you are unable to restore the distal pulse, splint the limb in the position that is most comfortable for the patient, and then provide prompt transport to the hospital. Notify medical oversight of the status of the distal pulse so that treatment can be arranged in advance.

Fractures Involving the Knee

Fractures around the knee may occur at the distal end of the femur, at the proximal end of the tibia, or in the patella. Because of local tenderness and swelling, it is easy to confuse a nondisplaced or minimally displaced fracture around the knee with a ligament injury. Likewise, a displaced fracture around the knee may produce significant deformity that makes it look like a dislocation. Manage these two types of injuries as follows:

- If there is an adequate distal pulse and no significant deformity, splint the limb with the knee straight.
- If there is an adequate pulse and significant deformity, splint the joint in the position of deformity.

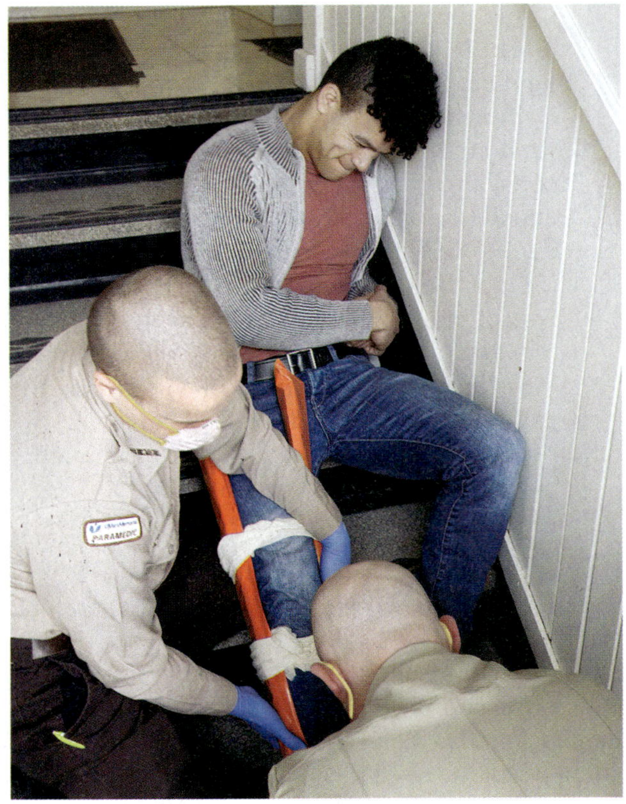

A

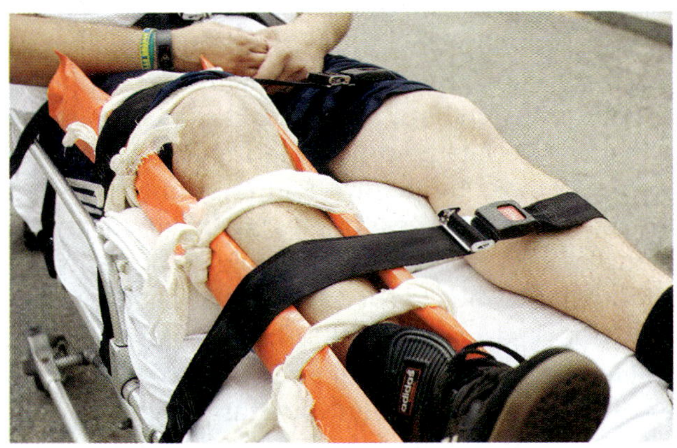

B

FIGURE 31-47 A. When the injured knee is straight, apply padded board splints extending from the hip to the ankle. **B.** If the knee is flexed and the foot has good pulses, apply padded board splints with the knee in the flexed position.

- If the pulse is absent below the level of the injury, suspect possible vascular damage, and contact medical oversight immediately for further instructions.
- Never use a traction splint if you suspect a fractured knee.

Dislocation of the Patella

A dislocated patella most commonly occurs in teenagers and young adults who are engaged in athletic activities. Some patients experience recurrent dislocations of the patella. As with recurrent dislocation of the shoulder, a minor twisting may be enough to produce the problem. Usually, the dislocated patella displaces to the lateral side. The displacement of the patella produces a significant deformity in which the knee is held in a moderately flexed position, and the patella is displaced to the lateral side of the knee (**FIGURE 31-48**).

Splint the knee in the position in which you found it; most often, this is with the knee flexed to a moderate degree. To stabilize the knee, apply padded board splints to the medial and lateral aspects of the joint, extending from the hip to the ankle. Use pillows to support the limb on the stretcher.

Occasionally, as you apply the splint, the patella will return to its normal position spontaneously. If this occurs, stabilize the limb as for a knee ligament injury in a padded long leg splint, and transport the patient to the ED. Report the spontaneous reduction as soon as you arrive at the hospital so that the medical staff is aware of the severity of the injury.

Injuries of the Tibia and Fibula

Fracture of the shaft of the tibia or the fibula may occur at any place between the knee joint and the ankle joint. Often both bones fracture at the same time. Even a single fracture may result in severe deformity, with significant angulation or rotation. Because the tibia is located just beneath the skin, open fractures of this bone are relatively common (**FIGURE 31-49**).

Fractures of the tibia and fibula should be stabilized with a padded rigid long leg splint or a vacuum splint that extends from the foot to the upper thigh. Once splinted, the affected leg should be secured to the opposite leg. Traction splints are not indicated for tibial fractures. As with most other fractures of the shaft of long bones, you should correct severe deformity before splinting by applying gentle longitudinal traction. The goal is to restore a position that will take a standard splint; it is not necessary to replace the fracture fragments in their anatomic position.

Fractures of the tibia and fibula are sometimes associated with vascular injury as a result of the distorted position of the limb following injury. Realigning the limb frequently restores an adequate blood supply to the foot. If it does not, transport the patient promptly and notify medical oversight while you are en route.

Ankle Injuries

The ankle is a commonly injured joint. Ankle injuries occur in people of all ages and range in severity from a simple sprain, which heals after a few days of rest, to severe fracture–dislocations that lead to permanent disability. As with other joints, it is sometimes difficult to tell a nondisplaced ankle fracture from a simple sprain

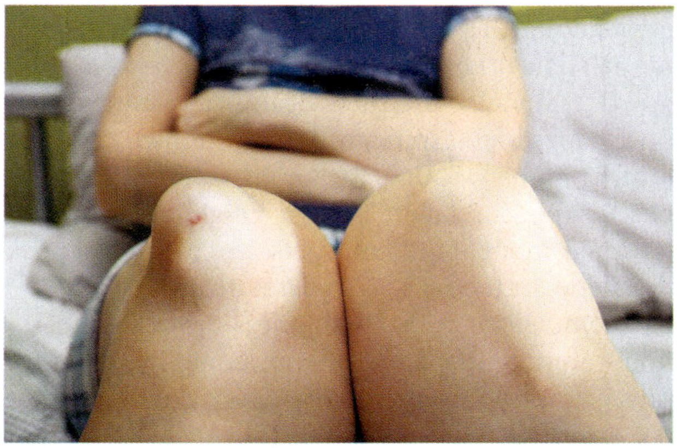

FIGURE 31-48 Usually, the dislocated patella displaces to the lateral side, and the knee is held in a partially flexed position.

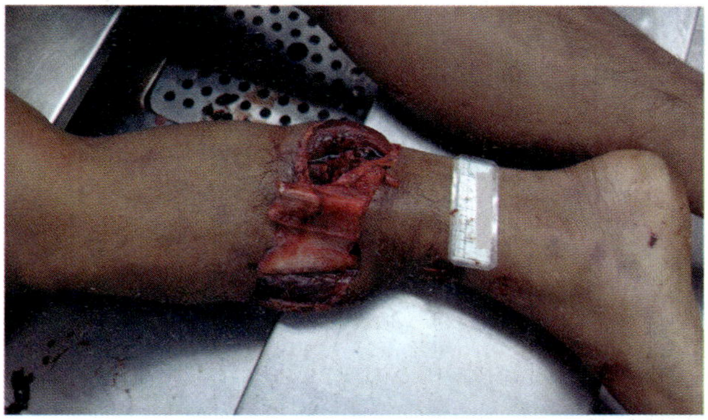

FIGURE 31-49 Because the tibia is so close to the skin, open fractures are relatively common.

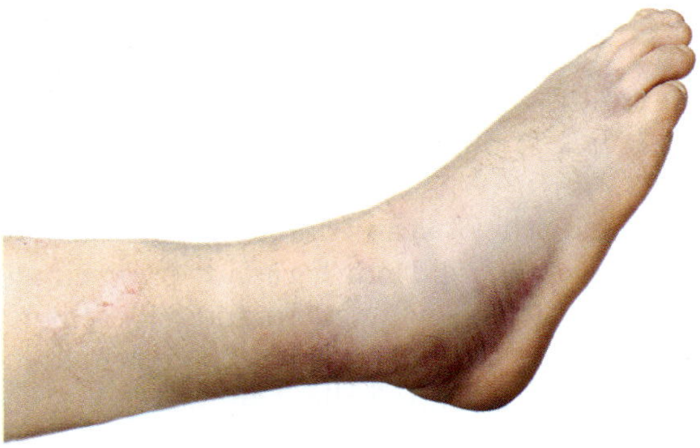

FIGURE 31-50 Swelling around the ankle is characteristic of sprains and fractures.

without radiograph examination (**FIGURE 31-50**). Therefore, any ankle injury that produces pain, swelling, localized tenderness, or the inability to bear weight must be evaluated by a physician. The most frequent mechanism of ankle injury is twisting, which stretches or tears the supporting ligaments. A more extensive twisting force may result in fracture of one or both malleoli. Dislocation of the ankle is usually associated with fractures of one or both malleoli.

You can manage the wide spectrum of injuries to the ankle in the same way, as follows:

1. Dress all open wounds.
2. Assess distal neurovascular function.
3. Correct any gross deformity by applying gentle longitudinal traction to the heel.
4. Before releasing traction, apply a splint.

You can use a padded rigid splint, a vacuum splint, or a pillow splint. Make sure it includes the entire foot and extends up the leg to the level of the knee joint.

Foot Injuries

Injuries to the foot can result in the dislocation or fracture of one or more of the tarsals, metatarsals, or phalanges of the toes. Toe fractures are especially common.

Of the tarsal bones, the calcaneus, or heel bone, is the most frequently fractured. Injury often occurs when the patient falls or jumps from a height and lands directly on the heel. The force of injury compresses the calcaneus, producing immediate swelling and ecchymosis. If the force of impact is great enough, as from a fall from a roof or tree, there may also be other fractures.

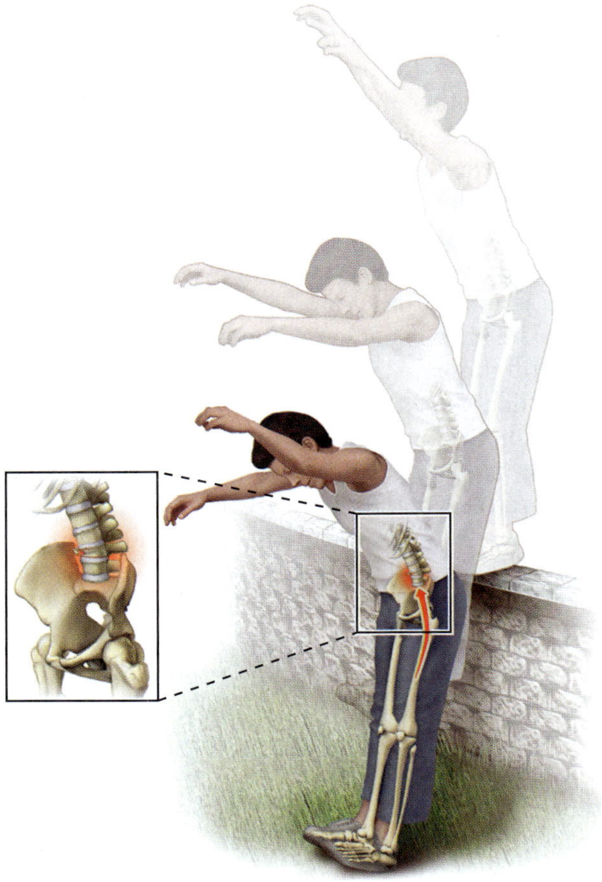

FIGURE 31-51 After a fall, the force of injury is transmitted up the legs to the spine, sometimes resulting in a fracture of the lumbar spine.

Occasionally, the force of injury is transmitted up the legs to the spine, producing a fracture of the lumbar spine (**FIGURE 31-51**). When a patient who has jumped or fallen from a height reports heel pain, ask them about back pain and carefully check the spine for tenderness and deformity.

If you suspect that the foot is dislocated, carefully remove the shoe and immediately assess for pulses and motor and sensory functions. Stabilize the extremity using a commercially available splint or a pillow splint, leaving the toes exposed so that you can periodically assess neurovascular function. Contact medical oversight and inform them if pulses are absent.

Injuries of the foot are associated with significant swelling but rarely with gross deformity. Vascular injuries are uncommon. As in the hand, lacerations involving the ankle and foot may damage important underlying nerves and tendons. Puncture wounds of the foot are common and may cause serious infection if not treated early. All of these injuries must be evaluated and treated by a physician.

To splint the foot, apply a rigid padded board splint, a vacuum splint, or a pillow splint, stabilizing the ankle joint and the foot (**FIGURE 31-52**). Leave the toes exposed so that you can periodically assess neurovascular function.

When the patient is lying on the stretcher, elevate the foot approximately 6 inches (15 cm) to minimize swelling. All patients with lower extremity injuries should be transported in the supine position to allow for elevation of the limb. Never allow the foot and leg to dangle off the stretcher onto the floor or ground.

If a patient has fallen from a height and reports heel pain, assess for the need to perform spinal motion restriction in addition to splinting the foot.

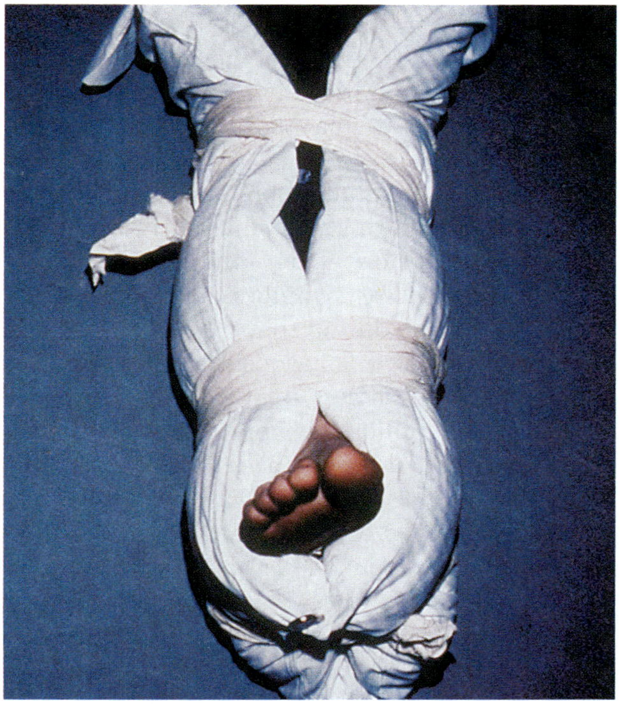

FIGURE 31-52 A pillow splint provides excellent stabilization of the foot.

Sprains and Strains

Because it may be difficult to differentiate among the various types of injuries in the field, it is best to err on the side of caution and treat every severe sprain as if it is a fracture. Therefore, general treatment of sprains and strains is similar to that of fractures and includes RICES (Rest, Ice, Compression, Elevation, and Splinting). In addition, reduce or protect the limb from weight-bearing activity. Manage pain as soon as is practical. RICES is described in Chapter 26, *Soft-Tissue Injuries*.

Amputations

You must control bleeding and treat for shock when dealing with traumatic amputations. Hemorrhage from complete or incomplete amputations can be severe and life threatening. Control any bleeding from the stump. If bleeding is severe, quickly apply a tourniquet. Complete traumatic amputations may occasionally not bleed much if the cut vessels go into spasm, reducing blood loss.

Surgeons can occasionally reattach amputated parts (**FIGURE 31-53**). However, correct prehospital care of the amputated part is vital to successful reattachment. With partial amputations, make sure to stabilize the part with bulky compression dressings and a splint to prevent further injury. Do not sever any partial amputations; doing so may complicate later reattachment.

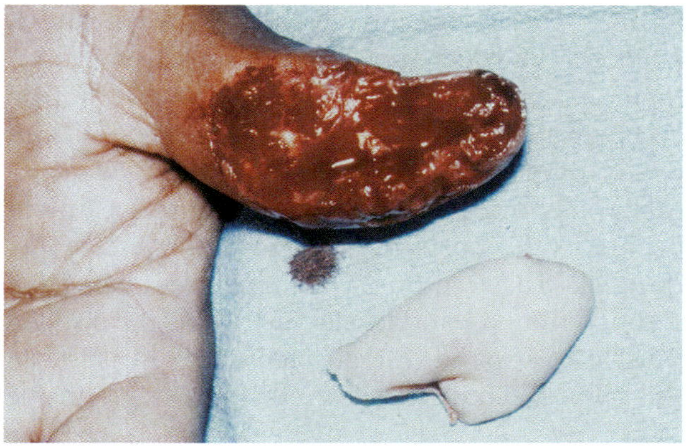

FIGURE 31-53 Amputated parts can occasionally be reattached, so make every attempt to find the part and transport it to the emergency department along with the patient.

With a complete amputation, wrap the clean part in a sterile dressing and place it in a plastic bag. Follow your local protocols regarding how to preserve amputated parts. In some areas, dry sterile dressings are recommended for wrapping amputated parts; in other areas, dressings moistened with sterile saline are recommended. Put the bag in a cool container filled with ice. Lay the wrapped part on a bed of ice; do not pack it in ice. The goal is to keep the part cool without allowing it to freeze or for frostbite to develop. The amputated part should be transported with the patient to the appropriate resource hospital.

Words of Wisdom

To prevent tissue damage from direct contact with the ice, never lay the part directly on ice without wrapping it first.

Compartment Syndrome

Muscles in the extremities are contained within the fascia, which divides the muscles into numerous compartments. Because fascia's ability to stretch or expand is limited, anything that increases pressure within the compartment, such as bleeding and swelling, has the potential to impede blood flow through the muscle inside. **Compartment syndrome** is a limb-threatening condition characterized by localized tissue swelling within a compartment. As blood flow decreases inside a muscle compartment, ischemia results and anaerobic metabolism compensates for the reduction in oxygen. This reduced oxygenation, in turn, damages and eventually kills the muscle cells. Definitive treatment occurs in the hospital, through a surgical procedure called a fasciotomy, which involves an incision through the skin and fascia that allows the swollen muscle to expand, thereby reducing pressure on the nerves, blood vessels, and other tissue inside the compartment. However, because compartment syndrome can be overlooked, some patients do not receive surgical intervention soon enough. In these unfortunate cases, it may become necessary for the surgeon to amputate the extremity.

Compartment syndrome often develops within 6 to 12 hours after injury, commonly subsequent to a crushing MOI or excessively tight placement of a cast. Early signs and symptoms of compartment syndrome include pain that is out of proportion to the injury, pain on passive stretch of muscles within the compartment, and altered sensation (abnormal, reduced, or absent). The soft tissue in the area may be very firm when palpated. Additional signs may include pallor and decreased power (ranging from decreased strength and movement of the limb to complete paralysis).

Compartment syndrome can occur with or without an accompanying bone fracture. However, when a fracture is involved, the most commonly occurring fracture site is the tibia for adults, and the forearm in children. If you have a patient with a fracture below the elbow or the knee, be on the lookout for extreme pain; decreased sensation, tingling, or numbness; pain on stretching of affected muscles; and decreased power/paralysis. If you suspect that a patient has compartment syndrome, splint the affected limb, keeping it at the level of the heart (but not above), and provide immediate transport, reassessing neurovascular status frequently during transport.

Be aware that another potential cause of compartment syndrome is a splint that has been applied too tightly. Therefore, after splinting an injured extremity, if signs or symptoms of compartment syndrome appear during transport, try loosening knots or other potentially constricting elements of the splint. Then reassess frequently to determine whether the condition has improved or worsened. It may be easy to dismiss a patient telling you how badly the injured extremity hurts as being consistent with a diagnosis of an underlying fracture. Consider the potential for compartment syndrome with all extremity injuries.

YOU are the EMT SUMMARY

1. Under which circumstances can orthopaedic injuries pose a threat to a patient's life?

Sprains, strains, and dislocations are rarely life threatening. Dislocations and isolated closed fractures can cause neurovascular damage and permanent disability if not treated promptly, but typically do not pose a threat to life. However, multiple closed long bone fractures, which can cause severe internal bleeding if bone fragments lacerate major blood vessels, can result in hypovolemic shock and death. Open fractures and extremity amputations (excluding fingers and toes) can also result in hypovolemic shock due to severe external bleeding. Amputation of a leg or arm can quickly lead to exsanguination (bleeding to death) if bleeding is not controlled. Contamination of the wound could also lead to an infection of the underlying tissue, even affecting bone. This infection can lead to gangrene or sepsis.

Pelvic fractures are potentially life threatening because the pelvic cavity can accommodate a large volume of blood. Patients can die of pelvic fractures because hypovolemic shock occurs secondary to severe internal bleeding when a fractured bone fragment or dislocated bone lacerates or severs a major artery or vein or there is significant bleeding from fractured bone ends.

2. Given the information you have, can you rule out a critical injury?

No. As concise as the dispatch information can sometimes be, you will not know the extent of a patient's injury (or injuries) until you arrive at the scene and perform a patient assessment. In this case, all you know is that the patient is conscious and alert and breathing and has a possible leg fracture. Although the dispatch information infers that this is an isolated injury secondary to a soccer-related incident, keep an open mind and avoid the preconceived notion that the leg injury is the only injury.

When you approach any patient, regardless of the nature of the call, you must perform a primary assessment to detect and correct immediate threats to the ABCs (XABCs if exsanguinating bleeding is present). Avoid tunnel vision when assessing and treating patients with orthopaedic trauma. A fractured leg may be the most obvious injury; however, it may not be the only injury. Also, it may not be the most life-threatening injury.

3. What initial treatment should you provide to this patient?

Because the patient denies having any other injuries (eg, a neck injury, which may require spinal motion restriction), your initial action, after taking standard precautions, should be to expose the injury site and perform manual stabilization. With an injury in the tibia–fibula area, you or your partner should manually stabilize above the ankle and below the knee. Manual stabilization will help minimize the potential for further injury by preventing movement of the leg.

After you expose and manually stabilize the injury site, assess the patient for obvious signs of injury, such as swelling, deformity, bruising, and open wounds. The absence of deformity does not rule out an underlying fracture, as the bone may be cracked without any displacement of the bone ends. Also, swelling often masks underlying deformity. Treat any extremity injury as though an underlying fracture is present and stabilize it appropriately.

4. What are some indicators of a fractured bone?

A fracture is defined as *any* break in the continuity of a bone and is classified as being open (overlying skin is not intact) or closed (overlying skin is intact). In many cases, the deformity is grossly obvious; in other cases, it is subtle. Signs of a fracture include deformity, point tenderness (pain on palpation directly over the injury), swelling, bruising, and crepitus.

5. How should you proceed with your assessment of this patient's injury?

This patient did not experience multisystem trauma or a significant MOI; therefore, a secondary assessment of the entire body is not indicated. Instead, focus on evaluating perfusion and sensory and motor functions distal to the injury. When you assess an extremity injury, remember the 6 Ps of musculoskeletal assessment: pain, paralysis, paresthesia, pulselessness, pallor, and pressure.

First, assess the patient's level of pain using a scale of 0 to 10. Next, assess perfusion. In some cases, a fractured bone end may compress or, in rare cases, sever a blood vessel, resulting in inadequate or absent perfusion distal to the fracture. Compare the color of the skin with that of the uninjured limb. If perfusion is adequate, the skin should be baseline color and warm. On general observation, the patient may appear ashen or gray. Palpate the dorsalis pedis pulse (on the top of the foot) and the posterior tibial

YOU are the EMT SUMMARY continued

pulse (on the posterior medial aspect of the ankle where the distal tibia ends). Pulses that are weak or absent in comparison with pulses in the uninjured limb also suggest compromised perfusion.

Next, use a blunt object, and stroke it up the bottom and sides of her foot. If she is unable to feel you touching her foot, you should suspect that a nerve has been compressed or otherwise injured by a fractured bone end. To test motor function, simply ask her to wiggle her toes; however, if this increases her pain, discontinue this part of the examination. Paresthesia (numbness or tingling) could indicate compromised perfusion and/or nerve injury. A feeling of pressure distal to the injury site could indicate elevated pressure within a fascial compartment due to internal bleeding; if this continues, it could result in compartment syndrome.

In addition to assessing perfusion and sensory and motor functions, assess the areas above and below the injury (the injury zone); in this case, the injury zone extends above her knee and below her ankle. Remember, her leg may be the most obvious injury, but it may not be the only injury.

6. How should you treat an injured extremity in which distal perfusion is absent?

In general, you should splint an orthopaedic injury in the position it was found, provided that distal perfusion is intact. If your assessment reveals that perfusion distal to the injury is compromised or absent (ie, pallor, absent distal pulses, cold skin), apply gentle longitudinal traction to realign the limb until perfusion is restored. The goal is *not* to return the extremity to its normal anatomic position, but rather to restore distal circulation. In many cases, gentle realignment of the limb restores adequate perfusion; however, if one attempt (local protocol may dictate more than one attempt) at realignment is unsuccessful, splint the injury, transport the patient as soon as possible, and notify the receiving facility early.

7. How should you splint this patient's injury?

Prior to splinting any extremity injury, assess the patient's distal perfusion and sensory and motor functions. Fractures of the tibia and fibula can be stabilized with a padded rigid leg splint; an air splint; or a vacuum splint that stabilizes the joints above and below the fracture site. In this case, stabilize the knee and ankle. As with most other fractures of the shaft of long bones, correct any severe deformity before applying the splint by applying gentle longitudinal traction. Restore the deformed limb to a position that will accommodate a splint—not necessarily to its normal anatomic position. The affected leg, once splinted, should be secured to the opposite leg.

Immediately after the splint is secured in place, reassess distal perfusion and sensory and motor functions. If perfusion is found to be inadequate, the splint should be loosened or reapplied as necessary to restore this vital function.

8. What are some methods for providing pain relief from orthopaedic trauma?

Pain relief is an important aspect in the overall care of a patient with orthopaedic trauma. Pain increases anxiety, which only adds to the patient's problems.

After you apply the splint, which should be padded for comfort, elevate the injured extremity above the level of the heart. This will help reduce pain and swelling by encouraging blood to drain from the extremity.

Chemical cold packs wrapped with gauze or some other type of insulating material can be applied directly over the injury site. A cold stimulus applied to the skin constricts the blood vessels; this can help reduce swelling and pain.

Certain medications can be administered to the patient by a paramedic. In some cases, especially during a prolonged transport, it may be helpful to request ALS intervention.

9. What is the most likely cause of the patient's complaint? What can you do to remedy the situation?

On the basis of the patient's complaint of numbness and tingling and your findings of pallor and weak pedal pulses, you should suspect that you applied the splint too tightly and that it is now impairing distal circulation.

Simply loosen the splint if it was applied too tightly. If you used padded board splints and triangular bandages (cravats), loosen the cravats. If you applied an air splint, release some of the air from the splint. If you applied a vacuum splint, gently attempt to spread the edges of the splint apart to the point at which the patient feels relief. If this is not possible and a prolonged transport time is anticipated, it would not be unreasonable to stop the ambulance and apply a different type of splint, provided that the patient's condition is stable. Regardless of the splint that you used, immediately reassess distal circulation after making any adjustments, and ask the patient whether the numbness and/or tingling has subsided. In most cases, these adjustments will lead to improvement.

YOU are the EMT SUMMARY continued

10. What factors increase the risk of complications following orthopaedic trauma?

Orthopaedic injuries can lead to systemic complications. Do not focus all of your attention on the skeletal injury; after all, there is a patient attached to the injured extremity! The risk of complications following orthopaedic trauma is increased by a variety of factors, such as the amount of force that caused the injury, the injury location, and the patient's overall health. Injuries in patients who smoke cigarettes or who have diabetes, for example, tend to heal poorly and complications are more common.

Any fracture, open or closed, is accompanied by a risk of bleeding. In general, the severity of bleeding is directly related to the force that caused the injury. A significant loss of tissue may occur at the fracture site if the muscle is severely damaged or if the bone's penetration of the skin causes a large wound.

Infection is another potential complication, especially in patients with open fractures or patients with other medical problems such as cigarette smoking or diabetes. To prevent contaminating an open fracture, and to minimize the risk of infection, brush away any obvious debris or rinse with normal saline on the skin surrounding the fracture before covering it with a moist sterile dressing.[10] Do not probe into an open fracture to retrieve debris. If a bone that is protruding through the wound retracts back into the wound during care, document that and report it to the receiving facility.

Long-term disability is one of the most devastating complications of orthopaedic trauma. In many cases, a severely injured limb can be successfully repaired; however, many patients may not be able to work for long periods because of severe, chronic pain and the extensive rehabilitation that is often required.

As an EMT, you can help reduce the risk of complications, thus reducing the risk or duration of long-term disability following orthopaedic trauma, by preventing further injury, properly splinting orthopaedic injuries, reducing the risk of wound infection, and transporting patients to an appropriate medical facility.

Prep Kit

Ready for Review

- Skeletal or voluntary muscle attaches to bone and forms the major muscle mass of the body. This muscle contains veins, arteries, and nerves.
- There are approximately 206 bones in the human body. When this living tissue is fractured, it can produce bleeding and significant pain.
- A joint is a junction where two bones come into contact. Joints are stabilized in key areas by ligaments.
- The body's physical development during childhood and the effects of aging during later adulthood present unique risk factors relating to musculoskeletal injury and disease.
- A fracture is a broken bone, a dislocation is a disruption of a joint, a sprain is a stretching injury to the ligaments around a joint, and a strain is a stretching of the muscle or tendons.
- Depending on the amount of kinetic energy absorbed by tissues, the zone of injury may extend beyond the point of contact. Always maintain a high index of suspicion for associated injuries.
- Fractures of the bones are classified as open or closed. Both are splinted in a similar manner, but remember to control bleeding and apply a sterile dressing to the open extremity injury before splinting.
- Fractures and dislocations are often difficult to diagnose without a radiographic examination. You will treat these injuries similarly. Stabilize the injury with a splint and transport the patient.

Prep Kit continued

- Signs of fractures and dislocations include pain, deformity, point tenderness, false motion, crepitus, swelling, and bruising.
- Signs of sprains include bruising, swelling, and an unstable joint.
- Compare the unaffected extremity with the injured extremity whenever possible.
- The main types of splints used by EMTs are rigid splints, traction splints, formable splints, and pelvic binders.
- For bone injuries, splint the injured extremity from the joint above to the joint below the injury site for complete stabilization. For joint injuries, splint the injured extremity from the bone above to the bone below the injury site.
- A sling and swathe are commonly used to treat shoulder dislocations and to secure injured upper extremities to the body. Lower extremities can be secured to the unaffected limb or to a backboard.
- The most common life-threatening musculoskeletal injuries are multiple fractures, open fractures with arterial bleeding, pelvic fractures, bilateral femur fractures, and limb amputations.

Vital Vocabulary

acromioclavicular (AC) joint A simple joint where the bony projections of the scapula and the clavicle meet at the top of the shoulder.

amputation An injury in which part of the body is completely severed.

articular cartilage A pearly white layer of specialized cartilage covering the articular surfaces (contact surfaces on the ends) of bones in synovial joints.

calcaneus The heel bone.

closed fracture Any break in a bone in which the overlying skin is not broken.

compartment syndrome Swelling in a confined space that produces dangerous pressure; may cut off blood flow or damage sensitive tissue.

crepitus A grating or grinding sensation or sound caused by fractured bone ends or joints rubbing together.

dislocation Disruption of a joint in which ligaments are damaged and the bone ends are no longer in contact.

displaced fracture A fracture in which bone fragments are separated from one another, producing deformity in the limb.

ecchymosis Bruising or discoloration associated with bleeding within or under the skin.

false motion Movement that occurs in a bone at a point where there is no joint, indicating a fracture; also called free movement.

fascia The fiberlike connective tissue that covers arteries, veins, tendons, and ligaments.

fibula The outer and smaller bone of the two bones of the lower leg.

fracture A break in the continuity of a bone.

glenoid fossa The part of the scapula that joins with the humeral head to form the glenohumeral joint.

hematuria Blood in the urine.

joint The place where two bones come into contact.

kyphosis A forward curving of the upper back caused by an abnormal increase in the curvature of the spine.

ligaments Bands of fibrous tissue that connect bones to bones. Ligaments support and strengthen a joint.

nondisplaced fracture A simple crack in the bone that has not caused the bone to move from its normal anatomic position; also called a hairline fracture.

open fracture Any break in a bone in which the overlying skin has been broken.

Prep Kit continued

osteoarthritis A progressive disease of the joints that destroys cartilage, promotes the formation of bone spurs in joints, and leads to joint stiffness.

osteoporosis A generalized bone disease, commonly associated with postmenopausal women, in which there is a reduction in the amount of bone mass leading to fractures after minimal trauma in either sex.

pelvic binder A device to splint the bony pelvis to reduce hemorrhage from bone ends, venous disruption, and pain.

point tenderness Tenderness that is sharply localized at the site of the injury, found by gently palpating along the bone with the tip of one finger.

position of function A hand position in which the wrist is slightly dorsiflexed and all finger joints are moderately flexed.

reduce To return a dislocated joint or fractured bone to its normal position; to set.

retroperitoneal space The space between the abdominal cavity and the posterior abdominal wall, containing the kidneys, certain large vessels, and parts of the gastrointestinal tract.

sciatic nerve The major nerve to the lower extremities; controls much of muscle function in the leg and sensation in most of the leg and foot.

sling A bandage or material that helps to support the weight of an injured upper extremity.

splint A flexible or rigid device used to protect and maintain the position of an injured extremity.

sprain A joint injury involving damage to supporting ligaments, and sometimes partial or temporary dislocation of bone ends.

strain Stretching or tearing of a muscle and/or tendon; also called a muscle pull.

swathe A bandage that passes around the chest to secure an injured arm to the chest.

tendons The fibrous connective tissue that attaches muscle to bone.

tibia The shinbone; the larger of the two bones of the lower leg.

tourniquet The bleeding control method used when a wound continues to bleed despite the use of direct pressure; useful if a patient is bleeding severely from a partial or complete amputation.

traction Longitudinal force applied to a structure.

zone of injury The area of potentially damaged soft tissue, adjacent nerves, and blood vessels surrounding an injury to a bone or a joint.

References

1. Fontánez R, Ramos-Guasp W, Ramírez H, De Jesús K, Conde JG, González J, Frontera WR. Musculoskeletal conditions in the emergency room: a teaching opportunity for medical students and residents. *P R Health Sci J.* 2021;40(2):68–74.
2. OA prevalence and burden. Osteoarthritis Action Alliance website. https://oaaction.unc.edu/oa-module/oa-prevalence-and-burden/. Accessed March 20, 2025.
3. Leland DP, Bernard CD, Keyt LK, et al. An age-based approach to anterior shoulder instability in patients under 40 years old: analysis of a US population. *Am J Sports Med.* 2020;48(1):56–62.
4. Prasetia R, Handoko HK, Rosa WY, Ismiarto AF, Petrasama, Utoyo GA. Primary traumatic shoulder dislocation associated with rotator cuff tear in the elderly. *Int J Surg Case Rep.* 2022;95:107200. doi:10.1016/j.ijscr.2022.107200
5. Doehrmann R, Frush TJ. Posterior shoulder instability. *StatPearls*. National Library of Medicine website. https://www.ncbi.nlm.nih.gov/books/NBK557648/. Updated July 10, 2023. Accessed March 20, 2025.
6. National Association of State EMS Officials. *National Model EMS Clinical Guidelines: Version 3.0.* https://nasemso.org/content.aspx?page_id=22&club_id=157064&module_id=701974. Updated March 2022. Accessed March 20, 2025.
7. Luokkala T, Laitinen MK, Hevonkorpi TP, Raittio L, Mattila VM, Launonen AP. Distal radius fractures in the elderly population. *EFORT Open Rev.* 2020;5(6):361–370.

Prep Kit continued

8. Lyng JW, Corsa JG, Nawrocki PS, Raetzke BD, Nackenson J, Bosson N. Prehospital Trauma Compendium: management of suspected femoral shaft fractures; a position statement and resource document of NAEMSP. *Prehosp Emerg Care*. Published online May 29, 2025. doi:10.1080/10903127.2025.2493846

9. Mohseni M, Mabrouk A, Simon LV. Knee dislocation. *StatPearls*. National Library of Medicine website. https://www.ncbi.nlm.nih.gov/books/NBK470595/. Updated February 27, 2024. Accessed March 20, 2025.

10. National Association of Emergency Medical Technicians. *PHTLS: Prehospital Trauma Life Support*. 10th ed. Burlington, MA: Jones & Bartlett Learning; 2023.

Additional Resources

Bangura A, Burke CE, Enobun B, et al. Are pelvic binders an effective prehospital intervention? *Prehosp Emerg Care*. 2023;27(1):24–30.

Berger-Groch J, Rueger JM, Czorlich P, et al. Evaluation of pelvic circular compression devices in severely injured trauma patients with pelvic fractures. *Prehosp Emerg Care*. 2022;26(4):547–555.

Gottfried A, Gendler S, Chayen D, et al. Hemorrhagic shock in isolated and non-isolated pelvic fractures: a registries-based study. *Prehosp Emerg Care*. 2024;28(4):589–597.

Nguyen P, Pokrzywa C, Figueroa J, et al. Predictive factors for the application of pelvic binders in the prehospital setting. *Prehosp Emerg Care*. 2024;28(2):425–430.

Philipsen SPJ, Vergunst AA, Tan ECTH. Traction splinting for midshaft femoral fractures in the pre-hospital and emergency department environment—a systematic review. *Injury*. 2022;53(12):4129–4138.

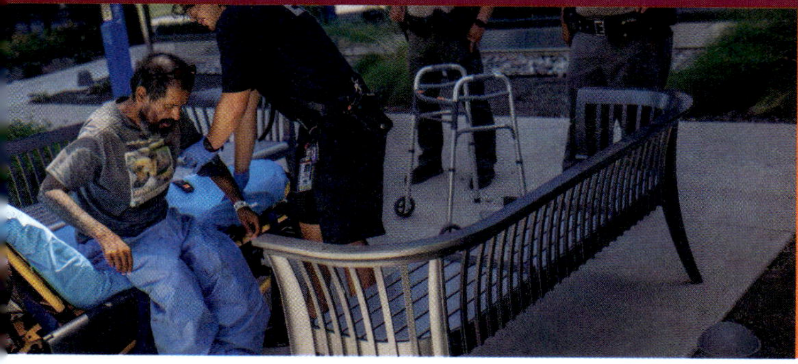

Chapter 32

Environmental Emergencies

NATIONAL EMS EDUCATION STANDARD COMPETENCIES

Trauma

Applies knowledge to provide basic emergency care and transportation based on assessment findings for an acutely injured patient.

Environmental Emergencies

- Submersion incidents (pp 1212–1218, 1221–1223)
- Temperature-related illness (pp 1194–1201, 1203–1208, 1210–1212)
- Bites and envenomation (pp 1225–1234)
- Lightning injury (pp 1224–1225)

KNOWLEDGE OBJECTIVES

1. Identify the four factors that affect how a person deals with exposure to a cold or hot environment. (pp 1194–1196)
2. Describe the five ways heat loss occurs in the body, and how the rate and amount of heat loss or gain can be modified in an emergency situation. (pp 1196–1197)
3. Describe the four general stages of hypothermia. (pp 1197–1199)
4. Describe local cold injuries and their underlying causes. (pp 1199–1201)
5. Describe the process of providing emergency care to a patient who has sustained a cold injury. (pp 1203–1205)
6. Explain the importance of following local protocols when rewarming a patient who is experiencing moderate or severe hypothermia. (p 1204)
7. Describe the three emergencies that are caused by heat exposure, including their risk factors, signs, and symptoms. (pp 1205–1208)
8. Describe the process of providing emergency care to a patient who is experiencing a heat emergency. (pp 1210–1212)
9. Describe drowning, including its incidence, risk factors, and prevention. (pp 1212–1217)
10. Describe conditions that may result in a spinal injury following a submersion incident and the steps for stabilizing a patient with a suspected spinal injury in the water. (pp 1213–1215)
11. List the basic rules of performing a water and ice rescue. (p 1214)
12. Explain why EMTs should have a prearranged rescue plan based on the environment in which they work. (p 1214)
13. Discuss how the body's protective mechanisms following submersion in cold water affect patient assessment and treatment. (pp 1215–1217)
14. Describe the three types of scuba diving emergencies, how they may occur, and their signs and symptoms. (pp 1217–1218)

15. Describe the process of providing emergency care to a patient who has been involved in a drowning or scuba diving emergency. (pp 1221–1223)
16. Discuss the types of dysbarism injuries, including their incidence, risk factors, signs and symptoms, and emergency medical treatment. (pp 1223–1224)
17. Discuss lightning injuries, including their incidence, risk factors, signs and symptoms, and emergency medical treatment. (pp 1224–1225)
18. Describe the process of providing emergency care to patients who have been bitten or stung by a venomous spider, Hymenoptera insect, snake, scorpion, or tick. (pp 1225–1234)
19. Describe the process of providing emergency care to a patient who has been injured by a marine animal. (p 1234)

SKILLS OBJECTIVES

1. Demonstrate the emergency medical treatment of local cold injuries in the field. (pp 1203–1205)
2. Demonstrate how to use a warm-water bath to rewarm the limb of a patient who has sustained a local cold injury. (pp 1204–1205)
3. Demonstrate how to treat a patient with heat cramps. (p 1210)
4. Demonstrate how to treat a patient with heat exhaustion. (p 1211; Skill Drill 32-1)
5. Demonstrate how to treat a patient with heatstroke. (p 1212)
6. Demonstrate how to stabilize a patient with a suspected spinal injury in the water. (p 1216; Skill Drill 32-2)
7. Demonstrate how to care for a patient who is suspected of having an air embolism or decompression sickness following a scuba diving emergency. (pp 1221–1223)
8. Demonstrate how to care for a patient who has been bitten by a venomous snake and is showing signs of envenomation. (pp 1228–1232)
9. Demonstrate how to care for a patient who has sustained a coelenterate envenomation. (pp 1234–1235)

Introduction

The human body functions best when all body systems operate in balance, a concept known as **homeostasis**. Environmental factors such as temperature and atmospheric pressure can overwhelm the body's ability to cope with its surroundings, potentially resulting in mental status changes, functional changes, and even death.

Environmental emergencies can occur in any setting and often accompany other illnesses and injuries that require treatment at the same time. For example, a trauma patient with hypothermia is at a higher risk of death than a patient with a normal body temperature. Children, older people, people with chronic illnesses, and young adults who overexert themselves are particularly susceptible to environmental factors. As an EMT, you can save lives by recognizing and responding properly to these emergencies, most of which require prompt treatment at the scene and in the hospital.

This chapter discusses the following types of environmental emergencies:

- The various forms of heat-, cold-, and water-related emergencies
- Pressure-related emergencies, or dysbarism injuries, caused by scuba diving and high altitude
- Injuries caused by lightning
- Injuries caused by bites and stings from spiders, Hymenoptera insects, snakes, scorpions, and ticks, and injuries from marine animals

You will learn how the body reacts to these injuries and how to diagnose and treat the resulting conditions.

Factors Affecting Exposure

The following four factors will affect how a person is able to maintain homeostasis, specifically their ability to maintain a normal body temperature.

When a person is exposed to excess heat or cold for a prolonged period, their body's ability to regulate its internal temperature is overwhelmed. When this happens, patients can become very ill and may die. Consider these factors when assessing patients, especially patients with an altered mental status:

1. **Physical condition.** Patients who are ill or in poor physical condition will not be able to tolerate extreme temperatures as well as those whose cardiovascular, metabolic, and nervous systems are all functioning well. For example, an athlete in peak physical condition performs better and is less likely to experience injury or illness than someone with a less active lifestyle. To maintain normal body temperature, the heart, blood vessels, and other organs must quickly respond to keep the body regulated. People who are not in good physical condition or those with chronic illnesses may have a limited ability to regulate their body temperature.
2. **Age.** Children and older adults are more likely to experience temperature-related illness. There are many reasons for this increased risk.
   - **Children.** Infants have poor thermoregulation (the body's ability to maintain normal temperature); the ability to shiver and generate heat when the body is cold does not develop until approximately 12 to 18 months. An infant's surface area–to–mass ratio is larger than an adult's, so infants heat up and cool down faster. When you get cold, you put on a sweater; a small child may not think to do this or may have difficulty finding and putting one on.
   - **Older adults.** People lose subcutaneous tissues as they age, reducing the amount of insulation they have. Poor circulation also contributes to increased heat loss. This is why older people often wear extra layers of clothing. Medications can also affect an older person's body thermostat, putting them at increased risk for temperature-related emergencies. Finally, older adults are at high risk for falls, and lying immobile on a hot or cold surface can rapidly lead to changes in body temperature.
3. **Nutrition and hydration.** Your body needs calories for metabolism. Staying well hydrated provides water as a catalyst for much of this metabolism. A lack of healthy food or water will aggravate both hot and cold stress. Calories provide fuel to burn, creating heat during the cold, and water provides sweat for evaporation and removing heat. Alcohol use may increase fluid loss and place the patient at greater risk for temperature-related emergencies; moreover, if a person is intoxicated, they may not realize they are too hot or too cold.
4. **Environmental conditions.** Factors such as air temperature, humidity level, and wind can complicate or improve environmental situations. A light breeze helps you stay cool when it is hot outside, but a cold wind when it is cold outside can be uncomfortable. Extremes in temperature and humidity are not needed to produce hot or cold injuries. Many hypothermia cases occur at temperatures between 30°F (–1°C) and 50°F (10°C). Most heatstroke cases occur when the temperature is above 80°F (26.7°C) and the humidity is 80% or higher. When evaluating your patient's condition, consider the environment and whether your patient is prepared for that situation. People with limited financial resources, such as older persons on a fixed income, may turn the heat down in the winter or neglect to use air conditioning

YOU are the EMT

At 1415 hours, you are dispatched to a farm at 1102 State Route 4 for a 55-year-old who fainted after working in the garden. The temperature is 98°F (36.7°C), and the humidity is high. You and your partner proceed to the scene; your response time is 7 minutes.

1. How does the body normally balance heat production and elimination?
2. What factors can decrease the body's ability to eliminate excess heat?

in the summer because of cost concerns. Some people may not open windows in a heat wave for fear of burglars. An understanding of the environmental conditions may help in your assessment and treatment decisions.

Cold Exposure

Normal body temperature is 98.6°F (37°C). Complicated regulatory mechanisms keep this internal temperature constant, regardless of the **ambient temperature**, which is the temperature of the surrounding environment. If the body, or any part of it, is exposed to cold environments, these mechanisms may be overwhelmed. Prolonged or extreme cold exposure may cause injury to individual parts of the body, such as the feet, hands, ears, or nose, or to the body as a whole.

Because heat always travels from a warmer place to a cooler place, body heat tends to move into the environment. Heat loss can occur in the following five ways:

- **Conduction** is the transfer of heat from a part of the body to a colder object or substance by direct contact, such as when a warm hand touches cold metal or ice, or is immersed in water with a temperature of less than 98°F (36.7°C). Heat can also be gained if the object or substance being touched is warm.
- **Convection** occurs when heat is transferred to circulating air, such as when cool air moves across the body surface. A person who stands outside in windy, wintry weather and wears only lightweight clothing is mainly experiencing heat loss by convection. A person can gain heat if the air moving across the person's body is hotter than the temperature of the environment, such as in deserts, industrial settings (eg, foundries), or a sauna.
- **Evaporation** is the conversion of any liquid to a gas, a process that requires energy, or heat. Evaporation is the natural mechanism by which sweating cools the body. This is why swimmers coming out of the water feel a sensation of cold as the water evaporates from their skin. People who exercise vigorously in a cool environment may sweat and feel warm at first, but later, as their sweat evaporates, they can become cold.
- **Radiation** is the transfer of heat by radiant energy. Radiant energy is a type of invisible light that transfers heat. Radiation causes heat loss, such as when a person stands in a cold room. Heat can also be gained by radiation, such as when a person stands by a fire.
- **Respiration** in most climates causes body heat loss as warm air in the lungs is exhaled into the atmosphere and cooler air is inhaled. The inhaled air cools the thorax and the blood traveling through the lungs, which can decrease body temperature. In climates where the ambient temperature is warmer than body temperature, the person inhales air that is warmer than the air they exhale, causing the body to gain heat with each breath.

Simple ways to modify the body's rate and amount of heat gain or loss include the following:

- **Increase or decrease heat production.** One way for the body to increase its heat production is to increase the rate of metabolism of its cells; the body can accomplish this through shivering (active movement of many muscles to generate heat). Also, people often have a natural urge to move around when they are cold. A person who is hot tends to reduce the level of activity, thus reducing heat production.
- **Move to an area where heat loss is decreased or increased.** The most obvious way to decrease heat loss from radiation and convection is to move out of a cold environment and seek shelter from the wind. The same holds true for a patient who is too hot. Simply moving the patient into the shade can reduce the ambient temperature by several degrees. If you cannot move the patient, create shade and increase air movement by fanning the patient. Patients with altered mental status may not recognize the need to move out of the hot or cold or may not be able to move.
- **Wear the appropriate clothing for the environment.** To avoid heat loss in cold environments, wear layers of clothing that provide good insulation, such as wool, down, and synthetic fabrics. Protective clothing traps perspiration and prevents evaporation, which prevents cooling. Keep the head, hands, and feet covered, and remove wet clothing if possible. To

encourage heat loss in hot environments, wear lightweight, loose-fitting clothing, particularly around the head and neck.

Hypothermia

Hypothermia means "low temperature." This condition is diagnosed when a person's **core temperature** (ie, the temperature of the heart, lungs, and vital organs) falls below 95°F (35°C).[1,2] The body can usually tolerate a drop in core temperature of a few degrees. However, below this critical point, the body cannot regulate its temperature and generate body heat. Progressive loss of body heat then begins.

To protect itself against heat loss, the body normally constricts blood vessels in the skin; this results in the characteristic appearance of blue lips and/or fingertips. The constricted blood vessels relocate the blood from the cold surface of the skin to the center, or core, of the body. This movement of blood away from the surface of the skin decreases the body's heat loss. As a secondary precaution against heat loss, the body tends to create additional heat by shivering. As cold exposure worsens and these mechanisms are overwhelmed, many body functions begin to slow down and mental status deteriorates, resulting in lethargy, confusion, and apathy. Eventually, the functioning of key organs such as the heart begins to slow. Untreated, this process can lead to death.

Hypothermia can develop either quickly, as when someone is immersed in cold water, or gradually, as when a person is exposed to the cold environment for several hours or more. Keep in mind that the temperature does not have to be below freezing for hypothermia to occur. Hypothermia may develop at temperatures well above freezing in people who are unresponsive for a prolonged period in a cool or even room-temperature environment, such as a person who has experienced a drug overdose or stroke. People who are experiencing homelessness are at especially high risk for hypothermia. Even in summer, swimmers who remain in the water for a long time are at risk of hypothermia. Like all heat- and cold-related conditions, hypothermia is more common among young and old people and those with illness, who are less able to adjust to temperature extremes.

Patients with injuries or illness, such as burns, shock, head injury, stroke, generalized infection, injuries to the spinal cord, diabetes, and hypoglycemia, are more susceptible to hypothermia, as are patients who have taken certain drugs or consumed alcohol. In patients who are bleeding excessively (hemorrhagic shock), the body's ability to clot is negatively affected by cold, thus worsening their condition.

Signs and Symptoms

Signs and symptoms of hypothermia generally become more severe as the core temperature falls. Hypothermia generally progresses through four stages, as shown in **TABLE 32-1**. Although there is no clear distinction among the stages, the different signs and symptoms of each will help you estimate the severity of the condition. When you assess a patient in the field, you should be able to distinguish between mild and severe hypothermia.

To assess the patient's core body temperature, pull back on your glove and place the back of your hand on the patient's skin at the abdomen (**FIGURE 32-1**). This area of the body is usually well protected and will give you a quick, general idea of the patient's core temperature. If the skin feels cool, the patient is likely experiencing a generalized cold emergency.

If you work in a cold environment, and/or depending on local protocols, you may carry a hypothermia thermometer, which registers lower core temperatures. It must be inserted in the rectum for an accurate reading. Regular thermometers will not register the temperature of a patient who has significant hypothermia.

Mild hypothermia occurs when the core temperature is between 89.8°F (32.1°C) and 95°F (35°C).[2] The patient is usually alert and shivering in an attempt to generate more heat through muscular activity. The patient may jump up and down and stamp their feet. Pulse rate and respirations are usually rapid. The skin may appear red or dark compared with the person's baseline skin tone but may eventually appear pale, then cyanotic. People in a cold environment may have blue lips or fingertips because of the body's constriction of blood vessels at the skin to retain heat.

Moderate hypothermia exists when the core temperature is between 82.5°F and 89.7°F (28.1°C to 32°C).[1] In the course of moderate hypothermia, shivering stops and muscular activity decreases.

TABLE 32-1 Characteristics of Systemic Hypothermia

Extent of Hypothermia	Mild	Moderate	Severe/Profound
Core temperature	**89.8°F to 95°F (32.1°C to 35°C)**	**82.5°F to 89.7°F (28.1°C to 32°C)**	**Severe: 75.2°F to 82.4°F (24°C to 28°C)** **Profound: <75.2°F (<24°C)**
Signs and symptoms	Shivering, foot stamping	Loss of coordination, muscle stiffness, shivering stops, progressing toward coma	Confusion, loss of coordination, inability to communicate, eventually apparent death
Cardiorespiratory response	Constricted blood vessels, rapid breathing	Slow respirations, slow and weak pulse, possibly dysrhythmias	Cardiac arrest
Level of consciousness	Withdrawn	Confused, lethargic, sleepy, progressing toward unresponsiveness	Unresponsive

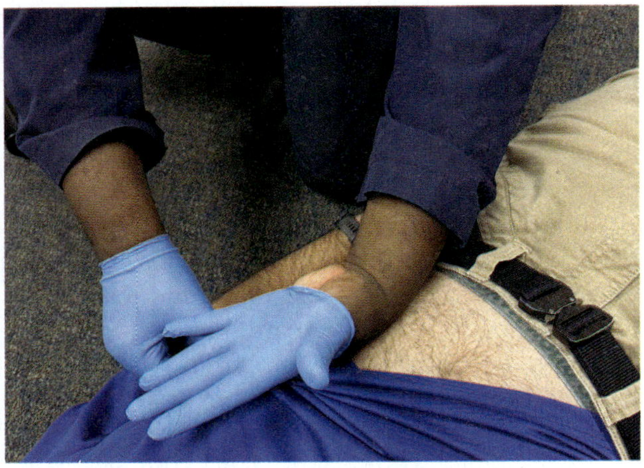

FIGURE 32-1 To assess a patient's core body temperature, pull back your glove and place the back of your hand on the patient's skin at the abdomen.

Courtesy of Rhonda Hunt.

At first, small, fine muscle activity such as coordinated finger motion ceases. Eventually, as the temperature falls further, all muscle activity stops and mental status deteriorates.

Severe hypothermia is considered to be a core temperature of less than 82.4°F (28°C).[1] As the core temperature reaches this point, the patient becomes lethargic and usually stops fighting the cold. The level of consciousness decreases, and the person may exhibit unexpected behaviors. For example, as the muscles that control vasoconstriction fatigue and stop working, blood may rush from the body's core to the extremities and cause the patient to feel hot instead of cold, prompting them to remove their clothes. Alternatively, the person may exhibit burrowing behavior in a last-ditch effort to maintain warmth. Poor coordination and memory loss follow, along with reduced or complete loss of sensation to touch, mood changes, and impaired judgment. The patient becomes less communicative, experiences joint or muscle stiffness, and has trouble speaking. The patient begins to appear stiff or rigid.

If the core temperature continues to fall, vital signs slow; the pulse becomes slower and weaker, and respirations become shallow or absent. Cardiac dysrhythmias may occur as the blood pressure decreases. Eventually, profound hypothermia, defined as a core temperature of less than 75.2°F (24°C), may develop. At this point, all cardiorespiratory activity may cease, pupillary reaction is slow, and the patient may appear dead (ie, cold to the touch and rigid, which may resemble rigor mortis). However, *never assume that a cold, pulseless patient is dead.* Patients may still survive if proper emergency care is provided. It is critical that you perform an extended pulse check (up to a full minute). Assess at the carotid or femoral pulse. A patient in apparent cardiac arrest from hypothermia should not be considered dead until aggressive rewarming has been attempted, along with resuscitation. Remember the saying: "No one is dead unless they are *warm* and dead." It is important to note that the "warm and dead" rule does not apply to patients who have died from a cause other than hypothermia; in these patients, the signs of death discussed elsewhere in this text still apply.

> **Words of Wisdom**
>
> It is not uncommon for some people to become hypothermic and be unaware they are cold. This situation may occur when patients have consumed alcohol or drugs. For example, a fan at a college football game may consume alcohol, feel warm and remove their shirt, and become hypothermic. These patients may present with altered mental status. Don't assume this presentation is just the alcohol; consider hypothermia even if the patient reports not feeling cold.

Local Cold Injuries

Most injuries from cold are confined to exposed parts of the body. The extremities, particularly the feet and hands, and the ears, nose, and face are especially vulnerable to cold injury (**FIGURE 32-2**). When exposed parts of the body become very cold but not frozen, injuries such as frostnip and immersion foot (also called trench foot) can result. When the parts become frozen, the injury is called **frostbite**.

If possible, determine the duration of the exposure, the temperature to which the body part was exposed, and the wind velocity during exposure. These important factors will help you determine the severity of a local cold injury. You should also investigate these potential underlying factors:

- Exposure to wet conditions
- Inadequate insulation from cold or wind
- Restricted circulation from tight clothing or shoes or circulatory disease
- Fatigue
- Poor nutrition
- Alcohol or drug abuse
- Hypothermia
- Diabetes
- Cardiovascular disease
- Age

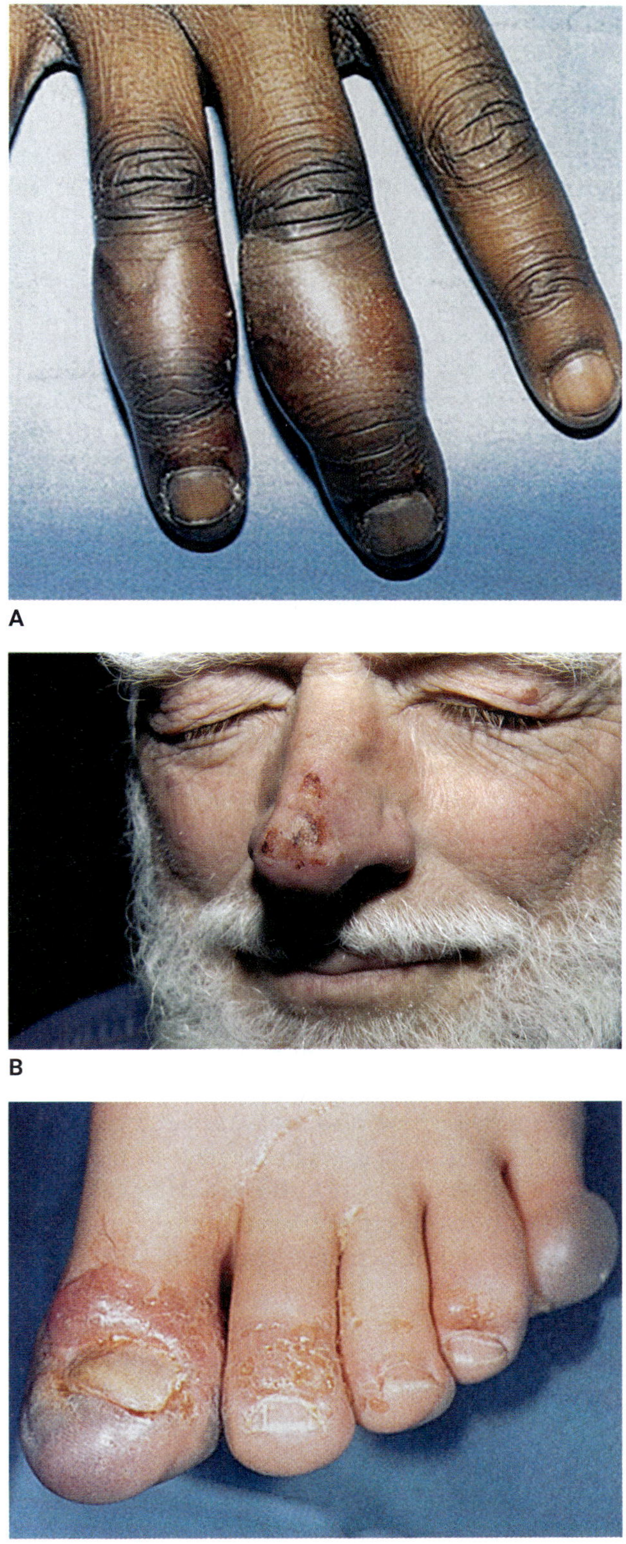

FIGURE 32-2 The (**A**) hands, (**B**) nose, and (**C**) feet are particularly susceptible to frostbite.

A: Courtesy of Neil Malcom Winkelmann; **B:** © Dr. P. Marazzi/Science Source; **C:** © Charles Stewart MD, EMDM MPH.

In hypothermia, blood is shunted away from the extremities to maintain the core temperature. This shunting of blood increases the risk of local cold injury to the extremities, ears, nose, and face. Thus, the patient with hypothermia should also be assessed for frostbite or other local cold injury. The reverse is also true. Remember, both local and systemic cold exposure injuries can occur in the same patient.

Frostnip and Immersion Foot

After prolonged exposure to the cold, the skin may freeze, whereas the deeper tissues are unaffected. This condition, which often affects the ears, nose, and fingers, is called frostnip. Because frostnip is usually painless, the patient often is unaware that a cold injury has occurred. Immersion foot occurs after prolonged exposure to cold water. It is particularly common in hikers or hunters who stand for a long time in a river or lake. With both frostnip and immersion foot, the skin is pale (blanched) and cold to the touch; baseline color does not return after palpation of the skin. In some cases, the skin of the foot will be wrinkled, but it can also remain soft. The patient reports loss of feeling and sensation in the injured area.

Frostbite

Frostbite is the most serious local cold injury because the tissues are actually frozen. Freezing permanently damages cells, although the exact mechanism by which damage occurs is unknown. The presence of ice crystals within the cells may cause physical damage. The change in the water content in the cells may also cause changes in the concentration of critical electrolytes, producing permanent changes in the chemistry of the cell. When the ice thaws, further chemical changes occur in the cell, causing permanent damage or cell death, called necrosis or gangrene (**FIGURE 32-3**). If gangrene occurs, the dead tissue may need to be surgically removed, sometimes by amputation. Following less severe damage, the exposed part will become inflamed, tender to touch, and unable to tolerate exposure to cold.

Frostbite can be identified by the hard, waxy feel of the affected tissues (**FIGURE 32-4**). The injured part feels firm to frozen as you gently touch it. If the frostbite is only skin deep, it will feel leathery or thick instead of hard. Blisters and swelling may be present. Maintain a high index of suspicion for potential frostbite in these patients if the exposure to cold has been substantial and the tissues feel abnormal. With a deep injury that has thawed or partially thawed, the skin may appear red or white, or it may be mottled and cyanotic (purple and blue). In patients with dark skin, these changes in color may be less apparent.

As with a burn, the depth of skin damage will vary. With superficial frostbite, only the skin is frozen; with deep frostbite, the deeper tissues are frozen as well. You may not be able to tell superficial from deep frostbite in the field. When possible, the

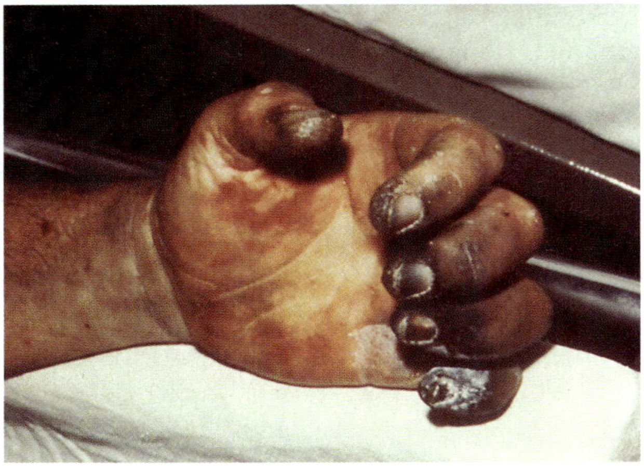

FIGURE 32-3 Gangrene (necrosis), or permanent cell death, occurs when tissue is frozen and destructive chemical changes occur in the cells.

Courtesy of Dr. Jack Poland/CDC.

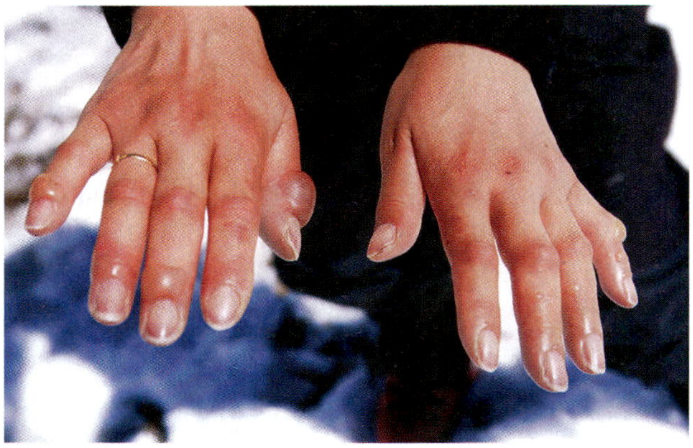

FIGURE 32-4 Frostbitten parts are usually hard and waxy to the touch.

Courtesy of Neil Malcom Winkelmann.

patient should be transported to a medical facility, such as a burn center, where physicians familiar with this injury can quickly make this distinction. Rapid initiation of thrombolytic therapy for severe frostbite can reduce the risk that amputation will be necessary.[3] EMTs should also be aware of centers in their area where the drug iloprost (Aurlumyn) is available for injection. This vasodilator was approved by the Food and Drug Administration specifically for treatment of severe frostbite injuries and has been shown to significantly reduce the need for finger or toe amputation.[4]

Assessment of Cold Injuries

Management of hypothermia in the field, regardless of the severity of the exposure, consists of stabilizing the ABCs and preventing further heat loss.

Scene Size-up

Typically, your scene assessment begins with information provided by dispatch. Note environmental conditions. Air temperature, wind chill, and whether it is wet or dry are important aspects of scene size-up and will likely affect the patient.

Ensure that the scene is safe for you and other emergency responders. Identify potential safety hazards, such as wet grass, mud, or icy streets. Cold environments may present special challenges both for you and your patient; consider special hazards such as avalanches. Take appropriate standard precautions and consider the number of patients you may have. Summon additional help, such as a search-and-rescue team, as quickly as possible.

As you observe the scene, look for indicators of the mechanism of injury (MOI). For example, if you find a vehicle in a secluded ditch off the highway and the vehicle's roof and hood are covered with fresh snow, then you may assume that the patient was in a motor vehicle crash and has been exposed to the cold for a long time.

Primary Assessment

In a cold emergency, your patient's chief complaint may be only that they are cold, or the cold may be an additional complication of an existing medical injury or trauma. Perform a rapid examination to determine whether a life threat exists, and if so, treat it. If the chief complaint is simply feeling cold, quickly assess the patient's core temperature by placing the back of your hand on the abdomen. Evaluate the patient's mental status quickly using the AVPU (Awake and alert, responsive to Verbal stimuli, responsive to Pain, Unresponsive) scale. An altered mental status indicates the intensity of the cold injury. Consider spinal motion restriction based on your scene size-up and the chief complaint.

Your assessment should account for the physiologic changes that occur as a result of hypothermia. If you believe the patient is in cardiac arrest, modify the ABC (Airway, Breathing, Circulation) sequence so that *C* comes first (CAB); thus, you will provide high-quality chest compressions, then address airway and breathing. Ensure the patient has an adequate airway and is breathing. If your patient's breathing is slow or shallow, ventilation with a bag-mask device may be necessary. Use warmed and humidified oxygen if it is available, because it helps to warm the patient from the inside out.

If you cannot feel a radial pulse, gently palpate for a carotid pulse. For a patient with hypothermia, this may require a prolonged pulse check of up to 60 seconds. Even a pulse rate of 1 or 2 beats/min indicates cardiac activity, and cardiac activity may spontaneously recover once the body core is warmed. However, there is evidence that cardiopulmonary resuscitation (CPR), when correctly done, will increase blood flow to the critical parts of the body. The American Heart Association recommends that CPR be started if the patient has no detectable pulse or breathing.

Perfusion will be compromised based on the severity of the cold exposure. Your assessment of the patient's skin will not be helpful in determining shock. Assume that shock is present and treat underlying conditions appropriately. Bleeding may be difficult to find because of the slow-moving circulation and thick clothing. If the scene size-up, MOI, or chief complaint suggests the potential for bleeding, look for it carefully, remembering internal bleeding will not be visualized.

Even mild hypothermia can have serious consequences and complications, including cardiac dysrhythmias and blood clotting abnormalities. Therefore, all patients with hypothermia require rapid transport for evaluation and treatment. Assess the scene for the safest way to quickly move your patient from the cold environment. As you package your patient for transport, work quickly, safely, and gently. Rough handling of a patient with hypothermia may cause a cold, slow, weak heart to twitch or fibrillate. If transportation is delayed, protect the patient from further heat loss.

History Taking

After the life threats have been managed during the primary assessment, investigate the chief complaint. Obtain a medical history and be alert for injury-specific signs and symptoms as well as any pertinent negatives.

Obtaining a patient's history in these situations may be difficult. If possible, find out how long your patient has been exposed to the cold environment, either from the patient or bystanders. Exposures may be short or prolonged in duration. For example, a patient may have acute hypothermia from sudden immersion in cold water or hypothermia that developed over the course of hours, as may be seen in persons experiencing homelessness. Your SAMPLE history (Signs and symptoms, Allergies, Medications, Pertinent past medical history, Last oral intake, Events leading up to the illness or injury) can provide important information affecting both your treatment in the field and the treatment your patient will receive in the hospital. Recall that medications and underlying medical conditions may have an impact on the way cold affects the patient's metabolism. The patient's last oral intake and activity prior to the exposure will help to determine the severity of the cold injury.

Secondary Assessment

The secondary assessment is used to uncover injuries that may have been missed during the primary assessment. In some instances, such as a critically injured patient or a short transport time, you may not have time to conduct a secondary assessment.

Focus your physical examination on the severity of hypothermia, assessing the areas of the body directly affected by cold exposure, and the degree of damage. Is the whole body cold (hypothermia) or just parts (frostbite)? These determinations will affect your treatment decisions. For example, a patient who stops shivering, but remains in a cold environment, will experience a rapid decrease in body temperature: a sign of severe hypothermia and a life-threatening emergency.

Determine the degree and extent of cold injury, as well as any other injuries or conditions that may not have been initially detected. The numbing effect of cold, both on the brain and on the body, may impair your patient's ability to tell you about other injuries or illnesses. Therefore, a careful examination of your patient's entire body will help you avoid missing important clues to your patient's condition.

Keep in mind that vital signs may be altered by the effects of hypothermia and can be an indicator of its severity. Respirations may become slow and shallow, resulting in low oxygen levels in the body. Low blood pressure and a slow pulse also indicate moderate to severe hypothermia. Carefully evaluate your patient for changes in mental status such as confusion, lethargy, and odd behavior.

Determine the body's core temperature using a hypothermia thermometer, if local protocols allow. Pulse oximetry will often be inaccurate or unobtainable due to the lack of perfusion in the extremities.

Reassessment

Repeat the primary assessment. Reassess vital signs and the chief complaint. Has the patient's condition improved with the interventions? Identify and treat changes in the patient's condition. Keep a close eye on your patient's level of consciousness and vital signs. As the body rewarms, the sudden redistribution of fluids and the release of built-up chemicals can have harmful effects, including cardiac dysrhythmias. Be vigilant even if the patient's condition appears to be improving.

Review all treatments that have been performed. In a cold-related emergency, depending on your local protocols, your treatment may only include oxygen delivery. Reassess oxygen delivery and continue to provide for a warm environment by removing any wet or frozen clothing. Do not remove any clothing frozen to the patient's skin.

Communicate all the information you have gathered to the receiving facility, which may be essential in evaluating and treating your patient in the hospital. Your documentation should always include the patient's physical status, the conditions at the scene, information gathered from bystanders, and any changes in the patient's mental status during treatment and transport.

Management of Cold Emergencies

In most cases, move the patient from the cold environment to prevent further heat loss. To prevent further damage to the feet, do not allow the patient to walk; maintain the patient in a supine position. Remove any wet clothing, and place dry blankets over and under the patient (**FIGURE 32-5**). If available, give the patient warm, humidified oxygen if you have not already done so as part of the primary assessment.

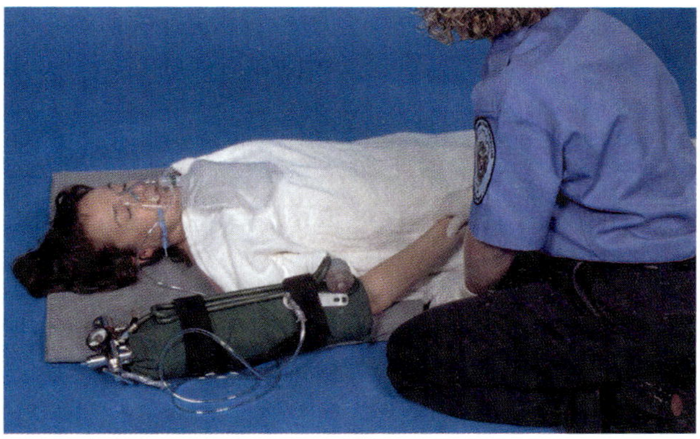

FIGURE 32-5 Place dry blankets over and under the patient with hypothermia; give warm, humidified oxygen, if available.

Always handle the patient gently so that you do not cause any pain or further injury to the skin. Rough handling of a patient with moderate to severe hypothermia may cause the heart to go into ventricular fibrillation, which may not respond to defibrillation. Patient exertion can also cause this condition, so move the patient, rather than having them exert themselves. Ventricular fibrillation is a condition characterized by uncontrollable twitching of the heart without effective pumping action. Do not massage the extremities. Do not allow the patient to eat or to use any stimulants, such as coffee, tea, soda, or tobacco products. Stimulants are vasoconstrictors, which may further impair circulation to affected areas.[5]

If the patient is alert, is shivering, responds appropriately, and has a core temperature of 89.8°F to 95°F (32.1°C to 35°C), then the hypothermia is mild. Begin passive rewarming slowly, which includes placing the patient in a warm environment and removing wet clothing. Turn the heat up high in the patient compartment of the ambulance. You may give sips of warm sweetened fluids by mouth, as allowed by local protocols, assuming the patient is alert and can swallow without difficulty, and may permit active movement.[5]

YOU are the EMT

You arrive at the scene and find the patient sitting under a tree in his garden; he is conscious but confused. His wife tells you that he has been working outside all day. She further states that despite her efforts, he refused to take a break and drink some water. As your partner opens the jump kit, you perform a primary assessment.

Recording Time: 0 Minutes	
Appearance	Flushed (compared with baseline)
Level of consciousness	Responds to voice, but confused.
Airway	Open, clear of secretions or foreign bodies
Breathing	Increased rate and depth
Circulation	Radial pulses weak and rapid; skin hot and moist; no gross bleeding

The patient's wife tells you that when she went to check on him, she found him sitting under a tree; initially, he did not respond to her. She further tells you that he has hypertension and angina, for which he takes furosemide (Lasix), potassium chloride (K-Dur), lisinopril (Prinivil), and nitroglycerin as needed. He also has insulin-dependent diabetes. They were up late at a party the prior evening. He drank quite a bit more alcohol than normal and vomited this morning.

3. What risk factors does this patient have that predispose him to a heat emergency?

4. What type of heat emergency do you suspect he is experiencing? Why?

For a patient with moderate or severe hypothermia, your goal is to prevent further heat loss. Remember to restrict movements and handle the patient gently to decrease the risk of ventricular fibrillation. In addition to removing their clothes and placing them in a warm environment, apply heat packs or hot water bottles to the groin, axillary, and cervical regions. To avoid burns, do not place heat packs directly on the skin. Emergency medical services (EMS) agencies located in cold climates may carry forced air warming systems that blow warm air through holes in a special blanket that is placed next to the patient's skin. When these systems are available, they should be used early to help rewarm the patient.

Other active rewarming methods are best accomplished in the emergency department (ED) utilizing aggressive strategies to introduce heat into the body's core. Such therapies might include warm intravenous (IV) fluids, lavage with warm fluids, and rewarming blood outside the body before reintroducing it (extracorporeal rewarming). Rewarming the patient too quickly, or from the extremities rather than the core, may cause a fatal cardiac dysrhythmia or other significant complications. Afterdrop is a condition in which the patient's core temperature continues to decrease after rewarming efforts have begun because colder blood from the extremities returns to the heart. For this reason, local protocols may dictate the appropriate type of rewarming strategies based on the patient's presentation.

If you cannot get the patient out of the cold immediately, move the patient out of the wind and away from contact with any object that will conduct heat away from the body. Place blankets and a waterproof protective cover on the patient. To prevent body heat loss from the head and neck, cover these areas with a towel. Regardless of the nature or severity of the cold injury, remember that even an unresponsive patient may be able to hear you. Some patients have reported hearing a clinician pronounce them dead; this clinician forgot the saying, "No one is dead unless they are warm and dead."

Emergency Care of Local Cold Injuries

The emergency treatment of local cold injuries in the field should include the following steps:

1. Remove the patient from further exposure to the cold.
2. Handle the injured part gently, and protect it from further injury.
3. Remove any wet or restricting clothing from the patient, especially over the injured part.

If there is no chance of reinjury or if transport to the ED will be significantly delayed, consider active rewarming if local protocols allow. Consult medical direction, if available. With frostnip, contact with a warm object may be all that the patient needs; you can use your hands or the patient's own body (eg, have the patient tuck their hands into their armpits). During rewarming, the affected part will often tingle and become red or purple, depending on the person's baseline skin color. With immersion foot, remove wet shoes, boots, and socks, and rewarm the foot gradually, protecting it from further cold exposure. Next, cover it loosely with a dry, sterile dressing. Never rub or massage injured tissues, which could cause further damage. Do not re-expose the injury to cold.

With a late or deep cold injury, such as frostbite, remove any jewelry from the injured part and cover the injury loosely with a dry, sterile dressing. Do not break blisters or rub or massage the area. It is commonly advised to not apply heat or rewarm the part. Unlike with frostnip and trench foot, rewarming of the frostbitten extremity is best accomplished in the ED. You can cause further injury to fragile tissues by attempting to rewarm a frostbitten part. Never apply something warm or hot, such as the exhaust from the ambulance engine or, even worse, an open flame. Do not allow the patient to stand or walk on a frostbitten foot. Evaluate the patient's general condition for the signs or symptoms of systemic hypothermia. Support the vital functions as necessary, and provide rapid transport to the hospital.

If prompt hospital care is unavailable and medical direction instructs you to begin rewarming in the field, use a warm-water bath. Immerse the frostbitten part in water with a temperature between 98.6°F and 102°F (37°C and 39°C).[2] Check the water temperature with a thermometer before immersing the limb, and recheck it frequently during the rewarming process. Stir the water continuously. Keep the frostbitten part in the water until it feels warm and sensation has returned to the skin. Dress the area with dry, sterile dressings, including placing them between injured fingers or toes. Expect the patient to report severe pain.

Never attempt rewarming if there is any chance that the part may freeze again before the patient reaches the hospital. Some of the most severe consequences of frostbite, including gangrene and amputation, have occurred when parts thawed and then were allowed to refreeze.

Cover the frostbitten part with soft, padded, sterile cotton dressings. If blisters have formed, do not break them. Remember, you cannot accurately predict the outcome of a case of frostbite early in its course. Even body parts that appear gangrenous may recover following proper treatment.

Cold Exposure and the EMS Clinician

As an EMT, you are also at risk for hypothermia if you work in a cold environment. If cold weather search-and-rescue operations are a possibility in your assigned areas, you should receive survival training and precautionary tips. Become familiar with local conditions. Be aware of existing and potential weather conditions, and monitor changes that are forecast for the area. Make sure to wear proper appropriate clothing. Your vehicle, too, must be properly equipped and maintained for a cold environment. You cannot help others if you do not protect yourself. Never allow yourself to become a victim!

Heat Exposure

Recall that normal body temperature is 98.6°F (37°C). In a hot environment or during vigorous physical activity, the body will try to rid itself of the excess heat. The two most efficient methods to decrease heat are sweating (and evaporation of the sweat) and dilation of skin blood vessels, which brings blood to the skin surface to increase the rate of heat radiation. In addition, a person who becomes overheated can remove clothing and seek a cooler environment.

Ordinarily, the heat-regulating mechanisms of the body work well, and people are able to tolerate significant temperature changes. When heat gain exceeds heat loss, hyperthermia can result. **Hyperthermia** is a high core temperature, usually 101°F (38.3°C) or higher.

When the body's mechanisms to decrease body heat are overwhelmed and the body is unable to tolerate the excessive heat, a heat emergency develops in the patient. High air temperature can reduce heat loss by radiation; high humidity reduces heat loss through evaporation. The inability to acclimate (adjust) to the heat is a risk factor. Another risk factor is vigorous exercise, during which sweat loss can exceed 1 liter per hour, causing loss of fluid and electrolytes.

A heat emergency can take the following three forms:

- Heat cramps
- Heat exhaustion
- Heatstroke

All three forms may be present in the same patient because untreated heat exhaustion may progress to heatstroke. Heatstroke is life threatening.

People at greatest risk for a heat emergency include the following[6]:

- Children
- Older adults
- People with preexisting medical conditions (eg, heart disease, chronic obstructive pulmonary disease, diabetes, dehydration, obesity)
- Pregnant persons
- People who work outdoors or who otherwise experience physical exertion in hot conditions, including emergency responders
- People living in urban areas (cities tend to be warmer due to decreased green areas and increased presence of materials such as asphalt that absorb and emit heat)
- People without the ability to adapt to and recover from heat exposure, including people with disabilities (whether from impaired thermoregulatory mechanisms or disruption to services they rely on, as may occur when community resources are overwhelmed during a heat wave)
- People experiencing homelessness
- Athletes

Older people, newborns, and infants exhibit poor thermoregulation. Newborns and infants are often dressed in too much clothing. Alcohol and certain

Words of Wisdom

It is important to keep yourself hydrated while on duty, especially during periods of heavy exertion or when working in the heat. The color of urine (usually darker with dehydration) and frequency of urination correlate directly with the body's hydration status.

medications such as diuretics taken by patients with heart failure dehydrate the body or decrease the body's ability to sweat, also making a person more susceptible to heat emergencies. When you are treating someone for a heat emergency, always obtain a medication history.

Heat Cramps

Heat cramps are painful muscle spasms that occur after vigorous exercise. They do not occur only when it is hot outdoors. They may be seen in factory workers and even well-conditioned athletes. The exact cause of heat cramps is not well understood. It is known that sweat produced during strenuous exercise, particularly in a warm environment, causes a change in the body's electrolyte balance. The result may be a loss of essential electrolytes from the cells. Dehydration may also play a role in the development of muscle cramps. Large amounts of water loss can result from excessive sweating. This loss of water may affect muscles that are being stressed and cause them to spasm.

Heat cramps usually occur in the leg or abdominal muscles. When the abdominal muscles are involved, the pain and muscle spasm may be so severe that the patient appears to have an acute abdominal condition. If a patient with a sudden onset of abdominal cramps has been exercising vigorously in a hot environment, suspect heat cramps.

Heat Exhaustion

Heat exhaustion is the most common heat emergency. Heat exposure, stress, and fatigue are causes of heat exhaustion. This condition occurs when the water and electrolytes lost through heavy sweating are so extensive that the fluids circulating through the vascular system become insufficient to meet the body's demands, resulting in a state similar to hypovolemic shock. Recall that for sweating to be an effective cooling mechanism, the sweat must be able to evaporate from the body. Otherwise, the body will continue to produce sweat, with further loss of body water. People standing in the hot sun, particularly those wearing several layers of clothing, such as sports fans or parade watchers, may sweat profusely but experience little body cooling. The sweat-soaked clothing will actually begin to trap heat, increasing body temperature. High humidity will also decrease the amount of evaporation that can occur. The heat index provided in **FIGURE 32-6** shows how high humidity increases the effects of ambient temperature. For example, if the temperature is 90°F (32.2°C) with 85% humidity, the effect of the atmosphere on a person would be the same is if the air temperature were 117°F (47.2°C).

Words of Wisdom

The wet bulb globe temperature (WBGT) is an alternative to the heat index, designed to more accurately measure the effects of environmental conditions on the human body. Where the heat index focuses on air temperature and humidity, the WBGT incorporates factors such as exposure to direct sunlight, wind, and heat-absorbing surfaces such as synthetic turfs.[7]

People working or exerting themselves in poorly ventilated areas are unable to release heat through convection. Thus, people who work or exercise vigorously and those who wear heavy clothing in a warm, humid, or poorly ventilated environment are particularly susceptible to heat exhaustion.

The signs and symptoms of heat exhaustion and those of associated hypovolemia are as follows:

- Dizziness, weakness, or syncope (a brief loss of consciousness) with accompanying nausea, vomiting, or headache. Muscle cramping may also be present, including abdominal cramping.
- Onset while working vigorously or exercising in a hot, humid, or poorly ventilated environment and sweating heavily.
- Onset, even at rest, in the older and infant age groups in hot, humid, and poorly ventilated environments or extended time in hot, humid environments. People who are not acclimatized to the environment may also experience onset at rest.
- Cold, clammy skin with ashen pallor.
- Dry tongue and thirst.
- Normal vital signs, although the pulse is often rapid and weak (an indication for use of pulse oximetry) and the diastolic blood pressure may be low.
- Normal or slightly elevated body temperature—on rare occasions, up to 104°F (40°C).

Temperature (°F)

Relative Humidity (%)	80	81	84	86	88	90	92	94	96	98	100	102	104	106	108	110
40	80	81	83	85	88	91	94	97	101	105	109	114	119	124	130	136
45	80	82	84	87	89	93	96	100	104	109	114	119	124	130	137	
50	81	83	85	88	91	95	99	103	108	113	118	124	131	137		
55	81	84	86	89	93	97	101	106	112	117	124	130	137			
60	82	84	88	91	95	100	105	110	116	123	129	137				
65	82	85	89	93	98	103	108	114	121	126	130					
70	83	86	90	95	100	105	112	119	126	134						
75	84	88	92	97	103	109	116	124	132							
80	84	89	94	100	106	113	121	129								
85	85	90	96	102	110	117	126	135								
90	86	91	98	105	113	122	131									
95	86	93	100	108	117	127										
100	87	95	103	112	121	132										

Likelihood of Heat Disorders With Prolonged Exposure or Strenuous Activity

Caution / Extreme Caution / Danger / Extreme Danger

FIGURE 32-6 High humidity increases the effects of ambient temperature.

Courtesy of the National Weather Service/NOAA.

Heatstroke

Heatstroke, the least common but most serious heat emergency, occurs when the body is subjected to more heat than it can handle and normal mechanisms for getting rid of the excess heat are overwhelmed. The body temperature then rises rapidly to the level at which tissues are destroyed. Untreated heatstroke always results in death.

Heatstroke can develop in patients during vigorous physical activity or when they are outdoors or in a closed, poorly ventilated, humid space. It also occurs during heat waves among people (particularly geriatric patients) who live in buildings with no air conditioning or with poor ventilation. It may also develop in children who are left unattended in a locked vehicle on a hot day.

The absence of perspiration is an important and classically described sign of heatstroke. When the patient no longer perspires, the body has lost its thermoregulatory mechanism. Many patients with heatstroke have hot, dry, flushed skin because their sweating mechanism has been overwhelmed. However, in the course of heatstroke, the skin may be moist or wet due to exertion by the patient. Consider the possibility that the patient only appears to still be sweating because their clothing became saturated before the onset of heatstroke. If you misinterpret their presentation, not only may you fail to realize their body has stopped compensating, but you may fail to consider the need to remove their saturated clothing, which is trapping heat and making the situation worse. Also keep in mind that a patient can have heatstroke even if they are still sweating. This presentation is often seen in endurance athletes, military personnel, or emergency clinicians who wear personal protective equipment, such as firefighters, SWAT team members, or hazardous materials workers. The body temperature rises rapidly in patients with heatstroke, reaching 104°F (40°C) or higher. As the body core temperature rises, the patient's level of consciousness decreases, resulting in unconsciousness.

Often, the first sign of heatstroke is confusion or a change in behavior. However, the patient often becomes unresponsive quickly and seizures may occur. The pulse is usually rapid and strong at first, but as the patient becomes increasingly unresponsive, the pulse becomes weaker and the blood pressure falls. The respiratory rate increases as the body attempts to compensate. As mentioned, absence of sweating is an ominous sign. If you are perspiring in the environment, your patient should also be perspiring. If any one of these signs is present, suspect heatstroke and act accordingly.

Assessment of Heat Emergencies

Scene Size-up

As part of your scene size-up, perform an environmental assessment. How hot is it outside? How hot is it in the room where your patient is located? How well is the patient tolerating the heat? Dispatch may report the call initially as a medical or trauma emergency. The heat emergency may be secondary. Always look for hazards as well as clues as to what may have caused your patient's emergency. If the patient is unconscious, has an altered mental status, or requires IV fluids to treat shock, consider calling for advanced life support (ALS) assistance as long as doing so does not delay access to aggressive cooling techniques.

As you observe the scene, look for indicators of the MOI. For example, you arrive on the scene at a shopping mall to find an older man with a decreased level of consciousness inside a parked vehicle on a warm, humid, sunny day. The MOI for this patient is sitting in a warm environment under direct sunlight with no ventilation. Expect that a child found in an enclosed car on a warm day who has an altered mental status is experiencing hyperthermia until proven otherwise.

Heat emergencies commonly occur in the context of athletic events and practices. They are one of the most frequent causes of sudden death in athletes.[8] Because athletic trainers are often present in these instances, you may find the patient placed in a cold-water immersion bath inside the athletic training room. It is harmful to allow heat to persist for any amount of time because critical cell damage occurs within 30 minutes; therefore, if heatstroke is present, cooling prior to transport is indicated if rapid cooling with an ice bath is indicated and available. If the patient is placed in a cold-water immersion bath on your arrival, monitor the patient in the water and assist as necessary. Do not remove the patient until the body temperature has normalized to the appropriate level, around 102.2°F (39°C).[2] Do not overcool the patient. Overcooling can lead to shivering, which generates more heat. When shivering occurs and ALS is present, medication can be given to stop it. Monitor the patient closely.

Finally, if you anticipate a prolonged scene time, protect yourself from the heat and remember to stay hydrated. Take appropriate standard precautions, including gloves and eye protection. Long-sleeved shirts and long pants may be uncomfortable in warm weather; however, they can help protect you from being splashed by blood or other body fluids.

Primary Assessment

As you approach your patient, observe how the patient interacts with you and the environment. This will help identify the patient's degree of distress. Introduce yourself and ask about the chief complaint. A heat emergency may be the primary problem or it may simply be aggravating a medical or trauma condition. Remember, prolonged heat exposure may stress the heart, causing a heart attack. Use this initial interaction to guide you in assessing for immediate life threats and related problems. Perform a rapid scan and avoid tunnel vision.

Assess the patient's mental status. Heatstroke is a life-threatening emergency. Gather clues about their mental status to identify the severity of your patient's condition. The more altered the patient's mental status is, the more serious the heat emergency.

Assess the patient's airway and breathing and treat any life threats. Unless the patient is unresponsive, the airway should be patent. Nausea and vomiting, however, may occur. Position the patient to protect the airway as necessary. If the patient is unresponsive, be cautious of how you open the airway; consider spinal motion restriction if trauma is a possibility. If your patient is unresponsive, insert an airway and provide bag-mask ventilations. Measure the blood glucose if the patient's mental status is altered.

If circulation is adequate, assess the patient for perfusion and bleeding. Assess the patient's skin condition carefully (**TABLE 32-2**). Treat the patient aggressively for shock by removing the patient from the heat and positioning the patient to improve circulation.

TABLE 32-2 Skin Condition

Skin Condition	Indication
Moist, pale, cool skin	Body is losing excessive fluid and salt.
Hot, dry skin	Body is unable to regulate core temperature.
Hot, moist skin	Body may be unable to regulate core temperature.

Words of Wisdom

If a commercial device for an ice bath or a tarp is not available, a body bag can provide a temporary container to serve as the tub.[8]

History Taking

After the life threats have been managed during the primary assessment, investigate the chief complaint. Obtain a medical history and be alert for specific signs and symptoms such as the absence of perspiration, decreased level of consciousness, confusion, muscle cramping, nausea, and vomiting.

Obtain a SAMPLE history if possible. Patients with inadequate oral intake or who are taking diuretics may have difficulty tolerating exposure to heat. Remember, many medications used by geriatric patients affect how well they tolerate heat. Be thorough in your questioning. Determine your patient's exposure to heat and humidity and activities prior to the onset of symptoms.

Secondary Assessment

The secondary assessment is used to uncover injuries that may have been missed during the primary assessment. In some instances, such as a critically injured patient or a short transport time, you may not have time to conduct a secondary assessment.

If your patient is unresponsive, perform a secondary assessment of the entire body, looking for problems or explanations as to what is wrong. Obtain the patient's vital signs to help understand the severity of the emergency.

If the patient is conscious, perform an assessment of specific areas of the body. Heat exposure has significant effects on the metabolism, muscles, and cardiovascular system. Assess the patient for muscle cramps or confusion. Examine the patient's mental status and take the patient's vital signs.

Perform a detailed examination if circumstances and time permit. Pay special attention to the patient's skin temperature, **turgor**, and level of moisture. Skin turgor is the ability of the skin to resist deformation. It is tested by gently pinching skin on the abdomen or back of the hand. Normally the skin will quickly flatten out. If the patient is dehydrated, the skin will remain tented (poor skin turgor). Perform a careful neurologic examination.

Patients with hyperthermia will often have tachycardia and tachypnea. As long as they maintain a normal blood pressure, their bodies will compensate for the fluid loss. Once their blood pressure begins to fall, it indicates they are no longer able to compensate for fluid loss and are going into shock. Your assessment of the patient's skin will help determine the severity of the emergency. For example, in heat exhaustion, the skin temperature may be normal or may even be cool and clammy; however, in heatstroke, the skin is hot.

If a thermometer is available, check the patient's body temperature. Your unit equipment may include disposable or oral thermometers with disposable covers, infrared digital skin thermometers, or tympanic (ear) thermometers. You may not use these devices routinely, so become familiar with how they work. In patients with a heat-related emergency, monitoring of pulse oximetry is also useful.

Reassessment

Watch your patient's condition carefully for deterioration. Remove your patient as quickly as possible from the hot environment. Patients with heat cramps or exhaustion usually respond well to passive cooling and fluids by mouth. Patients with symptoms of heatstroke who cannot be cooled on scene should be transported immediately in a cool ambulance, passively cooled with clothing removal, and actively cooled by spraying the patient with water and fanning to enhance evaporation. Any decline in level of consciousness is an ominous sign. Monitor the patient's vital signs at least every 5 minutes. Evaluate the effectiveness of your interventions.

TABLE 32-3 Symptoms of Heat Exhaustion and Heatstroke

Heat Exhaustion Symptoms	Heatstroke Symptoms (Medical Emergency)
Dizziness or fainting	Headache
Heavy sweating	Confusion or delirium
Cold, pale, and clammy skin	Possible loss of consciousness
Nausea or vomiting	Absence of sweating, or dry skin, except in exertional heatstroke
Fast, weak pulse	Hot, red/darkened skin
Weakness or muscle cramps	Nausea or vomiting
Excessive thirst	Rapid heart rate
	Body temperature above 104°F (40°C)

Be careful not to overcool a patient who is experiencing a heat emergency, but the risk of failing to reverse heatstroke by active cooling far exceeds the risk of overcooling. Remember, heatstroke is fatal if not reversed rapidly and effectively.

Inform the ED staff as soon as possible that your patient is experiencing heatstroke, because additional resources may be required. Document the environmental conditions and the activities the patient was performing prior to the emergency in your patient care report. Consider other possibilities of the altered mental status, such as traumatic brain injury, alcohol consumption, or a low blood glucose level (**TABLE 32-3**).

Management of Heat Emergencies

Heat Cramps

Take the following steps to treat heat cramps in the field (**FIGURE 32-7**):

1. Promptly remove the patient from the hot environment, including direct sunlight. Loosen or remove any tight clothing.

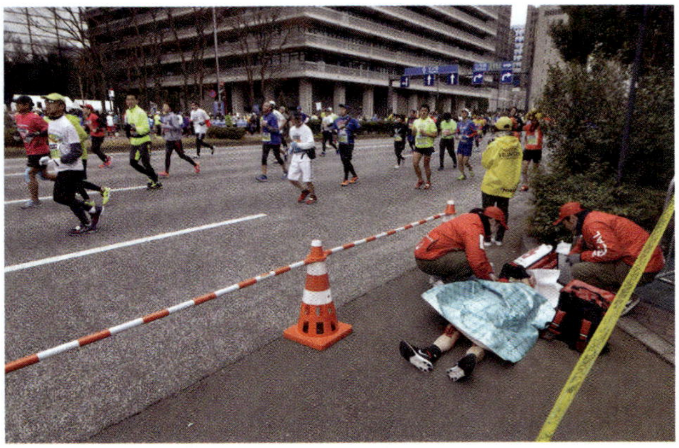

FIGURE 32-7 A patient with any heat emergency should be moved to a cool environment as you begin your assessment and treatment.

2. Administer high-concentration oxygen if the patient shows signs of hypoxia or respiratory distress.
3. Rest the cramping muscles. Have the patient sit or lie down until the cramps subside.
4. Replace fluids by mouth. Give water, juice, or a diluted (half-strength) balanced cool electrolyte solution, such as a sports drink. In most cases, plain water is the most useful. Do not give salt tablets or solutions that have a high salt concentration.
5. Cool the patient with cool water spray or mist, and add convection to the cooling method by manually or mechanically fanning the patient.

When the heat cramps are gone, the patient may resume activity. For example, an athlete can return to play once the heat cramps have disappeared. However, heavy sweating may cause the cramps to reoccur. The best strategy for treatment and prevention is hydration by drinking enough water.

If the cramps do not go away after these measures, transport the patient to the hospital. If you are uncertain that the patient's cramps were caused by the heat or you note anything out of the ordinary, contact medical direction or transport the patient to the hospital.

Heat Exhaustion

To treat the patient with heat exhaustion, follow the steps in **SKILL DRILL 32-1**:

1. Promptly remove the patient from the hot environment, preferably into the back of the

Skill Drill 32-1 Treating for Heat Exhaustion

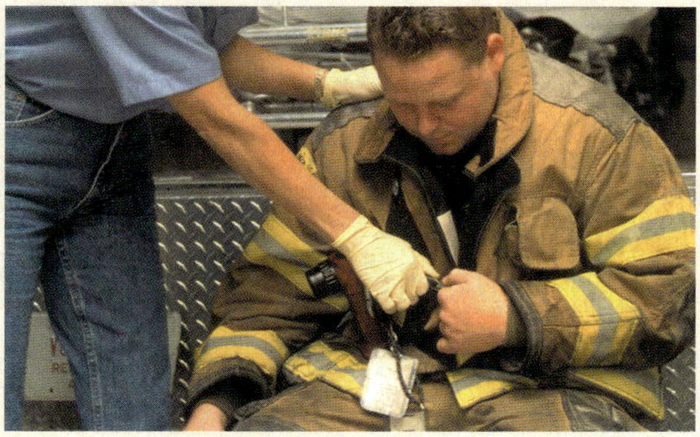

Step 1

Move the patient to a cooler environment. Remove extra clothing.

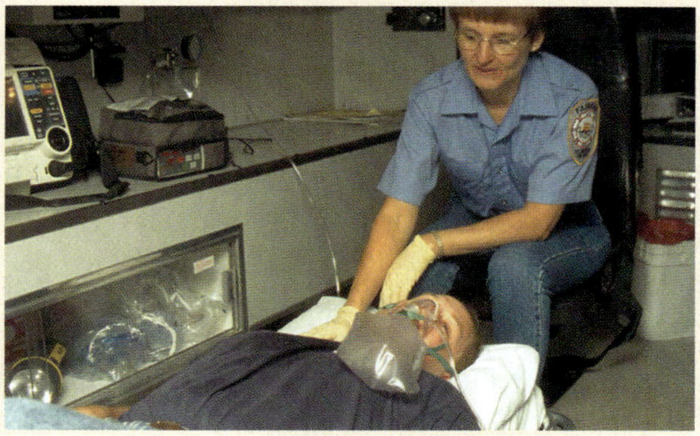

Step 2

Give oxygen if indicated. Check the patient's blood glucose level if mental status is altered. Perform cooling measures as available. Place the patient in a supine position and fan the patient.

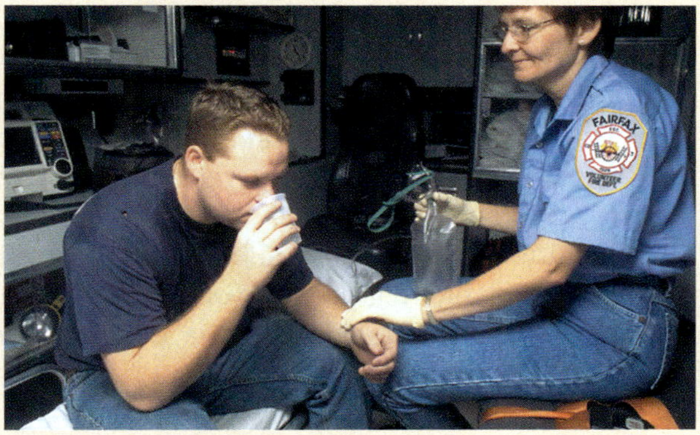

Step 3

If the patient is fully alert, give sips of water or electrolyte solution by mouth.

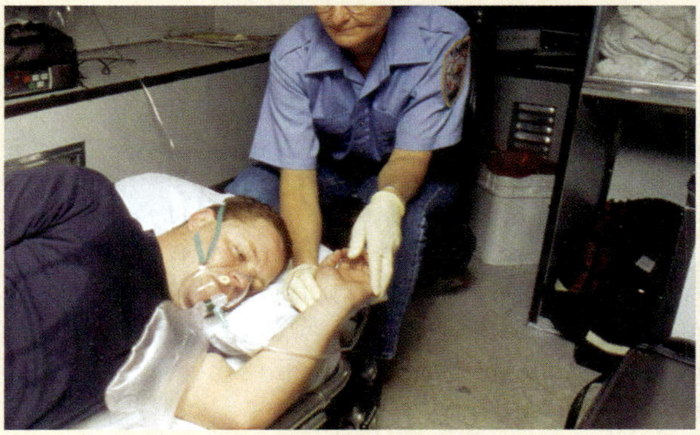

Step 4

If nausea develops, secure and transport the patient on their left side.

air-conditioned ambulance. If outdoors, move out of direct sunlight. Remove any excessive layers of clothing (**Step 1**).

2. Administer high-concentration oxygen if the patient is showing signs of hypoxia or respiratory distress.
3. If the patient has an altered mental status, check the blood glucose level.
4. Cool the patient with misting, fanning, and administration of ice packs to the trunk of the patient's body.
5. Encourage the patient to lie down. Loosen any tight clothing and cool the patient by manually or mechanically fanning them (**Step 2**).
6. If the patient is fully alert, encourage them to sit up and slowly drink water or an electrolyte

solution (eg, Gatorade, Powerade), as long as nausea does not develop. Never force fluids by mouth into a patient who is not fully alert, or allow the patient to drink while supine, because the patient could aspirate the fluid into the lungs. If the patient becomes nauseated, transport the patient on the left side to prevent aspiration (**Step 3**).

In most cases, these measures will reverse the symptoms, causing the patient to feel better within 30 minutes. Prepare to transport the patient to the hospital, and also consider a rendezvous with ALS for more aggressive treatment, such as IV fluid therapy and close monitoring, especially in the following circumstances:

- The symptoms do not clear up promptly.
- The level of consciousness decreases.
- The body temperature remains elevated.
- The person is very young, is older, or has any underlying medical condition, such as diabetes or cardiovascular disease.

7. Transport the patient on their left side if you think the patient may be nauseated, but make certain that the patient is secured (**Step 4**).

Heatstroke

Recovery from heatstroke is only possible if treatment is administered rapidly, so you must identify this patient quickly. Emergency treatment has one objective: lower the body temperature by any means available. Take the following steps when treating a patient with heatstroke:

1. Move the patient out of the hot environment and into the shade.
2. Remove the patient's clothing.
3. Administer high-concentration oxygen if indicated. If needed, assist the patient's ventilations with a bag-mask device and appropriate airway adjuncts as per your protocol. If the patient is unresponsive and unable to protect their airway, consider rapid transport and cooling en route. Consult medical direction if available.
4. Immerse the patient in an ice bath if available (**FIGURE 32-8**). If an ice bath is not possible, attempt the tarp-assisted cooling with oscillation (TACO) method. To implement the TACO method, place the patient on a tarp and pour ice water over them. Then move the tarp back and forth (oscillate it) to enhance the heat dissipation.[2] If neither of these options is available, cover the patient in towels or sheets that have been soaked in ice water. It is imperative to rotate the towels/sheets to avoid trapping heat. Continue cold-water immersion at the scene until the core temperature is less than 102.2°F (39°C).
5. Exclude other causes of altered mental status, and check blood glucose level.
6. Provide rapid transport to the hospital after initial cooling measures.
7. Notify the hospital as soon as possible.
8. Do not overcool the patient. Call for ALS assistance if the patient begins to shiver.

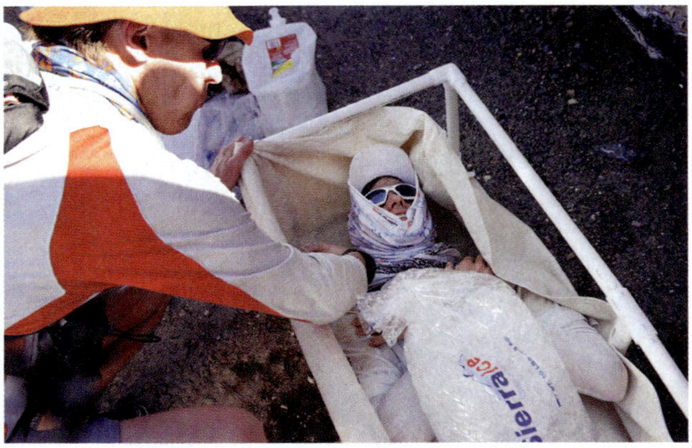

FIGURE 32-8 As part of treatment of heatstroke, if available, immerse the patient in an ice-water bath. Cooling should begin immediately and continue en route to the hospital

If your patient has any signs of heatstroke (eg, core temperature >104°F [40°C], altered mental status), begin emergent cooling measures. After performing rapid cooling, provide rapid transport.

Drowning

Drowning is the process of experiencing respiratory impairment from submersion or immersion in liquid. According to the Centers for Disease Control and Prevention, in the United States, more than 4,500 people died from drowning each year from 2020 through 2022, which is 500 more people than drowned in 2019.[11] In addition to those who die,

Special Populations

TEMPERATURE-RELATED EMERGENCIES IN GERIATRIC PATIENTS

Remember that the aging process alters the body's ability to compensate for its surroundings. Temperature-related emergencies can develop in older people over time, even in indoor environments that may not seem uncomfortable to you. Internal temperature regulation slows with age because function of the endocrine system declines. Heat gain or loss in response to environmental changes is delayed by impaired circulation and decreased sweat production in the skin. In addition, thermoregulation can be adversely affected by chronic disease, medication use, and alcohol use.

Approximately one-half of all deaths from hypothermia occur in people 65 years or older,[9] and approximately 60% of hyperthermia-related deaths occur in this population.[10] In some areas, temperature extremes combined with a large geriatric population can create a serious public health issue. For example, Arizona has an abnormally high rate of heat-related deaths due to its long, hot summers and large geriatric population. EMS agencies should be prepared to help reduce risk in their communities. Older people should be checked on during hot and cold spikes to ensure they are appropriately sheltered.

about 8,000 nonfatal drownings occur annually in the United States.[12] Drowning is the leading cause of death in children ages 1 to 4 years and the second leading cause of death for children 5 to 14 years, with motor vehicle collisions being the most common. Infants are most likely to drown in bathtubs or buckets, whereas preschoolers most commonly drown in swimming pools.[13] Teenagers and adults are also at risk of drowning. In fact, of the 4,500 drowning deaths in the United States in 2022, 70% of the victims were adults.[14] Alcohol consumption, preexisting seizure disorders, geriatric patients with cardiovascular disease, and unsupervised access to water are among the major risk factors.

Drowning is often the last in a cycle of events caused by panic in the water. It can happen to anyone who is submerged in water for even a short time. Struggling toward the surface or the shore, the person becomes fatigued or exhausted, which leads them to sink even deeper. Most people can hold their breath for about a minute when submerged under water. After that, water is inhaled and then the person coughs. Without rescue, the person continues to aspirate, becomes hypoxic, loses consciousness, and within a few minutes stops breathing and then experiences cardiac arrest. In cold water, this process is extended. However, drowning also occurs in buckets, puddles, bathtubs, toilets, and other places where the person is not completely submerged. This risk is of particular concern with young children, who can drown in as little as 1 inch (3 cm) of water; they do not need to be completely submerged, such as in a swimming pool.

Spinal Injuries in Submersion Incidents

Although rare, submersion incidents may be complicated by spinal fractures and spinal cord injuries. Assume that spinal injury exists with the following conditions:

- The submersion has resulted from a diving mishap or fall from a significant height.
- The patient is conscious but reports weakness, paralysis, or numbness in the arms or legs.
- Other signs of spinal cord injury are evident.

Words of Wisdom

Before using an automated external defibrillator (AED) on a pulseless drowning patient, ensure that the patient is not lying in a pool of water and the chest has been dried off. Use caution when operating an AED in this situation.

While they are very rare, most spinal injuries in diving incidents affect the cervical spine. When spinal injury is suspected, the neck must be protected from further injury; thus, you may need to stabilize the suspected injury while the patient is still in the water. It is recommended that, if possible, three people perform this procedure, with at least one having specific training; however, do not delay response if fewer than three people are available. If the situation does not indicate a possible spinal injury, stabilization is not recommended. To stabilize

Safety Tips

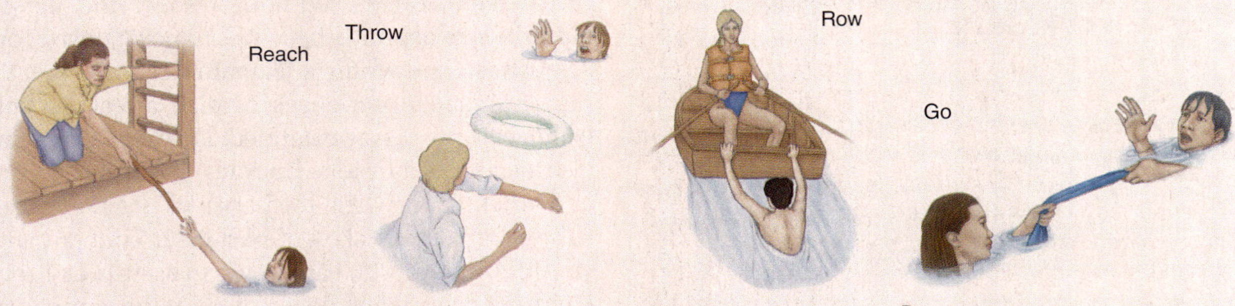

FIGURE 32-9 Basic rules of water rescue. **A.** Reach for the person from shore. If you cannot reach the person from shore, wade closer. **B.** If an object that floats is available, throw it to the person. **C.** Use a boat if one is available. **D.** If you must swim to the person, use a towel or board for the person to hold onto. Do not let the person grab you.

You must ensure the safety of rescue personnel and request additional rescue resources, as appropriate, before a water rescue can begin. Water rescue is typically handled by specialized rescue personnel, but you may be involved if you arrive first or if water rescue is included in your scope of practice per local protocols. If the patient is conscious and still in the water, and you have the proper equipment and training, perform a water rescue. The saying "Reach, throw, and row, and only then go" (**FIGURE 32-9**) sums up the basic rule of water rescue. First, try to reach for the patient. If that does not work, throw the patient a rope, a life preserver, or any floatable object that is available. For example, an inflated spare tire, rim and all, will float well enough to support two people in the water. Next, use a boat if one is available. Do not attempt a swimming rescue unless you are trained and experienced in the proper techniques. Even then, you should always wear a helmet and a personal flotation device (**FIGURE 32-10**). Too many well-meaning rescuers have themselves become victims while attempting a swimming rescue. In cold climates or cold-water locations, rapid hypothermia is also a concern for rescuers. Be prepared for this potential event.

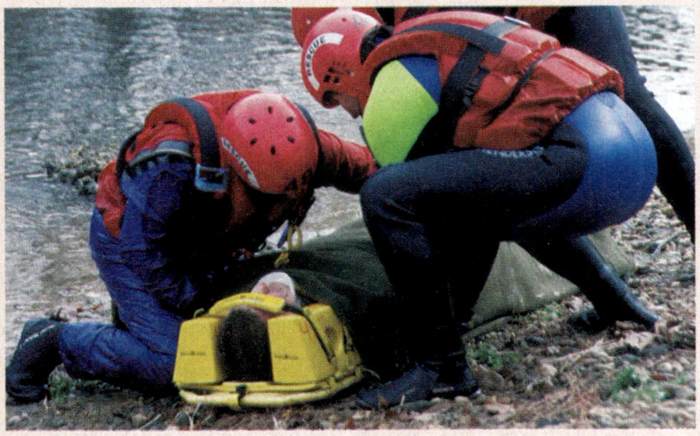

FIGURE 32-10 When performing a water rescue, you must be properly trained and must wear proper personal protective equipment, including a personal flotation device.

The steps for ice rescue are similar and may involve reaching with a pole or ladder or throwing a rope or flotation device. A victim who has fallen through the ice may also be coached into placing their arms out of the water and onto the ice, kicking and rolling out of the water, and crawling to safety.

If you work in a recreation area near lakes, rivers, or the ocean, you should have a prearranged plan for water rescue. For colder areas, a plan for ice rescue is also necessary. This plan should include access to and cooperation with local clinicians who are trained and skilled in water rescue; these clinicians should help to develop the protocol for water rescue. Because the success of any water rescue depends on how rapidly the patient is removed from the water and ventilated, make sure you always have immediate access to personal flotation devices and other rescue equipment. Survival rates drastically decline the longer a victim is immersed. Cold-water drowning survival rates are somewhat higher.

a suspected spinal injury in water, follow the steps in **SKILL DRILL 32-2**:

1. Turn the patient supine while maintaining alignment between the head and torso. Twisting only the head, for example, may aggravate any injury to the cervical spine (**Step 1**).
2. Open the airway and begin ventilation. Immediate ventilation is the primary treatment of all drowning patients as soon as the patient is faceup in the water. Use a pocket mask or bag-mask device if it is available or mouth-to-mouth ventilation, unless there is active community transmission of aerosolized or airborne respiratory illness. Have the other rescuer support the head and trunk as a unit while you open the airway and begin artificial ventilation (**Step 2**). Be prepared to manage vomiting; most drowning victims who require rescue breathing or chest compressions will vomit.[15]
3. Have the third rescuer float a buoyant backboard or spinal restriction device under the patient as you continue ventilation (**Step 3**).
4. Secure the trunk and head to the board or device to restrict spinal motion (**Step 4**).
5. Remove the patient from the water on the backboard (**Step 5**).
6. Cover the patient with a blanket. Give oxygen if the patient is breathing spontaneously. Begin CPR if there is no pulse. Effective cardiac compression or CPR is extremely difficult to perform when the patient is still in the water (**Step 6**).

Hypothermia in the Context of Submersion

When a person is submerged in water that is colder than body temperature, heat will be conducted from the body to the water. The resulting hypothermia can protect vital organs from the lack of oxygen. In addition, exposure to cold water will occasionally activate certain primitive reflexes, which may preserve basic body functions for prolonged periods.

Also, whenever a person dives or jumps into very cold water, the **diving reflex**, slowing of the heart rate caused by submersion in cold water, may cause immediate bradycardia, a slow heart rhythm. Loss of consciousness and drowning may follow. However, the person may be able to survive for an extended period under water, thanks to a lowering of the metabolic rate associated with hypothermia.

Because of these physiologic mechanisms, local protocols often dictate that resuscitation efforts continue for up to 1 hour after submersion, while simultaneously rewarming the patient. Pay close attention to the body temperature of a person who is rescued from cold water. Treat hypothermia caused

YOU are the EMT

You perform a secondary assessment, which does not reveal any gross signs of injury, while a firefighter goes to get the stretcher and your partner assesses the patient's vital signs.

Recording Time: 6 Minutes	
Respirations	24 breaths/min; adequate depth
Pulse	130 beats/mm; weak and regular
Skin	Hot, flushed, and moist
Blood pressure	88/66 mm Hg
Oxygen saturation (Spo_2)	95%
Temperature	105.4°F (40.8°C)

5. What specific treatment is required for this patient?
6. What is the most likely explanation for this patient's vital signs?

Skill Drill 32-2 Stabilizing a Suspected Spinal Injury in the Water

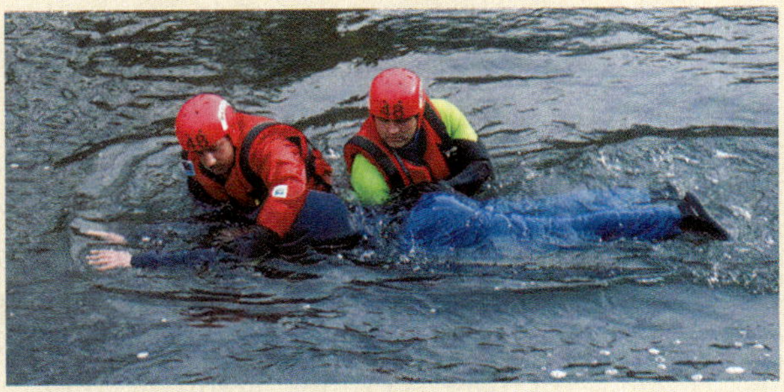

Step 1

Turn the patient to a supine position by rotating the entire upper half of the body as a single unit.

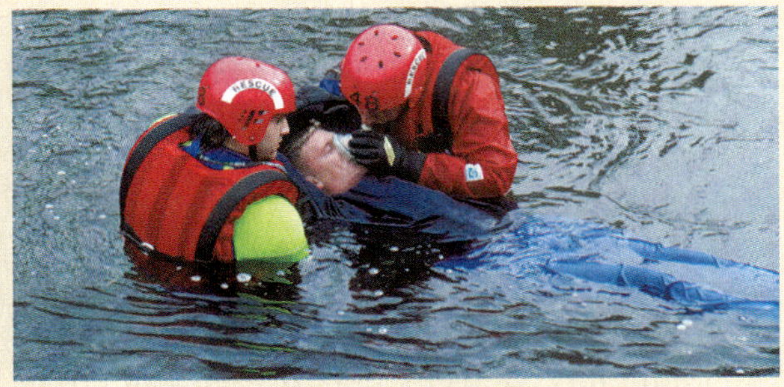

Step 2

As soon as the patient is turned, begin artificial ventilation using a pocket mask or bag-mask device if it is available or mouth-to-mouth ventilation.

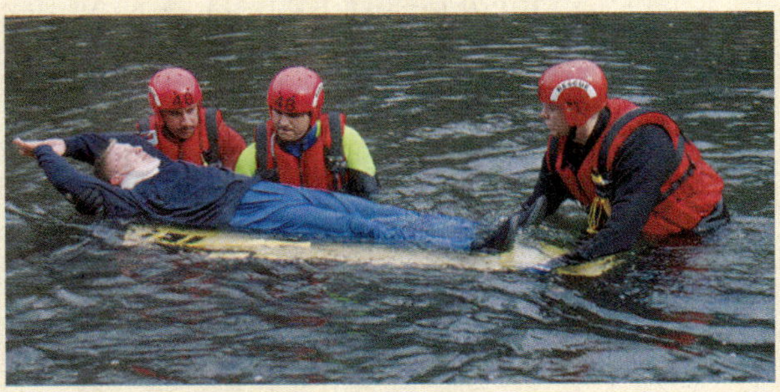

Step 3

Float a buoyant backboard or appropriate device under the patient.

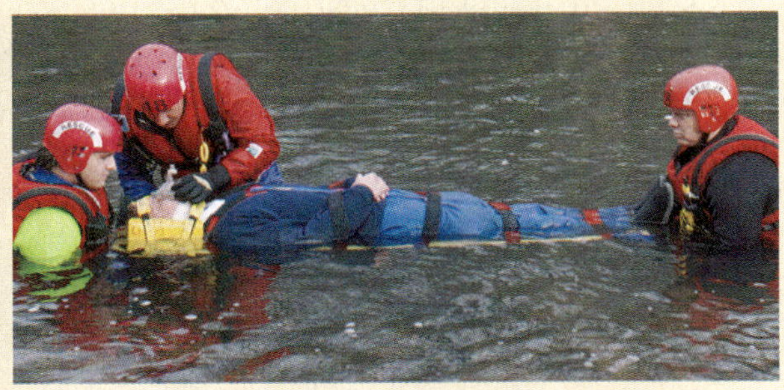

Step 4

Secure the patient to the backboard or device.

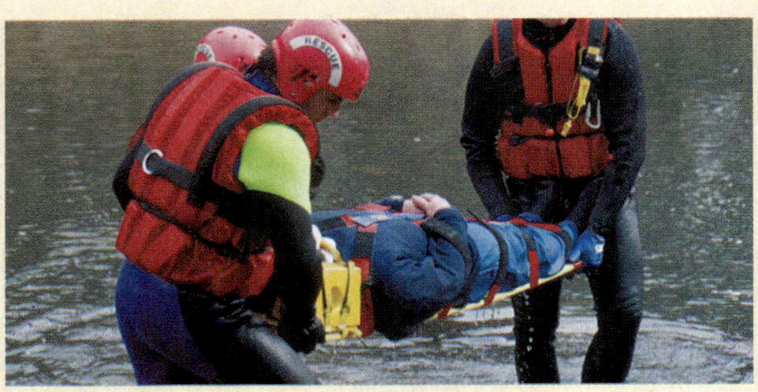

Step 5

Remove the patient from the water.

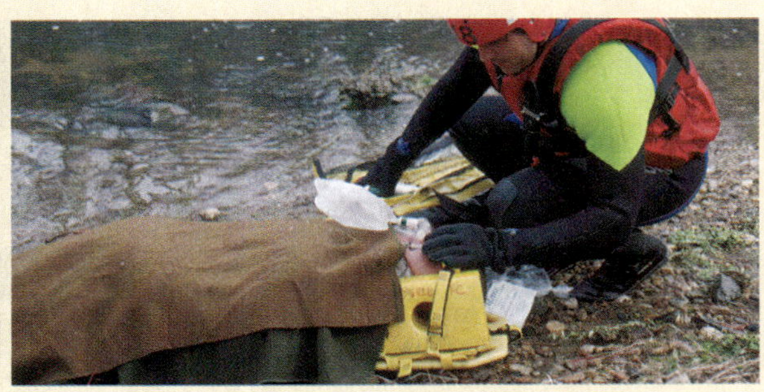

Step 6

Maintain the body's normal temperature and apply oxygen if the patient is breathing. Begin CPR if breathing and pulse are absent.

by immersion in cold water the same way you treat hypothermia caused by cold exposure. Prevent further heat loss from contact with the ground, stretcher, or air, and transport the patient promptly.

Scuba Diving Emergencies

In the United States, more than 1,300 injuries relating to scuba diving occur each year, with over 10% resulting in death.[16] Scuba, which is an acronym for self-contained underwater breathing apparatus, is a system that delivers air to the mouth and lungs at atmospheric pressures that increase with the depth of the dive. Most of these injuries relate to preexisting medical problems of the divers, procedural errors, a change in the environment, or problems with the equipment, such as running out of gas, which accounts for approximately 10% of incidents.[17]

With or without scuba gear, deep underwater dives can result in many types of serious water-related injuries. These injuries can happen even to the experienced diver or swimmer. To help describe the nature of these injuries, scuba diving can be thought of in three phases: descent, bottom, and ascent.

Descent Emergencies

Descent problems are usually caused by the sudden increase in pressure on the body as the person dives deeper into the water. Some body cavities cannot adjust to the increased external pressure of the water; the result is severe pain. The usual areas affected are the lungs, the sinus cavities, the middle ear, the teeth, and the area of the face surrounded by the diving mask. Usually, the pain caused by these "squeeze problems" forces the diver to return to the surface to equalize the pressures, and the problem clears up by itself. A diver who continues to report pain, particularly in the ear, after returning to the surface should be transported to the hospital.

A special problem may develop in a person with a perforated tympanic membrane (ruptured eardrum) while diving. If cold water enters the middle ear through a ruptured eardrum, the diver may sustain a loss of balance and orientation. The diver may then shoot to the surface and experience ascent problems.

Emergencies at the Bottom

Problems related to the bottom of the dive are rarely seen. They include inadequate mixing of oxygen and carbon dioxide in the air the diver breathes and accidental feeding of poisonous carbon monoxide into the breathing apparatus. Both are the result of faulty connections in the diving gear. These situations can cause drowning or rapid ascent; they require emergency resuscitation and transport of the patient. Most recreational certified divers are limited to 130 feet (40 m). Deeper dives require technical training.[18] If a recreational diver descends below 130 feet (40 m), they may experience equipment malfunction and gas compression injuries.

Ascent Emergencies

Most of the serious injuries associated with diving are related to ascending from the bottom and are referred to as ascent problems. These emergencies usually require aggressive resuscitation. Two particularly dangerous medical emergencies are air embolism and decompression sickness.

Air Embolism

The most dangerous, and most common, emergency in scuba diving is an **air embolism**, a condition involving bubbles of air in the blood vessels. An air embolism may occur on a dive as shallow as 6 feet (2 m). The problem starts when the diver holds their breath during a rapid ascent. The air pressure in the lungs remains at a high level while the external pressure on the chest decreases. As a result, the air inside the lungs expands rapidly, causing the alveoli in the lungs to rupture. The air released from this rupture can cause the following injuries:

- Air may enter the pleural space and compress the lungs (a pneumothorax).
- Air may enter the mediastinum (the space within the thorax that contains the heart and great vessels), causing a condition called pneumomediastinum.
- Air may enter the bloodstream and create bubbles of air in the vessels called air emboli.

Pneumothorax and pneumomediastinum both result in pain and severe dyspnea. An air embolus will act as a plug and prevent the normal flow of blood and oxygen to a specific part of the body. The brain and spinal cord are the organs most severely affected by air embolism because they require a constant supply of oxygen.

The following are potential signs and symptoms of an air embolism:

- Blotching (mottling of the skin)
- Froth (often pink or bloody) at the nose and mouth
- Severe pain in muscles, joints, or abdomen
- Dyspnea and/or chest pain
- Dizziness, nausea, and vomiting
- Dysphasia (difficulty speaking)
- Cough
- Cyanosis
- Difficulty with vision
- Paralysis and/or coma
- Irregular pulse and cardiac arrest

Decompression Sickness

Decompression sickness, commonly called the **bends**, occurs when bubbles of gas, especially nitrogen, obstruct the blood vessels. This condition results from too rapid an ascent from a dive, too long a dive at too great a depth, or repeated dives within a short time. During the dive, nitrogen that is being breathed dissolves in the blood and tissues because it is under pressure. When the diver ascends, the external pressure is decreased, and the dissolved nitrogen forms small bubbles within those tissues. These bubbles can lead to problems similar to those that occur in air embolism (blockage of tiny blood vessels, depriving parts of the body of their normal blood supply), but severe pain in certain tissues or spaces in the body is the most common problem.

Similarly, decompression sickness can occur in a person who has completed a safe dive then shortly after travels in a car up a mountain or flies in an unpressurized airplane that climbs too rapidly to a great height. However, this risk diminishes after 24 to 48 hours.

The most striking symptom is abdominal and/or joint pain so severe that the patient literally doubles over, or bends. Dive tables and diving computers are available to calculate and record the proper rate of ascent from a dive, including the number and length of pauses that a diver should make on the way up. However, even divers who stay within these limits can occasionally experience symptoms of the bends.

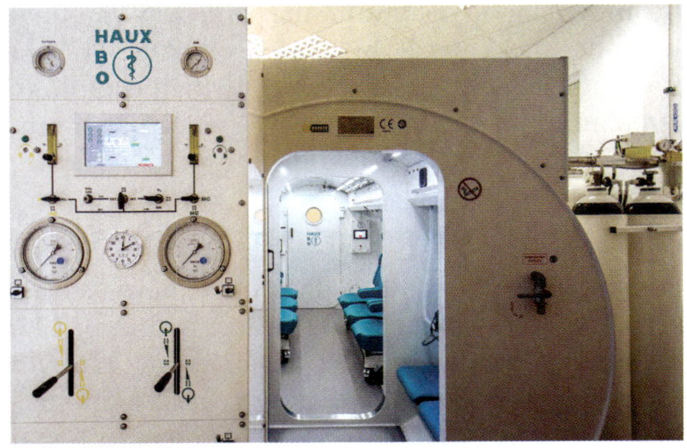

FIGURE 32-11 A hyperbaric chamber, usually a small room, is pressurized to a level higher than atmospheric pressure and used in the treatment of decompression sickness and air embolism.

© David Tanecek/CTK/Alamy Stock Photo.

You may find it difficult to distinguish between air embolism and decompression sickness. In general, air embolism occurs immediately on return to the surface, whereas the symptoms of decompression sickness may not occur for several hours. The emergency treatment is the same for both. It consists of basic life support (BLS), including supplemental oxygen, followed by recompression in a hyperbaric oxygen chamber: a chamber or a small room that has 100% oxygen pressurized to a level higher than atmospheric pressure (**FIGURE 32-11**). Recompression treatment improves tissue oxygenation, allows the bubbles of gas to dissolve into the blood, and equalizes the pressures inside and outside the lungs. Once these pressures are equalized, gradual decompression can be accomplished under controlled conditions to prevent the bubbles from re-forming.

Assessment of Drowning and Scuba Diving Emergencies

Scene Size-up

In managing water emergencies, your standard precautions should include gloves, mask, and eye protection at a minimum. Check for hazards to your crew. Never drive through moving water; even a small amount can cause the vehicle to be swept away. Use extreme caution when driving through standing water. Never attempt a water rescue without proper training and equipment. Call for additional resources early.

If your patient is still in the water, look for the best, safest means of removal. This may require additional help from search-and-rescue teams or special extrication equipment. Trauma and an associated need to provide spinal motion restriction must be considered when the scene is a recreational setting. Check for additional patients based on where and how the emergency occurred.

As you observe the scene, look for indicators of the MOI. As you put together information from dispatch and your observations of the scene, consider how the MOI produced the injuries suspected.

Primary Assessment

Use your evaluation of the patient's chief complaint to guide you in your assessment of life threats and determine whether spinal motion restriction is necessary. Pay particular attention to chest pain, dyspnea, and complaints related to sensory changes when a diving emergency is suspected. Determine the patient's level of consciousness using the AVPU scale. Be suspicious of drug and alcohol use and the effects on the patient's level of consciousness.

Standard measures should be taken for any patient found or injured while in the water. Begin with opening the airway and assessing breathing in unresponsive patients. If there is a high risk of spinal trauma, take appropriate actions and use the jaw-thrust maneuver to open the airway. The airway may be obstructed with water. Suction according to protocol if the patient has vomited and expect that the patient is likely to vomit during your care and resuscitation. Provide ventilations with a bag-mask device for inadequate breathing. Use an airway adjunct to facilitate bag-mask ventilations as necessary.

If the patient is responsive, provide high-concentration oxygen with a nonrebreathing mask if the oxygen saturation level is less than 92%; maintain an oxygen saturation level of 94% to 98%. If spinal injury is not suspected, position the patient to protect the airway from aspiration in the event of vomiting.

Auscultation and frequent reassessment of breath sounds in drowning patients is a key part of your assessment. You may hear diminished sounds or even gurgling sounds from water that has been inhaled. Provide this information, and any changes in the patient's lung sounds, to the ALS clinicians who may rendezvous with your unit as well as to the receiving facility. Breath sounds are also particularly significant for patients with scuba diving injuries; while the patients ascended to the surface, a pneumothorax or tension pneumothorax may have developed.

Check for a pulse. It may be difficult to find a pulse because of constriction of the peripheral blood vessels and low cardiac output, resulting in cyanosis. Nevertheless, if the pulse is unmeasurable, the patient may be in cardiac arrest. After administering two breaths, begin CPR and apply your AED according to BLS and the International Liaison Committee on Resuscitation guidelines.[19]

Evaluate the patient for adequate perfusion and treat for shock by maintaining normal body temperature and improving circulation through positioning. The patient's skin may be cold to the touch. If the MOI suggests trauma, assess for bleeding and treat appropriately.

Even if resuscitation in the field appears successful, always transport patients to the hospital. Inhalation of any amount of fluid can lead to delayed complications lasting for days or weeks. Patients with decompression sickness and air embolism must be treated in a recompression chamber. If you live in an area with a significant amount of scuba diving activity, you will have transport protocols for such cases. Usually, the patient will be stabilized in the nearest ED. Perform all interventions en route.

History Taking

After the life threats have been managed during the primary assessment, investigate the chief complaint. Obtain a medical history and be alert for injury-specific signs and symptoms as well as any pertinent negatives.

Obtain a SAMPLE history with special attention to the dive parameters. If possible, document the following details relating to the patient's diving history[2]:

- Number of dives completed in recent days
- "Bottom time" in dives (ie, how much time spent underwater)

- Dive profiles (ie, compliance with their dive tables)
- Maximum depth of the dive
- Rate of ascent
- Whether safety stops were used (and if so, the time and depth)
- Dive gas used (ie, air versus mixed gases such as Nitrox, Heliox, or Trimix)
- Water temperature
- Time of onset of symptoms

Also ask if the patient has traveled to high altitude or flown within 48 hours of their last dive, if they have consumed alcohol or drugs, and whether they have other medical conditions or recent illness. Do not adjust or turn off any of the patient's dive equipment, as it may provide important information about their dive.

Secondary Assessment

The secondary assessment is used to uncover injuries that may have been missed during the primary assessment. In some instances, such as a critically injured patient or a short transport time, you may not have time to conduct a secondary assessment.

If the patient is responsive, focus your physical examination on the basis of the chief complaint and the history obtained. This should include a thorough examination of the patient's lungs, including breath sounds.

Prolonged submersion typically results in an unresponsive patient. It is important to begin with a full-body scan in these situations to look for hidden life threats and potential trauma, even if trauma is not suspected. A scuba diver with a possible medical condition should be assessed for indications of decompression sickness or an air embolism. Focus on pain in the joints and the abdomen. Pay attention to whether your patient is getting adequate ventilation and oxygenation, and check for signs of hypothermia.

Time and personnel permitting, complete a detailed assessment en route to the hospital. A careful examination may reveal additional injuries not initially observable. Examine the patient for respiratory, circulatory, and neurologic compromise. A careful distal circulatory, sensory, and motor function examination will be helpful in assessing the extent of the injury. Assess for peripheral pulses, skin color and discoloration, itching, pain, and paresthesia (numbness and tingling). Palpate for the presence of subcutaneous emphysema, which may be present if there is a lung overpressurization injury.

Check the patient's pulse rate, quality, and rhythm. Pulse and blood pressure may be difficult to palpate in a patient with hypothermia. Check carefully for both peripheral and central pulses, and listen over the chest for a heartbeat if pulses are weak. Check the respiratory rate, quality, and rhythm and listen for breath sounds. Assess and document pupil size and reactivity.

Although it is a valuable tool, oxygen saturation readings may produce a false low reading because of hypoperfusion of the patient's monitoring finger. Shivering also can interfere with obtaining an accurate reading because of excessive movement.

Reassessment

Repeat the primary assessment. Reassess vital signs and the chief complaint. Are your treatments for problems with the ABCs still effective? Are there any new problems with the ABCs that must be corrected?

The condition of patients who have experienced submersion in water may deteriorate rapidly because of pulmonary injury, fluid shifts in the body, cerebral hypoxia, and hypothermia. Patients with pneumothorax, air embolism, or decompression sickness may decompensate quickly. Assess your patient's mental status constantly, and assess vital signs at least every 5 minutes. Pay particular attention to respirations and breath sounds.

Document the circumstances of the drowning and extrication. The receiving facility personnel will need to know how long the patient was submerged, the temperature of the water, the clarity of the water, and whether there was any possibility of cervical spine injury.

If you respond to a scuba diving incident, the receiving facility personnel will also need a complete dive profile to properly treat your patient. This information may be available in a dive log, on a dive computer, or from the patient's diving partners. If possible, bring all of the diver's equipment to the hospital. It will be helpful in determining the cause of the incident. Be sure to document the disposition of this equipment.

Emergency Care for Drowning or Scuba Diving Emergencies

Drowning Emergencies

Treatment for drowning begins with rescue and removal from the water. Provide spinal motion restriction when signs or symptoms of spinal cord injury are present or suspected. Artificial ventilation should be provided as soon as possible. If rapid removal from the water is not possible, provide artificial ventilation in the water, which has been shown to increase survival; however, this should occur only if it does not compromise the rescuer's own safety.[12] If it is indicated, spinal motion restriction should continue while artificial ventilation is being performed.

If the patient is not breathing, clear any vomit from the airway manually or with suction and assist ventilations with a bag-mask device or pocket mask with supplemental oxygen. Rolling patients onto their side or performing abdominal thrusts will not remove water from the lungs and should not be done unless the airway is obstructed. Frothy sputum in the patient's airway does *not* require removal with suctioning. When resuscitating a patient who has drowned, follow the usual ABC order. Address airway and breathing concerns first, beginning with five rescue breaths, then use compressions and the AED. Do not delay CPR to retrieve or apply an AED.[12] Hands-only CPR is not indicated in drowned patients who are in cardiac arrest.

Words of Wisdom

A person swimming in shallow water may experience **breath-holding syncope**, a loss of consciousness caused by a decreased stimulus for breathing. This happens to swimmers who breathe in and out rapidly and deeply before entering the water in an effort to expand their capacity to stay underwater. Whereas this technique increases the swimmer's oxygen level, the hyperventilation involved lowers the carbon dioxide level. Because an elevated level of carbon dioxide in the blood is the strongest stimulus for breathing, the swimmer may not feel the need to breathe even after using up all the oxygen in the lungs. This results in drowning. The emergency treatment for a patient with breath-holding syncope is the same as that for a drowning patient.

If the patient is breathing spontaneously, but has been submerged, administer oxygen if the oxygen saturation level is less than 92%; maintain an oxygen saturation level of 94% to 98% (if this was not done as part of the primary assessment).[12] Treat all drowning patients for hypothermia by removing wet clothing and wrapping them in warm blankets. Patients who need any type of resuscitation after drowning should be transported to an ED.[12]

Resuscitation efforts are not initiated for unwitnessed drowning victims who are found in a state of decomposition.

Scuba Diving Emergencies

When treating conscious patients who are suspected of having an air embolism or decompression sickness from scuba diving, follow these accepted treatment steps:

1. Remove the patient from the water. Try to keep the patient calm.
2. Administer high-concentration oxygen regardless of the initial oxygen saturation level to target a level of 94% to 98%.
3. Consider the possibility of pneumothorax and monitor the patient's breath sounds for development of a tension pneumothorax. Avoid the use of continuous positive airway pressure without direct medical oversight.
4. If an air embolism is suspected, place the patient in the left lateral recumbent position.
5. Provide prompt transport based on medical direction feedback to the ED or to the nearest facility with hyperbaric oxygen therapy capabilities for treatment, based on local protocols.

Injury from decompression sickness is often reversible with proper treatment. However, if the bubbles block critical blood vessels that supply the brain or spinal cord, permanent central nervous system injury may result. Therefore, the key in emergency management of serious ascent problems is to recognize that an emergency exists and treat as soon as possible. Depending on local protocols, consider transport to a facility with a hyperbaric chamber if there is one near your service area. Remember that air medical transport for someone who has sustained an injury in ascending from a dive can be dangerous because the decrease in air pressure may worsen the underlying decompression injury. If air medical transport is needed, the cabin should be pressurized to the lowest possible altitude. When helicopter EMS is used, the patient should be transported at the lowest possible altitude.[2]

Prevention

Each year, many young children drown in residential pools. The drowning chain of survival can reduce deaths associated with drowning (**FIGURE 32-12**).[12] The first link in the drowning chain of survival and most effective way to prevent deaths is prevention. One approach to prevention is regulatory efforts. Although regulations may vary by jurisdiction, typical residential codes state that swimming pools must be surrounded by a fence that is at least 6 feet (2 m) high, with slats no farther apart than 3 inches (8 cm), and self-closing, self-locking gates. The most common problem is a lack of adult supervision. An incident can occur when a child is unattended for only a few seconds.

Regulations concerning alcohol use in the context of water recreation are also important. Alcohol use is commonly a contributing factor in adult drownings and is particularly a concern in boating accidents. While alcohol intoxication is prohibited when operating a boat, and alcohol use is prohibited at many beaches, greater efforts may be required to teach the public about the effects of alcohol use, namely its effects on judgment and coordination, when participating in water-related recreation.

Swimming education is also key in preventing drowning deaths. The CDC reports that over 40 million adults in the United States do not know how to swim and over one-half of all adult Americans have never taken a swimming lesson.[11] This lack of swimming education is particularly common among minority groups, including Black, Hispanic, and American Indian or Alaska Native (AIAN) people. Rates of drowning deaths are particularly high among the AIAN and Black populations. Swimming education represents a health disparity requiring greater availability of training and education for these populations.[11]

As a health care professional, you can participate in prevention efforts by becoming involved in public education to make people aware of the hazards of swimming pools and water recreation. Signs promoting the use of life vests should be placed at public access to open water. The state of Alaska implemented a Kids Don't Float program that provides loaner life vests at points of public access to waterways.[20] Promotion of swimming lessons for communities can also help reduce the number of drownings. Educating the public about the dangers of leaving infants unattended in the bathtub is also an important public health message that EMS clinicians can help spread.

YOU are the EMT

You call for ALS assist as you place the patient in a body bag that the neighbors have filled with water and ice. You continue active cooling measures while maintaining the patient's airway and frequently reassessing his temperature. When you reassess the patient, you note that his level of consciousness has improved. When his temperature reaches 102.2°F (39°C), you remove him from the bath, place him on the stretcher, and begin transport.

Recording Time: 11 Minutes	
Level of consciousness	Responsive to voice, confused
Respirations	24 breaths/min; normal depth
Pulse	120 beats/min; regular
Skin	Less flushed (returning to baseline color), warm, and wet
Blood pressure	96/70 mm Hg
Oxygen saturation (Spo_2)	94%

7. What additional assessment should you perform on this patient?

8. What treatment should you provide en route to the hospital?

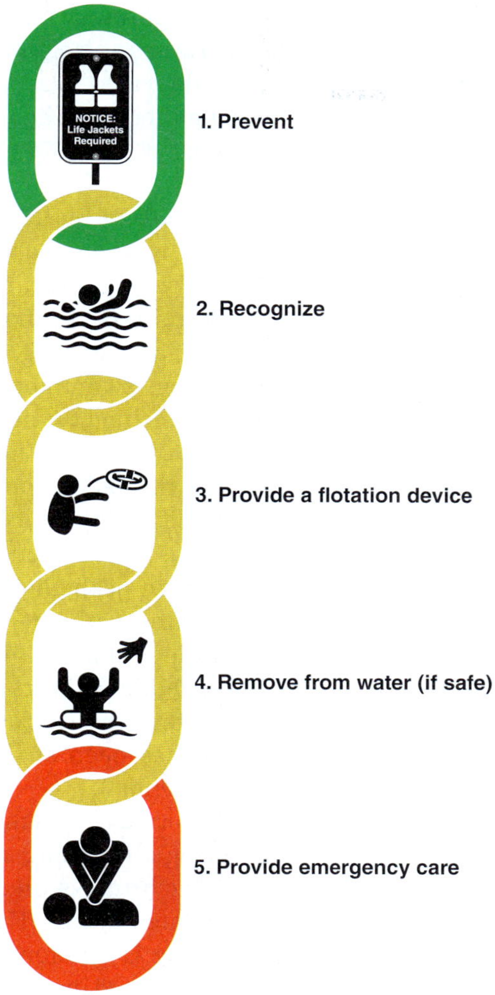

FIGURE 32-12 The drowning chain of survival.

The second link in the drowning chain of survival is recognition. Most people do not realize that drowning happens very quickly and it takes active observation to recognize that someone is in distress before they submerge and cannot be seen. Drowning victims often call for help or signal that they are in distress. Recognition is especially difficult in open bodies of water such as lakes.

The third link involves providing a flotation device until the fourth link, removal from the water, can be performed safety. When possible, unresponsive patients should be removed in the supine position; conscious patients can be removed in the Fowler position. The final step in the chain is early care by BLS and ALS, which is known to improve survival. Fortunately, less than 0.5% of those rescued after a drowning experience cardiac arrest.[12]

High Altitude

High altitudes can cause **dysbarism injuries**. Dysbarism injuries are any signs and symptoms caused by the difference between the surrounding atmospheric pressure and the total gas pressure in various tissues, fluids, and cavities of the body. Altitude illnesses occur when an unacclimated person is exposed to diminished oxygen pressure in the air at high altitudes. These illnesses affect the central nervous system and pulmonary system, and range from common acute mountain sickness to high-altitude cerebral edema (HACE) and high-altitude pulmonary edema (HAPE).

Acute mountain sickness is caused by diminished oxygen pressure in the air at altitudes above 6,500 feet (2,000 m), resulting in diminished oxygen in the blood (hypoxia). Acute mountain sickness most commonly occurs at elevations of 8,000 to 10,000 feet (2,400 to 3,000 m), with some symptoms beginning as early as 5,000 to 7,000 feet (1,500 to 2,100 m) in persons who are not acclimated.[2,21] Ascending too high too fast is another risk factor for this condition. The signs and symptoms include a headache, light-headedness, fatigue, weakness, loss of appetite, nausea, vomiting, difficulty sleeping,

Special Populations

PEDIATRIC RISK FACTORS FOR ALTITUDE ILLNESS

Children with any of the following conditions are at especially high risk of developing altitude illness[2]:

- Current upper or lower respiratory illness or otitis media
- Congenital heart disease
- Down syndrome (especially with obstructive sleep apnea)
- Preexisting lung disease such as bronchopulmonary dysplasia or cystic fibrosis
- Sickle cell anemia
- Diseases that impair ventilation such as severe scoliosis or neuromuscular diseases

Also at higher risk are term infants younger than 6 weeks and preterm infants younger than 10 weeks from the time of term pregnancy. Signs and symptoms in infants and young children include pallor, difficulty sleeping, and vomiting, and they may be less playful and fussy.[2]

shortness of breath during physical exertion, and a swollen face. Treatment primarily consists of stopping the ascent and descending to a lower altitude, and administering oxygen if the patient is dyspneic. Rapid improvement should occur when the patient rapidly descends 1,000 feet (300 m) or more.[21] However, consider other possible causes for the same symptoms, such as hypoglycemia or carbon monoxide poisoning from a camping stove.

With HAPE, fluid collects in the lungs, hindering the passage of oxygen into the bloodstream. It can occur at altitudes of 8,000 feet (2,400 m) or greater. The signs and symptoms include shortness of breath, crackles in the lungs, weakness, cough with pink sputum, cyanosis, and a rapid pulse. A child who lives at altitude is at risk of HAPE after they descend to a lower altitude and then return to the high altitude.[2]

HACE usually occurs in climbers ascending to more than 8,000 feet (2,400 m) and may accompany HAPE; it can quickly become life threatening. The signs and symptoms include a severe, constant, throbbing headache; ataxia (lack of muscle coordination and balance); extreme fatigue; vomiting; and loss of consciousness. The symptoms of HACE and HAPE may overlap.

In the field, treatment for HAPE and/or HACE consists of quickly but safely descending to an altitude of at least 500 to 1,000 feet (150 to 300 m) lower than the current altitude.[2] If descent is not possible, ALS should be contacted. During the descent, begin providing high-concentration oxygen, and promptly transport to an appropriate facility. For inadequate respirations, provide positive-pressure ventilation with a bag-mask device. If local protocols allow, continuous positive airway pressure may be helpful for a patient with respiratory distress from HAPE.

Lightning

According to the National Weather Service, there are an estimated 25 million cloud-to-ground lightning flashes in the United States each year. Lightning kills an average of 51 people per year in the United States based on documented cases.[22] This number has decreased over the past several years. Although documented lightning injuries in the United States average approximately 300 per year, undocumented lightning injuries are likely much higher.

The energy associated with lightning comprises direct current of up to 200,000 amps and a potential of 100 million volts or more delivered over a very short time. Temperatures generated from lightning vary between 20,000°F and 60,000°F (11,000°C and 33,000°C).

Most deaths and injuries caused by lightning occur during the summer months when people are enjoying outdoor activities, although approximately one-third of those struck by lightning were indoors.[23] Activities most commonly associated with lightning injuries include boating, fishing, swimming, and playing sports. Farmers sustain the highest number of work-related lightning injuries. If there are no witnesses to the event, it may not be readily apparent that the person has sustained a lightning injury.[2]

Whether a lightning strike is fatal depends on whether the person is in the path of the lightning discharge. The current associated with the lightning discharge travels along the ground. Although some people are injured or killed by a direct lightning strike, many people are indirectly struck when standing near an object that has been struck by lightning, such as a tree (splash effect).

The cardiovascular and nervous systems are most commonly injured during a lightning strike; therefore, respiratory or cardiac arrest is the most common cause of lightning-related deaths. The tissue damage caused by lightning is different from that caused by other electric-related injuries (ie, high-voltage power line injuries) because the tissue damage pathway usually occurs over the skin, rather than through it. During your assessment, look for not only the entrance wound but also the exit wound. The exit wound does not necessarily occur on the same side of the body. Additionally, because the duration of a lightning strike is short, skin burns are often superficial or partial thickness; full-thickness burns are rare. Burns may have a fernlike pattern. Lightning injuries are categorized as being mild, moderate, or severe[2]:

- **Mild.** Signs and symptoms include loss of consciousness, amnesia, anxiety, confusion, dizziness, tingling, weakness, and cool or mottled extremities. Burns, if present, are typically superficial. Hypertension may occur and is usually temporary.
- **Moderate.** Signs and symptoms include seizures, respiratory arrest or agonal breathing,

dysrhythmias that spontaneously resolve, paralysis, and superficial burns.

- **Severe.** Cardiopulmonary arrest may occur with fixed, dilated pupils. Because resuscitation may be delayed when the strike occurs in a remote location, many of these patients do not survive.

Emergency Medical Care

As with any scene response, your priority is safety. Take measures to protect yourself and your partner from being struck by lightning, especially if the thunderstorm is still in progress. Contrary to popular belief, lightning can, and does, strike in the same place twice. Move the patient to a place of safety, preferably in a sheltered area.

If you are in an open area and adequate shelter is unavailable, it is important to recognize the signs of an impending lightning strike and take immediate action to protect yourself, as repeated strikes are not uncommon. If you suddenly feel a tingling sensation or your hair stands on end, the area around you has become charged, which is a sure sign of an imminent lightning strike. Make yourself as small a target as possible by squatting down into a ball, with as little of your body as possible touching the ground. If you are in a group, people should spread out. If you are standing near a tree or other tall object, move away as fast as possible, preferably to a low-lying area. Lightning tends to strike objects that project from the ground (ie, trees, fences, buildings).

The process of triaging multiple victims of a lightning strike is different than the conventional triage methods used during a mass-casualty incident. When a person is struck by lightning, respiratory or cardiac arrest, if it occurs, usually occurs immediately. Delayed respiratory or cardiac arrest is much less likely to develop in those who are conscious following a lightning strike; most of these people will survive. Therefore, you should focus your efforts on those who are in respiratory or cardiac arrest because immediate treatment is associated with positive outcomes. This process, called **reverse triage**, differs from conventional triage, where such patients would ordinarily be classified as deceased. See Chapter 38, *Incident Management*, for further discussion of triage.

A person struck by lightning may fall from a height or be thrown. Though rare, this can result in fractures of long bones and spinal vertebrae. Therefore, if it appears the patient has fallen or been thrown, manually stabilize the patient's head in a neutral in-line position and open the airway with the jaw-thrust maneuver. If the patient is in respiratory arrest with a pulse, follow the ABC sequence: begin immediate bag-mask ventilations with 100% oxygen. If the patient is in cardiac arrest, follow the CAB sequence: begin CPR, attach an AED as soon as possible, and provide defibrillation if indicated. Spontaneous respirations may be delayed after return of spontaneous circulation.

Transport the patient to the closest appropriate facility. If CPR or ventilations are not required, address other injuries (ie, splint fractures, dress and bandage burns) and provide continuous monitoring while en route to the hospital. A patient with signs and symptoms of a lightning strike, but no obvious life threats, should still be transported to the ED for evaluation.

Bites and Envenomation

This section discusses bites and stings from spiders, Hymenoptera insects, snakes, scorpions, and ticks, and injuries from marine animals.

Spider Bites

Spiders are numerous and widespread in the United States. Many species of spiders bite. However, only two species native to the United States are able to deliver serious, even life-threatening bites: the female black widow spider and the brown recluse spider. When you care for a patient who has had some type of bite, be alert to the possibility that the spider may still be in the area, although it is unlikely. Remember that your safety is of paramount importance.

Black Widow Spider

The female black widow spider (*Latrodectus*) is fairly large, measuring approximately 2 inches (5 cm) long with its legs extended. It is usually black and typically has a distinctive, bright red-orange marking in the shape of an hourglass on its abdomen (**FIGURE 32-13**). The female black widow spider is larger and more toxic than the male. Black widow spiders are found in every state except Alaska. They

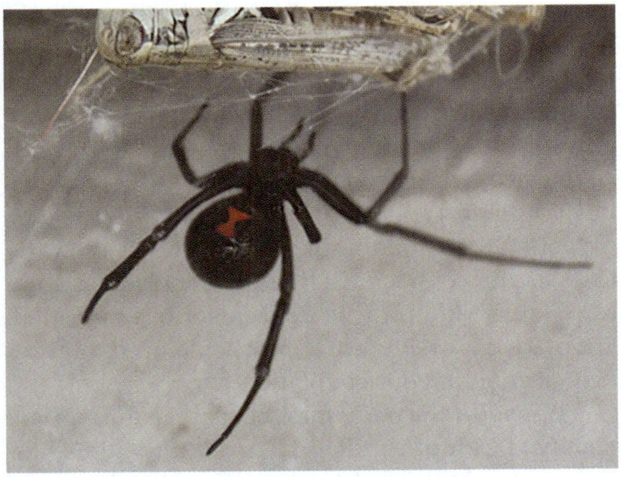

FIGURE 32-13 Black widow spiders are distinguished by their glossy black color and bright red-orange hourglass marking on the abdomen.

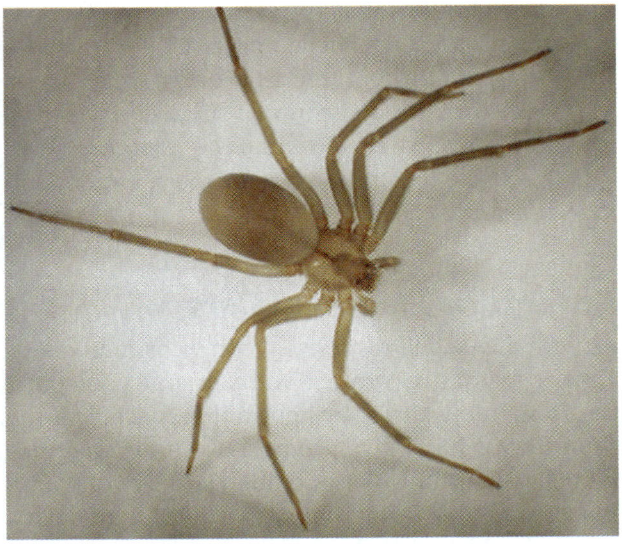

FIGURE 32-14 Brown recluse spiders are dull brown and have a dark, violin-shaped mark on the back.

prefer dry, dim places around buildings, in woodpiles, and among debris.

The bite of the black widow spider is sometimes overlooked. If the site becomes numb right away, the patient may not even recall being bit. However, most black widow spider bites cause localized pain and symptoms, including agonizing muscle spasms. In some cases, a bite on the abdomen causes muscle spasms so severe that the patient may be thought to have an acute abdominal condition, possibly peritonitis. The main danger with this type of bite, however, is that the black widow's venom can damage nerve tissues (it is a neurotoxin). Other systemic symptoms include dizziness, sweating, nausea, vomiting, and rashes. Tightness in the chest and difficulty breathing develop within 24 hours, as well as severe cramps, with boardlike rigidity of the abdominal muscles. Generally, these signs and symptoms subside over 48 hours.

If necessary, a physician can administer an **antivenin**, a serum containing antibodies that counteract the venom, but because of a high incidence of side effects, its use is reserved for severe bites, for older or particularly vulnerable patients, and for children younger than 5 years. In children, these bites can be fatal. In general, emergency treatment of a black widow spider bite consists of BLS for the patient in respiratory distress. More often, the patient will require only pain relief. Transport the patient to the ED as soon as possible for treatment. If possible, safely bring the spider to the hospital or take a photo of the spider with a cell phone and send it to the hospital ahead of time so that it can be definitively identified.

Brown Recluse Spider

The brown recluse spider (*Loxosceles*) is dull brown and, at 1 inch (3 cm), smaller than the black widow (**FIGURE 32-14**). The short-haired body has a violin-shaped mark, brown to yellow in color, on its back. Although the brown recluse spider lives mostly in the southern and central parts of the country, it may be found throughout the continental United States. The spider takes its name from the fact that it tends to live in dark areas: in corners of old, unused buildings, under rocks, and in woodpiles. In cooler areas, it moves indoors to closets, drawers, cellars, and clothing.

In contrast to the venom of the black widow spider, the venom of the brown recluse spider is not neurotoxic but cytotoxic; that is, it causes severe local tissue damage. Typically, the bite is not painful at first but becomes so within hours. The area becomes swollen and tender, developing a pale, mottled, cyanotic center and possibly a small blister (**FIGURE 32-15**). Over the next several days, a scab of dead skin, fat, and debris forms and digs down into the skin, producing a large ulcer that may not heal

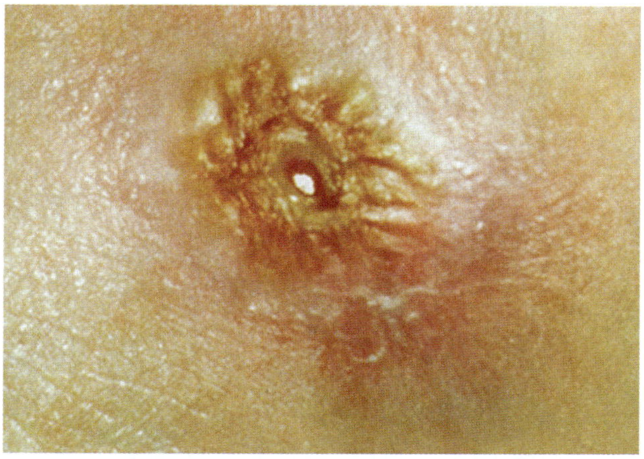

FIGURE 32-15 The bite of a brown recluse spider is characterized by swelling, tenderness, and a pale, mottled, cyanotic center. There may also be a small blister on the bite.

Courtesy of Department of Entomology, University of Nebraska.

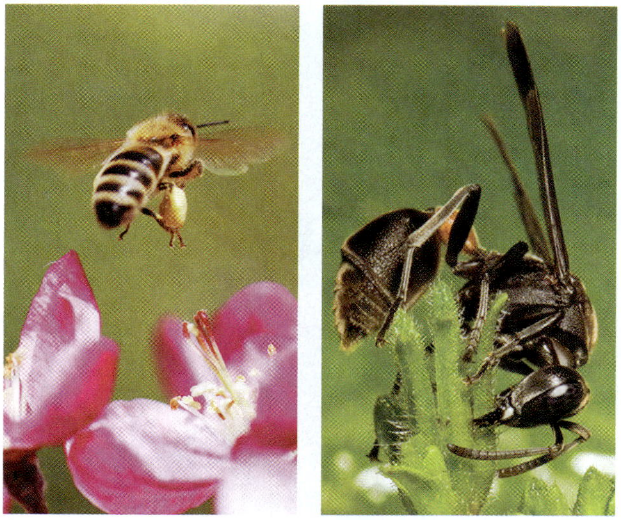

A B

FIGURE 32-16 Most stinging insects inject venom through a small, hollow spine that projects from the abdomen. **A.** The stinger of the honeybee is barbed; the honeybee cannot withdraw its stinger once it has stung someone. **B.** The wasp's stinger is unbarbed, meaning that it can inflict multiple stings.

A: © manfredxy/ShutterStock; **B:** © Heintje Joseph T. Lee/ShutterStock.

unless treated promptly. Transport patients with such symptoms as soon as possible.

Rarely, systemic signs and symptoms of a brown recluse spider bite may occur, including fever, chills, nausea, vomiting, and rash; more serious effects may include severe anemia, clotting problems, kidney failure, and death.[24] Your role in this situation is to provide BLS and prompt transport to the ED. Again, it is helpful if you can identify the spider and either safely bring it to the hospital with the patient, or take a picture of the spider and send it to the hospital ahead of time. Because symptoms do not typically develop for hours after the bite occurs, this is usually not possible.

Hymenoptera Stings

Up to 5% of the global population may experience a systemic allergic reaction to insect stings in their lifetime.[25] Each year hornet, wasp, and bee stings account for approximately 72 deaths in the United States. Most of these individuals (84%) are male.[26]

The **Hymenoptera** order of insects includes bees, wasps, yellowjackets, and ants. Typically, stings from these insects are painful but are not a medical emergency. The stinging organ of most bees, wasps, and hornets is a small, hollow spine projecting from the abdomen. Venom can be injected through this spine directly into the skin. The stinger of the honeybee is barbed, which prevents the bee from withdrawing it (**FIGURE 32-16A**). Consequently, the bee leaves a part of its abdomen embedded with the stinger and dies shortly after flying away. If the stinger is not removed from the skin, it can continue to inject venom for up to 20 minutes. Wasps and hornets do not have this handicap; they can sting repeatedly (**FIGURE 32-16B**). Because these insects usually fly away after stinging, it is often impossible to identify which species was responsible for the injury.

Some ants, especially the fire ant (**FIGURE 32-17A**), also strike repeatedly, injecting a particularly irritating **toxin**, or poison, at the bite sites. It is not uncommon for a patient to rapidly sustain multiple ant bites, usually on the feet and legs (**FIGURE 32-17B**).

Signs and symptoms of an insect sting include sudden pain, swelling, localized heat, widespread urticaria, and skin discoloration near the site (typically redness in people with light skin or darker skin in patients with dark skin). If the patient is allergic to the venom, then anaphylaxis may occur. The signs and symptoms of anaphylaxis are flushed skin, low blood pressure, and difficulty breathing that is usually associated with reactive airway sounds such as wheezes, or in severe cases, diminished or absent

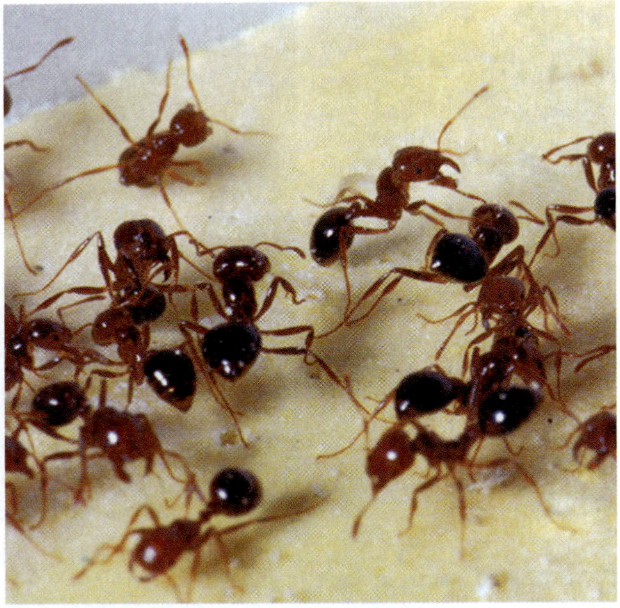

A

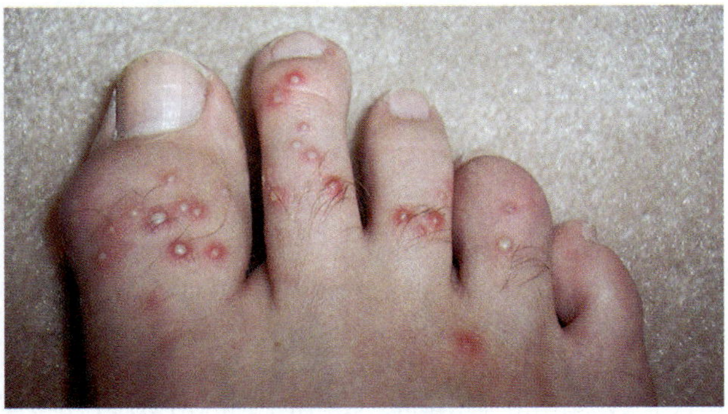

B

FIGURE 32-17 **A.** The fire ant. **B.** Fire ants inject an irritating toxin at multiple sites. Bites are generally found on the feet and the legs and appear as multiple small, raised pustules.

breath sounds. Hives (urticaria) may develop near the site of envenomation or centrally on the body. The patient can also have swelling to the face, throat, and tongue. Anaphylaxis is a true emergency and can be fatal if not recognized and treated quickly with epinephrine. If anaphylaxis develops, be prepared to administer epinephrine or to assist the patient in administering an epinephrine auto-injector (EpiPen). Also be prepared to support the airway and breathing should the patient experience significant respiratory compromise. Chapter 21, *Allergy and Anaphylaxis*, contains a detailed discussion of anaphylaxis treatment.

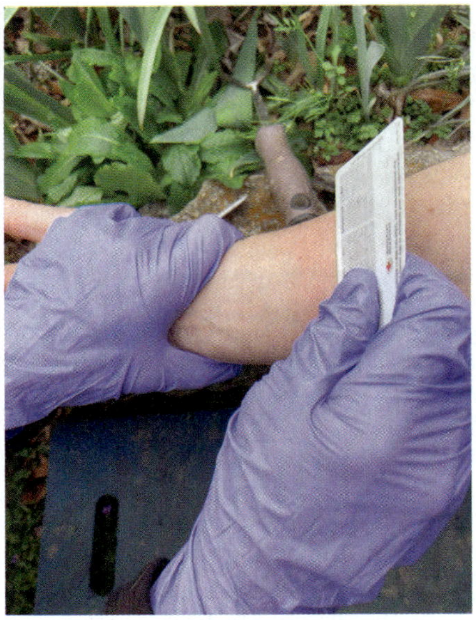

FIGURE 32-18 To remove the stinger of a honeybee, gently scrape the skin with the edge of a sharp, stiff object such as a driver's license.

If the allergic reaction was caused by an insect sting and the stinger is still in place, attempt to remove the stinger by scraping the skin with the edge of a sharp, stiff object such as a credit card (**FIGURE 32-18**). Do not use tweezers or forceps to remove the stinger because doing so may squeeze more venom into the wound. Gently wash the area with soap and water or a mild antiseptic. Try to remove any jewelry from the area before swelling begins. Position the patient with the injection site slightly below the level of the heart.[2]

Snake Bites

Snake bites are a worldwide problem. According to the World Health Organization, approximately 5.4 million people are bitten by snakes each year. Of these, 81,410 to 137,880 are killed, and many more experience amputation or permanent disability.[27] However, snake bite fatalities in the United States are extremely rare: approximately 5 per year for the entire country.[28]

Of the approximately 115 different species of snakes in the United States, only 19 are venomous. These include the rattlesnake (*Crotalus*); the copperhead (*Agkistrodon contortrix*); the cottonmouth, or water moccasin (*Agkistrodon piscivorus*); and the coral snakes (*Micrurus fulvius* and *Micruroides euryxanthus*) (**FIGURE 32-19**). At least one of these venomous species is found in every state except Alaska,

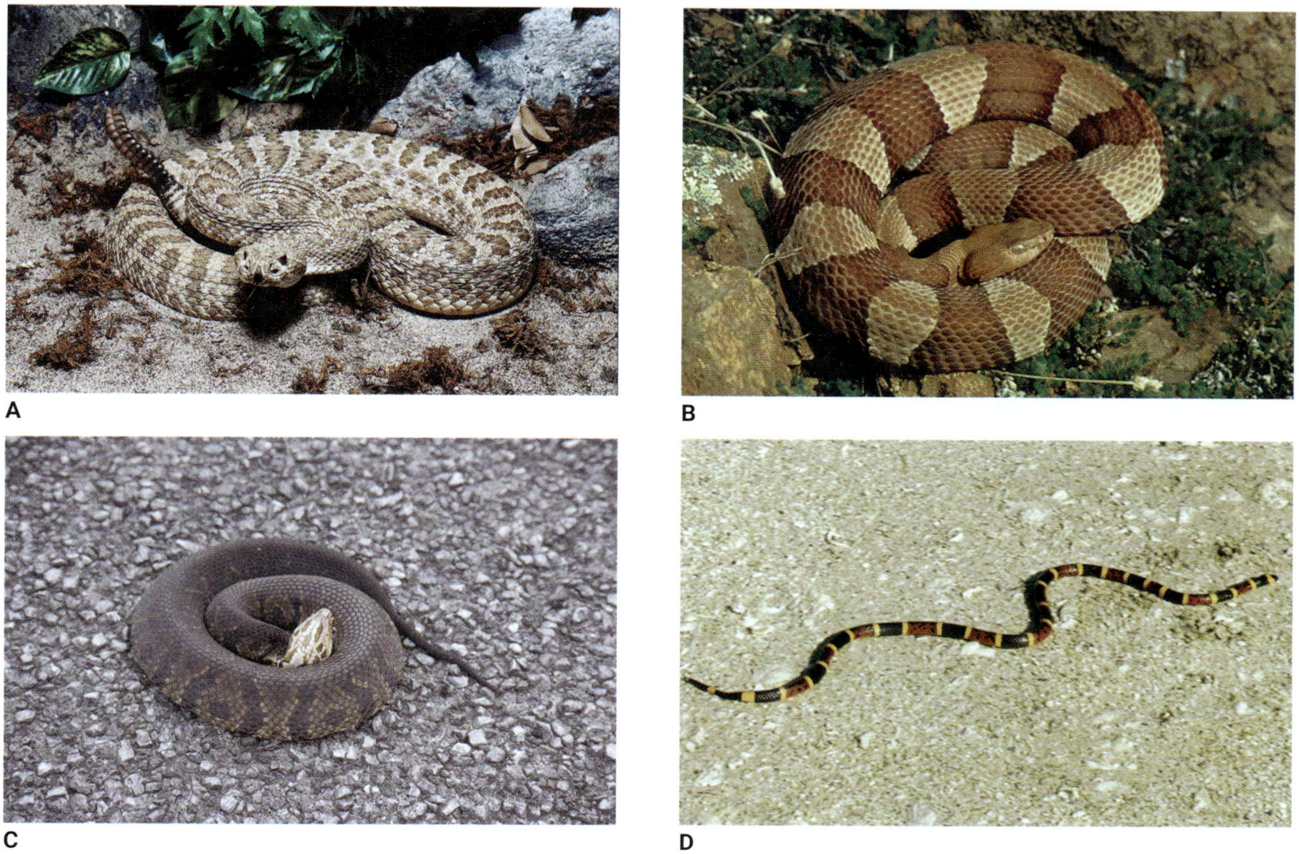

FIGURE 32-19 A. Rattlesnake. **B.** Copperhead. **C.** Cottonmouth (water moccasin). **D.** Coral snake.

A: © Photos.com; **B:** Courtesy of Ray Rauch/US Fish & Wildlife Service; **C:** © SuperStock/Alamy Stock Photo; **D:** Courtesy of Luther C. Goldman/US Fish & Wildlife Service.

Hawaii, and Maine. As a general rule, these snakes are timid. They usually do not bite unless provoked or accidentally injured, as when they are stepped on. There are a few exceptions to these rules. Cottonmouths are often aggressive, and rattlesnakes are easily provoked. Coral snakes, in contrast, usually bite only when they are being handled.

Most snake bites occur between April and October, when the animals are active. Texas reports the largest number of bites. Other states with a major concentration of snake bites are Louisiana, Georgia, Oklahoma, North Carolina, Arkansas, West Virginia, and Mississippi. If you work in one of these areas, you should be thoroughly familiar with the emergency handling of snake bites. Remember, almost any time you are caring for a patient with a snake bite, another snake may be in the area and create a second victim—you. Therefore, use extreme caution on these calls and be sure to wear the proper protective equipment for the area.

In general, only one-third of snake bites result in significant local or systemic injuries. Often, envenomation does not occur because the snake has recently struck another animal and exhausted its supply of venom for the time being.

Venomous snakes native to the United States have hollow fangs in the roof of the mouth that inject the venom from two sacs at the back of the head. The classic appearance of the venomous snake bite, therefore, is two small puncture wounds, usually approximately 0.5 inch (1 cm) apart, with discoloration and swelling, and the patient usually reports pain surrounding the bite (**FIGURE 32-20**). Fang marks are a clear indication of a venomous snake bite. In rare cases, the skin may only be scratched with a broken fang, but it is still possible for the patient to experience signs of envenomation or for the wound to later develop an infection. A snake bite with other tooth marks may be from a nonvenomous snake. If you are unsure whether the snake was

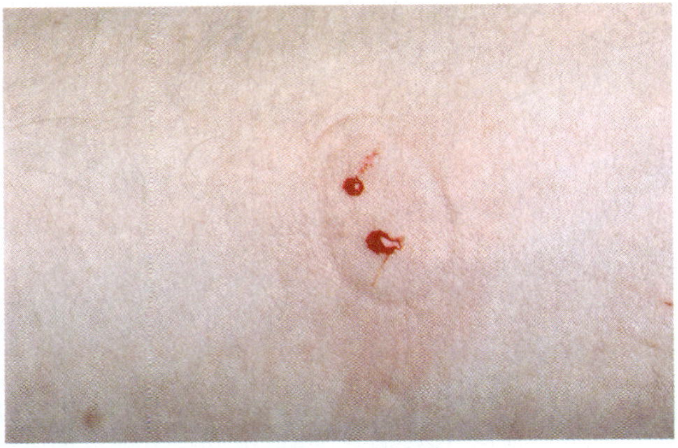

FIGURE 32-20 A snake bite wound from a poisonous snake typically has characteristic markings: two small puncture wounds approximately 0.5 inch (1 cm) apart, discoloration, and swelling.

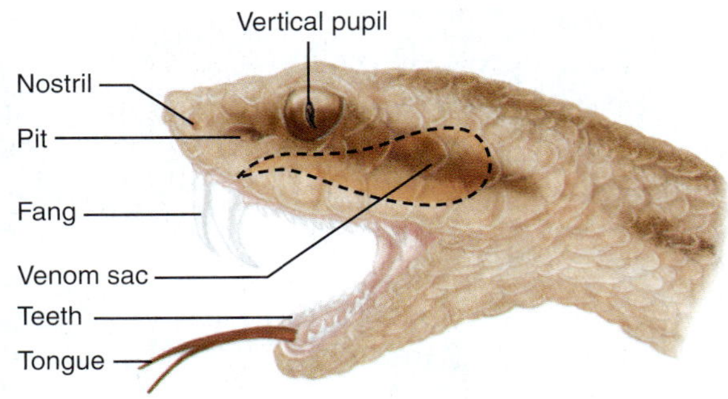

FIGURE 32-21 Pit vipers have small, heat-sensing organs (pits) located in front of their eyes that allow them to strike at warm targets, even in the dark.

venomous, proceed as if it was, especially if the patient exhibits other signs and symptoms.

A person who has been bitten by any venomous snake needs prompt transport. Also, notify the hospital as soon as possible if a patient has been bitten by a pit viper or coral snake. Some venoms can cause paralysis of the nervous system, and hospitals may not have appropriate antivenin on hand.

Words of Wisdom

Most pet snakes are nonvenomous. Even so, if a person was bitten by a pet snake, you should ask the owner the type of snake and then contact poison control for treatment advice.

Pit Vipers

Rattlesnakes, copperheads, and cottonmouths are all pit vipers, with triangular-shaped, flat heads (**FIGURE 32-21**). They take their name from the small pits located just behind each nostril and in front of each eye. The pit is a heat-sensing organ that allows the snake to strike accurately at any warm target, especially in the dark, when it cannot see through its vertical, slit-like pupils.

The fangs of the pit viper normally lie flat against the roof of the mouth and are hinged to swing back and forth as the mouth opens. When the snake strikes, the mouth opens wide and the fangs extend; in this way, the fangs penetrate whatever the mouth strikes. The fangs are hollow teeth that act like hypodermic needles. They are connected to a sac containing a reservoir of venom, which in turn is attached to a poison gland. The gland itself is a specifically adapted salivary gland, which produces enzymes that digest and destroy tissue. The primary purpose of the venom is to kill small animals and facilitate the digestive process.

In the United States, the most common form of pit viper is the rattlesnake. Several different species of rattlesnake can be identified by the rattle on the tail. The rattle is numerous layers of dried skin that were shed but failed to fall off, coming to rest against a small knob on the end of the tail. Rattlesnakes have many patterns of color, often with a diamond pattern. They can grow to 6 feet (2 m) or longer.

Copperheads are smaller than rattlesnakes, usually 2 to 3 feet long (60 to 90 cm) with a red-copper color crossed with brown or red bands. These snakes typically inhabit woodpiles and abandoned dwellings, often close to areas of habitation. Although they account for most of the venomous snake bites in the eastern United States, copperhead bites are almost never fatal; however, note that the venom can cause significant damage to tissues in the extremities.

Cottonmouths grow to approximately 4 feet (1 m) in length. Also called water moccasins, these snakes are olive or brown, with black cross-bands and a yellow undersurface. They are water snakes and have a particularly aggressive pattern of behavior. Although fatalities from these snake bites are rare, tissue destruction from the venom may be severe.

The signs of envenomation by a pit viper are severe burning pain at the site of the injury, followed by swelling and a blue discoloration (ecchymosis) that signals bleeding under the skin. This blue discoloration may be more difficult to see in people with dark skin. These signs are evident within 5 to 10 minutes after the bite has occurred and last over the next 36 hours. In addition to destroying tissues locally, the venom of the pit viper can interfere with the body's clotting mechanism and cause bleeding at various distant sites. This toxin affects the entire nervous system. Other systemic signs, which may or may not occur, include weakness, nausea, vomiting, sweating, seizures, fainting, vision problems, changes in level of consciousness, and shock. If swelling has occurred, use a pen to mark its edges on the skin. This will allow physicians to assess the timing and extent of the swelling with greater accuracy. If the patient has no local signs an hour after being bitten, it is likely that envenomation did not take place.

The toxicity is related to the amount of toxin injected. A bite will affect children more than adults because there is less body mass to absorb the toxin. The same principle holds true for a small adult.

In treating a snake bite from a pit viper, follow these steps:

1. Calm the patient; assure them that venomous snake bites are rarely fatal. Place the patient in a supine position and explain that staying still will slow the spread of any venom through the system. Determine the approximate time of the bite and document your time en route to a receiving facility. This time from onset to evaluation at the facility is one of the criteria used in grading the severity of the incident and in determining the amount of antivenin to be used.
2. Locate the bite area; clean it gently with soap and water or a mild antiseptic. Do not apply ice to the area.
3. If the bite occurred on an arm or leg and the transport time to the hospital is anticipated to exceed 2 hours, place the affected extremity slightly below the level of the heart.
4. If an anaphylactic reaction to the venom occurs, treat with an epinephrine.
5. Do not give anything by mouth, and be alert for vomiting.
6. If, as rarely happens, the patient was bitten on the trunk, keep the patient supine and calm and transport as quickly as possible.
7. Monitor the patient's vital signs and mark the skin with a pen proximal to the area that is swollen to monitor whether swelling is spreading.
8. If there are any signs of shock or hypoxia, administer oxygen.
9. If the snake has been killed, as is often the case, bring it with you in a secure, hard-sided container so that physicians can identify it and administer the proper antivenin. Alternatively, take a picture of the snake with a cell phone and send it to the hospital ahead of time.
10. Notify the hospital that you are bringing in a patient who has a snake bite; if possible, describe the snake.
11. Transport the patient promptly to the appropriate hospital.

If the patient shows no sign of envenomation, provide BLS as needed, place a sterile dressing over the suspected bite area, and limit movement of the injury site. All patients with a suspected snake bite should be taken to the ED, regardless of whether they show signs of envenomation. Treat the wound as you would any deep puncture wound to prevent infection.

Familiarize yourself with the venomous snakes in your region, as well as local protocols for treating snake bites. There may be specific hospitals where antivenin is more readily available, either in the facility or through zoos, health departments, or other services.

Words of Wisdom

In the United States, antivenin is available for the black widow spider, bark scorpions, crotalid snakes (rattlesnake, copperhead), and coral snakes; however, not all hospitals carry them. If your protocols do not specify the hospital, poison control can assist you to determine which hospital in your area has the appropriate antivenin for your patient.

Coral Snakes

The coral snake is a small reptile with a series of bright red, yellow, and black bands completely encircling the body. Many harmless snakes have similar coloring, but only the coral snake has red and yellow bands next to one another, as this helpful rhyme suggests: "Red on yellow will kill a fellow; red on black, venom will lack."

A rare creature that lives in most southern states and in the Southwest, the coral snake is a relative of the cobra. It has tiny fangs and injects the venom with its teeth by a chewing motion, leaving behind one or more puncture or scratch-like wounds. Because of its small mouth and teeth and limited jaw expansion, the coral snake usually bites its victims on a small part of the body, such as a finger or toe.

Coral snake venom is a powerful toxin that causes paralysis of the nervous system. Within a few hours of being bitten, a patient may exhibit bizarre behavior, followed by progressive paralysis of eye movements and respiration. Often, there are limited or no local symptoms.

Successful treatment, either emergency or long term, depends on positive identification of the snake and support of respiration. Antivenin is also available for coral snake bites, but most hospitals do not stock it. Therefore, you should contact poison control and notify the receiving hospital of the need for it as soon as possible. The steps for emergency care of a coral snake bite are the same as a pit viper bite.

Scorpion Stings

Scorpions are eight-legged arthropods from the class Arachnida. They have a venom gland and a stinger at the end of their tail (**FIGURE 32-22**). Scorpions are rare; they live primarily in the southwestern United States and in deserts. With one exception, a scorpion's sting is usually very painful but not dangerous, causing localized swelling and discoloration. The exception is the *Centruroides sculpturatus.* Although it is found naturally in Arizona and New Mexico, as well as parts of Texas, California, and Nevada, it may be kept as a pet in other locations. The venom of this particular species may produce a severe systemic reaction that leads to circulatory collapse, severe muscle contractions,

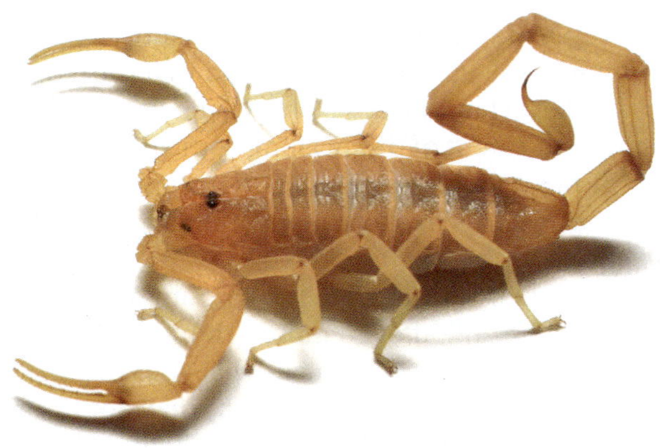

FIGURE 32-22 The sting of a scorpion is usually more painful than it is dangerous, causing localized swelling and discoloration. This photo shows a *Centruroides sculpturatus*, the venom of which may produce a severe systemic reaction.

YOU are the EMT

The patient's level of consciousness has improved and he is asking what happened. You begin transport because ALS has a delayed response. You reassess his vital signs and clinical condition every 5 minutes. His temperature continues to drop and is now 101.6°F (38.7°C). You will arrive at the hospital in approximately 35 minutes.

Recording Time: 16 Minutes	
Level of consciousness	Alert and oriented
Respirations	22 breaths/min; normal depth
Pulse	120 beats/min and regular; appears to be stronger
Skin	Less flushed, moist
Blood pressure	98/58 mm Hg
Oxygen saturation (Spo_2)	96%

9. What other conditions should you consider as potential causes of the patient's altered mental status?

excessive salivation, hypertension, convulsions, and cardiac failure. Antivenin is available but must be administered by a physician. If you are called to care for a patient with a suspected sting from *C sculpturatus*, notify the receiving hospital as early as possible to facilitate the availability of this antivenin. Administer BLS and provide rapid transport to the ED.

Tick Bites

Found most often on brush, shrubs, trees, sand dunes, or other animals, ticks usually attach themselves directly to the skin (**FIGURE 32-23**). Only a fraction of an inch (approximately 3 mm) long, they can easily be mistaken for a freckle, especially because their bite is not painful. Indeed, the danger with a tick bite is not from the bite itself, but from the infecting organisms that the tick carries. While some ticks do not carry disease, approximately 50,000 cases of bacterial, viral, and parasitic disease are transmitted to humans by ticks every year in the United States.[29] Rocky Mountain spotted fever and Lyme disease are two of the diseases spread by ticks. Both are spread through the tick's saliva, which is injected into the skin when the tick attaches itself. The longer a tick stays embedded, the greater the chance that a disease will be transmitted.

Rocky Mountain spotted fever, which is not limited to the Rocky Mountains area, occurs within 7 to 10 days after a bite by an infected tick. Its symptoms include nausea, vomiting, headache, weakness, paralysis, and possible cardiorespiratory collapse.

Lyme disease has received extensive publicity. Lyme disease was originally seen only in the town of Lyme, Connecticut. According to the Centers for Disease Control and Prevention, it has now been reported in all states except for Hawaii. It occurs most commonly in the Northeast and the Great Lakes states; Pennsylvania reported the largest number of cases from 2011 to 2013. The first symptoms are generally fever and flulike symptoms, sometimes associated with a bull's-eye rash that may spread to several parts of the body (**FIGURE 32-24**). After a few days or weeks, painful swelling of the joints, particularly the knees, occurs. Lyme disease may be confused with rheumatoid arthritis and, like that

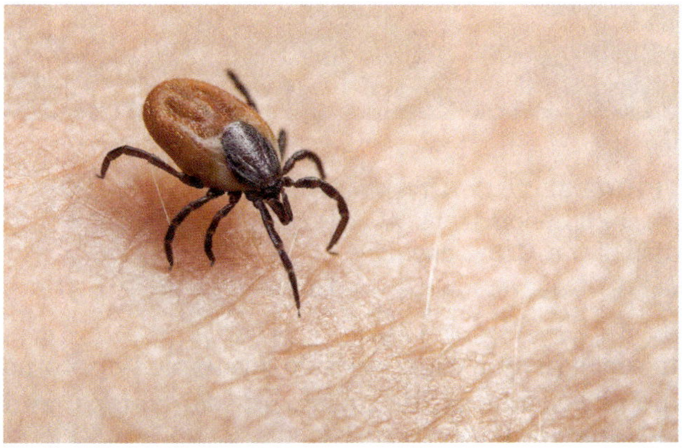

A

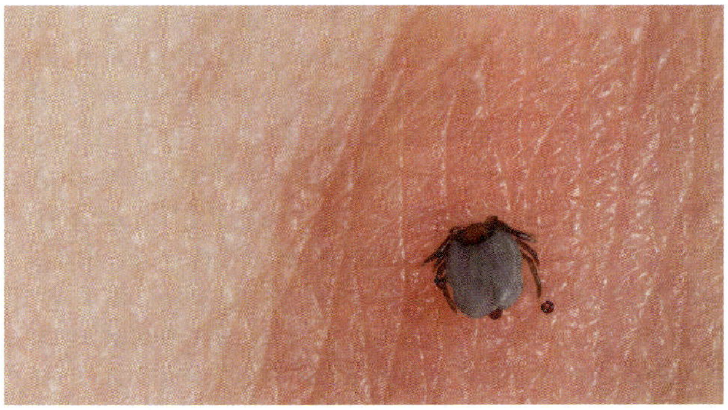

B

FIGURE 32-23 Ticks typically attach themselves directly to the skin. **A.** The deer tick (*Ixodes scapularis*) is common in North America and known to transmit Lyme disease. **B.** The tick has embedded itself in the person's skin.

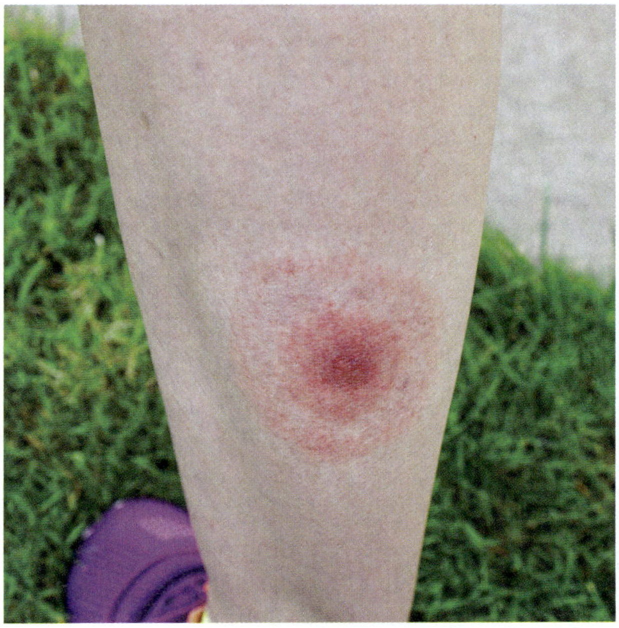

FIGURE 32-24 The rash associated with Lyme disease has a characteristic bull's-eye pattern.

disease, may result in permanent disability. However, if it is recognized and treated promptly with antibiotics, the patient may recover completely.

Tick bites occur most commonly during the summer months, when people are out in the woods wearing little protective clothing. Do not attempt to suffocate the tick with gasoline or petroleum jelly, or burn it with a lighted match; you will only increase the risk of infection or burn the patient. For patients in conventional EMS settings with signs and symptoms of Lyme disease, provide any necessary supportive emergency care and transport the patient for further evaluation. In a situation (such as wilderness EMS) where access to care is delayed, remove the tick from the patient. Using fine tweezers, grasp the tick by the head, as close to the skin as possible, and pull gently but firmly straight up so that the skin is tented. Hold this position until the tick releases.[30] Special tweezers are available for this, but are unnecessary. This method will usually remove the whole tick. (Partial removal can lead to infection.) Cleanse the area with antiseptic and save the tick in a glass jar or other container so that it can be identified. Do not handle the tick with your fingers. The patient should follow up with their health care clinician as soon as possible.

Words of Wisdom

Alpha-gal syndrome is an allergy to mammalian meat, especially red meat, that develops within a week to several months in some patients after a tick bite infection (usually from a lone star tick). A person with alpha-gal syndrome who eats meat may experience an anaphylactic reaction and need emergency treatment with epinephrine.[31]

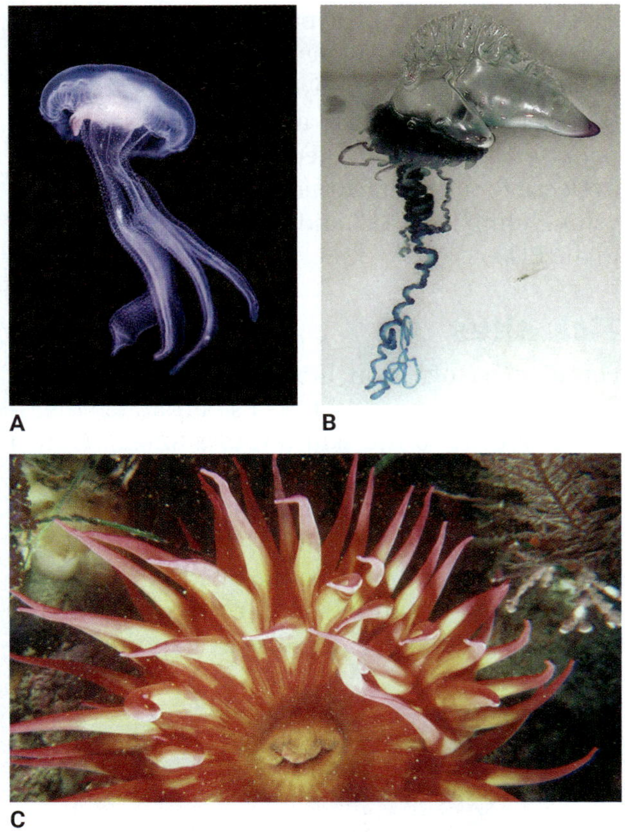

FIGURE 32-25 Coelenterates are responsible for many marine envenomations. **A.** Jellyfish. **B.** Portuguese man-of-war. **C.** Sea anemone.

Injuries From Marine Animals

Coelenterates, including fire coral, Portuguese man-of-war, sea wasp, sea nettles, true jellyfish, sea anemones, true coral, and soft coral, are responsible for more envenomations than any other marine animals (**FIGURE 32-25**). The stinging cells of the coelenterate are called nematocysts, and large animals may discharge hundreds of thousands of them. Envenomation causes very painful, red lesions in people with light skin extending in a line from the site of the sting. These lesions may be more difficult to see in people with dark skin. Systemic symptoms include headache, dizziness, muscle cramps, and fainting.

To treat a sting from the tentacles of a jellyfish, a Portuguese man-of-war, various anemones, corals, or hydras, remove the patient from the water and remove the tentacles by scraping them off with the edge of a stiff object, such as a credit card. Do not try to manipulate the remaining tentacles; doing so will only cause further discharge of the nematocysts. Once jellyfish tentacles are removed, vinegar can be applied to the affected area (avoid applying vinegar for sea nettle stings).[2] On rare occasions, a patient may have a systemic allergic reaction to the sting of one of these animals. Treat this patient for anaphylactic shock and provide rapid transport to the hospital.

Toxins from the spines of urchins, stingrays, and certain spiny fish such as the lionfish, scorpion fish, or stonefish are also heat sensitive. Therefore, the best treatment for such injuries is also to soak the affected extremity in hot water (113°F [45°C]) for 30 minutes. Doing so will often provide dramatic relief from local pain. However, the patient still needs to be transported to the ED because an allergic reaction or infection, including tetanus, could develop.

If you work near the ocean, you should be familiar with the marine life in your area. The emergency treatment of common coelenterate envenomations consists of the following steps:

1. Limit further discharge of nematocysts by avoiding fresh water, wet sand, showers, or careless manipulation of the tentacles. Keep the patient calm, and reduce motion of the affected extremity.
2. Remove the remaining tentacles by scraping them off with the edge of a stiff object such as a credit card. Do not use your ungloved hand to remove the tentacles, because self-envenomation will occur. Persistent pain may respond to immersion in hot water (113°F [45°C]) for 30 minutes. If available, immersion in vinegar may also help alleviate the symptoms (except for sea nettle stings).
3. Provide transport to the ED.

YOU are the EMT SUMMARY

1. How does the body normally balance heat production and elimination?

Normal core temperature—that of the heart, lungs, and other vital organs—is usually around 98.6°F (37°C). A series of regulatory mechanisms keep this internal temperature constant, regardless of the ambient temperature (the temperature of the surrounding environment). However, heat elimination must balance heat production; if it does not, a temperature-related emergency occurs.

There are several ways the body removes excess heat, the most efficient of which are sweating (especially through evaporation of the sweat) and dilation of the blood vessels. Ordinarily, the heat-regulating mechanisms of the body work very well and people are able to tolerate significant temperature changes. People can also assist their bodies with heat elimination by removing heat-retaining clothing or by moving to a cooler environment.

2. What factors can decrease the body's ability to eliminate excess heat?

Several factors can decrease a person's ability to eliminate excess heat. If air temperature is high, heat loss by radiation is reduced. Heat travels from a warmer place to a cooler place; if the ambient temperature is higher than body temperature, heat will move from the environment and into the body. If the relative humidity, the amount of moisture in the air, is high, heat loss by evaporation is reduced. Heat elimination is most impaired when both the air temperature and relative humidity are high.

Vigorous exercise causes a loss of fluids and electrolytes, resulting in dehydration. People who have an inadequate intake of water can also become dehydrated. Dehydration decreases heat loss through sweating and evaporation.

Small children and older adults exhibit poor thermoregulation; therefore, they are less able to eliminate excess body heat. Additionally, the body's water content decreases with age, which reduces the ability to sweat.

Certain medical conditions, such as heart disease, chronic obstructive pulmonary disease, diabetes, dehydration, and obesity, interfere with the process of body heat elimination. In addition, alcohol and certain drugs, including medications that dehydrate the body (ie, diuretics) or decrease the ability of the body to sweat, reduce heat elimination from the body.

3. What risk factors does this patient have that predispose him to a heat emergency?

Your patient has several risk factors for a heat emergency, the single most significant of which is prolonged exertion in a hot, humid environment. Also, the patient has not been drinking any water. Combining his inadequate intake of fluid with the profuse sweating that occurs during exposure to a hot environment, you should suspect that he is dehydrated.

The patient's past medical history also predisposes him to a heat emergency. Diabetes is a systemic condition that impairs many body functions, including thermoregulation, as well as fluid regulation if blood sugar levels are high. The patient also has hypertension, for which diuretics, such as the furosemide in this case, are often prescribed. Diuretics promote urination, further contributing to his dehydration.

YOU are the EMT SUMMARY continued

4. What type of heat emergency do you suspect he is experiencing? Why?

There are several clinical findings that indicate your patient is experiencing the most serious heat illness, heatstroke. Unlike other less severe forms of heat illness (eg, heat cramps, heat exhaustion), patients with heatstroke have an altered level of consciousness, ranging from confusion to coma, and flushed, hot skin. Your patient has both of these. Untreated heatstroke causes permanent brain and tissue damage; in most cases, it causes death.

5. What specific treatment is required for this patient?

Because your patient has clear signs of heatstroke (eg, core temperature >104°F [40°C], altered mental status), begin emergent cooling measures. Immerse the patient in an ice bath if available. If an ice bath is not possible, attempt the TACO method: Place the patient on a tarp and pour ice water over them. Then move the tarp back and forth (oscillate it) to enhance the heat dissipation. If neither of these options is available, cover the patient in towels or sheets that have been soaked in ice water. It is imperative to rotate the towels/sheets to avoid trapping heat. Stop cooling measures when the patient's temperature reaches 102.2°F (39°C) to prevent overcooling. After performing rapid cooling, provide rapid transport. Any delays in providing treatment increase the potential for permanent brain and tissue damage or death.

Continue to monitor the patient and notify the receiving facility early so the facility can continue treatment immediately on your arrival.

6. What is the most likely explanation for this patient's vital signs?

Your patient's vital signs—tachypnea, tachycardia, and hypotension—indicate shock. This is because heatstroke is associated with a severe loss of fluids and electrolytes, which results in hypovolemia. You should expect that patients with heatstroke will be tachypneic and tachycardic because of all the heat energy they have in their body. This response alone may enable patients to start to compensate for the severe fluid loss that occurs with heatstroke. The presence of hypotension, however, indicates that the body's compensatory mechanisms have failed (decompensated shock).

Patients with hypovolemic shock associated with heatstroke will need IV fluids and other treatment aimed at correcting electrolyte abnormalities at the hospital. Consider an ALS intercept, but do not delay cooling or transport to do this. AEMTs and paramedics are able to establish IV lines and administer fluids, but these interventions are less urgent than cooling. Otherwise, closely monitor the patient.

7. What additional assessment should you perform on this patient?

Your patient's level of consciousness has deteriorated, and he has a history of type 1 diabetes. Blood glucose should be assessed to ensure he is not hypoglycemic. His temperature should be reassessed every 5 minutes.

8. What treatment should you provide en route to the hospital?

Ideally, you should monitor the patient's core temperature; this is most reliably obtained by assessing the patient's rectal temperature, if local protocols allow. It is important to note that the core temperature increases rapidly in patients with heatstroke, but does not decrease as quickly, even with aggressive cooling measures. If the patient's temperature reaches 102.2°F (39°C) stop cooling measures as the temperature may continue to decline.

If your protocols do not allow you to monitor a patient's core temperature rectally, an axillary temperature should be assessed, although it is less accurate and will not be possible when the patient is immersed in ice water.

When actively cooling a patient with heatstroke, do not cool to the point of shivering. Shivering generates more heat and can occur when cooling is not monitored closely.

9. What other conditions should you consider as potential causes of the patient's altered mental status?

Altered mental status may be associated with heatstroke alone or could be the result of a completely different problem. An increase in heat energy causes the body to expend a lot of glucose; therefore, consider the possibility of hypoglycemia, especially because this patient has diabetes, which increases that risk. You should also consider the possibility of a head injury. Recall that the patient apparently fainted. When this occurred, he may have fallen and struck his head, resulting in a concussion or intracranial hemorrhage. Do not rule out an occult head injury in the absence of obvious signs of trauma.

Prep Kit

Ready for Review

- Cold-related emergencies can be either a local or a systemic problem.
- Local cold injuries include frostbite, frostnip, and immersion foot. Frostbite is the most serious because the tissues freeze. All patients with a local cold injury should be removed from the cold and protected from further exposure.
- If instructed to do so by medical direction, rewarm frostbitten parts by immersing them in water at a temperature between 98.6°F and 102°F (37°C and 39°C).
- The key to treating patients with hypothermia is to stabilize vital functions and prevent further heat loss. Do not attempt to rewarm patients who have moderate to severe hypothermia because they are susceptible to the development of dysrhythmias.
- Do not consider a patient dead until the person is "warm and dead." Local protocols will dictate whether such patients receive CPR or defibrillation in the field.
- The body's regulatory mechanisms normally maintain body temperature within a very narrow range around 98.6°F (37°C). Body temperature is regulated by heat loss to the atmosphere via conduction, convection, evaporation, radiation, and respiration.
- Heat emergencies can take three forms: heat cramps, heat exhaustion, and heatstroke.
  - Heat cramps are painful muscle spasms that occur with vigorous exercise. Treatment includes removing the patient from the heat, resting the affected muscles, and replacing fluid loss.
  - Heat exhaustion is essentially a form of hypovolemic shock caused by dehydration. Symptoms include cold and clammy skin, weakness, confusion, headache, and rapid pulse. Body temperature can be high, and the patient may or may not still be sweating. Treatment includes removing the patient from the heat and treating for mild hypovolemic shock.
  - Heatstroke is a life-threatening emergency and is usually fatal if untreated. Patients with heatstroke are often dry and will have body temperatures up to 104°F (40°C) or greater. Patients who have heatstroke due to exertion may have wet skin. Changes in mental status can include coma. Rapid lowering of the body temperature in the field is critical.
- The first rule in caring for drowning victims is to avoid becoming a victim yourself. Protect the spine when removing patients from the water because spinal cord injuries often occur in drownings. Be alert for hypothermia.
- Injuries associated with scuba diving may be immediately apparent or may show up hours later. Patients with an air embolism or decompression sickness may have pain, paralysis, or an altered mental status. Be prepared to transport such patients to a recompression facility with a hyperbaric chamber.
- Venomous spiders native to the United States are the black widow spider and the brown recluse spider.
- Venomous snakes found in the United States include pit vipers and coral snakes.
- A person who has been bitten by a venomous snake needs prompt transport; clean the bite area and keep the patient calm to slow the spread of venom.
- Notify the hospital as soon as possible if a patient has been bitten by a pit viper or coral snake. Some venoms can cause paralysis of the nervous system, and hospitals may not have appropriate antivenin on hand.
- Patients who have been bitten by ticks may be infected with Rocky Mountain spotted fever or Lyme disease and should see a doctor within a day or two. Remove the tick using tweezers, and save it for identification.
- Always provide prompt transport to the hospital for any patient who has been bitten by a venomous insect or animal. Remember that vital signs can deteriorate rapidly. Carefully monitor the patient's vital signs en route, especially for airway compromise.

Prep Kit continued

Vital Vocabulary

air embolism The presence of air in the veins, which can lead to cardiac arrest if it enters the heart.

ambient temperature The temperature of the surrounding environment.

antivenin A serum that counteracts the effect of venom from an animal or insect.

bends A common name for decompression sickness.

breath-holding syncope Loss of consciousness caused by a decreased breathing stimulus.

conduction The loss of heat by direct contact (eg, when a body part comes into contact with a colder object).

convection The loss of body heat caused by air movement (eg, a breeze blowing across the body).

core temperature The temperature of the central part of the body (eg, the heart, lungs, and vital organs).

decompression sickness A painful condition seen in divers who ascend too quickly, in which gas, especially nitrogen, forms bubbles in blood vessels and other tissues; see *bends*.

diving reflex The slowing of the heart rate caused by submersion in cold water.

drowning The process of experiencing respiratory impairment from submersion or immersion in liquid.

dysbarism injuries Any signs and symptoms caused by the difference between the surrounding atmospheric pressure and the total gas pressure in various tissues, fluids, and cavities of the body.

evaporation The conversion of water or another fluid from a liquid to a gas.

frostbite Damage to tissues as the result of exposure to cold; frozen body parts; frozen or partially frozen body parts are frostbitten.

heat cramps Painful muscle spasms usually associated with vigorous activity in a hot environment.

heat exhaustion A heat emergency in which a significant amount of fluid and electrolyte loss occurs because of heavy sweating.

heatstroke A life-threatening condition of severe hyperthermia caused by exposure to excessive natural or artificial heat, marked by warm, dry skin; severely altered mental status; and often irreversible coma.

homeostasis A balance of all systems of the body.

Hymenoptera An order of insects that includes bees, wasps, ants, and yellowjackets.

hyperthermia A condition in which the body core temperature rises to 101°F (38.3°C) or more.

hypothermia A condition in which the body's core temperature falls below 95°F (35°C).

radiation The transfer of heat to colder objects in the environment by radiant energy; for example, heat gain from a fire.

respiration The inhaling and exhaling of air; the physiologic process that exchanges carbon dioxide from fresh air.

reverse triage A triage process used in treating multiple victims of a lightning strike, in which efforts are focused on those who are in respiratory and cardiac arrest. Reverse triage is different from conventional triage, where such patients would be classified as deceased.

toxin A poison or harmful substance.

turgor The ability of the skin to resist deformation; tested by gently pinching skin on the forehead or back of the hand.

Prep Kit continued

References

1. Duong H, Patel G. Hypothermia. *StatPearls*. National Library of Medicine website. https://www.ncbi.nlm.nih.gov/books/NBK545239/. Updated January 19, 2024. Accessed March 31, 2025.
2. National Association of State EMS Officials. *National Model EMS Clinical Guidelines: Version 3.0.* https://nasemso.org/content.aspx?page_id=22&club_id=157064&module_id=701974. Updated March 2022. Accessed March 31, 2025.
3. Wexler A, Zavala S. The use of thrombolytic therapy in the treatment of frostbite injury. *J Burn Care Res*. 2017;38(5):e877–e881. doi:10.1097/BCR.0000000000000512
4. FDA approves first medication to treat severe frostbite. US Food and Drug Administration website. https://www.fda.gov/news-events/press-announcements/fda-approves-first-medication-treat-severe-frostbite. Published February 14, 2024. Accessed May 20, 2025.
5. European Resuscitation Council. Accidental hypothermia. *Resuscitation* website. https://www.resuscitationjournal.com/cms/10.1016/j.resuscitation.2021.02.011/asset/ce160958-00c1-469a-9155-3cd91e032bfa/main.assets/gr5_lrg.jpg. Accessed March 31, 2025.
6. Who is most at risk to extreme heat? Heat.gov website. https://www.heat.gov/pages/who-is-at-risk-to-extreme-heat. Accessed March 31, 2025.
7. Arif S. Heat index vs wet bulb globe temperature: all you need to know. Perry Weather website. https://perryweather.com/resources/heat-index-wet-bulb-globe-temp/. Published June 13, 2024. Accessed May 20, 2025.
8. Belval LN, Casa DJ, Adams WM, et al. Consensus statement—prehospital care of exertional heat stroke. *Prehosp Emerg Care*. 2018;22(3):392–397.
9. Li J. Hypothermia. Medscape website. https://emedicine.medscape.com/article/770542-overview?form=fpf#a6. Updated October 21, 2021. Accessed March 31, 2025.
10. QuickStats: percentage distribution of heat-related deaths, by age group—National Vital Statistics System, United States, 2018–2020. *MMWR Morb Mortal Wkly Rep*. 2022;71:808.
11. Drowning increases in the US. Centers for Disease Control and Prevention website. https://www.cdc.gov/vitalsigns/drowning/index.html. Updated June 18, 2024. Accessed March 31, 2025.
12. McCallin TE, Dezfulian C, Bierens J, et al. 2024 American Heart Association and American Academy of Pediatrics focused update on special circumstances: resuscitation following drowning: an update to the American Heart Association Guidelines for Cardiopulmonary Resuscitation and Emergency Cardiovascular Care. *Circulation*. 2024;154(6). https://doi.org/10.1542/peds.2024-068444
13. Denny SA, Quan L, Gilchrist J, et al. Prevention of drowning. *Pediatrics*. 2019;143(5). doi:10.1542/peds.2019-0850
14. Westly E. Adult drowning deaths are increasing. Scientific American website. https://www.scientificamerican.com/article/adult-drowning-deaths-are-increasing-swimming-lessons-and-reduced-alcohol/. Published August 27, 2024. Accessed March 31, 2025.
15. Parenteau M, Stockinger Z, Hughes S, et al. Drowning management. *Milit Med*. 2018;183(2):172–179.
16. Buzzacott P, Schiller D, Crain J, Denoble PJ. Epidemiology of morbidity and mortality in US and Canadian recreational scuba diving. *Public Health*. 2018;155:62–68.
17. Penrice D, Cooper JS. Diving casualties. *StatPearls*. National Library of Medicine website. https://www.ncbi.nlm.nih.gov/books/NBK459389/. Updated November 28, 2022. Accessed March 31, 2025.
18. Technical diving. National Oceanic and Atmospheric Association website. https://oceanexplorer.noaa.gov/technology/technical/technical.html. Published November 3, 2023. Accessed March 31, 2025.
19. CPR with rescue breaths vital to resuscitation after drowning, new guidelines say. American Heart Association website. https://www.heart.org/en/news/2024/11/12/cpr-with-rescue-breaths-vital-to-resuscitation-after-drowning. Published November 12, 2024. Accessed March 31, 2025.
20. About kids don't float. Alaska Department of Natural Resources website. https://dnr.alaska.gov/parks/boating/kdfhome.htm. Accessed March 31, 2025.
21. Hackett P, Shlim D. High elevation travel and altitude illness. *CDC Yellow Book 2024*. Centers for Disease Control and Prevention website. https://wwwnc.cdc.gov/travel/yellowbook/2024/environmental-hazards-risks/high-elevation-travel-and-altitude-illness. Reviewed May 1, 2023. Accessed March 31, 2025.
22. Lightning safety awareness week. National Weather Service website. https://www.weather.gov/iln/lightning-safetyweek. Accessed March 31, 2025.
23. Lightning strike victim data. Centers for Disease Control and Prevention website. https://www.cdc.gov/lightning/data-research/index.html. Published April 15, 2024. Accessed March 31, 2025.
24. Anoka IA, Robb EL, Baker MB. Brown recluse spider toxicity. *StatPearls*. National Library of Medicine website. https://www.ncbi.nlm.nih.gov/books/NBK537045/. Updated August 7, 2023. Accessed March 31, 2025.
25. Ludman SW, Boyle RJ. Stinging insect allergy: current perspectives on venom immunotherapy. *J Asthma Allergy*. 2015;8:75–86.
26. National Center for Health Statistics. Number of deaths from hornet, wasp, and bee stings among males and females—National Vital Statistics System, United States, 2011–2021. Centers for Disease Control and Prevention website. https://www.cdc.gov/mmwr/volumes/72/wr/pdfs/mm7227a6-H.pdf. Accessed March 31, 2025.

Prep Kit continued

27. Snakebite envenoming. World Health Organization website. https://www.who.int/news-room/fact-sheets/detail/snakebite-envenoming. Published September 12, 2023. Accessed March 31, 2025.
28. Venomous snakes. Centers for Disease Control and Prevention website. https://www.cdc.gov/niosh/topics/snakes/default.html. Reviewed June 28, 2021. Accessed March 31, 2025.
29. Tickborne disease surveillance data summary. Centers for Disease Control and Prevention website. https://www.cdc.gov/ticks/data-research/facts-stats/tickborne-disease-surveillance-data-summary.html. Updated July 15, 2024. Accessed March 31, 2025.
30. What to do after a tick bite. Centers for Disease Control and Prevention website. https://www.cdc.gov/ticks/after-a-tick-bite/index.html. Published June 11, 2024. Accessed March 31, 2025.
31. Alpha-gal syndrome and meat allergy. Allergy and Asthma Network website. https://allergyasthmanetwork.org/food-allergies/alpha-gal-syndrome-and-meat-allergy/. Accessed March 31, 2025.

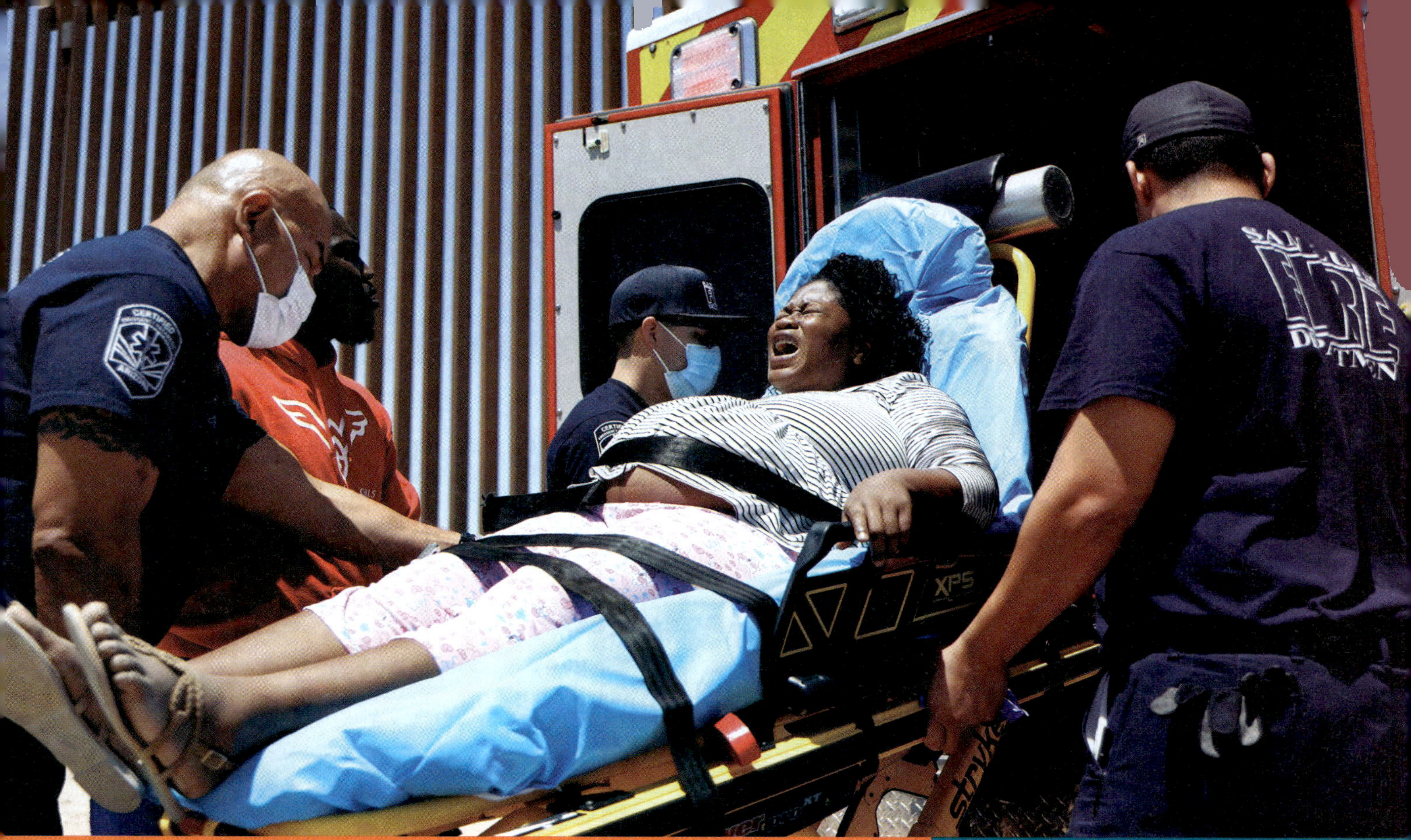

Special Patient Populations

SECTION

8

33 Gynecologic Emergencies

34 Obstetrics and Neonatal Care

35 Patients With Special Challenges

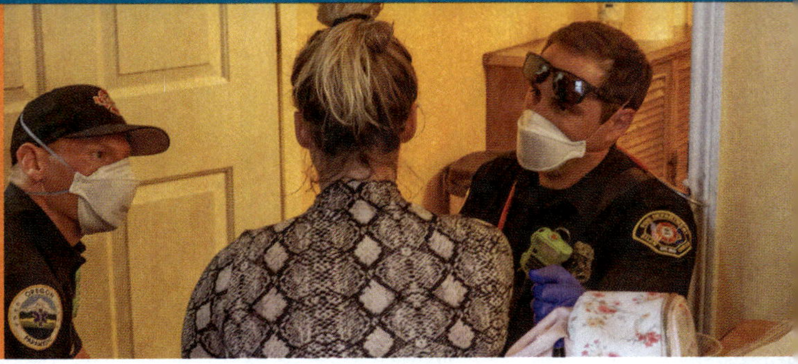

Chapter 33

Gynecologic Emergencies

NATIONAL EMS EDUCATION STANDARD COMPETENCIES

Special Patient Populations

Applies knowledge of growth, development and aging, and assessment findings to provide basic emergency care and transportation for a patient with special needs.

Gynecology

- Vaginal bleeding (p 1247)
- Infections (pp 1245–1247)

KNOWLEDGE OBJECTIVES

1. Describe the anatomy and physiology of the female reproductive system; include the developmental changes that occur during puberty and menopause. (pp 1243–1245)
2. Discuss the special, age-related patient management considerations emergency medical technicians (EMTs) should provide for both younger and older patients who are experiencing gynecologic emergencies. (pp 1244, 1246)
3. List common examples of gynecologic emergencies; include the causes, risk factors, assessment findings, and patient management considerations. (pp 1245–1247)
4. Explain how an EMT would recognize conditions associated with hemorrhage during pregnancy. (p 1247)
5. Discuss the assessment and management of a patient who is experiencing a gynecologic emergency; include a discussion of specific assessment findings. (pp 1247–1252)
6. Explain the general management of a patient who is experiencing a gynecologic emergency in relation to privacy and communication. (pp 1248–1249)
7. Give examples of the personal protective equipment EMTs should use when treating patients with gynecologic emergencies. (pp 1251–1252)

SKILLS OBJECTIVES

There are no skills objectives for this chapter.

Introduction

The female body is uniquely formed to conceive and give birth. This difference makes females susceptible to many conditions that do not occur in males. This chapter examines a few of those conditions. Female anatomy is discussed first, followed by conditions that may be encountered in the prehospital setting. Vaginal bleeding causes are reviewed. Health concerns specific to the very young and the very old are discussed. The principles of treating a patient who has been the victim of sexual assault or rape, as well as recognizing the potential use of date rape drugs, are discussed in Chapter 35, *Patients With Special Challenges*.

Words of Wisdom

Providers should be mindful that a patient who does not identify as female can have gynecologic issues. Thus, the EMS clinician must consider conditions relating to the female reproductive system regardless of the patient's perceived gender.

Because there are unique medical risks associated with being a genotypic male or female, it is important to know this information for the medical record, but it should be ascertained in a sensitive manner. For instance, you may use questions such as, "What gender do you currently identify yourself as?", "What gender were you identified as at birth?", or "Have you had any gender-specific surgeries?"

Anatomy and Physiology

The female reproductive system includes internal and external structures. The external female genitalia consist of the vaginal opening just posterior to the urethral opening (**FIGURE 33-1**). The **labia majora** and **labia minora** are folds of tissue that surround the urethral and vaginal openings. At the anterior end of the labia is the clitoris, and at the posterior end is the anus. The **perineum** is the area of tissue between the vagina and the anus. The labia are extremely vascular and can be injured, but because of their location, they seldom are damaged except in cases of sexual abuse.

In terms of internal structures, the **ovaries** are the primary female reproductive organs (**FIGURE 33-2**). The ovaries are located on each side of the lower abdomen and produce an ovum, or egg, that, if fertilized, will develop into a fetus. The **fallopian tubes** transport the ovum from the ovary to the uterus. The **uterus** is the muscular organ where the fetus grows during pregnancy. The narrowest portion of the uterus, the **cervix**, opens into the vagina. The **vagina** is the outermost cavity of a woman's reproductive system and forms the lower part of the birth canal.

When females reach puberty, they begin to ovulate and experience menstruation. **Ovulation** is the cycle in which the ovum is released. The onset of menstruation is called *menarche* and usually occurs between the ages of 11 and 16 years, although it can occur earlier or later. Any female who has reached

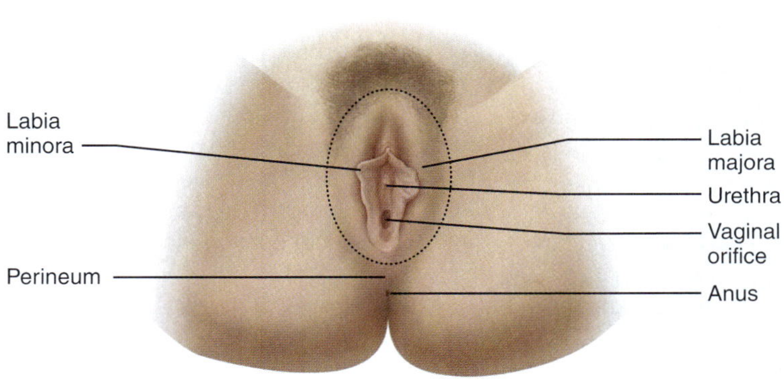

FIGURE 33-1 The external genitalia of the female reproductive system.

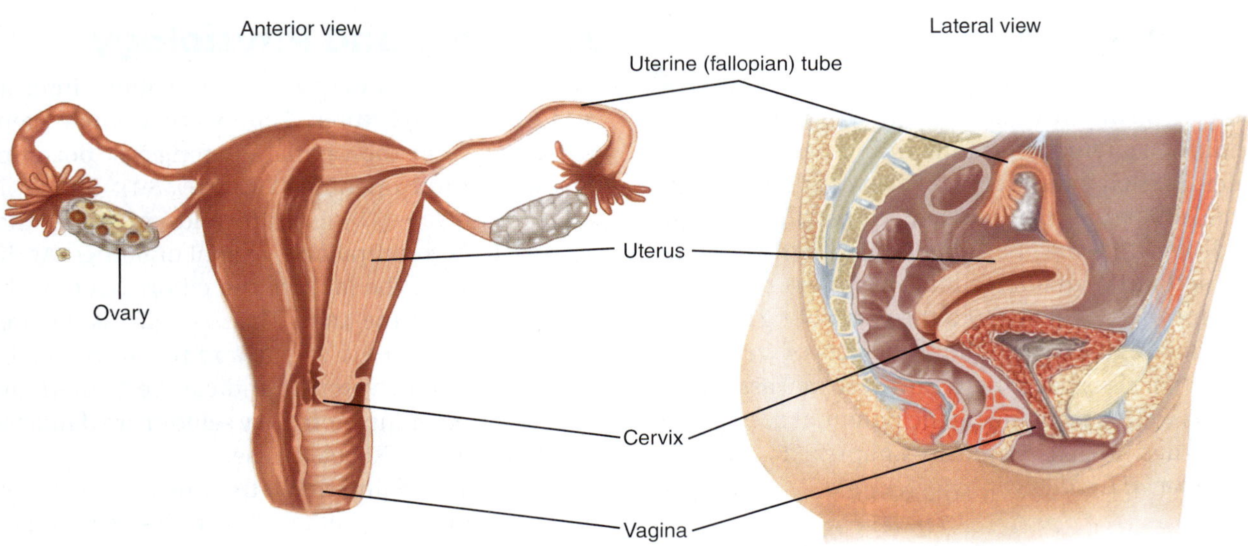

FIGURE 33-2 Anterior and lateral views of the female reproductive system.

menarche is capable of becoming pregnant. Women continue to experience the cycle of ovulation and menstruation until they reach *menopause,* which marks the end of menstrual activity. Women reach menopause at widely varying ages, but it commonly occurs around the age of 50 years.

Special Populations

UNDERSTANDING MENARCHE

The onset of menarche in females can be an emotionally and physically disturbing event. It is not uncommon for this event to be preceded by cramping pain that can be misinterpreted by the child who has not yet experienced menstruation. Most young females will have learned about the menstrual process from their parents, peers, social media, or school health classes, but some are still unprepared when it occurs. Young females from low-income families may be less prepared for the onset of their menstruation.[1] Parents may also be in denial, insisting that their child is too young to be experiencing menstruation.

Approach the patient (and parents) in the most professional manner possible. It is essential to be comfortable speaking to patients about gynecologic illnesses. The EMT should communicate in a direct and professional manner using appropriate terms. Empathize with their concerns.

Special Populations

UNDERSTANDING MENOPAUSE

Menopause is the permanent cessation of the menstrual cycle. It typically occurs between 45 and 58 years of age.[2] The process of menopause is complicated. As menopause approaches, menstrual periods may become irregular and vary in severity. It is not uncommon for women at this stage to continue to have irregular menstrual periods for several months to 1 year as the process progresses. It is important to recognize that during this time it is still possible for women to become pregnant. If a couple no longer uses birth control methods because they believe pregnancy cannot occur, they may be in denial when they see signs of pregnancy. Treat patients with compassion and reassure them, but also transport them for examination by a physician to determine if this or something else (such as a tumor or cyst) is causing the problem.

Be sensitive that individuals often struggle emotionally as well as physically with the changes that occur during menopause.

Each ovary produces an ovum during each menstrual cycle. Usually, only one ovum is released into the fallopian tube. The ovaries do not necessarily alternate each menstrual cycle with regard to which ovary's ovum is released. Some women experience minor cramping pain during ovulation when an ovum is released. The pain is sometimes described as a dull pain on one side of the lower abdomen. The quality and severity of the pain vary for each woman.

The process of fertilization begins in the vagina, where sperm from the male penis are deposited in the female reproductive tract. The sperm pass through the cervix into the uterus and eventually up the fallopian tubes. As the ovum moves slowly down the fallopian tube, sperm moving up the tube can surround it. The goal is for a sperm to fertilize the ovum. When an ovum is fertilized in the fallopian tube, the developing embryo travels into the uterus, where the lining of the walls of the uterus has become engorged with blood in anticipation of receiving a fertilized ovum. Here, the embryo attaches to the uterine wall and continues to grow.

If the ovum is not fertilized in the fallopian tube, it continues to travel into the uterus. The period of ovulation during which fertilization may occur is about 14 days. If the ovum is not fertilized in this time, the lining of the uterus begins to separate and menstruation occurs. The menstrual flow consists of blood from the separated lining of the uterus and typically lasts 2 to 7 days.[3] Female hormones produced primarily in the ovaries control the process of ovulation and menstruation.

Pathophysiology

The causes of gynecologic emergencies are varied and range from sexually transmitted infections (STIs) to trauma. You should recognize and properly treat female patients with any kind of abdominal or pelvic pain and consider problems that could be potentially life threatening.

Pelvic Inflammatory Disease

Pelvic inflammatory disease (PID) is an infection of the upper female reproductive organs—specifically, the uterus, ovaries, and fallopian tubes—that occurs almost exclusively in sexually active women. Disease-causing organisms enter the vagina during sexual activity and migrate through the opening of the cervix and into the uterine cavity. The infection may then expand to the fallopian tubes and cause scarring that increases the risk of sterility or life-threatening events such as ectopic pregnancy. Ectopic pregnancy is a pregnancy that develops outside the uterus, most often in the fallopian tube. If the ovaries are affected, PID can lead to the development of a life-threatening abscess.

The most common presenting sign of PID is generalized lower abdominal pain. The pain generally starts during or after normal menstruation, so inquiring about the date of the patient's last menstrual period is an important detail of the patient's history. The pain may be described as achy and may be made worse by walking, possibly causing the patient to walk with a shuffling gait.

Other signs and symptoms include an abnormal and often foul-smelling vaginal discharge, increased pain during sexual intercourse, fever and chills, general malaise, pain or burning on urination, and nausea and vomiting. Risk factors associated with PID include having multiple sex partners and/or a partner who has had sex with multiple people, having an untreated STI, having a past history

YOU are the EMT

At 1355 hours, you are dispatched to the middle school at 4300 West Avenue for a female patient presenting with abdominal pain. You and your partner respond to the scene, which is located about 4 miles away. While you are en route, dispatch notifies you that the patient is located in the Student Health Office. The weather is overcast, the temperature is 78°F (26°C), and the traffic is light.

1. What medical problems come to mind based on this dispatch information?
2. What questions will be important to ask on this call?

of PID, being younger than 26 years, douching, and using an intrauterine device for birth control.[4]

Sexually Transmitted Infections

STIs can lead to more serious conditions. For example, untreated gonorrhea and chlamydia often progress to PID.

> **Special Populations**
>
> **PREVALENCE OF STIS AMONG GERIATRIC PATIENTS**
>
> Your differential diagnosis should include STIs even if your patient is older. Older adults remain sexually active into their 70s and often later. The incidence of STIs is increasing in patients older than 65 years and is outpacing the increase in the general population. Reasons for this include underestimation of risk, use of erectile dysfunction drugs, hormone therapy in women, and lack of education about STIs.[5,6]

Chlamydia is caused by the bacterium *Chlamydia trachomatis.* According to the Centers for Disease Control and Prevention (CDC), chlamydia is currently the most commonly reported STI in the United States.[7] Although the symptoms of chlamydia are usually mild or absent, some women may report lower abdominal pain, low back pain, nausea, fever, pain during sexual intercourse, and/or bleeding between menstrual periods. Chlamydial infection of the cervix can spread to the rectum, leading to rectal pain, discharge, or bleeding. If it is left untreated, the disease can progress to PID. In rare cases, chlamydia causes arthritis that may be accompanied by skin lesions and inflammation of the eye and urethra.

Bacterial vaginosis is the most common vaginal infection in women age 15 to 44 years, according to the CDC.[8] In this infection, normal bacteria in the vagina are replaced by an overgrowth of other bacterial forms. Symptoms may include itching, burning, or pain and may be accompanied by a "fishy," foul-smelling discharge. Pregnant women with bacterial vaginosis may have premature babies or babies born with low birth weight. If it is left untreated, bacterial vaginosis can lead to more serious infections or result in PID.

Gonorrhea is caused by *Neisseria gonorrhoeae,* a bacterium that can grow and multiply rapidly in the warm, moist areas of the reproductive tract, including the cervix, uterus, and fallopian tubes in

YOU are the EMT

You arrive at the scene and find the patient, a 14-year-old female, lying on her side with her knees flexed on a cot in the health office. She is conscious and alert but is crying. After introducing yourself and your partner, you perform a primary assessment.

Recording Time: 0 Minutes	
Appearance	Obvious distress
Level of consciousness	Conscious and alert
Airway	Open; clear of secretions and foreign bodies
Breathing	Normal rate; adequate depth
Circulation	Radial pulses slightly increased and strong; skin is baseline color, warm, and moist; no obvious bleeding

The patient tells you that her pain started suddenly after lunch. She is normally healthy, has no previous medical problems, and takes no medications. The patient points to the right lower quadrant of her abdomen when asked the location of her pain. She says that lying on her side seems to make it a little bit better and that she feels slightly nauseated but has not vomited.

3. What immediate medical treatment, if any, does this patient require?

4. On the basis of this initial information, what additional specific questions should you ask?

women and in the urethra in women and men. The bacterium can also grow in the mouth, throat, eyes, and anus. Symptoms, which are generally more severe in men than in women, appear approximately 2 to 10 days after exposure. Women may be infected with gonorrhea for months but not have any symptoms, or only mild ones, until the infection has spread to other parts of the reproductive system. If untreated, gonorrheal infection can lead to infertility or ectopic pregnancy, or the bacteria can spread to the joints, skin, heart, or even meninges.[9]

When symptoms do appear in women, they generally present as painful urination, with associated burning or itching; a yellowish or bloody vaginal discharge, usually with a foul odor; and blood associated with vaginal sexual intercourse. More severe infections may present with cramping and abdominal pain, nausea and vomiting, and bleeding between menstrual periods; these symptoms indicate that the infection has progressed to PID. Rectal infections generally present with anal discharge and itching and occasional painful bowel movements with fecal blood spotting. Infection of the throat (for which oral sex is the introducing factor) usually results in mild symptoms consisting of painful or difficult swallowing, sore throat, swollen lymph glands, and fever. Headache and nasal congestion may also be present. If the infection is not treated, in rare cases the bacterium may enter the bloodstream and spread to other parts of the body, causing sepsis.[10]

Safety Tips

Remember that many STIs can also be transmitted by contact with blood. Some examples of these diseases include syphilis, many types of hepatitis, and human immunodeficiency virus.

Vaginal Bleeding

Because menstrual bleeding occurs monthly in most women, vaginal bleeding that is the result of other causes may initially be overlooked. Some possible causes of vaginal bleeding include abnormal menstruation, vaginal trauma, ectopic pregnancy, spontaneous abortion (miscarriage), cervical polyps, and cancer. Trauma to the internal female genitalia from any cause other than vaginal penetration is rare because these organs are located deep within the pelvis. Injuries to the vagina and external genitalia are painful and serious because of the large number of nerves and blood vessels in this area. In contrast, internal bleeding from polyps or cancer, while also serious, may be relatively painless.

Ectopic pregnancy and spontaneous abortion are two conditions that can cause vaginal bleeding in women early in pregnancy who may not realize they are pregnant. All cases of vaginal bleeding should be taken seriously, and the patient should be evaluated by a physician for a thorough gynecologic examination. Ectopic pregnancy and spontaneous abortion, both potentially life-threatening conditions, are covered in Chapter 34, *Obstetrics and Neonatal Care.*

Patient Assessment

Obtaining an accurate and detailed patient assessment is critically important when dealing with gynecologic issues. You will be able to gain only a primary impression of the problem in the field, yet a thorough patient assessment will help determine just how sick the patient is and whether you should initiate lifesaving measures. This is especially true when dealing with abdominal pain.

Women experience many of the same conditions that cause abdominal pain in men, such as ulcers and appendicitis. In addition, there are numerous gynecologic causes of abdominal pain. Examples include ectopic pregnancy, ovarian cyst, endometriosis (the growth of uterine tissue outside of the uterus), pelvic inflammatory disease, and miscarriage. Missing the diagnosis may be fatal for the patient, especially in the case of ectopic pregnancy.

Words of Wisdom

Gynecologic emergencies can occur at any age. Focus on assessing and correcting the patient's ABCs (Airway, Breathing, and Circulation), and prioritize rapid transport.

Scene Size-up

Every emergency call, including calls involving gynecologic emergencies, begins with a thorough scene size-up. Is the scene safe? Will you need

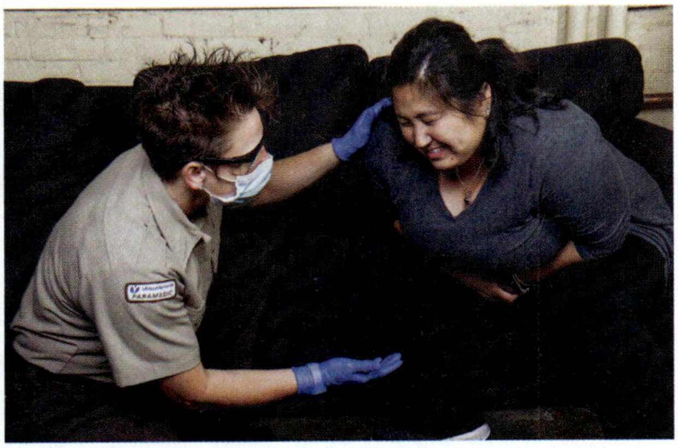

FIGURE 33-3 Note the position of the patient during your assessment.

assistance? How many patients do you have? What is the nature of illness (NOI) or mechanism of injury (MOI)? Have you taken standard precautions? Gynecologic emergencies can be messy, sometimes involving significant amounts of blood and body fluids contaminated with organisms that can potentially cause communicable diseases.

Where and in what position is the patient found (**FIGURE 33-3**)? If the patient is at home, what is the condition of the residence? All of the information you obtain contributes to your assessment of the patient's overall health and the safety of the scene. Your documentation needs to be accurate and thorough. Involve law enforcement if any type of assault is suspected.

Often, the NOI or MOI in patients with gynecologic emergencies will be understood from the dispatch information, such as in cases of sexual assault. In many patients, the exact nature of the condition will not emerge until you gather patient history information. For example, your patient may present with vague symptoms such as abdominal pain, and you will not be able to determine the exact nature of the problem until you gather more information during the patient history.

Primary Assessment

The general impression is an important aspect of all patient assessments. As you approach the patient, you should quickly determine if the person's condition is stable or unstable. Use this information to help you as you proceed further with the assessment. Use the AVPU scale to determine the patient's level of consciousness.

Always evaluate the airway and breathing immediately to ensure they are adequate, and treat any airway or breathing problem that is identified according to established guidelines and local protocol. Identifying and treating life threats takes precedence over all other assessment and treatment.

It is important to carefully assess circulation in all patients. Palpate a pulse and evaluate skin color, temperature, and moisture to help identify the patient who might have blood loss. Because skin paleness can be difficult to detect in patients with dark skin, look for pale mucous membranes inside the inner lower eyelid or check for slow capillary refill. On general observation, the patient may appear ashen or gray. A patient who has experienced significant blood loss because of vaginal bleeding may not demonstrate obvious signs of shock but may still be hypovolemic. If the patient has a weak or rapid pulse or has pale, cool, or diaphoretic skin, place the patient in a supine position. Cover the patient to keep them warm, and then transport to the nearest appropriate hospital for treatment.

Most gynecologic emergencies are not life threatening; however, if signs of shock exist because of bleeding, then rapid transport is necessary. The remainder of the assessment can be performed en route to the hospital.

History Taking

Begin by asking about the patient's chief complaint, but realize some of the questions you must ask may be considered extremely personal. Be sensitive to the patient's feelings and ensure privacy and dignity are protected. Gynecologic emergencies can be highly embarrassing for patients, and many people are extremely uncomfortable discussing their sexual history in front of strangers or even close family members. Adolescent patients may want to keep their sexual history from their parents.

For a report of abdominal pain, ask specific questions about the current event. OPQRST (Onset, Provocation/palliation, Quality, Region/radiation, Severity, Timing) is a good guide to help with your questioning. When was the onset of the discomfort? Is there anything that makes the pain better or worse? Ask the patient to describe the pain. It may be dull and cramping or sharp and stabbing in nature. Also ask if the pain moves or is recognized anywhere else. Establishing a pain scale (ie, severity) can help gauge illness progression and the effects of treatment and determine how long the patient has been experiencing pain. Associated symptoms such as syncope, light-headedness, nausea, vomiting, and fever are also relevant. For a report of vaginal bleeding, ask about onset, duration, quantity (number of sanitary pads or tampons soaked), and associated symptoms such as syncope and light-headedness.

Obtain a SAMPLE (Signs and symptoms, Allergies, Medications, Pertinent past medical history, Last oral intake, Events leading up to the illness or injury) history beginning with the current symptoms. Note any allergies the patient has or any over-the-counter or prescription medications the patient is taking, such as drugs to reduce the risk of acquiring human immunodeficiency virus (HIV) or birth control pills, or any other birth control method being used. Ask the patient about medical conditions. Also ask specifically about the last menstrual period, which will help determine if the patient is possibly pregnant. Not every woman has a menstrual cycle every month, which may make determining the possibility of pregnancy challenging. Do not let your guard down by ruling out pregnancy as a possibility. Ask about the possibility of STIs and the possibility of pregnancy. Find out when the patient last ate or drank and what events led up to the calling for EMS. Use the history of events, chief complaint, and answers to your other questions to lead further questioning. For example, if the patient reports having intercourse, ask about birth control and about symptoms of pregnancy. If the patient has vaginal bleeding, ask how many sanitary pads or tampons are being used per hour. This information can help create an estimate of blood loss.

Secondary Assessment

The secondary assessment may be performed on scene, en route to the emergency department (ED), or, in some instances, not at all. If the patient is critically ill or injured or the transport time is short, you may not have time to conduct this part of the patient assessment process.

Pertinent secondary assessment findings should include:

- **Vital signs.** Blood pressure, pulse, skin color, orthostatic vital signs
- **Abdomen.** Distention and tenderness
- **Genitourinary.** Visible bleeding
- **Neurologic.** Mental status

Your physical examination of a gynecologic patient should be limited and professional. Examine the genitalia only if doing so is necessary to treat the patient. Protect the patient's privacy during the physical examination; however, having a chaperone

YOU are the EMT

The patient remains anxious and alert but is still in obvious pain. She gives you consent to take her vital signs. She tells you she has never had sex, that her menstrual period ended last week and was normal, and that she noticed a small amount of vaginal bleeding after the pain began that has not even soaked a mini-pad.

Recording Time: 8 Minutes	
Respirations	14 breaths/min; adequate depth
Pulse	100 beats/min; strong and regular
Skin	Baseline color, warm, and moist
Blood pressure	102/70 mm Hg
Oxygen saturation (Spo_2)	98% (on room air)

5. What additional assessment should you perform on this patient?

6. What must you do prior to transporting this patient?

is advised. Few people are comfortable with having their body exposed to a crowd of family, neighbors, EMTs, police officers, or firefighters. Limit the personnel present to only those required to perform the necessary tasks; show patients you respect them by being an advocate for their modesty. You also serve as a role model for other EMS clinicians when you act this way.

Street Smarts

If it is absolutely necessary to assess the patient's genital area, it is advised to ask the patient's permission as with all interventions, and have another crew member chaperone the examination. While some patients prefer to have a caregiver of the same gender care for them when sensitive gynecologic or genitourinary conditions are present, this is not always possible, especially in the prehospital setting. Data show that in 2017 only 35% of EMTs were female, and there is little information regarding gender diversity in EMS.[11,12]

The population of women older than 65 years is increasing, and although they are past their childbearing years, many will have other gynecologic problems. They may have concerns specific to hormone replacement therapy, may have an increased risk of cancer, or could be experiencing internal physical changes in the female organs associated with aging (eg, pelvic floor prolapse, urinary incontinence). Although these problems cannot be treated in the prehospital environment, perform and record a thorough assessment and treat any of the patient's immediate needs.

Focus your physical examination on the history of events and the patient's chief complaint. If vaginal bleeding is present, you should ask about its quality and quantity. You need to look at vaginal bleeding when it is sufficient to cause shock. If questioning suggests less aggressive bleeding and no evidence of shock, privacy takes precedence, and examination is deferred to the ED. Use external sanitary pads to absorb the bleeding and keep the possibility of hypoperfusion or shock in mind. Always ask if there is pain associated with the vaginal bleeding or discharge. Never insert anything, including a tampon, into the vagina to control bleeding.

Vaginal discharge does not need to be visualized if the patient reports that no bleeding is present and if the vital signs are normal. Ask the patient to describe the characteristics and history of the discharge, and document this information. A transport decision is based on the patient's vital signs.

Fever, nausea, and vomiting are common with many medical conditions but should be considered especially significant with gynecologic emergencies. Fever should always be considered a sign of an infectious process. Any report of syncope from the patient, especially if the patient reports vaginal

YOU are the EMT

When you palpate the patient's abdomen, you note rebound tenderness in the right lower quadrant. The patient and her parents wish for her to be transported to a nearby hospital. You secure her to the stretcher, reassess her vital signs, and begin transport. You also bring along health information the school has provided.

Recording Time: 28 Minutes	
Level of consciousness	Conscious and alert
Respirations	14 breaths/min; adequate depth
Pulse	98 beats/min; strong and regular
Skin	Baseline color, warm, and dry
Blood pressure	104/68 mm Hg
Oxygen saturation (Spo_2)	99% (on room air)

7. Why is it important to continuously reassess this patient's vital signs if they are stable?

8. What information is important to share with the hospital?

bleeding, is considered significant. Treat the patient reporting this symptom as being in shock until proven otherwise.

Street Smarts

As EMS clinicians, even though we are there to help patients, we are "invading" their personal space. During the assessment, explain to patients what you are about to do and why. This will help gain their trust and confidence.

Assess the patient's vital signs, including heart rate, rhythm, and quality; respiratory rate, rhythm, and quality; skin color, temperature, and condition; capillary refill time; and blood pressure. Consider obtaining orthostatic vital signs if bleeding is known or suspected. Pay special attention to the presence of tachycardia and hypotension, which could be early indicators of hemorrhagic shock.

Monitor the patient's condition frequently to watch for changes in vital signs and mental status. Consider using noninvasive blood pressure monitoring to continuously track the patient's blood pressure. Remember, pulse oximetry readings may not be accurate in the setting of hypovolemia.

Reassessment

Repeat the primary assessment. Reassess the patient's vital signs and the chief complaint. Reassess the patient's vital signs every 5 minutes to identify hypoperfusion from excessive blood loss. If the patient shows signs of shock, begin treatment and rapid transport.

How is the patient's condition improving with the interventions? Identify and treat any changes in the patient's condition. For example, a patient who appears to be losing consciousness should be positioned in the supine position and reassessed. Finally, pay specific attention to your patient's needs and respect the person's desire for conversation or silence. Provide the patient with calm reassurance. Explain that the hospital staff will be well qualified to provide treatment.

Emergency Medical Care

There are few interventions that can or should be done for a patient with a gynecologic emergency. Patients with vaginal bleeding should be treated for hypoperfusion or shock. Keep them warm, place them in a supine position, and provide supplemental oxygen even if they are not experiencing

YOU are the EMT

You reassess the patient en route to the hospital; her mental status and vital signs indicate that she is stable. You call your radio report to the receiving facility and give them your estimated time of arrival.

Recording Time: 38 Minutes	
Level of consciousness	Conscious and alert
Respirations	16 breaths/min; adequate depth
Pulse	98 beats/min; strong and regular
Skin	Baseline color, warm, and dry
Blood pressure	102/70 mm Hg
Oxygen saturation (Spo_2)	99% (on room air)

You learn later that the hospital determined from diagnostic testing that she had an ovarian cyst. She was later discharged home with her family

9. Why is it important to transport a patient who has this type of abdominal pain to the hospital, even if the individual is in stable condition?

difficulty breathing. Consider advanced life support intercept for fluid replacement depending on transport times and local protocols, then transport to the nearest appropriate receiving facility.

Use sanitary pads on the external genitalia to absorb the blood. Tampons that are already in place do not need to be removed. If the bleeding relates to sexual trauma, be aware that the genitals have a rich nerve supply, making injuries very painful. Treat any external lacerations, abrasions, and tears with sterile compresses, using local pressure to control bleeding and a diaper-type bandage to hold the dressings in place. Leave any foreign bodies in place after stabilizing them with bandages. Under no circumstances should you pack or place dressings inside the vagina.

Continue to assess patients while transporting them to the ED. Contusions and other blunt trauma will require careful in-hospital evaluation. Notify staff at the receiving hospital of all relevant information, including the possibility of pregnancy, so a proper response can be prepared. Carefully document the patient's condition and chief complaint, the scene details, and all interventions, especially in cases of sexual assault.

Street Smarts

Ectopic pregnancy is a life-threatening condition that may present with only a small amount of vaginal bleeding. This is a case where the amount of bleeding you observe externally may mislead you. Carefully observe for signs of shock in any patient who has vaginal bleeding and abdominal pain.

Safety Tips

Gynecologic emergencies may involve significant blood and body fluids. PPE, including gloves, eye protection, and a mask, must be considered.

YOU are the EMT SUMMARY

1. What medical problems come to mind based on this dispatch information?

Abdominal pain can signal a wide range of problems, including trauma; GI problems such as gastroenteritis, appendicitis, inflammatory bowel diseases, and constipation; gynecologic illnesses such as pelvic inflammatory disease, ovarian cyst, and endometriosis; or pregnancy-related problems.

2. What questions will be important to ask on this call?

Questions should include:

- How old is the patient?
- What are the characteristics of the pain? Specifically, where is the pain located? What does it feel like? When did it start? What was happening when it started? What makes it better or worse?
- What other signs or symptoms are present?
- When was the last meal, bowel movement, and menstrual period? Is there a chance of pregnancy?
- What past illnesses does the patient have, and what medications does she take?

3. What immediate medical treatment, if any, does this patient require?

No immediate interventions are indicated at this time. A full set of vital signs should be obtained.

4. On the basis of this initial information, what additional specific questions should you ask?

While maintaining the patient's privacy, at this point you should ask:

- When was your last bowel movement and was it normal?
- When was your last menstrual period and was it normal? Is there any chance you could be pregnant, or have you ever had sex?
- Do you have any vaginal bleeding? If yes, how much (eg, spotting or heavy bleeding that soaks a specific number of sanitary napkins/pads)?
- Do you have any unusual vaginal discharge? If yes, what color, when did it start, and does it smell bad?

YOU are the EMT SUMMARY continued

5. What additional assessment should you perform on this patient?

You should palpate the patient's abdomen, beginning in the area farthest from her pain. You should not examine her perineum, as there is no apparent reason to do so.

6. What must you do prior to transporting this patient?

Prior to transport, you should ask the patient for her assent to do so and then contact her parents to explain the situation, ask their preference of hospital, and get their consent for transport. If time permits, allow the child to briefly speak to her parents.

7. Why is it important to continuously reassess this patient's vital signs if they are stable?

Repeat vital signs are essential for this patient because, despite her denial of pregnancy, there is a small chance she is not being truthful; if she were pregnant, her signs and symptoms would suggest ectopic pregnancy and she could deteriorate rapidly.

8. What information is important to share with the hospital?

You must report the patient's age, sex, menstrual history, and the characteristics of her pain. Additionally, state the present vital signs and note that they have remained stable.

9. Why is it important to transport a patient who has this type of abdominal pain to the hospital, even if the individual is in stable condition?

EMTs should transport this patient because they lack the diagnostic tools to rule out life-threatening causes of abdominal pain.

Prep Kit

Ready for Review

- The female body is uniquely formed to conceive and give birth. This difference makes females susceptible to a number of conditions that do not occur in males.
- If fertilization of the ovum does not occur within about 14 days of ovulation, the lining of the uterus begins to separate and menstruation occurs and lasts for about 1 week.
- When females reach puberty, they begin to ovulate and experience menstruation. They continue to experience the cycle of ovulation and menstruation until they reach menopause.
- The causes of gynecologic emergencies are varied and range from STIs to trauma.
- Pelvic inflammatory disease (PID) is an infection of the upper female reproductive organs: the uterus, ovaries, and fallopian tubes. PID can lead to an ectopic pregnancy or an abscess, which can cause death.
- STIs can lead to more serious conditions, such as pelvic inflammatory disease.
- Because menstrual bleeding occurs every month in most women, vaginal bleeding that is the result of other causes may initially be overlooked. Some possible causes of vaginal bleeding include abnormal menstruation, vaginal trauma, ectopic pregnancy, spontaneous abortion, cervical polyps, ectopic pregnancy, miscarriage, and even cancer.
- There are few interventions that can or should be done in the prehospital setting to treat a gynecologic emergency.
- Whenever you care for patients who have a gynecologic emergency, you must maintain the patients' privacy as much as possible.

Prep Kit continued

Vital Vocabulary

bacterial vaginosis An overgrowth of bacteria in the vagina; characterized by itching, burning, or pain, and possibly a "fishy"-smelling discharge.

cervix The lower third, or neck, of the uterus.

chlamydia A sexually transmitted infection caused by the bacterium *Chlamydia trachomatis.*

fallopian tubes The tubes that connect each ovary with the uterus and are the primary location for fertilization of the ovum.

gonorrhea A sexually transmitted infection caused by *Neisseria gonorrhoeae.*

labia majora Outer fleshy "lips" covered with pubic hair that protect the vagina.

labia minora Inner fleshy "lips" devoid of pubic hair that protect the vagina.

ovaries The primary female reproductive organs that produce an ovum, or egg, that, if fertilized, will develop into a fetus.

ovulation The process in which an ovum is released from a follicle.

pelvic inflammatory disease (PID) An infection of the fallopian tubes and the surrounding tissues of the pelvis.

perineum The area of skin between the genitals and the anus.

uterus The muscular organ where the fetus grows, also called the womb; responsible for contractions during labor.

vagina The outermost cavity of a woman's reproductive tract; the lower part of the birth canal.

References

1. Herbert AC, Ramirez AM, Lee G, et al. Puberty experiences of low-income girls in the United States: a systematic review of qualitative literature from 2000 to 2014. *J Adolesc Health*. 2017;60(4):363–379.
2. Menopause basics. Office on Women's Health website. https://www.womenshealth.gov/menopause/menopause-basics. Updated January 6, 2023. Accessed August 8, 2024.
3. Heavy and abnormal periods. The American College of Obstetricians and Gynecologists website. Reviewed April 2024. Accessed February 11, 2025.
4. Division of STD Prevention, National Center for HIV, Viral Hepatitis, STD, and TB Prevention, Centers for Disease Control and Prevention. About pelvic inflammatory disease (PID). Centers for Disease Control and Prevention website. https://www.cdc.gov/pid/about. Updated December 13, 2023. Accessed August 8, 2024.
5. Gangestad, A. Why STIs are on the rise in older adults. University Hospitals website. https://www.uhhospitals.org/blog/articles/2023/07/why-stis-are-on-the-rise-in-older-adults. Published July 11, 2023. Accessed August 8, 2024.
6. Harvard Health Publishing. Sexually transmitted disease? At my age? Harvard Health Publishing website. https://www.health.harvard.edu/diseases-and-conditions/sexually-transmitted-disease-at-my-age. Published February 1, 2018. Accessed August 8, 2024.
7. Division of STD Prevention, National Center for HIV, Viral Hepatitis, STD, and TB Prevention, Centers for Disease Control and Prevention. Sexually transmitted infections treatment guidelines, 2021. Chlamydial infections. Centers for Disease Control and Prevention website. https://www.cdc.gov/std/treatment-guidelines/chlamydia.htm. Updated July 22, 2021. Accessed August 8, 2024.
8. Division of STD Prevention, National Center for HIV, Viral Hepatitis, STD, and TB Prevention, Centers for Disease Control and Prevention. Bacterial vaginosis—CDC basic fact sheet. Centers for Disease Control and Prevention website. https://www.cdc.gov/bacterial-vaginosis/about. Updated December 11, 2023. Accessed August 8, 2024.
9. Li R, Hatcher JD. Gonococcal arthritis. *StatPearls*. National Library of Medicine website. https://www.ncbi.nlm.nih.gov/books/NBK470439/. Updated May 29, 2023. Accessed February 11, 2025.
10. Complications: gonorrhoea. National Health Service website. https://www.nhs.uk/conditions/gonorrhoea/complications/. Reviewed September 15, 2021. Accessed August 8, 2024.
11. Crowe RP, Krebs W, Cash RE, Rivard MK, Lincoln EW, Panchal AR. Females and minority racial/ethnic groups remain underrepresented in emergency medical services: a ten-year assessment, 2008–2017. *Prehosp Emerg Care*. 2020;24(2):180–187.
12. Rudman JS, Farcas A, Salazar GA, et al. Diversity, equity, and inclusion in the United States emergency medical services workforce: a scoping review. *Prehosp Emerg Care*. 2023;27(4):385–397.

Prep Kit continued

Additional Resources

Ecochard R, Gougeon A. Side of ovulation and cycle characteristics in normally fertile women. *Hum Reprod*. 2000;15(4):752–755.

National Association of State EMS Officials. *National Model EMS Clinical Guidelines: Version 3.0.* https://nasemso.org/wp-content/uploads/National-Model-EMS-Clinical-Guidelines_2022.pdf. Updated March 2022. Accessed August 8, 2024.

National Highway Traffic Safety Administration. *National Emergency Medical Services Education Standards*. https://www.ems.gov/assets/EMS_Education-Standards_2021_FNL.pdf. Published January 2021. Accessed August 8, 2024.

Zink N. CE article: sensitive subject. EMS World website. https://www.hmpgloballearningnetwork.com/site/emsworld/education/ce-article-sensitive-subject. Published October 2021. Accessed August 8, 2024.

Chapter 34

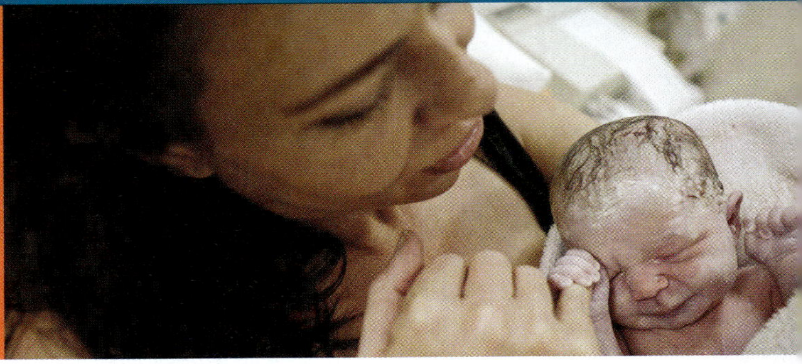

Obstetrics and Neonatal Care

NATIONAL EMS EDUCATION STANDARD COMPETENCIES

Special Patient Populations

Applies knowledge of growth, development, and aging and assessment findings to provide basic emergency care and transportation for a patient with special needs.

Obstetrics

- Normal delivery (pp 1271–1282)
- Vaginal bleeding in the pregnant patient (pp 1262–1264)
- Normal pregnancy (anatomy and physiology) (pp 1260–1261)
- Pathophysiology of complications of pregnancy (pp 1261–1267)
- Assessment of the pregnant patient (pp 1267–1270)
- Abnormal delivery
  - Nuchal cord (p 1279)
  - Prolapsed cord (pp 1288–1289)
  - Breech delivery (pp 1287–1289)
  - Shoulder dystocia (p 1287)
  - Prematurity (p 1290)
  - Multiparity (pp 1289–1290)
- Third-trimester bleeding and antepartum bleeding
  - Placenta previa (pp 1263–1264)
  - Abruptio placentae (pp 1263–1264)
- Spontaneous abortion/miscarriage (p 1264)
- Ectopic pregnancy (p 1263)
- Preeclampsia/eclampsia (pp 1261–1262)
- Postpartum complications (p 1291)

Neonatal Care

- Newborn stabilization (pp 1276–1280)
- Neonatal resuscitation (pp 1282–1283)

Trauma

Applies knowledge to provide basic emergency care and transportation based on assessment findings for an acutely injured patient.

Special Considerations in Trauma

- Pregnant patient (pp 1265–1267)
- Pediatric patient (Chapter 35, *Patients With Special Challenges*)
- Geriatric patient (Chapter 35, *Patients With Special Challenges*)
- Cognitively impaired patient (Chapter 35, *Patients With Special Challenges*)

KNOWLEDGE OBJECTIVES

1. Identify the anatomy and physiology of the female reproductive system. (pp 1258–1260)
2. Explain the normal changes that occur in the body during pregnancy. (pp 1260–1261)

3. Recognize complications of pregnancy including abuse, substance misuse, hypertensive disorders, bleeding, spontaneous abortion (miscarriage), and gestational diabetes. (pp 1261–1267)
4. Discuss the need to consider two patients—the mother and the unborn fetus—when treating a pregnant trauma patient. (pp 1265–1267)
5. Discuss special considerations involving pregnancy in different cultures and with teenage patients. (p 1267)
6. Explain assessment of the pregnant patient. (pp 1267–1270)
7. Explain the significance of meconium in the amniotic fluid. (p 1269)
8. Differentiate among the three stages of labor. (pp 1270–1271)
9. Describe the indications of an imminent delivery. (pp 1271–1272)
10. Explain the steps involved in normal delivery management. (pp 1271–1282)
11. List the contents of an obstetrics kit. (pp 1272–1273)
12. Explain the necessary care of the fetus as the head appears. (p 1279)
13. Describe the procedure followed to clamp and cut the umbilical cord. (p 1279)
14. Describe delivery of the placenta. (pp 1281–1282)
15. Explain the steps to take in neonatal assessment and resuscitation. (pp 1282–1287)
16. Recognize complicated delivery emergencies, including shoulder dystocia, breech presentations, limb presentations, umbilical cord prolapse, spina bifida, multiple gestation, preterm birth, postterm pregnancy, and fetal demise. (pp 1287–1291)
17. Describe postpartum complications and how to treat them. (p 1291)

SKILLS OBJECTIVES

1. Demonstrate how to prepare the delivery area, including donning sterile gloves (p 1274; Skill Drill 34-1)
2. Demonstrate the procedure to assist in a normal cephalic delivery. (pp 1276–1278; Skill Drill 34-2)
3. Demonstrate how to clamp and cut the umbilical cord. (pp 1278–1279)
4. Demonstrate the steps to follow in postdelivery care of the newborn. (pp 1280–1282)
5. Demonstrate how to assist in delivery of the placenta. (pp 1281–1282)
6. Demonstrate the postdelivery care of the mother. (p 1280)
7. Demonstrate procedures to follow for complicated delivery emergencies, including vaginal bleeding, shoulder dystocia, breech presentation, limb presentation, and prolapsed umbilical cord. (pp 1287–1291)

Introduction

While most childbirths in the United States occur in a health care setting with trained medical personnel in attendance, the rate of births occurring in out-of-hospital settings has increased in recent decades. During 2018 and 2019, there were 8,614 out-of-hospital deliveries, with emergency medical services (EMS)-assisted delivery in 3,515 of these and 1,712 delivery complications.[1] Care was more often provided by a basic life support (BLS) crew when these calls originated from counties with greater racial or ethnic diversity, as is more common in urban areas. Unplanned in-home deliveries are associated with a higher complication rate and higher neonatal mortality rate.[1]

Words of Wisdom

The United States has experienced significant growth in the number of rural areas with no obstetric services, which has created "maternity care deserts."[2] An increase in out-of-hospital and preterm births has been observed when rural areas lose hospital-based obstetric services.[3]

When responding to an obstetric emergency, the EMT is faced with a critical decision: delay transport and assist with the delivery on scene or initiate transport with minimal delay and plan for delivery at the hospital. Multiple factors affect this decision, such as trauma, weather, and distance to the hospital. This chapter explains how to make this decision and how to proceed if on-scene delivery is necessary. It describes the anatomy and physiology of a normal pregnancy and the normal process of childbirth. Also discussed are common complications, including trauma in a pregnant patient, so that you will be prepared to handle normal and abnormal deliveries. Finally, the chapter discusses the evaluation and care of the newborn and neonatal resuscitation.

> **Words of Wisdom**
>
> Documentation of the last menstrual period (often noted as LMP) should be included in the history section of the patient's chart. The last menstrual period is documented as the first day of the patient's last menstrual bleeding. Documentation should also include the average number of days that the patient experiences bleeding and the average number of days between the start of each cycle. For individuals who have experienced **menopause**, the month and year of the last known menstrual period should be charted, if possible, particularly when relevant to the chief complaint (eg, vaginal bleeding, abdominal pain).

Anatomy and Physiology of the Female Reproductive System

The female reproductive system includes the ovaries, fallopian tubes, uterus, cervix, vagina, and breasts. The ovaries are two glands located on either side of the uterus that are similar in function to the male testes. Each ovary contains thousands of follicles, and each follicle contains an egg. Females are born with all the eggs they will release in their lifetime.

During puberty, the maturing female body undergoes multiple physical and hormonal changes, ultimately leading to **menarche**. After the first menstrual bleeding occurs, periods begin occurring with more regularity. Ultimately, a routine cycle is established, with a mean duration of 28 days between menstrual periods. During the typical menstrual cycle, only one follicle (of 10 to 20 that attempt the process each month) will mature and release an egg. The remaining follicles die and are reabsorbed by the body. The processes that the follicle goes through and the actual release of the egg (ovulation) are stimulated by the release of specific hormones in the female body. Ovulation occurs approximately 2 weeks prior to menstruation. Immediately following ovulation, the **endometrium** (the lining of the inside of the uterus) begins to thicken in preparation for the potential implantation of a fertilized egg. If the egg is not fertilized within 12 to 24 hours after it has been released from the follicle, it will simply die, and the thickened endometrium will be shed because it is not needed. This shedding (or bleeding) occurs on the first day of the menstrual cycle.

The fallopian tubes extend out laterally from the uterus, with one tube associated with each ovary. When an egg is released from the ovary, it travels through the fallopian tube to the uterus. Fertilization, which occurs when a sperm meets an egg, usually takes place when the egg is inside the fallopian tube. The fertilized egg then continues to the uterus where, if implantation occurs, the fertilized egg develops into an **embryo** (the stage from 0 to 10 weeks after fertilization) and then a **fetus** (the stage from 10 weeks until delivery) and grows until the time of delivery at approximately 9 months (40 weeks) of gestation (**FIGURE 34-1**). The uterus is a muscular organ that encloses and protects the developing fetus. During labor, it produces

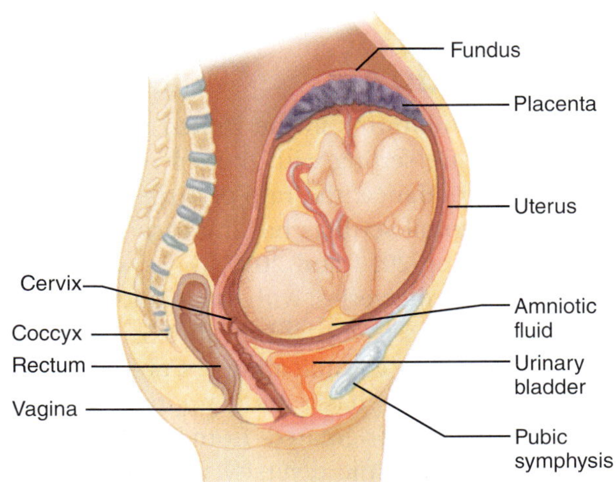

FIGURE 34-1 Anatomic structures of the pregnant person.

contractions and ultimately helps to push the fetus through the **birth canal**. The birth canal is made up of the vagina and the lower third, or neck, of the uterus, called the **cervix**. During pregnancy, the cervix contains a mucus plug that seals the uterine opening, preventing contamination from the outside. When the cervix begins to dilate, this plug is discharged into the vagina as pink-tinged mucus, sometimes called **bloody show**. This small amount of bloody discharge often signals the beginning of labor.

The vagina is the outermost cavity of the female reproductive system and forms the lower part of the birth canal. It is approximately 3 to 5 inches (8 to 12 cm) in length, beginning at the cervix and ending as an external opening of the body. The vagina completes the passageway from the uterus to the outside world for the newborn. The area between the vagina and the anus is called the **perineum**.

The breasts are also a part of the female reproductive system. Early signs of pregnancy include increased size and tenderness in the breasts. Shortly after the baby is born, mammary glands within the breasts begin to produce milk, which is carried through small ducts in the nipples.

As the fetus continues to develop, it requires increasingly more nourishment and support. The **placenta** is a disk-shaped structure attached to the uterine wall that provides nourishment to the fetus through the umbilical cord. The **umbilical cord** connects the mother and fetus through the placenta. The developing fetus depends on this connection for oxygenation, nutrition, and waste removal. The umbilical cord contains two arteries and one vein. The umbilical vein carries oxygenated blood from the placenta to the heart of the fetus, and the umbilical arteries carry deoxygenated blood and waste products from the aorta of the fetus to the placenta. Blood normally does not mix between the fetus and the pregnant mother because of the placental barrier (**FIGURE 34-2**). This barrier consists of two layers of cells, keeping the circulations of the mother and the fetus separated but allowing nutrients, oxygen, waste, and carbon dioxide to pass between them to support the fetus as it grows. Many drugs and toxins are also able to pass through this barrier. Anything ingested by a pregnant person therefore has the potential to affect the fetus.

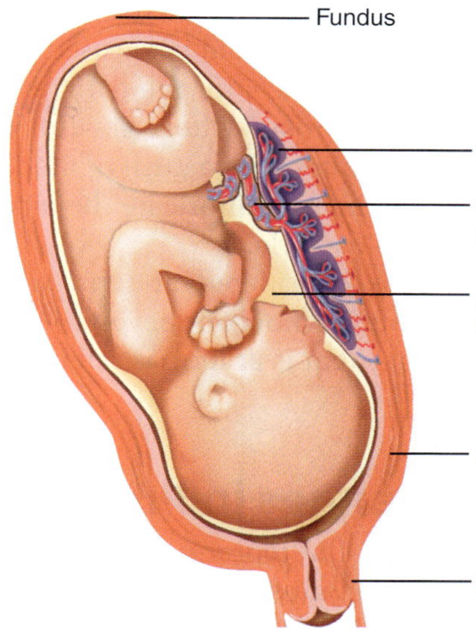

FIGURE 34-2 The placental barrier keeps the maternal and fetal blood separate but allows nutrients, oxygen, waste, carbon dioxide, toxins, and most medications to pass between the fetus and mother.

After delivery of the newborn, the placenta separates from the uterus and is delivered. The flow of oxygen through the fetal circulation is altered while in the womb and transitions to normal physiology within minutes after birth.

The fetus develops inside a fluid-filled, baglike membrane called the **amniotic sac**, or bag of waters. The sac contains approximately 500 to 1,000 mL of amniotic fluid, which helps insulate and protect the

Words of Wisdom

A baby's "due date" is the predicted date of delivery based on the first day of a pregnant person's last menstrual period. Although many pregnant individuals have a general idea of the date their last menstrual cycle began, those who are young, have irregular cycles, and did not know they were pregnant may have difficulty determining when their last menstrual period started. Also, some calculate their due date based on the number of weeks from conception rather than last menstrual period. It is important to remember that the due date is only a prediction of when a pregnant person is likely to deliver the baby, and many factors can cause the actual date of delivery to be earlier or later than anticipated.

fetus. When the sac ruptures, usually at the beginning of labor, the amniotic fluid is released (sometimes in a gush). It is typical for the patient to tell you that their "water broke." Often, patients experience a small leak rather than a gush of fluid. This clear, odorless fluid helps to lubricate the birth canal and remove any bacteria.

A pregnancy is considered at term when it reaches 39 weeks but has not gone beyond 40 weeks, 6 days. A pregnancy that is at term is referred to as **term gestation**.

Normal Changes in Pregnancy

Four body systems—the reproductive, respiratory, cardiovascular, and musculoskeletal systems—undergo major physiologic and anatomic changes during pregnancy. Understanding these changes is important when assessing and treating a pregnant patient.

In the reproductive system, hormone levels increase to support fetal development and prepare the body for childbirth. These increased hormone levels and the changes they produce also put the pregnant patient at an increased risk for complications from trauma, bleeding, and some medical conditions. As the fetus develops, the uterus grows, stretching to accommodate a term fetus. As the size of the uterus increases, so does the amount of fluid it contains. These factors eventually result in displacement of the uterus out of its well-protected position within the pelvic area and may expose it to injury. By the 20th week of pregnancy, the top of the uterus is at or above the belly button. This positioning increases the chance of direct fetal injury in trauma.

In the second trimester of pregnancy, the rapid growth of the uterus leads to changes in the respiratory system. As the uterus grows, it pushes up on the diaphragm, displacing it from its normal position and leading to reduced tidal volume with each breath. To make up for this, the pregnant person's respiratory rate must increase. Pregnancy also increases the patient's overall demand for oxygen as the metabolic demands and workload increase to support the developing fetus. These changes lead to an overall reduction in respiratory reserve and decreased ability to compensate during times of respiratory distress.

Changes also occur in the cardiovascular system. Overall blood volume gradually increases throughout the pregnancy to allow for adequate perfusion of the uterus as the fetus grows and to prepare for the blood loss that will occur during childbirth. Blood volume may increase by as much as 50% by the end of the pregnancy. The number of red blood cells also increases, which increases the need for iron. During pregnancy, patients often take prenatal vitamin supplements containing iron to avoid becoming anemic. **Anemia** is a condition in which the bloodstream does not contain enough red blood cells to effectively transport oxygen throughout the body. Blood clotting factors also change as the body prepares for childbirth. The speed of clotting increases to protect against excessive bleeding during delivery. By the end of the pregnancy (third trimester), the pregnant patient's heart rate increases by up to 20% (approximately 12 to 20 more beats per minute) to accommodate the increase in blood volume. Cardiac output is significantly increased by the end of the pregnancy. Although an otherwise healthy person may tolerate increased cardiovascular demand without issue, pregnant patients with underlying medical conditions may be more susceptible to cardiac compromise.

YOU are the EMT

At 0625 hours, you are dispatched to a residence at 2505 Landa Park Boulevard for a woman in labor. You and your partner proceed to the scene, which is located a short distance away. While en route, dispatch advises you that the patient is 38 weeks pregnant and her contractions are 3 minutes apart.

1. What anatomic and physiologic changes occur during pregnancy? How will they affect your assessment of the patient?
2. How will you determine whether delivery is imminent or if there is enough time to transport the pregnant patient?

During pregnancy there is an increased risk for gastroesophageal reflux, nausea, vomiting, and potential aspiration. The filling and emptying of the stomach into the small intestine are controlled by key hormones and the nervous system. Changes in these systems and the displacement of the stomach upward because of the increased size of the uterus significantly increase the chance that a pregnant patient will vomit and aspirate. You should be prepared to quickly manage the patient's airway if needed.

Weight gain during pregnancy is normal; however, the increase in body weight eventually challenges the heart and affects the musculoskeletal system. Certain hormones affect the musculoskeletal system by relaxing ligaments that stabilize bones and joints. Individuals in the third trimester of pregnancy also experience a change in the body's center of gravity, making them susceptible to slipping and falling.

Complications of Pregnancy

Although most patients who are pregnant are healthy, some may have preexisting medical conditions when they conceive or become ill during pregnancy. Administering oxygen to a pregnant patient with respiratory distress and/or cardiovascular compromise is safe and can reduce fetal distress.

Note that in discussing many of the conditions that follow, it is advised that the pregnant patient be transported on the left side. This recommendation is not intended to treat the patient's underlying condition, per se, but to avoid introducing a different complication: **supine hypotensive syndrome**. Supine hypotensive syndrome is caused by compression of the inferior vena cava by the pregnant uterus when the patient lies supine, reducing the amount of blood that is returned to the heart. Hypotension (low blood pressure) may result from this compression. To prevent this complication, any patient in the third trimester of pregnancy should always be positioned leaning at least slightly to the left side during transport, except during delivery.

Diabetes

Diabetes will develop in more than 8% of pregnant patients in the United States.[4] This condition, called **gestational diabetes**, typically resolves after delivery. Treatment of a pregnant patient with diabetes is the same as treatment for any patient who has diabetes. Pregnant individuals can control their blood glucose level with diet and exercise or take medication. In some cases, they will have to manage their condition with insulin injections. If gestational diabetes is not managed properly, it can cause complications such as preeclampsia, large fetal size, or premature birth.

A pregnant patient experiencing hyperglycemia or hypoglycemia should be cared for in the same manner as any patient with diabetes. If a pregnant patient has an altered level of consciousness, your assessment should include determining whether the patient has a history of diabetes, and you should check the blood glucose level if local protocols permit.

Many pregnant patients experience nausea before labor and may not have eaten recently. These factors can lead to hypoglycemia and weakness. Consult with medical direction if delivery is imminent.

Hypertension in Pregnancy

Hypertension in pregnancy generally manifests as one of three conditions: gestational hypertension, preeclampsia, or eclampsia. Elevated blood pressure is a feature of all three conditions; however, the degree of hypertension and the presence of systemic effects, such as protein in the urine, altered mental status, or seizures, will aid in determining the patient's specific condition. All three of these conditions pose risks to the mother and fetus.

Gestational hypertension is the presence of high blood pressure in the absence of other systemic effects. High blood pressure in this context is defined as systolic blood pressure higher than 140 mm Hg and diastolic blood pressure higher than 90 mm Hg. The condition is considered severe when the systolic blood pressure is higher than 160 mm Hg and/or the diastolic blood pressure is higher than 110 mm Hg.

Preeclampsia, a condition that occurs in the second half of pregnancy (after 20 weeks' gestation), involves new-onset hypertension along with other systemic effects, such as protein in the urine. This condition occurs in approximately 3% to 8% of pregnancies worldwide.[5] In the United States, incidence is particularly high among African American patients.[6] Other risk factors for preeclampsia include chronic high blood pressure or kidney disease prior to pregnancy, preeclampsia in a previous pregnancy, obesity, age greater than 40 years, multiple gestation, and family history of preeclampsia.[7] Preeclampsia is characterized by the following signs and symptoms:

- Hypertension (systolic blood pressure >140 mm Hg, diastolic blood pressure >90 mm Hg)
- Severe or persistent headache
- Visual abnormalities such as seeing spots, blurred vision, or sensitivity to light
- Swelling in the hands and feet (edema)
- Upper abdominal or epigastric pain
- Dyspnea and/or retrosternal chest pain
- Anxiety
- Altered mental status

A related condition, **eclampsia**, is characterized by the presence of seizures. To treat a patient having seizures caused by eclampsia, lay the patient on the left side, maintain the airway, and administer supplemental oxygen. If vomiting occurs, suction the airway. Provide rapid transport for a pregnant patient having seizures, and call for an advanced life support (ALS) intercept, if available.

Street Smarts

Differentiating between gestational hypertension, preeclampsia, and eclampsia can be difficult, but good clinical decision-making (or critical thinking) skills can help. It may be helpful to think of the conditions as existing along a spectrum of the same disease process. For example, if you are transporting a pregnant patient who has a blood pressure of 148/96 mm Hg, but no other signs or symptoms are present at your initial examination, the patient's condition suggests gestational hypertension. During reassessment, the patient reports blurred vision, a severe headache, and abdominal pain. The condition has worsened and progressed from gestational hypertension into preeclampsia. As you pull into the ambulance bay of the hospital, the patient begins to experience active seizures. The condition is now eclampsia, because seizure activity is present. This example underscores the importance of continually reassessing your patient, listening to your patient, and communicating changes in the patient's condition to hospital personnel.

Bleeding

Vaginal bleeding during pregnancy can be the result of a number of conditions (**TABLE 34-1**). The timing of the bleeding along with the presence

YOU are the EMT

When you arrive at the scene, you are greeted at the door by the patient's husband. He is obviously anxious and tells you, "She's having the baby! I thought I could get her to the hospital in time, but I was wrong." You find the patient, a 28-year-old woman, lying supine in her bed. You introduce yourself and your partner and perform a primary assessment.

Recording Time: 0 Minutes	
Appearance	Diaphoretic; in obvious pain
Level of consciousness	Conscious and alert
Airway	Open; clear of secretions and foreign bodies
Breathing	Increased rate; adequate depth
Circulation	Increased pulse rate; strong and regular; no gross bleeding

The patient tells you that she feels as if she needs to move her bowels and that her contractions are now about 2 minutes apart and last about 45 seconds. A brief visual examination of the vaginal area does not reveal crowning. According to the patient's husband, this is her third delivery, and she has had gestational diabetes and preeclampsia with this pregnancy. Her amniotic sac ruptured about 5 hours ago.

3. What are gestational diabetes and preeclampsia? How can they affect this delivery?

4. Is there time to transport this patient, or should you prepare for imminent delivery?

TABLE 34-1 Conditions That Can Cause Vaginal Bleeding

Condition	Timing	Pain	Bleeding
Ectopic pregnancy	Early pregnancy—generally 6 to 8 weeks after last missed period.	Severe lower abdominal pain, typically unilateral. May radiate to one shoulder.	Ranges from scant brown spotting to profuse bright red.
Abruptio placentae	Later pregnancy—usually after 20 weeks.	Lower abdominal and/ or back pain. May be associated with contractions.	Moderate vaginal bleeding. Most bleeding is internal.
Placenta previa	Later pregnancy—usually after 20 weeks.	Relatively painless.	May present as moderate bleeding to life-threatening hemorrhage.

and location of pain can help identify the patient's condition.

An **ectopic pregnancy** is when an embryo develops outside of the uterus, most often in a fallopian tube. A patient with an ectopic pregnancy may present with signs of shock related to internal bleeding when the fallopian tube ruptures (**FIGURE 34-3**). It is estimated that ectopic pregnancies account for 1% to 2% of reported pregnancies in the United States.[8] Sudden onset of severe abdominal pain and vaginal bleeding in the first trimester of pregnancy should be considered ectopic pregnancy until proven otherwise. It is also important to consider the possibility of an ectopic pregnancy in a patient who has missed a menstrual cycle and reports sudden, severe, usually unilateral pain in the lower abdomen. A history of pelvic inflammatory disease, tubal ligation, or previous ectopic pregnancies should heighten your suspicion of a possible ectopic pregnancy. Vaginal bleeding in early pregnancy may also be a sign of a spontaneous abortion, which is discussed in more detail in the following section.

In the later stages of pregnancy, vaginal bleeding may indicate a serious condition involving the placenta. In **abruptio placentae**, the placenta separates prematurely from the wall of the uterus (**FIGURE 34-4**). The most common causes are hypertension and trauma. A patient with abruptio placentae often reports severe pain; however, vaginal bleeding may not be heavy. The patient may also present with signs of shock such as weak, rapid pulse and pale, cool, diaphoretic skin. In **placenta previa**, the placenta develops over and covers part of or the entire cervix (**FIGURE 34-5**). When early labor begins and the cervix begins to dilate, the pregnant patient may experience heavy vaginal bleeding, often without significant pain. Both abruptio placentae and placenta previa are life-threatening conditions for both the mother and fetus and require immediate rapid transport.

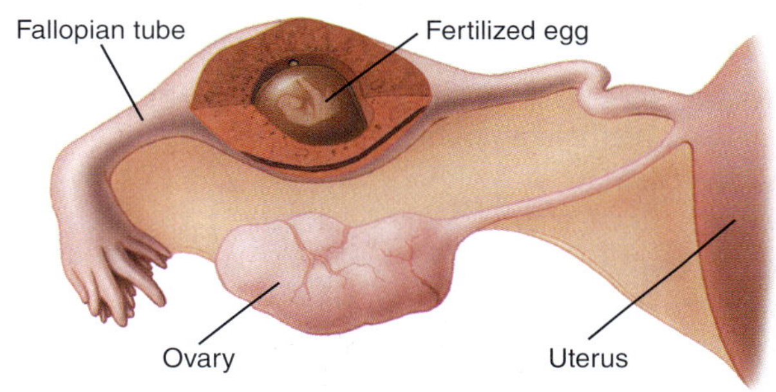

FIGURE 34-3 In an ectopic pregnancy, a fertilized egg implants somewhere other than in the uterus. Here, it is implanted in one of the fallopian tubes, the most common location for an ectopic pregnancy.

Street Smarts

Regardless of the cause of the bleeding, the pregnant patient may be emotional and very concerned about the baby. Your professional approach in communicating with the patient will play a crucial part in calming the patient's emotions and gaining control of the situation. Decreasing the patient's anxiety can affect how the patient and the fetus respond during this emergency.

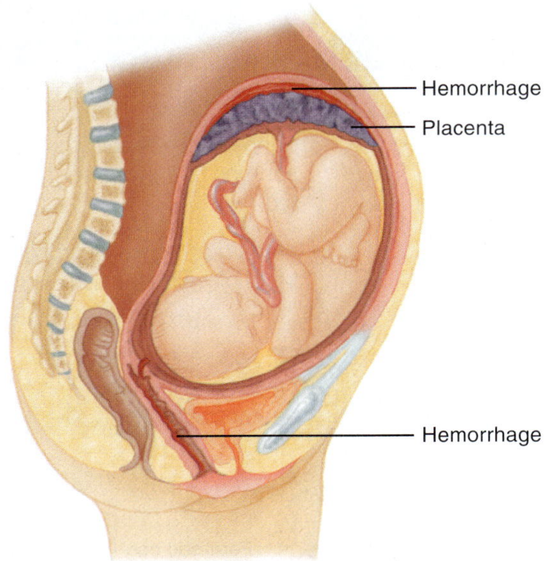

FIGURE 34-4 In abruptio placentae, the placenta separates prematurely from the wall of the uterus.

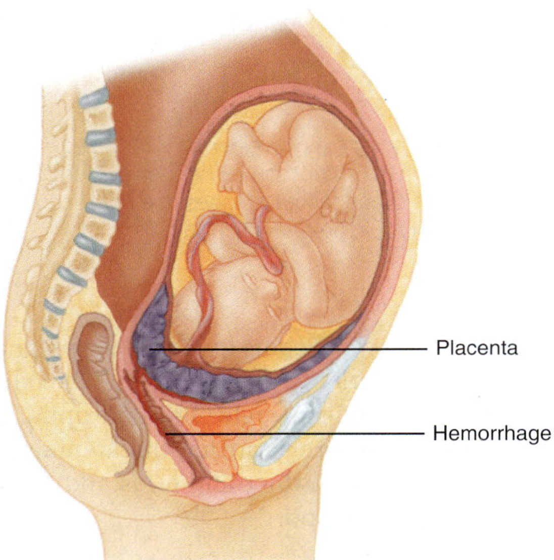

FIGURE 34-5 In placenta previa, the placenta develops over and covers the cervix.

Any bleeding from the vagina in a pregnant patient is a serious sign and should be treated promptly in the hospital. If the patient shows signs of shock, position the patient on the left side and administer high-concentration oxygen per local protocols. Place a sterile pad or sanitary pad over the vagina, and replace it as often as necessary. Save the pads so that hospital personnel can estimate how much blood loss the patient experienced. Also save any tissue that may be passed from the vagina. Do not put anything into the vagina to control bleeding.

Abortion

Spontaneous abortion is the loss of a pregnancy prior to 20 weeks of gestation without any preceding surgical or medical intervention. The term is often used interchangeably with **miscarriage**. Spontaneous abortion is frequently associated with abdominal cramping and vaginal bleeding. Although chromosomal abnormality, trauma, drug use, underlying medical conditions, and certain sexually transmitted diseases may increase the risk of experiencing miscarriage, the direct cause is often unknown.

An **induced abortion** is the elective termination of a pregnancy prior to the time of viability. Induced abortions are typically performed by a licensed health care clinician by using a medication or performing a surgical procedure. The abortion may also be induced illegally by an untrained person or by the patient, at risk of great harm to the patient. Regardless of the reason or the cause of the abortion, complications are possible.

The most serious complications of abortion, whether it be spontaneous or induced, are bleeding and infection. Bleeding can result when portions of the fetus or placenta remain inside the uterus (incomplete abortion) or when the wall of the uterus is injured (perforation of the uterus and possibly the adjacent bowel or bladder). Infection can result from perforation and from the use of nonsterile instruments. If the patient is in shock, treat and provide prompt transport to the hospital. Collect and bring to the hospital any tissue that passes through the vagina. Never try to pull tissue out of the vagina. Place a sterile pad or sanitary pad on the vagina. In rare cases, massive bleeding may occur and cause severe hypovolemic shock. In these cases, treat for shock and provide immediate transport.

Substance Use Disorder

Overall, use of prescription opioids, marijuana, or illicit drugs by pregnant people and the hospitalization of newborns who need care due to intrauterine drug exposure are on the rise in the United States. Individuals with substance use disorders often have had little or no prenatal care.[9] The effects of the substance use on the fetus can include prematurity, low birth weight, and severe respiratory depression. Some of these infants will die.

Opioid use disorder, particularly among teen mothers, has become a serious public health threat.[10] It should be considered while obtaining the patient history. Patients who have disclosed their opioid use to their physician may be taking an opioid antagonist to treat their disorder and prevent ongoing use during their pregnancy. It is essential to report this history to the receiving facility.

Examples of other substances used during pregnancy that may harm fetal development include alcohol and tobacco. **Fetal alcohol syndrome** is a condition seen in infants born to mothers who have alcohol use disorder. This condition places the child at greater risk for cognitive, social, and developmental disorders.[11]

If you are assisting at a delivery and suspect the patient has a substance use disorder, pay special attention to your own safety. Take standard precautions. As with all imminent deliveries, personal protective equipment (PPE) should include eye protection, a face mask, and gloves. Clues that the patient may have a substance use disorder include the presence of drug paraphernalia, empty wine or liquor bottles, and statements made by the patient or by family members or bystanders. This newborn is more likely to need immediate resuscitation. Assist with the delivery, and be prepared to support the newborn's respirations and administer oxygen if indicated during transport. Do not judge or lecture the patient. Your job is to help with the delivery, provide treatment to the mother and the newborn, and transport both to the hospital.

Maternal Cardiac Arrest

The most common causes of maternal cardiac arrest in the United States include hemorrhage, heart failure, amniotic fluid embolism, and sepsis. Cardiac arrest occurs in 1 in every 36,000 pregnancies.[12] Survival of the pregnant patient is much lower in the out-of-hospital setting than in the hospital.[13] One of the key tenets in resuscitation of the pregnant patient is that saving the mother provides the best chance for saving the fetus. Resuscitation efforts should focus on aggressively treating the pregnant patient with high-quality cardiopulmonary resuscitation (CPR) and rapid transport to the closest appropriate facility.

Treatment of cardiac arrest in a pregnant patient may require modifications, depending on how far along the pregnancy is. If the patient is in the third trimester, manual displacement of the uterus toward the patient's left side may be necessary to facilitate blood return to the right side of the heart.[14] High-quality, minimally interrupted CPR is essential for the pregnant patient, as is early use of an automated external defibrillator. Remember, the baby has the best chance to survive if the mother is resuscitated. Use of mechanical CPR devices has not been tested and is not advised in pregnant individuals. Chapter 14, *BLS Resuscitation*, describes how to perform manual displacement of the uterus.

Notify personnel at the receiving facility as soon as possible that you are en route with a pregnant trauma patient in cardiac arrest so they will have time to prepare. It is possible that a cesarean section may be performed on arrival to the hospital in order to save the fetus. Performing a cesarean section is not within the scope of practice for nonphysician EMS clinicians.

Trauma and Pregnancy

When you are dispatched to a trauma call that involves a pregnant person, you have two patients to consider: the mother and the unborn fetus. Causes of trauma in pregnant patients, as in any other patient, may be unintentional (eg, motor vehicle crash) or intentional (eg, assault). Any of these events can affect the developing fetus.

The leading causes of trauma in pregnant people are motor vehicle crashes, falls, and intimate partner violence.[15] Contributing factors include hormonal changes that loosen the joints and the increased weight of the uterus and displacement of abdominal organs, which shift the patient's center of gravity. Increased blood volume and elevated resting heart rate, both normal changes during pregnancy, may mask the signs and symptoms of shock until a significant amount of blood has been lost. Fetal distress may also be present well before signs of shock are evident in the pregnant patient. In the case of serious trauma, the blood supply to the fetus is often actively reduced as a physiologic reflex so that the mother receives an adequate amount of blood.

When called to a trauma patient who is pregnant, be alert to additional concerns and be ready to assess and manage unique types of injuries. For example, as a pregnancy progresses, the uterus enlarges substantially, making it especially vulnerable to penetrating trauma and blunt injuries. The fetus may be injured directly from penetrating types of trauma such as gunshot wounds and stabbings. A traumatic injury to the abdomen can be life threatening to the mother and fetus because the pregnant uterus has a rich blood supply. If the mother is hypoxic, is in shock, or has hypovolemia, the fetus will be in distress. In most cases, the only chance to save the fetus is to adequately resuscitate the mother.

Words of Wisdom

By 20 weeks of gestation, the top of the uterus has grown to the level of the patient's belly button. That position makes the fetus more susceptible to injury. This is important to remember when caring for a pregnant patient who has sustained trauma and to aid in your assessment of a pregnant patient's abdomen.

When a pregnant person is involved in a motor vehicle crash, a fall, or other trauma with a significant mechanism of injury (MOI), severe hemorrhage may result from injuries to the pregnant uterus. Severe injuries have been shown to have a six-fold increase in the incidence of abruptio placentae. This condition results in significant intrauterine hemorrhage that can cause life-threatening hypovolemic shock in the mother and also increases the chance of fetal death. In a pregnant trauma patient, suspect abruptio placentae when the MOI is blunt trauma to the abdomen and the patient's signs and symptoms suggest shock. Common symptoms include vaginal bleeding and severe abdominal pain. In this situation, quickly assess and transport the patient, support the airway, administer high-flow oxygen, place sanitary pads on the vagina, position the patient on the left side, and call for ALS backup.

Improper positioning of the seat belt can result in injury to the pregnant patient and the fetus if they are involved in a motor vehicle crash. The lap belt should be placed under the abdomen and over the pelvis (iliac crests), and the shoulder belt should be positioned between the breasts. Carefully assess a pregnant patient's abdomen and chest for seat belt marks, bruising, and obvious trauma. Maintain a high index of suspicion for internal abdominal bleeding in the mother and possible direct injury to the fetus, regardless of seat belt placement.

Physical Abuse

Intimate partner violence often begins or worsens during pregnancy, with an estimated 324,000 pregnant people experiencing physical abuse each year in the United States.[16] Abuse during pregnancy increases the risk of spontaneous abortion, preterm delivery, and low birth weight. The patient is at risk of bleeding, infection, and uterine rupture. Homicide is a leading cause of maternal death in the United States.[17] A calm, professional approach is especially important if you suspect your patient has been abused. Pay attention to the environment for any signs of abuse. Your attention to detail will be helpful in your documentation and in informing the physicians and staff who will be caring for the patient at the hospital.

Pregnant patients who are abused may be reluctant to explain how their injuries occurred. If possible, talk to the patient in a private area, away from the potential abuser. Suspect abuse when the story of how an injury happened does not make sense. An abused patient who is pregnant will be concerned about the developing baby. The best way for you to care for the fetus is to treat the pregnant patient. Reassure the patient as you provide treatment. Support the patient's airway, breathing, and circulation (ABCs), control any bleeding, stabilize extremity injuries, treat for shock, and keep the patient warm.

Caring for the Pregnant Trauma Patient

Although you have two patients to care for when your patient is pregnant, your focus should be on assessing and treating the mother. It is difficult to assess the extent of internal blood loss in a pregnant patient. When the pregnant patient has sustained trauma, the MOI should be the basis for suspicion of shock because the physiologic changes that occur with pregnancy can hide the typical signs and symptoms of shock. As you assess and treat the patient, be prepared for vomiting, and anticipate the need to manage the airway to protect the patient from aspirating. Attempt to determine the gestational age (in number of weeks). This will help you determine the size of the fetus and the position of the uterus in the patient's abdominal cavity. It is nearly impossible for you to accurately assess or determine the status of the fetus, so you should aggressively provide emergency medical care to the patient to provide the best possible outcome for the fetus.

Follow these guidelines when treating a pregnant trauma patient:

1. **Maintain an open airway.** A pregnant patient has an increased risk of vomiting and aspiration. Be prepared for and anticipate vomiting; keep your suction unit readily available.
2. **Administer high-concentration oxygen.** Remember that the patient's body is also supplying oxygen to the fetus. Keep the oxygen saturation level high and administer high-concentration oxygen by nonrebreathing mask.
3. **Ensure adequate ventilation.** Listen to breath sounds, and confirm that bilateral breath sounds are present. If the patient's ventilations are inadequate, provide or assist ventilation with a bag-mask device and high concentration oxygen.
4. **Assess circulation.** Control any external bleeding with direct pressure. Maintain a high index of suspicion for internal bleeding and shock based on the MOI. Keep the patient warm.
5. **Consider transport needs.** Transport the patient on the left side. If the patient is on a long backboard, the entire board can be tilted to the side. Call early for ALS assistance or a medical helicopter for significant MOIs or major traumatic injuries. Transport the patient to a specialty obstetric center or trauma center if one is available in your area; give early notification that you have a pregnant trauma patient in transport.

Cultural Value Considerations

Cultural sensitivity is important when you are assessing and treating a pregnant patient. Some cultures may have a value system that will affect the choice of how individuals care for themselves during pregnancy and how they have planned the childbirth process. Some cultures may not permit a male health care clinician, especially in the prehospital setting, to assess or examine a female patient. Some cultures may view pregnancy differently than you do in terms of social, psychological, and emotional issues. Some may see pregnancy as a means of achieving status and recognition within the family unit, whereas others may experience a drop in self-esteem. Respect these differences and honor requests from the patient. Always remember that your responsibility is to the patient and is limited to providing care and transport. In addition, keep in mind that an informed adult with decision-making capacity has the right to refuse all or any part of your assessment or care. Ask permission before performing assessments or treatments, and even before cutting the umbilical cord.

Teenage Pregnancy

Although teenage pregnancy rates have been declining in the United States, teenage pregnancy is still a common occurrence.[18,19] A pregnant teenager may be unaware of the pregnancy, may be in denial about it, or may be afraid to seek prenatal care. As you begin to assess any female teenager, you should remember that pregnancy is a possibility, even if the patient denies being sexually active. Respect the teenager's privacy and need for independence. If possible, perform your assessment and obtain the history away from the teenager's parents. Consider the possibility that the pregnancy resulted from rape or incest. Be aware that in most states, a teenager who becomes pregnant is considered emancipated, meaning the teenager has the rights of an adult, at least as they relate to giving or refusing consent for medical treatment. Become familiar with the laws in your state so that you will know when pregnant teenagers can give or refuse consent for themselves.

Patient Assessment

Childbirth is seldom an unexpected event, but there are occasions when it becomes an emergency. Dispatch protocols usually include the dispatcher asking simple questions to determine whether birth is imminent. Some of this information passed to you from dispatch may help you prepare for the situation. Remember, trauma or medical conditions may result in unpredicted complications.

Scene Size-up

Take standard precautions; gloves and eye and face protection are a minimum if delivery has already begun or is complete. If the call is going to result in a field delivery and if time allows, a gown should also be used. Do not be lax in your safety observations and precautions because a delivery is in progress or the family is anxious. Rushing may endanger not only you but also the fetus and pregnant patient. Remain calm and professional. Consider calling for additional or specialized resources.

Not every call to a pregnant patient will be because the patient is in labor, of course, so it is important to determine the MOI or nature of illness in a pregnant patient. Do not develop tunnel vision during a call, assuming that because the patient is pregnant, that is the reason for the call! Because a pregnant patient's balance may be altered, trauma from falls and the need for spinal motion restriction must be considered.

Safety

When caring for a person in active labor, you will likely be in close quarters with a patient who is breathing heavily. As with any other emergency, if you suspect the patient is infected with an airborne communicable disease, wear an N95 mask. In this case, standard PPE will also include protective eyewear, a gown, and gloves.

Primary Assessment

Form a general impression as to whether the patient is in active labor and, if so, whether you have time to assess for imminent delivery and address other possible life threats. Perform a rapid examination of the patient to assess for airway, breathing, or circulation problems. The chief complaint may be, "The baby is coming!" Take a moment to confirm whether the fetus will be delivered in the next few minutes or whether you have time to continue to evaluate the situation. When trauma or medical problems such as vaginal bleeding or seizures are the presenting complaint, evaluate these first and then assess the effect of these problems on the fetus.

During an uncomplicated birth, life-threatening conditions involving the patient's airway and breathing usually are not an issue. However, a motor vehicle crash, an assault, or any number of medical conditions in a pregnant patient may cause a life threat to exist and may result in a complicated delivery. In these situations, assess the airway and breathing to ensure they are adequate. If needed, provide airway management and administer high-concentration oxygen.

External and internal bleeding are potential life threats to the patient and should be assessed early. Blood loss after delivery is expected, but significant bleeding is not. Recall that normal changes in pregnancy result in increased overall blood volume, increased heart rate, and changes in blood clotting. These changes can have a significant effect on a pregnant patient who is bleeding, regardless of the cause. Quickly assess for any potential life-threatening bleeding, and begin treatment immediately. Assess the skin for color, temperature, and moisture, and check the pulse to determine whether it is too fast or too slow. Because skin pallor can be difficult to detect in patients with dark skin, you may need to check for pale mucous membranes inside the inner lower eyelid or slow capillary refill. If there are signs of shock, control the bleeding, administer oxygen, and keep the patient warm.

By gathering this initial information, you should be able to determine whether a patient who is experiencing active labor can be transported to the hospital for delivery or whether delivery is imminent, requiring on-scene delivery. Differentiating between *active labor* and *imminent delivery* is discussed further under "Normal Delivery Management."

History Taking

Regardless of whether the patient is in active labor, is having an obstetric emergency, or is a pregnant patient with another complaint (eg, trauma), obtain a thorough history. Obtain a SAMPLE (Signs and symptoms, Allergies, Medications, Pertinent past medical history, Last oral intake, Events leading up to the illness or injury) history. Some pregnant patients will have a history of medical problems for which they take prescription medications. Some individuals with no history of medical problems will require medications during pregnancy. Pertinent history should include questions related specifically to prenatal care, including whether the patient has been receiving prenatal care. Identify any complications the patient may have had during the pregnancy or potential complications expected during delivery that the patient's physician has identified. These complications may include the size or position of the fetus or the position and health of the placenta. Determine the due date, fetal movement, frequency of contractions, and history of previous pregnancies and deliveries and their complications, if any. Determine whether there is a possibility of more than one fetus. Ask whether the patient has taken any drugs or medications during the pregnancy or has used any opioids or illicit drugs recently. If the patient's water has broken, ask whether the fluid was green or had any odor. Green fluid is due to staining from **meconium** (fetal stool). The presence of meconium can indicate newborn distress.

Understanding certain terms unique to pregnancy will allow you to more accurately communicate the patient's obstetric history with other health care clinicians. Gravida is a term used to describe the number of times a person has been pregnant. Para is a term used to describe the number of times a pregnant person has delivered a viable newborn, one carried for more than 20 weeks' gestation. For example, a person who has been pregnant twice, resulting in one healthy delivery and one miscarriage, would be described as gravida 2, para 1. A person who is pregnant for the first time would be described as gravida 1, para 0. After delivering a viable baby, this person's description would be gravida 1, para 1.

Pregnancy history may be documented with G (gravida), P (para), and A (abortive history). For example, if a person has had two pregnancies, resulting in one a viable newborn and one miscarriage, the documentation would be G2P1A1.

It is also useful to understand the following commonly encountered obstetric terms:

- *Primigravida* describes a person who is pregnant for the first time.
- *Primipara* describes a person who has had only one delivery.
- *Multigravida* describes a person who has been pregnant two or more times, irrespective of the outcome.
- *Nullipara* describes a person who has never delivered a viable newborn, although she may have been pregnant before.
- *Multipara* describes a person who has delivered two or more viable newborns.
- *Grand multipara* describes a person who has delivered five or more viable newborns.

Secondary Assessment

Perform a complete assessment of the major body systems as needed, with emphasis on the patient's chief complaint. Ask if the patient can feel the fetus moving. If the patient is in labor, the physical

YOU are the EMT

Shortly after your partner assesses the patient's vital signs, you observe the fetus's head crowning at the vaginal opening. As the head delivers, you can feel the umbilical cord wrapped around the fetus's neck.

Recording Time: 7 Minutes (Mother)	
Respirations	24 breaths/min; adequate depth
Pulse	110 beats/min; strong and regular
Skin	Baseline color, warm, and moist
Blood pressure	122/82 mm Hg
Oxygen saturation (Spo_2)	98% (on room air)

5. How should you manage the umbilical cord?

6. What would you do if the amniotic sac was still intact?

examination should focus on contractions and possible delivery. Assessing contractions is described later in the chapter under "The Delivery."

The secondary assessment of a pregnant patient should include a complete set of vital signs and pulse oximetry. Vital signs should include pulse; respirations; skin color, temperature, and condition; and blood pressure. Be especially alert for tachycardia and hypotension (which could mean hemorrhage or compression of the inferior vena cava) or hypertension (possibly indicating preeclampsia). Blood pressure typically decreases slightly during the first two trimesters of pregnancy but returns to normal during the third trimester. Compare your findings with previous blood pressure readings the patient may know of from prenatal visits. Hypertension, even when mild, may indicate more serious problems.

Reassessment

As time allows, repeat the primary assessment with a focus on the patient's ABCs and vaginal bleeding, particularly after delivery. Obtain another set of vital signs and compare the results with those obtained earlier. Frequent reassessment of vital signs may identify hypoperfusion from excessive blood loss as a result of delivery. Recheck interventions and treatments to determine whether they were effective.

If your assessment determines that delivery is imminent, notify staff at the receiving hospital. Provide an update on the status of the mother and newborn after delivery. On the rare occasion that the delivery of the placenta does not occur within 30 minutes or you determine that a complication is occurring that cannot be treated in the field, notify the hospital staff of your findings as you transport. Be sure to notify staff at the receiving hospital of all relevant information so they have time to prepare. The information you provide may help the hospital staff determine whether the patient will be seen in the emergency department or the labor and delivery unit. When a pregnant patient has problems unrelated to childbirth (such as trauma or difficulty breathing), be sure to include the patient's pregnancy status in your radio report. The hospital staff will want to know the patient's number of weeks of gestation, due date, and any known complications of the pregnancy.

Thorough documentation is essential, especially in the case of a newborn where delivery occurred in the field. In this situation, you will have two patient care reports to complete. Obstetrics is among the most litigated specialties in medicine; therefore, scrupulous documentation is essential.

Stages of Labor

The three stages of labor are (1) dilation of the cervix, (2) delivery of the fetus, and (3) delivery of the placenta. The first stage begins with the onset of contractions and ends when the cervix is fully dilated. Because the cervix has to be stretched thin by uterine contractions until the opening is large enough for the fetus to pass through into the vagina, the first stage of labor is usually the longest. In **primigravida** patients, the first stage of labor lasts a mean duration of 12 to 18 hours, compared to a mean duration of 6.5 to 13 hours for **multigravida** patients. You will usually have time to transport a patient who is in the first stage of labor.

The onset of labor starts with contractions of the uterus. Other signs of the beginning of labor are the bloody show (blood-streaked mucus) and the rupture of the amniotic sac (water breaking). These events usually occur near the first contraction or early in the first stage of labor. Initially, the uterine contractions may not occur at regular intervals. The patient may mistake the symptoms for nagging backache. In true labor, the frequency and intensity of contractions increase with time. The uterine contractions become more regular and last approximately 30 to 60 seconds each. The length of labor varies greatly.

TABLE 34-2 lists characteristics of true labor versus false labor, or Braxton-Hicks contractions. With false labor, you should provide transport for the patient. With true labor, you may need to prepare for a delivery, depending on the stage of labor, the patient's condition, and transport time.

Some patients experience a premature rupture of the amniotic sac, before the fetus is ready to be born. When this occurs, the patient may or may not go into labor. Some patients may experience this premature rupture as long as several months before they are due to deliver. In this situation, you will need to provide supportive care and transport to the hospital. These patients are usually placed on bed rest and followed up closely by an obstetrician.

TABLE 34-2 False Labor Versus True Labor

False Labor (Braxton-Hicks Contractions)	True Labor
Contractions are not regular and do not increase in intensity or frequency. Contractions come and go.	Contractions, once started, consistently get stronger and closer together.
Pain and contractions start and stay in the lower abdomen.	Pain and contractions may start in the lower back and "wrap around" to the lower abdomen.
Physical activity or a change in position may alleviate the pain and contractions.	Physical activity may intensify the contractions. A change in position does not relieve contractions.
Bloody show, if present, is brownish.	The bloody show is pink or red and generally accompanied by mucus.
If leakage of fluid occurs, it is usually urine. It will be in small amounts and smell of ammonia.	The amniotic sac may have broken just before the contractions started or it may break during contractions. A moderate amount of fluid that may smell sweet will be present, and fluid will continue to leak.

Toward the end of the third trimester of pregnancy, the head of the fetus normally descends into the mother's pelvis as the fetus positions for delivery. This movement down into the pelvis is called **lightening**. Some patients will report feeling this movement and may describe it as a relief because once the fetus has moved from under their rib cage, breathing becomes easier. Lightening may also occur gradually and not be noticed by some patients.

The second stage of labor begins when the fetus enters the birth canal, and it ends with delivery of the newborn (spontaneous birth). During this stage, you will have to decide whether to help the patient deliver at the scene or provide transport to the hospital. Because the fetus goes through positional changes as it moves through the birth canal during this stage, the uterine contractions are usually closer together and last longer. Pressure on the rectum may make the patient feel the need to have a bowel movement. Under no circumstances should you let the patient sit on the toilet. The patient may also have the uncontrollable urge to push down. The perineum will begin to bulge significantly. When the top of the fetus's head begins to appear at the vaginal opening, this is called **crowning**.

The third stage of labor begins with the birth of the newborn and ends with the delivery of the placenta. During this stage, the placenta must separate completely from the uterine wall. Contractions continue, assisting the separation process and clamping down and closing the blood vessels that connected the placenta to the uterine lining. This may take up to 30 minutes.

Normal Delivery Management

As part of your assessment, you should determine whether delivery is imminent. If delivery is imminent, you must prepare to deliver the baby at the scene. If the delivery is not imminent, prepare the patient for transport and perform the remainder of the assessment en route to the hospital.

Preparing for Delivery

Consider delivery at the scene when delivery is imminent (will occur within a few minutes) or when a natural disaster, inclement weather, or other environmental factor makes it impossible to reach the hospital. A patient who has delivered before may be able to tell you whether delivery is about to happen. Otherwise, asking the following questions will help you determine whether delivery is imminent:

- How long have you been pregnant?
- When are you due?
- Is this your first pregnancy?
- Are you having contractions? How far apart are the contractions? How long do the contractions last?
- Have you had any spotting or bleeding?

- Has your water broken?
- Do you feel as though you need to have a bowel movement?
- Do you feel the need to push?

Ask the following questions to help determine any potential complications:

- Were any of your previous deliveries by cesarean section?
- Have you had any problems in this or any previous pregnancy?
- Do you use drugs, drink alcohol, or take any medications?
- Is there a chance you are having more than one baby?
- Does your physician expect any other complications?

Keep in mind that *active labor* is not necessarily the same as *imminent delivery* (**TABLE 34-3**). When delivery becomes imminent, the patient will present with the signs and symptoms of active labor (ie, contractions, rupture of membranes, bloody show), but also later developments in the labor process. If the patient reports being about to deliver, needing to move the bowels, or feeling the need to push, immediately prepare for a delivery and consider calling for additional resources. The fetus's head is probably pressing on the rectum, and delivery is about to occur. Otherwise, does the patient have an extremely firm abdomen? Visually inspect the vagina to check for crowning. Crowning is an indication that the delivery is occurring. Do not touch the vaginal area until you have determined that delivery is imminent. In general, you should touch the vaginal area only during the delivery and when your partner is present. Gently spread the pregnant patient's legs apart, explaining that you are doing so to decide whether the baby should be delivered immediately or whether to initiate transport to the hospital for the delivery.

Once labor has begun, it cannot be slowed or stopped. Never attempt to hold the patient's legs together; doing so will only complicate the delivery. Do not allow the patient to sit on the toilet. Instead, offer reassurance that the sensation of needing to move the bowels is normal and that it means the baby is coming.

TABLE 34-3 Recognizing Imminent Delivery

When you encounter	
Active labor, which includes:	Contractions, rupture of membranes, and bloody show
and	
These additional signs and symptoms:	Crowning of the head or other body part, or mother's report of urge to push, urge to move bowels, or feeling that delivery is near
delivery is imminent!	

Street Smarts

When a patient pushes during labor, it is not uncommon for a bowel movement to occur. If this happens, discreetly and rapidly remove the feces and place clean towels under the patient's perineum.

If your decision is to deliver the baby at the scene, remember that you are only assisting the patient with the delivery. Your part is to help, guide, and support the baby as it is born. Use standard precautions at all times. Administer oxygen to the patient if indicated. Limit distractions for yourself and the patient. You want to appear calm and reassuring while protecting the patient's privacy. Most important, recognize when the situation is beyond your level of training. If there is any doubt, contact medical direction for further guidance. Always recognize your own limitations. If you are unsure about what to do, transport the patient even if delivery might occur during transport.

The ideal place to deliver the baby is in your ambulance or the privacy of the patient's home. The area should be warm and private, with plenty of room to move around. Your emergency vehicle should always be equipped with a sterile emergency obstetric (OB) kit containing the following items (**FIGURE 34-6**):

- Surgical scissors or a scalpel
- Umbilical cord clamps
- Towels, drapes, or sheets
- 4 × 4–inch (10 × 10–cm) gauze sponges and/or 2 × 10–inch (5 × 25–cm) gauze sponges

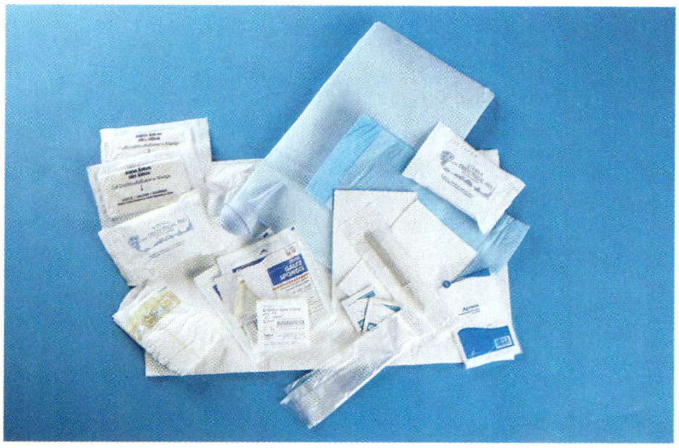

FIGURE 34-6 Your unit should contain a sterile obstetric kit.

- Sterile gloves
- Infant blanket
- Sanitary pads
- A plastic bag

In addition, you should have appropriate PPE and equipment such as an infant bag-mask device to resuscitate the newborn if needed.

Once you have determined that delivery is imminent and you have positioned the patient in an acceptable location, open the OB kit and continue to prepare for the delivery.

Patient Position

The patient's clothing and undergarments should be removed or pushed up to the waist. Preserve the patient's privacy as much as you can while helping to position the patient. If the emergency delivery is occurring at home, move the patient to a sturdy, flat surface or the floor if the patient will allow it. You will find it easier to work with the patient on a firm surface that is padded with blankets, folded sheets, or towels rather than on a bed. Put a pillow or blankets beneath the hips to elevate them approximately 2 to 4 inches (5 to 10 cm). It is sometimes more comfortable for the patient to put a pillow under one hip to allow the body to turn to one side. Allow the patient to get comfortable. Support the patient's head, neck, and upper back with pillows and blankets. The legs and hips should be flexed, with the feet flat on the surface beneath and the knees spread. Patients who have delivered before may prefer another delivery position, such as on the side. Another position is acceptable if both you and the patient are comfortable with it. You should also begin preparing for the newborn's arrival.

Track the progression of the delivery closely at all times. You want to avoid an explosive delivery, in which the crowning head pops out too quickly and uncontrollably.

Street Smarts

If you are the team leader during a situation where birth is imminent, communication with your crew members is essential. Do not assume that other members on the crew know what you expect them to do. Communicate effectively and give clear instructions, such as, "I will assist with the delivery of the baby. I want you to stay by the mother's head." Directly point to crew members and address them by name so there is no ambiguity about whom you are speaking to. Communicate with your crew, and have a plan for where you will place the newborn after delivery, who will be responsible for drying the newborn and keeping the newborn warm, and who will be responsible for caring for the mother and the newborn after delivery. Effective communication and strong leadership will go a long way toward calming the nerves of your patient and the crew.

Preparing the Delivery Field

Take the following steps to prepare the area where the delivery will occur:

1. Put on a protective face shield and gown. As time allows, place towels or sheets on the floor around the delivery area to help soak up body fluids and to protect the mother and the newborn.
2. Carefully open the OB kit so its contents remain sterile.
3. Put on the sterile gloves (**SKILL DRILL 34-1**). Once they are on, handle only sterile materials.
4. Use the sterile sheets and drapes from the OB kit to make a sterile delivery field. Place one drape under the patient's buttocks, and unfold it toward the feet. Wrap another behind the patient's back and drape it over each thigh (**FIGURE 34-7A**). Finally, drape a third sheet across the abdomen (**FIGURE 34-7B**).

Skill Drill 34-1 Putting on Sterile Gloves

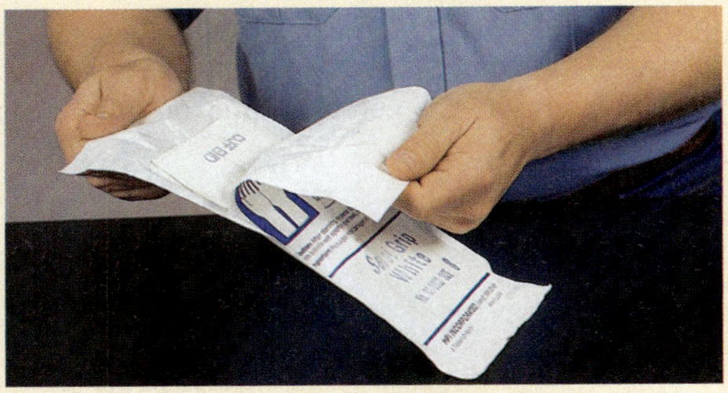

Step 1

Carefully open the sterile glove package without touching the gloves.

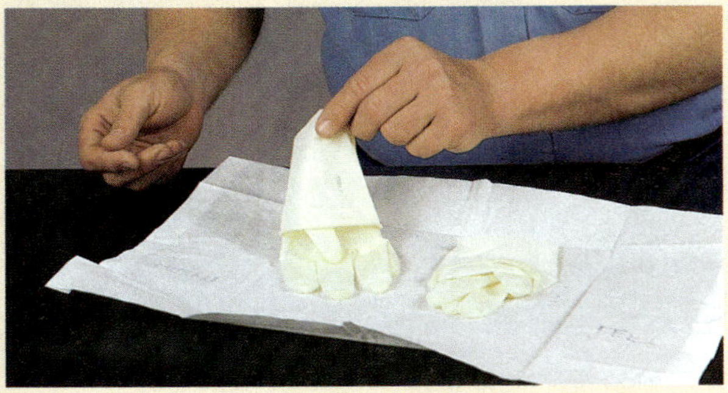

Step 2

Pick up the first glove by grasping one edge.

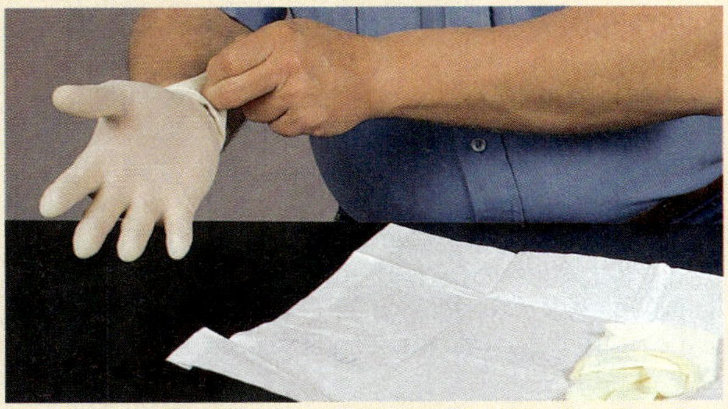

Step 3

Pull on the first glove, being careful not to touch the outside of the glove.

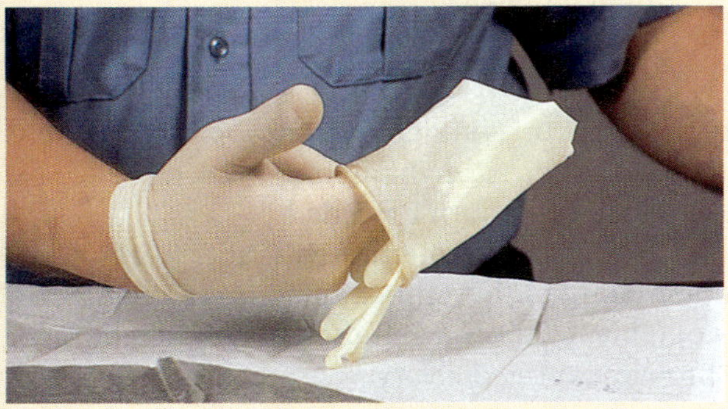

Step 4

Grasp the second glove by sliding two fingers of your gloved hand inside the rolled edge.

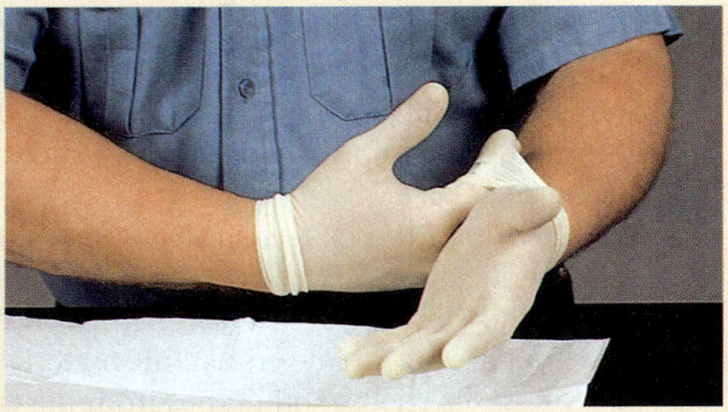

Step 5

Put on the second glove.

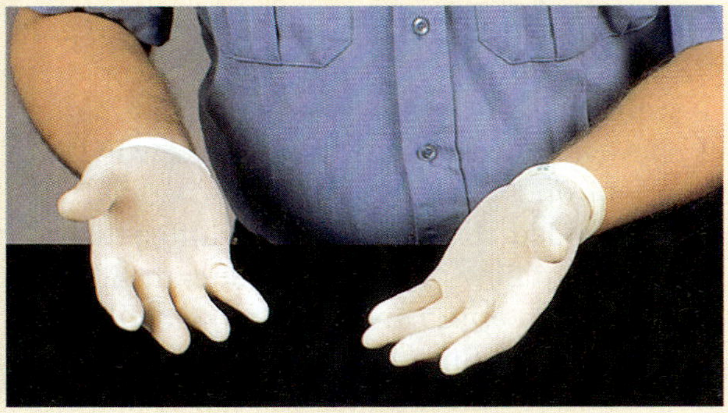

Step 6

Keep the gloves as sterile as possible.

The Delivery

Your partner should be at the patient's head to provide comfort and reassurance during the delivery. The patient may want to grip someone's hand and may yell, cry, or say nothing at all. It is common for patients to become nauseated during delivery, and some may vomit. If this occurs, have your partner assist the patient and ensure that the airway remains clear.

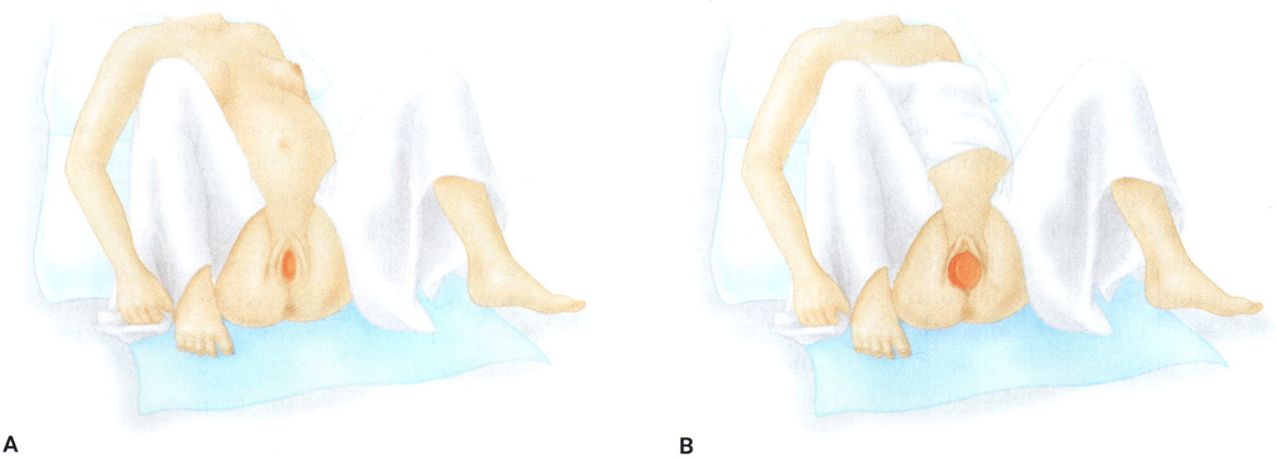

FIGURE 34-7 Preparing the delivery field. **A.** Use sterile sheets and drapes from the OB kit to make a clean delivery field. Place one sheet under the patient's buttocks. Wrap another sheet behind the back with either end draped over the thighs. **B.** Drape another sheet over the abdomen.

YOU are the EMT

You have successfully slipped the umbilical cord from around the neck and have completed delivery of the rest of the body. It is a girl! As you assess the newborn, your partner reassesses the patient's vital signs.

Recording Time: 12 Minutes (Mother)	
Level of consciousness	Conscious and alert
Respirations	22 breaths/min; adequate depth
Pulse	114 beats/min; strong and regular
Skin	Baseline color, warm, and moist
Blood pressure	130/60 mm Hg
Oxygen saturation (Spo_2)	98% (on room air)

Meanwhile, you assess the newborn.

Recording Time: 0 Minutes (Newborn)	
Level of consciousness	Whimpering with limited movement of extremities
Respirations	38 breaths/min
Pulse	80 beats/min
Skin	Cyanosis on the face, trunk, and extremities

7. What is involved in the routine postdelivery care of a newborn?

8. What immediate treatment is indicated for this newborn?

You must continually check for crowning. Some patients, especially those who have previously had children, may experience precipitous (fast) labor and birth. When labor is too fast, the tissues do not have time to stretch, and the patient is at risk for tears in the perineal area (see "Delivering the Head" in this chapter). Position yourself so that you can see the perineal area at all times. Time the patient's contractions, starting at the beginning of one and ending with the beginning of the next, to determine the frequency of the contractions. In addition, time the duration of each contraction by feeling the patient's abdomen from the moment the contraction begins (uterus and abdomen tightening) to the moment it ends (uterus and abdomen relaxing). Remind the patient to take quick, short breaths during each contraction but not to strain. Encourage the patient to rest and breathe deeply through the mouth between contractions.

Follow the steps in **SKILL DRILL 34-2** to deliver the newborn:

1. Crowning is the definitive sign that delivery is imminent and transport should be delayed until after the child has been born (**Step 1**).
2. Allow the patient to push the head out. Use your hands to support the bony parts of the head as it emerges. The child's body will naturally rotate to the right or left at this point in the delivery. Continue to support the head by grasping it with your hands over its ears to allow it to turn in the same direction. Avoid the eyes and fontanelles (soft spots on the newborn's skull). Feel at the neck to determine whether the umbilical cord is wrapped around it. If it is, gently lift it over the head without pulling hard on the cord (**Step 2**).
3. Once the head is delivered, it will rotate on its own to one side. At the next contraction, the upper shoulder will be visible. Guide the head down slightly to help the upper shoulder deliver (**Step 3**).
4. Support the head and upper body as the shoulders deliver. You may need to guide the head up slightly to help deliver the lower shoulder (**Step 4**).
5. Once the body is delivered, support the newborn firmly but gently. The newborn will be

Skill Drill 34-2 Delivering the Newborn

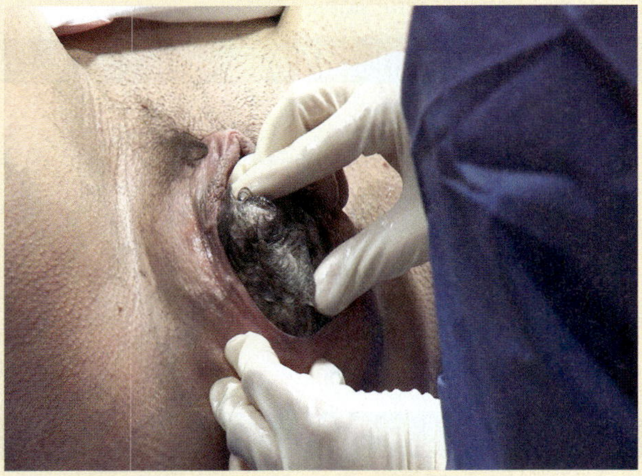

Step 1

Crowning is the definitive sign that delivery is imminent and transport should be delayed until after the child has been born.

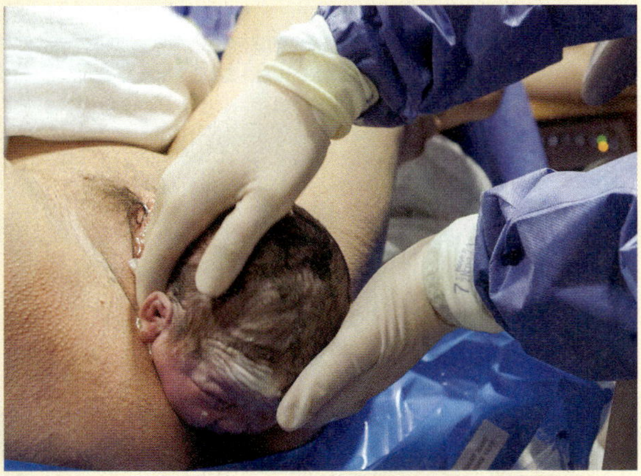

Step 2

Use your hands to support the bony parts of the head as it emerges. The child's body will naturally rotate to the right or left at this point in the delivery. Continue to support the head to allow it to turn in the same direction.

Skill Drill 34-2 Delivering the Newborn continued

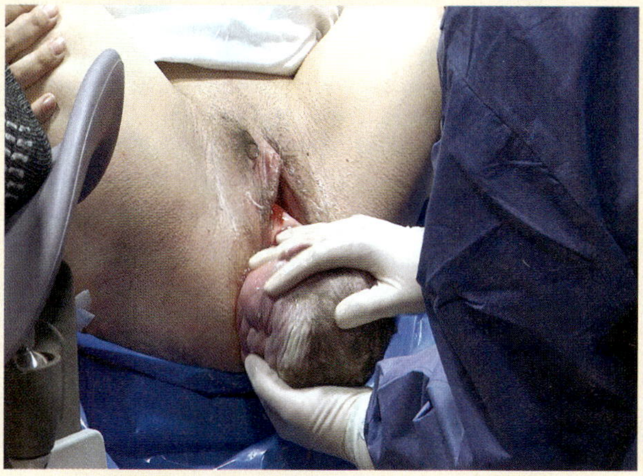

Step 3

As the upper shoulder appears, guide the head down slightly to deliver the shoulder.

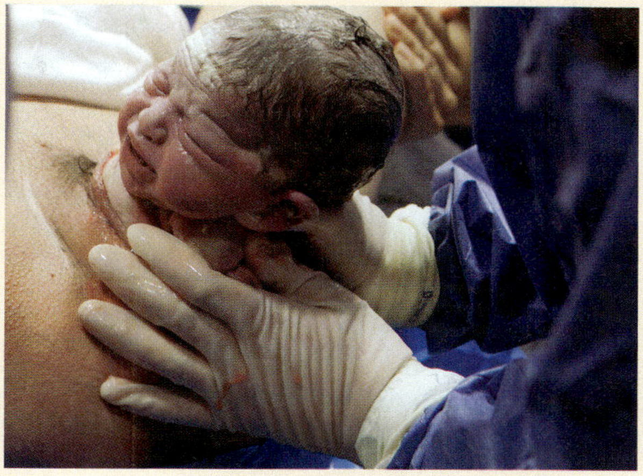

Step 4

Support the head and upper body as the lower shoulder delivers, guide the head up if needed.

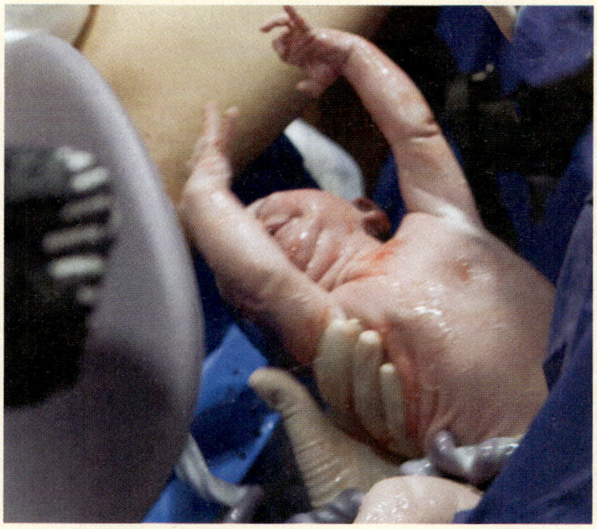

Step 5

Handle the newborn firmly but gently, support the head, and keep the neck in a neutral position to maintain the airway. Consider placing the newborn on the mother's abdomen with the umbilical cord still intact, allowing skin-to-skin contact to warm the newborn. Otherwise, keep the newborn approximately at the level of the vagina until the cord has been cut.

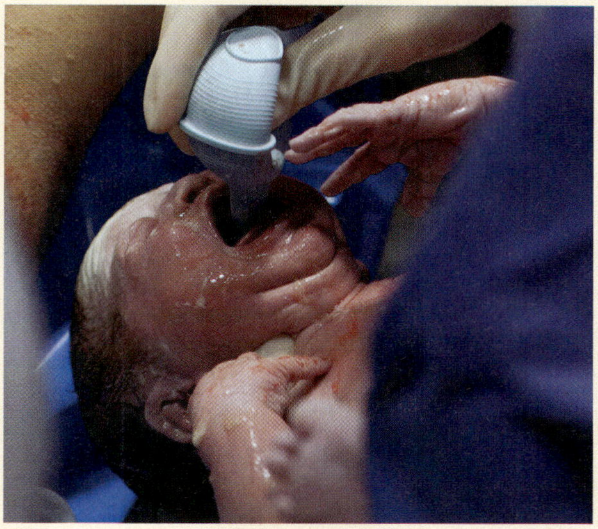

Step 6

After delivery and prior to cutting the cord, if the child is gurgling or shows other signs of respiratory distress, suction the mouth and then the nose gently with a bulb syringe to clear any amniotic fluid and ease the newborn's initiation of air exchange.

(continues)

Skill Drill 34-2 Delivering the Newborn continued

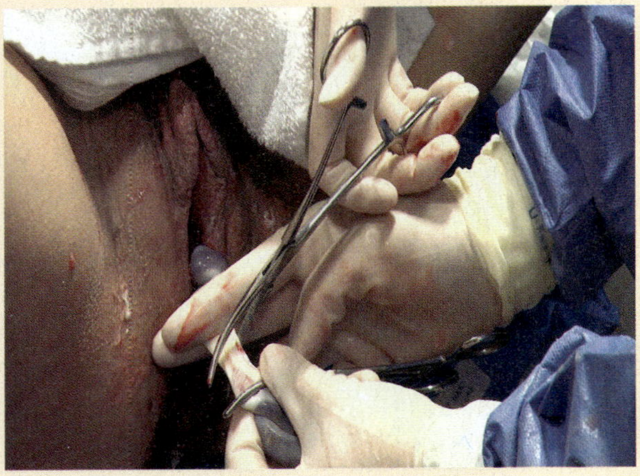

Step 7

Wait 60 seconds for the umbilical cord to stop pulsing. Place a clamp on the cord. Place a second clamp 2 to 3 inches (5 to 8 cm) away from the first.

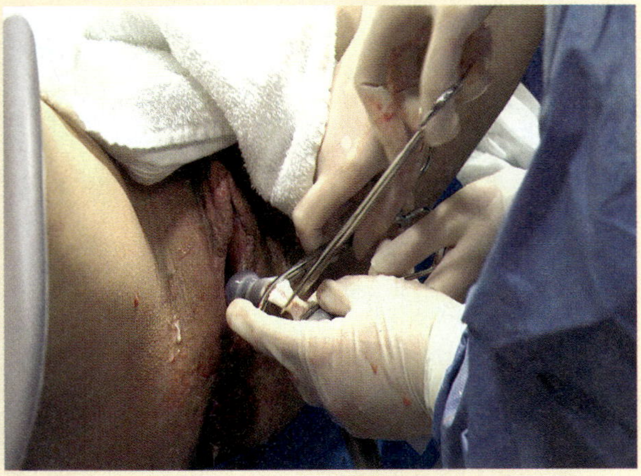

Step 8

Cut between the clamps.

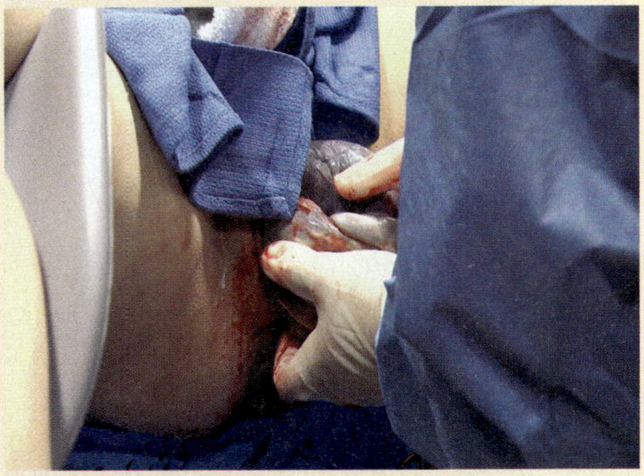

Step 9

Allow the placenta to deliver itself. Do not pull on the cord to speed delivery.

very slippery. Support the newborn's head with the neck in a neutral position to keep the airway open (**Step 5**).

6. If the mother is willing and able, place the newborn directly on the mother's abdomen, with the cord still intact. This skin-to-skin technique keeps the newborn warm and perfused; the mother's skin provides warmth while the placental perfusion continues until the pulsations in the cord stop.
7. After delivery and prior to cutting the cord, it is not necessary to suction the mouth and oropharynx to clear any amniotic fluid if the newborn is vigorous unless the airway is obstructed by secretions. Remove visible secretions from the nose and mouth using a cloth.

If secretions are obstructing the airway, clear them by gently suctioning the mouth and then the nose using a bulb syringe (**Step 6**).

8. After at least 60 seconds, place a clamp on the umbilical cord. Then place a second clamp 2 to 3 inches (5 to 8 cm) away from the first (**Step 7**).
9. Cut between the two clamps (**Step 8**).
10. The placenta will deliver itself, usually within 30 minutes of birth. Never pull on the end of the umbilical cord in an attempt to speed delivery of the placenta (**Step 9**).

Delivering the Head

Observe the head as it begins to exit the vagina so you can provide support as it emerges. It may take many contractions from the time the head begins to crown until the head delivers. Once it is obvious that the head is coming out farther with each contraction, place your sterile gloved hand over the emerging bony parts of the head, avoid the eyes and fontanelles, and, by exerting minimal pressure, control the delivery of the head. This will allow the head to come out smoothly and prevent it and the rest of the newborn from suddenly popping out during a strong contraction, possibly causing injury to the patient's perineal area and/or to the newborn. Continue to support the head as it rotates.

The risk of perineal tearing during labor can be reduced by applying gentle pressure across the perineum with a sterile gauze pad. Also be prepared for the possibility of the patient having a bowel movement because of the increased pressure on the rectum.

As you assist with the delivery of the head, be careful that you do not poke your fingers into the newborn's eyes or the fontanelles. The fontanelles are soft spots on the newborn's skull that will eventually become covered with bone. At birth, the brain is covered only with skin and membranes at these areas. There are two primary fontanelles, one on the top of the head and one near the back of the head.

Unruptured Amniotic Sac

The amniotic sac will usually rupture at the beginning of labor; if not, it may rupture during contractions. If the amniotic sac has not ruptured by the time the fetal head is crowning, it will appear as a fluid-filled sac (comparable to a water balloon) emerging from the vagina. This situation is potentially life threatening for the fetus because the sac will suffocate the fetus if it is not removed.

If the sac has not ruptured spontaneously by the time the fetus's head begins crowning, you may puncture the sac with a clamp or tear it by twisting it between your fingers. Make sure the puncture site is away from the fetus's face, and perform this procedure only as the head is crowning. As the sac is punctured, amniotic fluid will gush out. Push the ruptured sac away from the fetus's face as the head is delivered. Wipe the mouth and nose with gauze. If the airway is obstructed with fluid, clear the newborn's mouth and nose using the bulb syringe. If the amniotic fluid is greenish (indicating meconium staining) instead of clear or has a foul odor, notify the receiving hospital. Meconium in the amniotic fluid may result in respiratory distress or an airway obstruction in the newborn.

Umbilical Cord Around the Neck

As soon as the head is delivered, use one finger to feel whether the umbilical cord is wrapped around the neck. This condition, called a **nuchal cord**, occurs in approximately one-fourth of births.[20,21] A nuchal cord that is wound tightly around the neck could strangle the fetus, in which case it must be released immediately from the neck. Usually, you can slip the cord gently over the delivered head (or over the shoulder, if necessary). If this is not possible and the cord is tightening or impeding delivery,[22] you must cut the cord by placing two clamps approximately 2 inches (5 cm) apart on the cord and cutting between the clamps. Once the cord is cut, you must attempt to speed the delivery by encouraging the patient to push harder and possibly more often because the fetus will now have no oxygen supply until it is delivered and breathing spontaneously. Handle the cord very carefully; it is fragile and easily torn.

Delivering the Body

Once the head has been delivered, it usually rotates to one side or the other. This rotation places the body in a better position for delivery. By this time, the patient will most likely be ready to push again, and the upper shoulder will be visible in the vagina. The head is the largest part of the fetus. Once it is delivered, the body usually delivers easily. Support

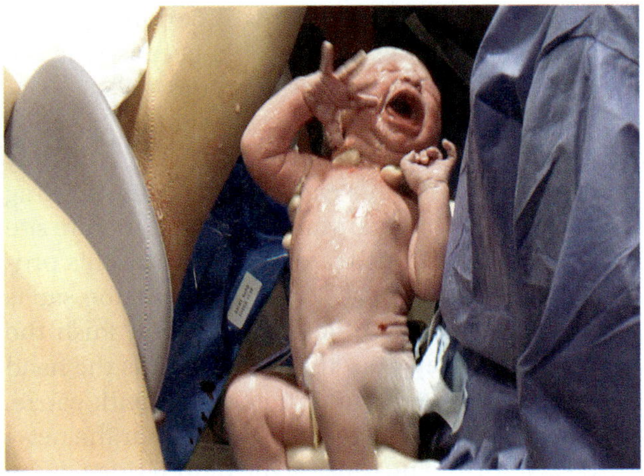

FIGURE 34-8 When you are holding the newborn, use two hands to support the entire body, including the head. One hand should support the back, chest, and head without squeezing or otherwise placing excess pressure on the neck. The second hand should support the buttocks.

the head and upper body as the shoulders deliver. Make sure to always support the head with one hand. Lower the head a little to deliver the upper shoulder, and then very gently raise it to deliver the lower shoulder. Do not pull the fetus from the birth canal. Once the shoulders deliver, the abdomen and hips will appear and will slide out easily. The newborn will be extremely slippery, so make sure to support the body with your other hand as it delivers. The newborn may be covered with a white, cheesy substance called **vernix caseosa**. Support and hold the newborn with both of your hands. Handle the newborn firmly but carefully (**FIGURE 34-8**).

Street Smarts

With the delivery of a newborn, you must divide your attention between two patients. This can keep two EMTs busy, even when things go well. To ensure that possible special care needs do not result in neglect of one of the patients, designate one member of the crew to pay primary attention to each patient. Call for additional help early if you suspect that both will need special care or that one will require resuscitation.

Postdelivery Care

As soon as the newborn is delivered, if the mother is able and willing, hand the newborn to the mother or place the newborn on the mother's chest or abdomen with skin-to-skin contact and cover with a blanket. As described earlier, this helps keep the newborn warm and may improve perfusion. Dry and stimulate the newborn, then wrap the baby in a clean, dry blanket or towel to maintain warmth. Newborns are very sensitive to temperature, so warm the blanket or towel, if possible, before you use it. Wrap the newborn so that only the face is exposed, making sure the top of the head is covered. Keep the neck in a neutral position so the airway remains open. Consider placing the newborn on one side. If circumstances prevent placing the newborn on the mother, cradle the newborn in your arms. Use a sterile gauze pad to wipe secretions from the newborn's mouth and nose as needed. If your local protocols specify, keep the newborn at the same level as the mother's vagina until the umbilical cord has been cut.

Words of Wisdom

Recording the time of birth is important because this information is needed for the birth certificate. It also provides you with a starting point from which to time the intervals for Apgar scores. This is even more important with multiple births. You will be busy, so you might consider asking a family member to act as "timekeeper."

Postdelivery care of the umbilical cord is important because infection is easily transmitted through the cord to the newborn. In a term newborn who is vigorous and not showing signs of respiratory distress, it has become generally accepted practice to place the newborn on the mother's chest and delay cord clamping until it has stopped pulsing, which typically occurs within 60 seconds.[22,23] In any newborn who requires immediate care for respiratory distress or other complication, prompt care takes priority over delayed cord clamping. Using the two clamps in the OB kit, clamp the cord between the mother and the newborn, preferably 5 to 6 inches (13 to 15 cm) from the newborn's body.[24] Place the clamps approximately 2 to 3 inches (5 to 8 cm) apart. When they are firmly in place, carefully cut the cord between them with sterile scissors or a scalpel. Remember, the cord is fragile; if handled roughly, it could be torn from the newborn's abdomen, resulting in a fatal hemorrhage. Once the clamps are in place, there is no need to rush.

Words of Wisdom

The American Heart Association suggests that when the infant does not need urgent resuscitation and delayed cord clamping is not possible, a technique called milking the cord may be beneficial in newborns 28 weeks' gestation and older.[25] This measure involves gently squeezing the cord to direct blood from the cord into the newborn, thereby increasing the newborn's blood volume. This technique is not used in younger newborns because of the increased risk that it may cause hemorrhage in the ventricle of the brain. Milking the cord requires special training, and state and medical director approval will be needed to determine if it is within the EMT's scope of practice.

Once the newborn has begun to breathe, the skin color should change from a dark-red or purple to a lighter red or pink color. At this time, evaluate the newborn for term gestation, good muscle tone, and breathing/crying; also obtain the 1-minute Apgar score (see "The Apgar Score" in this chapter). If the mother is alert and in stable condition and you have not done so already, hand the newborn to the mother so that skin-to-skin contact can begin while you dry and wrap the newborn. If this is not possible, give the newborn, wrapped in a warm blanket, to your partner, who can monitor the newborn and complete the initial care. You need to return your attention to the mother and the delivery of the placenta.

Delivery of the Placenta

The placenta is attached to the end of the umbilical cord, which is coming out of the patient's vagina. The placenta usually delivers within a few minutes of the birth, although it may take as long as 30 minutes, so do not delay transport waiting for the placenta to deliver. As with delivering the newborn, your job is only to assist. Never pull on the end of the umbilical cord in an attempt to speed delivery of the placenta. You may tear the cord, the placenta, or both and cause serious or perhaps life-threatening hemorrhage. A gush of bloody fluid, usually less than 500 mL, occurs before the placenta delivers and is normal and expected.

The normal placenta is round, approximately 7 inches (18 cm) in diameter, and approximately 1 inch (2.5 cm) thick. One surface is smooth and covered with a shiny gray membrane. The other surface is rough, divided into lobes, and is a dark red-brown color similar to raw liver. Wrap the entire placenta and cord in a towel, place them into a plastic bag, and take them to the hospital. Hospital personnel will examine the placenta and the cord to make certain that the entire placenta has been delivered. If a piece of the placenta has been retained inside the patient, it could cause persistent bleeding or infection.

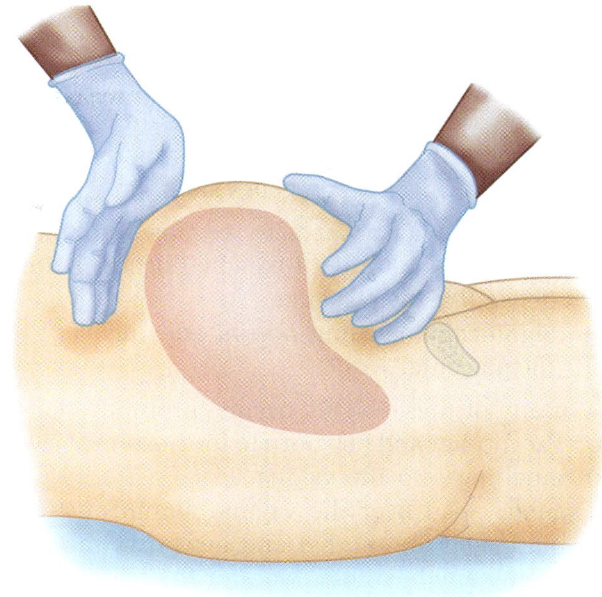

FIGURE 34-9 After delivery, massage the fundus (the upper end of the uterus) in a firm, circular motion.

After delivery of the placenta and before transport, place a sterile pad or sanitary pad over the vagina and straighten the patient's legs. You can help to slow bleeding by massaging the patient's abdomen using a firm, circular, kneading motion with one hand cupped over the top of the fundus and the other above the pubic bone (**FIGURE 34-9**). The **fundus** is the upper end of the uterus and will present as a firm, grapefruit-size mass in the lower abdomen. The abdominal skin will be wrinkled and very soft. As you massage the fundus, the uterus will contract and become firmer. This may be uncomfortable for the patient. Provide reassurance and explain that it is necessary to help control the bleeding. Breastfeeding also stimulates the uterus to contract because, like massaging the uterus, it causes the production of oxytocin, a hormone that helps to contract the uterus and slow bleeding.

Take a moment to congratulate the new mother and thank anyone who assisted. Be sure to record the time of birth in your patient care report.

The following are emergency situations:

- The placenta has not delivered after 30 minutes.
- More than 500 mL of bleeding occurs before delivery of the placenta.
- Significant bleeding occurs after delivery of the placenta.

If any of these events occurs, promptly transport the mother and newborn to the hospital. Never put anything into the vagina. Place a sterile pad or sanitary pad over the vagina, administer oxygen, and keep the mother and newborn warm by preventing any heat loss. Monitor the mother's vital signs closely. Ensure that both the mother and newborn are properly restrained prior to transport. The baby may be secured to the mother with an approved neonatal restraint system, in a car seat, or in an isolette, unless resuscitation is needed.

Neonatal Assessment and Resuscitation

The American Heart Association and American Academy of Pediatrics have published guidelines on the routine care and resuscitation of newborns. The first minute after birth is often referred to as the "golden minute," and during this time all newborns should be assessed to determine the need for resuscitation. Take standard precautions, and always wear gloves when handling a newborn.

During the first minute of life, perform the following four initial steps of newborn care:

- Airway positioning and suctioning, if needed
- Drying
- Warming
- Tactile stimulation

These initial steps of newborn care should be carried out in all newborns. If signs of good tone and adequate ventilation are not present after performing the initial steps for approximately 30 seconds, then positive-pressure ventilation with a bag-mask device may be necessary. If the newborn is vigorous with good tone and has adequate respirations (good color, strong cry, and spontaneous respirations) in the first minute of life, then note the Apgar score and place the baby onto the mother's chest for skin-to-skin bonding and routine care. The normal respiratory and cardiovascular physiologic responses expected are that the newborn will begin breathing spontaneously within 30 seconds after birth, and the heart rate will be 100 beats/min or higher.

Many newborns require some form of stimulation that will encourage them to breathe air and begin circulating blood through the lungs (**TABLE 34-4**). The following list provides additional details regarding the initial steps of newborn care.

- Position the newborn on the back with a towel or blanket under the shoulders so that the neck is slightly extended in a neutral or sniffing position.
- If the newborn has an obvious airway obstruction or needs positive-pressure ventilation, suction the mouth and then the nose using a bulb syringe or suction device with an 8 French or 10 French catheter.[24] Suction both sides of the back of the mouth, where secretions tend to collect, but avoid deep suctioning of the mouth and throat, which can cause the heart rate to slow.

TABLE 34-4 Initial Steps for Newborn Care and Resuscitation

Assess and support	• Airway (position and suction if needed) • Breathing (tactile stimulation) • Circulation (heart rate and skin color) • Temperature (warm) and skin (dry)
Basic life support interventions	• Dry and warm the newborn. • Provide tactile stimulation while actively drying and warming. • Open the airway and suction only if needed. • Use a bag-mask device to ventilate the newborn if needed. This is seldom required. • Perform chest compressions if there is no pulse or if the heart rate is <60 beats/min after 30 seconds of ventilation and is not increasing.

- In addition to vigorously drying the newborn's head, back, and body with dry towels, you may rub the newborn's back and gently flick or slap the soles of the feet.

If the newborn does not breathe after 30 seconds of stimulation, begin positive-pressure ventilation with room air, using an appropriate-size bag-mask device.

You should be properly equipped for resuscitation measures in case the newborn is in distress. Most of the equipment and supplies needed to resuscitate a newborn can be found in your OB kit. Other items you may need are clean, dry towels; an infant blanket; a bag-mask device with a 450-mL reservoir; and masks in both newborn and preterm sizes.

Additional Resuscitation Efforts

Observe the newborn for spontaneous respirations, skin color, and movement of the extremities. If the respiratory effort appears appropriate, evaluate the heart rate by palpating the pulse at the brachial artery or listening to the newborn's chest with a stethoscope. It should be at least 100 beats/min. The heart rate is the most important measure in determining the need for further resuscitation (**FIGURE 34-10**).

If chest compressions are required, use the hand-encircling technique for two-person resuscitation (**FIGURE 34-11**). Perform bag-mask ventilation during a pause after every third compression. Avoid giving a compression and a ventilation simultaneously, because one will decrease the effectiveness of the other. Cardiac arrest in newborns is nearly always the result of ventilation compromise. Use a compression-to-ventilation ratio of 3:1, which will yield a total of 120 actions per minute (90 compressions and 30 ventilations). Hands-only CPR is not as effective as ventilation with CPR. Remember that adequate ventilation is absolutely critical to the successful resuscitation of the newborn.

Transport any newborn who requires more than routine resuscitation to a hospital with a level III neonatal intensive care unit, if available in your area. This type of unit is designed for newborns who require specialized care. If a level III neonatal intensive care unit is not available in your area, provide rapid transport to the closest appropriate facility.

Meconium-stained amniotic fluid is seen in approximately 17% of term births. The risk of meconium-stained amniotic fluid generally increases with gestational age, and postterm newborns (42 weeks' gestation and beyond) are at highest risk. Meconium can be thick or thin. If the newborn aspirates thick meconium, significant lung disease and even death can occur. If you see meconium in the amniotic fluid or meconium staining and the newborn is not breathing adequately, consider quickly suctioning the newborn's mouth and then nose after delivery before providing rescue ventilations.[26]

The Apgar Score

The **Apgar score** is the standard scoring system used to assess the status of a newborn. The last name of the scoring system's creator, Virginia Apgar, serves as a mnemonic to help remember the five areas of activity that are tested.

- **Appearance.** Shortly after birth, the skin of a light-skinned newborn and the mucous membranes of a dark-skinned newborn should turn pink. Newborns often have cyanosis of the extremities for a few minutes after birth, but hands and feet should "pink up" quickly. Blue skin all over or blue mucous membranes signal central cyanosis.
- **Pulse.** Measure the pulse by chest auscultation. If a stethoscope is not available, you can measure pulsations with your fingers at the brachial pulse. A newborn with no pulse requires immediate CPR.
- **Grimace or irritability.** Grimacing, crying, or withdrawing in response to stimuli is normal and indicates that the newborn is doing well. Test this by snapping a finger against the sole of the newborn's foot.
- **Activity or muscle tone.** The degree of muscle tone indicates the oxygenation of the tissues. Normally, the hips and knees are flexed at birth, and, to some degree, the newborn will resist attempts to straighten them. A newborn should not be floppy or limp.
- **Respirations.** Normally, a newborn's respirations are regular and rapid, with a good strong cry. If the respirations are slow, shallow, or labored, or if the cry is weak, the newborn may have respiratory insufficiency and need assistance with ventilation. Complete absence of respirations or crying is obviously a very serious sign; in addition to assisted ventilation, CPR may be necessary.

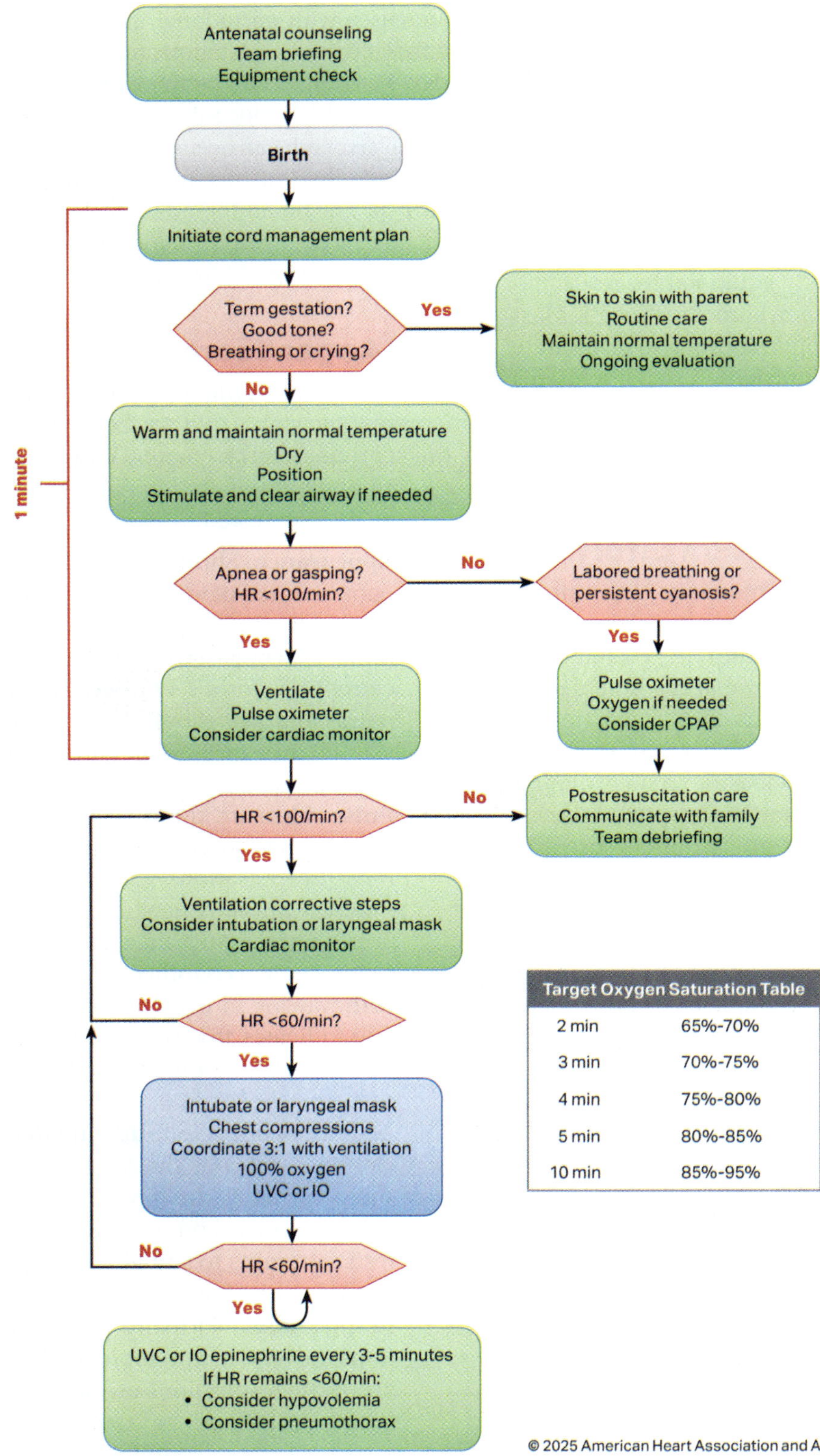

Target Oxygen Saturation Table	
2 min	65%-70%
3 min	70%-75%
4 min	75%-80%
5 min	80%-85%
10 min	85%-95%

FIGURE 34-10 Basic Neonatal Resuscitation Program algorithm.

Abbreviations: CPAP, continuous positive airway pressure; HR, heart rate; IO, intraosseous; UVC, umbilical venous catheter

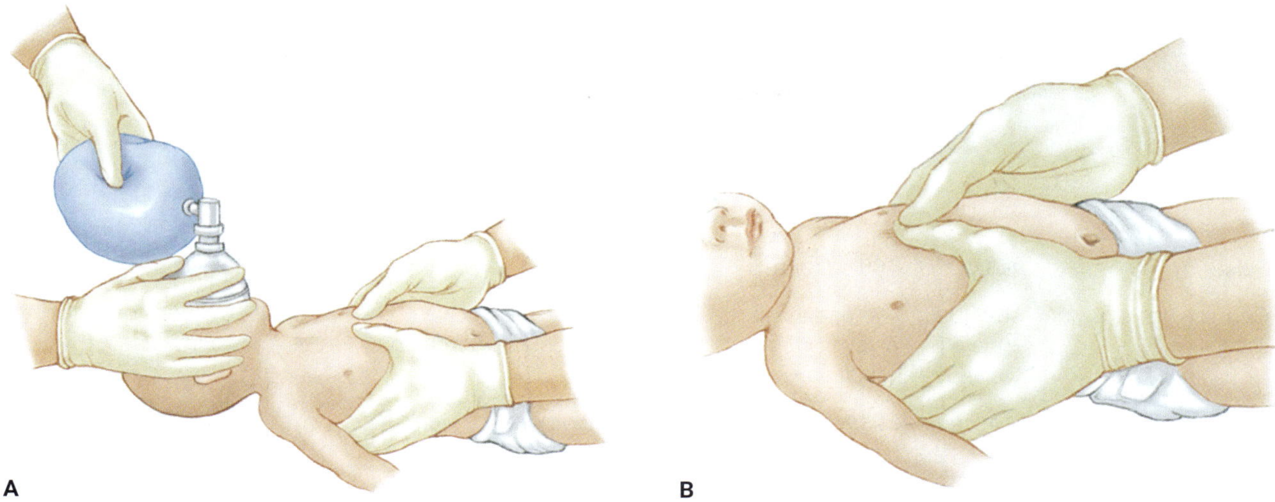

FIGURE 34-11 A. Chest compressions should be given with the hands encircling the newborn and thumbs side by side. **B.** In very small newborns, you may need to overlap the thumbs.

YOU are the EMT

After 30 seconds of ventilation with a bag-mask device, you reassess the newborn.

Recording Time: 5 Minutes (Newborn)	
Level of consciousness	Crying and moving all extremities
Respirations	60 breaths/min
Pulse	120 beats/min
Skin	Mucous membranes, pink; hands and feet, cyanotic
Oxygen saturation (Spo_2)	94% (on room air)

You swaddle the newborn, then hand the newborn to the mother. The placenta delivers and is appropriately cared for. You reassess the mother's vital signs and then prepare for transport by securing the mother and newborn in appropriate restraint systems.

Recording Time: 20 Minutes (Mother)	
Level of consciousness	Conscious and alert
Respirations	20 breaths/min; adequate depth
Pulse	98 beats/min; strong and regular
Skin	Baseline color, warm, and moist
Blood pressure	126/60 mm Hg
Oxygen saturation (Spo_2)	97% (on room air)

En route to the hospital, you reassess the newborn and mother. The mother remains conscious and alert and has mild vaginal bleeding. The newborn's mucous membranes are pink, but her hands and feet remain cyanotic; her heart rate is 130 beats/min, and her respirations are rapid; she pulls her foot away when you flick the sole; and she resists your attempts to straighten her knees. You call the receiving hospital and give your radio report; your estimated time of arrival is 6 minutes.

9. What further treatment is indicated for the mother?
10. What Apgar score should you assign to this newborn at 5 minutes after birth?

TABLE 34-5 Apgar Scoring System

Area of Activity	Score 2	Score 1	Score 0
Appearance	Entire newborn is pink.[a]	Body is pink, but hands and feet remain blue.	Entire newborn is blue or pale.
Pulse	More than 100 beats/min	Fewer than 100 beats/min	Absent pulse
Grimace or irritability	Newborn cries and tries to move foot away from finger snapped against sole of foot.	Newborn gives a weak cry in response to stimulus.	Newborn does not cry or react to stimulus.
Activity or muscle tone	Newborn resists attempts to straighten hips and knees.	Newborn makes weak attempts to resist straightening.	Newborn is completely limp, with no muscle tone.
Respiration	Rapid respirations	Slow respirations	Absent respirations

[a]The colors stated here reflect the traditional wording of this scoring system. "Pink" and "blue" should be understood to represent the newborn's perfusion status, with respect to baseline skin color.

As shown in **TABLE 34-5**, each of these five areas receives a numeric value (0, 1, or 2). The total of the five values is the Apgar score. The highest possible score is 10.

Words of Wisdom

Some researchers have found that newborns who have darker skin color are much more likely than those who have light skin color to receive an Apgar score of less than 10. They suggest that that this disparity reflects systemic bias and that the Apgar score should be revised to eliminate color.[27]

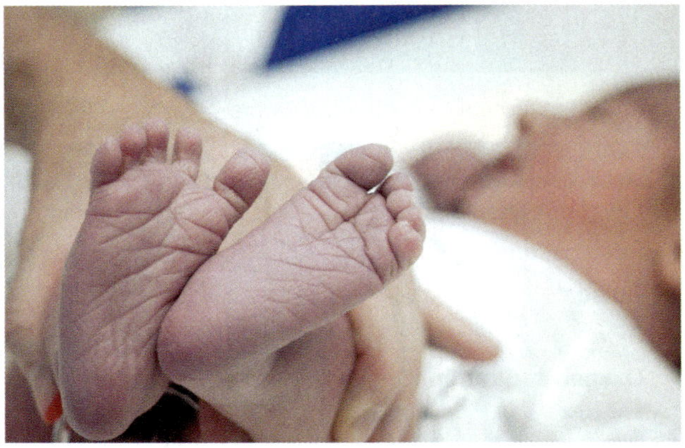

FIGURE 34-12 Newborns who have cyanosis limited to the extremities immediately after delivery would receive only 1 point for "Appearance" on the Apgar scale.

The Apgar score should be calculated at 1 minute and again at 5 minutes after birth. Calculation of the Apgar score should not delay resuscitation efforts and is generally deferred when resuscitation is required. A score of 7 or higher is generally considered reassuring. **FIGURE 34-12** shows a photo of a newborn with an Apgar score of less than 10.

Follow these steps when assessing a newborn:

1. One minute after the newborn is delivered, quickly calculate the Apgar score to establish a baseline on the newborn's status.
2. Stimulation should result in an immediate increase in respiration rate. If not, you must begin ventilations with a bag-mask device at a rate of 40 to 60 breaths/min. Unlike adults, in whom sudden cardiac arrest may precede respiratory arrest, newborns who are in cardiac arrest usually have had a respiratory arrest first. Therefore, it is essential to keep the newborn ventilating and oxygenating well.
3. If the newborn is breathing well, check the pulse rate by feeling the brachial pulse or auscultating the chest with a stethoscope. The pulse rate should be at least 100 beats/min. If it is less than 100 beats/min, begin ventilations with a bag-mask device. Begin ventilations

without oxygen attached, as the 21% oxygen in the atmosphere is often sufficient and a rapid change from the prebirth saturation levels may slow the newborn's circulatory transition. Ventilation alone may increase the newborn's heart rate. Reassess respirations and heart rate at least every 30 seconds to make sure the pulse rate is increasing and respirations are becoming spontaneous and normalizing.

4. Assess the newborn's oxygenation via pulse oximetry, which is best taken at the right wrist, and observe for central cyanosis. The oxygen saturation does not usually reach the 85% to 95% range until approximately 10 minutes after birth. If central cyanosis is present or the oxygen saturation does not improve but breathing is adequate, administer blow-by oxygen by holding oxygen tubing or an oxygen mask close to the newborn's face. Set the oxygen flow rate at 5 L/min.
5. Remember that you now have two patients. Request a second unit as soon as possible if you determine that the newborn is in any distress and will require resuscitation.

For newborns who do not begin breathing on their own or do not have an adequate heart rate, continue CPR and rapidly transport. Once CPR has been started, do not stop until the newborn responds with adequate respirations and heart rate or is pronounced dead by a physician. Do not give up! If the newborn presents in distress, do not take time to assess the Apgar score—begin resuscitation immediately.

Special Populations

INFANT CPR VERSUS _NEWBORN_ CPR

Current information on neonatal resuscitation may vary from what you learned in your class on CPR, which usually does not differentiate between CPR for an infant and CPR for a newborn. Know your specific local protocols on neonatal resuscitation. If the heart rate is less than 60 beats/min despite at least 30 seconds of positive-pressure ventilation, increase the oxygen concentration to 100% and begin CPR. Likewise, if the newborn is not breathing and has no pulse, begin CPR. The compression-to-ventilation ratio for a newborn is 3:1; that is, you should provide three compressions using the hand-encircling technique followed by one ventilation, then repeat.[14] When performed at this rate, you will deliver 90 compressions and 30 breaths per minute.

Words of Wisdom

Since the rate of newborn positive-pressure ventilation is quite fast, it may help to say, "Breathe, two, three; breathe, two, three . . ." to assure you ventilate at an adequate rate.

Complicated Delivery Emergencies

Shoulder Dystocia

Shoulder dystocia is a condition that occurs when the shoulders are unable to clear the pelvic opening after the newborn's head delivers. When shoulder dystocia occurs, after the head clears the vaginal opening, instead of the shoulders delivering, the head pulls back tightly against the mother's perineum (known as the turtle sign). Until maneuvers are performed to allow the shoulders to move past the pelvis, delivery cannot occur.

Shoulder dystocia is associated with significant complications, including possible fetal death if delivery cannot be completed in a timely manner. If the shoulders do not deliver within a minute or two after the head, attempt the following maneuver with the mother supine[24]:

1. Hyperflex the mother's hips, pulling her thighs toward her abdomen while abducting them away from the body in an exaggerated supine knee–chest position.
2. Apply firm pressure above the pubic symphysis to attempt to free the first shoulder.
3. Attempt to angle the baby's head posteriorly as far as possible, but *never* pull on it.
4. Continue the delivery as usual once the first shoulder is free.

If these actions fail to release the shoulders, contact medical direction and prepare for urgent transport.

Breech Delivery

The position in which an infant is born or the body part that is delivered first is called the **presentation**.

Most infants are born head first, in what is called a **vertex presentation**. Occasionally, the buttocks are delivered first. This is called a **breech presentation** (**FIGURE 34-13**). With a breech presentation, the fetus is at great risk for trauma from the delivery. In addition, a prolapsed cord is more common in a breech delivery. Breech deliveries usually take longer than a normal delivery, so there may be time to get the pregnant patient to the hospital. If the buttocks have already passed through the vagina, however, the delivery has begun. You should provide emergency care and call for ALS backup. In general, if the patient does not deliver within 10 minutes of the buttocks' presentation, provide prompt transport. Consult medical direction to guide you in this difficult situation.

Preparing for a breech delivery is the same as for a normal childbirth. Position the pregnant patient, prepare the OB kit, and place yourself and your partner as you would for a normal delivery. Allow the buttocks and legs to deliver spontaneously, supporting them with your hand to prevent rapid expulsion. The buttocks will usually come out easily. If necessary, rotate the baby's trunk clockwise or sweep the legs from the vagina. After the legs have delivered, let them dangle on either side of your arm as you support the body to prevent the head from hyperextending. Be mindful to keep the fetus raised off of the umbilical cord.

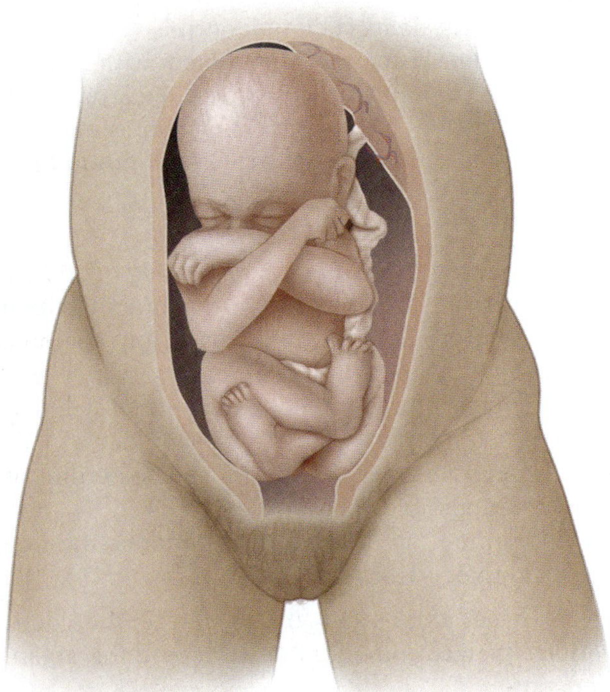

FIGURE 34-13 In a breech presentation, the buttocks are delivered first. Breech deliveries are usually slow, so you will often have time to transport the patient to the hospital.

The head is almost always facedown and should be allowed to deliver spontaneously. If it does not deliver immediately, you will need to perform a potentially lifesaving procedure to manage the newborn's airway. Make a "V" with your gloved fingers and position them inside the vagina over the baby's cheeks, without blocking the baby's mouth, to keep the walls of the vagina from compressing the baby's airway. Allow the chin to tilt toward the chest, slightly flexing the neck.

Note that this situation and a prolapsed cord are the only two circumstances in which you should insert your fingers into the vagina. Also note that when assisting a breech delivery, as with a shoulder dystocia, you should never pull on the baby's body; just support it when the mother is ready to push.

Presentation Complications

On rare occasions, the presenting part of the fetus is neither the head nor the buttocks but a single arm or leg. This is called a **limb presentation** (**FIGURE 34-14**). You cannot successfully deliver a fetus with a limb presentation in the field. These fetuses usually must be delivered surgically. If you are faced with a limb presentation, you must transport the patient to the hospital immediately. If a limb is protruding, cover it with a sterile towel. Never try to push it back in, and never pull on it. Place the patient supine, with the head down and pelvis elevated. Because the mother and fetus are likely to be physically stressed, remember to administer high-flow oxygen to the mother.

Prolapse of the umbilical cord, a situation in which the umbilical cord comes out of the vagina before the fetus (**FIGURE 34-15**), is another rare presentation that must be treated in the hospital. This situation is dangerous because the fetus's head will compress the cord during birth and cut off circulation, depriving the fetus of oxygenated blood. Do not attempt to push the cord back into the vagina. Prolapse of the umbilical cord usually occurs early in labor when the amniotic sac ruptures. There is usually time to get the patient to the hospital. Your

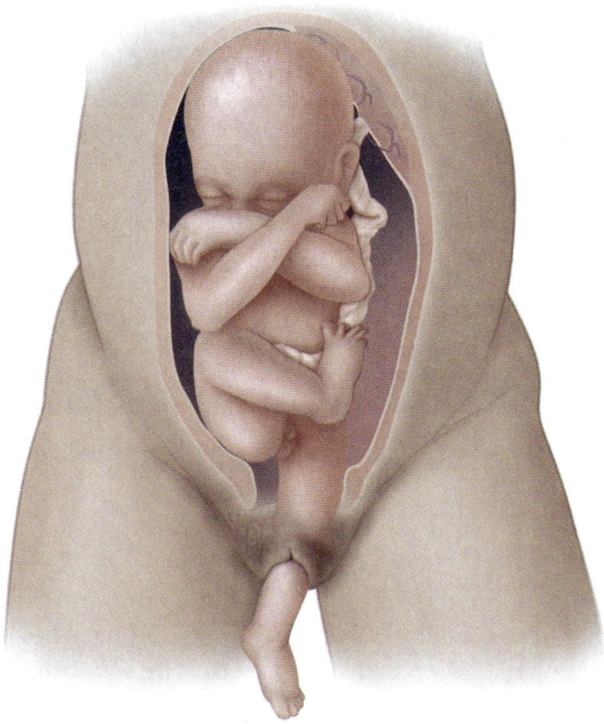

FIGURE 34-14 In rare cases, a limb, usually a single arm or leg, presents first. This is a life-threatening situation, and you must provide prompt transport for hospital delivery.

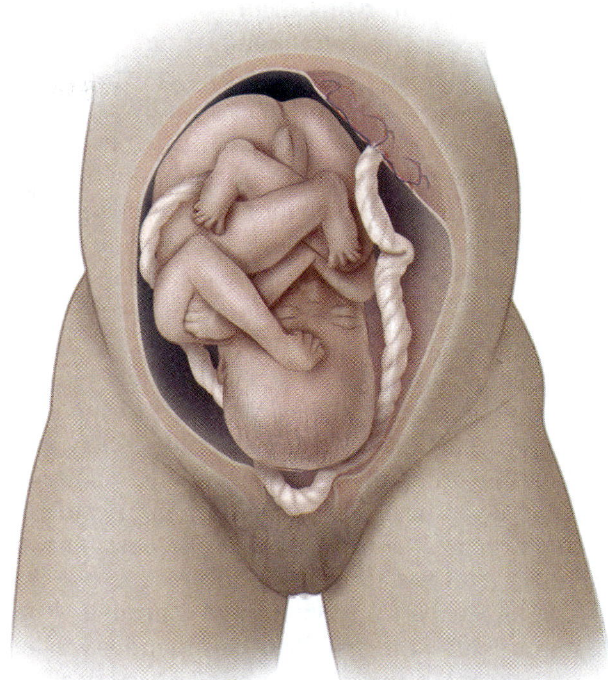

FIGURE 34-15 A prolapsed umbilical cord is a life-threatening situation for the fetus and must be treated at the hospital.

job is to try to keep the fetus's head from compressing the cord.

Place the pregnant patient supine with the foot end of the stretcher raised 6 to 12 inches (15 to 30 cm) higher than the head, with the hips elevated on a pillow or folded sheet. Alternatively, the patient may be placed in the knee–chest position: kneeling and bent forward, facedown. Either of these positions will help keep the weight of the fetus off the prolapsed cord. Carefully insert your sterile gloved hand into the vagina, palpate for pulsations in the cord, and gently push the presenting part (usually the fetus's head) away from the umbilical cord. Remember that this is one of only two situations (the other being a breech presentation) in which you should place a hand or finger into the vagina. Maintain this position and continue to keep the pressure off of the cord continuously throughout the transport to the hospital and possibly until the patient is in the operating room. Wrap a sterile towel, moistened with saline, around the exposed cord. Administer high-flow oxygen, and transport rapidly.

Spina Bifida

Spina bifida is a developmental defect in which a portion of the spinal cord or meninges may protrude outside of the vertebrae and possibly outside of the body. When it protrudes outside the body, the protrusion is seen on the newborn's back, usually in the lumbar area. It is important to cover the open area of the spinal cord with a moist, sterile dressing and then an occlusive dressing to seal the area immediately after birth to help prevent a potentially fatal infection. This treatment will have a positive effect on the newborn's outcome. Maintenance of the newborn's body temperature is important, so if you must use moist dressings, which can lower the body temperature, have someone hold the newborn against their body. Chapter 35, *Patients With Special Challenges*, discusses spina bifida in greater detail.

Multiple Gestation

Multiple births represent approximately 3% of births in the United States. Approximately 97% of multiple births are twins, with triplets or greater multiples occurring infrequently.[19] Pregnant individuals usually know if they are carrying multiple fetuses. Sometimes, there is a family history of twins or patients suspect they are having twins because they have an unusually large abdomen. Usually, however, the identification of multiple fetuses is made early in pregnancy with modern ultrasonographic techniques. With multiple fetuses, always be prepared for more than one resuscitation, and call for assistance.

Twins are usually smaller than single fetuses, and delivery is typically not difficult. Consider the possibility that you are dealing with twins any time the first newborn is small or the patient's abdomen remains fairly large and firm after the birth. You should also ask the patient about the possibility of multiples. If twins are present, the second one will usually be born within 45 minutes of the first. About 10 minutes after the first birth, contractions will begin again, and the birth process will repeat itself.

The procedure for delivering twins is the same as that for a single fetus; however, you will need some supplies from an additional OB kit. Clamp and cut the cord of the first newborn as soon as it has been delivered and before the second newborn is delivered. The second fetus may deliver before or after the first placenta. There may be only one placenta, or one for each fetus. When the placenta has been delivered, check whether there is one umbilical cord or two. If you see only one umbilical cord coming out of the first placenta, another placenta is still to be delivered. If both cords are attached to one placenta, the delivery is complete. Identical twins are always the same sex; fraternal twins may be the same or different sexes.

Record the time of birth of each twin separately. Twins may be so small that they appear to have been born preterm; handle them carefully and keep them warm. Identify the first newborn delivered as "Baby A." With the delivery of two or more newborns, you can indicate the order of delivery by writing on a piece of tape and placing it on the blanket or towel that is wrapped around each newborn.

Preterm Birth

Term gestation is considered to be between 39 weeks and 40 weeks, 6 days, which is approximately 9 calendar months. A normal, single newborn at term will weigh approximately 7 lb (3 kg) at birth. Any birth that occurs before 37 weeks of gestation have been completed is considered preterm. In the United States, approximately 10% of births are preterm.[28] This determination is not always easy to make. Often, the exact gestation time cannot be determined. A preterm newborn is smaller and thinner than a term newborn at term, and the head is proportionately larger in comparison with the rest of the body (**FIGURE 34-16**). The vernix caseosa will be absent or minimal on a preterm newborn. There will also be less body hair.

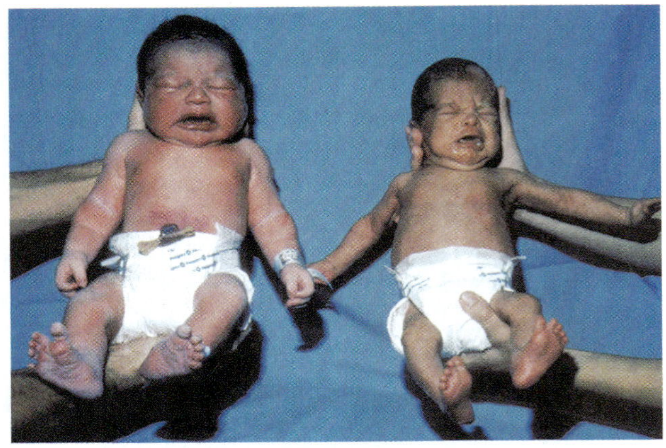

FIGURE 34-16 Preterm newborns (right) are smaller and thinner than term newborns.

Preterm newborns need special care to survive. They often require resuscitation, which should be performed unless physically impossible. With such care, preterm newborns as small as 1 lb (0.5 kg) have survived.

Postterm Pregnancy

Approximately 5% of deliveries occur postterm in the United States.[28] Postterm means the gestation period is longer than 41 completed weeks of gestation. The rate of postterm pregnancies has been steadily declining for the past decade.

A true postterm pregnancy can lead to complications in both the mother and fetus. Postterm fetuses can be larger than a typical 40-week fetus, sometimes weighing more than 10 lb (5 kg), which can lead to a more difficult labor and delivery and an increased chance of injury to the fetus as it travels through the birth canal. The likelihood of a cesarean section being required is increased. The mother is also at increased risk for perineal tears and infection. Postterm newborns have an increased risk of meconium aspiration, infection, and being stillborn and may not have developed normally because of the restricted size of the uterus. Be prepared to resuscitate the newborn, as respiratory and neurologic functions may have been affected. The larger size of the fetus causes it to take up more space inside the uterus, resulting in compression of the structures, including the blood vessels of the placenta and the umbilical cord.

Fetal Death

Unfortunately, you may find yourself delivering a fetus that died in the uterus before labor began. This situation will test your medical, emotional, and social abilities. Grieving parents will be emotionally distraught and may be hostile, requiring all of your professionalism and support skills. Chapter 4, *Communications and Documentation*, discusses how to handle the death of a child in detail.

The onset of labor may be premature, but labor will otherwise progress normally in most cases. If an intrauterine infection has caused the death of the fetus, you may note an extremely foul odor. Depending on the stage of decomposition, the delivered fetus may have skin blisters, skin sloughing, and a dark discoloration. The head will be soft and perhaps grossly deformed.

Do not attempt to resuscitate an obviously dead newborn. However, do not confuse this situation with that in which a newborn is in cardiopulmonary arrest as a complication of the birthing process. You must attempt to resuscitate newborns if there is any question about viability.

Postpartum Complications

Some bleeding always occurs with delivery, but bleeding that exceeds approximately 1,000 mL is considered high risk for maternal mortality and morbidity.[29] If bleeding continues after delivery of the placenta, continue to massage the uterus, but check your technique and hand placement. If the patient appears to be in shock, treat accordingly and transport, massaging the uterus en route. Excessive bleeding after birth is usually caused by the muscles of the uterus not fully contracting, which may occur following the birth of more than one newborn, a long labor process that leaves the uterus too "tired" to contract, or a delivery in which parts of the placenta remain inside the uterus. This condition is potentially life threatening for the mother. Cover the vagina with a sterile pad, changing the pad as often as necessary. Do not discard any blood-soaked pads; hospital personnel will use them to estimate the amount of blood loss. Also save any tissue that may have passed from the vagina.

Administer oxygen if necessary, monitor vital signs frequently, and transport the patient immediately to the hospital. Never hold the patient's legs together or pack the vagina with gauze pads in an attempt to control bleeding.

Postpartum patients are also at increased risk of a venous embolism. One reason is the increased clotting ability that is a normal change of pregnancy. Also, a pregnant patient who has been on bed rest for any length of time is more susceptible to clots. The most common embolism seen in postpartum patients is a pulmonary embolism, which is a clot that travels through the bloodstream and becomes lodged in the pulmonary circulation. This obstruction will block blood flow to the lungs and is potentially life threatening. If you deliver a newborn in the field and the mother begins to report sudden difficulty breathing or shortness of breath, consider the possibility that the patient has a pulmonary embolism.

You should also suspect a pulmonary embolism in patients with respiratory complaints who have recently delivered, especially with the sudden onset of difficulty breathing or altered mental status. Individuals have died of a postpartum pulmonary embolism anywhere from days to several weeks or months after childbirth. Provide supportive care of the ABCs with high-flow oxygen and rapid transport to the hospital.

YOU are the EMT SUMMARY

1. What anatomic and physiologic changes occur during pregnancy? How will they affect your assessment of the patient?

Most pregnancy-related changes are observed in the respiratory and cardiovascular systems. As the uterus enlarges during pregnancy, it is displaced upward from the pelvic cavity, where it is normally protected, and is therefore exposed to potential injury. The enlarged uterus pushes upward on the diaphragm. This decreases the ability to breathe deeply, so the respiratory rate increases slightly to maintain adequate minute volume. Pregnancy also increases maternal oxygen demand and consumption, and the body compensates with increased respiratory rate as well. Blood volume increases throughout pregnancy. To accommodate the increase in total blood volume, heart rate increases up to 20%, or approximately 20 beats/min, by the third trimester of pregnancy.

Vital signs changes during pregnancy, such as an increase in heart rate and respiratory rate, should not be assumed to be pregnancy related if the patient experiences an acute illness or injury. Instead, assume these changes to be signs of shock until proven otherwise.

2. How will you determine whether delivery is imminent or if there is enough time to transport the pregnant patient?

Ask the patient how long she has been pregnant, when she is due to deliver, and if this is her first pregnancy. *As a general rule*, labor is longer in patients who are pregnant for the first time (primigravida). If the patient is experiencing contractions, ask her how far apart they are and how long they last. Ask if her bag of waters (amniotic sac) has ruptured. This typically occurs toward the end of the first stage of labor, but may not occur until the delivery itself. Ask her if she is experiencing any vaginal spotting or bleeding; during the first stage of labor a plug of mucus, sometimes mixed with blood (bloody show), is expelled from the dilating cervix and discharged from the vagina. Ask the patient if she feels the urge to push or move her bowels as the pressure of the baby's head on the perineum may be misinterpreted as the need to have a bowel movement. The presence of crowning is an obvious indicator that delivery is in progress. Perhaps one of the most reliable indicators of imminent delivery is when the patient states, "I'm having this baby now!" This is especially true in patients who have given birth before.

3. What are gestational diabetes and preeclampsia? How can they affect this delivery?

Gestational diabetes, or diabetes of pregnancy, is a condition that develops during pregnancy and typically resolves on its own after delivery. Gestational diabetes is associated with newborns who are large for their gestational age, which could lead to shoulder dystocia, a condition in which the fetus's shoulders are too broad to fit through the mother's pelvic opening, or other delivery complications caused by the fetus's size. In addition, many patients experience nausea before labor and have not eaten recently, factors that could lead to hypoglycemia and weakness in the mother and fetus.

Preeclampsia is characterized by hypertension; edema of the hands, feet, and face; and protein in the urine. Other symptoms may include visual disturbances (eg, seeing spots, blurred vision), headache, and anxiety.

Untreated preeclampsia may lead to eclampsia, which is characterized by life-threatening seizures. The presence of preeclampsia, as with gestational diabetes, increases the risk of fetal distress, which may necessitate resuscitation of the newborn after delivery.

4. Is there time to transport this patient, or should you prepare for imminent delivery?

The patient is experiencing frequent (every 2 minutes) contractions that are lasting 45 seconds, and she has the urge to move her bowels, which indicates that the fetus is in the birth canal. On the basis of these factors, delivery will likely occur within the next few minutes; therefore, you and your partner should prepare for imminent delivery.

5. How should you manage the umbilical cord situation?

As soon as the head has delivered, you should assess for the location of the umbilical cord. If wrapped around the newborn's neck, an umbilical cord must be managed immediately because if the cord is wrapped tightly around the newborn's neck, the airway could be constricted. Usually, you can slip the cord gently over the head (or shoulders, if necessary). If not and the cord is tightening or impeding delivery, place two clamps on the cord approximately 2 inches (5 cm) apart and cut between them. Delivery must proceed quickly if this is necessary, as the newborn is no longer receiving oxygen from the mother once the cord is clamped. Handle the cord very carefully; it is fragile and easily torn.

YOU are the EMT SUMMARY continued

6. What would you do if the amniotic sac was still intact?

If you notice that the amniotic sac seems to be intact after the head delivers or as the head is crowning, immediately puncture the membrane and allow the fluid to drain. Avoid using sharp objects to puncture the membrane; first attempt to use your gloved fingers to tear the membrane. Once the membrane ruptures and the fluid drains, wipe the traces of the membrane away from the newborn's mouth and nose and continue with the delivery.

7. What is involved in the routine postdelivery care of a newborn?

Immediate postdelivery care of a newborn, regardless of the newborn's appearance, involves keeping the newborn dry and warm and facilitating effective breathing. The need for further treatment is based on assessment of the newborn's respiratory effort, heart rate, and skin color.

8. What immediate treatment is indicated for this newborn?

The newborn is breathing; however, her heart rate is low (80 beats/min) and her trunk and extremities are cyanotic. These clinical signs indicate that she is hypoxemic and will require additional resuscitative measures. Begin positive-pressure ventilations with a bag-mask device. Newborn bradycardia is almost always the result of hypoxemia.

Ventilate the newborn at a rate of 40 to 60 breaths/min for 30 seconds with room air, and then reassess the heart rate. In most cases, a brief period of positive-pressure ventilation is all that is needed to increase the newborn's heart rate. If the heart rate is still less than 100 beats/min after 30 seconds of positive-pressure ventilation, continue ventilations, slowly add oxygen, keep the newborn warm, and transport at once.

9. What further treatment is indicated for the mother?

After delivery and before transport, place a sterile pad or sanitary pad over the vaginal opening and straighten the mother's legs. *Never place any pads or dressings into the vagina.* Gently massage the mother's abdomen with a firm, circular kneading motion to cause the uterus to contract and help control bleeding.

If severe bleeding occurs after placental delivery, transport immediately and treat the mother for shock. Place additional sterile pads or sanitary pads over the mother's vaginal opening, administer high-flow oxygen if necessary, and keep her warm with blankets. Closely monitor her vital signs en route.

10. What Apgar score should you assign to this newborn at 5 minutes after birth?

This newborn has pink mucous membranes but cyanotic hands and feet; therefore, you should assign a score of *1* for appearance. Her heart rate is 120 beats/min; therefore, assign a score of *2* for the pulse. She moves her foot away when you flick the soles; therefore, assign a score of *2* for grimace. She resists your attempts to straighten her knees, which indicates good muscle tone; therefore, assign a score of *2* for activity. Finally, her respirations are rapid (40 to 60 breaths/min is a normal newborn respiratory rate); therefore, assign a score of *2* for respirations. On the basis of your assessment findings, you should assign the newborn an Apgar score of 9 at 5 minutes. Since you were busy with resuscitative measures at 1 minute, no Apgar score would likely have been obtained at that time, but because of the low heart rate and generalized cyanosis, it would have been lower than the 5-minute score.

Prep Kit

Ready for Review

- Inside the uterus, the developing fetus is within the amniotic sac. The umbilical cord connects the mother and fetus through the placenta. Eventually, contractions of the uterus will propel the fetus through the birth canal.
- Throughout pregnancy, the body changes to accommodate the fetus. The primary systems involved with these changes are the respiratory, cardiovascular, and musculoskeletal systems.

Prep Kit continued

- As a result of enlargement of the uterus, a pregnant patient's respiratory capacity changes with increased respiratory rates and decreasing minute volumes.
- A pregnant person's blood volume increases by as much as 50%, and the heart rate increases by 20%.
- Increased hormone levels affect the musculoskeletal system by making the joints looser, or less stable.
- Complications of pregnancy include hypertensive disorders, bleeding, and diabetes.
- During a trauma call that involves a pregnant person, you have two patients to consider: the mother and the unborn fetus. Trauma to the mother may have a direct effect on the condition of the fetus.
- The first stage of labor, dilation, begins with the onset of contractions and ends when the cervix is fully dilated. The second stage of labor, expulsion of the fetus, begins when the cervix is fully dilated and the fetus enters the birth canal; it ends with delivery of the newborn. The third stage of labor, delivery of the placenta, begins with the delivery of the newborn and ends with the delivery of the placenta.
- Once labor has begun, it cannot be slowed or stopped; however, there is usually time to transport the patient to the hospital during the first stage of labor. During the second stage of labor, you must decide whether to deliver at the scene or transport the patient. During the third stage of labor, after delivery of the newborn, anticipate delivery of the placenta. This may occur after transport has been initiated and usually is within 30 minutes of delivery of the newborn. Warm, dry, and stimulate the newborn after birth.
- Abnormal or complicated deliveries include shoulder dystocia, breech deliveries (buttocks first), limb presentations (arm or leg first), and prolapse of the umbilical cord (umbilical cord first). Quickly transport the patient with a limb presentation or prolapsed umbilical cord to the hospital.
- You should place a finger or hand into the vagina for only two reasons: to keep the walls of the vagina from compressing the fetus's airway during a breech presentation or to push the fetus's head away from the cord when the cord is prolapsed.
- Assess a newborn for term gestation, good muscle tone, and breathing/crying to determine whether resuscitation is needed. Also obtain an Apgar score 1 minute and 5 minutes after birth.
- Excessive bleeding after delivery is a serious emergency. Begin fundal massage. Cover the vagina with a sterile pad. Change the pad as often as necessary and take all used pads to the hospital for examination.

Vital Vocabulary

abruptio placentae Premature separation of the placenta from the wall of the uterus.

amniotic sac The fluid-filled, baglike membrane in which the fetus develops.

anemia A condition in which the bloodstream does not contain enough red blood cells to effectively transport oxygen throughout the body.

Apgar score A scoring system for assessing the status of a newborn that assigns a number value to each of five areas.

birth canal The vagina and cervix.

bloody show A small amount of blood in the vagina that appears at the beginning of labor and may include a plug of pink-tinged mucus that is discharged when the cervix begins to dilate.

breech presentation A delivery in which the buttocks come out first.

cervix The lower third, or neck, of the uterus.

crowning The appearance of the fetus's head at the vaginal opening during labor.

Prep Kit continued

eclampsia A pregnancy complication that is characterized by new-onset hypertension (systolic blood pressure >140 mm Hg or diastolic blood pressure >90 mm Hg) with seizure activity and preceding systemic effects, such as blurred vision, headache, or protein in the urine. It is differentiated from preeclampsia by the presence of seizure activity.

ectopic pregnancy A pregnancy that develops outside the uterus, typically in a fallopian tube.

embryo The early stage of development after the fertilization of the egg (first 10 weeks).

endometrium The lining of the inside of the uterus.

fetal alcohol syndrome A condition caused by the consumption of alcohol by a pregnant person; characterized by growth and physical problems, intellectual disability, and a variety of congenital abnormalities in the child.

fetus The developing, unborn offspring inside the uterus, from 10 weeks after fertilization until birth.

fundus The dome-shaped top of the uterus.

gestational diabetes Diabetes that develops during pregnancy in individuals who did not have diabetes before pregnancy.

gestational hypertension A blood pressure greater than or equal to 140 mm Hg systolic or 90 mm Hg diastolic in a pregnant person in whom hypertension has not previously been diagnosed.

induced abortion The elective termination of a pregnancy prior to the time of viability.

lightening The movement of the fetus down into the pelvis late in pregnancy.

limb presentation A delivery in which the presenting part is a single arm or leg.

meconium Fetal stool. When appearing as a dark green material in the amniotic fluid, it can indicate distress or disease in the newborn; it can be aspirated into the fetus's lungs during delivery.

menarche The first menstrual cycle or onset of the first menstrual bleeding in females.

menopause The cessation of menstruation, typically in the fourth or fifth decade of life.

miscarriage The spontaneous passage of the fetus and placenta before 20 weeks; also called spontaneous abortion.

multigravida A person who has had previous pregnancies.

nuchal cord An umbilical cord that is wrapped around the fetus's neck.

perineum The area of skin between the genitals and the anus.

placenta The tissue attached to the uterine wall that nourishes the fetus through the umbilical cord.

placenta previa A condition in which the placenta develops over and covers the cervix.

preeclampsia A pregnancy complication that is characterized by new-onset hypertension (systolic blood pressure >140 mm Hg or diastolic blood pressure >90 mm Hg) along with systemic effects, such as blurred vision, headache, or protein in the urine. It is differentiated from eclampsia by the lack of seizure activity.

presentation The position in which an infant is born; defined by the part of the body that appears first.

primigravida A person who is experiencing their first pregnancy.

prolapse of the umbilical cord A situation in which the umbilical cord comes out of the vagina before the fetus.

spina bifida A developmental defect in which a portion of the spinal cord or meninges may protrude outside of the vertebrae and possibly even outside of the body, usually at the lower third of the spine in the lumbar area.

spontaneous abortion The loss of a pregnancy prior to 20 weeks of gestation without any preceding surgical or medical intervention. Often called a miscarriage.

supine hypotensive syndrome Low blood pressure resulting from compression of the inferior

Prep Kit continued

vena cava by the weight of the pregnant uterus when the person is supine.

term gestation A pregnancy that is at term, between 39 weeks and 40 weeks, 6 days.

umbilical cord The structure that connects the pregnant person to the fetus via the placenta; contains two arteries and one vein.

vernix caseosa A white, cheesy substance that covers the body of the fetus.

vertex presentation A delivery in which the head of the newborn comes out first.

References

1. Cash RE, Kaimal AJ, Samuels-Kalow ME, Boggs KM, Swanton MF, Camargo CA Jr. Epidemiology of emergency medical services-attended out-of-hospital deliveries and complications in the United States. *Prehosp Emerg Care*. 2024;28(7):890–897.
2. Sonenberg A, Mason DJ. Maternity care deserts in the US. *JAMA Health Forum*. 2023;4(1):e225541. doi:10.1001/jamahealthforum.2022.5541
3. Kozhimannil KB, Hung P, Henning-Smith C, Casey MM, Prasad S. Association between loss of hospital-based obstetric services and birth outcomes in rural counties in the United States. *JAMA*. 2018;319(12):1239–1247.
4. QuickStats: percentage of mothers with gestational diabetes, by maternal age—National Vital Statistics System, United States, 2016 and 2021. *MMWR Morb Mortal Wkly Rep*. 2023;72(1):16.
5. Rybak-Krzyszkowska M, Staniczek J, Kondracka A, et al. From biomarkers to the molecular mechanism of preeclampsia: a comprehensive literature review. *Int J Mol Sci*. 2023;24(17):13252.
6. Dawson EL. Preeclampsia, genomics, and public Health. Centers for Disease Control and Prevention website. https://blogs.cdc.gov/genomics/2022/10/25/preeclampsia/. Published October 25, 2022. Accessed April 14, 2025.
7. Who is at risk of preeclampsia. National Institutes of Health website. https://www.nichd.nih.gov/health/topics/preeclampsia/conditioninfo/risk. Reviewed June 14, 2022. Accessed April 14, 2025.
8. Sepilian VP. Ectopic pregnancy: practice essentials. Medscape website. https://emedicine.medscape.com/article/2041923-overview?form=fpf#showall. Updated August 9, 2024. Accessed April 14, 2025.
9. Simmons E, Austin AE. Association of prenatal substance use with prenatal and postpartum care: evidence from the Pregnancy Risk Assessment Monitoring System, 2016–2019. *Prev Med*. 2022;159:107065.
10. Substance use during pregnancy. Centers for Disease Control and Prevention website. https://www.cdc.gov/maternal-infant-health/pregnancy-substance-abuse/index.html. Published May 15, 2024. Accessed April 14, 2025.
11. About fetal alcohol spectrum disorders (FASDs). Centers for Disease Control and Prevention website. https://www.cdc.gov/fasd/about/index.html. Published March 6, 2025. Accessed April 14, 2025.
12. Pawar SJ, Anjankar VP, Anjankar A, Adnan M. Cardiopulmonary arrest during pregnancy: a review article. *Cureus*. 2023;15(2):e35219. doi:10.7759/cureus.35219
13. Berteloot K, Sabbe M. Challenges during cardiac arrest in pregnancy. *Resusc Plus*. 2024;21:100855. doi:10.1016/j.resplu.2024.100855
14. Berg KM, Bray JE, Ng K-C, et al. 2023 international consensus on cardiopulmonary resuscitation and emergency cardiovascular care science with treatment recommendations: summary from the Basic Life Support; Advanced Life Support; Pediatric Life Support; Neonatal Life Support; Education, Implementation, and Teams; and First Aid Task Forces. *Circulation*. 2023;148(24):e187–e280. doi:10.1161/CIR.0000000000001179
15. Chang AK. Pregnancy trauma. Medscape website. https://emedicine.medscape.com/article/796979-overview?form=fpf. Updated July 15, 2024. Accessed April 14, 2025.
16. Intimate partner violence endangers pregnant people and their infants. National Partnership for Women and Families website. https://nationalpartnership.org/report/intimate-partner-violence/. Published May 2021. Accessed April 14, 2025.
17. Wallace M, Gillispie-Bell V, Cruz K, Davis K, Vilda D. Homicide during pregnancy and the postpartum period in the United States, 2018–2019. *Obstet Gynecol*. 2022 Feb 1;139(2):347.
18. US teen birth rate reached another historic low in 2022. Centers for Disease Control and Prevention website. https://www.cdc.gov/nchs/pressroom/nchs_press_releases/2023/20230601.htm. Reviewed June 1, 2023. Accessed April 14, 2025.
19. Osterman MJK, Hamilton BE, Martin JA, Driscoll AK, Valenzuela CP. Births: final data for 2022. *Natl Vital Stat Rep*. 2024 Apr;73(2):1–56.
20. Młodawska M, Młodawski J, Świercz G, Zieliński R. The relationship between nuchal cord and adverse obstetric

Prep Kit continued

and neonatal outcomes: retrospective cohort study. *Pediatr Rep*. 2022;14(1):40–47.

21. Vasa R, Dimitrov R, Patel S. Nuchal cord at delivery and perinatal outcomes: single-center retrospective study, with emphasis on fetal acid-base balance. *Pediatr Neonatol*. 2018 Oct;59(5):439–447.
22. Beaird DT, Ladd M, Jenkins SM, et al. EMS prehospital deliveries. *StatPearls*. National Library of Medicine website. https://www.ncbi.nlm.nih.gov/books/NBK525996/#. Updated October 26, 2023. Accessed May 20, 2025.
23. Wyckoff MH, Singletary EM, Soar J, et al. 2021 international consensus on cardiopulmonary resuscitation and emergency cardiovascular care science with treatment recommendations: summary from the Basic Life Support; Advanced Life Support; Neonatal Life Support; Education, Implementation, and Teams; First Aid Task Forces; and the COVID-19 Working Group. *Resuscitation*. 2021;169:229–311.
24. National Association of State EMS Officials. *National Model EMS Clinical Guidelines: Version 3.0*. https://nasemso.org/wp-content/uploads/National-Model-EMS-Clinical-Guidelines_2022.pdf. Updated March 2022. Accessed April 14, 2025.
25. American Heart Association, European Resuscitation Council, International Liaison Committee on Resuscitation. *2025 International Liaison Committee on Resuscitation Consensus on Science With Treatment Recommendations: Executive Summary*. https://ilcor.org/uploads/PLS-2025-COSTR-Full-Chapter.pdf. Published 2025. Accessed July 16, 2025.
26. American Academy of Pediatrics. To suction or not to suction: the meconium debate continues. *NRP*. 2019;28(1).
27. Grünebaum A, Bornstein E, Dudenhausen JW, et al. Hidden in plain sight in the delivery room: the Apgar score is biased. *J Perinat Med*. 2023;51(5):628–633.
28. Martin JA, Osterman MJK. Shifts in the distribution of births by gestational age: United States, 2014–2022. *Natl Vital Stat Rep*. 2024 Jan;73(1):1–11.
29. Committee on Practice Bulletins-Obstetrics. Practice bulletin no. 183: postpartum hemorrhage. *Obstet Gynecol*. 2017;130(4):e168–e186. doi:10.1097/AOG.0000000000002351

Additional Resources

American Academy of Pediatrics Committee on Fetus and Newborn, American College of Obstetricians and Gynecologists Committee on Obstetric Practice. The Apgar score. *Pediatrics*. 2015;136(4):819–822.

Dombrowski MP, Bottoms SF, Saleh AA, Hurd WW, Romero R. Third stage of labor: analysis of duration and clinical practice. *Am J Obstet Gynecol*. 1995;172(4 Pt 1): 1279–1284.

Haydon ML, Gorenberg DM, Nageotte MP, et al. The effect of maternal oxygen administration on fetal pulse oximetry during labor in fetuses with nonreassuring fetal heart rate patterns. *Am J Obstet Gynecol*. 2006;195(3):735–738.

Jeejeebhoy FM, Zelop CM, Lipman S, et al. Cardiac arrest in pregnancy. *Circulation*. 2015;132(18):1747–1773.

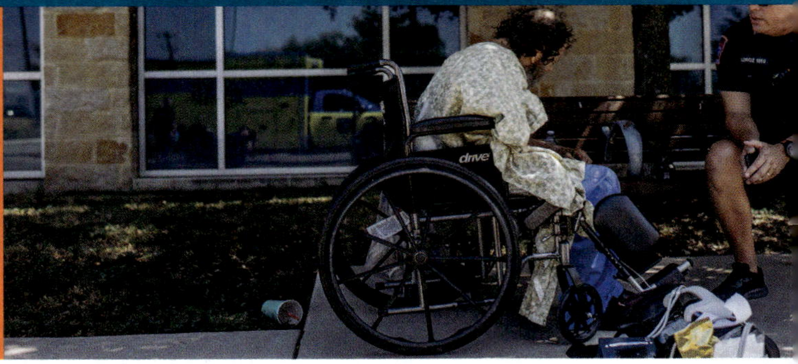

Chapter 35

Patients With Special Challenges

NATIONAL EMS EDUCATION STANDARD COMPETENCIES

Special Patient Populations

Applies knowledge of growth, development, and aging and assessment findings to provide basic emergency care and transportation for a patient with special needs.

Patients With Special Challenges

Recognizing and reporting abuse and neglect (pp 1318–1326)

- Abuse/intimate partner violence (pp 1318–1326)
- Neglect (pp 1318–1326)
- Child/dependent adult maltreatment (pp 1317–1326)
- Homelessness (pp 1329–1330)
- Poverty (pp 1329–1330)
- Bariatrics (pp 1308–1309)
- Technology dependent (pp 1309–1316)
- Hospice/terminally ill (pp 1328–1329)
- Tracheostomy care/dysfunction (p 1310; Chapter 11, *Airway and Ventilation Management*)
- Home care (p 1328)
- Sensory deficit/loss (pp 1303–1306)
- Developmental disability (pp 1300–1303)
- Autism spectrum disorder (p 1301)
- Orthotics/prosthetics (p 1308)

Trauma

Applies knowledge to provide basic emergency care and transportation based on assessment findings for an acutely injured patient.

Special Considerations in Trauma

- Pregnant patient (Chapter 34, *Obstetrics and Neonatal Care*)
- Pediatric patient (pp 1318–1320)
- Geriatric patient (pp 1321–1323)
- Cognitively impaired patient (pp 1300–1303)

KNOWLEDGE OBJECTIVES

1. Give examples of patients with special challenges EMTs may encounter during a medical emergency. (pp 1299–1300)
2. Explain the special patient care considerations required when providing emergency medical care to patients with intellectual disabilities, including patients with autism spectrum disorder (ASD), Down syndrome, or prior brain injuries. (pp 1300–1303)
3. Describe the different types of visual impairments and the special patient care considerations required when providing emergency medical care for visually impaired patients, depending on the level of their disability. (pp 1303–1304)
4. Describe the various types of hearing impairments and the special patient care considerations required when providing

emergency medical care for hard-of-hearing patients, including tips for effective communication. (pp 1304–1306)

5. Describe the various types of hearing aids worn by patients; include strategies to troubleshoot a hearing aid that is not working. (pp 1305–1306)
6. Explain the special patient care considerations required when providing emergency medical care to patients with physical disabilities, including cerebral palsy, spina bifida, paralysis, and orthotics/prosthetics. (pp 1306–1308)
7. Define obesity. (p 1308)
8. Explain the special patient care considerations required when providing emergency medical care to bariatric patients; include the best way to move bariatric patients. (pp 1308–1309)
9. Explain the special patient care considerations required when providing emergency medical care to patients who rely on a form of medical technology assistance, including the following:
   - Tracheostomy tube (p 1310)
   - Home oxygen (p 1310)
   - Mechanical ventilator (pp 1310–1312)
   - Apnea monitor (pp 1312–1313)
   - Internal cardiac pacemaker (p 1313)
   - Ventricular assist device (VAD) (pp 1313–1314)
   - External defibrillator vest (p 1314)
   - Central venous catheter (pp 1314–1315)
   - Gastrostomy tube (p 1315)
   - Ventricular peritoneal shunt (p 1315)
   - Vagus nerve stimulator (p 1316)
   - Colostomy bag, ileostomy bag, or urostomy bag (p 1316)
10. Discuss emergencies involving infants, including sudden unexpected infant death (SUID), unexplained sudden death in infancy (USDI), brief resolved unexplained event (BRUE). (pp 1316–1318)
11. Describe child abuse and neglect and its possible indicators, including the medical and legal responsibilities of EMTs when caring for a pediatric patient who is a possible victim of child abuse. (pp 1318–1321)
12. Explain the assessment and care of a geriatric patient who has potentially been abused or neglected. (pp 1321–1323)
13. Discuss the special considerations when caring for a patient who has reportedly been sexually abused or raped. (pp 1323–1326)
14. Describe care for patients living in assisted-living facilities or at home. (pp 1326–1328)
15. Contrast hospice and palliative care with curative care. (pp 1328–1329)
16. Explain the responsibilities of EMTs when responding to calls for terminally ill patients who have do not attempt resuscitation (DNAR) or physician orders for life-sustaining treatment (POLST) medical documentation. (p 1329)
17. Discuss the issues of poverty and homelessness in the United States, their negative effects on a person's health, and the role of EMTs as patient advocates. (pp 1329–1330)

SKILLS OBJECTIVES

1. Demonstrate different strategies to communicate effectively with a patient who has a hearing impairment. (pp 1304–1306)

Introduction

In the United States, medical advancements have allowed many patients to receive improved health care in the out-of-hospital environment. As a result, the number of children and adults with chronic diseases and injuries who live at home or other community settings continues to grow. As an EMT, you will sometimes be called to assist these patients and should understand the special challenges that caring for them may present. Some examples of patients with special health care challenges include the following:

- Children who were born prematurely and who have associated respiratory problems
- Infants or small children with congenital heart disease

- Patients with neurologic disease (occasionally caused by hypoxia at the time of birth, as with cerebral palsy)
- Patients with congenital or acquired diseases resulting in altered body function that requires medical assistance for breathing, eating, urination, or bowel function
- Patients with sensory deficits such as hearing or visual impairments
- Geriatric patients with chronic diseases requiring visitation from a home health care service

These patients may depend on specialized equipment, such as mechanical ventilators, intravenous pumps, or other devices, to maintain their lives. Do not be distracted by the noise and mechanics of the medical equipment; focus on the patient the medical equipment may be assisting.

In addition, you may be called to care for patients who present special challenges relating to abuse or neglect, or you may otherwise encounter these individuals while working in your community. These calls will involve unique emotional and psychological considerations and may present criminal implications. Regardless of the circumstances that make a call "special," you should assess and care for these patients the same way you would care for your other patients.

Street Smarts

During stressful emergency events, it is imperative to use the TEAM approach (Trust Every Available Member). Collaboration, including with the patient's family or other home caregivers, leads to a better standard of care and patient outcome.

Words of Wisdom

Primary caregivers of patients at high risk for cardiac arrest should be trained in cardiopulmonary resuscitation (CPR). You should advocate for this as part of your community engagement efforts.

Developmental Disability

The term **developmental disability** refers to a group of conditions that may impair development in the areas of physical ability, learning, language development, or behavioral coping skills. **Intellectual disability** is a subset of developmental disability, where patients have significant limitations in both intellectual functioning and skills needed for daily living. The diagnosis of intellectual disability is made by before age 22 years, which is considered the approximate age by which intellectual development has ended.[1] Intellectual disability spans a spectrum from mild to profound. The level of care and support these patients may need varies greatly.

Street Smarts

Until 2010, the term "mental retardation" was sometimes used to describe patients with intellectual disabilities. That term is no longer appropriate. You should use the term *intellectual disability* when documenting interactions and during verbal interactions with patients and other health care professionals.

Developmental disabilities, including intellectual disabilities, may be caused by genetic factors, congenital factors (eg, prenatal infections, prenatal

YOU are the EMT

At 1435 hours, you are dispatched to a residence at 575 Ranger Drive for a 19-year-old man with a fever. You recognize the address because you have responded to this patient on several occasions. He has quadriplegia and is ventilator dependent because of a spinal injury that occurred 2 years ago. You and your partner proceed to the scene; your response time is 5 minutes.

1. How will your assessment and treatment of this patient differ from that of a patient who is not dependent on a ventilator?
2. What role do the parents or caregivers of patients with special health care needs have in the prehospital setting?

exposure to drugs or alcohol), complications at birth, malnutrition, or environmental factors. Other causes that may occur after birth include traumatic brain injury and poisoning (such as from lead or other toxins).

Patients with intellectual disabilities are susceptible to the same disease processes as other patients, including diabetes, heart attack, and respiratory difficulties. Assess and treat the patient according to the chief complaint. During transport, keep the patient as calm as possible.

Autism Spectrum Disorder

Autism spectrum disorder (ASD) is a neurodevelopmental disorder characterized by deficits in social communication and social interaction, along with restricted, repetitive patterns of behavior, interests, or activities.[2] The causes of ASD are not completely understood and likely multifactorial. In the United States, approximately 1 in 31 children experiences ASD.[3] It is three times more common in males than in females and in those who have an older sibling with the condition.[4]

Patients with autism often have abnormal sensory responses. They may not feel cold, heat, or pain as others do. They may respond to pain by laughing, humming, singing, or removing clothing. Likewise, applying bandages or tape can cause anxiety or aggression. When possible, examine the patient beginning at the feet and moving upward, while explaining each step of your exam. Even when these patients cannot speak, they often understand speech.

Patients with autism may have increased sensitivity to noise or physical stimulation. Keep the transport environment calm and minimize stimulation to help with these issues. Limit the use of emergency lights and siren when practical and safe. Allowing a patient to wear sound-dampening devices may also help.

The use of distraction techniques while applying a blood pressure cuff or listening with a stethoscope may be necessary. Patients may have a short phrase, item, or particular routine they use that provides comfort. Allowing their routine to be carried out when practical may avoid triggering outbursts or escalating behavior. If departmental policy permits, allow a family member or trusted caregiver to ride in the transport compartment with the patient to facilitate care. Demonstration of examination techniques on a trusted individual may help comfort the patient. Use short, direct, and simple phrases when communicating, and allow extra time for the patient to process the communication if possible.

Street Smarts

When caring for a patient with autism, maintain a calm demeanor, provide clear and simple instructions, create a safe space, and reduce overwhelming stimuli. Remember that the patient's behavior may be a result of feeling overwhelmed by the situation.

Street Smarts

Some EMS systems have begun carrying special kits, such as Carter Kits Sensory Bags, that contain items known to comfort and focus the attention of children with autism and other patients who may become overwhelmed by an emergency. These kits contain items such as fidget toys, noise-canceling earmuffs, a weighted blanket, nonverbal communication cards, and sunglasses.

Down Syndrome

Down syndrome is characterized by a genetic chromosomal defect resulting in mild to severe intellectual impairment (**FIGURE 35-1**). The normal human somatic cell contains 23 pairs of chromosomes. In most cases, Down syndrome, also known as trisomy 21,

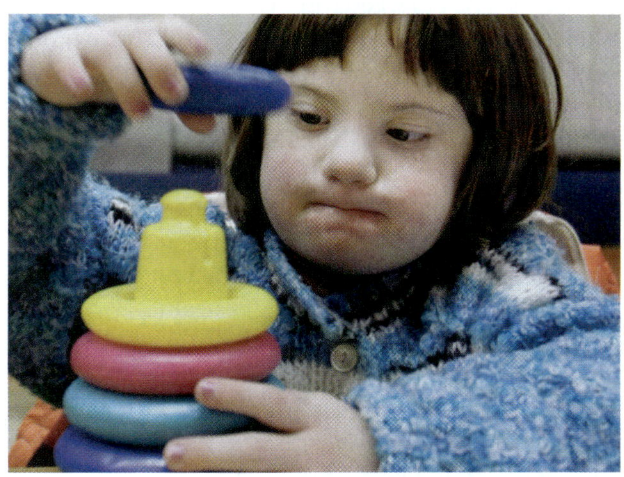

FIGURE 35-1 A child with Down syndrome.

occurs when the pair of 21st chromosomes fail to separate, so that the ovum or sperm contains 24 chromosomes. When fertilization occurs, a triplication (trisomy) of chromosome 21 occurs. The extra chromosome disrupts the normal course of development.

Increased maternal age and a family history of Down syndrome are known risk factors for this condition. Various physical characteristics are associated with Down syndrome: a round head with a flat occiput; an enlarged, protruding tongue; slanted, wide-set eyes; folded skin on either side of the nose, covering the inner corners of the eye; short, wide hands; and a small face and features. People with Down syndrome usually do not have all of these signs, but a diagnosis can be made at birth because several of the signs can be seen. Depending on their level of intellectual disability, people with Down syndrome may lead independent lives. They may be employed, vote, and get involved in their communities.

Patients with Down syndrome are at increased risk for medical complications, including leukemia and conditions that affect the cardiovascular, sensory, endocrine (eg, hypothyroidism), musculoskeletal, dental, and gastrointestinal systems as well as neurologic development. Approximately one-half of these patients have heart conditions and vision problems, and as many as three-quarters experience hearing loss.[5]

Because people with Down syndrome often have large tongues and small oral and nasal cavities, airway management may be difficult. These patients may also have misaligned teeth and other dental problems. The enlarged tongue and dental problems can lead to speech abnormalities as well. In an emergency situation, if airway management is necessary, bag-mask ventilation can be challenging. In the case of airway obstruction, a jaw-thrust maneuver may be all that is needed to clear the airway. In an unconscious patient, either the jaw-thrust maneuver or a nasopharyngeal airway may be necessary. The airway should also be a prime consideration in behavioral emergencies requiring restraint.

Some people with Down syndrome have epilepsy. Most of the seizures are generalized. Patient care is the same as for other patients with seizures. Chapter 18, *Neurologic Emergencies,* discusses the emergency management of seizures in detail.

Instability of the atlantoaxial joint, where the first two cervical vertebrae meet, is common in people with Down syndrome.[6] This is termed atlantoaxial instability. Most patients with atlantoaxial instability do not show symptoms; however, they are at increased risk of complications when they experience trauma. Keep this in mind when you receive a call for a musculoskeletal problem or possible neurologic problem in a patient with Down syndrome. If the atlantoaxial joint becomes dislocated, as may occur with trauma, the patient may experience difficulty walking, neck pain or decreased neck mobility, and sensory deficits. Such a dislocation can even cause spinal cord injury. Atlantoaxial instability is diagnosed using a radiograph of the cervical vertebrae.

Brain Injury

A patient with a prior brain injury may be difficult to assess and treat. Patients with brain injuries may face a complex array of challenges related to the injury. In such cases, gathering a complete medical history from the patient, family, and friends will be helpful. Your interaction with patients with brain injuries should be tailored to their specific abilities. Take the time to speak with the patient and family to establish what is considered normal for the patient; for example, determine whether the patient has cognitive, sensory, communication, motor, behavioral, or psychological deficits.

When you care for a patient with a prior brain injury, talk in a calm, soothing tone, and watch the patient closely for signs of anxiety or aggression. In some cases, the patient may need to be specifically positioned or restrained to ensure your safety and the safety of the patient. Do not expect the patient to walk to the ambulance or stretcher. As always, treat the patient with respect, use their name, explain procedures, and reassure the patient throughout the process.

Chapter 28, *Head and Spine Injuries,* discusses traumatic brain injuries in detail.

Interacting With Patients Who Have a Developmental Disability

It is normal to feel uncomfortable when initiating contact with a patient with an intellectual disability, especially if you have not encountered such situations frequently. The best plan of action is to treat the patient as you would any other patient.

Approach the patient in a calm, friendly manner, watching for signs of increased anxiety or fear.

Remember, you are a stranger and are approaching with a group of people. The patient may not understand your uniform or realize that you and your team are there to help. It may be helpful to have your team members wait until you can establish a rapport with the patient. You can then introduce the team members and explain what they are going to do as you slowly bring them forward.

You might interact with a patient with an intellectual disability as follows: "Hello, Mr. Pemberton. My name is Jerry Booker." Shake Mr. Pemberton's hand if he will allow it. "We're here to help you. Your sister called us. She says you're not feeling well today, and we're here to help you feel better. My partner, Tina, is going to take your blood pressure. Do you remember having that done before?" Allow Mr. Pemberton to see and touch the blood pressure cuff as your partner moves forward. Move slowly but deliberately. Explain beforehand what you are going to do, just as with any other patient. Watch carefully for signs of fear or reluctance from the patient. Make sure you are at eye level with the patient. If the patient is sitting, kneel or sit down. This is important in communicating with all patients; however, it is even more important in making the patient with special challenges comfortable.

If communication is particularly difficult, consider asking family members or caregivers what methods the patient uses to communicate. Some patients may communicate verbally, whereas others may use pictures or be completely noncommunicative. These individuals may be able to describe how the patient communicates feelings of pain or discomfort and provide you with additional information regarding the patient's medical history.

Do your best to soothe the patient's anxiety and discomfort as you work through your assessment and provide treatment. By initially establishing trust and communication, you will have a much better chance for a successful outcome.

Street Smarts

Because patients with intellectual disabilities may have difficulty adjusting to change or a break in routine, an emergency call that generates a roomful of strangers can be overwhelming. Patients may become more difficult to interact with as their anxiety level increases. Make every effort to respect the patient's wishes and concerns. Take as much time as necessary to calmly and clearly explain the treatment the patient is about to receive.

Sensory Disabilities

Visual Impairment

Visual impairments may result from many different causes, including a congenital defect, disease, injury, or degeneration of the eyeball, optic nerve, or nerve pathway (eg, with aging). The degree of visual impairment may range from partial to total. Some patients have a loss of peripheral or central vision; others can distinguish light from dark or identify general shapes.

Visual impairments may be difficult to recognize. During your scene size-up, look for signs that indicate the patient is visually impaired, such as the presence of eyeglasses, a cane, or a service animal (**FIGURE 35-2**). Immediately introduce yourself

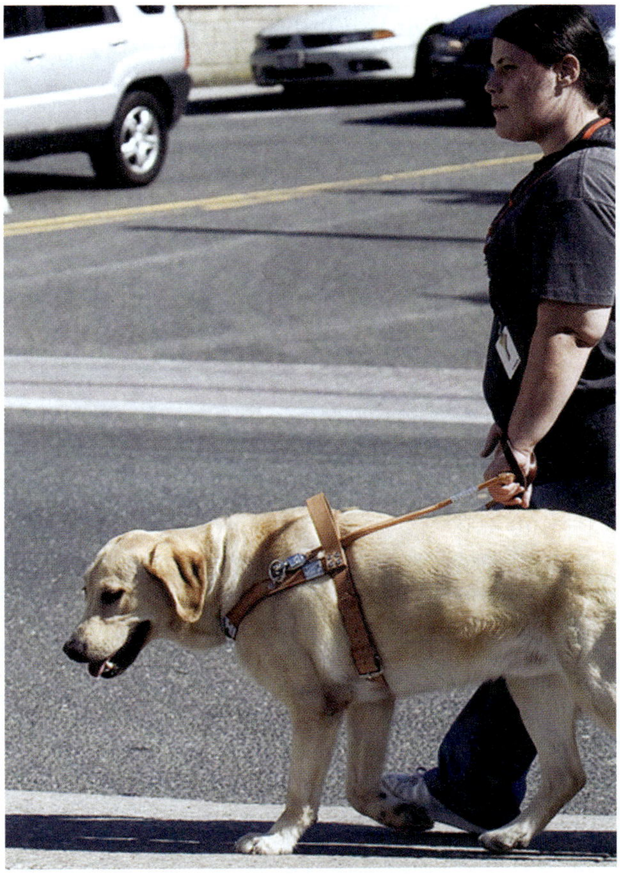

FIGURE 35-2 Service dogs can often be identified by their harnesses or other special devices such as a vest.

Courtesy of the Guide Dog Foundation for the Blind. Photographed by Christopher Appoldt.

when you enter the room. Have your team members introduce themselves so that the patient can identify their voices and locations. In addition, retrieve any visual aids and give them to your patient to make the interaction more comfortable.

A visually impaired patient may feel vulnerable, especially during the chaos of a crash scene. The patient may have learned to use other senses such as hearing, touch, and smell to compensate for the loss of sight, and the sounds and smells of the scene may be disorienting. Remember to tell the patient what is happening, identify noises, and describe the situation and surroundings, especially if you must move the patient.

The patient may use a cane or walker to ambulate safely. Even if the patient will be carried on a gurney, remember to take the patient's cane or walker. Unless the patient is in critical condition, a service animal should remain with the patient in the patient compartment of the ambulance and will provide reassurance for the patient and prevent delays in transport; however, in some cases you may need to make arrangements for the care or accompaniment of the animal. A friend of the patient or an animal control officer can be helpful in this situation. You should avoid separating the patient and the animal whenever possible, however. If it is necessary to move furniture in the patient's home to access the patient, it should be moved back to its original position before leaving the scene.

An ambulatory patient may be led by a light touch on the arm or elbow. Alternatively, you may allow the patient to rest a hand on your shoulder, as this may enhance the patient's sense of balance and security while moving. Ask patients which method they prefer to use. Patients should be gently guided but never pulled or pushed. Obstacles need to be communicated in advance. Statements such as "You're approaching the stairs. We're going to take five steps down," will allow the patient to anticipate and navigate the obstacles safely.

Words of Wisdom

Service animals are not classified as pets and are, by law, permitted to accompany the patient unless the animal is injured or out of control. Review the Service Animals section in the Americans With Disabilities Act for further information.[7]

Hearing Impairment

Hearing impairment can range from a slight hearing loss to total deafness. Patients who are hard of

YOU are the EMT

You arrive at the scene and find the patient lying supine in a hospital-style bed in the living room. He immediately looks at you when you approach him but does not talk to you. The patient's mother tells you that he began running a fever earlier in the day. She further advises you that the patient's home health nurse was present earlier and contacted his physician, who requested that EMS transport him to the hospital. While your partner gathers additional information, you perform a primary assessment.

Recording Time: 0 Minutes	
Appearance	Eyes open
Level of consciousness	Conscious and alert; this is his baseline mental status
Airway	Tracheostomy tube in place; upper airway clear of secretions and foreign bodies
Breathing	14 breaths/min via mechanical ventilator
Circulation	Increased pulse rate (strong and regular); skin is baseline color, hot, and moist; no gross bleeding

3. What are some conditions that would cause a patient to become dependent on a mechanical ventilator?

4. How does a tracheostomy tube affect a patient's ability to communicate? How can you determine whether your patient is alert?

hearing may have difficulty with pitch, volume, and speaking distinctly. Some patients learn to speak even though they have never heard sounds. Other patients may have heard speech and learned to speak, but have since sustained partial or total hearing loss. Many older people will have some degree of hearing loss. Chapter 4, *Communications and Documentation*, discusses hearing loss in further detail.

The two most common forms of hearing loss are sensorineural deafness and conductive hearing loss. **Sensorineural deafness**, or nerve damage, results from a lesion or damage to the inner ear. **Conductive hearing loss** is caused by a faulty transmission of sound waves, which can occur when a person has an accumulation of wax inside the ear canal or a perforated eardrum.

Words of Wisdom

As with all interventions for barriers to communication, you should document the use of an interpreter. Also remember that conclusions based on the information from interpreters may not be valid. Ask the interpreter to report exactly what the patient signs and not to add any commentary, however well intentioned.

During your scene size-up, look for clues that a person could be hard of hearing, including the presence of hearing aids, poor pronunciation of words, or failure to respond to your presence or questions. Patients may not have their hearing aids in place. Assist the patient with finding and inserting any hearing aids as appropriate, or ask family members to help you. It may be helpful to communicate by writing until the hearing aids are located. If none of these options is possible, placing your stethoscope in the patient's ears and speaking through the diaphragm may amplify your voice sufficiently to be understood by the patient. Many patients who are hard of hearing can also read lips to some extent. Therefore, face the patient while you communicate so that they can see your mouth; do not exaggerate your lip movements or look away. Position yourself approximately 18 inches (46 cm) in front of the patient. Because patients who are hard of hearing typically have more difficulty hearing higher frequency sounds, never shout; instead, try lowering the pitch of your voice.

Ask the patient, "How would you like to communicate with me?" Some patients may prefer written communication or the use of gestures or pictures; others may prefer use of American Sign Language. An interpreter, family member, or friend may be a valuable teammate. If needed, ask the interpreter to accompany the patient to the hospital, because this may decrease the stress of communication on the patient, EMS crew, and the hospital staff. If an interpreter is not readily available, call the receiving facility to request one as soon as you are aware of the need.

Depending on the nature of the patient's hearing impairment, the following tips may help you communicate with the patient:

- Speak slowly and distinctly into the less impaired ear, or position yourself on that side.
- Change speakers. Given that 80% of hearing loss is related to an inability to hear high-pitched sounds, it may be helpful to have a team member with a low-pitched voice communicate with the patient.
- Provide paper and a pencil so that you can write your questions and the patient can write responses.
- Have only one EMT ask interview questions, to avoid confusing the patient.

Hearing Aids

A hearing aid is essentially a device that makes sound louder. Hearing aids cannot restore hearing to normal, but they do improve hearing and listening ability. Hearing aids can be either external or internal, depending on the type of hearing damage. Several types of hearing aids are available (**FIGURE 35-3**):

- **Behind the ear.** The working parts are contained in a plastic case that rests behind the ear.
- **In the canal and completely in the canal.** These hearing aids are contained in a tiny case that fits partly or completely into the ear canal.
- **In the ear.** All parts are contained in a shell that fits in the outer part of the ear.

You may also encounter an older style of hearing aid in which the earpiece is wired to a microphone and processor unit that typically fits in the patient's pocket. Finally, implantable hearing aids are an option for patients with less profound hearing loss.

When assisting a patient to insert a hearing aid, look to see which ear the device is indicated for. The device needs to fit snugly without forcing. If you hear a whistling sound, the hearing aid may not be in far enough to create a seal or the volume may be too loud. Try repositioning the hearing aid, or remove it and turn down the volume. If the hearing aids are transported, document the transport and transfer of hearing aids to hospital personnel, noting the name of the person to whom they were transferred. Prescription hearing aids cost several thousand dollars and are easy to lose during transport. Give them to the family when possible. Never try to clean hearing aids, and do not get them wet.

If the hearing aid can be installed but it is not working, try troubleshooting the problem. First, make sure the hearing aid is turned on. Try a fresh battery, and check the tubing to make sure it is not twisted or bent. Ensure that the switch is set on M (microphone), not T (telephone). Many new hearing aids are controlled using a smartphone app that the patient should know how to control. For an older wired hearing aid, try a spare cord; the old one may be broken or shorted. Finally, make sure the ear mold is not clogged with wax.

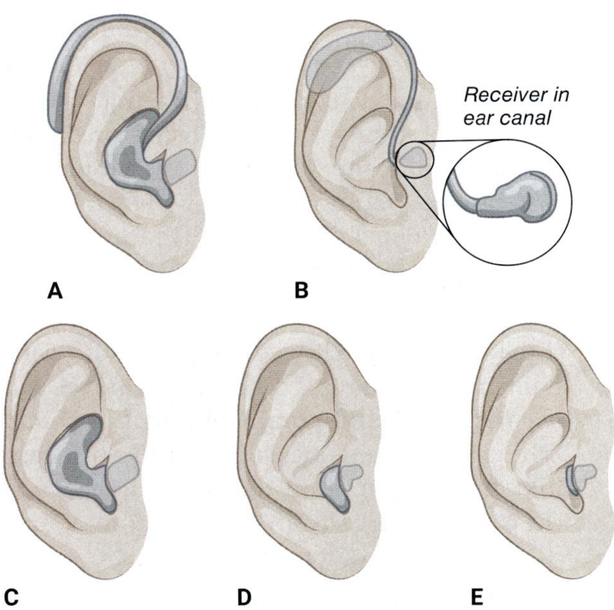

FIGURE 35-3 Different types of hearing aids. **A.** Behind the ear. **B.** Miniature behind the ear. **C.** In the ear. **D.** In the canal. **E.** Completely in the canal.

Words of Wisdom

Many patients with borderline hearing impairments may not be aware of the extent of their problem. The distracting and noisy EMS environment may worsen the situation. If a patient frequently asks you to repeat things, suspect a hearing impairment.

Words of Wisdom

Some patients who are hard of hearing are sensitive to loud noises close to their ears. Remember to use a normal tone of voice when speaking to these patients.

Physical Disabilities

Cerebral Palsy

Cerebral palsy is a term for a group of disorders characterized by poorly controlled body movement (**FIGURE 35-4**). This disorder is a result of damage to the developing fetal brain while in utero, oxygen deprivation at birth, a traumatic brain injury at birth, or infection such as meningitis during early childhood. Patients with cerebral palsy can have symptoms that range from mild to severe, involving poor posture and uncontrolled, spastic movements of the limbs.

Cerebral palsy is also associated with other conditions such as visual and hearing impairments, difficulty communicating, epilepsy, and intellectual

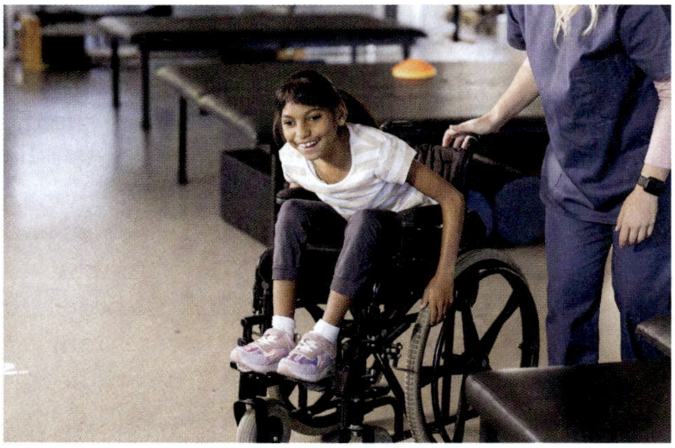

FIGURE 35-4 A person with cerebral palsy.

disabilities. Many patients with cerebral palsy possess some degree of intellectual impairment, whereas others have a normal intelligence level and are able to live independently with minimal support. Patients with cerebral palsy may have an unsteady gait (ataxia) and may require the assistance of a wheelchair or walker. Transport this type of equipment with the patient, provided it can be secured properly in the ambulance.

As with all patients, assessing the Airway, Breathing, and Circulation (ABCs) is of the utmost importance when treating a patient with cerebral palsy. Closely observe the airway status of a patient with cerebral palsy because these patients may have increased secretion production and difficulty swallowing (dysphagia), requiring aggressive suctioning to clear the airway.

When you care for a patient with cerebral palsy, note the following:

- Do not assume that patients with cerebral palsy have an intellectual disability. Although 30% to 50% of patients have some intellectual disability, many people with cerebral palsy have a normal intelligence level or only slight intellectual impairment.[8]
- Limbs are often underdeveloped and are susceptible to injury (eg, a fall from a wheelchair).
- Patients who are able to walk may have an unsteady gait and be susceptible to falls.
- If the patient has a specifically made pillow or chair (as many pediatric patients do), the patient may prefer to use it during transport. Remember to pad the patient to ensure their comfort, and never force a patient's extremities into any position.
- Whenever possible, transport walkers or wheelchairs with the patient.
- Up to 50% of children with cerebral palsy experience seizures.[8] Be prepared to address a seizure if one occurs, and keep a suction unit available.

Spina Bifida

The spinal canal is typically closed by birth and must grow and expand as the child grows. Neural tube deformities can result in serious birth defects. The most common neural tube deformity is **spina bifida**, in which the lower portion of the spine does not close during embryonic or fetal development, resulting in an exposed portion of the spinal cord (**FIGURE 35-5**). The opening can be closed surgically, but the child is often left with spinal and neurologic damage. Adequate maternal intake of vitamin B_9 (folic acid) reduces the risk of spina bifida. Most defects occur before the woman knows she is pregnant, so since 1992, the US government has mandated that foods such as breads, cereals, and grains be fortified with vitamin B_9. This effort has decreased the incidence of spina bifida, but, unfortunately, it is still one of the most common disabling birth defects in the United States. As such, it is likely that you will care for someone who has spina bifida.

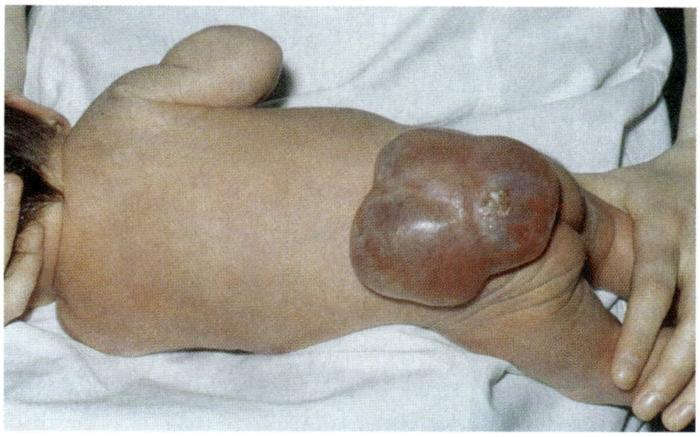

FIGURE 35-5 Spina bifida is one of the most common disabling birth defects in the United States.

Some patients with spina bifida also have hydrocephalus, which requires the placement of a shunt to drain excessive amounts of cerebrospinal fluid from the brain.[9] Other conditions associated with spina bifida include partial or full paralysis of the lower extremities, loss of bowel and bladder control, and an allergy to latex products. Latex-free products should be kept on the ambulance to avoid an anaphylactic reaction in patients with spina bifida. While most EMS supplies were latex-free prior to the coronavirus disease 2019 (COVID-19) pandemic, the supply shortages during the pandemic resulted in latex supplies reappearing in many systems.

Patients with spina bifida will benefit from the same considerations that you offer when you treat a patient with paralysis or a patient who has difficulty moving. Ask patients how to best move them before you transport them.

Paralysis

Paralysis is the inability to voluntarily move one or more body parts. It may be caused by stroke, trauma, or birth defects. Paralysis does not always involve a loss of sensation. Some patients will have normal sensation or even hyperesthesia (increased sensitivity), which may cause the patient to experience touch as pain in the affected area. Paralysis of one side of the face may cause communication challenges.

The diaphragm of some paralyzed patients may not function correctly, requiring the use of a ventilator. Patients may also rely on specialized equipment such as urinary catheters, tracheostomy tubes, colostomy bags, or feeding tubes, which are discussed later in this chapter. Some patients may have difficulty swallowing, creating the need for suctioning. Each type of spinal cord paralysis requires its own equipment and may have its own complications.

Patients who have partial or total loss of sensation in a limb cannot tell you when you are injuring them. Always use a gentle touch and take great care when lifting or moving a paralyzed patient. Ask patients how best to move them before you transport them.

Orthotic and Prosthetic Devices

Orthotics and prosthetics are both devices that help a person improve body movement and function. An **orthotic device** is externally applied to support a body part or improve its function. For example, braces and splints are used to support the limbs or spine. A **prosthetic device** (also called a prosthesis) is used to partially or wholly replace an absent or deficient body part. Possible causes of functional impairments that may cause a person to need a prosthetic or orthotic device include injuries, congenital conditions, neurologic problems such as stroke, joint problems, infection or medical conditions, and amputation.

When transporting a patient who uses an orthotic or prosthetic device, if time permits, the EMT should ask the patient if they would like their device transported with them. If the EMT notices that a patient's device no longer serves its intended function, such as if the patient has lost weight and the device no longer fits properly, the patient should be directed to the appropriate resource to refit or replace their device.[10]

Bariatric Patients

Obesity in adults is generally defined as a body mass index (BMI) of 30 or greater. For children, it is defined relative to the child's age group, sex, and growth charts.[11] These definitions are general guidelines only and do not take into consideration factors such as the person's muscle mass. In an adult with

YOU are the EMT

The patient's axillary temperature reads 101.2°F (38.4°C). The patient has a gastrostomy tube and his mother tells you that she administered an appropriate dose of acetaminophen through the tube about an hour ago. Your partner assesses the patient's vital signs while you perform a physical examination, which reveals no obvious abnormalities. You note that the patient has a colostomy bag and an indwelling urinary catheter.

Recording Time: 5 Minutes	
Respirations	14 breaths/min; provided by mechanical ventilator
Pulse	110 beats/min; strong and regular
Skin	Baseline color, hot, and moist
Blood pressure	118/62 mm Hg
Oxygen saturation (Spo_2)	99% (on oxygen)

5. What are some potential complications that may result from your patient's condition? What can you do to prevent them or minimize the risks?
6. What do you suspect is the patient's underlying problem? What specific treatment should you provide to him?

severe obesity (sometimes called extreme or morbid obesity), the BMI is 40 or greater. In the United States, over 40% of adults 20 years or older have obesity, and nearly 10% have severe obesity.[12] Approximately 20% of children have obesity.[13]

While at the simplest level, obesity may be considered an effect of excess calorie consumption, there are numerous other factors at play, such as low metabolic rate or genetic predisposition. Health literacy and access to healthy, affordable food choices are also important factors. In the United States, non-Hispanic Black adults and adults with a lower education level are more likely to experience obesity.[12]

Obesity negatively affects the person's quality of life, and the extra weight can cause a variety of problems, such as mobility difficulties, diabetes, hypertension, heart disease, and stroke.

Interacting With Patients Who Have Obesity

People with obesity sometimes become targets of public ridicule and discrimination. They may be embarrassed by their condition or fearful of scorn as a result of past experiences. Some of those negative interactions may have occurred with an insensitive health care professional. As with any patient, work hard to put these patients at ease. Establish the patient's chief complaint and then communicate your plan to help. Many patients with severe obesity have a complex and extensive medical history, so mastering the art of conducting a patient interview will serve you well in your patient interactions.

As always, treat the patient with dignity and respect. Consider whether you have a bias toward people with obesity. Recognizing this bias can help ensure you deliver the same care for these patients as you would for others.

Transporting a Patient With Obesity

If transport is necessary, plan early for extra help and do not be afraid to call for additional clinicians and/or specialized equipment if necessary. In particular, send a member of your team to find the easiest and safest exit to use. Remember, everyone's safety is at stake! You do not want to risk dropping the patient or injuring a team member by trying to lift too much weight. Moves, no matter how simple they may seem, become far more complex when handling a patient with obesity.

Patients with severe obesity may overcome mobility difficulties by pulling, rocking, or rolling into a position. The constant strain on their body's structures may leave them with chronic joint injuries or osteoarthritis. When you move a patient with severe obesity, follow these tips:

- Ask the patient how best to move them before attempting to do so.
- Avoid lifting the patient by only one limb, which would risk injury to overtaxed joints.
- Coordinate and communicate all moves to all team members prior to starting to lift.
- If the move becomes uncontrolled at any point, stop, reposition, and resume.
- Look for pinch or pressure points from equipment because this could cause significant soft-tissue injuries or deep vein thrombosis.
- Large patients will often have difficulty breathing in a supine position. When safe and appropriate to do so, elevate the head of the stretcher when transporting patients with obesity.
- There are many types of specialized equipment for patients with obesity, and some areas have specifically equipped bariatric ambulances for such patients. Become familiar with the resources available in your area.
- Plan egress routes to accommodate large patients, equipment, and the lifting team members. Remember: Do no harm!
- Notify the receiving facility early to allow special arrangements to be made prior to your arrival to accommodate the patient's needs.

For further discussion of the equipment used to transport a patient with obesity, see Chapter 8, *Lifting and Moving Patients*.

Patients With Medical Technology Assistance

When assessing a patient whose survival depends on medical technology, keep in mind that the parents, caregivers, or home health care staff members have become experts on the patient's condition. They are trained to use and troubleshoot problems with this medical equipment and may provide invaluable insights. Assess the patient's baseline vital signs, and note any allergies (eg, to medications or latex), medications, and other pertinent medical history. You must first determine the patient's normal baseline status before an assessment of the current condition can be made. It is often helpful to ask the patient or caregivers, "What is different today?"

Tracheostomy Tubes

Tracheostomy tubes ensure a patent airway in patients who have anatomic abnormalities, require long-term mechanical ventilation, require frequent tracheal suctioning, or have recurrent pulmonary infections. As an EMT, you may be called to assist a patient or caregiver in managing a tracheostomy site and related equipment. See Chapter 11, *Airway and Ventilation Management*, for a detailed discussion of tracheostomy care.

Home Oxygen

Patients with certain chronic lung diseases (such as chronic obstructive pulmonary disease) may require long-term home oxygen use. Two types of oxygen delivery systems are used for these patients. The first option is the use of oxygen from compressed gas cylinders, similar to what is available on an ambulance, only smaller and more convenient for home use. The second option is to use a machine that concentrates oxygen from the ambient air and then compresses it for delivery to the patient.

Compressed oxygen cylinders do not require electricity or complex machinery. If the power is out, the oxygen from a compressed cylinder will still flow, as long as the supply in that cylinder remains adequate. Additionally, the liter flow per minute of oxygen cylinders is limited only by the regulator attached to the cylinder and the amount of gas left in the cylinder. The drawbacks of using compressed gas cylinders mainly center around portability and limited supply. Oxygen cylinders can be heavy, bulky, and difficult to transport. Although small cylinders are available that can be carried more easily, the amount of oxygen available in these small cylinders may be suitable for a short duration only. Additionally, regardless of the size of the oxygen cylinder, it will run out of oxygen eventually. Thus, patients using compressed gas cylinders must have multiple cylinders in the home and must coordinate with an oxygen supplier for regular delivery and pickup of these cylinders. Although oxygen is not flammable, it will cause items that are already on fire to burn at much higher temperatures and with much greater intensity.

A home oxygen concentrator takes ambient air and scrubs the nitrogen from the atmospheric air, leaving behind almost 100% oxygen (**FIGURE 35-6A**). After the oxygen has been concentrated, it is compressed so that it can be delivered to the patient via an oxygen delivery device, such as a nasal cannula or face mask. The compression that home oxygen concentrators are able to achieve varies by machine but is generally limited to 10 L/min. The main benefit of the oxygen concentrator machine is that it can provide an unlimited supply of oxygen as long as it is functioning properly and has a reliable source of electrical power. There are also smaller, more portable oxygen concentrators that can provide patients with increased mobility and freedom of travel, although these units are usually able to provide only 1 to 3 L/min of flow in most cases (**FIGURE 35-6B**). In the event of a power failure, the patient must have a backup compressed gas cylinder to use until power is restored.

When caring for patients who are on home oxygen, you should ask them why they are on home oxygen, how long they have been on home oxygen, what their baseline home oxygen requirement is (ie, how many liters per minute, how many hours per day), and whether their home oxygen requirement has changed recently. It is also important to establish these patients' baseline oxygen saturation levels. Many patients with chronic lung disease will have baseline oxygen saturations that are lower than normal. Regardless of their baseline oxygen saturation level, any patient who is in respiratory distress should be placed on supplemental oxygen at a level appropriate for their level of distress and work of breathing.

Mechanical Ventilators

Some patients who are on a mechanical ventilator at home cannot breathe without assistance (**FIGURE 35-7**). Others may use the ventilator only while sleeping or during physical exertion. Patients requiring a mechanical ventilator may not have an underlying respiratory drive because of a congenital defect or a chronic lung disease process. Other

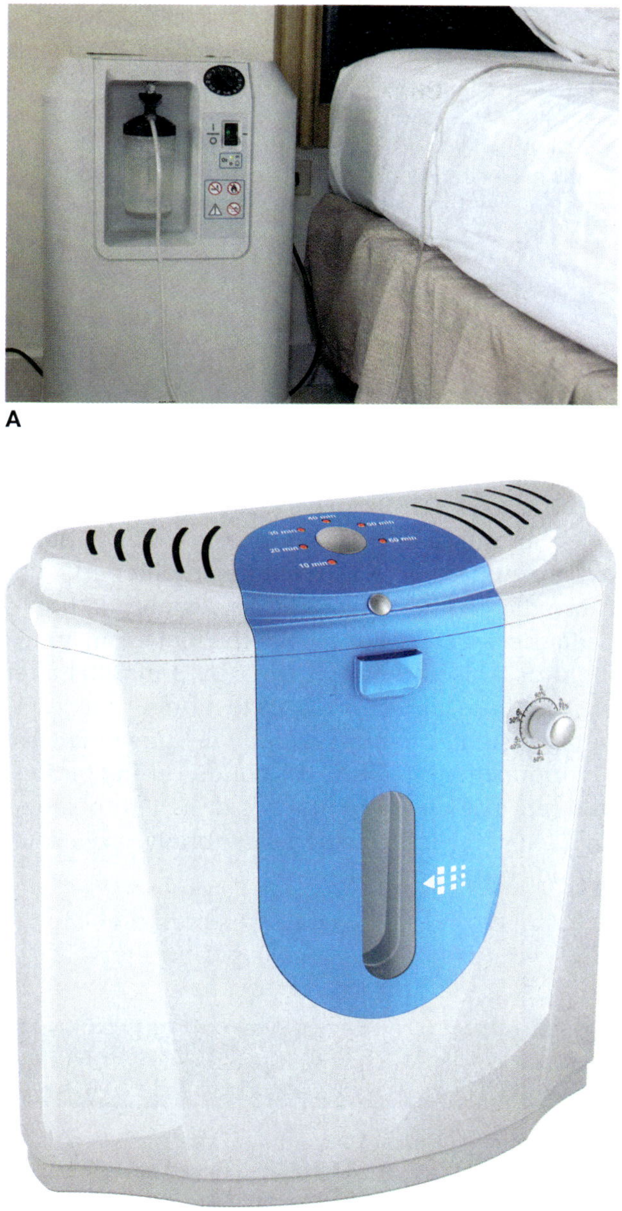

A

B

FIGURE 35-6 A. Home oxygen concentrator. **B.** Portable oxygen concentrator.

A: © abalcazar/iStock/Getty Images Plus/Getty Images; B: © natatravel/Shutterstock.

patients may have a traumatic brain injury, muscular dystrophy, or another disease process that weakens their ability to breathe and requires a permanent tracheostomy and mechanical ventilator.

Remember that patients with tracheostomies typically do not breathe through the mouth and nose; therefore, a face mask or nasal cannula cannot be used to treat them. If the ventilator malfunctions and the patient can breathe on their own, remove the patient from the ventilator and apply a tracheostomy collar. This oxygen-delivery device is specifically designed to cover the tracheostomy **stoma** and features a strap that goes around the neck. Tracheostomy collars are usually available in hospitals, where many patients have tracheostomies, and may not be available in a prehospital setting. If you do not have a tracheostomy collar, you can improvise by placing a face mask over the stoma (**FIGURE 35-8**). Even though the mask is shaped to fit the face, you can usually achieve an adequate fit over the patient's neck by adjusting the strap. If the

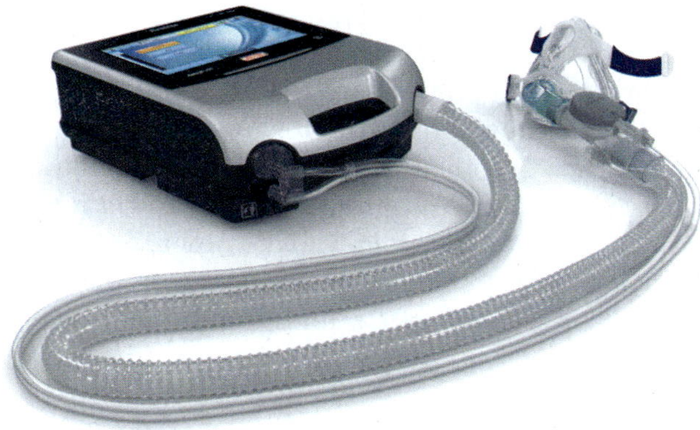

FIGURE 35-7 The ResMed Astral home ventilator shown provides mechanical ventilation to both ventilation dependent and nondependent patients.

© ResMed 2025. Used with permission.

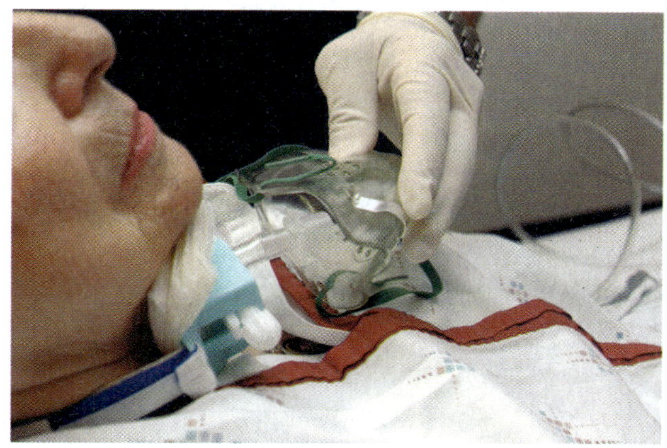

FIGURE 35-8 When caring for a person with a tracheostomy, if the ventilator fails and you do not have a tracheostomy collar, use a face mask instead.

© Jones & Bartlett Learning.

patient's own ventilations are absent or inadequate, ventilate the patient using a bag-mask device.

Patients on home mechanical ventilators may require assisted ventilation throughout transport. Remember that the patient's caregivers will know how the mechanical ventilator works and can help you attach the bag and valve from a bag-mask device to the tracheostomy tube in preparation for transport. When troubleshooting a ventilator problem, it may be helpful to use the DOPE mnemonic:

- **D** Displacement. Has the tracheostomy tube been partially or even completely displaced?
- **O** Obstruction. Is there material in the tube that needs to be suctioned, or does the tracheal tube need to be replaced because it is completely blocked?
- **P** Pneumothorax. Are breath sounds present on both sides of the chest?
- **E** Equipment. Does the ventilator have power? Is there water or a kink in the ventilator tubing that is preventing airflow? Is the tubing connected properly?

Management of a patient's tracheostomy tube is discussed further in Chapter 11, *Airway and Ventilation Management*.

Words of Wisdom

Several states have adopted laws that require a backup generator or other devices to prevent the loss of electric supply to the homes of families or institutions that have patients using mechanical ventilators.

Apnea Monitors

While caring for an infant with special challenges, you may come across an apnea monitor (**FIGURE 35-9**). The apnea monitor is typically used when an infant is born prematurely, needs home oxygen, or has a serious breathing problem.[14,15] Because the central nervous system is not mature in pediatric patients with special challenges, an apnea monitor is used for approximately 3 months after birth of these high-risk infants to monitor the respiratory system. A typical episode of apnea may last for approximately 15 to 20 seconds, during periods of sleep. The apnea monitor is designed to sound an alarm if the infant experiences bradycardia or an episode of apnea occurs.

YOU are the EMT

You consult with medical direction and receive instructions on how to proceed. The mechanical ventilator is too large to fit in your ambulance, so you prepare the bag-mask device, detach the ventilator circuit from the tracheostomy tube, and begin manual ventilations at 12 breaths/min. You request advanced life support (ALS) support, which is severely delayed due to traffic. You carefully move the patient to your stretcher, secure him properly, and load him into the ambulance. Following medical direction's instructions, you continue to manually ventilate the patient, reassess his vital signs, and begin transport to the hospital.

Recording Time: 15 Minutes	
Level of consciousness	Conscious and alert
Respirations	12 breaths/min; provided by bag-mask device
Pulse	118 beats/min; strong and regular
Skin	Baseline color, hot, and dry
Blood pressure	120/60 mm Hg
Oxygen saturation (Spo_2)	98% (on oxygen)

7. What is the benefit of allowing the patient's mother to accompany her son to the hospital?

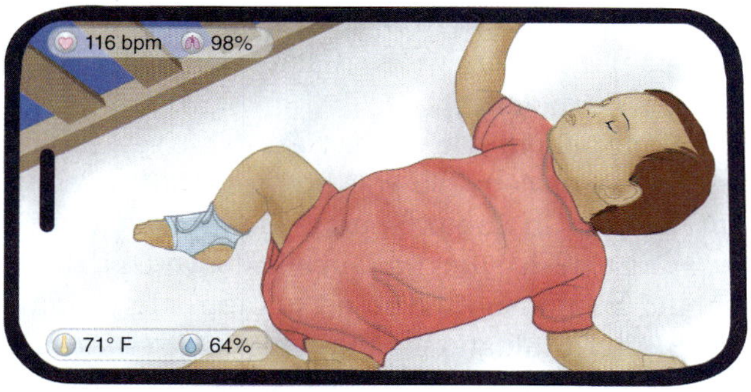

FIGURE 35-9 Infant apnea monitors can provide information about the infant's sleep state and vital signs. In the system shown here, the infant wears a sensor "sock," and a camera is positioned outside the crib. The data and video are sent to the caregiver's smartphone via Bluetooth.

The apnea monitor is attached with electrodes or a belt wrapped around the infant's chest or stomach. A pulse oximeter may also be used. The apnea monitor will provide a pulse oximetry reading that will help you assess the patient's respiratory status.

The parents or caregivers of pediatric patients with special challenges will be a useful resource when obtaining the patient's medical history and a history of the events leading to the call for assistance. Parents and caregivers become knowledgeable regarding the use of apnea monitors and may be able to provide you and your partner with a computerized printout to share with ALS clinicians or emergency department (ED) personnel. If possible, bring the apnea monitor to the receiving hospital with the infant so that it may be evaluated and any stored information may be retrieved for further analysis.

Internal Cardiac Pacemakers and Defibrillators

An internal cardiac pacemaker is a device implanted under the patient's skin or, more recently, directly in the heart, to regulate the heart rate. When placed under the skin, these devices are typically located on the nondominant side of the patient's chest so that normal activities are not hindered. In small or extremely thin patients, the device may be implanted in the abdomen. For patients with heart failure or a history of extremely rapid heart rates that require defibrillation, an internal pacemaker may include an implanted cardioverter-defibrillator (ICD), which monitors the patient's heart rhythm and is able to slow accelerated heart rates using pacing or defibrillation.[16]

When using an automated external defibrillator (AED) to resuscitate a person with an implanted device, never place the defibrillator pads directly over the device; doing so interferes with conduction of the AED.

It can be helpful for the hospital staff if you gather information about an implanted device while you obtain the patient's history during the patient assessment process. Consider asking these questions:

- What type of heart disorder do you have?
- How long has this device been implanted?
- What is your normal baseline rhythm and heart rate?
- If the implant is an ICD:
  - Do you know at what heart rate will the defibrillator fire?
  - How many times has the defibrillator delivered a shock?

Sometimes a patient will have a pacemaker identification card in their wallet that contains information specific to the device.

Ventricular Assist Devices

A ventricular assist device (VAD) is a special piece of medical equipment that takes over the function of one or both heart ventricles. These devices are typically used as a bridge to heart transplantation while a donor heart is being located or as a permanent solution for patients who do not qualify for a transplant. A left ventricular assist device (LVAD) is the most common type of VAD.

If you encounter a patient with a VAD, you will primarily provide supportive measures and basic care. The parents or caregivers should be knowledgeable about the device, so use them as a resource during transport. The patient should have a "go bag" containing extra batteries and other supplies that must always be transported with the patient. Be prepared to provide CPR if there is no evidence of perfusion. Keep in mind that the VAD may be functioning in the absence of a palpable pulse, so you will have to use other assessment techniques to determine adequate perfusion. Assess perfusion by noting level of consciousness; skin color, temperature, and moisture; and capillary refill.

If you encounter a patient with this device, call the number of the patient's support team, contact medical direction, or follow your local protocols. If the device's alarm is sounding, check all connections and be sure the batteries are fully charged. Notify ALS personnel as soon as possible so that other supportive measures may be initiated.

VAD technology has advanced significantly over the past decade. While you may be called for a crisis involving the VAD itself, it is far more likely that emergency medical services (EMS) will be called for medical emergencies related to VAD implantation. The most common of these emergencies is bleeding, often nosebleeds or gastrointestinal bleeding.[17] Because VAD patients are anticoagulated (taking blood thinners), bleeding can be significant. Infection, usually of the drive line that connects the VAD controller to the patient, is another reason patients may require transport. Both of these emergencies should be treated in the same manner as you would treat bleeding or sepsis in a patient without a VAD.

Words of Wisdom

Special equipment such as a VAD often includes a phone number to call for information specific to patient care. Patients and family members typically carry identification cards with necessary phone numbers and may be able to share this information with you. Make every reasonable effort to bring these patients to the hospital where the VAD was implanted to facilitate management of any problems with the device. This decision will obviously be a function of distance and patient condition. Seek online medical direction early, as these patients' needs may exceed the capabilities of some receiving facilities. Helpful apps are available for download to smartphones that provide VAD troubleshooting assistance and contact as well as transport information.[18]

External Defibrillator Vest

This device is a vest with built-in monitoring electrodes and defibrillation pads, which is worn by the patient under their clothing. The vest is attached to a monitor that provides alerts and voice prompts when it recognizes a dangerous rhythm and before it delivers a shock. The device uses high-energy shocks similar to an AED, so avoid contact with the patient if the device warns that it is about to deliver a shock.

If the patient is in cardiac arrest, the vest should remain in place while you perform CPR unless it interferes with compressions. Any patient who is wearing a device that has already delivered a shock should be transported to an appropriate hospital for further evaluation. See Chapter 17, *Cardiovascular Emergencies*, for further discussion of external defibrillator vests.

Words of Wisdom

If the patient is unresponsive and you are unsure whether the external defibrillator vest has already delivered a shock, look for blue gel on the patient's upper back. The electrodes on the vest release the gel immediately before the first shock is delivered. Do not delay care waiting for a defibrillator vest to provide treatment.

Central Venous Catheter

A central venous catheter, or central line, is a catheter that has its tip placed in the superior vena cava to provide venous access. It is used for many types of home care patients, including those receiving chemotherapy, long-term antibiotic therapy, pain management, total parenteral nutrition, and hemodialysis (**FIGURE 35-10**). Central venous catheters are often located in the chest, upper arm, or subclavicular area.

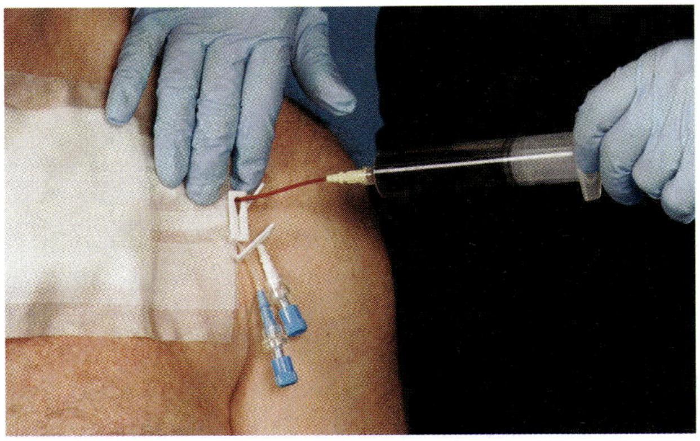

FIGURE 35-10 Patients who require frequent intravenous medications may have a central line in place.

Problems associated with central venous catheters include broken lines, infections around the lines, clotted lines, and bleeding around the line or from the tubing attached to the line. If bleeding occurs, apply direct pressure to the tubing and provide prompt transport to the hospital.

Gastrostomy Tubes

Gastrostomy tubes, sometimes referred to as gastric tubes or G-tubes, are placed into the stomach of patients who cannot adequately ingest fluids, food, or medication by mouth. These tubes may be inserted through the nose or mouth into the stomach (using a nasogastric or orogastric tube) or inserted surgically directly into the stomach through the abdominal wall (**FIGURE 35-11**). Gastric tubes may become dislodged during the patient's normal daily activities. If such a situation arises, immediately stop the flow of any fluids being infused through the tube, and assess the patient for signs or symptoms of bleeding into the stomach, such as vague abdominal discomfort, nausea, and vomiting (especially emesis with a "coffee-ground" appearance [older bleeding] or with bright red blood [more recent bleeding]).

Patients who have a gastric tube in place may still be at increased risk of aspiration. Always have suction readily available to clear any materials from the patient's mouth. Stop the flow of any fluids if signs of aspiration are present. Patients with gastric tubes who have difficulty breathing should be transported while sitting or lying on the right side with the head elevated 30° to prevent the contents of the stomach from passing into the lungs.

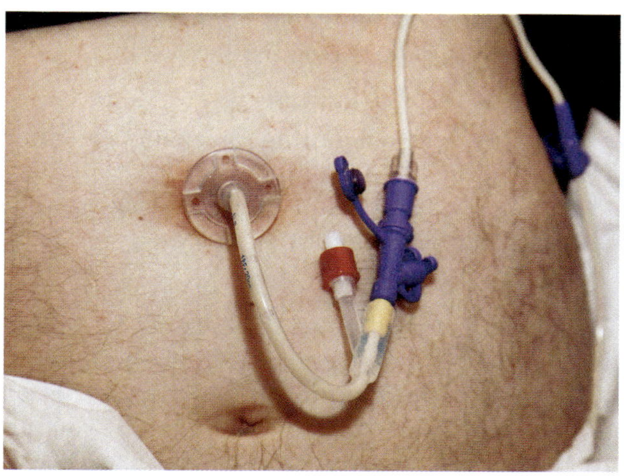

FIGURE 35-11 Gastric tubes may be placed through the skin into the stomach for children or adults who cannot be fed by mouth.

Patients with diabetes who receive insulin and gastric tube feedings may become hypoglycemic quickly if the gastric tube feedings are discontinued for any reason. Be alert for an altered mental status or a change in the baseline behavior of your patient. Unless the tube is dysfunctional, dislodged, or partially dislodged, continue the tube feeding and transport the pump with you.

Shunts

Some patients with chronic neurologic conditions may have shunts in place. For example, a patient with hydrocephalus will have a shunt. **Shunts** are tubes that drain excess cerebrospinal fluid from the ventricles of the brain to keep pressure from building up in the brain.

During your assessment of a patient with a shunt, you will likely feel a device beneath the skin on the side of the head, behind the ear. The device is a fluid reservoir, and its presence should alert you to the possibility that the patient has an underlying shunt. There are different types of shunts, including a ventriculoperitoneal (VP) shunt and a ventriculoatrial (VA) shunt. A VP shunt drains excess fluid from the ventricles of the brain into the peritoneum of the abdomen. A VA shunt drains excess fluid from the ventricles of the brain into the right atrium of the heart. A shunt may become blocked or an infection may result in the surrounding tissue. Infections as a result of shunt placement may occur within the first 2 months after shunt insertion. A blocked shunt may present as a medical emergency. If the shunt is unable to drain properly, intracranial pressure may increase, affecting the patient's mental status, and respiratory arrest may occur.

The signs that a patient is in distress include a high-pitched cry or bulging fontanelles (in infants), headache, projectile vomiting, altered mental status, irritability, fever, nausea, difficulty with coordination (walking), blurred vision, seizures, redness along the shunt tract, bradycardia, and heart dysrhythmias. Emergency medical care includes airway management and artificial ventilation during transport.

Vagus Nerve Stimulators

Nearly 3 million US adults (approximately 1% of the population) and 500,000 children have active epilepsy.[19] Vagus nerve stimulation is a form of treatment used for seizures that are not controlled with antiepileptic medications or if the patient is not a good candidate for brain surgery. Vagus nerve stimulators stimulate the vagus nerve at predetermined intervals to prevent seizure activity. Some devices deliver an extra burst if an impending seizure is detected. These devices are used in conjunction with medication to reduce the frequency of seizures. They are not meant to replace medications and are not currently used in children younger than 4 years. Further studies are being done regarding their effectiveness for seizure disorders. The device, which is approximately the size of a silver dollar, is surgically implanted under the patient's skin. The stimulator can last for up to 6 years or until the battery runs out. If you encounter a patient with this device, contact medical direction or follow your local protocols.

Colostomies, Ileostomies, and Urostomies

A **colostomy** or **ileostomy** is a surgical procedure that creates an opening from the large or small intestine to the surface of the body that allows for elimination of waste products. The special opening is referred to as a stoma. Feces are expelled and collected into a clear external bag or pouch, which is emptied or changed frequently.

If you encounter a patient with a colostomy or ileostomy bag, assess for signs and symptoms of dehydration if the patient reports diarrhea or vomiting. The area around the stoma is susceptible to infection, so patients and caregivers must be diligent with daily hygiene. Signs of infection include redness, warm skin around the stoma, and tenderness with palpation over the colostomy or ileostomy site.

A **urostomy** is a surgically created connection from the urinary system to the surface of the skin that allows urine to drain through a stoma in the abdominal wall instead of through the urethra. For example, a patient who has had their bladder removed due to cancer requires a urostomy.

Contact medical direction or follow your local protocols for the care of a patient with a colostomy, ileostomy, or urostomy bag.

Emergencies Involving Infants

Sudden Unexpected Infant Death

The term **sudden unexpected infant death (SUID)** refers to a sudden unexpected death of a child younger than 1 year where the cause is either known or not known.[20] Causes of death may include suffocation, infection, poisoning, cardiac problems, and trauma. One of the causes of SUID has long been known as sudden infant death syndrome (SIDS), which results in the death of a child younger than 1 year that cannot be explained by another cause after thorough investigation. However, some pediatric groups and investigative officials are replacing the use of SIDS with **unexplained sudden death in infancy (USDI)**.

USDI is thought to result from a combination of factors, including vulnerability (eg, underlying medical conditions), developmental stage, and environmental stressors (eg, sleeping position, exposure to smoke, excessive warmth).[21] In 2022, there were approximately 3,700 SUIDs in the United States, more than 1,500 of which were classified as USDI.[22] To reduce the risk of USDI, the American Academy of Pediatrics recommends placing infants (younger than 1 year) on their back on a firm mattress to sleep, in a crib that is free of bumpers, blankets, and toys. The Centers for Disease Control and Prevention recommends having the baby sleep in the same room, but not in the same bed, chair, or sofa, as an adult. Breastfeeding and use of a pacifier are also associated with a lower risk of USDI.

Although it is impossible to predict USDI, the following are several known risk factors:

- Mother younger than 20 years
- Mother smoked during pregnancy or after birth
- Mother used alcohol or illicit drugs during pregnancy or after birth
- Low birth weight

Deaths as the result of USDI can occur at any time of the day; however, these children are often discovered in the morning when the parents or caregivers go in to check on the infant. If you are the first clinician at the scene of suspected USDI, you will face three tasks: assessment of the scene, assessment and treatment of the patient, and communication and support of the family.

Patient Assessment and Treatment

USDI is a diagnosis of exclusion. All other potential causes must first be ruled out, a process that can be time-consuming for physicians. An infant who has been a victim of USDI will be pale or blue, not breathing, and unresponsive. Other causes for SUID include the following:

- Overwhelming infection
- Child maltreatment
- Airway obstruction from a foreign object or as a result of infection
- Meningitis
- Accidental or intentional poisoning
- Hypoglycemia (low blood glucose level)
- Congenital metabolic defects

Regardless of the cause, assessment and treatment of the infant remain the same. Remember that what you find in assessing the infant and the scene may provide important diagnostic information.

Begin with an assessment of the ABCs, and provide interventions as necessary. Depending on how much time has passed since the child was discovered, postmortem changes may have occurred. These signs include stiffening of the body, called rigor mortis, and dependent lividity, which is the pooling of blood in the lower parts of the body or those that are in contact with the floor or bed.

If the child shows such signs, call medical direction. In some EMS systems, a victim of SUID who has obvious signs of death may be declared dead on the scene. Deciding whether to start CPR on a child who shows clear signs of rigor mortis or dependent lividity can be difficult. Family members may consider anything less as withholding critical care. In this situation, the best course of action may be to contact medical direction. In cases where there is clear evidence of rigor mortis, medical direction typically advises that resuscitation be withheld to avoid disturbing the death investigation unless the safety of the crew would be compromised. If there is any question of the potential for survival, resuscitation is performed and the patient is transported to the hospital, where the family can receive more extensive support. Follow local protocols. If there is no evidence of postmortem changes, begin CPR immediately.

As you assess the infant, pay special attention to any marks or bruises on the child before performing any procedures, including CPR. Also note any intervention such as CPR that was done by the parents or caregivers before you arrived.

Scene Assessment

Carefully inspect the environment, following local protocols, noting the condition of the scene where the parents or caregivers found the infant. Your assessment of the scene should concentrate on the following:

- Signs of illness, including medications, humidifiers, or thermometers
- The general condition of the house
- Signs of poor hygiene
- Family interaction. Do not allow yourself to be judgmental about family interactions at this time. Note and report any behavior that is clearly not within the acceptable range, such as physical and verbal abuse.
- The site where the infant was discovered. Note all items in the infant's crib or bed, including pillows, stuffed animals, toys, and small objects.

The death of a child is a devastating event for a family and tends to evoke strong emotional responses among the EMS clinicians involved. Communication relating to the death and dying of a child is discussed in Chapter 4, *Communications and Documentation.*

Brief Resolved Unexplained Event

Occasionally, clinicians responding to a call for a possible pediatric cardiac arrest arrive to find an apparently healthy, normal infant. When this circumstance remains unexplained, even after a thorough medical examination, it is referred to as a **brief resolved unexplained event (BRUE)**, formerly called an apparent life-threatening event (ALTE). BRUE is defined as an event that occurs in an infant younger than 1 year of age that lasts less than 1 minute and includes at least two of the following signs or symptoms[23]:

- Absent, slow, or irregular respirations
- Pale or cyanotic skin
- Decreased level of consciousness
- Altered muscle tone (limp or rigid)

Parents or caregivers may report these signs and symptoms as well as others such as choking, gagging or seizing.

On assessment, the EMT will often find an infant who appears healthy and shows no signs of illness, distress, or other abnormalities. You should assess the infant's history and, if possible, the environment. Be aware the incident might be the result of maltreatment or another medical condition. Any abnormal finding on examination, such as fever, vomiting, signs of trauma, or abnormal breathing, would not be classified as BRUE. Significant past medical conditions such as seizure, congenital heart disorders, pulmonary diseases, or the presence of a VP shunt would also exclude a BRUE diagnosis.

Despite the appearance of an apparently normal infant after the prehospital exam, transport is required so the infant can have a full evaluation to rule out any possible life-threatening conditions. During transport monitor the infant carefully. Pay strict attention to assessment of the airway and breathing. Allow parents or caregivers to ride in the ambulance, if appropriate. Reassure the caregivers and explain that you cannot say what caused the event and that the physicians will have to determine the cause at the hospital.

If after a thorough workup at the hospital there is no explanation for the signs and symptoms reported by the caregiver, the infant's diagnosis will be BRUE.

Patients Who Have Experienced Abuse or Neglect

Child Abuse and Neglect

The term **child maltreatment** includes all forms of physical and emotional abuse, sexual abuse, neglect, and exploitation. The intentional injury of a child, whether physical or emotional, unfortunately is not rare in our society. In 2022, nearly 560,000 children were victims of child maltreatment in the United States.[24] Maltreatment is one of the leading causes of death in infants younger than 12 months of age. If suspected child maltreatment is not reported, the child is likely to be abused again, which can lead to permanent injury or death. Therefore, you must be aware of the signs of child maltreatment. As an EMT, you are a mandatory reporter and are legally required to report suspected maltreatment to law enforcement or child protection agencies. Be familiar with the specific details of your state's laws.

Signs of Child Maltreatment

As an EMT, you will be called to homes because of a reported injury to a child. Child maltreatment occurs in every socioeconomic status, so be aware of the patient's surroundings and document your findings objectively. EMTs are commonly called to testify in maltreatment cases, so it is essential to record all findings, including any statements made by parents or caregivers or others on the scene. Although it is your duty to report, not investigate, physical or sexual abuse, you can learn more about the situation by asking yourself the following questions:

- Is the injury typical for the developmental level of the child?
- Is the method of injury reported by the parent or caregiver consistent with the child's injury?
- Is the parent or caregiver behaving appropriately (concerned about the child's well-being)?
- Is there evidence of drinking or drug use at the scene?
- Was there a delay in seeking care for the child?
- Is there a good relationship between the child and the parent or caregiver?
- Does the child have multiple injuries at different stages of healing?
- Does the child have any unusual marks or bruises that may have been caused by cigarettes, heating grates, or branding injuries?
- Does the child have several types of injuries, such as burns, fractures, and bruises?
- Does the child have any burns on the hands or feet that involve a glove distribution (marks that encircle a hand or foot in a pattern that looks like a glove)?
- Is there an unexplained decreased level of consciousness?
- Is the child clean and an appropriate weight for their age?
- Is there any rectal or vaginal bleeding?
- What does the home look like? Clean or dirty? Is it warm or cold? Is there adequate food?

Your assessment in the field will allow a better assessment by the medical staff later. An easy way to remember these points for the pediatric population is the mnemonic CHILD ABUSE:

C Consistency of the injury with the child's developmental age
H History inconsistent with injury
I Inappropriate parental concerns

- **L** Lack of supervision
- **D** Delay in seeking care
- **A** Affect (body language)
- **B** Bruises of varying ages
- **U** Unusual injury patterns
- **S** Suspicious circumstances
- **E** Environmental clues

As you assess the pediatric patient, be alert to signs of abuse, such as those described in the following sections (**FIGURE 35-12**).

Bruises

In children, bumps and bruises occur commonly as the result of play and exploration. However, you must be able to differentiate these normal bruises from those commonly associated with physical abuse. Observe the color and location of any bruises. New bruises appear pink or red in patients with light skin tone; in patients with darker skin tone, they may appear red or purple. Over time, bruises turn blue, then green, then yellow-brown and faded. Note the location. Bruises to the back, buttocks, ears, or face are suspicious and are usually inflicted by a person. The TEN-4-FACESp decision tool can be used to help identify bruising that is consistent with abuse in children younger than 4 years.[25]

- **TEN** indicates bruising on the Torso, Ears, or Neck.
- **4** indicates bruising anywhere on an infant who is 4 months of age or less.
- **FACES** indicates bruising on the Frenulum (narrow strip of tissue that joins the upper lip to the gums), Angle of the jaw, Cheeks, Eyelids, or Subconjunctivae.
- **p** indicates the presence of Patterned bruising such as belt, hand, or other tool marks.

Burns

Burns to the penis, testicles, vagina, or buttocks are usually inflicted by someone else, as are burns

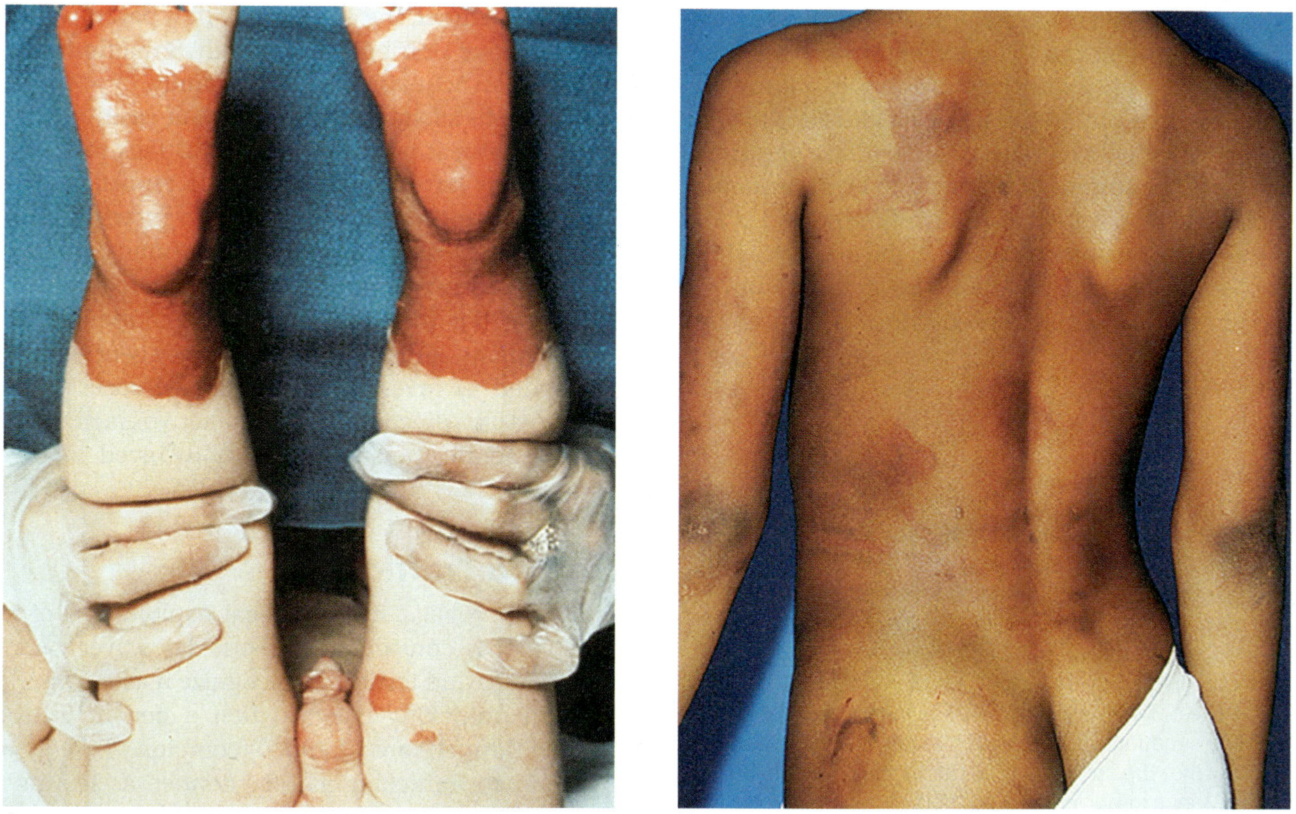

A B

FIGURE 35-12 Signs of child abuse. **A.** A scald. **B.** Multiple injuries at different stages of healing.

Courtesy of Ronald Dieckmann, MD.

that encircle a hand or foot to look like a glove. You should suspect abuse if the child has cigarette burns or grid pattern burns.

Fractures

Fractures of the humerus or femur do not normally occur without major trauma, such as a fall from a high place or a motor vehicle crash. Falls from a bed are not usually associated with fractures. Maintain an index of suspicion if an infant or young child sustains a femur fracture or a complete fracture of any bone. As discussed, children are more likely to experience greenstick (incomplete) fractures, as opposed to complete fractures, due to their soft and pliable bones. A complete fracture in a pediatric patient indicates that the child was exposed to significant traumatic force.

Shaken Baby Syndrome

Infants may sustain life-threatening head trauma by being shaken or struck on the head, a condition called **shaken baby syndrome**, a subset of abusive head trauma. With this condition, there is bleeding within the head and damage to the cervical spine as a result of intentional, forceful shaking. The infant will often be found unconscious, often without evidence of external trauma. The call for help may be for an infant who has stopped breathing or is unresponsive. The infant may appear to be in cardiopulmonary arrest, but what has likely occurred is that the shaking tore blood vessels in the brain, resulting in bleeding around the brain. The pressure from the blood results in an increased intracranial pressure, and in many cases leads to severe disability, coma and/or death.

> **Words of Wisdom**
>
> It is normal to have concerns about the care of children, but do not let your personal judgments cloud the true nature of a situation. You may feel upset by challenging socioeconomic factors that affect where a child lives, the condition of the home environment, and the child's sources of food. However, the parents or caregivers may have the best of intentions and may be doing everything possible for the child. In these situations, let the hospital staff or a supervisor know that the child and their family may need some assistance or community support. When in doubt, report the situation to the appropriate abuse and neglect authorities and the receiving facility.

Signs of Child Neglect

Neglect is refusal or failure on the part of the parent or caregiver to provide life necessities, such as food, water, clothing, shelter, personal hygiene, medicine, comfort, and personal safety.

Children who are neglected are often dirty or too thin or appear developmentally delayed because of a lack of stimulation. You may observe such children when you are making calls for unrelated problems. Report all cases of suspected neglect.

Symptoms and Other Indicators of Maltreatment

An abused child may appear withdrawn, fearful, or hostile. Be particularly concerned if the child refuses to discuss how an injury occurred. Occasionally, the parent or caregiver will reveal a history of several "accidents." Be alert for conflicting stories or a marked lack of concern from the parents or caregiver. Remember, the abuser may be a parent, caregiver, relative, or friend of the family. Sometimes the abuser is an acquaintance of the family.

EMTs in all states must report all cases of suspected maltreatment, even if the ED fails to do so. Most states have special forms for reporting. Supervisors are generally forbidden to interfere with the reporting of suspected maltreatment, even if they disagree with the assessment. You do not have to prove that there has been maltreatment. Law enforcement and child protection agencies are mandated to investigate all reported cases. Take all necessary precautions to protect yourself, your team, and the pediatric patient involved in this situation.

Human Trafficking

Human trafficking is the illegal exploitation of a person. It is considered modern-day slavery, and all 50 states and territories recognize it as a crime.[26] Human trafficking occurs when a person is exploited through force, fraud, or coercion.

Human trafficking may be defined as sex trafficking (91%) or forced labor (9%).[27] It can happen in urban, suburban, and rural areas and involve people of any gender (although more than three-quarters are women) and any age or nationality.[28] Traffickers may be strangers or acquaintances, such as family members, gang members, intimate partners, or employers. According to the organization Polaris, risk factors for becoming a victim of human trafficking include a history of having experienced poverty, abuse, substance use disorder, or mental health illness (or having lived with someone who was experiencing these conditions). Further, persons of color and persons who identify as a sexual minority are more likely to become victims of human trafficking.[29]

EMS clinicians are in a position to detect and report cases of suspected human trafficking, as they may encounter people being exploited in public settings such as truck stops, rest areas, or workplaces, or in private homes. Signs of human trafficking are subtle and may include the following[30]:

- A person who has recently been disconnected from their family or social network
- A child who stops attending school
- A person who is involved in commercial sex acts
- Signs of mental or physical abuse
- A person who seems fearful, timid, or submissive
- Signs of physical or medical neglect
- Brands or tattoos

Questions you might consider when evaluating a person whom you suspect is involved in human trafficking include the following:

- Does the person appear to be controlled by another person?
- Does the person seem to be coached about what to say?
- Are the living conditions inappropriate?
- Does the person appear to lack personal possessions?
- Does the person not appear to be free to move about or leave (ie, existence of surveillance equipment or unusual locks or security measures)?

Safety

If you encounter a person whom you suspect to be a trafficker, do not confront the person; instead notify law enforcement as soon as possible.

Care of the patient should focus on their medical needs, not in-depth questioning to determine whether they have been trafficked. Employ the following skills[31]:

- Use a caring, nonjudgmental communication style.
- When possible, interview and transport the patient without the suspected trafficker or any companion.
- Ask open-ended questions in a sensitive manner.
- Be attentive to verbal and nonverbal cues.
- Discreetly offer information about how the patient can access help when they are ready.

The Department of Homeland Security has developed awareness and educational materials through its Blue Campaign. It also provides support hotlines. To report suspected human trafficking, the number is 1-866-347-2423. To ask for help, the number is 1-888-373-7888, or the person may text HELP or INFO to BeFree (233733).

Elder Abuse and Neglect

Trauma in older people can also be caused by abuse. **Elder abuse** is defined as any action on the part of an older person's family member, caregiver, or other associated person that takes advantage of the older person's person (eg, physical abuse), property, or emotional state. Abuse can result from acts of commission (words or actions that cause harm), such as verbal, physical, or sexual assault. Abuse can also result from acts of omission (failure to act), such as denying an older person adequate nutrition or medical care.

The exact extent of elder abuse is often not known for several reasons, including the following:

- Elder abuse is a problem that has been largely hidden from society.
- The definitions of abuse and neglect among the geriatric population vary.
- Victims of elder abuse are often hesitant to report the problem to law enforcement agencies or human and social welfare personnel.

Nonetheless, elder abuse is known to be a significant problem in the United States, with approximately 1 in 10 older adults who live at home experiencing some form or maltreatment.[32]

The abused person may feel traumatized by the situation or be afraid that the abuser will punish them for reporting the abuse. The abused person may be frail and have multiple chronic medical conditions or dementia. The person may sleepwalk, have an impaired sleep cycle, and periodically shout at others. The person may also be incontinent and may depend on others for activities of daily living (ADLs).

The physical and emotional signs of abuse, such as rape, spousal physical abuse, and nutritional deprivation, are often overlooked or not accurately identified. Older women are particularly not likely to report incidents of sexual assault to law enforcement agencies. Patients with sensory deficits, dementia, and other forms of altered mental status, such as drug-induced depression, may not be able to report abuse.

Abusers of older people are sometimes products of child abuse, and the abuse that is inflicted on the older person may be retaliatory. Most of these abusers are not trained in the particular care that older people require and have little relief time from the constant care demands of their own family, children, and spouse. Their lives are significantly complicated by the constant, demanding needs of the older person they have to care for.

The abuser may also have marked fatigue, be unemployed with financial difficulties, or abuse one or more substances. With a careful eye, you can recognize the clues to these stressful situations and help guide the family toward programs in their community that are geared to helping the whole family. Programs such as adult day care, Meals on Wheels, and many local individualized programs help to decrease the stress put on the family and lower the chances of abuse. Refer the family to the 2-1-1 hotline to identify key supportive resources in their community.

Abuse is not restricted to the home. Environments such as nursing and convalescent homes and continuing care centers are also sites where older people sustain physical, psychological, financial, or pharmacologic harm. Care providers in these environments can consider older people to be management problems or categorize them as obstinate and undesirable patients. Consult local authorities, but in general you should assume that you have the same obligation to report suspected elder abuse as you do suspected child abuse. Notify receiving hospital personnel of your concerns, report to the proper authorities based on local protocols, and factually document your findings. If you are in doubt, err on the side of caution and make a report. Note that it is not your responsibility to prove that the abuse occurred, only to report your findings according to protocols.

Assessment of Elder Abuse

Abuse comes in many forms and may include physical assault. Be aware of the environment and conditions a patient lives in, and take note of soft-tissue injuries that cannot be explained by the person's lifestyle and physical condition.

While assessing the patient, try to obtain an explanation of what happened. You should suspect abuse when answers to questions about what caused the injury are concealed or avoided or inconsistent with medical findings.

You must also suspect abuse when you are given unbelievable answers. Be suspicious if you think "Does this make sense?" or "Do I really believe this story?" while reviewing the patient's history. As an EMT, you may be the first health care clinician to observe the signs of possible abuse. Information that may be important in assessing possible abuse includes the following:

- Caregiver apathy about the patient's condition
- Overly defensive reaction by the caregiver to your questions
- Caregiver does not allow the patient to answer questions
- Repeated visits to the ED or clinic
- A history of being accident-prone
- Unexplainable soft-tissue injuries
- Unbelievable, vague, or inconsistent explanations of injuries
- Psychosomatic complaints
- Chronic pain without medical explanation
- Self-destructive behavior
- Eating and sleep disorders
- Depression or a lack of energy
- A history of substance and/or sexual abuse

You should remember that patients who are being abused may be so afraid of retribution that they make false statements. A geriatric patient who is being abused by family members may lie about the origin of abuse for fear of being thrown out of the home. In other cases of elder abuse, sensory deprivation or dementia may hinder adequate explanation.

TABLE 35-1 Categories of Elder Abuse

Physical	• Assault • Neglect or abandonment • Dietary (malnutrition) • Poor maintenance of home • Poor personal hygiene • Sexual assault
Psychological	• Benign neglect • Verbal • Treating the person as an infant • Deprivation of sensory stimulation
Financial	• Theft of valuables • Embezzlement

Repeated abuse can lead to a high risk of death. As an EMT, you can help to reduce additional maltreatment of the patient by identifying the abuse (**TABLE 35-1**). This important measure may allow for referral to services of human, social, and public safety agencies and your state ombudsman.

Signs of Elder Abuse

Signs of abuse can be obvious or subtle. Injuries may be the result of acute or chronic abuse or neglect. Inflicted bruises are usually found on the buttocks and lower back, genitals and inner thighs, cheeks or earlobes, neck, upper lip, and inside the mouth. Pressure bruises caused by the human hand may be identified by oval grab marks, pinch marks, or handprints. Human bites are typically inflicted on the upper extremities and can cause lacerations and infection. You should inspect the patient's ears for indications of twisting, pulling, or pinching and evidence of frequent blows to the outer ears. You should also investigate multiple bruises in various states of healing by asking the patient and reviewing the patient's ADLs.

Burns are a common form of abuse. If you see burns, especially cigarette burns or physical marks that indicate that certain parts of the patient's body have been scalded systematically, you must suspect abuse. Typical abuse from burns is caused by contact with cigarettes, matches, heated metal, forced immersion in hot liquids, chemicals, and electrical power sources.

It may be difficult to see a failure to thrive in an older patient who has been abused. You should observe the patient's weight and try to determine whether the patient appears undernourished or has been unable to gain weight in the current environment. Does the patient have a ravenous appetite? Has medication been withheld? Is money being withheld, so the patient cannot buy food or medicine? You should also check for signs of neglect, such as evidence of a lack of hygiene, poor dental hygiene, poor temperature regulation, or lack of reasonable amenities in the home.

Words of Wisdom

As with other legally complex and emotionally charged issues, the possibility of elder abuse demands particularly careful documentation. Be thorough, objective, and factual, avoiding unsupported opinions and personal judgments. You may be called on to explain your report in a legal proceeding. Report your suspicions to the appropriate authorities and follow local protocols. Typically, the authorities will want to know specifics (eg, name, contact information) about the person you suspect is being abused and why you suspect abuse.

Sexual Assault and Rape

Unfortunately, **sexual assault** and **rape** are crimes that are all too common. The definition of rape, sexual assault, and similar terms differs by state. Although an estimated 82% of juvenile victims and 90% of adult victims are female, males are also victimized.[33] Approximately 1 in 4 women and 1 in 26 men in the United States experience attempted or completed rape in their lifetime.[34] Transgender individuals are also at higher risk of victimization. EMTs called to treat a victim of sexual assault, sexual abuse, or actual or alleged rape face many complex issues, ranging from obvious medical problems to serious psychological and legal issues. You may be the first person the victim has contact with after the encounter, and how you manage the situation from first contact throughout treatment and transport may have a lasting effect for the patient and you. Being professional, respectful, and empathetic is important.

When performing your assessment, be aware of findings suggesting the potential use of date rape or club drugs. The patient may or may not be aware of the use of drugs in the assault, but an inability to remember the event should create suspicion. While alcohol is the most frequently used date rape drug, drugs such as Rohypnol (flunitrazepam), known as roofies; GHB (gamma-hydroxybutyric acid), known as Liquid Ecstasy; Ketalar (ketamine), known as Special K; Klonopin (clonazepam); MDMA, known as Ecstasy; and Xanax (alprazolam) may be used to incapacitate a person to enable sexual assault and rape.

Drugs that are added into a person's drink may go undetected because they often do not have a color, smell, or taste. The effects may be immediate and can be enhanced with alcohol. The person may become weak and confused and may even have a loss of consciousness. These drugs cause muscle relaxation and loss of muscle compliance, which may make the victim more compliant during a sexual assault. If these drugs are still in the patient's system, during your assessment you may see hypotension, bradycardia, abdominal complaints, difficulty breathing, seizures, coma, and even death.

Because sexual assault and rape are crimes, you can generally expect law enforcement to be involved early in the situation. In many cases, EMS may be called by law enforcement. Police officers generally have basic medical training; many states require at least basic training at the first responder (emergency medical responder) level. Nevertheless, primary training for police officers focuses on crime investigation, not patient care.

A person who has been raped has just experienced a major trauma of the body and mind. The last thing this person wants to do is give a concise, detailed report of what has just occurred. If you attempt to gather patient information in this manner, it will most likely cause the victim to shut down. Having an EMT of the same gender as the patient providing assessment and care may be helpful in reducing anxiety.

The job of law enforcement is to solve the crime, arrest the perpetrator, and see justice served. Your job, as the EMT, is to handle the medical and psychological aspects of the case and to act as the patient advocate. In this capacity, it is important for you to focus on several key components.

The first component is the medical treatment of the patient. Is the victim physically injured? Are any life-threatening injuries present? On some occasions, patients will have sustained multiple-system trauma and will also need treatment of shock. Does the patient report any pain?

The second component is your psychological care of the patient. Do not cross-examine the patient or attempt to obtain information for the benefit of the police. These issues will be handled later by the hospital staff and police. Do not pass judgment on the patient, and protect the patient from the judgment of others on the scene. A crime may have been committed, and you need to remain aware of that fact. Many people report feeling violated when subjected to interrogation, criticism, or disbelief.

Last, remember that you are at a crime scene and the victim's body is part of that crime scene. Although your job is to treat the medical aspects of the incident and not to collect evidence, you still have a responsibility to preserve evidence. Do not cut through any clothing or throw away anything from the scene. Place bloodstained clothing and anything else that could be evidence in separate paper (not plastic) bags. Obtain evidence bags from the police if necessary. Paper bags allow wet items to dry naturally, whereas plastic allows mold to grow and may destroy biologic evidence.

It may be necessary to gently discourage patients from cleaning themselves. Victims tend to want to wash away not just the physical effects but also the humiliation and embarrassment of the assault. Valuable evidence can be destroyed in this process. Also discourage patients from urinating, changing clothes, moving their bowels, or rinsing out their mouth. If a patient insists on urinating, have the patient do so in a sterile urine container (if available). Also, have the patient deposit the toilet paper in a paper bag. Seal and label the bag for the police because these items can be critical evidence.

They will be photographed and examined by nurses trained in sexual assault examination and management (sometimes called sexual assault nurse examiners [SANE nurses])[35] or law enforcement personnel as well, and the evidence needs to be as accurate as possible. If you cannot discourage patients from taking these actions, respect their feelings. Some patients may refuse transport altogether, and they have the right to do so. In such cases, follow your system's refusal of treatment policy or procedure for sexual assault victims without judging or talking down to the patient. Your compassion is the best tool you have to gain the patient's confidence and encourage the person to get help.

If the patient refuses transport, offer to call the local rape crisis center for the person. Many communities have rape crisis centers with victim advocacy hotlines. Having a professional advocate at the scene may help the patient deal with the trauma, and the advocate can better explain in more compassionate detail the necessity of preserving evidence. Many victim advocates are rape-trauma survivors themselves. They can provide support to the patient in the hospital during any additional physical examinations.

Street Smarts

Keep a list of local resources that you can provide to individuals who have experienced a sexual assault. Remember men, women, children, transgender persons can be sexually assaulted. Although your patient may not feel comfortable speaking at the moment, knowing there are people who can help when they are ready can provide reassurance and courage at a later time.

Take the patient's history and limit any physical examination to a brief survey for life-threatening injuries. Treat all other injuries such as contusions or lacerations according to the appropriate procedures and protocols for your EMS system. Take standard precautions. Expose and examine the genitalia only if there is evidence of bleeding that needs to be treated. Cover and protect the patient from curious onlookers. Examine and interview the patient with a minimum of people present; move the patient to the ambulance if necessary.

The patient report is a legal document and may be subpoenaed, should the case result in an arrest and subsequent trial. Because you may have to appear in court, possibly several years later, document in detail the patient's history, assessment, treatment, and response to treatment. Keep the report concise and record any patient statements as exact quotes. Use quotation marks to indicate you are reporting the patient's version of events. Do not insert your own opinion as to whether the patient was sexually assaulted or raped or offer any conclusions that would prove or disprove the patient's account of the event. Focus on the facts. Record all of your observations during the physical examination: the patient's emotional state, the condition of clothing, obvious injuries, and so forth. Remember that rape is a legal term, not a medical diagnosis. A court must decide whether sexual intercourse was forcibly inflicted against the person's will. **TABLE 35-2**

TABLE 35-2 Treatment Principles for Sexual Assault

In addition to the usual treatment principles that apply to all victims, follow these special steps when treating patients who have been sexually assaulted:

1. Document the patient's history, assessment, treatment, and response to treatment in detail because you may have to appear in court many years later. Do not speculate. Record only the facts.
2. Complete the SAMPLE (Signs and symptoms, Allergies, Medications, Pertinent past medical history, Last oral intake, Events leading up to the illness or injury) history objectively.
3. Follow any crime scene policy established by your system to protect the scene and any potential evidence for police, particularly policies regarding evidence collection. If the patient is unclothed and will tolerate being wrapped in a sterile burn sheet, this may help investigators find any hair, fluid, or fiber from the alleged offender.
4. Do not examine the genitalia unless there is major bleeding. If an object has been inserted into the vagina or rectum, do not attempt to remove it.
5. Using an EMT who is the same gender as the patient may be helpful in reducing the patient's anxiety.
6. If possible, discourage the patient from bathing, voiding, or cleaning any wounds until after the hospital staff has completed an assessment. Handle the patient's clothes as little as possible, placing clothing and any other evidence in paper bags. If the patient insists on urinating, ask the patient to do so in a sterile urine container (if available). Also, deposit the toilet paper in a paper bag. Seal and label the bag for law enforcement. This can be critically important evidence.
7. If possible, transport the patient to a hospital with specialized staff such as SANE nurses who can fully evaluate these patients, perform medical and forensic examinations, and provide all aspects of medical and supportive care for these patients.

lists the treatment principles you should use when caring for a victim of sexual assault.

Often the most important intervention for sexual assault patients is comforting reassurance and transport to a facility that has employees who are certified to perform the proper physical examination in this type of case. Reminding patients that they are safe with you and that the hospital staff and the police will take good care of them may help provide reassurance. Sometimes just the presence of an EMT of the same gender as the patient can be emotionally helpful. Do not insist that the patient talk to you, but listen carefully and do not be judgmental if they do want to talk. Remember that victims of sexual assault may also need medical assistance; therefore, treat the medical injuries, but also remember to ensure the patient's privacy and provide emotional support.

Although most cases of sexual assault are on women by men, it is important to remember that it is possible for a man to be sexually assaulted or for the assailant to be either a woman or a man. The preceding principles of care still apply, and the likelihood of psychological trauma is just as strong.

Pediatric Sexual Abuse

Children of any age or gender can be victims of sexual abuse. Maintain an index of suspicion regardless of the patient's social or economic situation. This type of sexual abuse is often the result of long-standing abuse by relatives.

Your assessment of a child who has been sexually abused should be limited to determining the type of dressing any injuries require. Sometimes, a sexually abused child has also been beaten. Therefore, treat any bruises or fractures as well. Do not examine the genitalia of a young child unless there is evidence of bleeding or there is an injury that must be treated.

In addition, if you suspect that a child is a victim of sexual abuse, encourage the child not to wash, urinate, or defecate before a physician completes a physical examination. Although this step can be difficult for the victim, it is important to preserve evidence. If possible, ensure that an EMT or police officer of the same gender remains with the child, unless locating one will delay transport.

You must maintain professional composure the entire time you are assessing and caring for a sexually abused child. Maintain a concerned, caring approach, and shield the child from onlookers and curious bystanders. Obtain as much information as possible from the child and any witnesses. The child may be hysterical or unwilling to say anything at all, especially if the abuser is a relative or family friend. You are in the best position to obtain the most accurate firsthand information about the incident. Therefore, record any information carefully and completely on the patient care report. Transport all children who are victims of sexual assault. Sexual abuse of a child is a crime. Cooperate fully with law enforcement officials in their investigations.

Geriatric Sexual Abuse

Remember that geriatric patients, particularly those dependent on others for help with their ADLs, are at a heightened risk of abuse by caregivers. They may be unable to defend themselves or to report the crime, such as if they have an altered mental status. Moreover, they may fear the consequences of reporting the crime. In addition, many women do not report cases of sexual abuse because of shame and the pressure to remain silent and forget. As with any other patient, you must regard injuries to the genitals or rectum with no reported trauma as a sign of sexual abuse and report it to the appropriate authority.

Care for Patients in Special Settings

Nursing and Skilled Care Facilities

For many of the geriatric patients with whom you interact, the call will occur at a nursing home or other skilled care facility. Relatively healthy and active seniors often live in age-restricted active adult communities. A less expensive option is age-restricted apartments that provide seniors with the physical and emotional security that comes with living with other seniors. A similar type of facility, but one that also provides communal meals, social events, and other types of support, is an independent living facility. Assisted-living residential facilities support residents with ADLs and provide 24-hour assistance. Residents get assistance with daily medication administration, and some facilities address specialized patient issues such as Alzheimer disease and other types of dementia.

Nursing homes, also called skilled nursing facilities or long-term care facilities, are facilities that serve patients who need 24-hour care and are sometimes a step down from an acute care hospital. Patients require assistance with daily living and need therapeutic or rehabilitation services.

Calls to these types of facilities can sometimes be challenging. Patients often have a baseline altered level of consciousness and may not be able to tell you the nature of their illness or cause of their injury. The staff is usually spread thin and may not be familiar with what needs to be done to assist you when transport is necessary. The most important piece of information you need to establish immediately is, "What is wrong with the patient that is new or different today that made you call 9-1-1?" As soon as possible, establish the baseline status of the patient by talking to the staff who directly care for the patient on a daily basis.

With potentially limited information, you need to do an assessment to determine if the patient's problem is life threatening and/or requires ALS-level care. Optimally, the facility will provide you with a transfer record that provides critical information on the patient's history, medications, allergies, and current complaint. This information is critical because the ED staff need to know how to best treat the patient. Ideally, and when appropriate, transport the patient to the acute care facility where the patient has been treated before and where their records will be readily available.

Infection control needs to be a high priority when you visit these facilities. You not only need to protect yourself, but good handwashing and standard precautions can inhibit the spread of infectious pathogens to older people who already have compromised immune systems. You should also be cognizant of potential airborne pathogens. Something as simple as a cold or flu virus could result in a life-threatening pneumonia for a compromised older adult. An infection in an older patient can lead to life-threatening sepsis. Be sure to mask yourself if you have an upper respiratory infection, and mask the patient if they have one. Some risks to these patients and EMTs are described next.

Methicillin-resistant *Staphylococcus aureus* (MRSA) infections are common among people who live in close quarters such as nursing homes. The organism can be found in decubitus ulcers (bedsores), on feeding tubes, and on indwelling urinary catheters. The symptoms of MRSA depend on the type of infection. It can cause mild infections on the skin or invade the bloodstream, lungs, or urinary tract. MRSA is primarily spread by broken skin-to-skin contact but is also acquired by touching objects that have the bacteria on them. To protect yourself and reduce the spread of MRSA infections, you should wash your hands before and after every patient contact, properly dispose of or disinfect all medical equipment, and take appropriate standard precautions with every patient.

Similarly, many infections in hospitals are caused by **vancomycin-resistant enterococci (VRE)**. Enterococci are bacteria that are normally present in the human intestines and the female reproductive tract. Under the right circumstances, these bacteria can cause infection. Some of the enterococci have become resistant to vancomycin, the antibiotic commonly used to treat these infections.

The **respiratory syncytial virus (RSV)** causes an infection of the upper and lower respiratory tracts. Although more typically seen in children, the virus can also cause serious illness in older people, especially those with lung disease or weakened immune systems. The symptoms are similar to the common cold but can be more severe and last longer. The virus is highly contagious and is found in discharges from the nose and throat of an infected person. RSV is also transmitted by direct contact with droplets from coughs or sneezes and by touching a contaminated surface.

MRSA and RSV infections can be life threatening, especially in an immunocompromised patient. Look for isolation signs or ask about contagious disease when you approach a patient. Be sure to wear appropriate personal protective equipment and decontaminate your ambulance and diagnostic equipment after contact with nursing home residents whether a history of infectious disease is known or not. Be sure to document the infection control issue; advise the receiving facility;

and, depending on local protocol, report an infectious disease to your company or the local health department.

Clostridioides difficile (sometimes referred to as *C diff*) is a bacterium responsible for the most common cause of hospital-acquired infectious diarrhea, and it regularly causes sporadic cases of diarrhea in nursing homes. It is a bacterium that normally grows in the intestines. Antibiotic use may account for the rapid increase in toxic strains that ultimately cause illness. Health care workers may carry this bacterium following contact with contaminated feces. It can also be found on environmental surfaces such as furniture, floors, toilets, sinks, and bedding. The symptoms from the resultant colitis can range from minor diarrhea to a life-threatening inflammation of the colon. Typical alcohol-based hand sanitizers do not inactivate or kill *C difficile*. Contact precautions with gowns and gloves and handwashing with soap and water after each patient contact are essential to prevent transmission.

SARS-CoV-2 (severe acute respiratory syndrome coronavirus 2) is a strain of coronavirus that causes the disease COVID-19, a respiratory illness that may affect older, more vulnerable people, especially those living in communal settings such as long-term care facilities and those with preexisting medical conditions such as diabetes.

Home Care

Home care occurs within a patient's home environment. Patients requiring home services represent a spectrum of special health care populations, including infants and older adults, patients with chronic illnesses, and patients with developmental disabilities. These services are commonly needed among older patients with mobility problems.

Services offered by home care agencies include, but are not limited to, meal delivery, house cleaning, laundry, yard maintenance, physical therapy, and personal care, including bathing and wound care. Often, EMS is called to a residence when a home care provider has found the patient injured or has recognized a change in the patient's health status. Home care personnel are an important resource for you when you are obtaining the patient's baseline health status and the history of the present illness or condition. Home care personnel are usually familiar with the patient's surroundings and can obtain any health care documentation or medications that need to be transported with the patient to the hospital.

Hospice Care and Terminally Ill Patients

Unfortunately, not all illnesses can be cured. As health care clinicians, you and your team may be called on to assist a patient who has a terminal illness. The patient may be receiving hospice care at a hospice facility or at home.

Patients receiving hospice care are terminally ill, commonly with diseases such as cancer, heart or lung failure, end-stage dementia, or end-stage kidney or liver disease. The patient's physician will have determined that the illness is terminal, and in most cases has completed a do-not-attempt-resuscitation (DNAR) order or given physician orders for life-sustaining treatment (POLST) medical orders. This documentation outlines the scope of treatment and the interventions agreed on by the patient and/or the family. Hospice care provides comfort care, or palliative care (eg, treatment for pain, nausea, difficulty breathing), during a person's last days. Comfort care improves the patient's quality of life before death and allows the patient to be with family and friends. If you are called to a facility that provides hospice care or a home with a patient receiving hospice care, you will need to follow your local protocols, the patient's wishes, or legal documents such as a DNAR or POLST order. All necessary documentation must be brought to the hospital if the patient is to be transported to the hospital and must be noted in the patient care report.

If you are called to the home of a terminally ill patient, the care you give will have a lasting effect on the family. This is a time when respect, empathy, and sensitivity are most needed. Some homes with patients receiving hospice care may be chaotic. Family members may be having a difficult time coping with the situation, and they may be angry and hostile. Treat everyone with compassion and understanding. Members of your team may be able to separate family members to speak with them privately to defuse intense emotions and restore order.

Some terminally ill patients who are at home may be receiving outpatient care from a hospice or a home health nurse. You may be called to the home because of a delay in the arrival of the regular care provider or for transport so that a physician can address an immediate need, such as increasing pain. Because terminally ill patients may use a complex variety of pain medications, transdermal patches, or self-administered pain management devices, you may need to consult medical direction for guidance.

Even if a DNAR order is in place, family members may not understand what to do, and they may not be ready to face the death of a loved one. In such cases, obtain a thorough history and compassionately discuss the patient's wishes. Ask to review the DNAR order, and contact medical direction.

Ascertain the patient's and family's wishes about having the patient remain in the home or having the patient transported to the hospital. A family member who asks to accompany the patient should be allowed to do so. If the patient wishes to remain at home, this request should be honored, provided it is in accordance with your local or state protocol.

Local protocols for handling the death of a patient vary, so be familiar with your local or state regulations. The protocols identify whether the coroner needs to be called to report the death and, if so, who is responsible for contacting the coroner. Also determine whether a pronouncement of death is required and, if so, who is responsible for the determination.

Poverty and Homelessness

In 2023, 11.1% of the overall US population lived in poverty. In the United States, a significant racial disparity exists, with African American, Hispanic, and American Indian and Alaska Native populations at far greater risk of experiencing poverty.[36] People who live in poverty are often unable to provide for all of their own basic needs such as housing, food, child care, health insurance, and medication. An impoverished person or family may have housing but may go without food or medication in order to pay for that housing. Disease prevention strategies such as dental care, good nutrition, and exercise are often lacking, which increases the probability of disease.

Homelessness occurs when people are unable to acquire and/or maintain affordable housing. According to the National Alliance to End Homelessness, more than 500,000 people experience homelessness on any given night in the United States.[37] Individual persons make up more than 70% of the homeless population in the United States, with families making up the remaining population. In 2023, more than 140,000 people experienced chronic homelessness, defined as homelessness for an extended time or repeated homelessness. This population and the population of military veterans experiencing homelessness have both been steadily increasing in recent years. As with poverty risk, racial minorities are proportionally overrepresented among the homeless population in comparison to their numbers in the general population. Other subgroups at high risk for homelessness include members of the LGBTQIA+ community, survivors of domestic violence, people exiting the criminal legal system, and young adults who have aged out of the foster care system. The homeless population also includes people with mental illness, people

Street Smarts

Some patients experiencing homelessness may be uncomfortable with certain portions of the physical examination because of shame or embarrassment over their appearance or poor hygiene. It is important to communicate therapeutically with these individuals and use language and terms that normalize their condition. For example, using phrases such as "This is a safe place and I'll take care of you no matter how you are dressed" may reassure these patients that you will care for them regardless of how they appear. Some patients experiencing homelessness may have an odor because of an inability to access hygiene supplies or facilities. Some will have poor dentition and may mumble or not speak because of embarrassment about how their teeth look. It is important to consider these factors while caring for them. Allow these patients to guide what level of care and examination they are comfortable with when appropriate. Most importantly, reassure them that they are in a safe place and have no need to be apologetic or embarrassed about their condition or appearance.

with prior brain trauma, and people with addiction disorders.

The groups most likely to experience homelessness also tend to experience *unsheltered* homelessness at a disproportionate rate. Unsheltered homelessness refers to living in areas not intended for human habitation. These areas may not provide basic needs such as protection from the weather or clean water and may expose individuals to environmental risks such as traffic and acts of violence.[37]

Individuals experiencing homelessness are significantly more likely to use EMS and the ED than are individuals who have secure housing.

You are an advocate for all patients. Your job is to provide emergency medical care and transport patients to the appropriate facility. Remember that under the Emergency Medical Treatment and Active Labor Act, all hospital emergency departments *must* provide a medical assessment and required treatment, regardless of the patient's ability to pay. You can also be an advocate by becoming familiar with the social services resources within your community so you can refer patients to these lifelines. Depending on the community in which you work, there may be alternatives to the ED for transport consideration. Some hospitals have set up partnerships with area shelters to provide routine medical care and treatment for non–life-threatening conditions at the shelter in order to avoid tying up ED resources. Your knowledge of these community resources is crucial to facilitating efficient flow of the EMS network, as EMS is often the first to encounter patients experiencing homelessness on their way to the ED.

The Expanding Role of EMS in Addressing Special Populations

The evolution of mobile integrated health care and community paramedicine will benefit many patient populations, including patients with special challenges. As EMS systems around the United States continue to implement these positions, clinicians may be able to assess and treat more patients with low-acuity (nonemergency) conditions on scene without transport. In addition, they may be able to expand their roles in providing preventive care, chronic disease management, and postdischarge follow-up. Further, telemedicine options may continue to evolve, allowing EMS clinicians to provide care remotely, such as by giving advice to 9-1-1 callers over the phone.

YOU are the EMT

You call in your radio report to the ED. During your reassessment, you note that the patient is moving his head around and appears to be fighting your attempts to assist ventilations. You also note an acute change in his vital signs. His mother, who is riding in the back of the ambulance with you, asks you if you know what to do.

Recording Time: 25 Minutes	
Level of consciousness	Conscious; moving his head around; mother advises that he is agitated
Respirations	12 breaths/min; provided by bag-mask device
Pulse	130 beats/min; strong and regular
Skin	Baseline color, hot, and moist
Blood pressure	134/74 mm Hg
Oxygen saturation (Spo_2)	87% (on oxygen)

8. What has most likely happened to your patient? What should you do next?

YOU are the EMT SUMMARY

1. How will your assessment and treatment of this patient differ from that of a patient who is not dependent on a ventilator?

The principles of patient assessment and treatment are the same, regardless of the patient's special health care needs and any medical equipment that they require to function or live. As with any patient you encounter, your goal is to maintain the ABCs and safely transport the patient to an appropriate medical facility.

2. What role do the parents or caregivers of patients with special health care needs have in the prehospital setting?

When you care for a patient with special health care needs, it is imperative to listen to the people who take care of the patient. The parents or caregivers provide for the medical needs of the patient every day; therefore, they are aware of the patient's medical and/or surgical history, the patient's baseline mental status, and the names and doses of any medications the patient may be taking.

Parents or caregivers of this patient population are also trained and experienced in the use of any special equipment the patient requires. In many cases, the parent or caregiver will have performed certain interventions prior to calling 9-1-1. It is important to determine what interventions were performed, why they were performed, and what effect they had on the patient's condition.

3. What are some conditions that would cause a patient to become dependent on a mechanical ventilator?

A person who has any acute or chronic condition that impairs the respiratory muscles or injures the respiratory centers in the brain will require the use of a mechanical ventilator.

Your patient has quadriplegia secondary to a spinal injury. If the spinal cord is injured above the level of the fourth cervical vertebra (C4), paralysis of the respiratory muscles will also occur. Without a mechanical ventilator, your patient is unable to breathe at all.

Other conditions that often require mechanical ventilation include traumatic brain injury, muscular dystrophy, cystic fibrosis, and spina bifida. Regardless of why a patient requires mechanical ventilation, the most important thing for you to remember is that without it, the person is unable to breathe!

4. How does a tracheostomy tube affect a patient's ability to communicate? How can you determine whether your patient is alert?

Most patients with tracheostomy tubes are unable to speak. This is especially true if the patient requires mechanical ventilation, because they will be unable to breathe if the ventilator is detached from the tracheostomy tube. Patients with a tracheostomy tube who are not dependent on ventilators may be able to speak, although not as clearly, if they occlude the opening of the tube or use a special valve that fits over the end of the tracheostomy.

If patients cannot speak, they may communicate in other ways, such as by nodding the head or blinking the eyes. The parent or caregiver should be able to tell you whether the patient is communicating and responding as they normally do. A patient who responds to questions appropriately can be described as alert.

5. What are some potential complications that may result from your patient's condition? What can you do to prevent them or minimize the risks?

Patients with quadriplegia who are dependent on a ventilator are typically confined to a bed for prolonged periods. Prolonged immobilization can cause potentially serious complications, including pressure sores and pulmonary embolism.

Patients who are paralyzed are particularly susceptible to urinary tract infections and pneumonia. Urinary tract infections are typically related to indwelling urinary catheters (Foley catheters). Pneumonia often occurs because of decreased or absent cough reflexes and prolonged immobilization, which increases the risk of pulmonary secretions settling in the lungs and becoming infected.

In patients with indwelling urinary catheters, always maintain the catheter collection bag below the level of the bladder; this position will prevent urine from flowing back into the bladder and therefore minimizes the risk of infection.

Thick mucus plugs can develop in the tubes of patients with tracheostomy tubes, such as your patient, which can impair oxygenation and ventilation. Ask the parent or caregiver when the tube was last suctioned and observe for signs that indicate it may need to be suctioned (eg, restlessness, signs of hypoxemia). Many mechanical ventilators will sound an alarm if there is any obstruction in the ventilator circuit, such as a mucus plug in the tracheostomy tube.

YOU are the EMT SUMMARY continued

After you have transferred the patient to the ambulance stretcher, ensure that there are no wrinkles or lumps in the sheet or blanket under the patient. This simple step can help prevent pressure sores.

6. What do you suspect is the patient's underlying problem? What specific treatment should you provide to him?

The presence of fever suggests infection. In this patient, the infection could have several causes. Furthermore, it may be the result of more than one underlying problem.

Fever is often the only presenting sign of pneumonia in paralyzed patients. This is especially true in patients with quadriplegia because their respiratory muscles are also paralyzed; therefore, outward signs of respiratory distress, such as retractions, are not present. Another possibility is a urinary tract infection.

Infection requires antibiotic therapy, which can be administered only in a hospital setting. Treatment of a patient with a possible infection is mainly supportive: monitor the patient's ABCs, take standard precautions (eg, gloves, mask if necessary), and transport the patient to the hospital.

7. What is the benefit of allowing the patient's mother to accompany her son to the hospital?

The patient's mother should be allowed to accompany her son in the ambulance if she prefers. She can continue to be a source of information en route to the hospital, and could alert you to any changes in the patient's status, which may be obvious only to her.

The patient's mother can also bring supplies that the patient needs that you may or may not carry on your ambulance.

You must also consider the emotional needs of the patient. Unnecessarily separating a patient with special health care needs from their primary caregiver can be a source of emotional distress for the patient and the caregiver.

If the mother prefers to follow the ambulance in her own vehicle, assure her that you will take good care of her son.

8. What has most likely happened to your patient? What should you do next?

Your patient's clinical condition has changed. He appears to be fighting the ventilator, which is a sign of agitation. Furthermore, his heart rate has increased and his oxygen saturation level has decreased. You should suspect that he is not receiving adequate ventilation.

Tracheostomy tube obstruction is an emergency that requires immediate intervention; suction the tube and reassess the patient for signs of adequate oxygenation and ventilation.

The DOPE mnemonic can be used to troubleshoot acute deterioration in a patient with a tracheostomy tube. It is critical for you to recognize which problems you can correct and which problems require ALS. For example, if the tracheostomy tube has become dislodged, it must be replaced. If the patient has a pneumothorax, the patient may require a needle chest decompression, which EMTs are not trained to perform, although nothing in the history suggests that this is the case.

Prep Kit

Ready for Review

- Medicine and medical technology continue to improve, and the number of children and adults with chronic diseases or injuries who are living at home or in environments outside of the hospital setting continues to grow.
- You may find children and adults who are living at home who are dependent on mechanical ventilators, intravenous pumps, or other medical devices to maintain their lives.
- The basic principles of assessing and caring for patients with special challenges are the same as for all other patients.
- Developmental disabilities, including intellectual disabilities, may be caused

Prep Kit continued

by genetic factors, congenital factors, complications at birth, malnutrition, or environmental factors. Individuals with these disabilities may be unable to learn and socially adapt at a normal developmental rate.

- People with Down syndrome often have large tongues and small oral and nasal cavities, so intubation of these patients may be difficult.
- Visual impairments may be difficult to recognize. During your scene size-up, look for signs that indicate the patient is visually impaired, such as the presence of eyeglasses, a cane, or a service animal. Immediately introduce yourself when you enter the room, and have your team members introduce themselves so that the patient can identify their locations and voices.
- Hearing impairment may range from a slight hearing loss to total deafness. Clues that a person could be hard of hearing include the presence of hearing aids, poor pronunciation of words, or failure to respond to your presence or questions.
- Cerebral palsy is associated with other conditions such as visual and hearing impairments, difficulty communicating, epilepsy, and intellectual disability. Patients may also have an unsteady gait (ataxia) and may require the assistance of a wheelchair or walker.
- Spina bifida is associated with hydrocephalus, which requires the placement of a shunt to drain excessive amounts of cerebrospinal fluid from the brain. Other conditions associated with spina bifida include partial or full paralysis of the lower extremities, loss of bowel and bladder control, and an allergy to latex products.
- Patients with obesity may be embarrassed by their condition or fearful of scorn as a result of past experiences. If transport is necessary, plan early for extra help and do not be afraid to call for more clinicians or special equipment if necessary. In particular, send a member of your team to find the easiest and safest exit.
- Patients who depend on home ventilators or those who have chronic pulmonary medical conditions may breathe through a tracheostomy tube.
- When caring for patients who are on home oxygen, you must be able to assess their oxygen needs with consideration of their baseline status.
- Patients who are on a mechanical ventilator at home may not be able to breathe without assistance. If the ventilator malfunctions, remove the patient from the mechanical ventilator and assist ventilations with a bag-mask device.
- An apnea monitor is typically used when an infant is born prematurely, requires home oxygen, or has a serious breathing problem. The apnea monitor is designed to sound an alarm if the infant experiences bradycardia or if apnea occurs.
- An internal cardiac pacemaker is a device implanted under the patient's skin to regulate the heart rate. An automatic implanted cardioverter defibrillator (AICD) is also implanted under the skin and often has a pacemaker as well.
- A ventricular assist device (VAD) is a special piece of medical equipment that takes over the function of one or both heart ventricles. These devices are used as a bridge to transplantation while a donor heart is being located or as a permanent solution for patients who do not qualify for a transplant.

Prep Kit continued

- External defibrillation vests are worn under a patient's clothing. They monitor the patient's cardiac rhythm and provide an audible warning before administering a shock to correct the dysrhythmia.
- Gastrostomy tubes are placed into the stomach for feeding in patients who cannot ingest fluids, food, or medication by mouth. These tubes may be inserted through the nose or mouth or placed through the abdominal wall surgically.
- Shunts are tubes that extend from the ventricles in the brain to the abdomen to drain excess cerebrospinal fluid that may accumulate near the brain.
- A colostomy or ileostomy is a surgical procedure that creates an opening from the small or large intestine to the surface of the body to allow for elimination of waste products. Feces are expelled and collected into a clear external bag or pouch, which is emptied or changed frequently. Similarly, a urostomy drains urine.
- Emergencies involving infants include sudden unexpected infant death (SUID), unexplained sudden death in infancy (USDI), brief resolved unexplained event (BRUE).
- Carefully inspect the environment where a USDI victim was found, looking for signs of illness, abusive family interactions, and objects in the child's crib.
- Be aware of signs of abuse or neglect when caring for vulnerable populations such as children and older adults who depend on others for ADLs. Carefully document these signs, and report them according to your local protocols.
- Human trafficking occurs when a person is exploited through force, fraud, or coercion. It involves people of any gender, age, or nationality. When human trafficking is suspected, the paramedic should notify law enforcement.
- EMTs called to treat a victim of sexual assault, sexual abuse, or actual or alleged rape face many challenges, ranging from obvious medical problems to serious psychological and legal issues. You may be the victim's first contact after the encounter, and how the situation is managed from first contact throughout treatment and transport may have lasting effects for the patient and you. It is very important to always be professional, sensitive, and empathetic.
- You and your team may be called on to assist a patient who is terminally ill. Terminally ill patients may be in a hospice facility or at home.
- Under the Emergency Medical Treatment and Active Labor Act, all health care facilities *must* provide a medical assessment and required treatment, regardless of the patient's ability to pay.

Vital Vocabulary

autism spectrum disorder (ASD) A group of complex disorders of brain development, characterized by difficulties in social interaction, repetitive behaviors, and verbal and nonverbal communication.

brief resolved unexplained event (BRUE) An event that occurs in an infant lasting less than 1 minute and including two of the following: absent or abnormal respirations, pale or cyanotic

Prep Kit continued

skin, decreased level of consciousness, and altered muscle tone.

cerebral palsy A group of disorders characterized by poorly controlled body movement.

child maltreatment A general term applying to all forms of physical and emotional abuse, sexual abuse, neglect, and exploitation of children.

colostomy A surgical procedure to create an opening (stoma) between the colon and the surface of the body.

conductive hearing loss Hearing loss caused by a faulty transmission of sound waves.

developmental disability A group of conditions that may impair development in the areas of physical ability, learning, language development, or behavioral coping skills.

Down syndrome A genetic chromosomal defect that can occur during fetal development and that results in intellectual impairment as well as certain physical characteristics, such as a round head with a flat occiput and slanted, wide-set eyes.

elder abuse Any action on the part of an older person's family member, caregiver, or other associated person that takes advantage of the older person's person, property, or emotional state.

human trafficking The illegal exploitation of a person.

ileostomy A surgical procedure to create an opening (stoma) between the small intestine and the surface of the body.

intellectual disability A subset of developmental disability characterized by significant limitations in both intellectual functioning and skills needed for daily living.

methicillin-resistant *Staphylococcus aureus* (MRSA) A bacterium that causes infections in different parts of the body and is often resistant to commonly used antibiotics; can be found on the skin and in surgical wounds, the bloodstream, lungs, and urinary tract.

neglect Refusal or failure on the part of the parent or caregiver to provide life necessities.

obesity A complex condition in which a person has an excessive amount of body fat.

orthotic device An externally applied device that modifies the structural and functional characteristics of the neuromuscular and skeletal systems often used to support or brace the limbs or spine.

prosthetic device An externally applied device used to partly or wholly replace an absent or deficient limb segment.

rape A term often used in a legal context to refer to the crime of sexual penetration without consent; rape is a form of sexual assault, but not all sexual assaults are rape.

respiratory syncytial virus (RSV) A virus that causes an infection of the lungs and breathing passages; can lead to other serious illnesses that affect the lungs or heart, such as bronchiolitis and pneumonia; it is highly contagious and spread through droplets.

sensorineural deafness A permanent lack of hearing caused by a lesion or damage of the inner ear.

sexual assault The act of subjecting a person to sexual contact or behavior without the person's explicit consent.

shaken baby syndrome A syndrome seen in abused infants and children; the patient has been subjected to violent, whiplash-type shaking injuries inflicted by the abusing individual that may cause coma, seizures, and increased intracranial pressure due to tearing of the cerebral veins with consequent bleeding into the brain.

Prep Kit continued

shunts Tubes that drain excess cerebrospinal fluid from the brain to another part of the body outside of the brain, such as the abdomen, thus lowering pressure in the brain.

spina bifida A developmental defect in which a portion of the spinal cord or meninges may protrude outside of the vertebrae and possibly even outside of the body, usually at the lower third of the spine in the lumbar area.

stoma An opening through the skin and into an organ or other structure.

sudden unexpected infant death (SUID) A sudden unexpected death of a child younger than 1 year where the cause is either known or not known after investigation.

unexplained sudden death in infancy (USDI) Death of an infant or young child that remains unexplained after a complete autopsy; also called sudden infant death syndrome (SIDS).

urostomy A surgical procedure to create an opening (stoma) that connects the urinary system to the surface of the skin and allows urine to drain through the abdominal wall.

vancomycin-resistant enterococci (VRE) A bacterium that is normally present in the human intestines and the female reproductive tract, but which can cause infection and which is resistant to the antibiotic vancomycin.

References

1. FAQs on intellectual disability. American Association of Intellectual and Developmental Disabilities website. https://www.aaidd.org/intellectual-disability/faqs-on-intellectual-disability. Accessed April 18, 2025.
2. American Psychiatric Association. Autism spectrum disorder. In *Diagnostic and Statistical Manual of Mental Disorders*. 5th ed. Arlington, VA: American Psychiatric Association; 2013:50.
3. Autism prevalence rises to 1 in 31 in the US. Autism Speaks website. https://www.autismspeaks.org/what-autism. Published April 15, 2025. Accessed April 18, 2025.
4. Loomes R, Hull L, Mandy WPL. What is the male-to-female ratio in autism spectrum disorder? A systematic review and meta-analysis. *J Am Acad Child Adolesc Psychiatry*. 2017;56(6):466–474.
5. What conditions or disorders are commonly associated with Down syndrome? National Institutes of Health website. https://www.nichd.nih.gov/health/topics/down/conditioninfo/associated. Reviewed November 30, 2023. Accessed April 18, 2025.
6. Shimony N. Atlantoaxial instability in Down syndrome. Medscape website. https://emedicine.medscape.com/article/1180354-overview?form=fpf. Updated January 3, 2022. Accessed April 18, 2025.
7. Service animals. Americans With Disabilities Act website. https://www.ada.gov/topics/service-animals/. Accessed April 18, 2025.
8. Cerebral palsy. National Institutes of Health website. https://www.ninds.nih.gov/health-information/disorders/cerebral-palsy. Accessed April 18, 2025.
9. Sgouros S. Spina bifida hydrocephalus and shunts. Medscape website. http://emedicine.medscape.com/article/937979-overview. Updated May 16, 2023. Accessed April 18, 2025.
10. *WHO Standards for Prosthetics and Orthotics*. Geneva: World Health Organization; 2017.
11. Data, trends, and maps definitions and sources: obesity and weight status. Centers for Disease Control and Prevention website. https://www.cdc.gov/dnpao-data-trends-maps/database/definitions.html. Published October 21, 2024. Accessed April 18, 2025.
12. Adult obesity facts. Centers for Disease Control and Prevention website. https://www.cdc.gov/obesity/adult-obesity-facts/index.html. Published May 14, 2024. Accessed April 18, 2025.

Prep Kit continued

13. Childhood obesity facts. Centers for Disease Control and Prevention website. https://www.cdc.gov/obesity/childhood-obesity-facts/childhood-obesity-facts.html. Published April 2, 2024. Accessed April 18, 2025.
14. Kondamudi NP, Krata L, Wilt AS. Infant apnea. *StatPearls*. National Library of Medicine website. https://www.ncbi.nlm.nih.gov/books/NBK441969/. Updated August 12, 2023. Accessed April 18, 2025.
15. Jiang H. Prediction of cardiorespiratory events in preterm infants [thesis]. University of Tasmania website. https://figshare.utas.edu.au/articles/thesis/Prediction_of_cardiorespiratory_events_in_preterm_infants/25662768/1?file=45797802. Published 2023. Accessed April 18, 2025.
16. Sahu P, Acharya S, Totade M. Evolution of pacemakers and implantable cardioverter defibrillators (ICDs) in cardiology. *Cureus*. 2023;15(10):e46389. doi:10.7759/cureus.46389
17. McKillip RP, Gopalsami A, Montoya M, et al. Analysis of patients with ventricular assist devices presenting to an urban emergency department. *West J Emerg Med*. 2018;19(6):907–911.
18. EMS field guides. MyLVAD website. https://www.mylvad.com/medical-professionals/resource-library/ems-field-guides. Accessed April 18, 2025.
19. Epilepsy facts and stats. Centers for Disease Control and Prevention website. https://www.cdc.gov/epilepsy/data-research/facts-stats/index.html. Published May 15, 2024. Accessed April 18, 2025.
20. Moon RY, Carlin RF, Hand I; Task Force on Sudden Infant Death Syndrome and the Committee on Fetus and Newborn. Sleep-related infant deaths: updated 2022 recommendations for reducing infant deaths in the sleep environment. *Pediatrics*. 2022;150(1):e2022057990. doi:10.1542/peds.2022-057990
21. Vincent A, Chu NT, Shah A, et al. Sudden infant death syndrome: risk factors and newer risk reduction strategies. *Cureus*. 2023;15(6):e40572. doi:10.7759/cureus.40572
22. Data and statistics for SUID and SIDS. Centers for Disease Control and Prevention website. https://www.cdc.gov/sudden-infant-death/data-research/data/index.html#:~:text=These%20deaths%20occur%20among%20infants,1%2C529%20deaths%20from%20SIDS. Published September 17, 2024. Accessed April 18, 2025.
23. National Association of State EMS Officials. *National Model EMS Clinical Guidelines: Version 3.0*. https://nasemso.org/content.aspx?page_id=22&club_id=157064&module_id=701974. Updated March 2022. Accessed March 31, 2025.
24. US Department of Health and Human Services. *Child Maltreatment 2022*. Administration for Children and Families website. https://www.acf.hhs.gov/sites/default/files/documents/cb/cm2022.pdf. Published 2024. Accessed April 18, 2025.
25. Pierce MC, Kaczor K, Lorenz DJ, et al. Validation of a clinical decision rule to predict abuse in young children based on bruising characteristics. *JAMA Network Open*. 2021;4(4):e215832–e215832. doi:10.1001/jamanetworkopen.2021.5832
26. 2022 trafficking in persons report: United States. US Department of State website. https://www.state.gov/reports/2022-trafficking-in-persons-report/united-states/. Accessed April 18, 2025.
27. Feehs K, Wheeler AC. *2020 Federal Human Trafficking Report*. Human Trafficking Institute website. https://traffickinginstitute.org/wp-content/uploads/2022/01/2020-Federal-Human-Trafficking-Report-Low-Res.pdf. Published 2021. Accessed April 18, 2025.
28. World Day Against Trafficking in Persons statements. World Day Against Trafficking in Persons website. https://www.unodc.org/endht/en/statements.html. Published July 30, 2020. Accessed April 18, 2025.
29. National Survey Study. Polaris website. https://polarisproject.org/national-survivor-study/. Accessed April 18, 2025.
30. Indicators of human trafficking. US Department of Homeland Security website. https://www.dhs.gov/blue-campaign/indicators-human-trafficking. Updated May 30, 2024. Accessed April 18, 2025.
31. Miller R, Tharayil A, Miller B, Morshedi B. Human trafficking. In: Cone DC, Brice JH, Delbridge TR, Myers JB, eds. *Emergency Medical Services: Clinical Practice and Systems Oversight*. 3rd ed. Vol 1. Wiley-Blackwell; 2021:502–518.
32. About abuse of older persons. Centers for Disease Control and Prevention website. https://www.cdc.gov/elder-abuse/about/index.html. Published November 7, 2024. Accessed April 18, 2025.
33. Victims of sexual violence: statistics. RAINN website. https://www.rainn.org/statistics/victims-sexual-violence. Accessed April 18, 2025.
34. About sexual violence. Centers for Disease Control and Prevention website. https://www.cdc.gov/sexual-violence/about/index.html. Published January 23, 2024. Accessed April 18, 2025.
35. What is a SANE/SART? RAINN website. https://www.rainn.org/articles/what-sanesart. Accessed April 18, 2025.

Prep Kit continued

36. Shrider EA. Poverty in the United States: 2023. US Census Bureau website. https://www2.census.gov/library/publications/2024/demo/p60-283.pdf. Issued September 2024. Accessed April 18, 2025.
37. State of homelessness: 2024 edition. National Alliance to End Homelessness website. https://endhomelessness.org/homelessness-in-america/homelessness-statistics/state-of-homelessness/. Accessed April 18, 2025.

Additional Resources

American Academy of Pediatrics. *Pediatric Education for Prehospital Professionals (PEPP)*. 4th ed. Burlington, MA: Jones and Bartlett Learning, 2020.

Carter Kits Sensory Bags. Carter Kits website. https://carterkits.org. Accessed May 20, 2025.

National Association of State EMS Officials. *National EMS Scope of Practice Model 2019*. Washington, DC: National Highway Traffic Safety Administration; February 2019. Report No. DOT HS 812-666. https://www.ems.gov/assets/National_EMS_Scope_of_Practice_Model_2019.pdf. Accessed April 18, 2025.

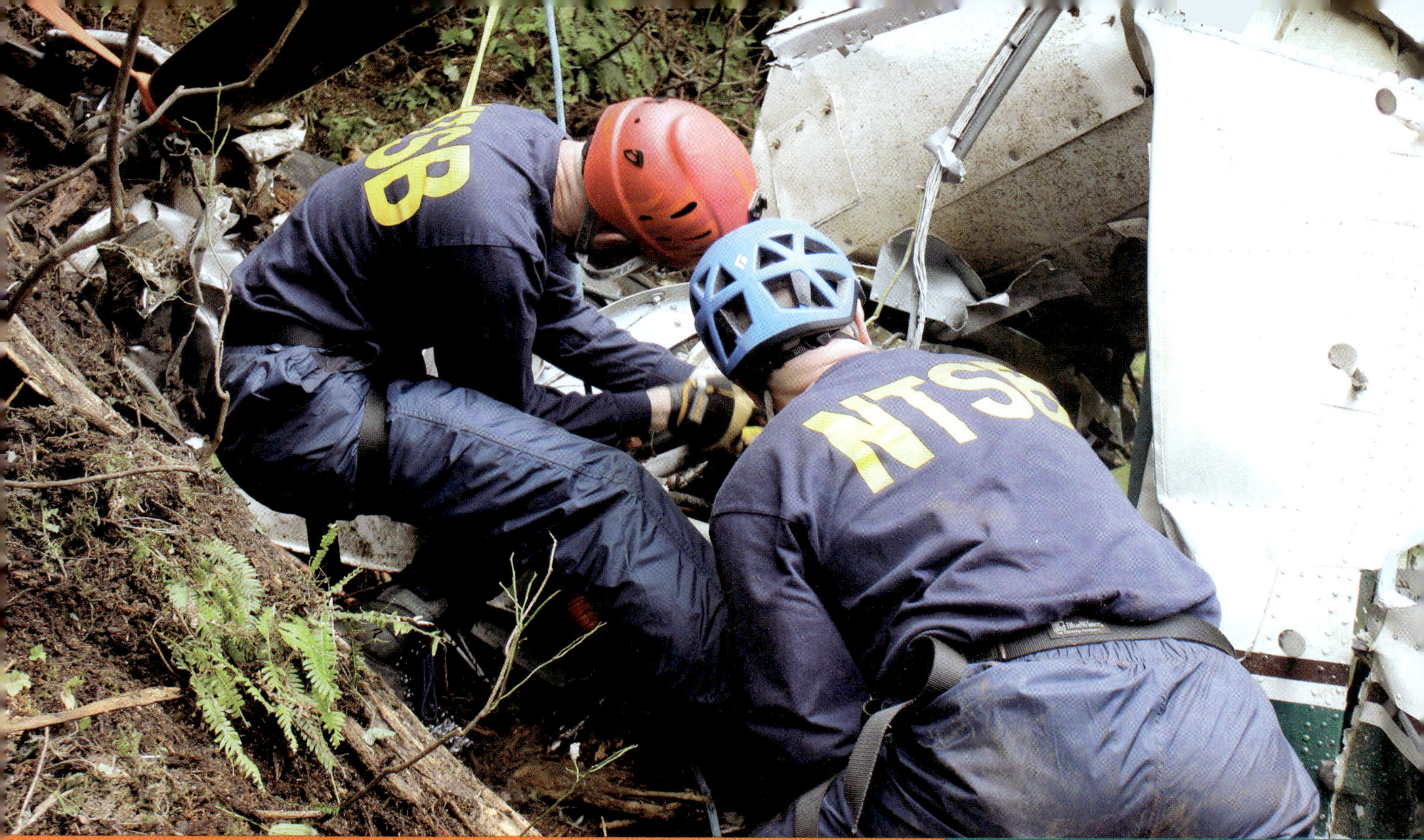

SECTION

9

EMS Operations

36 Transport Operations

37 Vehicle Extrication and Special Rescue

38 Incident Management

39 Terrorism Response and Disaster Management

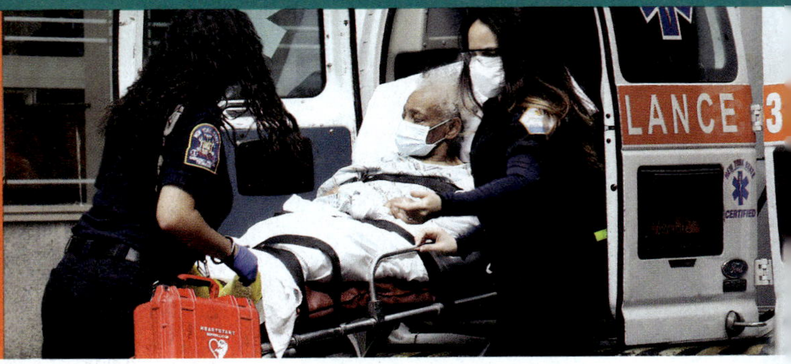

Chapter 36

Transport Operations

NATIONAL EMS EDUCATION STANDARD COMPETENCIES

EMS Operations

Knowledge of operational roles and responsibilities to ensure patient, public, and personnel safety.

Emergency Response Vehicles

- Risks and responsibilities of emergency response and radio communications (pp 1341–1351)
- Risks and responsibilities of operating emergency vehicles (pp 1360–1368)
- Pediatric transport considerations (pp 1361–1362)
- Risks and responsibilities of transport (pp 1357–1358)

Air Medical

- Safe air medical operations (pp 1370–1376)
- Criteria for utilizing air medical response (pp 1371–1372)
- Medical risks/needs/advantages (pp 1370–1376)

Medicine

Applies knowledge to provide basic emergency care and transportation based on assessment findings for an acutely ill patient.

Infectious Diseases

- Assessment and management of a patient who may have an infectious disease (Chapter 2, *Workforce Safety and Wellness*)
- How to decontaminate the ambulance and equipment after treating a patient (p 1359)
- Sepsis and septic shock (Chapter 13, *Shock*)

KNOWLEDGE OBJECTIVES

1. List the nine phases of an ambulance call; include examples of key tasks emergency medical technicians (EMTs) perform during each phase. (pp 1344–1359)
2. Name the medical equipment and supplies carried on an ambulance. (p 1346)
3. Describe the safety and operations equipment carried on an ambulance. (pp 1345–1349)
4. Name the specific parts of an ambulance that should be inspected daily. (p 1351)
5. List the minimum dispatch information required by emergency medical services (EMS) to respond to an emergency call. (p 1352)
6. Describe some high-risk situations and hazards during both pretransport and transport that may affect the safety of the ambulance and its passengers. (pp 1353–1358, 1360–1370)
7. Discuss the specific considerations required to ensure scene safety, including personal safety, patient safety, and traffic control. (pp 1354–1357)
8. Describe the key elements that must be included in the written patient care report upon patient delivery to the hospital. (p 1358)
9. Summarize the tasks EMTs must complete in the postrun phase. (p 1359)
10. Describe the concepts relating to decontamination, including cleaning, disinfection, high-level disinfection, and sterilization. (p 1359)

11. Discuss the guidelines for safely operating an ambulance. (pp 1360–1370)
12. Explain the factors that dictate the use of lights and siren to the scene and to the hospital (pp 1364–1366)
13. Describe the specific, limited privileges that are provided to emergency vehicle operators by most state laws and regulations. (p 1368)
14. Explain the additional risks and special considerations posed by the use of police escorts. (p 1369)
15. Describe the hazards and special considerations posed by specific driving situations, such as crossing intersections or driving on the highway. (pp 1369–1370)
16. Describe the capabilities, protocols, and methods for accessing air medical services. (pp 1370–1376)
17. Describe key scene safety considerations when preparing for helicopter emergency medical services, including establishing a landing zone, securing loose objects, reducing onsite hazards, and approaching the aircraft. (pp 1370–1376)

SKILLS OBJECTIVES

1. Demonstrate how to perform a daily inspection of an ambulance. (p 1351)
2. Demonstrate how to clean and disinfect the ambulance and equipment during the postrun phase. (pp 1344–1359)

Introduction

During the late 1700s, Napoleon Bonaparte commissioned the development of horse-drawn carts and a corps of soldiers trained to remove injured personnel from the battlefield and initiate treatment, establishing what was one of the more advanced professional emergency medical patient care systems in the world. Horse-drawn ambulances were also being used in major cities throughout the United States (**FIGURE 36-1**). American hospitals initiated their own professional ambulance services during the late 1860s. Ambulance attendants traveled with limited medical supplies, including brandy, a few tourniquets, several assorted bandages and sponges, basic splinting material, and blankets.

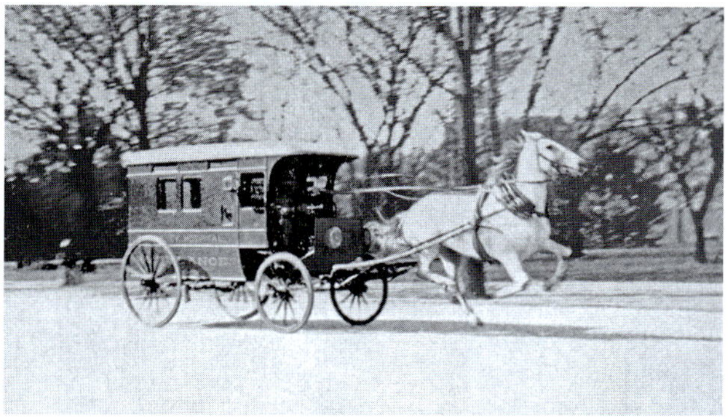

FIGURE 36-1 Horse-drawn ambulances were used in major cities throughout the United States during the 1800s.

Many of today's ambulances are equipped with state-of-the-art technology, including defibrillators and monitors that can transmit information directly to the emergency department (ED), video-assisted equipment for use with airway management or telemedicine, blood and oxygen testing equipment, ultrasonography equipment, mechanical ventilators, automated chest compression machines, global positioning systems (GPS), and computer-aided dispatch consoles. Even when following all safety guidelines, the emphasis on decreasing response times for time-critical conditions places the EMT in great danger while responding to calls. Although technology can greatly aid in directing the route and providing important information from the scene, it is also distracting and, therefore, potentially places the crew at higher risk for crashes. The driver who is operating the ambulance should focus solely on the road and maintaining safe driving habits, especially during lights and siren responses. In addition to assisting the driver, the EMT in the passenger's seat should be the person responsible for operating communication and navigation devices while en route to the scene. Anything that takes the driver's attention away from the road for even a second greatly increases the risk of a crash.

This chapter discusses ambulance design and the process of equipping and maintaining an ambulance. It focuses on the techniques and judgment that you will need to drive an ambulance or other emergency vehicle. Topics covered include parking considerations, emergency vehicle control and operation, the effects of weather on driving, and common hazards that are encountered while driving an ambulance. Finally, the chapter describes how to work safely with air medical services.

Safety Tips

The dangers of texting and driving are well known. However, we often downplay the cognitive workload placed on emergency responders who are operating a vehicle. We ask responders to safely operate the vehicle in an emergency situation, but we place multiple distractors within arm's reach that could draw their focus away from their primary role. From reading call notes from a computer-aided dispatch to requesting information regarding scene safety over the radio, these necessary distractions can all prove dangerous, if not fatal.

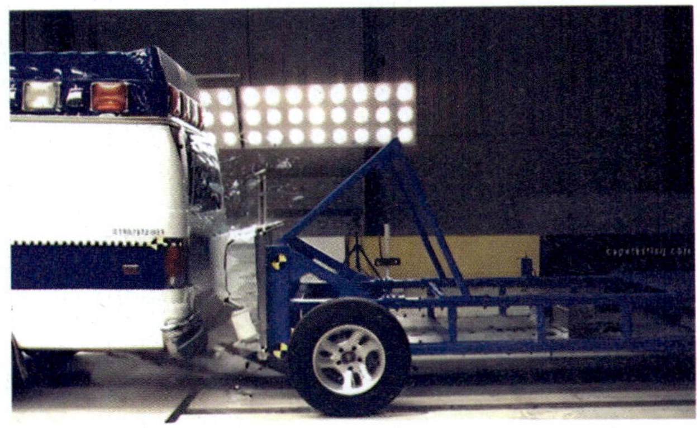

FIGURE 36-2 Ambulances are crash tested by manufacturers while being designed.

Courtesy of CDC.

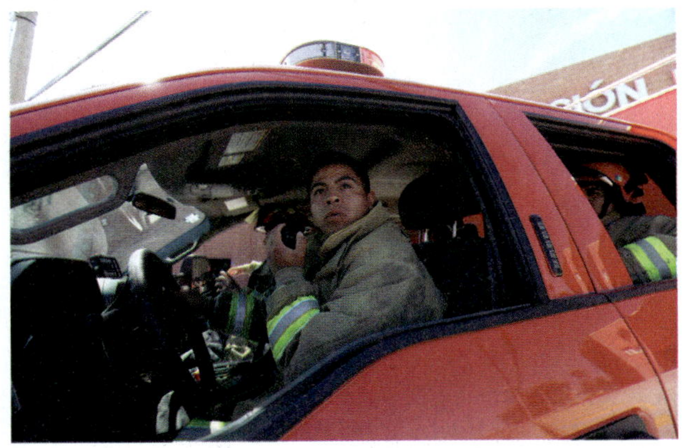

A

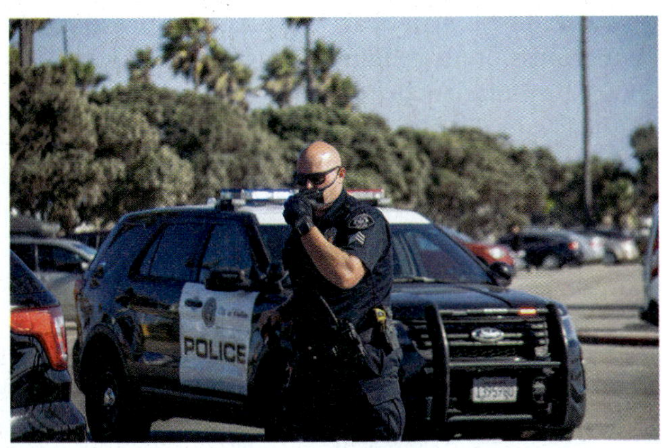

B

FIGURE 36-3 First responders, such as firefighters (**A**) and law enforcement personnel (**B**), are often the first to arrive at a scene.

(A) © JORGE ALVARADO/AP Photo; **(B)** © Glenn Highcove/Shutterstock.

Emergency Vehicle Design

An **ambulance** is a vehicle that is used for treating and transporting patients who need emergency medical care. The first use of motor-powered ambulances occurred in the late 1800s. For many decades after that, a hearse was the vehicle typically used as an ambulance. While a hearse had enough room for someone to lie down, it left little room for supplies or medical attendants.

Currently, ambulance designs are based on NFPA 1900, *Standard for Aircraft Rescue and Firefighting Vehicles, Automotive Fire Apparatus, Wildland Fire Apparatus, and Automotive Ambulances.* This standard was developed with consideration of Federal KKK-A-1822 standards and suggestions from the ambulance industry and emergency medical services (EMS) personnel (**FIGURE 36-2**).[1] One of the most significant developments in ambulance design has been the emphasis on creating the safest environment possible in the driver's compartment and the patient compartment. Another development is the use of **first-responder vehicles** (**FIGURE 36-3**), which respond initially to the scene with personnel and equipment to treat the sick and injured.

The modern ambulance is a vehicle for emergency medical care that has the following features:

- A driver's compartment
- A patient compartment that can accommodate two EMTs and at least one patient in a supine position (Additional patients may be seated on a bench seat or swivel seat with appropriate safety restraints.)

- Equipment and supplies to provide emergency medical care at the scene and during transport, to safeguard personnel and patients from hazardous conditions, and to carry out light extrication procedures
- Two-way radio communication so ambulance personnel can speak with the dispatcher, the hospital, public safety authorities, and online medical direction
- Design and construction that ensure maximum safety, efficiency, and comfort

Each state establishes its own standards for licensing or certifying ambulances. Many agencies now use the federal specifications (NFPA 1900) that cover the three types of basic ambulance designs (**FIGURE 36-4** and **TABLE 36-1**).

The six-pointed **Star of Life** emblem (**FIGURE 36-5**) identifies vehicles as ambulances. It is often affixed to the sides, rear, and roof of the ambulance. Local or state regulatory authorities determine what emblems may be displayed on the side of a prehospital care ambulance. Warning lights and public address

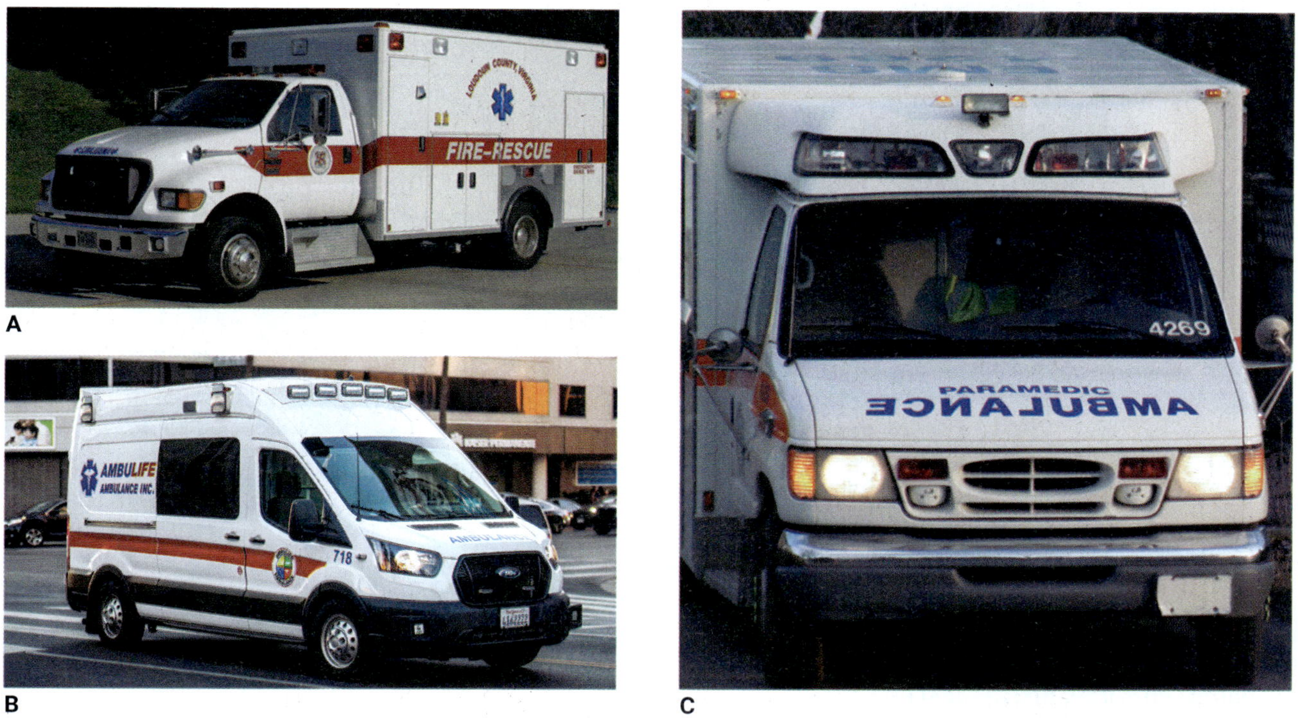

FIGURE 36-4 **A.** The conventional, truck cab-chassis has a modular ambulance body that can be transferred to a newer chassis (type I). **B.** The standard van ambulance has a forward-control integral cab body (type II). **C.** The specialty van ambulance has a cab that is mounted on a cut-away van chassis (type III).

YOU are the EMT

You are completing your morning vehicle checkoff. This is your first shift at your new station following successful completion of your new hire orientation, which included your mandatory emergency vehicle operator course. At 0800 hours, you are dispatched to 5220 Pacific Concourse Drive for an "assault." It is a cold, rainy morning, and there is heavy traffic in front of your station. You pull the ambulance out of the bay. Your partner informs you that the scene of the call is only a few miles away from your station.

1. What attributes should an emergency vehicle operator possess?
2. What factors should you consider before responding to the scene?

TABLE 36-1 Basic Ambulance Designs

Type I	Conventional, truck cab-chassis with a modular ambulance body that can be transferred to a newer chassis as needed
Type II	Standard van, forward-control integral cab-body ambulance
Type III	Specialty van cab with a modular ambulance body that is mounted on a cut-away van chassis

TABLE 36-2 Phases of an Ambulance Call

1. Preparation for the call
2. Dispatch
3. En route
4. Arrival at scene
5. Transfer of the patient to the ambulance
6. En route to the receiving facility (transport)
7. At the receiving facility (delivery)
8. En route to the station
9. Postrun

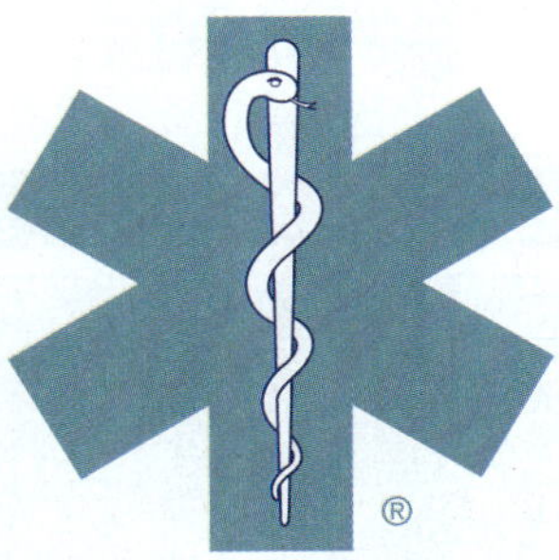

FIGURE 36-5 The Star of Life.

Courtesy of National Highway Traffic Safety Administration.

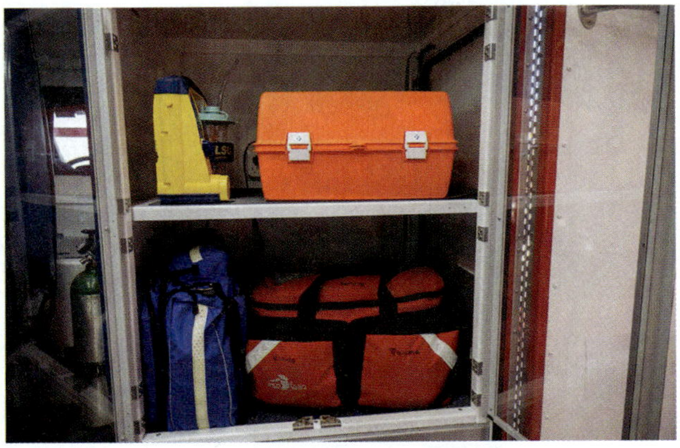

FIGURE 36-6 Store equipment and supplies in the ambulance according to how urgently and how often they are used.

Courtesy of Beulah Fire Protection District.

systems are necessary on licensed or certified ambulances.

Phases of an Ambulance Call

An ambulance call has nine phases: preparation, dispatch, en route, arrival at scene, transfer of patient to ambulance, en route to receiving facility (transport), at receiving facility (delivery), en route to station, and postrun, as shown in **TABLE 36-2**. These nine phases address the vehicle and its crew and their roles when responding to a medical emergency. The details of patient care are not included in these nine phases.

The Preparation Phase

During the preparation phase, you will check to make sure all of your equipment is functional and the appropriate supplies are in their proper place on the vehicle. Getting into the habit of performing a thorough vehicle checkoff will ensure you have the necessary supplies to respond to any call and will familiarize you with where items are kept so that you may quickly provide appropriate care without having to search for equipment. New equipment should be placed on an ambulance only after proper training is given on its use and care, and, additionally, after approval by the medical director.

Equipment and supplies should be durable and, to the extent possible, standardized. This makes it easy to quickly exchange equipment with other ambulances or restock after responding to a call.

Store equipment and supplies in the ambulance according to how urgently and how often they are used (**FIGURE 36-6**). Consider grouping equipment required for critical interventions in a similar location so that you do not have to waste valuable time retrieving these items from multiple locations. For example, package equipment for airway management, artificial ventilation, and oxygen delivery together and within easy reach of the head of the primary stretcher. Place items for cardiac care, control of external bleeding, and monitoring blood pressure at the side of the stretcher. Make sure batteries are fresh and equipment is functioning properly. The most common cause of automated external defibrillator (AED) malfunction is a dead battery.

Storage cabinets and kits should be held shut with a latch so they do not open while the ambulance is in motion. During this phase, all hard equipment and gear bags should be securely fastened in an appropriate mounting bracket or secured with webbing or straps. Loose items in the back of an ambulance can become dangerous projectiles in the event of a collision.

Medical Equipment

As an EMT, you have access to a large variety of medical equipment and supplies, far more than can be described here. Certain items on the ambulance must be available at all times, as dictated by state and jurisdictional requirements.

Basic Supplies

TABLE 36-3 lists the common supplies carried on ambulances. These include basic items such as personal protective equipment (PPE) and sharps containers, airway and ventilation equipment, basic wound care and bleeding control supplies, splinting supplies, childbirth supplies, an AED, patient transfer equipment, medications, communication equipment, and other regionally appropriate supplies.

Airway and Ventilation Equipment

It is important that two portable artificial ventilation devices that operate independently of an oxygen supply be carried on the ambulance: one for use in the ambulance and one for use outside the ambulance or as a spare. These devices include bag-mask devices capable of oxygen enrichment and, when attached to an oxygen supply with the oxygen reservoir in place, capable of supplying almost 100% oxygen. Masks for these devices come in a variety of sizes, from neonatal to adult, and are necessary materials to carry on the ambulance. Oxygen-powered devices are also available to provide ventilation to a patient but may quickly deplete available oxygen sources. You should follow local guidelines to identify the specific ventilation equipment carried on the ambulance.

The ambulance should carry portable and mounted suctioning units (**FIGURE 36-7**). These units must be powerful enough to generate a vacuum of 300 mm Hg when the tube is clamped. The suctioning force must be adjustable for use on infants and children. The units should include large-bore suction tubing, with semirigid tips available. The installed unit should include a suction yoke, a durable collection canister, suction catheters,

YOU are the EMT

Law enforcement officials have arrived on scene and it is safe for you to enter. On arrival, you are led to the back porch of a house where a 42-year-old woman is lying at the base of a set of three steps, holding her left knee. She tells you that her neighbor struck her in the left leg with a baseball bat following a verbal disagreement. You see obvious swelling and deformity to the patient's left knee.

Recording Time: 0 Minutes	
Appearance	Appears healthy; holding left leg; grimacing in pain
Level of consciousness	Alert and oriented
Airway	Open; clear of secretions or foreign bodies
Breathing	Increased rate; adequate depth
Circulation	Increased pulse rate, but strong and regular; skin is baseline color, warm, and dry

3. Based on the mechanism of injury and patient presentation, what equipment do you anticipate needing?

TABLE 36-3 Ambulance Equipment Checklist

Basic Supplies

- Pillows and pillowcases
- Sterile sheets
- Blankets
- Towels
- Disposable emesis bags or basins
- Boxes of disposable tissue
- Bedpan (optional)
- Urinals (one each for men and women; optional)
- Blood pressure cuffs (pediatric, adult, large adult)
- Blood glucose monitor
- Stethoscope
- Wet wipes
- Chemical cold/hot packs
- Sterile irrigation fluid
- Restraining devices
- Biohazard bags
- Hypoallergenic nitrile, vinyl, or other disposable hypoallergenic gloves (various sizes)
- Sharps container
- Set of hearing protectors and eye protection

Airway and Ventilation Equipment

- Infection control kits (goggles, masks, waterproof gowns)
- Oropharyngeal airways and nasopharyngeal airways of various sizes
- Continuous positive airway pressure (CPAP) equipment
- Advanced airway supplies, if local protocol permits (laryngeal mask airway, i-gel), with secondary placement confirmation devices
- Bag-mask devices (adult, child, and infant)
- Mounted suction unit and portable suction unit
- Assorted oxygen delivery devices (adult and pediatric)
- Oxygen supply units (both portable and installed)
- Pulse oximeter

Basic Wound Care Supplies

- Trauma shears
- Sterile sheets
- Sterile burn sheets
- Adhesive tape in several widths
- Self-adhering, soft roller bandages, 4 in. × 5 yd (10 cm × 5 m)
- Self-adhering, soft roller bandages, 2 in. × 5 yd (5 cm × 5 m)
- Sterile dressings, gauze, 4 × 4 in. (10 × 10 cm)
- Sterile dressings, abdominal or laparotomy pads, usually 6 × 9 in. (15 × 23 cm) or 8 × 10 in. (20 × 25 cm)
- Sterile universal trauma dressings, usually 10 × 36 in. (25 × 91 cm), folded into 9 × 10 in. (23 × 25 cm) packages
- Sterile, occlusive, nonadherent dressings (aluminum foil sterilized in original package)
- Occlusive dressings or chest seals
- Assortment of adhesive bandages
- Wound packing, hemostatic gauze
- Tourniquets

Splinting Supplies

- Adult-size traction splint
- A variety of arm and leg splints, such as vacuum, cardboard, plastic, foam-covered wire-ladder or aluminum alloy, or padded board (the number and type of splints should be determined by state regulations and your medical director)
- A variety of triangular bandages and roller bandages
- Long backboard, vacuum mattress, or scoop stretcher
- Cervical collars in an adjustable size or a variety of sizes
- Head stabilization devices

Childbirth Supplies

Emergency obstetric kit, including:

- Surgical scissors
- Hemostats or special cord clamps
- Small rubber bulb syringe
- Towels
- Gauze sponges
- Sterile gloves
- Sanitary napkins
- Plastic bag
- Baby blanket
- Baby stocking cap

Automated External Defibrillator

Semiautomated defibrillation equipment

Patient Transfer Equipment

- Wheeled ambulance stretcher
- Wheeled stair chair
- Other devices also carried on ambulances include:
  - Binder Lift
  - Portable/folding stretcher
  - Flexible stretcher
  - Transfer tarp or slide board
  - Basket stretcher

Medications and Other Supplies

- Oral glucose
- Oxygen
- Supplies for irrigating the skin and eyes
- Aspirin
- Epinephrine
- Nitroglycerin
- Inhaled beta agonist/bronchodilator/anticholinergic with small-volume nebulizer
- Naloxone (Narcan)
- DuoDote or other regional equipment, depending on the area and local protocol
- Portable radio or cell phone

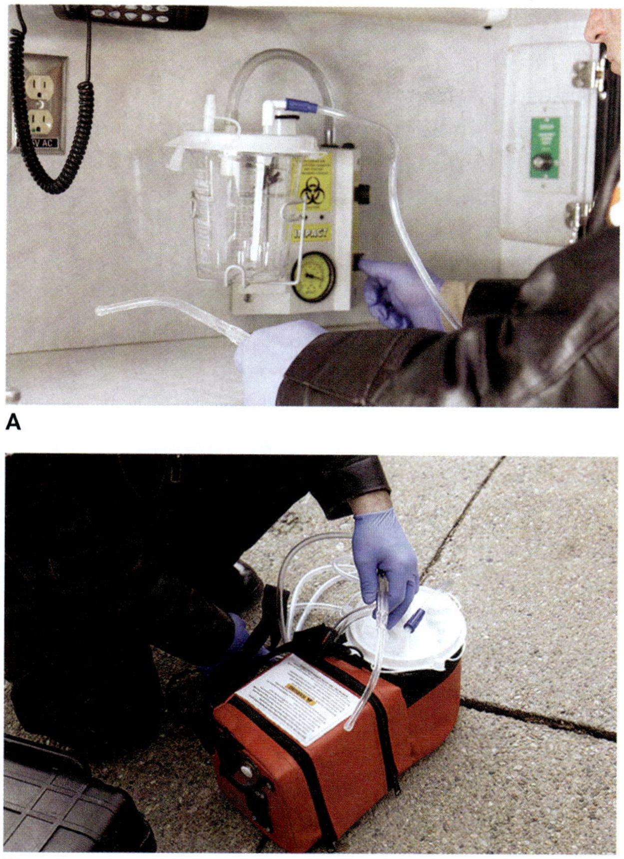

A

B

FIGURE 36-7 The ambulance should carry both a mounted suctioning unit (**A**) and a portable unit (**B**).

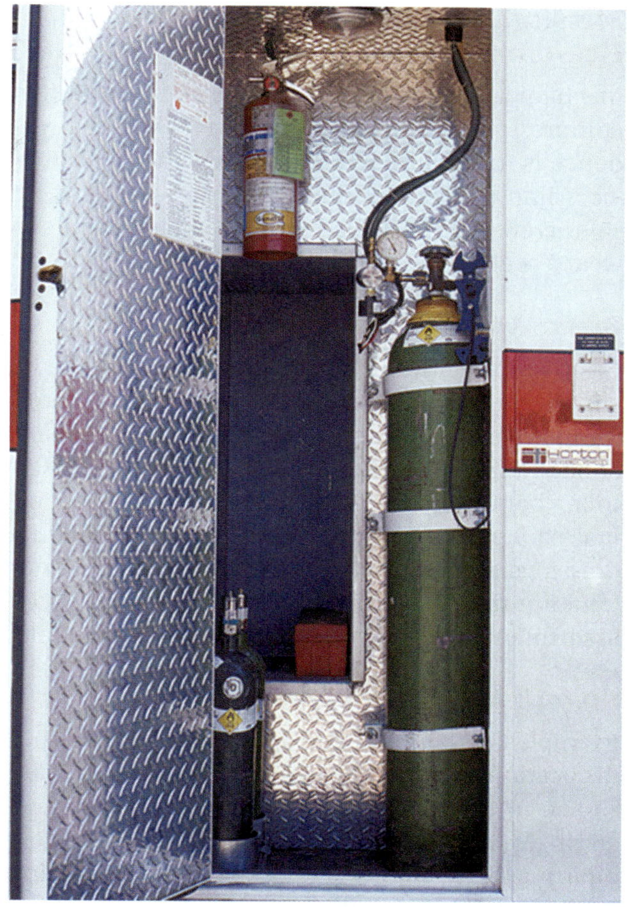

FIGURE 36-8 An oxygen unit with a capacity of 3,000 L of oxygen should be mounted on the ambulance.

sterile water for rinsing the suction tips, and suction tubing. As mentioned earlier, this equipment should be easily accessible when you are sitting at the head of the stretcher. The tubing must reach the patient's airway, regardless of the patient's position. All components of the suctioning unit must be disposable or made of material that is easy to clean and decontaminate.

The ambulance should carry at least two oxygen supply units: one portable and one installed on board. The portable unit should be located near a door or in the jump kit, for easy use outside the ambulance. While specific requirements for ambulance equipment vary by state, typically, an oxygen cylinder must have a minimum capacity of 425 L and be equipped with a yoke, pressure gauge, flowmeter, oxygen supply tubing, nonrebreathing mask, and nasal cannula. This unit must be able to deliver oxygen at a variable rate between 1 and 15 L/min. At least one extra portable 300- to 500-L cylinder should be kept on the ambulance. Many services equip the backup cylinder with its own yoke, gauge, regulator, and tubing so it can be used for a second patient.

Most mounted oxygen units have a capacity of 3,000 L of oxygen (**FIGURE 36-8**). It should also be equipped with visible flowmeters capable of delivering 1 to 15 L/min that are accessible from the head of the stretcher. Oxygen masks, with and without nonrebreathing bags, should be transparent, disposable, and in sizes for adults, children, and infants.

Words of Wisdom

Regardless of their location, portable oxygen tanks must always be secured by fixed clasps or housings to prevent accidental damage and to prevent the cylinder from becoming a projectile.

Mechanical Chest Compression Equipment

Mechanical chest compression devices operate on compressed gas or battery power. While the evidence is inconclusive regarding whether these devices improve patient outcomes, they do allow for safer crew transport, as they allow all occupants to wear a seat belt.

Basic Wound Care Supplies

Basic supplies for dressing open wounds should be carried on the ambulance. These include a pair of trauma shears; sterile sheets; sterile burn sheets; adhesive tape in several widths; self-adhering, soft roller bandages; sterile dressings; gauze; abdominal or laparotomy pads; sterile universal trauma dressings; sterile, occlusive, nonadherent dressings (aluminum foil sterilized in original package); an assortment of adhesive bandages; and tourniquets.

Splinting Supplies

Examples of supplies for splinting fractures and dislocations that may be carried on ambulances are shown in **FIGURE 36-9**. These supplies include an adult-size and a child-size traction splint; a variety of arm and leg splints, such as inflatable, vacuum, cardboard, plastic, foam wire-ladder, or padded board; a variety of triangular bandages and roller bandages; a short backboard; a long backboard; head stabilization devices; and cervical collars that are adjustable in size or a variety of sizes.

Childbirth Supplies

You must carry at least one sterile emergency obstetric kit that includes the supplies listed in Table 36-3, including a pair of scissors, hemostats or special cord clamps, umbilical tape or sterilized cord, a small rubber bulb syringe, towels, gauze sponges, pairs of sterile gloves, plastic wrap, sanitary napkins, a plastic bag, a baby stocking cap, and a baby blanket.

Automated External Defibrillator

Now a prehospital standard of care, semiautomated defibrillation equipment or manual monitor/defibrillators that have AED capability, as permitted by regulation and the local medical director, should always be carried on the ambulance (**FIGURE 36-10**).

Patient Transfer Equipment

Each ambulance should carry the following patient transfer equipment:

- A primary wheeled ambulance stretcher (**FIGURE 36-11**)
- A wheeled stair chair for use in narrow spaces
- A long backboard, vacuum mattress, or scoop stretcher

Stretchers must be provided with fasteners to secure them firmly to the floor or side of the ambulance during transport. Locking mechanisms should be capable of holding the stretcher in place in case the vehicle rolls over. Some ambulances

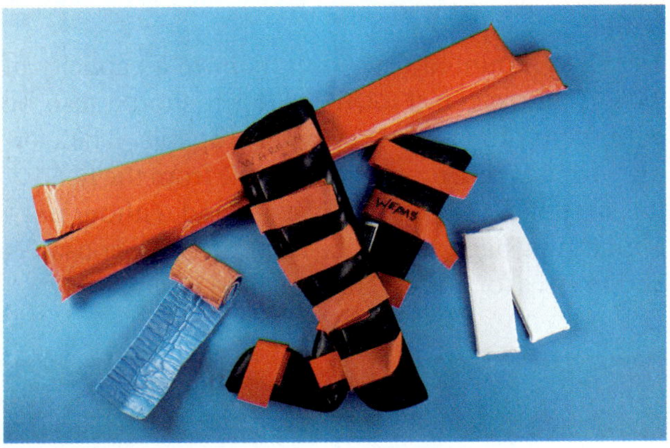

FIGURE 36-9 Supplies for splinting fractures and dislocations should be carried on the ambulance.

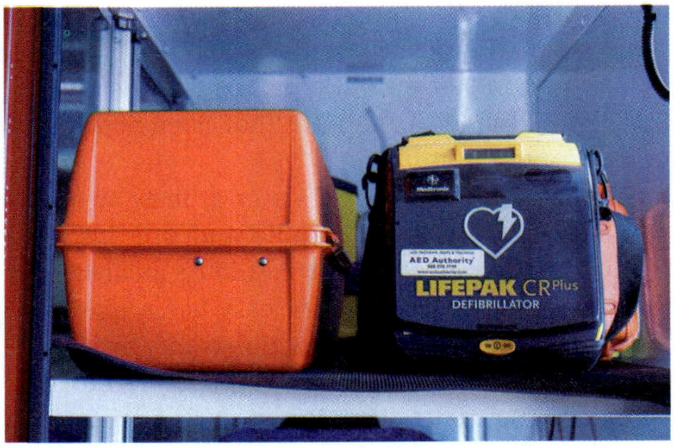

FIGURE 36-10 Every ambulance should carry an automated external defibrillator.

are equipped with systems that load the stretcher into the patient compartment automatically, helping decrease the strain that is placed on crew members' knees, legs, and backs. Make certain the wheeled stretcher is properly locked into position, because injuries can occur to both you and the patient if the stretcher becomes loose while the ambulance is in motion. Make sure there are at least three restraining devices for the patient, with deceleration or stopping straps over the shoulders, to prevent the patient from continuing to move forward in case the ambulance suddenly slows or stops. Regardless of the equipment used, it is important to use proper lifting techniques to avoid injuries. Chapter 8, *Lifting and Moving Patients*, discusses proper lifting and moving of patients.

Other patient transfer devices that can be used include the following:

- Scoop stretcher
- Vacuum mattress
- Portable/folding stretcher
- Flexible stretcher
- Basket stretcher
- Binder Lift

Street Smarts

In some cases, it may seem inconvenient or time consuming to apply shoulder straps when securing the patient to the ambulance stretcher. While you are securing the patient, explain how important it is for the person's safety. Using all straps to secure the patient is an essential habit, much like applying your own seat belt when riding in the cab. If a collision occurs and the patient sustains injuries from not having shoulder straps on, the EMT can be found liable.

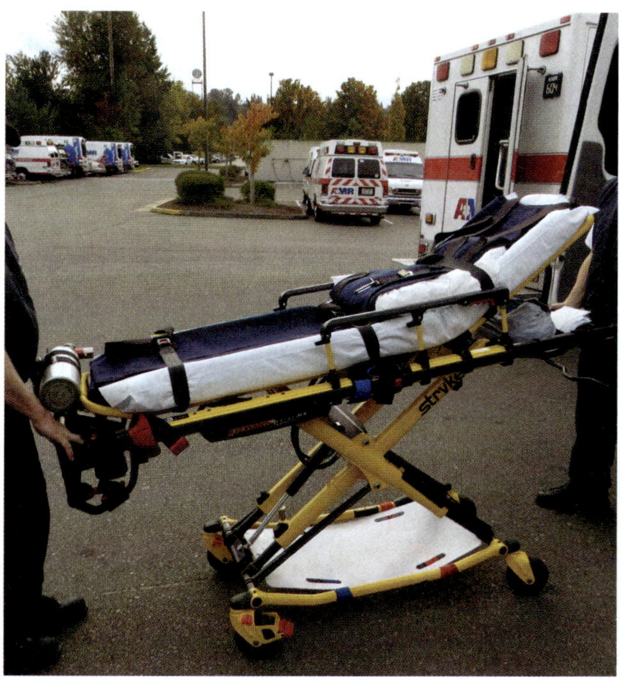

FIGURE 36-11 The wheeled ambulance stretcher should be locked into place at an appropriate height.

Medications

It is important that the ambulance carry appropriate, unexpired medications. Keep the telephone number and radio frequency of online medical direction or the local poison control center with you on the ambulance.

The Jump Kit

The ambulance must be equipped with a portable, durable, and waterproof **jump kit** that you can carry to the patient on every call (**FIGURE 36-12**). **TABLE 36-4** lists the items that are typically contained in a jump kit.

Safety and Operations Equipment

In addition to medical equipment, a properly stocked ambulance carries several kinds of equipment for ensuring responder safety, managing the

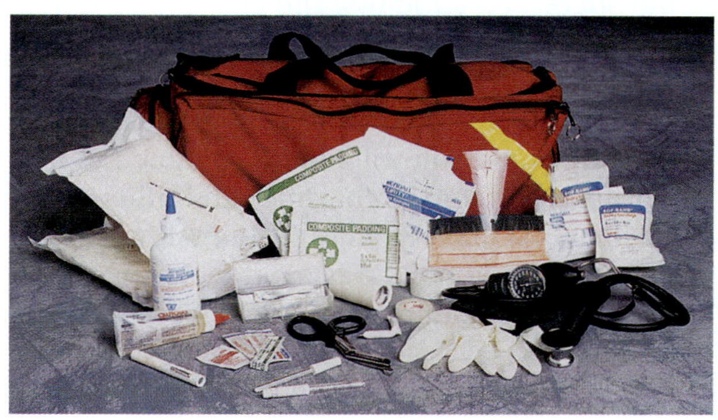

FIGURE 36-12 A portable jump kit should contain practically anything you will need during the first 5 minutes with the patient.

TABLE 36-4 Items Carried in a Jump Kit

- Nitrile, vinyl, or other disposable gloves
- Face shield or mask with goggles
- Triangular bandages
- Tourniquet
- Trauma shears
- Adhesive tape in various widths
- Universal trauma dressings
- Self-adhering soft roller bandages, 4 in. × 5 yd (10 cm × 5 m) and 2 in. × 5 yd (5 cm × 5 m)
- Oropharyngeal and nasopharyngeal airways in adult, child, and infant sizes[a]
- Bag masks for adults, children, and infants[a]
- Blood pressure cuff
- Stethoscope
- Penlight
- Sterile gauze dressings, 4 × 4 in. (10 × 10 cm)
- Sterile dressings (abdominal pads), 6 × 9 in. (15 × 23 cm) or 8 × 10 in. (20 × 25 cm)
- Adhesive strips
- Medications allowed by local protocols
- Oxygen saturation monitor[a]
- Blood glucose monitor

[a] These might be carried in a separate airway kit, along with the portable oxygen cylinder.

work area at an emergency scene, and locating emergency scenes.

Personal Safety Equipment

Along with your ANSI Class 2 reflective vest, you should always carry PPE that allows you to work safely in a limited variety of hazardous or contaminated situations. These situations include working at the edges of a structural fire or explosion, near the scene of a vehicle extrication or mass shooting, and in crowds. The equipment should protect you from exposure to blood and other potentially infectious body fluids. You will not be equipped to face all hazardous materials (hazmat) and other exposure situations that you may encounter; this is the job of specifically trained hazmat technicians and response teams. Your equipment might include the following:

- Face shields
- N95 masks
- Gowns, shoe covers, caps
- Turnout gear
- Helmets with face shields or safety goggles
- Safety shoes or boots
- Tactical vest and helmets

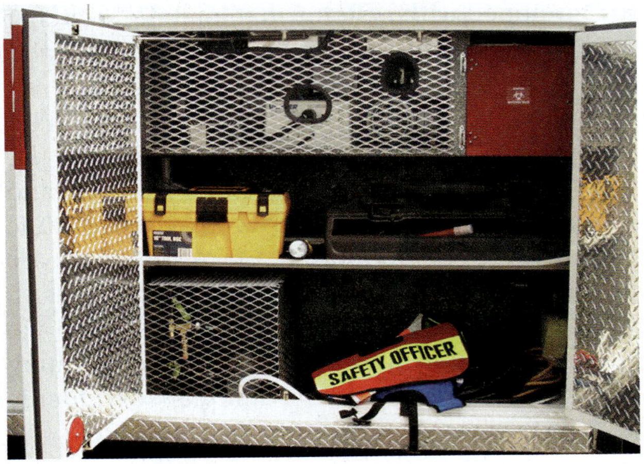

FIGURE 36-13 The ambulance should have a weatherproof compartment that can be reached from outside the patient compartment. It should hold equipment for safeguarding patients and EMTs, controlling traffic, and illuminating work areas.

Equipment for Work Areas

A weatherproof compartment that you can reach from outside the patient compartment should hold equipment for safeguarding patients and EMTs, controlling traffic and bystanders, and illuminating work areas (**FIGURE 36-13**). The following items are recommended:

- Warning devices that flash intermittently or have reflectors (Road flares can pose an additional hazard, such as ignition of flammable liquids or gases.)
- Two high-intensity flashlights of the recharging battery-powered, standup type
- Fire extinguisher, type ABC, dry chemical, 5-lb (2.3 kg) minimum
- Hard hats or helmets with face shields or safety goggles
- Portable floodlights, if applicable

Preplanning and Navigation Equipment

GPS devices and mobile data computers (MDCs), sometimes referred to as mobile data terminals (MDTs), are standard equipment in modern ambulances. The addresses of area hospitals and nursing homes should be stored for easy access.

Enter the location of the hospital into the GPS device before initiating transport to the hospital and review the route that you plan to take. You should never turn your attention away from driving to use a device of any type. Your partner should assist with providing updates from the MDC or GPS devices when responding to a call, especially when using lights and siren. Make sure you also have detailed street and area maps in the driver's compartment of the ambulance. Maps can serve as a backup if there are any technical issues with the GPS device or data transmission.

Familiarize yourself with the roads and traffic patterns in your town or city so you can plan alternate routes to frequent destinations. Pay particular attention to alternate routes that may provide you with ways around frequently raised bridges, congested traffic, and blocked railroad crossings. Often, switching to an alternate route will save more time than driving faster. You should be familiar with special facilities and locations within your regional operating area, such as other medical facilities, airports, arenas and stadiums, detention facilities, and chemical or research facilities that might pose unusual problems (staging areas may be predefined for emergency operations).

Personnel

Every ambulance must be staffed with at least one EMT in the patient compartment whenever a patient is being transported. Certain situations may require more assistance, such as providing assisted ventilations to a patient. Some states' EMS systems may allow non-EMT drivers to operate the ambulance when warranted by patient condition with two EMTs in the patient compartment. In these instances, the driver is usually a firefighter or law enforcement officer who is properly trained to operate the vehicle in emergency situations.

Daily Inspections

Being fully prepared means you and your team must inspect both the ambulance and equipment daily to ensure all items are in proper working order. Because your vehicle may be required to operate during bad weather or during emergency situations, you must ensure it is in proper working condition at all times. There is no margin for error when it comes to vehicle performance in an emergency. Inspections can help to minimize the risk that your ambulance experiences a preventable mechanical failure. The ambulance inspection should include the following:

- Fuel level
- Oil level
- Transmission fluid level
- Engine cooling system and fluid levels
- Batteries
- Brake fluid
- Engine belts
- Wheels and tires, including the spare, if there is one. Check inflation pressure and look for signs of unusual or uneven wear.
- All interior and exterior lights
- Windshield wipers and fluid
- Horn
- Siren
- Air conditioners and heaters
- Ventilating system
- Doors. Make sure they open, close, latch, and lock properly.
- Communication systems, vehicle and portable
- All windows and mirrors. Check for cleanliness and position.

Check all medical equipment and supplies daily, including all the oxygen supplies; the jump kit; splints, dressings, and bandages; spinal motion restriction equipment; and the emergency obstetrics kit. Is the equipment functioning properly? Are the supplies clean? Are there enough of them? All battery-operated equipment, including the defibrillator, should be operated and checked each day (**FIGURE 36-14**). Rotate the batteries according to an established schedule and ensure that any charging cables are connected.

Safety Precautions

A final part of the preparation phase is reviewing safety precautions. These precautions, which include standard traffic safety rules and regulations, should be followed on every call. Check safety devices, such as seat belts (in the cab and patient compartment), to ensure they are in proper working order. All equipment in the cab and in the patient compartment needs to be secured appropriately.

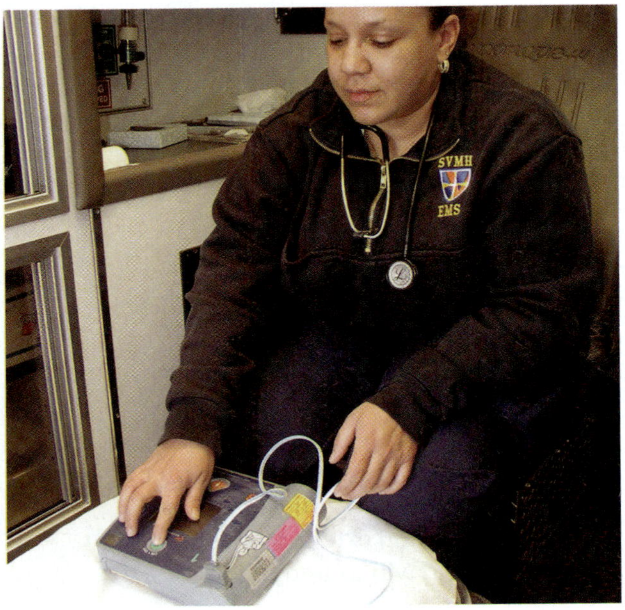

FIGURE 36-14 Always check the defibrillator at the beginning of each day.

Words of Wisdom

Because mechanical aspects of emergency work such as driving and moving patients strongly affect your safety and that of others, your service should have specific procedures for daily inspections. Following them protects you physically, and documenting your compliance is an important legal protection. Procedures should call for dating and either signing or initialing the check sheets and for storing them where they can be found later if needed.

The Dispatch Phase

Dispatch must be easy to access and in service 24 hours per day. It may be operated by the local EMS or by a shared service that also covers law enforcement and the fire department. The dispatch center might serve only one jurisdiction, such as a single city or town, or it might be an area or regional center serving several communities or an entire county. In either case, it should be staffed by trained personnel who are familiar with the agencies they are dispatching and the geography of the service area. For every emergency request, the dispatcher should gather and record the following minimum information:

- The nature of the call
- The name, current location, and call-back telephone number of the caller
- The location of the patient or patients
- The number of patients and some idea of the severity of their conditions
- Any other special problems or pertinent information about hazards or weather conditions

YOU are the EMT

After assessing the patient, you determine that she is hemodynamically stable. She did not have a loss of consciousness. She has deformity to her left knee with severe pain and tenderness on palpation. She has a history of hypertension and is allergic to penicillin. There was no fall associated with the event, and she was struck only once on the knee. There is no need for spinal motion restriction.

Recording Time: 5 Minutes	
Respirations	20 breaths/min; adequate depth
Pulse	98 beats/min; strong and regular
Skin	Baseline color, warm, and dry
Blood pressure	138/86 mm Hg
Oxygen saturation (Spo_2)	99% (on room air)

4. What assessment and treatment should be performed on scene and what should be delayed until you are in the ambulance and en route to the hospital?
5. How would you determine whether to use lights and siren during transport of this patient?

Many areas implement emergency medical dispatching, which provides the caller with prearrival instructions for patient care before the ambulance arrives. The emergency medical dispatcher follows a set of guidelines to determine the type of information given and then guides the caller through basic care such as bleeding control or initiating cardiopulmonary resuscitation (CPR).

Words of Wisdom

Your local telecommunicators and dispatchers are a valuable resource. They work hard to determine the exact circumstances of the incident to which you are responding and relay that information to you. However, their ability to provide useful information is limited by the person calling 9-1-1. Irrelevant or inaccurate information may be obtained and relayed to emergency responders. Take note of all information provided to you, but do not allow yourself to develop tunnel vision or decrease your level of situational awareness. There may be more patients than originally reported or a medical patient could have also sustained a traumatic injury. There is no replacement for your critical thinking skills and situational awareness on scene.

En Route to the Scene

In many ways, the en route or response phase of the call is the most dangerous for responders. Crashes between motor vehicles and emergency vehicles cause many serious injuries among EMS personnel. As you and your partner prepare to respond to the scene, make sure you fasten your seat belts and shoulder harnesses before you move the ambulance. Quickly review the most appropriate route that you intend to travel while responding to the call. You should also consider what alternate routes are available if your ambulance should encounter a raised bridge or traffic congestion. You should inform dispatch that your unit is responding and confirm the nature and location of the call. This is also an excellent time to ask for any other available information about the location. For example, you might learn that the patient is on the third floor or that the best door to use is around the side of the house.

When you are dispatched to the call, you must know whether to respond emergently (ie, with lights and siren) or nonemergently. This decision is based on the call information provided by the communications center and your local policy. Many emergency medical dispatching systems will classify the call using a code designator of *alpha* for low-priority, non-life-threatening emergencies or *echo* for critical, life-threatening emergencies. These designators, along with your local policy, hospital availability, and road conditions, can help you determine if it is necessary for your unit to respond emergently. Most EMS vehicle crashes occur when driving with lights and siren.[2] Data show that the use of lights and siren saves anywhere from 42 seconds to 3.8 minutes and few medical emergencies benefit from these time savings.[3] You and your crew must again determine whether to use lights and siren once you are ready to transport the patient to the hospital based on the patient's condition and your department protocols. Three basic principles govern the use of warning lights and siren on an ambulance:

1. The unit, to the best of your knowledge, must be responding to a true emergency call as defined by local protocol.
2. Audible and visual warning devices must be used simultaneously.
3. The unit must be operated with due regard for the safety of all others, on and off the roadway.

Always ask yourself, will the benefit of running lights and siren outweigh the three-fold risk of crashing during patient transport?[2]

In the event that you are responding to a violent crime or your dispatcher has detected the possibility that the scene is not safe for you to enter, you may be requested to stage your ambulance away from the scene while law enforcement officers respond to secure the scene. If you are requested to stage your ambulance, make sure it is a safe distance away from the scene. Bystanders or family members who see your ambulance stopped and not proceeding immediately to the scene may become agitated or violent because they want you to respond and render immediate care, even if the scene is not safe. Stage out of sight of the scene, even a few streets away. If there is only one road into or out of the neighborhood to which you are responding, do not stage on that road. If the person who originally assaulted a patient is fleeing the scene, you do not want to provide this person with the opportunity to delay or harm emergency responders. Follow local protocols and be aware of how your agency responds to possible unsafe scenes.

While en route to the call, the team should prepare to assess and care for the patient. Review dispatch information about the nature of the call and the location of the patient. Assign specific initial duties and scene management tasks to each team member and determine what type of equipment you will take with you when you first arrive on scene. Depending on the location of the patient, you may choose to take your primary stretcher or another patient transfer device with you immediately if access to the patient is limited. Make sure you follow your local operating procedures regarding the minimum equipment required for every call.

If the location of the patient changes or there are obstacles along your primary response route that could cause a significant delay, the person who is not operating the ambulance should be responsible for using the GPS or a map book to help determine an alternate route. Arriving at the scene safely and safely transporting the patient are two of the most challenging aspects of being an EMT. Refer to the "Safe Emergency Vehicle Operation" section in this chapter for techniques on safely driving and operating an ambulance.

Arrival at the Scene

On arrival at the incident, you will perform a scene size-up. This size-up starts while you are still inside the ambulance. You begin by evaluating the safety and stability of the scene. Do you see any hazards, or is the scene safe? Is this a medical call with only one patient who is sitting in clear view on the front porch? Is this a traffic accident with people entrapped in a vehicle? Is there a fight erupting on scene? As you gather more information, provide a brief report to your dispatch center with an update of the incident to which you have responded. This update will help to ensure that the appropriate resources are responding to the incident or possibly cancel additional resources that are not needed.

Report any unexpected situations, such as the need for specialized units, animal control for aggressive animals, a heavy rescue unit, or a hazardous materials (hazmat) team (**FIGURE 36-15**). Do not enter the scene if there are any hazards to you. If there are hazards at the scene, the patient should be moved somewhere safe before you begin care. The patient may have to be moved by others if you are not appropriately equipped.

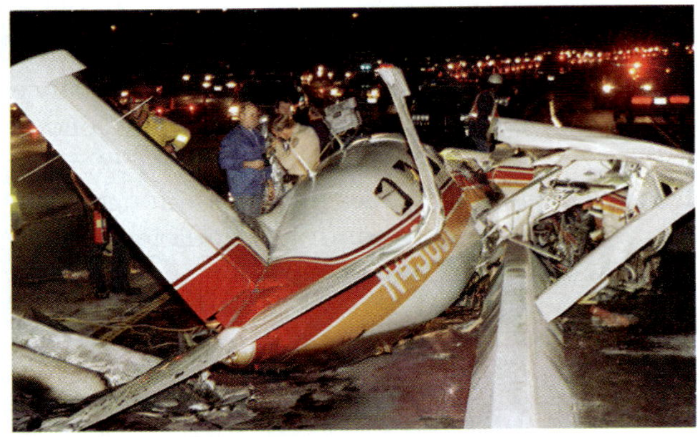

FIGURE 36-15 If you are the first to arrive on the scene of a mass-casualty incident, you should report to dispatch and ask for additional units, such as heavy rescue or hazmat units as needed.

Safety Tip

Patients may have pet dogs or other animals in the home when you arrive. Even if they tell you their pet has never bitten or harmed anyone, keep in mind that this same pet may have never seen a stranger touch their owner as you and the other EMS clinicians are about to do. The patient may be in pain and these observations by their pet may cause the animal to act aggressively to protect their loved one. If there is another family member on the scene, politely ask that they secure the animal in another area of the house and explain it is for everyone's safety.

Immediately size up the scene by using the following guidelines:

- Look for safety hazards to yourself, your partner, bystanders, and your patient or patients.
- Evaluate the need for additional units or other assistance.
- Determine the mechanism of injury in trauma patients or the nature of the illness on medical calls.
- Evaluate the need to perform spinal motion restriction.
- Take standard precautions. The type of care that you expect to give will dictate the PPE you should wear.

If you are the first EMT at the scene of a mass-casualty incident, quickly estimate the number of

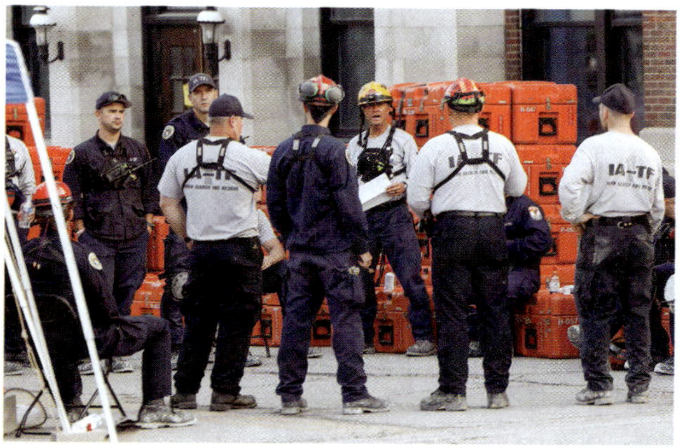

FIGURE 36-16 At a mass-casualty incident, follow instructions from the incident commander assigning your roles, which may include assisting with triage, treating patients, or loading patients for transport to the hospital.

patients, and communicate with your dispatch center or the incident commander if this person has arrived simultaneously (**FIGURE 36-16**). An accurate estimation of the number of patients will help to mobilize the appropriate number of resources to the scene. Remember that your initial estimation will be revised throughout the evolution of the incident. Mass-casualty incidents involve complex organization of personnel under the incident command system. In this system, individual EMTs may be assigned roles, such as beginning the triage process, assisting in treating patients, and loading patients for transport to a hospital. Chapter 38, *Incident Management*, discusses mass-casualty incidents in greater detail.

Safe Parking

In assessing the situation, you must decide where to park the ambulance. When parking, always use your parking brake. Pick a position that will allow for safe operations on scene, efficient traffic control, and a clear path for departing the scene. Always remember to leave yourself an exit. Whether initiating transport or retreating from a violent scene, you should park your vehicle with a clear departure path. It is best to park uphill and/or upwind of the scene if smoke or hazardous materials are present. Always leave your warning lights or devices engaged, and use extra caution if you must park on the back side of a hill or curve.

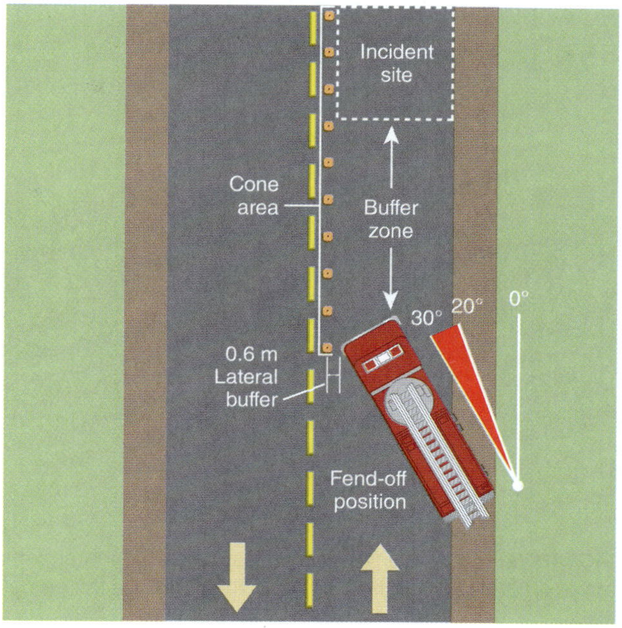

FIGURE 36-17 The fend-off position.

When operating on a roadway, the first emergency vehicle, whether ambulance, fire truck, or law enforcement vehicle, should create a barrier between the scene and traffic traveling in the same direction as the lane of traffic you are occupying. If you are the first vehicle to arrive on scene, you should park approximately 100 ft (30 m) before the scene on the same side of the road in the fend-off position (**FIGURE 36-17**). In the fend-off position, the ambulance is parked at a diagonal angle with the front wheels turned away from the scene. This position helps to block the scene and create a safety barrier within which you can operate. If a vehicle strikes the rear of an ambulance parked in the fend-off position, it is more likely to be deflected outward than directly into the area of the crash, where emergency personnel are working. Distracted drivers or poor weather conditions may create dangerous scenarios in which a vehicle may inadvertently drive into the scene at full speed. Assume someone may collide with your vehicle and strike personnel on the scene. Having a large emergency vehicle as a safety barrier may provide you with a cushion of space that could save your life.

If arriving after other emergency vehicles, the ambulance should be positioned approximately 100 ft (30 m) beyond the scene, thereby preventing

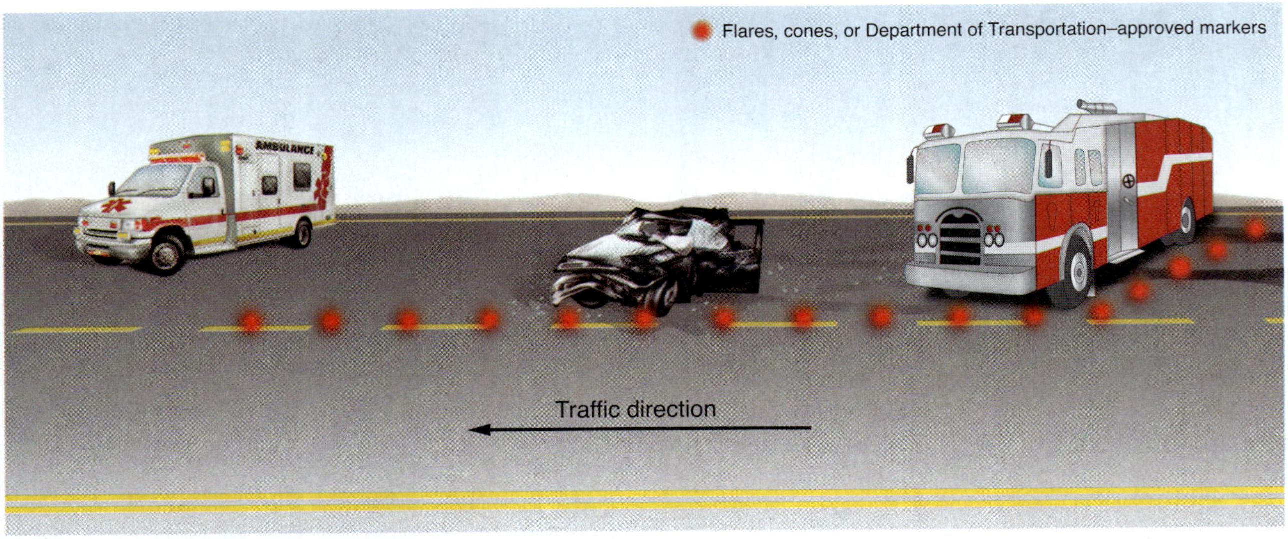

FIGURE 36-18 If other responders, such as firefighters or law enforcement officers, are on scene first, park the ambulance approximately 100 feet (30 m) past the scene on the same side of the road to allow an unobstructed departure path.

your vehicle from being blocked in when transporting a patient (**FIGURE 36-18**). If the street has not been completely closed and there is a driveway or parking lot adjacent to the scene, consider parking the ambulance there.

Stay away from any fires, explosive hazards, downed wires, and structures that might collapse. Be sure to set the parking brake. If your vehicle is blocking part of the roadway, leave on the emergency warning lights. Some motorists tend to drive toward emergency vehicles with flashing red or red and white lights. When possible, turn off headlights and fog lights at night scenes to prevent impairing the vision of oncoming traffic, but leave on other warning devices, especially amber lighting, until good traffic control is established surrounding the incident. Within these safety guidelines, you should try to park your ambulance as close to the scene as possible to facilitate emergency medical care. If necessary, you can temporarily block traffic to unload equipment and to load patients quickly and safely. If you must do this, try to do it quickly so traffic is not blocked any longer than necessary. Depending on the incident, lock the ambulance doors and ensure the designated driver has the keys. Doing so may prevent someone from stealing items from the ambulance or theft of the vehicle itself.

Safety Tips

When operating at an incident on any roadway, use caution when exiting the ambulance, wear protective equipment, and maintain a high level of situational awareness. Even with all of the emergency vehicles parked appropriately on a scene, distracted drivers may still drive straight into an emergency vehicle. Try to operate primarily within safe areas that use signage and large vehicles as barriers from the flow of traffic. Minimize your time on the scene. Whenever you are on a roadway, it is important to wear reflective safety vests or turnout gear. If you are retrieving equipment from the side compartment of your ambulance, you may be virtually invisible if you do not have a reflective vest on. Even attentive drivers may have difficulty seeing areas around the emergency vehicles that have all warning lights on.

Traffic Control

After you ensure your safety, your next responsibility at a crash scene is to care for the patients. Only after all the patients have been treated and the emergency situation is under control should you be concerned with restoring the flow of traffic. If the police have a delayed response to the scene, you might then need to take action to control the scene and limit access by other vehicles. It is important to ensure a safe environment for your crew and your patients.

The purposes of traffic control are to ensure an orderly traffic flow and to prevent a secondary crash. Under ordinary circumstances, traffic control is difficult. A crash or disaster scene presents serious additional problems. Passing motorists often slow down and stare, paying little attention to the roadway in front of them. Some curiosity seekers may park down the road and return on foot, creating additional hazards. As soon as possible, place appropriate warning devices, such as reflectors or LED traffic flares, on both sides of the crash.

Remember, the main objectives in directing traffic are to warn other drivers, to prevent secondary crashes, and to keep vehicles moving in an orderly manner so care of injured people is not interrupted.

The Transfer Phase

During the transfer phase, you must package the patient for transport, safely securing the patient to the wheeled ambulance stretcher, and then move to the ambulance and properly lift the patient into the patient compartment. Some scene conditions, such as steep embankments or unstable ground conditions, may make it unsafe for the wheeled ambulance stretcher to be moved with only two attendants. If additional rescuers are needed to move the patient, such as in a four-point movement, then be sure to request such assistance before attempting to move the patient.

No matter how careful the ambulance driver may be, riding to the hospital while lying down on a stretcher can be uncomfortable and even dangerous. Be sure to secure the patient with all manufacturer-approved straps (**FIGURE 36-19**). Use deceleration or stopping straps over the shoulders to prevent the patient from continuing to move forward in case the ambulance suddenly slows or stops. This is especially important if the patient is supine.

The Transport Phase

Inform dispatch when you are ready to leave with the patient. Report the number of patients you have, the name of the receiving hospital, and, in some jurisdictions, the beginning mileage of the ambulance. Even though you have already assessed and treated the patient, you should continue to monitor the patient's condition en route. These ongoing assessments may reveal changes in the patient's vital signs and overall condition. Recheck the patient's vital signs en route. The frequency of checking vital signs depends on the patient's acuity, but checking them every 15 minutes for a stable patient and every 5 minutes for an unstable patient is a practice that many services use. In addition, it is important that you continually reassess the patient's

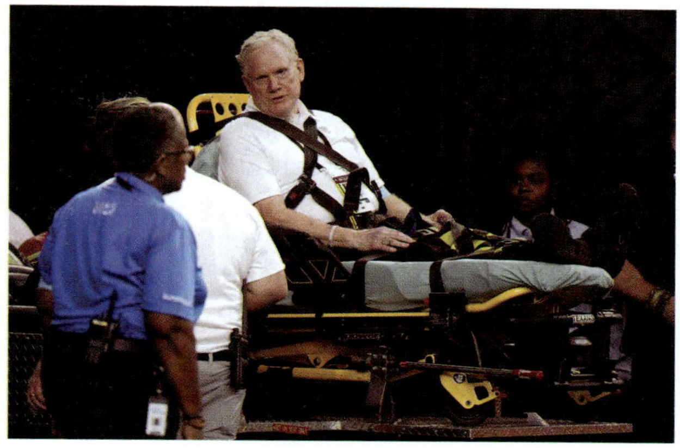

FIGURE 36-19 Secure the patient appropriately for protection during transport.

Words of Wisdom

When responding to a nursing home or assisted living facility, several actions can ensure smoother access to the facility and more efficient transfer of care. First, ask dispatch to instruct you to the specific location to enter the facility for easiest access to your patient. If it is after hours, obtain the door code or ask for a staff member to meet you at the entrance. When you arrive, determine who called 9-1-1; ask this person why the ambulance was called, and obtain other pertinent patient information. While receiving the patient handoff report, if the patient is confused or nonverbal, ask others on scene about the patient's normal mental status. Request transfer documentation, which typically includes a demographic sheet with the patient's personal information, a medical history sheet that lists medications and pertinent past medical history, and the patient's advance directive, if there is one. If this call is a nonemergency transfer, you will often need a physician's certification statement or a certificate of medical necessity form. Consult your local protocols.

clinical situation, address new problems, and note the patient's responses to earlier treatment.

During the transport phase, contact the receiving hospital. Inform online medical direction about the patient or patients and the nature of the problem or problems. Depending on the number of EMTs and how much care the patient needs, you may be able to begin documenting your patient care report while en route to the hospital.

Most important, do not abandon the patient emotionally. Do not become so involved in paperwork and ongoing assessments that you ignore the patient. The prehospital phase may be the only time that the patient will have one clinician dedicated solely to their care. Remember that you may be caring for the patient immediately after a tragic event or during life-threatening illness. Do not ignore how important compassion and caring can be during this phase. You are there to help the patient, so use this time to reassure the person. Sometimes small talk and conversation are appropriate, while other times just a quiet presence may be appreciated. Some patients, such as the very young or older people, may benefit from added attention during transport. Be aware of your patient's level of need.

The use of lights and siren when transporting a patient to the hospital should be evaluated before you start the transport process, as discussed earlier in this chapter. Many jurisdictions and medical directors specifically define which situations warrant use of emergency lights and siren for transport. Ignoring those directives could result in penalties or liability for any injuries caused.

Use common sense and defensive driving techniques at all times. In almost every case, you will provide any necessary lifesaving care right where you find the patient. You may perform less critical measures, such as bandaging and splinting, en route to the hospital.

The Delivery Phase

Inform dispatch as soon as you arrive at the hospital and, depending on your jurisdiction, identify your ending mileage as well. Then follow these steps to transfer the patient to the receiving hospital:

1. Report your arrival to the triage nurse or other arrival personnel.
2. Physically transfer the patient from the stretcher to the bed directed for your patient.
3. Present a complete verbal handoff report at the bedside to the nurse or physician who is taking over the patient's care. Include all pertinent information regarding your assessment and treatment. Answer any questions from the receiving staff.
4. Complete a detailed written report, obtain the required signatures, and leave a copy with an appropriate staff member. Electronic reports are commonly used. Your service should have a method for printing or sending electronic reports as well as obtaining electronic signatures.

See Chapter 4, *Communications and Documentation*, for a detailed review of information included in the patient care report.

Following the call, assess your current supply levels on the ambulance and determine if you need to return to your station or base before returning to service for the next call.

Street Smarts

As a prehospital emergency clinician, your verbal report and written documentation provide a vital portion of the patient's story. You hold the key to unlocking details of everything that occurred prior to the patient arriving at the hospital. You are the only one who can help provide details from the prehospital environment that can have a significant effect on the patient's course of care at the hospital. Never forget the importance of your role in the continuum of care.

En Route to the Station

Once you leave the hospital, inform dispatch whether you are in service and your intended destination. Depending on the call you just completed, your ambulance may not be prepared for another call until you return to your station. As soon as you are back at the station, you should do the following:

- Clean and disinfect the ambulance and any equipment that was used, if you did not do so before leaving the hospital (**FIGURE 36-20**).
- Restock any supplies you did not get at the hospital.

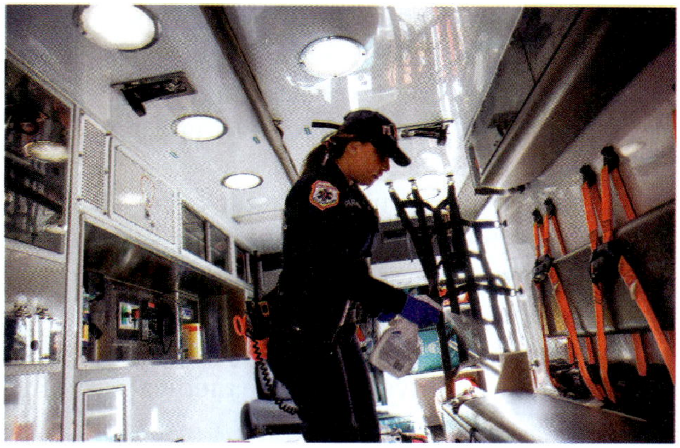

FIGURE 36-20 Clean and disinfect the ambulance and equipment at the station if you did not do so at the hospital.

The Postrun Phase

During the postrun phase, complete and file any additional reports and again inform dispatch of the unit status, location, and availability. This is also the appropriate time to debrief following the call. You should discuss the initial situation encountered on scene, strengths identified by the team's performance during the call, and opportunities for improvement regarding clinical knowledge, assessment, and skill proficiency. This debriefing process ideally should occur following every call in a professional, nonjudgmental manner while respecting each team member's input.

Each crew member is responsible for maintaining the ambulance so it is available at a moment's notice. This responsibility involves performing routine inspections and refueling the vehicle. Use a written checklist to document needed repairs or replacement of equipment and supplies.

Decontamination of the ambulance and equipment is vital to maintaining response readiness. The following processes are all types of decontamination:

- **Cleaning**. The process of removing dirt, dust, blood, or other visible contaminants from a surface or equipment
- **Disinfection**. The killing of pathogenic agents by directly applying a chemical made for that purpose to a surface or equipment
- **High-level disinfection**. The killing of pathogenic agents by using potent means of disinfection and use of thorough application processes
- **Sterilization**. A process, such as the use of heat, which removes all microbial contamination

A basic rule is to do the following after every call:

1. Immediately strip used linens from the stretcher after use, and place them in a plastic bag or in the designated receptacle in the ED.
2. Discard in an appropriate receptacle all disposable equipment used for care of the patient that meets your state's definition of medical waste. Most items will be considered general trash. Discard disposable equipment that is bloody or contaminated by body fluids in an OSHA-approved biohazard container. Discard noncontaminated disposable equipment used for care of the patient following OSHA and local guidelines.
3. Wash contaminated areas with soap and water or a cleaning solution. For disinfection to be effective, cleaning must be done first.
4. Disinfect all nondisposable equipment used in the care of the patient. For example, properly clean and disinfect stethoscopes, nondisposable blood pressure cuffs, pulse oximetry probes, and other reusable equipment.
5. Clean the stretcher with an EPA-registered germicidal/virucidal solution or bleach and water at 1:100 dilution. Follow manufacturer recommendations on minimum contact time, as most will require the surface to remain visibly wet with a solution for a specified amount of time.
6. Clean up any spillage or other contamination that occurred in the ambulance with the same germicidal/virucidal or bleach/water solution.

Words of Wisdom

Complete your daily duties, such as cleaning quarters, after the ambulance has been checked, cleaned, and restocked. Once these tasks are completed, there is usually downtime between calls. This is an excellent time to review local protocols, become familiar with your local response area, or train with ancillary services. Many EMTs also use this time to study for upcoming skills assessments or other courses required for recertification.

Safe Emergency Vehicle Operation

According to the National Highway Traffic Safety Administration, there has been an annual average of 29 fatal accidents involving an ambulance from 2012 to 2018. Of the crashes reviewed, 92.6% resulted from ambulance operator/driver error.[4,5] These statistics show the effect of these crashes on pedestrians, motorists, ambulance passengers, and EMS personnel (**FIGURE 36-21**). Learning how to properly operate your vehicle is just as important as learning how to care for patients when you arrive on the scene. An ambulance that is involved in a crash delays patient care, at a minimum, and may take the lives of the EMTs, patients in the ambulance, other motorists, or pedestrians.

The following section is provided to introduce you to safe driving techniques; however, you cannot become a proficient and safe ambulance driver without specialized training and practice. You are strongly encouraged to participate in a certified defensive driving program, such as those offered through your EMS organization, before attempting to operate an emergency vehicle. **TABLE 36-5** lists some general guidelines to follow when en route to a call.

Mental and Emotional Fitness

Not everyone who drives a motor vehicle is qualified to drive an emergency vehicle. In some states, you must successfully complete an approved emergency vehicle operations course before you are allowed to drive the ambulance on emergency calls. In any state, due diligence and caution are important characteristics, as are a positive attitude about your ability and tolerance of other drivers.

A crash may occur as a result of physical impairment of the driver. Do not drive if you are taking medications that may cause drowsiness or slow your reaction time. These include cold remedies, and analgesic and anxiolytic drugs. And, of course, you should never drive or provide medical care after

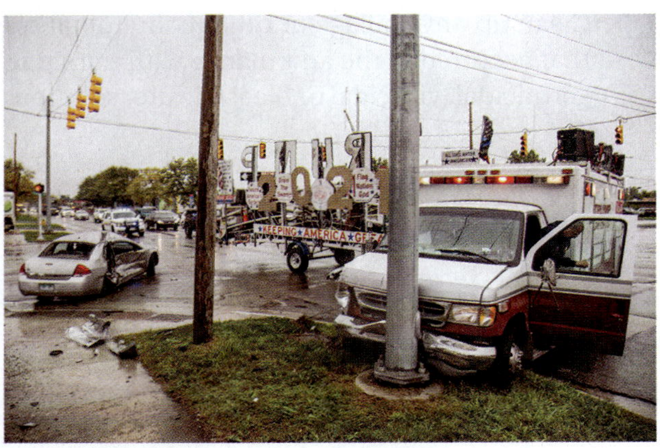

FIGURE 36-21 Each year, ambulance crashes are the cause of thousands of injuries to pedestrians, motorists, ambulance passengers, and EMS personnel.

TABLE 36-5 Guidelines for Safe Ambulance Driving

1. Select the shortest and least congested route to the scene at the time of the dispatch.
2. Avoid routes with heavy traffic congestion; know alternate routes to each hospital during rush hours.
3. Avoid one-way streets; they may become clogged. Do not go against the flow of traffic on a one-way street, unless absolutely necessary.
4. Watch carefully for bystanders as you approach the scene. Curious bystanders may be focused on the scene and not aware of approaching vehicles.
5. Park the ambulance in a safe place once you arrive at the scene. If you park facing into traffic, turn off your headlights so they do not blind oncoming motorists unless they are needed to illuminate the scene. If the vehicle is blocking part of the road, keep your warning lights on to alert oncoming motorists.
6. Drive within the speed limit while transporting patients, except in the rare extreme emergency.
7. Go with the flow of the traffic.
8. Always drive defensively.
9. Always maintain a safe following distance. Use the 4-second rule: stay at least 4 seconds behind another vehicle in the same lane. When you encounter adverse road or weather conditions, increase your following distance.
10. Maintain an open space or cushion in the lane next to you as an escape route in case the vehicle in front of you stops suddenly.
11. Use your siren if you turn on the emergency lights.
12. Always assume other drivers will not hear the siren or see your emergency lights.
13. Always exercise due regard for person and property.

drinking alcohol or using any other mind-altering substance. Although most employers have guidelines that require an employee to stop drinking at least 10 to 12 hours prior to the start of a shift, many factors affect the rate of alcohol metabolism, so it is possible to stop drinking for this length of time and still be impaired.

Fatigue has many causes, such as stress and lack of quality sleep in accordance with your body's circadian rhythms, as may occur when working the night shift. Operating an emergency vehicle while fatigued creates a dangerous risk to yourself and others. When fatigued, you may experience delayed reaction time or fall asleep behind the wheel. Although many services have regulations against working beyond a specific number of hours, all services do not take into consideration EMTs who may work for more than one service. It is your responsibility to notify your employer if you have previously worked a shift and feel unable to safely operate an emergency vehicle. Do not be ashamed to admit fatigue to yourself, your partner, or your supervisor. If you feel fatigued, you may be placed out of service for the remainder of the shift or until the fatigue has passed and you feel capable of safely operating the vehicle.

Words of Wisdom

Driving an ambulance does not automatically give you the authority to ignore basic traffic laws or operate the vehicle without due regard for the safety of others. The good judgment needed to drive an ambulance requires practice, even for the best drivers.

Another requirement is emotional fitness. Emotions should not be taken lightly. Other drivers can behave unpredictably. Whether through blatant disregard or a panicked response to an emergency vehicle behind their vehicle, other drivers on the road may have wildly different reactions when they encounter your ambulance. It is up to you to operate the vehicle in a safe fashion and never make any judgments or maneuvers based on an emotional response. Emotional maturity and stability are closely related to the ability to operate under stress.

Ambulance drivers should never adopt the attitude that an emergency response gives them the right to drive however they wish. The ambulance is likely much larger than your personal vehicle, and it will handle much differently, even under the best driving conditions. You must operate the vehicle with due regard for the safety of others and preservation of property. A greater responsibility is placed on the driver of an ambulance, and generally a lower burden of proof is needed to find that an EMT has caused a crash. As a rule, whenever lights and siren are used on an emergency call and there is a crash, the actions of the emergency vehicle operator fall under the most scrutiny.

Words of Wisdom

Ambulance crashes that kill EMTs, patients, or occupants of other vehicles are not uncommon. Many of them could have been prevented by the driver of the ambulance. Thoroughly attending to your own driving skills, driving according to established standards, and addressing any obvious lack of skills in your partner's driving all are crucial to your safety on the job.

Safety Restraints

Occupant and equipment restraints are the most important safety items on every ambulance. You should wear restraints en route to the scene and whenever you are not performing direct patient care that requires you to get out of your seat. If you must remove your seat belt to care for the patient, fasten the belt again as soon as possible.

Manufacturers continue to develop new ways to secure crew members in the patient compartment, enabling them to provide direct patient care while remaining restrained in a harness. Most recently, ambulance manufacturers have included airbags built into the shoulder straps in the crew seats.[6] Unfortunately, a report from the National Highway Traffic Safety Administration revealed that 84% of EMS clinicians involved in a serious crash were not wearing a seat belt at the time.[7] While most patients involved in these crashes were restrained in the back of the ambulance, only 33% were properly restrained with both lap and shoulder belts.[7]

Also, unrestrained or improperly restrained patients and medical equipment (especially defibrillators and portable oxygen tanks) may become airborne during a crash and place you and your patient at an additional risk (**FIGURE 36-22**). All equipment and cabinets must be secured.

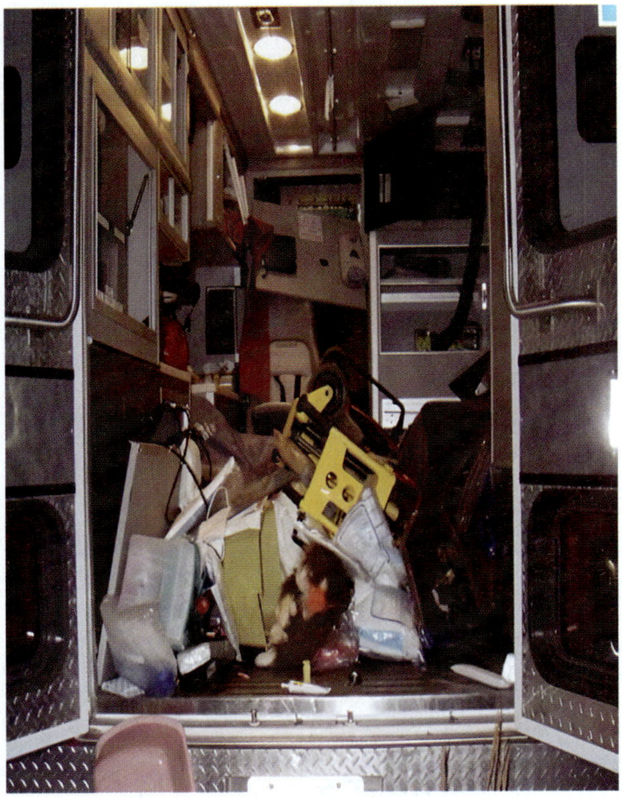

FIGURE 36-22 Patient compartment following a crash. The disarray suggests objects were not properly secured and could have injured the patient or EMS clinicians in the back of the ambulance.

Courtesy of National Institute for Occupational Safety and Health.

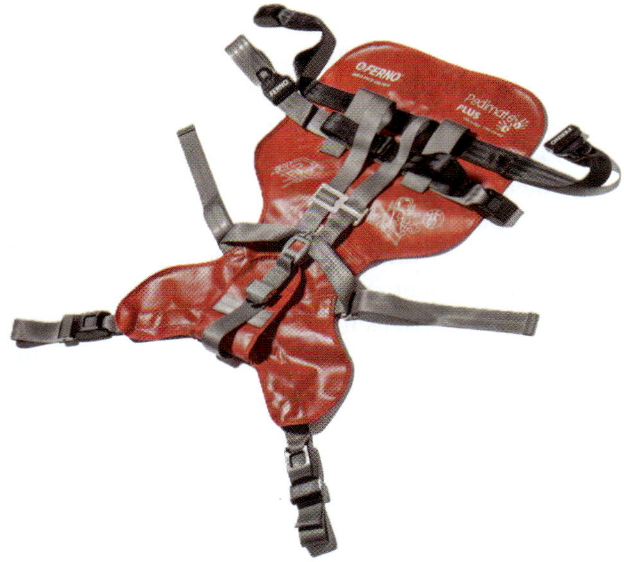

FIGURE 36-23 The Pedi-Mate Plus shown here attaches to the ambulance stretcher and is designed for children less than 100 pounds (45 kg). Use the pediatric patient restraint method approved by your agency.

Courtesy of Ferno-Washington, Inc. www.ferno.com.

Patients and any passengers accompanying the patient should also be properly restrained. As part of your daily ambulance inspection, ensure that you have the necessary equipment to transport an infant or child. Children weighing less than 40 pounds (18 kg) who do not require spinal motion restriction should be transported in a car seat or restrained to the ambulance stretcher using an appropriate-size device.[8] A car seat should be chosen according to the pediatric patient's weight and should meet the applicable standards set by the EMS agency's governing authority (**FIGURE 36-23**). At no time is it acceptable to transport a parent or caregiver holding an infant or child. If responding to a child's home, parents or caregivers can provide the child safety seat used in their vehicle. Alternatively, some agencies may carry inflatable car seats or child seats that are built into the ambulance airway chairs. Commercial devices are available to secure newborns to their mother's chest. Regardless of the device used, ensure that it is secured for transport.

There are only a few locations to place a car seat in an ambulance. Car seats are designed to be either forward-facing or rear-facing; they cannot be mounted sideways on a bench seat. To mount a car seat to the stretcher, place the head of the stretcher in an upright position. Place the seat so it is against the back of the stretcher. Secure one of the stretcher straps from the upper portion of the stretcher through the seat belt positions on the seat and strap it tightly to the stretcher. Repeat on the lower portion of the stretcher. Push the car seat into the stretcher tightly and retighten the straps. Car seats should not be mounted in the front of an ambulance.

For pediatric patients who require spinal motion restriction, secure the child on a suitable device. A patient in unstable condition who requires airway or ventilatory support should be positioned to allow maximum access for airway and ventilatory requirements. While rare, pediatric patients in cardiopulmonary arrest should be placed on a device that can be secured to the stretcher. Follow local protocols when transporting pediatric patients.

In a situation where the car seat has been physically damaged, do not use the patient's own car seat. Instead, transfer the patient to the ambulance's car seat or suitable restraining device.

Words of Wisdom

The first rule of safe driving in an emergency vehicle is that speed does not save lives; good care does. The second rule is that the driver and all passengers must wear seat belts and shoulder restraints at all times.

Vehicle Handling

Learn how your vehicle accelerates, corners, sways, and stops. Understand exactly how each particular vehicle will respond to steering, braking, and accelerating under various conditions.

Braking

Getting a feel for the proper brake pressure comes with experience and practice. Each vehicle has a different braking action. For example, the brakes on types I and III vehicles have a heavier feel than the brakes on a type II vehicle. The braking system on a diesel-powered unit will be different from the braking system on an identically equipped gasoline-powered unit. Certain heavy vehicles use air brakes, which have yet another feel. Get to know each vehicle you drive. It is important to understand the braking characteristics under various conditions.

Road Positioning and Cornering

Road position means the position of the vehicle on the roadway relative to the inside or outside edge of the paved surface. To corner efficiently, you must know the vehicle's current position and its projected path. The aim is to take the corner at the speed that will put you in the proper road position as you exit the curve (**FIGURE 36-24**). When driving an ambulance, focus on safely maneuvering through a corner as opposed to taking the fastest route. The safest path is to enter high in the lane (to the outside) and exit low (to the inside). This allows room for error if you enter the turn too fast.

When driving an ambulance during an emergency response on a multilane highway, you should usually stay in the extreme left-hand (fast) lane. This allows other motorists to move over to the right when they see or hear the ambulance approach.

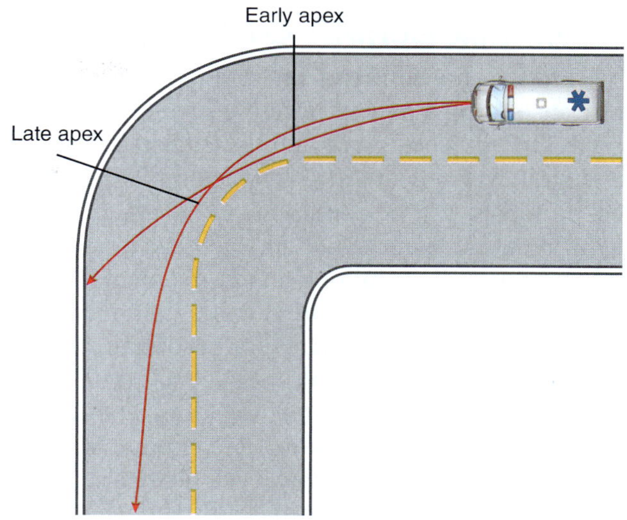

FIGURE 36-24 To keep the ambulance in the proper lane on a curve, you must know the vehicle's current position and projected path and take the corner at the correct speed.

Vehicle Size and Distance Judgment

Vehicle length and width are critical factors when maneuvering, driving, and parking an emergency vehicle. They are especially important with types I and III vehicles, which are wider than they look from behind the steering wheel. To brake and pass effectively, you must know the width and length of your vehicle. Vehicle size and weight greatly influence acceleration, braking, and stopping distances. Preventable accidents often occur when the driver is backing up the vehicle. Use someone outside the ambulance as a spotter when you are backing up to avoid any incidents. Good peripheral vision and depth perception will help you judge distances, but they are no substitute for intensive training, experience, and frequent evaluation of the vehicle.

Words of Wisdom

Centrifugal force is the tendency for objects to be pulled outward when rotating around a center. Vehicles are subject to this force when making a turn. If you must brake on a turn, brake gently while making the turn.

Siren Risk-Benefit Analysis

As discussed previously, whether responding to a call or transporting a patient from the scene to the hospital, the decision to activate the emergency lights and siren will depend on several factors, such as local protocols, patient condition, and the anticipated clinical outcome of the patient. We have to remember that our role is but one link in the chain of survival. Our goal should always be to do no harm and to safely deliver the patient to the appropriate facility.

As an EMT, you should also consider the patient's condition before activating emergency lights and siren. Emergency lighting and siren noise may increase the patient's anxiety level. If you are transporting a patient having a heart attack who is already anxious, the use of lights and siren could lead to more anxiety and an increase in heart rate, blood pressure, and oxygen demand. In such cases, it may be better to transport your patient without lights and siren activated to minimize external stimuli and to prevent worsening your patient's condition. If you do have to turn on the siren, tell the patient before you do so to prevent unnecessary anxiety.

Driver Anticipation

Never assume other drivers see you or will respond predictably when they encounter an emergency vehicle. As mentioned previously, people's responses can vary widely when they see an emergency vehicle approaching. Learn to expect the unexpected. Motorists may indeed pull over to the right and stop or drive as close to the curb as possible, but you cannot take this behavior for granted. Operate the ambulance in a manner that allows you adequate time and space to safely maneuver around vehicles that may have suddenly stopped or pulled over in the wrong direction. Look at the direction of the other vehicle's front tires to get an early indication of which way the vehicle will turn. Aggressive ambulance driving is never appropriate. You may not allow enough time for motorists to respond to your vehicle, or they may become nervous and not react in a rational manner.

Thanks to advances in automotive design, including soundproofing, motorists who drive at the speed limit with the windows up and the radio on may not hear noises from outside of the vehicle, such as emergency sirens or instructions called out over the ambulance's public address (PA) system, until the ambulance is very close. If the radio is loud, they may not hear the siren at all. Effective siren distances are much shorter than you might think. Keep in mind that as you increase the speed of your ambulance, you decrease the amount of time and space that people in vehicles in front of

YOU are the EMT

The hospital you are transporting to is 12 miles away. The patient's vital signs are normal. She states her pain is a 5 on a scale of 1 to 10. After traveling approximately 5 miles, you realize the ambulance is slowing down. Your partner tells you he has just heard on the radio that there is a motor vehicle crash a couple of miles ahead, and traffic is at a standstill. He says he can turn on the lights and siren and try to get through.

Recording Time: 12 Minutes	
Level of consciousness	Alert and oriented
Respirations	18 breaths/min; adequate depth
Pulse	98 beats/min; strong and regular
Skin	Baseline color, warm, and dry
Blood pressure	136/88 mm Hg
Oxygen saturation (Spo_2)	100% (on room air)

6. What should you consider when deciding whether it is appropriate to turn on the lights and siren to maneuver through traffic?
7. If you are in an unfamiliar area and do not know an alternate route, what are your options?

you have to hear your siren and react appropriately. Some ambulances are equipped with a specialized siren (eg, the Rumbler) that emits low-frequency siren sound waves that produce a vibration and may penetrate vehicles better than traditional sirens, allowing motorists to feel the siren.

Use of the PA system may actually worsen the situation because motorists may hesitate or make unexpected moves while attempting to hear or follow instructions. Moreover, an ambulance driver who is shouting to motorists and pedestrians over the PA system is distracted from the business of driving and forced to handle the microphone when both hands should be on the steering wheel. You should avoid using the ambulance's PA system during emergency driving.

Most important, you must always drive defensively. Never rely on what another motorist will do unless you get a clear visual signal. Even then, you must be prepared to take defensive action in the case of a misunderstanding, panic, or careless driving on the part of the other driver.

The Cushion of Safety

To safely operate an emergency vehicle, you must maintain a safe distance between your vehicle and any vehicles around you, referred to as a **cushion of safety**. The primary considerations in ensuring this cushion are keeping a safe distance between your vehicle and the one in front of you, checking for tailgaters behind the ambulance, and remaining aware of vehicles potentially hiding in the mirrors' **blind spots**.

To ensure you have enough reaction time and stopping distance from the vehicle in front of you, follow at a safe distance, which can be defined as driving approximately 4 or 5 seconds behind a vehicle traveling at an average speed. This distance allows the motorist enough time to move over to the right. If the motorist does not move, you will need to allow for enough time to avoid the vehicle.

While operating in emergency mode, tailgaters may follow your vehicle dangerously close in congested areas simply to use your ambulance to get through traffic. Doing so poses a threat to the crew and patient. If the ambulance has to slow down or stop suddenly to avoid a crash, the tailgating vehicle could collide with the rear of the ambulance, possibly causing you to lose control and strike other vehicles or pedestrians. Always scan the mirrors for vehicles following too closely. Instruct your partner in the rear compartment rendering care to stay alert for such vehicles and to inform you about any tailgaters.

If you are being tailgated, never speed up to create more distance. The tailgater may also speed up to continue to follow you through traffic. Your increased speed will be counterproductive as it will increase the distance needed to avoid a crash, thereby decreasing your cushion of safety and reaction time. Slamming on your brakes to scare the other driver usually does not work either and may also cause a crash. The best method for distancing yourself from the vehicle is to slow down. Generally, tailgaters are impatient and will speed up to pass you. You can also have your dispatcher contact the local police to let them know that someone is driving recklessly behind you.

Never, under any circumstance, get out of the ambulance to confront a driver. This will only delay your response or transport of the patient and can lead to a dangerous situation. It is also unprofessional for you to become involved in a verbal argument with any member of the public and may lead to disciplinary actions or termination, depending on your service's conduct regulations.

Finally, to avoid blind spots, adjust your vehicle's side mirrors to help see vehicles or pedestrians on either side of the ambulance. Even with well-positioned mirrors, however, there are three blind spots around the ambulance that you cannot see with side or rearview mirrors:

- The rearview mirror creates a blind spot, obstructing the view ahead and preventing the driver from seeing objects such as a pedestrian or vehicle. Many new ambulance drivers will not be used to the larger mirrors on ambulances, which create a special hazard of which the driver should be aware. If your ambulance has a GPS, MDC, or dash camera mounted near the dashboard, this may also contribute to a blind spot. To eliminate this blind spot, you should lean forward in your seat, so the equipment does not obstruct the view, especially when making turns at intersections.
- The rear of the vehicle cannot be seen fully through the mirror and is therefore a blind spot. Because of the configuration of today's ambulances and the relative height of the vehicle, the rearview mirror generally gives

the driver only a view of the patient compartment. It is not intended to be used for alerting the driver of a vehicle behind the ambulance. Because of this blind spot, many crashes occur when the ambulance driver is backing up. It is highly recommended, and required in many jurisdictions, that a **spotter** be used to help when backing up the vehicle. Rear-facing cameras are also helpful and much more common; however, these cameras may still have a limited view and be unable to provide an adequate view of the corners of the back of the ambulance. For this reason, rear-facing cameras do not replace the use of a spotter if one is available.

- The side of the vehicle often cannot be seen through the side view mirrors at a certain angle. Even when mirrors are adjusted properly, there will be spots around the sides of the vehicle that you cannot see. Entire vehicles may not be seen in the mirror, even though they are right next to the ambulance. To eliminate this problem, many EMS systems have smaller convex spot mirrors in addition to the side mirrors to help you see this blind spot. However, if these mirrors are not available, you need to lean forward or backward in the seat to help eliminate the blind spot. This is an especially important technique to use when shifting lanes or making turns. When making a turn from an appropriate lane or across multiple lanes, be aware that other motorists, bicyclists, or pedestrians may have traveled alongside the ambulance as you are beginning your turn.

Scan your mirrors frequently for any new hazards and maintain your cushion of safety. Keep in mind that the mirrors can provide a misleading view and may block people or vehicles. Properly adjust the mirrors before operating the vehicle, and adjust your position in the driver's seat to avoid blind spots. Always use a spotter whom you can see from the driver's side mirror and agreed-on hand signals when backing up the ambulance.

The Problem of Excessive Speed

Even in extreme life-and-death emergencies, excessive speed is not indicated. In most cases, if you properly assess and render appropriate treatments at the scene, speeding during transport is unnecessary, undesirable, and unsafe. No matter what the situation, you should never travel at a speed that is unsafe for the given road conditions. In almost every situation, slower means safer.

Excessive speeds do not increase a patient's chance of survival. More often, using excessive speed while driving to and from the scene has resulted in crashes in which the EMT, the patient, and occupants of other vehicles have been killed. It also makes it very difficult for the EMT attending to the patient to be able to provide any level of care because of the rough ride typically created by the excessive speed and maneuvering. Excessive speed also cuts down on the driver's reaction time and increases the time and distance needed to stop the ambulance. Operating at or beyond the speed limit can be viewed as operating the vehicle recklessly and without due regard. Although many state laws allow emergency vehicles to travel slightly faster than the posted speed limits in emergencies, they offer little or no protection against prosecution should the driver become involved in a motor vehicle crash. The legal ramifications of driving an emergency vehicle will be covered later in this section.

Recognition of Siren Syndrome

The siren may have a physiologic and a psychological effect on EMS clinicians as well as on other drivers. Driving emergently in an ambulance with the lights and siren activated, at least in the early phases of your career, will likely cause you to experience a rush of adrenaline. Your respiratory rate and heart rate will increase, and your palms may become sweaty. This physiologic response is natural, but it may limit your focus and also interfere with your ability to judge distance or the potential actions of others. Understanding your body's response to driving with lights and siren can help you to mitigate the associated risks. Take a deep breath and proceed with caution, remembering the guidelines for safe ambulance operation.

The siren may also increase the anxiety of other drivers or other drivers' tendencies to drive faster in the presence of sirens. Although a siren signifies a request for drivers to yield the right-of-way, drivers do not always do so. One of the biggest mistakes you can make as an EMT is to assume motorists will hear the siren and take proper action.

Weather and Road Conditions

Certain conditions can limit your ability to control the vehicle and can contribute to a crash. Ambulances do not handle the same as small motor vehicles. Ambulances are heavier than most vehicles and will have a longer braking time and stopping distance. In addition, the weight of the ambulance is unevenly distributed, which makes it more susceptible to rolling over. These factors, in addition to bad environmental conditions, greatly increase the chance that a crash may occur. Therefore, you should remain alert to changing weather, road, and driving conditions (**FIGURE 36-25**). Whether traveling to or from an emergency, you must modify your speed according to road conditions. Take warnings of ice or hazardous conditions seriously, and be prepared to take an alternate route, if necessary. If you run into unexpected traffic congestion or deteriorating travel conditions, notify the dispatcher so other emergency vehicles can select alternate routes. In the event of a major disaster or severe weather events, all public safety and emergency services should be coordinated.

Even the most careful drivers will occasionally run into unexpected situations that may require special driving skills. However, if you drive at a speed that is appropriate for the weather and road conditions and maintain an adequate cushion of safety, you will minimize the occurrence of crashing during these situations. You should decrease your speed in bad weather conditions such as fog, rain, snow, or ice. The following are examples of conditions that require the emergency vehicle operator to decrease speed, increase following distance, and be alert.

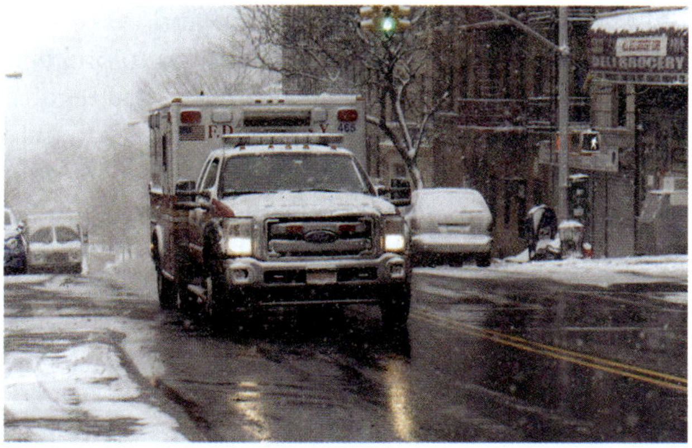

FIGURE 36-25 Modify your speed according to changing weather, road, and driving conditions.

Hydroplaning

On a wet road surface, tires are designed to move the water out of the way and stay in direct contact with the road. However, at speeds in excess of 30 mph, tires may be lifted off the road as water accumulates underneath; the vehicle may then feel as if it is floating. This problem is known as **hydroplaning**. At higher speeds on wet roadways, the front wheels may be riding on a sheet of water, robbing the driver of directional control of the vehicle. If hydroplaning occurs, you should gradually slow down without jamming on the brakes.

Water on the Roadway

Wet brakes will not slow the vehicle as efficiently as dry brakes, and the vehicle may pull to one side or the other. If you encounter a large pool of standing water, you will likely be unable to determine how deep the water is. You should avoid traveling through standing water if at all possible. If you must drive through standing water, slow down and turn on the windshield wipers. After driving out of the water, lightly tap the brakes several times until they are dry. If the vehicle is equipped with antilock brakes, apply a steady, light pressure to dry the brakes. Driving through moving water should be avoided at all times.

Decreased Visibility

In areas where there is fog, smog, snow, or heavy rain, slow down to a safe operating speed. Be cautious with activating your emergency lights, as they may be disorienting to you or other motorists. At night, use only low headlight beams for maximum visibility without reflection. You should always use headlights during the day to increase your visibility to other drivers. Also, watch carefully for stopped or slow-moving vehicles.

Ice and Slippery Surfaces

A light mist on an oily, dusty road can be just as slippery as a patch of ice. Good all-weather tires and an appropriate speed will significantly reduce traction problems. If you are in an area that often has snowy or icy conditions, consider using studded snow tires or tire chains, if they are permitted by law. You should be especially careful on bridges and overpasses when temperatures are close to freezing. These road surfaces will freeze much faster than surrounding road surfaces because they lack the warming effect of the ground underneath.

Although preventing skids and sliding is ideal, you are likely to skid or slide occasionally, especially if you live in climates with ice and snow. Your training should include the technique for correcting slides during turns. If you are likely to drive on ice and snow, practice control maneuvers until they become automatic—at low speeds in an area where there is no danger of crashes. Remember that four-wheel-drive and front-wheel-drive vehicles behave differently than rear-wheel-drive vehicles when sliding. It is also important to remember that although four-wheel-drive vehicles have better traction for acceleration in slippery conditions, they do not stop any faster than two-wheel-drive vehicles.

Laws and Regulations

Regulations regarding vehicle operations vary by state and by city, but some regulations are the same regardless of location. Drivers of emergency vehicles have certain limited privileges in every state. However, these privileges do not reduce their liability in a crash. In many cases, the driver is presumed to be guilty if a crash occurs while the ambulance is operating with warning lights and a siren. Many lawsuits against EMS personnel and services involve motor vehicle crashes.

While on an emergency call, emergency vehicles typically are exempt from laws pertaining to normal vehicle operations as long as you continue to operate the vehicle with due regard. If you are on an emergency call and you are using your warning lights and siren, you may be allowed to do the following:

- Park or stand in an otherwise illegal location
- Proceed through a red traffic light or stop sign, but never without stopping first
- Drive above the posted speed limit
- Drive against the flow of traffic on a one-way street or make a turn that is normally illegal
- Travel left of center to make an otherwise illegal pass

Remember that these exemptions vary by state and local jurisdiction. Therefore, you should check the local statutes or regulations in your area.

An emergency vehicle is *never* allowed to pass a school bus that has stopped to load or unload children and is displaying its flashing red lights or extended stop arm. If you approach a school bus that has its lights flashing, you should stop before reaching the bus and turn off your siren. Next, you should wait for the bus driver to make sure the children are safe, close the bus door, and turn off the flashing lights. Only then may you carefully proceed past the stopped school bus.

Right-of-Way Privileges

State motor vehicle statutes or codes often grant an emergency vehicle such as an ambulance the right to disregard the rules of the road when responding to an emergency. However, the operator of an emergency vehicle must still continue to operate in a safe fashion so as not to endanger people or property under any circumstances.

Consider this case: An ambulance is approaching an intersection that is controlled by a four-way stop sign. The ambulance, with lights and siren turned on, proceeds through the intersection without slowing or stopping and crashes into a vehicle coming from its right. Did the operator of the ambulance act appropriately by going through the intersection in this manner?

Right-of-way privileges for ambulances vary by state. Some states allow you to proceed through a red light or stop sign after you stop and make sure it is safe to go on. Other states allow you to proceed through a controlled intersection with due regard, using flashing lights and siren. This means you may proceed only if you consider the safety of all people who are using the highway. If you fail to use due regard, your service may be sued. If you are found to be at fault, you may personally have to pay punitive damages or face civil and criminal sanctions.

Get to know your local right-of-way privileges. Exercise them only when it is absolutely necessary for the patient's well-being. The use of lights and audible warning devices is a matter of state and local practice and protocol.

Use of Escorts

Using a police escort is an extremely dangerous practice. When other motorists hear a siren and see a police vehicle passing, they might assume the police vehicle is the only emergency vehicle and not see the ambulance. The only time an escort is justified is when you are in an unfamiliar area and truly need a guide more than an escort. In such cases, vehicles using warning lights or siren should use different tones to alert other motorists and be prepared to stop if needed. If you are being guided, follow at a safe distance. Assume nearby traffic will not be aware of your presence.

Specific Driving Situations

Intersection Hazards

Intersection crashes are the most common and usually the most serious type of crash in which ambulances are involved. Always be alert and careful when approaching an intersection. Change the siren tone before you reach the intersection. If you are on an urgent call and cannot wait for traffic lights to change, you should still come to a brief stop at the light; look around for other motorists and pedestrians before proceeding into the intersection. Scan the intersection and your mirrors for hazards and clear each lane before you proceed. Direct your full attention to the road while proceeding through the intersection; this is not the time to talk on the radio or consult the automatic vehicle location system map.

Motorists who time the traffic lights present a serious hazard. You may arrive at an intersection while the light is green. At the same time, a motorist who is timing the lights on the cross street arrives at the intersection. The motorist has a red light but knows it is about to turn green and is expecting to go through. This creates the possibility for a serious crash to occur.

Another common intersection hazard occurs when multiple emergency vehicles are responding through the same intersection. Having convoys of emergency vehicles is not uncommon because multiple resources respond from a similar location. This is a dangerous practice. A motorist who has yielded the right of way to the first vehicle may proceed into the intersection without expecting a second vehicle. You should exercise extreme caution in these situations. To signal motorists that a second unit is approaching, use a siren tone that is different from that of the first vehicle.

You must also be aware that additional emergency vehicles responding to the same call or to a different emergency call may be coming through the same intersection from a different direction. Serious accidents could occur when two emergency vehicles enter the same intersection unless both of the drivers are operating with due regard, allowing them the time to recognize the other vehicle and safely proceed through the intersection.

Highways

When you are responding to an emergency call and you must travel on the highway, you should turn off your emergency lights and siren until you have reached the far left lane. Turning off your emergency devices minimizes the possibility that other drivers will get confused and not know what to do or where to go.

When driving on a highway with your emergency devices activated, you should travel in the far left-hand lane, also known as the "passing lane." This allows the ambulance to safely pass vehicles, while still leaving a safety corridor on the left side of the ambulance in case of emergency or unexpected obstacles.

When you exit the highway, you should follow the same procedures as when you entered the highway: turn off all emergency devices, move onto the off-ramp, and then turn on the emergency lights and siren if necessary.

Unpaved Roadways

When you are required to drive the ambulance on an unpaved roadway, special care must be taken. Unpaved roadways often have uneven surfaces, loose gravel, and large potholes. While responding on this type of roadway, operate the vehicle at a lower speed and maintain a firm grip on the steering wheel to maintain complete control of the ambulance at all times. During the transport phase, these practices will help to provide a smoother ride for the EMT and patient on the stretcher.

School Zones

When you respond through a school zone with your emergency lights turned on, it is important to remember that the lights and siren tend to attract children to the roadway and create a potential hazard. In many states, it is unlawful for an emergency vehicle to exceed the speed limit in school zones, regardless of the condition of the patient.

Distractions

As technology progresses, so will the distractions you will face while operating the ambulance. Although MDCs and GPS devices are necessary to assist EMTs in determining the location of the call, these devices, along with using the vehicle's mounted mobile radio, listening to the stereo, talking on your cell phone, and eating or drinking, create additional driving hazards. While the ambulance is in motion, you should focus solely on driving and anticipate roadway hazards. Your partner should operate the MDC, GPS device, and portable radios or turn on the siren. Minimizing distractions allows for a safer response and minimizes the potential for mishaps.

Driving Alone

Although driving alone is not a standard practice or even allowable in certain systems, there may be an occasion when you need to respond to a scene by yourself in the ambulance and meet your partner at the scene. When presented with this situation, you have additional duties and responsibilities, such as figuring out the safest route to the call, operating the radios and emergency warning devices, and mentally preparing for the call. Situations such as these demand your complete attention and focus.

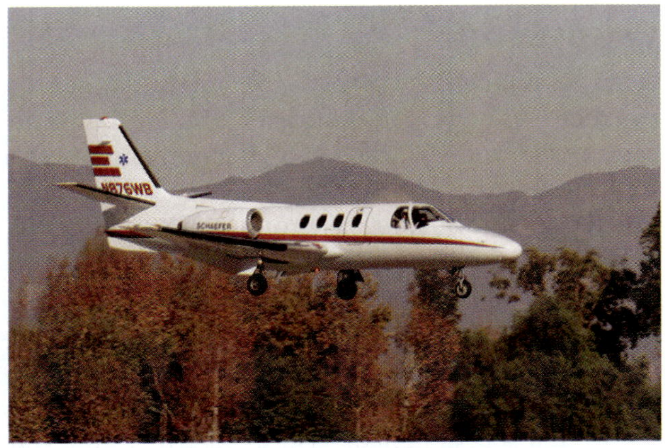

A

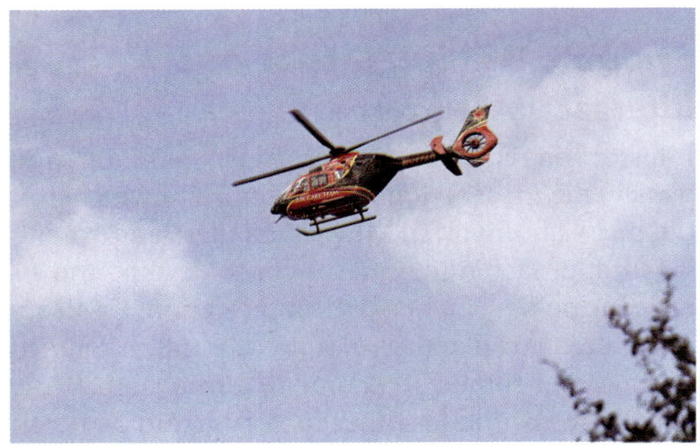

B

FIGURE 36-26 A. Fixed-wing aircraft are generally used to transfer patients from one hospital to another over distances greater than 200 to 250 miles. **B.** A rotary-wing aircraft, or helicopter, is used to help provide emergency medical care to patients who need to be transported quickly over shorter distances.

Air Medical Services

Air medical services are used to evacuate medical and trauma patients. They are capable of landing at or near the scene to provide rapid transport of patients to an appropriate hospital, including trauma centers, stroke centers, or cardiac centers. There are two basic types of air medical units: fixed-wing and rotary-wing, otherwise known as helicopters (**FIGURE 36-26**). Fixed-wing aircraft generally are used for interhospital patient transfers over distances greater than 200 to 250 miles. For shorter distances, rotary-wing aircraft are more efficient.

Specifically trained medical flight crews accompany all air medical services flights. Your role in fixed-wing aircraft transfers probably will be limited to providing ground transport for the patient and medical flight crew between the hospital and the airport.

Rotary-wing aircraft have become an important tool in providing emergency medical services that are otherwise not possible by local EMS responses. Air medical services can provide or sustain a higher level of care; deliver specialized supplies, such as blood products; expedite patient delivery to definitive care for time-critical interventions; and access patients from remote settings that other EMS agencies cannot reach in a timely manner.[9] Trauma patient survival is directly related to the time that elapses between injury and definitive treatment. Most helicopters that are used for emergency medical operations fly well in excess of 100 mph in a straight line, without road or traffic hazards, straight to a hospital helipad. The crew may include flight paramedics, flight nurses, specialty clinicians such as respiratory therapists, perfusionists, or physicians.

Familiarize yourself with the capabilities, protocols, and methods for accessing helicopters in your area. Most rural and suburban EMS jurisdictions and many urban systems have the capability to perform helicopter patient evacuations or have a mutual aid agreement with another agency such as police or hospital-based air medical service. The following discussion provides some general guidelines that you should be familiar with when considering whether to initiate an air medical services operation. It is an introduction to safe operations and is not intended to be substituted for the more extensive courses available locally. Helicopter services provide training in ground operations and safety for EMS systems, fire services, and first responders.

Words of Wisdom

Air medical services are commonly called **medevac** in wilderness and military settings and *HEMS* (which stands for helicopter EMS) in other EMS or interfacility responses.

Calling for Air Medical Services

Every agency has specific criteria for the type of patient who may receive medical evacuation and how and when to call for air medical services. These basic guidelines will help you understand the process better.

- **Why call for air medical services?**
  - The transport time to the hospital by ground ambulance is too long considering the patient's condition. This benefit in transport time could be greater in mountainous areas or other difficult terrain.
  - The patient requires urgent initiation of specialized treatment that is not locally available. The helicopter may be called to the scene or to the initial receiving hospital to transfer a patient to a facility that can provide definitive care.
  - The patient requires advanced care that you are unable to provide, such as inserting advanced airways or placing a chest tube.
  - A ground ambulance is unable to reach the patient in a timely manner, possibly because of road, traffic, or environmental conditions. However, the helicopter may respond directly to the scene.
  - There are multiple patients who will overwhelm local prehospital resources or the resources at the hospital reachable by ground transport.
- **Who receives air medical services?**
  - Medical evacuations should be used for patients with time-dependent injuries or illnesses. Patients suspected of having a stroke, heart attack, or serious traumatic injuries may benefit from evacuation via helicopter.
  - Serious conditions that may require the use of a helicopter may be found in remote areas and involve scuba diving accidents, near drownings, or skiing and wilderness accidents.
  - Other patients who may require medical evacuation are high-risk obstetric patients, candidates for limb replantation (for amputations), and patients requiring air transport to a burn center, a hyperbaric chamber center, or a venomous bite center. Because specific criteria vary by service, familiarize yourself with the criteria in your system used to call for this lifesaving service.
- **Whom do you call?**
  - Generally, your dispatcher must be notified first.
  - In some regions, after air medical services have been initiated, the ground EMS crew may be able to access the flight crew on a specifically designated radio frequency for one-on-one communications. If available, it is important to keep this frequency clear of chatter and lengthy communications. You may be asked to give a brief report including the patient's weight, clinical condition, and an update on the patient's condition. In this case, you should gather your thoughts and speak clearly and concisely, avoiding information that is not pertinent. Another important topic of communication between the ground and flight EMS crews will be where to land the helicopter. This will be covered in the next section.

Words of Wisdom

When you request air medical services, the pilot and crew will look at the call location, evaluate the weather patterns between you and them, and decide whether the flight can be made safely. Air medical services may be located more than 30 miles (48 km) from the call location, meaning the weather at their base or en route may be different than the weather at the scene. Understand that while it may be sunny and calm at your location, weather conditions may cause the flight crew to determine that it is unsafe to fly to your location or to the receiving hospital.

Safety Tips

The most dangerous phases of air transport are the takeoff and landing. It is essential that at least one person be dedicated to tasks associated with these phases of flight. This person should have access to the channel being used for radio communications and should not have patient care responsibilities. The person overseeing the landing of the aircraft should be communicating landing zone information such as obstacles, wind direction and speed, and any specialized information needed for a safe landing. Patient information should not be communicated during this phase; the flight crew will be able to communicate face to face with the patient care team after landing. EMS crews should cancel the helicopter response if there is evidence that the conditions would place the flight crew or the ground crew in danger or if the reasons for helicopter transport no longer exist.[9] In the event that several air medical organizations serve an area, helicopter shopping should be avoided. Helicopter shopping is the practice of calling multiple air medical services to take a call when one has refused the job because of safety concerns. Central coordinating centers can help avoid this problem.

Establishing a Landing Zone

A benefit of helicopter response is that helicopters do not need an airport to land. An important part of conducting a helicopter response is choosing the best location to establish a landing zone. Establishing a landing zone is the responsibility of either the ground EMS crew or a local fire department. It involves more than simply looking for a clear space. You must be prepared to take action to ensure the flight crew is able to land and take off safely. Similar to an airplane, a helicopter's approach and departure involve the aircraft descending or climbing at a consistent rate at a slight angle. Keeping in mind that the helicopter is unlikely to fly straight down or straight up, you should consider the following when selecting and establishing a landing zone:

- Ensure the area is a hard or grassy level surface that measures 100 × 100 ft (30 × 30 m) (recommended) and no less than 60 × 60 ft (18 × 18 m) (**FIGURE 36-27**). If the site is not level, notify the flight crew of the steepness and direction of the slope. The slope should not exceed 5 to 7 degrees.
- Ensure the area is clear of any loose debris that could become airborne and strike the helicopter, the patient, bystanders, or the EMS crew. This includes branches, trash bins, flares, sheets, caution tape, and medical equipment.
- Examine the immediate area for any overhead or tall hazards such as power lines, telephone cables, antennas, and tall or leaning trees. If you see any of these hazards, immediately inform the flight crew because an alternative landing site may be required. It is imperative to communicate what you can see from the ground. Low-altitude hazards should not be overlooked by ground contact. Such items as guardrails and reflective delineator posts can be a dangerous obstacle for the aircraft. At altitude, the flight crew may not be able to see hazards that you can see easily from the ground, especially at night. The flight crew may request that the hazard be marked or illuminated by weighted cones or that an emergency vehicle

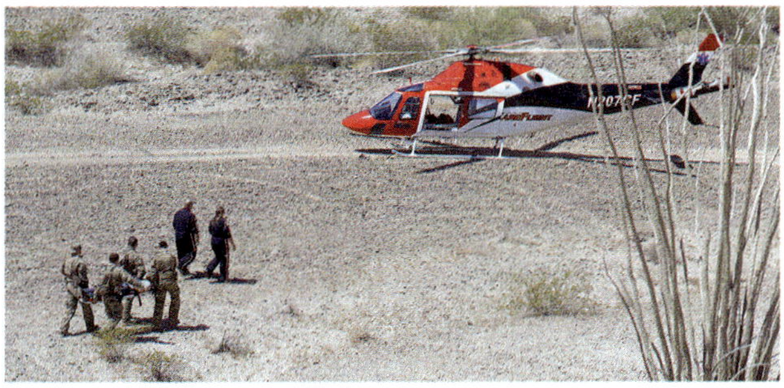

FIGURE 36-27 A landing area for an EMS helicopter should be a level surface measuring 100 ft × 100 ft (30 m × 30 m).

with its lights turned on be positioned next to or under the potential hazard.

- To mark the landing site, use weighted cones or lights designed for air operations, or position emergency vehicles at the corners of the landing zone with the headlights facing inward to form an "X." This procedure may be valuable during night landings as well. It is common for fire suppression personnel to help mark the landing site because they are often called to the scene to stand by. Never use caution tape or people to mark the site. Flares should not be used because they can become airborne, and they have the potential to start a fire or cause an explosion.
- Move all nonessential people and vehicles to a safe distance outside of the landing zone.
- Both the approach and departure will be performed into the wind. If the wind is strong, communicate the direction of the wind to the flight crew. They may request that you create some form of wind directional device to aid their approach.

Words of Wisdom

Consider working with local helicopter programs to establish predesignated landing zones. Requesting a helicopter can be much less stressful if your service has already identified several places that are suitable for a helicopter landing zone.

Ensuring Safety During Landing and Patient Transfer

Helicopter safety is a combination of using good sense and maintaining a constant awareness of the need for personal safety. You should stay away from the helicopter and go only where the pilot or flight crew member directs you. The most important rule is to keep a safe distance from the aircraft whenever it is on the ground. The engines may stay on and the rotor blades remain spinning if the flight crew does not expect to remain on the ground for a long time. However, this practice of "hot loading" and "hot unloading" is going out of favor due to safety concerns and the speed at which the helicopter can start up and slow down. If the helicopter is running, EMTs should stay outside the landing zone perimeter unless directed to come to the aircraft by the pilot or a member of the flight crew. Usually, the flight crew will come to the EMTs; they will carry their own equipment and do not require any assistance inside the landing zone. If you are asked to enter the landing zone, stay away from the rear of the aircraft, where the tail rotor is located; the tips of its blades move so rapidly that they are essentially invisible. Remove any loose items from yourself or the stretcher, including baseball hats, sheets, or loose medical supplies. Always approach a helicopter from the front, even if it is not running, and you should approach only after the pilot or a flight crew member signals it is clear to do so. If you imagine the front of the helicopter as the number 12 on a clock, then you should enter only the area between the 10 o'clock and 2 o'clock positions (**FIGURE 36-28**). If you must move from one side of the helicopter to another, go around the front. Never duck under the body, the tail boom, or the rear section of the helicopter. The pilot cannot see you in these areas.

Another area of concern is the height of the main rotor blade. On many aircraft, it is flexible and may dip as low as 4 ft (1.2 m) off the ground (**FIGURE 36-29**). When you approach the aircraft, walk in a crouched position. Wind gusts can alter the blade height without warning, so protect yourself and your equipment as you carry it under the blades.

When accompanying a flight crew member, you must follow directions exactly. Never open any

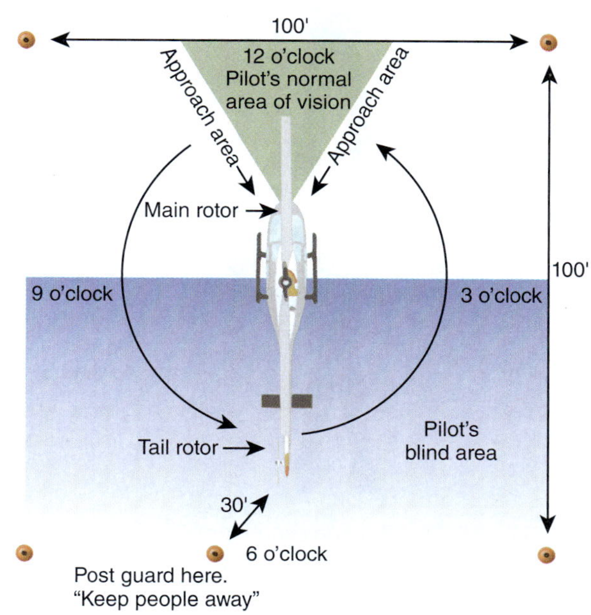

FIGURE 36-28 Safe-approach zone.

aircraft door or move equipment unless instructed by a crew member. When told to approach the aircraft, use extreme caution and pay constant attention to hazards.

Keep the following guidelines in mind when operating at a landing zone:

- Familiarize yourself with helicopter hand signals used within your jurisdiction (**FIGURE 36-30**).

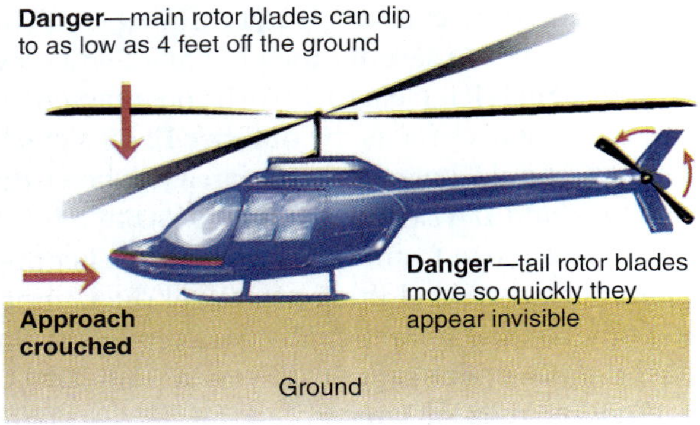

FIGURE 36-29 The main rotor blade of the helicopter is flexible and may dip as low as 4 feet (1.2 m) off the ground depending on the type of helicopter.

- Do not approach the helicopter unless instructed and accompanied by flight crew.
- Ensure all patient care equipment is properly secured to the stretcher and that the patient is fastened as well. This includes oxygen tanks, cervical collars, and head stabilizers. Any loose articles or belongings such as hats, coats, or bags that belong to the patient or crew should not be brought into the landing zone and will likely need to be transported to the hospital by ground.
- Be aware that some helicopters may load patients from the side, whereas others have rear-loading doors. Regardless of where the patient is being loaded, always approach the aircraft from the front unless otherwise instructed by the flight crew. It is very important that the pilot be able to see anyone who comes near the aircraft. Always take the same path when exiting and moving away from the helicopter, and move the patient headfirst unless otherwise instructed based on the aircraft type.
- Smoking, open flames, and flares are prohibited within 50 ft (15 m) of the aircraft at all times.
- Wear eye protection during approach and takeoff.

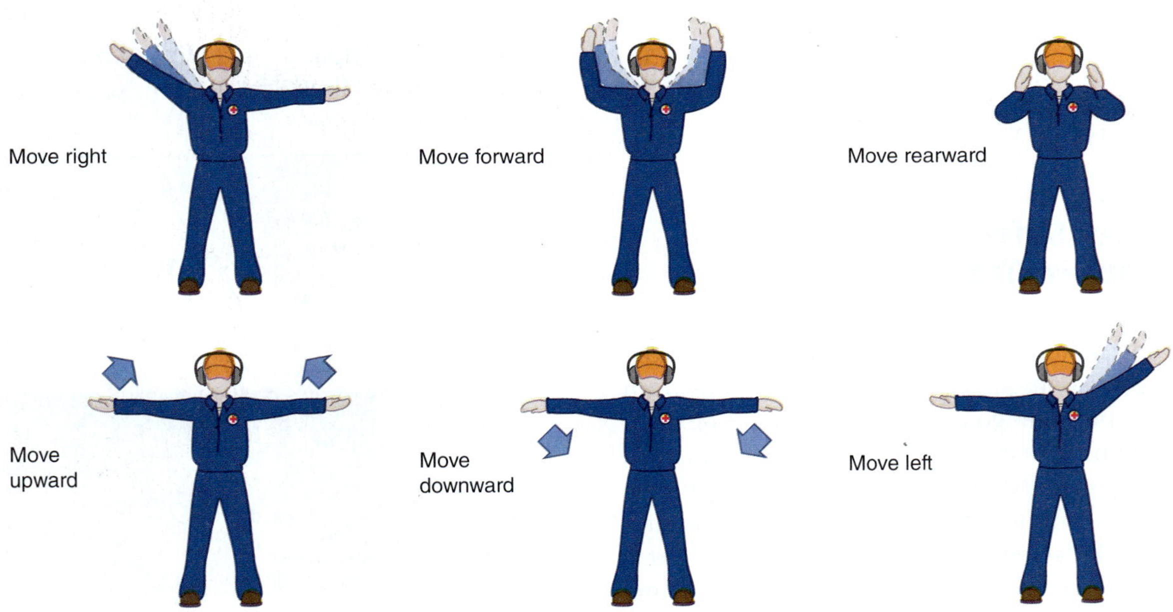

FIGURE 36-30 Some examples of helicopter hand signals. Be familiar with those used within your jurisdiction. The person giving the hand signals is facing the pilot, and their movements are described from the pilot's perspective. For example, in the first image, the person points to their own left to indicate movement to the pilot's right. In the third image, the person appears to be shoving an object away to indicate rearward motion by the pilot.

Avoiding Communication Issues

When interacting with other agencies, there is always the possibility of communication issues. Responses involving air medical services are no exception. Although the typical EMS system has a specific and well-defined jurisdiction, air medical services respond to requests throughout a large, multijurisdictional area. Because of this large area with numerous jurisdictions, the air medical service interacts with many services on a multitude of different radio frequencies.

To prevent miscommunication, a request for air medical services should include a ground contact radio channel (typically a preestablished mutual aid channel), as well as a call sign of the unit with which the flight crew should make contact.

Special Considerations

Night Landings

Nighttime operations are considerably more hazardous than daytime operations because of the darkness. Always make certain the flight crew is aware of any overhead hazards or obstructions and illuminate these if possible. Remember that what is easy for you to see from the ground may not be visible at all from the aircraft. The pilot will generally fly over the area at least twice at varying altitudes with the helicopter's lights on in order to confirm potential obstacles and overhead wires. Pilots and flight crew members often use night-vision goggles during nighttime landing zone operations. Do not shine spotlights, flashlights, or any other lights in the air; they may temporarily blind the pilot. Instead, direct low-intensity headlights or lanterns toward the ground at the landing site from opposite corners to form an "X" at the center of the landing zone.

Landing on Uneven Ground

If the helicopter must land on a grade (uneven surface), extra caution is advised. The slope should not exceed 5° to 7°. The main rotor blade will be closer to the ground on the uphill side. In this situation, approach the aircraft only from the downhill side or as directed by the flight crew (**FIGURE 36-31**). Do not move the patient to the helicopter until the crew has signaled that they are ready to receive you.

Limiting Factors for Air Medical Services

When making the decision to request air medical services, several important factors need to be taken into consideration, including weather, the environment/terrain, altitude, airspeed limitations, and cabin size. Helicopters are unable to operate in severe weather conditions such as thunderstorms,

YOU are the EMT

After turning around and determining a new route, your partner advises you there is now a 25-minute transport time. Your partner also warns that you are approaching a stopped school bus with its stop sign out, and children are exiting the bus.

Recording Time: 22 Minutes	
Level of consciousness	Alert and oriented
Respirations	20 breaths/min; adequate depth
Pulse	94 beats/min; strong and regular
Skin	Baseline color, warm, and dry
Blood pressure	142/90 mm Hg
Oxygen saturation (Spo_2)	97% (on room air)

8. When traveling in the emergency mode, how do you respond to a stopped school bus?

9. Where do most serious ambulance crashes occur, and what should you do to help avoid a crash?

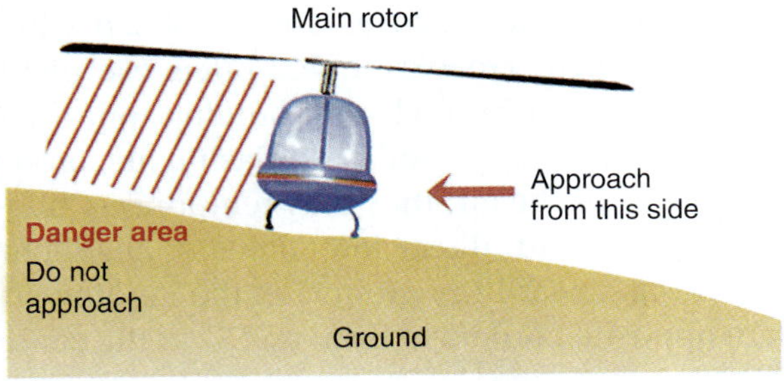

FIGURE 36-31 Approach a helicopter on a grade only from the downhill side.

Words of Wisdom

Disadvantages of using air medical services include the financial cost and the safety risk (ie, helicopter and plane crashes are more likely to be fatal). Although these considerations are important, if the patient's needs warrant air medical services and the circumstances allow for this response mode, then air medical services should be requested.

blizzards, and heavy rain. The environment may pose a risk as well. In mountainous or desert terrain, there may be too many hazards in the immediate vicinity to safely land the helicopter in the desired location.

Because of the helicopter cabin's confined space, helicopters are limited in the number of patients who can be safely transported and by the size of the patient whom they can safely transport. Although a helicopter may be able to safely lift off with a 500-pound (227-kg) patient, because of the person's size and girth, it may be impossible to safely fit and secure the patient into the cabin area. Some systems have access to bariatric helicopters, which can accommodate greater weight; EMTs should become familiar with the resources available in their area.

YOU are the EMT SUMMARY

1. What attributes should an emergency vehicle operator possess?

The EMT who is serving as an emergency vehicle operator should possess good situational awareness, be able to make reasonable decisions, and maintain a calm demeanor in stressful situations. Operating an emergency vehicle requires the driver's undivided attention and constant awareness of possible dangers. From deteriorating weather conditions to inattentive drivers on the roadway, many threats may be encountered while responding to an emergency. The driver will have to account for all of these factors while ensuring safe operation of the vehicle. Emergency vehicle operator courses are often required before personnel are cleared to operate an emergency vehicle. These courses are beneficial in teaching best practices specific to ambulance operation, including maintaining a safe distance from other vehicles, passing through an intersection, and driving with lights and siren activated. You must always operate the vehicle in a safe fashion. Remember, you will be unable to help anyone if you do not reach the scene or the hospital safely.

2. What factors should you consider before responding to the scene?

Before you begin your response, you need to consider several factors to ensure a safe, quick response. First, you must identify the location of the scene and the route you intend to take. Notify your dispatch center that you are responding. Given that the nature of the call involves the potential for violence (assault), you should ask your dispatch center if the scene has been secured by law enforcement officers and is safe for you to enter. With the scene being close to your station, you want to take the time to make sure the scene is safe. You do not want to rush into the scene only to realize you are in imminent danger. Stage your ambulance in a safe location that is close to the scene, but far enough away from any danger, until law enforcement has secured the scene.

You must also consider the weather conditions and traffic when deciding how you will respond to the scene. When there are poor weather conditions or heavy traffic, you will need to be extra vigilant and cautious when responding. It may be most appropriate to respond without lights and siren due to the weather conditions and the need to wait for law enforcement to secure the scene. It may be appropriate to respond cautiously with lights and siren if the scene has already been secured by law enforcement and there is heavy traffic through which you will need to travel. You must make a reasonable decision after looking at the specific circumstances and factors involved in the call. Remember that safety should always remain at the forefront.

YOU are the EMT SUMMARY continued

3. Based on the mechanism of injury and patient presentation, what equipment do you anticipate needing?

For this patient, you would need the jump kit, which should contain anything you might need within the first 5 minutes after making contact with any patient, including splinting and bandaging supplies. If she were unstable, splinting and bandaging would be delayed until you are en route and all other necessary assessments and treatments are completed.

4. What assessment and treatment should be performed on scene and what should be delayed until you are in the ambulance and en route to the hospital?

This patient is stable, with only an isolated injury to the left lower extremity. There was no loss of consciousness, and vital signs are within normal limits. Because this is not a priority load-and-go patient, you should complete your secondary assessment on scene and take the time to splint her leg.

Once you are en route to the hospital, repeat the primary assessment, including taking vital signs, and reassess the effectiveness of any interventions. Now would also be the time to treat any minor secondary injuries. Remember that stable patients should be reassessed every 15 minutes, and critical or unstable patients should be reassessed every 5 minutes.

5. How would you determine whether to use lights and siren during transport of this patient?

The transport mode (ie, lights and siren [emergency mode] versus no lights and siren [nonemergency mode]) is determined by the patient's current condition and anticipated clinical outcome. In this case, the patient is stable; she is alert and oriented, her vital signs are stable, and she has no life-threatening conditions (ie, airway problems, uncontrolled bleeding). Therefore, the use of lights and siren during transport is not indicated.

6. What should you consider when deciding whether it is appropriate to turn on the lights and siren to maneuver through traffic?

Regulations regarding vehicle operations vary by state and by city, but some regulations are the same regardless of location. Emergency vehicle operators have certain limited privileges in every state. However, these privileges do not reduce your liability in the event of a crash.

Three basic principles govern the use of warning lights and siren on an ambulance:

1. The unit must be, to the best of your knowledge, on a true emergency call.
2. The use of lights and siren must be authorized by your agency and medical director for the category and condition of the patient you are transporting.
3. Audible and visual warning devices must be used simultaneously.

The unit must be operated with due regard for the safety of all others, on and off the roadway.

In this situation, the patient's condition clearly does not warrant the use of lights and siren. If you choose to use an emergency transport, you will put yourself, your partner, your patient, and other motorists at risk. You could also face possible litigation. You have time to take an alternate route and avoid creating more hazards as other drivers try to move out of the way.

7. If you are in an unfamiliar area and do not know an alternate route, what are your options?

The best option would be to use a GPS device to navigate through an unfamiliar area. Another option is to call the dispatcher via radio and ask for street-by-street directions. As a last resort, you can wait for the traffic to clear.

8. When traveling in the emergency mode, how do you respond to a stopped school bus?

Although state motor vehicle statutes or codes often grant an emergency vehicle certain privileges when responding to an emergency, special privileges are not given to emergency vehicles when driving through a school zone or approaching a stopped school bus that is loading or unloading children. In these situations, the emergency vehicle operator is required to obey the law like any other motorist.

An emergency vehicle operator is never allowed to pass a school bus that has stopped to load or unload children and is displaying its red warning lights and extended stop arm. If you approach a school bus that is loading or unloading children, you should stop before you reach the bus and turn off your siren. Wait for the bus driver to make sure the children are safe, the bus door has been closed, and its red warning lights are turned off. Only then may you cautiously proceed past the stopped school bus.

YOU are the EMT SUMMARY continued

9. Where do most serious ambulance crashes occur, and what should you do to help avoid a crash?

Intersection crashes are the most common and usually the most serious type of crash involving ambulances. Therefore, the emergency vehicle operator must be especially careful and alert when approaching an intersection. If you are operating the vehicle in emergency mode and cannot wait for traffic lights to change, you should still come to a complete stop, look around for other motorists and pedestrians, and then cautiously proceed. The same applies if you approach an intersection with stop signs.

Prep Kit

Ready for Review

- Today's ambulances are designed according to strict government regulations based on national standards.
- The six-pointed Star of Life emblem identifies vehicles that meet federal specifications as licensed or certified ambulances.
- An ambulance call has nine phases:
  - Preparation for the call
  - Dispatch
  - En route
  - Arrival at scene
  - Transfer of the patient to the ambulance
  - En route to the receiving facility (transport)
  - At the receiving facility (delivery)
  - En route to the station
  - Postrun
- Certain items, such as sterile gloves, must be available on the ambulance at all times, as dictated by state and jurisdictional requirements.
- Every ambulance must be staffed with at least one EMT in the patient compartment whenever a patient is being transported. However, two EMTs are strongly recommended. Some services may operate with a non-EMT driver and a single EMT in the patient compartment.
- Check all medical equipment and supplies daily, including all the oxygen supplies, the jump kit, splints, dressings and bandages, backboards and other spinal stabilization equipment, and the emergency obstetric kit.
- During the postrun phase, you should complete and file any additional written reports and inform dispatch of your status, location, and availability. Perform a routine inspection to ensure the ambulance is ready to respond to the next call.
- Learning how to properly operate your vehicle is just as important as learning how to care for patients when you arrive on the scene.
  - The first rule of safe driving in an emergency vehicle is that speed does not save lives; good care does.
  - The second rule is that the operator and all passengers must wear seat belts and shoulder restraints at all times.
- Air medical services are used to evacuate medical and trauma patients. There are two basic types of air medical units: fixed-wing and rotary-wing, otherwise known as helicopters.

Vital Vocabulary

air medical services Fixed-wing and rotary-wing (known as helicopters) aircraft that have been modified for medical care; used to evacuate and transport patients with life-threatening injuries to treatment facilities.

ambulance A specialized vehicle for treating and transporting sick and injured patients.

blind spots Areas of the road that are blocked from your view by your vehicle or mirrors.

Prep Kit continued

cleaning The process of removing dirt, dust, blood, or other visible contaminants from a surface.

cushion of safety A safe distance between your vehicle and any vehicles around you.

decontamination The process of cleaning, disinfecting, and/or sterilizing clothing, equipment, vehicles, and personnel; may involve removing or neutralizing radiation, chemical, or other hazardous material.

disinfection The killing of pathogenic agents by direct application of chemicals.

first-responder vehicles Specialized vehicles used to transport EMS equipment and personnel to the scenes of medical emergencies.

high-level disinfection The killing of pathogenic agents by using potent means of disinfection.

hydroplaning Occurs when the tires of a vehicle are lifted off the road surface as a result of water piling up underneath them, making the vehicle feel as though it is floating.

jump kit A portable kit containing items that are used in the initial care of the patient.

medevac A term primarily used in wilderness and military settings to describe medical evacuation of a patient by helicopter.

spotter A person who assists a driver in backing up an ambulance to help adjust for blind spots at the back of the vehicle.

Star of Life The six-pointed star emblem that identifies vehicles that meet federal specifications as licensed or certified ambulances.

sterilization A process, such as heating, that removes microbial contamination.

References

1. National Fire Protection Association. *NFPA 1900: Standard for Aircraft Rescue and Firefighting Vehicles, Automotive Fire Apparatus, Wildland Fire Apparatus, and Automotive Ambulances*. Quincy, MA: NFPA; 2024.
2. Kupas DF, Zavadsky M, Burton B, et al. Joint statement on lights and siren vehicle operations on emergency medical services responses. *Prehosp Emerg Care*. 2022;26(3):459–461.
3. Neulander MJ, Siddiqui DI, Mountfort S. EMS lights and sirens. *StatPearls*. National Library of Medicine website. https://www.ncbi.nlm.nih.gov/books/NBK482203/. Updated September 12, 2022. Accessed May 5, 2025.
4. National Highway Traffic Safety Administration, US Department of Transportation. Analysis of ground ambulance crash data from 2012 to 2018. EMS.gov website. https://www.ems.gov/assets/Analysis-of-Ground-Ambulance-Crash-Data-From-2012-to-2018_FINAL.pdf. Published July 2023. Accessed May 5, 2025.
5. NHTSA publishes an analysis of 7 years of national ambulance crash data. US Fire Administration website. https://www.usfa.fema.gov/blog/nhtsa-publishes-data-on-ground-ambulance-crashes/. Published October 5, 2023. Accessed May 5, 2025.
6. Matthews P. Horton, IMMI rollout airbags for ambulance crew safety in patient compartment. Firehouse website. https://www.firehouse.com/apparatus/type/ambulance/news/53028988/horton-immi-rollout-mbrace-airbags-for-ambulance-crew-safety-in-patient-compartment. Published March 20, 2023. Accessed May 5, 2025.
7. de Anda HH, Moy HP. EMS Ground transport safety. *StatPearls*. National Library of Medicine website. https://www.ncbi.nlm.nih.gov/books/NBK558971/. Updated May 8, 2023. Accessed May 5, 2025.
8. US Department of Transportation, National Highway Traffic Safety Administration. Working group best-practice recommendations for the safe transportation of children in emergency ground ambulances. National Child Safety Passenger Board website. https://www.cpsboard.org/wp-content/uploads/2016/03/Safe-Transportation-of-Children-in-Ambulances.pdf. Published September 2012. Accessed May 5, 2025.
9. Lyng JW, Braithwaite S, Abraham H, et al. Appropriate air medical services utilization and recommendations for integration of air medical services resources into the EMS system of care: a joint position statement and resource document of NAEMSP, ACEP, and AMPA. *Prehosp Emerg Care*. 2021;25(6):854–873.

Additional Resources

Murray B, Kue R. The use of emergency lights and sirens by ambulances and their effect on patient outcomes and public safety: a comprehensive review of the literature. *Prehosp Disaster Med*. 2017;32(2):209–216.

National Association of State EMS Officials. *National EMS Scope of Practice Model 2019: Including Change Notices 1.0 and 2.0.* Washington, DC: National Highway Traffic Safety Administration; August 2021. Report No. DOT HS 813-151.

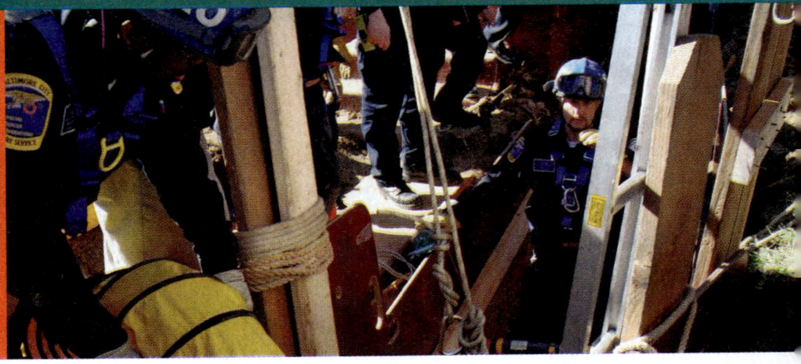

Chapter 37

Vehicle Extrication and Special Rescue

NATIONAL EMS EDUCATION STANDARD COMPETENCIES

EMS Operations

Knowledge of operational roles and responsibilities to ensure patient, public, and personnel safety.

Rescue Operations

- Safety principles of rescue operations (pp 1393–1397)

KNOWLEDGE OBJECTIVES

1. Explain the responsibilities of an emergency medical technician (EMT) in patient rescue and vehicle extrication. (p 1382)
2. Discuss how to ensure safety at the scene of a rescue incident, including scene size-up and the selection of the proper personal protective equipment and additional necessary gear. (pp 1382–1386)
3. Describe examples of vehicle safety components that may be hazardous to both EMTs and patients following a collision and how to mitigate their dangers. (pp 1386–1388)
4. Define the terms extrication and entrapment. (pp 1382–1383)
5. Describe the 10 phases of vehicle extrication and the role of the EMT during each one. (pp 1383–1392)
6. Discuss the various factors related to ensuring situational safety at the site of a vehicle extrication, including controlling traffic flow, performing a 360° assessment, stabilizing the vehicle, dealing with unique hazards, and evaluating the need for additional resources. (pp 1384–1388)
7. Describe the special precautions the EMT should follow to protect the patient during a vehicle extrication. (pp 1388–1389)
8. Explain the different factors that must be considered before attempting to gain access to the patient during an incident that requires extrication. (pp 1388–1389)
9. Explain the difference between simple access and complex access in vehicle extrication. (pp 1389–1391)
10. Discuss patient care considerations related to assisting with rapid extrication, providing emergency care to a trapped patient, and removing and transferring a patient. (pp 1391–1392)
11. Describe examples of situations that would require special technical rescue teams and the EMT's role in these situations. (pp 1393–1397)

SKILLS OBJECTIVES

There are no skills objectives for this chapter.

Introduction

As an EMT, you will usually not be responsible for rescue, though you may assist with extrication. Rescue involves many different processes and environments, including vehicle, water, structural collapse, and wilderness rescue. These incidents require training beyond the level of the EMT. You must understand the basic concepts of extrication in order to function effectively as part of a team during a rescue incident. In some cases, you may be the first emergency unit to arrive at the scene, and your initial actions may determine how efficiently the rescue is completed.

This chapter begins with a discussion of safety at the scene of a rescue incident, followed by the 10 phases of extrication. In most cases, once you have reached the patient, extrication will occur around you and the patient. Communication between you and the personnel performing the extrication is vital.

Safety

You must always be prepared, mentally and physically, for any incident that requires rescue or extrication. Your priority as an EMT is to provide patient care. However, your personal safety and the safety of your team are paramount and must be addressed before patient care is initiated. Safety begins with the proper mindset and the proper protective equipment.

The equipment you use and the gear you wear will depend on the hazards you expect to encounter, as well as what you observe during your scene size-up (**FIGURE 37-1**). Such protective gear may include turnout gear, a helmet, hearing protection, and a fire extinguisher. However, the importance of wearing blood- and fluid-impermeable gloves at all times during patient contact cannot be overemphasized. If you will be involved with extrication, wear a pair of leather gloves over your disposable gloves to protect you from injury when handling ropes, tools, broken glass, hot or cold objects, or sharp metal.

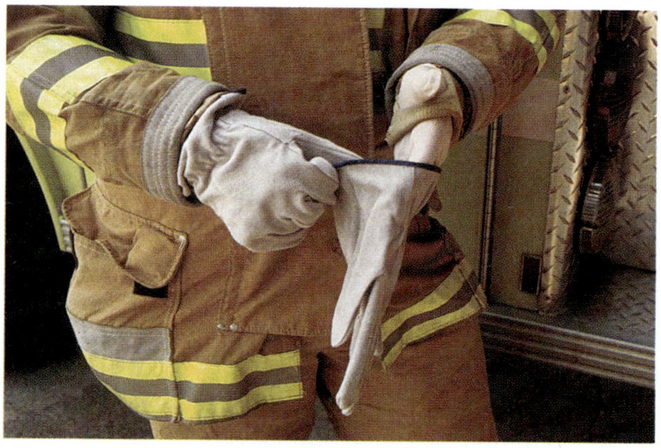

FIGURE 37-1 Proper protective equipment varies depending on the anticipated hazards.

Vehicle Safety Systems

A variety of safety systems are used in modern vehicles. Although many of these devices are useful when the vehicle is in motion, they can become hazards after the vehicle has been involved in a crash.

Shock-absorbing bumpers provide vehicle protection from low-speed impact. Following a frontal or rear-end crash, the shock absorbers within these bumpers may be compressed or loaded. Avoid standing directly in front of such bumpers, and

YOU are the EMT

It is 1400 hours and your unit is dispatched to a local beach access where callers have reported an aircraft has crashed. A small plane with two passengers onboard was flying over a popular tourist attraction when it began to experience a loss of power and crashed near a beach access. On your arrival, the local fire department has already completed a 360° assessment of the scene, and the captain advises you that the scene is safe for you to approach. You find that the pilot has sustained massive trauma to the head and chest that is incompatible with life. You note that firefighters are attempting to access a passenger who is entangled in the wreckage located just behind the pilot's seat.

1. What information is obtained from a 360° assessment of an aircraft crash?
2. How would your approach change if leaking fuel were present?

always approach vehicles from the side, because the shock absorbers can release and injure your knees and legs.

Manufacturers are mandated to incorporate supplemental restraint systems, or airbags, into all vehicles. These airbags fill with a nonharmful gas on impact and quickly deflate after the crash. Although they were present in some older vehicles, federal legislation mandated in 1998 that newly manufactured cars and light trucks be equipped with front airbags. Since that time, additional airbags have been added as standard or optional equipment on passenger vehicles. In addition to the standard front airbags located in the steering wheel and upper dashboard, it is important to remember that there may be airbags located at multiple points inside of the passenger compartment. Side airbags may be located in the door or the roof rail with the intention of protecting occupants in the event of a side-impact collision. The lower portion of the dashboard may have airbags designed to lessen the extent of injury to the patient's lower extremities and pelvis. Some vehicles even have airbags located in the seat belts or the front middle area to lessen seat belt injuries or injuries occurring when two front occupants strike one another.

Airbags should normally deploy and deflate before your arrival on the scene. However, airbags that have not deployed may spontaneously inflate while you or other rescue personnel are in the vehicle, injuring you and the patient. Use caution when working in damaged vehicles in which airbags have not inflated. Generally, you should maintain at least a 5-inch (13-cm) clearance around side-impact airbags, a 10-inch (25-cm) clearance around driver-side airbags, and a 20-inch (51-cm) clearance around passenger-side airbags. Many airbags are designed to be able to deploy up to 30 minutes after the engine has been turned off. Even if rescue workers disconnect the battery, there is still the possibility of airbag deployment while you are extricating the patient. Be aware of airbag locations while in the vehicle (**FIGURE 37-2**).

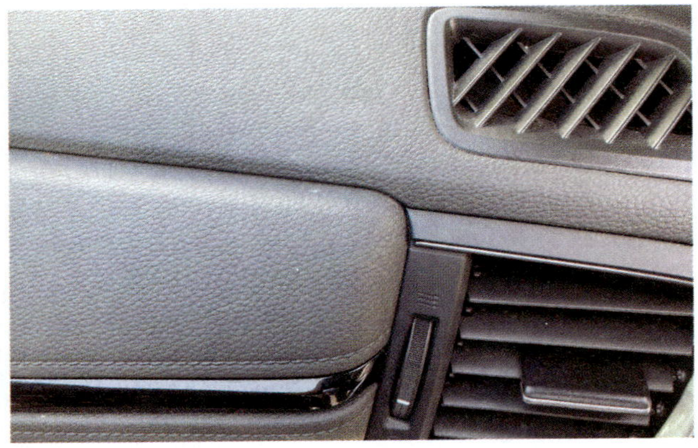

FIGURE 37-2 The presence of airbags will be marked on the vehicle's interior, as shown here on the passenger-side dashboard.

You may notice a haze similar to smoke inside vehicles in which airbags have deployed. This haze is caused by the cornstarch or talcum powder that manufacturers may place on the airbags to prevent the bag from sticking to itself before and during deployment. Patients may be anxious, mistaking the powder from the bag for smoke and thinking their vehicle is on fire. Be thorough in your assessment and reassure patients. Appropriate protective gear, including eye protection, should be worn during all roadway operations.

Words of Wisdom

A vehicle crash scene can present many hazards to emergency responders and patients, including fuel spills that pose fire and explosion risks, downed power lines that pose electric hazards, exposed high-voltage electrical lines in alternative-fuel vehicles, broken glass and torn metal, and exposure to potentially infectious body fluids. Your safety at every type of emergency scene begins with, and depends on, your scene size-up. What you see at the scene helps you determine which personal protective equipment to use and whether to call for additional resources or specialized assistance.

Fundamentals of Extrication

As an EMT, your primary concern during all phases of a rescue is safety, and your primary roles are to provide emergency medical care and prevent further injury to the patient. You will provide care to the patient as extrication goes on around you unless this proves to be too dangerous for you or the patient. **Extrication** is the removal from entrapment or from a dangerous situation or position (also called disentanglement).

Entrapment is a condition in which a person is caught within a closed area with no way out or has a limb or other body part trapped. In the context of this chapter, extrication means removal of a patient from a wrecked vehicle. However, the same principles and concepts apply to other situations, such as a collapsed building.

Words of Wisdom

Extended entrapment of a limb or other body part can lead to crush syndrome in a patient. Crush syndrome requires specific and specialized care. This condition is discussed in greater detail in Chapter 26, *Soft-Tissue Injuries*.

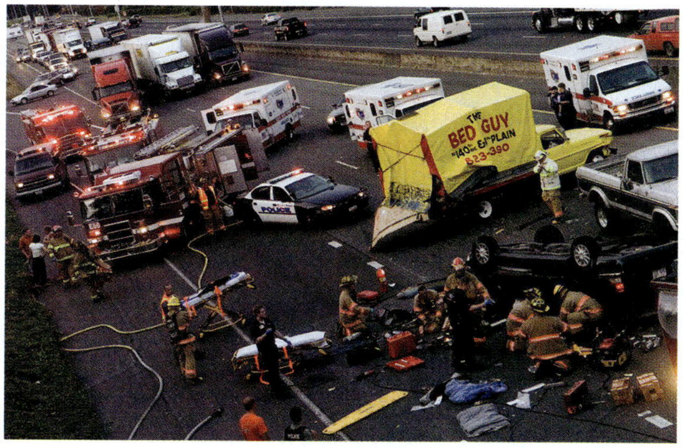

FIGURE 37-3 EMS clinicians, the rescue team, law enforcement officers, and firefighters have distinct responsibilities at a rescue scene and must cooperate to manage the incident.

Each emergency responder has a distinct role at a vehicle extrication scene. Emergency medical services (EMS) clinicians assess patients, provide immediate medical care, triage and package patients, provide additional assessment and care as needed once patients are removed, and provide transport to the emergency department.

The rescue team secures and stabilizes the vehicle, provides safe entrance and **access** to the patients (the ability to reach the patients), safely extricates patients, and provides adequate room so that patients can be removed properly.

Law enforcement officers control traffic, maintain order at the scene, establish and maintain a perimeter so that bystanders are kept at a safe distance, and ultimately investigate the crash or crime scene. Firefighters extinguish fire, prevent additional ignition, ensure that the scene is safe, and remove spilled fuel (**FIGURE 37-3**).

Roles and responsibilities often vary based on jurisdiction and the available agencies. For example, the fire department may take primary responsibility for traffic control in certain situations. An incident commander should take command of the scene and coordinate the response, ensuring the agencies work seamlessly together. Good communication among team members and clear leadership are essential to safe, efficient provision of proper emergency care.

There are 10 phases of the extrication process:

1. Preparation
2. En route to the scene
3. Arrival and scene size-up
4. Hazard control
5. Support operations
6. Gaining access
7. Emergency care
8. Removal of the patient
9. Transfer of the patient
10. Termination

Many of these phases are similar to the phases of an ambulance call. Each will be discussed, with emphasis on the phases in which you will participate.

Safety Tips

Just as in patient care, the first priority in rescue is *personal safety*. The scene of an extrication is dynamic, meaning it constantly changes. Oncoming vehicles often present the largest hazard at a crash scene. Be alert to new dangers, and plan an escape route.

Preparation

Preparing for an incident requiring extrication involves preincident training with rescue personnel for the various types of rescue situations to which you might respond. Tabletop discussions and mock scenarios conducted during training evolutions offer valuable insight and practice so that all personnel understand the operational capabilities and tactics that may be used during a real rescue. Just

TABLE 37-1 Extrication Equipment

- 12-in. (30.5-cm) wrench, adjustable, open-end
- 12-in. (30.5-cm) screwdriver, standard square bar
- 8-in. (20-cm) screwdriver, Phillips head #2
- Hacksaw with 12-in. (30.5-cm) carbide wire blades
- Vise-grip pliers, 10 in. (25 cm)
- 5-lb. (2.3-kg) hammer with 15-in. (38-cm) handle
- Fire axe, butt, 24-in. (61-cm) handle
- Wrecking bar with 24-in. (61-cm) handle. This may be a combination tool with a hammer and axe.
- 51-in. (130-cm) crowbar, pinch point
- Bolt cutter with 1- to 1.25-in. (25- to 32-mm) jaw opening
- Folding shovel, pointed blade
- Tin snips, double action, 8 in. (15-cm) minimum
- Gauntlets (reinforced leather covering past midforearm), one pair per crew member
- Rescue blanket
- Ropes, 5,400-lb. (2,449-kg) tensile strength in 50-ft. (15-m) lengths in protective bags
- Mastic knife (able to cut seat belt webbing)
- Spring-loaded center punch
- Roll of duct tape (for window application prior to center punch use)
- Pruning saw
- Heavy-duty 2 × 4–in. (5 × 10–cm) and 4 × 4–in. (10 × 10–cm) shoring (cribbing) blocks, various lengths

as they must check the equipment carried on the ambulance, rescue personnel must also check their extrication tools and response vehicles to ensure proper operation on a daily basis (**TABLE 37-1**). If you notice that any of the extrication equipment on your ambulance is damaged or nonfunctional, find an appropriate replacement or request one from your service. Such preparations reduce the possibility of equipment failure at an emergency scene.

En Route to the Scene

Procedures and safety precautions similar to those discussed in the phases of an ambulance call are used when responding to a rescue incident. Review dispatch information about the nature of the call and the location of the patient. If initial dispatch information includes keys that specialized resources may be necessary, ensure with your dispatcher that those resources have been assigned to the incident. Assign specific initial duties and scene management tasks to each team member and determine what type of equipment you will take with you when you first arrive on scene.

Words of Wisdom

Your dispatcher may be busy fielding multiple calls and assigning resources to separate events. If you identify the need for additional resources early in your response, ensure that those resources are en route. This is a team response, and your vigilance can help identify information that may have slipped through the cracks. Early recognition and mobilization of resources can make a huge difference for the patient.

Arrival and Scene Size-up

If you are the first unit to arrive on the scene, position the ambulance to block traffic and create a safety barrier within which you can safely begin to assess the scene. Use only essential warning lights, because too many lights tend to distract or confuse motorists. Many emergency responders have been injured on scenes when they were struck by passing vehicles. In some areas, policies indicate that emergency lighting for stationary vehicles can be reduced or turned off after the scene is secured, leaving only the first vehicle parked before the incident with emergency lighting activated; this practice may reduce the risk of a secondary crash.

If you are not the first to arrive, choose a location that will allow safe access to the scene while leaving an exit path for your vehicle. Avoid parking alongside the incident on an active roadway; doing so could increase the risk of your vehicle or responders being struck. See Chapter 36, *Transport Operations*, for further discussion of parking on scene.

Sometimes the scene at a crash is complicated by the presence of **hazardous materials**. A hazardous material is any substance that is toxic, poisonous, radioactive, flammable, or explosive and can cause injury or death with exposure. If there is a hazardous material present at the scene, always park uphill and upwind from the hazard and at a safe distance.

Before exiting your vehicle at an emergency scene, put on proper protective gear. At a minimum, this should include a high-visibility reflective safety vest. Be alert for any vehicles that might

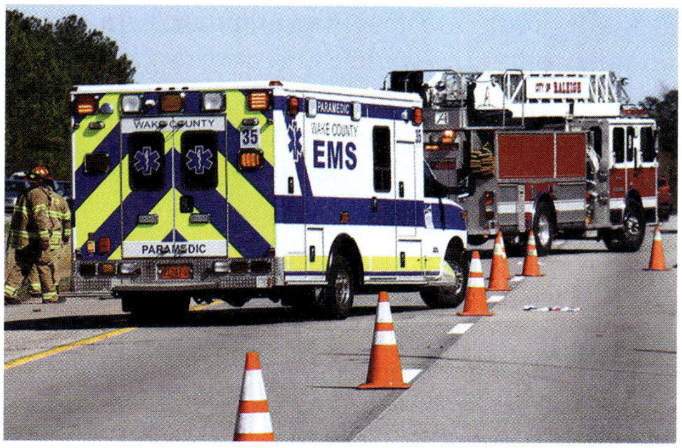

FIGURE 37-4 The scene of a crash should be marked properly, and traffic should be diverted so that responders have enough room to work.

cause injury to you. Do not assume that motorists will see you or heed the warning lights. Even during daylight hours, drivers may be distracted by the warning lights or trying to catch a glimpse of the scene. Inattentive drivers pose a serious threat to you, your partner, the patients, and all emergency responders working the scene.

Before proceeding, make sure the scene is properly marked and protected. Request assistance from law enforcement and/or fire personnel (**FIGURE 37-4**), who should close the road or divert traffic safely around the scene with cones, flares, or barricade tape. Remember, your job is to provide patient care. You may be forced to direct traffic until other units arrive, but ultimately, traffic control is usually handled by other public safety units.

Words of Wisdom

When responding to incidents at night, use your headlights and spotlights to illuminate the scene. Wear a high-visibility reflective safety vest so that you will be seen by fellow emergency responders and motorists.

Size-up is the ongoing process of information gathering and scene evaluation to determine appropriate strategies and tactics to manage an emergency, while paying attention to hazards such as downed power lines, leaking fluids, fire, and broken glass. One of the important responsibilities of scene size-up is to determine what, if any, additional resources will be needed. If you are first on the scene, you may need to initiate a rescue response or call for additional EMS units, law enforcement, utility departments, or specialized crews such as hazardous materials (hazmat) personnel.

A 360° walk-around of the scene will allow you to evaluate the hazards and potential injuries and determine the number of patients. If there is a large group of patients, implement local mass-casualty incident protocols as necessary. During your walk-around, look for the following:

- The mechanism of injury
- Vehicle stability
- Downed power lines
- Leaking fuels or fluids
- Smoke or fire
- Broken glass
- Trapped or ejected patients
- The number of patients and vehicles involved

Words of Wisdom

Practice situational awareness. Situational awareness is the ability to understand and react to the threats around you. Remember that scenes are dynamic; you should remain alert for changing situations. Consider weather and environmental conditions, and be aware of traffic, patients, and bystanders.

On the scene of a motor vehicle crash, it is important to note the physical damage to the structure of the vehicle or vehicles. A bent steering wheel is a mechanism of injury for significant face and/or thoracic trauma. Imprints in the dashboard, which are usually the result of the knees striking it, indicate the potential for serious lower extremity injuries such as hip dislocations and fractures. Determine if the patient was restrained or not. An unrestrained patient may have contact injuries as well as secondary injuries. This person may strike the windshield with the head, resulting in a spiderweb pattern of shattered glass and possible head, face, or neck injuries. Include any findings in your documentation and maintain a high index of suspicion, even if the patient does not present with significant obvious injuries. For a detailed discussion of the kinematics of trauma, see Chapter 24, *Trauma Overview*.

Use the information you have gathered to evaluate the need for additional resources such as the following:

- Extrication equipment
- Fire department
- Law enforcement
- Hazmat unit
- Utility company
- Advanced life support unit or units
- Air transport

Look for spilled fuel and other flammable substances. Motor vehicles carry a variety of fuels and lubricants that pose a fire hazard. Sometimes postcrash fires are started when sparks created during the crash ignite spilled fuel. A short in a vehicle's electric system or a damaged battery may also cause a postcrash fire. These fires may trap the occupants of the vehicle and require fire suppression. Rescue operations may also create sparks that could ignite spilled fuel. It is important to recognize these hazards as soon as possible during your scene size-up.

Environmental conditions can lead to unique hazards at a crash scene. Crashes that occur in rain, sleet, or snow, for example, present an added hazard for rescue personnel and patients. Crashes that occur on hills are harder to handle than those that occur on level ground. Uneven terrain increases the potential for the vehicle to roll over, requiring stabilization of the vehicle prior to gaining access. Remember that the conditions responsible for the crash may also cause other motorists to lose control of their vehicles and injure you.

Some crash scenes may present threats of violence if the vehicle's occupants are intoxicated, have an altered mental status, or are upset with other motorists. If they suddenly regain consciousness or are significantly confused, patients may perceive a threat during rescue operations. This may pose a threat to you or to others on the scene. Be alert for weapons that are carried in civilian vehicles.

You will need to coordinate your efforts with the rescue teams and with law enforcement officials. You should communicate with members of the rescue team throughout the extrication process. Report to the incident commander as soon as you arrive at the scene. Under the incident command system, rescue operations are integrated as a separate group. You become a member of this group and may enter the vehicle and provide care for the patient or patients when approved by the incident commander. The incident command system is described in Chapter 38, *Incident Management*.

Words of Wisdom

When people are entrapped, whether in a vehicle or a structure, their pets may also become injured. In any accident, be prepared to encounter an injured pet that may be trying to protect its owner. As an EMS clinician, you should become familiar working alongside your local animal control officers.

Hazard Control

A variety of hazards may be present at the extrication scene. Downed power lines are a common example. Never attempt to move downed power lines. If power lines are touching or located in proximity to a vehicle involved in the crash, patients should be instructed to remain in the vehicle until power is shut off by a utility company representative.

If you are not the first on scene, in most incidents, there will be an area designated as the **safe zone**. You and the ambulance should remain in that area, outside of the danger zone (**FIGURE 37-5**). The **danger zone (hot zone)** is an area where people can be exposed to sharp metal edges, broken glass, toxic substances, radiation, or explosion of hazardous materials.

Bystanders and family members can also create hazards. If they are allowed to get too close, they are at risk of injury and may also interfere with the overall management of the incident. For these reasons, the danger zone is off-limits to bystanders

Safety Tips

Always assume that oncoming traffic cannot see you and take appropriate steps to keep yourself safe. It is common for other drivers to slow down, focus on the collision, and even take photos. This unpredictable driving increases the risk of another collision. Up to 15% of vehicle crashes are secondary to a primary crash.[1] Awareness of other traffic is always a priority.

(**FIGURE 37-6**). You should help to set up and enforce this zone. If you arrive before the rescue team, coordinate crowd control with law enforcement officials.

The vehicle itself can be a hazard. Prior to attempting to gain access to the vehicle, the vehicle gear should be set in park with the parking brake set and the ignition turned off. Both battery cables should be disconnected, negative side first, to minimize the possibility of sparks or fire. A vehicle that came to rest on its side or roof is unstable and can be particularly dangerous. Rescue personnel can stabilize the vehicle with a variety of jacks or cribbing (wooden blocks). EMS clinicians should never

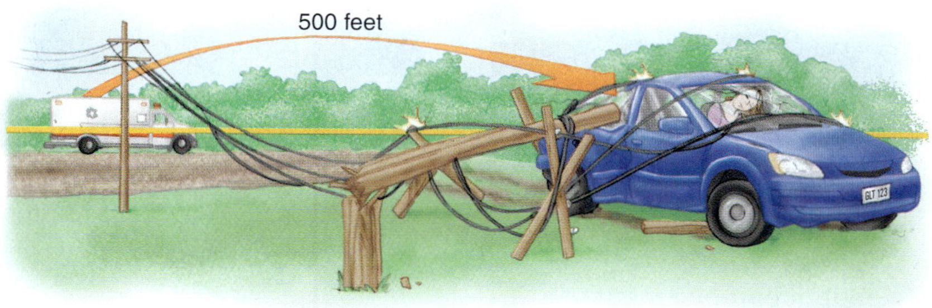

FIGURE 37-5 Remain outside the danger zone (hot zone).

YOU are the EMT

As you approach the wreckage of the aircraft, you see a badly damaged aluminum body with a twisted tubular frame protruding through sections of the aircraft body. There is a single small door at the front of the aircraft with additional aluminum bars over the top of the passenger compartment. The door is bent and cannot be opened manually. A rescue team member is able to cut through the bars with bolt cutters and use a hydraulic cutter to allow better access to the patient. You access the patient through the opposite side and perform a primary assessment. The patient appears to be an approximately 55-year-old woman and is unresponsive but breathing. Her legs and chest are pinned by twisted aluminum bars, and she has large lacerations to her left temple and right arm. The bones at the elbow are exposed.

Recording Time: 0 Minutes	
Appearance	Unresponsive with snoring respirations
Level of consciousness	Unresponsive
Airway	Open with a modified jaw thrust; clear of secretions or foreign bodies
Breathing	Decreased rate; shallow depth
Circulation	Radial pulses weak and rapid; skin cool, clammy, and pale (compared with baseline color); laceration to the forehead from the temple through the left orbit with minimal bleeding; laceration to right arm with the bones of the elbow exposed and bleeding controlled

Because of the mechanism of injury, the patient's clinical condition, and the possibility of a prolonged extrication, you request air transport to respond to the scene and to transport the patient to a trauma center located 35 miles away. You and your partner insert an oropharyngeal airway, assist her ventilations with a bag-mask device on high-flow oxygen, cover the laceration on her forehead, apply a cervical collar, and attempt to shield the patient from debris during the extrication process.

3. How should you initially attempt to gain access to a crash victim?

4. What treatment should you provide to a patient who is entrapped in wreckage?

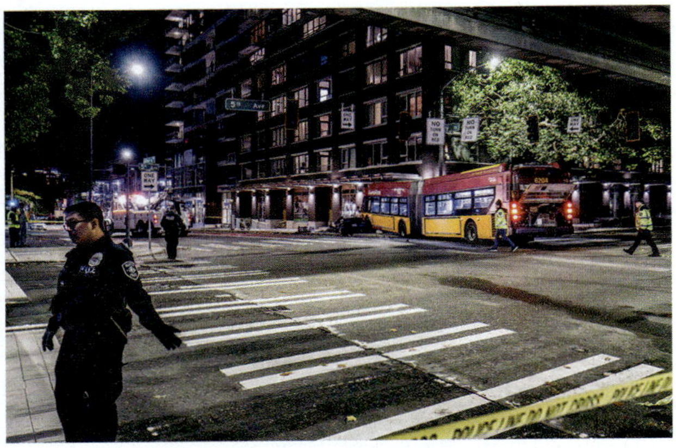

FIGURE 37-6 Establish a danger zone to prevent bystanders from entering the incident area.

attempt to access the patient compartment of a vehicle that is not on all four wheels until stabilization has been completed.

Alternative-Fuel Vehicles

It is increasingly common to encounter vehicles that use alternative fuels. Vehicles may be powered by electricity or electricity/gasoline hybrids, hydrogen fuel cells, or, less often, fuels such as propane, natural gas, or methanol. One feature is common throughout all alternative-fuel vehicles: the need for rescue personnel to disconnect the battery to prevent further fire or explosion. In many alternative-fuel vehicles, the batteries are not located in the engine compartment, but in other areas, such as the trunk or under the seats. Furthermore, there may be more than one battery or capacitor present used to store energy. Be aware that tanks used to store alternative fuels may be located in different places than in traditional gas-powered vehicles.

You must remain vigilant when presented with alternative-fuel vehicles and be aware of their inherent dangers. For example, hybrid batteries have a higher voltage than traditional automotive batteries, and it may take up to 10 minutes for a high-voltage system to deenergize after the main battery is turned off. Avoid contact with high-voltage cables (typically orange) and components throughout the rescue (**FIGURE 37-7**). After a crash, a high-voltage lithium-ion battery can off-gas or ignite suddenly, creating both a very hot fire and toxic gas hazard.[2]

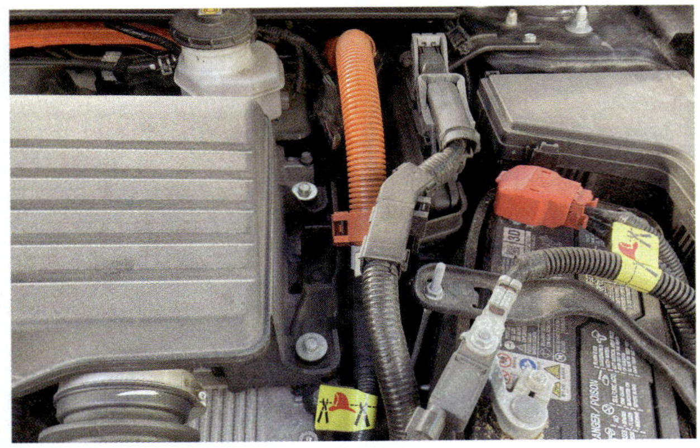

FIGURE 37-7 In alternative-fuel vehicles, such as the hybrid vehicle shown here, high-voltage cables will typically be covered in orange shielding, and additional markings may be present to warn against improper handling.

Do not approach the vehicle if you detect an unusual odor. If you experience burning in your eyes or throat, retreat to an area uphill and upwind until the scene is safe. Roll down the windows and open the doors if you observe fluids, sparks, flames, increasing temperature, or gurgling, popping noises. If not previously notified, call dispatch to request additional assistance from the fire department and/or hazmat team. If rescue or fire agencies are not on the scene, take these initial steps:

1. Approach the vehicle from the side, as it may be difficult to hear if the engine is running.
2. Chock the wheels or deflate the tires to prevent vehicle movement.
3. Put the vehicle in park, set the parking brake, and activate the hazard lights. Turn off the engine and move the vehicle key at least 16 feet (5 m) away from the vehicle.
4. Disconnect the vehicle's 12-volt battery if you have been trained to do so.

Support Operations

Support operations include lighting the scene, establishing tool and equipment staging areas, and marking helicopter landing zones. Fire and rescue personnel will work together on these functions.

Gaining Access

A critical phase of extrication is gaining access to the patient. Remember, do not attempt to gain access

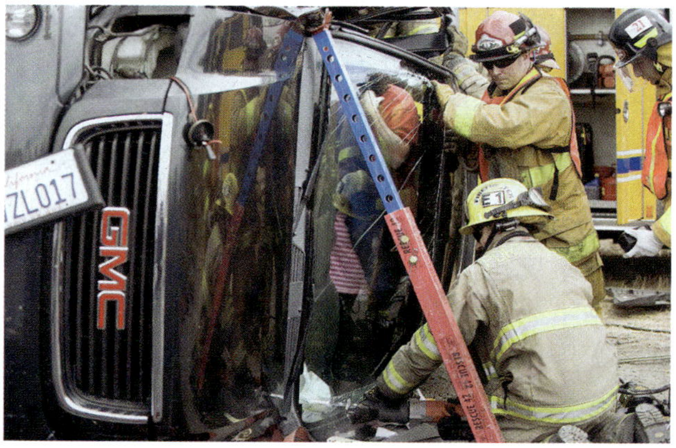

FIGURE 37-8 The exact way to gain access depends on many factors, including the terrain, the way in which the vehicle is situated, and the weather.

to the patient or enter the vehicle until you are sure the vehicle is stable and any hazards have been identified and properly controlled or eliminated. When an incident commander is present, you will be authorized to enter the scene or the vehicle only when these conditions have been met.

The safest, most efficient way to reach the patient or patients depends on the situation. It is up to you and the team to identify the best way to gain access. Darkness, uneven terrain, tall grass, shrubbery, and wreckage may make patients hard to find (**FIGURE 37-8**). Multiple vehicles with multiple patients may be involved. If this is the situation, you should locate and rapidly triage each patient to determine who needs urgent care before you proceed with any treatment and patient packaging. Triage is discussed in Chapter 38, *Incident Management*.

Words of Wisdom

Remember that scene size-up is an ongoing process, because the situation often changes. As a result, you may need to adjust your plans for gaining access and providing treatment.

To determine the exact location and position of the patient, consider the following questions:

- Is the patient in a vehicle or in some other structure?
- Is the vehicle or structure severely damaged?
- What hazards exist that pose a risk to the patient and responders?
- In what position is the vehicle? On what type of surface? Is the vehicle stable or is it likely to roll over?

You must also consider the severity of the patient's injuries and change your course of action as you learn more about the patient's condition. What if you have to quickly remove a patient from a vehicle because the environment is threatening or you need to perform cardiopulmonary resuscitation (CPR)? Chest compressions and airway management may be ineffective if the patient is upside down or pinned to the seat by the dashboard. Depending on the patient's condition and scene safety, you and your team may have to use the rapid extrication technique to move a patient who is not entrapped from a sitting position inside a vehicle to a supine position on a long backboard. A team of experienced EMTs should be able to perform rapid extrication of an untrapped patient in 1 minute or less.

During the access and extrication phases, make sure the patient remains safe. For example, cover the patient with a heavy, fire-resistant blanket or place a backboard between the windshield and the patient to protect the patient from breaking glass, flying particles, tools, or other hazards. In addition, maintain good communication with the patient. Reassure the patient that everything possible is being done to remove them from the situation. Always describe what you are going to do before you do it and as you are doing it, even if you think the patient is unresponsive (**FIGURE 37-9**).

In some cases, you or your partner may need to begin treatment during extrication. The rescue team should try to keep heat, noise, and force to a minimum and use only what is necessary to extricate the patient safely.

Simple Access

The first step is **simple access**, trying to get to the patient as quickly and simply as possible without using any tools or force. Motor vehicles are built for easy entry and exit; however, it may be necessary to use forcible entry methods. The rescue team is responsible for providing the entrance you need to gain access to the patient. In situations where the rescue team has not yet arrived and delayed access

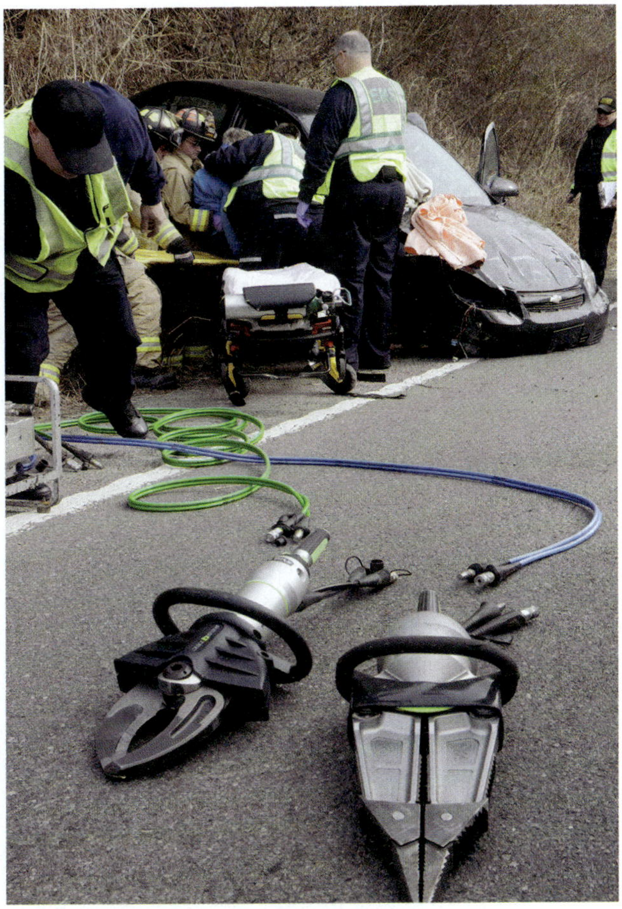

FIGURE 37-9 Always explain to the patient why you are there and what you are doing.

to the patient could be life threatening, simple hand tools, such as hammers, center punches (to break side or rear windows), pry bars, and hacksaws, are usually stored on the ambulance for you to use. Whenever possible, you should first try to unlock the doors (or ask the patient to unlock them) or roll down the windows. Try to open every door using the door handles to gain access before breaking any windows or using other methods of forced entry (**FIGURE 37-10**).

Street Smarts

Always try before you pry. Just like when resuscitating a patient, start with the basics. Try to open the door before resorting to the use of large hydraulic devices.

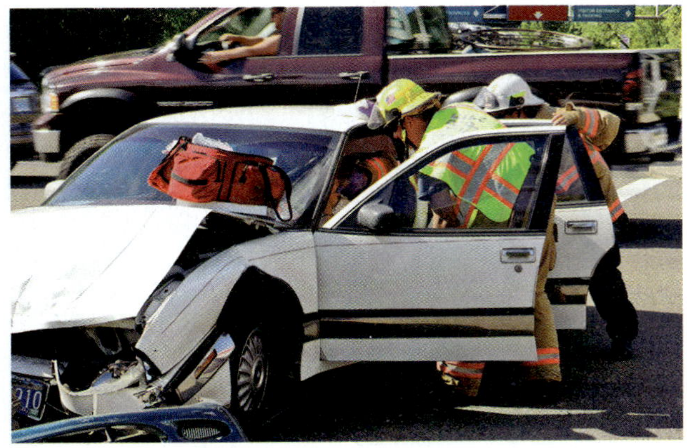

FIGURE 37-10 Get to the patient as quickly and simply as possible by opening the door without using tools or breaking any glass.

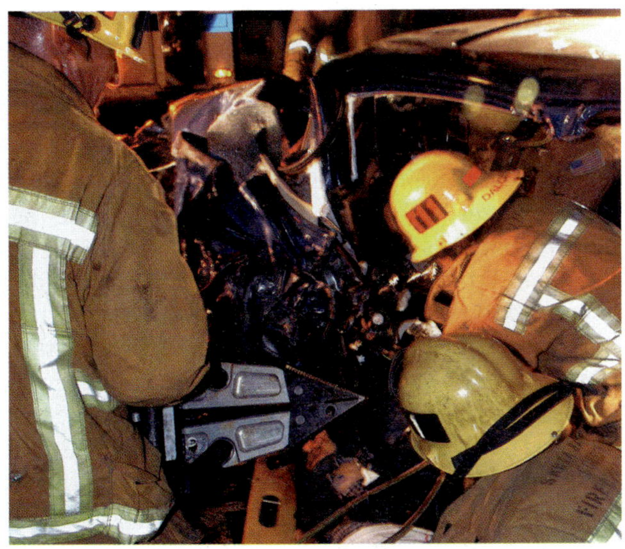

FIGURE 37-11 Complex access often requires the use of pneumatic and/or hydraulic devices.

Complex Access

Complex access requires the use of special tools, such as pneumatic and/or hydraulic devices, and special training that includes breaking the windshield or removing the roof (**FIGURE 37-11**). These advanced skills are typically performed by a specialized team rather than EMS clinicians and include the following:

- Brake and gas pedal displacement
- Dashboard roll-up

- Door removal
- Roof opening and removal
- Seat displacement
- Steering column displacement
- Steering wheel cutting

Emergency Care

Providing medical care to a patient who is trapped in a vehicle is essentially the same as for any other patient. Unless there is an immediate threat of fire, explosion, or other danger, once entrance and access to the patient have been provided and the scene is safe, you should perform a primary assessment and provide care before further extrication begins, as follows:

1. Assess and manage the patient's Airway, Breathing, and Circulation (ABCs).
2. If the patient presents with shock, cover them in warm blankets after your assessment.
3. If spinal motion restriction is indicated, apply a cervical collar.

Removal of the Patient

In the case of vehicle extrication, work with rescue personnel to determine the best route to remove the patient from the vehicle. This should be a collaborative effort with consideration given to the specific details of the entrapment, the patient's condition, and the expertise of the crews on scene. Whereas one crash may require removal of the patient through the driver's door, a similar crash may require complete removal of the vehicle's roof. Removal of a patient from a motor vehicle is a multistep process that is intensive in the number of rescue personnel involved, the equipment used, and the effort required to prevent further injury or harm.

As a part of your assessment, participate in the preparation for patient removal. Determine how urgently the patient must be extricated, where you should be positioned to best protect the patient during extrication, and, once the patient has been freed, how you will best move the patient from within the vehicle onto the backboard and onto the stretcher. Carefully examine the exposed area of the limb or other part of the patient that is trapped to determine the extent of injury and whether there is a possibility of hidden bleeding. If you have concerns about significant hemorrhage from a peripheral vascular injury, apply a tourniquet to control the hemorrhage. If possible, evaluate sensation in the trapped area so that you will know whether increased pain indicates that an object is pressing on or has impaled the patient during extrication.

YOU are the EMT

As your partner assesses the patient, she becomes responsive, responding to voice and moaning loudly. You remove the oropharyngeal airway and reassess her breathing. As the rescue team prepares to remove enough wreckage to allow her to be pulled free, you quickly assess the patient's vital signs.

Recording Time: 7 Minutes	
Respirations	15 breaths/min; shallow
Pulse	138 beats/min; weak at the radial artery
Skin	Cool, clammy, and pale
Blood pressure	98/40 mm Hg
Oxygen saturation (Spo_2)	93% (on oxygen)

A rescue team member informs you that the medical helicopter will arrive in approximately 4 minutes. A landing zone has been established approximately 500 yards (457 m) away. The patient is breathing on her own, and you administer a nonrebreathing mask and discontinue ventilations.

5. Is it appropriate to obtain the vital signs of a patient who is entrapped? Why or why not?

6. What should you do as the patient is being extricated from the wreckage?

During this time, the rescue team assesses exactly how the patient is trapped and determines the safest, easiest means of extrication. Your input is essential so that the rescue team plans an extrication that protects the patient from further harm. Reevaluate whether the patient needs to be immediately removed by using manual stabilization and the rapid extrication technique, or whether a spinal motion restriction device (such as a vest-style extrication device or short backboard) can be applied before the patient is moved further. In most cases, it is impractical and difficult to properly apply extremity splints within the vehicle. Extremity injuries can generally be rapidly supported and stabilized while the patient is being removed by securing an injured arm to the body and, if a leg is injured, securing one leg to the other. This will be adequate until the patient is placed on the stretcher or until time permits a more detailed assessment and splinting of each injury.

Once the extrication plan has been devised and everyone understands what will be done, determine how best to protect the patient. Often, you or your partner will be placed in the vehicle alongside the patient to monitor the individual's condition as the vehicle is being forcibly cut, bent, or disassembled. Be sure to wear proper protective clothing. You should have a helmet on with an impact-resistant visor down to protect your face.

Remember, your safety and that of the patient are paramount during this process. Extrication is often extremely noisy, and appropriate hearing protection should be worn by you and the patient. Be sure you can communicate effectively with the patient and the rescue team so that you can instantly let the rescue personnel know if they need to stop.

Transfer of the Patient

Once the patient has been freed, rapidly assess any other patients who were previously inaccessible, and then perform a complete primary assessment. Provide critical interventions, if required. Make sure to apply a cervical collar if this was not previously done.

To avoid injuring yourself, your team members, or the patient, ensure that each EMT is positioned to lift and carry properly at all times. Move the patient in a series of smooth, slow, controlled steps, with designated stops to allow for repositioning and adjustments. Make sure sufficient team members are available for the move. One EMT should be in charge; this EMT will plan and verbalize the exact steps that you will follow to move the patient from a sitting position in the vehicle to lying supine on the backboard or stretcher. The team should take the path that requires the least manipulation of the patient and equipment. Before beginning, the team leader will check that everyone understands the steps and is ready. Move only on the team leader's command and move the patient as a unit. While transferring the patient, continue to protect the patient from any hazards.

Once the patient has been placed on the stretcher, continue with any additional critical assessment and treatment that was deferred. If it is extremely cold or hot, raining, or snowing, load the stretcher and patient into the climate-controlled ambulance before continuing assessment and treatment. If the patient's condition requires immediate transport, provide only the additional care that is necessary to package the patient. Perform the remaining steps en route to the hospital.

Street Smarts

There are often several different ways a patient can be extricated from a vehicle or other entrapment. The team leader must determine the appropriate method. Team members should listen to determine their individual roles; offer closed-loop communication, acknowledging they understand their roles; and bring to the team leader's attention any circumstance that could injure the team or further injure the patient.

Street Smarts

Remember, bystanders may use the cameras on their phones to record the extrication. Be respectful of your patient's privacy as you transfer the patient from the entrapment into the back of the ambulance.

Termination

Termination involves returning the emergency units to service. For rescue units, this process may be time-consuming. All equipment used on the scene, including hydraulic, electric, and hand tools, must be cleaned, repacked, and checked before reloading them onto the vehicle.

You will also be required to check the ambulance thoroughly, replacing used supplies and decontaminating the unit as required by bloodborne pathogen standards.

Finally, rescue units and medical units will be required to complete all necessary reports.

Specialized Rescue Situations

On most calls, you can drive the ambulance to or within a short distance of the patient's location. However, in some situations, the patient can be reached only by teams trained in special technical rescues. Specialized skills of these teams include the following:

- Cave rescue
- Confined space rescue
- Cross-field and trail rescue (park rangers)
- Dive rescue
- Missing person search and rescue
- Mine rescue
- Mountain-, rock-, and ice-climbing rescue
- Ski slope and cross-country or trail snow rescue (ski patrol)
- Structural collapse rescue
- Tactical emergency medical support
- Technical rope rescue (low- and high-angle rescue)
- Trench rescue
- Water and small craft rescue
- White water rescue

The following sections discuss basic principles of selected specialized rescue operations. Some of these situations are covered in greater detail in Chapter 32, *Environmental Emergencies*.

Technical Rescue Situations

A **technical rescue situation** requires specialized skills and equipment to gain entry and enough room to operate. These situations may contain hidden dangers, and it is unsafe to include personnel who do not have the necessary training and experience. A **technical rescue group** is made up of people from one or more departments in a region who are trained and on call for certain types of technical rescues. Many members of a technical rescue group are also trained as emergency medical responders (EMRs) or EMTs so that they can provide the necessary immediate care when they safely reach the patient. Even when the technical rescue group includes a paramedic or physician, generally only essential care is provided until the group members can bring the patient to the nearest safe and stable setting, known as the staging area.

If a technical rescue group is necessary but is not present when you arrive, immediately check with the **incident commander** to make sure the group has been summoned and is en route to your location. The incident commander is the individual who has overall command of the scene in the field (**FIGURE 37-12**). Although every team member's input at the scene is important, one person must be clearly in charge. A lack of identifiable leadership at the scene hinders the rescue effort and patient care. The incident commander's assessment of the scene and the input from the medical crew regarding the patient's needs will dictate how medical care, packaging, and transport will proceed. Usually, the senior medical official is responsible for this role. Chapter 38, *Incident Management*, discusses this in more detail.

When you arrive at a scene where a technical rescue is in progress, you will usually be met by a member of the technical rescue group and directed or led to the staging area. If the staging area is some distance from the road, you may need to leave the ambulance on the road. Using the ambulance stretcher is impractical in these situations; instead,

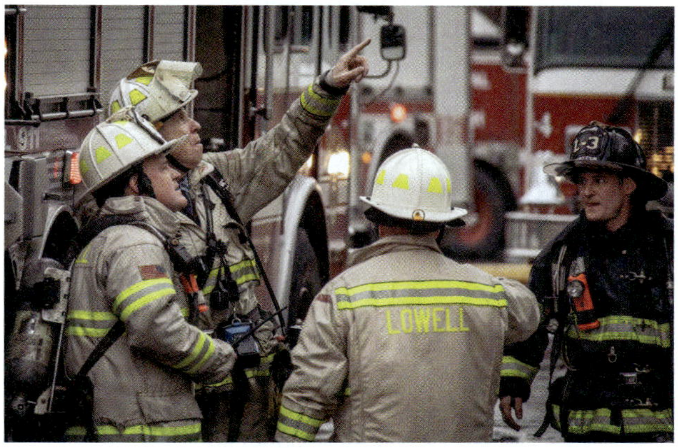

FIGURE 37-12 The incident commander is the individual who has overall command of the scene.

take a backboard and/or basket stretcher (or flexible stretcher) to carry the patient back to the ambulance. Be sure you take all of the jump kits and other equipment you may need to treat and stabilize the patient at the staging area.

When you arrive at the rescue site, identify the designated staging area and set up your equipment there. As soon as the technical rescue group brings the patient to the staging area, perform a primary assessment and, after providing the treatment indicated, package the patient without delay. Although you are responsible for the patient's care, it usually requires a cooperative effort by the technical rescue group and the EMTs to carry the patient to the waiting ambulance. Consider using air transport if the patient will need to be carried or transported an extensive distance.

Safety Tips

Do not endanger yourself, your partner, or the patient by attempting a technical rescue if you do not have the appropriate training and equipment. Await the arrival of appropriately trained resources to implement the rescue. You are not helping the patient by getting yourself into danger (and potentially needing to be rescued yourself).

Search and Rescue

When someone is missing outdoors and a search effort is initiated, an ambulance is usually summoned to the incident **command post** (location of the incident commander) or staging area. Each search team will be organized to include a member who is trained at the EMR or EMT level and who carries the essential equipment to provide immediate care. Your role, and that of the other EMTs who arrive with the ambulance, is to stand by at the command post until the missing person or people have been found.

As soon as you arrive at the scene and have been briefed on the situation, you should isolate and prepare the equipment you will need to carry to the patient's location; this will save time once the patient has been found or if a member of the search team is injured. The carry-in equipment, including a backboard or other devices you will need to perform spinal motion restriction (if needed), should be left in the back of the ambulance until it is needed so that it is protected from the weather. In addition, if the ambulance must be relocated, the equipment will not need to be reloaded and will not be left behind. You will usually be given a portable radio that is tuned to the search frequency so that you can monitor the progress of the search and communicate with those in charge of the search operation.

YOU are the EMT

The side of the plane has been cut away using hydraulic tools, and the patient's seat has been cut to allow access. The patient's legs are freed by moving the back of the seat. You remove the patient from the wreckage using the rapid extrication technique and perform a rapid secondary assessment as your partner reassesses her vital signs.

Recording Time: 18 Minutes	
Level of consciousness	Responsive to voice
Respirations	14 breaths/min
Pulse	148 beats/min; weak radial pulses
Skin	Cool, clammy, and pale
Blood pressure	80/58 mm Hg
Oxygen saturation (Spo_2)	94% (on oxygen)

You note a large, open wound just distal to her right knee with obvious deformity of the tibia. There is no active bleeding. After securing the patient on the gurney, you cover her with a blanket and continue treating her for shock.

7. How does the rapid extrication technique differ from other methods of patient removal? When is it indicated?

Sometimes, you may be asked to stay with relatives of the missing individual who are at the scene. Find out from relatives whether the missing person has any medical history that may need to be addressed and pass this information on to those who are in charge of the search. Unless you have been instructed otherwise, only the incident commander should communicate any news or progress of the search to the family. For this reason, be sure your radio is set at a discreet volume.

Once the missing person has been found, you will be guided by search personnel to that location or to a prearranged meeting point where the patient will be carried, which allows you to begin treatment more quickly. Consider relocating the ambulance or, if one is available, using a four-wheel drive, all-terrain vehicle (ATV), or snowmobile to decrease the time and effort needed to reach and carry out the patient. In some cases, helicopter rescue may be the best method of removing the patient to a safe location. Be sure equipment is evenly distributed among personnel and the pace is such that all can stay together easily. Remember that although EMS will assume the responsibility for patient care once they are at the patient's side, a cooperative effort between the EMS and search teams is necessary to safely carry the patient to the staging area and waiting ambulance.

Trench Rescue

Because of the physical forces involved, many cave-ins and trench collapses have poor outcomes for victims. Collapses usually involve large areas of falling dirt that weighs approximately 100 pounds per cubic foot (1,602 kg per cubic meter). Victims with thousands of pounds of dirt resting on their chests cannot fully expand their lungs and will become hypoxic.

The risk of a secondary collapse during the rescue operation is a concern for rescue personnel and EMTs. Safety measures can reduce the potential for injury from this and other hazards. When arriving on the scene of a cave-in or trench collapse, response vehicles should park at least 500 feet (150 m) from the scene. Because vibration is a primary cause of secondary collapse, all vehicles, including on-scene construction equipment, should be turned off. In addition, all road traffic should be diverted from the 500-foot (150-m) safety area. Other hazards include exposed or downed electric wires and broken gas or water lines. In addition, construction equipment at the collapse may be unstable and could fall into the cave-in or trench site.

Identify any witnesses to the incident. They may provide valuable information on the number of victims and their location within the collapsed area. Assist all uninjured people and nonessential personnel away from the area. At no time should medical or rescue personnel enter a trench deeper than 4 feet (1 m) without proper shoring (temporary supports to prevent collapse) in place.

During the extrication of any survivors from a cave-in or trench collapse site, trained rescue personnel will stabilize the scene and perform the rescue, while medical clinicians will provide patient care when it is safe to do so. Be prepared to receive patients once they have been extricated from the site.

Tactical Emergency Medical Support

A steady increase in violence throughout the United States has resulted in EMTs taking precautions to ensure personal safety. Normally, when the potential for violence exists, as in shootings, stabbings, and attempted suicides, responding units should wait until the scene is secured by law enforcement officers. However, some calls pose an increased risk to emergency responders. Incidents involving hostages, active shooters, barricaded subjects, and snipers require the use of specialized law enforcement tactical units or a **special weapons and tactics (SWAT) team**.

Because of the increased potential for injuries at these volatile incidents, many communities have incorporated specially trained EMTs, paramedics, nurses, and even physicians into their SWAT units (**FIGURE 37-13**). These EMS clinicians provide a special level of care to the sick and injured, and their training goes well beyond the practices seen in standard emergency medical care. Thus, the techniques used may seem inappropriate or inadequate. For example, spinal motion restriction is not used within an unsecured area where gunfire is a risk. The time and manpower necessary to perform this intervention may expose EMS clinicians and SWAT officers to injury or death from gunfire. Such altered standards of care are similar to those used by military EMS clinicians on the battlefield and are *not* used in the standard situations you will encounter as an EMT.

When called to the scene of a law enforcement **tactical situation**, determine the location of the command post and report to the incident commander for instructions or a designated staging area where ambulances will be held to await patients. Lights and siren should be turned off when nearing the scene, and outside radio speakers should not be used. The command post is usually located in an area that cannot be seen by the suspect and is out of range of possible gunfire. Remain in this area and do not roam beyond this site unless directed to do so by incident command. Nearby areas may be visible to the suspect, and you could be injured.

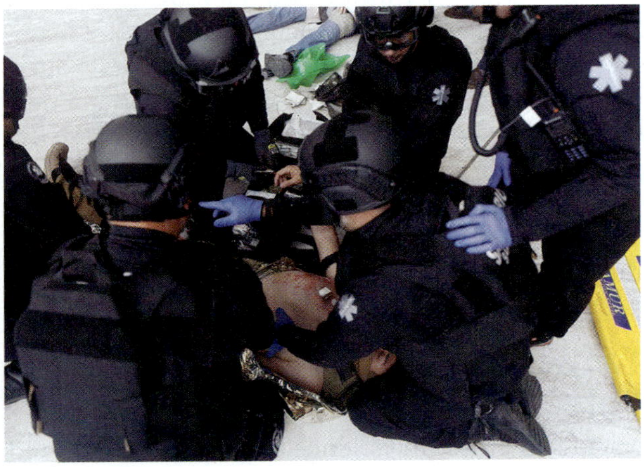

FIGURE 37-13 Tactical EMS clinicians undergo specialized training to provide patient care at potentially violent scenes.

Several planning measures will reduce the potential for chaos should a mass-casualty incident occur at the scene. First, have the incident commander identify the specific location of the incident, including the street address and the side of the street on which the house or building is located. The incident commander should determine a safe location (staging area) where you can meet SWAT team members or tactical EMS clinicians should an injury occur. The incident commander should also determine a safe route to this point. Tactical EMS clinicians or officers will remove the patient to this area for continued treatment and transport to a medical facility.

To save valuable time in critical situations, designate primary and secondary helicopter landing zones if your region uses aeromedical evacuation. The closest hospital, burn center, and trauma center should be identified. The route of travel to these facilities should also be noted. Many of these measures are incorporated into the operational plan

YOU are the EMT

A rescue team member drives the ambulance to the landing zone as your partner applies a rigid splint to the patient's right leg and covers the open wounds with a bulky dressing. You continue to attempt to obtain a brief medical history while you reassess her vital signs.

Recording Time: 40 Minutes	
Level of consciousness	Responsive to voice
Respirations	16 breaths/min; adequate
Pulse	128 beats/min; weak radial pulse
Skin	Cool, clammy, and pale
Blood pressure	84/60 mm Hg
Oxygen saturation (Spo_2)	96% (on oxygen)

The medical helicopter is waiting, and you give a verbal report to the flight paramedic. You assist in the loading of the patient onto the helicopter. You then return to the scene to retrieve any equipment you may have left and to assist with removal of the pilot's body from the wreckage.

8. What are your considerations when calling for air transport?

used by tactical EMS clinicians. If tactical EMS clinicians are used in your jurisdiction, coordinate with them on your arrival at the command post.

Words of Wisdom

Active shooter and mass-casualty incidents have increased in frequency in recent decades. Many agencies, recognizing the need to begin treatment immediately rather than wait outside, are being trained to enter the area directly surrounding the hazard (the warm zone) with appropriate law enforcement teams. These teams, called rescue task forces (RTFs), are crucial to patient survival in large-scale events. Their role is to identify patients, provide targeted lifesaving interventions, and perform extraction. Because it is impractical for EMS clinicians to carry large bags or heavy equipment, they generally provide only essential care, including applying tourniquets, sealing open chest wounds, or maintaining open airways with basic airway adjuncts and maneuvers. Such policies should be implemented in collaboration with local law enforcement and must include appropriate training.

Words of Wisdom

F-A-I-L-U-R-E

The reasons for rescue failure can be summarized by the mnemonic FAILURE:

F Failure to understand the environment or underestimating it
A Additional medical problems not considered
I Inadequate rescue skills
L Lack of teamwork or experience
U Underestimating the logistics of the incident
R Rescue versus recovery mode not considered
E Equipment not mastered

Structure Fires

In most areas, an ambulance is dispatched with the fire department to any **structure fire**, whether or not injuries are reported. A fire in a house or other building is considered a structure fire. When responding to a major fire scene, determine whether any special route will be necessary to reach the scene. Once you arrive at the scene, ask the incident commander where the ambulance should be staged. It is essential that the ambulance be staged in a visible location but parked far enough from the active scene to be safe from the fire itself or a collapsing building. You must also ensure that the ambulance will not block other arriving units or be blocked in by other equipment or hose lines. The fire officer who is the incident commander will help to determine this location.

After parking your ambulance, your next step is to determine whether there are any injured patients at the scene or whether you have been called to stand by. When you check in with the incident commander, you should be able to obtain this information. It is common for multiple ambulances to be dispatched to a structure fire. This practice allows for transport of any patients who are immediately found to require medical attention, as well as a resource to stand by during the firefighting operations. An ambulance should be available to assist with any rehabilitation efforts for firefighters. The National Fire Protection Association (NFPA) Standard 1584, *Standard on the Rehabilitation Process for Members During Emergency Operations and Training Exercises*, helps EMS clinicians understand the acceptable vital signs for rescuers who are coming through rehabilitation.[3] For further discussion of scene management, such as rehabilitation considerations for clinicians, see Chapter 38, *Incident Management*.

As with other specialized rescue situations, search and rescue in a burning building requires special training and equipment. Search and rescue operations are performed by teams of firefighters wearing full turnout gear and **self-contained breathing apparatus (SCBA)** and carrying tools and fully charged hose lines. These teams will bring patients out of the burning building to the area where the ambulance is staged. Therefore, unless otherwise ordered, you should always stay with the ambulance. The ambulance should leave the scene only if transporting a patient or if the incident commander has released it.

Sometimes the scene at a fire is complicated by the presence of hazardous materials. In addition to posing a threat to you and others at the immediate scene, hazardous materials may pose a threat to a larger population. Whenever there is a possibility that a hazardous material is involved, you will have to follow several additional special procedures. Chapter 38, *Incident Management*, covers the specifics of hazardous material procedures.

YOU are the EMT SUMMARY

1. What information is obtained from a 360° assessment of an aircraft crash?

The 360° assessment of an aircraft crash focuses on hazards unique to this type of incident. Common safety hazards include leaking fuels or other fluids, smoke or fire, broken glass, twisted metal, and aircraft instability. Safety issues must be addressed by the appropriate personnel before anyone attempts to gain access to the patient or patients.

Other information obtained during the 360° assessment of a plane crash includes the mechanism of injury, the position of the patient or patients in the aircraft, and whether patients are entrapped or have been ejected.

2. How would your approach change if leaking fuel were present?

A scene with leaking fuel cannot be made 100% safe unless the plane's fuel tank can be emptied. Safely emptying a fuel tank may not be possible before the patient's condition deteriorates. Therefore, it is imperative that you understand the capabilities of the fire department and rescue team and that all efforts be efficiently coordinated. The approach to extricating the patient and the speed with which this is accomplished may change based on the hazards present and the capabilities of the resources. Your safety and the safety of fellow responders comes first. Understand the risks of attempting such a rescue and plan an exit route in the event the scene becomes more unstable. Fuel spills must also be handled appropriately by qualified personnel. Rescue attempts may ignite the fuel. If the fuel spills onto the patient, they will have to be decontaminated prior to transport. Avoid walking through fuel spills, which will contaminate your own boots and then the ambulance.

3. How should you initially attempt to gain access to a crash victim?

Do not attempt to gain access to the patient until you are sure the wreckage is stable and any hazards have been identified and properly controlled or eliminated. The incident commander will inform you when it is safe to gain access to the patient.

Whenever possible, you should use simple access techniques to get to the patient. Try to unlock and open all of the doors, starting with the least damaged door. Using simple techniques can often save you valuable time, as extrication with hydraulic tools can take several minutes or longer. If the patient's condition requires immediate care and you cannot access the passenger compartment, attempt to provide basic care through windows or openings as the extrication is performed. Be on constant alert for dangers to yourself, your partner, and the patient.

If you must break a window to gain access, try to break one that is farthest away from the patient. However, if the patient's condition warrants immediate entry (ie, airway compromise, severe bleeding), do not hesitate to break the closest window. If you cannot gain access to the patient by opening a door or breaking a window, pneumatic and/or hydraulic rescue tools will be necessary to gain access to the patient and allow extrication of the patient from the vehicle.

4. What treatment should you provide to a patient who is entrapped in wreckage?

Treatment should occur only if there is no immediate threat of fire, explosion, or other danger. Once entry and access to the patient have been provided, perform a primary assessment and begin immediate emergency care before the process of extrication begins. Focus on identifying and correcting immediate life threats. A lengthy, detailed assessment is inappropriate because this delays the process of patient extrication. Pass on any information that you obtain about the type or degree of entrapment to the extrication team.

In the case of this patient, you can access only her head and upper extremities. Her legs and torso are pinned by the wreckage. Your partner is manually stabilizing the patient's head and maintaining an open airway with a modified jaw thrust. The airway is clear, and she is breathing, although the rate is a little slow and shallow. Due to the shallow respirations, you have begun to assist her ventilations with a bag-mask device. You have already determined that her pulse is weak and rapid, and her skin is cool, clammy, and pale. You note lacerations to her forehead and right arm.

On the basis of your findings, you should assist her ventilations, direct a fire responder or other clinician on the scene to control the bleeding from her forehead and arm, and control any other bleeding to the areas of her body that you can access. It would be appropriate to apply a cervical collar (after assessing the back of the neck for any deformities) to help maintain cervical spine alignment and stability. Cover as much of the patient as you can with a blanket to preserve body heat and to protect the patient from broken glass or metal fragments during the extrication process.

YOU are the EMT SUMMARY continued

The patient is showing signs of shock; therefore, after correcting problems with airway, breathing, and circulation, she must be extricated so that you can complete your assessment and provide additional treatment including spinal motion restriction.

5. Is it appropriate to obtain the vital signs of a patient who is entrapped? Why or why not?

It is not always appropriate or practical to obtain a complete set of vital signs while a patient is entrapped. Your primary focus should be to provide immediate lifesaving care and then have the patient extricated as quickly and safely as possible. While providing lifesaving care or if extrication is delayed, it is reasonable to obtain pertinent vital signs to help you determine the patient's status and overall acuity. For example, you may be able to palpate a radial pulse or note whether the patient is breathing slowly or rapidly as well as the quality of the respirations and presence of any respiratory distress. Noting a weak, rapid pulse in this scenario may help strengthen your suspicions of hemorrhagic shock. This check will not constitute a complete set of vital signs; however, it may help to identify acute changes in the patient's condition throughout extrication.

Do not delay extrication to assess the patient's vital signs. The longer the patient remains trapped in the vehicle, the longer the delay to definitive care.

6. What should you do as the patient is being extricated from the wreckage?

During the coordinated extrication process, your input is essential. Communication with the patient and fellow rescuers is extremely important. If you notice that the patient has life-threatening hemorrhage after her legs are freed from underneath the wreckage, you should communicate the need for immediate treatment before allowing further efforts at removing the patient. If the patient suddenly screams in pain, instruct the rescue team to stop extrication if possible while you determine where the patient is hurting; it may be necessary for the rescue team to take a different extrication approach.

Once a plan has been devised and all team members understand what will be done, you have a role in protecting the patient. Be sure you are all wearing the appropriate protective clothing (ie, a bunker coat, heavy-duty gloves [over your exam gloves], a rescue helmet with goggles and mask or full face shield, and hearing protection). You may also be able to shield the patient with a fire safety blanket. When possible, position yourself alongside the patient to monitor their condition as the wreckage is being cut, bent, or disassembled. In the case of this patient, you and your partner are positioned on opposite sides of the aircraft. Your partner should continue to provide manual stabilization of the cervical spine if it can be managed safely while you continue assessment and treatment of life-threatening injuries.

7. How does the rapid extrication technique differ from other methods of patient removal? When is it indicated?

The main difference between the rapid extrication technique and other methods of patient removal is that it is fast and requires minimal preparation of the patient in the vehicle before removal. For example, it takes between 6 and 8 minutes—and in some cases, even longer—to properly apply a spinal motion restriction device. This is clearly too long when your patient is critically injured and needs immediate treatment and transport. The rapid extrication technique can be performed in 1 minute or less, but should be done carefully with as little neck and back movement as possible while moving the patient onto a backboard or scoop stretcher for transfer to the ambulance stretcher.

8. What are your considerations when calling for air transport?

Air transport is an excellent consideration when a patient is in critical condition, there is an immediate need for a higher level of care, or the distance or road conditions would make transport lengthy. Patients with time-sensitive conditions or who require a higher level of care, such as advanced airway management or blood product administration in trauma, may benefit from the expertise and available resources that can be provided by a critical care flight team. Medical helicopters can quickly access remote locations and provide rapid transport to definitive care. You must locate an area that is large enough and obstacle-free to allow for a landing zone. If the rescue site is not accessible as a landing zone, identify the nearest safe location and transport the patient by ambulance to the alternative location. To save valuable time in critical situations, designate primary and secondary helicopter landing zones.

Prep Kit

Ready for Review

- You must always be prepared, mentally and physically, for any incident that requires rescue or extrication.
- As an EMT, your first priority in a rescue incident is personal safety.
- EMS personnel are responsible for the assessment, care, triage, packaging, and transport of patients.
- The rescue team secures and stabilizes the vehicle, provides safe access to patients, and safely extricates patients.
- Law enforcement officers control traffic, maintain order at the scene, establish and maintain a perimeter, and ultimately investigate the crash or crime scene.
- Firefighters extinguish fire, prevent additional ignition, ensure scene safety, and remove spilled fuel. Variations in responsibilities are possible, depending on jurisdictional protocols.
- Vehicle safety systems, such as shock-absorbing bumpers and airbags, protect your patients but also have the potential to injure you.
- Simple access is easily achieved without the use of tools or force. Complex access requires heavy-duty tools and special training.
- The 10 phases of extrication are:
  - Preparation
  - En route to the scene
  - Arrival and scene size-up
  - Hazard control
  - Support operations
  - Gaining access
  - Emergency care
  - Removal of the patient
  - Transfer of the patient
  - Termination
- In some situations, the patient can be reached only by teams trained in special technical rescues. As an EMT, you will need to understand your role in these situations and the special safety and procedural considerations.

Vital Vocabulary

access The act of gaining entry to an enclosed area and reaching a patient.

command post The location of the incident commander at the scene of an emergency and where command, coordination, control, and communication are centralized.

complex access Entry that requires special tools and training and includes the use of force.

danger zone (hot zone) An area where people can be exposed to hazards such as electric wires, sharp metal edges, broken glass, toxic substances, radiation, or fire.

entrapment The situation of being caught (trapped) within a vehicle, room, or container with no way out or of having a limb or other body part trapped.

extrication Removal of a patient from entrapment or a dangerous situation or position, such as removal from a wrecked vehicle, industrial incident, or collapsed building.

hazardous materials Any substances that are toxic, poisonous, radioactive, flammable, or explosive and cause injury or death with exposure.

incident commander The individual who has overall command of the incident in the field.

safe zone An area of protection providing safety from the danger zone (hot zone).

self-contained breathing apparatus (SCBA) A respirator with an independent air supply used by firefighters to enter toxic and otherwise dangerous atmospheres.

simple access Entry that is easily achieved without the use of tools or force.

size-up The ongoing process of information gathering and scene evaluation to determine

Prep Kit continued

appropriate strategies and tactics to manage an emergency.

special weapons and tactics (SWAT) team A law enforcement tactical unit with specialized training in situations involving armed conflict and potential violence.

structure fire A fire in a house, apartment building, office, school, plant, warehouse, or other building.

tactical situation A hostage, robbery, or other situation in which armed conflict is threatened or shots have been fired and the threat of violence remains.

technical rescue group A team of emergency responders from one or more departments in a region who are trained and on call for certain types of technical rescue.

technical rescue situation A rescue that requires special technical skills and equipment in one of many specialized rescue areas, such as technical rope rescue, cave rescue, and dive rescue.

References

1. Sarker AA, Paleti R, Mishra S, Golias MM, Freeze PB. Prediction of secondary crash frequency on highway networks. *Accid Anal Prev*. 2017;98:108–117.
2. EMS guidance for responding to crashes and fires involving electric and hybrid-electric vehicles equipped with high-voltage batteries. EMS.gov website. https://www.ems.gov/assets/EMS-Electric-Vehicle-Resource-Page-R4.pdf. Published February 2024. Accessed May 6, 2025.
3. National Fire Protection Association (NFPA). *NFPA 1584: Standard on the Rehabilitation Process for Members During Emergency Operations and Training Exercises*. 2022 Edition. Quincy, MA: NFPA.

Additional Resources

National Highway Traffic Safety Administration. Air bags. https://www.nhtsa.gov/vehicle-safety/air-bags. Accessed May 6, 2025.

National Highway Traffic Safety Administration. *National Emergency Medical Services Education Standards*. https://www.ems.gov/assets/EMS_Education-Standards_2021_FNL.pdf. Published January 2021. Accessed January 24, 2024.

Teixeira PGR, Brown CVR, Emigh B, et al. Civilian prehospital tourniquet use is associated with improved survival in patients with peripheral vascular injury. *J Am Coll Surg*. 226(5);2018:769–776.

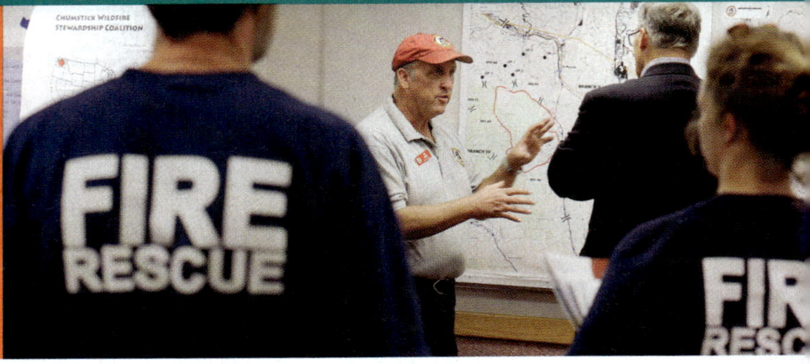

Chapter 38

Incident Management

NATIONAL EMS EDUCATION STANDARD COMPETENCIES

EMS Operations

Knowledge of operational roles and responsibilities to ensure patient, public, and personnel safety.

Incident Management

- Establish and work within the incident management system (p 1404)
- Understand the principles of crew resource management (see Chapter 9, *The Team Approach to Health Care*)

Multiple-Casualty Incidents*

- Operational goals (p 1407)
- Field triage principles (pp 1415–1420)
- Destination determination (p 1420)
- Treatment principles (p 1414)

Hazardous Materials

- Risks and responsibilities of operating on the scene of a hazardous materials incident (pp 1422–1437)

KNOWLEDGE OBJECTIVES

1. Describe the purpose of the National Incident Management System (NIMS) and its major components. (p 1404)
2. Describe the purpose of the incident command system (ICS) and its organizational structure. (pp 1404–1409)
3. Explain the role of emergency medical services (EMS) response within the ICS. (pp 1409–1411)
4. Describe how the ICS assists EMS in ensuring both personal safety and the safety of bystanders, health care professionals, and patients during an emergency. (pp 1409–1411)
5. Describe the role of the emergency medical technician (EMT) in establishing command under the ICS. (p 1411)
6. Describe the purpose of the medical branch of the ICS and its organizational structure. (pp 1411–1414)
7. Describe the specific conditions that would define a situation as a mass-casualty incident (MCI); include examples. (p 1414)
8. Describe what occurs during primary and secondary triage, how triage categories are assigned to patients on the scene, and how destination decisions regarding triaged patients are made. (pp 1415–1420)
9. Explain how to perform various triage methods. (pp 1417–1419)
10. Contrast a disaster with a mass-casualty incident. (pp 1420–1421)
11. Describe the role of EMTs during a disaster operation. (pp 1420–1421)
12. Recognize the entry-level training or experience requirements identified by the HAZWOPER regulation for EMTs to respond to a hazardous materials (hazmat) incident. (pp 1421–1422)
13. Define *hazardous material*; include the classification system used by the National Fire Protection Association (NFPA). (pp 1421, 1434–1437)

*This text uses the term mass-casualty incident.

14. Discuss the specific reference materials that EMTs use to recognize a hazmat incident. (pp 1422–1426)
15. Explain the role of EMTs during a hazmat incident both before and after the hazmat team arrives, including precautions to ensure the safety of civilians and responders. (pp 1426–1432)
16. Describe how the three control zones are established at a hazmat incident, the characteristics of each zone, and the responders who work within each one. (pp 1432–1434)
17. Describe the four levels of personal protective equipment (PPE) required at a hazmat incident to protect responders from injury by or contamination from a particular substance. (p 1435)
18. Explain patient care at a hazmat incident, including the special considerations for patients who require immediate treatment and transport prior to full decontamination. (pp 1435–1437)

SKILLS OBJECTIVES

1. Demonstrate how to perform triage based on a fictional scenario that involves a mass-casualty incident. (pp 1414–1419)
2. Using a reference, correctly identify Department of Transportation (DOT) labels, placards, and markings that are used to designate hazardous materials. (pp 1426–1430)
3. Demonstrate the ability to use a variety of reference materials to identify a hazardous material. (pp 1422–1426)

Introduction

Some of the most challenging situations you will encounter are disasters and mass-casualty incidents. In this text, a disaster refers to any situation, human-made or natural, that overwhelms your resources. Emergency medical services (EMS), in collaboration with other agencies, plays a key role in the medical aspects of any disaster and should participate in all phases of disaster management within their community.[1] A single incident with two critical patients can constitute a disaster if there is only one EMS unit available to respond. A **mass-casualty incident (MCI)** refers to any call that involves three or more patients, any situation that places such a great demand on available equipment or personnel that the system would require a **mutual aid response** (an agreement between neighboring EMS systems to respond when local resources are insufficient to handle the response), or any incident that has the potential to create one of the previously mentioned situations. Bus or train crashes and earthquakes are obvious examples of MCIs. These incidents can be overwhelming because you will encounter a large number of patients and not have enough resources.

When you respond to an event with a large number of patients, you must use a systematic approach to manage the incident efficiently. By learning to use the principles of the incident command system (ICS), you will be able to do the greatest good for the greatest number of people. As an EMT, you will typically be assigned to work within the EMS/medical branch under an ICS, but you may be asked to function in other areas, which will be discussed later in this chapter. The National Incident Management System (NIMS) was developed to promote more efficient coordination between emergency responders at the regional, state, and national levels. To reduce on-scene problems and to increase your efficiency, you need a solid understanding of the basics of the NIMS. Training courses may be accessed through the Federal Emergency Management Agency (FEMA) website.

Words of Wisdom

As an EMS clinician, you may be the first person to arrive to an MCI. It is imperative that you understand the roles of the ICS within your coverage area, as you might have to be the initial incident commander until more help arrives. The initial steps that you take will set the tone for the incident's success.

National Incident Management System

The Department of Homeland Security implemented the **National Incident Management System (NIMS)** in 2004. Most incidents are handled at the local level, but major incidents require the involvement of multiple jurisdictions, agencies, and emergency response disciplines. The NIMS provides a comprehensive framework to enable federal, state, and local governments, as well as private-sector and nongovernmental organizations, to work together effectively. The NIMS is used to prepare for, prevent, respond to, mitigate, and recover from domestic incidents, regardless of cause, size, or complexity, including acts of catastrophic terrorism and hazardous materials (hazmat) incidents.

Two important underlying principles of the NIMS are flexibility and standardization. The organizational structure must be flexible enough to be rapidly adapted for use in any situation. The NIMS provides standardization in terminology, resource classification, personnel training, certification, and more. This standardization allows for unity of effort, which is a third guiding principle of NIMS. Unity of effort allows various agencies to achieve common objectives by supporting each other while maintaining individual authorities. In other words, multiple agencies can work together toward the same goal, while maintaining their autonomy. The unity of effort is possible due, in part, to the NIMS concept of interoperability, which refers to the ability of agencies of different types or from different jurisdictions to communicate with each other. Interoperability can be accomplished by maintaining a shared frequency or by having radio systems programmed to other agencies' frequencies.

The ICS is one component of the NIMS. The three major NIMS components are as follows:

1. **Communications and information management.** Effective communications, information management, and information sharing are critical aspects of domestic incident management. The NIMS communications and information management systems enable the essential functions needed to assess available information, provide interoperability, and ensure appropriate communication of decisions.
2. **Resource management.** The NIMS sets up mechanisms to describe, inventory, track, and dispatch resources before, during, and after an incident. The NIMS also defines standard procedures to recover equipment used during the incident.
3. **Command and coordination.** The NIMS standardizes incident management for all hazards and across all levels of government. It provides comprehensive frameworks and recommended organizational structures. The NIMS standard incident command structures are based on three key constructs: ICS, multiagency coordination systems, and public information systems.

Incident Command System

It is important for you to be familiar with the terminology and concepts of the **incident command system (ICS)** (referred to by some agencies as the incident management system). The purpose of the ICS is to ensure responder and public safety, achieve incident management goals, and ensure the efficient use of resources.

As you know, communication is the building block of good patient care. Common terminology and the use of clear text communications (plain English as opposed to 10-codes) help responders from multiple agencies work efficiently together.

Using the ICS gives you a modular organizational structure that can be applied to all hazards. The ICS can be activated for incidents ranging from a single vehicle crash with one patient to a natural gas pipeline explosion involving multiple communities and numerous injuries. The goal of the ICS is to make the best use of your resources to manage the environment around the incident and to treat patients during an emergency. The ICS is designed to avoid duplication of effort and **freelancing**, in which individual units or different organizations make independent and often inefficient decisions about the next appropriate action. Follow your local standard operating procedures for establishing the ICS.

One of the organizing principles of the ICS is to limit the **span of control** of any one individual. This principle refers to keeping the supervisor-to-worker ratio at one supervisor for five subordinates. If more than five people are reporting to the

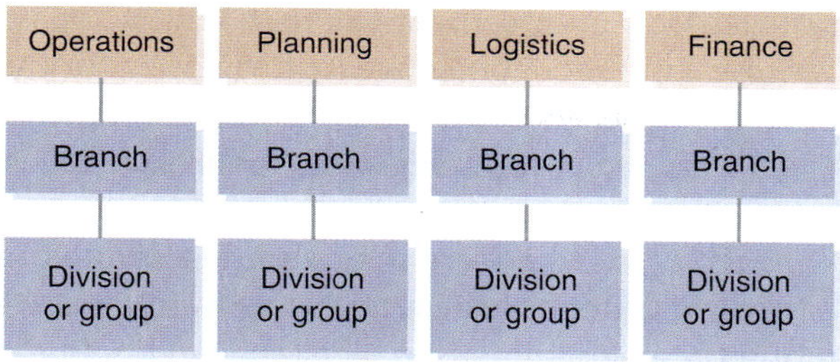

FIGURE 38-1 The incident command system's organizational structure may include sections, branches, divisions, and groups.

same supervisor, the span of control is being exceeded and the supervisor needs to divide tasks and delegate the supervision of some tasks to another person. The NIMS does acknowledge that this is a guideline. Incident personnel may evaluate the actual incident and use their best judgment to determine the appropriate span of control.

The organizational levels may include sections, branches, divisions, and groups **FIGURE 38-1**:

- **Sections** are responsible for a major functional area such as finance/administration, logistics, planning, or operations. Each section's chief (lead) reports directly to the incident commander (IC).
- **Branches** are managed by the branch director and may be functional or geographic in nature. These tend to be established when span of control is a problem, such as at larger incidents, where more oversight may be needed. Branches are in charge of activities directly related to the section (eg, fire, law enforcement, EMS, rescue).
- **Divisions and groups** serve to align resources and/or crews under one supervisor. Divisions usually refer to crews working in the same geographic area. Groups usually refer to crews working in the same functional area, but possibly in different locations. To better visualize how divisions and groups work, consider an incident involving a midair collision between two commercial aircraft. With two scenes separated by almost 1 mile, Division A, composed of a fire suppression group, a rescue group, and an EMS group, may be assigned to work the site where the first aircraft came down, and Division B, composed of similar groups, works the site of the second aircraft.

Generally, the larger the incident, the more divisions there will be. A small incident may require only an IC and support from fire, EMS, and law enforcement. An incident on a much larger scale, such as Hurricane Helene in 2024, will require massive efforts and many agencies working together.

In some regions, emergency operations centers may exist. The centers are usually operated by the city, state, or federal government. These centers will usually be activated only in a large-scale or complex event that may go on for multiple operational periods, or a pandemic that may be problematic for weeks or months. Such events can involve hundreds of patients and tax the entire system. Many community-based emergency operations centers were activated during the COVID-19 pandemic to coordinate resources between government resources and prehospital care, health care, and public health.[2]

The responders who will participate in an MCI or a disaster should use the ICS. When an incident occurs, find out from your service who is in charge, how it is activated, and what your expected role will be.

ICS Roles and Responsibilities

There are many roles defined in the ICS. The general staff includes **command** and, depending on the

YOU are the EMT

Your unit is dispatched to a crash just outside a local amusement park involving an open-air tram transporting guests from the parking lot to the front gate, and a passenger bus that swerved out of control while making a turn. Dispatch advises there have been multiple calls reporting the crash with varied reports of injuries.

1. How will you decide whether to declare this an MCI?
2. How will the ICS facilitate operations at this scene?

situation, possibly finance/administration, logistics, operations, and planning. It is important for you to understand the specific duties of each and how they work to coordinate the response.

Command

The **incident commander (IC)** is the person in charge of the overall incident. The IC will assess the incident, establish the strategic objectives and priorities, and develop a plan to manage the incident (**FIGURE 38-2**). The number of command duties the IC takes on often varies by the size of the incident. Small incidents often mean the IC will assume responsibility for all command duties. In an incident of medium size or complexity, the IC may delegate some functions but retain others. For example, at a motor vehicle crash site with multiple patients, the IC may designate a safety officer or a public information officer but maintain responsibility for the other command functions. In a complex situation, the IC may appoint team members to all command roles.

Large MCIs, such as a hazmat incident or active shooter, require a multiagency or multijurisdictional response and need to use a **unified command system**. In this case, plans are drawn up in advance by all agencies that assume a shared responsibility for decision making. The response plan should designate the lead and support agencies in several types of MCIs. For example, it may specify that the hazmat team will take the lead in a chemical leak, the medical team will take the lead in a multivehicle crash, and law enforcement will take lead in a mass shooting. One set of objectives is developed for the entire incident. A collective approach is made to develop strategies to achieve incident objectives. Agencies that share a border should train often with each other to ensure that a unified command system will function well and that communication among the responders is well established before a real incident occurs.

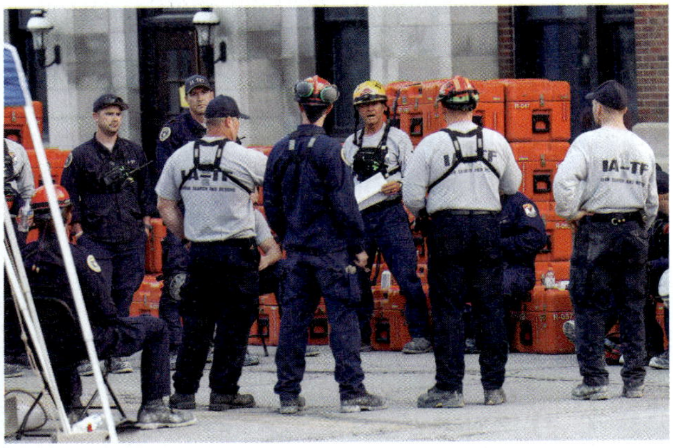

FIGURE 38-2 The person in command at a mass-casualty incident oversees the incident and develops a plan for the response.

A **single command system** is one in which one person is in charge, even if multiple agencies respond. It is generally used with incidents in which one agency has the most responsibility for incident management. Ideally, it is used for short-duration, limited incidents that require the services of a single agency.

Your IC should be on or near the scene to enable easy communication with all emergency responders. It is important that you know who the IC is, how to communicate with the IC, and where the **command post** is located. If the incident is very large, you will report to a supervisor working under the IC. This will help to maintain a manageable span of control. To make the IC easily identifiable, some type of garment is worn, such as a brightly colored vest labeled with the word COMMAND. The command post may be set up at a vehicle, and it may be identified by a placard or unique color strobe (green is commonly used to identify a command post). Make sure your supervisor or the IC knows of any plans or operations before they are initiated.

Communication is particularly important if a transfer of command takes place. Because an incident can rapidly change in size and complexity, an IC may turn over command to someone with more experience in a critical area. This change, or transfer of command, must take place in an orderly manner and, if possible, face to face. In extreme situations, it could be done by phone, radio, or email, although these methods are not recommended. It is imperative that the transfer of command be communicated to those involved in the incident, especially the command staff and general staff. Your agency should have standard operating procedures that govern the transfer of command. Make certain to follow the standard operating procedures. When an incident draws to a close, there should be a **termination of command**. Your agency should implement **demobilization** procedures as the situation deescalates or comes to an end.

The sections required for a response are designated by command based on the needs of the situation. As mentioned, they may include finance/administration, logistics, operations, and planning. Each is led by a section chief.

Finance/Administration

The **finance/administration** section chief is responsible for documenting all expenditures at an incident for reimbursement. Finance personnel are not usually needed at smaller incidents, but at larger incidents it is necessary to keep track of personnel hours and expenditures for materials and supplies. Ultimately, that information is reported at meetings of the general staff. Responding agencies and organizations may be eligible for reimbursement after the incident, and an efficient finance/administration section chief will help your agency to succeed in the reimbursement process. Finance personnel should be trained in the process of assessing expenditures long before an actual incident.

The various functions within the finance/administration section include (1) the time unit, (2) the procurement unit, (3) the compensation and claims unit, and (4) the cost unit. The time unit is responsible for ensuring the daily recording of personnel time and equipment use. The procurement unit deals with all matters concerning vendor contracts. The compensation and claims unit has two major purposes: dealing with claims as a result of the incident, and injury compensation. Finally, the cost unit is responsible for collecting, analyzing, and reporting the costs related to an incident.

Logistics

The **logistics** section is responsible for communications equipment, facilities, food and water, fuel, lighting, and medical equipment and supplies for patients and emergency responders. Local standard operating procedures will list the medical equipment needed for the incident, depending on the type of incident. Logistics personnel are trained to find food, shelter, fuel, and health care for you and the other responders at the scene of an MCI. In a large incident, it is often necessary for many people to handle logistics, but only the section chief will report to the IC.

Operations

At a large or complex incident, the IC should appoint an **operations** section chief, who is responsible for managing the tactical operations usually handled by the IC on routine EMS calls. This frees the IC to coordinate with other agencies and the media, engage in strategic planning, and ensure that logistics are functioning effectively. The operations section chief will supervise the people working at the scene of the incident, who will be assigned to branches, divisions, and groups. Operations personnel often have experience in management within EMS.

Planning

The **planning** section solves problems as they arise during the incident. Planners obtain data about the problem, analyze the previous incident plan, and predict what or who is needed to make the new plan work. They need to work closely with the operations, finance/administration, and, especially, logistics sections. Planners can and should call on technical experts to help with the planning process. They should document their decisions and what they learned from the incident and set out a course for demobilizing the response when necessary.

Another function of the planning section is the development of an **incident action plan (IAP)**, which is the central tool for planning during a response to a disaster emergency. The IAP is prepared by the planning section chief with input from the appropriate sections and units of the incident command team. The purpose of an IAP is to provide clear, concise information about incident activities, including objectives, tactics, and assignments. It should be written at the outset of the response and revised continually throughout the response. In an initial response for an incident that is readily controlled, a written plan may not be necessary. Larger, more complex incidents will require an IAP to coordinate activities. The level of detail required in an IAP will vary according to the size and complexity of the response.

Command Staff

Three important positions that help the general staff (eg, section chiefs) and the IC are the safety officer, the public information officer, and the liaison officer.

The **safety officer** monitors the scene for conditions or operations that may present a hazard to responders and patients. The safety officer may need to work with environmental health and hazmat specialists. The importance of the safety officer cannot be underestimated; this individual has the authority to stop an emergency operation whenever an unsafe situation is detected. A safety officer should remove hazards to EMS personnel and patients before the hazards cause injury.

> **Words of Wisdom**
>
> While large or complex incidents may have a designated incident safety officer, remember that every responder at an incident must act as a safety officer and call out unsafe practices to ensure that everyone goes home at the end of the day.

The **public information officer (PIO)** provides the public and media with clear information. The designated PIO may cooperate with PIOs from other agencies in a **joint information center (JIC)**. In some circumstances, the PIO/JIC may be responsible for distributing a message designed to improve a situation, prevent panic, and provide evacuation directions. A wise PIO positions the JIC well away from the incident command post and, most importantly, away from the incident, to minimize distractions. Also, the PIO must keep the media safe and from becoming part of the incident.

The **liaison officer** relays information and concerns among command, the general staff, and other agencies. If an agency is not represented in the command structure, questions and input should be given through the liaison officer. For example, if the incident involves an airline crash, the liaison officer may interact with the National Transportation Safety Board, airline officials, and airport staff.

Communications and Information Management

Communications has historically been the weak point at most major incidents. To minimize the effects of communications problems, it is recommended that communications be integrated. This means that all agencies involved should be able to communicate quickly and effortlessly via radios on designated channels. Effective communication allows for accountability throughout the incident and instant interaction among responders. As always, and more so during a large incident, you must maintain professionalism on all radio communications, and remember to communicate clearly and concisely using plain language (not 10-codes or language specific to your system). When possible, face-to-face communication is helpful to avoid excessive radio traffic.

Mobilization and Deployment

When the need for additional resources (eg, EMS personnel) has been identified, a request is made and these resources are mobilized and deployed to the scene. To minimize the potential for freelancing, responders should not depart for the scene until this request has been made. As initial resources are deployed, a staging area is often designated, slightly removed from the incident to prevent traffic congestion until specific needs can be determined.

Check-in at the Incident

On arrival at an incident, first check in with the IC at the base, staging area, or other location designated by the IC. If the incident is large or complex, you will be assigned to a supervisor working under the IC. Check-in also allows for personnel tracking throughout the incident and ensures that costs, wages, and reimbursement can be calculated accurately. Should a building collapse or secondary incident occur, it is vital for the IC to have an accurate report of what resources and personnel were on scene prior to that secondary event.

Initial Incident Briefing

After the check-in process is complete, report to your supervisor for an initial briefing that will allow you to obtain information regarding the incident, as well as your specific job functions and responsibilities. You may also obtain radio frequencies during this briefing, which will enable you to communicate with the incident team.

Incident Record Keeping

Record keeping is important for financial reasons and for documentation purposes. If a large piece of equipment becomes inoperable, it may be possible for the agency to be reimbursed for replacement costs. Record keeping also allows for tracking of time spent on the incident for reimbursement purposes.

Accountability

Because of the large number of responders at a large incident, accountability is important. Accountability means keeping your supervisor advised of your location, actions, and completed tasks. It also includes advising your supervisor of the tasks that you have been unable to complete and what tools you need to complete them.

Incident Demobilization

Once the incident has been stabilized and all of the hazards mitigated, the IC will determine which resources are needed or not needed and when to begin demobilization. This process allows for a prompt return of resources to their parent organizations to be placed back in service.

Words of Wisdom

Preplanning is crucial to the success of an MCI response, as is participating in mock or practice MCI drills. Once a disaster plan is in place, it should be run as a simulation event (**FIGURE 38-3**). Multiple agencies should be invited to participate, including police, fire, EMS, helicopter services, and hospitals. After the drill, a debriefing allows responders to review the plan's effectiveness and make any necessary changes.

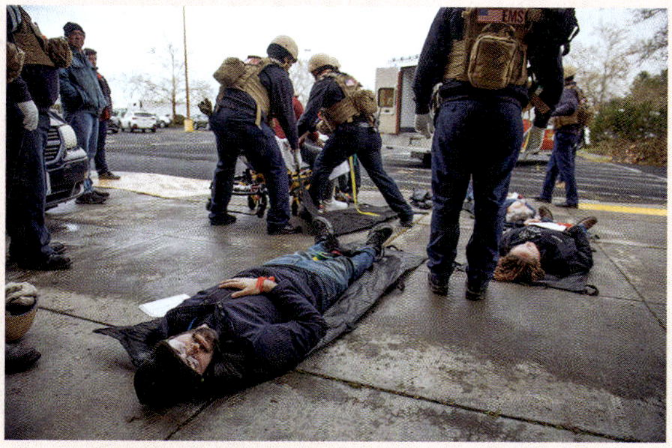

FIGURE 38-3 Interagency planning and practice are crucial to a successful MCI response. Active shooter training, conducted in Walla Walla, Washington, is shown here.

EMS Response Within the ICS

Preparedness

Preparedness involves the decisions made and basic planning done before an incident occurs. Every state is at risk for natural disasters, such as hurricanes, tornadoes, earthquakes, and wildfires. Therefore, preparedness in a given area involves anticipating the most likely natural disasters for that specific area, among other disasters.

Your EMS agency should have written disaster plans that you are regularly trained to carry out. A copy of the disaster plan should be accessible to EMS crews at all times. EMS facilities should have disaster supplies for at least a 72-hour period of self-sufficiency. Your EMS agency should have mutual aid agreements with surrounding organizations; these will facilitate requests for help in an emergency. All groups with mutual aid agreements should practice using the plans frequently. Organizations should share a list of resources with each other so they will know early on what they can access. Many regions have large caches of emergency supplies that can be quickly deployed in large-scale incidents. Also, your local EMS organizations should develop an assistance program for the families of EMS responders. If EMS responders have concerns about their families during a disaster, their effectiveness on the job could be diminished.

Words of Wisdom

Developing a plan that includes an evacuation center for first responders' families (separate from the public) in the event of an evacuation order will help ease the minds of those working the incident. This designated location allows families of first responders to support each other and keeps them from being bothered by the public for information. Members of the public often mistakenly assume that a first responder's family members have information that has not been shared with the public.

Scene Size-up

Remember that scene size-up starts with dispatch. If dispatch information indicates a possible unsafe scene, stay away from the scene or get only close enough to make an assessment without putting yourself in harm's way. When you arrive first on the scene of an incident, you will make an initial assessment and some preliminary decisions. The size-up will be driven by three basic questions that you must ask yourself:

- *What do I have?*
- *What do I need?*
- *What do I need to do?*

These questions have a symbiotic relationship. The answer from one helps to answer the others, and each answer represents a piece to the puzzle. Work as a team when you answer these questions because overlooking just one safety issue early on can start a chain reaction of problems.

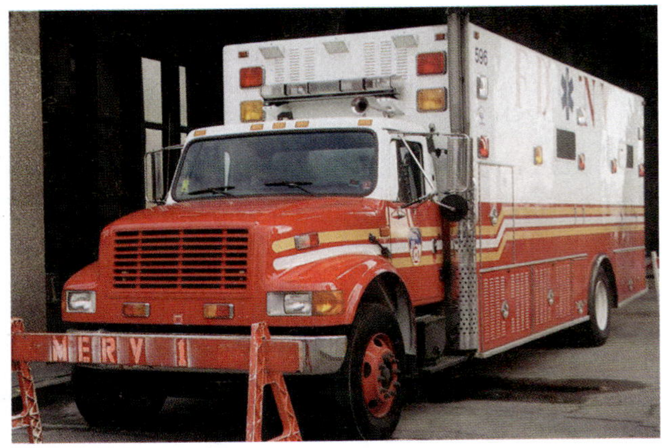

FIGURE 38-4 This mobile emergency room is staffed by EMTs, paramedics, and physicians who are able to provide advanced life support to multiple patients simultaneously on the scene of a mass-casualty incident.

What Do I Have?

Start with scene safety. First, assess the scene for hazards. Warn all other responders about hazardous materials, fuel spills, electrical hazards, or other safety concerns as soon as possible. Confirm the incident location.

Establish whether the incident is open or closed. An **open incident** is one that is not yet contained; there may be patients who are yet to be located and the situation may be ongoing, producing even more patients. A **closed incident** is one that is contained and in which all casualties are accounted for. However, as with any situation, a closed incident may quickly become an open incident as situations change.

Estimate the number of casualties. Immediately provide a brief incident report to dispatch. An example of such a report would be: "EMT unit number one arriving on scene, multiple vehicles involved, eight casualties visible, full road blockage, no apparent hazards at this time, EMT unit number one is assuming command."

What Do I Need?

Decide what resources are needed. You may need more EMS responders, ambulances, or other forms of transportation. If extrication is required, a rescue unit and fire department response may be needed. If there are hazardous materials, request a hazmat team immediately (discussed later in the chapter). Many large EMS systems deploy specialized MCI units or mobile emergency room vehicles that have the capacity to treat dozens of patients at the scene (**FIGURE 38-4**).

What Do I Need to Do?

Keep the following priorities, in this order, in mind:

- Safety
- Incident stabilization
- Preservation of life, property, and the environment

YOU are the EMT

On reaching the scene, you see utter chaos. Your unit is the first to arrive, and the large crowd makes it virtually impossible to determine the number of patients or the extent of injuries. The dispatcher advises that law enforcement, fire department, and additional EMS units are en route.

3. How should you and your partner proceed?

4. Once command has been established, what are your duties?

Safety is paramount. Safety includes your life, your partner's life, and other responders' lives. Then, consider the safety of the patients and any bystanders. Putting yourself and your partner first will be difficult for anyone dedicated to saving lives, but the situation will only worsen if you become victims. You have the skills, and bystanders usually do not. Further, if a responder is injured, other responders may focus on "their own," removing critical resources from the incident.

Initially, you may have to work to isolate or stabilize the incident before providing care to injured people. This is another difficult concept for all emergency workers. Remember, you cannot help the injured if the scene is unstable. An unstable scene can lead to an injured EMT or additional bystanders becoming injured, thereby making your job much more difficult.

Establishing Command

Once you have performed a good scene size-up and answered the three basic questions, command should be established by the most senior official or the most qualified responder, notification to other responders should go out, and necessary resources should be requested. Recall that a command system ensures that resources are effectively and efficiently coordinated. Command must be established early, preferably by the first-arriving, most experienced public safety official from the most relevant service. These officials may include police, fire, or EMS personnel.

Communications

As discussed earlier, communication is often the key problem at an MCI or a disaster. The infrastructure may be damaged, or communications capabilities may be overwhelmed. If possible, use face-to-face communications to limit radio traffic. Some organizations responding to a disaster might not know how to use a radio. As mentioned previously, if you communicate via radio, do not use 10-codes or language specific to your EMS system. Doing so could be confusing for ancillary services and other personnel who are responding. Most communications problems should be worked out before a disaster happens by designating channels strictly for command during a disaster.

Whatever form of communications equipment is used, it must be reliable, durable, and field-tested. Be sure there are backups in place if the primary communications system does not work. Some regions have mobile self-contained communications centers, whereas others use local radio groups such as ham radio operators to assist with communications. Most important, your plan should include a "plan B" in case of communications failure.

The Medical Branch of Incident Command

What has traditionally been referred to as medical incident command is more commonly known as the medical (or EMS) branch of the ICS (**FIGURE 38-5**). At incidents that have a significant medical factor, the IC will designate someone as the director of the medical branch under the operations section. This person will supervise the primary roles of the medical branch: triage, treatment, and transport of injured people. The medical branch director helps to ensure that EMS units responding to the scene are working within the ICS, each medical division or group receives a clear assignment before beginning work at the scene, and personnel remain with their vehicle in the staging area until they are assigned their duties.

Triage Supervisor

The **triage supervisor** is ultimately in charge of counting and prioritizing patients. During large incidents, a number of triage personnel may be needed. The primary duty of the triage division or group is to ensure that all patients receive initial assessment of their condition. One of the most difficult parts of working as triage personnel is that you must not begin treatment until all patients are triaged, with the exception of specific, limited lifesaving interventions, or you will compromise your triage efforts.

Treatment Supervisor

The **treatment supervisor** will locate and set up the **treatment area** with a tier for each priority of patient. The treatment supervisor ensures that secondary triage of patients is completed and that adequate patient care is provided as resources allow. The treatment supervisor also assists with moving

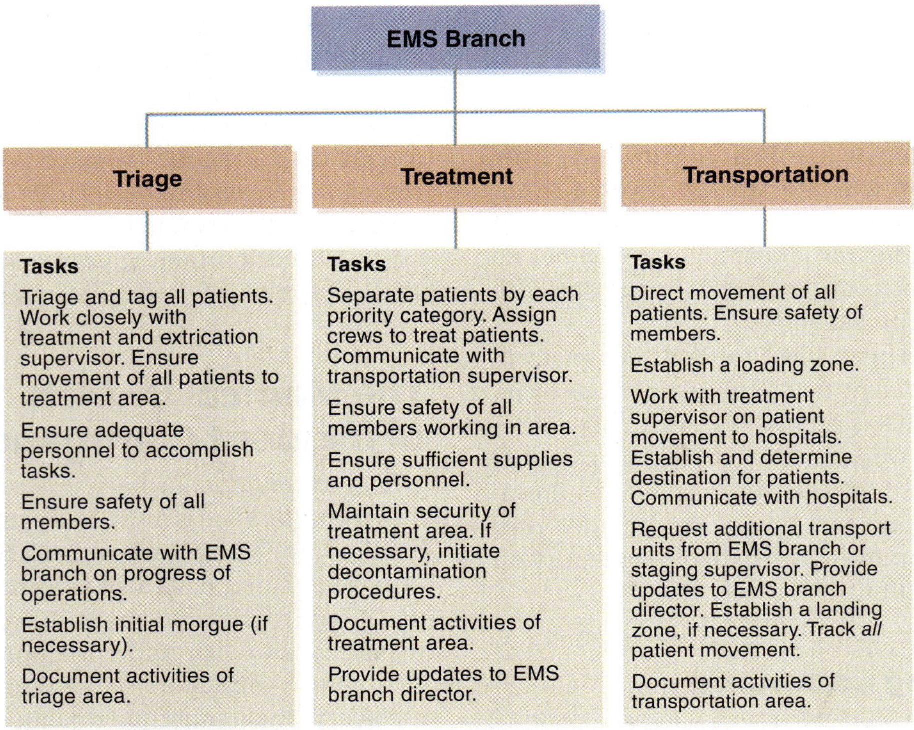

FIGURE 38-5 Components of the medical branch within the incident command system.

patients to the **transportation area**. While supervising the responders, the treatment supervisor must communicate with the medical branch director to request sufficient quantities of supplies, including bandages, burn supplies, airway and respiratory supplies, and patient packaging equipment.

Transportation Supervisor

The **transportation supervisor** coordinates the transportation and distribution of patients to appropriate receiving hospitals and helps to ensure that hospitals do not become overwhelmed by a patient surge. The transportation supervisor coordinates with the IC to ensure that enough personnel and ambulances are in the staging area or have been requested. Some regions may plan for a designated hospital to coordinate with area hospitals on destination decisions. An MCI typically disrupts the everyday functioning of the region's trauma system, so good coordination is needed. The transportation supervisor documents and tracks the number of transport vehicles, patients transported, and the facility destination of each vehicle and patient.

Staging Supervisor

A **staging supervisor** is assigned when an MCI or disaster requires a multivehicle or multiagency response. Emergency vehicles receive direction from the staging supervisor to enter an MCI scene and should drive only in the directed area. The staging area should be established away from the scene so that the parked vehicles are not in the way. If a staging area is located too close to a chaotic scene, patients or fellow responders may see the number of ambulances waiting and bring patients directly to the staging area as opposed to the triage area. The staging supervisor locates an area to stage equipment and responders, tracks unit arrivals, and releases vehicles and supplies when ordered by command. This position plans for efficient access to and exit from the scene and prevents traffic congestion among responding vehicles.

Physicians on Scene

In an MCI or disaster, some areas have plans in place for physicians to respond to the scene. Sometimes this includes the EMS medical director or another physician who regularly works, trains, and interacts with your agency. Sometimes, even without a plan, the enormity of the situation may require physicians on scene. EMS physicians, especially, will have the training to make difficult triage decisions. They also provide secondary triage decisions in the treatment area, deciding which priority patients are to be transported first. Physicians can provide on-scene medical direction for EMTs, and they can provide care as appropriate. Like other fire and EMS clinicians, there is the possibility that physicians who are nearby may self-dispatch to respond to the scene to help. If you encounter a physician, you should ensure that this person is assigned to the incident. This precaution will verify the physician's credentials and ensure this new resource is factored into the ICS. As mentioned previously, the IC must be able to account for all people on scene should a secondary event occur.

Rehabilitation Supervisor

In disasters or MCIs that will last for extended periods, a rehabilitation section for the responders should be established. The **rehabilitation supervisor** establishes an area that provides protection for responders from the elements and the situation. The **rehabilitation area** should be located away from exhaust fumes and crowds (especially members of the media) and out of view of the scene itself. Rehabilitation is where a responder's needs for rest, fluids, food, and protection from the elements are met.

The rehabilitation supervisor must also monitor responders for signs of stress. These signs may include dehydration, fatigue, confusion, and complete collapse. NFPA 1584, *Standard on the Rehabilitation Process for Members During Emergency Operations and Training Exercises*, helps guide EMS on rehab operations. EMS agencies should preplan with other local responders to establish these guidelines.[3] Remember that all EMS personnel must be aware of signs of stress. Your service might consider having a defusing team in this area to support the team's emotional needs. Responders should be encouraged to take advantage of these services but should never be forced to participate.

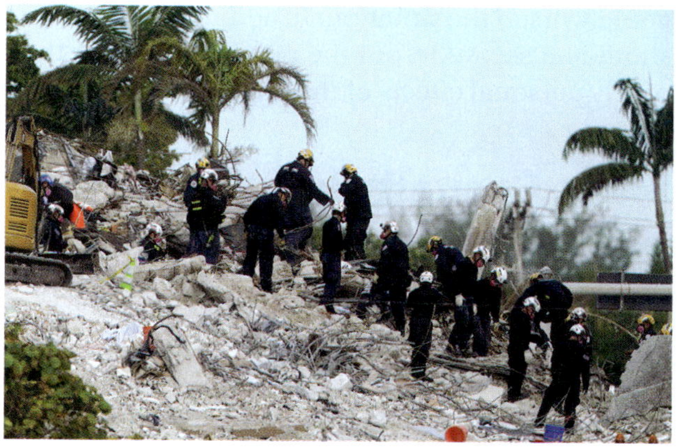

FIGURE 38-6 Some disasters will involve search and rescue or extrication. Shown here, rescue crews work at the site of a collapsed condominium in Surfside, Florida, in 2021.

Extrication and Special Rescue

Some MCIs or disasters require search and rescue or extrication of patients (**FIGURE 38-6**). A unit leader may need to be appointed. For example, an **extrication supervisor** may be needed to oversee the removal of patients trapped in vehicles or structures, or a **rescue supervisor** may be needed to ensure resources are available for specialized rescue situations. In some incidents, victims may need to be extricated or rescued by specifically trained personnel before they can be triaged and treated. Extrication and rescue can be dangerous, so team member safety is of utmost importance.

Morgue Supervisor

In some MCIs or disasters, there will be many dead patients. The **morgue supervisor** will work with area medical examiners, coroners, disaster mortuary assistance teams, and law enforcement agencies to coordinate removal of the bodies and even, possibly, body parts. The morgue supervisor should attempt to leave the dead victims in the location found, if possible, until a removal and storage plan can be determined. The location of victims may help in the identification of the dead victims in mass-fatality situations, or there may be crime scene considerations. If it is determined that a morgue area is needed, the morgue supervisor should ensure that the morgue is out of view of the living patients and other responders because the psychological impact could worsen the situation. In addition, the morgue should be secured from the public to prevent theft of any personal effects of the dead victims.

Mass-Casualty Incidents

As discussed earlier, an MCI is an emergency situation that involves three or more patients, places great demands on the EMS system, and/or has the potential to produce multiple casualties. However, other causes of MCIs are far more common than disasters and are usually much smaller in scope. **FIGURE 38-7** is a diagrammed example of a residential building fire confined to one apartment that may produce only one patient but that has the potential to generate dozens of patients from the responders and residents. Loss of power to a hospital or nursing home with ventilator-dependent and nonambulatory victims is considered an MCI, although no one is injured. By using the ICS and the NIMS and understanding the various roles and responsibilities of each position, the responders and/or IC can scale the plan to manage the incident in a smooth, organized manner.

All systems have different protocols for when to declare an MCI and initiate the ICS; however, as an EMT, ask yourself the following questions when considering whether the call is an MCI:

- How many seriously injured or ill patients can I care for effectively and transport in the ambulance? One? Two?
- What happens when I have three patients to manage?
- How long will it take for additional help to arrive?
- What happens if the number of patients exceeds the number of available ambulances?

Obviously, you and your team cannot treat and transport all injured patients at the same time. At an MCI, you will often experience an increased demand for equipment and personnel. For example, you may realize that you are the only ambulance crew currently at the scene and there is a wait of 15 or more minutes before the next ambulance arrives. Never begin transporting patients if there are still other patients present who are sick or wounded before another responding agency has arrived to continue triage and care. Doing so would leave patients at the scene without medical care and can be considered abandonment. If there are multiple patients and not enough resources to handle them without abandoning victims, you should declare an MCI (at least for the present time), request additional resources, and initiate the ICS and triage procedures (discussed next) (**FIGURE 38-8**). Although this may cause some delay in initiating treatment of all patients, it will not adversely affect the patient care. Always follow your local protocol. Many large EMS systems deploy specialized MCI units or mobile emergency room vehicles that have the capacity to treat dozens of patients at the scene.

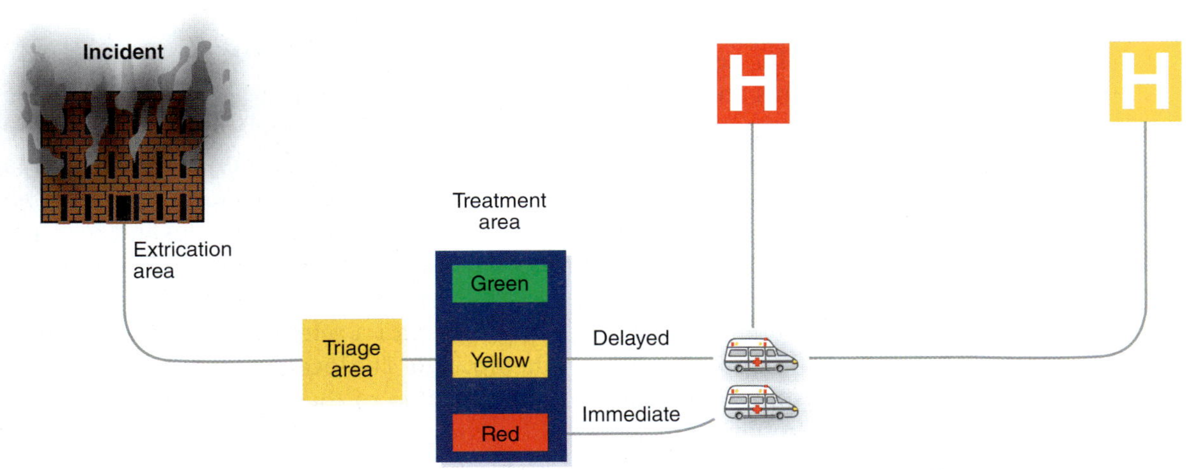

FIGURE 38-7 Diagram of a mass-casualty incident. The incident command system established at the scene of a building fire may look similar to this diagram. Hospital destination depends on the number of patients and local resources.

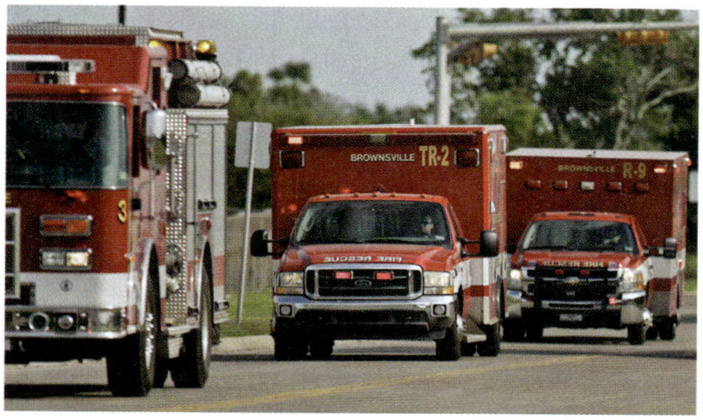

FIGURE 38-8 Mass-casualty incidents require additional ambulances and EMS clinicians from the immediate region.

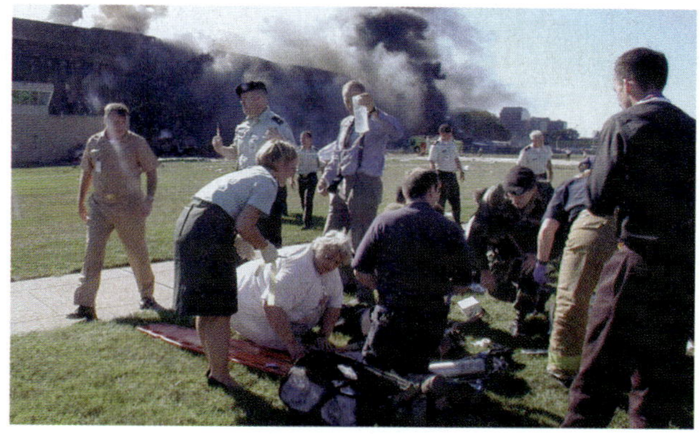

FIGURE 38-9 Triage is the process of sorting and prioritizing patients based on severity of conditions. Shown here, medical personnel and volunteers work the first medical triage area set up outside the Pentagon after a hijacked commercial airliner crashed into the southwest corner of the building on September 11, 2001.

Triage

Triage is the process of sorting patients based on the severity of their injuries (**FIGURE 38-9**). The goal of doing the greatest good for the greatest number means the triage assessment is brief, and you will group the patients into basic categories. **Primary triage** is the initial triage done in the field, allowing you to quickly and accurately categorize the patient's condition and transport needs, whereas **secondary triage** is done as patients are brought to the treatment area. During primary triage, patients are briefly assessed and then identified in some way, such as by attaching a triage tag or colored triage tape. The main information needed on the tag is a unique number and a triage category. Rapid and accurate triage will help bring order to the chaos of the MCI scene and allow the most critical patients to be transported first. After the primary triage, the triage supervisor should communicate the following information to the medical branch director:

- Total number of patients
- Number of patients in each of the triage categories
- Recommendations for extrication and movement of patients to the treatment area
- Resources needed to complete triage and begin movement of patients

When the initial triage has been completed, secondary triage, or retriage, can occur, allowing you to reassess all remaining patients and, if necessary, to upgrade their triage category. In smaller MCI events, this step may not be necessary if enough resources have arrived on the scene.

Words of Wisdom

For multiple victims of a lightning strike, you should use the reverse triage method. With traditional triage, an apneic and pulseless patient would typically be triaged as "black" or "expectant." In the case of a lightning strike, however, treat cardiac or respiratory arrest victims first. Lightning strike injuries are covered in detail in Chapter 32, *Environmental Emergencies*.

Triage Categories

There are four common triage categories. You can remember them using the mnemonic IDME, which stands for Immediate (red), Delayed (yellow), Minor or Minimal (green; hold), and Expectant (black; likely to die or dead) (**TABLE 38-1**). This is the order of priority for treatment and transport of the patients at an MCI.

Immediate (red-tag) patients are your first priority. They need immediate care and transport. They usually have problems with the Airway, Breathing, and Circulation (ABCs), head trauma, or signs and symptoms of shock.

Delayed (yellow-tag) patients are the second priority and need treatment and transport, but it can be delayed. These patients usually have multiple injuries to bones or joints, including back injuries with or without spinal cord injury.

TABLE 38-1 Triage Priorities

Triage Category	Typical Injuries
Red tag: first priority (immediate) Patients who need immediate care and transport Treat these patients first, and transport as soon as possible	• Airway and breathing compromise • Uncontrolled or severe bleeding • Severe medical problems • Signs of shock (hypoperfusion) • Severe burns • Open chest or abdominal injuries
Yellow tag: second priority (delayed) Patients whose treatment and transport can be temporarily delayed	• Burns without airway compromise • Major or multiple bone or joint injuries • Back injuries with or without spinal cord damage
Green tag: third priority, minimal (walking wounded) Patients who require minimal or no treatment and transport can be delayed until last	• Minor fractures • Minor soft-tissue injuries
Black tag: fourth priority (expectant) Patients who are already dead or have little chance for survival Treat salvageable patients before treating these patients	• Obvious death • Obviously nonsurvivable injury, such as major open brain trauma • Respiratory arrest (if limited resources) • Cardiac arrest

Minimal (green-tag) patients are the third priority. These patients may require no field treatment or only minimal treatment. In some parts of the world, this is the hold category. These patients are the "walking wounded" at the scene. If they have any apparent injuries, they are usually soft-tissue injuries such as contusions, abrasions, and lacerations.

The last priority is the expectant (black-tag) patients who are dead or whose injuries are so severe that they have, at best, a minimal chance of survival. This category may include patients who are in cardiac arrest or who have an open head injury, for example. If you have limited resources, this category may also include patients in respiratory arrest. Patients in this category receive treatment and transport only after patients in the other three categories have received care.

Words of Wisdom

You may encounter exceptions to the four-color system described here. A fifth triage category, the orange-tag category, is sometimes added. This category represents an intermediate category between the critical (red tag) and noncritical, nonambulatory (yellow tag) categories of patients. During a true MCI, there may be patients who require prompt evaluation and treatment for symptoms that are the result of medical comorbidities and not the acute traumatic injuries associated with the initial event. Consider patients who are having nontraumatic chest pain or shortness of breath following the event. If placed in this intermediate category, these patients could be more appropriately prioritized for treatment and transport because their condition may be treated by a specific destination that is not a trauma center (eg, cardiac catheterization center, hyperbaric chamber). The Fire Department of the City of New York's Simple Triage and Rapid Treatment (FDNY-START) system now incorporates the orange-tag category, and there may be ongoing developments as other systems adopt similar classifications.

Some branches of the military use both a black triage color (deceased) and a blue triage color (unlikely to survive transport). If you have military installations in your response area, you should coordinate with them to determine which color triage tags they are using to avoid confusion in the event of an MCI.

Triage Tags

Whatever triage system is used, it is vital that a patient has a tag or some type of label. Tagging patients early assists in tracking them and keeping an accurate record of their condition. Triage tags should be waterproof and easy to read (**FIGURE 38-10**). The patient tags or tape should be color-coded and should clearly show the category of the patients. The use of both symbols and colors to indicate the triage categories is important in case some responders are color-blind.

The tags will become part of the patient's medical record. Most have a tear-off receipt with

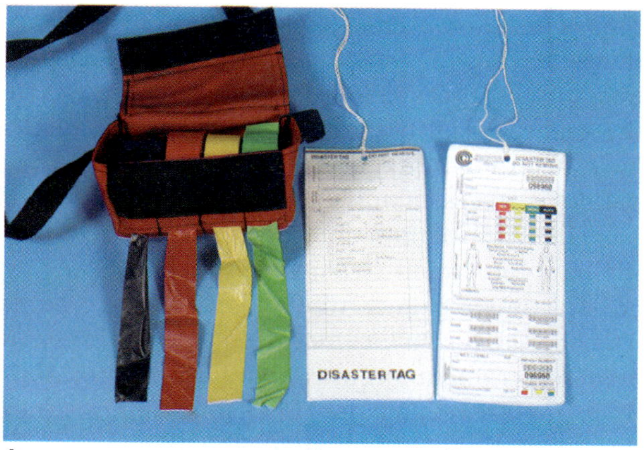

A B C

FIGURE 38-10 Triage tags (from left to right). **A.** Waterproof triage tape. **B.** Triage tag: back. **C.** Triage tag: front.

a number correlating with the number on the tag. When torn off by the transportation officer, it will assist in tracking the patient. If the patient is unconscious and cannot be identified at the scene, the tag will be an identifier for tracking purposes. Some areas use digital photography to assist in identifying patients later. The photograph is catalogued with the patient's tag number, and the patient's location is tracked with this information. When family members are brought to crisis centers to help locate loved ones, the pictures may be of assistance. This technique has been used effectively in Europe and Israel with Polaroid or digital photos. Another way of tracking and accounting for patients is to issue only 20 to 25 cards or tags at a time, with a scorecard to mark how patients are triaged and their priority. When the responder returns for more tags, the scorecard will provide a patient count to help command and the staff to develop a plan to respond and ensure that appropriate resources are either available or summoned. Whatever labeling system is used, it is imperative for the transportation officer to be able to identify which patient was transported by which unit and to which destination, and the priority of the patient's condition.

Triage Systems

Simple Triage And Rapid Treatment (START)

START triage is one of the easiest methods of triage. START stands for Simple Triage And Rapid Treatment. The staff members at Hoag Memorial Hospital, Newport Beach, California, developed this method of triage. It is easily mastered with practice and enables responders to rapidly categorize patients at an MCI. START triage uses a limited assessment of the patient's ability to walk, respiratory status, hemodynamic status (pulse), and neurologic status.

The first step of the START triage system is performed on arrival at the scene by calling out to patients at the disaster site, "If you can hear my voice and are able to walk . . ." and then directing patients to an easily identifiable landmark. You should pick a landmark that is away from your ambulance. Bringing a large number of patients toward you and your ambulance will hinder your ability to properly triage all of the patients. You can send the ambulatory patients toward a landmark, such as a lamp pole or the corner of a street. This will help to manage the chaos of an MCI. The injured people in this group are the walking wounded and are considered minimal (green) priority, or third-priority, patients.

The second step in the START process is directed toward nonwalking patients. Move to the first nonambulatory patient and assess the respiratory status. If the patient is not breathing, open the airway by using a simple manual maneuver. A patient who still does not begin to breathe is triaged as expectant (black). If the patient begins to breathe, tag the person as immediate (red), place in the recovery position, and move on to the next patient (**FIGURE 38-11**).

If the patient is breathing, quickly estimate the respiratory rate. A patient who is breathing faster than 30 breaths/min or slower than 10 breaths/min is triaged as an immediate priority (red). If the patient is breathing from 10 to 29 breaths/min, move to the next step of the assessment.

The next step is to assess the hemodynamic status of the patient by checking for bilateral radial pulses. An absent radial pulse implies the patient is likely hypotensive; tag this person as an immediate priority (red). If the radial pulse is present, go to the next assessment.

The final assessment in START triage is to assess the patient's neurologic status, which simply means to assess the patient's ability to follow simple commands, such as "Show me three fingers." This assessment establishes that the patient can understand and follow commands. A patient who is

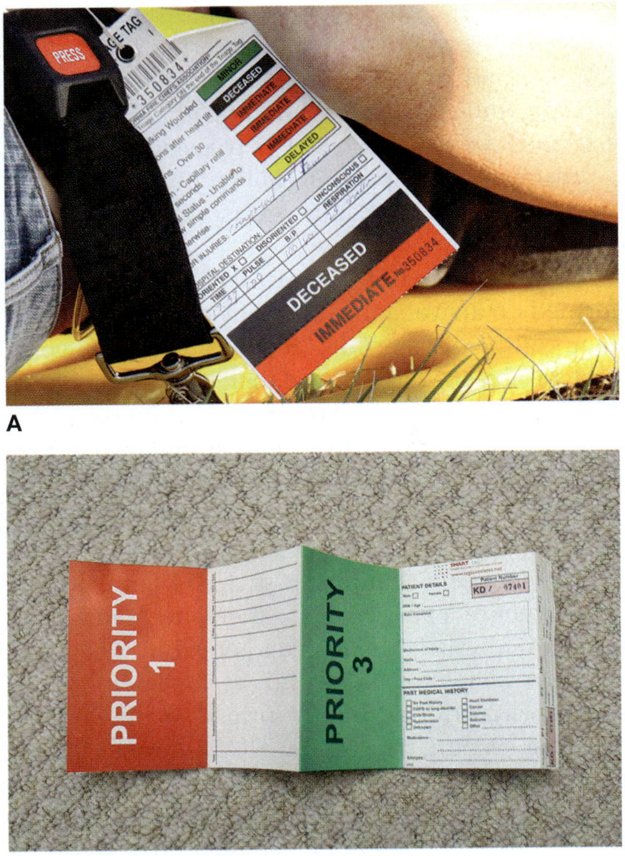

A

B

FIGURE 38-11 A. A START triage tag is ripped to the level of severity. **B.** A SMART triage tag folds to the level of severity. (SMART is a series of triage products that can be used in support of specific triage systems, including START.)

A: Nancy G Fire Photography, Nancy Greifenhagen/Alamy Stock Photo; **B:** Courtesy of Richard Pilbery.

unconscious or cannot follow simple commands is an immediate priority patient (red). A patient who complies with a simple command should be triaged in the delayed category (yellow).

Sort, Assess, Lifesaving interventions, and Treatment and/or Transport (SALT)

Another triage method is the Sort, Assess, Lifesaving interventions, and Treatment and/or Transport (SALT) triage system. This triage system begins with a global sorting of patients. This step identifies the patients who are able to understand verbal instructions and are therefore likely to have good systemic perfusion. Patients who can walk are asked to move to a designated area and are assigned last priority. This is an attempt to decrease the number of patients leaving the scene and overwhelming local hospital resources before EMS can begin to move the highest priority patients. Once those patients have been identified and moved, each remaining patient is assessed individually.

The SALT method differs from others in its lifesaving intervention steps, which include bleeding control, opening the airway, and two rescue breaths for children. It also includes needle decompression for tension pneumothorax and auto-injector antidotes for ALS clinicians. These interventions may be all that is needed to upgrade the patient's condition on the SALT triage scale.

The SALT system includes a gray category for expectant and reserves black for patients who are deceased. This gray category is for patients whose survival requires resources that are not currently available on scene but who may be retriaged if those resources become available. For example, a patient with agonal breathing following multiple penetrating chest traumas or a patient with extensive burns may be placed in the gray category.

The final step is treatment and/or transport.

Words of Wisdom

The Model Uniform Core Curriculum (MUCC) was written to identify key elements of an effective triage system.[4] It was designed to offer uniform triage criteria so that emergency personnel responding to an MCI from different jurisdictions would have a simple, easy-to-use system that promotes a shared understanding of the triage levels. SALT triage is the only MUCC-compliant triage system, although many other triage systems are used throughout the country.

JumpSTART Triage for Pediatric Patients

Lou Romig, MD, recognized that the START triage system does not take into account the physiologic and developmental differences of pediatric patients (**FIGURE 38-12**). Thus, she developed the **JumpSTART triage** system for pediatric patients. JumpSTART is intended for use in children younger than 8 years or who appear to weigh less than 100 pounds (45 kg). As in START, the JumpSTART system begins by identifying the walking wounded.

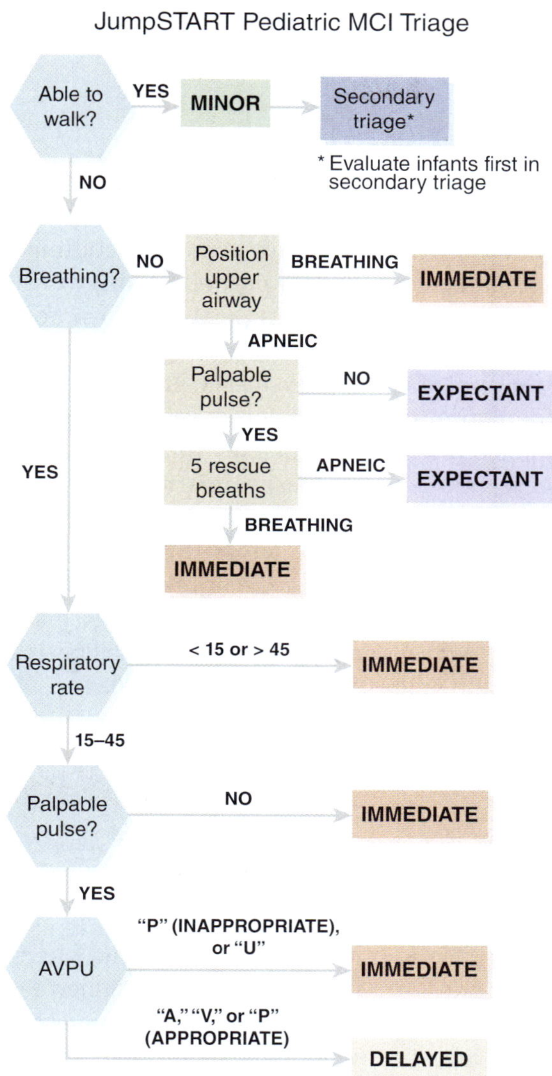

FIGURE 38-12 The JumpSTART triage system.

Infants or children not developed enough to walk or follow commands (including children with special needs) should be taken as soon as possible to the treatment area for immediate secondary triage. This action assists in getting children who cannot take care of their own basic needs to a health care clinician. There are several differences within the respiratory status assessment compared with that in START. First, if you find that a pediatric patient is not breathing, open the airway. If the patient begins breathing, they receive an immediate (red) tag. If they do not start spontaneously breathing, check the pulse. If there is no pulse, label the patient as expectant (black). If the patient has a pulse, provide five rescue breaths. A child who does not breathe after five rescue breaths should be labeled expectant; if they do breathe, they are labeled immediate. The primary reason for this difference is that the most common cause of cardiac arrest in children is respiratory arrest.

The next step of the JumpSTART process is to assess the approximate rate of respirations. A child who is breathing fewer than 15 breaths/min or more than 45 breaths/min is tagged as an immediate priority (red), and you move on to the next patient. If the respirations are within the range of 15 to 45 breaths/min, the patient is assessed further.

The next assessment in JumpSTART triage is also the hemodynamic status of the patient. Just like in START, you are simply checking for a distal pulse. This does not need to be the brachial pulse; assess the pulse that you feel the most competent and comfortable checking. If a distal pulse is not felt, label the child as an immediate priority and move to the next patient. If the child has a distal pulse, move on to the next assessment.

The final assessment is for neurologic status. Because of the developmental differences in children, their responses will vary. For JumpSTART, a modified AVPU score is used. A child who is unresponsive or responds to pain by posturing or with incomprehensible sounds or is unable to localize pain is tagged as an immediate priority. A child who responds to pain by localizing it or withdrawing from it or is alert is considered a delayed-priority patient (yellow).

Triage Special Considerations

There are a few special situations in triage. Patients who are hysterical and disruptive to rescue efforts may need to be handled as an immediate priority and transported off the site, even if they are not seriously injured. Panic breeds panic, and this type of behavior could have a negative effect on other patients and on the responders.

A responder who becomes seriously ill or injured during the rescue effort should be handled as an immediate priority and be transported off the site as soon as possible to avoid negative effect on the morale of remaining responders.

Hazmat and weapons of mass destruction incidents force the hazmat team to identify patients as contaminated or decontaminated before the regular triage process. Contamination by chemicals or biologic weapons in a treatment area, hospital, or trauma center could obstruct all systems and organizations coping with the MCI or disaster. Bear in mind that some incidents may require multiple triage areas or teams because the victims are located far apart.

Destination Decisions

All patients triaged as immediate (red) or delayed (yellow) should preferably be transported by ground ambulance or air ambulance, if available, to the most appropriate facility (trauma, burn, or pediatric center). In extremely large situations, a bus may transport the walking wounded. If a bus is used for minimal-priority patients, it is strongly suggested that they be transported to a hospital or clinic distant from the MCI or disaster site to avoid overwhelming the local area hospital resources. If a bus is used, plan for at least one EMT or paramedic to ride on board and to have an ambulance follow the bus. If a minimal-priority patient's condition worsens, the patient could be moved to the ambulance and transported to a closer facility. The EMT or paramedic can stay with the minimal-priority patients until their arrival at the designated hospital. Any worsening of a patient's condition must be relayed to the receiving hospital as soon as possible in whatever manner the incident dictates. Refer to the Centers for Disease Control and Prevention's 2021 decision scheme for field triage of injured patients. This scheme is presented in Chapter 24, *Trauma Overview*.

Immediate-priority patients should be transported two at a time until all are transported from the site. Then patients in the delayed category can be transported two or three at a time until all are at a hospital. Finally, the walking wounded are transported. Expectant patients who are still alive would receive treatment and transport at this time. Dead victims are handled or transported according to local standard operating procedures.

It is important to remember that during an MCI, local hospitals may have their resources overwhelmed. Early notification to receiving facilities will allow for hospitals to increase staffing and move patients within their facility as required. Typically, EMS agencies will know a hospital's surge capacity, which will tell the agency how many patients of each category the hospital is able to safely handle and care for.

Disaster Management

The term **disaster** is a designation made by an elected official to describe a widespread event that disrupts functions and resources of a community and threatens lives and/or property. Many disasters do not necessarily result in personal harm; for example, a drought that causes widespread crop damage may not affect the physical health of those living in the community. However, many disasters such as floods, fires, and hurricanes will result in widespread injuries and even secondary problems such as increased incidence of medical emergencies and disease transmission. Unlike an MCI, which generally lasts no longer than a few hours, emergency responders will generally be on the scene of a disaster for days to weeks and sometimes months (as in the events following Hurricane Helene in 2024).

Words of Wisdom

Although you can declare an MCI as an EMT, only an elected official can declare a disaster.

Your role in a disaster is to respond when requested and to report to the IC for assigned tasks. In a disaster with an overwhelming number of casualties, area hospitals may decide that they cannot treat all patients at their facility. In this case, they may mobilize medical and nursing teams with equipment and set up a **casualty collection area** at a facility near the disaster scene, such as a warehouse. Once at the casualty collection area, the teams can perform triage, provide medical care, and transport patients to the hospital on a priority basis.

If a casualty collection area is established, it will be coordinated through the ICS in the same way as all other branches and areas of the operation. This is usually done only in a major disaster such as an earthquake when transportation to a hospital facility is impossible or involves prolonged delays. It may take several hours to establish a casualty collection area.

In smaller incidents, where there is an immediate threat in the initial incident area, patients may be brought to a designated casualty collection point where secondary triage and treatment can be performed. This strategy is used in active military combat and in mass shooting incidents when the perpetrator has not yet been apprehended.

Street Smarts

MCIs and disasters take a physical and emotional toll on emergency responders. Seek medical evaluation if you have been injured, come in contact with any hazardous substance, or inhale any dust, fumes, or smoke. Often the health effects of such exposures do not manifest for years and are difficult to link back to a specific event. In addition, you should be aware of the signs of stress in yourself and in your coworkers. Consider taking advantage of support opportunities, such as critical incident stress debriefing (CISD), critical incident stress management (CISM), and peer support programs, after an incident if you feel they may be valuable. Chapter 2, *Workforce Safety and Wellness*, covers stress and CISD/CISM in detail.

Words of Wisdom

Urban Search and Rescue teams (USARs) and Disaster Medical Assistance Teams (DMATs) may be mobilized in the event of a natural disaster or MCI. USARs typically provide rescue and initial medical stabilization to patients entrapped in confined spaces, such as from a structural collapse. DMATs provide medical care during an incident; they include clinicians such as physicians, paramedics, nurses, and EMTs who work at the federal level. DMATs are typically activated for periods of 2 weeks, and they arrive with sufficient supplies and equipment to provide care for 3 days.

Introduction to Hazardous Materials

Your training has taught you that rapid response to the scene of a crash can save lives. However, when you arrive at the scene of a possible hazmat incident, you must first step back and assess the situation. It can be very difficult to stop yourself from immediately engaging in patient care, particularly if you can see a patient. However, rushing into an unsafe scene can have catastrophic results. If you are overcome by a hazardous substance, not only will patients suffer because you will be unable to assist them, but you will also place a strain on the system because you will require emergency care.

Because of the unique aspects of responding to and working at a **hazardous materials (hazmat) incident**, the Occupational Safety and Health Administration (OSHA) has published a set of guidelines known as the Hazardous Waste Operations and Emergency Response (HAZWOPER). All clinicians, including EMTs, must meet specific additional training requirements before becoming involved in hazmat incidents. As an EMT, you need training at the First Responder Awareness Level. This text does not include the skills and information necessary to meet those requirements. You need to check with your agency for information about specific awareness-level training.

On the basis of the HAZWOPER regulation, first responders at the awareness level should have sufficient training or experience to demonstrate the following competencies:

- An understanding of what hazardous substances are and the risks associated with them
- An understanding of the potential outcomes of an incident

YOU are the EMT

Using the ambulance's public address system, you ask for anyone who can walk to come to the front gate, where a bus will be positioned to transport them. Next, you approach a supine middle-aged woman who is unresponsive with slow respirations. She has weak radial pulses. The next patient you encounter is a teenage boy who is apneic with a weak carotid pulse and no radial pulses. You note exposed brain matter. The third patient is an older woman with a severe laceration through the neck and chest; the neck injury has caused near-decapitation. She is apneic and pulseless.

5. What are your considerations in determining whether you should stop and provide treatment for the first patient?

6. What triage categories should you assign to the second and third patients?

- The ability to recognize the presence of hazardous substances
- The ability to identify the hazardous substances, if possible
- An understanding of the role of the awareness-level first responder in the emergency response plan
- The ability to determine the need for additional resources and to notify the communications center

Recognizing a Hazardous Material

A **hazardous material** is any material that poses an unreasonable risk of damage or injury to people, property, or the environment if it is not properly controlled during handling, storage, manufacture, processing, packaging, use and disposal, and transportation. Recognizing a hazmat incident, determining the identity of the material or materials, and understanding the hazards involved often require some detective work. You must train yourself to take the time to look at the whole scene so that you can identify the critical visual indicators and fit them into what you know about the problem.

Hazardous materials may be involved in any of the following situations (**FIGURE 38-13**):

- A truck or train crash in which a substance is leaking from a tank truck or railroad tank car
- A leak, fire, or other emergency at an industrial plant, refinery, or other complex where chemicals or explosives are produced, used, or stored
- A leak or rupture of an underground natural gas pipe
- Deterioration of underground fuel tanks and seepage of oil or gasoline into the surrounding ground
- Buildup of methane or other by-products of waste decomposition in sewers or sewage-processing plants
- A motor vehicle crash in which a gas tank has ruptured

Initially, it is important to approach the scene from a safe location and direction. The traditional rules of staying uphill and upwind are a good place to start. In addition, it may be wise to use binoculars

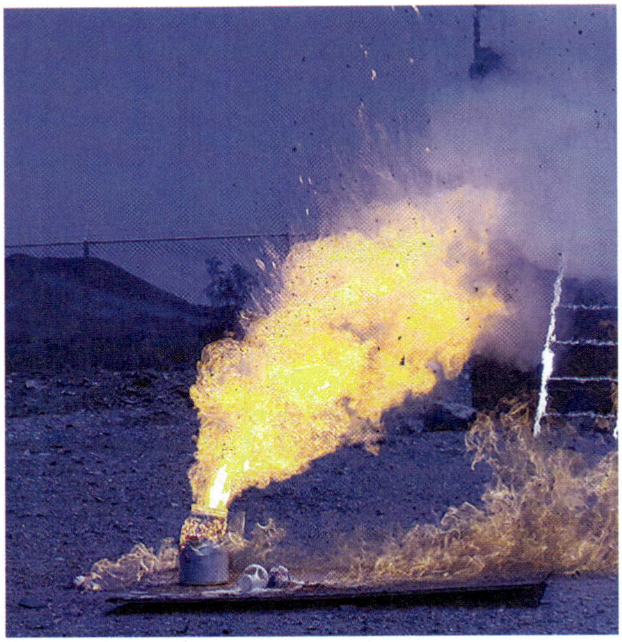

A

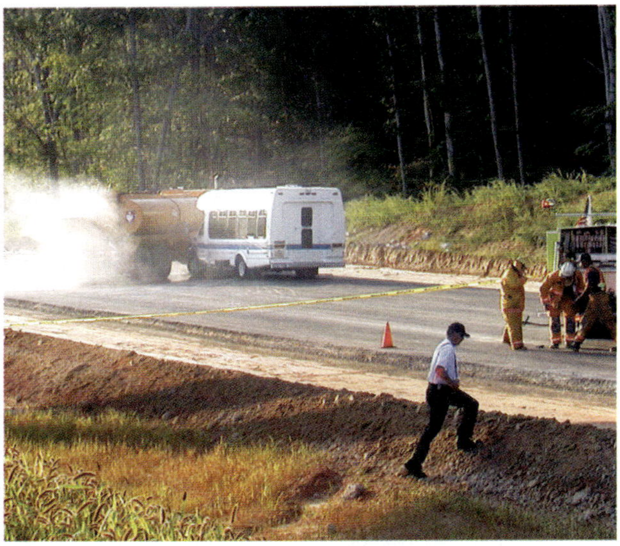

B

FIGURE 38-13 Two examples of hazardous materials incidents. **A.** Burning container of flammable liquid. **B.** Crashed tanker truck.

A: Courtesy of Rob L. Jackson/US Marines; **B:** Courtesy of George Roarty/Virginia Department of Emergency Management.

and view the scene from a safe distance. Be sure to question anyone involved in the incident; a wealth of information may be available to you if you simply ask the right person. Take enough time to assess the scene and interpret other clues such as dead animals near the point of release, discolored pavement, dead grass, visible vapors or puddles, or labels that may help identify the presence of a hazardous material. Once you have a basic idea of what happened or determine that danger may be present, you can begin to formulate a plan for addressing the incident.

Occupancy and Location

A wide variety of chemicals are stored in warehouses, hospitals, laboratories, industrial complexes, residential garages, bowling alleys, home improvement centers, garden supply stores, restaurants, and scores of other facilities or businesses in your response area. So many different chemicals exist in so many different locations that you could encounter almost anything during any type of emergency situation. The location and type of building are two good indicators of the possible presence of a hazardous material. For example, a biomedical laboratory is more likely than a preschool to have chemicals that could be hazardous on site. However, it is important to remember that many common buildings may have materials, like large amounts of cleaning supplies, that could be hazardous in the right scenario.

Senses

Another way to detect the presence of hazardous materials is to use your senses, although this technique must be used carefully to avoid exposure. The senses you can safely use are sight and sound. As a general rule, the farther you are from the incident, the safer you will be. When it comes to hazmat incidents, "leading with your nose" is not a good tactic, but using binoculars from a distance is.

Clues that are seen or heard from a distance may enable you to take precautionary steps. Vapor clouds at the scene, for example, are a signal to move yourself and others away to a place of safety; the sound of an alarm from a toxic gas sensor in a chemical storage room or laboratory may also serve as a warning to retreat. Some highly vaporous and odorous chemicals (eg, chlorine and ammonia) may be detected by smell a long way from the actual point of release.

> **Words of Wisdom**
>
> If you have accidentally become exposed to a hazardous material by getting in too far, own it. For your safety, and the safety of your crew and patients, it is imperative that you advise command of your exposure and receive the proper decontamination and treatment. Do not feel embarrassed and try to hide the accidental exposure. Your life is more important than your ego.

Containers

In basic terms, a **container** is any vessel or receptacle that holds a material. Often the container's type, size, and material of construction provide important clues about the nature of the substance inside. Nevertheless, do not rely solely on the type of container when making a determination about hazardous materials.

Red phosphorus from a drug laboratory, for example, might be found in an unmarked plastic container. In this case, there may not be legitimate markings to alert you to the possible contents. Gasoline or waste solvents may be stored in 55-gallon (208-L) steel drums. Sulfuric acid, at 97% concentration, could be found in a polyethylene drum that might be colored black, red, white, or blue. In most cases, there is no correlation between the color of the drum and the possible contents. The same sulfuric acid might also be found in a 1-gallon (3.8-L) amber glass container. Steel or polyethylene drums, bags, high-pressure gas cylinders, railroad tank cars, plastic buckets, aboveground and underground storage tanks, cargo tanks, and pipelines all are examples of how hazardous materials are packaged, stored, and transported (**FIGURE 38-14**).

Some recognizable chemical containers, such as 55-gallon (208-L) drums and compressed gas cylinders, can be found in almost every type of manufacturing facility. Materials stored in a cardboard drum are usually in solid form. Stainless steel containers hold particularly dangerous chemicals, and cold liquids are kept in containers designed to maintain the appropriate temperature (**FIGURE 38-15**).

One way to distinguish containers is to divide them into two categories based on their capacity: bulk and nonbulk storage containers.

Container Volume

Bulk storage containers include fixed tanks, highway cargo tanks, rail tank cars, totes, and intermodal

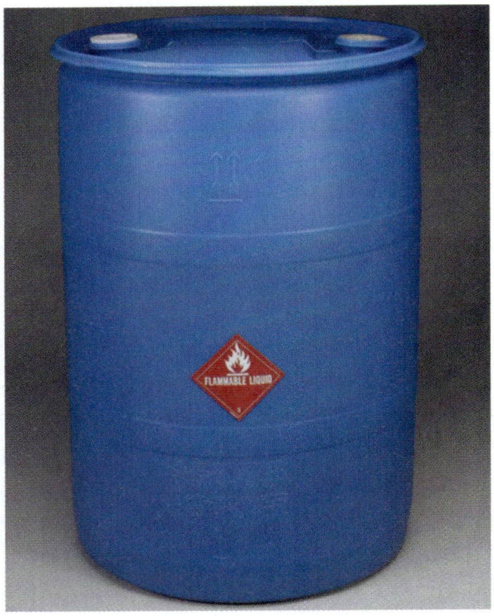

FIGURE 38-14 Drums may be constructed of many different types of materials, including cardboard, polyethylene, and stainless steel. The drum shown here is made of polyethylene.

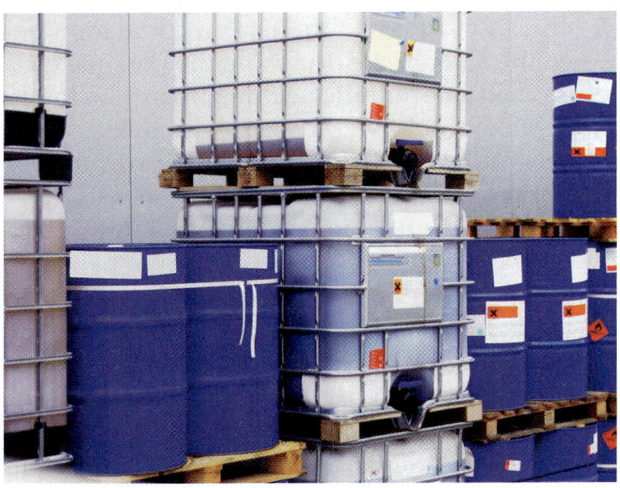

FIGURE 38-15 A series of chemical storage containers.

Safety Tips

When you consider locations for possible hazardous materials incidents, do not limit your thinking. You may be surprised at how many different kinds of containers you may find in your area.

tanks. In general, bulk storage containers are found in buildings that rely on and need to store large quantities of a particular chemical. Most manufacturing facilities have at least one type of bulk storage container. Often these bulk storage containers are surrounded by a secondary containment system to help control an accidental release. **Secondary containment** is an engineered method to control spilled or released product if the main containment vessel fails. A 5,000-gallon (18,927-L) vertical storage tank, for example, may be surrounded by a series of short walls that form a catch basin around the tank.

Large-volume horizontal tanks are also common. When stored above ground, these tanks are referred to as aboveground storage tanks; if they are placed underground, they are known as underground storage tanks. These tanks can hold a few hundred gallons to several million gallons of product and are usually made of aluminum, steel, or plastic.

Another commonly encountered bulk storage vessel is the tote, also referred to as an intermediate bulk container. Totes are found in a variety of shapes and sizes, with the most common sizes being 275 and 330 gallons (1,041 and 1,249 L). These portable plastic tanks are surrounded by a stainless steel web that adds both structural stability and protection to the container. They can contain any type of chemical, including flammable liquids, corrosives, food-grade liquids, or oxidizers (**FIGURE 38-16**).

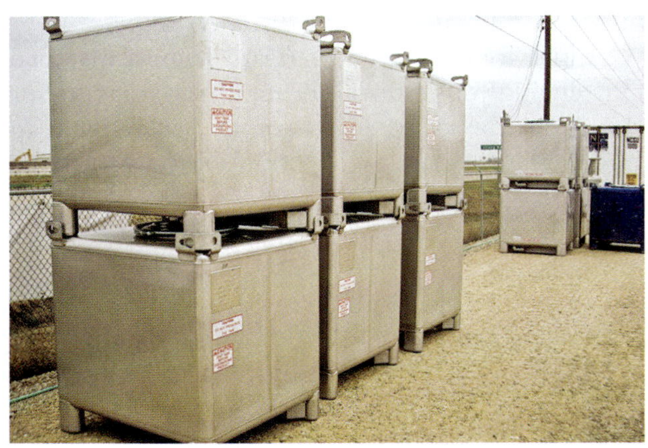

FIGURE 38-16 A tote is a commonly encountered bulk storage vessel.

Shipping and storing totes can be hazardous. These containers often are stacked atop one another and moved with a forklift, and a mishap with the loading or moving process can damage the tote. Because totes have no secondary containment system, any leak has the potential to create a large puddle. In addition, the steel webbing around the tote may make it difficult to access and patch leaks.

Intermodal tanks are both shipping and storage vessels. They hold between 4,000 and 6,000 gallons (15,142 and 22,712 L) of product and can be pressurized or nonpressurized. Intermodal tanks can also be used to ship and store gaseous substances that have been chilled until they liquefy, such as liquid nitrogen. In most cases, an intermodal tank is shipped to a facility, where it is stored and used and then returned to the shipper for refilling. Intermodal tanks can be shipped by all methods of transportation: air, sea, and land (**FIGURE 38-17**).

Nonbulk Storage Vessels

Essentially, **nonbulk storage vessels** are all types of containers other than bulk containers. Nonbulk storage vessels can hold a few ounces to 119 gallons (450 L) of product and include vessels such as drums, bags, compressed gas cylinders, cryogenic containers, and more. Nonbulk storage vessels hold commonly used commercial and industrial chemicals such as solvents, industrial cleaners, and compounds. This section describes the most commonly encountered types of nonbulk storage vessels.

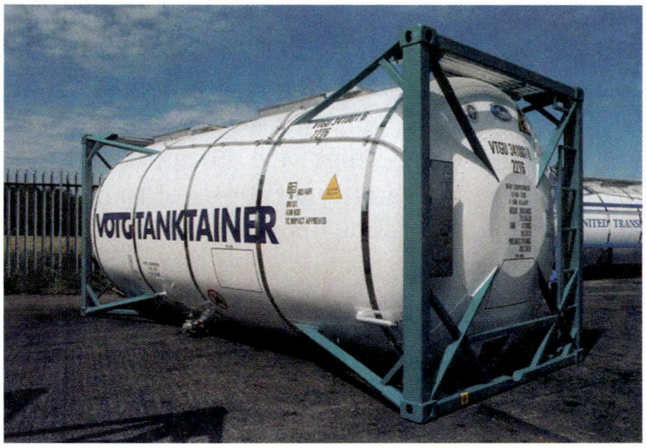

FIGURE 38-17 An intermodal tank.

Courtesy of UBH International Ltd.

Drums

Drums are easily recognizable, barrel-like containers. They are used to store a wide variety of substances, including food-grade materials, corrosive substances, flammable liquids, and grease. Drums may be constructed of low-carbon steel, polyethylene, cardboard, stainless steel, nickel, or other materials. Generally, the nature of the chemical determines the construction of the storage drum. Steel utility drums, for example, hold flammable liquids, cleaning fluids, oil, and other noncorrosive chemicals. Polyethylene drums are used for corrosives such as acids, bases, oxidizers, and other materials that cannot be stored in steel containers. Cardboard drums hold solid materials such as soap flakes, sodium hydroxide pellets, and food-grade materials. Stainless steel or other heavy-duty drums generally hold materials too aggressive (ie, too reactive) for either plain steel or polyethylene.

Bags

Bags are commonly used to store solids and powders such as cement powder, sand, pesticides, soda ash, and slaked lime. Storage bags may be constructed of plastic, paper, or plastic-lined paper. Bags come in different sizes and weights, depending on their contents.

Pesticide bags must be labeled with specific information (**FIGURE 38-18**). You can learn a great deal from the label, including the following details:

- Name of the product
- Active ingredients
- Hazard statement

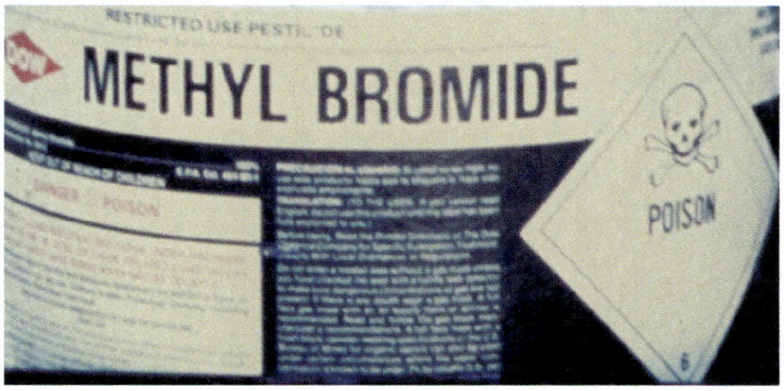

FIGURE 38-18 A pesticide bag must be labeled with the appropriate information.

Courtesy of the USDA.

- The total amount of product in the container
- The manufacturer's name and address
- The Environmental Protection Agency (EPA) registration number, which provides proof that the product was registered with the EPA
- The EPA establishment number, which shows where the product was manufactured
- Signal words to indicate the relative toxicity of the material:
  - Danger—Poison: Highly toxic by all routes of entry
  - Danger: Severe eye damage or skin irritation
  - Warning: Moderately toxic
  - Caution: Minor toxicity and minor eye damage or skin irritation
- Practical first-aid treatment description
- Directions for use
- Agricultural use requirements
- Precautionary statements such as mixing directions or potential environmental hazards
- Storage and disposal information
- Classification statement on who may use the product

In addition, every pesticide label must carry the statement, "Keep out of reach of children."

Carboys

Some corrosives and other types of chemicals are transported and stored in **carboys** (**FIGURE 38-19**). A carboy is a glass, plastic, or steel container that holds 1 to 15 gallons (4 to 57 L) of product. Glass carboys are often placed in a protective wood, foam, fiberglass, or steel box to help prevent breakage. For example, nitric acid, sulfuric acid, and other strong acids are often transported and stored in thick glass carboys protected by a wooden or polystyrene (Styrofoam) crate to shield the glass container from damage during normal shipping.

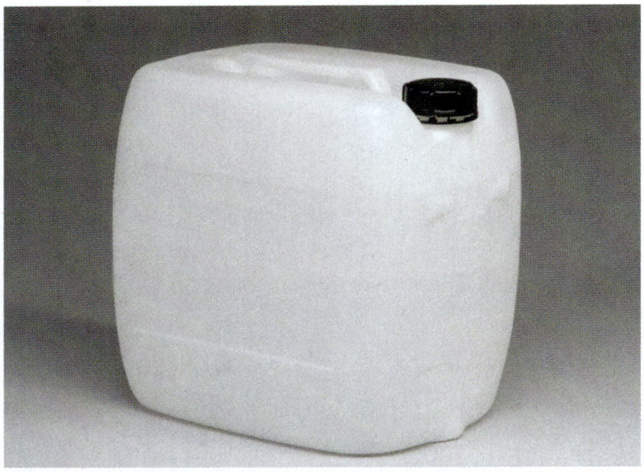

FIGURE 38-19 A carboy is used to transport and store corrosive chemicals.

Courtesy of EMD Chemicals, Inc.

Cylinders

Several types of **cylinders** are used to hold liquids and gases. Uninsulated compressed gas cylinders are used to store substances such as nitrogen, argon, helium, and oxygen. They come in a range of sizes. As an EMT, you are already familiar with the shape of a cylinder; it holds the oxygen for your patients.

The Department of Transportation Marking System

The presence of labels, placards, and other markings on buildings, packages, boxes, and containers can often enable you to identify a released chemical. When used correctly, marking systems indicate the presence of a hazardous material from a safe distance and provide clues about the substance.

The US Department of Transportation (DOT) marking system is an identification system characterized by labels, placards, and markings (**FIGURE 38-20**). This marking system is used in the United States when materials are being transported from one location to another. The same marking system is also used in Canada by Transport Canada.

Placards are diamond-shaped indicators (at least 9.8 inches [250 mm] per side) that are placed on all four sides of highway transport vehicles, railroad tank cars, and other forms of transportation carrying hazardous materials (**FIGURE 38-21**). Labels are smaller versions (3.9 inches [100 mm] per side) of placards; they are placed on the four sides of individual boxes and smaller packages being transported.

Placards, labels, and markings are intended to give a general idea of the hazard inside each container or cargo tank. A placard identifies the broad hazard class (flammable, poison, corrosive) to

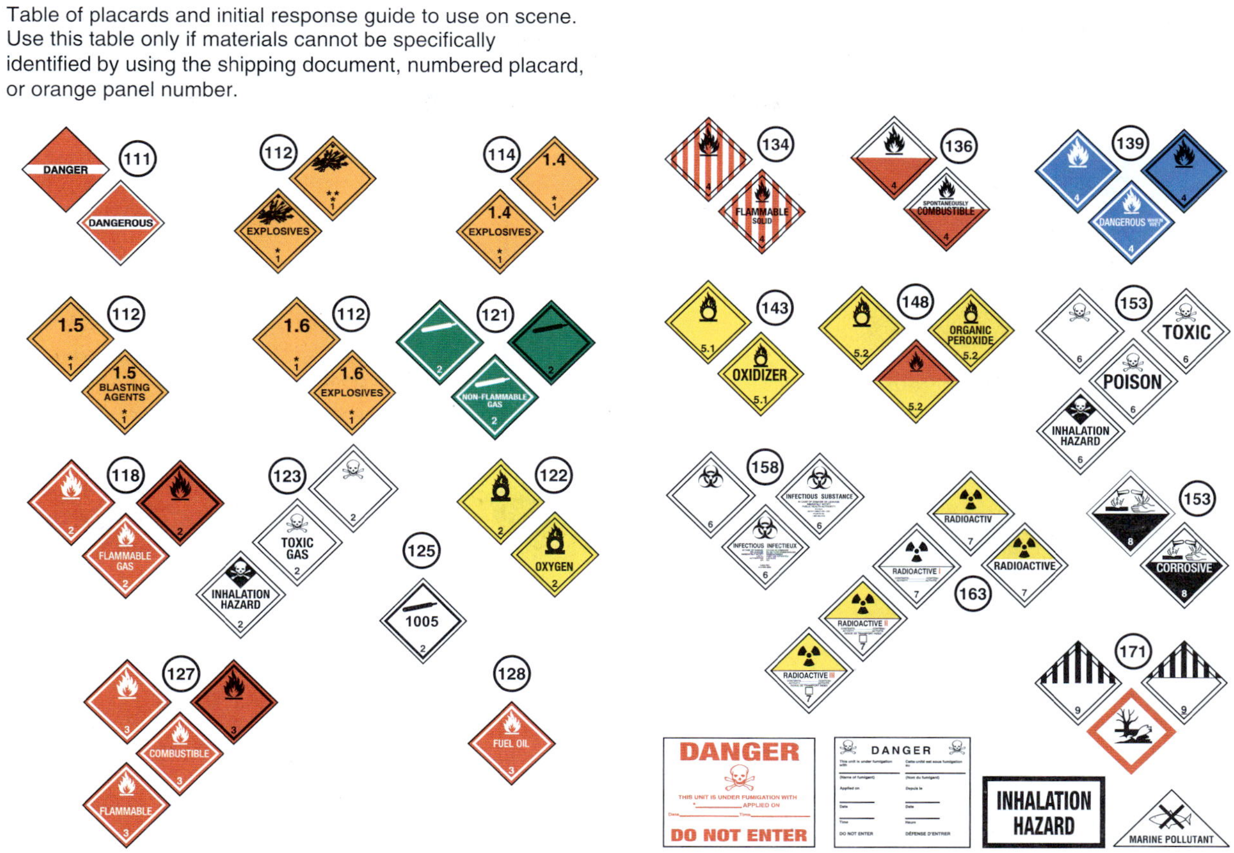

FIGURE 38-20 The Department of Transportation uses labels, placards, and markings (such as these found in the *Emergency Response Guidebook*) to give a general idea of the hazard inside a particular container or cargo tank.

Courtesy of the US Department of Transportation.

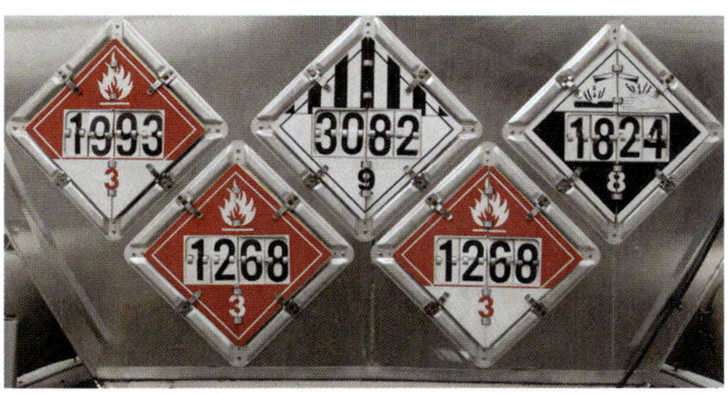

FIGURE 38-21 A placard is a large diamond-shaped indicator that is placed on all sides of transport vehicles that carry hazardous materials.

which the material inside belongs. A label on a box inside a delivery truck, for example, relates only to the potential hazard inside that particular package (**FIGURE 38-22**).

Other Considerations

The DOT system does not require that all chemical shipments be marked with placards or labels. In most cases, the package or cargo tank must contain a certain amount of hazardous material before a placard is required. For example, the "1,000-pound rule" applies to blasting agents (a substance that contains a fuel and oxidizer that is intended for blasting, but is not classified as an explosive), flammable and nonflammable gases, flammable/combustible liquids, flammable solids, air-reactive solids, oxidizers and organic peroxides, poison solids, corrosives, and miscellaneous (class 9) materials. Placards are required for these materials only when the shipment weighs more than 1,000 pounds (454 kg). Commercial package delivery services often carry small amounts of hazardous materials that fall below that weight limit. The vehicle exterior will not display placards to warn you of the danger.

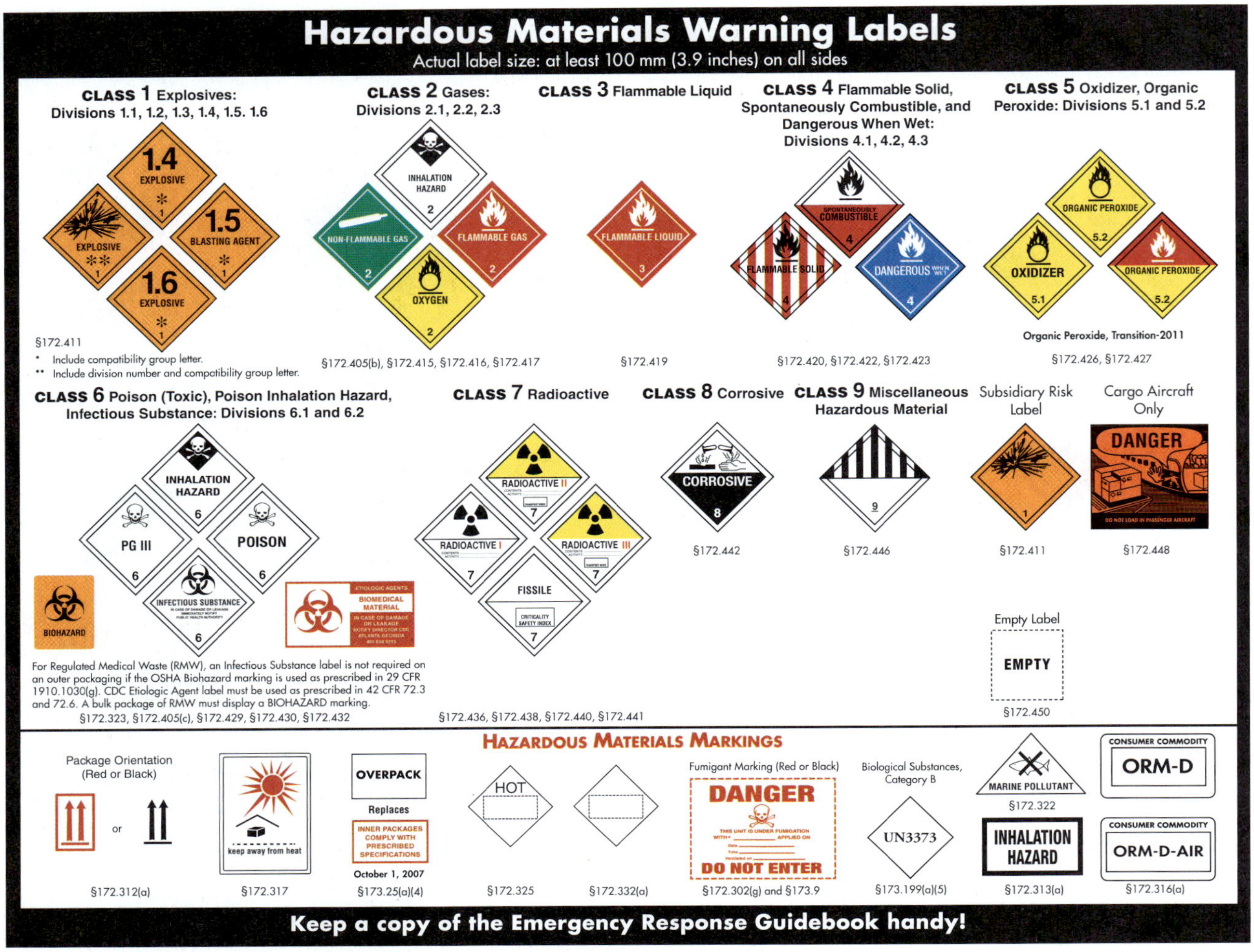

FIGURE 38-22 A label is a smaller version of the placard and is placed on boxes or smaller packages that contain hazardous materials.

Conversely, some chemicals are so hazardous that shipping any amount of them requires the use of labels or placards. These materials include explosives, poisonous gases, water-reactive solids, and high-level radioactive substances. A four-digit United Nations number may be required on some placards. This number identifies the specific material being shipped; a list of United Nations numbers is included in the *Emergency Response Guidebook*.

The Emergency Response Guidebook

The DOT's ***Emergency Response Guidebook (ERG)*** offers a certain amount of guidance for responders operating at a hazmat incident (**FIGURE 38-23**). This guide is updated every 3 to 4 years and provides information on approximately 4,000 chemicals. The US DOT and the Secretariat of Communications and Transportation of Mexico, along with Transport Canada, jointly developed the *ERG*. You can download a free copy or the mobile app of the *ERG* via the Pipeline and Hazardous Materials Safety Administration website.

Safety Data Sheets

A common source of information about a particular chemical is the **safety data sheet (SDS)**. Essentially, the SDS provides basic information about the chemical makeup of a substance, the potential hazards it presents, appropriate first aid in the event of an exposure, and other pertinent data for safe

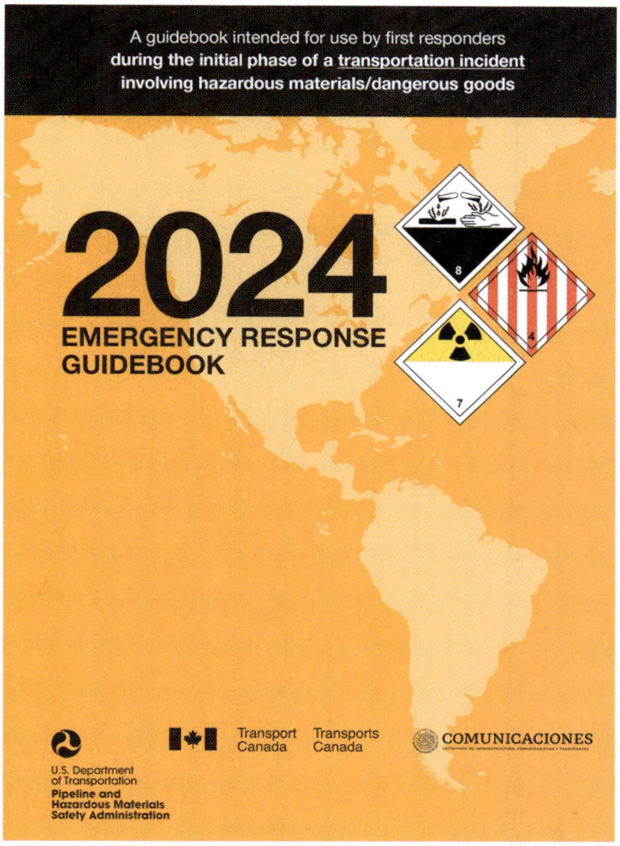

FIGURE 38-23 The *Emergency Response Guidebook* is a reference used as a base for your initial actions at a hazardous materials incident.

Courtesy of the US Department of Transportation.

handling of the material (**FIGURE 38-24**). It will typically include the following details:

- The name of the chemical, including any synonyms for it
- Physical and chemical characteristics of the material
- Physical hazards of the material
- Health hazards of the material
- Signs and symptoms of exposure
- Routes of entry
- Permissible exposure limits
- Responsible-party contact
- Precautions for safe handling (including hygiene practices, protective measures, and procedures for cleaning up spills or leaks)
- Applicable control measures, including personal protective equipment
- Emergency and first-aid procedures
- Appropriate waste disposal

All facilities that use or store chemicals are required by law to have an SDS on file for each chemical used or stored in the facility. Many sites, especially those that stock many different chemicals, may keep this information archived on a computer database. Although the SDS is not a definitive response tool, it is a key piece of the puzzle. The SDS can also be obtained from the transporting vehicle.

Shipping Papers

Shipping papers are required whenever hazardous materials are transported from one place to another. They include the names and addresses of the shipper and the receiver, identify the material being shipped, and specify the quantity and weight of each part of the shipment. Shipping papers for road and highway transportation are called **bills of lading** or **freight bills** and are located in the cab of the vehicle (**FIGURE 38-25**). Drivers transporting chemicals are required by law to have a set of shipping papers on their person or within easy reach inside the cab at all times.

CHEMTREC

Operated by the American Chemistry Council, the **Chemical Transportation Emergency Center (CHEMTREC)**, is an agency that provides invaluable technical information for first responders of all disciplines who are called on to respond to chemical incidents. The toll-free number for CHEMTREC is 1-800-262-8200. CHEMTREC can provide you with technical chemical information via telephone, fax, or other electronic media. It also offers a phone conferencing service to connect you with thousands of shippers, subject matter experts, and chemical manufacturers.

When you call CHEMTREC, be sure to have the following basic information ready:

- The name of the chemical(s) involved in the incident (if known)
- Name of the caller and callback telephone number
- Location of the incident or problem
- Shipper or manufacturer of the chemical (if known)
- Container type
- Railcar or vehicle markings or numbers
- The shipping carrier's name

SAFETY DATA SHEET
ANHYDROUS AMMONIA

TI

DISTRIBUTORS:

TANNER INDUSTRIES, INC.

DIVISIONS:

NATIONAL AMMONIA	NORTHEASTERN AMMONIA
HAMLER INDUSTRIES	BOWER AMMONIA & CHEMICAL

735 Davisville Road, Third Floor, Southampton, PA 18966; 215-322-1238
CORPORATE EMERGENCY TELEPHONE NUMBER: 800-643-6226 CHEMTREC: 800-424-9300

DESCRIPTION

CHEMICAL NAME: Ammonia, Anhydrous — **CAS REGISTRY NO**: 7664-41-7
SYNONYMS: Ammonia — **CHEMICAL FAMILY**: Inorganic Nitrogen Compound
FORMULA: NH_3 — **MOL. WT**: 17.03 (NH_3) — **COMPOSITION**: 99+% Ammonia

STATEMENT OF HEALTH HAZARD

HAZARD DESCRIPTION:
Ammonia is an irritant and corrosive to the skin, eyes, respiratory tract and mucous membranes. Exposure to liquid or rapidly expanding gases may cause severe chemical burns and frostbite to the eyes, lungs and skin. Skin and respiratory related diseases could be aggravated by exposure.
Not recognized by OSHA as a carcinogen.
Not listed in the National Toxicology Program.
Not listed as a carcinogen by the International Agency for Research on Cancer.

EXPOSURE LIMITS FOR AMMONIA: Vapor

OSHA	50 ppm,	35 mg / m³ PEL	8 hour TWA
NIOSH	35 ppm,	27 mg / m³ STEL 15 minutes	
	25 ppm,	18 mg / m³ REL	10 hour TWA
	300 ppm,	IDLH	
ACGIH	25 ppm,	18 mg / m³ TLV	8 hour TWA
	35 ppm,	27 mg / m³ STEL 15 minutes	

TOXICITY: LD 50 (Oral / Rat) 350 mg / kg

PHYSICAL DATA

BOILING POINT: -28°F at 1 Atm.
PH: N/A
SPECIFIC GRAVITY OF GAS (air = 1): 0.596 at 32°F
SPECIFIC GRAVITY OF LIQUID (water = 1): 0.682 at 28°F (Compared to water at 39°F).
PERCENT VOLATILE: 100% at 212°F
APPEARANCE AND ODOR: Colorless liquid or gas with pungent odor.
CRITICAL TEMPERATURE: 271.4°F
GAS SPECIFIC VOLUME: 20.78 Ft³/Lb at 32°F and 1 Atm.
VAPOR DENSITY: 0.0481 Lb/Ft³ at 32°F
LIQUID DENSITY: 38.00 Lb/Ft³ at 70°F
APPROXIMATE FREEZING POINT: -108°F
WEIGHT (per gallon): 5.15 pounds at 60°F
VAPOR PRESSURE: 114 psig at 70°F
SOLUBILITY IN WATER (per 100 pounds of water): 86.9 pounds at 32°F, 51 pounds at 68°F
SURFACE TENSION: 23.4 Dynes / cm at 52°F
CRITICAL PRESSURE: 111.5 atm

Revision: September 2024 — Page 1 of 4 — Prepared By: JRP

FIGURE 38-24 An example of a safety data sheet for anhydrous ammonia.

Courtesy of Tanner Industries, Inc., Southampton, PA.

- Recipient of material
- Local conditions and exact description of the situation

When you are speaking with CHEMTREC personnel, spell out all chemical names; if using a third party, such as a dispatcher, it is vital that you confirm all spellings to avoid misunderstandings. One number or letter out of place could throw off all subsequent research. When in doubt, obtain clarification.

Identification

Unfortunately, even with all of these resources, identifying materials can still be difficult. Little consistency is used on labels and placards, and sometimes dishonest transporters will not label containers or vessels appropriately. The laws and regulations that cover labeling of packages and transport vehicles can also be misleading. As discussed previously, in most cases, the package or tank must contain a certain amount of a hazardous material before a placard is required. For example, a truck may be carrying various types of hazardous materials, but each in small enough quantity that it is not required by law to display any labels or placards. The truck may show only a “Please drive carefully” placard, implying that it does not carry hazardous materials. Therefore, a crash involving this truck is a serious situation, but you would not

STRAIGHT BILL OF LADING
ORIGINAL - NOT NEGOTIABLE

BOL/Reference No.
RSI82715

CARRIER: NORFOLK SOUTHERN

Date: 12/23/2024

Shipper: RSI LOGISTICS, INC (OKEMOS, MI US)

The property described below, in apparent good order, except as noted (contents and condition of packages unknown), marked, consigned, and destined as indicated below, which said carrier (the word carrier being understood throughout this contract as meaning any person or corporation in possession of the property under the contract) agrees to carry to its usual place of delivery at said destination, if on its route, otherwise to deliver to another carrier on the route to said destination. It is mutually agreed, as to each carrier of all or any said property, that every service to be performed hereunder shall be subject to all the terms and conditions of the Uniform Domestic Straight Bill of Lading set forth (1) in Offcial, Southern, Western and Illionis Freight Classification in effect on the date hereof, if this is a rail or a rail-water shipment, or (2) in the applicable motor carrier classification or tariff if this is a motor carrier shipment
Shipper herby certifies that he is familiar with all the terms and conditions or the said bill of lading, including those on the back thereof, set forth in the classification or tariff which governs the transportation of this shipment, and the said terms and conditions are hereby agreed to by the shipper and accepted for himself and his assigns.

Consignee Information: CONSIGNEE DEER PARK, TX Address: City: DEER PARK, TX US	
Route: NS-ESTL-BNSF	
Origin Switch Route:	
Destination Switch Route: HUSTN-PTRA	Rail Car No: GATX290861

For assistance in any transportation emergency involving chemicals, phone CHEMTREC, day or night, Toll Free 1-800-424-9300

DESCRIPTION		*THGIEW
ONE TANK CAR	Contains: Methyl Esters STCC#2899415 BIODIESEL-15, Biodiesel Sales Order Contract No: RSI82715 Sales Order Contract No: AAT122308-4 Purchase Order Contract No: AAT122308-4	(Sub. To Correction) 204400 Lbs.

SEAL NUMBERS:

Gross

Tare

Net

Weighed By: ____________________

If charges are to be prepaid, write or stamp here, "To be Prepaid"
Prepaid

Subject to Section 7 of the conditions of applicable bill of lading, if this shipment is to be delivered to the consignee witho ut recourse on the consignor, the consignor shall sign the following statement:: *The carrier shall not make delivery of this shipment without payment of freight and all other lawful charges.*

Not In Effect

* This is to certify that the above named materials are properly classified, described, packaged, marked, and labeled, and are in proper condition for transportation, according to the applicable regulations of the Department of Transportation.

FIGURE 38-25 A bill of lading or freight bill.

Courtesy of RSI Logistics.

necessarily know this if you relied only on labels and placards. Always maintain a high index of suspicion when approaching the scene of a truck or train tanker crash.

Some substances are not hazardous; however, when mixed with another substance, they may become highly toxic. There may not be regulations against carrying such substances together on one truck or railroad car (or adjacent tank cars). The driver of a commercial truck and the conductor of a train, however, must carry shipping papers that identify what is being transported in their care. These shipping papers may be your first clue that there is a possible hazmat problem, although, depending on the nature of the incident, the papers may not be available to you.

YOU are the EMT

While you are triaging the patients, several other ambulances and other pieces of fire department equipment arrive on the scene, as well as a battalion chief who assumes command. You update him on your findings and the status of your EMS personnel and ambulances. There are 37 walking wounded (green) patients who will need to be loaded onto a bus for transport. Of the three remaining patients, two have been tagged expectant (black) and one is immediate (red).

7. What changes, if any, should you make in your initial triage assignments with the arrival of additional responders?

8. What should you consider in deciding whether to set up a treatment area at this incident?

In the event of a leak or spill, a hazmat incident is often indicated by the presence of the following:

- A visible cloud or strange-looking smoke resulting from the escaping substance
- A leak or spill from a tank, container, truck, or railroad car with or without hazmat placards or labels
- An unusual, strong, noxious (harmful), harsh odor in the area

To indicate the presence of normally odorless toxic gases or fluids during a leak or spill, manufacturers may add a substance that produces a strong noxious odor. However, a large number of hazardous gases and fluids are essentially odorless (or do not have a distinctive unpleasant smell) even when a substantial leak or spill has occurred. In some incidents, many people are exposed and may be injured or killed before the presence of a hazmat incident is identified. If you approach a scene where more than one person has collapsed or is unconscious or in respiratory distress, you should assume that there has been a hazmat leak or spill and that it is unsafe to enter the area.

It is important for you to understand the potential danger of hazardous materials and know how to operate safely at a hazmat incident. If you do not follow the proper safety measures, you and many others could end up needlessly injured or dead. The safety of you and your team, the other responders, and the public must be your most important concern.

There will be times when the ambulance is the first to arrive at the scene. As you approach, if any signs suggest that a hazmat incident has occurred, stop at a safe distance and park upwind or uphill from the incident. After rapidly sizing up the scene, call for a hazmat team. If you are already too close by the time you first recognize the danger, immediately leave the area. Once you have reached a safe place, try to rapidly assess the situation and provide as much information as possible when calling for the hazmat team, including your specific location, the size and shape of the containers of the hazardous material, and what you have observed and have been told has occurred. Do not reenter the scene, and do not leave the area until you have been cleared by the hazmat team, or you may contribute to the situation by spreading hazardous materials. Finally, do not allow civilians to enter the scene, if possible. No one should enter the area without the proper protective equipment, respiratory protection, or training.

Above all, avoid any contact with the material!

Words of Wisdom

Safety considerations at hazmat scenes differ considerably from those involved in emergency response in general. A hazmat scene requires you to have an even higher degree of alertness than usual to avoid entering a dangerous environment and to help others avoid it. There is also a need to prevent the spread of contamination to yourself and your ambulance. Understanding these two concepts is a good start toward safe operations in the presence of hazardous materials.

Hazmat Scene Operations

Once you have recognized the incident as one involving hazardous materials and have called for the hazmat team, focus your efforts on activities that will ensure the safety and survival of the greatest number of people. Use the ambulance's public address system to alert people who are near the scene and direct them to move to a location where they will be sufficiently far from danger. With the aid of others on your team, try to set up a perimeter to stop traffic and people from entering the area.

Establishing Control Zones

Setting control zones and limiting access to the incident site helps reduce the number of civilians and responders who may be exposed to the released substance. **Control zones** are established at a hazmat incident based on the chemical and physical properties of the released material, the environmental factors at the time of the release, and the general layout of the scene. Of course, isolating a city block in the busy downtown area of a large city presents far different challenges than isolating the area around a rolled-over cargo tank on an interstate highway. Each situation is different, requiring flexibility and thoughtfulness. Securing access to the incident helps ensure that no one will accidentally enter a contaminated area.

If the incident takes place inside a structure, the best place to control access is at the normal points of ingress and egress (entry and exit): the doors. Once the doors are secured so that no unauthorized personnel can enter, appropriately trained emergency response crews can begin to isolate other areas as appropriate.

The same concept applies to outdoor incidents. The goal is to secure logical access points around the hazard. Begin by controlling intersections, on and off ramps, service roads, and other access routes to the scene. Law enforcement officers should assist by diverting traffic at a safe distance outside the hazard area. They should block off streets, close intersections, and redirect traffic as needed.

During a long-term incident, highway department or public works department employees may be called on to set up traffic barriers. Whatever methods or devices are used to restrict access, they should not limit or prevent a rapid withdrawal of responders from the area.

It is not uncommon to set large control zones at the onset of an incident, only to discover that the zones may have been established too liberally. At the same time, control zones should not be defined too narrowly (**FIGURE 38-26**). As the IC gets more information about the specifics of the chemical or material involved, the control zones may be expanded or reduced. Ideally, the control zones will be established in the right place the first time. Wind shifts are a common reason why control zones are modified during the incident. If there is a prevailing wind pattern and you are in the area, that should be factored into any decision making when it comes to control zones.

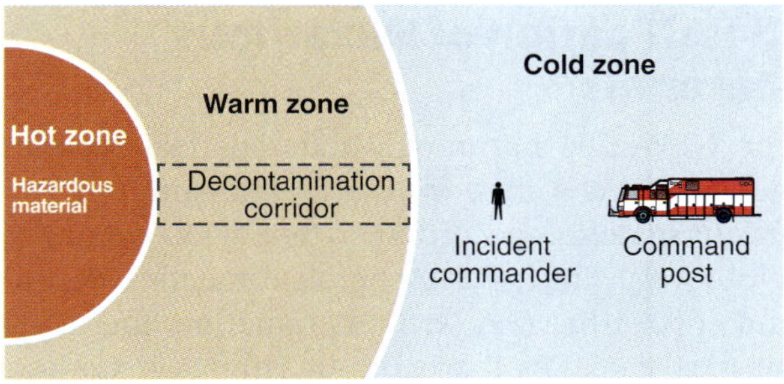

FIGURE 38-26 Control zones spread outward from the center of a hazardous materials incident.

Typically, control zones at hazmat incidents are labeled as *hot, warm,* or *cold.* You may also discover that other terms are used, such as *exclusionary zone* (hot zone), *contamination reduction zone* (warm zone), and *outer perimeter* (cold zone). In any case, make sure you understand the terminology used in your jurisdiction. Be aware that different jurisdictions may use terminology and setup procedures unlike the ones used in your agency. As long as you understand the concepts behind the actions and remember that safety is the main focus, the act of setting up and naming zones can remain flexible.

The **hot zone** is the area immediately surrounding the release, which is also the most contaminated area. Its boundaries should be set large enough that adverse effects from the released substance will not affect people outside of the hot zone. An incident involving a gaseous substance or a vapor, for example, may require a larger hot zone than one involving a solid or nonvolatile liquid leak. In some cases, atmospheric monitoring, plume modeling, or reference sources such as the *ERG* may prove useful in helping to establish the perimeters of a hot zone. Specifically trained responders, in accordance with their level of training, should be tasked with using these tools. Keep in mind that the physical characteristics of the released substance will significantly affect the size and layout of the hot zone. In addition, all specifically trained responders entering the hot zone should avoid contact with the product to the greatest extent possible. Adhering to this important policy makes the job of decontamination easier and reduces the risk of cross-contamination.

Personnel accountability is important, so access into the hot zone must be limited to only the responders necessary to control the incident. All personnel and equipment must be decontaminated when they leave the hot zone. This practice ensures that contamination is not inadvertently spread to clean areas of the scene.

The **warm zone** is where personnel and equipment transition into and out of the hot zone. It contains control points for access to the hot zone as well as the decontamination area. Only the minimum number of personnel and the equipment necessary to perform decontamination or support those operating in the hot zone should be permitted in the warm zone.

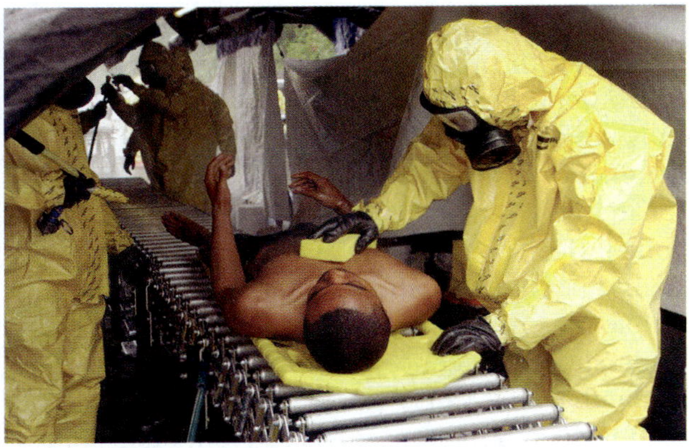

FIGURE 38-27 Patients should be decontaminated before they are taken to treatment areas.

A patient's skin and clothing may contain hazardous material, so the **decontamination area** is set up in the warm zone, near the exit point into the cold zone for EMS handoff. The decontamination area is the designated area where contaminants are removed before an individual can go to another area. **Decontamination**, in the context of a hazmat incident, is the process of removing or neutralizing and properly disposing of hazardous materials from equipment, patients, and rescue personnel. The decontamination area must include special containers for contaminated clothing and special bags to isolate each patient's personal effects safely until they can be decontaminated. The area will also contain several special facilities to thoroughly wash and rinse patients and backboards (**FIGURE 38-27**). The water that is used must be captured and delivered into special sealable containers.

Anyone who leaves the hot zone must pass through the decontamination area. Firefighters' and hazmat team members' outer protective gear is rinsed and washed in the decontamination area before it is removed (**FIGURE 38-28**). To prevent needless contact and transmission of splash or residues, different personnel are used in the decontamination and treatment areas. Do not move into the decontamination area unless you are properly trained and equipped. Wait for the patients to be brought to you.

Beyond the warm zone is the **cold zone**. The cold zone is a safe area where personnel do not need to wear any special protective clothing for safe operation. Personnel staging, the command post,

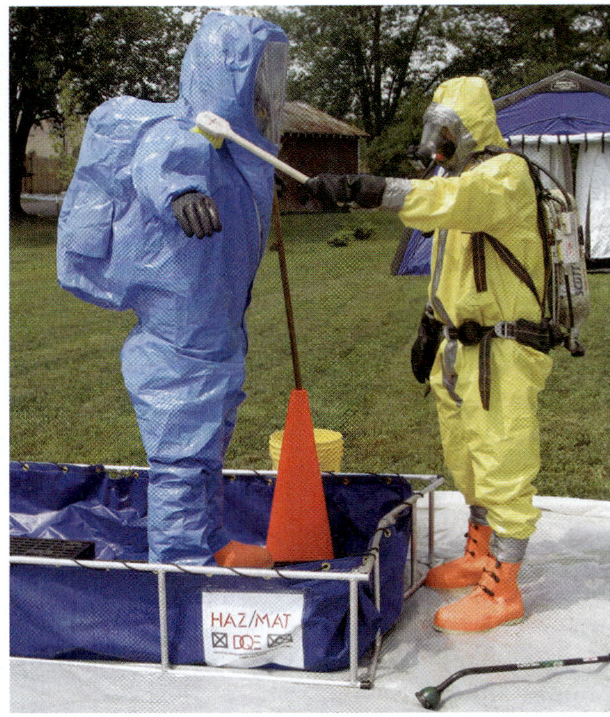

FIGURE 38-28 The decontamination zone is where firefighters' and hazmat team members' outer protective gear is rinsed and washed before removal.

EMS clinicians, and the area for medical monitoring, support, and/or treatment after decontamination are all located in the cold zone.

Role of the EMT

As an EMT, your job is to report to a designated area outside of the hot and warm zones and provide triage, treatment, transport, or rehabilitation when hazmat team members bring patients to you.

Classification of Hazardous Materials

The NFPA 704 hazardous materials classification standard is a system for the identification of hazardous materials according to health hazard or toxicity levels, fire hazard, chemical reactive hazard, and special hazards (such as radiation and acids) for fixed facilities that store hazardous materials.[5] Toxicity protection levels are also classified according to the level of personal protection required. For your safety, you must know the type and degree of health, fire, and reactive hazard protection you need to operate safely near these substances before you enter the scene.

Toxicity Level

Toxicity levels are measures of the health risk that a substance poses to someone who comes in contact with it. There are five toxicity levels: 0, 1, 2, 3, and 4. The higher the number, the greater the toxicity, as follows:

- **Level 0** includes materials that would cause little, if any, health hazard if you came in contact with them.
- **Level 1** includes materials that would cause irritation on contact but only mild residual injury, even without treatment.
- **Level 2** includes materials that could cause temporary damage or residual injury unless prompt medical treatment is provided. Both levels 1 and 2 are considered slightly hazardous but require use of self-contained breathing apparatus (SCBA) if you are likely to come in contact with them.
- **Level 3** includes materials that are extremely hazardous to health. Contact with these materials requires full protective gear so that none of your skin surface is exposed.
- **Level 4** includes materials that are so hazardous that minimal contact will cause death. For level 4 substances, you need specialized gear that is designed for protection against that particular hazard.

Note that all health hazard levels, with the exception of 0, require respiratory and chemical protective gear that is not standard on most ambulances and specialized training. **TABLE 38-2** further describes the four hazard classes.

TABLE 38-2 Toxicity Levels of Hazardous Materials

Level	Health Hazard	Protection Needed
0	Little or no hazard	None
1	Slightly hazardous	SCBA (level C suit) only
2	Slightly hazardous	SCBA (level C suit) only
3	Extremely hazardous	Full protection, with no exposed skin (level A or B suit)
4	Minimal exposure causes death	Special hazmat gear (level A suit)

Personal Protective Equipment Level

Personal protective equipment (PPE) levels indicate the amount and type of protective gear that you need to prevent injury from a particular substance. The four recognized protection levels, A, B, C, and D, are as follows (**FIGURE 38-29**):

- **Level A**, the most hazardous, requires fully encapsulated, chemical-resistant protective clothing that provides full body protection, as well as SCBA and special, sealed equipment.
- **Level B** requires nonencapsulated protective clothing or clothing that is designed to protect against a particular hazard (**FIGURE 38-30**).
- **Level C**, like Level B, requires the use of nonpermeable clothing and eye protection. In addition, face masks that filter all inhaled outside air must be used.
- **Level D** requires a work uniform, such as coveralls, that affords minimal protection.

Usually, this clothing is made of material that will allow only limited amounts of moisture and vapor to pass through (nonpermeable). All levels of protection require the use of gloves. Two pairs of rubber gloves are needed for protection in case one pair must be removed because of heavy contamination. Level B also requires eye protection and breathing devices that contain their own air supply, such as SCBA.

Caring for Patients at a Hazmat Incident

Generally, hazmat team members who are trained in prehospital emergency care will initiate emergency care for patients who have been exposed to a hazardous material. However, because of the dangers, time constraints, and bulky protective gear that team members wear, it is practical only to provide the simplest assessment and essential care

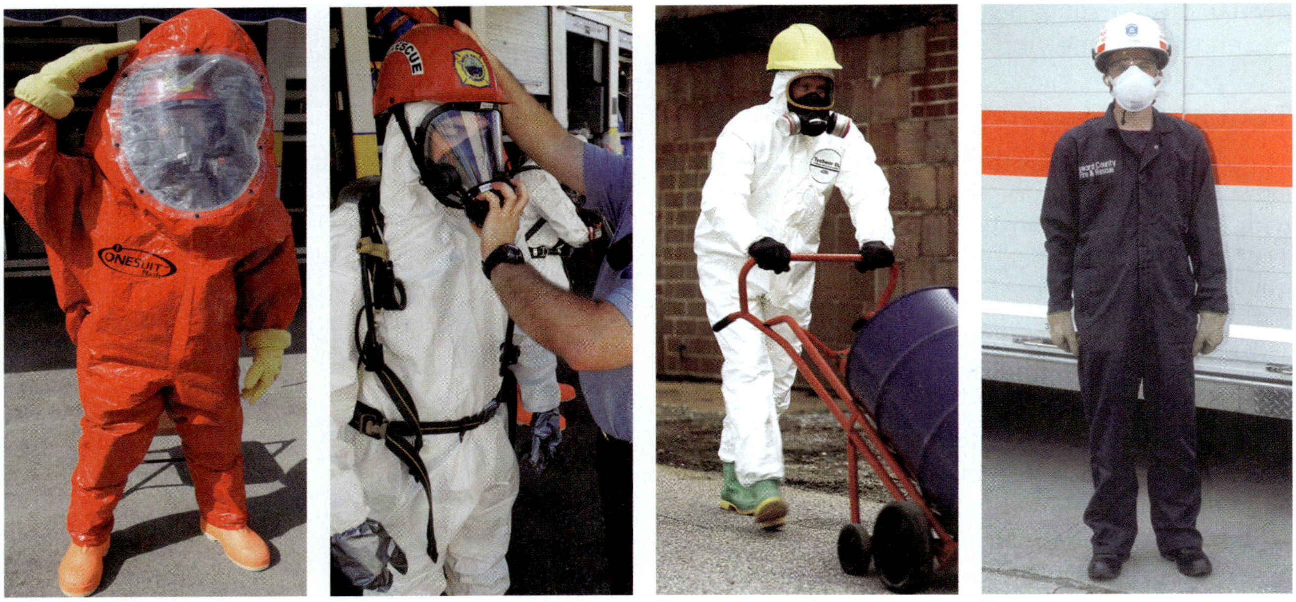

A B C D

FIGURE 38-29 Four levels of protection. **A.** Level A protection. **B.** Level B protection. **C.** Level C protection. **D.** Level D protection.

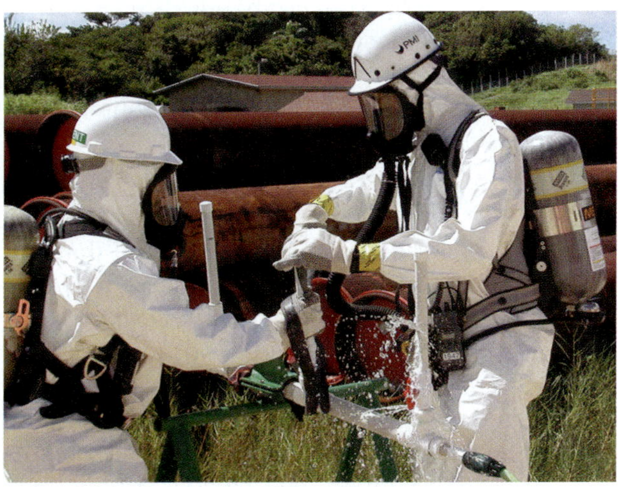

FIGURE 38-30 Workers in Level B protection.

in the hazard zone and the decontamination area. In addition, to avoid entrapment and spread of contaminants, no bandages or splints are applied—except for pressure dressings that are needed to control bleeding—until the clean (decontaminated) patient has been moved to the treatment area. Therefore, when you are providing care in the treatment area, assess and treat the patient in the same way as you would a patient who has not been previously assessed or treated.

Your care of patients at a hazmat incident must address the following two issues:

- Any trauma that has resulted from other related mechanisms, such as vehicle crash, fire, or explosion
- Injury and harm that have resulted from exposure to the hazardous substance

Most serious injuries and deaths from hazardous materials result from airway and breathing problems. Therefore, be sure to maintain the airway, and, if the patient appears to be in distress, give oxygen at 12 to 15 L/min with a nonrebreathing mask. Monitor the patient's breathing at all times. If you see signs that indicate respiratory distress is increasing, you may need to provide assisted ventilation with a bag-mask device and high-flow oxygen.

Treat the patient's injuries in the same way that you would treat any injury. There are few specific antidotes or treatments for exposure to most hazardous materials. Different people may respond differently to contact with the same hazardous material. Therefore, your treatment for the patient's exposure to the toxic substance should focus mainly on supportive care and initiating prompt transport to the hospital.

If antidotes or other special treatments need to be initiated in the field, they will be ordered by medical direction and relayed to the officer in charge of EMS operations at the scene. If special treatment includes medications, intravenous fluids, or other advanced care, paramedics or other advanced personnel will be sent to work with you at the treatment area.

Special Care

In some cases, before the decontamination area has been completely set up, the hazmat team will find one or two patients who need immediate treatment and transport without delay if they are to survive. Even if the decontamination area is set up and functioning, some patients may have such respiratory distress or otherwise urgent critical condition that the time necessary for full decontamination may prove fatal. If additional delay for proper decontamination seems life threatening in nontoxic exposure situations, it may be necessary to simply cut away all of the patient's clothing and do a rapid rinse to remove the majority of the contaminating matter before transport.

If you must treat and transport a patient who has not been properly decontaminated, you will need to increase the amount of protective clothing you wear, including the use of SCBA. At the least, this should include two pairs of gloves, goggles or a face shield, a protective coat, respiratory protection, and a disposable fluid-impervious apron or similar outfit. Many hazmat teams carry lightweight, easy-to-use, disposable, fluid-impervious protective suits for such a purpose. Remember, however, that transporting a contaminated patient merely increases the scope of the event. The decision to transport even one patient with critical injuries rests with the IC, who bases the decision on recommendations made by the hazmat team.

Prior to your arrival on scene, there are steps you can take to make decontaminating the ambulance easier. First, tape the cabinet doors shut. Any equipment kits, monitors, and other items that will not be used en route should be removed from the patient compartment and placed in the front of the ambulance or in outside compartments. Before loading the patient, turn on the power vent ceiling fan and patient compartment air-conditioning unit fan. Unless the weather is too severe, the windows in the driver's area and sliding side windows in the patient compartment should also be partially opened to prevent creating a "closed box" inside the ambulance and to ensure that it is properly ventilated for the safety of the patient, you, and your team members.

When you leave the scene, inform the hospital that you are transporting a critically injured patient who has not been fully decontaminated at the scene. This will allow the hospital to prepare to receive the patient. Many emergency departments have decontamination facilities and trained personnel for such an event. You may be diverted to a facility with these capabilities if the receiving hospital is not so equipped. On arrival, one EMT enters the emergency department and, after giving hospital staff the report and advising them again of the incomplete decontamination, obtains directions before the patient is unloaded and brought inside. If there are enough ambulances at a hazmat scene, one may be isolated and used only to transport such patients. Remember, the ambulance needs to be decontaminated before transporting another patient.

YOU are the EMT

As the patients are being retriaged and treated, the IC contacts the local trauma center to advise staff of the situation and to determine how many of the walking wounded they can handle in addition to the one critically injured patient. Hospital staff advises him that they can handle 10 of the patients. You reassess a boy whom you originally triaged as expectant. He is now apneic and pulseless. Based on the patient's injuries, medical direction determines that resuscitation is not indicated.

9. What factors should be considered when determining the appropriate transport destination?

10. Why did medical direction advise termination of resuscitation?

YOU are the EMT SUMMARY

1. How will you decide whether to declare this an MCI?

In this case, you are responding to an incident potentially involving many patients, and the severity of their injuries is unknown. One ambulance and two EMTs can effectively treat and transport only two stable patients *or* one critical patient at a time. In addition, there will likely be a crowd at the scene, which may hinder responder access and pose a possible danger to them, so law enforcement should be dispatched to control bystanders.

An MCI involves three or more patients, places great demand on the equipment or personnel of the EMS system, or has the potential to produce multiple casualties. On the basis of the information provided by dispatch, you should request additional EMS units. It is arguably better to call for help earlier, rather than wait until you arrive at the scene and find yourself overwhelmed by patients—some of whom may be critically injured. This holds true for all types of resources. The longer it takes to call for help, the longer it will take for help to arrive. Some centralized dispatch systems automatically send multiple EMS units and fire or law enforcement units depending on the information received from callers. In other cases, however, dispatch is dependent on input from the first responding agency. Other dispatched units can be cancelled if you determine they are not needed after you arrive on scene.

2. How will the ICS facilitate operations at this scene?

You have requested the assistance of other EMS units because you have determined that there are more patients than you can effectively care for. When the other units arrive, the ICS will facilitate the processes of triage, treatment, and transport; it will also help control the duplication of efforts and freelancing, in which individual units or different organizations make independent and often inefficient decisions that could compromise the effectiveness of the entire operation.

3. How should you and your partner proceed?

Once you have conducted a good scene size-up and answered the three basic questions—*What do I have? What resources do I need? What do I need to do?*—command is established by the highest-ranking appropriate public safety provider present, notification to other responders goes out, and necessary resources are requested. In this instance, you and your partner will need to establish command until more senior personnel arrive. If not already done, one of your first actions as you establish command of the scene should be to immediately request additional resources. Keep in mind that this number may change throughout the evolution of the incident, but you should not delay requesting additional resources just to make sure you have an idea of the perfect number of resources needed.

4. Once command has been established, what are your duties?

Once an IC and safety officer have been identified, you and your partner should begin the process of locating the patients and triaging them.

Because you and your partner are the only EMTs at the scene, you will initially need to function as the triage and treatment officer, and the primary and secondary triage will likely occur in the same area. If you have triaged all patients and additional help has still not arrived, begin treating the most critically injured patients first. As additional EMTs and ambulances arrive, they should be assigned accordingly; again, priority is given to the most critically injured patients. Depending on which units have arrived and what has been accomplished already, you will typically pass command to another person and continue performing triage or begin treating patients. In some systems that have a well-developed ICS or MCI plan, these roles will automatically evolve as personnel arrive.

5. What are your considerations in determining whether you should stop and provide treatment for the first patient?

Major treatment is not allowed during the triage process; however, because this patient is breathing (although slowly) and has a pulse, it is acceptable to stop and roll her to the recovery position. This may facilitate her breathing and possibly improve her condition. Due to her altered mental status, respiratory status, and weak pulses, she should be categorized as immediate (red). You should return to treat her as soon as you have completed triage or assign her to one of the first units responding to the scene.

6. What triage categories should you assign to the second and third patients?

Both patients should be categorized as expectant (black tag). The boy is unresponsive; is not breathing; has a slow, weak carotid pulse; and has no radial

YOU are the EMT SUMMARY continued

pulses. He also has exposed brain matter indicating injury that is highly likely to be incompatible with life. The near-decapitation injury in the older woman is also likely to be incompatible with life. Compared with others encountered during your triage, these two patients are the least likely to survive. If you and your partner were to focus on treating these two patients, the condition of the patient you categorized as red could deteriorate further, potentially resulting in her death also.

7. What changes, if any, should you make in your initial triage assignments with the arrival of additional responders?

One patient was initially triaged as immediate (red tag); her triage category should stay the same.

When you and your partner were the only EMTs at the scene, you had to decide which patients were the most critical, yet the most likely to survive with immediate treatment and prompt transport. Patients triaged as red and yellow should still receive the most immediate treatment and transport.

If you leave the teenager in the expectant category, he will die. However, if you provide immediate treatment and prompt transport, there is a chance that he will survive. Because he is apneic, begin ventilations and if he loses his pulse, begin CPR and contact medical direction; treatment and transport may still be indicated. Because the third patient has already been pulseless for a while and had an injury incompatible with life, beginning treatment would be futile, so she should remain triaged as black.

8. What should you consider in deciding whether to set up a treatment area at this incident?

Initially, there were only two EMTs at the scene and three critically injured patients. It would be more practical and save time to triage and treat the patients in the same area. Taking the time to set up a treatment area would delay patient care and require more personnel. Once more EMS resources arrive at the scene, there may be a need for a designated treatment area if transport will be delayed for any of the patients or if any of the patients initially triaged as green begin to show symptoms or need treatment for minor injuries.

9. What factors should be considered when determining the appropriate transport destination?

As soon as you declare an MCI, area hospitals should be notified as early as possible, informing them of the situation and determining their surge capacity; this information will tell the IC how many patients in each category are able to receive safe and effective care. It will also allow the hospitals to increase their staffing and, if needed, move patients within the facility.

The basic principles of transport that apply to any other patient also apply to MCIs; the most critically injured (red-tagged) patients should be transported to a designated trauma center, whereas yellow-tagged patients can be transported to hospitals that are located farther away. In cases where the closest trauma center is located a great distance away, air medical transport should be considered. Incident command or a designated transport officer should coordinate the transport, particularly when many patients are being transported, to prevent one receiving site from being overwhelmed. The receiving hospital for each patient should be notified.

10. Why did medical direction advise termination of resuscitation?

He is a poor candidate because he is apneic and pulseless with exposed brain matter. A patient who is critically injured will require more resources than are available and will pull valuable resources from others who may benefit from less time-consuming care. Multiple other patients may be saved in the amount of time required to treat this one individual. Even though it would be ideal to save everyone, the purpose of triage is to do the most good for the greatest number.

However, once all other patients are treated, or if there is enough manpower, even those patients who are considered poor candidates may receive treatment. This patient's age is a consideration for attempting resuscitation. Although an older person is more likely to have a more extensive medical history, a younger person may respond well to minimal treatment. If you are unsure whether to resuscitate, it is acceptable to initiate treatment and contact medical direction for further direction, which in this case was to terminate the resuscitation.

YOU are the EMT SUMMARY continued

Patient No. 1
Triage Tag
No. 239351

Move the Walking Wounded — MINIMAL

NO respirations after head tilt — EXPECTANT

☐ Respirations–under 10 — IMMEDIATE

☐ Perfusion–capillary refill over 2 seconds /radial pulse absent — IMMEDIATE

☐ Mental status–unresponsive — IMMEDIATE

Otherwise — DELAYED

MAJOR INJURIES: None
HOSPITAL DESTINATION : Trauma Center
ORIENTED ×④ DISORIENTED ☐ UNCONSCIOUS ☒

TIME	PULSE	B/P	RESPIRATION
1425	132	N/A	6
N/A	N/A	N/A	N/A

PERSONAL INFORMATION:
NAME : Unknown
MALE ☐ FEMALE ☒ AGE: N/A WEIGHT : N/A
MEDICAL COMPLAINTS/HISTORY
Unknown medical history

EXPECTANT No 239351

IMMEDIATE No 239351

Patient No. 2
Triage Tag
No. 239352

Move the Walking Wounded. — MINIMAL

NO respirations after head tilt — EXPECTANT

☐ Respirations–under 10 — IMMEDIATE

☐ Perfusion–capillary refill over 2 seconds /radial pulse absent — IMMEDIATE

☐ Mental status–unresponsive — IMMEDIATE

Otherwise — DELAYED

MAJOR INJURIES: Open skull fx with exposed brain matter
HOSPITAL DESTINATION : No transport
ORIENTED × ☐ DISORIENTED ☐ UNCONSCIOUS ☒

TIME	PULSE	B/P	RESPIRATION
1427	174	N/A	0
N/A	N/A	N/A	N/A

PERSONAL INFORMATION:
NAME : Not available
MALE ☒ FEMALE ☐ AGE: N/A WEIGHT : N/A
MEDICAL COMPLAINTS/HISTORY
Apneic, absent radials/weak carotid pulse, exposed brain matter, unknown medical hx

EXPECTANT No 239352

Patient No. 3
Triage Tag
No. 239353

Move the Walking Wounded — MINIMAL

NO respirations after head tilt — EXPECTANT

☐ Respirations–under 10 — IMMEDIATE

☐ Perfusion–capillary refill over 2 seconds /radial pulse absent — IMMEDIATE

☐ Mental status–unresponsive — IMMEDIATE

Otherwise — DELAYED

MAJOR INJURIES: Chest and head
HOSPITAL DESTINATION : No transport
ORIENTED × ☐ DISORIENTED ☐ UNCONSCIOUS ☒

TIME	PULSE	B/P	RESPIRATION
1428	N/A	N/A	N/A
N/A	N/A	N/A	N/A

PERSONAL INFORMATION:
NAME : Not available
MALE ☐ FEMALE ☒ AGE: N/A WEIGHT : N/A
MEDICAL COMPLAINTS/HISTORY
Unconscious, apneic, pulseless, unknown medical history

EXPECTANT No 239353

Prep Kit

Ready for Review

- The NIMS provides a comprehensive framework to enable federal, state, and local governments, as well as private-sector and nongovernmental organizations, to work together effectively. The NIMS is used to prepare for, prevent, respond to, mitigate, and recover from domestic incidents, regardless of cause, size, or complexity, including acts of catastrophic terrorism and hazardous materials (hazmat) incidents.
- The three major NIMS components are command and coordination, communication and information management, and resource management.
- The purpose of the ICS is to ensure responder and public safety, achieve incident management goals, and ensure the efficient use of resources.
- Preparedness involves the decisions made and basic planning done before an incident occurs.
- Your agency should have written disaster plans that you are regularly trained to carry out.
- At incidents that have a significant medical factor, the IC will designate someone as the chief of the medical (or EMS) branch under the operations section. This person will supervise the primary roles of the medical group: triage, treatment, and transport of the injured.
- An MCI refers to any call that involves three or more patients, any situation that places so great a demand on available equipment or personnel that the system would require a mutual aid response, or any incident that has a potential to create one of the previously mentioned situations.
- The goal of triage is to do the greatest good for the greatest number of people. This means that the triage assessment is brief and the patient condition categories are basic.
- There are four basic triage categories, which can be recalled using the mnemonic IDME:
    - Immediate (red)
    - Delayed (yellow)
    - Minimal (green; hold)
    - Expectant (black; likely to die or dead)
- A disaster is a widespread event that disrupts functions and resources of a community and threatens lives and property.
- Many disasters, such as a drought, may not involve personal injuries.
- When you arrive at the scene of a hazmat incident, you must first step back and assess the situation. This can be very stressful, particularly if you see a patient.
- CHEMTREC is a valuable resource for identifying a hazardous material and determining the appropriate response.

Vital Vocabulary

bills of lading The shipping papers used for transport of chemicals over roads and highways; also referred to as freight bills.

bulk storage containers Any container other than nonbulk storage containers, such as fixed tanks, highway cargo tanks, rail tank cars, totes, and intermodal tanks. These are typically found in manufacturing facilities and are often surrounded by a secondary containment system to help control an accidental release.

carboys Glass, plastic, or steel containers, ranging in volume from 5 to 15 gallons (19 to 57 L).

casualty collection area An area set up by physicians, nurses, and other hospital staff near a major disaster scene where patients can receive further triage and medical care.

Chemical Transportation Emergency Center (CHEMTREC) An agency that assists emergency responders in identifying and handling hazardous materials transport incidents.

Prep Kit continued

closed incident An incident that is contained; all casualties are accounted for.

cold zone A safe area at a hazardous materials incident for the agencies involved in the operations. The incident commander, the command post, EMS clinicians, and other support functions necessary to control the incident should be located in this zone. Also referred to as the clean zone or the support zone.

command In incident command, the position that oversees the incident, establishes the objectives and priorities, and develops a response plan.

command post The designated field command center where the incident commander and support staff are located.

container Any vessel or receptacle that holds material, including storage vessels, pipelines, and packaging.

control zones Areas at a hazardous materials incident that are designated as hot, warm, or cold, based on safety issues and the degree of hazard found there.

cylinders Portable, compressed gas containers used to hold liquids and gases such as nitrogen, argon, helium, and oxygen. They have a range of sizes and internal pressures.

decontamination The process of removing or neutralizing and properly disposing of hazardous materials from equipment, patients, and responders.

decontamination area The designated area in a hazardous materials incident where all patients and responders must be decontaminated before going to another area.

demobilization The process of directing responders to return to their facilities when work at a disaster or mass-casualty incident has finished, at least for those particular responders.

disaster A widespread event that disrupts community resources and functions, in turn threatening public safety, citizens' lives, and property.

drums Barrel-like containers used to store a wide variety of substances, including food-grade materials, corrosives, flammable liquids, and grease. May be constructed of low-carbon steel, polyethylene, cardboard, stainless steel, nickel, or other materials.

Emergency Response Guidebook (ERG) A preliminary action guide for first responders operating at a hazardous materials incident in coordination with the US Department of Transportation's labels and placards marking system. Jointly developed by the DOT, the Secretariat of Communications and Transportation of Mexico, and Transport Canada.

extrication supervisor In incident command, the person appointed to determine the type of equipment and resources needed for a situation involving extrication or special rescue; also called the rescue officer.

finance/administration In incident command, the position in an incident responsible for accounting of all expenditures.

freelancing When individual units or different organizations make independent and often inefficient decisions about the next appropriate action.

freight bills The shipping papers used for transport of chemicals along roads and highways; also referred to as bills of lading.

hazardous material Any substance that is toxic, poisonous, radioactive, flammable, or explosive and causes injury or death with exposure.

hazardous materials (hazmat) incident An incident in which a hazardous material is no longer properly contained and isolated.

hot zone The area immediately surrounding a hazardous materials spill or incident site that endangers life and health. All responders working in this zone must wear appropriate protective clothing and equipment. Entry requires approval by the incident commander or other designated officer.

Prep Kit continued

incident action plan (IAP) An oral or written plan stating general objectives reflecting the overall strategy for managing an incident.

incident commander (IC) The overall leader of the incident command system to whom commanders or leaders of incident command system divisions report.

incident command system (ICS) A system implemented to manage disasters and mass-casualty incidents in which section chiefs, including finance/administration, logistics, operations, and planning, report to the incident commander.

intermodal tanks Shipping and storage vessels that can be either pressurized or nonpressurized.

joint information center (JIC) An area designated by the incident commander, or a designee, in which public information officers from multiple agencies distribute information about the incident.

JumpSTART triage A sorting system for pediatric patients younger than 8 years or weighing less than 100 pounds (45 kg). There is a minor adaptation for infants because they cannot ambulate on their own.

liaison officer In incident command, the person who relays information, concerns, and requests among responding agencies.

logistics In incident command, the position that helps procure and stockpile equipment and supplies during an incident.

mass-casualty incident (MCI) An emergency situation involving three or more patients or that can place great demand on the equipment or personnel of the EMS system or has the potential to produce multiple casualties.

morgue supervisor In incident command, the person who works with area medical examiners, coroners, and law enforcement agencies to coordinate the disposition of dead victims.

mutual aid response An agreement between neighboring EMS systems to respond to mass-casualty incidents or disasters in each other's region when local resources are insufficient to handle the response.

National Incident Management System (NIMS) A Department of Homeland Security system designed to enable federal, state, and local governments and private-sector and nongovernmental organizations to effectively and efficiently prepare for, prevent, respond to, and recover from domestic incidents, regardless of cause, size, or complexity, including acts of catastrophic terrorism.

nonbulk storage vessels Any container other than bulk storage containers, such as drums, bags, compressed gas cylinders, and cryogenic containers. These hold commonly used commercial and industrial chemicals such as solvents, industrial cleaners, and compounds.

open incident An incident that is not yet contained; there may be patients to be located and the situation may be ongoing, producing more patients.

operations In incident command, the position that carries out the orders of the commander to help resolve the incident.

personal protective equipment (PPE) levels A means of classifying the amount and type of protective equipment that an individual must use to avoid injury during contact with a hazardous material.

placards Signage required to be placed on all four sides of highway transport vehicles, railroad tank cars, and other forms of hazardous materials transportation; the sign identifies the hazardous contents of the vehicle, using a standardization system with diamond-shaped indicators.

planning In incident command, the position that ultimately produces a plan to resolve any incident.

primary triage A type of patient sorting used to rapidly categorize patients; the focus is on speed in locating all patients and determining an initial priority as their conditions warrant.

Prep Kit continued

public information officer (PIO) In incident command, the person who keeps the public informed and relates any information to the media.

rehabilitation area The area that provides protection and treatment to firefighters and other responders working at an emergency. Here, workers are medically monitored and receive any needed care as they enter and leave the scene.

rehabilitation supervisor In incident command, the person who establishes an area that provides protection for responders from the elements and the situation.

rescue supervisor In incident command, the person appointed to determine the type of equipment and resources needed for a situation involving extrication or special rescue; also called the extrication officer.

safety data sheet (SDS) A form, provided by manufacturers and compounders (blenders) of chemicals, containing information about chemical composition, physical and chemical properties, health and safety hazards, emergency response, and waste disposal of a specific material; also known as material safety data sheet (MSDS).

safety officer In incident command, the person who monitors the scene for conditions or operations that may present a hazard to responders and patients; this person may stop an operation when responder safety is an issue.

secondary containment An engineered method to control spilled or released product if the main containment vessel fails.

secondary triage A type of patient sorting used in the treatment area that involves retriage of patients.

single command system A command system in which one person is in charge; generally used with small incidents that involve only one responding agency or one jurisdiction.

span of control In incident command, the subordinate positions under the commander's direction to which the workload is distributed; the ideal supervisor/worker ratio is one supervisor for five subordinates.

staging supervisor In incident command, the person who locates an area to stage equipment and personnel and tracks unit arrival and deployment from the staging area.

START triage A patient sorting process that stands for Simple Triage And Rapid Treatment and uses a limited assessment of the patient's ability to walk, respiratory status, hemodynamic status, and neurologic status.

termination of command The end of the incident command structure when an incident draws to a close.

toxicity levels A means of classifying the risk that a hazardous material poses to the health of an individual who comes into contact with it.

transportation area The area in a mass-casualty incident where ambulances and crews are organized to transport patients from the treatment area to receiving hospitals.

transportation supervisor In incident command, the person in charge of the transportation sector in a mass-casualty incident who assigns patients from the treatment area to waiting ambulances in the transportation area.

treatment area The location in a mass-casualty incident where patients are brought after being triaged and assigned a priority, where they are reassessed, treated, and monitored until transport to the hospital.

treatment supervisor In incident command, the person, usually a physician, who is in charge of and directs EMS clinicians at the treatment area in a mass-casualty incident.

triage The process of sorting patients based on the severity of injury and medical need to establish treatment and transportation priorities.

triage supervisor In incident command, the person in charge of the incident command triage sector who directs the sorting of patients into triage categories in a mass-casualty incident.

Prep Kit continued

unified command system A command system used in larger incidents in which there is a multiagency response or multiple jurisdictions are involved.

warm zone The area located between the hot zone and the cold zone at a hazardous materials incident. The decontamination corridor is located in this zone.

References

1. Ely RM, Schwartz DS, Liu JM, et al. Role of EMS in disaster response: a position statement and resource document of NAEMSP. *Prehosp Emerg Care*. 2025;29(3):315–321.
2. How emergency operations centers are aiding the COVID-19 response. Gates Foundation website. https://www.gatesfoundation.org/ideas/articles/emergency-operations-centers. Accessed May 2, 2025.
3. National Fire Protection Association (NFPA). *NFPA 1584: Standard on the Rehabilitation Process for Members During Emergency Operations and Training Exercises*. NFPA website. https://www.nfpa.org/codes-and-standards/nfpa-1584-standard-development/1584. Published 2022. Accessed May 2, 2025.
4. US Department of Transportation, National Highway Traffic Safety Administration. *Model Uniform Core Criteria for Mass Casualty Incident Triage: Addendum to the Emergency Medical Technician Instructional Guidelines*. EMS.gov website. https://www.ems.gov/assets/MUCC_Addendum_EMT.pdf. Published December 2017. Accessed May 2, 2025.
5. National Fire Protection Association (NFPA). *NFPA 704: Standard System for the Identification of the Hazards of Materials for Emergency Response*. NFPA website. https://www.nfpa.org/product/nfpa-704-standard/p0704code#. Published 2022. Accessed May 2, 2025.

Additional Resources

Arshad FH, Williams A, Asaeda G, et al. A modified simple triage and rapid treatment algorithm from the New York City (USA) Fire Department. *Prehosp Disaster Med*. 2015;30(2):199–204.

Chemical Hazards Emergency Medical Management. START adult triage algorithm. US Department of Health and Human Services. https://chemm.hhs.gov/startalgotext.htm. Updated February 21, 2025. Accessed May 2, 2025.

Department of Homeland Security. *National Incident Management System*. Federal Emergency Management Agency website. https://www.fema.gov/emergency-managers/nims. Updated February 14, 2025. Accessed May 2, 2025.

National EMS Management Association. *Operational Templates and Guidance for EMS Mass Incident Deployment*. Emmitsburg, MD: US Fire Administration; 2012. https://www.usfa.fema.gov/downloads/pdf/publications/templates_guidance_ems_mass_incident_deployment.pdf. Accessed May 2, 2025.

SALT mass casualty triage: concept endorsed by the American College of Emergency Physicians, American College of Surgeons Committee on Trauma, American Trauma Society, National Association of EMS Physicians, National Disaster Life Support Education Consortium, and State and Territorial Injury Prevention Directors Association. *Disaster Med Public Health Prep*. 2008;2(4):245–246.

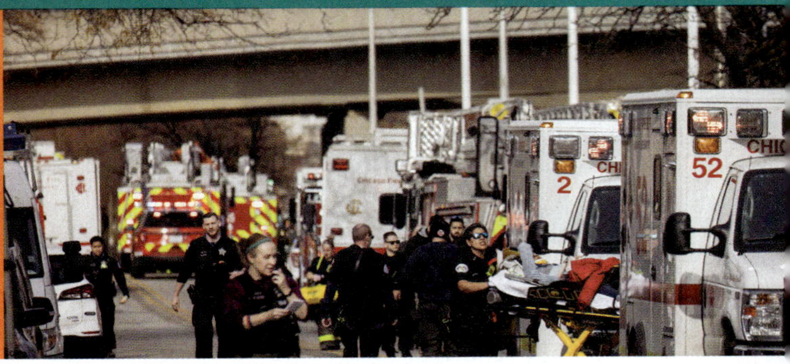

Chapter 39

Terrorism Response and Disaster Management

NATIONAL EMS EDUCATION STANDARD COMPETENCIES

EMS Operations

Knowledge of operational roles and responsibilities to ensure patient, public, and personnel safety.

Mass-Casualty Incidents Due to Terrorism and Disaster

- Risks and responsibilities of operating on the scene of a natural or man-made disaster (pp 1451–1454; see Chapter 38, *Incident Management*)

KNOWLEDGE OBJECTIVES

1. Discuss international terrorism and domestic terrorism. (pp 1447–1448)
2. Describe the different types of goals that commonly motivate terrorist groups to carry out terrorist attacks. (p 1448)
3. Describe different weapons of mass destruction (WMDs). (pp 1450–1451)
4. Explain how the Department of Homeland Security (DHS) National Terrorism Advisory System (NTAS) relates to the actions and precautions emergency medical technicians (EMTs) must take while performing their daily activities. (pp 1451–1452)
5. Name the key observations EMTs must make on every call to determine the potential of a terrorist attack. (p 1452)
6. Explain the critical response actions that EMTs must perform at a suspected terrorist event. (pp 1452–1454)
7. Discuss the history of chemical agents, their main classifications, their routes of exposure, and their effects on patient care. (pp 1454–1462)
8. Describe the different categories of biologic agents, their routes of exposure, and their effects on patient care. (pp 1463–1469)
9. Explain the role of emergency medical services (EMS) in relation to syndromic surveillance and points of distribution during a biologic event. (p 1469)
10. Discuss the history of nuclear/radiologic devices, sources of radiologic materials and dispersal devices, medical treatment of patients, and protective measures EMTs must take during a nuclear/radiologic incident. (pp 1469–1473)
11. Describe the different types of incendiary and explosive devices. (p 1473)

SKILLS OBJECTIVES

1. Demonstrate the steps EMTs can take to establish and reassess scene safety during a terrorist event. (p 1451)
2. Demonstrate the steps EMTs can take to care for a patient exposed to a chemical agent. (pp 1454–1462)
3. Demonstrate the use of the DuoDote Auto-Injector and/or the Antidote Treatment Nerve Agent Auto-Injector. (pp 1457–1460)

Introduction

With the incidence of terrorist attacks continuing to rise in the United States, you must be mentally and physically prepared for the possibility of a terrorist event. Both international groups and domestic terrorists have been responsible for these attacks, with an alarming trend toward targeting civilian populations. From coordinated attacks with firearms and homemade explosives to large-scale events targeting hundreds or thousands, it is no longer a question of *if* another attack will occur, but when and where it will occur.

The use of weapons of mass destruction (WMDs), or weapons of mass casualty (WMCs), further complicates the management of the terrorist incident and places you in greater danger. Although it is difficult to plan and anticipate a response to many terrorist events, there are several key principles that apply to every response. This chapter discusses the types of terrorist events, personnel safety, and patient treatments, and also gives you tools to prepare to respond to these events. You will learn the signs, symptoms, and treatment of patients who have been exposed to nuclear, chemical, or biologic agents or an explosive attack. At the end of this chapter, you will be able to answer the following key questions:

- What are my initial actions?
- Whom should I notify, and what should I tell them?
- What type of additional resources do I require?
- How should I proceed to address the needs of the victims?
- How do I ensure the safety of myself, my partner, and the victims?
- What is the clinical presentation of a victim exposed to a WMD?
- How do I assess and treat patients who have been affected by a WMD?
- How should I avoid becoming contaminated or cross-contaminated with a WMD agent?

For the EMT working in today's society, these new challenges all translate to the need to maintain a high degree of situational awareness, prepare yourself mentally and physically to respond to these types of events, and support educating immediate responders to assist in saving lives.

What Is Terrorism?

Although **terrorism** is often thought to be a more recent trend, terrorist attacks have been present for centuries and predate the United States. While much of our understanding of terrorism is based on past experience, it is important to recognize that the means and tactics employed by terrorists continuously evolve over time.

Historically, terrorism has been broadly categorized as international or domestic. **International terrorism** is thought to be inspired by, or associated with, designated foreign terrorist organizations or nations. **Domestic terrorism** is inspired by ideologic goals concerning the terrorist's own nation, such as political, religious, social, racial, or environmental beliefs. According to the US Department of Justice, both types are characterized as follows[1]:

- Involves violent acts or acts dangerous to human life that violate federal or state law
- Appears to be intended (i) to intimidate or coerce a civilian population; (ii) to influence the policy of a government by intimidation or coercion; or (iii) to affect the conduct of a government by mass destruction, assassination, or kidnapping

In the United States, there were over 231 domestic terrorist attacks between 2010 and 2021.[2] An example is the Boston Marathon bombing in 2013

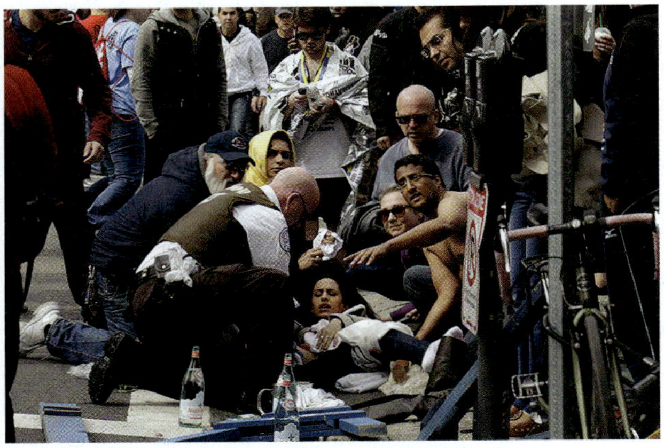

FIGURE 39-1 The bombing at the Boston Marathon in 2013 was an example of domestic terrorism.

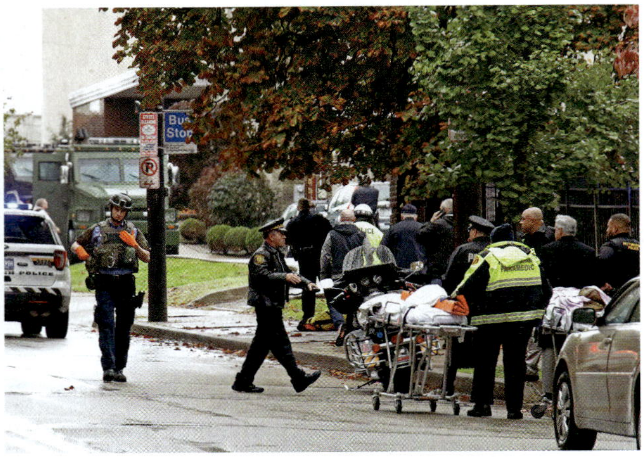

FIGURE 39-2 In 2018, a shooter, after posting antisemitic and anti-immigrant messages online, killed 11 worshippers at the Tree of Life synagogue in Pittsburgh, Pennsylvania.

(**FIGURE 39-1**). Terrorist organizations are often categorized based on their beliefs and goals:

- **Religious extremist groups/doomsday cults** include groups such as Aleph (formerly Aum Shinrikyo), which carried out chemical attacks in Tokyo in 1994 and 1995. Religious extremist groups may advocate the destruction of institutions and governments that do not align with their strict adherence to specific religious beliefs.
- **Extremist political groups** may include violent separatist groups and those who seek political, religious, economic, and social freedom.
- **Cyber terrorists** attack a population's technological infrastructure to draw attention to their cause or target financial centers to steal or divert funds. Recently, cyber terrorism has included hacking into hospital computer systems and barring access until a ransom is paid.
- **Single-issue groups** are motivated by a wide array of social causes. These groups include antiabortion groups, animal rights groups, anarchists, racists, and even ecoterrorists who threaten or use violence to protect the environment (**FIGURE 39-2**).

Active Shooter Events

An alarming new trend in domestic terrorism involves the concept of the **lone wolf terrorist attack**. This method has quickly become a frequent threat in the United States and has resulted in some of the most devastating attacks on US soil in recent years. In *Report: Lone Wolf Terrorism*, the National Security Critical Issue Task Force defines lone wolf terrorism as "the deliberate creation and exploitation of fear through violence or threat of violence committed by a single actor who pursues political change linked to a formulated ideology, whether his own or that of a larger organization, and who does not receive orders, direction, or material support from outside sources."[3]

The motives of the lone wolf terrorist are not always clear (**FIGURE 39-3**). These attacks may target schools, music festivals, or even shopping centers and have been difficult to predict. Examples of lone wolf terrorist attacks include the 2015 Emanuel Church shooting in Charleston, South Carolina; the Pulse nightclub shooting of 2016 in Orlando, Florida; the 2017 Las Vegas, Nevada, shooting at the Route 91 Harvest music festival; and the 2022 Robb Elementary School shooting in Uvalde, Texas. These four events alone accounted for more than 130 deaths and approximately 1,000 injuries.

Many lone wolf terrorist attacks involve firearms and not explosives; thus this type of event can be further classified as an **active shooter event**. Beginning in 2013, a committee of the American College of Surgeons that included law enforcement, emergency medical services (EMS), fire, military, and federal agencies produced recommendations for best practices aimed at improving survival during active shooter and intentional mass-casualty events. The committee's

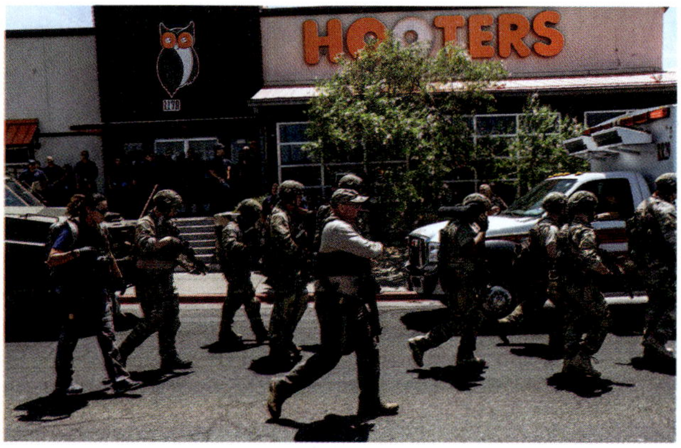

FIGURE 39-3 Law enforcement and EMS respond to a lone wolf shooting in El Paso, Texas, in 2019 that resulted in 23 deaths and 22 injuries.

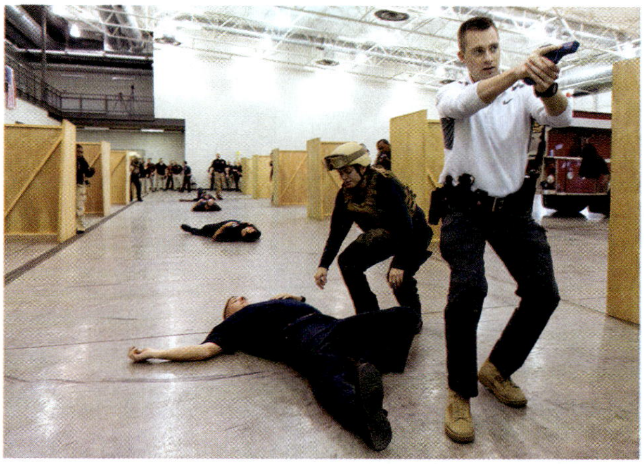

FIGURE 39-4 During interagency task force training, such as the session shown here in Omaha, Nebraska, EMS clinicians learn to work with law enforcement during an active shooter event.

recommendations are known as the Hartford Consensus. The Hartford Consensus consists of four reports that have helped to shape national policy and provides a framework for educating both the public and first responders.[4–6]

The Hartford Consensus recommends that a response plan designed for active shooter response should include the acronym THREAT: Threat suppression, Hemorrhage control, Rapid Extrication to safety, Assessment by medical clinicians, and Transport to definitive care. This plan encourages a continuum of care that begins with immediate responders: those who are present at the time and place of the attack. The continuum of care progresses with professional responders arriving at the scene and trauma professionals at the hospital.

The Hartford Consensus highlights the importance of early hemorrhage control. Although education and training can help immediate responders truly make a difference and improve survival, there may not always be uninjured people available to help the injured. The Hartford Consensus recommends reevaluating the practice of staging away from the scene and having patients brought to the ambulance. Traditionally, it may take a significant amount of time for professional responders to reach injured patients after the threat has been neutralized and the scene has been declared safe for all responders to enter. To provide care sooner, many EMS organizations have revised the roles and responsibilities of personnel responding to an active shooter event (**FIGURE 39-4**). EMS crews may be equipped with ballistic vests and helmets so that they can potentially be paired with law enforcement to assist with treatment and evacuation of injured people from an active scene. Such crews are referred to as rescue task forces.

Some EMS clinicians wear body armor while on duty for personal protection. Several types of body armor are available, offering different features and levels of protection. If your agency provides body armor, you should understand the level of protection your body armor provides. Ensure that it fits properly and is cleaned appropriately, and follow all manufacturer recommendations for its use.

Words of Wisdom

EMS agencies should remain mindful of the public perception of body armor. Recent literature has demonstrated the routine use of body armor by EMS systems increases the number of patients who refuse treatment and transport.[7]

The recommendations from the Hartford Consensus also paved the way for the Stop the Bleed campaign. Launched in 2015 by the Department of Defense, this nationwide campaign promotes offering education on hemorrhage control to the public to help improve the willingness and effectiveness

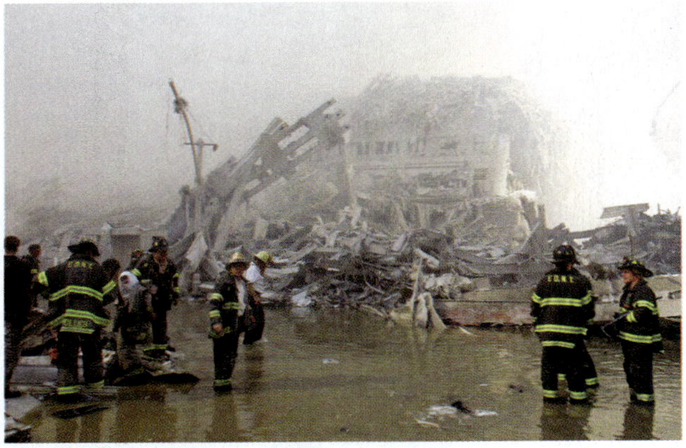

FIGURE 39-5 The September 11, 2001, attack on the World Trade Center in New York City accounted for most of the deaths caused by terrorists in 2001.

of immediate responders who are able to help save lives at the point of injury. Over four million people around the world have been trained to save a life through the Stop the Bleed campaign.[8]

When multiple "actors" (ie, people or groups) plan or engage in terrorism together, it is no longer a lone wolf event. Nineteen hijackers worked together to commit the worst act of terrorism in US history on September 11, 2001 (**FIGURE 39-5**). At least four terrorists worked together to commit the London Subway bombings on July 7, 2005. On October 7, 2023, approximately 3,000 Hamas-led terrorists crossed into Israel and killed nearly 1,200 people while injuring and abducting thousands more.[9]

Weapons of Mass Destruction

A **weapon of mass destruction (WMD)**, or **weapon of mass casualty (WMC)**, is any agent designed to bring about mass death, casualties, and/or massive damage to property and infrastructure (bridges, tunnels, airports, and seaports). To help remember the different kinds of weapons of mass destruction, use the mnemonic **B-NICE**: **bi**ologic, **n**uclear, **i**ncendiary, **c**hemical, and **e**xplosive weapons; or CBRNE for **c**hemical, **b**iologic, **r**adiologic, **n**uclear, and **e**xplosive weapons.

To date, the preferred WMD for terrorists has been explosive devices. Terrorist groups have favored tactics that use vehicle-borne explosives or pedestrian suicide bombers. While many previous attempts by terrorists to use either chemical or biologic weapons to their full capacity have been unsuccessful, these weapons still pose a meaningful threat; in 2024 alone, the US Department of Homeland Security reported 18 chemical or biologic incidents in the United States, with one death reported.[10] As an EMT, you must not underestimate the destructive potential of these weapons.

Words of Wisdom

While many of the acts of terrorism you may be familiar with occur in large cities or gatherings, terrorism can occur anywhere. Acts of terrorism have targeted car dealerships, shopping centers, places of worship, restaurants, and many other public locations.

YOU are the EMT

You and your partner are on standby at a local holiday parade. Due to many parades in the area, you are the only medical resource assigned to this parade. As the parade is nearing the midway point, your unit is requested to respond to an injured law enforcement officer who was found with multiple stab wounds in an alley along the parade route. As you near the officer's location, you suddenly see dozens of people frantically running away from the parade route. Your partner stops the ambulance immediately. A worker rushes up to your unit and says event staff had reports of a trash can that was smoking heavily about two blocks up. As he was walking to investigate the report, a man stepped out of the crowd and began to shoot a large rifle into the crowd. He said there were lots of people lying on the ground bleeding, and he believes the suspected shooter was shot and killed by police.

1. On the basis of the information you have received, how should you approach this incident?
2. What indicators suggest that an incident is the result of terrorism?

Although WMDs are not easy to obtain or create, doing so is not impossible. Use of the proper techniques during the 1995 Aum Shinrikyo attack on the Tokyo subway could have resulted in tens of thousands of casualties. Moreover, the technical recipes for making B-NICE weapons can be found on the Internet; in fact, they have even been published on terrorist group websites.

Chemical Terrorism/Warfare

Chemical agents are manufactured substances that can have devastating effects on living organisms. They can be produced in liquid, powder, or vapor form depending on the chemical compound, desired route of exposure, and dissemination technique. Developed during World War I (WWI), these agents have been implicated in thousands of deaths since being introduced on the battlefield, and they have been used to terrorize civilian populations. These agents consist of the following types:

- Vesicants (blister agents)
- Respiratory agents (choking agents)
- Nerve agents
- Metabolic agents (cyanides)

Biologic Terrorism/Warfare

Biologic agents are organisms that cause disease. They are generally found in nature; however, for terrorist use, they must be cultivated, synthesized, and mutated in a laboratory. The **weaponization** of biologic agents is performed to artificially maximize the target population's exposure to the germ, thereby exposing the greatest number of people and achieving the desired result.

The primary types of biologic agents that you may come in contact with during a biologic event include the following:

- Viruses
- Bacteria
- Toxins

Nuclear/Radiologic Terrorism

There have been only two publicly known uses of nuclear materials as weapons of war, both occurring during wartime. During World War II (WWII), Hiroshima and Nagasaki were devastated when they were targeted with nuclear bombs. The destructive power demonstrated by the attack ended WWII and has served as a deterrent to nuclear war.

There are nations that hold close ties with terrorist groups (known as **state-sponsored terrorism**) and have obtained some degree of nuclear capability. It is also possible for a terrorist to secure radioactive materials or waste to perpetrate an act of terror. These materials are far easier for a terrorist to acquire than are nuclear weapons and require less expertise to use. Radioactive materials such as those in radiologic dispersal devices (RDDs), also known as "dirty bombs," can cause widespread panic and civil disturbances. These devices are covered later in this chapter.

EMT Response to Terrorism

When you respond to a terrorist event, the basic foundations of patient care remain the same; however, the treatment can and will vary. Terrorist events can produce a single casualty, hundreds of casualties, or even thousands of casualties. In all cases, you must remember situational awareness is key. You must do everything in your power to be as safe as possible while caring for the sick and injured. Your response in one situation may not be appropriate for another situation. In mass-casualty terrorist events, it is important to use triage and base patient care on available resources.

Safety Tips

When preplanning for mass-casualty incidents, your agency should work with your community to ensure EMS is aware of any festivals, celebrations, gatherings, or events and prepare accordingly. Large crowds have been a focal point for terrorist attacks, so knowing their location, your means of ingress and egress, local hospitals, communication frequencies, and onsite resources will help ensure you can respond and help if called to do so. It is common for these large events to have a formal incident action plan to be prepared should an attack occur.

Recognizing a Terrorist Event (Indicators)

The planning of most acts of terror is **covert**, which means that the public safety community generally has no prior knowledge of the time, location, or nature of the attack. This element of surprise makes responding to an event more complex. You must constantly be aware of your surroundings and understand the possible risks for terrorism associated with certain locations, at certain times. Therefore, it is important that you know the current threat level issued by the federal government through the Department of Homeland Security (DHS).

The National Terrorism Advisory System (NTAS) is designed to communicate information about terrorist threats by providing timely, detailed information to the US public.[11] Alerts from the NTAS contain a summary of the threat and the actions that first responders, government agencies, and the public can take to maintain safety. On the basis of threat information, make sure you take the appropriate actions and precautions while you continue to perform your daily duties and respond to calls.

The DHS has not issued specific recommendations for EMS personnel to follow in response to specific threats. Follow your local protocols, policies, and procedures.

It is your responsibility to be aware of information sent out by the advisory system at the start of your workday. Daily newspapers, television news programs, and multiple websites (including the DHS website) all give up-to-date information. Understanding and being aware of the current threat is only the beginning of responding safely to calls.

To determine the potential for a terrorist attack, make the following observations on every call:

- **Type of location.** Is the location a monument, infrastructure, government building, or a specific type of location, such as a temple? Is there a large gathering? Is there a special event taking place?
- **Type of call.** Is there a report of an explosion or suspicious device nearby? Are there reports of people fleeing the scene?
- **Number of patients.** Are there multiple victims with similar signs and symptoms? This is probably the single most important clue that a terrorist attack or an incident involving a WMD has occurred.
- **Victims' statements.** This is probably the second-best indication of a terrorist or WMD event. Are the victims fleeing the scene giving statements such as "Everyone is passing out," "There was a loud explosion," or "There are a lot of people shaking on the ground"? If so, something is occurring that you do not want to rush into, even if it is questionable as to whether it is a terrorist event.
- **Preincident indicators.** Has there been a recent increase in violent political activism? Are you aware of any credible threats made against the location, gathering, or occasion?

Response Actions

Once you suspect that a terrorist event has occurred or a WMD has been used, there are certain actions you must take to ensure you will be safe and properly prepared to help the community.

Scene Safety

Remember to stage your vehicle a safe distance (usually 1 to 2 blocks) from the incident, and wait for law enforcement personnel to advise you that the scene has been made secure. If you think that it may not be safe, do not enter. When dealing with a WMD scene, assume you will not be able to enter the scene where the event has occurred; nor do you want to. You may be told where to stage. Generally, the best location for staging is upwind and uphill from the incident. Wait for assistance from those who are trained in assessing and managing WMD scenes. Expect that a perimeter will be created, usually by law enforcement personnel, to isolate the scene, prevent further contamination of evidence, and protect rescuers and the public from further danger. In addition, remember the following rules:

- Failure to park your vehicle at a safe location can place you and your partner in danger (**FIGURE 39-6**). Always have an escape plan determined beforehand, in case the scene becomes unsafe.

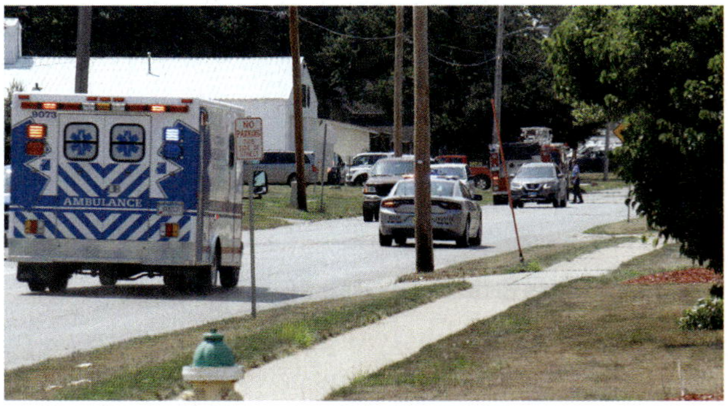

FIGURE 39-6 In the photo, an ambulance stops at a distance from an active shooting incident, where law enforcement is securing the scene.

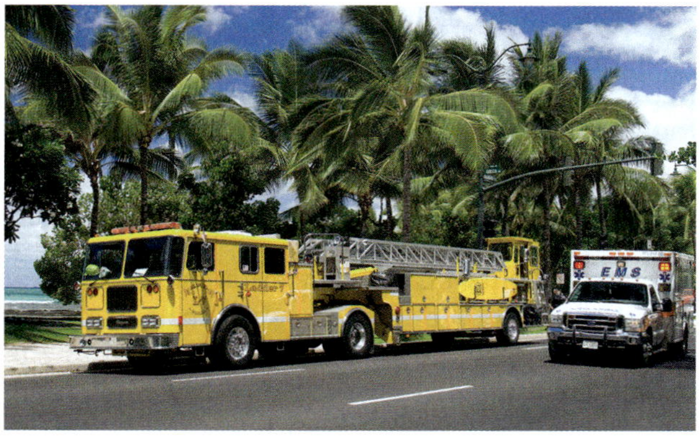

FIGURE 39-7 Make sure your vehicle is not blocked in by other emergency vehicles.

- If your vehicle is blocked in by other emergency vehicles or damaged by a secondary device (or event), you will be unable to escape or provide transportation for victims (**FIGURE 39-7**).

Terrorists have been known to plant additional explosives that are set to explode after the initial bomb. This type of **secondary device** is intended primarily to injure responders and to secure media coverage because the media generally arrive on scene just after the initial response. Secondary devices are often triggered by electronic equipment such as cell phones and are designed to detonate when triggered by the bomber.

Responder Safety (Personnel Protection)

The best form of protection from a WMD agent is to avoid contact with the agent. The greatest threats facing you in a WMD attack are contamination and **cross-contamination**. Contamination with an agent occurs when you have direct contact with the WMD or are exposed to it. Cross-contamination occurs when you come in contact with a contaminated person who has not yet been decontaminated.

If a defined command system has not been established early in an event, victims may be brought to you for care before a decontamination process is in place. At any scene where an agent may have been released that could cause patient contamination, ensure patients have gone through the proper decontamination process before you accept them for care.

Notification Procedures

When you suspect a terrorist or WMD event has taken place, notify the dispatcher. Vital information needs to be communicated effectively if you are to receive the appropriate assistance. Inform dispatch of the nature of the event, any additional resources that may be required, the estimated number of patients, and the upwind route of approach or optimal route of approach. See Chapter 4, *Communications and Documentation*, for information on effective communication.

It is extremely important to establish a staging area, where additional arriving units will converge. Be mindful of access and exit routes when you direct units to respond to a location. It is unwise to have units respond to the front entrance of a hotel or apartment building that has sustained an explosion. See Chapter 36, *Transport Operations*, for more on vehicle positioning.

Finally, trained responders in the proper protective equipment are the only people equipped to handle the WMD incident. These specialized units, traditionally hazardous materials (hazmat) teams, must be requested as early as possible because of the time required to assemble and dispatch the team and their equipment. Many jurisdictions share hazmat teams, so the team may have to travel a long distance to reach the location of the event. It is always better to be safe than sorry; call the team early, and the outcome of the call may be more favorable.

Keep in mind that there may be more than one type of device or agent present.

Words of Wisdom

On September 11, 2001, communications were severely affected by the collapse of the World Trade Center. The primary communications repeater was located on top of the North Tower and was the tallest antenna in the world. In addition, excess radio traffic made transmitting and receiving messages extremely difficult. Not only were radio communications affected, but most cell phones and most radio and television stations were disabled. The lesson learned from this event is to have multiple backups to your ability to communicate with your dispatcher. In the event of a terrorist or WMD event, follow best practices of radio communication.

Establishing Command

The first clinician on the scene must begin to sort out the chaos and define responsibilities under the incident command system (ICS). As the first person on scene, you may need to establish command until additional personnel arrive. Depending on the circumstances and stage of the operation, you and other EMTs may function as medical branch directors, triage supervisors, treatment supervisors, transportation supervisors, logistic officers, or command and general staff. If the initial ICS is already in place, then immediately find the medical staging officer to receive your assignment. Chapter 38, *Incident Management*, discusses in detail how to work within the ICS and the National Incident Management System.

Reassessing Scene Safety

Do not rely on others to secure your safety. It is your responsibility to constantly assess and reassess the scene for safety. This is an important component of situational awareness. It is easy to overlook a suspicious package while you are treating casualties. Stay alert. Something as subtle as a change in the wind direction during a gas attack or an increase in the number of contaminated patients can place you in danger. Never become so involved with the tasks you are performing that you do not look around and make sure the scene remains safe. Remember that as a responder, you may represent a prime target for those meaning to cause harm and incite chaos.

Words of Wisdom

Although it may be difficult for you because of ethical or moral reasons to treat a suspected criminal or suspected terrorist, it is important that this patient receive the normal standard of care. You are not the judge or jury. It is up to the legal system to prove in a court of law that someone is guilty.

Chemical Agents

Chemical agents are substances that are dispersed to kill or injure. Modern-day chemicals were first developed during WWI and WWII. During the Cold War, some of these agents were stockpiled, while others were banned due to their potential for harm. Whereas the United States has long renounced the use of chemical weapons, many nations still develop and stockpile them. These agents are deadly and pose a threat if they are acquired by terrorists.

Chemical weapons have several classifications. The properties or characteristics of an agent can be described as liquid, gas, or solid material. **Persistency** and **volatility** describe how long the agent will stay on a surface before it evaporates. Persistent, or nonvolatile, agents can remain on a surface for long periods, usually longer than 24 hours. Nonpersistent, or volatile, agents evaporate relatively quickly when left on a surface in the optimal temperature range. An agent that is described as highly persistent (such as VX, a nerve agent) can remain in the environment for weeks to months, whereas an agent that is highly volatile (such as sarin, also a nerve agent) will turn from liquid to gas (evaporate) within minutes to seconds.

Route of exposure is how the agent most effectively enters the body. Chemical agents can have either a vapor or contact hazard. Agents with a **vapor hazard** enter the body through the respiratory tract in the form of vapors. Agents with a **contact hazard** (or skin hazard) give off very little vapor or no vapors and enter the body through the skin.

YOU are the EMT

Several law enforcement officers run past your ambulance toward the scene of the shooting. You are told that the suspect is no longer a threat, and they need immediate assistance at the scene of the shooting. Two blocks away, additional officers are evacuating the area around the trash can that was smoking heavily.

3. What should you consider when determining if the scene is safe for you and other EMS personnel to enter?

4. What immediate actions should you perform prior to proceeding into the scene?

Vesicants (Blister Agents)

The primary route of exposure of blister agents, or **vesicants**, is the skin (contact) or eyes; however, if vesicants are left on the skin or clothing long enough, they produce vapors that can enter the respiratory tract. Vesicants cause burn-like blisters to form on the victim's skin and in the respiratory tract. The vesicant agents consist of sulfur mustard (H), lewisite (L), and phosgene oxime (CX) (the symbols H, L, and CX are military designations for these chemicals). The vesicants usually cause the most damage to damp or moist areas of the body, such as the eyes, armpits, groin, and respiratory tract. Signs of vesicant exposure on the skin include the following:

- Skin irritation, burning, and reddening
- Immediate, intense skin pain (with L and CX)
- Formation of large blisters
- Gray discoloration of skin (a sign of permanent damage seen with L and CX)
- Swollen and closed or irritated eyes
- Permanent eye injury (including blindness)

If vapors were inhaled, the patient may experience the following signs and symptoms:

- Hoarseness and stridor
- Severe cough
- Hemoptysis (coughing up blood)
- Severe dyspnea

Sulfur mustard (H), commonly known as mustard gas, is a brown-yellow oily substance that is generally considered very persistent. When released, mustard gas has the distinct smell of garlic or mustard and is quickly absorbed into the skin and/or mucous membranes. As the agent is absorbed into the skin, it begins an irreversible process of damage to the cells. Absorption through the skin or mucous membranes usually occurs within seconds, and damage to the underlying cells takes place within 1 to 2 minutes.

Mustard gas is considered a **mutagen**, which means that it mutates, damages, and changes the structures of cells. Eventually, cellular death will occur. On the surface, the patient will generally not show any signs or symptoms until 4 to 6 hours after exposure (depending on concentration and amount of exposure) (**FIGURE 39-8**).

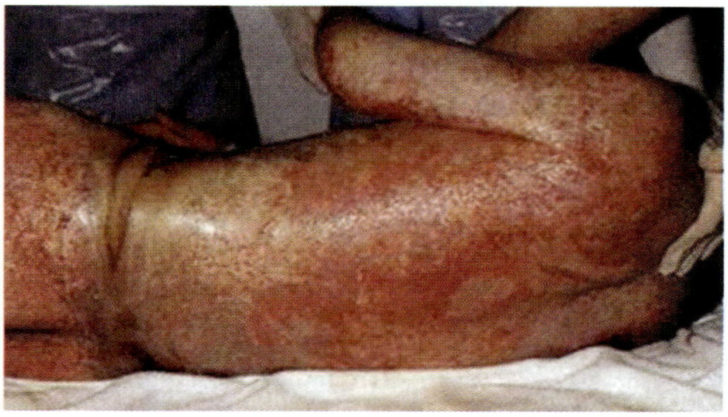

FIGURE 39-8 Skin damage resulting from exposure to sulfur mustard (H).

Courtesy of Dr. Saeed Keshavarz/RCCI, Research Center of Chemical Injuries/IRAN.

The patient will experience a progressive reddening of the affected area, which will gradually develop into large painful blisters. These blisters are very similar in shape and appearance to those associated with thermal partial-thickness (second-degree) burns. The fluid within the blisters does not contain any of the agent; however, the skin covering the area is considered contaminated until trained personnel have decontaminated the patient.

Mustard gas also attacks vulnerable cells within the bone marrow and depletes the body's ability to reproduce white blood cells. Like other burns, the primary complication associated with vesicant blisters is secondary infection. If the patient survives the initial direct injury from the agent, the depletion of the white blood cells leaves the patient with a decreased resistance to infections. Although sulfur mustard is regarded as persistent, the vapors it releases when dispersed can be inhaled. This creates upper and lower airway compromise. The result is damage and swelling of the airways. The airway compromise makes the patient's condition far more serious.

Lewisite (L) and **phosgene oxime (CX)** produce blister wounds very similar to those caused by mustard gas. They are highly volatile and have a rapid onset of symptoms, compared with the delayed onset seen with mustard gas. These agents produce immediate intense pain and discomfort when contact is made. The patient's skin may have a gray discoloration at the contaminated site. Although tissue damage also occurs with exposure to these agents, they do not cause the secondary cellular injury that is associated with mustard gas.

Vesicant Agent Treatment

There are no antidotes for mustard gas or CX exposure. British anti-lewisite is the antidote for agent L;

however, it is not carried by civilian EMS. Ensure the patient has been decontaminated before you initiate any treatment. If any agent has been inhaled, the patient may require prompt airway support as soon as decontamination is completed. Initiate transport as soon as possible. Generally, burn centers are best equipped to handle the wounds and subsequent infections produced by vesicants. Follow your local protocols when determining the transport destination.

Pulmonary Agents (Choking Agents)

The pulmonary agents are gases that cause immediate harm to people exposed to them and include chlorine (Cl) and phosgene. These agents produce respiratory-related symptoms such as dyspnea and tachypnea. The primary route of exposure for these agents is through the respiratory tract, which makes them an inhalation or vapor hazard. Once inside the lungs, they damage the lung tissue and fluid leaks into the lungs. Pulmonary edema develops in the patient, resulting in difficulty breathing because of severely impaired gas exchange.

Chlorine (Cl) was the first chemical agent ever used in warfare. It has a distinct odor of bleach and creates a green haze when released as a gas. Initially, it produces upper airway irritation and a choking sensation. The patient may later experience the following signs and symptoms:

- Shortness of breath
- Tightness in chest
- Hoarseness and stridor as the result of upper airway constriction
- Gasping and coughing
- Blurred vision and lacrimation

With serious exposures, patients may experience pulmonary edema, complete airway constriction, and death. The fumes from a mixture of household bleach and ammonia create an acid gas that produces similar effects. According to the American Association of Poison Control Centers' 2023 data report, after medications, household cleaning substances were the most common cause of poison exposure in adults; they were the leading cause in children.[12]

Do not confuse **phosgene** with phosgene oxime, a blistering agent, or vesicant. Not only has phosgene been produced for chemical warfare, but it is also a product of combustion that might be produced as a result of a fire involving other chemicals, such as at a textile factory or house, or from metalwork or burning Freon (a liquid chemical historically used in refrigeration). Therefore, you may encounter a victim of exposure to this gas during a call or at a fire scene. Phosgene is a very potent agent that has a delayed onset of symptoms, usually hours. Unlike Cl, when phosgene enters the body, it generally does not produce severe irritation that would possibly cause victims to leave the area or hold their breath. In fact, the odor produced by the chemical is similar to that of freshly mowed grass or hay. The result is that much more of the gas may enter the body unnoticed. Initially, a mild exposure may include the following signs and symptoms:

- Nausea
- Tightness in chest
- Severe cough
- Dyspnea on exertion

The victim of a severe exposure may present with dyspnea at rest and excessive pulmonary edema. The pulmonary edema may be so severe that the patient continually coughs up white or pink-tinged fluid. A severe exposure produces such large amounts of fluid in the lungs that the patient may become hypovolemic and subsequently hypotensive.

Pulmonary Agent Treatment

The best initial treatment of any patient who has been exposed to a pulmonary agent is to remove the patient from the contaminated atmosphere. This should be done by trained personnel wearing the proper personal protective equipment (PPE). Aggressively manage Airway, Breathing, and Circulation (ABCs), paying attention to oxygenation, ventilation, and suctioning, if required. Do not allow the patient to be active because this will worsen the condition. There are no antidotes to counteract the pulmonary agents. The primary goals for basic life support prehospital emergency care are to assess the ABCs, allow the patient to rest in a position of comfort with the head elevated, and initiate rapid transport. If the patient's condition does not improve with basic airway support, consider requesting an advanced life support (ALS) intercept. Continuous positive airway pressure may benefit some of these patients, but others will require more advanced airway management.

Nerve Agents

The **nerve agents** are among the deadliest chemicals developed. They are classified as WMDs. Nerve agents are not readily available to the general public and are extremely toxic and rapidly fatal with any route of exposure. Designed to kill a large number of people by using small quantities, nerve agents can cause cardiac arrest within seconds to minutes of exposure. Nerve agents, discovered while in search of a superior pesticide, are a class of chemical called organophosphates, which are found in some household bug sprays, agricultural pesticides, and some industrial chemicals at much lower strengths than in the weaponized form. Organophosphates block an essential enzyme in the nervous system, causing the body's organs to become overstimulated and burn out.

G agents came from the early nerve agents, the G-series, which were developed by German scientists (hence the G) in the period after WWI and during WWII. There are three G-series agents, which are all designed with the same basic chemical structure with slight variations to produce different properties. The two variations of these agents are lethality and volatility. The following G agents are listed from high volatility to low volatility:

- **Sarin (GB)**. Highly volatile colorless and odorless liquid. Turns from liquid to gas within seconds to minutes at room temperature. The lethal concentration of sarin in air is approximately 28 to 35 mg/m^3 per minute for a 2-minute exposure time by a healthy adult breathing normally. Sarin is primarily a vapor hazard, with the respiratory tract as the main route of entry. This agent is especially dangerous in enclosed environments such as office buildings, shopping malls, and subway cars. When this agent comes into contact with the skin, it is quickly absorbed and evaporates. When sarin is on clothing, it has the effect of **off-gassing**, which means that the vapors are continuously released over time (similar to perfume). This renders the victim and the victim's clothing contaminated.
- **Soman (GD)**. Twice as persistent as sarin and five times as lethal. It has a fruity odor as a result of the type of alcohol used in the agent and generally has no color. This agent is a contact and inhalation hazard that can enter the body through skin absorption and through the respiratory tract. A unique additive in GD causes it to bind to the cells that it attacks faster than any other agent. This irreversible binding is called **aging**, which makes it more difficult to treat patients who have been exposed.
- **Tabun (GA)**. Approximately one-half as lethal as sarin and 36 times more persistent. Under the proper conditions it will remain present for several days. It has a fruity smell and an appearance similar to sarin. The components used to manufacture GA are easy to acquire, and the agent is easy to manufacture, which makes it unique. GA is a contact and inhalation hazard that can enter the body through skin absorption and through the respiratory tract.
- **V agent (VX)**. Clear, oily agent that has no odor and looks like baby oil. V agent was developed by the British after WWII and has chemical properties similar to the G-series agents. The difference is that VX is more than 100 times more lethal than sarin and is extremely persistent (**FIGURE 39-9**). In fact, VX is so persistent that given the proper conditions, it will remain relatively unchanged for weeks to

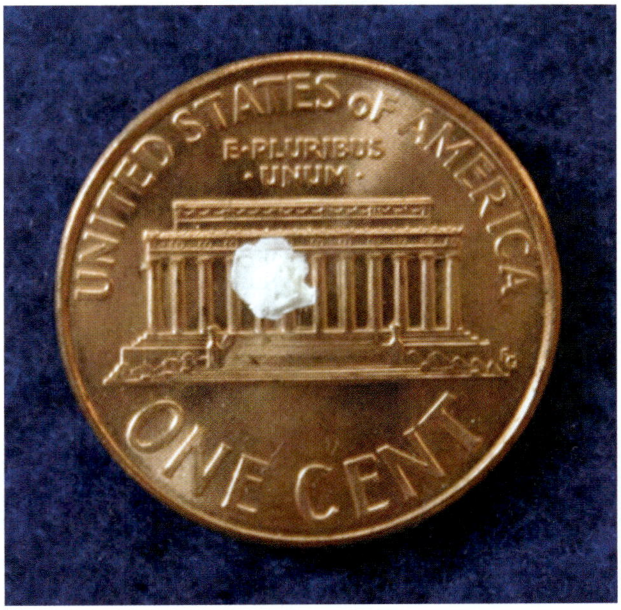

FIGURE 39-9 VX is one of the most toxic chemicals ever created. The dot on the penny demonstrates the amount needed to achieve the lethal dose.

months. These properties make VX primarily a contact hazard because it lets off very little vapor. It is easily absorbed into the skin, and the oily residue that remains on the skin's surface is extremely difficult to decontaminate.

Nerve agents all produce similar symptoms but have varying routes of entry. Nerve agents differ slightly in lethal concentration or dose and also differ in their volatility. Some agents are designed to quickly become a gas (nonpersistent or highly volatile), whereas others remain a liquid for a period of time (persistent or nonvolatile). These agents have been used successfully in warfare and, until recently, were the only type of chemical agent that had been used successfully in a terrorist act. Once the agent has entered the body through skin contact or through the respiratory system, the patient will begin to exhibit a pattern of predictable symptoms. Like all chemical agents, the severity of the patient's symptoms will depend on the route of exposure of the agent and the amount of exposure.

Safety Tips

The Federal Emergency Management Agency's Center for Domestic Preparedness programs offer both web-based and in-person training sessions that are often free of charge to the participants. These programs are offered to first responders and would greatly expand your knowledge and training in WMD responses.

The symptoms of nerve agent exposure are described in **TABLE 39-1** using the military mnemonic SLUDGEM and the medical mnemonic DUMBELS. The medical mnemonic is more useful to you because it lists the symptoms associated with exposure to nerve agents that pose the greatest threat of death to the patient. You may also hear the term "killer Bs," referencing the symptoms of bradycardia, bronchospasm, and bronchorrhea, which are the most likely causes of death to the patient.

There are only a handful of medical conditions that are associated with the bilateral pinpoint constricted pupils (**miosis**) seen with nerve agent exposure. Conditions such as a cerebrovascular accident, direct light to both eyes, and an opioid drug overdose all can cause bilaterally constricted pupils. Therefore, assess the patient for all of the SLUDGEM/DUMBELS signs and symptoms to

TABLE 39-1 Symptoms of Exposure to Nerve Agents

Military Mnemonic: SLUDGEM	Medical Mnemonic: DUMBELS (all age groups)
Salivation, Sweating, Seizures	Diarrhea
Lacrimation (excessive tearing) (also rhinorrhea)	Urination
Urination	Miosis (pinpoint pupils), Muscle weakness
Defecation, Drooling, Diarrhea	Bradycardia, Bronchospasm, Bronchorrhea
Gastric upset and cramps	Emesis (vomiting)
Emesis (vomiting)	Lacrimation (excessive tearing) (also rhinorrhea)
Muscle twitching/Miosis (pinpoint pupils)	Seizures, Salivation, Sweating

YOU are the EMT

As you approach the scene of the shooting, a law enforcement officer informs you that the source of the smoke from the trash can was a smoke grenade. That area has been secured by law enforcement and there are no additional patients at that location.

5. Given the situation, what are some unique concerns about this incident?

6. What types of injuries should you expect to encounter?

Safety Tips

The basic chemical ingredient in nerve agents is organophosphate. This is a common chemical that is used in lower concentrations for insecticides. Whereas industrial chemicals do not possess sufficient lethality to be effective WMDs, they are easy to acquire, are inexpensive, and have similar effects to the nerve agents. Crop-duster planes and drones could be used to disseminate these chemicals. Be cautious when responding to calls where insecticide equipment is stored and used, such as a farm or supply stores that sell these products. The symptoms and medical care of victims of organophosphate insecticide poisoning are identical to those for victims of the nerve agents.

determine whether the patient has been exposed to a nerve agent.

Miosis is the most common symptom of nerve agent exposure and can persist for days to weeks. This symptom, along with the others listed in Table 39-1, will help you recognize exposure to a nerve agent early. Miosis will be seen quickly in a vapor exposure but may occur later after an isolated skin exposure. In some cases, the patient may have been exposed to both.

The seizures that are associated with nerve agent exposure are unlike those found in patients with a history of seizure. The seizure will continue until the patient dies or until treatment is given with a nerve agent antidote kit (DuoDote Auto-Injector or Antidote Treatment Nerve Agent Auto-Injector [ATNAA]).

Nerve Agent Treatment

Fatalities from severe exposure to a nerve agent occur as a result of respiratory complications, which lead to respiratory arrest. Once the patient has been decontaminated, be prepared to treat aggressively, if the patient is to be saved. You can greatly increase the patient's chances of survival simply by providing airway and ventilatory support. As with all emergencies, securing the ABCs is the best and most important treatment that you can provide. Often in patients exposed to these agents, seizures will begin and will not stop. These patients will require administration of nerve agent antidote kits in addition to support of the ABCs.

Medical treatment for nerve agent exposure may include the **DuoDote Auto-Injector**. The DuoDote Auto-Injector contains 2.1 mg of atropine and 600 mg of pralidoxime chloride (2-PAM) and is delivered as a single dose through one needle. Atropine is used to block the nerve agent from binding with the body's receptor sites. However, because the nerve agent may remain in the body for long periods, pralidoxime chloride is used to eliminate the agent from the body. Many of the symptoms described in

Words of Wisdom

On March 20, 1995, members of Aum Shinrikyo, a Japanese cult, released sarin (GB) in the Tokyo subway, coordinating the release on multiple cars during the busy morning commute. The first arriving medical responders were met with chaos as thousands of people fled the subway system (**FIGURE 39-10**). Many were contaminated and showed signs and symptoms of nerve agent exposure. In the end, more than 5,000 people sought medical care for exposure to sarin, and 12 people died.

This attack illustrates a key objective of terrorism: panic. Most of the people who sought medical care had not been poisoned, but their fear created a burden for local resources. To mitigate the effects of panic, these events may require an additional form of triage to sort exposed individuals from panicked individuals who were not actually exposed. It should also be noted that during this response, none of the EMS personnel wore protective clothing, so most became cross-contaminated.

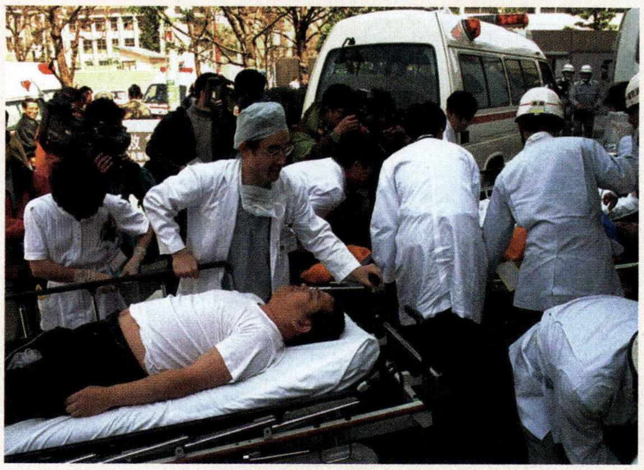

FIGURE 39-10 Medical professionals responding to an attack in 1995, where cult members released sarin in the Tokyo subway.

the DUMBELS mnemonic can begin to be reversed with the use of atropine; however, many doses may be necessary to see total cessation of the symptoms. The military form of this combination injector is the **Antidote Treatment Nerve Agent Auto-Injector (ATNAA)**.

In some regions, EMTs may carry DuoDote kits on the unit and will be called on to administer the antidotes to themselves or their patients. If your service carries a nerve agent antidote, refer to your local protocols for dosage and usage information. These medications are delivered using the same technique as the EpiPen auto-injector; however, multiple doses may need to be administered, thus requiring multiple kits. Activated antidote kits need to be properly disposed of in a sharps container.

TABLE 39-2 provides a quick reference and comparison of the nerve agents.

Special Populations

AGE-RELATED CONSIDERATIONS FOR DUODOTE ADMINISTRATION

The US Food and Drug Administration has approved Duodote administration for patients weighing more than 90 pounds (41 kg).[13] In children, an overdose of pralidoxime chloride may cause extreme muscular weakness, resulting in respiratory depression. Medical direction may approve the antidote's use in children who weigh less than 90 pounds (41 kg) and have serious signs of nerve agent poisoning, especially if atropine is not available in other forms. Pediatric autoinjectors (AtroPen) in 0.25-mg or 0.5-mg doses may be available and indicated in these situations. Pralidoxime chloride 600-mg autoinjectors may be administered to infants weighing more than 26 pounds (12 kg) if signs of severe poisoning are present.

Notify medical direction when caring for older adults known to have impaired kidney function or hypertension. Smaller doses of pralidoxime chloride are recommended in these patients.[14]

Metabolic Agents (Cyanides)

Hydrogen cyanide (AC) and cyanogen chloride (CK) are both agents that affect the body's ability to use oxygen. **Cyanide** is a colorless gas that has an odor similar to that of bitter almonds. The effects of the cyanides begin on the cellular level and are rapidly seen at the organ and system levels. Unlike nerve agents, however, these deadly gases are commonly found in many industrial settings. Cyanides are produced every year in massive quantities throughout the United States for industrial uses such as gold and silver mining, photography, and plastics

TABLE 39-2 The Nerve Agents

Name	Military Designation	Odor	Special Features	Onset of Symptoms	Volatility	Route of Exposure
Tabun	GA	Fruity	Easy to manufacture	Immediate	Low	Skin contact and vapor hazard
Sarin	GB	None (if pure) or strong	Will off-gas while on victim's clothing	Immediate	High	Primarily respiratory vapor hazard; skin exposure is extremely lethal
Soman	GD	Fruity	Ages rapidly; difficult to treat	Immediate	Moderate	Skin contact; minimal vapor hazard
V agent	VX	None	Most lethal chemical agent; difficult to decontaminate	Immediate	Very low	Skin contact; no vapor hazard (unless aerosolized)

processing. The combustion of household goods such as insulation, carpeting, upholstery, plastic, and synthetic rubber can release a significant amount of cyanide. Thus, a patient who has inhaled smoke at a fire may experience cyanide toxicity. A firefighter who is involved in overhaul after the fire may also be exposed to cyanide and must wear proper protective equipment.

There is very little difference in the symptoms found between AC and CK. In low doses, these chemicals are associated with dizziness, light-headedness, headache, and vomiting. Higher doses will produce symptoms that include the following:

- Shortness of breath and gasping respirations
- Respiratory distress or arrest
- Tachypnea
- Flushed skin (may be difficult to detect in dark-skinned people)
- Tachycardia
- Altered mental status
- Seizures
- Coma
- Apnea
- Cardiac arrest

The symptoms associated with the inhalation of a large amount of cyanide will all appear within several minutes. Death is likely unless the patient is treated promptly.

Words of Wisdom

Patients who are exposed to cyanide and who have shortness of breath will have a normal pulse oximetry reading. This is because cyanide impairs the body's ability to offload the oxygen molecules at a cellular level. Cyanide will create true hypoxia at a cellular level despite the presence of oxygen circulating through the bloodstream.

Cyanide Agent Treatment

Cyanide binds with the body's cells, preventing oxygen from being used. After trained personnel wearing the proper PPE have removed the patient from the source of exposure, even if there is no liquid contamination, all of the patient's clothes must be removed to prevent off-gassing in the ambulance. Trained and protected personnel must decontaminate any patients who may have been exposed to liquid contamination before you can initiate treatment. Then you can support the patient's ABCs. Mild effects of cyanide exposure will generally resolve by simply removing the victim from the source of contamination and administering supplemental oxygen. Severe exposure, however, will require aggressive oxygenation and perhaps ventilation with supplemental oxygen. Always use a bag-mask device or oxygen-powered ventilator device to ventilate a victim of a metabolic agent. The agent can easily be passed on from the patient to you through mouth-to-mouth or mouth-to-mask ventilations.

Hydroxocobalamin is a cyanide antidote included in an intravenous (IV) infusion kit (Cyanokit) that is carried by some ALS ambulances. Hydroxocobalamin binds to the cyanide, making a nontoxic byproduct. Initiate transport immediately if administration of an antidote by ALS is not available.

Words of Wisdom

Always make sure your patients have been thoroughly decontaminated by trained personnel before you come in contact with them. Chemical agents are primarily a vapor hazard, and all of the patient's clothing must be removed prior to treatment to prevent off-gassing to you. Protect yourself as you manage the airway of a patient exposed to a vapor hazard. Many of the vapors may linger in the patient's airway, and cross-contamination may occur.

TABLE 39-3 summarizes the chemical agents. The odors of the particular chemicals are provided for informational purposes only. The sense of smell is a poor tool to use to determine whether there is a chemical agent present. Many people are unable to smell the agents, and the odor could be derived from another source. This information is useful to you if you receive reports from victims who claimed to smell bleach or garlic, for example. Never enter a potentially hazardous area and "sniff the air" to determine whether a chemical agent is present.

TABLE 39-3 Chemical Agents

Name	Military Designations	Odor	Lethality	Onset of Symptoms	Volatility	Primary Route of Exposure
Nerve agents	Tabun (GA) Sarin (GB) Soman (GD) VX	Fruity or none	Highly lethal chemical agents; kill within minutes; effects are reversible with antidotes	Immediate	Moderate (GA, GD) Very high (GB) Low (VX)	GA—both GB—vapor hazard GD—both VX—contact hazard
Vesicants	Mustard (H) Lewisite (L) Phosgene oxime (CX)	Garlic (H) Geranium (L)	Cause large blisters to form; inhalation severely damages upper airway; severe, intense pain and gray skin discoloration (L, CX)	Delayed (H) Immediate (L, CX)	Very low (H, L) Moderate (CX)	Primarily contact, with some vapor hazard
Pulmonary agents	Chlorine (Cl) Phosgene (CG)	Bleach Cut grass (CG)	Cause irritation choking (Cl); severe pulmonary edema (CG)	Immediate (Cl) Delayed (CG)	Very high	Vapor hazard
Cyanide agents	Hydrogen cyanide (AC) Cyanogen chloride (CK)	Almonds (AC) Irritating (CK)	Highly lethal chemical gases; kill within minutes; effects are reversible with antidotes	Immediate	Very high	Vapor hazard

Words of Wisdom

Use of chemical agents for crowd control dates back more than 2,000 years, when the Chinese army placed ground red pepper onto rice paper and deployed it into the eyes of their adversaries. The chemical riot-control agent primarily used by law enforcement in the United States today is 2-chlorobenzalmalononitrile (CS). Chloroacetophenone (CN) may also be encountered, typically in consumer products such as "pepper spray," but its use by law enforcement is less common because it is more toxic than CS.[15] These agents, commonly referred to as tear gases, cause irritation to the eyes and respiratory tract. While they generally do not cause long-term effects, the hysteria that is often associated with their use in a crowd of people can resemble a chemical attack.

Patients who are at higher risk for adverse effects when exposed to these agents include children and individuals who have prior respiratory illness, are experiencing delirium with agitation, have used alcohol or other drugs, or have been sprayed multiple times.[16]

EMS clinicians should approach these scenes with appropriate PPE. EMS care should be focused on irrigating the skin and eyes (ask the patient to remove contact lenses, if possible) and removing the patients from the area to an environment with clean air. If the patient is wheezing, a bronchodilator agent may be administered. Monitor the patient's oxygen and ventilation status carefully and intervene as needed.

Biologic Agents

Biologic agents pose many difficult issues when used as WMDs. Biologic agents can be almost completely undetectable. Also, most of the diseases caused by these agents will be similar to the other minor illnesses commonly seen by EMS clinicians.

Biologic agents are grouped as viruses, bacteria, and neurotoxins and may be spread in various ways. **Dissemination** is the means by which a terrorist spreads the agent; for example, agents could be spread by poisoning the water supply or aerosolizing the agent into the air or ventilation system of a building. A **disease vector** is an animal that spreads disease, once infected, to another animal. For example, bubonic plague can be spread by infected rats; smallpox by infected humans; and West Nile virus by infected mosquitoes. How easily the disease spreads from one human to another human is called *communicability*. Some diseases, such as those caused by the human immunodeficiency virus (HIV), are difficult to spread by routine contact. Therefore, communicability is considered low. In other instances when communicability is high, such as with smallpox, the person is considered **contagious**. Typically, routine standard precautions are enough to prevent contamination from contagious biologic organisms.

Incubation is the time between the person becoming exposed to the agent and the appearance of the first symptoms. The incubation period is especially important for you to understand. Although patients may not exhibit signs or symptoms, they may be contagious.

Be aware of when you should suspect the use of biologic agents. If the agent is in the form of a powder, as was the case in the October 2001 terrorist attacks involving letters laced with anthrax powder and distributed via the US mail system, the incident must be handled by hazmat specialists. Patients who come in direct contact with the agent need to be decontaminated before you make any contact with them or initiate treatment. Fortunately, once recognized and identified, treatment is similar to that for other bacterial infections.

Viruses

Viruses are germs that require a living host to multiply and survive. A virus is a simple organism and cannot thrive outside of a host (living body). Once in the body, the virus invades healthy cells and replicates itself to spread through the host. As the virus spreads, so does the disease that it carries. Viruses spread from host to host by direct methods, such as through respiratory droplets, or through vectors. A *vector* is any agent that acts as a carrier or transporter.

Viral agents that may be used during a biologic terrorist release pose an extraordinary problem for health care clinicians, especially those in EMS. Although some viral agents do have vaccines, there is often no treatment for a viral infection other than antiviral medications for some agents. Because of this characteristic, the following viruses have the potential to be used as terrorism agents.

Smallpox

Smallpox is a highly contagious disease. If encountered, use all forms of standard precautions to prevent cross-contamination. Simply by wearing examination gloves, a HEPA-filtered respirator, and eye protection, you will greatly reduce your risk of contamination. The last natural case of smallpox in the world was seen in 1977. Before the rash and blisters show, the illness will start with a high fever and body aches and headaches. The patient's temperature is usually in the range of 101°F to 104°F (38.3°C to 40°C).

An easy, quick way to differentiate the smallpox rash from other skin disorders is to observe the size, shape, and location of the lesions. In smallpox, all the lesions are identical in their development. In other skin disorders, the lesions will be in various stages of healing and development. The rash is called a pustular rash, as the bumps are raised, fluid-filled lesions. Smallpox blisters begin on the face and extremities and eventually move toward the chest and abdomen. The disease is in its most contagious phase when the blisters begin to form (**FIGURE 39-11**). Unprotected contact with these blisters will promote transmission of the disease (**TABLE 39-4**). There is a vaccine to prevent smallpox; however, it has been linked to rare medical complications and, in rare cases, death. Should an outbreak occur, the US government has enough vaccine stockpiled to vaccinate every person in the United States.

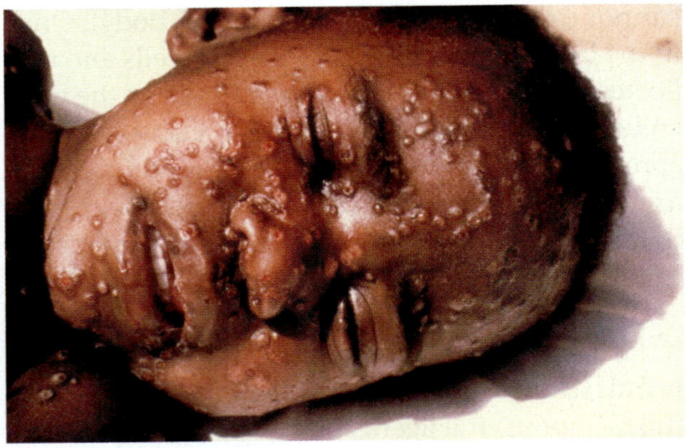

FIGURE 39-11 In smallpox, all the lesions are identical in their development. In other skin disorders, the lesions will be in various stages of healing and development.

Courtesy of CDC.

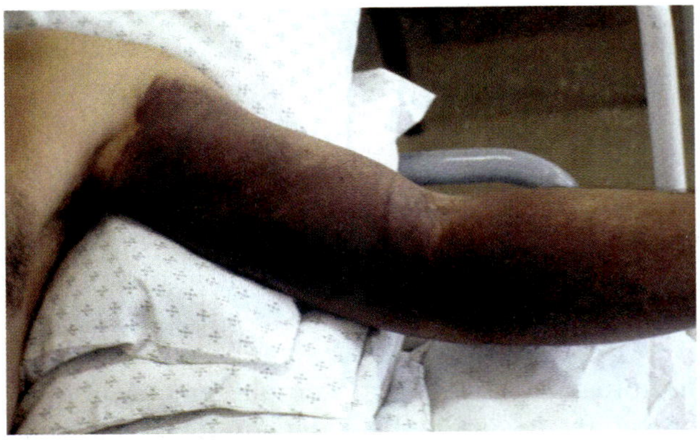

FIGURE 39-12 Viral hemorrhagic fevers cause the blood vessels and tissues to seep blood. The end result is ecchymosis, bloody sputum, and blood in the patient's stool. Notice the severe discoloration in the arm of this patient with Crimean Congo hemorrhagic fever, indicating internal bleeding.

Courtesy of Professor Robert Swanepoel/National Institute for Communicable Disease, South Africa.

TABLE 39-4 Characteristics of Smallpox

Dissemination	Aerosolized for warfare or terrorist uses
Communicability	High from infected patients or contaminated items (such as blankets); person-to-person transmission possible
Route of entry	Inhalation of coughed droplets or direct skin contact with blisters
Signs and symptoms	Severe fever, malaise, body aches, headaches, small blisters on the skin, bleeding of the skin and mucous membranes; incubation period 10 to 12 days; duration of the illness, approximately 4 weeks
Medical management	Standard precautions; no specific treatment; provide supportive care (ABCs)

Viral Hemorrhagic Fevers

Viral hemorrhagic fevers consist of a group of diseases caused by viruses that include the Ebola, Rift Valley, Marburg, Lassa, dengue, and yellow fever viruses, among others. This group of viruses causes the blood in the body to seep out from the tissues and blood vessels (**FIGURE 39-12**). Initially, the patient will have flulike symptoms, progressing to more serious symptoms such as internal and external hemorrhaging.

Viral hemorrhagic fevers can be found across the world and, depending on the disease, can be transmitted from person to person or through a zoonotic host. An Ebola outbreak in West Africa in 2014 resulted in imported cases in the United States. This was the largest Ebola outbreak reported and led to cases in 10 countries. While outbreaks in the United States are rare, a traveler in the United States died of Lassa fever in 2024, and several cases of dengue infection (spread by mosquitoes) were reported in San Diego, California, in the same year.[17]

Take all standard precautions when treating these illnesses or caring for someone with flulike symptoms and a recent travel history. Mortality rates can range from 5% to 90%, depending on the strain of virus, the victim's age and health condition, and the availability of a modern health care system (**TABLE 39-5**).

Bacteria

Unlike viruses, **bacteria** do not require a host to multiply and live. These single-celled microorganisms reproduce rapidly and are much more complex and larger than viruses. They can grow up to 100 times larger than the largest virus. Bacteria contain all the cellular structures of a normal cell and are completely self-sufficient. Most bacterial infections can be treated with antibiotics.

TABLE 39-5 Characteristics of Viral Hemorrhagic Fevers

Dissemination	Direct contact with infected body fluids; can be aerosolized for use in an attack
Communicability	Moderate from person to person, contaminated items, or zoonotic hosts
Route of entry	Direct contact with infected body fluids
Signs and symptoms	Sudden onset of fever, weakness, muscle pain, headache, and sore throat; all followed by vomiting and, as the virus runs its course, internal and external bleeding
Medical management	Standard precautions; no specific treatment; provide supportive care (ABCs) and treat for shock and hypotension, if present

Most bacterial infections will generally begin with flulike symptoms, which can make it quite difficult for health care clinicians to identify whether the cause is a biologic attack or a natural infection.

Words of Wisdom

Because humans are acceptable hosts and vectors for many viruses and bacteria, take standard precautions at all times. If you fail to take standard precautions, you may not only become a host for a virus, you may spread it as well. Remember, a virus spreads from person to person to survive, and many infectious diseases present in a manner similar to common colds.

Inhalation and Cutaneous Anthrax (*Bacillus anthracis*)

Anthrax is caused by deadly bacteria that lie dormant in a spore (protective shell). When exposed to the optimal temperature and moisture, the germ will be released from the spore. The routes of entry for anthrax bacteria are inhalation, cutaneous, and gastrointestinal (from consuming food that contains spores) (**FIGURE 39-13**). The inhalational form, or pulmonary anthrax, is the deadliest and often presents as a severe cold. Pulmonary anthrax is associated with a 90% death rate if untreated and presents with pneumonia. Antibiotics can be used to treat anthrax. There is also a vaccine to prevent anthrax infections (**TABLE 39-6**).

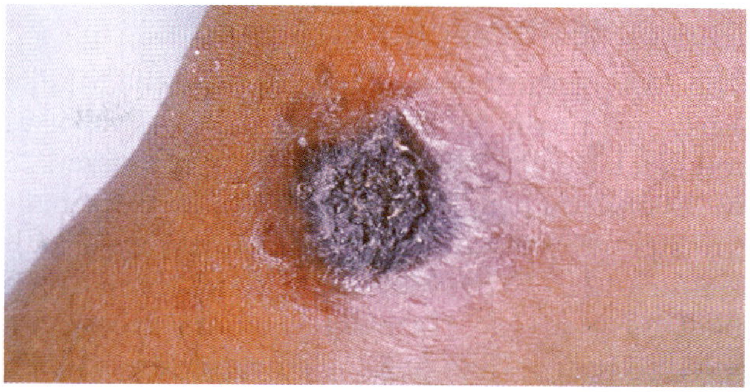

FIGURE 39-13 Cutaneous anthrax.

TABLE 39-6 Characteristics of Anthrax

Dissemination	Aerosol
Communicability	Only in the cutaneous form (rare)
Route of entry	Inhalation of spore, skin contact with spore, or direct contact with skin wound (cutaneous)
Signs and symptoms	Flulike symptoms, fever, respiratory distress with tachycardia, shock, pulmonary edema, and respiratory failure after 3 to 5 days of flulike symptoms
Medical management	Inhalation: Standard precautions, oxygen, ventilatory support if patient has pulmonary edema or respiratory failure, and transport Cutaneous: Standard precautions, apply dry sterile dressing to prevent accidental contact with wound and fluids

Plague (Bubonic/Pneumonic)

The 14th-century plague ravaged Asia, the Middle East, and finally Europe (where it was known as the Black Death). In total, it killed an estimated 75 to 200 million people; in Europe alone, it killed approximately 50% of the population. In the early 19th century, 12 to 15 million people in India and China died due to plague. The plague's natural vectors are infected rodents and fleas. When a person is bitten by an infected flea or comes in contact with an infected rodent (or the waste of the rodent), the person can contract bubonic plague.

Bubonic plague infects the **lymphatic system** (a passive circulatory system in the body that bathes the tissues in lymph and works with the immune system). When this occurs, the patient's **lymph nodes** (area of the lymphatic system where infection-fighting cells are housed) become infected with the bacteria and grow. The glands of the nodes will grow large (up to the size of a tennis ball) and round, forming **buboes** (**FIGURE 39-14**).

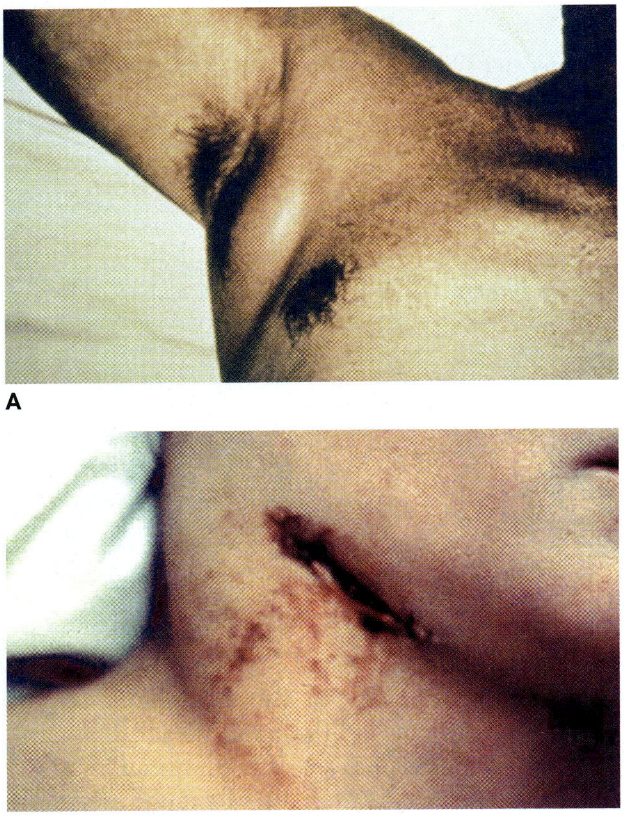

A

B

FIGURE 39-14 A. Plague bubo at lymph node under arm. **B.** Plague bubo at lymph node on neck.

Courtesy of CDC.

If left untreated, the infection may spread through the body, leading to sepsis and possibly death. This form of plague is not contagious and is not likely to be seen in a bioterrorist incident.

Pneumonic plague is a lung infection, also known as plague pneumonia, that results from inhalation of plague bacteria. This form of the disease is contagious and has a much higher death rate than the bubonic form (**TABLE 39-7**).

Neurotoxins

Neurotoxins are the most deadly substances known to humans. The strongest neurotoxin is 15,000 times more lethal than VX and 100,000 times more lethal than sarin. These toxins are produced from plants, marine animals, molds, and bacteria. The route of entry for these toxins is through ingestion, inhalation from aerosols, or injection. Unlike viruses and bacteria, neurotoxins are not contagious and have a faster onset of symptoms. Although these biologic toxins have immense destructive potential, they have not been used successfully as a WMD.

Botulinum Toxin

The most potent neurotoxin is **botulinum**, which is produced by bacteria. When introduced into the body, this neurotoxin affects the nervous system's ability to function. Voluntary muscle control diminishes as the toxin spreads. Eventually the toxin

TABLE 39-7 Characteristics of Plague

Dissemination	Aerosol
Communicability	Bubonic: Low, only from contact with fluid in buboes Pneumonic: High, from person to person
Route of entry	Ingestion, inhalation, or cutaneous
Signs and symptoms	Fever, headache, muscle pain and tenderness, pneumonia, shortness of breath, extreme lymph node pain and enlargement (bubonic)
Medical management	Standard precautions, provide supportive care (ABCs), oxygen if indicated, and transport

TABLE 39-8 Characteristics of Botulinum Toxin

Dissemination	Aerosol or food supply sabotage or injection
Communicability	None
Route of entry	Ingestion, inhalation
Signs and symptoms	Dry mouth, intestinal obstruction, urinary retention, constipation, nausea and vomiting, abnormal pupil dilation, blurred vision, double vision, drooping eyelids, difficulty swallowing, difficulty speaking, and respiratory failure as the result of paralysis
Medical management	Provide supportive care (ABCs), oxygen, and transport; provide ventilatory support in case of paralysis of the respiratory muscles; vaccine available

causes muscle paralysis that begins at the head and face and spreads downward throughout the body. The patient's accessory muscles and diaphragm will become paralyzed, and the patient will go into respiratory arrest. If detected, there is an antidote for botulism (**TABLE 39-8**).

Ricin

Although not as deadly as botulinum, **ricin** is still five times more lethal than VX. This toxin is derived from mash that is left over from processing castor beans (**FIGURE 39-15**). When introduced into the body, ricin causes pulmonary edema and respiratory and circulatory failure leading to death (**TABLE 39-9**).

The clinical picture depends on the route of exposure. The toxin is quite stable and extremely toxic by many routes of exposure, including inhalation. It is likely that 0.5 to 3 mg of ricin can kill an adult and that the ingestion of just one seed can kill a child.

Although all parts of the castor bean are poisonous, it is the seeds that are the most toxic. Castor bean ingestion causes a rapid onset of nausea, vomiting, abdominal cramps, and severe diarrhea, followed by vascular collapse. Death usually occurs on the third day in the absence of appropriate medical intervention.

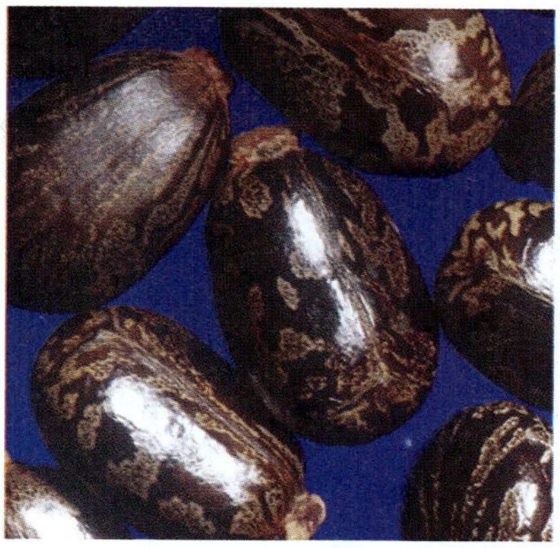

FIGURE 39-15 These seemingly harmless castor beans contain the key ingredient for ricin, one of the most potent toxins known to humans.

TABLE 39-9 Characteristics of Ricin

Dissemination	Released into indoor or outdoor air (aerosol) Food and water contamination
Communicability	None
Route of exposure	Inhalation, ingestion, injection
Signs and symptoms	Inhaled: Fever; chills; nausea; local irritation of the eyes, nose, and throat; profuse sweating; headache; muscle aches; nonproductive cough; chest pain; dyspnea; pulmonary edema; severe lung inflammation; cyanosis; seizures; respiratory failure Ingested: Fever; chills; headache; muscle aches; nausea and vomiting; diarrhea; severe abdominal cramping; dehydration; gastrointestinal bleeding; necrosis of the liver, spleen, kidneys, and gastrointestinal tract; and death Injected: No signs except swelling at the injection site and death
Medical management	Provide supportive care (ABCs); no treatment or vaccine available

Ricin is least toxic by the oral route. This is probably a result of poor absorption in the gastrointestinal tract, some digestion in the gut, and, possibly, some expulsion of the agent as caused by the rapid onset of vomiting. Ingestion causes local hemorrhage and necrosis of the liver, spleen, kidneys, and gastrointestinal tract. Signs and symptoms appear 4 to 8 hours after exposure.

Inhaling ricin will cause nonspecific weakness, cough, fever, hypothermia, and hypotension. Symptoms occur approximately 4 to 8 hours after inhalation, depending on the inhaled dose. The onset of profuse sweating some hours later signifies the termination of the symptoms.

Treat with both respiratory support and cardiovascular support as needed. ALS intervention along with rapid transport to the emergency department for early intubation and ventilation, combined with treatment of pulmonary edema, are appropriate. Paramedics can also initiate the IV fluids and electrolyte replacement that are essential to treat the dehydration caused by profound vomiting and diarrhea.

TABLE 39-10 summarizes the biologic agents.

TABLE 39-10 Biologic Agents

Disease	Person-Person Transmission	Incubation Period	Duration of Illness	Lethality (approximate case fatality rates)
Inhalation anthrax	No	1 to 6 d	3 to 5 d (usually fatal if untreated)	High
Pneumonic plague	Moderate	2 to 3 d	1 to 6 d (usually fatal)	High unless treated within 12 to 24 h
Smallpox	High	7 to 17 d (average, 12 d)	4 wk	High to moderate
Viral hemorrhagic fevers	Moderate	4 to 21 d	Death within 7 to 16 d	High to moderate, depending on type of fever
Botulinum poisoning	No	1 to 5 d	Death within 24 to 72 h; lasts months if patient does not die	High without respiratory support
Ricin poisoning	No	18 to 24 h	Death within 10 to 12 d for ingestion	High

YOU are the EMT

On arriving at the scene, you establish medical command. You see eight people lying in the street, including the suspect and two police officers. There are a few bystanders who are attempting to help the injured. You see several people applying makeshift tourniquets to bleeding extremities and one person performing cardiopulmonary resuscitation (CPR) on a teenage girl. After triaging the patients, you have three patients who are in the expectant category (black tags), three patients in the immediate category (red tags), and two patients in the delayed category (yellow tags).

7. On the basis of the number of patients and their apparent conditions, how many ambulances and EMTs should be present at the scene?

Words of Wisdom

In a mass-casualty incident, it is important to frequently communicate with your patient. Remember, your patient is probably scared and does not know what is going on. Explain to your patient any delays that are occurring, as well as the actions you are taking, so you may alleviate the patient's fears.

Other EMT Roles During a Biologic Event

Syndromic Surveillance

Syndromic surveillance is the monitoring, usually by local or state health departments, of patients presenting to emergency departments and alternative care facilities, EMS call volume, and the use of over-the-counter medications. More recently, syndromic surveillance through wastewater sampling has been used to detect community outbreaks of COVID-19. In some cases, the number of Internet searches or social media posts related to a disease have similarly been used to detect upticks of a disease in a community.[18] Monitoring signs and symptoms that resemble influenza is particularly important. Local and state health departments monitor for an unusual influx of patients with these symptoms in hopes of discovering an outbreak early. The role of EMS in syndromic surveillance is valuable in the overall tracking of a biologic terrorist event or infectious disease outbreak. Quality management and dispatch operations need to be aware of an unusual number of calls from patients with unexplainable symptom clusters coming from a particular region or community.

Points of Distribution (Strategic National Stockpile)

Points of distribution (PODs) are existing facilities that are used as mass distribution sites for antibiotics, antidotes, vaccinations, and other medications and supplies during an emergency.

These medications may be released in deliveries called "push packs" by the Centers for Disease Control and Prevention (CDC) Strategic National Stockpile (**FIGURE 39-16**). These push packs have a delivery time of 12 hours anywhere in the country and contain antibiotics, chemical antidotes, antitoxins, life-support medications, IV administration supplies, airway maintenance supplies, and medical/surgical items. In some regions, local and state municipalities have started to stockpile their own supplies to reduce the time delay.

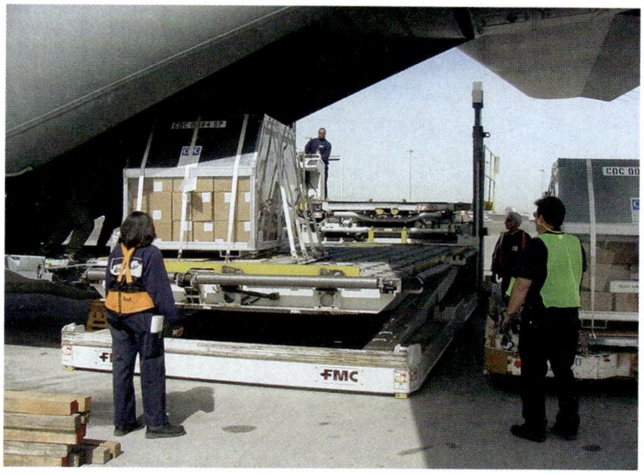

FIGURE 39-16 The Centers for Disease Control and Prevention Strategic National Stockpile can deliver one of many push packs to any location in the country within 12 hours of an emergency.

EMTs, AEMTs, and paramedics may be called on to assist in the delivery of the medications to the public (depending on local emergency management planning). Your role may include triage, disease testing, vaccination administration, treatment of seriously ill patients, and patient transport to the hospital. Most plans for PODs include at least one ambulance on standby to transport seriously ill patients.

Radiologic/Nuclear Devices

What Is Radiation?

Ionizing radiation is energy that is emitted in the form of rays, or particles. This energy can be found in **radioactive material**, such as rocks and metals. Radioactive material is any material that emits radiation. This material is unstable, and it attempts to stabilize itself by changing its structure in a natural process called **decay**. As the substance decays, it emits radiation until it stabilizes. The process of radioactive decay can take from as little as seconds to billions of years; meanwhile, the substance remains radioactive.

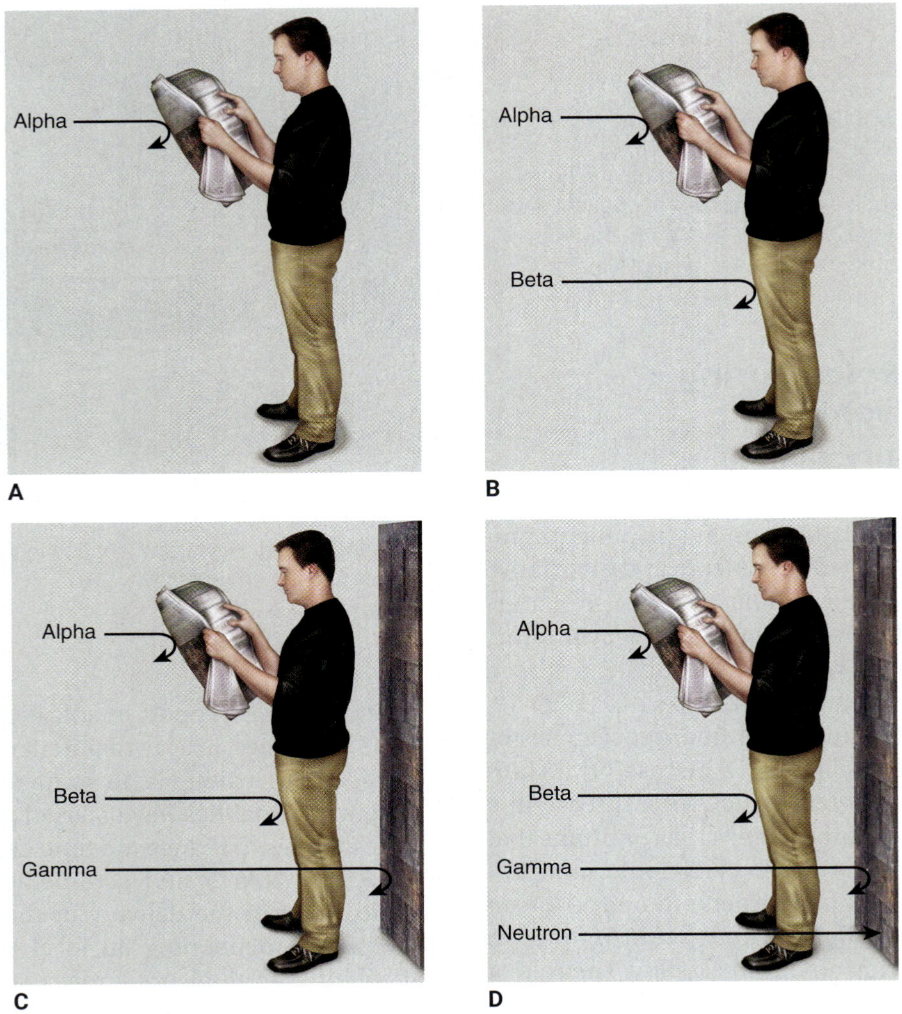

FIGURE 39-17 The penetrating potential of radiation. **A.** Alpha. **B.** Beta. **C.** Gamma. **D.** Neutron.

The energy that is emitted from a strong radiologic source is released in one or more of several forms, which are termed **alpha radiation**, **beta radiation**, **gamma (x-ray) radiation**, or **neutron radiation**. Alpha radiation is the least harmful penetrating type of radiation and cannot penetrate through most objects. In fact, a sheet of paper or the body's skin can easily stop it. Beta radiation is slightly more penetrating than alpha radiation and requires a layer of clothing to stop it. Gamma rays travel faster and have more energy than alpha and beta rays. These rays easily penetrate through the human body and require lead or several inches of concrete to prevent penetration. Neutron particles are among the most powerful forms of radiation. Neutrons easily penetrate through lead and require several feet of concrete to stop them (**FIGURE 39-17**).

Sources of Radiologic Material

There are thousands of radioactive materials found on the earth. These materials are generally used for purposes that benefit humankind, such as medicine, killing germs in food (irradiating), and construction. Once radiologic material has been used for its purpose, the material remaining is called radiologic waste. Radiologic waste remains radioactive but is no longer useful for its original purpose. These materials can be found at the following locations:

- Hospitals and other health care facilities with radiology departments
- Colleges and universities
- Nuclear power plants
- Chemical and industrial sites

Not all radioactive material is tightly guarded, and the waste is often not guarded at all. This makes radioactive material and substances appealing to terrorists.

Radiologic Dispersal Devices

A **radiologic dispersal device (RDD)** is any container that is designed to disperse radioactive material. Generally, a bomb is used to disperse the material. Such a weapon is often referred to as a **dirty bomb** because it pairs the effects of an explosion with the effects of contamination. Just the thought of an RDD creates fear in a population, and so the ultimate goal of some terrorists, fear, is accomplished. However, the actual destructive capability of a dirty bomb is limited to the size of the explosion. Thus, patients who are injured by a dirty bomb are most likely to present immediately with blast injuries rather than radiation burns or toxicity. Put simply, exposure to the radioactive material would require exposure to the explosion. There may be long-term injuries and illness associated with the use of an RDD, yet not much more than the bomb would create by itself. In short, the dirty bomb is an ineffective WMD.

Nuclear Energy

Nuclear energy is artificially made by altering (splitting) radioactive atoms. The result is an immense amount of energy that usually takes the form of heat. Nuclear material is used in medicine, weapons, naval vessels, and power plants. Nuclear material gives off all forms of radiation, including neutrons (the deadliest type). Like radioactive material, when nuclear material is no longer useful it becomes waste that remains radioactive.

Nuclear Weapons

The destructive energy of a nuclear explosion is unlike any other weapon in the world. That is why nuclear weapons are kept in only secure facilities throughout the world. There are nations that have ties to terrorists and that have actively attempted to build nuclear weapons. However, these nations do not have the capability to deliver a nuclear weapon, such as a missile or bomb.

There is also the deterrent of complete mutual annihilation. Therefore, the likelihood of a nuclear attack is extremely remote.

Unfortunately, since the collapse of the Soviet Union, the whereabouts of many small nuclear devices have become unknown. These small suitcase-size nuclear weapons are called **Special Atomic Demolition Munitions (SADM)**. The SADM, or "suitcase nuke," was designed to destroy individual targets, such as important buildings, bridges, tunnels, and large ships. Some of these are believed to be missing. Information or updates on the whereabouts of these devices has not been made public.

Symptomatology

Patients exposed to a known or suspected source of excessive radiation are considered victims of acute radiation toxicity. The effects of radiation exposure will vary depending on the amount of radiation received and the route of entry. Radiation can be introduced into the body by all routes of entry as well as through the body (irradiation). Patients can inhale radioactive dust from nuclear fallout or from a dirty bomb or have radioactive liquid absorbed into their body through their skin. Once inside the body, the radiation source will irradiate the person from within rather than from an external source (such as radiography equipment). Some common signs of acute radiation sickness are listed in **TABLE 39-11**. Additional injuries will occur with a nuclear blast,

TABLE 39-11 Common Signs of Acute Radiation Toxicity

Low exposure	Nausea, vomiting, diarrhea, dizziness, headache
Moderate exposure	Superficial burns, hair loss, compromised immune system (death of white blood cells), and cancer
Severe exposure	Partial- and full-thickness burns, cancer, and death

such as thermal and blast trauma, trauma from flying objects, and eye injuries.

Protective Measures

Individuals exposed to ionizing radiation simply through proximity to the source are unlikely to be contaminated or radioactive. However, when patients have a radioactive source on their bodies (such as debris from a dirty bomb), they are contaminated and must be initially cared for by a hazmat responder. Once the patient is decontaminated and there is no threat to you, you may begin treating the ABCs and treat the patient for any burns or trauma. The risk to rescuers wearing gloves, gown, N95 mask, and eye protection is low from most contaminated patients.[14] Any clothing or body fluids obtained from the patient should be secured in plastic bags. Place all body fluids in containers and properly dispose of them with other potentially radioactive waste. Do not eat or drink anything until you have been assured the patient has been fully decontaminated.

There are no suits or protective gear designed to completely shield you from radiation. The people who work in high-risk areas wear specific protection such as lead-lined suits; however, this equipment is not available to EMTs. The best ways to protect yourself from the effects of radiation are to use time and distance and to shield yourself using buildings and walls. Do not enter a hazmat area unless you are trained as a hazmat responder and have proper training in the use of self-contained breathing apparatus.

- **Time.** Radiation has a cumulative effect on the body. The less time that you are exposed to the source, the less the effects will be. If you realize the patient is near a radiation source, leave the area immediately.
- **Distance.** Radiation is limited as to how far it can travel. Depending on the type of radiation, moving only a few feet is often enough to remove you from immediate danger. Alpha radiation cannot travel more than a few inches but gamma rays can travel hundreds or thousands of meters. Take this into account when responding to a nuclear or radiologic incident and make certain that responders are stationed far enough away from the incident. Remember that when the distance from a radiation source is doubled, its intensity is reduced by one-fourth. See Chapter 26, *Soft-Tissue Injuries.*
- **Shielding.** Remember, the path of all radiation can be stopped by a specific object. It will be impossible for you to recognize the type of radiation being emitted or even from which direction it is coming. Therefore, always assume you are dealing with the strongest form of radiation and use concrete shielding (such as buildings or walls) between yourself and the incident. The importance of shielding cannot be overemphasized.

Medical Management

The highest priority when caring for a person who has been exposed to radiation is to find and treat any threats to the patient's life. Most of these patients will not exhibit signs and symptoms of the exposure immediately. Nausea, vomiting, and seizures suggest exposure to a high dose of radiation. Document the time of symptom onset, and manage the symptoms as you would for other patients.

YOU are the EMT

The patients have been triaged and appropriately treated. After the transportation officer notifies the receiving facilities about the patients' injuries, the final patient is transported. She is an unresponsive adult who is breathing and has no radial pulse. You glance at an adjacent patient with a large gunshot wound to the head and confirm that he is not breathing even after a head tilt. After decontaminating yourselves and the ambulance, you and your crew discuss the incident, including terrorism in general.

8. What type of terrorist group was most likely responsible for this incident?

9. What level of knowledge of terrorism and weapons of mass destruction should you possess?

In the event of a mass community exposure to radiation, EMTs may be called to help distribute potassium iodide pills. This drug reduces the risk of thyroid cancer after exposure to radioactive material.[14]

Incendiary and Explosive Devices

Incendiary and explosive devices come in various shapes and sizes. Incendiary devices are weapons used to start fires. Terrorists use flamethrowers, chemicals, Molotov cocktails, or other explosive devices for this purpose. Although you are not required to recognize all of the possible types of explosive devices, including improvised explosive devices, it is important for you to be able to identify an object you believe is a potential device, notify the proper authorities, and safely evacuate the area. Always remember that there is the possibility of a secondary device when you are responding to the scene of an incendiary or explosive device call.

The type and severity of wounds sustained from incendiary and explosive devices primarily depend on the patient's distance from the epicenter of the explosion. Patients close to the epicenter of the explosion are likely to sustain injury from all wound-causing agents of the munitions. Patients who are farther away from the epicenter are likely to experience a combination of blast injuries from the explosion and penetrating trauma injuries from primary and secondary projectiles created by the explosion. For a review of the types of blast injury (ie, primary, secondary, tertiary, quaternary, and quinary), their mechanisms of injury, and the types of injury sustained, see Chapter 24, *Trauma Overview*.

YOU are the EMT SUMMARY

1. On the basis of the information you have received, how should you approach this incident?

This incident calls for your highest level of alertness and vigilance. Your life and the lives of others depend on your ability to quickly and accurately sort through the information. You must process the information, determine what is pertinent, and create a plan of action. Given that frantic bystanders often provide some of the early reports in these types of incidents, it is reasonable to consider that some of the information may be confusing or inaccurate. Do not become distracted. Focus on reports that provide any information about immediate threats to your safety and the location of injured personnel.

From the information you have received, there has been a possible mass-casualty event involving multiple scenes within close proximity to your current location. You are not able to determine if there is a hazmat component to this call, but that thought should be in your mind, given the reports of smoke coming from a trash can followed by a shooting. While we often consider staging away from a dangerous scene, you have been thrust into the middle of this incident. You should make sure you are in a safe location. With possible multiple events and/or attackers in your proximity, retreating could be as dangerous as advancing toward the injured. Do your best to get your bearings and stay calm. Ensure that adequate resources are dispatched, including those with the capacity to assess and manage potential safety threats.

2. What indicators suggest that an incident is the result of terrorism?

Information from dispatch such as the location and type of incident, the number of patients, and victims' statements may be the first indicators that an incident is the result of terrorism. For example, is the incident location a government building, a festival, or a specific structure? Are there multiple patients with similar injuries or symptoms, such as difficulty breathing? Are victims fleeing the scene and making statements such as "There was a loud explosion?" There may be incidents involving terrorism that are on a small scale and some that are on a much larger scale. Some terrorist attacks may be designed in a strategic way to create maximum chaos or try to lure more people to a certain area to maximize the number of injured. If there are separate reports of multiple unusual events near each other, you must consider the possibility of terrorism. For example, if you are responding to reports of an unconscious person and separate 9-1-1 calls come in about an explosion at a church across the street from the initial dispatch location, you must consider the possibility of terrorism.

YOU are the EMT SUMMARY continued

3. What should you consider when determining if the scene is safe for you and other EMS personnel to enter?

Due to the unique circumstances of this incident, you will have to weigh the risks and benefits of continuing to stage versus continuing into the scene. You should evaluate the current threat level at your precise location. Can you hear active gunfire? Are you near the location of a recent explosion or active fire? Is there any threat of hazardous materials where you are or where you are planning to go? Are there any reports from law enforcement or bystanders that a threat is headed in your direction? Remember that there may be secondary devices that specifically target both responders rushing to help the injured and anyone who is fleeing the initial scene. A good resource in this incident would be the closest law enforcement official. This person should be able to provide current information about known or suspected threats to your safety and report whether the scene is secured for you to begin treating the injured.

4. What immediate actions should you perform prior to proceeding into the scene?

As discussed with regard to recommendations from the Hartford Consensus, EMS systems must reevaluate the practice of staging away from the scene and waiting for patients to be brought to the ambulance. You have already been thrust into the middle of this incident. While requesting additional resources, communicate your location to dispatch. Ask if they have any information about the scene. If your agency supplies any ballistic vests or helmets for EMTs, you should put this equipment on immediately. Find the closest law enforcement officer. This person may be able to provide some protection from threats as you maintain your current position or advance toward injured personnel when it is determined to be appropriate for you to do so. If you are going to move toward the injured, vdo not worry about bringing every piece of medical equipment. Your initial role will likely be triage and basic treatment to control life-threatening hemorrhage. Carry your triage tape or tags and basic trauma equipment. Do not weigh yourself down with unnecessary items. You want to be able to move quickly if another threat emerges.

5. Given the situation, what are some unique concerns about this incident?

Terrorists have been known to plant additional explosives (secondary devices) that are set to detonate after the initial device. Secondary devices are primarily intended to injure emergency responders or bystanders who have gathered in attempts to help or flee the scene. These devices may not be in the same location as the primary device. The secondary device could be a package or briefcase that has been planted across the street or it could be an electronic device, such as a cell phone, that is designed to detonate on activation.

Although the scene may be secured initially, you must realize that the scene can easily become unsafe. Do not rely on others to keep you safe; it is *your* responsibility to constantly reassess the scene for indicators of danger. A subtle change in wind direction during an incident involving radiation or an increase in the number of patients who are contaminated can place you in danger.

6. What types of injuries should you expect to encounter?

Given this scenario, you would expect to find that the majority of injuries involve penetrating trauma. The initial report of a police officer who was stabbed will present differently than someone who was shot with a high-velocity rifle, but both patients are at risk for catastrophic injuries and life-threatening hemorrhage. The severity of the injuries can depend on the type of gun that was used, the number of times the person was shot, and the anatomic location of the injuries. Penetrating trauma to the extremities may produce significant hemorrhage that may require the use of a tourniquet. Penetrating trauma to the head, neck, and chest is often rapidly fatal if not immediately treated with appropriate airway management, ventilatory support, and hemorrhage control.

7. On the basis of the number of patients and their apparent conditions, how many ambulances and EMTs should be present at the scene?

Your general impression of the scene has revealed that there are eight total patients, with five of them considered salvageable. Assume all five patients have critical injuries until they have been triaged and treatment has begun. One ambulance and two EMTs can effectively care for only one critically injured patient at a time. You will likely need at least five ambulances and 10 EMTs to transport the five critical patients. However, remember that some patients who were initially triaged in the expectant category may ultimately be upgraded to the immediate category as more resources arrive on scene. Therefore, there should be a total of eight ambulances and 16 EMTs at the scene: 2 EMTs and one ambulance per patient. It is better to have enough resources to treat

YOU are the EMT SUMMARY continued

every patient than to have a patient who requires treatment and no available resources.

In many communities, the EMT is asked simply to report the number of potential patients and the scene size-up details to dispatch, and dispatch will then deploy the appropriate number of ambulances and other resources.

This scenario demonstrates how the resources required to manage an incident due to terrorism could easily overwhelm the available sources for a single EMS system.

8. What type of terrorist group was most likely responsible for this incident?

In this incident, a single actor created a diversion to push the crowd in his direction before he began shooting into the crowd. This behavior suggests a lone wolf terrorist. The motive may not always be clear in these types of attacks. There may be a personal grievance or motive that relates to a larger group, but lone wolf terrorists, by definition, do not receive any assistance from outside sources in planning or implementing their attack.

9. What level of knowledge of terrorism and weapons of mass destruction should you possess?

You are not expected to be an expert in terrorism and weapons of mass destruction (WMDs). However, you are expected to be aware of the various types of threats and recognize certain indicators of terrorism when responding to an incident. As an EMT, you should possess a basic working knowledge of the different types of WMDs that terrorists could use, signs and symptoms and treatment of victims of WMDs, measures to take to ensure personal safety and safety of the patient, and knowledge of the incident command system.

Prep Kit

Ready for Review

- As a result of the increase in terrorist activity, it is possible that you, as an EMT, could witness a terrorist event. You must be mentally and physically prepared for the possibility of a terrorist event.
- Types of groups that tend to use terrorism include religious extremist groups/doomsday cults, extremist political groups, cyber terrorists, and single-issue groups.
- Lone wolf terrorist attacks, particularly active shooter events, are a growing threat in the United States. EMS systems should incorporate the Hartford Consensus recommendations to guide care at these scenes. The Stop the Bleed campaign has trained members of the public to help save lives in these situations.
- A weapon of mass destruction (WMD) is any agent designed to bring about mass death, casualties, and/or massive damage to property and infrastructure (bridges, tunnels, airports, and seaports). These can be biologic, nuclear, incendiary, chemical, and explosive weapons (B-NICE).
- Indicators that may give you clues as to whether the emergency is the result of a terrorist attack include the type of location, type of call, number of patients, victims' statements, and preincident indicators.
- If you suspect that a terrorist or an event involving a WMD has occurred, ensure that the scene is safe. If you have any doubt that it may not be safe, do not enter. Wait for assistance.
- Terrorists may set secondary devices that are designed to explode after the initial bomb, thus injuring responders and increasing media coverage. Constantly assess and reassess the scene for safety.
- Chemical agents are manufactured liquid, gas, or solid substances that can have devastating effects on living organisms.
- Persistency and volatility describe how long the agent will stay on the surface before it

Prep Kit continued

the agent most effectively enters the body.
evaporates, and the route of exposure is how the agent most effectively enters the body.

- Biologic agents include viruses such as smallpox and those that cause viral hemorrhagic fevers; bacteria such as those that cause anthrax and plague; and neurotoxins such as botulinum toxin and ricin.
- Nuclear or radiologic weapons produced from radioactive waste material can create a massive amount of destruction.
- Ionizing radiation is energy that can enter the human body and cause damage.
- Explosive and incendiary devices come in various shapes and sizes. It is important to be able to identify an object you believe is a potential device and notify the proper authorities, while safely evacuating the area.

Vital Vocabulary

active shooter event An act of terror in which firearms are used in an ongoing assault of multiple people.

aging The process by which the temporary bond between an organophosphate and acetylcholinesterase undergoes hydrolysis, resulting in a permanent covalent bond.

alpha radiation A type of energy that is emitted from a strong radiologic source; it is the least harmful penetrating type of radiation and cannot travel more than a few inches or penetrate most objects.

anthrax A disease caused by a deadly bacterium (*Bacillus anthracis*) that lies dormant in a spore (protective shell); the germ is released from the spore when exposed to the optimal temperature and moisture. The routes of entry are inhalation, cutaneous, and gastrointestinal (from consuming food that contains spores).

Antidote Treatment Nerve Agent Auto-Injector (ATNAA) A nerve agent antidote kit containing atropine and pralidoxime chloride; delivered as a single dose through one needle.

bacteria Microorganisms that reproduce by binary fission. These single-cell creatures reproduce rapidly. Some can form spores (encysted variants) when environmental conditions are harsh.

beta radiation A type of energy that is emitted from a strong radiologic source; it is slightly more penetrating than alpha radiation and requires a layer of clothing to stop it.

B-NICE A mnemonic for the types of weapons of mass destruction: biologic, nuclear, incendiary, chemical, and explosive.

botulinum Produced by bacteria, this is the most potent neurotoxin known. When introduced into the body, this neurotoxin affects the nervous system's ability to function and causes botulism.

buboes Enlarged lymph nodes (up to the size of a tennis ball) that are characteristic in people infected with the bubonic plague.

bubonic plague Bacterial infection that affects the lymphatic system. It is transmitted by infected rodents and fleas and characterized by acute malaise, fever, and the formation of tender, enlarged, inflamed lymph nodes that appear as lesions, called buboes. Also called the Black Death.

chlorine (Cl) The first chemical agent ever used in warfare. It has a distinct odor of bleach and creates a green haze when released as a gas. Initially it produces upper airway irritation and a choking sensation.

contact hazard The term used to describe the danger posed by a chemical whose primary route of entry into the body is through the skin; posed by a hazardous agent that gives off very little or no vapors; also called a skin hazard.

Prep Kit continued

contagious An infectious disease that spreads from one human to another; communicable.

covert An act in which the public safety community generally has no prior knowledge of the time, location, or nature of the attack.

cross-contamination Occurs when a person is contaminated by an agent as a result of coming in contact with another contaminated person.

cyanide An agent that affects the body's ability to use oxygen. It is a colorless gas that has an odor similar to almonds. The effects begin on the cellular level and are very rapidly seen at the organ and system levels.

decay A natural process in which a material that is unstable attempts to stabilize itself by changing its structure.

dirty bomb Name given to an explosive radiologic dispersal device.

disease vector An animal that, once infected, spreads a disease to another animal.

dissemination The means by which a terrorist will spread an agent; for example, by poisoning the water supply or aerosolizing the agent into the air or ventilation system of a building.

domestic terrorism Terrorism that is carried out by people in their own country.

DuoDote Auto-Injector A nerve agent antidote kit containing atropine and pralidoxime chloride; delivered as a single dose through one needle.

G agents Early nerve agents that were developed by German scientists in the period after World War I and into World War II. There are three such agents: sarin, soman, and tabun.

gamma (x-ray) radiation A type of energy that is emitted from a strong radiologic source that travels faster and has more energy than alpha and beta rays. These rays easily penetrate through the human body and require lead or several inches of concrete to prevent penetration.

incubation The period between exposure to an agent and onset of resulting symptoms.

international terrorism Terrorism that is carried out by people in a country other than their own; also known as cross-border terrorism.

ionizing radiation Energy that is emitted in the form of rays, or particles.

lewisite (L) A blistering agent that has a rapid onset of symptoms and produces immediate, intense pain and discomfort on contact.

lone wolf terrorist attack An act of terror carried out by a single person to further an ideologic goal.

lymphatic system A passive circulatory system in the body that transports a plasmalike liquid called lymph, a thin fluid that bathes the tissues of the body.

lymph nodes The area of the lymphatic system where infection-fighting cells are housed.

miosis Excessively constricted pupil; often bilateral after exposure to nerve agents.

mutagen A substance that mutates, damages, and changes the structures of DNA in the body's cells.

nerve agents A class of chemical called organophosphates; they function by blocking an essential enzyme in the nervous system, which causes the body's organs to become overstimulated and burn out.

neurotoxins Biologic agents that are the deadliest substances known to humans; they include botulinum toxin and ricin.

neutron radiation The type of energy that is emitted from a strong radiologic source, involving particles that are among the most powerful forms of radiation; the particles easily penetrate through lead and require several feet of concrete to stop them.

off-gassing The release of an agent after exposure—for example, from a person's clothes that have been exposed to the agent.

persistency How long a chemical agent will stay on a surface before it evaporates.

Prep Kit continued

phosgene A pulmonary agent that is a product of combustion, resulting from a fire at a textile factory or house, or from metalwork or burning Freon. It is a very potent agent that has a delayed onset of symptoms, usually hours.

phosgene oxime (CX) A blistering agent that has a rapid onset of symptoms and produces immediate, intense pain and discomfort on contact.

pneumonic plague A lung infection, also known as plague pneumonia, that is the result of inhalation of plague-causing bacteria.

points of distribution (PODs) Existing facilities used as mass distribution sites for antibiotics, antidotes, vaccinations, and other medications and supplies during an emergency.

radioactive material Any material that emits radiation.

radiologic dispersal device (RDD) Any container that is designed to disperse radioactive material.

ricin A neurotoxin derived from mash that is left over from processing castor beans; causes pulmonary edema and respiratory and circulatory failure leading to death.

route of exposure The manner by which a toxic substance enters the body.

sarin (GB) A nerve agent that is one of the G agents; a highly volatile colorless and odorless liquid that turns from liquid to gas within seconds to minutes at room temperature.

secondary device A secondary explosive used by terrorists, set to explode after the initial bomb.

smallpox A highly contagious viral disease; it is most contagious when blisters begin to form.

soman (GD) A nerve agent that is one of the G agents; twice as persistent as sarin and five times as lethal; it has a fruity odor as a result of the type of alcohol used in the agent, and is a contact and an inhalation hazard that can enter the body through skin absorption and through the respiratory tract.

Special Atomic Demolition Munitions (SADM) Small suitcase-size nuclear weapons that were designed to destroy individual targets, such as important buildings, bridges, tunnels, and large ships.

state-sponsored terrorism Terrorism that is funded and/or supported by nations that hold close ties with terrorist groups.

sulfur mustard (H) A vesicant; it is a brown-yellow oily substance that is generally considered very persistent; has the distinct smell of garlic or mustard and, when released, is quickly absorbed into the skin and/or mucous membranes and begins an irreversible process of damaging the cells. Also called mustard gas.

syndromic surveillance The monitoring, usually by local or state health departments, of patients presenting to emergency departments and alternative care facilities, the recording of EMS call volume, and the use of over-the-counter medications.

tabun (GA) A nerve agent that is one of the G agents; 36 times more persistent than sarin and approximately one-half as lethal; has a fruity smell and is unique because the components used to manufacture the agent are easy to acquire and the agent is easy to manufacture.

terrorism A violent and unlawful act dangerous to human life intended to intimidate or coerce a government, the civilian population, or any segment thereof, in furtherance of political or social objectives.

V agent (VX) One of the G agents; it is a clear, oily agent that has no odor and looks like baby oil; more than 100 times more lethal than sarin and extremely persistent.

vapor hazard The term used to describe danger posed by an agent that enters the body through the respiratory tract.

vesicants Blister agents; the primary route of entry for such agents is through the skin.

viral hemorrhagic fevers A group of diseases caused by viruses that include the Ebola, Rift Valley, and yellow fevers, among others. This

Prep Kit continued

group of viruses causes the blood in the body to seep out from the tissues and blood vessels.

viruses Germs that require a living host to multiply and survive.

volatility How long a chemical agent will stay on a surface before it evaporates.

weaponization The creation of a weapon from a biologic agent that is generally found in nature and that causes disease; the agent is cultivated, synthesized, and/or mutated to maximize the target population's exposure to the germ.

weapon of mass casualty (WMC) Any agent designed to bring about mass death, casualties, and/or massive damage to property and infrastructure (bridges, tunnels, airports, and seaports); also known as a weapon of mass destruction (WMD).

weapon of mass destruction (WMD) Any agent designed to bring about mass death, casualties, and/or massive damage to property and infrastructure (bridges, tunnels, airports, and seaports); also known as a weapon of mass casualty (WMC).

References

1. US Department of Homeland Security, Federal Bureau of Investigation. Domestic terrorism: definitions, terminology, and methodology. Pub. L. 116-92. National Defense Authorization Act for Fiscal Year 2020. US Department of Justice; 2020.
2. The rising threat of domestic terrorism in the US and federal efforts to combat it. US Government Accountability Office website. https://www.gao.gov/blog/rising-threat-domestic-terrorism-u.s.-and-federal-efforts-combat-it. Published March 2, 2023. Accessed May 5, 2025.
3. Alfaro-Gonzalez L, Barthelmes RJ, Bartol C, et al.; Security Studies Program. *Report: Lone Wolf Terrorism.* Georgetown Security Studies Review website. georgetownsecuritystudiesreview.org/wp-content/uploads/2015/08/NCITF-Final-Paper.pdf. Published June 27, 2015. Accessed May 5, 2025.
4. Jacobs LM, Wade D, McSwain NE, et al. Hartford Consensus: a call to action for THREAT, a medical disaster preparedness concept. *J Am Coll Surg.* 2014;218(3):467–475.
5. Jacobs LM Jr; Joint Committee to Create a National Policy to Enhance Survivability from Intentional Mass-Casualty and Active Shooter Events. The Hartford Consensus III. Implementation of bleeding control. *J Spec Oper Med.* 2015;15(4):136–141.
6. Jacobs LM; Joint Committee to Create a National Policy to Enhance Survivability from Intentional Mass Casualty and Active Shooter Events. The Hartford Consensus IV: a call for increased national resilience. *Bull Am Coll Surg.* 2016;101(3):17–24.
7. McGuire SS, Bellolio F, Sztajnkrycer MD, et al. Use of body armor by EMS clinicians, workplace violence, and racial and ethnic disparities in care. *JAMA Netw Open.* 2025;8(1):e2456528. doi:10.1001/jamanetworkopen.2024.56528
8. American College of Surgeons. Out of great tragedy, a life-saving response begins around the world. Stop the Bleed website. www.stopthebleed.org/our-story. Accessed May 5, 2025.
9. Goldman S, Lipsky AM, Radimislensky I, et al. October 7th mass casualty attack in Israel: injury profiles of hospitalized casualties. *Ann Surg Open.* 2024;5(3):e481. doi:10.1097/AS9.0000000000000481
10. *Office of Intelligence and Analysis: Homeland Threat Assessment 2025.* US Department of Homeland Security website. https://www.dhs.gov/sites/default/files/2024-10/24_0930_ia_24-320-ia-publication-2025-hta-final-30sep24-508.pdf. Published 2025. Accessed May 5, 2025.
11. National Terrorism Advisory System. Department of Homeland Security website. https://www.dhs.gov/national-terrorism-advisory-system. Updated April 14, 2022. Accessed May 5, 2025.
12. Poisoning statistics, 2023. Poison Control: National Capital Poison Center website. https://www.poison.org/poison-statistics-national. Accessed May 5, 2025.
13. Office of Clinical Pharmacology review. US Food and Drug Administration website. https://www.fda.gov/media/108679/download. Published December 7, 2016. Accessed May 5, 2025.
14. National Association of State EMS Officials. *National Model EMS Clinical Guidelines: Version 3.0.* https://nasemso.org/wp-content/uploads/National-Model-EMS-Clinical-Guidelines_2022.pdf. Updated March 2022. Accessed May 5, 2025.

Prep Kit continued

15. Horowitz BZ. Tear gas in America: cry the beloved country. *Toxicol Comm*. 2020;4(1):59–61.
16. Loren A, Hurst K. Pepper spray exposure: treatments and risk factors for severe reactions. JEMS website. https://www.jems.com/patient-care/pepper-spray-exposure-treatments-and-risk-factors-for-severe-reactions/. Published April 22, 2025. Accessed May 5, 2025.
17. Brown C, Choi MJ, McLellan S, Shoemaker T. Post-travel evaluation to rule out viral special pathogen infection. *Yellow Book*. Centers for Disease Control and Prevention website. https://wwwnc.cdc.gov/travel/yellowbook/2024/infections-diseases/viral-hemorrhagic-fevers. Published April 23, 2025. Accessed May 5, 2025.
18. Wilson AE, Lehmann CU, Saleh SN, Hanna J, Medford RJ. Social media: a new tool for outbreak surveillance. *Antimicrob Steward Healthc Epidemiol*. 2021;1(1):e50. doi:10.1017/ash.2021.225

Additional Resources

Center for Domestic Preparedness: training the best for the worst. US Department of Homeland Security website. https://cdp.dhs.gov. Accessed June 11, 2025.

Joint Committee to Create a National Policy to Enhance Survivability From Mass-Casualty Shooting Events. Improving survival from active shooter events: the Hartford Consensus. *Bull Am Coll Surg*. 2013;98(6):14–16.

More than 2 million people prepared to stop the bleed. https://www.facs.org/for-medical-professionals/news-publications/news-and-articles/bulletin/2022/june-2022-volume-107-number-6/more-than-2-million-people-prepared-to-stop-the-bleed/. American College of Surgeons website. Published June 1, 2022. Accessed May 5, 2025.

National Fire Protection Association (NFPA). *NFPA 3000: Standard for an Active Shooter/Hostile Event Response (ASHER) Program*. NFPA website. https://www.nfpa.org/product/nfpa-3000-standard/p3000code#. Published 2024. Accessed May 5, 2025.

Glossary

abandonment: Unilateral termination of care by the EMT without the patient's consent and without making provisions for transferring care to another medical professional with the skills and training necessary to meet the needs of the patient.

abdomen: The body cavity that contains many of the major organs of digestion and excretion. It is located below the diaphragm and above the pelvis.

abdominal thrust maneuver: The preferred method, in conjunction with back slaps, to dislodge a severe airway obstruction in adults and children; also called the Heimlich maneuver.

abduction: Motion of a limb away from the midline.

abrasion: Loss or damage of the superficial layer of skin as a result of a body part rubbing or scraping across a rough or hard surface.

abruptio placentae: Premature separation of the placenta from the wall of the uterus.

absorption: The process by which medications travel through body tissues until they reach the bloodstream.

accessory muscles: The secondary muscles of respiration. They include the neck muscles (sternocleidomastoids), the chest pectoralis major muscles, and the abdominal muscles.

access: The act of gaining entry to an enclosed area and reaching a patient.

acetabulum: The depression on the lateral pelvis where its three component bones join, in which the femoral head fits snugly.

acidosis: The buildup of excess acid in the blood or body tissues that can result from a primary illness.

acromioclavicular (AC) joint: A simple joint where the bony projections of the scapula and the clavicle meet at the top of the shoulder.

action: The therapeutic effect of a medication on the body.

active shooter event: An act of terror in which firearms are used in an ongoing assault of multiple people.

acute abdomen: A condition of sudden onset of pain within the abdomen, usually indicating peritonitis; immediate medical or surgical treatment is necessary.

acute coronary syndrome (ACS): A group of symptoms caused by myocardial ischemia; includes angina and myocardial infarction.

acute myocardial infarction (AMI): A heart attack; death of heart muscle following obstruction of blood flow to it. "Acute" in this context means "new" or "happening right now."

addiction: A state of overwhelming obsession or physical need to continue the use of a substance.

adduction: Motion of a limb toward the midline.

adenosine triphosphate (ATP): The nucleotide involved in energy metabolism; used to store energy.

adolescent: A young person age 12 to 18 years.

adrenal glands: Endocrine glands located on top of the kidneys that release adrenaline when stimulated by the sympathetic nervous system.

adrenergic: Pertaining to nerves that release the neurotransmitter norepinephrine, or noradrenaline (eg, adrenergic nerves, adrenergic response); also pertains to the receptors acted on by norepinephrine.

advanced emergency medical technician (AEMT): An individual who has training in specific aspects of advanced life support, such as intravenous therapy and the administration of certain emergency medications.

advance directive: Written documentation that specifies medical treatment for a competent patient should the patient become unable to make decisions; also called a living will or health care directive.

advanced life support (ALS): Advanced lifesaving procedures, such as advanced airway management, intravenous access, and medication administration.

adventitious breath sounds: Abnormal breath sounds such as wheezing, stridor, rhonchi, and crackles.

adverse effects: Any unwanted clinical results of a medication.

aerobic metabolism: Metabolism that can proceed only in the presence of oxygen.

aerosol-generating procedure (AGP): Any airway manipulation, such as CPR, that induces the production of aerosols that may present a risk for airborne transmission of pathogens.

afterload: The force or resistance against which the heart pumps.

ageism: The assumption that older people are less healthy or capable; can lead to poor patient assessment and care.

aging: The process by which the temporary bond between an organophosphate and acetylcholinesterase undergoes hydrolysis, resulting in a permanent covalent bond.

agonal breathing (or gasps): The reflexive, slow, and inadequate breathing that some patients in cardiac arrest exhibit as the brainstem becomes hypoxic.

agonist: A medication that causes stimulation of receptors.

airborne transmission: The spread of an organism via droplets or dust.

air embolism: The presence of air in the veins, which can lead to cardiac arrest if it enters the heart.

air medical services: Fixed-wing and rotary-wing (known as helicopters) aircraft that have been modified for medical care; used to evacuate and transport patients with life-threatening injuries to treatment facilities.

airway: The upper airway tract or the passage above the larynx, which includes the nose, mouth, and throat.

algor mortis: Cooling of the body after death until it matches the ambient temperature.

alkalosis: The buildup of excess base (lack of acids) in the body fluids.

allergen: A substance that causes an allergic reaction.

allergic reaction: The body's exaggerated immune response to an internal or surface agent.

alpha-adrenergic receptors: Portions of the nervous system that, when stimulated, can cause constriction of blood vessels.

alpha radiation: A type of energy that is emitted from a strong radiologic source; it is the least harmful penetrating type of radiation and cannot travel more than a few inches or penetrate most objects.

ALS assist: An intervention in which a clinician trained in basic life support provides assistance, while remaining within their scope of practice, to a clinician who is performing an advanced life support (ALS) procedure.

altered mental status: Any deviation from alert and oriented to person, place, time, and event, or any deviation from a patient's baseline mental status.

alveolar ventilation: The volume of air that reaches the alveoli. It is determined by subtracting the amount of dead space air from the tidal volume.

alveoli: The air sacs of the lungs in which the exchange of oxygen and carbon dioxide takes place.

ambient temperature: The temperature of the surrounding environment.

ambulance: A specialized vehicle for treating and transporting sick and injured patients.

American Standard Safety System: A safety system for large oxygen cylinders, designed to prevent the accidental attachment of a regulator to a cylinder containing the wrong type of gas.

Americans With Disabilities Act (ADA): Comprehensive legislation that is designed to protect people with disabilities against discrimination.

amniotic sac: The fluid-filled, baglike membrane in which the fetus develops.

amputation: An injury in which part of the body is completely severed.

anaerobic metabolism: The metabolism that takes place in the absence of oxygen; the main by-product is lactic acid.

anaphylactic shock: Severe shock caused by an allergic reaction.

anaphylaxis: An extreme, life-threatening, systemic allergic reaction that may include shock and respiratory failure.

anatomic position: The position of reference in which the patient stands facing forward, arms at the side, with the palms of the hands forward.

anatomy: The study of the physical structure of the body and its components.

anchoring: A decision-making error in which the clinician settles on one possible cause of the patient's problems early and fails to consider other options.

anemia: A condition in which the blood contains an abnormally low number of red blood cells, resulting in a decreased ability to transport oxygen throughout the body via the bloodstream.

aneurysm: A swelling or enlargement of a part of an artery, resulting from weakening of the arterial wall.

angina pectoris: Transient (short-lived) chest discomfort caused by partial or temporary blockage of blood flow to the heart muscle; also called angina.

angioedema: Localized areas of swelling beneath the skin, often around the eyes and lips, but can also involve other body areas.

anisocoria: Naturally occurring uneven pupil size.

antagonist: A medication that binds to a receptor and blocks other medications.

anterior: The front surface of the body; the side facing you in the standard anatomic position.

anterograde (posttraumatic) amnesia: Inability to remember events after an injury.

anthrax: A disease caused by a deadly bacterium (*Bacillus anthracis*) that lies dormant in a spore (protective shell); the germ is released from the spore when exposed to the optimal temperature and moisture. The routes of entry are inhalation, cutaneous, and gastrointestinal (from consuming food that contains spores).

antibiotic: A medication used to treat infections caused by a bacterium.

anticoagulant: A medication that impairs the ability of blood to clot.

antidote: A substance that is used to neutralize or counteract a poison.

Antidote Treatment Nerve Agent Auto-Injector (ATNAA): A nerve agent antidote kit containing atropine and pralidoxime chloride; delivered as a single dose through one needle.

antifungal: A medication used to treat infections caused by a fungus.

antiplatelet: A medication that prevents blood platelets from clumping or sticking together.

antipyretics: Medications that treat or reduce a fever.

antivenin: A serum that counteracts the effect of venom from an animal or insect.

aorta: The main artery that receives blood from the left ventricle and delivers it to all the other arteries that carry blood to the tissues of the body.

aortic aneurysm: A weakness in the wall of the aorta that makes it susceptible to rupture.

aortic valve: The one-way valve that lies between the left ventricle and the aorta and keeps blood from flowing back into the left ventricle after the left ventricle ejects its blood into the aorta; one of four heart valves.

apex: The pointed extremity of a conical structure; plural form: *apices*.

Apgar score: A scoring system for assessing the status of a newborn that assigns a number value to each of five areas.

aphasia: The inability to understand and/or produce speech.

apnea: Absence of spontaneous breathing.

apneic oxygenation: A technique in which oxygen via nasal cannula set at 15 to 25 L/min is left in place during an intubation attempt, allowing for continuous oxygen delivery into the airways during all phases of the intubation procedure.

apparent life-threatening event (ALTE): An event that causes unresponsiveness, cyanosis, and apnea in an infant, who then resumes breathing with stimulation.

appendicitis: Inflammation or infection of the appendix.

appendicular skeleton: The portion of the skeletal system that comprises the arms, legs, pelvis, and shoulder girdle.

appendix: A small, tubular structure that is attached to the lower border of the cecum in the lower right quadrant of the abdomen.

applied ethics: The manner in which principles of ethics are incorporated into professional conduct.

arterioles: The smallest branches of arteries leading to the vast network of capillaries.

artery: A blood vessel, consisting of three layers of tissue and smooth muscle, that carries blood away from the heart.

articular cartilage: A pearly white layer of specialized cartilage covering the articular surfaces (contact surfaces on the ends) of bones in synovial joints.

artifact: A tracing on an ECG that is the result of interference, such as patient movement, rather than the heart's electrical activity.

aspiration: A respiratory emergency that occurs when foreign material such as fluid or food enters the lungs and prevents effective breathing.

aspirin (acetylsalicylic acid or ASA): A medication that is an antipyretic (reduces fever), analgesic (reduces pain), anti-inflammatory (reduces inflammation), and potent inhibitor of platelet aggregation (clumping).

assault: Unlawfully placing a patient in fear of bodily harm.

asthma: An acute spasm of the smaller air passages, called bronchioles, associated with excessive mucus production and with swelling of the mucous lining of the respiratory passages.

asystole: The complete absence of all heart electrical activity.

ataxic respirations: Irregular, ineffective respirations that may or may not have an identifiable pattern.

atelectasis: Collapse of the alveolar air spaces of the lungs.

atherosclerosis: A disorder in which cholesterol and calcium build up inside the walls of blood vessels, eventually leading to partial or complete blockage of blood flow.

atrium: One of the two upper chambers of the heart.

aura: A sensation experienced before a seizure; serves as a warning sign that a seizure is about to occur.

auscultate: To listen to sounds within an organ with a stethoscope.

autism spectrum disorder (ASD): A group of complex disorders of brain development, characterized by difficulties in social interaction, repetitive behaviors, and verbal and nonverbal communication.

automated external defibrillators (AEDs): Devices that detect treatable life-threatening cardiac dysrhythmias (ventricular fibrillation and ventricular tachycardia) and deliver the appropriate electrical shock to the patient.

automatic transport ventilator (ATV): A ventilation device attached to a control box that allows the variables of ventilation to be set. It frees the EMT to perform other tasks while the patient is being ventilated.

automaticity: The ability of cardiac muscle cells to contract without stimulation from the nervous system.

autonomic nervous system: The part of the nervous system that controls the involuntary activities of the body such as the heart rate, blood pressure, and digestion of food.

autonomy: The right of a patient to make informed choices regarding health care.

AVPU scale: A method of assessing the level of consciousness by determining whether the patient is Awake and alert, responsive to Verbal stimuli or Pain, or Unresponsive; used principally early in the assessment process.

avulsion: An injury in which soft tissue is torn completely loose or is hanging as a flap.

axial loading injuries: Injuries in which load is applied along the vertical or longitudinal axis of the spine, which results in load being transmitted along the entire length of the vertebral column (eg, shallow-water diving accident, fall from height with feetfirst landing).

axial skeleton: The part of the skeleton comprising the skull, vertebral column, and rib cage.

axons: Extensions of a neuron that carry impulses away from the nerve cell body to the dendrites (receivers) of another neuron.

backboard: A long, flat board made of rigid, rectangular material that is used to provide support to a patient who is suspected of having a hip, pelvic, spinal, or lower extremity injury; also called a spine board, trauma board, and longboard.

bacteria: Microorganisms that reproduce by binary fission. These single-cell creatures reproduce rapidly. Some can form spores (encysted variants) when environmental conditions are harsh.

bacterial vaginosis: An overgrowth of bacteria in the vagina; characterized by itching, burning, or pain, and possibly a "fishy"-smelling discharge.

bag-mask device: A device with a one-way valve and a face mask attached to a ventilation bag; when attached to a reservoir and connected to oxygen, it delivers up to 95% supplemental oxygen.

ball-and-socket joints: Joints that allow internal and external rotation, as well as bending.

bariatrics: A branch of medicine concerned with the management (prevention or control) of obesity and allied diseases.

barotrauma: Injury caused by pressure to enclosed body surfaces, for example, from too much pressure in the lungs.

barrier device: A protective item, such as a pocket mask with a valve, that limits exposure to a patient's body fluids.

base station: Any radio hardware containing a transmitter and receiver that is located in a fixed place.

basic life support (BLS): Noninvasive emergency lifesaving care that is used to treat medical conditions, including airway obstruction, respiratory arrest, and cardiac arrest.

basilar skull fractures: Fractures that usually occur following diffuse impact to the head (eg, falls, motor vehicle crashes); generally result from extension of a linear fracture to the base of the skull.

basket stretcher: A rigid stretcher commonly used in technical and water rescues that surrounds and supports the patient yet allows water to drain through holes in the bottom; also called a Stokes basket or litter.

battery: Unlawfully touching a patient or providing emergency care without consent.

Battle sign: Bruising behind an ear over the mastoid process that may indicate a skull fracture.

behavior: The way in which individuals interact with their environment.

behavioral health emergency: A situation in which a person's behavior poses a threat to themselves or others or prevents them from caring for themselves or functioning effectively in their community.

bends: A common name for decompression sickness.

beta-adrenergic receptors: Portions of the nervous system that, when stimulated, can cause an increase in the force of contraction of the heart, an increased heart rate, and bronchial dilation.

beta radiation: A type of energy that is emitted from a strong radiologic source; it is slightly more penetrating than alpha radiation and requires a layer of clothing to stop it.

biases: Fixed beliefs that are not based on objective knowledge.

biceps: The large muscle that covers the front of the humerus.

bilateral: A body part or condition that appears on both sides of the midline.

bile ducts: The ducts that convey bile between the liver and the intestine.

bills of lading: The shipping papers used for transport of chemicals over roads and highways; also referred to as freight bills.

bioethics: The study of ethics related to issues that arise in health care.

bipolar disorder: A type of mental illness characterized by alternating periods of depression and manic episodes.

birth canal: The vagina and cervix.

blind spots: Areas of the road that are blocked from your view by your vehicle or mirrors.

bloodborne pathogens: Pathogenic microorganisms that are present in human blood and can cause disease in humans. These pathogens include, but are not limited to, hepatitis B virus and human immunodeficiency virus (HIV).

blood pressure (BP): The pressure that the blood exerts against the walls of the arteries as it passes through them.

bloody show: A small amount of blood in the vagina that appears at the beginning of labor and may include a plug of pink-tinged mucus that is discharged when the cervix begins to dilate.

blow-out fracture: A fracture of the orbit or of the bones that support the floor of the orbit.

blunt trauma: An impact on the body by objects that cause injury without penetrating soft tissues or internal organs and cavities.

B-NICE: A mnemonic for the types of weapons of mass destruction: biologic, nuclear, incendiary, chemical, and explosive.

body mechanics: The relationship between the body's anatomic structures and the physical forces associated with lifting, moving, and carrying; the ways in which the body moves to achieve a specific action.

botulinum: Produced by bacteria, this is the most potent neurotoxin known. When introduced into the body, this neurotoxin affects the nervous system's ability to function and causes botulism.

brachial artery: The major vessel in the upper extremities that supplies blood to the arm.

bradycardia: A slow heart rate, less than 60 beats/min.

brain: The controlling organ of the body and center of consciousness; functions include perception, control of reactions to the environment, emotional responses, and judgment.

brainstem: The area of the brain between the spinal cord and cerebrum, surrounded by the cerebellum; controls functions that are necessary for life, such as respiration.

breach of confidentiality: Disclosure of information without proper authorization.

breath-holding syncope: Loss of consciousness caused by a decreased breathing stimulus.

breath sounds: An indication of air movement in the lungs, usually assessed with a stethoscope.

breech presentation: A delivery in which the buttocks come out first.

bronchi: Hollow airway passages that branch to the right and left from the trachea and divide into smaller bronchioles.

bronchial breath sounds: Normal breath sounds made by air moving through the bronchi.

bronchioles: Subdivisions of the smaller bronchi in the lungs that terminate at alveoli; made of smooth muscle and dilate or constrict in response to various stimuli.

bronchiolitis: Inflammation of the bronchioles that usually occurs in children younger than 2 years and is often caused by the respiratory syncytial virus.

bronchitis: An acute or chronic inflammation of the lung that may damage lung tissue; usually associated with cough and production of sputum and, depending on its cause, sometimes fever.

buboes: Enlarged lymph nodes (up to the size of a tennis ball) that are characteristic in people infected with the bubonic plague.

bubonic plague: Bacterial infection that affects the lymphatic system. It is transmitted by infected rodents and fleas and characterized by acute malaise, fever, and the formation of tender, enlarged, inflamed lymph nodes that appear as lesions, called buboes. Also called the Black Death.

bulk storage containers: Any container other than nonbulk storage containers, such as fixed tanks, highway cargo tanks, rail tank cars, totes, and intermodal tanks. These are typically found in manufacturing facilities and are often surrounded by a secondary containment system to help control an accidental release.

burnout: A combination of exhaustion, cynicism, and reduced performance resulting from long-term job stresses in health care and other high-stress professions.

burns: Injuries in which soft-tissue damage occurs as a result of thermal heat, frictional heat, toxic chemicals, electricity, or nuclear radiation.

calcaneus: A large bone that forms the heel of the foot; also called the heel bone.

capillaries: The small blood vessels that connect arterioles and venules; various substances pass through capillary walls, into and out of the interstitial fluid, and then on to the cells.

capillary refill: A test that evaluates distal circulatory system function by squeezing (blanching) blood from an area such as a nail bed and watching the speed of its return after releasing the pressure.

capillary vessels: The tiny blood vessels between the arterioles and venules that permit transfer of oxygen, carbon dioxide, nutrients, and waste between body tissues and the blood.

capnography: A noninvasive method to quickly and efficiently provide information on a patient's ventilatory status, circulation, and metabolism. It effectively measures the concentration of carbon dioxide in expired air over time.

capnometry: The use of a capnometer, a device that measures the amount of expired carbon dioxide.

carbon dioxide: A component of air that typically makes up 0.03% of air at sea level; also a waste product exhaled during expiration by the respiratory system.

carbon dioxide retention: A condition characterized by a chronically high blood level of carbon dioxide in which the respiratory center no longer responds to high blood levels of carbon dioxide.

carbon monoxide: An odorless, colorless, tasteless, and highly poisonous gas that results from incomplete oxidation of carbon in combustion.

carboys: Glass, plastic, or steel containers, ranging in volume from 5 to 15 gallons (19 to 57 L).

cardiac arrest: An event in which the heart fails to generate effective and detectable blood flow; pulses are not palpable in cardiac arrest, even if muscular and electrical activity continues in the heart.

cardiac muscle: The heart muscle.

cardiac output (CO): A measure of the volume of blood circulated by the heart in 1 minute, calculated by multiplying the stroke volume by the heart rate.

cardiac tamponade (pericardial tamponade): Compression of the heart as the result of buildup of blood or other fluid in the pericardial sac, leading to decreased cardiac output.

cardiogenic shock: A state in which not enough oxygen is delivered to the tissues of the body, caused by low output of blood from the heart. It can be a severe complication of a large acute myocardial infarction, as well as other conditions.

cardiopulmonary resuscitation (CPR): The combination of chest compressions and rescue breathing used to establish adequate ventilation and circulation in a patient who is not breathing and has no pulse.

carina: The structure at which the trachea divides into the left and right main stem bronchi.

carotid artery: The major artery that supplies blood to the head and brain.

carpals: Small bones that compose the wrist.

cartilage: The smooth connective tissue that forms the support structure of the skeletal system and provides cushioning between bones; also forms the nasal septum and portions of the outer ear.

casualty collection area: An area set up by physicians, nurses, and other hospital staff near a major disaster scene where patients can receive further triage and medical care.

cavitation: A phenomenon in which speed causes a bullet to generate pressure waves, which cause damage distant from the bullet's path.

cecum: The first part of the large intestine, into which the ileum opens.

cells: The fundamental units of the human body.

cellular metabolism: A set of chemical reactions that supplies cells with energy. Includes both anaerobic and aerobic metabolism.

cellular respiration: Use of oxygen by the cells to carry out their specific activities; also called cellular metabolism.

cellular telephone: A low-power portable radio that communicates through an interconnected series of repeater stations called cells.

Centers for Disease Control and Prevention (CDC): The primary federal agency that conducts and supports public health activities in the United States. The CDC is part of the US Department of Health and Human Services.

central nervous system (CNS): The brain and spinal cord.

central neurogenic hyperventilation: An abnormal breathing pattern associated with increased ICP that is characterized by deep, rapid breathing; this pattern is similar to Kussmaul respirations, but without an acetone breath odor.

central pulses: Pulses that are closest to the core (central) part of the body where the vital organs are located; include the carotid, femoral, and apical pulses.

cerebellum: One of the three major subdivisions of the brain, sometimes called the little brain; coordinates the various activities of the brain, particularly fine body movements.

cerebral edema: Swelling of the brain.

cerebral palsy: A group of disorders characterized by poorly controlled body movement.

cerebrospinal fluid (CSF): Fluid produced in the ventricles of the brain that flows in the subarachnoid space and bathes the meninges.

cerebrovascular accident (CVA): An interruption of blood flow to the brain that results in the loss of brain function; also called a stroke.

cerebrum: The largest part of the three subdivisions of the brain, sometimes called the gray matter; made up of several lobes that control movement, hearing, balance, speech, visual perception, emotions, and personality.

certification: A process in which a person, an institution, or a program is evaluated and recognized as meeting certain predetermined standards to provide safe and ethical care.

cervical spine: The portion of the vertebral column consisting of the first seven vertebrae that lie in the neck.

cervix: The lower third, or neck, of the uterus.

channel: An assigned frequency or frequencies that are used to carry voice and/or data communications.

Chemical Transportation Emergency Center (CHEMTREC): An agency that assists emergency responders in identifying and handling hazardous materials transport incidents.

chemoreceptors: Receptors that monitor the levels of oxygen, carbon dioxide, and pH of the cerebrospinal fluid and then provide feedback to the respiratory centers to modify the rate and depth of breathing based on the body's needs at any given time.

chest compression fraction: The total percentage of time during a resuscitation attempt in which active chest compressions are being performed.

Cheyne-Stokes respirations: A cyclical pattern of abnormal breathing that increases and then decreases in rate and depth, followed by a period of apnea.

chief complaint: The reason a patient called for help; also, the patient's response to questions such as "What's wrong?" or "What happened?"

chief concern: The condition requiring the most urgent intervention as determined by the clinician's assessment of the patient; it is not always the same as the chief complaint.

child maltreatment: A general term applying to all forms of physical and emotional abuse, sexual abuse, neglect, and exploitation of children.

chlamydia: A sexually transmitted infection caused by the bacterium *Chlamydia trachomatis.*

chlorine (Cl): The first chemical agent ever used in warfare. It has a distinct odor of bleach and creates a green haze when released as a gas. Initially it produces upper airway irritation and a choking sensation.

cholecystitis: Inflammation of the gallbladder.

chordae tendineae: Thin bands of fibrous tissue that attach to the valves in the heart and prevent them from inverting.

chronic bronchitis: Irritation of the major lung passageways from long-term exposure to infectious disease or irritants such as smoke.

chronic obstructive pulmonary disease (COPD): A lung disease characterized by chronic obstruction of lung airflow that interferes with normal breathing and is not fully reversible.

chyme: The substance that leaves the stomach. It is a combination of all of the eaten foods with added stomach acids.

circulatory system: The complex arrangement of connected tubes, including the arteries, arterioles, capillaries, venules, and veins, that moves blood, oxygen, nutrients, carbon dioxide, and cellular waste throughout the body.

circumferential burns: Burns that go completely around a body part, such as an arm, a foot, or the chest.

cirrhosis: A chronic and progressive disease in which normal liver cells are replaced by fibrotic scar tissue.

clavicle: The collarbone; it is lateral to the sternum and anterior to the scapula.

cleaning: The process of removing dirt, dust, blood, or other visible contaminants from a surface.

closed abdominal injury: An injury in which there is soft-tissue damage inside the body but the skin remains intact.

closed chest injury: An injury to the chest in which the skin is not broken, usually caused by blunt trauma.

closed-ended questions: Questions that can be answered in short or single-word responses.

closed fracture: Any break in a bone in which the overlying skin is not broken.

closed head injury: Injury in which the brain has been injured but the skin has not been broken and there is no obvious bleeding.

closed incident: An incident that is contained; all casualties are accounted for.

closed injuries: Injuries in which damage occurs beneath the skin or mucous membrane but the surface of the skin remains intact.

coagulation: The formation of clots to plug openings in injured blood vessels and stop blood flow.

coccyx: The last three or four vertebrae of the spine, which are fused; the tailbone.

cognitive disabilities: Conditions that impair a person's ability to remember information, process information, make decisions, or communicate in a normal fashion.

cold zone: A safe area at a hazardous materials incident for the agencies involved in the operations. The incident commander, the command post, EMS clinicians, and other support functions necessary to control the incident should be located in this zone. Also referred to as the clean zone or the support zone.

colostomy: A surgical procedure to create an opening (stoma) between the colon and the surface of the body.

coma: A state of profound unconsciousness from which the patient cannot be roused.

combining vowel: The vowel used to combine two word roots or a word root and suffix.

command: In incident command, the position that oversees the incident, establishes the objectives and priorities, and develops a response plan.

command post: The designated field command center where the incident commander and support staff are located.

commotio cordis: A blunt chest injury caused by a sudden, direct blow to the chest that occurs only during the critical portion of a person's heartbeat.

communicable disease: A disease that can be spread from one person or species to another.

communication: The transmission of information to another person—verbally or through body language.

community paramedicine: A health care model in which experienced paramedics receive advanced training to equip them to provide additional services in the prehospital environment, such as health evaluations, monitoring of chronic illnesses or conditions, and patient advocacy.

compartment syndrome: Swelling in a confined space that produces dangerous pressure; may cut off blood flow or damage sensitive tissue.

compassionate persuasion: The act of guiding a person to accept an offer of treatment that they initially did not want while respecting patient autonomy.

compassion fatigue: A stress disorder characterized by gradual lessening of compassion over time.

compensated shock: The early stage of shock, in which the body can still compensate for blood loss.

compensatory damages: Damages awarded in a civil lawsuit that are intended to restore the plaintiff to the same condition that they were in prior to the incident.

competent: Legally able to make rational decisions about personal well-being.

complex access: Entry that requires special tools and training and includes the use of force.

compliance: The ability of the alveoli to expand when air is drawn in during inhalation.

concussion: A temporary loss or alteration of part or all of the brain's abilities to function without actual physical damage to the brain.

conduction: The loss of heat by direct contact (eg, when a body part comes into contact with a colder object).

conductive hearing loss: Hearing loss caused by a faulty transmission of sound waves.

conjunctiva: The delicate membrane that lines the eyelids and covers the exposed surface of the eye.

conjunctivitis: Inflammation of the conjunctiva.

consent: Permission to render care.

contact burn: A burn caused by direct contact with a hot object.

contact hazard: The term used to describe the danger posed by a chemical whose primary route of entry into the body is through the skin; posed by a hazardous agent that gives off very little or no vapors; also called a skin hazard.

contagious: An infectious disease that spreads from one human to another; communicable.

container: Any vessel or receptacle that holds material, including storage vessels, pipelines, and packaging.

contamination: The presence of infectious organisms or foreign bodies on or in objects such as dressings, water, food, needles, wounds, or a patient's body.

continuous positive airway pressure (CPAP): A method of noninvasive ventilation used primarily in the treatment of critically ill patients with respiratory distress; can prevent the need for endoracheal intubation.

continuum of care: The concept of consistent patient care across the entire health care team from first patient contact to patient discharge; working together with a unified goal results in improved individual and team performance, better patient and clinician safety, and improved patient outcome.

contraindications: Conditions that make a particular medication or treatment inappropriate because it would not help, or may actually harm, a patient.

contributory negligence: A legal defense that may be raised when the defendant thinks that the conduct of the plaintiff somehow contributed to any injuries or damages that were sustained by the plaintiff.

control zones: Areas at a hazardous materials incident that are designated as hot, warm, or cold, based on safety issues and the degree of hazard found there.

contusion: A bruise from an injury that causes bleeding beneath the skin without breaking the skin; also called ecchymosis.

convection: The loss of body heat caused by air movement (eg, a breeze blowing across the body).

conventional reasoning: A type of reasoning in which a child looks for approval from peers and society.

core temperature: The temperature of the central part of the body (eg, the heart, lungs, and vital organs).

cornea: The transparent tissue layer in front of the pupil and iris of the eye.

coronal (frontal) plane: An imaginary plane where the body is divided into front and back parts.

coronary arteries: The blood vessels that carry blood and nutrients to the heart muscle.

coronavirus disease 2019 (COVID-19): A respiratory disease caused by the virus SARS-CoV-2. The virus is a coronavirus, similar to the one that causes the common cold.

coup–contrecoup (brain) injury: A brain injury that occurs when force is applied to the head and energy transmission through brain tissue causes injury on the opposite side of original impact.

covert: An act in which the public safety community generally has no prior knowledge of the time, location, or nature of the attack.

coxae: The hip bones (singular: *coxa*).

crackles: A crackling, rattling breath sound that signals fluid in the air spaces of the lungs.

cranium: The part of the skull that encloses the brain and is composed of eight bones.

credentialing: An established process to determine the qualifications necessary to be allowed to perform a particular skill or role, or to function as an organization.

crepitus: A grating or grinding sensation or sound caused by fractured bone ends or joints rubbing together.

crew resource management (CRM): A set of procedures for use in environments where human error can have disastrous consequences. It empowers people within a team to communicate effectively with one another with a goal of improving team situational awareness, patient and crew safety, and overall communication.

cricoid cartilage: A firm ridge of cartilage that forms the lower part of the larynx.

cricothyroid membrane: A thin sheet of fascia that connects the thyroid and cricoid cartilages that make up the larynx.

critical incident stress management (CISM): A process that confronts the responses to critical incidents and defuses them, directing the emergency services personnel toward physical and emotional equilibrium.

cross-contamination: Occurs when a person is contaminated by an agent as a result of coming in contact with another contaminated person.

croup: A viral inflammatory disease of the upper respiratory system that may cause a partial airway obstruction and is characterized by a barking cough; usually seen in children.

crowning: The appearance of the fetus's head at the vaginal opening during labor.

crush injury: An injury that occurs when a great amount of force is applied to the body.

crush syndrome: Significant metabolic derangement that develops when crushed extremities or body parts remain trapped for prolonged periods. This can lead to kidney failure and death.

cultural competence: The ability to deliver care in a way that meets the social, cultural, and linguistic needs of patients.

cultural humility: The attribute of being curious about others and keeping an open mind when interacting with people from an unfamiliar culture.

cultural imposition: A type of bias in which individuals impose their beliefs, values, and practices on others because they believe their ideals are superior.

Cushing triad: Increased systolic blood pressure, decreased heart rate, and irregular respirations that result from increased intracranial pressure.

cushion of safety: A safe distance between your vehicle and any vehicles around you.

cyanide: An agent that affects the body's ability to use oxygen. It is a colorless gas that has an odor similar to almonds. The effects begin on the cellular level and are very rapidly seen at the organ and system levels.

cyanosis: A blue skin discoloration that is caused by a reduced level of oxygen in the blood. Although pallor, or a decrease in blood flow, can be difficult to detect in people with dark skin, it may be observed by examining mucous membranes inside the inner lower eyelid and capillary refill. On general observation, the patient may appear ashen or gray.

cylinders: Portable, compressed gas containers used to hold liquids and gases such as nitrogen, argon, helium, and oxygen. They have a range of sizes and internal pressures.

cystitis: Inflammation of the bladder.

danger zone (hot zone): An area where people can be exposed to hazards such as electric wires, sharp metal edges, broken glass, toxic substances, radiation, or fire.

DCAP-BTLS: A mnemonic for assessment in which each area of the body is evaluated for Deformities, Contusions, Abrasions, Punctures/penetrations, Burns, Tenderness, Lacerations, and Swelling.

dead space: Any portion of the airway that contains air but cannot participate in gas exchange, such as the trachea and bronchi.

decay: A natural process in which a material that is unstable attempts to stabilize itself by changing its structure.

deceleration: The slowing of an object.

decision-making capacity: Ability to understand and process information and make a choice regarding appropriate medical care.

decompensated shock: The late stage of shock when blood pressure is falling.

decompression sickness: A painful condition seen in divers who ascend too quickly, in which gas, especially nitrogen, forms bubbles in blood vessels and other tissues; also known as the bends.

decontamination: The process of cleaning, disinfecting, and/or sterilizing clothing, equipment, vehicles, and personnel; may involve removing or neutralizing radiation, chemical, or other hazardous material.

decontamination area: The designated area in a hazardous materials incident where all patients and responders must be decontaminated before going to another area.

dedicated line: A special telephone line that is used for specific point-to-point communications; also called a hotline.

deep: Farther inside the body and away from the skin.

deep partial-thickness burns: Burns that extend deeper into the dermis, destroying more of the blood vessels. They appear lighter in color than superficial partial-thickness burns and are dryer and less painful. Partial-thickness burns are also referred to as second-degree burns.

defamation: The communication of false information about a person that is damaging to that person's reputation or standing in the community.

defibrillate: To shock a fibrillating (chaotically shaking) heart with specialized electric current in an attempt to restore a normal, rhythmic beat.

dehydration: Loss of water from the tissues of the body.

delirium: An acute state of confusion, which occurs suddenly and may fluctuate over short periods. Rather than a disease itself, it is a sign of any number of underlying problems.

delirium tremens (DTs): A severe withdrawal syndrome seen in individuals with alcohol use disorder who are deprived of ethyl alcohol; characterized by restlessness, fever, sweating, disorientation, agitation, and seizures; can be fatal if untreated.

delusions: False beliefs that persist despite incontrovertible evidence to the contrary.

dementia: A slow, progressive decline in cognitive function that impairs memory function and leads to behavior change.

demobilization: The process of directing responders to return to their facilities when work at a disaster or mass-casualty incident has finished, at least for those particular responders.

denitrogenation: The process of replacing nitrogen in the lungs with oxygen to maintain a normal oxygen saturation level during advanced airway management.

dependent edema: Swelling in the part of the body closest to the ground, caused by collection of fluid in the tissues; a possible sign of heart failure.

dependent lividity: Blood settling to the lowest point of the body, causing discoloration of the skin; a definitive sign of death.

depositions: Oral questions asked of parties and witnesses under oath.

depression: A persistent mood of sadness, despair, and discouragement; may be a symptom of many different mental and physical disorders, or may be a disorder on its own.

dermis: The inner layer of the skin, containing hair follicles, sweat glands, nerve endings, and blood vessels.

designated officer: The individual in the department who is charged with the responsibility of managing exposures and infection control issues.

developmental disability: A group of conditions that may impair development in the areas of physical ability, learning, language development, or behavioral coping skills.

diabetes mellitus: A metabolic disorder in which the ability to metabolize carbohydrates (sugars) is impaired, usually because of a lack of insulin.

diabetic ketoacidosis (DKA): A form of hyperglycemia in uncontrolled diabetes in which certain acids accumulate when insulin is not available.

diamond carry: A carrying technique in which one clinician is located at the head end of the stretcher or backboard, one at the foot end, and one at each side of the patient; each of the two clinicians at the sides uses one hand to support the stretcher or backboard so that all are able to face forward as they walk.

diaphoretic: Characterized by light or profuse sweating.

diaphragm: A muscular dome that forms the undersurface of the thorax, separating the chest from the abdominal cavity. Contraction of the diaphragm (and the chest wall muscles) brings air into the lungs. Relaxation allows air to be expelled from the lungs.

diastole: The relaxation, or period of relaxation, of the heart, especially of the ventricles.

diastolic pressure: The pressure that remains in the arteries during the relaxing phase of the heart's cycle (diastole) when the left ventricle is at rest.

diffusion: Movement of a gas from an area of higher concentration to an area of lower concentration.

digestion: The processing of food that nourishes the individual cells of the body.

dilation: Widening of a tubular structure such as a coronary artery.

diphtheria: An infectious disease in which a pseudomembrane forms, lining the pharynx; this lining can severely obstruct the passage of air into the larynx.

direct contact: Exposure or transmission of a communicable disease from one person to another by physical contact.

direct laryngoscopy: Visualization of the airway with a laryngoscope.

dirty bomb: Name given to an explosive radiologic dispersal device.

disaster: A widespread event that disrupts community resources and functions, in turn threatening public safety, citizens' lives, and property.

discovery: The phase of a civil lawsuit where the plaintiff and defense obtain information from each other that will enable the attorneys to have a better understanding of the case and which will assist in negotiating a possible settlement or in preparing for trial. Discovery includes depositions, interrogatories, and demands for production of records.

disease vector: An animal that, once infected, spreads a disease to another animal.

disinfection: The killing of pathogenic agents by direct application of chemicals.

dislocation: Disruption of a joint in which ligaments are damaged and the bone ends are no longer in contact.

displaced fracture: A fracture in which bone fragments are separated from one another, producing deformity in the limb.

dissecting aneurysm: A condition in which the inner layers of an artery, such as the aorta, become separated, allowing blood (at high pressures) to flow between the layers.

dissemination: The means by which a terrorist will spread an agent; for example, by poisoning the water supply or aerosolizing the agent into the air or ventilation system of a building.

distal: Farther from the trunk or nearer to the free end of the extremity.

distracting injury: Any injury that prevents the patient from noticing other injuries, even severe injuries; for example, a painful femur or tibia fracture that prevents the patient from noticing back pain associated with a spinal fracture.

distraction: A spinal injury in which adjacent vertebrae are pulled apart from one another, such as may occur in hanging victims.

distress: A negative response to a stressor.

distributive shock: A condition that occurs when there is widespread dilation of the small arterioles, small venules, or both.

diverticula: Pouches that bulge out through weak places in the wall of the colon.

diverticulitis: Inflammation in small pockets at weak areas in the muscle walls of the intestines.

diverticulosis: A condition in which diverticula develop in the colon.

diving reflex: The slowing of the heart rate caused by submersion in cold water.

do not attempt resuscitation (DNAR) order: Written documentation by a physician giving permission to medical personnel not to attempt resuscitation in the event of cardiac arrest.

documentation: The recorded portion of the EMT's patient interaction, either written or electronic. This becomes part of the patient's permanent medical record.

domestic terrorism: Terrorism that is carried out by people in their own country.

dorsal: The posterior surface of the body, including the back of the hand.

dorsalis pedis artery: The artery on the anterior surface of the foot between the first and second metatarsals.

dose: The amount of medication given on the basis of the patient's size and age.

Down syndrome: A genetic chromosomal defect that can occur during fetal development and that results in intellectual impairment as well as certain physical characteristics, such as a round head with a flat occiput and slanted, wide-set eyes.

drowning: The process of experiencing respiratory impairment from submersion or immersion in liquid.

drums: Barrel-like containers used to store a wide variety of substances, including food-grade materials, corrosives, flammable liquids, and grease. May be constructed of low-carbon steel, polyethylene, cardboard, stainless steel, nickel, or other materials.

DuoDote Auto-Injector: A nerve agent antidote kit containing atropine and pralidoxime chloride; delivered as a single dose through one needle.

duplex: The ability to transmit and receive simultaneously.

durable power of attorney for health care: A type of advance directive executed by a competent adult that appoints another individual to make medical treatment decisions on their behalf, in the event that the person making the appointment loses decision-making capacity.

duration: The amount of time that clinical effects of a medication last.

duty to act: A medicolegal term relating to certain personnel who either by statute or by function have a responsibility to provide care.

dysarthria: Slurred speech.

dysbarism injuries: Any signs and symptoms caused by the difference between the surrounding atmospheric pressure and the total gas pressure in various tissues, fluids, and cavities of the body.

dyspnea: Shortness of breath.

dysrhythmia: An irregular or abnormal heart rhythm.

early adult: A young adult age 18 to 40 years.

ecchymosis: A buildup of blood beneath the skin that produces a characteristic blue or black discoloration as the result of an injury; also called a bruise or contusion.

eclampsia: A pregnancy complication that is characterized by new-onset hypertension (systolic blood pressure greater than 140 mm Hg or diastolic blood pressure greater than 90 mm Hg) with seizure activity and preceding systemic effects, such as blurred vision, headache, or protein in the urine. It is differentiated from preeclampsia by the presence of seizure activity.

ectopic pregnancy: A pregnancy that develops outside the uterus, typically in a fallopian tube.

edema: The presence of abnormally large amounts of fluid between cells in body tissues, causing swelling of the affected area.

elastic bougie: A flexible device that is inserted between the glottis under direct laryngoscopy; the endotracheal tube is threaded over the device, facilitating its entry into the trachea.

elder abuse: Any action on the part of an older person's family member, caregiver, or other associated person that takes advantage of the older person's person, property, or emotional state.

elimination: The process of removing a medication or chemical from within the body.

emancipated minor: A person who is under the legal age in a given state but, because of other circumstances, is legally considered an adult.

embolism: A condition in which a blood clot or other substance (embolus) in the circulatory system travels to a blood vessel, where it causes a blockage of blood flow.

embolus: A blood clot or other substance in the circulatory system that travels to a blood vessel, where it causes a blockage of blood flow.

embryo: The early stage of development after the fertilization of the egg (first 10 weeks).

emergency: A serious situation, such as injury or illness that threatens the life or welfare of a person or group of people and requires immediate intervention.

emergency doctrine: The principle of law that permits a health care clinician to treat a patient in an emergency situation when the patient is incapable of granting consent because of an altered level of consciousness, disability, the effects of drugs or alcohol, or the patient's age.

emergency medical care: Immediate care or treatment.

emergency medical responder (EMR): A professional, such as police officer, firefighter, lifeguard, or other rescuer, who may arrive first at the scene of an emergency to provide initial medical assistance and ensure access to EMS.

emergency medical services (EMS): A multidisciplinary system to provide out-of-hospital care to the sick and injured within communities.

emergency medical technician (EMT): An individual who has training in basic life support, including automated external defibrillation, use of a definitive airway adjunct, and assisting patients with certain medications.

emergency move: A move in which the patient is dragged or pulled from a dangerous scene before assessment and care are provided.

***Emergency Response Guidebook* (ERG):** A preliminary action guide for first responders operating at a hazardous materials incident in coordination with the US Department of Transportation's labels and placards marking system. Jointly developed by the DOT, the Secretariat of Communications and Transportation of Mexico, and Transport Canada.

emesis: Vomiting.

emotional intelligence: The ability to understand and manage one's own emotions and properly respond to the emotions of others.

emphysema: A disease of the lungs in which there is extreme dilation and eventual destruction of the pulmonary alveoli with poor exchange of oxygen and carbon dioxide; it is one form of chronic obstructive pulmonary disease.

EMT-administered medication: Administration of a medication by the EMT directly to the patient.

endocrine: A type of pancreatic gland that produces insulin and glucagon.

endocrine glands: Glands that secrete or release chemicals that are used inside the body.

endocrine system: The complex message and control system that integrates many body functions, including the release of hormones.

endometrium: The lining of the inside of the uterus.

endotracheal: Through the tracheal tube; a rarely used medication administration method.

endotracheal (ET) intubation: Insertion of an ET tube directly through the larynx between the vocal cords and into the trachea to maintain and protect an airway.

end-tidal carbon dioxide ($ETCO_2$): The amount of carbon dioxide present at the end of an exhaled breath.

enteral medications: Medications that enter the body through the digestive system.

entrapment: The situation of being caught (trapped) within a vehicle, room, or container with no way out or of having a limb or other body part trapped.

envenomation: The act of injecting venom.

enzymes: Substances designed to speed up the rate of specific biochemical reactions.

epidemic: A disease outbreak in which new cases of a disease in a human population substantially exceed the number expected based on recent experience.

epidermis: The outer layer of skin, which is made up of cells that are sealed together to form a watertight protective covering for the body.

epidural hematoma: An accumulation of blood between the skull and the dura mater.

epiglottis: A thin, leaf-shaped valve that allows air to pass into the trachea but prevents food and liquid from entering.

epiglottitis: A bacterial infection in which the epiglottis becomes inflamed and enlarged and may cause an upper airway obstruction.

epilepsy: A disorder in which abnormal electrical discharges occur in the brain, causing seizures and possible loss of consciousness.

epinephrine: A hormone produced by the body (commonly called adrenaline) and a drug produced by pharmaceutical companies that increases pulse rate and blood pressure; the drug of choice for an anaphylactic reaction.

epistaxis: A nosebleed.

esophageal intubation: Improper placement of an advanced airway device into the esophagus rather than into the trachea.

esophagus: A collapsible tube that extends from the pharynx to the stomach; muscle contractions propel food and liquids through it to the stomach.

ethics: The philosophy of right and wrong, of moral duties, and of ideal professional behavior.

ethmoid bone: A bone in the skull that separates the nasal cavity from the brain.

ethnocentrism: A type of bias in which individuals consider their own cultural values as more important when interacting with people of a different culture.

eustachian tube: A tube that connects the middle ear to the oropharynx.

evaporation: The conversion of water or another fluid from a liquid to a gas.

evidence-based medicine (EBM): An approach to medicine where decisions are based on well-conducted research that is integrated with the expertise of the EMS clinician and the patient's wishes and needs.

evisceration: The displacement of organs outside the body.

exhalation: The passive part of the breathing process in which the diaphragm and the intercostal muscles relax, forcing air out of the lungs.

exocrine: A type of gland, such as those in the pancreas, that produces enzymes for protein, carbohydrate, and fat breakdown within the duodenum.

expiratory reserve volume: The amount of air that can be exhaled following a normal exhalation.

exposure: A situation in which a person has had contact with blood, body fluids, tissues, or airborne particles in a manner that suggests disease transmission may occur.

expressed consent: A type of consent in which a patient gives verbal or nonverbal authorization for provision of care or transport.

extension: The straightening of a joint or backward bending of the spine.

external auditory canal: The ear canal; leads to the tympanic membrane.

external respiration: The exchange of gases between the lungs and the blood cells in the pulmonary capillaries; also called pulmonary respiration.

extremity lift: A lifting technique that is used for patients who are supine or in a sitting position with no suspected extremity or spinal injuries.

extrication: Removal of a patient from entrapment or a dangerous situation or position, such as removal from a wrecked vehicle, industrial incident, or collapsed building.

extrication supervisor: In incident command, the person appointed to determine the type of equipment and resources needed for a situation involving extrication or special rescue; also called the rescue officer.

eyes-forward position: A head position in which the patient's eyes are looking straight ahead and the head and torso are in line.

fallopian tubes: The tubes that connect each ovary with the uterus and are the primary location for fertilization of the ovum.

false imprisonment: The confinement of a person without legal authority or the person's consent.

false motion: Movement that occurs in a bone at a point where there is no joint, indicating a fracture; also called free movement.

family-centered care: An approach to health care in which patients of all ages and other stakeholders in the patient's well-being, often family members, are treated with respect and inclusion regarding the care of the patient.

fascia: The fiberlike connective tissue that covers arteries, veins, tendons, and ligaments.

febrile seizure: A seizure that results from sudden high fever; most often seen in children.

Federal Communications Commission (FCC): The federal agency that has jurisdiction over interstate and international telephone and telegraph services and satellite communications, all of which may involve EMS activity.

femoral artery: The major artery of the thigh, a continuation of the external iliac artery. It supplies blood to the lower abdominal wall, external genitalia, and legs. It can be palpated in the groin area.

femoral head: The proximal end of the femur, articulating with the acetabulum to form the hip joint.

femur: The thighbone; the longest and one of the strongest bones in the body.

fetal alcohol syndrome: A condition caused by the consumption of alcohol by a pregnant person;

characterized by growth and physical problems, intellectual disability, and a variety of congenital abnormalities in the child.

fetus: The developing, unborn offspring inside the uterus, from 10 weeks after fertilization until birth.

fibula: The smaller of the two bones that form the lower leg, located on the lateral side.

field impression: The conclusion about the cause of the patient's condition after considering the situation, history, and examination findings.

finance/administration: In incident command, the position in an incident responsible for accounting of all expenditures.

first-responder vehicles: Specialized vehicles used to transport EMS equipment and personnel to the scenes of medical emergencies.

flail chest: A condition in which two or more adjacent ribs are fractured in two or more places or in association with a fracture of the sternum so that a segment of the chest wall is effectively detached from the rest of the thoracic cage.

flame burn: A burn caused by an open flame.

flank: The region below the rib cage and above the hip.

flash burn: A burn caused by exposure to very intense heat, such as in an explosion.

flexible stretcher: A stretcher that is a rigid carrying device when secured around a patient but can be folded or rolled when not in use; also called a soft stretcher.

flexion: The bending of a joint or forward bending of the spine.

flutter valve: A one-way valve that allows air to leave the chest cavity but not return; may be part of a commercial vented occlusive dressing.

focal seizure: A seizure affecting a limited portion of the brain.

focused assessment: A type of physical assessment typically performed on patients who have sustained nonsignificant mechanisms of injury or on responsive medical patients. This type of examination is based on the chief complaint and focuses on one body system or part.

fontanelles: Areas where the newborn's or infant's skull has not fused together; usually disappear at approximately 18 months of age.

foodborne transmission: The contamination of food or water with an organism that can cause disease.

foramen magnum: A large opening at the base of the skull through which the brain connects to the spinal cord.

forcible restraint: The act of physically preventing an individual from initiating any physical action.

four-person log roll: The recommended procedure for moving a patient with a suspected spinal injury from the ground to a long backboard or other spinal precaution device.

Fowler position: An inclined position in which the head of the bed is raised.

fracture: A break in the continuity of a bone.

freelancing: When individual units or different organizations make independent and often inefficient decisions about the next appropriate action.

freight bills: The shipping papers used for transport of chemicals along roads and highways; also referred to as bills of lading.

frontal bones: The bones of the cranium that form the forehead.

frontal lobe: The brain area primarily responsible for personality, judgment, planning, problem solving, concentration, and self-awareness.

frostbite: Damage to tissues as the result of exposure to cold; frozen or partially frozen body parts are frostbitten.

full-thickness burns: Burns that affect all skin layers and may affect the subcutaneous layers, muscle, bone, and internal organs, leaving the area dry, leathery, and white, dark brown, or charred; often referred to as third-degree burns.

fundus: The dome-shaped top of the uterus.

G agents: Early nerve agents that were developed by German scientists in the period after World War I and into World War II. There are three such agents: sarin, soman, and tabun.

gag reflex: A normal reflex mechanism that causes retching; activated by touching the soft palate or the back of the throat.

gallbladder: A sac on the undersurface of the liver that collects bile from the liver and discharges it into the duodenum through the common bile duct.

gamma (x-ray) radiation: A type of energy that is emitted from a strong radiologic source that travels faster and has more energy than alpha and beta rays. These rays easily penetrate through the human body and require lead or several inches of concrete to prevent penetration.

gastric distention: A condition in which air fills the stomach, often as a result of high volume and pressure during artificial ventilation.

gastroesophageal reflux disease (GERD): A condition in which the sphincter between the esophagus and the stomach opens, allowing stomach acid to move up into the esophagus, usually resulting in a burning sensation within the chest; also called acid reflux.

gel: A semiliquid substance that is administered orally in capsule form or through plastic tubes.

gender identity: A personal sense of oneself as male or female (or, less commonly, both or neither).

general impression: The overall initial impression that determines the priority for patient care; based on the patient's surroundings, the mechanism of injury, signs and symptoms, and the chief complaint.

generalized seizure: A seizure characterized by severe twitching of all of the body's muscles that may last several minutes or more; formerly known as a grand mal seizure.

generic name: The original chemical name of a medication (in contrast with one of its proprietary or trade names); the name is not capitalized.

genital system: The reproductive system in men and women.

geriatrics: The assessment and treatment of disease in someone who is age 65 years or older.

germinal layer: The deepest layer of the epidermis where new skin cells are formed.

gestational diabetes: Diabetes that develops during pregnancy in individuals who did not have diabetes before pregnancy.

gestational hypertension: A blood pressure greater than or equal to 140 mm Hg systolic or 90 mm Hg diastolic in a pregnant person in whom hypertension has not previously been diagnosed.

Glasgow Coma Scale (GCS) score: An evaluation tool used to determine level of consciousness, which evaluates and assigns point values (scores) for eye opening, verbal response, and motor response, which are then totaled; it is effective in helping predict patient outcomes.

glenoid fossa: The part of the scapula that joins with the humeral head to form the glenohumeral joint.

globe: The eyeball.

glottis: The space in between the vocal cords that is the narrowest portion of the adult's airway; also called the glottic opening.

glucose: One of the basic sugars; it is the primary fuel, in conjunction with oxygen, for cellular metabolism.

Golden Period: The time from injury to definitive care, during which treatment of shock and traumatic injuries should occur because survival potential is best; also called the Golden Hour.

gonorrhea: A sexually transmitted infection caused by *Neisseria gonorrhoeae*.

good air exchange: A term used to distinguish the degree of distress in a patient with a mild airway obstruction. With good air exchange, the patient is still conscious and able to cough forcefully, although wheezing may be heard.

Good Samaritan laws: Statutory provisions enacted by many states to protect citizens from liability for errors and omissions in giving good-faith emergency medical care, unless there is wanton, gross, or willful negligence.

governmental immunity: Legal doctrine that can protect an EMS clinician from being sued or that may limit the amount of the monetary judgment that the plaintiff may recover; generally applies only to EMS systems that are operated by municipalities or other governmental entities.

greater trochanter: A bony prominence on the proximal lateral side of the thigh, just below the hip joint.

great vessels: The collective term for the venae cavae, aorta, and pulmonary arteries and veins.

gross negligence: Conduct that constitutes a willful or reckless disregard for a duty or standard of care.

grunting: A sign of increased work of breathing, heard as an *uh* sound during exhalation; reflects a pediatric patient's attempt to keep the alveoli open.

guarding: Muscle contractions of the abdominal wall to minimize the pain of abdominal movement. It may occur through conscious effort of the patient or involuntarily, in which case it is a sign of peritonitis.

hair follicles: The small organs that produce hair.

hallucinations: False perceptions involving the senses of sight, sound, taste, smell, or touch.

hallucinogen: An agent that produces false perceptions in any one of the five senses.

handoff: The transfer of pertinent patient information and the responsibility for the patient's care; often involves the physical movement of the patient and associated equipment; also known as handover.

hazardous material: Any substance that is toxic, poisonous, radioactive, flammable, or explosive and causes injury or death with exposure.

hazardous materials (hazmat) incident: An incident in which a hazardous material is no longer properly contained and isolated.

head tilt–chin lift maneuver: A combination of two movements to open the airway by tilting the forehead back and lifting the chin; not used for trauma patients.

health care directive: A written document that specifies medical treatment for a competent patient, should the individual become unable to make decisions. Also known as an advance directive or a living will.

health care proxy: A type of advance directive executed by a competent adult that appoints another individual to make medical treatment decisions on their behalf in the event that the person making the appointment loses decision-making capacity. Also known as a durable power of attorney for health care.

health equity: As defined by the World Health Organization, "the absence of unfair and avoidable or remediable differences in health among population groups defined socially, economically, demographically, or geographically."

health information exchange (HIE): A system that allows EMS clinicians to access relevant health data (eg, past medical problems, medications, allergies, end-of-life decisions), avoid unnecessary duplication of effort in data entry, and view patient outcomes related to hospital care.

heart: A hollow muscular organ that pumps blood throughout the body.

heart failure: A disorder in which the heart loses part of its ability to effectively pump blood, usually as a result of damage to the heart muscle and usually resulting in a backup of fluid into the lungs if the left ventricle is involved.

heart rate (HR): The number of heartbeats during a specific time (usually 1 minute).

heat cramps: Painful muscle spasms usually associated with vigorous activity in a hot environment.

heat exhaustion: A heat emergency in which a significant amount of fluid and electrolyte loss occurs because of heavy sweating.

heatstroke: A life-threatening condition of severe hyperthermia caused by exposure to excessive natural or artificial heat, marked by warm, dry skin; severely altered mental status; and often irreversible coma.

hematemesis: The vomiting of blood.

hematology: The study and prevention of blood-related disorders.

hematoma: A mass of blood that has collected within damaged tissue beneath the skin or in a body cavity.

hematuria: Blood in the urine.

hemiparesis: Weakness on one side of the body.

hemoglobin: An oxygen-carrying protein found in red blood cells.

hemophilia: A hereditary condition in which the patient lacks one or more of the blood's normal clotting factors.

hemopneumothorax: The accumulation of blood and air in the pleural space of the chest.

hemoptysis: The coughing up of blood.

hemorrhage: Bleeding.

hemorrhagic stroke: A type of stroke that occurs as a result of bleeding inside the brain.

hemostatic dressing: A dressing impregnated with a chemical compound that slows or stops bleeding by assisting with clot formation.

hemothorax: A collection of blood in the pleural cavity.

hepatitis: Inflammation of the liver, usually caused by a viral infection, that causes fever, loss of appetite, jaundice, fatigue, and altered liver function.

hernia: The protrusion of an organ or tissue through an abnormal body opening.

herpes simplex: A common virus that is asymptomatic in 80% of people carrying it, but characterized by small blisters on the lips or genitals in symptomatic infections.

high-level disinfection: The killing of pathogenic agents by using potent means of disinfection.

hinge joints: Joints that can bend and straighten but cannot rotate; they restrict motion to one plane.

histamines: Chemical substances released by the immune system in allergic reactions that are responsible for many of the symptoms of anaphylaxis, such as vasodilation.

history taking: A step within the patient assessment process that provides detail about the patient's chief complaint and an account of the patient's signs and symptoms.

hollow organs: Structures through which materials pass, such as the stomach, small intestines, large intestines, ureters, and urinary bladder.

homeostasis: A balance of all systems of the body.

hormones: Substances formed in specialized organs or glands and carried to another organ or group of cells in the same organism; they regulate many body functions, including metabolism, growth, and body temperature.

host: The organism or individual that is attacked by the infecting agent.

hot zone: The area immediately surrounding a hazardous materials spill or incident site that endangers life and health. All responders working in this zone must wear appropriate protective clothing and equipment. Entry requires approval by the incident commander or other designated officer.

human immunodeficiency virus (HIV): Acquired immunodeficiency syndrome (AIDS) is caused by HIV, which damages the cells in the body's immune system so that the body is unable to fight infection or certain cancers.

human trafficking: The illegal exploitation of a person.

humerus: The supporting bone of the upper arm.

hydroplaning: Occurs when the tires of a vehicle are lifted off the road surface as a result of water piling up underneath them, making the vehicle feel as though it is floating.

hydrostatic pressure: The pressure that a fluid exerts against the walls of its container.

Hymenoptera: An order of insects that includes bees, wasps, ants, and yellowjackets.

hypercapnia: An abnormally high level of carbon dioxide in the bloodstream.

hyperextension: Excessive extension of the spine.

hyperflexion: Excessive flexion of the spine.

hyperglycemia: An abnormally high blood glucose level.

hyperosmolar hyperglycemic state (HHS): A life-threatening condition resulting from high blood glucose that typically occurs in older adults and that causes altered mental status, dehydration, and organ damage; formerly called hyperosmolar hyperglycemic nonketotic syndrome.

hyper-rotation: Excessive rotation of the spine.

hypertension: Blood pressure that is higher than the normal range.

hypertensive emergency: An emergency situation created by excessively high blood pressure, which can lead to serious complications such as stroke or aneurysm.

hyperthermia: A condition in which the body core temperature rises to 101°F (38.3°C) or more.

hyperventilation: Rapid or deep breathing that lowers the blood carbon dioxide level below normal; may lead to increased intrathoracic pressure, decreased venous return, and hypotension when associated with bag-mask device use.

hyperventilation syndrome: This syndrome occurs in the absence of physical problems. The respiratory rate of a person who is experiencing hyperventilation syndrome may be as high as 40 shallow breaths/min or as low as only 20 very deep breaths/min. This syndrome is often associated with panic attacks.

hypnotic: A sleep-inducing effect or agent.

hypoglycemia: An abnormally low blood glucose level.

hypoperfusion: A condition in which the circulatory system fails to provide sufficient circulation to maintain normal cellular function; also called shock.

hypotension: Blood pressure that is lower than the normal range.

hypothermia: A condition in which the internal body temperature falls below 95°F (35°C).

hypovolemic shock: A condition in which low blood volume, due to massive internal or external bleeding or extensive loss of body water, results in inadequate perfusion.

hypoxia: A dangerous condition in which the body tissues and cells do not have enough oxygen.

hypoxic drive: A condition in which chronically low levels of oxygen in the blood stimulate the respiratory drive; seen in patients with chronic lung diseases.

ileostomy: A surgical procedure to create an opening (stoma) between the small intestine and the surface of the body.

ileus: Paralysis of the bowel, arising from any one of several causes; stops contractions that move material through the intestine.

ilium: One of three bones that fuse to form the pelvic ring.

immune: The state of being able to resist the adverse effects of an infectious exposure.

immune response: The body's response to a substance perceived by the body as foreign.

immune system: The body system that includes all of the structures and processes designed to mount a defense against foreign substances and disease-causing agents.

immunology: The study of the body's immune system.

impaled objects: Objects that penetrate the skin but remain in place.

implied consent: Type of consent in which a patient who is unable to give consent is given treatment under the legal assumption that this person would want treatment.

incident action plan (IAP): An oral or written plan stating general objectives reflecting the overall strategy for managing an incident.

incident command system (ICS): A system implemented to manage disasters and mass-casualty incidents in which section chiefs, including finance/administration, logistics, operations, and planning, report to the incident commander.

incident commander (IC): The overall leader of the incident command system to whom commanders or leaders of incident command system divisions report.

incision: A sharp, smooth cut in the skin.

incontinence: Loss of bowel and/or bladder control; may be the result of a generalized seizure.

incubation: The period between exposure to an agent and onset of resulting symptoms.

index of suspicion: Awareness that unseen life-threatening injuries or illness may exist when determining the mechanism of injury.

indications: The therapeutic uses for a specific medication.

indirect contact: Exposure or transmission of disease from one person to another by contact with a contaminated object.

induced abortion: The elective termination of a pregnancy prior to the time of viability.

infant: A young child age 1 month to 1 year.

infarction: Death of a body tissue, usually caused by interruption of its blood supply.

infection: The abnormal invasion of a host or host tissues by organisms such as bacteria, viruses, or parasites, with or without signs or symptoms of disease.

infection control: Procedures to reduce transmission of infection among patients and health care personnel.

infectious disease: A medical condition caused by the growth and spread of small, harmful organisms within the body.

inferior: Below a body part or nearer to the feet.

inferior vena cava: One of the two largest veins in the body; carries blood from the lower extremities and the pelvis and the abdominal organs to the heart.

influenza: A disease caused by a virus that has crossed the animal–human barrier and infected humans and that kills thousands of people every year.

influenza type A: Virus that has crossed the animal/human barrier and has infected humans, reaching a pandemic level in 2009 with the H1N1 strain.

informed consent: Permission for treatment given by a competent patient after the potential risks, benefits, and alternatives to treatment have been explained.

ingestion: Swallowing; taking a substance by mouth.

inhalation: The active, muscular part of breathing that draws air into the airway and lungs; a medication delivery route.

in loco parentis: Legal authorization for a person or organization to take on some of the functions and responsibilities of a parent.

inspiratory reserve volume: The amount of air that can be inhaled after a normal inhalation; the amount of air that can be inhaled in addition to the normal tidal volume.

insulin: A hormone produced by the islets of Langerhans (endocrine glands located throughout the pancreas) that enables glucose in the blood to enter cells; used in synthetic form to treat and control diabetes mellitus.

intellectual disability: A subset of developmental disability characterized by significant limitations in both intellectual functioning and skills needed for daily living.

intermodal tanks: Shipping and storage vessels that can be either pressurized or nonpressurized.

internal respiration: The exchange of gases between the blood and the tissue cells.

international terrorism: Terrorism that is carried out by people in a country other than their own; also known as cross-border terrorism.

interoperable communications system: A communication system that uses voice-over-Internet protocol (VoIP) technology to allow multiple agencies to communicate and transmit data.

interrogatories: Written questions that the defense and plaintiff send to one another.

interstitial space: The space in between the cells.

intervertebral disks: Tough, elastic structures between adjoining vertebrae that act as shock absorbers.

intracellular space: The space within a cell or cells.

intracerebral hematoma: Bleeding within the brain tissue (parenchyma) itself; also referred to as an intraparenchymal hematoma.

intracranial pressure (ICP): The pressure within the cranial vault.

intramuscular (IM) injection: An injection into a muscle; a medication delivery route.

intranasal (IN): A delivery route in which a medication is pushed through a specialized atomizer device called a mucosal atomizer device (MAD) into the naris.

intraosseous (IO) injection: An injection into the bone; a medication delivery route.

intrapulmonary shunting: Bypassing of oxygen-poor blood past nonfunctional alveoli to the left side of the heart.

intravenous (IV) injection: An injection directly into a vein; a medication delivery route.

involuntary activities: Actions of the body that are not under a person's conscious control.

involuntary muscle: Muscle over which a person has no conscious control. It is found in many automatic regulating systems of the body.

ionizing radiation: Energy that is emitted in the form of rays, or particles.

iris: The muscle and surrounding tissue behind the cornea that dilate and constrict the pupil, regulating the amount of light that enters the eye; pigment in this tissue gives the eye its color.

irreversible shock: A condition defined by the inability to successfully achieve resuscitation regardless of the methods employed.

ischemia: A lack of oxygen that deprives tissues of necessary nutrients, resulting from partial or complete blockage of blood flow; potentially reversible because permanent injury has not yet occurred.

ischemic stroke: A type of stroke that occurs when blood flow to a particular part of the brain is cut off by a blockage (eg, a blood clot) inside a blood vessel.

ischium: One of three bones that fuse to form the pelvic ring.

jaundice: Yellow skin or sclera that is caused by liver disease or dysfunction. In individuals with dark skin, the discoloration may be more evident in the sclera.

jaw-thrust maneuver: Technique to open the airway by placing the fingers behind the angle of the jaw and bringing the jaw forward; used for patients who may have a cervical spine injury.

joint: The place where two bones come into contact; also called an articulation.

joint capsule: The fibrous sac that encloses a joint.

joint information center (JIC): An area designated by the incident commander, or a designee, in which public information officers from multiple agencies distribute information about the incident.

jump kit: A portable kit containing items that are used in the initial care of the patient.

JumpSTART triage: A sorting system for pediatric patients younger than 8 years or weighing less than 100 pounds (45 kg). There is a minor adaptation for infants because they cannot ambulate on their own.

junctional tourniquet: A device that provides proximal compression of severe bleeding near the axial or inguinal junction with the torso.

Just Culture: An approach to quality management that strives to balance accountability and justice in a system that believes in learning from errors.

kidnapping: The seizing, confining, abducting, or carrying away of a person by force, including transporting a competent adult for medical treatment without the individual's consent.

kidney stones: Solid crystalline masses formed in the kidney, resulting from an excess of insoluble salts or uric acid crystallizing in the urine; may become trapped anywhere along the urinary tract.

kidneys: Two retroperitoneal organs that excrete the end products of metabolism as urine and regulate the body's salt and water content.

kinetic energy: The energy of a moving object.

Kussmaul respirations: Deep, rapid breathing; usually the result of an accumulation of certain acids when insulin is not available in the body.

kyphosis: A forward curving of the upper back caused by an abnormal increase in the curvature of the spine.

labia majora: Outer fleshy "lips" covered with pubic hair that protect the vagina.

labia minora: Inner fleshy "lips" devoid of pubic hair that protect the vagina.

labored breathing: Breathing that uses the muscles of the chest, back, and abdomen to assist in expanding the chest; occurs when air movement is impaired, may be slower or faster than normal, and is characterized by grunting, stridor, and use of accessory muscles

laceration: A deep, jagged cut in the skin.

lacrimal glands: The glands that produce fluids to keep the eye moist; also called tear glands.

lactic acid: A metabolic by-product of the breakdown of glucose that accumulates when metabolism proceeds in the absence of oxygen (anaerobic metabolism).

large intestine: The portion of the digestive tube that encircles the abdomen around the small bowel, consisting of the cecum, the colon, and the rectum. It helps regulate water balance and eliminate solid waste.

larynx: A complex structure formed by many independent cartilaginous structures that all work together; where the upper airway ends and the lower airway begins; also called the voice box.

lateral: Parts of the body that lie farther from the midline; also called outer structures.

lateral bending: A mechanism of injury whereby a segment of the spine is suddenly or excessively bent laterally.

length-based resuscitation tape: A tape used to estimate an infant's or child's weight on the basis of body length; appropriate drug doses and equipment sizes are listed on the tape.

lens: The transparent part of the eye through which images are focused on the retina.

lesser trochanter: The projection on the medial/superior portion of the femur.

leukotrienes: Chemical substances that contribute to anaphylaxis; released by the immune system in allergic reactions.

lewisite (L): A blistering agent that has a rapid onset of symptoms and produces immediate, intense pain and discomfort on contact.

liaison officer: In incident command, the person who relays information, concerns, and requests among responding agencies.

libel: False and damaging information about a person that is communicated in writing.

licensure: The process whereby a competent authority, usually the state, allows people to perform a regulated act.

life expectancy: The average number of years a person can be expected to live.

ligaments: Bands of fibrous tissue that connect bones to bones. Ligaments support and strengthen a joint.

lightening: The movement of the fetus down into the pelvis late in pregnancy.

limb presentation: A delivery in which the presenting part is a single arm or leg.

linear skull fractures: Fractures that commonly occur in the temporoparietal region of the skull and that are not associated with deformities to the skull; also referred to as nondisplaced skull fractures.

liver: A large, solid organ that lies in the right upper quadrant immediately below the diaphragm; it produces bile, stores glucose for immediate use by the body, and produces many substances that help regulate immune responses.

load-distributing band (LDB): A circumferential chest compression device composed of a constricting band and backboard that is either electrically or pneumatically driven to compress the heart by putting inward pressure on the thorax.

logistics: In incident command, the position that helps procure and stockpile equipment and supplies during an incident.

lone wolf terrorist attack: An act of terror carried out by a single person to further an ideologic goal.

lumbar spine: The lower part of the back, formed by the lowest five nonfused vertebrae; also called the dorsal spine.

lumen: The inside diameter of an artery or other hollow structure.

lymph: A thin, straw-colored fluid that carries oxygen, nutrients, and hormones to the cells and carries waste products of metabolism away from the cells and back into the capillaries so that they may be excreted.

lymph nodes: Tiny, oval-shaped structures located in various places along the lymph vessels that filter lymph.

lymphatic system: A passive circulatory system in the body that transports a plasmalike liquid called lymph, a thin fluid that bathes the tissues of the body.

malleolus: A rounded bony prominence on either side of the ankle; also called the ankle bone.

mandible: The bone of the lower jaw.

manic episode: A period of markedly elevated mood and increased activity and energy levels, often lasting 1 week or longer.

manubrium: The upper quarter of the sternum.

mass-casualty incident (MCI): An emergency situation involving three or more patients or that can place great demand on the equipment or personnel of the EMS system or has the potential to produce multiple casualties.

mastoid process: The prominent bony mass at the base of the skull approximately 1 inch (2.5 cm) posterior to the external opening of the ear.

mature minor: A child who is of adequate age and maturity to make health care decisions.

mature minor doctrine: Legal authorization for certain minors with adequate age and maturity to consent or refuse medical treatment.

maxillae: The upper jawbones that assist in the formation of the orbit, the nasal cavity, and the palate and hold the upper teeth.

mean arterial pressure (MAP): The average pressure in the circulatory system during one cardiac cycle.

mechanical piston device: A device that depresses the sternum via a compressed gas-powered or electric-powered plunger mounted on a backboard.

mechanism of injury (MOI): The forces, or energy transmission, applied to the body that cause injury.

meconium: Fetal stool. When appearing as a dark green material in the amniotic fluid, it can indicate distress or disease in the newborn; it can be aspirated into the fetus's lungs during delivery.

MED channels: VHF and UHF channels that the Federal Communications Commission has designated exclusively for EMS use.

medevac: A term primarily used in wilderness and military settings to describe medical evacuation of a patient by helicopter.

medial: Parts of the body that lie closer to the midline; also called inner structures.

mediastinum: Space within the chest that contains the heart, major blood vessels, vagus nerve, trachea, major bronchi, and esophagus; located between the two lungs.

medical director: The physician who authorizes or delegates to the EMT the authority to provide medical care in the field.

medical emergencies: Emergencies that are caused by disease (illnesses or conditions) rather than a physical force acting on the body (ie, trauma).

medical oversight: Supervision of an EMS system or education program that includes instructions given directly by radio or cell phone (online/direct) to those on scene or indirectly by protocol/guidelines (off-line/indirect); also includes credentialing EMS clinicians and overseeing quality improvement activities as authorized by the medical director of the service or program.

medication: A substance that is used to treat or prevent disease or relieve pain.

medication error: Inappropriate use of a medication that could lead to patient harm.

medicolegal: A term relating to medical jurisprudence (law) or forensic medicine.

medulla oblongata: Nerve tissue that is continuous inferiorly with the spinal cord; serves as a conduction pathway for ascending and descending nerve tracts; coordinates heart rate, blood vessel diameter, breathing, swallowing, vomiting, coughing, and sneezing.

melena: Dark, foul-smelling, tarry stool containing digested blood.

menarche: The first menstrual cycle or onset of the first menstrual bleeding in females.

meninges: Three distinct layers of tissue that surround and protect the brain and the spinal cord within the skull and the spinal canal.

meningitis: An inflammation of the meningeal coverings of the brain and spinal cord; usually caused by a virus or a bacterium.

meningococcal meningitis: An inflammation of the meningeal coverings of the brain and spinal cord; can be highly contagious.

menopause: The cessation of menstruation, typically in the fourth or fifth decade of life.

mental illness: A chronic health condition involving changes in behavior, thinking, and/or emotion, which significantly interferes with the patient's ability to function in daily life.

mental model: A person's perception of "what's going on" in a given situation.

metabolism: The biochemical processes that result in production of energy from nutrients within cells.

metacarpals: Bones of the hand, situated between the carpals and phalanges.

metatarsals: Bones of the foot, situated between the tarsals and phalanges.

metered-dose inhaler (MDI): A miniature spray canister used to direct medications through the mouth and into the lungs.

methicillin-resistant *Staphylococcus aureus* (MRSA): A bacterium that causes infections in different parts of the body and is often resistant to commonly used antibiotics; can be found on the skin and in surgical wounds, the bloodstream, lungs, and urinary tract.

midbrain: The part of the brain that is responsible for helping to regulate the level of consciousness.

middle adult: An adult age 40 to 65 years.

midsagittal (midline) plane: An imaginary vertical line drawn from the middle of the forehead through the nose and the umbilicus (navel) to the floor, dividing the body into equal left and right halves.

mild airway obstruction: Occurs when a foreign body partially obstructs the patient's airway. The patient is able to move adequate amounts of air, but also experiences some degree of respiratory distress.

minute alveolar ventilation: The volume of air moved through the lungs in 1 minute minus the dead space; calculated by multiplying tidal volume (minus dead space) and respiratory rate.

minute volume: The volume of air that moves into and out of the lungs per minute; calculated by multiplying the tidal volume and respiratory rate; also called minute ventilation.

miosis: Excessively constricted pupil; often bilateral after exposure to nerve agents.

miscarriage: The spontaneous passage of the fetus and placenta before 20 weeks; also called spontaneous abortion.

mission-critical communications: Any communications where disruption will result in the failure of the mission at hand.

mobile data terminal (MDT): A small computer terminal inside the ambulance that directly receives data from the dispatch center.

mobile integrated healthcare (MIH): A method of delivering health care that involves providing health care within the community rather than at a physician's office or hospital.

morality: A code of conduct that can be defined by society, religion, or a person, affecting character, conduct, and conscience.

morgue supervisor: In incident command, the person who works with area medical examiners, coroners, and law enforcement agencies to coordinate the disposition of dead victims.

Moro reflex: An infant reflex in which, when an infant is caught off guard, the infant opens their arms wide, spreads the fingers, and seems to grab at things.

motor nerves: Nerves that carry information from the central nervous system to the muscles of the body.

mucosal atomizer device (MAD): A device that is used to change a liquid medication into a spray and push it into a nostril.

mucous membranes: The lining of body cavities and passages that communicate directly or indirectly with the environment outside the body.

mucus: The watery secretion of the mucous membranes that lubricates the body openings.

multigravida: A person who has had previous pregnancies.

multiplex: The ability to transmit audio and data signals through the use of more than one communications channel.

multisystem trauma: Trauma that affects more than one body system.

musculoskeletal system: The bones and voluntary muscles of the body.

mutagen: A substance that mutates, damages, and changes the structures of DNA in the body's cells.

mutual aid response: An agreement between neighboring EMS systems to respond to mass-casualty incidents or disasters in each other's region when local resources are insufficient to handle the response.

myocardial contractility: The ability of the heart muscle to contract.

myocardial contusion: Bruising of the heart muscle.

myocardium: The heart muscle.

nasal cannula: An oxygen-delivery device in which oxygen flows through two small, tubelike prongs that fit into the patient's nostrils; delivers 24% to 44% supplemental oxygen, depending on the flow rate.

nasal flaring: Widening of the nostrils, indicating an airway obstruction.

nasopharyngeal airway: Airway adjunct inserted into the nostril of an unresponsive patient or a patient with an altered level of consciousness who is unable to maintain airway patency independently; also referred to as a nasal airway.

nasopharynx: The part of the pharynx that lies above the level of the roof of the mouth, or palate.

National EMS Education Standards: A set of professional standards published by the National Highway Traffic Safety Administration that define the knowledge and competencies that students should acquire to perform at entry level as an EMS clinician. Four levels are defined: emergency medical responder, emergency medical technician, advanced emergency medical technician, or paramedic.

National EMS Information System (NEMSIS): A system funded by the National Highway Traffic

Safety Administration that is responsible for developing and maintaining the national EMS data standard.

National EMS Scope of Practice Model: A document created by the National Highway Traffic Safety Administration (NHTSA) that outlines the minimum entry-level skills performed by EMS clinicians at each nationally recognized level.

National Incident Management System (NIMS): A Department of Homeland Security system designed to enable federal, state, and local governments and private-sector and nongovernmental organizations to effectively and efficiently prepare for, prevent, respond to, and recover from domestic incidents, regardless of cause, size, or complexity, including acts of catastrophic terrorism.

nature of illness (NOI): The general type of illness a patient is experiencing.

neglect: Refusal or failure on the part of the parent or caregiver to provide life necessities.

negligence: Failure to provide the same care that a person with similar training would provide.

negligence per se: A theory that may be used when the conduct of the person being sued is alleged to have occurred in clear violation of a statute.

nerve agents: A class of chemical called organophosphates; they function by blocking an essential enzyme in the nervous system, which causes the body's organs to become overstimulated and burn out.

nervous system: The system that controls virtually all activities of the body, both voluntary and involuntary.

neurogenic shock: Circulatory failure caused by paralysis of the nerves that control the size of the blood vessels, leading to widespread dilation; seen in patients with spinal cord injuries.

neurons: The functional units of the nervous system; also called nerve cells.

neurotoxins: Biologic agents that are the deadliest substances known to humans; they include botulinum toxin and ricin.

neutron radiation: The type of energy that is emitted from a strong radiologic source, involving particles that are among the most powerful forms of radiation; the particles easily penetrate through lead and require several feet of concrete to stop them.

newborn: A person age birth to 1 month.

nitroglycerin: A medication that increases cardiac perfusion by causing blood vessels to dilate; EMTs may be allowed to assist the patient to self-administer this medication.

noise: Anything that dampens or obscures the true meaning of a message.

nonbulk storage vessels: Any container other than bulk storage containers, such as drums, bags, compressed gas cylinders, and cryogenic containers. These hold commonly used commercial and industrial chemicals such as solvents, industrial cleaners, and compounds.

nondisplaced fracture: A simple crack in the bone that has not caused the bone to move from its normal anatomic position; also called a hairline fracture.

nonrebreathing mask: A combination mask and reservoir bag system that is the preferred way to give oxygen in the prehospital setting; delivers up to 90% inspired oxygen and prevents inhaling the exhaled gases (carbon dioxide).

norepinephrine: A hormone produced by the body and a drug sometimes used in the treatment of shock; produces vasoconstriction through its alpha-stimulator properties.

nuchal cord: An umbilical cord that is wrapped around the fetus's neck.

obesity: A complex condition in which a person has an excessive amount of body fat.

obstructive shock: Shock that occurs when there is a block to blood flow in the heart or great vessels, causing an insufficient blood supply to the body's tissues.

occipital bone: The most posterior bone of the cranium.

occipital lobe: The brain area primarily responsible for vision.

occlusion: A blockage, usually of a tubular structure such as a blood vessel.

occlusive dressing: An airtight dressing that protects a wound from air and bacteria; a commercial vented version allows air to passively escape from the chest, while an unvented dressing may be made of petroleum jelly–based (Vaseline) gauze, aluminum foil, or plastic.

Occupational Safety and Health Administration (OSHA): The federal regulatory compliance agency that develops, publishes, and enforces guidelines concerning safety in the workplace.

off-gassing: The release of an agent after exposure—for example, from a person's clothes that have been exposed to the agent.

older adult: An adult age 65 years or older.

oncotic pressure: The pressure of water to move, typically into the capillary, as the result of the presence of plasma proteins.

onset of action: The amount of time from the administration of a medication to the onset of clinical effects.

open abdominal injury: An injury in which there is a break in the surface of the skin or mucous membrane, exposing deeper tissue to potential contamination.

open-book pelvic fracture: A life-threatening fracture of the pelvis caused by a force that displaces one or both sides of the pelvis laterally and posteriorly.

open chest injury: An injury to the chest in which the chest wall itself is penetrated by a fractured rib or, more frequently, by an external object such as a bullet or knife.

open-ended questions: Questions for which the patient must provide detail to give an answer.

open fracture: Any break in a bone in which the overlying skin has been broken.

open head injury: Injury to the head often caused by a penetrating object in which there may be bleeding and exposed brain tissue.

open incident: An incident that is not yet contained; there may be patients to be located and the situation may be ongoing, producing more patients.

open injuries: Injuries in which there is a break in the surface of the skin or the mucous membrane, exposing deeper tissue to potential contamination.

open pneumothorax: An open or penetrating chest wall wound through which air passes during inspiration and expiration, creating a sucking sound; also referred to as a sucking chest wound.

operations: In incident command, the position that carries out the orders of the commander to help resolve the incident.

opioid: A synthetically produced medication, drug, or agent that acts as a central nervous system depressant and produces insensibility or stupor; used to relieve pain.

OPQRST: A mnemonic used in evaluating a patient's pain: Onset, Provocation/palliation, Quality, Region/radiation, Severity, and Timing.

optic nerve: A cranial nerve that transmits visual information to the brain.

oral: By mouth; a medication delivery route.

oral glucose: A simple sugar that is readily absorbed by the bloodstream; it is carried on the EMS unit.

orbit: The eye socket, made up of the maxilla and zygoma.

organs: Groups of tissues that perform similar or interrelated jobs.

orientation: The mental status of a patient as measured by memory of person (name), place (current location), time (current year, month, and approximate date), and event (what happened).

oropharyngeal airway: Airway adjunct inserted into the mouth of an unresponsive patient to keep the tongue from blocking the upper airway and to facilitate suctioning the airway, if necessary; also referred to as an oral airway.

oropharynx: A tubular structure that extends vertically from the back of the mouth to the esophagus and trachea.

orthopnea: Severe dyspnea experienced when lying down and relieved by sitting up.

orthotic device: An externally applied device that modifies the structural and functional characteristics of the neuromuscular and skeletal systems often used to support or brace the limbs or spine.

osteoarthritis: A progressive disease of the joints that destroys cartilage, promotes the formation of bone spurs in joints, and leads to joint stiffness.

osteoporosis: A generalized bone disease, commonly associated with postmenopausal women, in which there is a reduction in the amount of bone mass leading to fractures after minimal trauma in either sex.

ovaries: The primary female reproductive organs that produce an ovum, or egg, that, if fertilized, will develop into a fetus.

overconfidence: A decision-making error in which the clinician overestimates their ability and chooses the wrong treatment path or ignores others' input, resulting in harmful actions.

overdose: An excessive quantity of a drug that, when taken or administered, can have toxic or lethal consequences.

over-the-counter (OTC) medications: Medications that may be purchased directly by a patient without a prescription.

ovulation: The process in which an ovum is released from a follicle.

oxygen: A gas that all cells need for metabolism; the heart and brain, especially, cannot function without oxygen.

oxygen toxicity: A condition of excessive oxygen consumption resulting in cellular and tissue damage.

oxygenation: The process of delivering oxygen to the blood by diffusion from the alveoli following inhalation into the lungs.

paging: The use of a radio signal and a voice or digital message that is transmitted to pagers ("beepers") or desktop monitor radios.

palliative care: A specialized health care approach focused on treating pain and promoting comfort, rather than attempting to cure a disease or prolong life.

palmar: The anterior region of the hand (palm).

palmar grasp reflex: An infant reflex that occurs when something is placed in the infant's palm; the infant grasps the object.

palpate: To examine by touch.

pancreas: A flat, solid organ that lies below the liver and the stomach; it is a major source of digestive enzymes and produces the hormone insulin.

pancreatitis: Inflammation of the pancreas.

pandemic: A disease outbreak that occurs on a global scale.

paradoxical chest motion: Respirations in which the chest moves inward during inhalation and outward during exhalation, opposite of the chest wall's normal motion during breathing.

paramedic: An individual who has extensive training in advanced life support, including endotracheal intubation, emergency pharmacology, cardiac monitoring, and other advanced assessment and treatment skills.

parasympathetic nervous system: A subdivision of the autonomic nervous system, involved in control of involuntary functions, mediated largely by the vagus nerve through the chemical acetylcholine.

parenteral medications: Medications that enter the body by a route other than the digestive tract, skin, or mucous membranes.

parietal bones: The bones that lie between the temporal and occipital regions of the cranium.

parietal lobe: The brain area primarily responsible for processing sensory and spatial information.

parietal pleura: Thin membrane that lines the chest cavity.

paroxysmal nocturnal dyspnea: Severe shortness of breath, especially at night after several hours of reclining; the person is forced to sit up to breathe.

partial pressure: The term used to describe the amount of gas in air or dissolved in fluid, such as blood.

patella: The kneecap; a specialized bone that lies within the tendon of the quadriceps muscle.

patent: Open, clear of obstruction.

pathogen: A microorganism that is capable of causing disease in a susceptible host.

pathophysiology: The study of how normal physiologic processes are affected by disease.

patient-assisted medication: When the EMT assists the patient with the administration of their own medication.

patient care report (PCR): The legal document used to record all patient care activities. This report has direct patient care functions but also administrative and quality control functions. PCRs are also known as *prehospital care reports.*

peak: The point or period when the maximum clinical effect of a drug is achieved.

pectoral girdle: The supporting structure for the arms, which attaches the arms to the axial skeleton. It comprises the clavicles and scapulae; also called the shoulder girdle.

pediatric assessment triangle (PAT): A structured assessment tool used to rapidly form a general impression of the infant or child without touching them; consists of assessing appearance, work of breathing, and circulation to the skin.

pediatrics: A specialized medical practice devoted to the care of the young.

peer-assisted medication: When the EMT administers medication to self or to a partner.

pelvic binder: A device to splint the bony pelvis to reduce hemorrhage from bone ends, venous disruption, and pain.

pelvic girdle: The supporting structure for the legs, which serves to connect the legs to the axial skeleton.

pelvic inflammatory disease (PID): An infection of the fallopian tubes and the surrounding tissues of the pelvis.

penetrating trauma: Injury caused by objects, such as knives and bullets, that pierce the surface of the body and damage internal tissues and organs.

penetrating wound: An injury resulting from a sharp, piercing object.

perfusion: The circulation of oxygenated blood within an organ or tissue in adequate amounts to meet the cells' current needs.

pericardial effusion: A collection of fluid between the pericardial sac and the myocardium.

pericardium: The fibrous sac that surrounds the heart.

perineum: The area of skin between the genitals and the anus.

peripheral nervous system (PNS): The part of the nervous system that consists of 31 pairs of spinal nerves and 12 pairs of cranial nerves; these may be sensory nerves, motor nerves, or connecting nerves.

peristalsis: The wavelike contraction of smooth muscle by which the ureters or other tubular organs propel their contents.

peritoneal cavity: The abdominal cavity.

peritoneum: The membrane lining the abdominal cavity (parietal peritoneum) and covering the abdominal organs (visceral peritoneum).

peritonitis: Inflammation of the peritoneum.

per os (PO): Through the mouth; a medication delivery route; same as oral.

per rectum (PR): Through the rectum; a medication delivery route.

persistency: How long a chemical agent will stay on a surface before it evaporates.

personal protective equipment (PPE): Protective equipment that blocks exposure to a pathogen or a hazardous material.

personal protective equipment (PPE) levels: A means of classifying the amount and type of protective equipment that an individual must use to avoid injury during contact with a hazardous material.

pertinent negatives: Negative findings that warrant no care or intervention.

pertussis (whooping cough): An airborne bacterial infection that affects mostly children younger than 6 years. Patients will be feverish and exhibit a "whoop" sound on inspiration after a coughing attack; highly contagious through droplet infection.

petechiae: Small, flat, purple-red blotches on the skin that do not blanch when pressure is applied; may be seen in individuals with meningococcal infection.

phalanges: The bones of the fingers and toes.

pharmacodynamics: The process by which a medication works on the body.

pharmacokinetics: The processes that the body performs on a medication, including how it is absorbed, distributed, possibly changed, and eliminated.

pharmacology: The study of the properties and effects of medications.

pharynx: A muscular tube that allows air, liquid, and food to pass from the nose or mouth to the lower airways and esophagus; composed of the nasopharynx, oropharynx, and the laryngopharynx; commonly referred to as the throat.

phosgene: A pulmonary agent that is a product of combustion, resulting from a fire at a textile factory or house, or from metalwork or burning Freon. It is a very potent agent that has a delayed onset of symptoms, usually hours.

phosgene oxime (CX): A blistering agent that has a rapid onset of symptoms and produces immediate, intense pain and discomfort on contact.

phrenic nerves: The two nerves that innervate the diaphragm; necessary for adequate breathing to occur.

physiology: The study of the normal functions of living organisms and their parts.

pin-indexing system: A system established for portable cylinders to ensure that a regulator is not connected to a cylinder containing the wrong type of gas.

pinna: The external, visible part of the ear.

placards: Signage required to be placed on all four sides of highway transport vehicles, railroad tank cars, and other forms of hazardous materials transportation; the sign identifies the hazardous contents of the vehicle, using a standardization system with diamond-shaped indicators.

placenta: The tissue attached to the uterine wall that nourishes the fetus through the umbilical cord.

placenta previa: A condition in which the placenta develops over and covers the cervix.

planning: In incident command, the position that ultimately produces a plan to resolve any incident.

plantar: The bottom surface of the foot.

plasma: A sticky, yellow fluid that carries the blood cells and nutrients and transports cellular waste material to the organs of excretion.

platelets: Tiny, disc-shaped elements that are much smaller than the cells; they are essential in the initial formation of a blood clot, the mechanism that stops bleeding.

pleura: The serous membranes covering the lungs and lining the thorax, completely enclosing a potential space known as the pleural space.

pleural effusion: A collection of fluid between the lung and chest wall that may compress the lung.

pleural space: The potential space between the parietal pleura and the visceral pleura; described as "potential" because under normal conditions, the space does not exist.

pleuritic chest pain: Sharp, stabbing pain in the chest that is worsened by a deep breath or other chest wall movement; often caused by inflammation or irritation of the pleura.

pneumonia: An infectious disease of the lung that damages lung tissue.

pneumonic plague: A lung infection, also known as plague pneumonia, that is the result of inhalation of plague-causing bacteria.

pneumothorax: An accumulation of air or gas in the pleural cavity.

point tenderness: Tenderness that is sharply localized at the site of the injury, found by gently palpating along the bone with the tip of one finger.

points of distribution (PODs): Existing facilities used as mass distribution sites for antibiotics, antidotes, vaccinations, and other medications and supplies during an emergency.

poison: A substance whose chemical action could damage structures or impair function when introduced into the body.

polydipsia: Excessive thirst that persists for long periods despite reasonable fluid intake; often the result of excessive urination.

polyphagia: Excessive eating; in diabetes, the inability to use glucose properly can cause a sense of hunger.

polypharmacy: The use of multiple medications on a regular basis.

polyuria: The passage of an unusually large volume of urine in a given period; in diabetes, this can result from the wasting of glucose in the urine.

pons: An organ that lies below the midbrain and above the medulla and contains numerous important nerve fibers, including those for sleep, respiration, and the medullary respiratory center.

poor air exchange: A term used to describe the degree of distress in a patient with a mild airway obstruction. With poor air exchange, the patient often has a weak, ineffective cough, increased difficulty breathing, or possible cyanosis and may produce a high-pitched noise during inhalation (stridor).

portable stretcher: A stretcher with a strong, rectangular, tubular metal frame and rigid fabric stretched across it.

position of function: A hand position in which the wrist is slightly dorsiflexed and all finger joints are moderately flexed.

positional asphyxia: Restriction of chest wall movements and/or airway obstruction; can rapidly lead to sudden death.

postconventional reasoning: A type of reasoning in which a child bases decisions on their conscience.

posterior: The back surface of the body; the side away from you in the standard anatomic position.

posterior tibial artery: The artery just behind the medial malleolus; supplies blood to the foot.

postictal state: The period following a seizure that lasts 5 to 30 minutes; characterized by labored respirations and some degree of altered mental status.

posttraumatic stress disorder (PTSD): A delayed stress reaction to a prior incident. Often the result of one or more unresolved issues concerning the incident, and may relate to an incident that involved physical harm or the threat of physical harm.

potential energy: The product of mass, gravity, and height, which is converted into kinetic energy and results in injury, such as from a fall.

potentially psychologically traumatizing event: Any incident that deeply affects the mental and emotional well-being of an EMS clinician. These events have the potential to cause posttraumatic stress disorder and other mental health conditions.

power grip: A technique in which the stretcher or backboard is gripped by inserting each hand under the handle with the palm facing up and the thumb extended, fully supporting the underside of the handle on the curved palm with the fingers and thumb.

power lift: A lifting technique in which the EMT's back is held upright, with legs bent, and the patient is lifted when the EMT straightens the legs to raise the upper body and arms.

preconventional reasoning: A type of reasoning in which a child acts almost purely to avoid punishment or to get what they want.

preeclampsia: A pregnancy complication that is characterized by new-onset hypertension (systolic blood pressure greater than 140 mm Hg or diastolic blood pressure greater than 90 mm Hg) along with systemic effects, such as blurred vision, headache, or protein in the urine. Differentiated from eclampsia by the lack of seizure activity.

prefix: The part of a term that appears before a word root, changing the meaning of the term.

preload: The precontraction pressure in the heart as the volume of blood builds up.

preoxygenation: The process of providing oxygen, often in combination with ventilation, prior to intubation in order to raise the oxygen levels of body tissues; a critical step in advanced airway management. This extends the time during which an advanced airway can be placed in an apneic patient, because the more oxygen that is available in the alveoli, the longer the patient can maintain adequate gas exchange in the lungs during the procedure.

preschooler: A child age 3 to 6 years.

prescription medications: Medications that are distributed to patients only by pharmacists according to a physician's order.

presentation: The position in which an infant is born; defined by the part of the body that appears first.

primary assessment: A step within the patient assessment process that identifies and initiates treatment of immediate and potential life threats.

primary (direct) injury: An injury to the brain and its associated structures that is a direct result of impact to the head.

primary prevention: Efforts to prevent an injury or illness from ever occurring.

primary triage: A type of patient sorting used to rapidly categorize patients; the focus is on speed in locating all patients and determining an initial priority as their conditions warrant.

primigravida: A person who is experiencing their first pregnancy.

projectile: Any object propelled by force, such as a bullet by a weapon.

prolapse of the umbilical cord: A situation in which the umbilical cord comes out of the vagina before the fetus.

prone: Lying facedown.

prostate gland: A small gland that surrounds the male urethra where it emerges from the urinary bladder; it secretes a fluid that is part of the ejaculatory fluid.

prosthetic device: An externally applied device used to partly or wholly replace an absent or deficient limb segment.

protected health information (PHI): Any information about health status, provision of health care, or payment for health care that can be linked to an individual. This is interpreted rather broadly and includes any part of a patient's medical record or payment history.

proximal: Closer to the trunk.

proximate causation: Proof that a negligent act or lack of action caused an injury or worsened an existing injury.

psychiatric disorder: An illness with psychological or behavioral symptoms and/or impairment in functioning caused by a social, psychological, genetic, physical, chemical, or biologic disturbance.

psychosis: A mental disorder characterized by the loss of contact with reality; may be evidenced by hallucinations and/or delusions.

pubic symphysis: A hard, bony, and cartilaginous prominence found at the midline in the lowermost portion of the abdomen where the two halves of the pelvic ring are joined by cartilage at a joint with minimal motion.

pubis: One of three bones that fuse to form the pelvic ring.

public health: The branch of medicine that is focused on examining the health needs of entire populations with the goal of preventing health problems.

public information officer (PIO): In incident command, the person who keeps the public informed and relates any information to the media.

public safety access point (PSAP): A call center, staffed by trained personnel who are responsible for managing requests for police, fire, and ambulance services.

pulmonary artery: The major artery leading from the right ventricle of the heart to the lungs; carries oxygen-poor blood.

pulmonary blast injuries: Pulmonary trauma resulting from short-range exposure to the detonation of explosives.

pulmonary circulation: The flow of blood from the right ventricle through the pulmonary arteries and all of their branches and capillaries in the lungs and back to the left atrium through the venules and pulmonary veins; also called the lesser circulation.

pulmonary contusion: Injury or bruising of lung tissue that results in hemorrhage.

pulmonary edema: A buildup of fluid in the lungs, often as a result of heart failure.

pulmonary embolism: A condition in which a blood clot (embolus) breaks off from a large vein and travels to the blood vessels of the lung, causing obstruction of blood flow.

pulmonary veins: The four veins that return oxygenated blood from the lungs to the left atrium of the heart.

pulse: The wave of pressure created as the heart contracts and forces blood out the left ventricle and into the major arteries.

pulse oximetry: An assessment tool that measures oxygen saturation of hemoglobin in the capillary beds.

pulse pressure: The difference between the systolic and diastolic pressures.

punitive damages: Damages that are sometimes awarded in a civil lawsuit when the conduct of the defendant was intentional or constituted a reckless disregard for the safety of the public.

pupil: The circular opening in the middle of the iris that admits light to the back of the eye.

putrefaction: Decomposition of body tissues; a definitive sign of death.

quadrants: The sections of the abdominal cavity; a descriptive tool in which two imaginary lines intersect at the umbilicus, dividing the abdomen into four equal areas.

quality assurance (QA): A reactive process that involves monitoring compliance against a standard to identify problems that have already occurred.

quality improvement (QI): A proactive process that involves making changes to a system to improve performance.

rabid: Infected with the rabies virus.

raccoon eyes: Bruising under the eyes that may indicate a skull fracture.

radial artery: The major artery in the forearm; it is palpable at the wrist on the thumb side.

radiation: The transfer of heat to colder objects in the environment by radiant energy; for example, heat gain from a fire.

radioactive material: Any material that emits radiation.

radiologic dispersal device (RDD): Any container that is designed to disperse radioactive material.

radius: The bone on the thumb side of the forearm.

rape: A term often used in a legal context to refer to the crime of sexual penetration without consent; rape is a form of sexual assault, but not all sexual assaults are rape.

rapid extrication technique: A technique to move a patient from a sitting position inside a vehicle to supine on a backboard in less than 1 minute when conditions do not allow for standard methods of spinal motion restriction.

rapport: A trusting relationship that clinicians build with their patients.

reassessment: A step within the patient assessment process performed at regular intervals during the assessment process to identify and treat changes in a patient's condition. A patient in unstable condition should be reassessed every 5 minutes, whereas a patient in stable condition should be reassessed every 15 minutes.

recovery position: A side-lying position used to maintain a clear airway in unresponsive patients who are breathing adequately and do not have suspected injuries to the spine, hips, or pelvis.

rectum: The lowermost end of the colon.

red blood cells: Cells that carry oxygen to the body's tissues; also called erythrocytes.

reduce: To return a dislocated joint or fractured bone to its normal position; to set.

referred pain: Pain felt in an area of the body other than the area where the cause of pain is located.

rehabilitation area: The area that provides protection and treatment to firefighters and other responders working at an emergency. Here, workers are medically monitored and receive any needed care as they enter and leave the scene.

rehabilitation supervisor: In incident command, the person who establishes an area that provides protection for responders from the elements and the situation.

renal pelvis: A cone-shaped area that collects urine from the kidneys and funnels it through the ureter into the bladder.

repeater: A special base station radio that receives messages and signals on one frequency and then automatically retransmits them on a second frequency.

rescue supervisor: In incident command, the person appointed to determine the type of equipment and resources needed for a situation involving extrication or special rescue; also called the extrication officer.

residual volume: The air that remains in the lungs after maximal expiration.

resilience: The capacity of an individual to cope with and recover from distress.

res ipsa loquitur: A legal principle stating that a defendant may be held liable without direct evidence if they had exclusive control over the cause of harm, the injured person played no role in the harm, and the harm would not have occurred without negligent conduct.

respiration: The inhaling and exhaling of air; the physiologic process that exchanges carbon dioxide from fresh air.

respiratory arrest: Complete cessation of breathing (apnea) or agonal gasps that will lead to cardiac arrest if intervention does not occur immediately.

respiratory compromise: The inability of the body to move gas effectively.

respiratory distress: A condition marked by difficulty breathing and an abnormal respiratory rate or effort; can range from mild to severe and can progress to respiratory failure.

respiratory failure: A condition in which oxygen levels are too low to meet the body's needs and ventilation is impaired, leading to high carbon dioxide levels; accompanied by serious signs and symptoms and must be corrected quickly.

respiratory syncytial virus (RSV): A virus that causes an infection of the lungs and breathing passages; can lead to other serious illnesses that affect the lungs or heart, such as bronchiolitis and pneumonia; it is highly contagious and spread through droplets.

respiratory system: All the structures of the body that contribute to the process of breathing, consisting of the upper and lower airways and their component parts.

responsiveness: The way in which a patient responds to external stimuli, including verbal stimuli (sound), tactile stimuli (touch), and painful stimuli.

reticular activating system (RAS): Located in the upper brainstem; responsible for maintenance of consciousness, specifically one's level of arousal.

retina: The light-sensitive area of the eye where images are projected; a layer of cells at the back of the eye that changes the light image into electric impulses, which are carried by the optic nerve to the brain.

retinal detachment: Separation of the retina from its attachments at the back of the eye.

retractions: Movements in which the skin pulls in around the ribs during inspiration.

retrograde amnesia: The inability to remember events leading up to a head injury.

retroperitoneal: Behind the abdominal cavity.

retroperitoneal space: The space between the abdominal cavity and the posterior abdominal wall, containing the kidneys, certain large vessels, and parts of the gastrointestinal tract.

retroperitoneum: The potential space located posterior to the peritoneal cavity of the abdomen.

return of spontaneous circulation (ROSC): The return of a pulse and effective blood flow to the body in a patient who previously was in cardiac arrest.

reverse triage: A triage process used in treating multiple victims of a lightning strike, in which efforts are focused on those who are in respiratory and cardiac arrest. Reverse triage is different from conventional triage, where such patients would be classified as deceased.

Revised Trauma Score (RTS): A scoring system used for patients with head trauma.

rhonchi: Coarse, low-pitched breath sounds heard in patients with chronic mucus in the upper airways.

ricin: A neurotoxin derived from mash that is left over from processing castor beans; causes pulmonary edema and respiratory and circulatory failure leading to death.

rigor mortis: Stiffening of the body muscles; a definitive sign of death.

rooting reflex: An infant reflex that occurs when something touches an infant's cheek, and the infant instinctively turns their head toward the touch.

route of exposure: The manner by which a toxic substance enters the body.

rule of nines: A system that assigns percentages to sections of the body, allowing calculation of the amount of skin surface involved in the burn area.

sacroiliac joint: The connection point between the pelvis and the vertebral column.

sacrum: One of three bones (the others being the two pelvic bones) that make up the pelvic ring; consists of five fused sacral vertebrae.

safe zone: An area of protection providing safety from the danger zone (hot zone).

safety data sheet (SDS): A form, provided by manufacturers and compounders (blenders) of chemicals, containing information about chemical composition, physical and chemical properties, health and safety hazards, emergency response, and waste disposal of a specific material; also known as material safety data sheet (MSDS).

safety officer: In incident command, the person who monitors the scene for conditions or operations that may present a hazard to responders and patients; this person may stop an operation when responder safety is an issue.

sagittal (lateral) plane: An imaginary line where the body is divided into left and right parts.

salivary glands: The glands that produce saliva to keep the mouth and pharynx moist.

SAMPLE history: A brief history of a patient's condition to determine Signs and symptoms, Allergies, Medications, Pertinent past history, Last known status, and Events leading to the injury or illness.

sarin (GB): A nerve agent that is one of the G agents; a highly volatile colorless and odorless liquid that turns from liquid to gas within seconds to minutes at room temperature.

scald burn: A burn caused by hot liquids.

scalp: The thick skin covering the cranium, which usually bears hair.

scanner: A radio receiver that searches or scans across several frequencies until the message is completed; the process is then repeated.

scapula: The shoulder blade.

scene size-up: A step within the patient assessment process that involves a quick assessment of the scene and the surroundings to provide information about scene safety and the mechanism of injury or nature of illness before you enter and begin patient care.

schizophrenia: A complex, difficult-to-identify mental disorder whose onset typically occurs during early adulthood. Symptoms typically become more prominent over time and include delusions, hallucinations, a lack of interest in pleasure, and erratic speech.

school age: A person who is 6 to 12 years of age.

sciatic nerve: The major nerve to the lower extremities; controls much of muscle function in the leg and sensation in most of the leg and foot.

sclera: The tough, fibrous, white portion of the eye that protects the more delicate inner structures.

scoop stretcher: A stretcher that is designed to be split into two or four sections that can be fitted around a patient who is lying on the ground or other relatively flat surface.

scope of practice: A formal definition of the care that the EMT is authorized and expected to provide for a patient; most commonly defined by state law.

sebaceous glands: Glands that produce an oily substance called sebum, which discharges along the shafts of the hairs.

secondary assessment: A step within the patient assessment process in which a systematic physical examination of the patient is performed. The examination may be a systematic exam or an assessment that focuses on a certain area or region of the body, often determined through the chief complaint.

secondary containment: An engineered method to control spilled or released product if the main containment vessel fails.

secondary device: A secondary explosive used by terrorists, set to explode after the initial bomb.

secondary (indirect) injury: The aftereffects of the primary injury; includes abnormal processes such as cerebral edema, increased intracranial pressure, cerebral ischemia and hypoxia, and infection; onset is often delayed following the primary brain injury.

secondary prevention: Efforts to limit the effects of an injury or illness that has already occurred.

secondary triage: A type of patient sorting used in the treatment area that involves retriage of patients.

sedative: A substance that decreases activity and excitement.

seizure: A neurologic episode caused by a surge of electrical activity in the brain; can be a convulsion characterized by generalized, uncoordinated muscular activity, and can be associated with loss of consciousness.

self-contained breathing apparatus (SCBA): A respirator with an independent air supply used by firefighters to enter toxic and otherwise dangerous atmospheres.

semen: Fluid ejaculated from the penis and containing sperm.

seminal vesicles: Storage sacs for sperm and seminal fluid, which empty into the urethra at the prostate.

sensitization: Developing a sensitivity to a substance that initially caused no allergic reaction.

sensorineural deafness: A permanent lack of hearing caused by a lesion or damage of the inner ear.

sensory nerves: The nerves that carry sensations such as touch, taste, smell, heat, cold, and pain from the body to the central nervous system.

septic shock: Shock caused by severe infection, usually a bacterial infection.

severe airway obstruction: Occurs when a foreign body completely obstructs the patient's airway. The patient cannot breathe, talk, or cough.

sexual assault: The act of subjecting a person to sexual contact or behavior without the person's explicit consent.

sexual orientation: A person's emotional, romantic, or sexual attraction to other people.

shaken baby syndrome: A syndrome seen in abused infants and children; the patient has been subjected to violent, whiplash-type shaking injuries inflicted by the abusing individual that may cause coma, seizures, and increased intracranial pressure due to tearing of the cerebral veins with consequent bleeding into the brain.

shallow respirations: Respirations characterized by little movement of the chest wall (reduced tidal volume) or poor chest excursion.

shared decision making: A collaborative process in which the clinician works with the patient to come up with the optimal health care approach, accounting for the patient's unique situation, concerns, and values.

shock: A condition in which the circulatory system fails to provide sufficient circulation to maintain normal cellular functions; also called hypoperfusion.

shunts: Tubes that drain excess cerebrospinal fluid from the brain to another part of the body outside of the brain, such as the abdomen; lowers pressure in the brain.

sickle cell disease: A hereditary disease that causes normal, round red blood cells to become oblong, or sickle shaped.

sign: Objective finding that can be seen, heard, felt, smelled, or measured.

simple access: Entry that is easily achieved without the use of tools or force.

simple pneumothorax: Any pneumothorax that is free from significant physiologic changes and does not cause drastic changes in the vital signs of the patient.

simplex: Single-frequency radio; transmissions can occur in either direction but not simultaneously; when one party transmits, the other can only receive, and the party that is transmitting is unable to receive.

single command system: A command system in which one person is in charge; generally used with small incidents that involve only one responding agency or one jurisdiction.

situational awareness: A state of sustained knowledge and understanding of one's surroundings and of potential risks to the safety of the patient or EMS team.

size-up: The ongoing process of information gathering and scene evaluation to determine appropriate strategies and tactics to manage an emergency.

skeletal muscle: Muscle that is attached to bones and usually crosses at least one joint; striated, or voluntary, muscle.

skeletal system: The framework of the body, composed of bones and other connective tissues, that supports and protects internal organs and other body tissues.

slander: False and damaging information about a person that is communicated by spoken word.

sling: A bandage or material that helps to support the weight of an injured upper extremity.

small intestine: The portion of the digestive tube between the stomach and the cecum, consisting of the duodenum, jejunum, and ileum.

smallpox: A highly contagious viral disease; it is most contagious when blisters begin to form.

small-volume nebulizer: A respiratory device that holds liquid medicine that is turned into a fine mist. The patient inhales the medication into the airways and lungs as a treatment for conditions such as asthma.

smooth muscle: Involuntary muscle; it constitutes the bulk of the gastrointestinal tract and is present in nearly every organ to regulate automatic activity.

sniffing position: An upright position in which the patient's head and chin are thrust slightly forward to keep the airway open.

social drivers of health: The conditions in which people live, including the forces and systems shaping their daily lives.

solid organs: Solid masses of tissue where much of the chemical work of the body takes place (eg, liver, spleen, pancreas, kidneys).

solution: A liquid mixture that cannot be separated by filtering or allowing the mixture to stand.

soman (GD): A nerve agent that is one of the G agents; twice as persistent as sarin and five times as lethal; it has a fruity odor as a result of the type of alcohol used in the agent, and is a contact and an inhalation hazard that can enter the body through skin absorption and through the respiratory tract.

somatic nervous system: The part of the nervous system that regulates activities over which there is voluntary control.

span of control: In incident command, the subordinate positions under the commander's direction to which the workload is distributed; the ideal supervisor/worker ratio is one supervisor for five subordinates.

Special Atomic Demolition Munitions (SADM): Small suitcase-size nuclear weapons that were designed to destroy individual targets, such as important buildings, bridges, tunnels, and large ships.

special weapons and tactics (SWAT) team: A law enforcement tactical unit with specialized training in situations involving armed conflict and potential violence.

sphenoid bone: A bone in the skull that helps connect the neurocranium (the portion of the skull that protects the brain and sensory organs) to the facial skeleton.

sphincters: Muscles arranged in circles that are able to decrease the diameter of tubes. Examples are found within the rectum, bladder, and blood vessels.

sphygmomanometer: A device used to measure blood pressure.

spina bifida: A developmental defect in which a portion of the spinal cord or meninges may protrude outside of the vertebrae and possibly even outside of the body, usually at the lower third of the spine in the lumbar area.

spinal cord: An extension of the brain, composed of virtually all the nerves carrying messages between the brain and the rest of the body. It lies inside of and is protected by the spinal canal.

spinal motion restriction (SMR): Patient positioning and moving techniques that minimize unwanted movement of the potentially injured spine.

spleen: A solid lymphatic organ located in the left upper quadrant of the abdomen.

splint: A flexible or rigid device used to protect and maintain the position of an injured extremity.

spontaneous abortion: The loss of a pregnancy prior to 20 weeks of gestation without any preceding surgical or medical intervention. Often called a miscarriage.

spontaneous respirations: Breathing that occurs without assistance.

spotter: A person who assists a driver in backing up an ambulance to help adjust for blind spots at the back of the vehicle.

sprain: A joint injury involving damage to supporting ligaments, and sometimes partial or temporary dislocation of bone ends.

staging supervisor: In incident command, the person who locates an area to stage equipment and personnel and tracks unit arrival and deployment from the staging area.

stair chair: A lightweight folding device that is used to carry an alert, seated patient up or down stairs.

standard of care: Accepted levels of emergency care expected by reason of training and profession; written by legal or professional organizations so that patients are not exposed to unreasonable risk or harm.

standard precautions: Protective measures that have traditionally been developed by the Centers for Disease Control and Prevention (CDC) for use in dealing with objects, blood, body fluids, and other potential exposure risks of communicable disease.

standing orders: Written documents, signed by the EMS system's medical director, that outline specific directions, permissions, and sometimes prohibitions regarding patient care; also called *protocols*.

Star of Life: The six-pointed star emblem that identifies vehicles that meet federal specifications as licensed or certified ambulances.

START triage: A patient sorting process that stands for Simple Triage And Rapid Treatment and uses a limited assessment of the patient's ability to walk, respiratory status, hemodynamic status, and neurologic status.

state-sponsored terrorism: Terrorism that is funded and/or supported by nations that hold close ties with terrorist groups.

status asthmaticus: An emergency that occurs when standard treatments fail to relieve asthma symptoms, resulting in acute respiratory failure.

status epilepticus: A condition in which seizures recur every few minutes or last longer than 30 minutes.

statute of limitations: The time within which a case must be commenced.

steam burn: A burn caused by exposure to hot steam.

sterilization: A process, such as heating, that removes microbial contamination.

sternocleidomastoid muscles: The muscles on either side of the neck that allow movement of the head.

sternum: The breastbone.

stimulant: An agent that produces an excited state.

stoma: An opening through the skin and into an organ or other structure.

strain: Stretching or tearing of a muscle and/or tendon; also called a muscle pull.

strangulation: Complete obstruction of blood circulation in a given organ as a result of compression or entrapment; an emergency situation causing death of tissue.

stratum corneum: The outermost or dead layer of the skin.

stridor: A harsh, high-pitched, respiratory sound, generally heard during inspiration, that is caused by partial blockage or narrowing of the upper airway; may be audible without a stethoscope.

stroke: An interruption of blood flow to the brain that results in the loss of brain function; also called a cerebrovascular accident (CVA).

stroke volume: The volume of blood pumped forward with each ventricular contraction.

structure fire: A fire in a house, apartment building, office, school, plant, warehouse, or other building.

subarachnoid hemorrhage: Bleeding into the subarachnoid space, where the cerebrospinal fluid circulates.

subcutaneous emphysema: A crackling sensation felt on palpation of the skin indicating that air has become trapped beneath the skin.

subcutaneous injection: Injection into the fatty tissue between the skin and muscle; a medication delivery route.

subcutaneous tissue: Tissue, largely fat, that lies directly under the dermis and serves as an insulator of the body.

subdural hematoma: An accumulation of blood beneath the dura mater but outside the brain.

sublingual (SL): Under the tongue; a medication delivery route.

substance misuse: The use of any substance in a manner other than its intended design to produce a desired effect.

substance use disorders (SUDs): Chronic, treatable medical conditions characterized by the uncontrolled use of substances such as alcohol, opioids, stimulants, or other drugs, despite harmful consequences.

sucking chest wound: An open or penetrating chest wall wound through which air passes during inspiration and expiration, creating a sucking sound. See also *open pneumothorax*.

sucking reflex: An infant reflex in which the infant starts sucking when their lips are stroked.

suction catheter: A hollow, cylindrical device used to remove fluid from the patient's airway.

sudden unexpected infant death (SUID): A sudden unexpected death of a child younger than 1 year where the cause is either known or not known after investigation.

suffix: The part of a term that comes after the word root, at the end of the term.

sulfur mustard (H): A vesicant; it is a brown-yellow oily substance that is generally considered very persistent; has the distinct smell of garlic or mustard and, when released, is quickly absorbed into the skin and/or mucous membranes and begins an irreversible process of damaging the cells. Also called mustard gas.

superficial: Closer to or on the skin.

superficial burns: Burns that affect only the epidermis, characterized by skin that is red/darker but not blistered or actually burned through; also referred to as first-degree burns.

superficial partial-thickness burns: Burns that affect the epidermis and some portion of the dermis but not the subcutaneous tissue, characterized by blisters and skin that is discolored (ranging from lighter to red/darker compared to baseline skin color), moist, and mottled. Partial-thickness burns are also referred to as second-degree burns.

superior: Above a body part or nearer to the head.

superior vena cava: One of the two largest veins in the body; carries blood from the upper extremities, head, neck, and chest into the heart.

supine: Lying faceup.

supine hypotensive syndrome: Low blood pressure resulting from compression of the inferior vena cava by the weight of the pregnant uterus when the person is supine.

surfactant: A liquid protein substance that coats the alveoli in the lungs, decreases alveolar surface tension, and keeps the alveoli expanded; a low level in a premature infant contributes to respiratory distress syndrome.

surrogate decision maker: A person authorized to make health care decisions on behalf of a patient when the patient lacks decision-making capacity.

suspension: A mixture of ground particles that are distributed evenly throughout a liquid but do not dissolve.

sutures: Fibrous joints that connect the unfused cranial bones after birth.

swathe: A bandage that passes around the chest to secure an injured arm to the chest.

sweat glands: The glands that secrete sweat, located in the dermal layer of the skin.

sympathetic nervous system: The part of the autonomic nervous system that controls active functions such as responding to fear (also known as the fight-or-flight system).

symphyses: Joints that have grown together to form a very stable connection.

symptom: Subjective finding that the patient feels but that can be identified only by the patient.

symptomatic hyperglycemia: A hyperglycemic state resulting from several problems, including ketoacidosis, dehydration because of excessive urination, and hyperglycemia.

symptomatic hypoglycemia: Severe hypoglycemia resulting in changes in mental status.

syncope: A fainting spell or transient loss of consciousness.

syndromic surveillance: The monitoring, usually by local or state health departments, of patients presenting to emergency departments and alternative care facilities, the recording of EMS call volume, and the use of over-the-counter medications.

synovial fluid: The small amount of liquid within a joint used as lubrication.

synovial membrane: The lining of a joint that secretes synovial fluid into the joint space.

systemic circulation: The portion of the circulatory system outside of the heart and lungs.

systemic vascular resistance (SVR): The resistance that blood must overcome to be able to move within the blood vessels; related to the amount of dilation or constriction in the blood vessel.

systole: The contraction, or period of contraction, of the heart, especially that of the ventricles.

systolic pressure: The increased pressure in an artery with each contraction of the ventricles (systole).

tabun (GA): A nerve agent that is one of the G agents; 36 times more persistent than sarin and approximately one-half as lethal; has a fruity smell and is unique because the components used to manufacture the agent are easy to acquire and the agent is easy to manufacture.

tachycardia: A rapid heart rate, more than 100 beats/min.

tachypnea: Rapid respiratory rate.

tactical situation: A hostage, robbery, or other situation in which armed conflict is threatened or shots have been fired and the threat of violence remains.

talus: The bone that forms the lower portion of the ankle.

tarsals: The group of bones situated between the lower leg bones (ie, tibia and fibula) and the metatarsal bones of the foot.

team: In the context of EMS, a group of health care clinicians who are assigned specific roles and are working interdependently in a coordinated manner under a designated leader.

team leader: The team member who provides role assignments, coordination, oversight, centralized decision making, and support for the team to accomplish their goals and achieve desired results.

technical rescue group: A team of emergency responders from one or more departments in a region who are trained and on call for certain types of technical rescue.

technical rescue situation: A rescue that requires special technical skills and equipment in one of many specialized rescue areas, such as technical rope rescue, cave rescue, and dive rescue.

telemetry: A process in which electronic signals are converted into coded, audible signals; these signals can then be transmitted by radio or telephone to a receiver with a decoder at the hospital.

temporal bones: The lateral bones on each side of the cranium; the temples.

temporal lobe: The brain area primarily responsible for taste, hearing, and the ability to understand words.

temporomandibular joint: The joint formed where the mandible and cranium meet, just in front of the ear.

tendons: The fibrous connective tissues that attach muscle to bone.

tension pneumothorax: An accumulation of air or gas in the pleural cavity that progressively increases pressure in the chest and that interferes with cardiac function, with potentially fatal results.

term gestation: A pregnancy that is at term, between 39 weeks and 40 weeks, 6 days.

termination of command: The end of the incident command structure when an incident draws to a close.

terrorism: A violent and unlawful act dangerous to human life intended to intimidate or coerce a government, the civilian population, or any segment thereof, in furtherance of political or social objectives.

testicle: A male genital gland that contains specialized cells that produce hormones and sperm.

therapeutic communication: Verbal and nonverbal communication techniques that encourage patients to express their feelings and to achieve a positive relationship.

therapeutic effect: The desired or intended effect a medication is expected to have on the body.

thermal burn: A burn caused by heat.

thoracic cage: The chest or rib cage.

thoracic spine: The 12 vertebrae that lie between the cervical vertebrae and the lumbar vertebrae. One pair of ribs is attached to each of these vertebrae.

thorax: The chest cavity that contains the heart, lungs, esophagus, and great vessels.

thromboembolism: A blood clot that has formed within a blood vessel and is floating within the bloodstream.

thrombophilia: A tendency toward the development of blood clots as a result of an abnormality of the system of coagulation.

thrombosis: A condition in which a blood clot, either in the arterial or venous system, forms at the site of a damaged blood vessel (referred to as a thrombus) and obstructs blood flow.

thyroid cartilage: A firm prominence of cartilage that forms the upper part of the larynx; the Adam's apple.

tibia: The shinbone; the larger of the two bones of the lower leg.

tidal volume: The amount of air (in milliliters) that is moved into or out of the lungs during one breath.

toddler: A child age 1 to 3 years.

tolerance: The need for increasing amounts of a drug to obtain the same effect.

tonsil tips: Large, semi-rigid suction tips recommended for suctioning the pharynx.

topical medications: Lotions, creams, and ointments that are applied to the surface of the skin and affect only that area; a medication delivery route.

topographic anatomy: The superficial landmarks of the body that serve as guides to the structures that lie beneath them.

torts: Wrongful acts that give rise to a civil lawsuit.

tourniquet: The bleeding control method used when a wound continues to bleed despite the use of direct pressure; useful if a patient is bleeding severely from a partial or complete amputation.

toxicity levels: A means of classifying the risk that a hazardous material poses to the health of an individual who comes into contact with it.

toxicology: The study of toxic or poisonous substances.

toxidrome: A collection of signs and symptoms associated with a class of poison; aids in the identification of certain toxins.

toxin: A poison or harmful substance.

trachea: The windpipe; the main trunk for air passing to and from the lungs.

tracheostomy: A surgical procedure to create an opening (stoma) into the trachea; a stoma in the neck connects the trachea directly to the skin.

tracheostomy tube: A plastic tube placed within the tracheostomy site (stoma).

traction: Longitudinal force applied to a structure.

trade name: The brand name that a manufacturer gives a medication; the name is capitalized.

tragus: The small, rounded, fleshy bulge that lies immediately anterior to the ear canal.

trajectory: The path a projectile takes once it is propelled.

transdermal (transcutaneous): Through the skin; a medication delivery route.

transient ischemic attack (TIA): A disorder of the brain in which brain cells temporarily stop functioning because of insufficient oxygen, causing strokelike symptoms that resolve completely within 24 hours of onset.

transmission: The way in which an infectious disease is spread: contact, airborne, by vehicles, or by vectors.

transportation area: The area in a mass-casualty incident where ambulances and crews are organized to transport patients from the treatment area to receiving hospitals.

transportation supervisor: In incident command, the person in charge of the transportation sector in a mass-casualty incident who assigns patients from the treatment area to waiting ambulances in the transportation area.

transverse (axial) plane: An imaginary line where the body is divided into top and bottom parts.

trauma emergencies: Emergencies that are the result of physical forces applied to the body; injuries.

trauma score: A score calculated from 1 to 16, with 16 being the best possible score. It relates to the likelihood of patient survival with the exception of a severe head injury. It takes into account the Glasgow Coma Scale (GCS) score, respiratory rate, respiratory expansion, systolic blood pressure, and capillary refill.

traumatic asphyxia: A pattern of injuries seen after a severe force is applied to the chest, forcing blood from the great vessels back into the head and neck.

traumatic brain injury (TBI): Physical damage to the brain caused by an external force; can result in cognitive, movement, communication, behavioral, and emotional changes.

treatment area: The location in a mass-casualty incident where patients are brought after being triaged and assigned a priority, where they are reassessed, treated, and monitored until transport to the hospital.

treatment supervisor: In incident command, the person who is in charge of and directs EMS clinicians at the treatment area in a mass-casualty incident.

triage: The process of sorting patients based on the severity of injury and medical need to establish treatment and transportation priorities.

triage supervisor: In incident command, the person in charge of the incident command triage sector who directs the sorting of patients into triage categories in a mass-casualty incident.

triceps: The muscle in the back of the upper arm.

tripod position: An upright position in which the patient leans forward onto outstretched arms with the head and chin thrust slightly forward.

trunking: Telecommunication systems that allow a computer to maximize use of a group of frequencies.

trust versus mistrust: The stage of development from birth to approximately 18 months of age, during which infants gain trust in their parents or caregivers if their world is planned, organized, and routine.

tuberculosis: A chronic bacterial disease, caused by *Mycobacterium tuberculosis*, that usually affects the lungs but can also affect other organs such as the brain and kidneys; it is spread by cough and can lie dormant in a person's lungs for decades and then reactivate.

tunica media: The middle and thickest layer of tissue of a blood vessel wall, composed of elastic tissue and smooth muscle cells that allow the vessel to expand or contract in response to changes in blood pressure and tissue demand.

turbinates: Layers of bone within the nasal cavity.

turgor: The ability of the skin to resist deformation; tested by gently pinching skin on the forehead or back of the hand.

two- to three-word dyspnea: A severe breathing problem in which a patient can speak only two to three words at a time without pausing to take a breath.

tympanic membrane: The eardrum; a thin, semitransparent membrane in the middle ear that transmits sound vibrations to the internal ear by means of auditory ossicles.

type 1 diabetes: An autoimmune disorder in which the individual's immune system produces antibodies to the pancreatic beta cells, and therefore the pancreas cannot produce insulin; onset in early childhood is common.

type 2 diabetes: A condition in which insulin resistance develops in response to increased blood glucose levels; can be managed by exercise and diet modification, but is often managed by medications.

UHF (ultra-high frequency): Radio frequencies between 300 and 3,000 MHz.

ulna: The inner bone of the forearm, on the side opposite the thumb.

umbilical cord: The structure that connects the pregnant person to the fetus via the placenta; contains two arteries and one vein.

umbilicus: The navel; also called the belly button.

unconscious bias: Beliefs that a person holds about others that are not based on fact or objectively analyzed experiences and that the person is not consciously aware of holding.

unexplained sudden death in infancy (USDI): Death of an infant or young child that remains unexplained after a complete autopsy; also called sudden infant death syndrome (SIDS).

unified command system: A command system used in larger incidents in which there is a multiagency response or multiple jurisdictions are involved.

unintended effects: Actions that are undesirable but pose little risk to the patient.

untoward effects: Actions that can be harmful to the patient.

uremia: Severe kidney failure resulting in the buildup of waste products within the blood. Eventually, brain functions will be impaired.

ureter: A small, hollow tube that carries urine from the kidneys to the bladder.

urethra: The canal that conveys urine from the bladder to outside the body.

urinary bladder: A sac behind the pubic symphysis made of smooth muscle that collects and stores urine.

urinary system: The organs that control the discharge of certain waste materials filtered from the blood and excreted as urine.

urinary tract infection (UTI): An infection, usually of the lower urinary tract (urethra and bladder), that occurs when normal flora bacteria enter the urethra and grow.

urostomy: A surgical procedure to create an opening (stoma) that connects the urinary system to the surface of the skin and allows urine to drain through the abdominal wall.

urticaria: Small areas of generalized itching and/or burning that appear as multiple raised areas on the skin; also known as hives.

uterus: The muscular organ where the fetus grows, also called the womb; responsible for contractions during labor.

$\dot{V}/\dot{Q}$ ratio: A measurement that examines how much gas is being moved effectively and how much blood is flowing around the alveoli where gas exchange (perfusion) occurs.

V agent (VX): One of the G agents; it is a clear, oily agent that has no odor and looks like baby oil; more than 100 times more lethal than sarin and extremely persistent.

vagina: The outermost cavity of a woman's reproductive tract; the lower part of the birth canal.

vancomycin-resistant enterococci (VRE): A bacterium that is normally present in the human intestines and the female reproductive tract, but which can cause infection and which is resistant to the antibiotic vancomycin.

vapor hazard: The term used to describe danger posed by an agent that enters the body through the respiratory tract.

vasoconstriction: The narrowing of a blood vessel, such as with hypoperfusion or cold extremities.

vasoocclusive crisis: Ischemia and pain caused by sickle-shaped red blood cells that obstruct blood flow to a portion of the body.

vector-borne transmission: The use of an animal to spread an organism from one person or place to another.

veins: The blood vessels that carry blood from the tissues to the heart.

vented chest seal: An occlusive dressing designed to allow air to escape through the dressing but not be drawn back in.

ventilation: The exchange of air between the lungs and the environment; occurs spontaneously by the patient or with assistance from another person, such as an EMT.

ventral: The anterior surface of the body.

ventricle: One of the two lower chambers of the heart.

ventricular fibrillation (VF): Disorganized, ineffective quivering of the ventricles, resulting in no blood flow and a state of cardiac arrest.

ventricular tachycardia (VT): A rapid heart rhythm in which the electrical impulse begins in the ventricle (instead of the atria), which may result in inadequate blood flow and eventually deteriorate into cardiac arrest.

venules: Very small, thin-walled blood vessels.

vernix caseosa: A white, cheesy substance that covers the body of the fetus.

vertebrae: The bones of the vertebral column.

vertebral column: The structure formed by the 33 vertebrae, separated by intervertebral disks. It houses and protects the spinal cord; also called the spinal column.

vertex presentation: A delivery in which the head of the newborn comes out first.

vesicants: Blister agents; the primary route of entry for such agents is through the skin.

vesicular breath sounds: Normal breath sounds made by air moving into and out of the alveoli.

VHF (very high frequency): Radio frequencies between 30 and 300 MHz; the VHF spectrum is further divided into high and low bands.

video laryngoscopy: Visualization of the vocal cords, and thereby placement of the endotracheal tube, that is facilitated by use of a video camera and monitor.

viral hemorrhagic fevers: A group of diseases caused by viruses that include the Ebola, Rift Valley, and yellow fevers, among others. This group of viruses causes the blood in the body to seep out from the tissues and blood vessels.

virulence: The strength or ability of a pathogen to produce disease.

viruses: Germs that require a living host to multiply and survive.

visceral pleura: Thin membrane that covers the lungs.

vital capacity: The amount of air that can be forcibly expelled from the lungs after breathing in as deeply as possible.

vital signs: The key signs that are used to evaluate the patient's overall condition, including respirations, pulse, blood pressure, level of consciousness, and skin characteristics.

vocal cords: Thin white bands of tough muscular tissue that are lateral borders of the glottis and serve as the primary center for speech production.

volatility: How long a chemical agent will stay on a surface before it evaporates.

voluntary activities: Actions that we consciously perform, in which sensory input or conscious thought determines a specific muscular activity.

voluntary muscle: Muscle that is under direct voluntary control of the brain and can be contracted or relaxed at will; skeletal, or striated, muscle.

warm zone: The area located between the hot zone and the cold zone at a hazardous materials incident. The decontamination corridor is located in this zone.

weapon of mass casualty (WMC): Any agent designed to bring about mass death, casualties, and/or massive damage to property and infrastructure (bridges, tunnels, airports, and seaports); also known as a weapon of mass destruction (WMD).

weapon of mass destruction (WMD): Any agent designed to bring about mass death, casualties, and/or massive damage to property and infrastructure (bridges, tunnels, airports, and seaports); also known as a weapon of mass casualty (WMC).

weaponization: The creation of a weapon from a biologic agent that is generally found in nature and that causes disease; the agent is cultivated, synthesized, and/or mutated to maximize the target population's exposure to the germ.

wellness: The active pursuit of a state of good health.

wheal: A raised, swollen, well-defined area on the skin resulting from an insect bite or allergic reaction.

wheeled ambulance stretcher: A specially designed stretcher that can be rolled along the ground. A collapsible undercarriage allows it to be loaded into the ambulance; also called an ambulance stretcher.

wheezing: A high-pitched, whistling breath sound that is most prominent on expiration, and which suggests an obstruction or narrowing of the lower airways; occurs in asthma and bronchiolitis.

white blood cells: Blood cells that have a role in the body's immune defense mechanisms against infection; also called leukocytes.

word root: The main part of a term that contains the primary meaning.

work of breathing: An indicator of oxygenation and ventilation; reflects the patient's attempt to compensate for hypoxia.

xiphoid process: The narrow, cartilaginous lower tip of the sternum.

zone of injury: The area of potentially damaged soft tissue, adjacent nerves, and blood vessels surrounding an injury to a bone or a joint.

zygomas: The quadrangular bones of the cheek, articulating with the frontal bone, the maxillae, the zygomatic processes of the temporal bone, and the great wings of the sphenoid bone.

Index

Note: Locators followed by the letter '*f*' and '*t*' refer to figures and tables respectively.

A

abandonment, 80, 91
abbreviations, medical terminology, 155–156
ABCs assessment, 332
abdominal injuries. *See also specific abdominal injuries*
  assessment, 916, 1119–1124
  closed/blunt, 1115–1116, 1115*f*
  emergency medical care, 1115–1116, 1125*f*
  interventions, 1124
  open/penetrating, 1116–1117, 1116*f*, 1125–1126, 1125*f*
  from seat belts and airbags, 1115–1116, 1116*f*
  transport decisions, 1122
  wounds, emergency medical care, 973–974, 973*f*
abdominal-thrust maneuver (Heimlich maneuver)
  definition of, 609
  technique, 597–598
abduction, definition of, 153, 171, 1165
abortion, spontaneous. *See* miscarriage, spontaneous abortion
abrasion, 961–962, 962*f*, 996
abruptio placentae, 1263, 1263*f*, 1263*t*, 1264*f*, 1266
absorption, 493, 527
  of toxins, 841–842, 842*f*
access
  definition of, 1383, 1400
  for extrication, 1388–1391, 1389*f*
    complex, 1390–1391, 1390*f*, 1400
    simple, 1389–1390, 1390*f*
accessory muscles, 337, 394
acetabulum, 179, 223
acetaminophen poisoning, 859
acidosis, 678, 684, 804
  definition of, 418, 804, 813
  hyperventilation and, 678
  metabolic. *See* metabolic acidosis
acquired immunodeficiency syndrome (AIDS), 625–626
acromioclavicular (AC) joint, 1164, 1190
acromioclavicular joint separation, 1164
action, definition of, 490, 527
activated charcoal, 847–848, 859
active shooter, 1397
active shooter event, 1448, 1476
acute abdomen
  causes of, 768–773
  definition of, 766, 786
  gynecologic problems and, 774
  physical examination, 778
acute chest syndrome, 808
acute coronary syndrome (ACS), 699–702, 726
acute kidney injury (AKI), 773
acute myocardial infarction (AMI)
  consequences, 701
  definition of, 698, 726
  physical findings, 701
  signs/symptoms, 700
  silent, 700
acute psychosis, 877–878
Adam's apple, 1001
addiction, 848, 867
adduction, definition of, 153, 171
adenosine triphosphate (ATP), 216, 223
adolescents
  definition of, 243, 254
  interviews with, 245
  physical changes, 244, 244*f*
  psychosocial changes, 244, 244*f*
  suicide risk, 874
  vital signs, 244
adrenal glands, 212, 223
adrenaline. *See* epinephrine
adrenergic, 200, 223
adults
  early
    definition of, 246, 254
    physical changes, 246, 246*f*
    psychosocial changes, 246
    vital signs, 246
  middle
    definition of, 246, 254
    physical changes, 246–247, 247*f*
    psychosocial changes, 247
  older, 247
    cardiovascular system, 248
    definition of, 254
    depression, 872
    digestive systems, 249–250
    endocrine system of, 249
    nervous systems, 250–251, 250*f*
    psychosocial changes, 251–252
    renal systems, 250
    respiratory system, 249
    sensory changes, 251
    suicide risk, 875
Advair (fluticasone), 660*t*
advanced emergency medical technician (AEMT), 23
  definition of, 6
  training for, 7
advance directives, 71, 91
advanced life support (ALS), 7
  definition of, 7, 23, 562, 609
adventitious breath sounds, 653, 653*t*, 684
adverse effects, 491, 527
AEIOU TIPS mnemonic, 743
aerobic metabolism, 216, 223
  definition of, 481
  internal respiration and, 412–413
aerosol-generating procedure (AGP), 44, 57, 416, 481
afterload, definition of, 537, 558
age, nerve agents, 1457
ageism, 248
agonal breathing, 563, 609
agonal gasps, 418, 481
agonist, 490, 527
AIDS. *See* acquired immunodeficiency syndrome
air ambulances, definition of, 1378
airbags, 1382
  abdominal injuries from, 1115–1116, 1116*f*
  vehicular collisions and, 902–904
airborne transmission, 39, 57
air embolism
  in ascent injuries, 1217–1218
  causes, 1026
  definition of, 1030, 1217, 1238
  pathophysiology, 975, 975*f*
air medical services, 1370–1376, 1370*f*, 1378
  avoiding communication issues, 1375
  calling for, 1371–1372
  landing and patient transfer, ensuring safety during, 1373–1374, 1373*f*, 1374*f*
  landing zone, establishing, 1372–1373, 1372*f*
  special considerations, 1375–1376
    landing on uneven ground, 1375, 1376*f*
    limiting factors for, 1375–1376
    night landings, 1375

air splints, 1159–1160
airway
adjuncts, 431–436, 432*f*
anatomy, in adults, 249
artificial. *See* airway adjuncts
assessment, 416–424, 417*t*, 418*f*
assisting with ALS procedures, 469–476
definition of, 481
emergency medical care
head injuries, 1055
spinal injuries, 1058
evaluation/assessment, 336
inhalation injury, 983
lower, 641*f*
anatomy of, 404–407, 406*f*
infection of, 646*t*
inhalation injuries, 987–988
obstruction of, 648–649
management, 402, 436–437
management equipment, in ambulances, 1345–1347, 1346*t*, 1347*f*
in brain-injured patient, 1056
with continuous positive airway pressure or CPAP, 454–459
dentures and, 464
with gastric distention, 449
pediatric, 464–469
recovery position for, 436–437
stomas and, 459–461
supraglottic devices for, 475*f*
tracheostomy tubes and, 459–461, 460*f*
obstruction
causes, 676–677
from facial fractures, 1023–1024
from foreign body. *See* foreign bodies, airway obstruction
mild, 596–597
in responsive patients, 597
in unresponsive patients, 336, 426, 426*f*, 597, 599
opening, 424–428
in adults, 569–571, 569–570*f*
head tilt–chin lift maneuver for, 426, 569–570, 569–570*f*
jaw-thrust maneuver for, 427–428
in unresponsive patient, 425
problems, 336
suctioning
equipment for, 428–429, 428–429*f*
techniques for, 429–431
upper, 641, 641*f*
anatomy of, 402–404, 403*f*
infection of, 646*t*
obstruction of, 648–649
albuterol, indications/contraindications, 660*t*
alcohol
consumption, history taking, 353
intoxication, history taking and, 353
poisoning from, 849–850, 859
alcohol use disorder, 850
algorithms
neonatal resuscitation, 1284*f*
opioid-associated emergency for health care clinicians, 852*f*
algor mortis, 74, 91
alkalosis, 678, 684
causes of, 678
allergens, 817
categories of, 819–820
definition of, 671, 684, 833
allergic reactions, 817
definition of, 833
epinephrine administration for, 826–831
to medication, 819
severe, categories of, 541
signs/symptoms, 823*t*
source, 820
vs. anaphylaxis, 817
alpha-adrenergic receptors, 200, 223
alpha radiation, 1470, 1476
altered mental status, 335, 394, 743, 757, 760, 871, 892. *See also* mental status, alteration
alternative fuel vehicles, 1382, 1388, 1388*f*
alveolar ventilation, 409*t*, 481
alveoli, 186, 223, 641*f*
ambient temperature, 1196, 1238
ambulance calls, phases, 1344*t*
arrival at scene, 1354–1357, 1354*f*, 1355*f*
delivery, 1358
dispatch, 1352–1353
en route to scene, 1354–1355
en route to station, 1358, 1359*f*
postrun, 1359
preparation. *See* ambulances, preparation
safe parking, 1355–1356, 1355–1356*f*
traffic control, 1356–1357
transfer, 1357, 1357*f*
ambulances
air. *See* air ambulances
cleaning, 1359, 1379
daily inspections, 1351
definition of, 1342, 1378
designs, 1342, 1342*f*, 1344*t*
disinfection, 1359, 1379
features, 1342–1343
jump kit, 1349, 1349*f*, 1350*t*, 1379
licensing specifications, 1342*f*, 1343
personnel, 1351
preparation
mechanical chest compression equipment, 1348
medical equipment, 1344*f*, 1345–1349, 1346*t*, 1347–1350*f*, 1350*t*, 1352*f*
storage of equipment/supplies, 1344*f*, 1345
preplanning/navigation equipment, 1350–1351
safety/operations equipment, 1350
safety precautions, 1351
work areas, equipment for, 1350, 1350*f*
American Heart Association (AHA), basic life support standards, 78
American Sign Language, 1305
American Standard Safety System, 439, 481
Americans With Disabilities Act (ADA), 10, 23
amniotic fluid, 1258–1259
amniotic sac, 1259
definition of, 1259, 1294
unruptured, 1279
amphetamines, 855
amputations, 1151, 1190
bleeding control, 1185
definition of, 963, 996, 1185
anaerobic metabolism, 216, 223
definition of, 481
internal respiration and, 413
anaphylactic reactions, 675
anaphylactic shock
causes, 548*t*
definition of, 541, 558
signs/symptoms, 542*t*, 548*t*
treatment, 548*t*, 550
anaphylaxis, 541, 675, 684, 817
definition of, 558, 818, 833
epinephrine administration for, 826–831
sequence of events in, 818*f*
signs/symptoms, 646*t*, 823*t*
vs. allergic reaction, 817
anatomic position, 174
anchoring, 312, 316
anemia, 809, 813, 1260, 1294
aneurysms, 736, 760
definition of, 558
dissecting, 705
hemorrhagic stroke and, 735–736
syncope and, 542
angina pectoris
definition of, 699–700, 726
pain, 699
angioedema, 818, 833
angioplasty, 718
angular collision, motorcycle, 908
angulation, 1183
animal bites, 975–976, 976*f*
anisocoria, 376, 1003, 1030
ankle
bones, 1143, 1143*f*
injuries, 1183–1184, 1184*f*
antagonist, 490, 527
anterior, definition of, 153, 171
anterograde (posttraumatic) amnesia, 1044, 1082
anthrax, 1465, 1465*f*, 1465*t*, 1468*t*, 1476
antibiotic, 490, 527
antibody, 818*f*
anticholinergics, 838*t*
anticoagulant medications, 521, 521*t*
antidote, 838, 867

Antidote Treatment Nerve Agent Auto-Injector (ATNAA), 1459, 1476
antifungal, 490, 527
antigen, 818*f*
antiplatelet medications, 521, 521*t*
antipyretics, 493, 527
antivenin, 1226, 1238
ant stings, 1227
anus, 1243, 1243*f*, 1247
anxious-avoidant attachment, 238
aorta, 194, 223, 929, 953
  definition of, 689, 726
aortic aneurysm, 705, 726, 768*t*
aortic valve, 692, 726
apex portion, 153, 171
Apgar score, 1280–1287, 1286*t*, 1294
aphasia, 737, 760
apnea, 417, 418, 481
apnea monitors, 1312–1313, 1313*f*
apneic oxygenation, 470, 481
appendicitis, 768*t*, 769, 786
appendicular skeleton, 179
  definition of, 175–176
appendix, 208, 210, 223, 769
applied ethics, definition of, 87, 91
aqueous humor, 1002
arachnoid mater, 1034–1035
arm, anatomy, 1141
arteries, 194
  in extremities, 1140*f*
  function, 692
arterioles, 194, 223, 694, 930
articular cartilage, 177, 223, 1143, 1190
artifact, ECG, 714–715, 726
artificial eyes, 1019–1020
artificial ventilation
  gastric distention and, 571–572
  methods, order of preference, 446
  normal *vs.*positive-pressure ventilation, 446–448, 447*t*
  of pediatric patients, 449
  precautions, 446
aspiration, 364, 403, 481, 677, 684
aspirin, 507, 528
  poisoning, 859
assault, definition of, 80–81, 91
assessment. *See under specific emergencies*
  flowchart, 323, 325, 332, 348, 355, 388
  focused. *See* focused assessment
  history taking. *See* history taking
  overview, 324
  primary assessment. *See* primary assessment
  scene size-up. *See* size-up
  secondary assessment. *See* secondary assessment
asthma
  definition of, 684
  in geriatric patient, 674
  management, 674–675
  medications, 660*t*
  pathophysiology, 673, 673*f*
  in pediatric patient, 674
  signs/symptoms, 646*t*
asystole, 702, 726
ataxic respirations, 418, 481
atelectasis, definition of, 647, 684
atherosclerosis, 248
  definition of, 726, 735, 760
  ischemic stroke and, 735, 735*f*
  pathophysiology, 698–699, 698–699*f*
atrioventricular node (AV node), 691
atrium, 191, 223, 689, 726
attachment
  anxious-avoidant, 238
  secure, 238
aura, definition of, 739, 760
auscultation, 356, 394
autism spectrum disorder (ASD), 1301, 1334
automated external defibrillator (AED)
  in ambulances, 1346*t*, 1348, 1348*f*
  maintenance, 583
  overview of, 576–577, 576*f*
  with pacemaker, 579, 581
  patient care following, 581–583
  public access to, 15
  sample checklist, 584*f*
  special situations, 579, 581
  transdermal medication patches and, 581
  uses of, 577–581, 580*f*
  wet patients and, 581
automatic implantable cardiac defibrillator (AICD), 719–720, 720*f*
automaticity, 691, 726
automatic transport ventilator (ATV), 453–454, 481
autonomic nervous system (ANS), 201, 223
  definition of, 558, 694, 727
  functions, 535, 691, 931, 1036
  regulation of heart function, 691
  in shock, 535
autonomy, definition of, 91
AVPU test for responsiveness
  description, 334, 335*f*
  primary assessment and, 615–617
avulsions
  definition of, 997
  facial, 1009*f*
  pathophysiology, 962–963, 963*f*
axial loading injuries, 1045, 1082
axial skeleton, 177–179
  definition of, 175
axons, 205, 224

B

back, focused assessment, 382
backboard, 284, 284*f*, 297, 1056
  lifting and carrying patient, 284–287
  moving patient on stairs, 288, 289
  one-handed carry, 287
  placement for extrication, 1391–1392
  short, 293–294
bacteria, as biologic warfare agents, 1464–1466, 1476
bacterial vaginosis, 1246, 1254
bag-mask device, 416–417
  advantages, 448–453, 448*f*
  components, 449
  definition of, 448, 481
  pediatric, 449
  pediatric patient, 468–469
  technique
    two-person, 450, 452*f*
    using EC clamp, 450
bag-mask ventilation, for newborn, 1283
bags, for hazardous materials, 1425–1426, 1426F
ball-and-socket joints, 177, 224
balloon angioplasty, 718
bandages/bandaging, 992, 993*f*
barbiturates, 853
bariatric patients, 1308–1309
bariatrics, 278, 297
barotrauma, 236, 254
barrier devices
  definition of, 481
  for infectious disease risk reduction, 44–46, 45*f*
  types, 448, 448*f*
base stations
  definition of, 130, 143
  licensing, 134
basic life support (BLS), 7, 23
  adult procedures, review of, 571, 572*t*
  algorithm, 580*f*
  automated external defibrillation. *See* automated external defibrillator
  cardiopulmonary resuscitation. *See* cardiopulmonary resuscitation
  chain of survival, 564–566, 564*f*
  definition of, 562, 609
  elements, 563*f*, 564*f*
  external chest compressions, 568*f*
  for infants/children, 586–594, 587*t*
    responsiveness determination, 588, 588*f*
  principles of, 562–566
basilar skull fractures, 1020, 1040, 1040*f*, 1082
basket stretcher, 293, 293*f*, 297
bath salts, 856
battery
  definition of, 81, 91
  example of, 81
Battle sign, 1040, 1040*f*, 1083
beclomethasone (Beclovent), 660*t*
bee stings, 1227
behavioral health emergency, 870, 892
  assessment, 880–884
belly breathing (diaphragmatic breathing), 236, 405
bends, 1218, 1238
benzodiazepines, 853
beta-adrenergic receptors, 200, 224
beta radiation, 1470, 1476
biases, 312, 316
biceps muscle, 182, 224
bile ducts, 210, 224

bills of lading, 1429, 1431*f*, 1441
bioethics, definition, 86, 91
biologic terrorism/warfare
agents, 1451, 1468*t*
bacteria, 1464–1466, 1476
neurotoxins, 1466–1468, 1466*f*, 1467–1468*t*, 1477
viruses, 1463–1464, 1464*f*, 1464*t*, 1465*t*, 1478
bipolar disorder, 872, 892
birth canal, 1259, 1294
bites, 1225–1234
emergency medical care, 975–977
insect
allergens from, 819, 819*f*
allergic reactions to, 819
as poisoning by injection, 843–844
snake, 1228–1232, 1229–1230*f*
spider, 1225–1227, 1226*f*
tick, 1233–1234, 1233*f*
black eye, 1017*f*
black widow spider bites, 1225–1226, 1226*f*
bladder, urinary. *See* urinary bladder
blast injuries
categories of, 911–914
definition of, 911
eye, 1018
mechanism of injury, 965
mechanisms of, 911–913, 913*f*
primary blast injury, types of, 913–914
tissues at risk, 917–918
bleeding assessment, 936–939
in brain, 737–738
from capillary vessels, 934, 934*f*
control
in facial injuries, 1009*f*, 1024
in neck injuries, 1025–1026
in pelvic injuries, 1172–1173
definition of, 932, 953
from ears, 947–948
emergency medical care, 939–948
external
assessment of, 342–343
control of, 342–343
significance, 932–933
types of, 932–934, 934f
gastrointestinal, 769–770
internal
emergency care for, 948–951
mechanisms of injury/nature of illness, 935
signs/symptoms of, 935–936
from mouth, 947–948
from nose, 947–948
postpartum, 1281
safety precautions, 933
subarachnoid, 1044, 1083
transport decisions, 937
vaginal, 1262–1264
blind spots, 1378
cushion of safety, 1365
blister agents, 1455–1456, 1455*f*
blood
function of, 199–200
in perfusion triangle, 534, 535*f*
bloodborne pathogens, 39, 57
blood clotting, 539, 698
blood composition, 196
blood disorders emergencies. *See* hematologic emergencies
blood flow, regulation, 535
blood glucose
assessment, 385
determination methods, 384
levels, normal range, 792
monitor (glucometer), 801
self-monitoring, 794*f*
blood pressure (BP), 196, 224
in acute myocardial infarction, 701
of adolescents, 244
of adults, 246
of children, infants, 234
control, 535
decrease, 368
definition of, 394
diastolic, 369, 395
measurement, 356, 369
by auscultation, 370–372
by palpation, 370, 373
units of, 694
in shock, 543
systolic, 369, 397
blood supply, of musculoskeletal system, 1139
bloody show, 1259, 1294
blowout fracture, 1017, 1030
BLS. *See* basic life support
blunt myocardial injury, 1104
blunt trauma
to chest, 1087
definition of, 900, 925
eye, 1017–1018, 1018*f*
from falls, 908–909, 910*f*
as mechanism of injury, 328
neck, 1025, 1025*f*
in vehicular collisions, 901–907, 901–902*f*
B-NICE, 1450–1451, 1476
body heat loss, from cold exposure, 1196
body language
in dealing with patient, 105
as nonverbal communication, 100–101, 101*f*
body mechanics, 259, 297
body temperature
assessment, 1196
core, 1197, 1198*t*, 1238
body weight, of infants, 235
bonding, definition of, 238
bones. *See also specific types of bones*
in children, 1143-1144
fracture types, 1146-1147
in older adults, 1144-1145
skeletal system and, 175-176
botulinum, 1466, 1467*t*, 1468*t*, 1476
Bourdon-gauge flowmeter, 440
brachial artery pulse, 195*t*, 224
brachial plexus, 1036*f*
brachial pulse, palpation, 338–340, 339*f*
bradycardia
definition of, 368, 394, 702, 727
pulse rate, 368
bradypnea, in respiratory failure, 338*t*
brain, 201–203
age-related changes, 250, 250*f*
anatomy, 730–731, 731*f*, 1034, 1034*f*
bleeding in, 737–738
cerebrospinal fluid, 203
circulation in the head, 203
damage, from hypoglycemia, 798
depressed function, 375
left hemisphere problems, 737
physiology, 730–731, 731*f*
protective coverings, 1034–1035, 1035*f*
right hemisphere problems, 737
brain death, 73
brainstem, 202, 224
anatomy, 731, 731*f*, 1034
breach of confidentiality, 69, 91
breach of duty, 79
in determining negligence, 79
breath-holding syncope, 1221, 1238
breathing
adequate
recognition of, 416
signs of, 645
assessment, 336–338
in infants/children, 593, 593*f*
of quality of breathing, 364
of respiratory rate, 363, 363*f*, 363*t*
of respiratory rhythm, 363–364
bilateral, 473
diaphragmatic or belly, 236
emergency medical care
head injuries, 1056
spinal injuries, 1058
inadequate or hypoventilation
recognition of, 416–419
signs/symptoms of, 645*t*
labored, 417, 418*f*
physiology of, 407–413, 409–410*f*, 409*t*, 412–413*f*
breath sounds, 363
assessment, 364–366, 365*f*
in respiratory system emergencies, 652–653, 653*f*
wheezing, 366
breech presentation, 1287–1288, 1288*f*, 1294
brief resolved unexplained event (BRUE), 1317–1318, 1334
bronchi, 186, 224
bronchial breath sounds, 653, 684
bronchioles, 186, 224, 406, 481
bronchiolitis, 665–666, 684
signs/symptoms, 646*t*
bronchitis, 670, 684
dyspnea and, 646*t*
medications for, 660*t*
signs/symptoms, 646*t*

brown recluse spider bites, 1226–1227, 1227*f*
bruises, child abuse, 1319
bruising, as fracture signs, 1148, 1149*f*
buboes, 1466, 1466*f*, 1476
bubonic plague, 1466, 1466*f*, 1466*t*, 1476
bulk storage container, 1423–1424, 1441
bullets, penetrating trauma from, 910, 913*f*
burn depth, 978–979, 979*f*
burnout, definition of, 34, 57
burns
  assessment, 981–985
  child abuse, 1319–1320
  circumferential, compartment syndrome and, 978
  classification, 978–980, 979*f*, 980*f*
  complications, 977–978
  deaths from, 978–979
  definition of, 958, 997
  to eye, 1014–1015, 1014–1015*f*
  in infants/children, 980
  interventions, 985
  pathophysiology, 977
  thermal, emergency medical care, 987
  transport decisions, 983
bystanders, 79
  duty to act and, 79
  presence during patient interview, 104

C

calcaneus, 181, 224, 1143, 1143*f*, 1190
cannabis compounds, 856
capillaries, 194–195, 694
capillary refill time
  definition of, 394
  evaluation, 342
capillary vessels, 194, 224
capnography, 383–384, 394–395, 422, 481
capnometry, 422, 422*f*, 481
carbon dioxide
  definition of, 383, 395
  during inspiration, 641
  during respiration, 641, 645*f*
  retention
    definition of, 647, 684
    hypoxic drive and, 647
carbon monoxide, 679, 684
  intoxication, 987
  poisonings, 841, 845
carboys, 1426, 1426*f*, 1441
cardiac arrest, 698, 722
  definition of, 701, 727
  in pregnancy, 603
  sudden death and, 701–702
cardiac asthma, 671
cardiac compromise, physical findings, 701
cardiac cycle, 694
cardiac medications, overdose. *See also specific cardiac medications*
cardiac monitoring, 715–718
cardiac muscle, 182, 224, 1140
cardiac output, 193, 224, 537, 1089
  definition of, 537, 727
  formula, 695
cardiac surgery, for cardiovascular emergencies, 718–719, 719*f*
cardiac tamponade, 538, 558
  definition of, 1109
  pathophysiology, 538, 1100–1102, 1102*f*
  signs/symptoms, 1100–1102
  treatment, 549
cardiogenic shock
  causes, 537*t*, 547*t*
  definition of, 536, 558, 702, 727
  signs/symptoms, 547*t*, 702
  treatment, 547, 547*t*, 549, 702
cardiopulmonary resuscitation (CPR)
  airway opening in adults. *See* airway
  artificial ventilation, 571–572
  cardiac arrest in pregnancy, 603
  in chain of survival, 564–566, 564*f*
  for children, 586–594, 587*t*, 588
  compression technique, 567–568, 568*f*
  definition of, 562, 609
  education and training, 605
  external chest compressions, 568*f*
  feedback devices, 569*f*
  goal of, 562–563
  indications, 340
  for infants, 586–594, 587*t*
  interrupting, 594
  need for, 563–564
  when not to start, 594–595
  one-rescuer adult, 572, 573
  opioid overdose, 603
  performing, 566–572
  special circumstances, 603–604
  steps, 562–563
  stopping, 595–596
  switching positions during, 575–576
  timing, 562, 563*f*
  two-rescuer adult, 572, 574–575
cardiovascular assessment
  geriatric patients, 374–375
  pediatric patients, 374
cardiovascular emergencies
  assessment, 706–710
  atherosclerosis, 698–699, 698–699*f*
  cardiac arrest. *See* cardiac arrest
  cardiac surgery for, 718–719, 719*f*
  cardiogenic shock, 702
  hypertensive, 705–706
  interventions, 711
  pacemakers for, 718–719, 719*f*
  pathophysiology, 698–706, 698*f*
  pulmonary edema, 704
  sudden death, 701–702
  transport decisions, 708, 711
  vital signs, 711–712
cardiovascular system
  anatomy, 689–698, 690*f*, 692–693*f*
  breathing physiology and, 407–413, 409–410*f*, 409*t*, 412–413*f*
  focused assessment, 366–375
  of infants, 235
  medical emergencies, 613, 613*t*
  of older adults, 248
  perfusion triangle, 534, 535*f*
  physiology, 689–698, 690*f*, 692–693*f*
carina, 186, 224, 406, 406*f*, 481
carotid arteries, 1001
carotid artery pulse, 195*t*, 224
  in child, 339
  palpation of, 339, 339*f*
carpals, 179, 224
carpopedal spasm, 678
cartilage, 176, 176*t*, 224
  definition of, 1143
car-versus-bicycle collisions, 907, 907*f*
castor beans, ricin poisoning from, 861*f*, 1467–1468, 1467–1468*t*
casualty collection area, 1420, 1441
cathinones, synthetic, 856
cavitation, 910, 911*f*, 913*f*, 925, 1117
CBRNE mnemonic, 1450
cecum, 208, 224
cellular metabolism, 220, 224
cellular respiration, 408*t*, 482
cellular telephone, 132, 143
central cyanosis, 1283, 1287
central nervous system (CNS), 201, 224, 201–204. *See also specific central nervous system structures*
  anatomy, 1034–1035, 1034*f*
  definition of, 1033
  protection, 1034–1035
central neurogenic hyperventilation, 1042, 1083
central pulses, 345
central venous catheters, 1314–1315, 1314*f*
cerebellum, 202, 224
  anatomy, 731, 731*f*
  functions, 1034
cerebral cortex, 1043
cerebral edema, 1041, 1083
cerebral embolism, 735
cerebral palsy, 1306–1307, 1306*f*, 1335
cerebrospinal fluid (CSF), 189, 224, 1035
cerebrovascular accident (CVA), 734. *See also* stroke
cerebrum, 201, 224
  anatomy, 731, 731*f*, 1034, 1034*f*
  function, 1034
certification, 9–10, 23, 79
cervical collars, 1055–1066
cervical spine, 177–178, 224
  focused assessment, 379–380
  stabilization, 1057–1062
cervix, 1243, 1244*f*, 1245, 1246, 1254, 1259, 1294
chain of survival, 564–566, 564*f*
channel, radio, definition of, 130, 143
CHART method, 122
cheek injuries, 1024
chemical burns
  emergency medical care, 988–989, 988–989*f*
  eye, 1014–1015, 1014*f*

chemical mediators, 818*f*
chemicals, as allergens, 820
chemical terrorism/warfare, 1451
agents, 1451
biological, 1463–1469, 1464*f*, 1464*t*, 1465*t*
metabolic or cyanides, 1460–1462, 1462*t*
nerve agents, 1457–1460, 1457*f*, 1458*t*, 1459*f*, 1460*t*
respiratory/choking, 1456
vesicants, 1455–1456, 1455*f*
contact hazard, 1454
description, 1451
persistency, 1454
route of exposure, 1454
vapor hazard, 1454
volatility, 1454, 1478
Chemical Transportation Emergency Center (CHEMTREC), 1429, 1441
chemoreceptors
definition of, 413, 482
functions, in respiration, 413
chest
focused assessment, 380
injuries. *See* chest injuries
chest compression fraction, 594
chest compressions
external, 566, 567*f*, 568*f*
hand position, 567–568, 568*f*
technique, 567–568, 568*f*
fraction, 609
for infants, 588
for newborn, 1283
chest injuries. *See also specific chest injuries*
assessment, 914, 1092–1096
closed, 1089–1090, 1090*f*
emergency medical care, 1098
interventions, 1096
open, 1090, 1090*f*
pathophysiology, 1089–1091, 1090*f*
signs/symptoms, 1091–1092
transport decisions, 1094
chest pain
in angina pectoris, 699
pleuritic, 675–676, 686
chest thrusts, 598, 598*f*
Cheyne-Stokes respirations, 418, 418*f*, 482, 1042
chief complaint, 122, 143
definition of, 328, 395
investigation, 349–350, 349*f*
chief concern, 122, 143, 395
child abuse, signs, 1318–1320, 1319*f*
childbirth
abnormal/complicated, 1287–1291, 1288*f*
multiple births, 1289–1290
normal, 1271–1287
delivering the newborn, 1275–1280
delivery field preparation, 1271–1274, 1275*f*
preparation for delivery, 1271–1274, 1275*f*
stages of labor, 1270–1271
placenta, delivery of, 1281–1282
postdelivery care, 1280–1282
supplies, in ambulances, 1346*t*, 1348
child maltreatment, 1318, 1335
child neglect, signs of, 1320
children
adolescent. *See* adolescents
AED, 594
airway in, 190
airway opening
head tilt–chin maneuver, 593
jaw-thrust maneuver, 593
anatomy
airway, 405, 405*f*
basic life support, 586–594, 587*t*
blood loss, from skull region, 1049
cardiopulmonary resuscitation, 586–594, 587*t*, 588
communication with, 109–110, 110*f*
consent in critical situations, 65–66, 66*f*
CPR, 590–591
with diabetes, 793, 799
foreign body obstructions, 599–603, 600*f*
immunizations, recommended, 50
infants. *See* infants
musculoskeletal system, 1143
oropharyngeal airway insertion, 432
poisonings, 836
rescue breathing, 593
respiratory rates, 190
school-age. *See* school-age children
in shock
circulation emergencies and management, 543, 551–552
dehydration emergencies and management, 553
chlamydia, 1246, 1254
chlorine, in chemical terrorism/warfare, 1456, 1462*t*, 1476
choking agents, in chemical terrorism/ warfare, 1456
choking, universal sign for, 597, 597*f*
cholecystitis
definition of, 767, 786
localization of pain, 768*t*
referred pain from, 768*f*, 767
signs/symptoms, 769
cholinergic agents, 838*t*
chordae tendineae, 193, 224
chronic bronchitis, 670, 685
chronic diseases, 1299
chronic kidney disease, 773
chronic obstructive pulmonary disease (COPD), 670, 685
definition of, 685
management, 671
medications for, 660*t*
pathophysiology, 670–671, 670*f*
signs/symptoms, 670*f*
types, 670
vs. heart failure, 671, 672*t*
chyme, 209, 225
Cincinnati Prehospital Stroke Scale, 749, 750*t*
circulation
assessment, 338–342, 339*f*, 341–342*f*
capillary refill, 342, 342*f*
skin assessment and, 340–342, 342*f*
devices and techniques to assist, 583–586
fetal, 1259
circulatory compromise, 416
circulatory system
anatomy, 191–196
arteries, 194
blood composition, 196
capillaries, 194–195
heart, 191–194
spleen, 196
veins, 195–196
geriatric, 697
pediatric, 697–698
physiology, 196–201
blood, function of, 199–200
inadequate circulation, 198
nervous system control, CNS and, 200–201
normal circulation, 197–198
circumflex coronary arteries, 692*f*
cirrhosis, 786
civil lawsuit, 78
clavicle injuries, 179, 179*f*, 225, 1103, 1163–1164, 1164*f*
cleaning
of ambulance, 1359, 1379
disinfectant solution for, 48
clitoris, 1243
clonic phase, 739
closed-ended questions
definition of, 102, 143
in patient interview, 102, 103*t*
closed incident, 1410, 1442
closed injuries
abdominal, 1115–1116, 1116*f*
assessment, 965–972
chest, 1089–1090, 1090*f*, 1109
emergency medical care of, 972
fractures, 1146, 1190
Clostridioides difficile, 780, 1328
Clostridium botulinum, 859*t*
clothing, of toxin-exposed patient, 840
coagulation, 934, 953
cocaine, 855
coccyx, 178, 225
cognitive disabilities, 390, 395
cold injuries
assessment, 1201–1202
emergency medical care, 1203–1204, 1203*f*
hypothermia, 1197–1199, 1198*f*, 1198*t*
interventions, 1203–1204
local, 1199–1201, 1199*f*
prevention, 1203–1204
transport decisions, 1202
underlying factors, 1199
cold zone, 1432, 1433*f*, 1434, 1442

Colles fracture, 1170
colon, 765
colors, medical terminology, 150
colostomy, 1316, 1335
coma, 732, 760
combining form, medical terminology, 158–160*t*
combining vowels, medical terminology, 148–149, 171
command
  establishing, at terrorism event, 1454
  in incident command system, 1406–1407, 1406*f*, 1442
command post, 1394, 1396, 1397, 1400, 1406, 1442
commotio cordis, 1105, 1109
communicable disease, 623, 636
  definition of, 38, 57
  vs. infectious disease, 38
communication
  age and, 99–100
  with children, 109–110, 110*f*
  with critically ill or injured patient, 114–115
  culture and, 99–100
  death and dying, 115–118
  definition of, 97, 143
  with older adults, 107–109, 108*f*
  en route, 136*t*
  health literacy and, 99
  with hearing-impaired patients, 110, 111*f*
  importance of, 97
  during labor/delivery, 1273
  at mass-casualty incident, 1411
  with medical control and hospitals, 137–139, 137*f*
  medical fear and, 99
  noise and, 101
  with non–English-speaking patients, 111–112
  nonverbal
    body language, 100–101, 101*f*
    eye contact, 100–101
    facial expressions, 100–101
    physical factors and, 101–102, 102*t*
  with other health care professionals, 112, 114*f*
  patient care handoff, 112–114
  personal experience and, 99–100
  radio. *See* radio communications
  respect and, 99
  therapeutic, 98, 145
  verbal, 97, 102–106
  with visually impaired patients, 110–111
  written, 97, 118–129
    documenting refusal of care, 126–129, 127–128*f*, 127–128*t*
    special reporting situations, 129
communication systems
  base station radios, 130
  cellular/satellite telephones, 132
  digital equipment, 131–132
  equipment, 132–133
  mobile and portable radios, 130, 130–131*f*
  mobile data terminals, 133, 133*f*
  repeater-based, 131, 131*f*
communication techniques, 103*t*
community paramedicine, 302, 316
compartment syndrome, 960–961, 978, 1186, 1190
compassionate persuasion, 68, 91
compassion fatigue, 57
compensated (nonprogressive) shock, 543, 543*t*, 558
compensatory damages, 86, 91
competent, definition of, 72, 91
complex access, 1390–1391, 1390*f*, 1400
compliance, 454, 482
concussion
  definition of, 1083
  signs/symptoms, 1044
  spinal cord, 1045, 1083
conduction, 1196, 1238
conductive hearing loss, 1305, 1335
confidentiality, disclosure of information, 69
conjunctiva, 340, 395, 1002–1003, 1030
conjunctivitis, 1011, 1030
connecting nerves, 1036, 1036*f*
consent
  definition of, 62–63, 91
  expressed, 64, 92
  implied, 64–65, 93
  informed, 64, 93
  involuntary, 65
  minors and, 65–66, 66*f*
  for organ donation, 75, 76*f*
  refusal of, 67–69
contact burn, 987, 997
contact hazard, 1454, 1476
contact lenses, 1019–1020
contagious, 1463, 1477
containers, for hazardous materials, 1423–1426, 1424*f*
contamination
  definition of, 38, 57, 997
  in soft-tissue injuries, 961
  standard precautions, 40, 41*t*
continuous positive airway pressure (CPAP), 669, 685
  application, 456–459
  complications, 459
  for heart failure, 703*t*
  contraindications, 456
  definition of, 482
  indications, 446, 456
continuum of care, 301, 316
contractility, 695
contraindications, definition of, 491, 528
contributory negligence, 85
  decision-making capacity, definition, 91–92
controlled motorcycle crash, 908
control zones, 1432–1433, 1433–1434*f*, 1442
contusion, 959, 959*f*, 997
  brain, 1045
  definition of, 935, 953
  pulmonary, 1103
convection, 1196, 1238
conventional reasoning, 243, 254
COPD. *See* chronic obstructive pulmonary disease
coral snake bites, 1229*f*, 1231–1232
core temperature, 1197
  definition of, 1238
  falling, 1197
cornea, 1002*f*, 1003, 1030
coronal plane, definition of, 174–175
coronary arteries, 692, 727
coronary artery disease, 699
coronary sinus, 692*f*
coroner (medical examiner), 74, 75*f*
corticosteroids, 659
coughing techniques, to avoid contamination, 40, 40*f*
coup–contrecoup brain injury, 902, 902*f*, 930, 1041
cover, definition of, 1451, 1477
COVID-19, 631, 667, 685, 1469
  characteristics, 646*t*
  signs/symptoms, 646*t*
coxae, 179, 225
CPAP. *See* continuous positive airway pressure
CPR. *See* cardiopulmonary resuscitation
crackles (rales), 366, 395, 653*t*, 685
cranium, 177, 225
credentialing, 10–11, 23
crepitus, 356, 379, 395, 1109, 1148, 1190
crew resource management (CRM), 305, 316
cricoid cartilage, 186, 225, 1001–1002
cricothyroid membrane, 186, 225
critical incident stress management (CISM), 57
critically ill or injured patient, communication, 114–115
cromolyn (Intal), 660*t*
cross-contamination, 1453, 1477
croup
  characteristics, 646*t*, 664
  definition of, 685
  signs/symptoms, 646*t*
crowning, 1271, 1294
crush injury, 960, 997
crush syndrome, 960–961, 997
crying patients, history taking and, 390
cultural competence, 54, 57
cultural considerations, during pregnancy, 1267
cultural humility, 54–55, 57, 100, 143–144
cultural imposition, 100, 144
culture, communication and, 99–100
Cushing triad, 1042, 1057, 1083
cushion of safety, 1365–1366, 1379
custody, involuntary consent and, 65
cyanides
  in chemical terrorism/warfare, 1460–1462, 1462*t*, 1477
  poisonings, 845

cyanosis
in anaphylactic shock, 541
causes, 340, 340*f*
in chest injuries, 1092
definition of, 395, 558
skin color and, 617*f*
cylinders
gas, 437–438, 437*f*
for hazardous materials, 1426, 1442
cystic fibrosis (CF), 679–681
cystitis, 773, 786
localization of pain, 768*t*

D

danger zone (hot zone), 1386, 1387*f*, 1400, 1433, 1433*f*
date rape drugs, 853
DCAP-BTLS mnemonic
definition of, 356, 356*t*, 395
in trauma assessment, 1006
dead space, 191, 225, 409*t*, 410, 482
death/dying
communication, 115–118
child, 117–118
conveying news, 116
cultural implications, 117
EMT's role during, 116–117
definitive signs of, 74, 75*f*
hypothermia and, 73
medical examiner cases, 74–75, 75*f*
medical identification insignia and, 76, 76*f*
organ donation, consent for, 75, 76*f*
physical signs of, 73–75
presumptive signs of, 73, 74*t*
decay, of radiological material, 1469, 1477
deceleration, 930
decision-making capacity, definition, 63
decompensated shock, 543, 543*t*, 558
decompression sickness, 1218, 1238
decontamination, 1379
area, 1434, 1434*f*, 1442
definition of, 1442
equipment, 294
in hazmat incidents, 1434, 1434*f*
decreased visibility, 1367
dedicated line (hotline), 130, 144
deep partial-thickness burns, 978, 979, 997
deep, definition of, 152, 171
deep vein thrombosis, 809
de-escalation, 67, 100–101, 884–888, 885*t*
defamation, 81, 92
defendant, 84
defibrillation, 702, 727
defibrillators, 1313
deformity, as fracture signs, 1147, 1148*f*
dehydration, 542–543, 558
definition of, 542
signs and symptoms of, 553*t*
delirium, 744, 760, 876–877, 892
delirium tremens (DTs), 850, 867
delivery
abnormal/complicated, 1287–1291
preparation for, 1275*f*
delusions, 878, 892
dementia, 761, 876, 892
demobilization, 1406, 1442
denitrogenation, 453, 482
dental appliances
causing airway obstruction, 464
dentures, airway maintenance and, 464
dental injuries
emergency medical care, 1024
with facial fractures, 1024, 1024*f*
traumatic, 1024, 1024*f*
dentures, airway maintenance and, 464
Department of Homeland Security, 1321
Department of Transportation (DOT), marking system for hazardous materials, 1426–1427, 1427*f*
dependent edema, 727
dependent lividity, 74, 74*f*, 92, 595
depositions, definition, 85
depressed skull fracture, 1040, 1040*f*
depression, 871–872, 892
dermis, 205, 225
anatomy, 957–958, 957*f*
definition of, 957, 997
designated officer, 40, 57
developmental disabilities
autism spectrum disorder, 1301, 1335
characteristics, 1300–1301
definition of, 1300, 1335
patient interaction and, 1302–1303
Down syndrome, 1301–1302, 1301*f*, 1335
diabetes mellitus, 791
blood glucose self-monitoring, 794*f*
in children, 799
definition of, 813
insulin and, 791
pathophysiology, 793–796
type 1, 793–795
type 2, 795–796
diabetic ketoacidosis (DKA), 796–797, 814
dialysis, renal, 781–783
diamond carry, 285–286, 286*f*, 297
diaphoretic, 342, 395
diaphragm, 186–187, 187*f*, 225
during inspiration, 641
diaphragmatic breathing (belly breathing), 236
diastole, 196, 225, 694
diastolic pressure, 369, 395
dieffenbachia, 861*f*, 862
diet, healthy, 29, 29*f*
diffusion, 189, 225, 412, 482
definition of, 402
digestive system
anatomy, 206–210
abdomen, 206–208
appendix, 210
esophagus, 209
large intestine, 210
liver, 209–210
mouth, 208
oropharynx, 208–209
pancreas, 209
rectum, 210
small intestine, 210
stomach, 209
in older adults, 249–250
physiology, 210–211
digital equipment, for communication systems, 131–132
dilation, 692, 727
diphtheria
characteristics, 646*t*
definition of, 685
signs/symptoms, 646*t*
direct contact, 38, 39*f*, 57
directional terms. *See* medical terminology direct laryngoscopy, 470, 482
direct pressure
for external bleeding, 934, 940*f*
dirty bomb, 1477, 1551
disability
developmental, 1300
long-term, from musculoskeletal injuries, 1163
Disaster Medical Assistance Teams (DMATs), 1421
disasters
casualty collection area, 1420
definition of, 1403, 1420, 1442
management, 1420
discovery, definition, 85
disease prevention, wellness and, 32–33
disease vector, 1463, 1477
disinfection
of ambulance, 1359, 1379
high-level, 1359, 1379
dislocations
definition of, 1149, 1190
elbow, 1167, 1168*f*
knee, 1181–1182, 1182*f*
patellar, 1183, 1183*f*
shoulder, 1165–1166, 1168*f*
signs/symptoms, 1149, 1150*f*
dispatch phase of EMS, 134
displaced fracture, 1146, 1190
dissecting aneurysm, 705, 727
dissemination, 1463, 1477
distal, definition of, 152, 171
distal radius fractures, 1170, 1170*f*
distracting injury, 328, 395
distraction, spinal injury, 1045, 1083
distributive shock, 540–541, 558
diverticulitis, 767, 768*t*, 771–772, 786
diving reflex, 1215, 1238
documentation
of assessment findings. *See under specific emergency situations*
definition of, 97, 144
of refusal of care, 126–129, 127–128*f*, 127–128*t*
domestic terrorism, 1447, 1477
do not attempt resuscitation (DNAR) order, 71, 92

do-not-use abbreviations, 155, 156*t*
DOPE mnemonic, 1312
dorsalis pedis artery pulse, 195*t*, 225
dorsal, definition of, 153, 171
dose/doses, 490, 528
Down syndrome, 1301–1302, 1301*f*, 1335
dragging methods, moving of patients, 268, 268*f*
draw sheet method, 279, 279*f*
dressings
  bandaging and, 992, 993*f*
  occlusive, 973, 997
  sterile, 976, 992–993
driver anticipation, 1364–1365
driving alone, 1370
driving, of emergency vehicles
  cushion of safety for, 1379
drowning
  assessment, 1218–1220
  definition of, 1212, 1238
  events in, 1212–1217
  interventions, 1220
  prevention, 1222–1223
  transport decisions, 1220
  water rescue, 1214, 1214*f*
drug-related injuries, 84
drugs/medications
  absorption. *See* absorption
  administration, 489
    cross-check procedure, 500–501
    and EMT, 501–506, 502–505*t*
    error, 524
    steps, 498–500
  as allergens, 819
  allergic reaction to, 819
  in ambulances, 1346*t*, 1349
  definition of, 490
  gaseous, 498
  gel, 498
  metered-dose inhaler, 497, 497*f*
  names of, 492
  overdose, 859
  prescription, 492
  respiratory inhalation, 660*t*
  routes of administration, 492–495, 496*t*
    inhalation, 516–520
    intramuscular, 509–515
    intranasal, 515–516
    oral, 506–507, 528
    sublingual, 507–509
  solution, 497
  suspension, 497
  tablets/capsules, 495–497
  topical, 497
  transdermal, 497–498
drug use, history taking, 353
drums, for hazardous materials, 1425
DUMBELS mnemonic, 858, 1458t
duodenal ulcer, 768*t*
duodenum, 764
DuoDote kit, 858, 1459, 1477
duplex, 132, 144
durable power of attorney for health care, 71, 92
dura mater, 1035
duration, 491, 528
duty to act, 79, 92
dysarthria, 737, 761
dysbarism injuries, 1223, 1238
dysphagia, 1307
dyspnea
  causes, 647–648, 1091–1092
  definition of, 482, 640, 685
  paroxysmal nocturnal, 646*t*
  signs/symptoms, 411
dysrhythmia
  definition of, 727
  sudden death and, 701

E

ear
  anatomy, 1001, 1001*f*
  Battle sign, 1040, 1040*f*
  bleeding from, 947–948
  injuries, 1021–1022, 1022*f*
early adults. *See* adults, early
Ebola, 631
ecchymosis, 379, 395
  definition of, 953, 997, 1190
  as fracture sign, 1148
  internal bleeding and, 935
  pathophysiology, 959
eclampsia, 1262, 1295
ectopic pregnancy
  assessment, 1263
  definition of, 1295
  pathophysiology, 1245
  signs/symptoms, 1247–1248
edema
  definition of, 537, 558
  dependent, 704, 727
  pulmonary. *See* pulmonary edema
ejection
  in auto crashes, 900, 906
  in motorcycle collision, 908
elastic bougie, 471, 482
elbow
  dislocation, 1167–1168, 1168*f*
  injuries, 1167, 1168*f*
  sprain, 1168
elder abuse and neglect, 1335
  assessment of, 1322–1323
  categories of, 1323*t*
  signs of, 1323
electrical burns, 989–991, 990*f*
electrical conduction system, 690, 691*f*
electrocardiogram (ECG)
  electrodes, 714–715, 714*f*
  transmission over UHF frequencies, 132
electrolytes. *See also specific electrolytes*
elimination, 491, 528
emancipated minors, 65–66, 92
embolus, 677, 685, 735, 735*f*, 761
embryo
  definition of, 1258, 1295
  implantation, 1258
emergency, definition of, 77, 77*f*. *See also specific emergencies*
emergency doctrine, 64
emergency medical care. *See under specific emergencies*
  in absence of DNR orders, 75
  consent for, 64
  definition of, 62, 92
emergency medical dispatcher (EMD), paging of EMS personnel, 135
emergency medical responder (EMR)
  definition of, 6, 23
  training for, 7
emergency medical services (EMS)
  components of
    prevention, 19–20
    public education, 20
    research, 18
  definition of, 3, 23
  expanding role of, 1330
  history of, 3–5
  national levels of training, 6–7, 6*t*
  notification, 137
  purpose of, 3–5
  research, 18
  response, dispatch, 134
  standardization of, 5–6
Emergency Medical Services for Children (EMSC) program, 4
emergency medical technician (EMT)
  certification, 9–10
  credentialing, 10–11
  definition of, 3, 23
  education and training, 8–9
  effective performance, team, 303–308
  general description, 300
  licensure, 10
  professional attributes, 11–13, 12*t*, 12*f*
  and public health, 18–20
  roles/responsibilities, 11, 11*t*
  system overview, 13–14, 13*f*
  training for, 7
emergency move. *See* moving of patients
Emergency Response Guidebook (US DOT), 1428, 1428*f*
emergency vehicles
  ambulances. *See* ambulances
  first-responder, 1342, 1379
emesis, 766, 786, 850, 867
emotional intelligence, 106–107, 144
emphysema
  definition of, 685
  lung destruction in, 670–671
  signs/symptoms, 646*t*
employer, infection control responsibilities, 46–47
EMR. *See* emergency medical responder
EMT. *See* emergency medical technician
EMT-administered medication, 501–506, 502–505*t*, 528
endocrine emergencies
  assessment, 799–802
  communication, 811
  documentation, 802
  emergency medical care, 803–805
  medical emergencies, 613, 613*t*
  transport decisions, 800

endocrine glands, definition of, 790, 814
endocrine system, 211–212, 790, 814
  anatomy, 790–792, 791*f*
  in older adults, 249
  pathophysiology, 792–798
    diabetes. *See* diabetes mellitus
    symptomatic hypoglycemia, 798
  physiology, 790–792
endometrium, 1258, 1295
endotracheal (ET) intubation, 469, 482, 528
end-stage renal disease (ESRD), 781
end-tidal carbon dioxide ($ETCO_2$), 422, 482
energy
  kinetic, 898
  nuclear, 1471
  potential, 898
  trauma and, 897–899, 897*f*
en route communications, 136*t*
enteral medications, 492, 528
entrance wound, 910, 964
  electrical burns, 989–991, 990*f*
entrapment, 1382, 1400
envenomations, 819, 833, 1225–1234
environmental emergencies
  bites and envenomations, 1225–1234
  definition of, 1194
  exposure
    to cold temperatures, 1196–1197
    factors affecting, 1194–1196
  heat exposure. *See* heat exposure illnesses
  from high altitude, 1223–1224
  lightning injuries, 1224
  marine animal injuries, 1234–1235, 1234*f*
  radiation exposure, 1205
  risk factors, 1194
  water-related. *See* drowning
environmental exposure, factors affecting, 1194–1196
environmental/industrial exposures, 679
enzymes, 210, 225
epidemic, 624, 636
epidermis, 205, 225, 957, 957*f*, 997
epidural bleeding, 738, 738*f*
epidural hematoma, 1043, 1043*f*, 1083
epiglottis, 185, 225
  adult *vs.* child, 405, 405*f*
  function, 403
epiglottitis
  characteristics, 646*t*, 664–665
  definition of, 685
  signs/symptoms, 646*t*
epilepsy, 761
epinephrine (adrenaline), 200, 225, 512, 514–515, 514*f*, 528
  administration, 826–831
  contraindications, 826*t*
  definition of, 825, 833
  dosage/administration, 826–831
  effects, 535–536
  indications, 826*t*
  side effects, 826*t*
EpiPen administration, 826–828
epiphyseal (growth) plate
  fracture, 1147
  injuries, in children, 1169
epistaxis (nosebleeds), 1020–1021, 1021*f*
  controlling, 948
  definition of, 953
  emergency medical care, 1021
  nasal fractures and, 1021
errors, reporting of, 125–126, 126*f*
esophageal intubation, 474, 482
esophageal varices, 770–771
esophagitis, 770
esophagus, 209
  anatomy, 1088
  functions, 764
ethical responsibilities, for health care providers, 86–88
ethics
  applied, 87, 91
  definition of, 86, 92
  guidelines for decision making, 84
ethmoid bone, 177, 225
ethnocentrism, 99, 144
eustachian tube, 1021, 1030
evaporation, 1196, 1238
evidence-based medicine (EBM), 18, 23
evisceration
  abdominal, emergency medical care, 1125, 1126*f*
  definition of, 997, 1136
    abdominal, 1117, 1126*f*
  pathophysiology, 973, 973*f*
excessive speed, problem of, 1366
excited delirium, 965, 997
exercise, for wellness, 29–30, 29*f*
exhalation, 410, 482
exit wound, 910
exocrine, 211*t*, 225
expiration, 409, 641
expiratory reserve volume, 191, 225
exposure
  definition of, 38, 58
expressed consent, 64, 92
extension, 177, 225
  definition of, 153, 171
external auditory canal, 1021, 1022*f*, 1030
external chest compressions
  hand position, 567–568, 568*f*
  technique, 567–568, 568*f*
external defibrillator vest, 720, 1314
external genitalia
  female, injuries to, 1129
  male, injuries to, 1129
external respiration (pulmonary), 412, 412*f*, 482
extremities
  focused assessment, 381–382, 382*f*
  handling injured, 1157
  injuries, that impair circulation, 1155
  lower, anatomy of, 1141–1143
  upper, anatomy, 1141, 1142*f*
extremity lift, 275–276, 297
extrication
  definition of, 1382, 1400
  equipment, 1384, 1384*t*
  at mass-casualty incident, 1413, 1413*f*
  phases
    arrival and scene size-up, 1384–1386, 1385*f*
    emergency care, 1391
    en route to scene, 1384
    gaining access, 1388–1391, 1389*f*
    hazard control, 1386–1388, 1387*f*
    preparation, 1383–1384, 1384*t*
    removal of patient, 1391–1392
    support operations, 1388
    termination, 1392–1393
    transfer of patient, 1392
extrication supervisor, 1413, 1442
eye
  age-related changes, 251
  anatomy, 1002–1003, 1002*f*
  artificial, 1019–1020
  contact, as nonverbal communication, 100–101
  contact lenses, 1019–1020
  injuries, 1010–1020, 1010–1011*f*
    blast injuries, 1019
    blunt trauma, 1017–1018, 1018*f*
    burns, 1014–1015, 1014–1015*f*
    chemical agents in, 841, 842*f*
    chemical burns, emergency medical care, 988–989, 988*f*, 989*f*
    foreign objects, 1010–1014
    following head trauma, 1018–1019, 1018*f*
    impaled foreign object, 1010–1014
    initial examination, 1010*f*
    lacerations, 1016–1017, 1017*f*
  irrigation, 1011, 1014, 1015*f*
  orbit of, 1002
  postexposure management, 50–51
  protection, for risk reduction and prevention, 43, 45*f*
  raccoon, 1040, 1040*f*, 1083
eyelid, removal of foreign object from, 1011
eyes-forward position, 1058, 1083

F

face
  anatomy, 1000–1003, 1000*f*
  expressions
    as nonverbal communication, 100–101
facial injuries. *See also specific facial injuries*
  assessment, 1004–1008
  bleeding, causing airway obstruction, 464, 464*f*
  emergency medical care, 1008–1026, 1009*f*
  fractures, 1023–1024, 1024*f*
  interventions, 1007
  soft-tissue, 1004, 1004*f*
  transport decisions, 1006
fainting. *See* syncope

fallopian tubes, 215, 225
anatomy, 1243–1245, 1243*f*, 1258
definition of, 1254
falls, accidental
abdominal injuries from, geriatric patients, 1115
trauma from, 908–909, 910*f*
false imprisonment, 81, 92
false motion, 1149, 1190
as fracture sign, 1149
family
balancing with work and health, 33–34
presence during patient interview, 104
family-centered care, 109, 144
fascia, 962–963, 997
definition of, 1139, 1190
compartment syndrome and, 1186
febrile seizures, definition of, 740, 761
Federal Communications Commission (FCC), 133, 144
The Federal Food, Drug, and Cosmetic Act of 1938, 492
Federal Interagency Committee on Emergency Medical Services (FICEMS), 4
female reproductive system
anatomy, 765, 1127, 1128*f*, 1243–1245, 1243*f*, 1258–1260, 1258*f*
external genitalia, 1243*f*
genitalia injuries, 1129, 1133
pathophysiology, 1245–1246
physiology, normal, 1243–1245
femoral artery, 195*f*, 195*t*, 225
femoral head, 180, 226
femoral shaft fractures, 1175–1181
femur, 180, 226
fertilization, 1258–1259*f*
fetal alcohol syndrome, 1265, 1295
fetal death, 1291
fetal distress, 1265
fetus, 1258–1259, 1295
fibula, 181, 226, 1142*f*, 1143, 1190
injuries, 1183, 1183*f*
field impression, 324, 395
finance/administration, in incident command system, 1407, 1442
finger injuries, 1170, 1171*f*
fire ant stings, 819, 819*f*
first-responder vehicles, 1342, 1379
flail chest, 1102–1103, 1103*f*, 1109
flame burn, 987, 997
flank, of human body, 1123, 1136
flash burn, 987, 997
flexible stretcher, 292, 293*f*, 297
flexion, 177, 226
definition of, 153, 171
injuries, of spine, 1045
Flovent Diskus (fluticasone), 660*t*
flowchart, patient assessment, 325, 332, 348, 355, 388
fluticasone (Flovent Diskus), 660*t*
flutter valve, 1098, 1109
focal seizures, definition of, 739, 761
focused assessment
abdomen, 380–381, 381*f*
back, 382
cardiovascular system, 366–375
cervical spine, 379–380
chest, 380
in chief complaint investigation, 363*t*
definition of, 395
extremities, 381–382, 381–382*f*
geriatric patients, 386
head, 379–380, 380*f*
neck, 379–380, 380*f*
neurologic system, 375
neurovascular status, 377–379
respiratory system, 362–366
fontanelles, 184, 226
anatomy, 236*f*
definition of, 254
functions, 236
food, as allergen, 819
foodborne transmission, 40, 58
food poisoning, 859–860
foot
bones, 1142*f*, 1143
injuries, 1184–1185, 1185*f*
foramen magnum, 177, 226
force
causing musculoskeletal injuries, 1145
in determining mechanism of injury, 328
forcible restraint
definition of, 66, 92
local laws and, 66–67, 67*f*
forearm fractures, 1169–1170, 1170*f*
foreign bodies
airway obstruction
in infants/children, 599–603, 600*f*
recognizing, 461–464, 462*f*, 596–597, 597*f*, 677
removal, 597–603, 599*f*, 600*f*
in eye, 1010–1014
impaled
in abdomen, 1123
emergency medical care, 974–975
in eye, 1012
in vagina, 1251–1252
four-person log roll, 1062
Fowler position, 154*f*, 155, 171
fractures
blood loss from, 1172
child abuse, 1320
clavicle, 1103
closed, 1146, 1190
definition of, 1146, 1190
facial. *See* facial injuries, fractures
humerus, 1166–1167, 1166*t*
in child, through growth plate, 1160
injuries associated with, 1146–1149
linear, 1040, 1040*f*
open, 1146, 1190
osteoporosis and, 1175
pathologic, 1147
rib, 1102
signs/symptoms, 1148*f*, 1149
skull, 1037, 1040*f*
basilar, 1040, 1040*f*
depressed, 1040, 1040*f*
sternal, 1103
types, 1146, 1147*f*
Freedom House Ambulance Service, 4–5, 4*f*
freelancing, 1404, 1442
free movement, as fracture sign, 1149
freight bills, for hazardous materials, 1429, 1431*f*, 1442
French catheter, 429, 429*f*
frequency, definition of, 130
friends, presence during patient interview, 104
frontal bones, 177, 226
frontal lobe, 202, 226
frostbite, 342, 395
definition of, 1200–1201, 1238
emergency medical care, 1205
signs/symptoms, 1200, 1200*f*
frostnip, 1199–1200
full-thickness burns, 979, 997
fundus, 1258*f*, 1295

G

G agents, 1457, 1477
gag reflex, 432, 432*f*, 482
gallbladder, 210, 226
gallstones, 769
gamma (x-ray) radiation, 1470, 1477
gangrene, 1200, 1200*f*
gas cylinders
flowmeters, 439–440, 440*f*
pressure regulators, 439
safety considerations, 438
gastric distention, 482, 571
airway management and, 453
artificial ventilation and, 571–572
definition of, 609
gastroenteritis, 771
gastroesophageal reflux disease (GERD), 770, 786
gastrointestinal emergencies
assessment, 776–780
medical emergencies, 613, 613*t*
transport decisions, 777
gastrointestinal hemorrhage, 769–770
gastrointestinal system
anatomy, 764–765, 764*f*
pathophysiology, 766–776
gastrostomy tubes (gastric tubes; G-tubes), 1315, 1315*f*
GCS. *See* Glasgow Coma Scale
gel, definition of, 498, 528
GEMS diamond, 386, 387*t*
gender identity, 244, 254
general impressions. *See also under specific emergencies*
definition of, 333, 395
formation, 333–334, 334*f*
generalized seizures, definition of, 738–739, 761
generic name, definition of, 492, 528

genital system, 214–215
  female. *See also* female reproductive system
  male. *See also* male reproductive system
genitourinary injuries. *See also specific genitourinary injuries*
  anatomy, 1127–1129
  assessment, 1129–1132
  emergency medical care, 1132–1133
  interventions, 1132
  rape, 1133
  sexual assault, 1133
  transport decisions, 1131
  geriatric patient abdominal injuries from falls, 1115
  investigating chief complaint/chief concern, 351–352
  primary assessment, 346
geriatrics, 254
  definition of, 247
geriatric sexual abuse, 1326
germinal layer, 205, 226
gestation, 1260
gestational diabetes, 792, 1261, 1295
gestational hypertension, 1261, 1262, 1295
glands. *See specific glands*
Glasgow Coma Scale (GCS), 376*t*, 1052*t*
  definition, 926
  modified, 1052
  in neurologic emergencies, 753*t*
  scoring, 376*t*, 753*t*, 919, 920*t*
  trauma score and, 919–920, 921*t*
glenoid fossa, 1165, 1190
globe
  definition of, 1003, 1030
  laceration of, 1016
  rupture of, 1018
glottic opening, 404
glottis, 404, 482
gloves
  for cleaning/disinfecting, 42–43, 43*f*
  double, 42–43
  latex, 42
  removal technique, 43
  vinyl, 41
glucagon, 791
  for hypoglycemia, 798
glucometer (blood glucose monitor), 384, 801
glucose
  blood levels. *See* blood glucose
  definition of, 791, 814
  function, 791
  oral administration, 755, 803–804, 803*f*
Golden Period (Golden Hour), 347, 347*f*, 395, 547, 1153
gonorrhea, 1246–1247, 1254
good air exchange, 462, 464, 482
Good Samaritan laws, 81–82, 92
governmental immunity, definition, 82, 92
greater trochanter, 180, 226
great vessels, 195, 226
greenstick fractures, 1147, 1147*f*
GRIEVING mnemonic, 116
gross negligence, 82, 92
grunting, 685
guarding
  abdominal, 380
  definition of, 395, 786, 1136
  disorders associated with, 778
  as fracture sign, 1148
  signs/symptoms, 1121
gunshot wounds, penetrating trauma from, 898
gynecologic emergencies, 613*t*. *See also specific gynecologic emergencies*
  assessment, 1247–1251
  emergency medical care, 1251–1252
  interventions, 1251
  transport decisions, 1249

H

H1N1 virus (swine flu), 624
hair follicles, 205, 226
hallucinations, 877–878, 892
hallucinogens
  definition of, 857, 867
  overdose, 857
hand
  anatomy, 1142, 1142*f*
  injuries, 1170–1171, 1171*f*
handwashing, proper technique for, 40, 42, 42*f*
hazard control, at extrication scene, 1386–1388, 1387*f*
hazardous materials
  containers, 1423–1426, 1424*f*
  definition of, 1385, 1400, 1421
  Department of Transportation marking system, 1426–1427, 1427*f*
  detection by senses, 1423
  identification, 1430–1432
  occupancy/location, 1423
  references
    CHEMTREC, 1429, 1442
    Emergency Response Guidebook, 1428, 1428*f*
    safety data sheets, 1428–1429, 1430*f*
    shipping papers/bills of lading, 1429, 1431*f*, 1442
hazardous materials incidents (hazmat incidents)
  definition of, 1421, 1442
  examples, 1422–1423, 1422*f*
  scene operations, 1432–1434
    establishing control zones, 1432–1434, 1433–1434*f*
    patient care, 1435–1437
    personal protective equipment levels, 1435, 1436*f*
hazards, on-scene evaluation of, 326–327, 326*f*
HAZWOPER regulations, 1421
head
  anatomy, 1000–1003, 1000*f*
  focused assessment, 379–380, 380*f*
headache
  emergency medical care, 755–756
  types of, 756
head injuries. *See also* traumatic brain injury (TBI)
  assessment, 914, 1046–1051
  definition of, 1038
  emergency medical care, 1055–1057
  helmet removal, 1074–1079, 1076*f*
  interventions, 1050
  transport
    decision making for, 1049–1050
    of sitting patients, 1070–1072
    of standing patients, 1072
    of supine patients, 1062–1069
head-on collision, motorcycle, 908
head tilt–chin lift maneuver, 569–570, 569–570*f*
  definition of, 482, 609
  technique
    for adult, 426, 569–570, 569–570*f*
    for child, 593
health, balancing with work and family, 33–34
health care directive, 71, 92
health care proxy, 71, 92–93
health equity, 19, 24
health information exchange (HIE), 125
Health Insurance Portability and Accountability Act (HIPAA), 13, 69–70, 105
health literacy, 99
hearing, age-related changes, 251
hearing aids, 1305–1306, 1306*f*
hearing-impaired patients, 1304–1306, 1306*f*
  communication with, 110, 111*f*
  hearing aids for, 1305–1306, 1306*f*
heart, 191–194
  blood flow, 692*f*
  circulation, 691–697, 693*f*
  definition of, 689
  electrical conduction system, 690, 691*f*
  in perfusion triangle, 534, 535*f*
  structures of, 690*f*
  valves of, 690*f*
heart failure
  vs. chronic obstructive pulmonary disease, 671, 672*t*
  definition of, 702–703, 727
  left-side, 704
  right-side, 704
  signs/symptoms, 646*t*, 671, 703*t*
  treatment, 703*t*
heart rate (HR), 193, 226
heat cramps
  definition of, 1206, 1238
  emergency medical care, 1210, 1210*f*
  pathophysiology, 1206
heat exhaustion
  definition of, 1206, 1238
  emergency medical care, 1210–1212
  pathophysiology, 1206
  signs/symptoms, 1206

heat exposure illnesses
assessment, 1208–1210, 1209*t*
interventions, 1210
pathophysiology, 1206
transport decisions, 1209
types of. *See specific heat-related illnesses*
heat index, 1206, 1207*f*
heatstroke
definition of, 1207, 1238
emergency medical care, 1212, 1212*f*
pathophysiology, 1207–1208
signs/symptoms, 1207–1208
Heimlich maneuver. *See* abdominal-thrust maneuver
Helicobacter pylori, 768
helmets
motorcycle collisions and, 907
removal, 1074–1079, 1076*f*
car-versus-bicycle collision and, 907, 907*f*
in head and spinal injuries, 1074–1079
hematemesis, 768, 786, 850, 867, 935, 953
hematologic disorder, 806
hematologic emergencies. *See also specific hematologic emergencies*
assessment, 809–810
emergency medical care, 811
as medical emergencies, 613, 613*t*
pathophysiology, 806–809, 807*f*
transport decisions, 811
hematology, 806, 814
anatomy, 806–807, 807*f*
blood-forming organs, 806–807, 807*f*
definition of, 806
physiology, 806–807, 807*f*
hematoma, 379
definition of, 395, 953, 997
epidural, 1043, 1043*f*
facial, 1004, 1004*f*
internal bleeding and, 935
in older adults, 1043
pathophysiology, 959, 960*f*
subdural, 1043–1044, 1043*f*, 1083
hematuria, 936, 953
definition of, 1136, 1173, 1190
pelvic fractures and, 1173
urinary tract infections and, 773
hemiparesis
definition of, 761
hypoglycemia and, 743
postictal state and, 742
hemoglobin, 196, 226, 412
hemophilia, 808–809, 814, 934, 953
hemopneumothorax, 1101*f*, 1109
hemoptysis, 935, 953, 1092
hemorrhage. *See* bleeding
hemorrhagic shock, 542
hemorrhagic stroke
causes, 735–736
definition of, 761
hemorrhoids, 772
hemostatic dressing, 941–944, 953
hemothorax, 416, 482
definition of, 1100, 1109
pathophysiology, 1100
hepatitis
characteristics, 627*t*
definition of, 38, 58, 626
signs/symptoms, 626–628, 626*f*
transmission, 38, 627*t*
hepatitis A immunization, 50
herbicides, absorption of, 842
hernia, 772–773, 786
heroin, 851
herpes simplex, 625, 636
high-altitude pulmonary edema (HAPE), 1223–1224
high-level disinfection, 1359, 1379
highways, specific driving situations, 1369
hinge joints, 177, 226
HIPAA. *See* Health Insurance Portability and Accountability Act
hip dislocation, 1173–1174, 1174*f*
histamine, definition of, 817–818, 833
history taking, 348–354
confusing behavior and, 390
crying patients and, 390
definition of, 348, 395
identifying pertinent negatives, 352–354
language barrier in, 391
multiple symptoms and, 390
OPQRST, 350
for patients with limited cognitive abilities, 390
SAMPLE history. *See* SAMPLE history
on sensitive topics, 353–354, 353*f*
silent patients and, 389
HIV. *See* human immunodeficiency virus
hollow organs, 1114*f*, 1117–1118, 1136
home care, 1328
homelessness, 1329–1330
home of a terminally ill patient, 1328
homeostasis, 1194, 1238
definition of, 558
in shock, 533
home remedies, 709
honeybee stings, 819
hormones, 212, 226
definition of, 790, 814
hornet stings, 819
hospice care, 1328–1329
hospital, EMS communication with, 137–139, 137*f*
host, 48, 58
hot zone (danger zone), 1386, 1433, 1433*f*, 1442
human bite wounds, 976, 977*f*
human body. *See specific body systems*
pathophysiology, 217–220
planes of body, 174–175, 174*f*
topographic anatomy, 174–175
human immunodeficiency virus (HIV)
definition of, 39, 58
immune response, 50
signs/symptoms, 625–626
transmission of, 39
human trafficking, 1320–1321, 1335
humerus, 179, 226
distal, fracture of, 1166–1167
fracture, 1166–1167, 1166*t*
hydrocarbons, 854
hydroplaning, 1367, 1379
hydrostatic pressure, 199, 226
hymenoptera, 1227–1228, 1238
hypercapnia, definition of, 217, 226, 414, 482
hyperextension of spine, 1045, 1083
hyperflexion, 1045, 1083
hyperglycemia
characteristics, 793*t*
definition of, 740, 761, 792, 814
interventions, 801
signs/symptoms, 792, 793*t*
hyperosmolar hyperglycemic nonketotic syndrome (HHNS), 797
hyperrotation, 1045, 1083
hypersensitivity to drugs, 507
hypertension
definition of, 372, 396
during pregnancy, 1261–1262
hypertensive emergency
aortic/dissecting aneurysm, 705
definition of, 705, 727
hyperthermia, 1205, 1209, 1238
hyperventilation, 571, 609, 678–679, 685
hyperventilation syndrome (panic attack), 678, 685
hyphema, 1017, 1018*f*
hypnotic, 849, 867
hypoglycemia, 506, 528
altered mental state and, 743, 743*f*
characteristics, 793*t*
definition of, 740, 761, 814
emergency medical care, 805–806
interventions, 801
pathophysiology (symptomatic), 796
signs/symptoms, 792, 793*t*
hypoperfusion, 198, 226, 931, 953
hypotension, 372, 396, 1055
hypothermia, 342, 396
death and, 73
definition of, 558, 1197, 1238
emergency medical care, 1197–1205, 1203*f*
mild, 1197
neurogenic shock and, 541
prevention, 1203–1204
severe, 1198
signs/symptoms, 1197–1199, 1198*t*
submersion and, 1215–1217
hypothermia thermometer, 1197, 1202
hypovolemic shock, 542
causes, 542, 548*t*
circulatory compromise and, 416
definition of, 558, 953
development, 935
in open injuries, 973
signs/symptoms, 548*t*
treatment, 548*t*, 550–551

hypoxemia, 420
hypoxia, 217, 226
  death from, 410
  definition of, 482, 647, 685
  signs of, 108
hypoxic drive, 190, 226, 411
  carbon dioxide retention and, 647
  definition of, 482, 647, 685
  physiology, 410

I

ICP. *See* intracranial pressure
ICS. *See* incident command system
I-gel airway device, 476, 476*f*
ileostomy, 1316, 1335
ileus, 766, 786
ilium, 179, 226
immersion foot, 1200
immune response, 817, 833
immune system, 817
  definition of, 817, 833
  infants, 237
  pathophysiology, 817–819, 818*f*
  physiology, 817, 818*f*
immunity
  definition of, 48, 58
  Good Samaritan laws and, 81–82
  to infectious disease, 49*t*, 50
immunizations, 50
immunologic emergencies
  assessment, 820–821
  chief complaint investigation, 822
  communication/documentation of, 825
  emergency medical care, 825–831
  as medical emergencies, 613, 613*t*
  transport decisions, 825
immunology, 817, 833
impaled objects, 963, 997
implied consent
  definition of, 64, 93
  emergency doctrine of, 64
  for treating children in critical situations, 64
inadequate breathing, 191
incarcerated hernia, 773
incendiary and explosive devices, in terrorism, 1473
incident action plan, 1407, 1443
incident commander (IC)
  definition of, 1400, 1405–1406, 1443
  roles/responsibilities, 1393–1394, 1393*f*, 1405–1408
incident command system (ICS)
  command, 1406–1407, 1406*f*, 1443
  command staff, 1407–1408
  communications and information management, 1404, 1408
  definition of, 1404, 1443
  EMS branch
    communications, 1411
    establishing command, 1411
    preparedness of, 1409
    response within, 1409–1411, 1410*f*
  equipment, 1408–1409
  finance/administration, 1407, 1443
  logistics, 1407, 1443
  medical branch. *See* medical incident command
  mobilization/deployment, 1408–1409
  with multiple patients, 330, 330*f*
  operations, 1407
  organizational divisions, 1404, 1405*f*
  planning, 1407
  roles/responsibilities, 1405–1408
incident management, 1403–1437
incision, 962, 997
inclusive workplace
  cultural diversity, 54–55
  incivility, 53–54
  sexual harassment, 54
incomplete fracture, 1147
incontinence
  definition of, 739, 761
  generalized seizures and, 739
incubation period, 1463, 1477
index of suspicion, 615, 636, 898, 926
indications, definition of, 491, 528
indirect contact, 39, 58
induced abortion, 1264, 1295
industrial/environmental exposures, 679
infants
  AED, 594
  airway, 405, 405*f*
  bag-mask ventilation, 236
  basic life support, 586–594, 587*t*
  blood loss, from skull region, 1057
  cardiovascular system, 235
  chest compressions, 588
  CPR, chest compressions, 589–590
  definition of, 235, 235*f*, 254
  foreign body airway obstruction, 599–603, 600*f*
  immune system, 237
  immunizations, recommended, 50
  nervous system, 236–237
  physical changes, vital signs, 235
  psychosocial changes, 237–238, 237*t*
  pulmonary system, 235–236
  in shock
    circulation emergencies and management, 551–552
    dehydration emergencies and management, 553, 553*t*, 554*f*
  weight, 235
infarction, 698, 727
infection, definition of, 38, 58
infection control
  definition of, 47, 58
  employer responsibilities for, 46–47
  establishing routine for, 47–48
infectious disease, 624, 636
  AIDS, 625–626
  COVID-19, 631
  definition of, 38, 58
  Ebola, 631
  epidemic and pandemic considerations, 624
  general assessment principles, 623–624
  immunity to, 49*t*, 50
  management principles, general, 624
  postexposure management, 50–51
  risk reduction and prevention
    employer responsibilities, 46–47
    establishing infection control routine, 47–48
    eye protection, 43, 45*f*
    gloves, 42–43, 43*f*
    gowns, 43–44
    handwashing, proper technique for, 42
    masks, respirators, and barrier devices, 44–46, 45*f*
    sharps disposal, proper, 46, 46*f*
    standard precautions, 41*t*
  routes of transmission, 38–40, 38*f*
  standard precautions, 40
  travel medicine and, 631–632
  vs. communicable diseases, 38
inferior, definition of, 151–152, 171, 694, 727
inferior vena cava, 195, 226, 689, 690*f*, 694
influenza, 624–625, 636–637
  definition of, 624
  type A
    characteristics, 646*t*
    definition of, 667, 685
informed consent, 64, 93
ingestion, 867
  of toxins, 836, 839*f*
inhalation, 494, 528
  definition of, 408, 483
  physiology, 408–410
inhalation injury, 987–988
inhalation medications, 516–520
injuries, drug-related, 84
in loco parentis, definition, 66, 93
insecticides, absorption of, 842
insect stingsallergens from, 819
  allergic reactions to, 819
inspiration, 409, 641
inspiratory reserve volume, 191, 226
institutional standards, standards of care and, 77–78
insulin
  definition of, 791, 814
  diabetes mellitus and, 792
  pumps, for diabetes, 794
  role of, 791
Intal (cromolyn), 660*t*
integumentary system
  anatomy, 205–206
  physiology, 206
intellectual disability, 1300, 1335
intended effect. *See* therapeutic effect
intermodal tanks, 1425, 1425*f*, 1443
internal cardiac pacemakers, 1313
internal respiration, 412–413, 412–413*f*, 483
interoperable communications system, 133, 144

interrogatories, definition, 85, 93
intersection hazards, specific driving situations, 1369
interstitial space, 199, 226
intervertebral disks, 178, 226, 1038, 1083
interviews, patient
  with adolescents, 245
  communication techniques, 104
  with older adults, 107–109, 108*f*
  presence of family, friends or bystanders during, 104
  questions for, 102
  techniques to avoid, 104*t*
intestine, 765
intoxicated patients, history taking and, 390
intracellular space, 199, 226
intracerebral hematoma, 1044, 1044*f*, 1083
intracranial hemorrhage, 1042–1043
  epidural hematoma, 1043
  intracerebral hematoma, 1044, 1044*f*
  subarachnoid hemorrhage, 1044
  subdural hematoma, 1043–1044
intracranial pressure (ICP)
  definition of, 1042, 1083
  increased, in infant, 237
  increase, with hemorrhagic stroke, 733
  in traumatic brain injury, 1042
intramuscular (IM) injection, 494, 528
intramuscular medications, 509–515
intranasal (IN), 495
intranasal medications, 515–516
intraosseous (IO) injection, 494, 528
intrapulmonary shunting, 415, 483
intravenous (IV) injection, 494, 528
involuntary activities, 1036, 1083
involuntary consent, 65
involuntary muscle, 182, 226
ionizing radiation, 1469, 1477
ipratropium (Atrovent), 660*t*
iris, 1003, 1003*f*, 1030
irreversible shock, 543, 558
irrigation, of eye, 1011, 1014, 1015*f*
ischemia, 586–587, 609, 698, 727, 735, 761
ischemic stroke
  definition of, 735, 761
  pathophysiology, 735, 735*f*
ischium, 179, 227
islets of Langerhans
  definition of, 791
  function, 791

J

jaundice, 340–341, 396, 626, 626*f*
jaw-thrust maneuver, 570, 570*f*
  definition of, 483, 609
  purpose, 427–428
  technique, 570, 570*f*, 1048, 1058*f*
    for adult, 427–428
    for child, 593
jellyfish stings, 1234, 1234*f*
joint capsule, 176, 227
joint information center (JIC), 1408, 1443
joints, 176–177
  anatomy, 1142*f*, 1143
  definition of, 1143, 1190
  functions, 1142*f*
jugular venous distention (JVD), 1093
jump kit, 1349, 1349*f*, 1350*t*, 1379
JumpSTART triage system, 1418–1419, 1419*f*, 1443
junctional tourniquet, 946–947, 946*f*, 953
Just Culture, 17, 24

K

kidnapping, 81, 93
kidneys, 213, 227
  anatomy, 1118–1119
  definition of, 773
  infection, localization of pain, 768*t*
  injuries, 1118, 1132
kidney stones
  characteristics, 773
  definition of, 786
  localization of pain, 768*t*
kinetic energy, 898, 926
King LT airway device, 475, 475*f*
knee
  dislocation, 1181–1182
  ligament injuries, 1181
Kussmaul respirations, 419, 796, 800, 814
kyphosis, 1144

L

labels, for hazardous materials, 1426–1427, 1427*f*
labia majora, 1243, 1243*f*, 1254
labia minora, 1243, 1243*f*, 1254
labored breathing, 337, 396, 417, 418*f*, 483
labor, stages, 1270–1271
lacerations
  definition of, 997
  ear, 1021, 1022*f*
  emergency medical care, 1016–1017, 1017*f*
  eye, 1016–1017, 1017*f*
  facial, 1020
  fractures and, 1154
  pathophysiology, 962, 962*f*
  scalp, 1039, 1039*f*
lacrimal glands, 1003, 1003*f*, 1030
lactic acid, 216, 227, 1139
landline phone, 133
language
  barriers, in history taking, 391
  tone, pace and volume of, 100
  understandable, in dealing with patient, 105
large intestine, 207*f*, 210, 211*t*, 1114
laryngectomy, 459
laryngopharynx, 402, 403*f*
laryngospasm, 432
larynx
  anatomy, 404, 1002, 1002*f*
  definition of, 483
  fracture, 1026
  injuries, 1026
lateral bending, 1045, 1083
lateral, definition of, 152, 171
laws and regulations, 1368–1369
  right-of-way privileges, 1368
  use of escorts, 1369
laws/regulations, standards of care imposed by, 76–77
Lazarus syndrome, 603–604
left ventricular assist devices, 585, 720–722, 1313
leg, anatomy, 1142*f*, 1143
length-based resuscitation tape, 367, 396, 465
lens, 1002*f*, 1003, 1030
lesser trochanter, 180, 227
leukotrienes, 817–818, 833
level of consciousness
  AVPU test for, 334, 335*f*
  categories of, 334–336
lewisite (L), 1455, 1460*t*, 1477
liaison officer, 1408, 1443
libel, definition of, 81, 93
licensure
  definition of, 10, 24, 79
  requirements, 10
life expectancy, 248, 254
life support chain, 215–217
life threats
  identification, 332–333
  treatment, 332–333
  uncontrolled external bleeding, 334
lifting of patients, technique, 257–258, 277*f*
ligaments, 176, 176*t*
  definition of, 1143, 1190
light burns, to eye, 1016
lightening, of fetus, 1271, 1295
lightning injuries, 1224
limb lead placement, 714, 714*f*
limb presentation, 1288, 1289*f*, 1295
linear skull fracture, 1040*f*, 1041, 1083
liquid oxygen, 438
lithium, 848
liver, 209–210
  physiology, 764
living will. *See* advance directives
load-distributing band (LDB), 585–586, 586*f*, 609
locked joint, as fracture sign, 1149
logistics, in incident command system, 1407, 1443
log rolling, 279, 279*f*, 280
  for moving patients, technique, 1062
lone wolf terrorist attack, 1448, 1477
Los Angeles Prehospital Stroke Scale, 749, 751*t*
lower airway, 185–186
lower extremities, 180–181
lumbar spine, 178, 227
lumen, 698, 727

lungs
assessment, in respiratory system emergencies, 652–653
compliance, 454
wet *vs.* dry, 671
lung sounds, adventitious, 652, 653*t*
Lyme disease, 1233–1234
bull's-eye rash, 1233*f*
lymph, 211, 227
lymphatic system, 211
bubonic plague and, 1466
definition of, 1477
lymph nodes, 211, 227
bubonic plague and, 1466
definition of, 1477
lysergic acid diethylamide (LSD), 857

M

male reproductive system
anatomy, 765, 1127, 1127*f*
external genitalia, injuries to, 1129
genitalia injuries, emergency medical care, 1132–1133
malleolus, 181, 227
Mallory-Weiss tear, 771
mandatory reporting, 83–84
mandible, 177, 227
mandibular fractures, 1024
manic episode, 872, 892
manual left displacement of the uterus, 604*f*
manubrium, 179, 227
marijuana, 857
marine animal injuries, 1234–1235, 1234*f*
masks
for infectious disease risk reduction, 44–46, 45*f*
mass-casualty incidents (MCIs)
accountability, 1409
definition of, 1403, 1414, 1443
demobilization, 1409
diagram, 1414, 1414*f*
disasters, 1420
initial briefing, 1408
mutual aid response, 1403, 1443
record keeping, 1408–1409
reporting, 129
scene, check-in, 1408
transport decisions, 1420
mast cells, 818*f*
mastoid process, 1001, 1030
material safety data sheet. *See* safety data sheet
maternal cardiac arrest, 1265
mature minor, 66
mature minor doctrine, 66, 93
maxillae, 177, 227
maxillary fractures, 1024
MCIs. *See* mass-casualty incidents
MDI. *See* metered-dose inhaler
mean arterial pressure (MAP), 374, 396
mechanical chest compression equipment, 1348
mechanical piston device, 585, 585*f*, 609
mechanical ventilator, 1310–1312, 1311*f*
mechanics of breathing, 186–188
mechanism of injury (MOI)
in blunt *vs.* penetrating trauma, 327–328
definition of, 327, 396, 897, 926
determination, 327–328
profiles, 900
significant, 900
meconium, 1269, 1283, 1295
staining, 1283
medevac, 1371, 1379
medial, definition of, 152, 171
mediastinum, 406, 483, 1088–1089
definition of, 483
structures in, 406–407, 1099
medical
calling, 138–139
EMS communication with, 137–139, 137*f*
medical director, 16, 24
medical emergencies, 897, 926
assessment, 614–615
definition of, 613, 637
infectious diseases, 623–624
interventions, 613
transport, 620–623, 621–622*f*
decision making, 617
destination selection and, 622–623
time on scene and, 621
types, 621–622, 621–622*f*
types of, 613–614, 613*t*
medical equipment, in ambulances, 1344*f*, 1345–1349, 1346*t*, 1347–1350*f*, 1350*t*, 1352*f*
medical examiner (coroner), 74, 75*f*
medical fear, 99
medical identification insignia, 76, 76*f*
medical identification tags, 348
medical incident command, 1411, 1412*f*
extrication supervisor, 1413, 1443
morgue supervisor, 1413–1414, 1444
physicians on scene, 1413
rehabilitation supervisor, 1413, 1443
rescue supervisor, 1413, 1443
staging supervisor, 1412
transportation supervisor, 1412, 1444
treatment supervisor, 1411–1412, 1444
triage, 1415–1420, 1416*t*, 1417*f*
triage supervisor, 1411, 1444
medical necessity, 124
Medical Orders for Life-Sustaining Treatment (MOLST), 71
medical oversight, 16, 24
Medical Practices Act, 79
medical technology assistance, patients with
apnea monitors, 1312–1313, 1313*f*
central venous catheters, 1314–1315, 1314*f*
colostomy, 1316, 1335
external defibrillator vest, 1314
gastrostomy tubes, 1315, 1315*f*
home care, 1328
ileostomy, 1316, 1335
internal cardiac pacemakers, 1313
left ventricular assist devices, 585, 720–722, 1313
mechanical ventilator, 1310–1312, 1311*f*
shunts, 1315, 1335
tracheostomy tubes, 1310
urostomy, 1316
vagus nerve stimulators, 1316
medical terminology
abbreviations, 155–156, 163–169*t*
anatomy of, 148–149
in calling medical direction, 138–139
colors, 150
combining form, 158–160*t*
combining vowels, 148–149
components, 148–149
directional terms, 151–153, 152*f*, 152*t*
Fowler, 155
introduction, 148
master tables, 158–169*t*
movement terms, 153, 153*f*
pharmacology, related to abbreviations, 163–169*t*
plural endings, 149
position of the patient, 154–155, 154*f*
Fowler, 154*f*, 155
prone, 154, 154*f*
recovery position, 154*f*
supine, 154, 154*f*
prefixes, 148, 161*t*
medication administration, 161*t*
numerical, 150*t*
position, direction, and location, 150, 151*t*
suffixes, 148, 162*t*
symbols, 157, 157*t*
word roots, 148, 158–160*t*
medication error, 524, 528
medications. *See* drugs/medications
medicolegal, definition of, 64, 93
medulla oblongata, 202, 227
melena, 768, 786
definition of, 954, 1136
internal bleeding and, 935
menarche, 1243, 1258, 1295
meninges
anatomy, 1035, 1035*f*
definition of, 1083
meningitis
definition of, 637
diagnosis, 628–629
meningococcal meningitis, 628, 637
menopause, 1258, 1295
definition of, 1244
menstrual cycle, 1258, 1259, 1263
menstruation, 1243–1245, 1247
mental/emotional fitness, 1360–1361
mental health crisis care systems, 870–871
mental health problems
emergencies. *See* psychiatric/behavioral emergencies
involuntary consent for mentally ill patients, 65

mental illness, 870, 892
mental model, 112, 144
mental status, alteration
in acute myocardial infarction, 701
causes, 743–745
in hypoglycemia, 743, 743*f*
as neurologic emergency, 743–745, 743*f*
mescaline, 857*t*
mesentery, 114
metabolic acidosis, causes, 418
metabolic agents, in chemical terrorism/warfare, 1460–1462, 1460*t*, 1462*t*
metabolism, 216, 227, 383, 396, 411, 483
metacarpals, 179, 227
metatarsals, 181, 227
metered-dose inhaler (MDI), 497, 497*f*, 517–520, 517*f*, 528
administration, 800–801
contraindications, 659
definition of, 685
medications for, 658, 659, 660*t*
spacer, 661, 661*f*
methamphetamine, 855
methicillin-resistant *Staphylococcus aureus* (MRSA), 1327, 1335
definition of, 637
transmission, 631
midbrain, 202, 227
middle adults. *See* adults, middle
midsagittal (midline) plane, definition of, 175
migraine headaches, 756
mild airway obstruction, 462, 483
military time, 119*t*
ministroke. *See* transient ischemic attack
minute alveolar ventilation, 409*t*, 483
minute volume, 191, 227, 409*t*, 483, 1089
miosis, 1458–1459, 1477
miscarriages (spontaneous abortions), 1247, 1295
definition of, 1264
signs/symptoms, 1264
mission-critical communications, 112, 144
mitral valve, 690*f*
mobile data terminals, 133, 133*f*, 144
mobile integrated health care (MIH), 19, 24, 302, 316, 871, 893
mobile radio, 130, 130–131*f*
monitoring devices, for vital signs. *See* vital signs; specific monitoring devices
morality, 86, 93
morgue supervisor, 1413–1414, 1443
Moro reflex (startle reflex), 236, 254
morphine, 851, 851*t*
motorcycle crash, 907–908
motor function assessment, 382
motor nerves, 205, 1036
motor vehicle crashes
airbags and, 902–904
with bicycles, 907, 907*f*
crash scenes, 1382
extrication of passengers. *See* extrication
frontal collision injuries, 904, 905*f*
frontal impact, types of, 902*f*, 904
lateral, 904–905
motorcycle, 907–908
with pedestrians, 907
during pregnancy, 1265
rear-end, 904, 905*f*
rollover crashes, 905–906
rotational, 906–907
seat belts and, 904
"star" on windshield, 1046*f*
motor vehicles
alternative-fuel type, 1388
safety systems, 1381–1382, 1382*f*
mouth, 208
bleeding from, 947–948
mouth-to-mask ventilation
advantages, 448
barrier device, 448, 448*f*
technique, 448
moving of patients
anatomy and body mechanics, 258–265, 259*f*
geriatric considerations, 262
patient weight, 265
pediatric considerations, 262, 262*f*
safe lifting and carrying, 265, 265*t*
safe reaching and pulling, 263–265, 263–264*f*
backboard, 284, 284*f*
basket stretcher, 293, 293*f*
across bed, 279, 279*f*
binder lifts, 291
directions and commands, 265–266
emergency moves, 267–276
definition of, 267
dragging methods, 268, 268*f*
nonurgent moves, 275
one-person drags, carries, and lifts, 270, 270*f*
one-person technique, 268, 269*f*
urgent move, 270–271
flexible stretcher, 292, 293*f*
neonatal isolettes, 290–291, 291*f*
patient positioning, 266–267
personnel considerations, 267
portable/folding stretchers, 291–292, 292*f*
principles of, 258–267
short backboards, 293–294
Slipp patient mover, 291
stair chair, 288–290
vacuum mattresses, 284, 285*f*
wheeled ambulance stretcher, 276–284, 277*f*
electronic stretcher, 277, 278*f*
loading, 282–284
pushing, 280–282, 281–282*f*
transferring patient, 278–280
MRSA. *See* methicillin-resistant *Staphylococcus aureus*
mucosal atomizer device (MAD), 495, 528
mucous membranes, 205, 227, 958, 997
mucus, 206, 227
multigravida, 1269–1270, 1295
multiple births, 1289–1290
multiple-casualty incident. *See* mass casualty incidents
multiplex communications, 132, 144
multisystem trauma, 914, 926
muscles of breathing, 186–188
muscles, types, 1139, 1140*f*. *See also specific types of muscles*
muscular dystrophy, 1310–1311
musculoskeletal assessment, 6 Ps, 1155
musculoskeletal injuries
assessment, 1151–1156
in burn injuries, 984–985
emergency medical care, 1156–1163
interventions, 1155
mechanism of injury, 1145–1146
specific. *See specific musculoskeletal injuries*
transport
considerations for, 1156
decision making, 1152
musculoskeletal system, 182, 227
anatomy, 181–182, 1139–1140, 1140*f*
skeletal muscle, 182
blood supply, 1140
in children, 184
handling injured extremities, 1157
pathophysiology of
children, 1143
older adults, 1144–1145
physiology, 182
mustard (sulfur mustard), 1455, 1460*t*
mutagens, 1455, 1477
mutual aid response, 1403, 1443
Mycobacterium tuberculosis, 629
myocardial contractility, 537, 558
myocardial contusion, 1094*t*, 1104, 1109
myocardial ischemia, 699
myocardium, 191, 227, 691, 727

N

naloxone, 515–516, 516*f*
nasal cannulas, 443, 443*t*, 483
nasal flaring, 338, 396
nasopharyngeal (nasal) airway
contraindications, 435
definition of, 483
indications, 435
insertion, 435–436
in pediatrics, 466–467
types, 434–435, 434*f*
nasopharynx, 184, 227, 402–403, 403*f*, 483

National EMS Advisory Council (NEMSAC), 4
National EMS Education Standards, 6, 24
National EMS Information System (NEMSIS), 10, 24, 120
National EMS Scope of Practice Model, 6, 24
National Fire Protection Association (NFPA), 1434–1435
National Highway Traffic Safety Administration (NHTSA), 1361
National Incident Management System (NIMS)
  components, 1404
  definition of, 1404, 1443
  principles, 1404
National Registry of EMTs (NREMT), 5
nature of illness (NOI), 328, 396, 614, 637. *See also under specific illnesses/disorders*
nebulizers, small-volume, 658, 659
neck anatomy, 1001–1002, 1001*f*
neck injuries
  assessment, 914–916, 1004–1008
  emergency medical care, 1008, 1009*f*, 1024, 1025*f*
  interventions, 1007
  open wounds, emergency medical care, 973, 975*f*
  soft-tissue, 1004, 1004*f*
  transport decisions, 1006
neglect, 1318–1326, 1319*f*, 1323*t*, 1325*t*, 1335
negligence
  categories, 79
  contributory, 85
  definition of, 93
negligence per se, 80, 93
Neisseria gonorrhoeae, 1246
neonatal isolettes, 290–291, 291*f*
neonatal resuscitation
  algorithm, 1284*f*
  performing, 1282–1287
    chest compressions, 1283
    positive-pressure ventilation, 1282
    steps, 1282*t*
  rapid assessment, 1282–1287
nephrons, 250
nerve agents, 1457–1460, 1457*f*, 1458*t*, 1459*f*, 1460*t*, 1477
nervous system
  anatomy, 730–731, 732*f*
  anatomy and physiology
    central nervous system, 201–204
  brain, 201–203
    cerebrospinal fluid, 203
    circulation in the head, 203
  central, anatomy of, 1034–1035, 1034*f*, 1035*f*
  focused assessment, 375
  of infants, 236–237
  motor nerves, 205
  of older adults, 250–251, 250*f*
  pathophysiology, 731–732
    stroke, 734, 735*f*
  peripheral, anatomy of, 1035–1036, 1036*f*
  physiology, 730–731, 731*f*, 1033–1036
  sensory nerves, 204–205
  spinal cord, 204
neurogenic shock, 540–541
  causes, 548*t*
  definition of, 558
  signs/symptoms, 548*t*
  treatment, 548*t*, 550
neurologic emergencies
  altered mental state, 743–745, 743*f*
  assessment, 745–755
  communication, 755
  documentation, 754, 755
  emergency medical care, 755–757
  as medical emergencies, 613, 613*t*
  transport decisions, 745
neuromuscular growth, toddlers/preschoolers, 240
neurons, 201, 228
neurotoxins, as biological warfare agents, 1466–1468, 1468*t*, 1477
neurovascular compromise, 1163
neurovascular status assessment, 377–379, 1155
neutron radiation, 1470, 1477
newborn
  assessment, 1282–1287
  crying, 1283
  delivering, 1275–1280
    of body, 1279–1280
    of head, 1279
  preterm, 1290, 1290*f*
  pulmonary system, 235–236
  skin color, 1283
Newton's law, 899–900
9-1-1 calls, 135, 135*f*
nitroglycerin, 507–509, 508*f*, 528
  dosage/administration, 712–714
  forms of, 712
Nitrostat. *See* nitroglycerin
noise
  communication and, 101
  definition of, 101, 144
nonbulk storage vessels, 1425
nondisplaced fracture, 1146, 1190
nonhemorrhagic shock, 542
nonprogressive (compensated) shock, 543, 543*t*, 558
nonrebreathing masks
  definition of, 483
  pediatric patient, 467–468
  usage, 443–444, 443*f*
norepinephrine, 200, 228
  effects, 535–536
nose
  anatomy, 1020–1021, 1021*f*
  bleeding from, 947–948
  fractures, 1020–1021
  injuries, 1020–1021, 1021*f*
nosebleeds (epistaxis), 947–948, 953
notification
  of hospital, 137, 137*f*
  procedures, for terrorism events, 1453
nuchal cord, 1279, 1295
nuclear terrorism/warfare
  exposure
    medical management, 1472–1473
    protective measures, 1472
    symptomatology, 1471–1472, 1471*t*
  weapons/devices, 1471
nursing/skilled care facilities, 1326–1328
nutrition, for wellness, 28–29, 29*f*

O

obesity, 1308–1309, 1335
objective information, 118
oblique fracture, 1147, 1147*f*
obstetric kit, emergency, 1272–1273
obstructive shock, 537–540
  causes, 548*t*
  definition of, 558–559
  signs/symptoms, 548*t*
  treatment, 548*t*, 549
occipital bone, 177, 228
occipital lobe, 202, 228
occlusion
  of coronary artery, 698
  definition of, 727
occlusive dressings, 973, 997, 1098, 1109
Occupational Safety and Health Administration (OSHA), 40
off-gassing, 1457, 1477
older adults. *See* adults, older
olecranon process fracture, 1164
oncotic pressure, 199, 228
one-handed carry, 287
one-rescuer adult CPR, 572, 573
onset of action, 491, 528
onset of problem, in OPQRST, 350
open-book pelvic fracture, 947, 954
open-ended questions
  definition of, 102, 144
  in patient interview, 102, 103*t*
open fractures, 1146, 1149, 1149*f*, 1190
open incident, 1410, 1443
open injuries
  abdominal
    definition of, 1136
    emergency medical care, 1124–1126, 1125*f*
    signs/symptoms, 1116–1117, 1116*f*
  assessment, 965–972
  chest, 1090, 1090*f*, 1109
  definition of, 958, 997
  emergency medical care, 972–977, 975*f*
  head, 1041, 1083
  types of, 961–965, 962–965*f*
open pneumothorax, 1098, 1098*f*, 1110
open skull fractures, 1040*f*, 1041
operations, in incident command system, 1407, 1443

opioid
algorithm, life-threatening, 852*f*
CPR and, 603
definition of, 850–851, 867
poisonings, 850–853
OPQRST, 777–778, 1154
definition of, 350, 396
for pain assessment, 709, 710*t*
optic nerve, 1003, 1030
oral glucose, 506, 528, 755
oral medications, 506–507, 528
orbit, 177, 228, 1000–1001
organ donation, consent for, 75, 76*f*
organophosphates, 858
orientation, 335, 396
oropharyngeal (oral) airway
definition of, 431, 483
insertion
in adults, 432
in children, 432, 465–466
for unresponsive patients, 431, 432*f*
oropharynx, 208–209, 403, 403*f*, 483
orthopnea, 646*t*, 685
orthotic device, 1308, 1335
osteoarthritis, 1144–1145
osteoporosis, 1144
fracture risk, 1174
ovaries, 215, 228
anatomy, 1243–1245, 1243*f*, 1258
definition of, 1254
overconfidence, 312, 317
overdose
cardiac medications, 858
definition of, 837, 867
over-the-counter (OTC) medications, 492
definition of, 492
overdosage, 850
ovulation, 1243–1245, 1254, 1258
oxygen, 515–517, 516–517, 528
during inspiration, 409, 641
during respiration, 641, 645*f*
supplemental, 437–443
equipment for, 437*f*, 437–440, 438*t*
hazards, 442–443
nasal cannula, 444
supply units, in ambulance, 1345–1347, 1347*f*
oxygenation, 648, 670, 685
definition of, 408*t*, 483
physiology, 411
respiration and, 533
oxygen cylinders
flowmeters, 439–440, 440*f*
hazards, 442–443
pin-indexing system, 438–439, 439*f*
placing into service, 440–442
pressure regulators, 439
safety precautions/considerations, 438, 442
sizes, 437, 438*t*
oxygen-delivery devices, 443–445
nasal cannulas, 444, 444*f*
nonrebreathing mask, 443–444, 443*f*
oxygen humidifiers, 445, 445*f*
partial rebreathing mask, 444
tracheostomy mask, 445, 445*f*
Venturi mask, 444–445, 444*f*
oxygen humidifiers, 445, 445*f*
oxygen saturation (Spo_2), 420
oxygen toxicity, 443, 483

P

pacemakers
automated external defibrillation and, 579, 581
for cardiovascular emergencies, 718–719, 719*f*
paging, 135, 144
pain
of acute myocardial infarction, 700–701
in angina, 699
as fracture sign, 1149
localization
in appendicitis, 768*t*
in diverticulitis, 768*t*
in duodenal ulcer, 768*t*
quality, in OPQRST, 350
radiation, 350
referred, 767, 768*f*, 768*t*, 786
responsiveness to, 335*f*
palliating factors, in OPQRST, 350
palmar grasp reflex, 236, 254
palmar, definition of, 153, 171
palpate, 339, 396
pancreas, 209
physiology, 791
pancreatitis, 768*t*, 769, 786
pandemic, 624, 637, 667, 685
panic attack (hyperventilation syndrome), 678
paradoxical chest motion, 338, 380, 1093, 1102–1103, 1110
paralysis, definition of, 1308
paramedic
definition of, 6, 24
training for, 7, 8*f*
parasympathetic nervous system, 204, 228, 691, 727, 1037
parenteral medications, 493, 528
parietal bones, 177, 228
parietal lobe, 202, 228
parietal pleura, 406, 483
paroxysmal nocturnal dyspnea, 646*t*, 685
partial pressure of oxygen (Pao_2), 408
partial rebreathing mask, 444
partial-thickness burns, 978, 997
patella, 180, 228
dislocation, 1183, 1183*f*
patent airway, 410, 411*f*, 483
pathogen, definition of, 38, 58
pathologic fracture, 1147*f*
pathophysiology. *See under specific emergency disorders*
patient
assessment of. *See* assessment
autonomy, 63, 91
determining number at scene, 330, 330*f*
high-priority, 346–347
interviews with. *See* interviews, patient
moving. *See* moving of patients
nutrition/hydration, exposure and, 1195
physical condition, exposure and, 1195
transfer of. *See* transfer of patients
patient assessment flowchart, 325, 332, 348, 355, 388
patient-assisted medication, 501, 528
patient care handoff, 112–114
patient care report (PCR)
administration information gathered from, 118–119
CHART method, 122
confidentiality of, 124
data collection, 119–120
definition of, 118, 144
electronic, 121*f*
example of, 118*f*
functions, 118
legal issues, 119
narrative section, 121
patient information in, 119
purpose of, 118–120
quoting patient in, 120*t*
refusal form, 68
requirements for, 120, 120*t*
significant negative findings in, 121
SOAP method, 122–124
types of, 120–121
patient medications, 520–524
patient rights, to refuse treatment, 68
PCR. *See* patient care report
peak, 491, 529
pectoral girdle, 179, 228
anatomy, 1140, 1141*f*
pedestrians, collisions with vehicles, 907
pediatric airway management, 464–469
nasopharyngeal, 466–467
oropharyngeal, 465–466
oxygen delivery devices
bag-mask device, 468–469
nasal cannula, 467
nonrebreathing mask, 467–468
two-person bag-mask ventilation, 469
pediatric assessment triangle (PAT), 396
pediatric emergencies, abdominal injuries, 1112
pediatric patients
investigating chief complaint/chief concern, 351
primary assessment, 343–346
sexual abuse, 1326
PEEP *See* positive end-expiratory pressure
peer-assisted medication, 501, 529
pelvic binder, 947, 954, 1161, 1163*f*, 1191
pelvic compression device, 947
pelvic fractures
care of, 1172–1173, 1173*f*
open, 1172

types, 1172–1173
with urinary bladder injuries, 1129
pelvic girdle, 179, 228, 1142
pelvic inflammatory disease (PID)
cause, 1245–1246
definition of, 1254
pelvis, 179
focused assessment, 381, 382*f*
fractures, 1172–1173, 1173*f*
penetrating trauma
definition of, 900, 926
low-energy, 910, 910*f*
as mechanism of injury, 328
medium-velocity and high-velocity, 911
neck injuries from, 1025, 1026*f*
penetrating wound, 963, 964*f*, 997
peptic ulcer disease, 768
perfusion, 197, 228
components, 695
definition of, 336, 396, 533, 559, 695, 727, 931–932, 954
physiology, 533–536, 931–932, 932*f*
poor, 345, 345*f*
perfusion triangle, 534, 535*f*
pericardial effusion, 538, 559
pericardial tamponade. *See* cardiac tamponade
pericardium (pericardial sac)
definition of, 1110
function, 1101
perineum
anatomy, 1243, 1243*f*, 1259
definition of, 1254, 1295
peripheral nerve injury, 1035–1036
peripheral nervous system (PNS), 201, 228
anatomy, 1035–1036, 1036*f*
definition of, 1035
peristalsis, 214, 228, 765
peritoneal cavity, 1114, 1136
peritoneum, 766, 786, 1114, 1136
peritonitis, 766, 786, 1114, 1121, 1137
per os (PO), 493, 529
per rectum (PR), 493, 529
persistency, 1454, 1477
person-first language, 107
personal experience, communication and, 99–100
personal protective equipment (PPE), 1265
definition of, 38, 58, 396
face shields, 43
glasses, 43, 45*f*
gloves, 42–43, 43*f*
gowns, 43–44
levels for hazmat incidents, 1435, 1436*f*
masks, 44–46, 45*f*
as safety precaution, 329
personal safety equipment in ambulances, 1350
pertinent negatives, 352, 396
pertussis (whooping cough)
characteristics, 646*t*, 667
definition of, 685
signs/symptoms, 630, 646*t*
pesticides
absorption of, 842
bags for, 1425–1426, 1426*f*
petechiae, 629, 637
phalanges, 179, 228
pharmacodynamics, 490, 529
pharmacokinetics, 490–491, 529
pharmacology, principles of, 489–529
pharynx, 185, 228
phencyclidine (PCP), 857
phosgene oxime (CX), 1455, 1460*t*, 1478
phrenic nerve, 190, 228, 407, 483
physical abuse, 1266
burn injuries suggestive of, 981
history taking, 353, 353*f*
physical disabilities
cerebral palsy, 1306–1307, 1307*f*, 1335
muscular dystrophy, 1310–1311
paralysis, 1308
spina bifida, 1307, 1307*f*, 1335
physical factors, in nonverbal communication, 101–102, 102*t*
Physician Orders for Life-Sustaining Treatment (POLST), 71
physicians, at mass-casualty incident scene, 1413
pia mater, 1035
pin-indexing system, 438–439, 439*f*, 484
pinna, 1001, 1001*f*, 1030
pit vipers, 1230–1231, 1231*f*
placards, for hazardous materials, 1426–1427, 1427*f*
placenta
definition of, 1259, 1295
delivery of, 1281–1282
placenta previa, 1263, 1263*t*, 1264*f*, 1295
plaintiff, 79–80
planes of body, 174–175, 174*f*
planning, in incident command system, 1407, 1443
plantar portion, definition of, 171
plantar surface, definition of, 153
plants
as allergens, 819–820
poisonous, 860–862, 860*t*, 861*f*
plasma, 196, 228
components, 694
definition of, 807
platelets (thrombocytes), 196, 228
definition of, 807
functions, 694
play, importance for toddlers/preschoolers, 240
pleura, 186, 187*f*, 228
pleural effusion, 676, 676*f*, 685
pleural space, 186, 228–229, 1100
pleuritic chest pain, 675–676, 686
plural endings, medical terminology, 149
pneumonia
characteristics, 646*t*, 666
definition of, 686
pathophysiology, 670
signs/symptoms, 646*t*
pneumonic plague, 1466, 1466*t*, 1468*t*, 1478
pneumothorax
causes, 416
definition of, 484, 686
management, 676
open, 1098, 1098*f*, 1110
pathophysiology, 675, 676*f*
signs/symptoms, 646*t*
simple, 1099, 1110
spontaneous, 675–676, 1099, 1110
points of distribution (PODs), 1469, 1478
point tenderness, 1147, 1148*f*, 1191
poison centers, 840
poison, definition of, 836, 867
poisonings
by absorption, 841–842, 842*f*
food, 859–860
by ingestion, 839*f*, 842–843
by inhalation, 839–841
by injection, 843–844
from plant ingestions, 860–862, 860*t*, 861*f*
signs/symptoms, 843
treatment, 847
polydipsia, 795, 814
polyphagia, 795, 814
polypharmacy, 520, 529, 867
polyuria, definition of, 795, 814
pons, 202, 229
poor air exchange, 462, 484
portable/folding stretchers, 291–292, 292*f*, 297
portable radio, 130, 130–131*f*
Portuguese man-of-war stings, 1234, 1234*f*
positional asphyxia, 885, 893
position of function, 1191
positive end-expiratory pressure (PEEP), 449
positive–pressure ventilation
neonatal, 1284*f*
vs. normal ventilation, 446–448, 447*t*
postconventional reasoning, 243, 254
posterior, definition of, 153, 171, 694, 727
posterior tibial artery pulse, 195*t*, 229
postexposure management, general considerations for, 50–51
postictal state
definition of, 738, 761
hemiparesis and, 742
safety during, 742
postpartum complications, 1291
postterm pregnancy, 1290–1291
posttraumatic (anterograde) amnesia, 1044
posttraumatic stress disorder (PTSD), 875–876, 893
combat veteran, 876
definition of, 58
signs and symptoms of, 875–876
potential energy, 898, 926
potentially psychologically traumatizing event, 58
poverty, 1329–1330

power grip, 261–262, 262*f*, 297
power lift, 260, 261, 297
PPE. *See* personal protective equipment
preconventional reasoning, 243, 254
preeclampsia
  definition of, 1261–1262, 1295
  signs/symptoms, 1262
  transport precautions, 1262
  treatment, 1261
prefixes, medical terminology, 148, 161*t*, 171
  definition of, 148
  medication administration, 161*t*
  numerical, 150*t*
  position, direction, and location, 150, 151*t*
pregnancy emergencies, 1267–1270
  cardiac arrest in, 603
  cultural considerations, 1267
  ectopic, 1245, 1247, 1263, 1295
  emergencies, mechanism of injury/nature of illness, 1268
  fetal death, 1291
  hypertension during, 1261–1262
  interventions during, 1270
  normal maternal changes, 1260–1261
  pathophysiology, 1261–1267
  postpartum complications, 1291
  postterm, 1290–1291
  transport decisions, 1270
  trauma during, 1265–1267
  trauma patient, caring for, 1266–1267
preload, 537, 559, 695
premature rupture of the amniotic sac, 1270
preoxygenation, 469, 484
preschool-age children
  definition of, 239, 254
  examination of, 239–240
  physical changes, 239–240, 240*f*
  psychosocial changes, 240–241
  vital signs, 241
prescription medications, 492, 529
pressure regulators, for gas cylinders, 439
presumptive negligence, 77
preterm birth, 1290, 1290*f*
prevention
  primary, 20, 24
  secondary, 20, 24
primary assessment, 332–347
  of airway, 336
  bleeding control and assessment, 342–343
  of breathing, 336–338
  of circulation, 338–342, 339*f*, 341–342*f*
  definition of, 332, 396
  in determining patient care and transport priorities, 346–347, 347*f*
  general impression, 333–334, 334*f*
  geriatric patients, 346
  level of consciousness assessment, 334–336
  life threats identification, 332–333
  of orientation, 335
  pediatric patients, 343–346
  questions for, 335
  of responsive patients, 336
  of unresponsive patients, 336
primary blast injuries, 912, 913–914
primary brain injury, 1041, 1083
primary prevention, 20, 24
primary survey. *See* primary assessment
primary triage, 1415, 1443
primigravida, 1269, 1295
professional standards, standards of care and, 77–78
projectile, 910, 926
prolapsed umbilical cord, 1289*f*, 1295
prone
  definition of, 171
  position, 154, 154*f*
prostate gland, 214, 229
prosthetic device, 1308, 1335
protected health information, 69, 93
protocols, for forcible restraint, 67
provoking factors, in OPQRST, 350
proximal femur fractures, 1174–1175
proximal, definition of, 152, 171
proximate causation, 79, 93
pruritus, in anaphylaxis, 818*f*
psilocybin mushrooms, 855*t*
psychiatric/behavioral emergencies. *See also specific emergencies*
  as medical emergencies, 613, 613*t*
psychiatric disorder, 871, 893
psychological distress, 34–35, 58, 79, 876
psychosis, 893
pubic symphysis, 179, 229
pubis, 179, 229
public education, 20
public health, and EMS, 18, 24
  definition of, 18
  health equity, 19
  social drivers of health, 18
public information officer (PIO), 1407–1408, 1444
public safety access point (PSAP), 15, 24
pulmonary artery, 194, 229
pulmonary blast injuries, 914, 926
pulmonary circulation, 191, 229
pulmonary contusion, 1103, 1110
pulmonary edema, 537*f*, 704
  definition of, 686
  high-altitude, 1223–1224
  management, 668–670
  pathophysiology, 668–670, 669*f*
  respiration and, 416
pulmonary embolism
  definition of, 686
  management, 678
  pathophysiology, 677–678, 677*f*
  signs/symptoms, 646*t*, 678
pulmonary veins, 193, 229
pulmonic valve, 690*f*
pulsation, 695
pulse, 194, 229
  locations, 195*t*
  vital signs, 340
pulse oximetry
  in airway management, 419–420
  definition of, 396, 484
  description of, 383, 383*f*, 420, 421*f*
  performing, 420
  purpose, 383
pulse pressure, 559
  definition of, 535, 559
pulse rate
  of adolescents, 244
  of adults, 246
  of children, infants, 234
  normal ranges, 368*t*
pulses
  in acute myocardial infarction, 701
  checking for, 568*f*
  definition of, 338, 396
  distal, 382*f*
  palpation, 339
  quality of, 368
  rhythm, 368
punitive damages, 86, 93
pupils
  assessment
  definition of, 1030
putrefaction, 74, 93, 594

Q

quadrants, 154, 171
  abdominal, 1112–1113, 1113*f*
  definition of, 154
quality assurance (QA), 16, 24
quality improvement (QI), 16, 24
quaternary blast injuries, 912–913
quinary blast injuries, 913

R

rabid animals, 976, 997
raccoon eyes, 1039, 1040*f*, 1083
radial artery pulse, 195*t*, 229
radial head fracture, 1168
radial pulse palpation, 339, 339*f*
radiation, 1196, 1238
  body heat loss from, 1196
radiation burns, 991–992
radiation of pain, 350
radioactive material
  definition of, 1469, 1478
  sources, 1470–1471
radio communications, 133–134
  notification, 135
  systems
    base station radios, 130
    mobile and portable radios, 130, 130–131*f*
radio equipment
  licensing standards, 134
  maintenance, 139–140

radio frequencies, allocation of, 133–134
radiologic dispersal device (RDD), 1471, 1478
radiologic terrorism/warfare
devices, 1471
exposure
medical management, 1472–1473
protective measures, 1472
symptomatology, 1471–1472, 1471*t*
previous incidents, 1450
radius, 179, 229
anatomy, 1141, 1142*f*
rales (crackles), 653*t*, 685
rape, 1133
rapid extrication technique, 271–275, 297
rapport
definition of, 105, 144
therapeutic, Golden Rules for, 105–106
reassessment, 388, 396
rebound tenderness
in appendicitis, 769
assessment, 381, 1121
Recognition of EMS Personnel Licensure Interstate CompAct (REPLICA), 9
records/recordkeeping
legal considerations, 70
for mass-casualty incident, 1408–1409
recovery position, 154*f*, 570–571, 571*f*
definition of, 484, 609
purpose, 436–437, 570–571, 570*f*
rectum, 210
red blood cells (RBCs)
definition of, 196, 229
functions, 694
production, 806, 807*f*
red phosphorus, containers for, 1423
reducible hernia, 773
referred pain
in abdominal conditions, 767, 768*f*, 768*t*
definition of, 786
refusal form, 126, 127–128*f*, 127–128*t*
refusal of care, documenting, 126–129, 127–128*f*, 127–128*t*
rehabilitation area, 1413, 1444
rehabilitation supervisor, 1413, 1444
relaxation, for wellness, 29–30
renal dialysis, 781–783
renal pelvis, 214, 229
renal system
emergencies, 773–774
of older adults, 250
of toddlers/preschoolers, 240
repeaters, 131, 131*f*, 144
reports/reporting
of errors, 125–126, 126*f*
of evidence at scene of crime, 84
honesty in, 88
legal considerations, 70
mandatory requirements, 83–84
obligation for, 83
patient, standard format for, 137
special situations, 129
submission of, 129
rescue situations
extrication. *See* extrication
specialized
search and rescue, 1394–1395
structure fires, 1397
tactical, 1395–1396
technical rescue situations, 1393–1394, 1393*f*
trench rescue, 1395
rescue supervisor, 1413, 1444
residual volume, 191, 229, 409*t*, 484
resilience, definition of, 35, 58
res ipsa loquitur, 80, 93
respiration, 188–190
in acute myocardial infarction, 701
assessment, 419–424
body heat loss from, 1196, 1238
definition of, 188, 229, 408*t*, 484, 641, 686
external, 482
external or pulmonary, 412, 412*f*
factors affecting, 415
external, 415
internal, 415
oxygenation and, 533
pathophysiology, 413–416
physiology, 411–413, 412*f*, 643–644, 644–645*f*
respiration rate, normal range, 417*t*
respirators, for infectious disease risk reduction, 44–46, 45*f*
respiratory agents, in chemical terrorism/warfare, 1456, 1460*t*
respiratory arrest, 414, 484
respiratory compromise, 217, 229
respiratory distress, 414, 484
definition of, 338
signs/symptoms, 417–418
respiratory emergencies
airway obstruction, 676–677
anaphylactic reactions, 675
assessment, 649–657
asthma. *See* asthma
cystic fibrosis, 679–681
emergency medical care, 657–664
environmental/industrial exposure, 679
general care, 657–658
pleural effusion, 676, 676*f*
pulmonary edema, 668–670, 669*f*
spontaneous pneumothorax, 675–676, 676*f*
respiratory failure, 414, 484
definition of, 338
respiratory rate, 417*t*
of adolescents, 244
of adults, 246
determination, 363, 363*f*
of infants, 234
normal ranges, 363*t*
respiratory syncytial virus (RSV), 1327, 1335
characteristics, 646*t*, 665
definition of, 686
signs/symptoms, 646*t*
respiratory system
anatomy, 402–407, 403–407*f*, 644*f*
lower airway, 185–186
mechanics of breathing, 186–188
muscles of breathing, 186–188
upper airway, 184–185
geriatric, 249, 643
pathophysiology, 644–647
pediatric, 641–643
physical examination, in burn injuries, 984
physiology of breathing and, 407–413, 409–410*f*, 409*t*, 412–413*f*
inadequate breathing, 191
normal breathing, characteristics of, 191
respiration, 188–190
ventilation, 190–191
signs, of anaphylactic shock, 542*t*
responsiveness
definition of, 334, 396
determination, in infants/children, 588, 588*f*
restraint, 267, 879*t*, 884–888, 885*t*
reticular activating system (RAS), 202, 229
retina, 1002*f*, 1003, 1030
retinal detachment, 1003, 1030
retractions, 337, 396, 418, 484
retrograde amnesia, 1044, 1083
retroperitoneal organs, 208, 229
retroperitoneal space, 1172, 1191
retroperitoneal structures, 765
retroperitoneum, 1114–1115, 1137
return of spontaneous circulation (ROSC), 562, 609–610
reverse triage, 1238
revised Trauma Score, (RTS), 920–921, 921*t*, 926
rhonchi, 366, 396, 653*t*, 654, 686
rib fractures, 1102
RICES mnemonic, 972, 1185
ricin, 1467–1468, 1467–1468*t*, 1478
rigor mortis, 74, 93, 594
Rocky Mountain spotted fever, 1233
rooting reflex, 236, 254
route of exposure, 1454, 1478
RSV. *See* respiratory syncytial virus
rule of nines, 980, 980*f*, 997
rule of palms, 980

S

sacroiliac joint, 177, 229
sacrum, 178, 229
safe emergency vehicle operation, 1360*t*, 1360–1370, 1360*f*
cushion of safety, 1365–1366
distractions, 1370
driver anticipation, 1364–1365
driving alone, 1370

safe emergency vehicle operation (*Continued*)
  excessive speed, problem of, 1366
  laws and regulations, 1368–1369
    right-of-way privileges, 1368
    use of escorts, 1369
  mental and emotional fitness, 1360–1361
  safety restraints, 1361–1362, 1362*f*
  siren risk–benefit analysis, 1364
  siren syndrome, recognition of, 1366
  specific driving situations, 1369–1370
    highways, 1369
    intersection hazards, 1369
    school zones, 1369–1370
    unpaved roadways, 1369
  vehicle handling, 1363
    braking, 1363
    road positioning and cornering, 1363, 1363*f*
    vehicle size and distance judgment, 1363
  weather and road conditions, 1367–1368, 1367*f*
    decreased visibility, 1367
    ice and slippery surfaces, 1367–1368
    water on the roadway, 1367
safety
  with compressed gas cylinders, 438
  on-scene. *See under specific emergency situations*
  systems, for motor vehicles, 1381, 1381*f*
safety data sheet (SDS), 867, 1428–1429, 1430*f*, 1444
safety officer, 1407–1408, 1444
safety/operations equipment, in ambulances, 1350
safety restraints, 1361–1362, 1362*f*
safe zone, 1386, 1400
Sager splint, 1176
sagittal (lateral) plane, definition of, 175
SALAD technique, 473
salivary glands, 208, 229
salmeterol (Serevent), 660*t*
Salmonella food poisoning, 860
SALT triage, 1418
SAMPLE history
  definition of, 397
  information in, 350
  obtaining, 350
  as part of history taking. *See* history taking
sarin (GB), 1457, 1460*t*, 1478
SARS. *See* s evere acute respiratory syndrome
SARS-CoV-2. *See*s evere acute respiratory syndrome coronavirus 2
SBAT format, 113
scald burn, 987, 997
scalp, 205, 229
  lacerations
    description of, 1039, 1039*f*
    emergency medical care, 1056
scanner, radio receiver, 132, 144
scapula, 179, 179*f*, 229
  injuries, 1163–1164, 1164*f*
SCBA. *See* self-contained breathing apparatus
scene
  of crime, evidence, reporting on, 84
  environmental considerations, 326
  of mass-casualty incident, check-in at, 1408
  size-up of. *See* size-up
  traffic at, 327
scene safety considerations, 878, 879*t*
scene size-up, definition, 325, 397
schizophrenia, 873, 893
school-age children definition of, 242
  physical changes, 242–243, 243f
  psychosocial changes, 243
  vital signs, 241
school zones, specific driving situations, 1369–1370
sciatic nerve, 1174, 1191
sclera, 341, 397, 1002*f*, 1003, 1030
scoop stretcher, 284–285, 298, 1062
scope of practice, 6, 76, 93
scorpion stings, 1232–1233, 1232*f*
scuba diving emergencies
  upon ascent, 1217–1218
  assessment, 1217–1220
  at bottom, 1217
  descent problems, 1217–1218
  emergency medical care, 1221–1223
  prevention, 1222–1223
  transport decisions, 1221–1222
  water rescue, 1214
scuba gear, 1217
seat belts, 51, 51*f*
  abdominal injuries from, 1115–1116, 1116*f*
  in vehicular collisions, 904
sebaceous glands, 205, 229
secondary assessment. *See also specific emergencies*
  components, 355–387
  definition of, 355, 397
  focused assessment, 362–377. *See also* focused assessment
  Glasgow Coma Scale, 376*t*
  vital signs, monitoring devices for. *See specific monitoring devices*
secondary blast injuries, 912
secondary brain injury, 1041, 1083
secondary containment, 1424–1425, 1444
secondary device, 1453, 1478
secondary prevention, 20, 24
secondary triage, 1415, 1444
secure attachment, 238
sedative, 849, 867
sedative-hypnotics, 853–854
seizures, 738–740
  causes, 730
  definition of, 738, 761
  emergency medical care, 757
  recognizing, importance of, 741
  types of, 738–739, 740*t*
self-contained breathing apparatus (SCBA), 1397, 1400
semen, 215, 229
seminal vesicles, 214, 229
sensitization, 541, 559
sensorineural deafness, 1305, 1335
sensory disabilities, 1303–1306, 1303*f*
sensory function
  age-related changes, 251
  assessment, 382
sensory nerves, 204–205, 1036
separation anxiety
  in infants, 240
  in toddlers/preschoolers, 240
sepsis, 374
September 11, 2001, terrorism event, 1450*f*, 1453
septic shock
  causes, 548*t*
  definition of, 540, 559
  signs/symptoms, 548*t*
  treatment, 548*t*, 550
Serevent (salmeterol), 660*t*
service dogs, for visually impaired patients, 1303*f*
severe acute respiratory syndrome (SARS), 631
severe acute respiratory syndrome coronavirus 2 (SARS-CoV-2), 1328
severe airway obstruction, 462, 484
severity, in OPQRST, 350
sexual assault, 1323–1326, 1325*t*, 1335
sexual assault nurse examiners (SANEs), 1324
sexual development, adolescent, 244
sexual harassment
  avoiding, 54
  workplace, 54
sexual history, 354
sexually transmitted infections (STIs), 1246–1247
sexual orientation, 255
shaken baby syndrome, 1335
  child abuse, 1320
shallow respiration, 337, 397
shared decision making, 68
sharps, proper disposal of, 46, 46*f*
shipping papers, for hazardous materials, 1429, 1430*f*
shivering, 1196–1197, 1198*t*
shock, 198, 218–220, 230
  assessment, 544–546
  causes, 536, 536*f*
  definition of, 533, 559, 931, 954
  emergency medical care, 546–551
  fluid administration, 542
  hypovolemic, signs/symptoms of, 936
  interventions, 546
  neurogenic, 1055
  pathophysiology, 533–536, 534*f*, 535*f*
  progression, 543–544, 543*t*
    compensated, 543, 543*t*
    decompensated, 543
    irreversible, 543, 543*t*

signs/symptoms, 542*t*, 933
supportive measures, 547–548*t*
transport decisions, 545
types of, 536–543
short backboards, 293–294
shortening, as fracture signs, 1146–1147, 1148*f*
shoulder dystocia, 1287
shoulder joint, dislocation, 1165–1166, 1165*f*
shunts, 781, 1316, 1336
sickle cell disease, 807–808, 807*f*, 814
side effects. *See under specific drugs/medications*
sign language, for communicating with hearing-impaired patients, 110, 111*f*
signs. *See also under specific disorders*
definition of, 324, 397
vs. symptoms, 324
signs of death, 73–75
simple access, 1389–1390, 1390*f*, 1400
simplex system, 132, 144–145
single command system, 1406, 1444
Singulair (montelukast), 660*t*
sinoatrial (SA) node, 690–691
sinus headaches, 732
siren risk–benefit analysis, 1364
siren syndrome, 1366
situational awareness, 305, 317, 325, 397, 1385
6 Ps of musculoskeletal assessment, 1155
size, of extrication scene, 1384–1386
size-up
definition of, 1385, 1400
of emergency scene, 325–330
considering additional or specialized resources, 330–331
ensuring scene safety, 326–327, 327*f*
mechanism of injury/nature of illness determination, 327–328
number of patients, determination of, 330, 330*f*
questions, for mass-casualty incident, 1409–1411
standard precautions for, 329–330, 329*f*
of extrication scene, 1385*f*
skeletal system, 175–181
anatomy, 175–181, 1037–1038, 1037*f*, 1141–1143, 1141–1145*f*
appendicular skeleton, 179
axial skeleton, 177–179
bones, 175–176
joints, 176–177
lower extremities, 180–181
pelvis, 179
physiology, 181
skin. *See also* integumentary system
anatomy, 957–958, 957*f*
assessment, 340–342, 342*f*
color, 340–341, 341*f*, 616, 617*f*
condition, in heat exposure illnesses, 1209*t*
functions, 340, 956–958, 1146
moisture, 341–342
signs, of anaphylactic shock, 542*t*
temperature, 341
turgor, 1209, 1238
skin turgor, 1209
skull
anatomy, 1037–1038, 1037*f*, 1140
fractures, 1039–1041, 1041*f*
basilar, 1040, 1041*f*
depressed, 1040, 1041*f*
linear, 1039, 1041*f*
open, 1041, 1041*f*
slander, 81, 93
sleep, wellness and, 30–31
slings
application, 1164*f*, 1165, 1165*f*
definition of, 1164, 1191
Slipp patient mover, 291
Slishman splint, 1176, 1176*f*
SLUDGEM mnemonic, 858, 1458, 1458*t*
small intestine, 210
smallpox, 1463–1464, 1464*f*, 1464*t*, 1465*t*, 1468*t*, 1478
small-volume nebulizers (SVNs), 517–520, 517*f*, 520*f*
administration of, 659, 661–664
definition of, 659, 686
smoking cessation, wellness and, 32
smooth muscle, 182, 230, 1139–1140, 1140*f*
snake bites, 1228–1232, 1229–1230*f*
coral, 1229*f*, 1231–1232
pit vipers, 1230–1231, 1231*f*
types, 1229*f*
sneezing techniques, to avoid contamination, 40, 40*f*
sniffing position, 338, 397
newborns, 1282
SOAP method, 122–124
social drivers of health, 18, 24
soft-tissue injuries
assessment, 965–972
from blunt trauma, 959
burns. *See* burns
closed, 958
definition of, 958
emergency medical care of, 972
death from, 958
emergency medical care, 972–977
of face and neck, 1004, 1004*f*, 1009, 1009*f*
interventions, 970
open, 965
definition of, 965
emergency medical care of, 972–977, 975*f*, 976*f*
pathophysiology, 958–965
prevention, 956
solid organs. *See also specific solid organs*
abdominal, 1113–1115, 1114*f*
definition of, 1137
solution, 497, 529
soman (GD), 1457, 1460*t*, 1478
somatic (voluntary) nervous system, 201, 230, 1036–1037
sovereign immunity, 82
spacer, 661
span of control, 1404, 1444
Special Atomic Demolition Munitions (SADM), 1471, 1478
special K (ketamine), 853
special situations, calling medical control and hospitals, 139
special weapons and tactics (SWAT) teams, 1395, 1401
specific driving situations, 1369–1370
highways, 1369
intersection hazards, 1369
school zones, 1369–1370
unpaved roadways, 1369
sperm, 1258
sphenoid bone, 177, 230
sphincters, 210, 230, 535, 559
sphygmomanometer, 196, 230, 369, 369*f*
spice, synthetic marijuana, 857
spider bites, 1225–1227, 1226*f*
spina bifida, 1289, 1295, 1307, 1307*f*, 1336
spinal column anatomy, 1038, 1038*f*
vertebrae, 1038, 1038*f*
spinal cord, 204, 230
functions, 731, 732*f*
spinal cord injuries, 1038, 1045
assessment, 1046–1051
brain contusion, 1045
concussion, 1044–1045, 1083
emergency medical care, 1057–1061
with face and neck injuries, 1025–1026
helmet removal, 1074–1079
interventions, 1050
signs/symptoms, 1045
in submersion incidents, 1213–1215
transport decisions, 1049–1050
spinal motion restriction, 1046, 1083
spine injuries. *See* spinal cord injuries
spiral fracture, 1147
spleen, 196
splints/splinting
definition of, 1157, 1191
distal circulation and, 1161
formable, 1159–1162
general principles, 1158–1159
of hand and wrist, 1170–1171
improper, hazards of, 1162
in-line traction, 1176
pelvic binder, 1161, 1163*f*, 1191
with pillow, 1183, 1185*f*
purpose, to control bleeding, 943, 943*f*, 972
rigid, 1159
supplies, in ambulances, 1346*t*, 1348, 1348*f*
traction, 1175–1181, 1191
spontaneous abortion, 1264, 1295
spontaneous pneumothorax, 675–676, 1099
spontaneous respiration, 336, 397
spotter, 1379

spotter, cushion of safety, 1366
sprains
  definition of, 1150–1151, 1191
  elbow, 1168
  management, 1185
  signs/symptoms, 1150
sputum types, 655
staging supervisor, 1412, 1444
stair chair, 288–290, 289*f*, 298
standard of care
  definition of, 76–77, 93
  establishment of, 77–79
  minimum, 78
standard precautions
  definition of, 40, 58, 329, 397
  types of protection in, 41*t*, 329, 329*f*
standing orders, 76, 140, 145
Star of Life, 1343, 1344*f*, 1379
startle reflex (Moro reflex), 236, 254
START triage, 1417–1418, 1418*f*, 1444
state government, standard of care for, 79
state-sponsored terrorism, 1478, 1551
status asthmaticus, 675, 686
status epilepticus, 739–740, 761
statute of limitations, 85, 94
steam burn, 987, 997
sterile dressings, 976, 992–993, 1009
sterilization, 1359, 1379
sternal fracture, 1103
sternocleidomastoid muscles, 1002, 1030
sternum, 179, 230
stimulants, definition of, 855, 867
stings
  hymenoptera, 1227–1228, 1238
  scorpion, 1232–1233, 1232*f*
STIs (sexually transmitted infections), 1246–1247
stomach, 209, 764–765
stomas, 1316, 1336
  airway management and, 459–461
  artificial ventilation, 571–572
  catheters for, 429, 429*f*
  definition of, 484, 1336
strains, 1151, 1185, 1191
strangulation, 773, 786
stratum corneum, 205, 230
stress
  peer support, 37
  posttraumatic stress disorder, 58
stretchers
  basket, 293, 293*f*
  flexible, 292, 293*f*
  portable/folding, 291–292, 292*f*
  wheeled. *See* wheeled ambulance stretchers
striated muscle, 1139
stridor, 363, 366, 462, 484, 597, 610, 819
  definition of, 397, 686
  diseases associated with, 653*t*
  sound of, 336
stroke (cerebrovascular accident)
  assessment, 749–752, 750–751*t*, 750*t*
  conditions mimicking, 738
  death from, 730
  definition of, 761
  emergency medical care, 756–757
  ischemic, 735, 735*f*
  signs/symptoms, 737–738
stroke volume (SV), 193, 230, 692, 695
structure fires, 1397
study tips, 9*t*
subarachnoid hemorrhage, 1044, 1083
subcutaneous emphysema, 379, 380*f*, 397, 1025, 1030
subcutaneous injection, 494, 529
subcutaneous tissue, 205, 230
subdural bleeding, 738, 738*f*
subdural hematomas, 1043–1044, 1043*f*, 1084
sublingual (SL), 495, 529
sublingual medications, 507–509
submersion
  hypothermia and, 1215–1217
  with suspected spinal injury, 1213–1215
substance misuse, 837
substance use disorders (SUDs), 877, 893, 1264–1265
sucking chest wound, 1098, 1098*f*, 1110
sucking reflex, 236, 255
suction catheter, 429, 484
suctioning
  equipment, 428–429, 429*f*
  techniques, 429–431
suctioning units, in ambulances, 1345, 1347*f*
sudden death, 701–702
sudden unexpected infant death (SUID), 1316–1317, 1336
suffixes, medical terminology, 148, 162*t*, 171
  definition of, 148
suicide, 873–875, 874*t*
sulfuric acid, containers for, 1423
sulfur mustard (H), 1455, 1455*f*, 1460*t*, 1478
sunlight exposure, excessive, 1210
superficial burns, 978, 998
superior, definition of, 152, 171, 694, 727
superior portion, 151–152, 171
superior vena cava, 195, 230, 694
supine, definition of, 154, 171
supine hypotensive syndrome, 1129, 1261, 1295–1296
supine position, 154, 154*f*, 171
supplemental restraint systems, 902–904
supplies, medical. *See also specific medical supplies*
  in ambulances, 1345, 1346*t*
surfactant, 412, 484
surrogate decision maker, 64, 94
suspension, 497, 529
sutures, 184, 184*f*, 230
swathe, 1164, 1164*f*, 1191
sweat glands, 205, 230
swelling, as fracture signs, 1148
swine flu (H1N1 virus), 624
symbols, medical terminology, 157*t*
sympathetic nervous system, 204, 230, 691, 727, 1037
sympathomimetics, 838*t*, 855–856
symphyses, 176, 230
symptomatic hyperglycemia, 798, 814
  definition of, 798
symptomatic hypoglycemia, 796, 814
symptoms. *See also under specific disorders*
  definition of, 324, 397
  multiple, history taking and, 390
  vs. signs, 324
syncope, 700, 727
  breath-holding, 1221
  definition of, 542, 742, 761
syndromic surveillance, 1469, 1478
synovial fluid, 177, 230
synovial membrane, 177, 230
synthetic cathinones, 856
systemic circulation, 191, 230
systemic reaction, 824
systemic vascular resistance (SVR), 196, 230
systole, 196, 230, 694
systolic pressure, definition of, 369, 397

T

tabun (GA), 1457, 1460*t*, 1478
tachycardia, definition of, 368, 397, 702, 727
tachypnea, 686, 1091, 1110
  in chest injuries, 1091
  in respiratory failure, 338*t*
tactical situation, 1396, 1401
tactile stimulation, 1282
talus, 181, 230
tarsals, 181, 230
TBI. *See* traumatic brain injury
team, health care and
  assisting with ALS skills, 309–310
  behavioral health calls, 313
  BLS and ALS providers, 309
  conflicts, troubleshooting, 312–313
  critical thinking and clinical decision making, 310–312
  effective performance, team, 303–308
    collaboration and communication, 304–305
    crew resource management, 305
    diverse and competent skill sets, 303–304
    roles and responsibilities, 303
    shared goal, 303
    supportive and coordinated leadership, 305
    team membership, 305–306
  general description, 300
  mental health calls, 313
  transfer of patient care, 308–309
  types of, 302
team leader, 305, 317

technical rescue group, 1393–1394, 1401
technical rescue situation, 1393–1394, 1393*f*, 1401
teenage pregnancy, 1267
teenagers. *See* adolescents
teeth
  avulsed, 1024
  fractured, 1024
teething, 238
telemetry, 131, 145
telephones, cellular/satellite, 132
temporal bones, 177, 230
temporal lobe, 202, 230
temporomandibular joint (TMJ), 1001, 1030
tenderness, as fracture sign, 1147, 1148*f*
tendons, 176, 176*t*, 231, 1139
tension headache, 732
tension pneumothorax, 416, 484
  definition of, 538, 1110
  pathophysiology, 1099–1100, 1100*f*
  signs/symptoms, 646*t*, 1099–1100
  treatment, 549
term gestation, 1260, 1281, 1290, 1296
terminal illness, 1328
termination of command, 1406, 1444
terrorism
  biologic warfare. *See* biologic terrorism/warfare
  chemical warfare. *See* chemical terrorism/warfare
  definition of, 1447
  events
    establishing command, 1454
    indicators of, 1451–1452
    notification procedures, 1453
    scene safety, 1452–1453, 1452–1453*f*, 1454
  incendiary/explosive devices, 1473
  nuclear/radiologic warfare, 1469–1473
tertiary blast injuries, 912
testicle, 215, 231
tetanus, 975–976
therapeutic communication, 98, 145
therapeutic effect, 490, 529
therapeutic rapport, for patient interview, 105–106, 105*f*
thermal burns
  definition of, 987, 998
  to eye, 1015–1016, 1016*f*
third-degree burns, 979, 998
thoracic cage, 175
thoracic cavity
  anatomy, 404–407, 407*f*, 1088–1089, 1088*f*
  physiology, 1087–1088, 1088*f*
thoracic spine, 178, 231
thorax, 179, 231
throat injuries, assessment of, 915
thrombocytes (platelets), 807
thromboembolism, 698, 727
thrombophilia, 809, 814
thrombosis, 735, 761, 814
thyroid cartilage, 185, 231, 404
TIA. *See* transient ischemic attack
tibia, 180, 231, 1143, 1191
  injuries, 1183, 1183*f*
tick bites, 1233–1234, 1233*f*
TICLS mnemonic, 344*t*
tidal volume, 191, 231, 363, 397, 409*t*, 484
time/timing
  for cardiopulmonary resuscitation, 562, 563*f*
  in OPQRST, 350
toddlers
  definition of, 239, 255
  examination of, 239–240
  physical changes, 239–240, 240*f*
  psychosocial changes, 240–241
  vital signs, 241
tolerance, 848, 867
tonic-clonic seizures, 739
tonic phase, 739
tonsil-tip catheter, 429, 429*f*, 484
tonsil tips, 429
topical medications, 497, 529
topographic anatomy, 174–175, 231
tort, 80, 94
  definition of, 80
touch/touching
  using in patient interview, 103, 104*f*
tourniquet
  application method, 944–947, 945*f*
  definition of, 944, 954, 1152, 1191
toxicologic emergencies
  airway assessment, 848
  assessment, 844–847
  emergency medical care, 847–848
  medical, 613, 613*t*
  pathophysiology, routes of absorption, 838–844, 839*f*, 842*f*
  with specific poisons
    alcohol, 849–850
    cannabis compounds, 856
    hallucinogens, 857
    hypnotics, 853–854
    marijuana, 857
    narcotics, 851
    opiates, 851
    opioids, 850–853
    organophosphates, 858
    sedatives, 853–854
  transport decisions, 846
toxicology, 836, 867
toxidrome, 837
  definition of, 867
toxin-induced hepatitis, 627*t*
toxin/poison, 1227, 1231, 1232, 1234–1235, 1238
toxins
  absorption of, 841–842, 842*f*
  definition of, 833, 836, 867
  inhalation of, 839–841
trachea, 185, 231, 404, 1088
tracheostomy
  collar, 1311, 1311*f*
  definition of, 445, 484
  mask, 445, 445*f*
  tubes
    airway management and, 459–461, 459*f*
    definition of, 459
tracheostomy tube, 484
traction, 1175–1181
  applying, 1177–1178
  definition of, 1191
traction splint, 1175–1181
trade name, definition of, 492, 529
tragus, 1001, 1030
trajectory, 910, 926
transcutaneous (transdermal) medications, 495, 497–498, 529
  automated external defibrillation and, 581
transfer of patients
  to ambulance, 1357–1358
  equipment, in ambulances, 1346*t*, 1348–1349, 1349*f*
  during extrication, 1392
transient ischemic attack (TIA), 736, 756, 761
transmission
  communication, 97, 130–133, 136
  definition of, 38, 58
  routes, for infectious diseases, 38–40, 38*f*
transport
  decisions. *See* under specific emergencies
  in mass-casualty incident triage, 1420
  moving patients for. *See* moving of patients
  refusal of, 68
  of sitting patients, with head injuries, 1070–1072
  of supine patients, with head injuries, 1062–1069
  types of, 918
transportation area, 1411–1412, 1444
transportation supervisor, 1412, 1444
transverse fracture, 1147
transverse (axial) plane, definition of, 175
trauma centers, levels of, 917*t*
trauma emergencies
  blast injuries, 911–914, 913*f*
  blunt. *See* blunt trauma
  definition of, 613, 637
  destination selection, 916–918, 917*t*
  energy and, 897–899, 901*f*
  to face. *See* facial injuries
  mechanism of injury, 897, 926
  multisystem, 914, 926
  to neck. *See* neck injuries
  on-scene time, 916
  patient assessment, 914–916
  patients levels and, 916, 917*t*
  penetrating, 900, 909–911, 913*f*, 926
  during pregnancy, 1265–1267
  transport decisions, 914, 916
trauma score, 918–920, 926
traumatic asphyxia, 1104, 1110

traumatic brain injury (TBI)
assessment, 1046–1051
death from, 1041
definition of, 1041, 1084
intracranial hemorrhage, 1042–1043
epidural hematoma, 1043
intracerebral hematoma, 1044, 1044*f*
subarachnoid hemorrhage, 1044
subdural hematoma, 1043–1044
intracranial pressure, 1042
travel medicine, 631–632
treatment area, 1411, 1444
treatment, refusal rights, 68
treatment supervisor, 1411–1412, 1444
trench rescue, 1395
triage, 1411
categories, 1415–1416, 1416*t*
definition of, 1415
destination decisions, 1420
JumpSTART, 1418–1419, 1419*f*, 1443
primary, 1415, 1444
SALT, 1418
secondary, 1415, 1444
special considerations, 1419–1420
START, 1417–1418, 1444
supervisor, 1411, 1444
triceps muscle, 182, 231
tricuspid valve, 690*f*
tricyclic antidepressants, 857–858
trimesters, 1260–1261
tripod position, 338, 397, 686
trisomy 21. *See* Down syndrome
trunking, 132–133, 145
trust versus mistrust, 255
tuberculosis, 629–630
characteristics, 629–630, 668
definition of, 637, 686
signs/symptoms, 646*t*
transmission, 629–630
tunica media, 194, 231
turbinates
anatomy, 1020, 1021*f*
definition of, 1030
turgor, 1209
twin births, 1289–1290
211 call line, 99
two-person bag-mask ventilation
pediatric patient, 469
two-rescuer adult CPR, 572, 574–575
two- to three-word dyspnea, 337, 397
tympanic membrane, 913, 926, 1021, 1022*f*, 1030
type 1 diabetes, 793–795, 814
type 2 diabetes, 798, 814

U

ulcers, 768–769
ulna, 179, 231
anatomy, 1141, 1142*f*
olecranon process fracture, 1168
ultra-high frequency, 130, 145
umbilical cord
anatomy, 1259
clamping, 1279
definition of, 1259, 1296
around newborn's neck, 1279
prolapsed, 1288–1289, 1289*f*, 1296
umbilicus, 174
unconscious bias, 100, 145
uncontrolled external bleeding, 334
unexplained sudden death in infancy (USDI), 1316–1317, 1336
unified command system, 1406, 1445
unilateral structure, definition of, 153
unintended effects, 491, 529
unpaved roadways, specific driving situations, 1369
untoward effects, 492, 529
upper airway, 184–185
upper extremities, 179
Urban Search and Rescue teams (USARs), 1421
uremia, 773, 786
ureter, 214, 231, 765
urethra, 214, 231
anatomy, 765, 1243*f*
urinary bladder, 214, 231
anatomy, 765–766
definition of, 766
injuries, 1129, 1132
urinary retention, 774
urinary system, 213–214
anatomy, 765–766, 766*f*
urinary tract emergencies
assessment, 776–780
as medical emergencies, 613, 613*t*
transport decisions, 777
urinary tract infections (UTIs), 773, 786
urine, 766
urologic system. *See* urinary system
urostomy, 1316, 1336
urticaria, 818
characteristics, 818, 818*f*
definition of, 833
uterine rupture, 1266
uterus
anatomy, 1243*f*, 1245, 1258–1259
definition of, 1254
manual left displacement, 604*f*

V

vaccines, 515
vacuum mattresses, 1062
vacuum splints, 1159–1162
V agent (VX), 1457–1458, 1460*t*, 1478
vagina, 215, 231
anatomy, 1243*f*, 1245, 1258–1259
bleeding from
causes of, 1247
in pregnancy, 1247
definition of, 1254
vagus nerve stimulators, 1316
vancomycin-resistant enterococci (VRE), 1327, 1336
vapor hazard, 1454, 1478
vasoconstriction, 342, 397, 934
vasodilatory shock, 416. *See also* distributive shock
vasoocclusive crisis, 807, 814
vector-borne transmission, 40, 58
vehicle crashes, 901–902
vehicle handling, 1363
braking, 1363
road positioning and cornering, 1363, 1363*f*
vehicle size and distance judgment, 1363
veins, 195–196, 930, 954
functions, 694
vs. arteries, 1259
vented chest seal, 1093, 1110
ventilation, 190–191
alveolar, 481
definition of, 188, 231, 408*t*, 484, 571, 610, 686
equipment, in ambulances, 1345, 1346*t*, 1347
factors affecting, 414–415
mechanisms, 408–411, 409*f*
mouth-to-mouth, 448
normal, *vs.* positive-pressure ventilation, 447*t*, 446–448
physiology, 1087
regulation, 410–411
ventilation/perfusion mismatch, 218, 413–414
ventilation rates, for apneic patients, 448
Ventolin. *See* albuterol
ventral portion, 153, 171
ventricle, 191, 231, 689, 728
ventricular fibrillation (VF), 702, 728
ventricular tachycardia (VT), 702, 728
Venturi mask, 444–445, 444*f*
venules, 694, 930, 954
verbal report, 113
vernix caseosa, 1280, 1290, 1296
vertebrae, 177, 231
anatomy, 1038, 1038*f*
vertebral body, 1037
vertebral column, 177, 231
vertex presentation, 1288, 1296
vesicants, 1455–1456, 1455*f*, 1460*t*, 1478
vesicular breath sounds, 653, 686
video laryngoscopy, 470, 485
violent patients, 888–889, 889*f*
viral hemorrhagic fevers, 1464, 1465*t*, 1468*t*, 1478–1479
virulence, 628, 637
viruses, in chemical terrorism/warfare, 1463–1464, 1464*f*, 1479
visceral pleura, 406, 485
visually impaired patients
communication with, 110–111
interaction with, 1303–1304, 1303*f*
vital capacity, 409*t*, 485
vital signs. *See specific age groups and vital signs*
definition of, 397
documenting, 125

vitreous humor, 1002
vocal cords, 404, 485
volatility, 1454, 1479
Volmax. *See* albuterol
voluntary activities, 1036, 1084
voluntary muscle, 182, 231

W

warm zone, 1433*f*, 1445
wasp stings, 819, 1227
water rescue, 1214, 1214*f*
WBCs. *See* white blood cells
weaponization, 1451, 1479
weapon of mass casualty (WMC), 1450, 1479
weather/road conditions, 1367–1368, 1367*f*
  decreased visibility, 1367
  ice and slippery surfaces, 1367–1368
  water on the roadway, 1367
wellness, 58
  balancing work, family and health, 33–34
  definition of, 28
  disease prevention and, 32–33
  exercise, 29–30, 29*f*
  nutrition, 28–29, 29*f*
  relaxation for, 29–30
  sleep, 30–31
wet patients, automated external defibrillation and, 581
wheals, 819, 819*f*, 833
wheeled ambulance stretcher, 276–284, 277*f*, 298
  description, 276–284, 277*f*
  electronic stretcher, 277, 278*f*
  loading, 282–284
  patient transfer, 278–280
  pushing, 280–282, 281–282*f*
  rolling, 276–277, 277*f*
  transferring patient, 278–280
wheeled stair chair, 288, 289*f*
wheezing, 462, 485
  in allergic reactions, 819
  in asthma, 673
  definition of, 397, 686
  respiratory diseases associated with, 653*t*
white blood cells (leukocytes; WBCs), 196, 231
  definition of, 806
  functions, 694
whole blood transfusion, 543
whooping cough. *See* pertussis
WMD. *See* weapon of mass destruction
Wong-Baker FACES pain rating scale, 351, 351*f*
word roots, medical terminology, 148, 158–160*t*, 171
work, balancing with family and health, 33–34
work of breathing, 344, 397, 686
wound care supplies, in ambulances, 1346*t*, 1348
wound healing, pathophysiology of, 958–959
wrist
  anatomy, 1142, 1142*f*
  injuries, 1170–1171

X

XABC mnemonic, 937
xiphoid process, 179, 231
x-ray (gamma) radiation, 1470, 1477

Y

yellowjacket stings, 1227

Z

zone of injury, 1145, 1191
zygomas, 177, 231